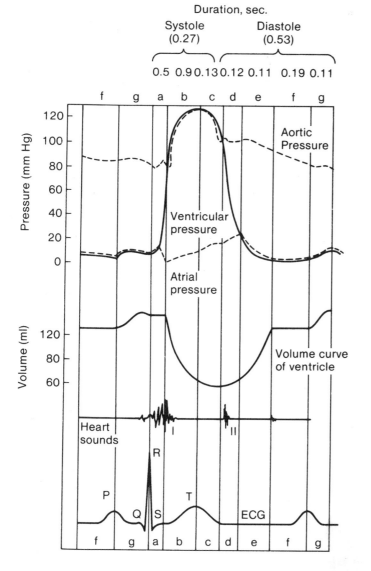

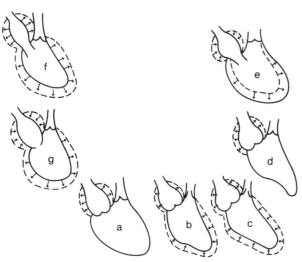

The cardiac cycle, illustrating the changes in aortic, left ventricular, and left atrial pressures, and in left ventricular volume, in relation to the phonocardiogram and the electrocardiogram. The duration of each phase at a heart rate of approximately 75 beats/min is indicated at the top of the figure. a, isovolumetric ventricular contraction; b, rapid ventricular ejection; c, slow ventricular ejection; d, isovolumetric relaxation; e, rapid ventricular filling; f, diastasis; g, atrial contraction; I, first heart sound; II, second heart sound. *Insets:* Changes in the configuration of the left atrium, mitral valve, left ventricle, and aortic valve during various phases of the cycle. (Adapted from Wiggens: Circulatory Dynamics. New York, Grune & Stratton, 1952.)

Cardiac Nursing

4TH EDITION

Cardiac Nursing

4TH EDITION

Susan L. Woods, RN, PhD
Professor and Associate Dean for Academic Programs
School of Nursing
University of Washington
Seattle, Washington

Erika S. Sivarajan Froelicher, RN, MA, PhD, MPH, FAAN
Professor
Department of Physiological Nursing
School of Nursing
and
Adjunct Professor
Department of Epidemiology and Biostatistics
School of Medicine
University of California, San Francisco
San Francisco, California

Sandra Adams (Underhill) Motzer, RN, PhD
Research Assistant Professor
Department of Biobehavioral Nursing and Health Systems
University of Washington
Seattle, Washington

With 36 Contributors

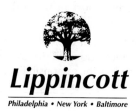

Lippincott

Philadelphia • New York • Baltimore

Acquisitions Editor: *Susan M. Glover, RN, MSN*
Assistant Editors: *Bridget Blatteau/Hilarie Surrena*
Project Editors: *Gretchen Metzger/Nicole Walz*
Senior Production Manager: *Helen Ewan*
Production Coordinator: *Nannette Winski*
Design Coordinator: *Brett MacNaughton*
Pre-press: *Jay's Publisher Services*
Compositor: *Shepherd, Inc.*
Printer: *Courier Westford*
Indexer: *Lynne Mahan*

4th Edition

Library of Congress Cataloging-in-Publication Data
Cardiac nursing / [edited by] Susan L. Woods, Erika S. Sivarajan Froelicher, Sandra Adams (Underhill) Motzer.—4th ed.
    p.   cm.
   Includes bibliographical references and index.
   ISBN 0-7817-1733-7
    1. Heart—Disease—Nursing. I. Woods, Susan L. II. Froelicher, Erica S. Sivarajan. III. Motzer, Sandra Adams.
    [DNLM: 1. Heart Diseases–nursing. 2. Heart Diseases—prevention & control–Nurses' Instruction. WY 152.5 C2672 2000]
   RC674.C3 2000
   610.73'691—dc21   99-030303

Dedication

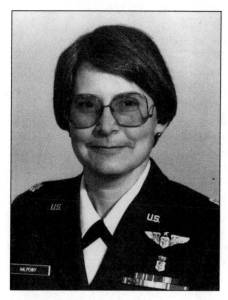

C. Jean Halpenny, RN, MA, Lt. Col. USAFR (Retired)
1941–1997

The 4th edition of *Cardiac Nursing* is dedicated to Jean Halpenny, our treasured friend and colleague. Jean died after a long and valiant struggle with breast cancer on August 23rd, 1997. Sue, Jean, and Sandy originally worked together in the cardiac care unit at the U.S. Public Health Service Hospital, while Erika worked in a cardiac care unit at the University of Washington Medical Center, all in Seattle, Washington. The four of us attended graduate school together and then taught cardiovascular nursing at the University of Washington. We decided there was a need for a comprehensive textbook in cardiac nursing. With the support and guidance of Susie Mansfield and Maxine Patrick, we launched the first edition in 1977, writing most of the chapters ourselves. As a result of our ongoing collaboration and friendship, that initial impetus of the 1st edition of Cardiac Nursing continues today.

As our way of honoring Jean, we want to tell you something about her life. Jean was born in Tucson, Arizona, on August 20th, 1941 to Corky and Leonard Halpenny. She was educated in Tucson through grade school. In early 1955 she moved with her parents and brother, Philip, to Mocamedes, Angola, Africa, where they lived for 2 years. During this period, Jean learned the Portuguese language and carried on her first 3 years of high school under University of Nebraska correspondence courses. Upon her return from Africa in late 1957, Jean completed her final year of high school in Tucson. In the Summer of 1960, before she entered the University of Michigan School of Nursing, Jean joined her parents in Lahore, West Pakistan. After 2 years at the University she withdraw, explaining that she did not have enough confidence in her abilities to be a nurse. In 1963 Jean enrolled in the foreign specialist program at the University of Arizona. But, while at the University, she served as a candy-striper volunteer St. Joseph's Hospital in Tucson. Upon graduation in 1965 with her BA in History, she realized that her true calling was nursing, and she returned to the Ann Arbor, Michigan campus and earned her BSN in 1967. Jean completed her MA, with a major in nursing and a minor in physiology and biophysics, at the University of Washington in 1975. In 1979 she was accepted into the predoctoral program in nursing science at the University of Washington, where she completed all coursework required for the PhD degree.

Jean's professional career spanned both military and civilian nursing. Jean enrolled in the U.S. Naval Reserve in 1966 and, in 1967, was accepted into the Officer Candidate School,

U.S. Women's Officer School in Newport, Rhode Island. She began her military nursing career at Naval Hospital, San Diego, in the intensive care unit, where she worked as a staff nurse for 2 years. In 1969 she was assigned to the U.S. Naval Hospital, Guam, Marianas Islands, where she served as charge nurse in military medical and newborn nursery. Jean moved to the Seattle area in 1971, continuing her military career in the Naval Reserve as a charge nurse, Naval Hospital, Whidbey Island. That reserve unit was disbanded in 1978, so Jean transferred to the U.S. Air Force Reserve at McChord AFB, where she served as flight nurse with the 40th Aeromedical Evacuation Unit for 11 years. After 23 years of distinguished military service, she retired in 1989 at the rank of Lieutenant Colonel.

Her civilian nursing career began in Seattle in 1971 when she began working at the U.S. Public Health Service Hospital cardiac care unit. In 1975 she accepted a faculty position in the Department of Physiological Nursing at the University of Washington School of Nursing, where she taught both undergraduate and graduate nursing students. In 1982 she began working for Group Health Cooperative of Puget Sound, first at the Eastside Hospital's intensive and coronary care units, and in 1990 at Eastside Home and Community Services. Jean also was an adjunct faculty member at Seattle Pacific University School of Health Sciences, where she served as a preceptor for students in community health nursing.

Jean devoted her life to the profession of nursing and to the love of family, friends, colleagues, and patients. Jean's love of learning, and joy of teaching, are well known to all who have worked with her, been her students, or benefited from her care. Her presence is missed.

Contributors to the 4th Edition

Margaret Wooding Baker, RN, MSN, C
Doctoral Student
School of Nursing
University of Washington
Seattle, Washington

Kathy Berra, RN, MSN, ANP
Clinical Trial Director
Stanford Center for Research in Disease Prevention
Stanford University
Palo Alto, California

Susan J. Blancher, RN, MN, ARNP
Clinical Nurse Specialist
Cardiology; Electrophysiology
Virginia Mason Medical Center
Seattle, Washington

Eleanor F. Bond, RN, PhD
Associate Professor
Department of Biobehavioral Nursing and Health Systems
University of Washington
Seattle, Washington

Debra Laurent-Bopp, MN, ARNP
Clinical Assistant Professor
Department of Biobehavioral Nursing and Health Systems
University of Washington
Seattle, Washington

Lieutenant Colonel Elizabeth J. Bridges, USAF NC, RN, PhD, CCRN
Director
Nursing Research
Lackland Air Force Base, 59th Medical Wing
San Antonio, Texas

Lora E. Burke, RN, PhD, MPH
University of Pittsburgh
Associate Professor
Department of Health and Community Systems
School of Nursing
Pittsburgh, Pennsylvania

Mary McMahan Busch, RN, MN
Field Clinical Representative
Guidant Corporation
Seattle, Washington

Ruth Craven, RNC, EdD
Assistant Dean, Educational Outreach
Associate Professor
Department of Biobehavioral Nursing and Health Systems
University of Washington
Seattle, Washington

Susanna Cunningham, RN, PhD
Professor
Department of Biobehavioral Nursing and Health Systems
University of Washington
Seattle, Washington

Michaelene Hargrove Deelstra, RN, MSN, ARNP
Cardiology/Acute Care Nurse Practitioner
Cardiology Summit
Clinical Facility
Department of Biobehavioral Nursing and Health Systems
University of Washington
Seattle, Washington

Sherri Del Bene, RN, MN
Nursing Manager, Cardiothoracic ICU
University of Washington Medical Center
Seattle, Washington

Joan M. Fair, RN, ANP, PhD
Research Project Director
Stanford Center for Research in Disease Prevention
School of Medicine
Palo Alto, California

Linda Felver, RN, PhD
Associate Professor
Department of Adult Health and Illness
School of Nursing
Oregon Health Sciences University
Portland, Oregon

Erika S. Sivarajan Froelicher, RN, MN, PhD, MPH, FAAN
Professor
Department of Physiological Nursing
School of Nursing;
Adjunct Professor
Department of Epidemiology and Biostatistics
School of Medicine
University of California, San Francisco
San Francisco, California

Polly E. Gardner, RN, MN, ARNP
Critical Care Clinical Nurse Specialist
Swedish Hospital Medical Center;
Clinical Instructor
Department of Biobehavioral Nursing and Health Systems
University of Washington
Seattle, Washington

Donna Gerity, RN, MN
Clinical Nurse Specialist, Cardiology
Minor & James Medical
Seattle, Washington

Margaret L. Hall, MD
Cardiologist
Summit Cardiology
Seattle, Washington

Jon S. Huseby, MD
Clinical Associate Professor of Medicine and Nursing
University of Washington;
Respiratory Disease Specialist
Polyclinic
Seattle, Washington

Carol Jacobson, RN, MN, CCRN
Clinical Instructor
Department of Biobehavioral Nursing and Health Systems
University of Washington;
Director
Quality Education Services
Seattle, Washington;
Critical Care Specialist
Swedish Medical Center
Seattle, Washington

Roxanne Juel, RN
Staff RN, Cardiac Center Lab
Virginia Mason Medical Center
Seattle, Washington

Holly Lea, RN
Former Research Assistant
School of Nursing
University of Washington
Seattle, Washington

Denise LeDoux, RN, MN, ARNP, CCRN
Clinical Nurse Specialist
Cardiac Surgery Services
Veterans Administration Medical Center;
Clinical Instructor
Department of Biobehavioral Nursing and Health Systems
University of Washington
Seattle, Washington

Kathryn A. Lee, RN, PhD, FAAN
Professor
Family Health Care Nursing
University of California, San Francisco
San Francisco, California

Barbara Levine, RN, PhD, CRNP
Clinical Director
Gerontological Nursing Practice;
Assistant Professor, University of Pennsylvania
University of Pennsylvania Health Systems
Philadelphia, Pennsylvania

Helen Luikart, RN, MS
Transport Coordinator/Nurse Educator
Department of Cardiothoracic Surgery
Stanford University Medical Center
Stanford, California

Carolyn Chandler Main, RN, MN, ARNP
Nurse Practitioner, Cardiology
Minor and James Medical;
Clinical Instructor
Department of Biobehavioral Nursing and Health Systems
University of Washington
Seattle, Washington

Kirsten M. Martin, RN, BSN, MS
Staff Nurse II
Intermediate Telemetry Care Unit
Alter Bates Medical Center
Berkeley, California

Major Margaret M. McNeill, USAF RN, MS, CCRN
Clinical Consultant
Defense Medical Standardization
Fort Detrick, Maryland

Nancy Houston Miller, BSN, RN
Associate Director
Stanford Cardiac Rehabilitation Program
Stanford University School of Medicine
Palo Alto, California;
Assistant Clinical Professor
Department of Physiological Nursing
University of California, San Francisco
San Francisco, California

Sandra Adams (Underhill) Motzer, PhD, RN
Research Assistant Professor
Department of Biobehavioral Nursing and Health Systems
University of Washington
Seattle, Washington

Jonathon Myers, PhD
Clinical Assistant Professor of Medicine
Cardiology Division
Palo Alto VA Health Care System
Stanford University
Palo Alto, California

Katherine M. Newton, RN, PhD
Assistant Scientific Investigator
Center for Health Studies
Group Health Cooperative of Pugent Sound
Seattle, Washington;
Affiliate Assistant Professor
Department of Biobehavioral Nursing and Health Systems
School of Nursing
Department of Epidemiology
School of Public Health and Community Medicine
University of Washington
Seattle, Washington

Deanna E. Ritchie, RN, MN, C, FAACVPR
Clinical Coordinator
Cardiac Rehabilitation
Northwest Hospital
Seattle, Washington

Julie Shinn, RN, MA, CCRN, FAAN
Cardiovascular Clinical Nurse Specialist
UCFS Stanford Health Center
Stanford University Medical Center
Stanford, California;
Assistant Clinical Professor
Department of Physiological Nursing
University of California, San Francisco
San Francisco, California

Ann Falsone Vaughan, RN, MSN, CCRN
Former Lecturer
Department of Behavioral Nursing and Health Sciences
University of Washington
School of Nursing
Seattle, Washington

Margaret Wallhagen
Associate Professor
Physiological Nursing
University of California, San Francisco
San Francisco, California

Susan L. Woods, RN, PhD
Professor and Associate Dean for Academic Programs
School of Nursing
University of Washington
Seattle, Washington

Brenda K. Zierler, RN, PhD
Research Assistant Professor
Department of Biobehavioral Nursing and Health Systems;
School of Nursing, and Adjunct Research Assistant Professor
Department of Surgery
School of Medicine
University of Washington
Seattle, Washington

Contributors to Previous Editions

Gaylene Altman, RN, MN

Gerard Bashein, MD, PhD

Kathy Berra, BSN, FAACVPR

Mary Boozer, RN, MN

Jenille Bradly, RN

Lynn Buchanan, RN, MSN

Evelyn Butera, RN, MS, CNN

Mary M. Canobbio, RN, MN

Karen K. Carlson, RN, MN, CCRN

Dianne J. Christopherson, RN, MN

Terry F. Cicero, RN, MN, CCRN

Barbara Bean Cochrane, PhD, RN

Marie Cowan, RN

Roberta S. Erickson, RN, PhD

Paul S. Fardy, PhD

Linda Ann Felthous, BS in Pharm, RPh

Joanne Gilbert, RN

Suan Boyce Gilmore, MN, RN

Mikell R. Goe, RN, MN, CCRN

Sheryl A. Greco, RN, MN

Ruth A. Gregersen, RN, MN, CCRN

Carlene M. Grim, RNC, MSN, SpDN

B. Lynn Grose, RN, MN CCRN

Janet B. Haskin, BSN, RN

Margaret M. Heitkemper, RN, PhD

Rose Homan, RN, MA, DDS

Patricia Hong, RN, MA

Sharon Jensen, MN, RN

Lucille T. Kadota, RN, MN, CCRN

Christine A. Kessler, RN, MN, CS

Sheila C. King, MS

Kathleen A. Kominski, RN, MN

Harriet W. LeClair, RN, MN

Barbara J. Loveys, RN, MN, CCRN

C. Kevin Malotte, DrPH

Mary S. McGregor, RN, MN

Pamela H. Mitchell, RN, MS, CNRN, FAAN

Lisa Monat, RN, MN

Carina K. Moravec, MA, RN, CCRN

Jan Muirhead, RN, MN

Patricia Mussnug, RN, MN, CCRN

Judith Rambeck Neufeld, RN, BS

Nancy A. Niles, RN, MA, CCRN

Roberta Oka, DNSc, RN

Susan G. Osguthorpe, MS, RN, CNA

Thomas A. Preston, MD

Wanda Roberts, RN, MN

Joanne Schnaidt Rokosky, RN, MN

Sarah J. Sanford, RN, MN, CCRN

Cynthia C. Scaizi, RN, MN

Mary F. Schmitz, RN, PhD

Joan Shaver, RN, PhD

Martha Shively, RN, PhD, CCRN

Brenda J. Siewicki, RN, MN

Phylita Skov, MS, RN

Margaret L. Snyder, RN, MN

Sandra D. Solack, RN, MSN

Margaret V. Sollek, RN, MN

Sharon A. Stephen, RN, MN, CCRN

Gene Trobaugh, MD

Martha Tyler, RN, MN

Deborah VanEtta, MN, RN, CCRN

Lorie R. Wild, RN, MN

Robert E. Willis, MD

Karen S. Wulff, RN, MN, CCRN

Preface to the 4th Edition

Cardiac Nursing continues to be *the* reference book for nurses caring for patients who have or are at risk for developing cardiac disease. *Cardiac Nursing, 4th Edition* provides the basic and advanced nurse with the most comprehensive evidence-based practice information.

New to This Edition

Many changes have occurred in the 4th edition. First, although Woods, Froelicher, and Underhill Motzer continue to edit Cardiac Nursing, any new contributions from our original co-author and editor, Jean Halpenny, are missing in this edition. Jean died of breast cancer in August 1997; this book is dedicated to her. Second, we have included information from a variety of different clinical practice guidelines to reflect the growing demand to provide evidence-based, cost-effective interventions when such data exist. Third, we have reorganized and revised the content to also meet the needs of adult nurse practitioners. Fourth, we have combined many chapters to provide a more comprehensive discussion of the topic, resulting in fewer chapter titles. Fifth, we have incorporated summary pharmacologic tables throughout the book. Sixth, for easy reference, inside covers now contain frequently used tables and illustrations. Last, we have broadened our focus to include a global perspective on cardiac disease and its management.

Organization

By reorganizing and revising the chapters and content, the 4th edition will help the nurse to provide care more confidently and effectively within the changing health care and economic environment across all practice settings. There are five parts to the 4th edition:

PART ONE: ANATOMY AND PHYSIOLOGY. Includes chapters on anatomy and physiology; systemic and pulmonary circulation and gas transport; and regulation of cardiac output and blood pressure.

PART TWO: PHYSIOLOGIC AND PATHOPHYSIO-LOGIC RESPONSES. Includes chapters on hematopoiesis, coagu-lation and bleeding; fluid and electrolyte balance and imbalance; acid-base balance and imbalance; sleep; and aging.

PART THREE: ASSESSMENT OF HEART DISEASE. Includes chapters on history taking and physical examination; laboratory tests; radiologic examination of the chest; electrocardiography; arrhythmias and conduction disturbances; cardiac electrophysiologic procedures; echocardiography, radioisotope studies, magnetic resonance imaging, phonocardiology; exercise testing; cardiac catheterization; and hemodynamic monitoring.

PART FOUR: TREATMENT OF HEART DISEASE. Includes chapters on myocardial ischemia and infarction; interventional cardiology techniques; heart failure; cardiac surgery; shock; sudden cardiac death and cardiac arrest; pacemakers and implantable defibrillators; acquired valvular heart disease and pericardial, myocardial, and endocardial disease.

PART FIVE: HEALTH PROMOTION AND DISEASE PREVENTION. Includes chapters on coronary heart disease risk factors and disease prevention; psychosocial interventions; smoking cessation and relapse prevention; hypertension; hyperlipidemia; activity and exercise; obesity; diabetes; and adherence.

The Tradition of Excellence

The 4th edition continues our tradition of excellence by having over 90 percent of the chapters written by cardiac nursing experts. It maintains our nursing philosophy by organizing the content within the framework of the nursing process, and includes numerous nursing care plans. Where possible, the rationale and evidence for treatments and interventions are included.

Without the initial support and encouragement from Louise "Susie" Mansfield and Maxine Patrick, the first edition may never have been written. We sincerely appreciate all the comments we received about the previous editions. We hope that you find that the 4th edition lives up to our tradition of excellence, and that the 4th edition becomes your primary reference source for cardiac nursing.

Susan L. Woods, RN, PhD
Erika S. Sivarajan Froelicher, RN, PhD, FAAN
Sandra Adams (Underhill) Motzer, RN, PhD

Table of Contents

PART I
Anatomy and Physiology 1

1   Cardiac Anatomy and Physiology   3
ELEANOR F. BOND

General Anatomic Description   3
Cardiac Structures   6
Cardiac Tissue   9
Coronary Circulation   12
Cardiac Innervation   16
Myocardial Cell Structure   17
Myocardial Cell Electrical Characteristics   18
Cardiac Action Potential   22
Sarcolemmal Ionic Currents   27
Factors Modifying Electrophysiologic Function   28
Propagation of the Cardiac Impulse   30
Mechanical Characteristics of Cardiac Cells   33
Mechanical Properties of the Myocardium   36
Myocardial Metabolism   42
Physiology of the Coronary Circulation   42
The Cardiac Cycle   44

2   Systemic Circulation   51
ELIZABETH J. BRIDGES

Structural Characteristics of the Vasculature and
   Lymphatics   55
Local Regulation   58
Vascular Smooth Muscle   58
Neurohumoral Stimulation   59
Calcium   59
Volume and Flow Distribution   59
The Arterial System   62
The Venous System   63
Microcirculatory Exchange   64
The Lymphatic System   66
Edema Formation   67

**3   The Pulmonary Circulation
and Gas Transport   73**
POLLY E. GARDNER

The Pulmonary Circulation   73
Structural Characteristics   75

Pulmonary Vascular Bed   75
Blood Reservoir   75
Effects of Lung Pressures   75
Alveolar—Capillary Transfer of Oxygen and Carbon
   Dioxide   76
Oxygen   78
Carbon Dioxide   78
Oxygen Delivery or Transport   78
Blood Oxygen Content   79
Measurement of Oxygen Delivery or Transport   79
Monitoring Tissue Oxygenation   80

**4   Control of Blood Pressure
and Cardiac Output   82**
ELIZABETH J. BRIDGES

Afferent Input and Receptors   82
Central Nervous System Regulation   84
Autonomic Nervous System Regulation   84
Systemic Hormones   88
Heart Rate   90
Intrinsic Cardiac Control   91
Extrinsic Control: Pericardial Limitation   92
Vascular Control   92
Long-Term Control of Blood Pressure   93
Local Regulation of Systemic Microvascular Beds   94
Venous System   96
Models of Cardiac Performance   97
Additional Effects of Respiration   99
Overall Control   101

PART II
Physiologic and Pathologic
Responses   107

5   Hematopoiesis and Coagulation   109
HOLLY LEA
BRENDA K. ZIERLER

Hematopoietic Cells   109
Hemostasis   112
Fibrinolysis   114
Bleeding Disorders   115
Clotting Disorders   121

6 Fluid and Electrolyte Balance and Imbalance   132
LINDA FELVER

Principles of Fluid Balance   132
Extracellular Fluid Volume Balance   134
Osmolality Balance   135
Principles of Electrolyte Balance   137
Electrolyte Imbalances   137
Summary   148

7 Acid-Base Balances and Imbalances   153
LINDA FELVER

Principles of Acid-Base Balance   153
Acid-Base Imbalances   155
Summary   160

8 Sleep   162
KATHRYN A. LEE

Nature of Sleep   162
Physiologic Responses During Sleep   166
Sleep and Cardiovascular Disease   167
Cardiac Events During Sleep   168
Cardiovascular Consequences of Breathing Disorders in Sleep   169
Nursing Management Plan   170
The Health Care Providers' Sleep   173
Summary   173

9 Physiologic Adaptions With Aging 180
RUTH F. CRAVEN

General Physiologic Changes   182
Cardiovascular Changes   182
Respiratory Changes   183
Renal Changes   184
Hepatic Changes   184
Drugs and the Elderly   184
Summary   185

PART III
Assessment of Heart Disease   187

10 History Taking and Physical Examination   189
BARBARA S. LEVINE
SANDRA UNDERHILL MOTZER

Cardiovascular History   189
Health History   190
Physical Assessment   195

11 Laboratory Tests Using Blood   227
MARGARET WOODING BAKER

Blood Specimen Collection   227
Cardiac Markers   230
Hematologic Studies   239
Arterial Blood Gases   243
Blood Chemistries   244
Serum Concentration of Selected Drugs   247

12 Radiologic Examination of the Chest   252
JON S. HUSEBY

How X-rays Work   252
Interpretation of Chest Radiographs   252
Chest Film Findings in Myocardial Infarction and Conditions That May Mimic Myocardial Infarction   254
Chest Film Findings in Complications of Acute Myocardial Infarction   258
Miscellaneous Uses of the Chest Radiograph   258

13 Electrocardiography   263
CAROL JACOBSON

Electrical Conduction Through the Heart   263
Basic Electrocardiography   266
The 12-Lead Electrocardiogram   268
Axis Determination   273
Intraventricular Conduction Abnormalities   276
Ischemia, Injury, and Infarction   282
Atrial and Ventricular Enlargement (Hypertrophy)   288
Electrolyte Imbalances   291

14 Arrhythmias and Conduction Disturbances   297
CAROL JACOBSON

Mechanisms of Arrhythmias   297
Basic Arrhythmias and Conduction Disturbances   302
Complex Arrhythmias and Conduction Disturbances   329

15 Cardiac Electrophysiology Procedures   363
SUSAN BLANCHER
CAROLYN CHANDLER MAIN

Diagnostic Electrophysiology Studies   363
Interventional Electrophysiology and Catheter Ablation   368
Nursing Care of the Patient Undergoing Electrophysiology Procedures   371

16 Echocardiography, Radioisotope Studies, Electron Beam Computed Tomography, Magnetic Resonance Imaging, and Phonocardiography   374
MARGARET HALL

Echocardiography   375
Stress Echocardiography   381
Transesophageal Echocardiography   381
Radioisotope Evaluation of the Heart   382
Positron Emission Tomography   383
Electron Beam Computed Tomography   383
Magnetic Resonance Imaging   383
Phonocardiology   384
Imaging in Cardiac Pathology   384
Conclusion   387

17 Exercise Testing   389
JONATHAN MYERS

Indications and Objectives   389
Safety and Personnel   389
Pretest Considerations   390
Exercise Test Selection   392
Interpretation of Exercise Test Responses   394
Test Termination   400
Recovery Period   401
Assessing Test Accuracy   401
Ancillary Methods for the Detection of Coronary
    Artery Disease   402
Gas Exchange Techniques   404
Prognosis   404
Exercise Testing in Special Populations   404
Summary   405

18 Cardiac Catheterization   409
MARY MCMAHON BUSCH
ROXANNE JUEL
KATHERINE M. NEWTON

Indications   409
Contraindications   410
Patient Preparation   410
Procedure   411
The Nurse in the Cardiac Catheterization
    Laboratory   418
Interpretation of Data   421

19 Hemodynamic Monitoring   427
ELIZABETH BRIDGES

Technical Aspects of Invasive Pressure
    Monitoring   427
Direct Arterial Pressure Monitoring   433
Central Venous Pressure Monitoring   436

Pulmonary Artery Pressure Monitoring   438
Cardiac Output Measurement   452
Continuous Cardiac Output   459
Bioimpedance Cardiac Output Measurements   461
Other Methods for Cardiac Output Measurement   462
Oxygen Supply and Demand   462

PART IV
Treatment of Heart Disease   479

20 Myocardial Ischemia Pathogenesis of Atherosclerosis   481
SUSANNA CUNNINGHAM
SHERRI DEL BENE
ANNE FALSONE VAUGHAN

Morphology of the Normal Arterial Wall   481
Cellular, Structural, and Molecular Components
    of Atherosclerotic Plaques   482
Morphology of the Atherosclerotic Lesion   487
Theories of Atherosclerosis Pathogenesis   489
Pathophysiology of Myocardial Ischemia and
    Infarction   495
        SUSANNA CUNNINGHAM

Causes and Classifications of Ischemia and
    Infarction   496
Alterations in Coronary Blood Flow   497
Endothelial and Blood Cell Interactions   497
Local Physiologic Alterations in Ischemia   498
Mechanisms for the Stress Response   501
Mechanisms for Pain   502
Circadian Rhythmicity   502
Consequences of Reperfusion   502
Restenosis and Reocclusion   503
Implications for Nursing   503
Diagnosis and Management of Myocardial
    Ischemia   508
        ANNE VAUGHAN

Epidemiology   508
Classification of Angina   508
Diagnosis   508
Medical Management   512
Prognosis   513
Nursing Management   513
Diagnosis and Management of Myocardial
    Infarction   515
        SHERRI DEL BENE
        ANNE VAUGHAN

Classification of Myocardial Infarctions   515
Diagnosis   516
Complications of Acute Myocardial Infarction   519
Medical Management   522
Pharmacologic Management   528
Nursing Management   531

**21 Interventional Cardiology
Techniques   541**
MICHAELENE HARGROVE DEELSTRA

Thrombolytic Therapy   541
Interventional Devices   544
Nursing Management   545

22 Heart Failure   560
DEBRA LAURENT-BOPP

Definition and Classifications   560
Pathophysiology   561
Clinical Manifestations   565
Medical Management   567
Nursing Management   574

23 Cardiac Surgery   580
DENISE LEDOUX
HELEN LUIKART

Evolving Trends in Cardiac Surgery   580
Preoperative Assessment and Preparation   580
Surgical Techniques   581
Cardiac Surgery Procedures for Coronary Artery
    Revascularization   584
Cardiac Surgery Procedures for Acquired Structural
    Heart Disease   587
Cardiac Transplantation   595

24 Shock   614
DEBRA LAURENT-BOPP
JULIE A. SHINN

Database for Nursing Management   614
Nursing Management Plan for the Patient in
    Shock   636

**25 Sudden Cardiac Death and Cardiac
Arrest   639**
CAROLYN CHANDLER MAIN
DONNA GERITY

Definition of Sudden Death   639
Pathology and Pathophysiology of Sudden Cardiac
    Arrest   639
Management of Sudden Cardiac Arrest   642
Survivors of Cardiac Arrest   653

**26 Pacemaker and Implantable
Defibrillators   661**
CAROL JACKSON
DONNA GERITY

Pacemakers   661
Implantable Cardioverter-Defibrillators   686

27 Acquired Valvular Heart Disease   699
DENISE LEDOUX

Database for Nursing Management   699

**28 Pericardial, Myocardial,
and Endocardial Disease   719**
MARGARET M. MCNEILL

Pericardial Disease   719
Cardiomyopathies   724
Endocardial Disease   729

**PART V
Health Promotion and Disease
Prevention   737**

**29 Coronary Heart Disease Risk
Factors   739**
KATHERINE M. NEWTON
ERIKA SIVARAJAN FROELICHER

Demographic Characteristics   740
Family History of Cardiovascular Disease   741
Cigarette Smoking   742
High Blood Pressure   743
Serum Lipids and Lipoproteins   743
Physical Activity   745
Diabetes Mellitus   747
Obesity, Weight Distribution, and Weight
    Change   748
Reproductive Hormones   750
Folate and Homocysteine   751
Antioxidants   751
Conclusions   752

30 Psychosocial Interventions   757
JOAN M. FAIR
ERIKA SIVARAJAN FROELICHER

Stress   757
Social Support   759
Personality Factors   759
Psychosocial Interventions   760

**31 Smoking Cessation: A Systematic
Approach to Managing Patients with
Coronary Heart Disease   764**
KRISTEN MARTIN
NANCY HOUSTON MILLER
ERIKA S. SIVARAJAN FROELICHER

Harmful Effects of Smoking   765
Benefits of Smoking Cessation   765
Theoretical Framework for Smoking Cessation   766

Smoking Cessation Interventions in the Coronary
    Heart Disease Population   766
General Trends in Smoking Cessation
    Interventions   767
Agency for Health Care Policy and Research
    Smoking Cessation Clinical Practice
    Guideline   767
Special Areas on Which to Focus   772

32 High Blood Pressure   777
    SUSANNA CUNNINGHAM

Database for Management   777
Management of High Blood Pressure   787

**33 Lipid Management and Coronary
     Heart Disease   819**
    JOAN M. FAIR
    KATHLEEN A. BERRA

Blood Lipids: Structure and Functions   819
Lipid Metabolism and Transport   820
Reverse Cholesterol Transport   821
Low-Density Lipoprotein Variants   821
Cholesterol and Endothelial Function   822
Dyslipidemic Disorders   822
Hypercholesterolemia   822
The Management of High Blood Cholesterol   823
Evaluation of the Patient with Elevated
    Cholesterol   824
Lipoprotein Measurement   824
Dietary Management of Hyperlipidemia   826
Weight Control and Lipid Management   828
Alcohol and Lipoproteins   829
Physical Activity and Lipoproteins   829
Hormones and Lipoproteins   829
Pharmacologic Management of Hyperlipidemia   829

34 Exercise and Activity   835
    DEANNA E. RITCHIE
    JONATHAN N. MYERS

Role of Exercise in Cardiovascular Health   835
Cardiac Rehabilitation   840

**35 Obesity: An Overview of
     Assessment and Treatment   860**
    LORA E. BURKE

Identification and Assessment of the Overweight or
    Obese Patient   861
Clinical Evaluation and Treatment Strategies   862
Treatment of Overweight and Obesity   863
Treatment Components   864
Summary   867

36 Diabetes Mellitus   869
    MARGARET I. WALLHAGEN

Definition, Prevalence, and Economic
    Consequences   869
Pathophysiology of Diabetes Mellitus   870
Complications of Diabetes Mellitus   871
Pathophysiology of Complications   872
Nursing Management of Diabetes   873
Health Screening and Monitoring   877
Summary   878

**37 Adherence to Cardiovascular
     Treatment Regimens   880**
    LORA E. BURKE

Significance of Nonadherence   880
Methods of Measurement   881
Determinants of Adherence   884
Models of Behavior Change   884
Adherence-Enhancing Strategies   885
Educational Strategies to Improve Adherence   887
Questionnaires Relevant to Adherence-Enhancing
    Interventions   888
Building a Therapeutic Relationship with the
    Patient   888
Summary   889

Index   893

Cardiac Nursing

4TH EDITION

Anatomy and Physiology

Cardiac Anatomy and Physiology

ELEANOR F. BOND*

An understanding of cardiac anatomy is helpful for understanding cardiac physiology and the functional consequences of disease. This chapter describes normal human adult gross cardiac and vessel anatomy, cellular structure, and ultrastructure. Contraction of the heart propels blood through the body, delivering nutrients and removing waste from all organs, including the heart itself. The chapter also describes the electrical, mechanical, and metabolic activities that underlie cardiac pump performance. Electrical, mechanical, and metabolic processes are integrated in the working heart and require constant perfusion. The coronary circulation is discussed in the context of its linkage to changing demands for nutrient delivery and waste removal. Finally, integrated cardiac performance is discussed.

GENERAL ANATOMIC DESCRIPTION

The heart, encased and cushioned in its own serous membrane, the pericardium, lies in the middle mediastinal compartment of the thorax between the two pleural cavities. Two thirds of the heart extends to the left of the body's midline (Fig. 1-1).

The heart consists of four muscular chambers, two atria and two ventricles, and associated structures. The right heart (right atrium and ventricle) receives blood from the body and pumps it into the low-pressure pulmonary arterial system, whereas the left heart (left atrium and ventricle) receives blood from the lungs and pumps it into the high-pressure systemic arterial system. Interatrial and interventricular septa separate the right and left atria and ventricles from each other.

The long axis of the heart is directed obliquely, leftward, downward, and forward. Any factor that changes the shape of the thorax changes the position of the heart and modifies the directional axis. Respiratory alterations in

*The material in this chapter was originally coauthored with Carol Jean Halpenny.

the level of the diaphragm or expansion of the rib cage change the cardiac axis. Thus, with a deep inspiration, the heart descends and becomes more vertical. Factors that may cause axis variations in healthy people include age, weight, pregnancy, body shape, and shape of the thorax. A tall, thin person usually has a more vertical heart, whereas a short, obese person usually has a more horizontal heart. Pathologic conditions of the heart, lungs, abdominal organs, and other structures influence the direction of the cardiac axis.

The surfaces of the heart are used to reference its position in relation to other structures and to describe the location of damage, as in a myocardial infarction. The right ventricle and parts of the right atrium and the left ventricle form the anterior (or sternocostal) cardiac surface (see Fig. 1-1; Fig. 1-2). The right atrium and ventricle lie anteriorly and to the right of the left atrium and ventricle in the frontal plane. Thus, when viewed from the front of the body, the heart appears to be lying sideways, directed forward and leftward, with the right heart foremost.

The small portion of the lower left ventricle that extends anteriorly forms a blunt tip composed of the apical part of the interventricular septum and the left ventricular free wall. Because of the forward tilt of the heart, movement of this apex portion of the left ventricle during cardiac contraction usually forms the *point of maximal impulse,* which can be observed in healthy people in the fifth intercostal space at the left midclavicular line, 7 to 9 cm from midline. The sternum, costal cartilages of the third to sixth ribs, part of the lungs, and, in children, the thymus, overlie the anterior cardiac surface.

The left atrium and a small section of the right atrium and ventricle comprise the base of the heart, which is directed backward and forms the posterior surface of the heart (Fig. 1-3). The thoracic aorta, esophagus, and vertebrae are posterior to the heart.

The inferior or diaphragmatic surface of the heart, comprising chiefly the left ventricle, lies almost horizontally on the upper surface of the diaphragm (Fig. 1-4). The right ventricle forms a portion of the inferior cardiac surface.

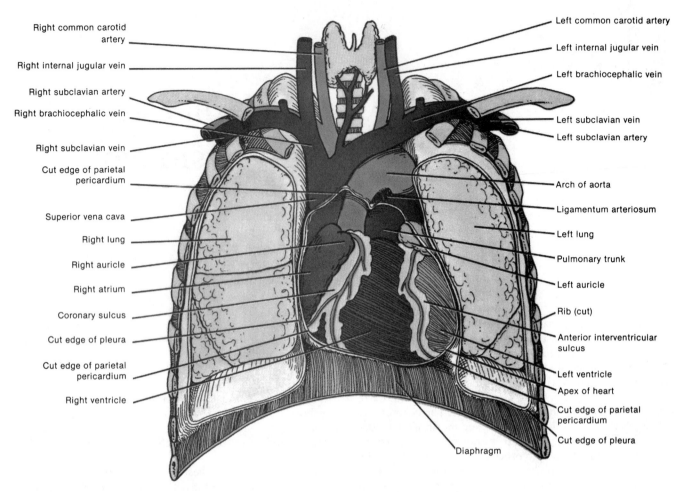

Right common carotid artery
Right internal jugular vein
Right subclavian artery
Right brachiocephalic vein
Right subclavian vein
Cut edge of parietal pericardium
Superior vena cava
Right lung
Right auricle
Right atrium
Coronary sulcus
Cut edge of pleura
Cut edge of parietal pericardium
Right ventricle

Left common carotid artery
Left internal jugular vein
Left brachiocephalic vein
Left subclavian vein
Left subclavian artery
Arch of aorta
Ligamentum arteriosum
Left lung
Pulmonary trunk
Left auricle
Rib (cut)
Anterior interventricular sulcus
Left ventricle
Apex of heart
Cut edge of parietal pericardium
Cut edge of pleura
Diaphragm

FIGURE 1-1 Anterior view of the heart, illustrating the position of the heart and associated structures in the thoracic cavity. (From Tortora GJ: Principles of Human Anatomy, 4th ed, p 302. New York, Harper & Row, 1986.)

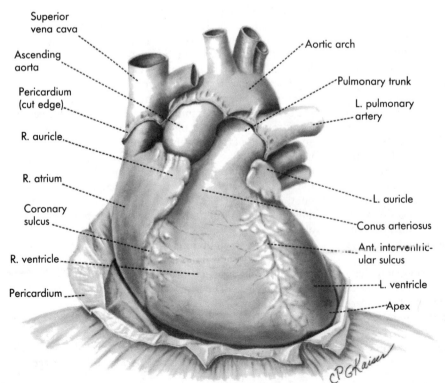

Superior vena cava
Ascending aorta
Pericardium (cut edge)
R. auricle
R. atrium
Coronary sulcus
R. ventricle
Pericardium

Aortic arch
Pulmonary trunk
L. pulmonary artery
L. auricle
Conus arteriosus
Ant. interventricular sulcus
L. ventricle
Apex

CPGKaiser

FIGURE 1-2 Anterior view of the heart, illustrating the cardiac structures. The pericardial sac has been cut open and reflected toward the diaphragm. (From Hollinshead WH, Rosse C: Textbook of Anatomy, 4th ed, p 523. Philadelphia, Harper & Row, 1985.)

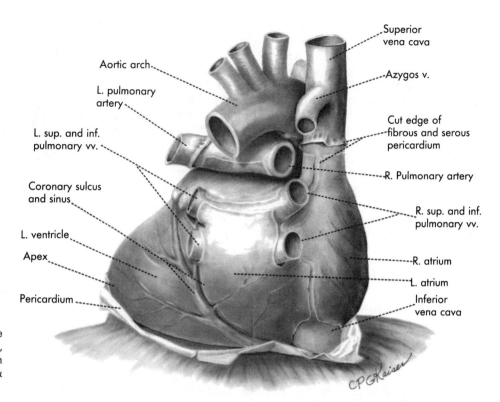

FIGURE 1-3 Posterior view of the heart. (From Hollinshead WH, Rosse C: Textbook of Anatomy, 4th ed, p 523. Philadelphia, Harper & Row, 1985.)

The right atrium forms the lateral right heart border, and therefore the right atrium and right lung lie close together. The entire right margin of the heart extends laterally from the superior vena cava along the right atrium and then toward the diaphragm to the cardiac apex. The lateral wall of the left ventricle and a small part of the left atrium form most of the left heart border. This portion of the left ventricle is next to the left lung and sometimes is referred to as the *pulmonary surface.*

The coronary (or atrioventricular [AV]) sulcus (groove) is the external landmark denoting the separation of the atria from the ventricles. The AV sulcus encircles the heart obliquely and contains coronary blood vessels, cardiac nerves, and epicardial fat. The aorta and pulmonary artery interrupt the AV sulcus anteriorly. The anterior and posterior interventricular sulci separate the right and left ventricles on the external heart surface. The crux of the heart is the point on the external posterior heart surface where the

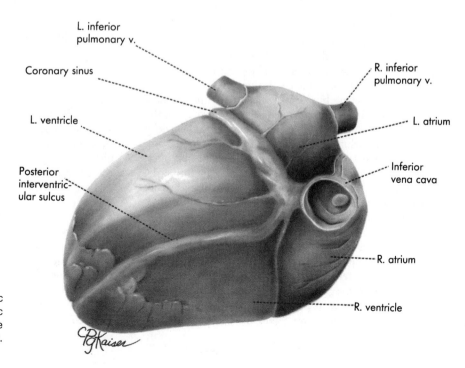

FIGURE 1-4 Inferior or diaphragmatic heart surface, with the pericardial sac reflected. (From Hollinshead WH, Rosse C: Textbook of Anatomy, 4th ed, p 524. Philadelphia, Harper & Row, 1985.)

posterior interventricular sulcus intersects the coronary (AV) sulcus externally and where the interatrial septum joins the interventricular septum internally.

The average adult heart is approximately 12 cm long from its base at the beginning root of the aorta to the left ventricular apex, 8 to 9 cm wide transversely at the widest part, and 6 cm thick anteroposteriorly. Tables have been derived to indicate normal ranges of heart size for various body weights and heights.[62]

The adult male heart comprises approximately 0.43% of body weight, 280 to 350 g, with an average of 300 g.[48,54] The adult female heart comprises approximately 0.40% of body weight, 230 to 300 g, with an average of 250 g.[48,54] Age, body build, frequency of physical exercise, and heart disease influence heart size and weight.

CARDIAC STRUCTURES

Fibrous Skeleton

Four adjacent, dense, fibrous connective tissue rings, the annuli fibrosi, surround the cardiac valves and provide an internal supporting structure for the heart. The annuli are attached together and connected by a central fibrous core (Fig. 1-5). Each annulus and valve has a different orientation, but the entire connective tissue structure, termed the *fibrous skeleton*, is oriented obliquely within the mediastinum.

The fibrous skeleton divides the atria from the ventricles. It provides the attachment site for some of the atrial and ventricular cardiac muscle fibers. An extension of the fibrous skeleton extends downward between the right atrium and left ventricle, forming the upper or membranous part of the interventricular septum.

Chambers

The wall thickness of each of the four cardiac chambers reflects the amount of pressure generated by the chamber. The two thin-walled atria serve functionally as reservoirs and conduits for blood that is being funneled into the ventricles; they add a small amount of force to the moving blood. The left ventricle, which adds the greatest amount of pressure to the flowing blood, is two to three times as thick as the right ventricle. The approximate wall thickness of the chambers are as follows: right atrium, 2 mm; right ventricle, 3 to 5 mm; left atrium, 3 mm; left ventricle, 13 to 15 mm.

The interatrial septum between right and left atria extends obliquely forward from right to left. The interatrial septum includes the fossa ovalis, a remnant of a fetal structure, the foramen ovale. The lower portion of the interatrial septum is formed by the lower medial right atrial wall on one side and the aortic outflow tract of the left ventricular wall on the other side. The lower muscular portion of the interventricular septum extends from the upper membranous part of the interventricular septum.

In considering the internal surfaces of the cardiac chambers, it is helpful to remember that blood flows more smoothly and with less turbulence across walls that are smooth than

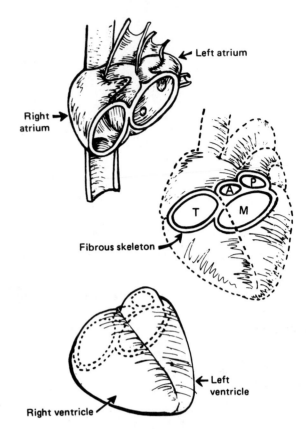

FIGURE 1-5 Schematic view of the fibrous skeleton, illustrating the attachment of the cardiac valves and chambers. The four annuli and their extensions lie in different planes, so it is impossible to depict them accurately on a plane surface. T, tricuspid valve; M, mitral valve; A, aortic valve; P, pulmonic valve. (Adapted from Rushmer RF: Cardiovascular Dynamics, p 77. Philadelphia, WB Saunders, 1976.)

across ridged walls. Blood pools more frequently in appendages or other areas out of the direct blood flow path.

RIGHT HEART

The posterior and septal walls of the right atrium are smooth, whereas the lateral wall and the right atrial appendage (auricle) have parallel muscular ridges, termed *pectinate muscles*. The right auricle extends over the aortic root externally.

The inferior wall of the right atrium and part of the superior wall of the right ventricle are formed by the tricuspid valve (Fig. 1-6). The anterior and inferior walls of the right ventricle are lined by muscle bundles, the trabeculae carneae, which form a rough-walled inflow tract for blood. One muscle group, the septomarginal trabecula or moderator band, extends from the lower interventricular septum to the anterior right ventricular papillary muscle.

Another thick muscle bundle, the christa supraventricularis, extends from the septal wall to the anterolateral wall of the right ventricle. The christa supraventricularis helps to divide the right ventricle into an inflow and outflow tract. The smooth-walled outflow tract, called the *conus arteriosus*, or *infundibulum*, extends to the pulmonary artery.

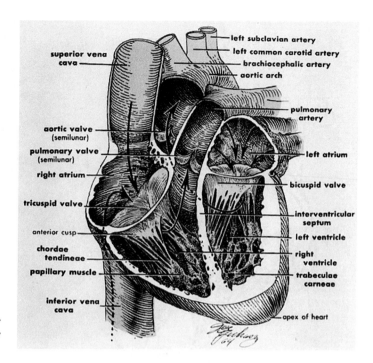

FIGURE 1-6 Schematic illustration of cardiac structures. (From Crouch JE: Functional Human Anatomy, 4th ed, p. 403. Philadelphia, Lea & Febiger, 1985.)

The concave free wall of the right ventricle is attached to the slightly convex septal wall. The internal right ventricular cavity is crescent or triangle shaped. The right ventricle also forms a crescent laterally around the left ventricle. Right ventricular contraction causes the right ventricular free wall to move toward the interventricular septum. This bellows-like action is effective in ejecting large and variable volumes into a low-pressure system (Fig. 1-7).

Venous blood enters the right atrium from the upper and lower posterior part of the atrium through the superior and inferior venae cavae. Most of the venous drainage from the heart enters the right atrium through the coronary sinus, which is located between the entrance of the inferior vena cava into the right atrium and the orifice of the tricuspid valve. Blood flows medially and anteriorly from the right atrium through the tricuspid orifice into the right ventricle.

Blood enters the right ventricle in an almost horizontal but slightly leftward, anterior, and inferior direction. It is ejected superiorly and posteriorly through the pulmonary valve (Fig. 1-8).

LEFT HEART

The left atrium is a cuboid structure that lies between the aortic root and the esophagus. The left atrial appendage, or auricle, extends along the border of the pulmonary artery. The walls of the left atrium are smooth except for pectinate muscle bundles in the atrial appendage.

The left ventricle's cone or oval shape is due to the generally concave left ventricular free wall and interventricular septum. The mitral valve and its attachments form the left ventricular inflow tract. The outflow tract is formed by the anterior surface of the anterior mitral valve cusp, the septum, and the aortic vestibule. The lower muscular interventricular

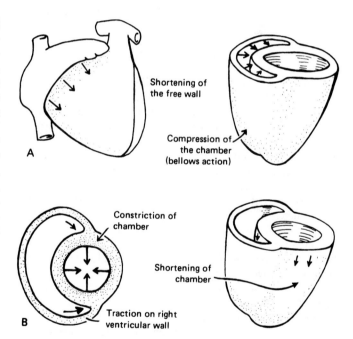

FIGURE 1-7 Right and left ventricular contraction. **(A)** Right ventricular contraction. Right ventricular ejection of blood is accomplished primarily by shortening and movement of the free wall toward the interventricular septum. Note the crescent shape of the right ventricle. **(B)** blood is ejected from the left ventricle primarily by a reduction in the diameter of the chamber. There is some ventricular shortening. (Adapted from Rushmer R: Cardiovascular Dynamics, p 92. Philadelphia, WB Saunders, 1976.)

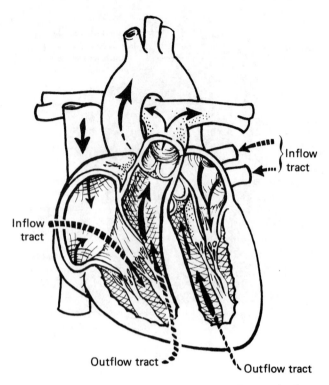

FIGURE 1-8 Blood flow through cardiac chambers and valves.

septum and free walls of the left ventricle are deeply ridged with trabeculae carneae muscle bundles, so most of the interior surface of the ventricle is rough. The upper membranous septum and aortic vestibule region have smooth walls.

The interventricular septum is functionally and anatomically a more integral part of the left ventricle than the right ventricle. The septum is triangle shaped, with its base at the aortic area. The upper septum separates the right atrium from the left ventricle and is often called the *AV septum*.

Blood is ejected from the left ventricle mainly by circumferential contraction of the muscular wall, that is, by decreasing the diameter of the cylinder (see Fig. 1-7). There is some longitudinal shortening. The ventricular cavity has a small surface area in relation to the volume contained, but high pressures can be developed because of the amount of ventricular muscle, the shape of the cavity, and the way the muscles contract.

Four pulmonary veins return blood from the lungs to openings in the posterolateral wall of the left atrium. Blood is directed obliquely forward out of the left atrium and enters the left ventricle in an anterior, leftward, inferior direction. Blood flows out of the ventricle from the apex toward the aorta in a superior and rightward direction (see Fig. 1-8).

Thus, blood flows from posterior orifices into both ventricles in a leftward direction and is ejected superiorly toward the center of the heart. The right ventricular tract is more tubular and the left ventricular tract more conical (see Fig. 1-8).

Valves

ATRIOVENTRICULAR VALVES

The AV tricuspid and bicuspid (mitral) valve complexes are composed of six components that function as a unit: the atria, the valve rings or annuli fibrosi of the fibrous skeleton,

the valve cusps or leaflets, the chordae tendineae, the papillary muscles, and the ventricular walls (see Fig. 1-6). The mitral and tricuspid valve cusps are composed of fibrous connective tissue covered by endothelium. They attach to the fibrous skeleton valve rings. Fibrous cords called *chordae tendineae* connect the free valve margins and ventricular surfaces of the valve cusps to papillary muscles and ventricular walls. The papillary muscles are trabeculae carneae muscle bundles oriented parallel to the ventricular walls, extending from the walls to the chordae tendineae (see Fig. 1-6). The chordae tendineae provide many cross-connections from one papillary muscle to two valve cusps or from trabeculae carneae in the ventricular wall directly to valves.

The adult tricuspid orifice is larger (approximately 11 cm in circumference, or capable of admitting three fingers) than the mitral orifice (approximately 9 cm in circumference, or capable of admitting two fingers). The combined surface area of the AV valve cusps is larger than the surface area of the valvular orifice because the cusps resemble curtain-like, billowing flaps.

Most commonly, there are three tricuspid valve cusps: the large anterior, the septal, and the posterior (inferior). There are usually two principal right ventricular papillary muscles, the anterior and the posterior (inferior), and a smaller set of accessory papillary muscles attached to the ventricular septum.

The arrangement of the two triangular bicuspid valve cusps has been compared with a bishop's hat, or miter. The smaller, less mobile posterior cusp is situated posterolaterally, behind and to the left of the aortic opening. The larger, more mobile anterior cusp extends from the anterior papillary muscle to the ventricular septum.

The left ventricle most commonly has two major papillary muscles: the posterior papillary muscle attached to the diaphragmatic ventricular wall, and the anterior papillary muscle attached to the sternocostal ventricular wall. Thus, the posteromedial papillary muscle extends to the posterolateral valve leaflet, and the anterolateral papillary muscle extends to the anteromedial valve leaflet. Chordae tendineae from each papillary muscle go to both mitral cusps.

During diastole, the AV valves open passively. Pressure in the atria exceeds that in the ventricles. The papillary muscles are relaxed. The valve cusps part, projecting into the ventricle, forming a funnel, which helps to promote blood flow into the ventricles (see Fig. 1-8). Toward the end of diastole, the deceleration of blood flowing into the ventricles, the movement of blood in a circular motion behind the cusps, and the increasing pressures in the ventricle compared with lessening pressures in the atria, help to close each valve. During systole, the free edges of the valve cusps are prevented from being everted into the atria by contraction of the papillary muscles and tension in the chordae tendineae. Thus, blood is prevented from flowing backward into the atria despite the high systolic ventricular pressures.

SEMILUNAR VALVES

The two semilunar (pulmonary [or pulmonic] and aortic) valves are each composed of three cup-shaped cusps of approximately equal size that attach at their base to the fibrous skeleton. The valve cusps are convex from below, with thickened nodules at the center of the free margins.

The cusps are composed of fibrous connective tissue lined with endothelium. The endothelial lining on the nonventricular side of the valves closely resembles and merges with that of the intima of the arteries beyond the valves. The aortic cusps are thicker than the pulmonic; both are thicker than the AV cusps.

The pulmonary valve orifice is approximately 8.5 cm in circumference, and the aortic valve is approximately 7.5 cm. The pulmonic valve cusps are termed *right anterior* (right), *left anterior* (anterior), and *posterior* (left); the positions of the cusps in the fetus are indicated parenthetically.

The sinuses of Valsalva are pouch-like structures immediately behind each semilunar cusp. The coronary arteries branch from the aorta from two of the pouches or sinuses of Valsalva. The aortic cusps are designated by the name of the nearby coronary artery: right coronary (right or anterior) aortic cusp, left coronary (left or left posterior) aortic cusp, and noncoronary (posterior or right posterior) aortic cusp. The specific cusp's position in the fetus and the adult, respectively, is indicated parenthetically.

The two semilunar valves are approximately at right angles to each other in the closed position. The pulmonic valve is anterior and superior to the other three cardiac valves.

When closed, the semilunar valve cusps contact each other at the nodules and along crescentic arcs, called *lunulae,* below the free margins. During systole, the cusps are thrust upward as blood flows from an area of greater pressure in the ventricle to an area of lesser pressure in the aorta or the pulmonary artery. The effect of the deceleration of blood in the aorta during late systole on small circular currents of blood in the sinuses of Valsalva helps passively to close the semilunar valve cusps. Backflow into the ventricles during diastole is prevented because of the cusps' fibrous strength, their close approximation, and their shape.

CARDIAC TISSUE

The heart wall is composed mainly of a muscular layer, the myocardium. The epicardium and the pericardium cover the external surface. Internally, the endocardium covers the surface.

Epicardium and Pericardium

The epicardium is a layer of mesothelial cells that forms the visceral or heart layer of the serous pericardium. Branches of the coronary blood and lymph vessels, nerves, and fat are enclosed in the epicardium and the superficial layers of the myocardium.

The epicardium completely encloses the external surface of the heart and extends several centimeters along each great vessel, encircling the aorta and pulmonary artery together. It merges with the tunica adventitia of the great vessels, at which point it doubles back on itself as the parietal pericardium. This continuous membrane thus forms the pericardial sac and encloses a potential space, the pericardial cavity (see Fig. 1-1). The serous parietal pericardium lines the inner surface of the thicker, tougher fibrous pericardial membrane. The pericardial membrane extends beyond the serous pericardium and is attached by ligaments and loose connections to the sternum, diaphragm, and structures in the posterior mediastinum.

The pericardial cavity is usually filled with 10 to 30 mL of thin, clear serous fluid. The main function of the pericardium and its fluid is to lubricate the moving surfaces of the heart. The pericardium also helps to retard ventricular dilation, helps to hold the heart in position, and forms a barrier to the spread of infections and neoplasia.

Pathophysiologic conditions such as cardiac tamponade or an exudate-producing pericarditis may lead to a sudden or large accumulation of fluid within the pericardial sac. This may impede ventricular filling (see Chapter 28). From 50 to 300 mL of pericardial fluid may be accumulated without serious ventricular impairment. When greater volumes accumulate, ventricular filling is impaired. If this happens slowly, the ventricles may be able to maintain an adequate cardiac output by contracting more vigorously. The pericardium is histologically similar to pleural and peritoneal serous membranes, so inflammation of all three membranes may occur with certain systemic conditions such as rheumatoid arthritis.

Myocardium

The myocardial layer is composed of cardiac muscle cells interspersed with connective tissue and small blood vessels. Some atrial and ventricular myocardial fibers are anchored to the fibrous skeleton (see Fig. 1-5). The thin-walled atria are composed of two major muscle systems: one that surrounds both of the atria, and another that is arranged at right angles to the first and that is separate for each atrium.

Each ventricle is a single muscle mass of nested figure-of-eight individual muscle fiber path spirals anchored to the fibrous skeleton.[50,59] Ventricular muscle fibers spiral downward on the epicardial ventricular wall, pass through the wall, spiral up on the endocardial surface, cross the upper part of the ventricle, and go back down through the wall (Fig. 1-9). This vortex arrangement allows for the circumferential generation of tension throughout the ventricular wall and thus is functionally efficient for ventricular contraction. Some fiber paths spiral around both ventricles. The fibers form a fan-like arrangement of interconnecting muscle fibers when dissected horizontally through the

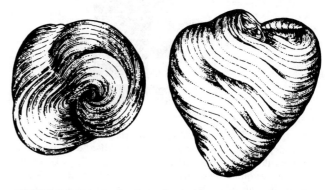

FIGURE 1-9 Schematic view of spiral arrangement of ventricular muscle fibers. (From Katz A: Physiology of the Heart, p 4. New York, Raven Press, 1977.)

ventricular wall.[59] The orientation of these fibers gradually rotates through the thickness of the wall (Fig. 1-10).

The myocardial tissue consists of several functionally specialized cell types:

> *Working myocardial cells* generate the contractile force of the heart. These cells have a markedly striated appearance owing to the orderly arrays of the abundant contractile protein filaments. Working myocardial cells make up the bulk of the walls of both atrial and both ventricular chambers.
>
> *Nodal cells* are specialized for pacemaker function. They are found in clusters in the sinus and AV nodes. These cells contain few contractile filaments, little sarcoplasmic reticulum (SR), and no transverse tubules. They are the smallest myocardial cells.
>
> *Purkinje cells* are specialized for rapid conduction of electrical impulses, especially through the thick ventricular wall. The large size, elongated shape, and

Endocardium

Midwall

100μm

Epicardium

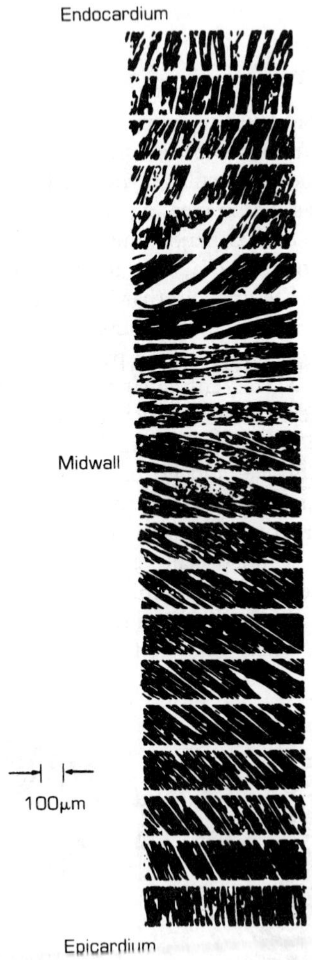

FIGURE 1-10 Changing ventricular muscle fiber angles at different depths. Reconstructed from a series of microphotographs. (From Streeter DD Jr, Spotnitz HM, Patel DP et al: Fiber orientation in the canine left ventricle during diastole and systole. Circ Res 24: 342, 1969. By permission of the American Heart Association, Inc.)

sparse contractile protein composition reflect this specialization. These cells are found in the common His bundle and in the left and right bundle branches as well as in a diffuse network throughout the ventricles. Purkinje cell cytoplasm is rich in glycogen granules, contributing to these cells' resistance to damage during anoxic periods. A secondary function of the Purkinje cells is to serve as a potential pacemaker locus. In the absence of an overriding impulse from the sinus node, Purkinje cells initiate electrical impulses.

In areas of contact between diverse cell types, there is usually an area of gradual transition in which the cells are intermediate in appearance.

Endocardium

The endocardium is composed of a layer of endothelial cells and a few layers of collagen and elastic fibers. The endocardium is in continuation with the tunica intima of the blood vessels.

Conduction Tissues

In the normal sequence of events, the specialized nodal myocardial cells depolarize spontaneously, generating electrical impulses that are conducted to the larger mass of working myocardial cells (Fig. 1-11). The sequential contraction of the atria and ventricles as coordinated units depends on the anatomic arrangement of the specialized cardiac conducting tissue. Small cardiac nerves, arteries, and veins lie close to the specialized conducting cells, providing neurohumoral modulation of cardiac impulse generation and conduction.

Keith and Flack[26] first described the sinus node in 1907. It lies close to the epicardial surface of the heart, above the tricuspid valve, near the anterior entrance of the superior vena cava into the right atrium. The sinus node is also referred to as the *sinoatrial node*. It is approximately 10 to 15 mm long, 3 to 5 mm wide, and 1 mm thick. Small nodal cells are surrounded by and interspersed with connective tissue. They merge with the larger working atrial muscle cells.

Bachmann[5] originally described an interatrial myocardial bundle conducting impulses from the right atrium to the left atrium. James[24] presented evidence for three *internodal conduction pathways* from the sinus node to the AV node. It is unclear whether the pathways are ever of functional significance.[51,55] It is generally concluded that the cardiac impulse spreads from the sinus node to the AV node by working atrial myocardial cell-to-cell conduction.[13]

Tarawa[60] initially described the AV node in 1906. It lies subendocardially on the right atrial side of the central fibrous body, in the lower interatrial septal wall. The node is close to the septal leaflet of the tricuspid valve and anterior to the coronary sinus. A group of fibers connects the node to working myocardial cells in the left atrium.[12] The AV node is approximately 7 mm long, 3 mm wide, and 1 mm thick.[61] Nodal fibers are interspersed with normal working myocardial fibers, which has led to difficulty in

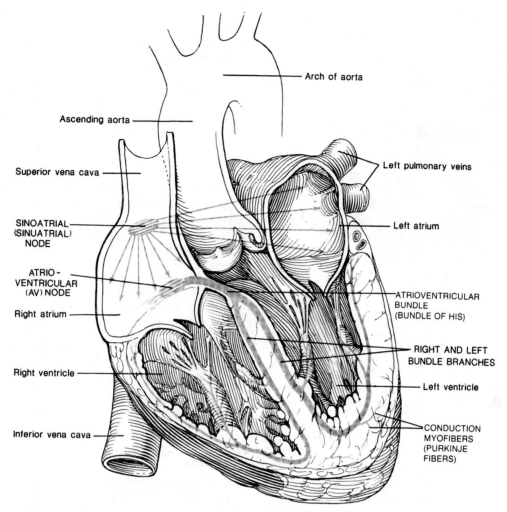

FIGURE 1-11 Schematic illustration of the human cardiac conducting system. (From Tortora GJ: Principles of Human Anatomy, 4th ed, p 311. New York, Harper & Row, 1986.)

identifying AV node boundaries. There are several zones of specialized conducting tissue in the AV junction area, including a transition zone between small nodal and larger working atrial myocardial cells, the compact AV node itself, the penetrating AV bundle, and the branching AV bundle.[2,17]

Fibers from the AV node converge into a shaft termed the *bundle of His* (also called the *penetrating AV bundle* or *common bundle*). It is approximately 10 mm long and 2 mm in diameter.[61] The bundle of His passes from the lower right atrial wall anteriorly and laterally through the central fibrous body, which is part of the fibrous skeleton.

As first noted by His[18] in 1893, the His bundle provides the only cellular connection between the atria and ventricles. The His bundle is of pivotal functional importance. Cardiac impulse transmission is slowed at this site, providing time for atrial contraction to dispel blood from the atria into the ventricles and thus to contribute to the subsequent cardiac output during ventricular contraction. At the membranous septal region of the heart, the right atrium and left ventricle are opposite each other across the septum, with

the right ventricle in close proximity. Three of the four cardiac valves are nearby[21] (Fig. 1-12). Thus, pathologic problems of the fibrous skeleton or of the tricuspid, mitral, or aortic valves may affect functioning of one or more of the other valves or may affect cardiac impulse conduction. Dysfunction of the AV conducting tissue may affect the coordinated functioning of the atria and ventricles.

Abnormal accessory pathways, termed *Kent bundles,* occasionally join the atria and ventricles through connections outside the main AV node and His bundle.[28,29] Tracts from the His bundle to upper interventricular septum (termed *paraspecific fibers of Mahaim*) are also abnormal but sometimes occur.[35,36] AV conduction is accelerated when impulses travel through these abnormal connections, bypassing the delay-producing AV junction. When this accelerated conduction occurs, cardiac output often falls because there is inadequate time for atrial contraction.[3]

The His bundle begins branching in the region of the crest of the muscular septum (see Fig. 1-11). The right bundle branch usually continues as a direct extension of the His bundle. The right bundle branch is a well defined,

Valve rings of heart

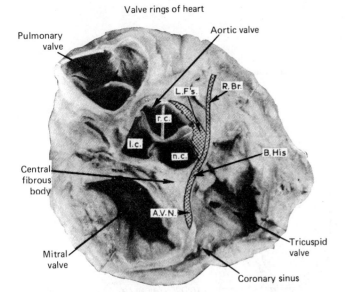

FIGURE 1-12 Schematic illustration of the relation of the atrioventricular conducting system to cardiac valves. Viewed from above. Note the proximity of the atrioventricular node (A.V.N.) to the aortic, mitral, and tricuspid valves and the proximity of the valves to each other. L.F., left ventricular conducting fiber; R. Br., right bundle branch; B. His, bundle of His; r.c., l.c., and n.c., right, left, and noncoronary cusps of the aortic valve. (From Hudson REB: Surgical pathology of the conducting system of the heart. Br Heart J 29: 652, 1967.)

single, slender group of fibers approximately 45 to 50 mm long and 1 mm thick. It initially courses downward along the right side of the interventricular septum, continues through the moderator band of muscular tissue near the right ventricular apex, and then continues to the base of the anterior papillary muscle. If a small segment of the bundle is damaged, the entire distal distribution is affected, owing to the right bundle's thinness, length, and relative lack of arborization.

The left bundle branch arises almost perpendicularly from the His bundle as the common left bundle branch. This common left bundle, approximately 10 mm long and 4 to 10 mm wide, then divides into two discrete divisions, the left anterior bundle branch and the left posterior bundle branch. The left anterior bundle branch, or left anterior fascicle, is approximately 25 mm long and 3 mm thick. It usually arises directly from the common left bundle after the origin of the posterior fascicle and close to the origin of the right bundle. It ramifies to the anterior septum and courses over the left ventricular anterior (superior) wall to the anterior papillary muscle, crossing the aortic outflow tract. Anterior and septal myocardial infarctions and aortic valve dysfunction often affect the left anterior bundle branch.

The large, thick, left posterior bundle branch, or left posterior fascicle, arises either from the first portion of the common left bundle or directly from the His bundle. The left posterior fascicle goes inferiorly and posteriorly across the left ventricular inflow tract to the base of the posterior papillary muscle, then spreads diffusely through the posterior inferior left ventricular free wall. It is approximately

20 mm long and 6 mm thick. This fascicle is often the least vulnerable segment of the ventricular conducting system because of its diffuseness, its location in a relatively protected nonturbulent portion of the ventricle, and its dual blood supply (Table 1-1).

Physiologic evidence exists for the trifascicular configuration of the bundles. Many conduction defects involving partial bundle-branch block may be explained on the basis of this model. Many investigators, however, have been unable to identify two discrete fascicular divisions of the left bundle branch and have found several variations in left bundle-branch configuration, such as the common left bundle fanning out diffusely along the septum and the free ventricular wall[38] (see Fig. 1-12). Three, rather than two, major divisions of the left bundle branch are frequently found, with a group of fibers ramifying from the left posterior fascicle and terminating in the lower septum and apical ventricular wall.[17]

Purkinje fibers, first described in 1845, form a complex network of conducting tissue ramifications that provide a continuation of the bundle branches in each ventricle.[45] They course down toward the ventricular apex and then up toward the fibrous rings at the ventricular bases. They spread over the subendocardial ventricular surfaces and then spread from the endocardium through the myocardium, thus spreading from inside outward, providing extensive contacts with working myocardial cells, and coupling myocardial excitation with muscular contraction.

CORONARY CIRCULATION

The heart is continuously active. Like all tissues, it must receive oxygen and metabolic substrates and have carbon dioxide and other wastes removed to maintain aerobic metabolism and contractile activity. However, unlike other tissues, it must generate the force to power its own perfusion. Perfusion needs of the heart are high.

Coronary Arteries

The major coronary arteries in humans are the right coronary artery and the left coronary artery, sometimes called the *left main coronary artery.* These arteries branch from the aorta in the region of the sinus of Valsalva (Figs. 1-13 and 1-14). They extend over the epicardial surface of the heart and branch several times. The branches usually emerge at a right angle from the parent artery.[10] The arteries plunge inward through the myocardial wall and undergo further branching. The epicardial branches exit first. The more distal branches supply the endocardial (internal) myocardium. The arteries continue branching and eventually become arterioles, then capillaries. Partially because the blood supply originates more distally, the endocardium is more vulnerable to compromised blood supply than is the epicardial (outer) myocardium.

There is much individual variation in the pattern of coronary artery branching. In general, the right coronary artery supplies the right atrium and ventricle. The left coronary artery supplies much of the left atrium and ventricle. The following discussion describes the most common

TABLE 1-1	Area Supplied by Common Arteries	
Structure	**Usual Arterial Supply**	**Common Variants**
Right atrium	Sinus node artery, branch of RCA (55%)*	Sinus node artery, branch of L circumflex (45%)
Left atrium	Major L circumflex†	Sinus node artery, branch of L circumflex (45%)
Right ventricle		
Anterior	Major RCA Minor LAD	
Posterior	Major RCA; posterior descending branch of RCA Minor LAD (ascending portion)	Posterior descending may branch from L circumflex (10%) LAD terminates at apex (40%)
Left ventricle		

Posterior (diaphragmatic)	Major L circumflex, posterior descending branch
	  of RCA
	Minor LAD (ascending portion)
		Posterior descending may branch from
		  L circumflex (10%)
		LAD terminates at apex (40%)

Anterior	L coronary artery; L circumflex and LAD	
Apex	Major LAD	

Intraventricular septum	Major septal branches of LAD
	Minor posterior descending branch of RCA
	  and AV nodal branch of RCA
		Minor posterior descending may branch from
		  L circumflex, and AV nodal may branch from
		  L circumflex

Left ventricular papillary muscles		
Anterior	Diagonal branch of LAD; other branches of LAD, other branches of L circumflex	Diagonal may branch from circumflex
Posterior	RCA and L circumflex	RCA and LAD
Sinus node	Nodal artery from RCA (55%)	Nodal artery from L circumflex (45%)
AV node	RCA (90%)	L circumflex (10%)
Bundle of His	RCA (90%)	L circumflex (10%)
Right bundle	Major LAD septal branches Minor AV nodal artery	
Left anterior bundle	Major LAD septal branches Minor AV nodal artery	
Left posterior bundle	LAD septal branches and AV nodal artery	

*Percentages in parentheses denote frequency of occurrence in autopsy studies.
†Major and minor refer to degree of predominance of an artery in perfusing a structure.
RCA, right coronary artery; LAD, left anterior descending artery; L, left; LV, left ventricle; AV, atrioventricular.
Data from James TN: Anatomy of the Coronary Arteries. New York, Paul B. Hoeber, 1961; and James TN; Anatomy of the coronary arteries and veins. In Hurst JW (ed): The Heart, 4th ed, pp 32–47. New York, McGraw-Hill, 1978.

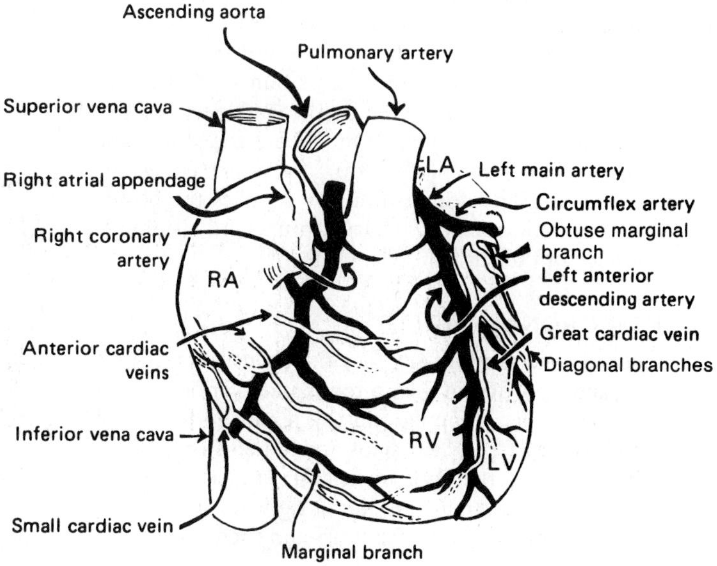

FIGURE 1-13 Principal arteries and veins on the anterior surface of the heart. Part of the right atrial appendage has been resected. The left coronary artery arises from the left coronary aortic sinus behind the pulmonary trunk. RA, right atrium; RV, right ventricle; LA, left atrium; LV, left ventricle. (Adapted from Walmsley R, Watson H: Clinical Anatomy of the Heart, p 203. New York, Churchill Livingston, 1978.)

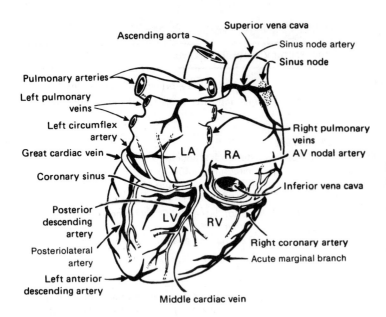

FIGURE 1-14 Principal arteries and veins on the infero-posterior surfaces of the heart. This schematic drawing illustrates the heart tilted upward at a nonphysiologic angle; normally, little of the inferior cardiac surface is visible posteriorly. The right coronary artery is shown to cross the crux and to supply the atrioventricular node. The artery to the sinus node in this figure arises from the right coronary artery. RA, right atrium; RV, right ventricle; LA, left atrium; LV, left ventricle. (Adapted from Walmsley R, Watson H: Clinical Anatomy of the Heart, p 205. New York, Churchill Livingston, 1978.)

pattern. Table 1-1 lists the major cardiac structures, their usual arterial supply, and some common variations (e.g., either the right or the left coronary artery may supply the AV node).

Individual anatomic variation should be considered in analyzing individual patient data. For example, angiographic visualization of the left circumflex artery might show severe stenosis. Although it is not likely that AV node and His bundle perfusion would be affected (because the right coronary artery typically perfuses these structures), in approximately 10% of cases the structures would be at risk. Thus, angiographic information is validated with clinical data. Also, apparently attenuated or narrowed vessels may be normal anatomic variants.

VESSEL DOMINANCE

Dominance (or *preponderance*), a term commonly used in describing coronary vasculature, refers to the distribution of the terminal portion of the arteries. The artery that reaches and crosses the *crux* (where the right and left AV grooves cross the posterior interatrial and interventricular grooves) is said to be *dominant*. In approximately 85% of cases, the right coronary artery crosses the crux and is dominant. The term can be confusing because in most human hearts, the left coronary artery is of wider caliber and perfuses the largest proportion of myocardium. Thus, the dominant artery usually does not perfuse the largest percentage of myocardial mass. The dominant artery supplies the posterior diaphragmatic interventricular septum and diaphragmatic surface of the left ventricle.

RIGHT CORONARY ARTERY

The right coronary artery supplies the right atrium, right ventricle, and a portion of the posterior and inferior surfaces of the left ventricle. It supplies the AV node and bundle of His in 90% of hearts, and the sinus node in 55% of hearts.[25] It originates behind the right aortic cusp and passes behind the pulmonary artery, coursing in the right AV groove laterally to the right margin of the heart and then posteriorly.

The major branches of the right coronary artery, in order of origin, are as follows:

1. Conus branch
2. Sinus node artery
3. Right ventricular branches
4. Right atrial branch
5. Acute marginal branch
6. AV nodal branch
7. Posterior descending branch
8. Left ventricular branch
9. Left atrial branch

The *conus branch* is small and exits within the first 2 cm of the right coronary artery in 60% of cases. It sometimes originates as a separate vessel with an ostium within a millimeter of the right coronary artery.[27] The branch proceeds centrally to the left of the pulmonic valve. It supplies the upper part of the right ventricle, near the outflow tract at the level of the pulmonic valve. When the conus branch anastomoses with a right ventricular branch of the left anterior descending artery, the resulting structure is called the *circle of Vieussens,* an important collateral link between left and right coronary arteries.

The sinus node artery arises from the right coronary artery in 55% of cases.[25] It proceeds in the opposite direction from the conus branch, coursing cranially and to the right, encircling the superior vena cava. It usually has two branches: one supplies the sinus node and parts of the right atrium, and the other branches to the left atrium.

The right coronary artery courses along the AV groove, giving rise next to one or more *right ventricular branches* that vary in length and distribute to the right ventricular wall.

The *right atrial branch* proceeds cranially toward the right heart border and perfuses the right atrium.

The *acute marginal branch* is a fairly large branch of the right coronary artery. It originates at the acute margin of the heart near the right atrial artery and courses in the opposite direction, toward the apex. It perfuses the inferior and diaphragmatic surfaces of the right ventricle and occasionally the posterior apical portion of the interventricular septum.

The *AV nodal branch* is slender and straight. It originates at the crux and is directed inward toward the center of the heart. It perfuses the AV node and the lower portion of the interatrial septum.

The *posterior descending branch* is an important branch of the right coronary artery. It supplies the posterosuperior portion of the interventricular septum. It exits at the crux and courses in the posterior interventricular sulcus.

The *left ventricular branch* originates just beyond the crux. It runs centrally in the angle formed by the left posterior AV groove and the posterior interventricular sulcus. It perfuses the diaphragmatic aspect of the left ventricle.

A *left atrial branch* may course along the posterior left AV groove and perfuse the left atrium.

LEFT CORONARY ARTERY

The left main coronary artery arises from the aorta in the ostium behind the left cusp of the aortic valve. This artery passes between the left atrial appendage and the pulmonary artery and then typically divides into two major branches: the *left anterior descending artery* and the *left circumflex artery*.

Left Anterior Descending Artery.
The left anterior descending artery supplies portions of the left and right ventricular myocardium and much of the interventricular septum. The left anterior descending artery appears to be a continuation of the left main coronary artery. It passes to the left of the pulmonic valve region, courses in the anterior interventricular sulcus to the apex, then courses around the apex to terminate in the inferior portion of the posterior interventricular sulcus. Occasionally, the posterior descending branch of the right coronary artery extends around the apex from the posterior surface; the left anterior descending artery ends short of the apex. The major branches of the left anterior descending artery, in the order in which they branch, are the following:

1. First diagonal branch
2. First septal branch
3. Right ventricular branch
4. Minor septal branches
5. Second diagonal branch
6. Apical branches

The *first diagonal branch* is usually a large artery. It originates close to the bifurcation of the left main coronary artery and passes diagonally over the free wall of the left ventricle. It perfuses the high lateral portion of the left ventricular free wall. Several smaller diagonal branches may exit from the left side of the left anterior descending artery and run parallel to the first diagonal branch. The one referred to as the *second diagonal branch* takes its origin approximately two thirds of the way from the origin to the termination of the left anterior descending artery. This second diagonal branch perfuses the lower lateral portion of the free wall to the apex.

A variable number of septal branches occur. The *first septal branch* is the first to exit the left anterior descending

artery. The others are referred to as *minor septal branches*. The septal branches exit at a 90-degree angle and course in the septum from the front to the back and caudally. Together, the septal branches perfuse two thirds of the upper portion of the septum and most of the inferior portion of the septum. The remaining superoposterior section of the septum is supplied by branches from the posterior descending artery, which usually derives from the right coronary artery.

One or more *right ventricular branches* may exist. One runs toward the conus branch of the right coronary artery and may anastomose into the circle of Vieussens.

The final branches are the *apical branches*. These perfuse the anterior and diaphragmatic aspects of the left ventricular free wall and apex.

Circumflex Artery.
The *circumflex artery* supplies blood to parts of the left atrium and left ventricle. In 45% of cases, it supplies the major perfusion of the sinus node; in 10% of cases, it supplies the AV node.[25] The circumflex artery exits from the left main coronary artery at a near right angle and courses posteriorly in the AV groove toward, but usually not reaching, the crux. If the circumflex reaches the crux, it gives rise to the posterior descending artery. In the 15% of cases in which this occurs, the left coronary artery supplies the entire septum and possibly the AV node.[12] The branches of the circumflex artery, in order of origin, are as follows:

1. Atrial circumflex branch
2. Sinus node artery
3. Obtuse marginal branches
4. Posterolateral branches

The *atrial circumflex branch* is usually small in caliber but may be as wide as the remaining portion of the circumflex. It runs along the left AV groove and perfuses the left atrial wall.

In 45% of cases, the *sinus node artery* originates from the initial portion of the circumflex; it runs cranially and dorsally, to the base of the superior vena cava in the region of the sinus node.[25,27] This artery perfuses portions of the left and right atria as well as the sinus node.

From one to four *obtuse marginal branches* may be seen. These vary greatly in size. They run along the ventricular wall laterally and posteriorly, toward the apex, along the obtuse margin of the heart. The marginal branches supply the obtuse margin of the heart and the adjacent posterior wall of the left ventricle above the diaphragmatic surface.

The *posterolateral branches* arise from the circumflex artery in 80% of cases.[27] These branches originate in the terminal portion of the circumflex artery and course caudally and to the left on the posterior left ventricular wall, supplying the posterior and diaphragmatic wall of the left ventricle.

The *posterior descending* and AV nodal arteries occasionally arise from the circumflex. When they do, the entire septum is supplied by branches of the left coronary artery.

Coronary Capillaries

Blood passes from arteries into arterioles, then into capillaries, where exchange of oxygen and other materials takes place. The heart has a dense capillary network with approximately 3,300 capillaries/mm², or approximately 1 capillary per muscle fiber.[63] Blood flow through coronary capillaries is regulated according to myocardial metabolic needs (see later).

When myocardial cells hypertrophy, the radius increases. The capillary network, however, does not appear to proliferate.[31] The same capillaries must perfuse a larger mass of tissue. The distance over which materials must diffuse is increased. Thus, with hypertrophy, the coronary circulation perfuses a larger tissue mass. At the same time, efficiency of exchange may be diminished.

Coronary Veins

Most of the venous drainage of the heart is through epicardial veins. The large veins course close to the coronary arteries. Two veins sometimes accompany an artery.[25] The major veins feed into the great cardiac vein, which runs alongside the circumflex artery, becomes the coronary sinus, and then empties into the right atrium (see Fig. 1-14). An incompetent (incompletely shut) semilunar valve called the valve of Vieussens marks the junction between the great cardiac vein and the coronary sinus. A similar structure, the thebesian valve, is also incompetent and is found at the entry of the coronary sinus into the right atrium. Venous blood from the right ventricular muscle is drained primarily by two to four anterior cardiac veins that empty directly into the right atrium, bypassing the coronary sinus (see Fig. 1-13).

Some veins, known as *thebesian veins,* empty directly into the ventricles (Fig. 1-15). They are more common on the right side of the heart, where the pressure gradient is favorable for such flow. Only a small amount of venous blood is returned directly to the left ventricle. When blood is returned to the left ventricle, it constitutes a component of physiologic shunt, or unoxygenated blood entering the systemic circulation. Many collateral channels are found in the venous drainage system.

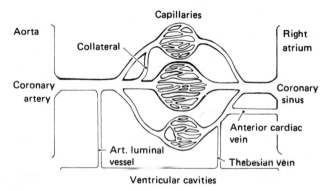

FIGURE 1-15 Schematic model of coronary circulation. As in other circulatory beds, the coronary circulation includes arteries, capillaries, and veins. Some veins drain directly into the ventricles. Collateral channels may link arterial vessels. Art, arterial. (Adapted from Ruch TC, Patton HD: Physiology and Biophysics 20th ed., Vol. 2, p 249. Philadelphia, WB Saunders, 1974.)

Lymph Drainage

Cardiac contraction promotes lymphatic drainage in the myocardium through an abundant system of lymphatic vessels, most of which eventually converge into the principal left anterior lymphatic. Lymph from this vessel empties into the pretracheal lymph node and then proceeds by way of two channels to the cardiac lymph node, the right lymphatic duct, and then into the superior vena cava.[40]

The importance of a normally functioning lymphatic system in maintaining an appropriate environment for cardiac cell function is frequently overlooked. Although complete cardiac lymph obstruction is rarely observed, experimental acute and chronic lymphatic impairment causes cellular myocardial and endocardial changes, particularly when occurring in conjunction with venous congestion.[40] Experimentally induced myocardial infarction in animals with chronically impaired lymphatic drainage causes more extensive cellular necrosis, an increased and prolonged inflammatory response, and a greater amount of fibrosis than infarction in animals without lymphatic obstruction.[40]

CARDIAC INNERVATION

Sensory nerve fibers from ventricular walls, the pericardium, coronary blood vessels, and other tissues transmit impulses by way of the cardiac nerves to the central nervous system. Motor nerve fibers to the heart are autonomic. Sympathetic stimulation accelerates firing of the sinus node, enhances conduction through the AV node, and increases the force of cardiac contraction. Parasympathetic stimulation slows the heart rate, slows conduction through the AV node, and may decrease ventricular contractile force.

Sympathetic preganglionic cardiac nerves arise from the first four or five thoracic spinal cord segments. The nerves synapse with long postganglionic fibers in the superior, middle, and cervicothoracic or stellate ganglia adjacent to the spinal cord. Most postganglionic sympathetic nerves to the heart travel through the superior, middle, and inferior cardiac nerves. However, several cardiac nerves with variable origins have been identified.[4,46] Parasympathetic preganglionic cardiac nerves arise from the right and left vagus nerves and synapse with postganglionic nerves close to their target cardiac cells.

Both vagal and sympathetic cardiac nerves converge in the cardiac plexus. The cardiac plexus is situated superior to the bifurcation of the pulmonary artery, behind the aortic arch, and anterior to the trachea at the level of tracheal bifurcation. From the cardiac plexus, the cardiac nerves course in two coronary plexuses along with the right and left coronary blood vessels.

Sympathetic fibers are richly distributed throughout the heart. Right sympathetic ganglia fibers most commonly innervate the sinus node, the right atrium, the anterior ventricular walls, and to some extent the AV node. Left sympathetic ganglia fibers usually extensively innervate the AV junctional area and the posterior and inferior left ventricle.[46]

A dense supply of vagal fibers innervates the sinus node, AV node, and ventricular conducting system; consequently, many parasympathetic ganglia are found in the region of the sinus and AV nodes. Vagal fibers also innervate both atria and, to a lesser extent, both ventricles.[46] Right vagal fibers have more effect on the sinus node; left vagal fibers have more effect on the AV node and ventricular conduction system. However, there is overlap. The clinical importance of vagal stimulation for ventricular function continues to be debated.

Although neurotransmitters from cardiac nerves are important modulators of cardiac activity, the success of cardiac transplantation illustrates the capacity of the heart to function without nervous innervation. (Chapter 23 discusses neurohumoral cardiac regulation in greater detail.)

MYOCARDIAL CELL STRUCTURE

Myocardial cells are long, narrow, and often branched. A limiting membrane, the sarcolemma, surrounds each cell. Specialized surface membrane structures include the intercalated disc, nexus, and transverse tubules (T-tubules). Major intracellular components are contractile protein filaments (called myofibrils), mitochondria, SR, and nucleus. There is a small amount of cytoplasm, called *sarcoplasm* (Fig. 1-16).

The *sarcolemma* is a thin phospholipid bilayer separating the intracellular and extracellular spaces. Across the barrier of the sarcolemma are marked differences in ionic composition and electrical charge. Proteins embedded in the sarcolemma serve multiple functions. Embedded receptors bind substances present in the extracellular space. That binding in turn activates or inhibits cell electrical, contractile, metabolic, or other functions. Embedded ion channels regulate ionic permeability and electrical function. Various carrier proteins facilitate the uptake of metabolic substrates such as glucose. Some sarcolemma proteins add structural stability.

Structurally, each myocardial cell is distinct. The *intercalated disc* forms a mechanical and electrical junction between adjacent cells. A specialized type of cell-to-cell connection, the *nexus* (sometimes called the *gap junction*), is present in the intercalated disc. The nexi are sites of direct exchange of small molecules. Nexi provide a low-resistance electrical path between cells, thus facilitating rapid impulse conduction. Physiologic conditions alter the permeability of the nexus. For example, two substances that vary with physiologic state are adenosine triphosphate (ATP) and cyclic adenosine monophosphate (cAMP) -dependent protein kinases. Both alter the permeability of the nexus.[8,58] Because of these junctions, the heart functions as a syncytium of coordinated cells, although anatomically the cells are discrete units.

Another specialized membrane structure, the *T-tubule system,* is an extensive labyrinthine network of membrane-lined tubes systematically tunneling inward throughout each cell. It is formed by invaginations of the sarcolemma, continuous with the surface membrane. The T-tubule lumen contains extracellular fluid. The T-tubular network carries electrical excitation to the central portions of myocardial cells, thus allowing near–simultaneous activation of deep and superficial parts of cells.

Myofibrils are long, rod-like structures that extend the length of the cell. They contain the contractile proteins, which convert the chemical energy of ATP into mechanical energy and heat. Contraction of the muscle involves the generation of force, shortening by the myofibrils, or both. The highly organized alignment of the contractile proteins in myofilaments gives the myocardial cell its striated (striped) appearance.

Mitochondria are small, rod-shaped membranous structures located within the cell. Breakdown of substrates and

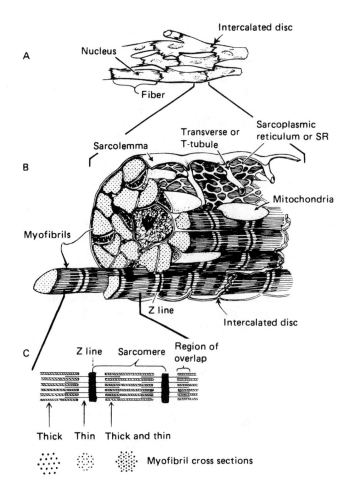

FIGURE 1-16 The microscopic structure of working myocardial cells. **(A)** Working myocardial cells as seen under the light microscope. Note the branching network of fibers and intercalated discs. **(B)** Schematic illustration of the internal structure of the working myocardial cell. Note the striated appearance of the myofibrils, the intimate association of the sarcoplasmic reticulum with the myofibrils, the presence of T-tubules, and the large number of mitochondria. **(C)** Structure of the sarcomere, illustrating alignment of thick and thin filaments. Cross-sections taken at three different positions along the sarcomere illustrate a region with only thick filaments, a region with only thin filaments, and a region of overlap where the thick and the thin filaments interdigitate. (Adapted from Braunwald E, Ross J, Sonnenblick E: Mechanisms of Contraction of the Normal and Failing Heart, 2nd ed, p 3. Boston, Little, Brown, 1976.)

synthesis of high-energy compounds occurs in the mitochondria. The relative abundance of mitochondria in cardiac muscle cells reflects the high level of biochemical activity required to support continuous contractile activity.

The *SR* is an extensive, self-contained internal membrane system. Both the T-tubules and SR contribute to linking of electrical depolarization of the membrane to the mechanical activity of the contractile protein filaments. This functional coordination is called excitation—contraction coupling. The SR is the major storage depot for calcium ion, releasing then taking up calcium ion with each contraction of the heart.

The *nucleus* contains the genetic material of the cell; it is the site where new proteins are synthesized.

MYOCARDIAL CELL ELECTRICAL CHARACTERISTICS

An electrical charge exists across the myocardial sarcolemma. The charge is called a *potential difference* and is measured in millivolts (mV). During the interim between excitations, the intracellular space of the cell is negative compared with the extracellular space. This potential difference is called the *membrane resting potential*. During excitation, the potential difference changes: the inside of the cell becomes less negative, or slightly positive compared with the extracellular space. This type of potential difference change is called *depolarization*. After depolarization, the membrane potential difference again becomes negative, returning to the membrane resting potential. This type of potential difference change is called *repolarization*. The depolarization–repolarization cycle is known as the *action potential*. The electrical excitation of the action potential is the signal that evokes contraction. Until the cell repolarizes sufficiently, there can be no action potential. If the potential difference becomes more negative than the usual resting potential, the membrane is said to be *hyperpolarized*. The more hyperpolarized the membrane, the more current is required to evoke an action potential.

Some myocardial cells have *automaticity*—that is, an intrinsic ability to depolarize spontaneously and initiate an action potential. The action potential generated in such a cell is then propagated throughout cardiac tissue. Depolarization of one cardiac cell initiates depolarization of adjacent cells and ultimately leads to cell contraction.

It is estimated that there are approximately 19 billion cells in the adult heart; these cells must depolarize in an orderly sequence if the heart is to undergo a coordinated contraction that is able to add force to moving blood. Impulses generated in ectopic sites in the heart are less likely to depolarize in an orderly sequence and less likely to contract in an orderly fashion that effectively pumps blood.

Basis for Myocardial Excitation: Characteristics of Biologic Membranes

Intracellular and extracellular spaces are separated by a thin insulating membrane, the sarcolemma. These spaces have very different ionic compositions. The intracellular space contains high concentrations of potassium ion (positively charged) and protein (negatively charged) and has low concentration of sodium ion (positively charged). The extracellular space consists of high concentrations of sodium ion and chloride ion (negatively charged); extracellular potassium ion concentration is low.

For each ion, concentration differences across the sarcolemma are determined by the sarcolemma's permeability to that ion and the strength of the forces moving the ion from one to the other side of the membrane. Electrical and concentration differences are maintained by a number of active and passive processes. Typical concentration differences are outlined in Table 1-2.

The sarcolemma is composed of phospholipid molecules. Each molecule consists of a charged hydrophilic (water-attracting) globular head and a noncharged

---

TABLE 1-2 Approximate Intracelluar and Extracellular Ion Concentrations and Activities in Cardiac Muscle*

Ion[†]	Extracellular Concentration[‡]	Intracellular Concentration[§11]	Ratio of Extracellular to Intracellular Concentration	E_1[¶]	Intracellular Activity[#]
Na^+	145 mM	15 mM	9.7	+60 mV	7.0 mM
K^+	4 mM	150 mM	0.027	−94 mV	125 mM
Cl^-	120 mM	5 mM	24	−83 mV	15 mM
Ca^{2+}	2 mM	10^{-4} M	2×10^4	+129 mV	8×10^{-6} mM

*Values given are approximations and vary according to the cardiac tissue, species, and method used for measurement.

[†]Na^+, sodium; K^+, potassium; Cl^-, chloride; Ca^{2+}, calcium.

[‡]mM, millimole per liter.

[11]Most of the intracellular calcium is bound to proteins or sequestered in intracellular organelles; thus, total intracellular calcium content approximates 1 to 2 mm·kg⁻¹ (2×10^{-3} M·kg⁻¹). During contraction, measurable intracellular calcium concentration approximates 10^{-5} M·kg⁻¹. Actual free intracellular sodium concentration may approach 1 mM because some intracellular sodium may be sequestered.

[¶]E_1, equilibrium potential; mV, millivolt.

[#]Median values from summarized data; these values should be considered as subject to revision.

Concentrations and equilibrium potentials from Sperelakis N: Origin of the cardiac resting potential. In Berne RM (ed): Handbook of Physiology, Section 2: The Cardiovascular System, vol 1, The Heart, p 193. Besthesda, American Physiological Society, 1979. Activities are approximations from Lee CO: Ionic activities in cardiac muscle cells and application of ion-sensitive microelectrodes, Am J Physiol 10: H461, H464, 1981; and Fozzard HA, Wasserstrom JA: Voltage dependence of intracellular sodium and control of contraction. In Zipes PP, Jalife J: Cardiac Electrophysiology and Arrhythmias, p 52. Orlando, Grune & Stratton, 1985.

hydrophobic (water-repelling) tail. The molecules organize into thin sheets, with the heads oriented in a consistent direction. Two sheets are aligned tail-to-tail to form a double layer (bilayer). The tails form the core of the sheet, and the heads are directed outward in both directions. The result is a 7- to 9-nm, high-resistance, insulated barrier to ionic movement.

Proteins are embedded within the phospholipid bilayer and may comprise more than half the mass of the membrane. The proteins act as receptors, channels, pumps, or structural stabilizers. They may be inserted into the intracellular or extracellular side of the bilayer or span its full thickness. Some of the proteins contain a water-filled pore that spans the membrane connecting the intracellular and extracellular spaces, forming a channel through which ions can pass. Membrane channels open and close in response to a stimulus (electrical, mechanical, or chemical), allowing passage of specific ions when open. The opening and closing properties of a channel are called its *gating* characteristics. The ability of a channel selectively to allow passage of certain ions while restricting other ions is called its *selectivity* property. Many ion channels are named after the ion for which they have selectivity. Some common types are sodium channels, potassium channels, and calcium channels (Fig. 1-17).

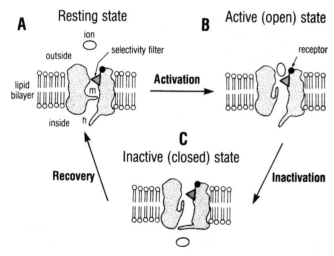

FIGURE 1-17 Schematic illustration of the three hypothetical states of voltage-dependent ion channels in cardiac cell membranes, such as those for sodium. In the resting state **(A)**, the activation (*m*) gate is closed and the inactivation (*h*) gate is open; ions are prevented from crossing the membrane through the channel. Depolarization to threshold activates the channel to the active state **(B)**, opening the activation gate and allowing ions to traverse the channel. Closure of the inactivation gate terminates the ion flux and inactivates the channel, **(C)**, Repolarization reactivates the channel to the resting, ready-to-be-activated state. Selectivity filters in the channel may determine the ion type or types admitted through the channel. (◄, selectivity filter.) (Adapted from Sperelakis N: Hormonal and neurotransmitter regulation of Ca^{++} influx through voltage-dependent slow channels in cardiac muscle membrane. Member Biochem 5: 134, 1984.)

Mechanisms of Ion Distribution Across the Myocardial Membrane

Ions are distributed across the membrane according to the membrane permeability to the ion and the electrical and diffusion forces on the ion. For each ion that can penetrate the membrane, there is a continual movement toward equilibrium. When equilibrium is reached, forces driving ion movement are balanced, and there is no additional net change in the ion distribution. The Nernst equation, discussed later, is useful in understanding the relationship between electrical and diffusional forces driving ion movement. It is useful to remember that the permeability properties of the living membrane change continually.

DIFFUSIONAL FORCE

Particles in solution move, or diffuse, from an area of higher concentration to an area of lower concentration. In the case of uncharged, soluble molecules, diffusion proceeds until there is a uniform distribution of the molecules within the solution. The solution is then said to be in equilibrium. At equilibrium, there is still particle movement within the solution, but no net change in overall distribution of particles. Charged particles also diffuse. The diffusion of charged particles is influenced not only by the concentration gradient but by electrical fields.

ELECTRICAL FORCE AND CURRENT

Like charges repel, opposite charges attract. Positively charged particles tend to flow toward negatively charged particles and regions; similarly, negatively charged particles are attracted to positive ions and regions. The electrical (or electromotive) force difference between regions is called the *potential difference* and is expressed in volts (1 mV = 0.001 V). The net flow of charges is called *current* (measured in amperes). *Resistance* is the opposition to the flow of current, measured in ohms. Ohm's law (electromotive force = current × resistance) describes the relation among current, voltage, and resistance.

When charged particles have different concentrations across a cell membrane, and some of the particles are able to permeate the membrane and others are not, an electrical force is established. This force influences the distribution of all other charged particles. The potential difference across biologic membranes is described by comparing the interior of the cell with the external solution. In the typical quiescent or resting myocardial cell, the potential difference is −70 to −90 mV; that is, the cell interior is negative with respect to the exterior (Fig. 1-18). When positively charged ions move from the extracellular fluid to the intracellular fluid, the current is said to be *inward*. With inward current, the cell interior becomes less negative, that is, it depolarizes. When positively charged ions flow into the extracellular space from the interior of the cell, the current is said to be *outward;* the cell repolarizes. Movement of negatively charged ions in one direction is electrically equivalent to an opposite-directed movement of positively charged ions. Thus, the inward movement of an anion such as chloride is called an outward current. This, too, causes repolarization.

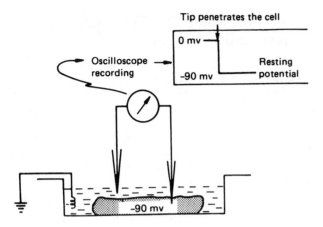

FIGURE 1-18 Schematic illustration of how intracellular electrical changes are recorded. When the tip of one microelectrode penetrates a cell, the oscilloscope trace shifts from the reference 0 potential and records the intracellular negative resting potential. (Adapted from Vassale M: Cardiac Physiology for the Clinician, p 2. New York, Academic Press, 1976.)

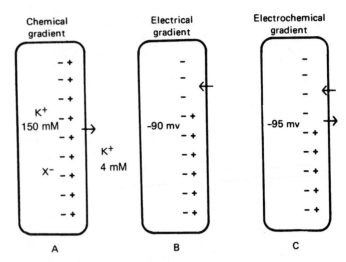

FIGURE 1-19 Development of potassium equilibrium potential. **(A)** The cell is assumed to have no intracellular electrical potential gradient because positive potassium (K⁺) ions are matched by negative protein (X–) charges. A chemical gradient directed outward favors the outflow of K⁺. **(B)** An electrical difference promotes the inward movement of potassium. **(C)** Potassium equilibrium is established when the inside of the cell has become sufficiently negative to oppose any further net potassium outflow. Note that the equilibrium potential for potassium (–95 mV) is slightly more negative than for the resting Purkinje cell (–90 mV). mM, millimoles; mV, millivolts. (Adapted from Vassale M: Cardiac Physiology for the Clinician, p 4. New York, Academic Press, 1976.)

Nernst Equation Calculation of Equilibrium Potential for Specific Ions. The Nernst equation is used to calculate the *equilibrium potential* for a particular ion. If that hypothetical voltage charged the membrane, then it would counterbalance the concentration difference. If the membrane were permeable to the ion, there would be no net ion movement. An understanding of the equilibrium potential is basic to an understanding of the electrical characteristics of biologic membranes.

Potassium is an important and useful example for discussion of the Nernst equation. Potassium, a positive ion, has a much higher concentration inside the myocardial cell than in the extracellular space. To balance the force of the concentration difference, the inside of the cell would need to be –94 mV compared with outside of the membrane. That charge, –94 mV, is known as the potassium equilibrium potential or the potassium Nernst potential for the cell. The resting myocardial membrane is permeable to potassium. The large concentration gradient is maintained because the actual voltage across the membrane between activation cycles, approximately –90 mV (inside negative), is nearly sufficient to hold the potassium inside the cell (Fig. 1-19). The slow outward trickle of potassium is corrected by a membrane pump that moves potassium back into the cell (and moves sodium out of the cell). If the resting potential were –94 mV, there would be no net potassium ion movement.

The following illustrates the Nernst equation calculation of the equilibrium potential for potassium ion:

$$E_K = \frac{RT}{FZ_K} \mathrm{Ln} \frac{[K^+]_o}{[K^+]_i}$$

Where E_K = equilibrium potential for K⁺

R = gas constant

T = absolute temperature

F = the Faraday (number of coulombs per mole of charge)

Z_K = the valence of K⁺ (+1)

$[K^+]_o$ = K⁺ concentration outside the cell (e.g., 4mM)

$[K^+]_i$ = K⁺ concentration inside the cell (e.g., 155mM)

Converting from the natural log to the base 10 log and replacing the constants measured at 37° C with numeric values, the equation becomes approximately

$$E_K = 61 \log_{10} \frac{[K^+]_o}{[K^+]_i}$$

$$E_K = 61 \log_{10} \frac{4}{155} = -97\,\mathrm{mV}$$

According to the Nernst equation, the higher the potassium ion concentration in the external solution, the more depolarized is the *potassium equilibrium potential.* If the resting membrane were highly permeable to potassium, then the higher the external potassium concentration, the more depolarized would be the *resting potential.* If one were to perform such an experiment, placing an intact muscle cell in a dish bathed in solutions with varying potassium concentrations, one would observe that this is the case. As the potassium concentration in the external solution is raised, the membrane becomes more depolarized. When the concentration of potassium ion in the extracellular fluid becomes equal to the concentration in the intracellular fluid, the membrane potential is 0 mV.

In cardiac surgery, when it is important to have a heart without electrical and mechanical activity, the organ is sometimes perfused with the cool cardioplegic solution.

The perfusate typically contains 15 to 35 mM potassium. As would be predicted from the Nernst equation, the cell membranes depolarize. The depolarized cells no longer experience an action potential, resulting in a motionless surgical field.

Each ion has a different equilibrium potential that depends on the relative concentration on the two sides of the membrane (see Table 1-2). In each case, the equilibrium potential is calculated using the Nernst equation. For example, given typical sodium ion concentrations as in Table 1-2, the equilibrium potential for sodium is approximately +60 mV. This means that if the membrane were permeable to sodium, then the membrane potential would have to be +60 mV to halt net inward sodium current. At typical resting potentials of –90 mV, a large electromotive force favors inward sodium current. The sodium concentration is markedly higher in the extracellular space than it is in the intracellular area. Thus, diffusion forces also favor inward sodium current. At rest, however, there is minimal net movement of sodium ion because the sodium channels are closed. When the channels open during activation, the diffusional and electrical forces combine to produce a large, but transient, inward current carried by sodium ion. The result is rapid depolarization.

The chloride ion concentration is higher in the extracellular space than in the intracellular space. Thus, diffusional force favors inward movement of chloride ion. However, the resting membrane potential is at approximately the chloride ion equilibrium potential. Thus, the negative potential opposes the net inward movement of chloride. The resting muscle membrane is permeant to chloride, but there is no net chloride movement.

The sarcoplasmic calcium ion concentration is extremely low. Calcium ion is actively removed from the sarcoplasm. It is taken up into the SR and pumped outward into the extracellular space. The extracellular calcium ion concentration is in the millimolar range, approximately 100,000 times higher than the intracellular concentration. Thus, a powerful concentration gradient would move calcium ion inward if a path were available. A powerful electrical force also favors inward movement. The calcium ion equilibrium potential calculated from the Nernst equation is more positive than +100 mV. However, the resting membrane is not permeant to calcium ion. As with the sodium ion, the opening of a channel for calcium ion movement evokes a large inward current. This happens during activation.

Calculation of the Membrane Resting Potential.
At high external potassium concentrations, the Nernst equation for potassium ion predicts resting membrane potential with good accuracy. In and below the physiologic range of external potassium ion concentrations, the membrane potential is slightly less negative than would be predicted based on potassium ion concentrations. This is because at very low external potassium concentrations, the membrane is slightly permeable to sodium ion. Because concentration and electrical gradients for sodium ion both favor inward movement of sodium ion, a slight sodium permeability results in a trickling inward of sodium ions (an inward current). The membrane depolarizes slightly, becoming several millivolts more positive than the potassium equilibrium potential. The ratio of potassium and sodium permeabilities determines the extent to which the resting membrane potential deviates from the potassium equilibrium potential. Equations have been developed to predict resting membrane potential based on permeabilities and concentrations of the permeating ions. These computations assume that the membrane is in a steady state and that there are no active ion pumps producing current.

Typically, cardiac muscle cells have a resting membrane potential of approximately –90 mV between excitations. Excitation and propagation of excitation depend on the resting membrane potential. The more negative the resting membrane potential, the more current is required to initiate excitation, but the speed and amplitude of depolarizing excitation are greater. The less negative the resting membrane potential, the less current required to initiate excitation; the speed and amplitude of depolarization are less. If the resting potential is depolarized a substantial amount, then the cell can be impossible to activate. The resting membrane potential is altered by changes in the ionic milieu on either side of the membrane and by hormones or drugs that alter the relative permeabilities of potassium or sodium ion. Factors that alter the action of the sodium–potassium pump alter the resting membrane potential. These include insulin and epinephrine (hyperpolarizing influences) and digoxin-like drugs (depolarizing influence).

Ionic Activity.
Although electrochemical gradients are most frequently explained in terms of chemical concentration gradients, it is actually each ion's chemical activity that affects most cellular functions. Ionic activity reflects interactions between ions as well as the ion concentration. An ion's activity is equal to its concentration times its activity coefficient. It is possible to make reasonably accurate measurements of ionic activities within cells. However, most descriptions of ion movements are based on ion concentration.

ION MOVEMENT ACROSS THE MYOCARDIAL CELL MEMBRANE

Passive Ion Movement. Ions traverse the sarcolemma passively through membrane-bound, water-filled pores called *channels*. When the channel is open, any ions that are able to pass through the channel move according to the concentration and electrical gradient, as constrained by the channel dimensions. When the channel is closed, ions do not penetrate. The opening and closing properties of an ion channel are referred to as its *gating* characteristics. The signal to open may be a change in the electrical field (voltage-gated channel) or a change in the chemical milieu (receptor-gated channel). Changes in the internal or external milieu may modify the gating of a channel. Further, there may be time-dependent effects. For example, a small depolarization opens the sodium channel; it closes after a few milliseconds.

An important channel characteristic is its ability to allow passage of some ions while excluding others. This is called *selective permeability*. A theoretical model of an ionic channel is given in Figure 1-17.

In Nobel prize-winning work, Hodgkin and Huxley[25] characterized the sodium current of the squid giant axon. The sodium channel is one of the most common in excitable cells and is well characterized. At rest, there is a negative resting membrane potential, perhaps −90 mV. Sodium ion concentration is high in the extracellular space, low intracellularly. Electrical and diffusion gradients both favor inward sodium ion movement, but there is no path for movement. The sodium channel is closed at the resting membrane potential. With a small electrical signal, the channel opens. The opening of the sodium channel in response to a small depolarizing current is sometimes described as opening of the *activation gate*. When the activation gate opens, the sodium channel is then open. Because the sodium channel is selectively permeable to sodium ion, sodium ions flow through the channel according to the electrical and concentration gradients. Both those forces favor the inward movement of sodium—an inward current. An intense current flows. After a few milliseconds, however, another gate (sometimes called the *inactivation gate* or *h gate*) closes, halting the current. The h gate remains closed until the membrane is restored to a negative voltage. At that time, the inactivation gate opens (but no current flows because the activation gate is closed). With the closing of either gate, current is halted. To summarize, then, the sodium channel is conceptualized as having two gates. At resting membrane potential, the channel is closed because the activation gate is closed. Depolarization opens that gate but, after a brief lag, the inactivation gate closes, again closing the channel. Repolarization opens the inactivation gate but closes the activation gate.

Scores of channels have been described, each with characteristic gating and selectivity profiles. The mixing of a selection of channel populations can produce a rich repertoire of biologic operating characteristics in various membranes. The membrane of vertebrate cardiac muscle is especially complex, with a diverse mix of channels. The result is a dynamic, responsive membrane that can be finely tuned to varying operating conditions. Some of the other major channels of the vertebrate heart are described later in this chapter.

Active Ion Transport. Any movement of ion against its electrochemical gradient is said to be *active movement* or *active transport*. To move any ion against its electrochemical gradient, energy must be used. The energy may be stored in ATP. In some cases, the energy stored in one ion's electrochemical gradient can be expended to power the movement of another ion against its electrochemical gradient. The former ion is said to be moving "downhill" or in the direction of a lower energy state. The ion that is moved against the gradient is said to be transported "uphill."

SODIUM–POTASSIUM-ADENOSINE TRIPHOSPHATASE PUMP. A slight trickling inward of sodium ions from the extracellular fluid occurs. In addition, with each activation, many cells experience a large transient inward sodium current. Were this not corrected, there would eventually be a loss of the concentration gradient for sodium ion. This does not happen because the cardiac muscle membrane (as well as many other types of membranes) has a pump that moves sodium ion out of the cell in exchange for an inward movement of potassium ions. In this case, both ions are moving uphill. The pump is powered by the energy stored in ATP; hence, the pump is known as the *sodium–potassium pump* or *sodium–potassium-ATPase*. This pump helps to reestablish the resting concentrations of intracellular sodium and potassium after cardiac depolarization. The ratio of sodium ions pumped out to potassium ions pumped in is usually 3:2. This ratio of 3:2 results in a net outward movement of charge and hyperpolarization of the resting membrane. A primary regulator of this pump is the intracellular concentration of sodium. Extracellular sodium concentration, intracellular potassium concentration, and particularly extracellular potassium concentration also influence pump activity. Digoxin-like drugs block the sodium–potassium pump[15]; epinephrine and insulin both stimulate the sodium–potassium pump, however, and are sometimes associated with hypokalemia, or lowering of the potassium concentration in the extracellular space due to inward pumping of potassium ion.

SODIUM–CALCIUM EXCHANGE. Another important cardiac membrane pump is the sodium–calcium pump. Calcium ion moves across the sarcolemma into the cell to activate contraction. It must be removed. Although there is some harvesting of calcium ion into the intracellular sequestering sites such as SR, the inward movement and storage cannot go on unopposed. Calcium ion is moved back into the extracellular space by means of an exchange pump. The energy stored in the sodium gradient powers the movement of calcium ion. In other words, sodium ion is moved downhill to pump calcium ion uphill.[31] Usually, this exchange mechanism transports three sodium ions into the cell for one calcium ion transported out of the cell. In this situation, the pump is electrogenic, but the direction or ratios of transmembrane ion exchanges may be reversed or changed. When the concentration of intracellular sodium ion is increased (e.g., when the use of digoxin-like drugs has partially blocked the sodium–potassium-ATPase pump), there is less energy stored in the sodium gradient. This exchange mechanism does not promote as great a sodium influx and calcium efflux. There is then more calcium ion stored in the SR and more calcium ion released during activation, with net positive inotropic effects.

CALCIUM ATPASE PUMPS. The cardiac SR actively pumps calcium ion uphill into its core in a process that hydrolyzes ATP as an energy source. An active calcium pump in the cardiac sarcolemma also extrudes calcium ion from the cell. The latter may be more important in vascular tissue than in cardiac muscle.

CARDIAC ACTION POTENTIAL

Each type of cardiac cell (e.g., working myocardial cells, nodal cells, Purkinje cells) has characteristic action potential features. In general, there are two types of action potentials, sometimes called *fast-* and *slow-response cells.* Fast-response cells, such as Purkinje cells and the working myocardial cells of the atrium and ventricle, have a rapid depolarization,

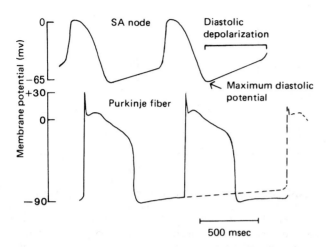

FIGURE 1-20 Action potentials of sinus node cells and Purkinje cells. Purkinje cell action potentials are usually elicited by propagated impulses. If Purkinje cells are not discharged by impulses from the sinus node or elsewhere, the Purkinje diastolic depolarization progresses enough to attain threshold. (Adapted from Vassale M: Cardiac Physiology for the Clinician, p 35. New York, Academic Press, 1976.)

then a period of sustained depolarization called the *plateau phase*. Conduction to adjacent cells is rapid. During the interim between action potentials, the resting potential is fairly constant. Slow-response cells, such as the sinus and AV node cells, spontaneously depolarize between action potentials, depolarize slowly during the action potential, and have a shorter, nonprominent plateau phase that

merges into a slower repolarization period. The latter conduct more slowly (Fig. 1-20). Differences in the ionic currents account for the differences in the shape of the action potential.

In the following sections, the action potential of a fast-response cell (the working myocardial cell) is characterized, and then the typical slow-responding cell is described. Finally, distinctive features of the other cell types are noted. Table 1-3 summarizes the electrophysiologic properties of the various tissue types.

Action Potential of Working Myocardial Cells

During the interim between contractions, the working myocardial cell has a resting membrane potential of approximately –90 mV. Excitation of the cell begins with a small depolarization to threshold potential, which is usually approximately –70 mV. This small depolarization evokes a large depolarization, the cardiac action potential upstroke. The action potential propagates the full length of the cell membrane and communicates to adjacent cells by means of current flow across the low-resistance path of the nexus. These cells are called *fast myocytes* because the initial depolarization rate is rapid.

The five phases of the cardiac action potential are summarized, then described in detail (Fig. 1-21). Briefly, phase 0 is the initial period of rapid depolarization, the action potential upstroke. The membrane potential changes from resting potential (approximately –90 mV) to a value positive to 0 mV (e.g., +30 mV). After this brief (<1 to 2 milliseconds) phase,

| TABLE 1-3 | **Cardiac Action Potential Properties*** |

	Fast-Conducting Tissue			**Slow-Conducting Tissue**	
	Purkinje	Atrial Muscle	Ventricular Muscle	Sinus Node	Atrioventricular Node
Resting potential	–90 to –95 mV	–80 to –90 mV	–80 to –90 mV	–50 to –60 mV	–60 to –70 mV
Activation threshold	–70 to –60 mV			–40 to –30 mV	
Action potential					
Rate of phase O (V_{max})	500 to 800 V/s	100 to 200 V/s	100 to 200 V/s	1 to 10 V/s	5 to 15 V/s
Amplitude	120 mV	110 to 120 mV	110 to 120 mV	60 to 70 mV	70 to 80 mV
Overshoot	30 mV	30 mV	30 mV	0 to 10 mV	5 to 15 mV
Duration	300 to 500 ms	100 to 300 ms	200 to 300 ms	100 to 300 ms	100 to 300 ms
Diastolic depolarization		Not prominent		Prominent	
Depolarizing current (major ion)		Na^+		Ca^{2+}	
Channel blocked by	Tetrodotoxin, type I antiarrhythmics, or sustained depolarization at –40 mV			Mn^{2+}, La^{3+}, verapamil, nifedipine, other inorganic substances, type IV antiarrhythmics	
Effect of adrenergic stimulation	Not pronounced			Pronounced	

*Values are approximations and vary with methods and specific tissue used.

Adapted from Bigger JT: Electrophysiology for the clinician, Eur Heart J 5(Suppl B): 2, 1984; Opie L: The Heart, p 44. Orlando, Grune & Stratton, 1984; Sperelakis N: Origin of the cardiac resting potential. In Berne RE (ed): Handbook of Physiology, Sec 2, The Cardiovascular System, vol 1, The Heart, p 190. Bethesda, MD, American Physiological Society, 1979; Zipes DP: Genesis of cardiac arrhythmias. In Braunwald E (ed): Heart Disease, 2nd ed, p 615. Philadelphia, WB Saunders, 1984.

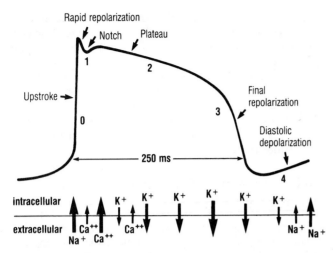

FIGURE 1-21 Schematic illustration of major ionic movements during a Purkinje cell action potential, with the cell depicted as exhibiting spontaneous depolarization. *Arrows* indicate approximate times when the indicated ion movement influences membrane potential. Pumps, exchanges, and leaks are not illustrated. Under normal physiologic conditions, Purkinje cells do not exhibit spontaneous depolarization. (Adapted from Ten Eick RE Baumgarten CM, Sunger DH: Ventricular dysrhythmia: Membrane basis of currents, channels, gates and cables. Prog Cardiovasc Dis 24: 159, 1981; Fozzard HA, Gibbons WR: Action potential and contraction of heart muscle. Am J Cardiol 31: 183, 1973.)

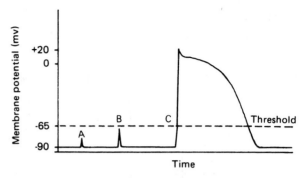

FIGURE 1-22 Schematic illustration of the initiation of an action potential when the membrane potential is depolarized to threshold. Small depolarizing stimuli (**A** and **B**) that fail to reach threshold (*dashed line*) are unable to initiate an action potential. When depolarization reaches threshold (**C**), a regenerative action potential is produced. Once the latter begins, further depolarization becomes independent of the initial stimulus. (From Katz AM: Physiology of the Heart, p 236. New York, Raven Press, 1977.)

there are three repolarizing phases. In phase 1, there is a small, early, rapid repolarization. Phase 2 is the so-called plateau phase. There is some minor additional depolarization and a prolonged slow repolarization. In phase 3, the repolarization becomes rapid, returning the membrane to resting potential. Phase 4 is not actually a part of the action potential but is used to describe the interval between action potentials. The membrane is in the repolarized state before another depolarization. The entire cardiac action potential may take hundreds of milliseconds. The duration and amplitude of each phase depends on the opening and closing of a variety of ion channel gates. This in turn depends on the ionic and neurohormonal milieu.

PHASE 0: ACTION POTENTIAL UPSTROKE

The working myocardial cell action potential is initiated by an inward current flowing primarily by way of the low-resistance nexus. This small current depolarizes the cell to threshold (approximately –70 mV; Fig. 1-22). Once threshold voltage is reached, the sodium channel activation gate opens, thus opening the sodium channel. There follows a large inward current carried by sodium ions. The depolarizing current opens more sodium channels, producing the propagating, regenerating, swift depolarization of the action potential upstroke. The peak voltages attained are +30 to +40 mV, approaching but not attaining the sodium equilibrium potential (which is approximately +65 mV). Depolarization closes the inactivation gate. The channel closes, halting the current, stopping depolarization.

The maximal velocity of phase 0 depolarization is sometimes called V_{max} (to be distinguished from the contractile variable, the maximal velocity of shortening, also called V_{max}).

The speed of impulse conduction through the myocardium depends on the V_{max} for the individual cells. V_{max} is a reflection of the operation of the sodium channels. Factors that alter the resting potential or the sodium gradient alter V_{max}. Such factors include ionic milieu and certain drugs, including many antiarrhythmic drugs. Class I antiarrhythmic agents (lidocaine, quinidine procainamide, others) block the fast sodium channel, slowing the rate of phase 0 depolarization.

The more negative the resting membrane potential, the faster is V_{max} and the greater is the amplitude of the depolarization. Hyperpolarization opens the inactivation gate. When depolarization opens the activation gate, the sodium channel is open, and the current is intense. Conversely, a less negative membrane voltage before threshold is associated with a slower V_{max} owing to failure adequately to remove inactivation (i.e., failure to open the inactivation gate). Hyperkalemia causes such depolarization; the condition is associated with arrhythmias.

PHASE 1: EARLY REPOLARIZATION

The rapid upstroke ceases when sodium channels close spontaneously after a few milliseconds (due to inactivation). Another transient current is activated—the transient outward current. This outward current is carried primarily by potassium ion and results in the slight repolarization of the cell to approximately +10 mV. Some chloride ions also flow. When the voltage is positive, both the concentration gradient and the electrical force (inside positive repels the positive potassium ion) favor outflow of potassium ion from the cell. This is an outward current. Similarly, with chloride ion, when the membrane potential is positive, the electrical gradient amplifies the concentration gradient, both favoring the inward movement of the negatively charged chloride ion. The inward movement of negative ions is electrically indistinguishable from an outward movement of positive ions; both are called *outward current.*

Phase 1 ends with the closure of the current-bearing channels. A "notch" appears on the action potential profile.

The voltage of the notch region has important effects on subsequent gating of other channels and can affect the shape of the remainder of the action potential.

PHASE 2: ACTION POTENTIAL PLATEAU

During the plateau, little net current flows. Inward (depolarizing) and outward (repolarizing) currents are nearly balanced; thus, there is little change in membrane voltage. Inward currents are carried by sodium and calcium ions. Calcium ion in turn evokes additional calcium ion release from internal stores, and contraction ensues. Outward currents are carried by potassium ions. Over time the calcium channels slowly inactivate; the repolarizing outward potassium current predominates; the membrane slowly repolarizes. The phase ends when the calcium channels are closed.

The sodium currents of the plateau may travel through a few fast sodium channels that failed to inactivate. At least two types of calcium channels are active. Both types of calcium channels open with depolarization, then close spontaneously after a certain period of time. β-Adrenergic agonists potentiate calcium currents, thus increasing the amplitude and duration of the plateau. The increase in calcium ion in turn has a positive inotropic effect on contraction. Calcium channel blockers, acidosis, and ATP depletion diminish calcium currents, diminish the plateau, and are negative inotropes.

The counterbalancing outward current is carried by potassium ion through multiple channel types. One type of potassium channel that is important in disease is the ATP-sensitive potassium current. This potassium channel is activated or opened when the ATP concentration falls, such as during ischemia. This in turn greatly shortens the duration of the plateau and hastens the onset of rapid repolarization phase. Shortened depolarization diminishes the calcium current and thus the contractile force.

The plateau phase distinguishes cardiac muscle from skeletal muscle or nerve tissue. The plateau provides for greater inward calcium currents in cardiac muscle. Because the tissue is refractory to stimulation for the duration of phase 2 and much of phase 3, cardiac muscle cannot be tetanically stimulated.

PHASE 3: LATE RAPID REPOLARIZATION

The calcium currents that sustained the plateau eventually stop. The calcium channels close, and repolarization proceeds unopposed, with outward movement of potassium ion. As the membrane voltage becomes increasingly negative, sodium channel inactivation is removed. The sodium channel can once again be excited or activated (as soon as a small depolarization opens the activation gate).

PHASE 4: INTERIM BETWEEN ACTION POTENTIALS

During rapid repolarization (phase 3), the membrane potential is restored to the resting potential. Phase 4 is the interim between the end of rapid repolarization and the start of the next action potential. During this phase, the membrane is permeable to potassium ion. The membrane voltage is close to the potassium equilibrium potential. The type of potassium channel open during this phase is called the *inward rectifier* (so called because it allows inward current more readily than outward current). Because the membrane potential is slightly more positive than the potassium equilibrium potential, potassium trickles outward.

Action Potential of Sinus Node-Type Cells

Sinus node-type cells are called *slow myocytes* because phase 0 depolarization is slower than in fast myocytes. Phase 1 is absent, phase 2 is abbreviated. Phase 3 is similar to that in fast myocytes, although slow myocytes repolarize to a less negative voltage than fast myocytes. Maximal negative voltage at the start of phase 4 is approximately –60 mV. During phase 4, there is spontaneous depolarization (see Fig. 1-20).

Phase 0 depolarization in slow myocytes is carried primarily by calcium ion rather than sodium ion. There is a less abrupt transition in the rate of depolarization before and after reaching threshold in sinus node cells.

Phase 1 is absent. There is no notch, and there is no large transient outward potassium current.

Phase 2 is present but abbreviated. Slow repolarization begins after the maximal positive voltage is reached. As in other cells, potassium efflux evokes repolarization in slow myocytes.

Phase 3, rapid repolarization, is similar to that in fast myocytes. The rate of repolarization is slower and the maximal diastolic potential attained is less negative than in fast-response cells.

During phase 4, the slow-response cells continually depolarize toward threshold. Because phase 4 coincides with the diastolic phase of the cardiac cycle, the membrane potential during phase 4 is frequently termed the *diastolic potential change* in automatic cells. The voltage at the start of phase 4 is the most negative voltage attained in these cells and is termed *maximal diastolic potential*.

Phase 4 spontaneous depolarization is due to the following sequence of currents: a nonselective channel opens, allowing inward sodium current; outward potassium current declines after some depolarization; transient (T)-type calcium channels open, allowing inward calcium current; and long-lasting (L)-type calcium channels open, allowing the full action potential depolarization.

Cells in the sinus node spontaneously depolarize to threshold more rapidly than do other automatic cardiac cells. Thus, the slope of phase 4 is steeper in sinus node cells than in other automatic cells. The ion current changes that account for the diastolic depolarization include a decrease in a stabilizing potassium current, an increase in a sodium current, some ongoing leakage of sodium ions, and eventually opening of the T-type calcium channels.[23,39]

Ionic currents flowing in slow-type myocytes are modulated by autonomic innervation. Adrenergic stimulation increases the potassium current, causing the cell to repolarize to a more negative potential, and the action potential to proceed more swiftly. Acetylcholine, the parasympathetic mediator, modifies the pacemaker currents to produce slowing.

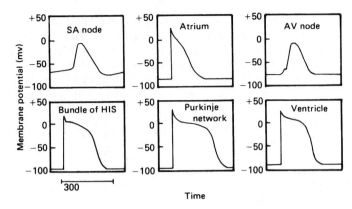

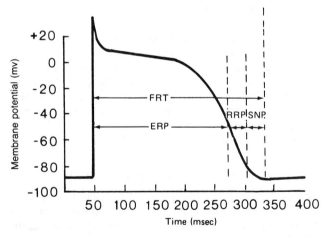

FIGURE 1-23 Characteristic action potentials in different regions of the heart. See text for description. (From Katz AM: Physiology of the Heart, p 251. New York, Raven Press, 1977.)

Action Potential of Purkinje-Type Cells

The action potential of the Purkinje cell is similar to that of the working myocardial cell, although somewhat prolonged in duration of the plateau. Hypoxia and acidosis in ischemic Purkinje cells may produce conditions in which the fast sodium channel is not opened. Phase 0 depolarization is then due to slow channel activation, carried primarily by calcium ion.

Action Potential of Atrial Cells

Atrial working myocardial cells undergo rapid depolarization. These cells have essentially no plateau period, but repolarization is slower than in Purkinje cells (Fig. 1-23). The total action potential duration of atrial cells is shorter than that of Purkinje cells. Atrial muscle cells do not spontaneously depolarize under physiologic conditions, but under some nonphysiologic conditions, spontaneous depolarization can occur.

Cells in the Atrioventricular Node

In general, spontaneously depolarizing cells of the AV node show similarities to sinus node cells in terms of rate of phase 0 depolarization and of maximal repolarization voltage (see Fig. 1-23).

Figure 1-24 illustrates the different electrophysiologic characteristics of cells termed *atrionodal, nodal,* and *nodal-His;* these action potentials have been identified as originating from the upper, middle, and lower junctional areas,

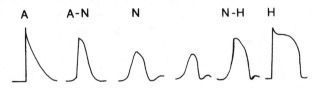

FIGURE 1-24 Schematic illustration of action potentials from atrial (*A*), atrionodal (*A-N*), nodal (*N*), nodal-His (*N-H*), and His bundle (*H*) cells. See text for discussion. (From Myerburg R, Lazzara R: Electrophysiologic basis of cardiac arrhythmias and conduction disturbances. Cardiovasc Clin 5: 9, 1973.)

respectively.[42] Other investigators contend that the electrophysiologic properties of atrionodal, nodal, and nodal-His cells are not correlated with definite anatomic areas.[17]

Cells in the Bundle of His

The electrophysiologic characteristics of His bundle cells closely resemble those of Purkinje cells in the distal conducting system. The duration of the His bundle action potential, however, is slightly less than that of cells in the Purkinje network. The most rapid period of depolarization and the longest period of repolarization occur in Purkinje cells at the distal end of the conducting system (see Fig. 1-23).

Refractory Periods

The period after depolarization, during which it is difficult or impossible to reexcite the cell, is termed the *refractory period* (Fig. 1-25). Refractoriness reflects the effects on depolarization of time and voltage requirements for the activation, inactivation, and recovery of ion channels.

During the *effective refractory period,* no action potential can be initiated by an external electrical stimulus. The duration of this period depends on the time it takes to remove inactivation from the sodium and calcium channels. The effective refractory period extends from phase 0 through the middle of phase 3.

During the *relative refractory period,* only a stimulus greater than normal can initiate an action potential. The relative refractory period occurs during the latter part of repolarization (late phase 3).

FIGURE 1-25 Excitability during the cardiac action potential. The effective refractory period (*ERP*), during which electrical stimuli of any strength are unable to initiate a propagated action potential, is followed by the relative refractory period (*RRP*), during which only stimuli greater than those that normally reach threshold can cause a propagated action potential. This is followed by the supernormal period (*SNP*), during which stimuli slightly less than those that normally reach threshold can cause a propagated action potential. The action potentials generated during the *RRP* and *SNP* usually propagate slowly. Full recovery time (*FRT*) is the interval after depolarization, after which threshold returns to normal and stimulation produces a normally propagated action potential. (Adapted from Katz AM: Physiology of the Heart, p 248. New York, Raven Press, 1977.)

The entire period between depolarization and complete repolarization is termed the *full recovery time*. Under normal conditions, cardiac cells are not depolarized until they have had time to recover fully from the previous depolarization. Usually, cells with long refractory periods have long action potential durations. The upper limits of normal heart rate responses and the time allowed for ventricular filling depend on normal cardiac electrical refractoriness.

Under certain conditions, a stimulus can initiate an action potential during the last part of phase 3 and the beginning of phase 4. Cardiac arrhythmias may occur during this period, especially when pathophysiologic situations such as ischemia promote abnormal refractory periods (see Chapter 14).

SARCOLEMMAL IONIC CURRENTS

The currents that combine to orchestrate the action potential can be studied independently. Neurohormonal and ionic milieu, pharmacologic agents, and pathologic processes variably influence each current. Powerful techniques using the patch clamp and molecular biology have

extended our understanding of the individual channels and hold the promise of increasing our understanding of important issues such as the generation of arrhythmias in disease states. New treatments are being developed. Some of the major channels are discussed individually (Table 1-4).

Inward Currents

The inward currents are carried by sodium or calcium ions moving into the cell. For each ion, there are several different types of channels, each with its own gating characteristics.

FAST INWARD CURRENT, I_{NA}

The fast sodium current is activated to cause rapid depolarization in phase 0 of fast-response cells. It was discussed in some detail previously. Briefly, the sodium channel opens with depolarization to threshold (−70 to −60 mV) but quickly closes owing to inactivation. Repolarization is necessary to remove the inactivation.[19] The fast sodium current is blocked by the puffer fish poison tetrodotoxin. Many antiarrhythmic agents, particularly class I agents, alter this current.

TABLE 1-4	**Cardiac Ionic Currents**		
Current*	Charge Carrier	Activation Mechanism	Function
Inward Currents			
I_{Na}	Na+	Voltage	AP upstroke
I_{Ca} (I_{Si}; I_{Ca_f} and I_{Ca_s})	Ca2+	Voltage	AP plateau E–C coupling AP upstroke Sinus pacemaker
I_f (I_h)	Na+ and K+	Voltage	Spontaneous depolarization
I_{ti} ($I_{t'}$ $I_{Na,K}$)	Na+ and K+	?(Ca2+)$_i$ [ ]	After-depolarization
Outward Currents			
I_K ($I_{x'}$ I_{x1} and I_{x2})	K+ (Na+)	Voltage	Repolarization
I_{to}	K+	Voltage, ?(Ca2+) [ ]	Early repolarization
I_{K1}	K+	Voltage	Resting potential Repolarization ?Plateau potential
$I_{K_{Ca}}$	K+	(Ca2+)$_i$ [ ]	Repolarization
$I_{K_{ACh}}$	K+	ACh, ? voltage	Inhibition
Pump/Exchange Currents			
I_p	Na+, K+	(K+), Na+) [ ], [ ]	Na+–K+-ATPase pump
$I_{Na, Ca}$	Na+, Ca2+	(Ca2+), (Na+) [ ], [ ]	Na+–Ca2+ exchange
Background Currents			
$I_{b_{Na}}$	Na+	?	Inward leakage
$I_{b_{Ca}}$	Ca2+	?	? Inward leakage
? $I_{b_{Cl}}$	Cl−	?	?

*Currents identified in multicellular preparations are labeled *I* and currents identified in single-cell preparations are labeled *i*. Some of these currents are speculative (see text).

Ach, acetylcholine; AP, action potential; E–C, excitation–contraction; [ ], concentration of ion indicated.

Adapted from Brown HF: Electrophysiology of the sinoatrial node. Physiol Rev 62: 506, 1982; Nobel D: The surprising heart, J Physiol 353: 43, 1984; Opie L: The Heart, p 47. Orlando, Grune & Stratton, 1984; and Reuter H: Ion channels in cardiac cell membranes. Annu Rev Physiol 46: 474, 1984.

CALCIUM CURRENTS

The two major types of calcium channels are termed L (long-lasting) and T (transient). The L current activates with depolarizations beyond –40 mV and then slowly inactivates. The T current activates at –70 mV and rapidly decays. Both channels probably contribute to the plateau of the cardiac action potential. The T channels contribute to phase 0 spontaneous depolarization in pacemaking cells and the L channels to the action potential in these cells. These currents may be potentiated by β-adrenergic (catecholamine) stimulation and diminished by acetylcholine and acidosis[57] (see later discussion). The current is blocked by inorganic compounds such as lanthanum, cobalt, nickel, and manganese. Organic, charged tertiary amines, such as verapamil, block the slow channel at the inner membrane. The block depends on membrane potential and the rate of stimulation. Organic dihydropyridines, such as nifedipine, also block the channel.

PACEMAKER CURRENT

Pacemaking results from the combining of at least four currents. There is a time-dependent inactivation of the potassium current, and thus a loss of outward current (which would tend to hyperpolarize). This alone does not produce depolarization: channels that carry ions with an equilibrium potential positive to the membrane potential also must open. The currents involved are I_h, I_{Ca}, and a background sodium current. I_h channels open at negative potentials (hence the designation "h"), close at positive potentials, and allow passage of both sodium (hence a depolarizing influence) and potassium. Gating is slow. Similarly, a sodium leak current occurs and is a depolarizing influence. Calcium channels are activated with depolarization. With increasing depolarization, the calcium T channels open, carrying inward depolarizing calcium current (I_{Ca}).[9]

TRANSIENT DIASTOLIC INWARD CURRENT, I_{ti}

The transient diastolic inward current is a nonselective current that carries both sodium and potassium and may be activated by intracellular calcium. It is not normally active but may be involved in initiating delayed depolarizations and triggering arrhythmias in Purkinje and ventricular muscle cells, particularly in situations of extracellular hypokalemia.

Other inward currents have been identified. Sodium and calcium "leak" currents and the sodium–calcium exchange mechanisms can generate small inward currents.

Outward Currents

A cell can experience outward current in two primary ways: (1) potassium can flow out of the cell, or (2) chloride can flow inward. Both tend to repolarize the membrane that had been depolarized. Both tend to stabilize the resting membrane potential. There are many types of potassium currents in cardiac muscle.

OUTWARD RECTIFYING CURRENT, I_K

The outward rectifying current causes repolarization after an action potential. It opens slowly after depolarization, so it is also called the *delayed rectifying current*. It carries potassium, and it closes with repolarization. It also may be labeled I_x, and has been subdivided into an I_{x1} early, rapid component and an I_{x2} late, slower component.

BACKGROUND OUTWARD CURRENT, I_{K1}

This potassium current closes with depolarization and opens with repolarization. Thus, when the cell is depolarized during the plateau phase, the channel is closed. Were the channel open, potassium would flow outward, resulting in a repolarization. This would abort the plateau and halt the calcium current, which activates contraction. Hence, it is efficient that this channel is closed during depolarization. It is open with repolarization and serves to stabilize the membrane potential close to the potassium equilibrium potential. It is sometimes called the *inward rectifier* because it is highly permeant to inward potassium currents. When the membrane is depolarized and potassium can flow outward, the channel closes. It is sensitive to the extracellular potassium concentration.

TRANSIENT OUTWARD CURRENT, I_{to}

This potassium current is linked with early (phase 1), rapid repolarization. It opens when a cell is depolarized after a period of hyperpolarization, and it closes quickly.

OTHER POTASSIUM CURRENTS

A non–voltage-dependent potassium current that is activated by an increase in the intracellular calcium concentration, I_{Kca}, may participate in the maintenance of the plateau and in repolarization. This current may be the same as or similar to the transient outward current (I_{to}).

Of potential importance in the diseased heart is the newly described ATP-dependent potassium channel. This channel opens when the ATP concentration falls to 10% to 20% of normal.[42] The action potential becomes abbreviated during ischemia. This channel may account for such a phenomenon. It would open when the ATP level dropped, shorten the action potential duration, and result in less contraction when the substrate needed for contraction was unavailable.[41]

Acetylcholine has been shown to activate potassium channels whose outward currents decrease during depolarization. Although this phenomenon may be related to potentiation of the background outward potassium current (I_{K1}), there is evidence for a separate voltage-responsive potassium current, I_{KACh}, whose channels are regulated by muscarinic cholinergic receptors.

Other outward currents have been identified. The sodium–potassium-ATPase pump usually generates a small outward current, I_p.

FACTORS MODIFYING ELECTROPHYSIOLOGIC FUNCTION

Factors that alter cardiac cell depolarization and repolarization do so by affecting the rates of voltage changes, the magnitudes of voltage changes, or the timing of the phases of the cardiac action potential. Such changes affect cardiac impulse generation, impulse conduction, or both, and reflect the effects of environmental alterations on transcellular ionic fluxes.

Impulse generation, or automaticity, is influenced by a cardiac cell's maximal diastolic repolarization, threshold level, and rate of spontaneous depolarization to threshold (slope of phase 4). If maximal diastolic repolarization becomes more negative, if threshold becomes less negative, or if the slope of phase 4 becomes less steep, the rate at which the entire cell is spontaneously depolarized can become slower; opposite effects can lead to a more rapid rate of spontaneous depolarization (see Chapter 14).

Cardiac impulse conduction velocity is influenced by the rate of depolarization (slope of phase 0), the magnitude of depolarization (amplitude of phase 0), the distance from resting potential to threshold level, the action potential and refractory period durations, and the resistance to current flow. If the rate or amplitude of phase 0 is decreased, the difference between resting potential and threshold is increased, the action potential or refractory periods are lengthened, or the resistance to current flow is increased, the rate of conduction can slow. For example, Purkinje cells have faster conduction velocities than nodal cells because the Purkinje cells have rapid sodium channels that create fast and large amplitudes of depolarization, Purkinje cells are large, and they are arranged in fascicles.

The responsiveness of cardiac cells is described by the relation between the membrane potential before rapid depolarization and the maximal velocity of conduction during rapid depolarization. Cardiac cell excitability is described by the current required to alter the membrane potential from resting to threshold.[53] Although once threshold is reached, the cell completely depolarizes, the amplitude of the action potential can be decreased if the distance between the resting potential and the threshold potential is less than usual. Stimuli that do not depolarize a cell to threshold are not effective in initiating action potentials, but such stimuli can have an effect on ionic movements, and in pathophysiologic situations, these stimuli may influence cardiac arrhythmias (see Chapter 14).

Cardiac impulse generation, conduction, or both can be altered by the effects on cardiac cells of changes in the ratio of extracellular to intracellular ionic concentrations,

acid–base changes, sympathetic and parasympathetic stimulation, myocardial stretch, cooling, ischemia, and heart rate changes. These factors often affect different cardiac cells in different ways; the following section discusses general selected examples of some of these alterations. (The effects of alterations in extracellular ionic concentrations on cardiac electrical and mechanical functions are discussed in Chapters 6 and 7.)

Adrenergic and Cholinergic Effects

CATECHOLAMINES

Although there are specific differences in the effects of different adrenergic substances, catecholamines generally have similar effects whether they are secreted by sympathetic nerve endings, are endogenous hormones, or are adrenergic drugs. The catecholamines have multiple and sometimes conflicting effects on cardiac cell action potentials. Catecholamines increase the magnitude and rate of diastolic depolarization in both Purkinje and sinus nodal cells. Repolarization becomes faster, and the action potential duration is shortened. The increased rate of sinus node spontaneous depolarization (slope of phase 4) appears to be the most important mechanism by which adrenergic effects increase heart rate (Fig. 1-26). Catecholamines increase the amplitude and rate of rise of phase 0 in junctional cells, which increases conduction velocity through the AV node. Catecholamines also increase myocardial contractility. Most of these catecholamine effects have been shown to be due to β-adrenergic stimulation and cAMP mediation.

ACETYLCHOLINE

The cholinergic effects of parasympathetic (vagal) nerve stimulation are more pronounced on the sinus node, the AV node, and atrial muscle than on ventricular muscle because parasympathetic nerve distribution is more sparse in ventricular muscle. The rate of diastolic depolarization (slope of phase 4) is decreased in sinus node cells, and the maximal diastolic potential becomes more negative as a result of vagal stimulation; thus, heart rate is slowed (Fig. 1-27). The sinus node action potential duration and refractory period are both shortened. There is a decreased rate of rise and amplitude of phase 0 in AV nodal cells in response to acetylcholine, which

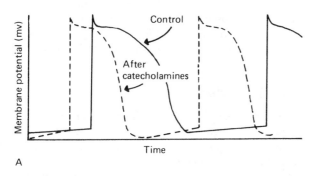

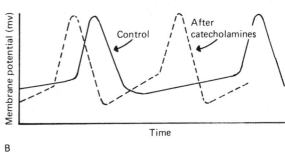

A

B

FIGURE 1-26 Schematic illustration of the general electrophysiologic effects of catecholamines on **(A)** Purkinje cells and **(B)** sinus node cells. (From Katz AM: Physiology of the Heart, pp 366, 367. New York, Raven Press, 1977.)

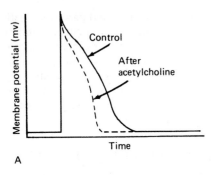 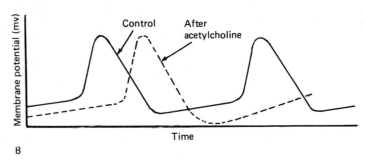

FIGURE 1-27 Schematic illustration of the general electrophysiologic effects of acetylcholine (vagal stimulation) on **(A)** atrial muscle cells and **(B)** sinus node cells. (From Katz AM: Physiology of the Heart, pp 362, 363. New York, Raven Press, 1977.)

leads to a slowing of AV conduction. The AV refractory period may also be prolonged. Atrial contractile strength is decreased. Most of these effects are related to cholinergically induced increases in potassium cellular efflux (see earlier) and decreases in calcium influx.[57] Cholinergic cardiac receptor stimulation has also been shown to result in the inhibition of cardiac catecholamine effects by inhibiting the β-adrenergic effects of cAMP and inhibiting prejunctional norepinephrine release.

Effects of Acidosis and Alkalosis

Acidosis slows repolarization and prolongs the action potential duration in Purkinje fibers. Cardiac calcium channels are blocked by acidosis, so slow action potentials exhibit a decreased rate of rise, amplitude, and duration.[57] Acidosis induces decreased contractility by decreasing calcium ion influx and decreasing the sensitivity of the myofibrils to calcium ion.[10] The sodium–potassium-ATPase pump is inhibited by acidosis.

Alkalosis can shorten the action potential duration. Purkinje automaticity is increased owing to an increased rate of diastolic depolarization.[53]

Other Effects

The action potential duration is related to the length of the preceding diastolic interval. When heart rate increases and the interval between successive cardiac impulses decreases, repolarization is faster in most cardiac cells and there is a shorter action potential duration. At slower heart rates, the action potential duration lengthens.

In experimental situations, the effects of *warming the heart* are somewhat similar to adrenergic effects (e.g., diastolic depolarization is increased in automatic fibers). *Cooling the heart* depresses spontaneous depolarization in automatic cells. Repolarization is delayed, and conduction is decreased. Arrhythmias may occur during cooling, which is clinically relevant for the cardiac surgical patient who has been subjected to hypothermia (see Chapter 23).

Stretching cardiac fibers increases the rate of diastolic depolarization and makes the maximal diastolic potential less negative in automatic fibers. Myocardial fiber stretch may cause arrhythmias during heart failure. The effects of *hypoxemia* and *ischemia* on the action potential are discussed in Chapter 20.

PROPAGATION OF THE CARDIAC IMPULSE

The spread of the cardiac impulse through the heart reflects (1) the anatomic characteristics of the conducting system; (2) structural characteristics of cells (e.g., cardiac cell type and diameter, arrangement of low-resistance intercalated discs, and contiguity to other cells capable of conducting current); and (3) electrophysiologic state of the cell membrane (i.e., resting potential, ionic concentrations and conductances, threshold membrane potential, rate and magnitude of depolarization, rate and magnitude of repolarization, duration of the action potential, and the refractory period). As in a battery, there is energy stored across the cell membrane. When one segment of the membrane depolarizes, positive charge enters the cell, and an electrical circuit is established along the cell.[57]

In general, current flows more easily inside the cell and to adjacent cells across the intercalated discs at tight junctions than laterally across adjacent, highly resistant areas of cell membranes. If the current is sufficient to depolarize adjacent cells, a wave of depolarization is propagated that spreads rapidly from cell to cell. Thus, the cardiac tissue behaves essentially as a syncytium, although propagation may be somewhat discontinuous.[56]

As the impulse spreads through the heart, it depolarizes tissue that has recovered and is excitable, but it cannot depolarize tissue that is still refractory. Because the cardiac impulse spreads rapidly through the atria, slowly through the AV junction, and then rapidly through the ventricles, both atria contract almost synchronously, the ventricles have time to receive blood from the contracting atria, and then both ventricles contract almost synchronously.

Atrial Conduction

Sinus node cells normally have the fastest rate of spontaneous depolarization and thus set the pace of cardiac excitation. The sinus node normally initiates the electrical impulse that is conducted to other areas of the myocardium, depolarizing other cells of the conducting system before those cells have time to depolarize spontaneously to threshold. The electrical impulse appears to spread outward in relatively concentric circles from the sinus node through the atria, moving in

TABLE 1-5	**Normal Cardiac Activation Sequence**		
Normal Sequence of Activation	Conduction Velocity (m/s)	Time for Impulse to Traverse Structure (s)	Rate of Automatic Discharge (per minute)
Sinoatrial node	—	} ~0.15	60–100
Atrial myocardium			None
AV node	0.02–0.05	}	See text
AV bundle	1.2–2		40–55
Bundle branches	} 2–4	} ~0.08	
Purkinje network			} 25–40
Ventricular myocardium	} 0.3–1	~0.08	} None

AV, atrioventricular; m, meters; s, second; ~, approximately.
    Adapted from Katz AM: Physiology of the Heart, p 259. New York, Raven Press, 1977.

approximately 0.1 second from the upper right atrium to the posterior left atrium. Conduction velocity (speed with which the impulse spreads) through the atria is approximately 0.8 to 1 m/s (Table 1-5). Conduction velocities are not equal through the atria; conduction is more rapid by way of the Bachman bundle into the left atrium than in other areas of the interatrial septum. Controversy about radial spread of the atrial impulse versus conduction by way of specialized atrial pathways may be explained by the orientation of atrial muscle fiber bundles. Atrial repolarization appears to spread in the same direction as depolarization.

Junctional Conduction

The cardiac impulse is not conducted through the connective tissue of the cardiac skeleton, so cardiac muscle tissue in the AV junction provides the only pathway for electrical conduction from the atria to the ventricles. Conduction velocity through the AV node is approximately 0.05 m/s, although in some areas it has been found to be as slow as 0.02 m/s.

The rate of impulse conduction through the AV junction is influenced by the atrial site at which the impulse enters the junctional area.[39] An initial normal slowing of conduction through the AV junction with a later increase in the speed of conduction is correlated with electrophysiologic differences in atrionodal, nodal, and nodal-His cells[43] (see Fig. 1-24). Other mechanisms have been postulated for the slowing of conduction through the junction, including the small size of the junctional conducting cells and the amounts of connective tissue interspersed among conducting cells.

The property of a propagating impulse becoming successively weaker is termed *decremental conduction*. The extent to which this occurs in the AV junction under normal circumstances continues to be debated. Extreme decremental conduction leads to AV blocks (see Chapter 14).

The slowing of the cardiac impulse at the AV junction prevents the atria and ventricles from contracting at the same time and protects the ventricles from the abnormally fast heart rates that can be generated in the atria under abnormal situations. Preexcitation syndromes can be explained on the basis of accessory junctional pathways[3] (see Chapter 14).

Ventricular Conduction

Cells in the His-Purkinje system have the most rapid conduction velocities in the heart, approximately 1.5 to 2 m/s in the His bundle and 2 to 4 m/s in the Purkinje system.[53] The cardiac impulse spreads in a rapid (approximately 0.08 second), sequential manner from the common His bundle through the bundle branches, then through the extensive ramifications of the Purkinje fiber system, and finally through ventricular muscle. Three general phases of ventricular activation may be described: septal depolarization, apex depolarization, and basal depolarization (Fig. 1-28; see Chapter 14).

The middle left septal area and the anterior and posterior left paraseptal areas are depolarized within the first 0 to 10 milliseconds.[11] The major wave of septal depolarization is from left to right.

Most of the left and right ventricular cavities are depolarized within 20 to 40 milliseconds.[11] Activation spreads from the endocardium toward the epicardium. The first epicardial depolarization is usually in the lower right ventricular wall because of its thinness, even though the internal left ventricular cavity is depolarized more rapidly than the right.

Purkinje fibers are sparsely distributed in the basal (upper) sections of the ventricles and septum, particularly in the right ventricle and the septum. The basal and posterior portions of both ventricles and the basal interventricular septum are the last areas to be activated, at approximately 80 milliseconds.[11]

Although Purkinje fibers conduct the cardiac impulse more rapidly than other cardiac cells, Purkinje cells in the distal terminations of the conducting system have longer action potential durations and refractory periods than do ventricular muscle fibers (see earlier). Because conduction is slower in cells with longer action potential durations and refractory periods, the conduction velocity of the cardiac impulse is slowed at the point where Purkinje fibers connect with ventricular muscle cells. In theory, the distal Purkinje fibers then function like a gate, the length of the refractory period in distal Purkinje fibers normally controlling the rate at which ventricular muscle fibers depolarize.[64] Excitation—contraction coupling and the rate of cardiac contraction

A

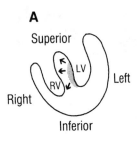

B

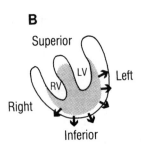

C

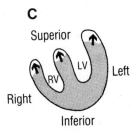

FIGURE 1-28 Schematic illustration of the sequence of ventricular depolarization. See text for description. RV, right ventricle; LV, left ventricle. (Adapted from Katz AM: Physiology of the Heart, pp 275, 276. New York, Raven Press, 1977.)

may be controlled by this gating mechanism. The existence and clinical importance of this gating mechanism have been questioned, however.[32]

Ventricular repolarization proceeds in general from the epicardium to the endocardium and spreads from the ventricular bases to the apices.[7] Thus, ventricular repolarization proceeds in a direction that is opposite to the direction of depolarization, and all portions of the ventricle recover at approximately the same time. However, ventricular repolarization is not homogeneous; under pathophysiologic conditions, this may help create situations that promote ventricular arrhythmias (see Chapter 14).

Excitation–Contraction Coupling

Electrical excitation (i.e., evoking of an action potential) causes cardiac muscle contraction. Calcium ion flows inward across the cell membrane during the action potential. Intracellular calcium stimulates release of calcium from internal stores. Intracellular calcium ion is the key unlocking the resting inhibition to contraction. The linking of electrical activity to mechanical activity is called *excitation–contraction coupling*. Removal of calcium from the myoplasm evokes relaxation. The mechanisms by which ionic fluxes across the sarcolemma evoke contraction and relaxation are illustrated in Figure 1-29.

In cardiac cells, calcium binding with troponin removes inhibition by tropomyosin and allows myosin to interact with actin, activate actomyosin-ATPase, and form crossbridges. As identified by Ringer more than 100 years ago, an increase in the cytosolic calcium concentration is necessary to trigger this process.[49]

Calcium influx across the sarcolemma in response to cardiac membrane depolarization triggers the release of calcium by the SR.[12] The terminal cisternae of the SR

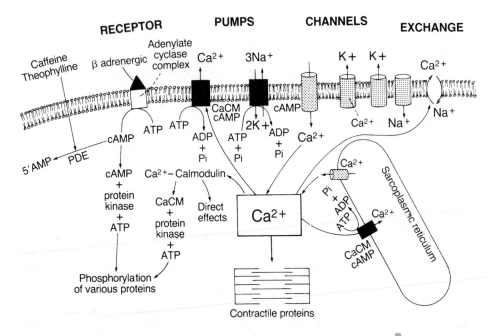

FIGURE 1-29 Schematic illustration of cardiac membrane transport processes and excitation–contraction coupling. CaCM, calcium–calmodulin; cAMP, cyclic adenosine monophosphate; ADP, adenosine monophosphate; ATP, adenosine triphosphate; PDE, phosphodiesterase. (Adapted from Shamoo AE, Ambudkar IS: Regulation of calcium transport in cardiac cells. Can J Physiol Pharmacol 62:13, 1984; Sperelakis N: Hormonal and neurotransmitter regulation of Ca++ influx through voltage-dependent slow channels in cardiac membrane. Mem Biochem 5(2): 153, 1984; and Tibbits GF, unpublished diagram.)

■ membrane pump; () exchange mechanism; ⌂ recepton-operated channel; ▯ voltage-gated channel; | diffusion; ▤ actin-myosum interaction

press closely on the T-tubule. Electron-dense bridges or "feet" are visible with electron microscopy spanning the distance between the two membrane systems.[14] These structures, the so-called *ryanodine receptors* (because of binding properties), communicate the signal for SR calcium ion release.

Calcium exerts several of its internal effects through combining with an intracellular protein called *calmodulin*. In cardiac myocardial cells, the calcium–calmodulin complex promotes calcium ion binding to troponin and thus promotes contraction. Calcium–calmodulin also may stimulate the calcium pumps on the SR and the sarcolemma and may stimulate sodium–calcium exchange; all these actions help remove calcium ion from the cytosol. Calcium–calmodulin influences the synthesis and breakdown of cAMP and may help promote sarcolemmal calcium influx. Calcium may exert several other effects, either directly or by combining with other intracellular proteins, and thus may modulate myocardial cell contraction and relaxation through several different mechanisms.

Stimulation of β-adrenergic receptors on the cardiac cell membrane influences transmembrane calcium fluxes and cardiac contraction through the intracellular production of cAMP from ATP, which in turn initiates several series of reactions involving intracellular protein phosphorylation (transfer of high-energy phosphates) by protein kinases. The metabolic actions of cAMP help to provide energy substrates for cardiac muscle contraction and relaxation. Phosphorylation of a sarcolemmal calcium channel membrane protein by cAMP creates a conformation or pore diameter change that places the calcium channel in a functional state available for voltage activation.[58] cAMP may also facilitate the SR release of calcium. Both actions promote an increased cytosolic calcium concentration and thus promote muscle contraction.

Phospholamban is an SR membrane protein that activates the SR calcium pump. Phosphorylation of phospholamban by cAMP, and by calmodulin at a different site, stimulates the calcium pump, increases SR calcium uptake, and promotes relaxation. cAMP phosphorylation of troponin influences the interaction between troponin and calcium, which also promotes relaxation.

Although uptake of calcium into the SR promotes relaxation, mechanisms that increase the amount of calcium in the SR promote increased calcium availability for tension generation during subsequent contractions. Thus, the increased rate and strength of contraction produced by β-adrenergic stimulation and other combined chronoinotropic mechanisms appear to be matched by mechanisms that enhance the rate of cardiac relaxation.[58]

Calcium, through its role as a regulator of contraction and its possible role as an initiator of contraction, is the major link between excitation and contraction. The intracellular calcium concentration is directly and indirectly influenced by the amount of calcium transported in and out of the cell across the sarcolemma.[58] Calcium sarcolemmal fluxes are affected by the membrane potential and by sodium and potassium concentrations and transcellular

fluxes. Conversely, potassium flux through the calcium-regulated potassium channel and sodium flux during sodium–calcium exchange are affected by the intracellular concentration of calcium.

MECHANICAL CHARACTERISTICS OF CARDIAC CELLS

Overview of Contraction

As seen in Figure 1-16, the myofibril is composed of a series of repeating units, called *sarcomeres*. Sarcomeres are the basic functional and structural units of the myofibril. Dark-staining Z lines mark the ends of the sarcomere. Attached to the Z line are the thin filaments. The center of the sarcomere is composed of the dark-appearing thick filaments. Interdigitating thin and thick filaments overlap to a variable extent. The amount of overlap is altered during shortening, when thick and thin filament proteins interact, and the filaments slide past one another.

The individual thick and thin filaments do not themselves change in length; the sarcomere (and the muscle as a whole) shortens. If shortening of the sarcomere (or the muscle cell) is prevented, the interaction of thick and thin filaments is manifested as tension or force generation. Such a contraction is termed *isometric*. When a stimulated muscle is allowed to shorten, tension is not increased, and the contraction is said to be *isotonic* (Figs. 1-30 and 1-31). In the heart, early systolic contraction is primarily isometric: tension increases, and muscle length remains fairly constant. Later in systole, the contraction is primarily isotonic: the heart muscle shortens, and the blood is expelled into the aorta. Little additional tension is developed.

Molecular Basis for Contraction

The *thick filaments* are composed primarily of the protein myosin. Myosin is large, consisting of six subunits: two heavy chains and four light chains per molecule. The two heavy chain subunits are coiled to form a long, rod-like tail at one end. At the opposite end of the long myosin heavy chain, a head protrudes from each subunit. Groups of myosin tails are arranged to form the rigid backbone of the thick filament. The heads are the site of ATP breakdown and interaction with the thin filaments. Heads project outward in a spiral along the length of the thick filament. At the center of the filament, the molecules reverse direction, leaving a bare region from which no heads protrude. The small light chains are nestled in the angle between head and tail, two per heavy chain. Both heavy and light chains are members of multigene families and exist in several forms, called *isoforms*. Variation in isoform composition may modify the rate or intensity of myosin chemical activity. This in turn may modify the contractile properties of the tissue. Age, mechanical loading, or metabolic or hormonal state may modify isoform composition.

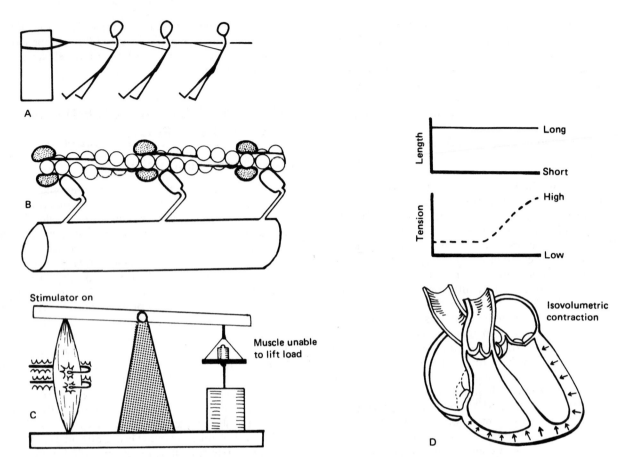

FIGURE 1-30 Isometric contraction. **(A)** In an isometric contraction, force is generated while muscles are held at a constant length. Schematically, this is analogous to the stick men pulling a load they cannot dislodge: A large force is generated, but no movement takes place. **(B)** At the molecular level, myosin heads attach to actin and pull, but filaments do not slide significantly past one another. **(C)** An experimental preparation producing isometric contraction consists of a muscle mounted on a lever with a very large load as counterweight. The muscle generates a force when stimulated, but the load is so great that the muscle cannot lift it. **(D)** In the heart, ventricular contraction is primarily isometric before the opening of the semilunar valves: Tension increases but no major shortening takes place. (**A** and **B** adapted from Katz AM: Physiology of the Heart, p 118. New York, Raven Press, 1977.)

The *thin filaments* are composed primarily of bead-shaped molecules of the protein actin arranged in an intercoiled, double-stranded chain. Two other proteins, troponin and tropomyosin, are located on the thin filaments at periodic intervals (Fig. 1-32). Actin interaction with the thick-filament protein, myosin, results in the transduction of the chemical energy of ATP into mechanical energy. Troponin and tropomyosin are called *regulatory proteins* because they modify the interaction of actin and myosin.

Myosin is an enzyme that breaks down the high-energy ATP molecule. During the resting state, the products of ATP breakdown remain bound to the myosin head. When myosin interacts with actin, the rate of ATP turnover is greatly increased. The chemical energy released from ATP is converted to the mechanical energy of contraction and heat.

According to the *cross-bridge theory,* a bond or cross-bridge forms during muscle contraction, linking thick and thin filaments. The protuberant myosin head contains an actin-binding site and forms the cross-bridge. This cross-bridge is capable of binding, flexing, releasing, and binding again, thus pulling the thin filament toward the center of the sarcomere in an isotonic contraction. If the muscle is held at a fixed length and is unable to shorten (an isometric contraction), tension is generated by the pulling of the cross-bridge.

When the muscle is relaxed during diastole, the interaction of myosin and actin is inhibited by tropomyosin and troponin. Electrical signals across the cell membrane trigger the release of calcium ion into the sarcoplasm from within the SR and from extracellular fluid by way of the sarcolemma and T-tubule membranes. This increase in intracellular calcium ion concentration is in turn a trigger for contraction. Calcium ion binds troponin; tropomyosin rotates in a manner such that resting inhibition to cross-bridge formation is removed, and cross-bridges form (see Fig. 1-32).

At relaxation, calcium ion concentration is very low in the sarcoplasm. When calcium ion concentration rises, contrac-

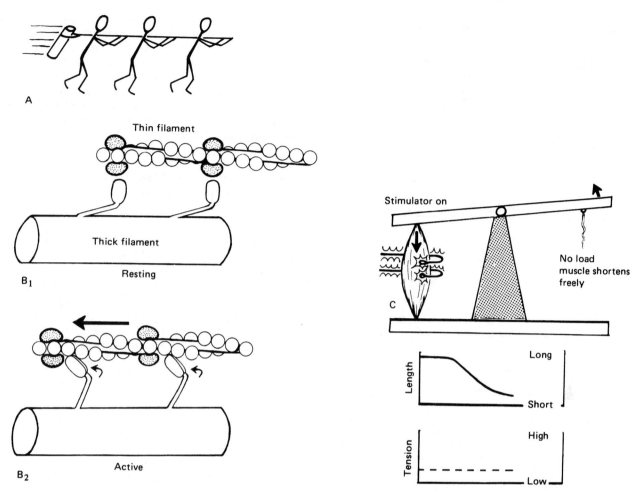

FIGURE 1-31 Isotonic contraction. **(A)** In an isotonic contraction, muscles shorten freely, and little tension is developed. Schematically, this is analogous to the stick men running with a very small load. Little force is generated, but movement takes place. **(B)** At the molecular level, myosin heads attach briefly to actin and pull the thin filament, then release in a cyclic fashion. The sarcomere shortens. **(C)** An experimental preparation producing isotonic contraction consists of a muscle mounted on a lever without significant counterload. The stimulated muscle shortens freely, not increasing its tension. (**A** and **B** adapted from Katz AM: Physiology of the Heart, pp 87, 112. New York, Raven Press, 1977.)

tion occurs. The sarcoplasmic calcium ion concentration determines the forcefulness of contraction. Figure 1-33 illustrates the relation: the higher the sarcoplasmic calcium ion concentration, the greater is the tension or pull the heart muscle can generate until a saturating concentration is attained.

Molecular Basis for Relaxation

Contraction ceases when calcium ion is removed from the sarcoplasm. Troponin releases its bound calcium ion; tropomyosin returns to the position in which actin and myosin interaction was blocked. The cell relaxes again (see Fig. 1-32).

Removal of calcium ion is essential in this sequence. Two mechanisms are important in this process. The SR pumps calcium ion into its core. This is an active process and requires chemical energy from ATP breakdown. Also, calcium ion is pumped outward across the sarcolemma. This, too, is an active process because calcium ion must be

moved against electrical and concentration gradients. Rather than using ATP directly, this process uses the energy stored in the sodium ion gradient. In conjunction with sodium ion moving inward down its concentration gradient, calcium ion is forced outward. The sodium ion gradient, in turn, is maintained by the sodium–potassium pump, which is powered by ATP.

The ATP required for the removal of calcium ion from the cell and for the cycling of cross-bridges may be depleted, for example, in myocardial ischemia. When this happens, cross-bridges form and are not broken; the muscle is stiff.

Modulation of Sarcoplasmic Calcium Ion Concentration

Interventions that alter the sarcoplasmic calcium ion concentration alter the force generated in a contraction. For example, β-adrenergic drugs such as epinephrine may increase

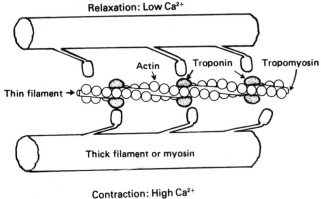

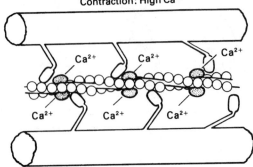

FIGURE 1-32 Molecular interactions during relaxation and contraction proposed by the cross-bridge theory of muscle contraction. During relaxation, when calcium ion (Ca^{2+}), concentration is low, no cross-bridges form. When intracellular Ca^{2+} concentration rises as it does after the action potential, troponin combines with Ca^{2+}, and the tropomyosin–troponin system changes in such a way as to allow attachment and pulling by cross-bridges. Adapted from Alpert NR and Hamrell BB: Cardiac hypertrophy: A compensatory and anticompensatory response to stress. In Vassalle M [ed]: Cardiac Physiology for the Clinician, p 196. New York, Academic Press, 1976.)

inward calcium current through calcium channels opened during the action potential, increasing sarcoplasmic calcium ion concentration and, thus, force of contraction. Certain antiarrhythmic drugs such as procainamide are associated with decreased calcium ion release from the SR and, thus, decreased systolic tension generation and blood pressure.[22]

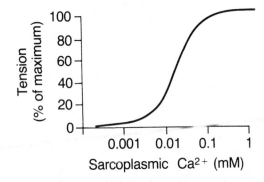

FIGURE 1-33 The calcium ion (Ca^{2+}) concentration versus tension relation. The higher the sarcoplasmic Ca^{2+} concentration, the more tension the heart muscle is able to generate until a maximum level is attained. Note the range of intracellular Ca^{2+} concentrations is significantly lower than the 1- to 2-mM concentration in the extracellular space.

Digitalis-like drugs increase the force of contraction. A prominent theory postulates that this effect is mediated by changes in the sarcoplasmic calcium ion concentration. Digitalis-like drugs partially block the sodium–potassium pump. As the transmembrane sodium ion gradient decreases, less calcium ion is pumped out across the sarcolemma. The intracellular calcium ion stores and calcium ion level during contraction increase. The end result is augmented contractile strength.

MECHANICAL PROPERTIES OF THE MYOCARDIUM

The heart is a pump. Its function is to add energy to the flowing blood, thus propelling it through the systemic and pulmonary circulations. The performance of the heart as a pump can be described in terms of the cardiac output (CO). This is the volume of blood pumped by one ventricle in 1 minute. It is equal to the stroke volume (SV), or volume of blood pumped with each beat, times the number of cardiac contractions (heart rate, HR) in 1 minute: ($CO = SV \times HR$). Typical normal values in a 70-kg man at rest (HR: 68 beats/min; SV: 80 mL) produce a cardiac output of 5,440 mL/min or 5.4 L/min.

The stroke volume is determined by the degree of ventricular filling during diastole, or preload, the force against which the ventricle must pump, or afterload, the contractile state of the myocardium, and by the heart rate. In the remainder of this section, these factors are discussed in more detail, and the manner in which they interact to influence the mechanical function of the heart is described.

Preload and Afterload

PRELOAD

Preload is the distending force that stretches the ventricular muscle immediately before electrical excitation and contraction. Figure 1-34 further defines preload and illustrates the role of preload in the contraction of a simple muscle preparation and in the heart. Left ventricular end-diastolic pressure is the left ventricular preload. In the absence of pathologic changes in the mitral valve or pulmonary hypertension, left atrial pressure and pulmonary artery wedge pressure are useful indices of left ventricular preload. Central venous pressure, in the absence of tricuspid valve disease, is an index of right ventricular preload (see Chapter 19).

AFTERLOAD

A related term often used to describe cardiac mechanical function is *afterload*. This is the force that opposes ventricular ejection (i.e., the load the muscle must move during contraction). Figure 1-35 illustrates the role of afterload in a simple muscle preparation and in the heart.

Left ventricular afterload is determined by the volume and mass of blood ejected by the ventricle, by the cross-sectional area of the vascular space into which the blood is being ejected, and by the ease with which that vascular space stretches. Total systemic vascular resistance (SVR) is the best clinical indicator of left ventricular afterload. SVR

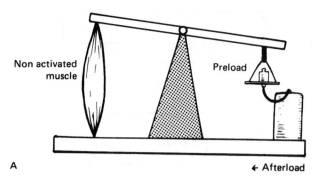

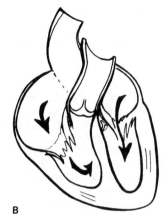

Preload = load stretching the
resting ventricle to its end-
diastolic volume

FIGURE 1-34 Preload. **(A)** In the isolated muscle preparation, preload is the load stretching the resting muscle. Thus, preload determines the resting length of the muscles. **(B)** In the heart, the ventricular preload is determined by the volume of blood stretching the resting ventricles.

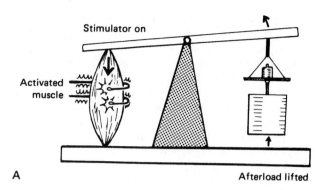

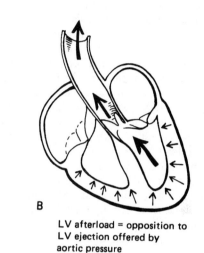

LV afterload = opposition to
LV ejection offered by
aortic pressure

FIGURE 1-35 Afterload. **(A)** In the isolated muscle preparation, afterload is the force opposing shortening. The muscle must generate enough tension to lift the afterload before it can shorten. **(B)** In the heart, the afterload is the force opposing ventricular ejection.

is derived from the force the heart muscle has added to the flowing blood: mean arterial pressure minus central venous pressure divided by the volume pumped (cardiac output). Mean arterial pressure is sometimes used as an approximate index of left ventricular afterload (see Chapter 19).

PRELOAD ROLE: LENGTH–TENSION RELATIONSHIP

Early in this century, Starling observed that, within limits, an increase in the volume of the left ventricle at the end of diastole results in the generation of increased active pressure and increased volume pumped during the ensuing contraction. Beyond a certain volume, this mechanism is no longer operational; increased end-diastolic volume results instead in decreased pressure developing and a decreased volume of blood being ejected.[44] This property is known as *Starling's law of the heart* or the *length–tension relation of cardiac muscle* (or sometimes, the *Frank-Starling law of the heart*). It is commonly illustrated in a graph (Fig. 1-36). Although the increment in active pressure generated is related to volume of the ventricle and consequently to the length of the ventricular muscle fibers, it is common to use preload (i.e., filling pressure) as an index of ventricular volume (see section on Compliance, later).

The length–tension mechanism is a functional one; it is thought to help maintain overall matching between left and right ventricular output. For instance, if a person reclines after being in a standing position (or elevates the legs when in a reclining position), the volume of blood returning to

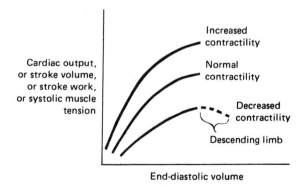

FIGURE 1-36 The length–tension relation of the heart. End-diastolic volume determines the end-diastolic length of the ventricular muscle fibers and is proportional to tension generated during systole as well as to cardiac output, stroke volume, and stroke work. A change in cardiac contractility causes the heart to perform on a different length–tension curve.

the heart transiently increases. The right ventricle is stretched and increases its force of contraction, pumping a larger stroke volume to the lungs and generating higher pressures. Pulmonary vascular pressures rise. This raises the left ventricular filling pressure or preload. Left ventricular filling volume increases. The left ventricle generates increased active pressure and pumps a larger stroke volume, and arterial vascular pressures rise (see Chapter 4).

The patient with a cardiac transplant becomes more dependent on the length–tension relation to increase cardiac output, particularly early in exercise.

Some forms of therapy are designed to take advantage of the length–tension characteristics of the heart. Examples of this are leg raising and intravascular volume expansion in the patient with shock. These therapies increase central blood volume and improve cardiac contractile force; they are easily and rapidly accessible. They are, however, associated with an increase in myocardial oxygen consumption and should be used carefully in the patient at risk for myocardial ischemia. These patients should be monitored for electrocardiographic signs of myocardial ischemia and for symptoms such as chest pain when interventions may result in increased preload.

The mechanical function of the heart is not characterized by a single curve describing the length–tension relation, but rather by a number of curves (see Fig. 1-36). Positive inotropic factors, that is, factors that increase the contractility of the heart, such as sympathetic stimulation, alter the length–tension relation, so that a higher tension is generated at the same left ventricular end-diastolic volume.

In heart failure, the heart length–tension relation again is altered. At each length, less tension is generated. In addition, with heart failure, the heart may become refractory to inotropic stimulation; it may be said that the Starling curve is reduced. Furthermore, in the failing heart, increases in length may result in decreases in force generated. Thus, the "descending limb" of the Starling curve is observed. Patients in severe failure may experience a vicious cycle wherein increased dilation of the heart reduces the contractile force, less blood is pumped, and still greater dilation occurs.

The cross-bridge theory of muscle contraction partly accounts for the length–tension relation of cardiac muscle (Fig. 1-37). Tension generated by muscle is proportional to the number of cross-bridges formed. At short lengths, thin filaments overlap one another and interfere with cross-bridge formation. Maximal tension development occurs in the range of muscle lengths at which the myosin cross-bridge regions maximally overlap the thin filaments without the thin filaments overlapping one another. If the muscle is stretched still further, the region of cross-bridge overlap is diminished; less tension is developed.[16]

Other factors also contribute to the shape of the Starling curve. For example, when the heart is stretched, more cells may be brought into parallel with the axis of shortening and may be able to contribute more effectively to the total development of force within the ventricle. Calcium ion, which grades the force of contraction, may enter the sarcoplasm in larger quantities for longer periods of time. Contractile filaments may be more sensitive to calcium ion at longer sarcomere lengths.

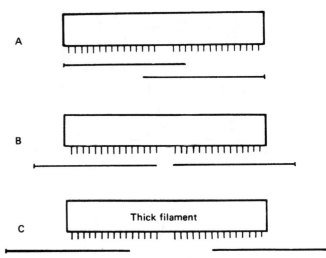

FIGURE 1-37 Schematic view of variations in overlap between the thick and thin filaments that account for the length–tension relation of cardiac muscle. **(A)** Sarcomere on ascending limb of length–tension curve. The thin filaments begin overlapping, interfering with attachment by cross-bridges. **(B)** Sarcomere with maximal effective overlap of thin and thick filaments and hence at the peak of the length–tension curve. **(C)** Sarcomere stretched beyond maximal overlap and hence on the descending limb of the length–tension curve. As the actin chains are pulled farther out, fewer actin sites are available for cross-bridge attachment. **(A and B** adapted from Katz AM: Physiology of the Heart, pp 129, 130. New York, Raven Press, 1977.)

Compliance. Starling's law of the heart relates end-diastolic length, rather than end-diastolic pressure, to the strength of contraction. End-diastolic length and pressure are, however, related. *Compliance* is the term used to describe that relation. Compliance (C) is the change in volume (ΔV) that results for a given change in pressure (ΔP): $C = \Delta V/\Delta P$. Stiffness (S) is the inverse of compliance ($S = \Delta P/\Delta V$). Increased stiffness is the same as decreased compliance.

Compliance of the heart is determined by inherent properties of the cardiac muscle tissue, by cardiac chamber geometry, and by the state of the pericardium. The myocardial tissue is stiffer with hypoxia, ischemia, and scarring, such as after a myocardial infarction[34] (curve 2 in Fig. 1-38). Infiltrative myocardial diseases such as amyloidosis increase muscle stiffness. Geometry changes that result in increased stiffness include hypertrophy. When operating at a more distended volume, the heart is invariably stiffer: it requires larger increments in filling pressure to achieve a given increment in volume (see Fig. 1-38). Pericardial conditions that increase cardiac stiffness include pericarditis and tamponade.

Implications for Patient Care. It is important to consider left ventricular compliance in patient care. In monitoring preload, the nurse commonly measures indices of left ventricular end-diastolic *pressure.* Yet, therapeutic goals are related to achieving an end-diastolic *volume* change that will take advantage of the length–tension relation of the

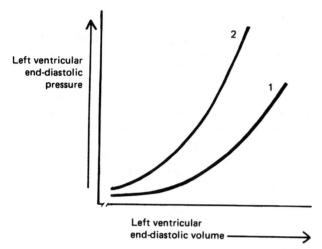

FIGURE 1-38 The stiffness of the left ventricle. Stiffness is the slope of the pressure–volume relation. Curve 1 represents normal stiffness; curve 2 represents an increase in stiffness such as that which might occur after a myocardial infarction. In both cases, increases in volume result in increased pressure and an increased increment in pressure for a given increment in volume. Compliance is the inverse of stiffness. (Adapted from Forrester JS, Diamond GA: Clinical application of left ventricular pressures. In Corday E, Swan HJC [eds]: Myocardial Infarction: New perspectives in diagnosis and management, pp 143–148 Baltimore, Williams & Wilkins, 1973.)

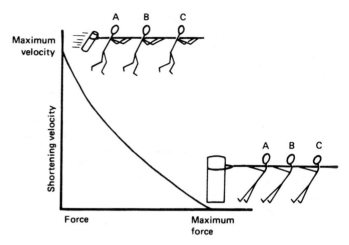

FIGURE 1-39 Approximation of the force–velocity of shortening relation of cardiac muscle. Velocity of shortening is maximal with extremely light afterload. Shortening is impossible with large afterloads. (Adapted from Katz AM: Physiology of the Heart, pp 87, 126. New York, Raven Press, 1977.)

heart to maintain or increase cardiac output. The pressure change is important, too, because elevated left ventricular filling pressures result in pulmonary congestion and edema.

For example, the first few days after a myocardial infarction are usually characterized by an increase in myocardial stiffness[20] (see Fig. 1-38). The same end-diastolic volume may be accompanied by such a markedly increased end-diastolic pressure that signs of left ventricular failure such as crackles appear (see Chapter 10). In this case, inotropic agents (which increase the force of contraction) would be of little or no benefit. Unloading therapies, however, that may decrease the end-diastolic volume can eliminate the damaging elevation in end-diastolic pressures. Furthermore, lowered ventricular pressures throughout diastole may improve coronary arterial filling. Better perfusion can improve tissue oxygenation and further diminish stiffness.

AFTERLOAD ROLE: FORCE–VELOCITY RELATIONSHIP

The heart's ability to contract is influenced by the amount of pressure above the preload it must actively generate. With a smaller afterload, the heart is able to contract more rapidly. Against very large afterload, contraction is much slower. This is often referred to as the *force–velocity of shortening relation,* or simply the *force–velocity relation* (Fig. 1-39). Changes in the initial muscle length or changes in contractility can alter the force–velocity relation.

An intuitive understanding of the force–velocity relation can be gained by reviewing the stick-figure cartoons in Figure 1-39. The lighter the load, the faster A, B, and C run; the heavier the load, the slower they can move. If the load

they are trying to pull is sufficiently heavy, they are unable to move it at all.

At the molecular level, the rate of cycling of cross-bridges may be equated to the speed of shortening. Generation of tension may be equated to attachment and pulling by the cross-bridges. The amount of tension the muscle can generate is determined by the number of cross-bridges the muscle is able to form. This is determined in part by the preload, or the amount of diastolic stretch placed on the muscle. Once a critical amount of force equivalent to the afterload, or force opposing ejection, is generated, the muscle shortens. The speed of that shortening may be equated with the speed of cycling of cross-bridges and is determined in part by the afterload.

Effect of Afterload on the Volume Ejected by the Ventricle. In addition to influencing the speed of shortening, afterload is related to extent of shortening. Increases in SVR, at a constant end-diastolic pressure, result in decreased volume pumped by the left ventricle. When pumping against decreased aortic pressure, the left ventricle pumps a larger volume.

Implications for Patient Care. It is important to consider the force–velocity relation in myocardial performance. Vasopressors that increase the SVR increase the afterload. Because of the inverse nature of the force–velocity relation, the development of greater force is accompanied by a slower velocity of shortening. There may be a concomitant fall in stroke volume and cardiac output. Further, there is an increase in the oxygen requirements of the cardiac tissue when afterload is increased.

Conversely, therapies that decrease the afterload are associated with faster and more extensive shortening and a larger volume pumped. The cardiac output increases. Increases in cardiac output achieved in this manner have the unique advantage of decreasing myocardial oxygen consumption. Reduction of afterload, however, is associated with decreased coronary perfusion pressure. Signs of myocardial ischemia may develop in patients with partially obstructed coronary arteries.

Contractility of Cardiac Muscle

Contractility describes the heart's ability to contract: it describes the ability of the heart muscle to shorten, develop tension, or both. Altered contractility is a change in the ability of the heart to contract independent of variations induced by altering either preload or afterload (see Fig. 1-36; Fig. 1-40). In Figure 1-36, the curves other than "normal" represent alterations in contractility.

Contractility is a property intrinsic to the muscle. Its physiologic basis is not yet understood. Although contractility is difficult to define or measure, it is a property of critical importance because abnormalities in contractility are a major problem in the failing heart. Many therapies are designed to enhance contractility.

Contractility is not equivalent to cardiac performance, which can be influenced by valvular function and circulating blood volume as well as by myocardial contractility.

Factors that affect the contractility of the heart are called *inotropic agents*. Positive inotropic agents increase contractility. These include sympathetic stimulation, excess thyroid hormone, epinephrine, norepinephrine, dopamine, dobutamine, isoproterenol infusion, and calcium salt infusion. Digitalis-like drugs have positive inotropic action. Negative inotropic agents decrease contractility; these include myocardial hypoxia, ischemia, acidosis, barbiturates, alcohol, procainamide and quinidine, propranolol, and possibly lidocaine.

Therapies that increase contractility increase myocardial oxygen consumption. Agents such as catecholamines increase both contractility and afterload and result in substantial increase in myocardial oxygen consumption.

Treppe

Heart rate is the fourth major determinant of the force of contraction. Alteration in the force of contraction with heart rate is called the *Treppe* or *staircase phenomenon*. In an experimental preparation with the preload held constant, the faster the rate of stimulation, the stronger is the force of contraction. Conversely, in the same preparation, slower rates of stimulation result in less forceful contraction. In the intact organism, as heart rate increases, there is decreased time for filling. The Treppe phenomenon provides some compensation for the decrement (Fig. 1-41).

Treppe is an intrinsic property of the heart muscle, independent of hormones or innervation. It is present in the transplanted heart. The physiologic basis for Treppe may be rate-driven variations in sarcoplasmic calcium ion concentration.

Two other types of rate-related alterations occur in force of contraction. A pause augments the force of the ensuing beat. This is called *rest potentiation*. After an extra beat, the force of the ensuing contraction is increased. This effect is called *postextrasystolic potentiation*.

The manner in which variations in cardiac rate or rhythm induce changes in cardiac output in the intact heart is complex. Rate-related variations in force of contraction and filling interact; the amount pumped depends on that complex interaction.

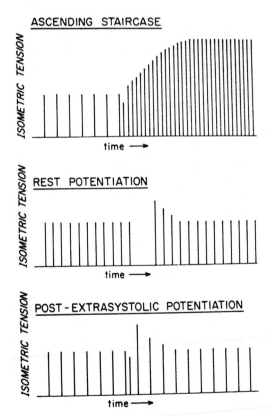

FIGURE 1-41 Changes in isometric force generated in cardiac muscle when the stimulation frequency is altered. (From Feigl EO: Physiology and Biophysics, 20th ed, vol 2, p 37. Philadelphia, WB Saunders, 1974.)

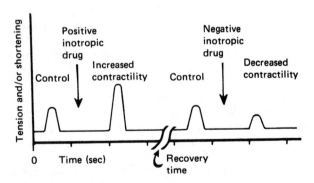

FIGURE 1-40 Positive and negative inotropic effects on tension development or myocardial shortening. An increase in myocardial contractility enhances the amount of tension developed, the rate of shortening, or both, without an increase in initial cardiac muscle length. A decrease in myocardial contractility reduces the amount of tension developed, the rate of shortening, or both, without a decrease in initial cardiac muscle length. (Adapted from Katz AM: Physiology of the Heart, p 166. New York, Raven Press, 1977.)

Cardiac Reserve

The interaction of the mechanical properties of the heart can be illustrated by considering the reserve capacity of the heart. *Cardiac reserve* refers to the ability of the heart to increase its output. In the healthy person, the reserve capacity is used to meet demands for increased blood flow, such as during exercise. Normal cardiac output is 5.5 L/min in a healthy, 70-kg man. Use of cardiac reserve typically increases cardiac output with activity to 18 L/min. Heart disease often limits the total possible output, and the patient may have to rely on reserve capacity simply to maintain a normal cardiac output at rest. The two components of cardiac reserve are increases in heart rate and stroke volume (Fig. 1-42).

Increases in heart rate increase the cardiac output. As the heart beats more rapidly, there is less time for filling. The rate-related increase in force of contraction partially compensates for the lower end-diastolic filling. At rates higher than approximately 180 beats/min, however, diastole is so shortened that diastolic filling is reduced. Stroke volume is then diminished, as predicted by the Starling relation. Furthermore, the coronary arteries are perfused during diastole, and fast heart rates diminish coronary blood flow. This may result in ischemia, which in turn diminishes myocardial compliance and contractility. The stiff ventricle requires greater filling pressures to expand it to the same diastolic volume and may well operate at a smaller volume, further diminishing stroke volume, again as defined by the Starling relation. Beyond a certain point, increasing the heart rate so decreases the volume pumped per beat that cardiac output falls.

During diastole, the heart can fill to a larger volume than usual, thereby increasing its stroke volume as defined by the Starling relation. This is sometimes called the *diastolic cardiac reserve.* Increases in diastolic volume are accompanied by increases in end-diastolic pressure. Left ventricular end-diastolic pressures beyond approximately 20 to 25 mm Hg typically result in pulmonary congestion and edema. The more dilated the ventricle, the more oxygen it requires (discussed later); this may be a limiting problem in the patient with coronary artery disease.

The heart is capable of ejecting a larger portion of its volume than it normally does; that is, it can contract to a smaller end-systolic volume. This is sometimes called the *systolic reserve;* it comes into play when the afterload is decreased (force–velocity relation) or contractility is increased. Increases in the velocity of contraction or contractility also make extra demands on the heart in terms of oxygen requirements and may be intolerable for the patient with coronary artery disease.

Factors involved in mechanical performance interact continuously. For example, an increase in afterload may result in a decrease in the stroke volume ejected. This in turn results in a larger volume of blood in the heart at end systole. The addition of an unchanged amount of blood during the subsequent diastole increases the end-diastolic volume. The ensuing contraction is more forceful, and stroke volume is increased owing to the Starling effect.

In hemorrhage, the filling pressure may diminish; the stroke volume decreases as predicted by the Starling relation. However, the afterload may also decrease. This tends to raise the stroke volume. Adrenergic outflow also contributes to increased stroke volume. The cardiac output may increase despite lowered filling pressures.

This section has discussed means by which the heart can increase its output. Just as a budget deficit can be corrected either by increasing income or by carefully managing spending, the cardiovascular system can meet demands for increased perfusion both by increasing output and by more efficiently using its present output. It can, for instance, shift blood flow to more active regions and extract more oxygen from the blood (see Chapter 4).

Assessment of the Patient's Pump Performance

Assessment of the patient includes the evaluation of numerous indices of overall pump performance:

- ◆ Urine output, mental status, skin color, and temperature are indices of the adequacy of cardiac output to various organs and tissues.
- ◆ Cardiac output may be measured directly.
- ◆ Left ventricular preload is estimated from the pulmonary artery wedge pressure.
- ◆ SVR (index of left ventricular afterload) is calculated.
- ◆ Blood pressure is the product of cardiac output and SVR.

These observations measure end products of many complexly interacting variables that together compose the reserve capacity of the cardiovascular system. In making

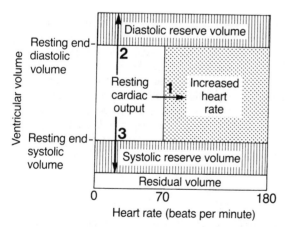

FIGURE 1-42 Cardiac reserve describes the ability of the heart to increase its output. Increases in heart rate increase the cardiac output (*arrow 1*). Stroke volume increases also increase the cardiac output. This can be accomplished by an increase in preload (diastolic reserve, *arrow 2*) or by contracting to a smaller end-systolic volume (systolic reserve, *arrow 3*). (From Rushmer RF: Cardiovascular Dynamics, p 274. Philadelphia, WB Saunders, 1976.)

these assessments, the nurse not only should ask whether blood flow and pressure are adequate, but should probe more deeply:

- How much of the patient's reserve capacity must be used to maintain the current level of functioning?
- Is the patient already tachycardiac, with a dilated left ventricle?
- Is the patient's heart already receiving a high level of endogenous catecholaminergic outflow?
- How much of the patient's reserve capacity is left? Of that left, how much can be used in planning the patient's care?
- What is the cost of the patient's current functional state in terms of myocardial oxygen consumption?

MYOCARDIAL METABOLISM

The chemical energy of ATP powers myocardial contraction, ion pumping, and many other activities. ATP is broken down (hydrolyzed) into adenosine diphosphate and inorganic phosphate. With hydrolysis, chemical energy is transformed into mechanical energy and heat. Because the heart is continuously active, ATP must be continuously available. The usual intramyocardial cellular concentrations of ATP (estimated at 5 mM) are sufficient to power contraction mechanical activity for only a few beats.

Creatine phosphate is a backup source of high-energy phosphate to replenish the ATP supply. However, energy stores in ATP and creatine phosphate together supply enough energy only for several minutes of activity. Thus, the heart depends on ongoing ATP synthesis. This occurs in a series of efficient, but complex, enzyme-dependent reactions. The bulk of myocardial ATP is synthesized in an aerobic environment. The presence of large amounts of mitochondria, the sites of aerobic synthesis of ATP in the myocardial cell, attest to the need for oxygen as an energy substrate. The myocyte contains more mitochondria than any other type of muscle cell.

Free fatty acids are the preferred myocardial fuel, particularly when the patient is in the fasting state. *Glucose* or its storage form, glycogen, can serve as an additional substrate for energy metabolism. Whereas glucose contributes only 15% to myocardial ATP synthesis in the fasting patient, its role increases to nearly 50% in the postprandial state. *Amino acids* play a minor role in energy metabolism of the heart. In starvation, however, amino acid intermediates may be metabolized to maintain energy stores.

PHYSIOLOGY OF THE CORONARY CIRCULATION

Under normal conditions at rest, the heart extracts a large amount of oxygen from the blood perfusing it: the difference in oxygen content between the arterial and coronary sinus blood is approximately 11.4 mL O_2/100 mL blood.[47] It is difficult to extract much more oxygen than this, yet the oxygen requirement of the heart may increase manyfold.

This additional oxygen can be supplied only by increasing the coronary blood flow. Coronary blood flow increases proportionately to myocardial metabolism and oxygen consumption.

Determinants of Myocardial Oxygen Consumption

Some oxygen is used in the "housekeeping" activities of the heart cells. This refers to those activities that are independent of contraction and includes such functions as maintenance of the proper ionic environment and repair or replacement of intracellular proteins. The amount of oxygen used in these functions is relatively small and stable.

Each contraction of the heart involves movements of ions across the cell membranes. By removing calcium ion from the fluid bathing the heart cells, the heart can be excited without actively developing tension. Experiments have shown that the cost of electrical depolarization and repolarization is small.[30] It is possible that cycling of pumps that maintain sodium and potassium ion concentrations is responsible for this oxygen requirement.

In addition to these two fairly constant and low requirements for oxygen, there are factors related to activity and the state of the heart that determine how much oxygen the heart needs. These constitute the major determinants of myocardial oxygen consumption ($M\dot{V}O_2$) and include intramyocardial tension, heart rate, shortening, and contractile state.

INTRAMYOCARDIAL TENSION

The *law of Laplace* is used to calculate intramyocardial tension. This law states

$$T \propto \frac{P \times R}{Th}$$

where T = intramyocardial wall tension, P = internal pressure within the ventricular cavity, R = radius of the ventricular cavity, Th = thickness of the ventricular wall, and $\propto$ signifies "proportional to." An increase in the afterload of the left ventricle causes the left ventricle to develop more pressure during the systolic period, thereby increasing intramyocardial tension and oxygen consumption. A rise in the preload or filling pressures of the left ventricle increases tension because both internal pressure and the radius of the ventricular cavity are increased and the thickness is decreased. Again, $M\dot{V}O_2$ is increased.

HEART RATE

Increased heart rate (at the same preload and afterload) increases the $M\dot{V}O_2$. Each beat represents the generation of tension by the myocardium.

SHORTENING

In an *isotonic twitch*, there is a component of the oxygen consumption that is proportional to the amount of shortening by a muscle. That is, there is a metabolic cost that is related to shortening. This is sometimes called the *Fenn effect* and is a characteristic of cardiac as well as of skeletal muscle. In cardiac muscle, a contraction with a large amount of shortening is one that expels a large stroke volume.

CONTRACTILE STATE

Contractility correlates with the amount of oxygen consumed by the heart. Positive inotropic factors increase the $M\dot{V}O_2$. Negative inotropic agents diminish $M\dot{V}O_2$.

PRESSURE VERSUS VOLUME WORK

Work done by the heart is proportional to the pressure generated times the volume pumped (stroke work = [mean arterial pressure – left atrial pressure] – stroke volume). Pressure generated is a component of the intramyocardial tension as described by the Laplace relation and thus contributes to the overall $M\dot{V}O_2$. The size of the stroke volume is related to the amount of myocardial shortening, and thus it too contributes to the $M\dot{V}O_2$. Although equal amounts of work can be obtained by altering pressure or volume, the cost in terms of $M\dot{V}O_2$ is much greater for high-pressure work than for high-volume work. Thus, cardiac work is poorly correlated with $M\dot{V}O_2$.

INDICES OF MYOCARDIAL OXYGEN CONSUMPTION

No single indicator of the oxygen requirements of the myocardium is available. Ideally, such an indicator would take into account all major determinants of the $M\dot{V}O_2$. The pressure–rate product and the tension–time index are two commonly used methods of estimation that have been validated.[7] Each takes into account one of the major determinants of the $M\dot{V}O_2$, the heart rate. Another major determinant, tension, is also considered in these indices. What is actually measured, however, is pressure. For pressure to be an indicator of tension, the other factors in the Laplace equation, that is, radius of the ventricular cavity and thickness of the ventricular wall, must be constant.

The pressure–rate product is calculated by multiplying the heart rate by either systolic or mean arterial pressure and dividing by 100.

The tension–time index more appropriately may be called the pressure–time index. It is calculated by multiplying the area under the left ventricular pressure curve by the heart rate.

Myocardial Oxygen Supply

CONTROL OF CORONARY BLOOD FLOW

Flow of blood in the coronary circulation is, as in all vascular beds, proportional to the perfusion pressure and inversely proportional to the resistance of the bed. Resistance in the coronary bed is altered by compression on it during systole and by metabolic, neural, and hormonal factors. Coronary artery disease can impose significant resistance.

The pressure difference that drives cardiac perfusion is the gradient between aortic pressure and the pressure in the right atrium, into which most of the coronary perfusion

ultimately returns. The coronary circulation, however, is autoregulated. This means that changes in the perfusion pressure over a range of pressures (approximately 60 to 180 mm Hg) make little difference in the amount of blood flowing to the heart if the other factors influencing perfusion are held constant.

Because the heart develops its own perfusion pressure, a fall in aortic pressure can reduce coronary perfusion, which in turn may further decrease cardiac function and pressure development. A cycle of deterioration may result.

During systole, the tension in the myocardial wall is high. This compresses the coronary arteries and prevents perfusion. Thus, the heart has the unique property of receiving most of its blood flow during diastole (Fig. 1-43). Rapid heart rates decrease the time spent in diastole and may impinge on coronary perfusion.

Intramyocardial tension tends to be highest in the subendocardial regions of the left ventricle. Thus, $M\dot{V}O_2$ is probably highest in this region; yet systolic compression is also greatest here. This in part explains why this area has an increased incidence of infarction. In transmural infarctions (i.e., ones that involve the full thickness of the left ventricular wall), the area of involvement is typically greater on the subendocardial surface than on the subepicardial surface (see Chapter 20). A factor that also contributes to this pattern of involvement in infarction is the pattern of coronary artery distribution. Because arteries enter the myocardium on the epicardial surface and plunge inward through the wall, the most easily compromised distal segments of the coronary arteries perfuse the endocardium.

The coronary arteries are innervated by α-sympathetic and parasympathetic fibers. The direct effects of neural outflow are the same in the coronary bed as in other systemic beds. α-Adrenergic stimulation (or norepinephrine) constricts arteries, and parasympathetic (vagal) stimulation dilates them. Pharmacologic doses of the β-adrenergic drug isoproterenol dilate the coronary artery bed. Often,

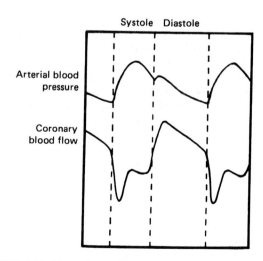

FIGURE 1-43 Effect of systolic compression on coronary blood flow. Note the decrease in flow during systole and the increase during diastole. (From Folkow B, Neil E: Circulation, p 421. Oxford, Oxford University Press, 1971.)

however, the direct effect of neural outflow on the coronary bed is masked because the autonomic nervous system also affects myocardial metabolism and contractility, and the effect of these latter factors predominates.

Local metabolic conditions are the predominant determinants of coronary perfusion. Increased metabolism or hypoxia leads to vasodilation and increased myocardial blood flow. The mechanism that mediates this effect is unknown. One hypothesis suggests that adenosine is released from myocardial tissue in proportion to the amount of oxygen being consumed, and that perfusion correlates with the amount of adenosine released.[1]

With atherosclerosis, significant resistance can develop in the coronary arteries. Lesions that occupy more than two thirds of the vessel's cross-sectional area may impinge significantly on flow at rest. Such lesions can prevent the increases in flow necessary when myocardial oxygen demand increases.

COLLATERAL CIRCULATION

Collateral arteries are interarterial vessels that can connect two branches of a single coronary artery or connect branches of the right coronary artery with branches of the left. In the human heart, collaterals are found through the full thickness of the myocardium, with the highest density near the endocardial surface. Although they are present at birth, collaterals do not become functionally significant unless the myocardium experiences hypoxic or ischemic insult. Before transformation, the collateral arteries are very narrow. They are devoid of smooth muscle and therefore are unable to respond to pharmacologic or metabolic vasoactive substances. After being stimulated to develop, the collateral tracts increase in diameter and develop a smooth muscle layer until, ultimately, the vessels are histologically similar to arterioles. When fully developed, these vessels are able to vasodilate when nitrates are administered and may autoregulate.[7] The time course from ischemic insult until significant enlargement is seen may be as short as 9 days.[52]

Three conditions are correlated with collateral development: coronary artery disease, chronic myocardial hypoxia, and myocardial hypertrophy. In coronary artery disease, the collateral diameter increases in proportion to the severity of coronary artery narrowing. Functionally significant increases in collateral structure are seen with a 75% or greater reduction in the luminal diameter of a major vessel. Chronic hypoxic myocardium is seen in patients with anemia, cyanotic heart disease, and chronic obstructive pulmonary disease.[65] There is also an increase in collateral diameter in hypertrophied hearts.[6] Attempts to stimulate development of collaterals with exercise programs have not been successful.[7] Collaterals frequently disappear after successful aortocoronary bypass grafting.[33]

Blood flow through collateral vessels may contribute significantly to myocardial perfusion. Patients with similar coronary occlusions have smaller areas of infarction when collateral development has occurred. Patients with abundant and well developed collaterals sometimes have a totally occluded coronary artery but no evidence of infarction. Blood flow through collateral vessels may be insufficient to meet increased demand, such as during exercise, and is insufficient to prevent necrosis in most cases.

Clinical Implications

It is important to analyze the effect of altered clinical states on the myocardial oxygen need. It is useful to consider the Laplace relation when evaluating oxygen demand in clinical states. For example, *hypertrophy of ventricular muscle* results in an increase in the thickness of the ventricular wall. This is advantageous in that wall tension is lower for the same left ventricular cavity size (the same end-diastolic volume); hence, oxygen consumption is decreased. However, development of hypertrophy is a two-edged sword. At the same time that wall tension is decreased, the mass of tissue requiring oxygen is increased; the net result may well be a greater demand by the heart for oxygen. Furthermore, because hypertrophy tends to increase the size of the muscle cells without increasing the tissue capillarity,[14] diffusional distances are increased. The supply of oxygen to the interior of the fiber may be significantly impaired.

With *cardiac dilation,* the radius of the left ventricle is increased. A larger end-diastolic volume is associated with higher end-diastolic pressure and increased pressure generation during systole, according to the Starling law. The Laplace relation predicts that both factors lead to increased intramyocardial wall tension. The stretching out of the heart wall is associated with decreased wall thickness, further increasing intramyocardial wall tension. The increase in oxygen demand can be significant.

THE CARDIAC CYCLE

Every ventricular contraction that propels blood to the body or the lungs is the result of the sequential activation of the cardiac chambers through the coordinated functioning of the electrical and mechanical factors. This section describes the changing cardiac pressures and volumes that coincide with the time sequence of cardiac events. An understanding of normal or abnormal cardiac functioning depends on familiarity with the cardiac cycle, which is represented graphically in Figure 1-44.

For the sake of simplicity, the description of events that occur during the cardiac cycle begins with events in the left heart. Figure 1-44 should be referred to frequently to obtain an understanding of what is occurring concurrently with respect to electrical activity; atrial, ventricular, and aortic pressures; atrial and ventricular volumes; valvular activity; and heart sounds.

Some general points about pressures and timing should be remembered during the following discussion. Blood flows from a chamber with a greater pressure to a chamber with a lower pressure. When valves are open between two chambers, pressures in both chambers change until they are approximately equal. When valves between two chambers are closed, the pressures in the chambers change relatively independently of each other.

Ventricular systole and diastole divide the cardiac cycle into two major phases. The cardiac cycle can be further

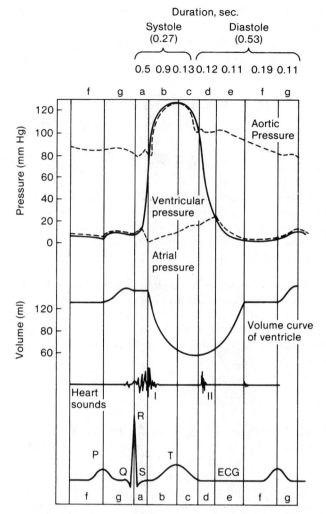

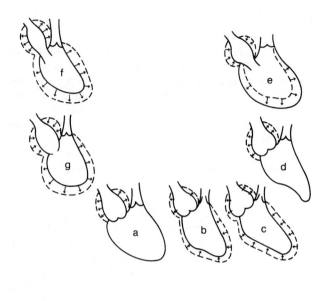

FIGURE 1-44 The cardiac cycle, illustrating the changes in aortic, left ventricular, and left atrial pressures, and in left ventricular volume, in relation to the phonocardiogram and the electrocardiogram. The duration of each phase at a heart rate of approximately 75 beats/min is indicated at the top of the figure. a, isovolumetric ventricular contraction; b, rapid ventricular ejection; c, slow ventricular ejection; d, isovolumetric relaxation; e, rapid ventricular filling; f, diastasis; g, atrial contraction; I, first heart sound; II, second heart sound. *Insets:* Changes in the configuration of the left atrium, mitral valve, left ventricle, and aortic valve during various phases of the cycle. (Adapted from Wiggens: Circulatory Dynamics. New York, Grune & Stratton, 1952.)

subdivided into several separate periods during systole and diastole. Because the cardiac cycle is continuous, the description of these periods can begin at any point.

Left Ventricular Cardiac Events

VENTRICULAR SYSTOLE

Isovolumic Ventricular Contraction (Period a, Fig. 1-44). Ventricular contraction follows ventricular depolarization (reflected by the electrocardiographic QRS wave). Ventricular pressure increases rapidly. At the onset of this period, pressures in the atrium and ventricle are approximately equal, but atrial pressure decreases with atrial muscle relaxation. Closure of the mitral valve buffers the atria from the high ventricular pressures.

The mitral valve closes when the ventricle contracts. Pressure in the ventricle becomes higher than in the atrium. The aortic valve remains closed until left ventricular pressure becomes greater than aortic pressure. Bulging of the cardiac valves due to abrupt ventricular pressure increases may cause slight increases in atrial and aortic pressures recorded during this period.

During the brief time when both mitral and aortic valves are closed, there are no actual changes in ventricular volume because no blood is flowing into or out of the ventricle. The ventricle changes shape during this period. The apparent increase in ventricular volume recorded on the ventricular volume curve in Figure 1-44 occurs when ventricular volume is calculated from the ventricular circumference.

Besides being called the *isovolumic* or *isovolumetric period*, this time has been termed the *isometric phase* of ventricular contraction because tension is increasing rapidly, whereas the muscle fibers do not shorten much until they overcome the afterload of aortic pressure. Muscle contraction is not completely isometric, however, because the ventricles change dimensions.

Rapid Ventricular Ejection (Period b, Fig. 1–44). Ventricular muscle contraction continues, and the aortic valve opens as long as left ventricular pressure exceeds aortic pressure. The aorta and left ventricle are essentially a common cavity at this time. Ventricular pressure continues to rise rapidly during the initial part of this period, then rises less rapidly during the latter part of the period to approximately the systolic pressure (120 mm Hg in the figure).

Ventricular volume decreases rapidly during ventricular ejection; two thirds or more of the stroke volume is ejected during this approximately 0.09-second period (Table 1-6). Aortic flow reaches peak velocity during the early part of the rapid ejection period before the point of maximal ventricular pressure. Aortic pressure may actually slightly exceed ventricular pressure during the latter period of rapid ventricular ejection, but blood continues to flow into the aorta because of the forward momentum of the blood. Much of the stroke volume is accommodated in the elastic proximal aorta.

The left atrium is relaxed at this time. Atrial pressure slowly begins to rise as blood from the lungs accumulates in the atrium. Ventricular repolarization begins.

Reduced Ventricular Ejection (Period c, Fig. 1–44). Ventricular and aortic pressures begin to decrease approximately 0.13 second before the end of ventricular contraction. During this time, ventricular muscle fibers are no longer contracting as forcefully as during the previous period. The fibers have reached a shorter length. Ventricular volume continues to fall, although at a slower rate than during rapid ejection, and blood continues to flow into the aorta. This period of reduced ventricular ejection comprises

TABLE 1-6	**Duration of Cardiac Cycle Periods* (in seconds)**
Isometric contraction	0.05
Maximal ejection	0.09
Reduced ejection	<u>0.13</u>
Total systole	0.27
Protodiastole	0.04
Isometric relaxation	0.08
Rapid inflow	0.11
Diastasis	0.19
Atrial systole	<u>0.11</u>
Total diastole	0.53

*Heart rate is approximately 75 beats/min.
From Scher AM: Mechanical events of the cardiac cycle. In Ruch TC, Patton, HD (eds): Physiology and Biophysics 20th ed., Vol. II, pp 102–116. Philadelphia, WB Saunders, 1974.

approximately the latter two thirds of the total ejection period (see Table 1-6).

Atrial pressure and volume continue to increase. Ventricular repolarization is usually complete by this time, as indicated by the end of the T wave.

VENTRICULAR DIASTOLE

Protodiastole (Initial Part of Period d, Fig. 1–44). As ventricular muscle relaxation begins, there is a brief period before ventricular pressure becomes lower than aortic pressure when no blood is being ejected from the ventricle. Blood flow momentarily reverses. This backflow at a time when ventricular pressure is becoming less than aortic pressure facilitates the closure of the aortic valve. The second heart sound occurs. During this time, a slight transient decrease in atrial pressure may occur, reflecting the effect of ventricular relaxation.

Isovolumic Ventricular Relaxation (Latter Part of Period d, Fig. 1–44). Ventricular pressure decreases rapidly as the ventricle relaxes. There is no change in ventricular volume during this period when all the cardiac valves are closed. After closure of the aortic valve, aortic pressure increases by a few millimeters of mercury, and the incisura or dicrotic notch is inscribed on the aortic pressure tracing. Atrial pressure continues to increase as the atrium continues to receive pulmonary venous blood.

Rapid Ventricular Filling (Period e, Fig. 1–44). The AV (mitral) valve opens when atrial pressure exceeds ventricular pressure. The ventricle fills rapidly with blood that has been accumulating in the atrium, but ventricular pressure continues to decrease during this period because ventricular relaxation continues. Most of the blood that was sequestered in the atrium during systole is emptied into the ventricle by the time the ventricle reaches maximal diastolic size. Atrial pressure decreases as the atria empty but remains slightly greater than ventricular pressure throughout this period.

Late Diastole (Diastasis; Period f, Fig. 1–44). The mitral valve remains open, and pressures in the atrium and ventricle equilibrate in the time after rapid ventricular filling and before the beginning of atrial contraction. Blood from the lungs continues to enter the left ventricle passively, so ventricular volume and pressure slowly increase. Coronary artery blood flow usually is maximum during late diastole. The beginning of atrial depolarization is indicated by the upstroke of the electrocardiographic P wave.

Atrial Contraction (Period g, Fig. 1–44)

Atrial muscle contraction follows atrial depolarization and results in an increase in left atrial pressure. Ventricular volume and pressure are increased slightly as the atrium forces most of its remaining blood into the ventricles.

Between 15% and 25% of the end-diastolic ventricular volume consists of blood that has been ejected from the atrium during atrial contraction. The contribution of atrial contraction to total ventricular volume depends on venous return and heart rate; it is greater at faster heart rates. This atrial contribution to ventricular volume may be lost when the atria and ventricles are electrically and mechanically dissociated, such as during atrial fibrillation or complete heart block (see Chapter 14). Aortic pressure continues to decrease as blood in the aorta flows into the periphery.

Toward the end of this period, the ventricles begin to depolarize. Diastole ends with the onset of ventricular contraction. The cardiac cycle is repeated.

Right Ventricular Cardiac Cycle

The sequence of events in the right ventricle during the cardiac cycle is exactly the same as in the left ventricle, but the timing of events in the two ventricles is slightly different. Right ventricular and pulmonary artery pressures are much lower than left ventricular and aortic pressures, and right atrial pressures are usually slightly less than left atrial pressures.

Several factors lead to differences in the timing of events between the right and left heart. Contraction of the left ventricle begins before contraction of the right ventricle. Left ventricular isovolumetric contraction and relaxation last longer than right ventricular isovolumetric contraction and relaxation, presumably because the left ventricle must develop more contractile force to overcome higher systemic pressures. Right ventricular ejection begins before, lasts longer than, and ends after left ventricular ejection, possibly because pressures in the pulmonary artery are lower than in the aorta. Thus, right ventricular filling and ejection periods are longer than left ventricular periods, but the durations of left and right ventricular electromechanical systole are almost equal.

Cardiac Valvular Events and Normal Heart Sounds

VALVULAR EVENTS

The differences in timing of right and left ventricular events lead to differences in timing of right and left valvular events. The AV valves close at the onset of ventricular systole. The mitral valve normally closes before the tricuspid valve because left ventricular contraction begins before right ventricular contraction.

The aortic and pulmonic valves open when ventricular pressures exceed arterial pressures. The pulmonic valve opens before the aortic valve. Right ventricular isovolumetric contraction is shorter than left ventricular isovolumetric contraction.

The aortic and pulmonic valves close when ventricular pressures fall below arterial pressures. The aortic valve closes before the pulmonic valve. The right ventricular ejection period is longer than the left.

The AV valves open during diastole when ventricular pressures are lower than atrial pressures. The tricuspid valve opens before the mitral valve because of the more rapid isovolumetric right ventricular relaxation.

NORMAL HEART SOUNDS

The specific mechanisms responsible for heart sounds continue to be disputed. Sudden accelerations and decelerations of blood, turbulent blood flow, and the movements of valves, heart walls, and blood vessels may all contribute to the production of vibrations and sounds audible at the body surface.

First Heart Sound. Closure of the mitral valve and oscillations in the movement of blood in the ventricles are associated with vibrations of the entire valvular apparatus and of atrial and ventricular walls. This creates the early components of the first heart sound. Later components of the first heart sound may be due to the acceleration of blood ejected into the aorta.

Second Heart Sound. The second heart sound actually appears to begin before semilunar valve closure. The mechanisms responsible for the second heart sound appear to include arterial blood flow decelerations due to ventricular relaxation, blood vessel wall vibrations, and semilunar valvular vibrations.

The closure of the pulmonic valve after the aortic valve leads to a two-component sound, which is accentuated during inspiration (see Chapter 10). During inspiration, the time between closure of the aortic and pulmonic valves is increased, probably because a fall in pulmonary vascular impedance leads to a longer right ventricular ejection time.

Clinical Applications of Cardiac Events

SYSTOLIC EVENTS

The stroke volume is the volume ejected by the ventricle in a single contraction. Stroke volume multiplied by the number of cardiac cycles per minute (heart rate) equals the cardiac output. A typical volume ejected by the ventricle is 60 to 130 mL/m²2 body surface area (BSA)/s, illustrated by the ventricular volume downstroke of Figure 1-44. The stroke volume is the difference between the ventricular end-diastolic and end-systolic volume. Approximately 24 to 36 mL/m² BSA/s remains in the ventricle at the end of systole.

The *ejection fraction* is the percentage of total ventricular volume ejected during each contraction (i.e., the stroke volume divided by end-diastolic volume). The ejection fraction is a frequently used index of ventricular function; normally, it is greater than 55% and usually is approximately 65% (see Chapters 18 and 19).

The maximal rate of left ventricular force development and rise of left ventricular pressure over time (peak dP/dt) occurs during isovolumic ventricular contraction. Peak dP/dt is sometimes used as a clinical measure of ventricular contractility.

Specific phases of the left ventricular systolic time intervals, such as the pre-ejection period, left ventricular ejection time, total electromechanical systole (Q-S), and the pre-ejection period/left ventricular ejection time ratio are derived from simultaneous noninvasive electrocardiogram, phonocardiogram, and carotid artery pulse tracing recordings. The value of systolic time interval measurements in the diagnosis and prognosis of ventricular dysfunction due to ischemic heart disease continues to be debated.[1,37] The tension–time index is also used to assess ventricular function. These intervals vary with heart rate.

DIASTOLIC EVENTS

Diastole comprises a greater portion of the cardiac cycle (approximately 65%) than does systole (approximately 35%) at normal heart rates (see Table 1-6). At faster heart rates, both systole and diastole are shortened, diastole proportionally more so than systole. For example, at a heart rate of 180 beats/min, diastole comprises approximately 40% and systole approximately 60% of the cardiac cycle. At faster heart rates, diastolic filling is increasingly important in terms of the decreased amount of time available for ventricular and coronary artery filling, which may lead to impaired myocardial functioning.

The jugular venous and the carotid arterial pulses normally reflect right and left heart events, respectively. All cardiovascular assessment and treatment plans intimately depend on an appreciation of the cardiac cycle.

REFERENCES

1. Ahmed SS, Levinson GE, Schwartz CJ et al: Systolic time intervals as measures of the contractile state of the left ventricular myocardium in man. Circulation 46: 559–571, 1972
2. Anderson RH, Becker AE, Brechenmacher C et al: The human atrioventricular junctional area: A morphological study of the AV node and bundle. Eur J Cardiol 3: 11–25, 1975
3. Anderson RH, Becker AE, Brechenmacher C et al: Ventricular preexcitation: A proposed nomenclature for its substrates. Eur J Cardiol 3: 27–36, 1975
4. Armour JD, Hopkins DA: Anatomy of the efferent autonomic nerves and ganglia innervating the heart. In Randall WC (ed): Nervous Control of Cardiovascular Function, pp 20–45. New York, Oxford University Press, 1984
5. Bachmann G: The inter-auricular time interval. Am J Physiol 41: 309–320, 1916
6. Barmeyer J: Postmortem measurement of intracoronary anastomotic flow in normal and diseased hearts: A quantitative study. Vasc Surg 5: 239–248, 1971
7. Cohen MV: Coronary Collaterals: Clinical and Experimental Observations. Mt. Kisco, NY, Futura, 1985
8. DeMello NW: Effect of isoproterenol and 3-isobutyl-1-methylxanthine on junctional conductance in heart cell pairs. Biochim Biophys Acta 1012: 291–298, 1990
9. DiFrancesco D: A new interpretation of the pace-maker current in calf Purkinje fibres. J Physiol (Lond) 314: 359–376, 1981
10. Donaldson SK, Bond E, Seeger L et al: Intracellular pH vs. MgATP^{2+} concentration as determinants of Ca^{2+} activated force generation of disrupted rabbit cardiac cells. Cardiovasc Res 15: 268–275, 1981
11. Durrer D, van Dama RT, Freud GE et al: Total excitation of the isolated human heart. Circulation 61: 899–912, 1970
12. Fabiato A: Calcium-induced release of calcium from the cardiac sarcoplasmic reticulum. Am J Physiol 245: C1–C14, 1983
13. Fawcett DW: Bloom & Fawcett: A Textbook of Histology, 11th ed, pp 296–310. Philadelphia, WB Saunders, 1986
14. Franzini-Armstrong C: Studies of the triad: Structure of the junction in frog twitch fibers. J Cell Biol 47: 488–499, 1970
15. Glynn IM: Annual review prize lecture: All hands to the sodium pump. J Physiol (Lond) 462: 1–30, 1993
16. Gordon AM, Huxley AF, Julian FJ: The variation in isometric tension with sarcomere length in vertebrate muscle fibres. J Physiol (Lond) 184: 170–192, 1966
17. Hecht HH, Kossmann CE, Childers RW et al: Atrioventricular and intraventricular conduction: Revised nomenclature and concepts. Am J Cardiol 31: 232–244, 1973
18. His W Jr: Die Thatigkeit des embryonalen Herzens und deren Bedeutung für die Lehre von der Herzbewegung beim Erwachsenen. Arbeiten aus der Med Klin zu Leipzig 1: 14–50, 1893
19. Hodgkin AL, Huxley AF: Currents carried by sodium and potassium ions through the membrane of the giant axon of *Loligo*. J Physiol (Lond) 116: 449–472, 1952
20. Hood WB Jr, Bianco JA, Humar R et al: Experimental myocardial infarction: Compliance in the healing phase. J Clin Invest 49: 1316–1323, 1970
21. Hudson REB: Surgical pathology of the conducting system of the heart. Br Heart J 29: 646–670, 1967
22. Hunter DR, Haworth RA, Berkoff HA: Cellular calcium turnover in perfused rat heart. Circ Res 51: 363–370, 1982
23. Irisawa H, Noma A: Pacemaker currents in mammalian nodal cells. J Mol Cell Cardiol 16: 777–781, 1984
24. James TN: The connecting pathways between the sinus node and AV node and between the right and the left atrium in the human heart. Am Heart J 66: 498–508, 1963
25. James TN: Anatomy of the Coronary Arteries. New York, Paul B Hoeber, 1961
26. Keith A, Flack M: The form and nature of the muscular connections between the primary divisions of the vertebrate heart. Journal of Anatomy and Physiology 41: 172–189, 1907
27. Kelly AE, Gensini GG: Coronary arteriography and left heart studies. Heart Lung 4: 85–98, 1975
28. Kent AFS: The right lateral auriculo-ventricular junction of the heart. J Physiol (Lond) 48: 22–24, 1914
29. Kent AFS: Researches on the structure and function of the mammalian heart. J Physiol (Lond) 14: 233–254, 1893
30. Klocke FJ, Braunwald E, Ross J Jr: Oxygen cost of electrical activation of the heart. Circ Res 18: 357–365, 1966
31. Langer GA: Sodium-calcium exchange in the heart. Annu Rev Physiol 44: 435–449, 1982
32. Lazzara R, El-Sherif N, Befeler FB et al: Regional refractoriness within the ventricular conduction system. Circ Res 39: 254–262, 1976
33. Levin DC, Beckmann CF, Sos TA et al: The effect of coronary artery bypass on collateral circulation. Radiology 141: 317–322, 1981
34. Lewis BS, Gotsman MS: Current concepts of left ventricular relaxation and compliance. Am Heart J 99: 101–112, 1980
35. Mahaim I: Kent's fibers and the A-V paraspecific conduction through the upper connections of the bundle of His-Tawara. Am Heart J 33: 651–653, 1947
36. Mahaim I, Winston T: Recherches d'anatomie comparee et de pathologie experimentale sur les connexions hautes du faisceau de His-Tawara. Cardiologia 5: 189–260, 1941
37. Mangschau A, Karlsen RL, Lippestad CT et al: Systolic time intervals and ejection fraction in assessing left ventricular performance following acute myocardial infarction. Acta Medica Scandinavica 215: 341–347, 1984
38. Massing GK, James TN: Anatomical configuration of the His bundle and bundle branches in the human heart. Circulation 53: 609–621, 1976
39. Maylie J, Morad M: Ionic currents responsible for the generation of pace-maker current in the rabbit sino-atrial node. J Physiol (Lond) 355: 215–235, 1984
40. Miller AJ: Lymphatics of the Heart, pp 107–164, 262–334. New York, Raven Press, 1982
41. Nichols CG, Ripoli C, Lederer WJ: ATP-sensitive potassium channel modulation of the guinea pig ventricular action potential and contraction. Circ Res 68: 280–287, 1991
42. Noma A, Shibasaki T: Membrane current through adenosine-triphosphate-regulated potassium channels in guinea pig ventricular cells. J Physiol (Lond) 363: 463–480, 1985

43. Paes de Carvalho A, de Almeida DF: Spread of activity through the atrioventricular node. Circ Res 8: 801–809, 1960

44. Patterson SW, Per HP, Starling EH: The regulation of the heart beat. J Physiol (Lond) 48: 465–513, 1914

45. Purkinje JE: Mikroskopisch-neurologische beobachtungen. Arch Anat Physiol Wiss Med 12: 281, 1845

46. Randall WC: Selective autonomic innervation of the heart. In Randall WC (ed): Nervous Control of Cardiovascular Function, pp 46–67. New York, Oxford University Press, 1984

47. Regan TJ, Frank MJ, Lehan PH et al: Myocardial blood flow and oxygen uptake during acute red blood cell volume increments. Circ Res 13: 172–181, 1963

48. Reiner L, Mazzoleni A, Rodriguez FL et al: The weight of the human heart. Arch Pathol 68: 58–73, 1959

49. Ringer S: A further contribution regarding the influence of the different constituents of the blood on the contraction of the heart. J Physiol (Lond) 4: 29–42, 1883

50. Robb JA, Robb JS, Robb RC: The normal heart. Heart J 23: 455–467, 1942

51. Scher AM, Spach MS: Cardiac depolarization and repolarization and the electrocardiogram. In Berne RM (ed): Handbook of Physiology. Section 2: The Cardiovascular System, vol 1, The Heart, pp 357–392. Bethesda, MD, American Physiological Society, 1979

52. Siepser SL, Kaltman AJ, Mills N et al: Coronary collateral flow after traumatic fistula between the right coronary artery and right atrium. N Engl J Med 287: 754–756, 1972

53. Singer DH, Baumgarten CM, Ten Eick RE: Cellular electrophysiology of ventricular and other dysrhythmias: Studies on diseased and ischemic heart. Prog Cardiovasc Dis 24: 97–156, 1981

54. Smith HL, Smith HL: The relation of the weight of the heart to the weight of the body and of the weight of the heart to age. Am Heart J 4: 79–93, 1928

55. Spach MS, Barr RC: Cardiac anatomy from an electrophysiological viewpoint. In Nelson CV, Geselivitz DB (eds): The Theoretical Basis of Electrocardiology, pp 3–20. Oxford, Clarendon Press, 1976

56. Spach MS, Lootsey JM: The nature of electrical propagation in cardiac muscle. Am J Physiol 244: H3–H22, 1983

57. Sperelakis N: Hormonal and neurotransmitter regulation of Ca^{++} influx through voltage-dependent slow channels in cardiac muscle membrane. Membrane Biochemistry 5: 131–166, 1984

58. Sperelakis N: Propagation mechanisms in the heart. Annu Rev Physiol 41: 441–457, 1979

59. Streeter DD Jr, Spotnitz HM, Patel DP et al: Fiber orientation in the canine left ventricle during diastole and systole. Circ Res 24: 339–347, 1969

60. Tarawa S: Das Reizleitungs system des Saugetierherzens [Monograph]. Jena, Germany, G Fischer, 1906

61. Titus JL, Daugherty GW, Edwards JE: Anatomy of the normal human atrioventricular conduction system. Am J Anat 113: 407–415, 1963

62. Ungerleider HE, Clark CP: A study of the transverse diameter of the heart silhouette with prediction table based on the teleoroentgenogram. Am Heart J 17: 92–102, 1939

63. Wearn JT: Morphological and functional alterations of the coronary circulation. Harvey Lect 35: 243–270, 1940

64. Weidmann S: Cardiac cellular physiology and its contribution to electrocardiology. Jpn Heart J 23(Suppl): 12–16, 1982

65. Zimmerman HA: The coronary circulation in patients with severe emphysema, cor pulmonale, cyanotic congenital heart disease, and severe anemia. Diseases of the Chest 22: 269–273, 1952

2

The Systemic Circulation

ELIZABETH J. BRIDGES*

The structural and functional characteristics of the systemic circulation determine the continuous adjustments in flow, pressure, and resistance that occur in each vascular bed and that are vital determinants of tissue function. The combined regulation of cardiac output, blood pressure, and systemic vascular resistance (SVR) determines tissue blood flow and ultimately determines the survival of each organ system and the body as a whole. Blood flow and nutrient exchange in various vascular beds are affected by the structural and metabolic characteristics of the vascular bed, the physical factors that affect vascular flow and the exchange of materials across the blood vessel wall, the local factors originating from the metabolically active cells and vascular endothelium that regulate flow to individual vascular beds, and local and systemic neuroendocrine regulation. This chapter describes the basic anatomy and physiology of the systemic circulation; Chapter 4 describes the overall regulation of cardiac output and blood pressure.

STRUCTURAL CHARACTERISTICS OF THE VASCULATURE AND LYMPHATICS

Blood vessels are usually classified in the following manner: aorta, large arteries; main arterial branch, small arteries, arterioles; terminal arterioles, capillaries, postcapillary venules; venules, small veins, main venule branch, large veins, and the vena cava.[126,128,175] These classifications are

*The views expressed in this chapter are those of the author and do not reflect the official policy of the Department of Defense or other departments of the United States Government.

The author thanks Dr. Loring Rowell for his expert consultation and assistance with the development of this chapter.

based on structural characteristics such as diameter, wall thickness, and the presence of muscle (Fig. 2-1). Although vessel sizes are given in Figure 2-1, blood vessel diameter is not an appropriate criterion to use for classification because differences in vessel size reflect the state of vessel contraction as well as differences between organ systems and species.[125,126]

With the exception of the capillaries, the systemic vasculature is composed of three layers: the tunica intima or internal layer, which consists of the endothelium and the basal membrane; the tunica media, which consists of smooth muscle and a matrix of collagen, elastin, and glycoproteins; and the tunica adventitia, which consists of connective tissue[127] (Fig. 2-2). In the larger arteries and veins, the tunica adventitia also contains blood vessels that supply the vessel wall (vasa vasorum).[107,126] The vascular endothelium has gained importance as a primary mediator of vascular function and is discussed in detail.

Arteries

Arteries with large diameters, in which the media contains smooth muscle and elastin, are called elastic arteries.[126] Because of the considerable amount of elastin, these large conducting arteries are able to distend to twice their unloaded length. As the arteries approach the periphery, they become smaller in diameter, and in the tunica media there is a relative decrease in elastin and a relative increase in smooth muscle.[98] These arteries are referred to as the muscular arteries.

The small arteries (prearteriolar vessels with a diameter less than 500 μm) receive nervous stimulation primarily from noradrenergic stimuli, with the nerve terminals located in the adventitia. Unlike the larger arteries, in which sympathetic neural constriction is activated by both α_1

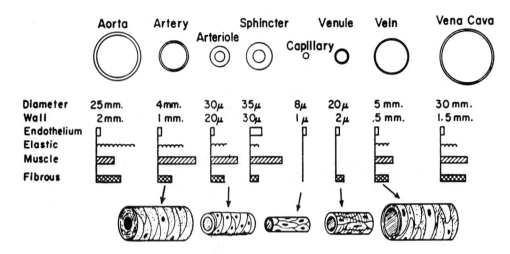

FIGURE 2-1 Schematic drawing of the major structural characteristics of the principal segments of blood vessels. The relative amounts of elastic tissue and fibrous tissues are largest in the aorta and least in small branches of the arterial tree. Small vessels have more prominent smooth muscle in the media. Capillaries consist only of endothelial cells. The walls of the veins are much like the arterial walls, but are thinner in relation to their caliber. (From Rushmer RF: Cardiovascular Dynamics, 4th ed, p 135. Philadelphia, WB Saunders, 1976.)

and postsynaptic α_2 receptors, the small arteries are noradrenergically constricted mainly by the postsynaptic α_2 receptors.[30,98] The small arteries are also sensitive to endothelium-derived relaxing and contracting factors.

Microvascular Bed

The term *microcirculation* denotes the vascular and lymphatic microcirculation. The vascular microcirculation consists of (1) large and small arterioles (*precapillary resistance vessels*); (2) terminal arterioles, which in many tissue serve as so-called precapillary sphincters[27,28]; and (3) other precapillary structures such as capillaries and nonmuscular venules, known collectively as the exchange vessels, and muscular venules (postcapillary resistance vessels). The term *lymphatic microvasculature* refers specifically to the terminal lymphatic vessels.[121,125]

ARTERIOLES

As the vessel diameter decreases from the small arteries to the arterioles, the number of smooth muscle layers decreases from approximately six layers in the 300-μm vessels to a single layer of irregularly dispersed smooth muscle in the 30- to 50-μm vessels.[98] At this point, the vessels are referred to as *arterioles*. In the proximal arterioles, noradrenergic sympathetic nerves activate presynaptic α_2 fibers, inhibiting further norepinephrine release from sympathetic vesicles (negative feedback). The postsynaptic α_1 and α_2 adrenoreceptors in the terminal arterioles[30,122] are responsible for the control of total blood flow to the exchange vessels.

The smallest arteriolar branches (8 to 20 μm in diameter) are called the *terminal arterioles*.[122] In some cases, smooth muscle extends beyond the intersection of the terminal arterioles with the nonmuscular capillaries into structures known as *precapillary sphincters*.[121] The terminal arterioles and precapillary sphincters control the distribution of blood supply to the exchange vessels.[1,2,27,28,122]

CAPILLARIES

Capillaries branch from terminal arteriolar segments. The capillary wall consists of endothelial cells and basal lamina; there is no tunica media or adventitia. Capillary diameter is

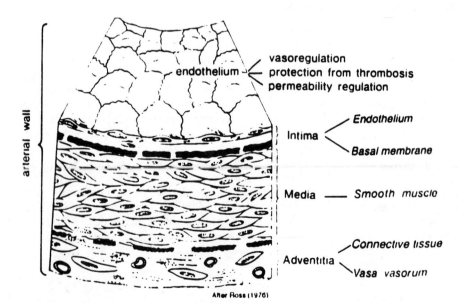

FIGURE 2-2 Histologic structure of the normal muscular artery demonstrating the different roles of the endothelium, smooth muscle, and fibrous tissue. (Adapted from Ross RM, Glomset J: The pathogenesis of atherosclerosis. N Engl J Med 295: 369–377, 1976. In Opie LH: The Heart: Physiology from Cell to Circulation, p. 234. Philadelphia, Lippincott–Raven, 1998.

4 to 8 μm, which is just large enough to allow the deformable red blood cells to pass through.[122,146] Not all exchange vessels in an area are simultaneously open. During periods of increased metabolism, capillary recruitment increases the number of open and perfused exchange vessels, thereby decreasing the distances for diffusion between exchange blood vessels and cells, as well as increasing the total surface area for exchange between the capillaries and cells.[122]

In microvascular beds located in the ears, fingers, and toes in humans and many other mammals, there are arteriovenous vascular channels that bypass the exchange vessels and allow blood to flow directly from arterioles to venules.[122,126] These arteriovenous anastomoses, which are richly innervated by the sympathetic nervous system, can be important in local temperature control in these areas, and even of the whole body in some conditions.[57]

EXCHANGE VESSEL ENDOTHELIUM

The endothelium of exchange vessels in various organs contains at least four different structures that determine the rate of filtration and bulk transport of water and solutes, as well as the exchange of larger molecules. The structure of the membrane (continuous, fenestrated, discontinuous, or tight junction) varies depending on the location of the vascular bed.[122,123,146] All four types of endothelium have a continuous basement membrane, with the exception of the discontinuous endothelium.

Continuous endothelium is found in skin; skeletal, smooth, and cardiac muscle; and the lungs. There are several mechanisms by which substances pass through continuous endothelium. Water and solutes pass through intercellular junctions (40Å to 1Å) driven predominantly by a pressure gradient (ΔP) driving fluid out of the vessels. This outward flow is partly counterbalanced by forces drawing water back into the vessels. Lipid-soluble substances (CO_2, O_2) pass directly through the cell by diffusion; cytoplasmic vesicles transport solutes and water back and forth through the endothelium; and vesicles intermittently fuse to create channels in the cell. The junctions between the cells are responsible for the high permeability of the membrane to "ultrafiltrate" or protein-free fluid, and for the rapid diffusion of small ions. The continuous endothelium is relatively impermeable to plasma proteins and large molecules.

Fenestrated vascular endothelium is located in the gastrointestinal mucosa, glands, renal glomerular capillaries, and peritubular capillaries. The endothelium has openings (fenestrae) that expose the basement membrane (renal glomerular capillaries) or are covered by a thin diaphragm (gastrointestinal mucosa, renal peritubular capillaries). The fenestrated endothelium has a higher permeability to water and small solute molecules than continuous endothelium, whereas its permeability to plasma proteins is low, similar to continuous endothelium.[122]

Discontinuous endothelium is located in the hepatic cells, bone marrow, and splenic sinusoids. Discontinuous endothelium contains gaps in both the endothelium and basement membrane, and is permeable to proteins and other large molecules.[44]

Tight-junction endothelium is located in the central nervous system and retina, and is the least permeable. The endothelial cells are connected by tight junctions that effectively restrict passage of all substances. Water and lipid-soluble molecules pass directly through the endothelium, whereas ions and lipid-insoluble substances, such as glucose and amino acids, are transported by membrane carriers.[23]

Venules

Venous capillaries extend to the postcapillary venules (nonmuscular, 7 to 50 μm) and collecting venules. Along with the capillaries, the nonmuscular venules act as exchange vessels. Smooth muscle reappears in venules that are approximately 30 to 50 μm in diameter. These venules, which receive adrenergic innervation, are referred to as the muscular venules, postcapillary resistance vessels, or capacitance vessels.[121,122,126,128,145] As is discussed in the section on microcirculation, postcapillary resistance tends to be far less than precapillary resistance and has almost no effect on overall SVR. The veins contain approximately 70% of total blood volume, with approximately 25% of this volume in the venules.[128]

Lymphatics

The lymphatics are a system of thin-walled vessels that collect and conduct lymph from the microvasculature to the central circulation. Lymph consists primarily of ultrafiltrate and proteins that have been filtered from exchange vessels. The initial lymphatic vessels (also known as terminal lymphatics or lymph capillaries), which consist of endothelialized tubes, originate in large, blind-terminal bulbs located in the connective tissue of most organ systems.[122,136] A very small and transient pressure gradient between the interstitium and the terminal lymphatics promotes fluid movement into the lymphatics.[2,136] The exact mechanism involved in the creation of the pressure gradient remains under investigation.[2,73] The lymphatic capillaries empty into collecting lymphatics, which in turn empty into transporting lymphatic vessels (Fig. 2-3). Beginning at the level of the collecting capillaries, there are bicuspid valves, and the larger lymphatics contain smooth muscle that contracts rhythmically. These characteristics facilitate the unilateral direction of lymph flow. Lymphatic flow may also be indirectly facilitated by rhythmic motion (i.e., walking, foot flexing) and respiration.[2,134,136] The central lymphatic vessels empty into the left and right lymphatic ducts, which empty into the subclavian veins.

Veins

In general, veins have a larger diameter and thinner, more compliant walls than arteries at equivalent branches of the vascular tree[128] (see Fig. 2-1). However, the thickness of the venous walls is variable, and in tall animals like humans and giraffes, the thickness depends on the location of the vein in the body. For example, the veins in the legs and feet, which withstand the high hydrostatic pressure associ-

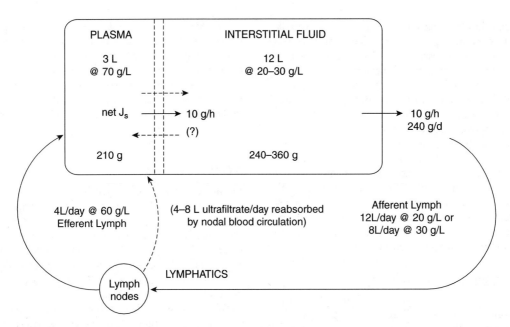

FIGURE 2-3 Steady-state distribution and circulation of fluid (ultrafiltrate) and plasma proteins in a normal human (weight, 65 kg). The *double dashed line* between plasma and interstitial fluid represents exchange vessel endothelium. The weights at the bottoms of the boxes represent the total content of each. (Renkin, EM: Some consequences of capillary permeability to macromolecules: Starling's hypothesis reconsidered. Am J Physiol 250: H706–H710, 1986)

ated with standing, are thick walled, whereas the veins near or above the level of the heart are thin walled.[22,130] The veins contain all three vascular layers found in the arteries; however, these layers are often indistinct.[126] Superficial veins form a rich anastomosis with deeper veins via vessels that perforate the muscles. These perforating veins allow venous return from cold skin to be diverted to warm muscle, providing a thermal short circuit, and they are particularly important for function of the muscle pump, which is described in Chapter 4.

VENOUS VALVES

With the exception of the intrathoracic and intracerebral veins, the medium-sized veins contain valves that are oriented in the direction of blood flow, thus preventing retrograde blood flow into the muscle.[128] The presence of competent valves is crucial to the ability to stand erect and in maintaining a reasonably low capillary pressure, because the valves interrupt the hydrostatic column that extends from the right atrium to the feet after each leg muscle contraction. After humans with normal valvular function stand up, the valves in dependent veins initially interrupt the hydrostatic column. However, over a period of approximately 2 to 3 minutes, as the veins fill with blood, the valves can no longer interrupt the hydrostatic column as volume continues to accumulate. At this time, there is a displacement of approximately 600 mL of blood from the central circulation into the legs and pelvic organs.[129] In conditions where blood flow is high, the hydrostatic effects associated with the loss of valvular function occur within 2 to 3 seconds. If the hydrostatic effects are not overcome by the muscle pump in the lower extremities (see Chapter 4), arterial hypotension and syncope result. This phenomenon is readily seen in the soldier who faints while standing motionless at attention.

The importance of the venous valves is also manifest in patients with incompetent (due to pregnancy) or congenitally absent valves in the deep veins. These patients may have severe orthostatic intolerance.[7,45] When valvular function is impaired or absent, the uninterrupted hydrostatic column between the right atrium and the feet causes pooling of blood in the dependent veins and an acute drop in end-diastolic volume and cardiac output. Wearing tight leotards counteracts this effect by reducing venous transmural pressure and venous volume in the legs.

VENOCONSTRICTION

In contrast to the arteries, not all veins constrict when exposed to norepinephrine (noradrenergic stimulation). For example, the postcapillary venules ranging from 0.007 to 2 mm in diameter do not have smooth muscle and therefore cannot constrict.[130] Most larger venules and small veins (including veins in the skeletal muscle) contain some smooth muscle,[128] but are sparsely innervated and are not considered sites of vasoconstriction. The lack of venoconstriction in the skeletal muscle is important because the leg veins do not constrict in orthostasis. The splanchnic organs (liver, gastrointestinal tract, pancreas, and spleen), however, are the exception because they are richly innervated by sympathetic noradrenergic fibers and are capable of venoconstriction. In addition, the veins in the skin respond to thermoregulatory reflexes. In humans, significant venoconstriction occurs only in the splanchnic circulation, and in response to thermoregulatory reflexes, the veins in the skin constrict and dilate.[51,130,132]

LOCAL REGULATION

In addition to the systemic factors that affect vascular resistance, there are local factors that control resistance, including autacoids, endothelium-derived vasoactive substances, local metabolic factors that match blood flow (oxygen transport) to metabolism, autoregulation (see Chapter 4), and local heating and cooling (as described in the section on venoconstriction).

Autacoids

The autacoids (vasoactive substances) include histamine, serotonin, prostaglandin, and bradykinin.[130] These factors most often compete with adrenergic (vasoconstrictive) effects and exert a local vasodilatory effect, which can improve tissue perfusion. The autacoids are not involved in systemic regulation of blood pressure or total peripheral resistance.

Endothelium-Derived Vasoactive Substances

The vascular endothelium, a single layer of squamous cells in the tunica intima, modulates vascular tone by secreting dilator and constrictor substances.[161] In addition, the endothelium affects platelet adhesion and aggregation and the regulation of vascular smooth muscle proliferation.[3,90,102,119,159] The proposed functions of the vascular endothelium are outlined in Table 2-1. As first demonstrated by Furchott and Zawadzki,[41] an intact endothelium is essential to these functions.

The endothelium-produced vasodilator substances include endothelium-derived relaxing factors (EDRF), prostaglandins, and endothelium-derived hyperpolarizing factor (EDHF). In addition, the endothelium produces endothelium-derived vasoconstrictor substances, including endothelin-1 (ET_1), the most potent vasoconstrictor

known; prostanoids (end products of the cyclooxygenase metabolism of arachidonic acid) such as thromboxane A_2 (TXA_2) and prostaglandin H_2; and superoxide anions.[171] A discussion of each of these factors follows, and a summary of the stimuli that cause the release of each of the factors is presented in Table 2-2.

ENDOTHELIUM-DERIVED RELAXING FACTORS

The endothelial cells primarily release factors that cause vascular relaxation. The major EDRF is nitric oxide (NO), but other relaxing factors include prostacyclin (prostaglandin I_2 [PGI_2]) and EDHF.[157,161] The formation and release of these relaxing factors is the result of endothelial agonist—receptor interaction. The agonists activate the endothelial cells, which increase cytoplasmic calcium through the inositol triphosphate cascade.[6] The increased cytoplasmic calcium initiates a cascade that stimulates the synthesis of NO, PGI_2, and EDHF.

Nitric Oxide. Nitric oxide, the first identified EDRF, is a gas with an extremely short half-life (seconds) that diffuses into vascular smooth muscle cells and causes vasodilation[76,94,112] (Fig. 2-4). Factors that stimulate release of NO are summarized in Table 2-2. Clinically, the pharmacologic

TABLE 2-1 Functions of the Vascular Endothelium Related to Vasomotor Function

Action	Factors Responsible
Release of vasodilatory agents	Endothelium-derived relaxing factor
	Nitric oxide
	Prostacyclin
	Endothelium-derived hyperpolarizing factor
	Bradykinin
Release of vasoconstrictor agents	Endothelin-1
	Angiotensin I/angiotensin II
	Prostacyclin
	Thromboxane A_2
	Superoxide anions
Antiaggregatory effects	Nitric oxide
	Prostacyclin
	Thromboresistant endothelium

TABLE 2-2 Stimuli for the Release of Endothelium-Mediated Vasoactive Substances

Factors	Stimuli
Vasodilating Factors	
Nitric oxide	Acetylcholine, histamine, arginine vasopressin, epinephrine, norepinephrine, bradykinin, adenosine diphosphate, serotonin (from aggregating platelets), thrombin (from coagulation cascade)
Endothelium-derived relaxing factor	
Prostacyclin	
Endothelium-derived hyperpolarizing factor	Shear stress, hypoxemia, pulsatile stretching of the vessel wall[15,58,61,89,116,133,162]
Bradykinin	
Vasoconstricting Factors	
Endothelium-derived contracting factor	Physical stimuli (mechanical stretch), arachidonic acid (endothelial injury and platelet aggregation), serotonin, adenosine diphosphate[162]
Endothelin-1	Thrombin, interleukin-1, epinephrine, angiotensin II, arginine vasopressin[13,77,178]
Prostanoids	Endothelin-1, endothelial membrane damage[178]
Superoxide anions	Physical stress (e.g., shear stress, postischemic reperfusion) Chemical endothelial stimulants (bradykinin, cytokines)[59,69,159,164]

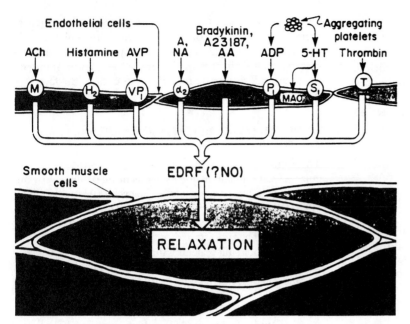

FIGURE 2-4 Schematic showing formation of vasoactive factors by vascular endothelium. Various substances may, by activation of specific receptors on endothelial cells, evoke release of relaxing factor(s) (endothelium–derived relaxing factors [EDRF]; nitric oxide?) that in turn causes relaxation of arterial vessels. ACh, acetylcholine; M, muscarinic receptors; H_2, histaminergic receptors; AVP, arginine vasopressin; VP_1, vasopressinergic receptors, P_1, purinergic receptors; A, adrenaline (norepinephrine); alpha$_2$, alpha$_2$–adrenergic receptor; AA, arachidonic acid; ADP, adenosine diphosphate; MAO, monoamine oxidase; 5–HT, 5–hydroxytryptamine (serotonin); S_1, serotonergic receptors, T, thrombin receptors. (From Vanhoutte PM: Endothelium and control of vascular function: State of the art lecture. Hypertension 13: 660, 1989.)

agents nitroglycerin and sodium nitroprusside cause vasodilation by the donation of NO or an NO-like compound[64,83]; however, nitroglycerin-induced coronary artery vasodilation does not require the presence of an intact endothelium.

After forming in the endothelial cells, NO diffuses into the smooth muscle cells, where it stimulates the formation of cyclic guanosine monophosphate, which leads to smooth muscle relaxation (see Fig. 2-4). NO also directly activates the vascular smooth muscle potassium channels.[9] The activation of the potassium channels hyperpolarizes the cell and inhibits the voltage-sensitive calcium channels, thereby decreasing calcium influx into the cell. NO also has secondary vasodilatory effects through the inhibition of endothelial synthesis of the vasoconstrictor ET_1.[12]

In addition to its effects on vasomotion, NO inhibits platelet aggregation and adhesion,[3,4,118,157,161] and smooth muscle proliferation.[25,137,138] Of importance, the protective effects of NO against platelet aggregation and vasoconstriction decrease naturally with aging and are also diminished with disease processes (e.g., hypertension, diabetes, postmyocardial infarction reperfusion injuries) and procedures (e.g., balloon angioplasty) that result in endothelial damage.[77,78,115] The loss of the protective endothelium and decreased NO production may foster increased platelet aggregation and vascular proliferation, which are keys to the development of atherosclerosis.[38,165] Decreased NO synthesis may also contribute to the pathologic vasoconstriction observed in response to an increase in serotonin after platelet aggregation.[25,85]

Endothelium-Derived Hyperpolarizing Factors.
In some cases, vasodilation mediated by endothelial factors may involve hyperpolarization of the cell (inside of the cell becomes more negative).[10,18,41] In response to shear stress and receptor stimulation from a variety of agonists (see Table 2-2), the hyperpolarization augments calcium influx into the cell, and, through a positive feedback loop, the increase in intracellular calcium augments the formation of the yet to be identified hyperpolarizing substance or substances known as EDHF, as well as NO.[19,34,35,93,166]

Of possible clinical importance, in some abnormal vascular responses observed with aging and in diseases such as diabetes and hypertension, there is a decrease in EDHF-mediated hyperpolarization, which may contribute to the pathologic changes associated with these processes.[156] However, the EDHF response may be enhanced by drugs such as the angiotensin-converting enzyme inhibitors,[163,169,170] exercise, and omega-3 unsaturated fatty acids,[35,93,101,143] which may potentially inhibit or reverse the age- and disease-related changes.

ENDOTHELIUM-DERIVED CONTRACTING FACTORS

The endothelium-derived contracting factors include ET_1, the vasoconstrictor prostanoids TXA_2 and prostaglandin H_2, superoxide anions, and components of the renin—angiotensin system. These substances are released in response to vasoconstrictive stimuli[13,107,119,159,164] (Fig. 2-5). Vasoconstriction also occurs as a result of a decrease in endothelial production of NO.

Endothelin-1.
Endothelin-1 is an amino acid peptide that binds to vascular smooth muscle membrane receptors. Under normal resting conditions, the circulating plasma level of ET_1 is very low and it acts locally, in a paracrine fashion, to cause vasodilation through the endothelial synthesis of NO, PGI_2, and EDHF.[173,176] Conversely, at increased levels, ET_1 directly stimulates the vascular smooth muscle and is the most potent vasoconstrictor known.[177]

From a clinical perspective, the effects of ET_1 are important for at least two reasons. First, in pathologic conditions, such as chronic heart failure, the plasma level of ET_1 is increased and may play an important role in the disease

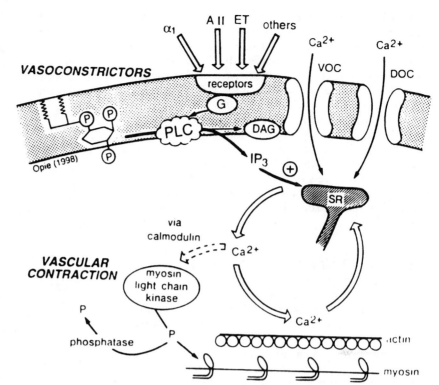

FIGURE 2-5 Vasoconstrictory mechanisms. Several act by releasing calcium from the sarcoplasmic reticulum (SR). For example, stimulation of vascular receptors by endothelin (ET), angiotensin II (AII), or norepinephrine (NE) leads to increased activity of phospholipase C (PLC), which splits phosphatidyl inositol into two messengers: IP_3 (inositol triphosphate) and 1,2–DAG (1, 2–diaclyglycerol). IP_3 promotes the release of calcium from the SR. Membrane–bound DAG activates protein kinase C. Vasoconstriction also occurs in response to enhanced activity of the calcium channels. (From Opie LH: The Heart: Physiology from Cell to Circulation, 3rd ed, p 239. Philadelphia, Lippincott–Raven, 1998.)

process.[17] For example, ET_1 enhances the conversion of angiotensin I to angiotensin II, causing a synergistic augmentation of vasoconstriction and sodium retention. In addition, the plasma level of ET_1 is inversely related to exercise capacity.[63,75] Second, identification of receptor subtype function (vasodilator vs. vasoconstrictor) may play an important role in developing therapies that target specific receptor subtypes for the treatment of disease processes such as hypertension, proliferative renal disease, myocardial infarction, and heart failure.[36,75,139,176]

Prostanoids. In response to both ET_1 and endothelial membrane damage by diseases such as diabetes, hypertension, and hypercholesterolemia, the vascular smooth muscle is exposed to vasoconstrictive substances such as serotonin (released from aggregating platelets) and the vasoconstrictor prostanoids TXA_2 and prostaglandin H_2. These substances, which interfere with the normal vasodilatory, antithrombotic, and homeostatic functions of the endothelium, act directly on the vascular smooth muscle, causing adherence and aggregation of platelets as well as vasoconstriction.[13,79,165,168,171]

Thromboxane A_2 is thought to play an important role in the pathogenesis of myocardial infarction.[179] Research related to the development of TXA_2 receptor antagonists is ongoing. These TXA_2 antagonists are also used in conjunction with glycoprotein IIb/IIIa receptor blocking antibodies (e.g., C7E3 Fab, abciximab) to enhance thrombolysis and decrease the incidence of coronary reocclusion.[20,21,178]

Superoxide Anions. In response to physical stresses, such as shear stress and postischemic reperfusion, and to chemical endothelial stimulants (bradykinin, cytokines), the endothelium produces oxygen-derived free radicals and hydrogen peroxide. The superoxide anions inactivate NO and cause vasoconstriction.[59,69,159,164] In contrast, superoxide dismutase (an enzyme system that breaks down the free radicals into nontoxic substances and inhibits the breakdown of NO by superoxide anions) inhibits pathologic ET_1 production and augments endothelial relaxation.[59,77,97]

LOCAL METABOLIC CONTROL OF BLOOD FLOW

Local metabolic factors that control resistance play a role in matching blood flow (oxygen transport) to metabolism. There is a long list of potential vasoactive factors. These factors may accumulate in low-flow conditions and cause vasodilation by inhibition of basal tone (Fig. 2-6). The

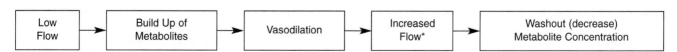

*Increased flow called reactive hyperemia.

FIGURE 2-6 Mechanism of local metabolic control of resistance. (Courtesy of Loring B. Rowell, University of Washington, Seattle, WA, 1998)

increased flow that occurs as a result of the vasodilation is referred to as *reactive hyperemia*. These local metabolic factors include hydrogen, potassium, phosphate, carbon dioxide, adenosine, adenine nucleotides, lactic acid, intermediates of the Krebs cycle, vasoactive peptides, osmolarity, and a local decrease in oxygen.[54,129,142,151,167] Many of these factors (i.e., potassium, osmolarity, PO_2) appear to play a role in the initiation of exercise-induced hyperemia, but other factors are responsible for sustained vasodilation. Some of these factors may exert their vasodilator effects through EDRF or NO.[94] An increase in flow-dependent shear stress on the endothelium has also been shown to cause vasodilation in skeletal muscle.[61] This vasodilation is mediated by the endothelial release of prostaglandin.[62]

VASCULAR SMOOTH MUSCLE

Vascular smooth muscle differs from striated muscle (e.g., skeletal, cardiac) muscle in that it does not have organized contractile filaments and thus lacks the striations (organized contractile filaments) seen in skeletal and cardiac muscle.[43] Although the sarcoplasmic reticulum is not as prominent in vascular smooth muscle as in cardiac muscle, it serves as the primary intracellular source of calcium.[148] In addition, the amount of myosin in smooth muscle is approximately one fifth of that found in striated muscle. Despite this relatively lower amount of myosin, smooth muscle develops higher force per cross-sectional area than striated muscle. Also, vascular smooth muscle usually contracts more slowly than striated muscle, and it maintains tonic contractions with lower energy (adenosine triphosphate [ATP]) expenditure.[99,100]

Smooth muscle throughout the body is characterized as "phasic" and "tonic." Phasic vascular smooth muscle, which is capable of high shortening velocities, is located in the portal veins. Tonic vascular smooth muscle is located in most of the small arteries and arterioles, has a slower shortening velocity, but is capable of maintaining sustained vascular tone.[53] As in cardiac and skeletal muscle, contraction of vascular smooth muscle is related to the formation and release of cross-bridges by the cyclic attachment and detachment of the heads of the contractile protein myosin with the double-helical filament actin (see Chapter 1). Tonic contractions allow for the maintenance of a basal vascular tone that is crucial for the maintenance of arterial blood pressure. The vasodilation and vasoconstriction of arterioles in response to neural and chemical stimuli occur around this level of basal tone (see Chapter 4), and may be viewed as modulating vascular tone.

Tonic contractions are the result of "latch bridges" or a "latch state," which is a decrease (or cessation) in the cross-bridge cycling rate. The exact mechanism of the latch bridge has yet to be elucidated,[48–50,70,99,100] although it is known that in this state, vascular tone is maintained despite a decrease in phosphorylation and ATP consumption.[70,80,95,96,99,100]

NEUROHUMORAL STIMULATION

In addition to stimulation by endothelium-derived vasodilating and vasoconstricting factors, neurohumoral factors bind with receptors on vascular smooth muscle. The effects of this stimulation vary throughout the vascular system.

Adrenergic Stimulation

α-ADRENERGIC STIMULATION

The primary neurotransmitter that affects the vascular smooth muscle is norepinephrine. The α_1-adrenergic receptors are located in arteries, arterioles, and cutaneous and visceral veins.[37] The α_1 receptor of the arterioles is the primary site for the control of peripheral resistance.[98] Binding of norepinephrine to the receptors initiates a cascade of events that increases cytoplasmic calcium, which in turn causes vasoconstriction.[90,153,154] The α_2 vascular smooth muscle receptors are present in large arteries, but are located with greater density on the terminal arterioles, which act as precapillary sphincters to control the number of open capillaries and total capillary blood flow.[30,106] Unlike stimulation of the presynaptic α_2 receptors, which inhibit the release of norepinephrine from the nerve terminal, stimulation of the postsynaptic α_2 receptors located on the vascular smooth muscle causes norepinephrine release and subsequent vasoconstriction. However, the α_2-mediated vasoconstriction is attenuated by the α_2 presynaptic inhibition of norepinephrine release. In addition, in contrast to α_1 receptor stimulation, the effect of norepinephrine on α_2 in terminal arterioles is inhibited by metabolites, thus fostering metabolic vasodilation even when vasoconstrictor tone to blood vessels in the skeletal muscle is high.

ß-ADRENERGIC STIMULATION

There are two major ß-adrenergic receptors. The ß-adrenergic receptors in the heart are predominantly of the β_1 receptor subtype, although there are also a smaller number of β_2 receptors, which play a role in coronary vasodilation.[26,33,158] ß-adrenergic receptors on the vascular smooth muscle are of the β_2 subtype.[67]

β_2-adrenergic stimulation of the vascular smooth muscle cell is associated with vascular smooth muscle relaxation, rather than the contraction (increased contractility) that occurs in the cardiac cell. Activation of β_2-adrenergic receptors on the vascular smooth muscle cell membrane activates cyclic adenosine monophosphate (cAMP), which in turn activates a protein kinase that phosphorylates (adds a phosphate) the myosin light-chain kinase enzyme (Fig. 2-7). Phosphorylation inactivates the enzyme, and as a result the myosin light-chain kinase is unable to participate in the phosphorylation of the myosin and the promotion of the active myosin kinase–calmodulin–calcium complex. Failure to form the complex causes inhibition of cross-bridge formation. ß-adrenergic stimulation also decreases intracellu-

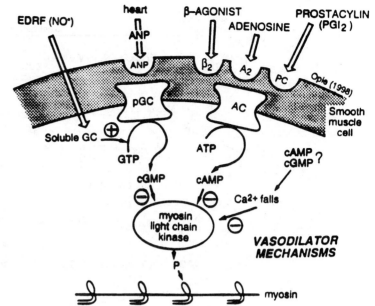

FIGURE 2-7 Vasodilatory mechanisms. Most act by formation of cyclic nucleotides, cyclic guanosine monophosphate (cGMP) and cyclic adenosine monophosphate (cAMP), both of which are vasodilatory, possibly through inhibition of myosin light-chain kinase. GMP is the messenger for guanylate cyclase (GC), which in turn is stimulated by atrial natriuretic polypeptide (ANP) or by factor (EDRF); i.e., nitric oxide. Vasodilatory cAMP is formed by stimulation of adenylate cyclase (AC) in response to β–stimulation or by adenosine (A) stimulation through A$_2$ receptors, or by prostacyclin (PO; PGI$_2$) receptor. ATP, adenosine triphosphate; pGC. (Opie, LH: The Heart: Physiology from Cell to Circulation, 3rd ed, p 240. Philadelphia, Lippincott–Raven, 1998.)

lar calcium by hyperpolarization of the vascular smooth muscle, which decreases the influx of calcium into the cell, increases cAMP-mediated extrusion of calcium from the cell, and promotes calcium uptake by the sarcoplasmic reticulum.[154]

CALCIUM

The major end point of extrinsic neurohormonal factors and local regulation of vascular tone involves a cascade of messengers that influence calcium movement in and out of the cell or sarcoplasmic reticulum, thus influencing the contractile process.[6,53] Knowledge of the role of calcium is important because the modulation of calcium flux is the focus of pharmacologic control of vascular resistance.

As with cardiac and skeletal muscle, the changes in intracellular calcium are responsible for vascular smooth muscle contraction and relaxation.[53,98,149] However, unlike skeletal and cardiac muscle, in which calcium reverses the inhibitory effect of troponin on the actin–myosin interaction, vascular smooth muscle cross-bridge formation and muscle contraction result from the indirect activation of myosin by calcium.

Sources of Calcium

The increased intracellular calcium comes from an influx of calcium across the sarcolemma and from the sarcoplasmic reticulum.[149,150] The calcium influx across the sarcolemma is through voltage-gated ion channels,[82,98,103] whereas the calcium released from the sarcoplasmic reticulum is the result of activation of the inositol 1,4,5-triphosphate–regulated channels, or calcium-induced calcium release.[6,38,53,56]

Calcium Signaling

The increased intracellular calcium binds with calmodulin, a small protein found in the cytosol of vascular smooth muscle (Fig. 2-8). The calcium–calmodulin complex activates the enzyme myosin light-chain kinase, which in turn phosphorylates the light protein chains of the myosin head. The phosphorylation activates the myosin (increases the ATPase activity), such that the myosin can interact with actin.[55] The process of phosphorylation is considered the primary mechanism of smooth muscle contraction.

Conversely, a decrease in the cytoplasmic calcium concentration inactivates the myosin light-chain kinase and permits dephosphorylation of myosin by the enzyme myosin light-chain phosphatase. The dephosphorylation facilitates the detachment of myosin from actin, resulting in relaxation.[149] The cytoplasmic calcium concentration is decreased through uptake of calcium into the sarcoplasmic reticulum,[11] transport out of the cell across the plasma membrane by Ca^{2+}-ATPase exchanger or a probable Na$^+$/Ca^{2+} exchanger,[53,81] and through closure of the membrane calcium channels through hyperpolarization or calcium channel blockers.[8,152]

VOLUME AND FLOW DISTRIBUTION

Resistance

As demonstrated in Figure 2-9, the pressure drop from the aorta to the small arteries is relatively small, approximately 25 mm Hg.[141] As much as 50% of the peripheral resistance appears to occur proximal to vessels with diameters of

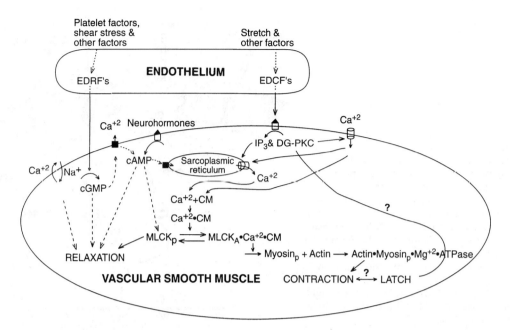

FIGURE 2-8 Hypothetical simplified illustration of interactions between endothelial and vascular smooth muscle cells. Physical forces or circulating factors from nerves, platelets, or other sources trigger the endothelial cell to produce endothelium–derived relaxing (EDRFs) and contracting factors (EDCFs), which diffuse into vascular smooth muscle or stimulate membrane receptors (▲). Calcium enters the cell through voltage–operated channels (▯) and may be released from intracellular stores such as sarcoplasmic reticulum (SR). Calcium (Ca^{+2}) interacts with calmodulin (CM), and together they activate myosin light-chain kinase (MLCK), which in turn phosphorylates (P) myosin so it can react with actin and cause vascular smooth muscle contraction. EDCFs activate inositol triphosphate (IP_3), which may promote the release of calcium from SR, and diacylglycerol (DG), which activates protein kinase C (PKC). PKC may influence the contractile proteins or promote the latch state. Cyclic guanosine monophosphate (cGMP), initiated by EDRFs, or cyclic adenosine monophosphate (cAMP), initiated by adrenergic and other vascular smooth muscle cell membrane receptor stimuli, may promote calcium cellular extrusion or uptake by the SR through activating membrane pumps. (▪).

100 μm. This finding indicates the primary sites for peripheral vascular resistance are the small arteries and the arterioles.[98,122,132]

Alterations in the diameter of the terminal arterioles or precapillary blood vessels control capillary and venous pressures, microvascular blood flow and exchange, and postcapillary venous volume.[27,28] Although the radius of the capillaries is considerably smaller than the radius of the arterioles, the resistance is lower because of the increase in cross-sectional area, as described later.

Volume Distribution

At rest, the systemic veins contain as much as 60% to 80% of the total blood volume, with 25% to 50% of this volume in the small veins (<1 mm in diameter). One-fourth of the total blood volume is in the capacious splanchnic circulation. Although the cross-sectional area is largest at the end of the capillaries, the largest volume of blood, as demonstrated in Figure 2-9, is in the veins because of the combination of cross-sectional area and the length of the veins.[135] The remainder of the blood is distributed in the aorta and systemic arteries (10%), the capillaries (5%), and the pulmonary bed and heart (15% to 25%).[128,179]

Blood Flow

DEFINITION OF FLOW

Blood flow ($\dot{Q}$) is expressed in terms of volume of blood per unit of time (volume/time). For example, the cardiac output, which is defined as the liters of blood pumped out of the left ventricle into the systemic circulation each minute, is usually expressed as liters per minute.[52]

DETERMINANTS OF FLOW

Nonturbulent flow ($\dot{Q}$) in a segment of an isogravitational blood vessel (i.e., a blood vessel on the same horizontal level) is determined by the pressure difference (ΔP) between the inflow and outflow ends of that segment divided by the resistance (R) to flow provided by that segment. The relationship is expressed in the following equation:

$$\dot{Q} = \Delta P/R$$

Substituting physiological values into this equation gives:

$$CO = \frac{MAP - RAP}{SVR}$$

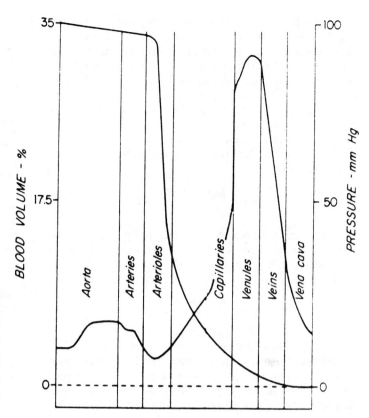

FIGURE 2-9 Changes in estimated blood volume (%) and blood pressure in consecutive segments of the systemic blood vessels. Note that the volume is predominantly in the venules. The pressure is high in the aorta and arteries, falls rapidly in the arterioles, and then falls more slowly from the capillaries to the vena cava. (From Scher AM: The veins and venous return. In Patton HD, Fuchs A, Hille B et al (eds): Textbook of Physiology, Vol 2, 21st ed, p 880. Philadelphia, WB Saunders, 1989.)

where MAP – RAP is the difference between the mean arterial pressure (MAP; as an indicator of aortic or upstream pressure) and right atrial pressure (RAP; downstream pressure) divided by the SVR, all of which determine the overall blood flow to the body.

Pressure. Blood pressure is the force exerted by the blood in a blood vessel. Clinically, pressure is expressed as millimeters of mercury, torr, or centimeters of H_2O. The relationship between these various measures is:

$$1 \text{ mm Hg} = 1 \text{ torr} = 1.36 \text{ cm } H_2O$$

Pressure in blood vessels has three components: (1) static pressure, which is related to the fullness of the vascular system at zero flow; (2) hydrostatic pressure, which is equal to the height of the column of liquid (h) times the density of the liquid (p) times the gravitational force (g): hydrostatic pressure = pgh; and (3) dynamic pressure, which is the pressure generated by the heart and is equal to flow times resistance (pressure = flow × resistance). The static pressure and the hydrostatic pressure are added to the dynamic pressure to give blood pressure. The hydrostatic pressure, and particularly the effect of the height of the fluid column, is especially important in the upright position, because the fluid column between the heart and the feet may add an additional 100 mm Hg of hydrostatic pressure to the dynamic pressure (100 mm Hg).

In the systemic circulation, blood flows from the aorta, where the MAP is 100 mm Hg, to the right atrium (mean

pressure = 0 to 6 mm Hg). The right atrial pressure depends on posture, state of hydration, rate and depth of breathing, and cardiac output. In the pulmonary circulation, the entire cardiac output flows from the pulmonary artery (pressure ranges from 7 to 18 mm Hg) to the left atrium (pressure ranges from 2 to 12 mm Hg, mean = 8 mm Hg), with a change in pressure of only approximately 10 mm Hg. The total pulmonary vascular resistance (PVR) is approximately 10% of the SVR. Changes in the PVR, however, may occur with changes in gravity, body position, lung volume, alveolar and intrapleural pressures, intravascular pressures, and right ventricular output without any change in pulmonary vascular tone.[74] Thus, changes in PVR must be interpreted with caution.

Resistance. Based on an analogy to Ohm's law, resistance (R) is equal to a pressure gradient (ΔP) divided by blood flow ($\dot{Q}$):

$$R = \Delta P / \dot{Q}$$

According to Poiseuille's law for streamlined nonpulsatile flow of a substance with uniform viscosity,[113] vascular resistance is proportional to a constant ($8/\pi$), the viscosity of the blood (η), and the length of the vessel (l); and is inversely proportional to the fourth power of the radius (r^4):

$$R = \frac{8/\eta}{\pi r^4}$$

The radius of the blood vessel is the principal factor determining resistance in the vascular system. For example, if all other factors are constant, decreasing the radius of the vessel by 50% causes resistance to increase 16-fold, because resistance is inversely proportional to the fourth power of the radius. An increase in blood viscosity causes resistance to increase, although this increased viscosity is seldom an acute event.[16,179] However, an increase in the hematocrit (e.g., polycythemia due to high altitude) can raise blood viscosity, causing resistance to rise.[104]

The units of resistance are dyne · sec/cm^5, dyne · sec · cm^{-5}, and mm Hg · L^{-1} · min^{-1}. SVR is calculated by the following equation:

$$SVR = \frac{MAP - RAP}{CO} \times 80$$

In this equation, 80 is a conversion factor for adjusting mm Hg·L^{-1}· min^{-1} to dyne · sec/cm^5.[29] The normal SVR ranges from 800 to 1,200 dynes · sec/cm^5.

Pulmonary vascular resistance is calculated:

$$PVR = \frac{\overline{PA} - PAWP}{CO} \times 80$$

where PA is mean pulmonary artery pressure and PAWP is pulmonary artery wedge pressure. The PVR ranges from 20 to 120 dynes · sec/cm^5, with an average of 100 dynes · sec/cm^5 (see Chapter 3).[140,174] As discussed, numerous factors other than vascular tone can alter the PVR; thus, an absolute value or a change in the PVR must be interpreted cautiously.

THE ARTERIAL SYSTEM

Arterial Pressure

Systolic and diastolic blood pressures describe the high and low values of pressure fluctuations around the mean of the arterial pressure wave.[42] The MAP in the ascending aorta depends on the cardiac output and SVR:

$$MAP = CO \times SVR$$

whereas arterial distensibility and left ventricular stroke volume determine the amplitude and contour of the pressure wave.[42] The peak systolic pressure is determined by the volume and velocity of left ventricular ejection (i.e., the larger the stroke volume, the larger the pulse pressure at any given distensibility), peripheral arterial resistance, the distensibility of the arterial wall, the viscosity of blood, and the end-diastolic volume in the arterial blood.[105,111] During diastole, arterial pressure decreases until the next ventricular contraction, so the minimal diastolic pressure is determined by factors that affect the magnitude and rate of the diastolic pressure drop. Factors that affect diastolic blood pressure include blood viscosity, arterial distensibility, peripheral resistance, and the length of the cardiac cycle.[109]

Arterial distensibility is affected by the elastic modulus of the arterial wall, which is the ratio between the force acting to deform the wall (stress) to the actual deformation produced (strain).[112] Distensibility is also affected by the geometry of the arterial wall, in accordance with a modified Laplace equation:[111]

Tension = pressure × radius/wall thickness

During systole, the elastic walls of the aorta and large arteries stretch as more blood enters than runs off into the periphery. Thus, a portion of the stroke volume is stored in the relatively distensible aorta during systole. During diastole, there is passive elastic recoil of the arterial walls, causing continued, but declining, ejection of blood out of the aorta and into the peripheral arteries. The elastic recoil transforms pulsatile flow into more continuous flow in the smaller vessels, and explains why the blood pressure does not drop to zero during periods of no flow (e.g., diastole).[32]

Pulse pressure is the difference between the systolic and diastolic pressures. A normal pulse pressure at the brachial artery is approximately 40 mm Hg. A higher pulse pressure may reflect where the pressure is measured in the body (increased pulse pressure in the periphery), and physiologically an increased pulse pressure is usually the result of increased stroke volume and ejection velocity. An increased pulse pressure is commonly seen with fever, anemia, exercise, and hyperthyroidism. In addition, aortic regurgitation is associated with an increased pulse pressure.[60] In this case, the increased pulse pressure is caused by the rapid ejection of a large stroke volume, which increases the systolic blood pressure ("water-hammer pulse"), and a rapid and marked decrease in diastolic pressure ("collapsing pulse") secondary to flow back through the insufficient valve and peripheral vasodilation.[71,111] An increase in pulse pressure also occurs with bradycardia because of an increase in stroke volume.[105,111] Finally, with aging the arterial tree stiffens, and the pulse pressure increases because of an increase in pressure wave reflection from the periphery and the subsequent increase in systolic blood pressure.[39,40,65] The increase in pulse pressure is particularly noticeable after the age of 50 to 60 years.[40,65] An acute decrease in pulse pressure is not a normal finding and may indicate an increase in vascular resistance, which is not an expected age-related change; decreased stroke volume (e.g., aortic stenosis); or decreased intravascular volume.[105,111]

Arterial Pressure Wave

The arterial system acts as both a conduit and cushion. The conduit function can be assessed by comparison of the mean pressure at various points in the arterial tree, whereas the cushioning function can be assessed by analyzing the pulsations (systolic and diastolic pressures) about the mean.[42,108] The latter effect can best be assessed by evaluating an arterial pressure waveform.

The contour or the aortic pressure wave is illustrated in Figure 2-10. The initial sharp upstroke reflects the pressure increase during the rapid ejection phase of ventricular systole and a slower rise during later systole. The upstroke of the waveform is referred to as the anacrotic limb. The downstroke of the pressure wave corresponds to the decrease in aortic pressure during decreased ventricular ejection, and the continued flow of blood into the periphery. The downstroke of the wave is interrupted by a sharp notch or incisura, denoting a transient reversal of blood flow just before aortic valve closure.[172] The interval following the incisura when the aortic pressure continues to

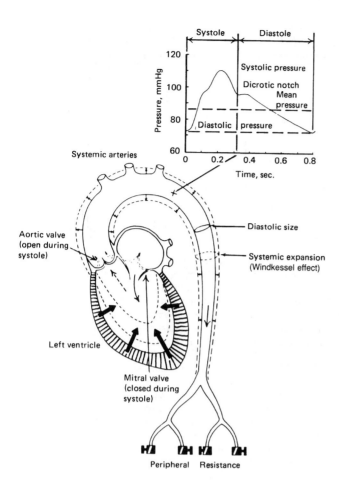

FIGURE 2-10 Schematic illustration of changes in aortic pressure during the cardiac cycle and the dampening role of the aorta and large arteries on the pulsatile flow from the heart during systole (sometimes termed the *Windkessel effect*). (From Shepherd JT, Vanhoutte PM: The Human Cardiovascular System: Facts and Concepts, p 78. New York, Raven Press, 1979.)

decrease is referred to as the diastolic runoff period.[32] There may be a second positive wave during the diastolic runoff that is referred to as the diastolic wave. This wave is related to the reflection of pressure pulse wave in the periphery.[111] As discussed later, the timing of the return of the reflected pressure wave from the periphery is important because if the reflected wave arrives during systole, it increases the workload of the left ventricle. Conversely, arrival of the reflected wave during diastole is beneficial because it augments the diastolic filling of the coronary arteries.

The systolic pressure in the brachial and femoral arteries may be as much as 5 to 20 mm Hg greater than central aortic pressure[46,120,131] (see Figure 19-7). As the arterial pressure pulse travels to the periphery, the shape and amplitude of the pulse change.[108,111] The pulse pressure and the systolic pressure increase, the ascending limb of the pulse wave becomes steeper, and the incisura or the aortic wave is replaced with a slightly later dicrotic notch.[111] The change in amplitude and contour of the arterial waveform is primarily the result of peripheral reflection. Reflection occurs when flow is impeded (primarily when low-resistance arteries terminate in high-resistance vessels) and the pressure wave is reflected in a retrograde (backward) fashion. This retrograde pressure wave combines with the antegrade (forward) pressure pulse, and the arterial pressure (primarily systolic pressure) is augmented.[14,46,108]

With aging, there is an increase in systolic blood pressure and pulse pressure, which is explained by the stiffening of the vessels that occurs with aging.[160] The stiffening causes increased peripheral reflection, with the retrograde pressure wave arriving back at the heart during systole, which increases the systolic blood pressure.[110] The increase in the systolic and pulse pressures is important because these findings may be predictive of cardiovascular risk.[147,160] An important point is that the vascular resistance does not normally increase with age and is not a dominant factor in the rise in the systolic blood pressure after age 60 years.[40] However, some people have an increase in vascular resistance with aging, which explains the increase in mean pressure observed.[65]

The relation between the central and peripheral arterial pressure is also altered in conditions such as exercise, shock, and the administration of vasodilators. In shock, the peripheral systolic pressure may overestimate the ascending aortic pressure by as much as 20 mm Hg.[110] In exercise, the peripheral systolic pressure may be as much as 80 mm Hg greater than central aortic pressure.[131] This finding has important clinical implications for exercise in patients who have undergone surgery on the aorta, because the peripheral pressure is not necessarily reflective of the pressure stress being applied to the aorta.

THE VENOUS SYSTEM

The venous system transports blood back to the heart from the microcirculation of each organ system and plays a crucial role in the maintenance of thoracic intravascular volume. The veins also serve as a low-pressure reservoir with the capacity to contain a large and variable volume of blood (similar to a giant capacitor sitting next to the right ventricle).

Venous Pressure and Resistance

In the supine position, the pressure generated by the heart in the large arteries is approximately 100 mm Hg. However, as demonstrated in Figure 2-11, the pressure decreases across the arterioles and capillaries, with a resultant pressure in the small veins of only 15 to 20 mm Hg. The right atrial pressure is approximately 0 to 5 mm Hg (depending on position, the state of hydration, and cardiac output). Thus, the pressure driving blood flow from the left side of the heart to the capillaries is approximately 80 mm Hg, whereas the driving pressure from the postcapillary vessels to the right atrium is only 15 to 20 mm Hg (difference between the postcapillary vessels and the right atrium). Interestingly, in the upright position, despite the addition of hydrostatic pressure (determined by the height of a continuous column of blood between any given point and the heart), this gradient is unchanged.

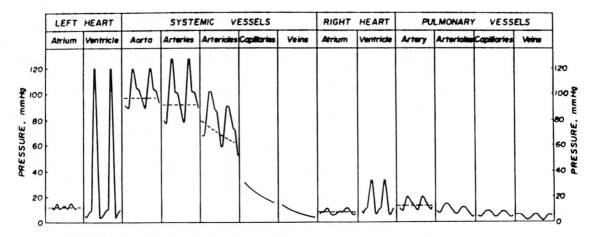

FIGURE 2-11 Pressure changes in the human cardiovascular system. In the left atrium, the pressure is low but pulsatile because of the rhythmic contractions of the atrial muscle. The main generator of pressure is the muscle of the left ventricle; in the latter cavity, the pressure alternates with each cardiac cycle from near 0 (diastole) to approximately 120 mm Hg (systole). When the pressure in the ventricle exceeds that in the aorta, the aortic semilunar valve opens, the ventricle and aorta become a common chamber, and the pressure in both rises in unison. The rise in aortic pressure causes an expansion of the aorta and the large arteries because of their elasticity and because blood enters the arterial trees faster than it leaves it through the small–bore arterioles. When the ventricle starts to relax, the aortic valve closes. As the ventricle continues to relax, the pressure within it drops quickly to near 0, but the pressure in the aorta falls slowly throughout ventricular diastole as the distended arterial tree recoils and blood continues to flow to the capillaries through the arterioles. The major loss of pressure occurs at the arterioles because of the high resistance to flow that they offer. The pressure in the capillaries and veins decreases further to approximately 0 in the great veins entering the right atrium; the flow in the systemic capillaries and veins is relatively nonpulsatile. The right side of the heart generates a pressure pattern similar to that in the systemic circulation, but the systolic pressure in the pulmonary artery is approximately six times less than that of the aorta, and the flow in the pulmonary capillaries is pulsatile. Mean pressures are indicated by dotted lines. In large arteries, the mean pressure is lower than in the aorta, although the systolic pressure is higher because of reflection of the pulse waves. (From Shepherd JT, Vanhoutte PM: The Human Cardiovascular System: Facts and Concepts, p 78. New York, Raven Press, 1979.)

Skeletal muscle contractions in the extremities (the muscle pump) and respiration (respiratory pump) play an essential role in propelling venous blood from the veins to the right atrium (see Chapter 4). In addition, the venous valves prevent backward flow into the muscle. Valvular function is particularly important during standing and exercise.[7,45] The valves also promote the one-way flow of blood through perforating veins that lie between the superficial and deep veins.

Venous Compliance

When empty, the thin walls of the veins are flattened and the vessels are elliptical in shape. As the veins fill with blood, they passively change to a circular shape. Because of this passive accommodation to an increase in volume, the veins are capable of receiving large volumes of fluid with only small increases in transmural pressure; that is, they are compliant. At increased pressures, the veins become distended and less compliant; thus, any given pressure change is associated with a smaller change in volume.[130] Because of the compliant nature of the veins, the venous system plays an important role in increasing and decreasing thoracic intravascular volume[51] (see Chapter 4).

MICROCIRCULATORY EXCHANGE

Flow Through the Microvascular Circulation

Blood flow ($\dot{Q}$) through the microcirculation (or any organ) is directly related to the difference in pressure between the arterial end of the vascular segment (P_A) and venous pressure (P_V), and is inversely related to vascular resistance (R_T)[72,122]:

$$Flow = (P_A - P_V)/R_T$$

In the absence of changes in arterial pressure (P_A), changes in local vascular resistance and intravascular pressure are caused by vasodilation and vasoconstriction of the arterioles. Any alteration in the tone of the muscular venules contributes little to the change in resistance.

Microvascular Transport Mechanisms

Solutes and water passively move across the endothelium as the result of two processes, diffusion and ultrafiltration. Diffusion is the result of the random kinetic motion of ions and molecules. Diffusion results in the net transport of substances along a concentration gradient from high to low concentration. Ultrafiltration is the combined movement of fluid and solutes in a unilateral direction through a membrane, except that the movement of the solutes is restricted by the membrane.[122] The driving force for ultrafiltration is the difference between hydrostatic pressure and oncotic pressure across the membrane.[122] Ultrafiltration is the primary mechanism for controlling plasma and interstitial fluid volume.[122]

DIFFUSION

Concentration gradients, created by the production or consumption of specific substances, are the primary driving forces for diffusion (with the exception of the tight-junction capillaries, which are affected by electrical gradients).[23,121] Because diffusion in or out of a blood vessel creates a concentration gradient along the vessel, diffusion exchange is strongly influenced by blood flow, particularly, as discussed later, for those substances that rapidly diffuse through the membrane wall.[23,121]

The rate of diffusion of a solute across the capillary wall (J_s) is proportional to the concentration gradient, that is, the difference between the concentration in the plasma (C_p) and interstitial concentration (C_i), the permeability (P_s) of the endothelium to the solute, and the surface area (A) available for exchange.

$$J_s = P_s A (C_p - C_i)$$

For substances that diffuse rapidly through the capillary endothelium (e.g., O_2, CO_2), the transport of the solute depends on the concentration gradient and blood flow (through the delivery or removal of the substance), and the rate of diffusion (J_s) is described as *flow-limited*.

$$J_s = (C_a - C_i)\dot{Q}$$

where C_a is the concentration of the substance in the arterial blood, C_i is the concentration of the substance in the interstitium, and $\dot{Q}$ is the rate of blood flow. Flow-limited diffusion has potentially important implications for oxygen delivery in the setting of decreased oxygen delivery (e.g., cardiogenic shock or during severe exercise when flow rates are so high that diffusion is limited). However, most substances have intermediate endothelial permeability, and the rate of diffusion depends on both endothelial permeability and flow.[122]

Most solutes, including small lipophilic and hydrophilic molecules and macromolecules, move through membranes of exchange vessels by diffusion. The route of diffusion depends on the type of membrane (continuous, fenestrated, discontinuous, and tight junction) and the characteristics of the substance (e.g., lipid soluble, ionic, large macromolecule). Water diffuses through the endothelium primarily through intercellular clefts.[24,86,87] Lipid-soluble substances, such as O_2, CO_2, and anesthetic gases, which pass easily through the lipid bilayer of the microvascular wall, diffuse relatively rapidly through the endothelium. Small hydrophilic solutes, such as ions and simple sugars, pass primarily through fenestrae, junctions between cells, or cell membrane protein-lined channels.[24,146] Macromolecular transport pathways include endothelial cell vesicles, fenestrae, intercellular junctions, and possibly temporary changes in the extracellular fiber matrix. Albumin, which accounts for 50% of colloid osmotic pressure, crosses most microvascular walls more readily than the globulins or fibrinogen.[72,86] The transport or movement of the macromolecules into the interstitium contributes to interstitial oncotic pressure.

ULTRAFILTRATION

The rate of fluid movement across a short segment of exchange vessel (J_v/A) is proportional to the net pressure difference across the vessel wall.[72] The net pressure difference reflects the algebraic sum of four pressures: intravascular (capillary) pressure (P_c), interstitial fluid pressure (P_i), plasma oncotic pressure (π_p), and interstitial oncotic pressure (π_i). The interstitium is the space between the capillary wall and cells. The interstitial space is filled with a collagen fiber framework and a gel made up of glycosaminoglycans, a salt solution, and proteins from the plasma.[2] The difference between plasma and interstitial oncotic pressure is referred to as colloid osmotic pressure (that portion of the osmotic pressure due to molecules that do not move freely across the membrane), to differentiate it from the total osmotic force, which is affected by all solute particles.[91]

Under normal conditions, intravascular hydrostatic pressure is higher than interstitial hydrostatic pressure; thus, the balance of the forces favors the movement of fluid and solutes out of the vessel (filtration). Conversely, the concentration of nonpermeating large molecules (permeating molecules do not contribute to the oncotic gradient) is higher in the plasma than in the interstitial fluid, and facilitates the movement of fluid and solutes into the vessel (reabsorption). The balance between the hydrostatic and oncotic forces determines the direction of fluid and solute movement across the vessel wall.

The primary direction of ultrafiltration is out of the vessel (filtration). The primary force behind filtration is capillary pressure (P_c). The true pressure opposing filtration (P_o) is not simply plasma oncotic pressure, but oncotic plasma pressure minus interstitial oncotic pressure plus interstitial hydrostatic pressure, and the reflection coefficient:

$$P_o = \sigma(\pi_p - \pi_i) + P_i$$

In general, the forces opposing filtration do not exceed capillary pressure, and filtration occurs along the entire length of the exchange vessel.[72,73]

In addition to the hydrostatic and oncotic forces, two other factors affect fluid movement across the exchange vessel: the hydraulic conductivity of the wall (L_p) and the reflection coefficient (σ). Hydraulic conductivity is a measure of the permeability of the exchange vessel to fluid, with the highest L_p values for fenestrated endothelia and lowest for tight-junction endothelia.[88,122,123] Hydraulic conductivity is difficult to measure and is estimated by the capillary filtration coefficient. The capillary filtration coefficient, which is equal to the product of hydraulic conductivity and the available area (L_pA), is expressed as milliliters of net filtrate formed in 100 g of tissue per minute for each milliliter increase in mean capillary filtration pressure ($ml \cdot min^{-1}$ mm Hg^{-1} 100 g^{-1}). The capillary filtration coefficient is a useful indicator of capillary permeability.[1,2] A decrease in the capillary filtration coefficient, for example by a reduction in the area available for exchange, reduces the rate of net capillary filtration for any given net filtration pressure. The second factor, the reflection coefficient (σ), represents the osmotic pressure exerted by a difference in the concentration gradient of a substance across a membrane (oncotic effect of the concentration gradient), and is affected by the ratio of the solute size to pore size—the greater the ratio, the greater the reflection coefficient.[72] The reflection coefficient is close to 1 for tight-junction endothelium, which is completely impermeable to protein. In normal systemic exchange vessels in the skin and skeletal muscle, with continuous or fenestrated endothelium, the reflection coefficient ranges from 0.8 to 0.95 for albumin and total protein,[2,73] which indicates that these vessels are not completely impermeable to proteins.[72,86,122] In the lungs, the reflection coefficients are in general lower for albumin (0.5 to 0.6) and protein (0.5 to 0.7).[2] In cases of injury to the endothelium, the reflection coefficient is markedly reduced, allowing increased movement of large molecules (e.g., protein) out of the exchange vessels. The relationship between edema and alterations in the factors that affect fluid flux, as described by Starling's equation, is discussed next.

The relationship between these factors is described by a modified version of Starling's initial equation for fluid flux[66,72,124,155]:

$$J_v = L_p A([P_c - P_i] - \overline{\sigma}[\pi_p - \pi_i])$$

Insertion of the following average values for systemic exchange vessels:

$L_p A = 6$ mL/h $\times$ mm Hg $\cdot$ kg
$P_c = 14$ mm Hg (average pressure)
$P_i = -2$ mm Hg
$\sigma = 0.95$
$\pi_p = 25$ mm Hg
$\pi_i = 10$ mm Hg

into the Starling equation results in fluid filtration from the plasma into the interstitium of approximately 300 mL/h or 7 L/d for a 65-kg person.[1,121] The net filtration is necessary to wash out the proteins that are continuously diffusing out of the vessels into the interstitium.[2,73] The ultrafiltrate and proteins that cross the vessel wall into the interstitial fluid are subsequently removed by the lymphatic system.[2,72,117,122,136]

In the initial conceptualization by Starling[155] and validation by Landis[66] of Starling's equation, it was thought that at the arterial end of the capillary the net forces favored the movement of fluid out of the vessel (filtration), somewhere in the middle of the vessel an equilibrium point was reached where there was neither a gain nor loss of fluid, and finally, on the venous end of the exchange vessel, the net forces favored reabsorption.[122] Although the validity of Starling's equation has been repeatedly confirmed,[87] the conceptualization of upstream filtration and downstream reabsorption has now been called into question.[72,73] With the exception of exchange vessels in intestinal mucosa, renal peritubular capillaries, and lymph nodes, which demonstrate continuous reabsorption,[87] the forces promoting fluid movement out of the vascular exchange vessels (filtration) are greater than the forces promoting fluid movement back into the vascular system (reabsorption). Therefore, the net fluid movement along the entire exchange vessel is in the direction of filtration.[72,73,88] In the tissues where there is net filtration, the lymphatic system plays an important role in the maintenance of tissue fluid balance.[1]

The net filtration over the entire length of the exchange vessel may be explained by the finding that the interstitial protein concentration varies inversely with the filtration rate.[72,73] An increase in filtration rate decreases the interstitial plasma concentration (π_i). The decrease in interstitial plasma concentration opposes filtration and a new steady state is reached. The dynamic interaction between filtration and oncotic pressure provides a buffer against excessive edema in situations such as heart failure, where there is an increase in intravascular pressure.[31,87]

In addition to the sustained reabsorption that occurs in the gastrointestinal mucosa and peritubular capillaries,[73] transient reabsorption (an "autotransfusion") occurs in the setting of the sustained vasoconstriction that occurs with hypovolemic hypotension.[68] This autotransfusion is the result of a change in the ratio of the precapillary to postcapillary resistance on mean capillary pressure. An alteration in microvascular pressure is a key component in the control of fluid flux into and out of the exchange vessels.

Mean capillary pressure (P_c) is determined by the arterial and venous pressures and the ratio of postcapillary resistance (R_a) to precapillary resistance (R_v), as described by the following equation derived by Pappenheimer and Soto-Rivera[114]:

$$P_c = \frac{(P_v + P_a) \times (R_v / R_a)}{1 + (R_v / R_a)}$$

where P_v is venous pressure, P_a is arterial pressure, R_v is postcapillary midpoint resistance, and R_a is precapillary midpoint resistance (where $R_v + R_a = R_{Total}$). An increase in either P_a or P_v results in an increase in P_c, unless counteracted by a decrease in the R_v/R_a ratio. The lower the R_v/R_a ratio (increased precapillary resistance or decreased postcapillary resistance), the lower the capillary pressure. It is this adjustment in R_v/R_a ratio, primarily through regulation of precapillary resistance (R_a) in the skeletal muscle and skin, that constitutes the primary effector mechanism for the central nervous system–mediated control of plasma volume.[1,84] The centrally mediated decrease in mean capillary pressure occurs only to the extent allowed by local autoregulatory adjustments, however.

In response to hypovolemic hypotension, compensatory precapillary vasoconstriction (increased R_a) decreases the mean P_c,[1,84] and the net pressure in the downstream (venous) segment of the exchange vessel favors reabsorption (Fig. 2-12). The transient reabsorption may also be aided by an arteriovenous gradient for permeability (i.e., permeability in the downstream exchange vessels is greater than in upstream exchange vessels).[72,86] As a result of this gradient, the decrease in capillary pressure on the venous end is offset by the increase in permeability, and filtration continues. Eventually the autotransfusion is opposed by the increase in interstitial oncotic pressure (π_i), and within a short time, a new steady state favoring filtration is again established.[1,72]

THE LYMPHATIC SYSTEM

Removal of fluid and plasma proteins from the interstitium by the terminal lymphatics is essential in the maintenance of an equilibrium in microvascular–interstitial exchange.[72] Depending on the protein concentration in the lymph, 8 to

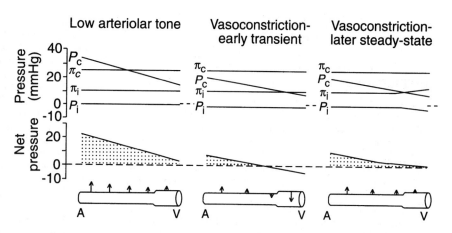

FIGURE 2-12 (Top) Axial gradient of four Starling pressures. **(Middle)** Net pressure. **(Bottom)** Direction of fluid flux. **(Left)** Control values. **(Middle)** Precapillary constriction lowers capillary pressure, resulting in transient fluid absorption. **(Right)** Final steady state (filtration) after interstitial fluid pressure and oncotic pressure have readjusted. P_c, capillary hydrostatic pressure; P_i, tissue hydrostatic pressure, π_c, capillary oncotic pressure; π_i, tissue oncotic pressure; A, arterial end of capillary; V, venular end of capillary. (From Levick JR: Capillary filtration–absorption balance reconsidered in light of dynamic extravascular factors. Exp Physiol 76: 846, 1991.)

12 L/d of lymph, which reflects net filtration due to movement of fluid out of the vascular bed, is removed from the interstitium by the lymphatic system[72,124] (see Fig. 2-3). Approximately 4 to 8 L of the ultrafiltrate is directly reabsorbed from the lymphatic vessels back into the blood vessels, and the remaining 4 L of efferent lymph, which includes all of the filtered protein, is delivered back to the central circulation.[2,124] These findings are relatively new and indicate that lymph flow is two times greater than previously thought. This high level of lymphatic flow supports the idea that filtration (return of lymph to the systemic vasculature) occurs along the entire length of lymphatic bed and not just in the central circulation.

EDEMA FORMATION

Edema, which is an abnormal increase in the volume of interstitial fluid in a tissue or organ,[122] occurs as the result of an imbalance in one or more of the factors described by the Starling equation for fluid flux.[1,2,31,87,114] The effects of a change in hydrostatic and oncotic forces on the net direction of fluid filtration were discussed previously.

Another important factor in the cause or prevention of edema is lymphatic flow. Normally, an increase in fluid filtration and interstitial volume is matched by an increase in lymphatic drainage.[1,47,122] However, edema may develop in cases where lymphatic drainage is obstructed or limited (e.g., postmastectomy lymphedema or an immobilized and dependent extremity).

There are numerous factors that prevent or limit edema formation. Centrally mediated as well as more local myogenic or metabolic mechanisms (see Chapter 4) play an important role in the control of precapillary resistance and mean capillary pressure, and thus fluid filtration.[2] In addition, three local interstitial-lymphatic buffering mechanisms play an equally important role in the local control of interstitial fluid volume. The three mechanisms—(1) hydrostatic buffering, due to a change in P_c or P_i; (2) oncotic buffering, due primarily to a change in π_i; and (3) lymphatic buffering—limit filtration and increase interstitial fluid volume by negative feedback.[1,2,31] The potential causes of edema, such as increased capillary pressure, a decrease in plasma oncotic pressure, or increased endothelial permeability, and the compensatory interstitial-lymphatic buffering mechanisms are summarized in Table 2-3. Because P_i increases by less than

	Edema Formation		
Factors	**Mechanism**	**Prevention of Edema Limitation or Mechanism**	
Venous congestion due to venous obstruction or volume overload	↑ P_c	Precapillary vasoconstriction (↑ R_a) will: Limit increase in P_c and decrease net filtration pressure	
Arteriolar vasodilation (↓ R_a) or venular constriction (↑ R_v)	↑ P_c d/t ↓ R_v/R_a ratio	?↓ Capillary filtration coefficient (L_pA) ↑ Lymph flow (?)	
Hypoproteinemia or hypoalbuminemia	↓ π_p	Secondary to increased filtration and interstitial fluid volume: ↓ π_i and ↑ P_i	
Increased endothelial permeability to proteins (inflammation/burns)	↓ σ, ↑ π_i ↓ P_i (?) ↑ Net filtration pressure	↑ Lymph flow	
Decreased Lymphatic Function			
Lymphedema (e.g., mastectomy)	↑ π_i	↑ P_i may increase flow into lymphatics	
Immobilization of dependent limb	↓ Lymphatic flow	?↓ Capillary filtration coefficient (L_pA)	

TABLE 2-3 Factors Associated with the Formation and Prevention of Edema[1,2,5,31,122,136]

R_a, precapillary (arteriolar) resistance; R_v, postcapillary (venular) resistance; P_c, capillary pressure; P_i, interstitial pressure; π_i, interstitial oncotic pressure; σ, coefficient of reflection; ↑, increased; ↓, decreased; ?, speculative effect.

5 mm Hg even in large edema, the decrease in π_i is the main mechanism to counteract edema in humans.[2]

REFERENCES

1. Aukland K, Nicolaysen G: Interstitial fluid volume: Local regulatory mechanisms. Physiol Rev 61: 556–643, 1981
2. Aukland K, Reed R: Interstitial-lymphatic mechanisms in the control of extracellular fluid volume. Physiol Rev 73: 1–78, 1993
3. Azuma H, Ishikawa M, Sekizaki S: Endothelium-dependent inhibition of platelet aggregation. Br J Pharmacol 88: 411–415, 1986
4. Bassenge E: Antiplatelet effects of endothelium-derived relaxing factor and nitric oxide donors. Eur Heart J 12(Suppl E): 12–15, 1991
5. Bates D, Levick J, Mortimer P: Starling pressures in the human arm and their alteration in postmastectomy oedema. J Physiol (Lond) 477: 355–363, 1994
6. Berridge M: Inositol triphosphate and calcium signaling. Nature 361: 315–325, 1993
7. Bevegård S, Lodin A: Postural circulatory changes at rest and during exercise in five patients with congenital absence of valves in the deep veins of the legs. Acta Medica Scandinavica 172: 21–29, 1962
8. Blaustein M, Ambesi A, Bloch R et al: Regulation of vascular smooth muscle contractility: Roles of sarcoplasmic reticulum (SR) and the sodium/calcium exchanger. Jpn J Pharmacol 58(Suppl II): 107P–114P, 1992
9. Bolotina V, Najibi S, Palacino J et al: Nitric oxide directly activates calcium-dependent potassium channels in vascular smooth muscle. Nature 368: 850–853, 1994
10. Bolton T, Lang R, Takewaki T: Mechanism of action of noradrenaline and carbachol on smooth muscle guinea-pig anterior mesenteric artery. J Physiol (Lond) 351: 549–572, 1984
11. Bond M, Kitazawa T, Somlyo AP et al: Release and recycling of calcium by the sarcoplasmic reticulum in guinea-pig portal vein smooth muscle. J Physiol, 355: 677–95, 1984
12. Boulanger C, Luscher T: Endothelin is released from the porcine aorta: Inhibition by endothelium-derived nitric oxide. J Clin Invest 85: 587–590, 1990
13. Boulanger E, Vanhoutte P: G proteins and endothelium-dependent relaxation. J Vasc Res 34: 175–185, 1997
14. Bridges E, Middleton R: Direct arterial vs oscillometric monitoring of blood pressure: Stop comparing and pick one (a decision making algorithm). Crit Care Nurs 17 (3): 58–72, 1997
15. Busse R, Mülsch A, Fleming I et al: Mechanisms of nitric oxide release from the vascular endothelium. Circulation 87(Suppl V): V18–V25, 1993
16. Chien S, Usami S, Skalak R: Blood flow in small tubes. In Renkin E, Michel C (eds): Handbook of Physiology, Vol Section 2, Vol IV, Microcirculation. Bethesda, MD, American Physiological Society, 1984
17. Clavell A, Stingo A, Margulies K et al: Physiological significance of endothelin: Its role in congestive heart failure. Circulation 87(Suppl V): V45–V50, 1993
18. Cohen D, Kemper M, Weissman C: Comprehensive physiological changes in the open heart patients, during the simple supine to lateral move. Crit Care Med 22: A35, 1994
19. Cohen R, Vanhoutte P. Endothelium-dependent hyperpolarization: Beyond nitric oxide and cyclic GMP. Circulation 92: 3337–3349, 1995
20. Coller B: GPIIb/IIIa antagonists: Pathophysiological and therapeutic insights from studies of c7E3Fab. Thromb Haemost 78: 730–735, 1997
21. Coller B: Platelets and thrombolytic therapy. N Engl J Med 322: 33–42, 1990
22. Conrad M: Functional Anatomy of the Circulation of the Lower Extremities. Chicago: Year Book, 1971
23. Crone E, Levitt D: Capillary permeability to small solutes. In Renkin E, Michel C (eds): Handbook of Physiology, Vol Section 2, Vol IV, Microcirculation, pp 411–466. Bethesda, MD, American Physiological Society, 1984
24. Curry R: Mechanics and thermodynamics of transcapillary exchange. In Renkin E, Michel C (eds): Handbook of Physiology, Vol Section 2, Vol IV, Microcirculation, pp 309–374. Bethesda, MD, American Physiological Society, 1984
25. de Belder A, Radomski M: Nitric oxide in the clinical arena. J Hypertens 12: 617–624, 1994
26. del Monte F, Kaumann A, Poole-Wilson P: Coexistence of functioning beta-1 and beta-2 adrenoreceptors in single myocytes from human ventricle. Circulation 88: 854–863, 1993
27. Duling B: Coordination of microcirculatory function with oxygen demand in skeletal muscle. In Kovach A, Hamar J, Szabo L (eds): Advances in Physiology: Cardiovascular Physiology: Microcirculation and Capillary Exchange, Vol 7, pp 1–16. Budapest: Akademiai Kaido, 1981
28. Duling B: Local control of microvascular function: Role in tissue oxygen supply. Annu Rev Physiol 42: 373–382, 1980
29. Eidelman L, Sprung C: Direct measurements and derived calculations using the pulmonary artery catheter. In Sprung C (ed): The Pulmonary Artery Catheter, 2nd ed, pp 101–118. Closter, NJ, Critical Care Research Associates, 1993
30. Faber J: In situ analysis of alpha-adrenoreceptors on arteriolar and venular smooth muscle in rat skeletal muscle microcirculation. Circ Res 62: 37–50, 1988
31. Fauchald P: Colloid osmotic pressure, plasma volume and interstitial fluid volume in patients with heart failure. Scand J Clin Lab Invest 45: 701–706, 1985
32. Feigl E: The arterial system. In Patton H, Fuchs A, Hille B et al (eds): Textbook of Physiology, Vol 2, 21st ed, pp 849–859. Philadelphia, WB Saunders, 1989
33. Feigl E: Neural control of coronary blood flow. J Vasc Res 35: 85–92, 1998
34. Félétou M, Vanhoutte P: Endothelium-dependent hyperpolarization of canine coronary smooth muscle. Br J Pharmacol 93: 515–524, 1988
35. Félétou M, Vanhoutte P: Endothelium-derived hyperpolarizing factor. Clin Exp Pharmacol Physiol 23: 1082–1090, 1996
36. Ferro C, Webb D: The clinical potential of endothelin receptor antagonists in cardiovascular medicine. Drugs 51: 12–27, 1996
37. Flavahan N, Cooke J, Shepherd J et al: Human postjunctional alpha-1 and alpha-2 adrenoreceptors: Differential distribution in arteries and limbs. J Pharmacol Exp Ther 241: 361–365, 1987
38. Flavahan N, Vanhoutte P: Endothelial cell signaling and endothelial dysfunction. Am J Hypertens 8: 28S–41S, 1995
39. Folkow B, Svanborg A: Physiology of cardiovascular aging. Physiol Rev 73: 725–764, 1993
40. Franklin S, Gustin W, Wong N et al: Hemodynamic patterns of age-related changes in blood pressure: The Framingham Heart Study. Circulation 96: 308–315, 1997
41. Furchott R, Zawadzki J: The obligatory role of endothelial cells in the relaxation of arterial smooth muscle by acetylcholine. Nature 288: 373–376, 1980
42. Gallagher D, O'Rourke M: What is the arterial pressure? In O'Rourke M, Safar M, Dzau V (eds): Arterial Vasodilation: Mechanisms and Therapy, pp 134–148. Philadelphia, Lea & Febiger, 1993
43. Gordon A: Contraction in smooth muscle and nonmuscle cells. In Patton H, Fuchs A, Hille B et al (eds): Textbook of

Physiology, Vol 1, 21st ed, pp 214–229. Philadelphia, WB Saunders, 1989

44. Granger D, Perry M: Permeability characteristics of the microcirculation. In Mortillaro N (ed): The Physiology and Pharmacology of the Microcirculation, Vol 1, pp 157–208. New York, Academic Press, 1983

45. Grimby G, Nilsson J, Sanne H: Cardiac output during exercise in patients with varicose veins. Scand J Clin Lab Invest 16: 21–30, 1964

46. Grossman W: Pressure measurement. In Baim DS, Grossman W (eds): Cardiac Catheterization, Angiography, and Intervention, 5th ed, pp 125–141. Baltimore, Williams & Wilkins, 1996

47. Guyton A, Granger H, Taylor A: Interstitial fluid pressure. Physiol Rev 51: 527–563, 1971

48. Hai C, Murphy R: Ca^{2+}, crossbridge phosphorylation, and contraction. Annu Rev Physiol 51: 285–291, 1989

49. Hai C, Murphy R: Cross-bridges phosphorylation and regulation of latch state in smooth muscle. Am J Physiol 254: C99–C106, 1988

50. Hai C, Rembold C, Murphy R: Can different four-state crossbridge models explain latch and the energetics of vascular smooth muscle? Adv Exp Med Biol 304: 159–170, 1991

51. Hainsworth R: Vascular capacitance: Its control and importance. Rev Physiol Biochem Pharmacol 105: 101–173, 1986

52. Hales S: Statistical essays containing haemastatics, or, an account of some hydraulic and hydrostatical experiments made on the blood and blood vessels of animals. In Willius F, Keys T (eds): Cardiac Classics, pp 127–155. St. Louis, CV Mosby, 1941

53. Horowitz A, Menice C, Laporte R et al: Mechanisms of smooth muscle contraction. Physiol Rev 76: 967–1003, 1996

54. Hudlicka O: Regulation of muscle blood flow (Editorial). Clin Physiol 5: 201–229, 1985

55. Ito M, Hartshorne D: Phosphorylation of myosin as a regulatory mechanism in smooth muscle. Prog Clin Biol Res 5 (327): 57–72, 1990

56. Ito T, Ikemoto T, Takadura S: Involvement of Ca^{+2} influx-induced Ca^{+2} release in contraction of intact vascular smooth muscles. Am J Physiol 261: H1464–H1470, 1991

57. Johnson J: Circulation to the skin. In Patton H, Fuchs A, Hille B et al (eds): Textbook of Physiology, Vol 2, 21st ed, pp 898–910. Philadelphia, WB Saunders, 1989

58. Joyner M, Dietz N: Nitric oxide and vasodilation in human limbs. J Appl Physiol 83: 1785–1796, 1997

59. Katusic Z, Vanhoutte P: Superoxide anion is an endothelium-derived contracting factor. Am J Physiol 257: H33–H37, 1989

60. Kern M, Aguirre F: Aortic regurgitation. In Kern M (ed): Hemodynamic Rounds: Interpretation of Cardiac Pathophysiology from Pressure Waveform Analysis, pp 17–25. New York, Wiley-Liss, 1993

61. Koller A, Kaley G: Endothelium regulates skeletal muscle microcirculation by a blood flow velocity sensing mechanism. Am J Physiol 258: H916–H920, 1990a

62. Koller A, Kaley G: Prostaglandins mediate arteriolar dilation to increased blood flow in skeletal muscle microcirculation. Circ Res 67: 529–534, 1990

63. Krum H, Goldsmith R, Wilshire-Clement M et al: Role of endothelin in the exercise intolerance of chronic heart failure. Am J Cardiol 75: 1282–1283, 1995

64. Kukovetz W, Holzmann S, Schmidt K: Cellular mechanisms of action of therapeutic nitric oxide donors. Eur Heart J 12(Suppl E): 16–24, 1991

65. Lakatta E: Cardiovascular system. In Masoro E (ed): Handbook of Physiology: Aging, pp 413–474. Bethesda, MD, American Physiological Society, 1995

66. Landis E: Micro-injection studies of capillary permeability II. Am J Physiol 82: 217–238, 1927

67. Lands A, Arnold A, McAuliff J et al: Differentiation of receptor systems activated by sympathomimetic amines. Nature 214: 597–598, 1967

68. Länne T, Lundvall J: Very rapid net transcapillary fluid absorption from skeletal muscle and skin in man during pronounced hypovolaemic circulatory stress. Acta Physiol Scand 136: 1–6, 1989

69. Laurindo F, Pedro M, Barbeiro H et al: Vascular free radical release: Ex vivo and in vivo evidence for a flow-dependent endothelial mechanism. Circ Res 74: 700–709, 1994

70. Lazalde C, Barr L: Identification of four state models of regulation of contraction of smooth muscle. Prog Clin Biol Res 5 (327): 51–56, 1990

71. LeDoux D: Acquired valvular heart disease. In Woods S, Sivarajan Froelicher E, Halpenny C et al (eds): Cardiac Nursing, 3rd ed, pp 798–819. Philadelphia, JB Lippincott, 1995

72. Levick J: Capillary filtration-absorption balance reconsidered in light of dynamic extravascular factors. Exp Physiol 76: 825–857, 1991

73. Levick J: Fluid exchange across the endothelium. Int J Microcirc Clin Exp 17: 241–247, 1997

74. Levitzky M: Pulmonary Physiology, 4th ed. New York, McGraw-Hill, 1995

75. Love M, McMurray J: Endothelin in chronic heart failure: Current position and future prospects. Cardiovasc Res 31: 665–674, 1996

76. Lüscher T: Endothelium-derived nitric oxide: The endogenous vasodilator in the human cardiovascular system. Eur Heart J 12(Suppl E): 2–11, 1991

77. Lüscher T, Boulanger C, Yang Z et al: Interactions between endothelium-derived relaxing and contracting factors in health and cardiovascular disease. Circulation 87(Suppl V): V36–V44, 1993

78. Lüscher T, Dohi Y, Tschudi M: Endothelium-dependent regulation of resistance arteries: Alterations with aging and hypertension. J Cardiovasc Pharmacol 19(Suppl 5): 534–542, 1992

79. Lüscher T, Vanhoutte P: The Endothelium: Modulation of Cardiovascular Function. Boca Raton, FL, CRC Press, 1990

80. Marston S: What is a latch? New ideas about tonic contraction in smooth muscle. J Muscle Res Cell Motil 10: 97–100, 1989

81. Matlib M: Role of sarcolemmal membrane sodium-calcium exchange in vascular smooth muscle tension. Ann NY Acad Sci 657: 531–542, 1991

82. McDonald T, Pelzer S, Trautwien W et al: Regulations and modulation of calcium channels in cardiac, skeletal, and smooth muscle cells. Physiol Rev 74: 365–507, 1994

83. McHugh J, Cheek D: Nitric oxide and regulation of vascular tone: Pharmacological and physiological considerations. Am J Crit Care 7: 131–140, 1998

84. Mellander S: On the control of capillary fluid transfer by precapillary and postcapillary vascular adjustment. Microvasc Res 15: 319–330, 1978

85. Meridith I, Yeung A, Weidinger F et al: Role of impaired endothelium-dependent vasodilation in ischemic manifestations of coronary artery disease. Circulation 87(Suppl V): V56–V66, 1993

86. Michel C: Capillary permeability and how it may change. J Physiol (Lond) 404: 1–29, 1988

87. Michel C: Fluid movements through capillary walls. In Renkin E, Michel C (eds): Handbook of Physiology, Vol Section 2, Vol IV, Microcirculation, pp 375–409. Bethesda, MD, American Physiological Society, 1984

88. Michel C, Phillips M: Steady-state fluid filtration at different capillary pressures in perfused frog mesenteric capillaries. J Physiol (Lond) 388: 421–435, 1987

89. Miller V, Vanhoutte P: Enhanced release of endothelium-derived factor(s) by chronic increases in blood flow. Am J Physiol 255: H4R46–H4R51, 1988

90. Miller W, Burnett J: Blood vessel physiology and pathophysiology. Rheum Dis Clin North Am 16: 251–260, 1990

91. Mohrman D, Heller L: Cardiovascular Physiology, 4th ed. New York, McGraw-Hill, 1997

92. Mombouli J, Nakashima M, Hamra M et al: Endothelium-dependent relaxation and hyperpolarization evoked by bradykinin in canine coronary arteries: Enhancement by exercise-training. Br J Pharmacol 117: 413–418, 1996

93. Mombouli J, Vanhoutte P: Endothelium-derived hyperpolarizing factor(s): Updating the unknown. Trends Pharmacol Sci 18: 252–256, 1997

94. Moncada S, Palmer R, Higgs E: Nitric oxide: Physiology, pathophysiology, and pharmacology. Pharmacol Rev 43: 109–142, 1991

95. Moreland R, Cilea J, Moreland S: Calcium dependent regulation of vascular smooth muscle contraction. Adv Exp Med Biol 308: 81–94, 1991

96. Morgan J, Perreault C, Morgan K: The cellular basis of contraction and relaxation in cardiac and vascular smooth muscle. Am Heart J 3: 961–968, 1991

97. Mügge A, Elwell J, Peterson T et al: Release of intact endothelium-derived relaxing factor depends on endothelial superoxide dismutase activity. Am J Physiol 260: C219–C225, 1991

98. Mulvany M, Aalkjeër C: Structure and function of small arteries. Physiol Rev 70: 922–961, 1990

99. Murphy R: What is special about smooth muscle? The significance of covalent crossbridge regulation. FASEB J 8: 311–318, 1994

100. Murphy R, Rembold C, Hai C: Contraction in smooth muscle: What is a latch? Prog Clin Biol Res 5 (327): 39–50, 1990

101. Nagao T, Nakashima M, Smart F et al: Potentiation of endothelium-dependent hyperpolarization to serotonin by dietary intake of NC 020, a defined fish oil, in the porcine coronary artery. J Cardiovasc Pharmacol 26: 679–681, 1995

102. Nayler W: The Endothelins, pp 139–147. Berlin, Springer-Verlag, 1990

103. Nelson M, Patlak J, Worley J et al: Calcium channels, potassium channels, and voltage dependence of arterial smooth muscle tone. Am J Physiol 259: C3–C18, 1990

104. Nichols W, O'Rourke M: McDonald's Blood Flow in Arteries, 3rd ed, pp 251–269. Philadelphia, Lea & Febiger, 1990

105. Nutter D: Measurement of the systolic blood pressure. In Hurst J (ed): The Heart, Arteries, and Veins 5th ed, p 182. New York, McGraw Hill, 1982.

106. Ohyanagi M, Faber J, Nishigaki K: Differential activation of alpha$_1$- and alpha$_2$-adrenoreceptors on microvascular smooth muscle during sympathetic nerve stimulation. Circ Res 68: 232–244, 1991

107. Opie L: The Heart: Physiology from Cell to Circulation. Philadelphia, Lippincott–Raven, 1998

108. O'Rourke M: Wave travel and reflection in the arterial system. In O'Rourke M, Safar M, Dzau V (eds): Arterial Vasodilation: Mechanisms and Therapy, pp 10–22. Philadelphia, Lea & Febiger, 1993

109. O'Rourke M: What is blood pressure? Am J Hypertens 3: 803–810, 1990

110. O'Rourke M, Avolio A, Kelly R et al: Difference between central and upper limb pressure wave forms in man. In O'Rourke M, Safar M, Dzau V (eds): Arterial Vasodilation: Mechanisms and Therapy, pp 117–133. Philadelphia, Lea & Febiger, 1993

111. O'Rourke R: The measurement of systemic blood pressure: normal and abnormal pulsations of the arteries and veins. In Hurst J, Schlant R (eds): The Heart, Arteries, and Veins, 7th ed, pp 149–162. New York, McGraw-Hill, 1990

112. Palmer R, Ferrige A, Moncada S: Nitric oxide release accounts for the biological activity of endothelium-derived relaxing factor. Nature 327: 524–526, 1987

113. Pappenheimer J: Contributions to microvascular research of Jean Leonard Marie Poiseuille. In Renkin E, Michel C (eds): Handbook of Physiology, Vol Section 2, Vol IV, Microcirculation (Part 1), pp 1–10. Bethesda, MD, American Physiological Society, 1984

114. Pappenheimer J, Soto-Rivera A: Effective osmotic pressure of the plasma proteins and other quantities associated with capillary circulation in the hindlimbs of cats and dogs. Am J Physiol 152: 471–491, 1948

115. Pearson P, Schaff H, Vanhoutte P: Long-term impairment of endothelium-dependent relaxations to aggregating platelets after reperfusion injury in canine coronary arteries. Circulation 81: 1921–1927, 1990

116. Pohl U, Holtz J, Busse R et al: Crucial role of endothelium in the vasodilator response to increased flow in vivo. Hypertension 8: 37–44, 1986

117. Price J: Influence of pressure and flow on constriction of blood vessels. J Fla Med Assoc 78: 825–827, 1991

118. Radomski M, Moncada S: Regulation of platelet function by nitric oxide. Thromb Haemost Disorders 7: 1–7, 1993

119. Reid J: Modulation of vascular reactivity by endothelium derived factors. Proc West Pharmacol Soc 36: 81–87, 1993

120. Remington J, O'Brien L: Construction of aortic flow pulse from pressure pulse. Am J Physiol 218: 437–447, 1970

121. Renkin E: Control of microcirculation and blood-tissue exchange. In Renkin E, Michel C (eds): Handbook of Physiology, Vol IV (Part 2), pp 627–687. Bethesda, MD, American Physiological Society, 1984

122. Renkin E: Microcirculation and exchange. In Patton H, Fuches A, Hille B et al (eds): Textbook of Physiology, Vol 2, 21st ed, pp 860–878. Philadelphia, WB Saunders, 1989

123. Renkin E: Multiple pathways of capillary permeability. Circ Res 41: 735–743, 1977

124. Renkin E: Some consequences of capillary permeability to macromolecules: Starling's hypothesis reconsidered. Am J Physiol 250: H706–H710, 1986

125. Rhodin J: Anatomy of the microcirculation. In Effros R, Schmid-Schonbein H, Ditzel J (eds): Microcirculation, pp 11–17. New York, Academic Press, 1981

126. Rhodin J: Architecture of the vessel wall. In Bohr D, Somlyo A, Sparks H (eds): Handbook of Physiology, Section 2, Vol 2, pp 1–31. Bethesda, MD, American Physiological Society, 1980

127. Ross R, Glomset J: The pathogenesis of atherosclerosis. N Engl J Med 295: 369–377, 1976

128. Rothe C: Venous system: Physiology of the capacitance vessels. In Shepherd J, Abboud F (eds): Handbook of Physiology: The Cardiovascular System, Peripheral Circulation and Organ Blood Flow, Vol Section 2, Vol III (Part 1), pp 397–452. Bethesda, MD, American Physiological Society, 1983

129. Rowell L: Human Cardiovascular Control, p 500. New York, Oxford University Press, 1993

130. Rowell L: Human Circulation: Regulation During Physical Stress. New York, Oxford University Press, 1986

131. Rowell L, Brengelmann G, Blackmon J et al: Disparities between aortic and peripheral pulse pressures induced by upright exercise and vasomotor changes in man. Circulation 37: 954–964, 1968

132. Rowell LB, O'Leary DS, Kellogg DLJ: Integration of cardiovascular control systems in dynamic exercise. In Rowell L, Sheperd J (eds): Handbook of Physiology, Exercise: Regulation and Integration of Multiple Systems, Vol Section 12, pp 770–838. Bethesda, MD, Oxford University Press, 1996

133. Rubanyi G, Romero J, Vanhoutte P: Flow-induced release of endothelium-derived relaxing factor. Am J Physiol 250: H1145–H1149, 1986

134. Schad H, Flowaczny H, Brechtelsbauer H et al: The significance of respiration on thoracic duct flow in relation to other driving forces of lymph flow. Pflugers Arch 378: 121–125, 1978

135. Scher A: The veins and venous return. In Patton H, Fuchs A, Hille B et al (eds): Textbook of Physiology, Vol 2, 21st ed, pp 879–886. Philadelphia, WB Saunders, 1989

136. Schmid-Schonbein G: Microlymphatics and lymph flow. Physiol Rev 70: 987–1028, 1990

137. Scott-Burden T, Vanhoutte P: The endothelium as a regulator of smooth muscle proliferation. Circulation 87(Suppl V): V51–V55, 1993

138. Scott-Burden T, Vanhoutte P: Regulation of vascular smooth muscle cell proliferation: Role of endothelium-derived relaxing factor (nitric oxide). J Vasc Biol 3: 445–446, 1991

139. Seo B, Oemar B, Siebenmann R et al: Both ETA and ETB receptors mediate contraction to endothelin-1 in human blood vessels. Circulation 89: 1203–1208, 1994

140. Sharkey S: A Guide to Interpretation of Hemodynamic Data in the Coronary Care Unit. Philadelphia, Lippincott–Raven, 1997

141. Sheperd J, Vanhoutte P: The Human Cardiovascular System: Facts and Concepts. New York, Raven Press, 1979

142. Shepherd J: Circulation to skeletal muscle. In Shepherd J, Abboud F, Geiger S (eds): Handbook of Physiology: The Cardiovascular System: Peripheral Circulation and Organ Blood Flow, Vol Section 2, Vol III (Part 1), pp 319–370. Bethesda, MD, American Physiological Society, 1983

143. Shimokawa H, Lam J, Chesebro J et al: Effects of dietary supplementation with cod-liver oil on endothelium-dependent response in porcine coronary arteries. Circulation 76: 898–905, 1987

144. Siegel F, Mironneau J, Schnalke F et al: Vasodilation evoked by K+ channel opening. Prog Clin Biol Res (5)327: 299–306, 1990

145. Simionescu M, Simionescu N: Ultrastructure of the microvascular wall: Functional correlations. In Renkin E, Michel C (eds): Handbook of Physiology: Microcirculation, Vol Section 2, Vol IV, pp 41–101. Bethesda, MD, American Physiological Society, 1984

146. Simionescu M, Simionescu N: Ultrastructure of the microvascular wall: Functional correlations. In Renkin E, Michel C (eds): Handbook of Physiology, Vol Section 2, Vol IV, Microcirculation, pp 41–101. Bethesda, MD, American Physiological Society, 1984

147. Smulyan H, Safar M: Systolic blood pressure revisited. J Am Coll Cardiol 29: 1407–1413, 1997

148. Somlyo A, Himpens B: Cell calcium and its regulation in smooth muscle. FASEB J 3: 2266–2276, 1989

149. Somlyo A, Somlyo A: Signal transduction and regulation in smooth muscle. Nature 372: 231–236, 1994

150. Somylo A, Somylo A: Principles of membrane biochemistry and their application to the pathophysiology of cardiovascular disease. In Fozzard H, Haber E, Jennings R et al (eds): The Heart and Cardiovascular System, pp 839–860. New York, Raven Press, 1991

151. Sparks HJ: Effect of local metabolic factors on vascular smooth muscle. In Bohr D, Somlyo A, Sparks H (eds): Handbook of Physiology: The Cardiovascular System: Vascular Smooth Muscle, Vol Section 2, Vol II, pp 475–513. Bethesda, MD, American Physiological Society, 1980

152. Spedding M, Paoletti R: Classification of calcium channels and the sites of action of drugs modifying channel function. Pharmacol Rev 44: 363–376, 1992

153. Sperelakis N, Ohya Y: Cyclic nucleotide regulation of Ca^{2+} slow channels and neurotransmitter release in vascular muscle. Prog Clin Biol Res 5 (327): 277–298, 1992

154. Sperelakis N, Tohse N, Ohya Y: Regulation of calcium slow channels in cardiac muscle and vascular smooth muscle cells. Adv Exp Med Biol 311: 163–187, 1992

155. Starling E: On the absorption of fluids from the connective tissue spaces. J Physiol (Lond) 19: 312–316, 1896

156. Taddei S, Virdis A, Mattei P et al: Aging and endothelial function in normotensive subjects and patients with essential hypertension. Circulation 91: 1981–1987, 1995

157. Thomas G, Ramwell P: Endothelium-derived relaxing factor and the vascular role of guanidino compounds. Transplant Proc 25: 2057–2060, 1993

158. Trivella M, Broten T, Feigl E: Beta-receptor subtypes in the canine coronary circulation. Am J Physiol 259: H1575–H1585, 1990

159. Vallance P: Endothelial regulation of vascular tone. Postgrad Med J 68: 697–701, 1992

160. van Bortel L, Spek J: Influence of aging on arterial compliance. J Hum Hypertens 12: 583–586, 1998

161. Vane J, Anggard E, Botting R: Regulatory functions of the vascular endothelium. N Engl J Med 323: 27–36, 1990

162. Vanhoutte P: Endothelium and control of vascular function. State of the art lecture. Hypertension 13: 658–667, 1989

163. Vanhoutte P: Endothelium-dependent responses and inhibition of angiotensin-converting enzyme. Clin Exp Pharmacol Physiol 23(Suppl 1): S23–S29, 1996

164. Vanhoutte P: Endothelium-derived relaxing and contracting factors. Adv Nephrol 19: 3–16, 1990

165. Vanhoutte P: Hypercholesterolaemia, atherosclerosis and release of endothelium-derived relaxing factors by aggregating factors. Eur Heart 12(Suppl E): 3E–12E, 1991

166. Vanhoutte P: Other endothelium-derived vasoactive factors. Circulation 87(Suppl V): V9–V17, 1993

167. Vanhoutte P: Vasodilatation: Vascular Smooth Muscle, Peptides, Autonomic Nerves, and Endothelium. New York, Raven Press, 1988

168. Vanhoutte P, Boulanger C: Endothelium dependent responses in hypertension. Hypertens Res 18: 87–98, 1995

169. Vanhoutte P, Boulanger C, Illiano S et al: Endothelium-dependent effects of converting-enzyme inhibitors. J Cardiovasc Pharmacol 22(Suppl 5): S10–S16, 1993

170. Vanhoutte P, Boulanger C, Mombouli J: Endothelium-derived relaxing factors and converting enzyme inhibition. Am J Cardiol 76: E3–E12, 1995

171. Vanhoutte P, Mombouli J: Vascular endothelium: Vasoactive mediators. Prog Cardiovasc Dis 49: 229–238, 1996

172. Varon A: Arterial, central venous, and pulmonary artery catheters. In Civetta J, Taylor R, Kirby R (eds): Critical Care, pp 847–865. Philadelphia, Lippincott–Raven, 1997

173. Wagner O, Christ G, Wojta J et al: Polar secretion of endothelin-1 by cultured endothelial cells. J Biol Chem 267: 16066–16068, 1992

174. West J: Respiratory Physiology, 5th ed. Baltimore, Williams & Wilkins, 1990

175. Wiedeman M: Dimensions of blood vessels from distributing artery to collecting vein. Circ Res 12: 375–378, 1963

176. Yanigasawa M: The endothelin system: A new target for therapeutic intervention. Circulation 89: 1320–1322, 1994

177. Yanigisawa M, Kurihara H, Kimura S: A novel potent vasoconstrictor peptide produced by vascular endothelial cells. Nature 332: 411–415, 1988

178. Zusman R: Eicosanoids: Prostaglandins, thromboxane, and prostacyclin. In Fozzard H, Haber E, Jennings R et al (eds): The Heart and Cardiovascular System, Vol 2, pp 1797–1815. New York, Raven Press, 1992

179. Zweifach B, Lipowsky H: Pressure-flow relations in blood and lymph microcirculation. In Renkin E, Michel C (eds): Handbook of Physiology, Vol Section 2, Vol IV, Microcirculation, pp 251–307. Bethesda, MD, American Physiological Society, 1984

3

The Pulmonary Circulation and Gas Transport

POLLY E. GARDNER

The pulmonary circulation removes oxygen from the atmosphere, transfers the oxygen to the blood in the alveoli, and exchanges carbon dioxide. Once oxygen has diffused from the alveoli to the pulmonary blood, the systemic circulation transports oxygen and nutrients from the gastrointestinal tract to the various tissues of the body. The systemic circulation also transports electrolytes, hormones, cells, and immune substances and carries waste products to the excretory organs for disposal. The principal functions of the pulmonary circulation (i.e., exchanges gases with outside environment) and systemic circulation (i.e., exchanges gases with inside environment, tissue, and cells) render them indispensable. Their primary purpose is to maintain homeostasis.

Each tissue controls its internal environment depending on its specific needs. The amount of oxygen released into the tissues and the amount of carbon dioxide released from the tissues are regulated by tissue activity. Oxygen delivery or transport to a particular tissue depends on the amount of oxygen inspired during ventilation, the adequacy of pulmonary gas exchange, perfusion of blood flow to the tissues, and the capacity of the blood to carry oxygen.[21] The blood flow to a particular vascular bed depends on the cardiac output and the degree of tone of the vascular bed. Thus, the chief aim of both circuits is to maintain a balance between oxygen consumption and demand for the various tissues of the body.[11,31]

The systemic circulation was discussed in Chapter 2. This chapter addresses the structural and functional characteristics of the pulmonary circulation, pulmonary gas exchange, and the transport of oxygen and carbon dioxide.

THE PULMONARY CIRCULATION

The pulmonary circulation is in series with the systemic circulation and receives the same cardiac output, approximately 5 to 6 L/min at rest for an adult, 70-kg man. The pulmonary circulation has only 10% the capacity of the systemic circulation, yet it must accommodate the same ejected volume. The primary function of the pulmonary circulation is to expose the blood to alveolar air so that oxygen can be taken up by the blood and carbon dioxide can be excreted.

Pulmonary Gas Exchange

Pulmonary gas exchange is the end product of respiration; its goal is to maintain arterial oxygen partial pressure (PaO_2) and arterial carbon dioxide partial pressure ($PaCO_2$) in normal ranges. Gas exchange of oxygen uptake and carbon dioxide elimination can be divided into four subgroups: ventilation, diffusion, perfusion, and work of breathing.[15]

Ventilation is the process of the exchange of air between the atmosphere (external environment) and alveoli. It involves the distribution of air into the pulmonary structures of the tracheobrachial tree to the alveoli of the lung. Lung volumes can be measured to assess the static properties of the lung, described in Table 3-1.[15] *Diffusion* is the movement of oxygen and carbon dioxide across the alveoli to the pulmonary capillaries. Gases move by diffusion from an area of high partial pressure to an area of low partial pressure.

Perfusion occurs when mixed venous blood flows from the peripheral circulation and distributes across the pulmonary capillaries. The *work of breathing* is the process of ventilation that adjusts to metabolic demands. The exchange of gases at the tissue level is known as the process of respiration.

Nonpulmonary Functions

Lung capillary endothelial cells produce, remove, modify, or inactivate certain bioactive substances such as prostaglandins, angiotensin, bradykinin, and norepinephrine.[24] During passage through the lungs, these substances can be partially or

TABLE 3-1 Lung Volumes and Capacities		
	Typical Values in Liters	
Lung Volumes and Capacities	**Men***	**Women†**
TV (tidal volume)	0.5	0.5
Amount of air that enters the lung with each normal breath. This value is reported as part of vital capacity or inspiratory capacity.		
TLC (total lung capacity)	6.4	4.9
Amount of gas volume the lungs contain when fully expanded.		
VC (vital capacity)	1.7	1.4
Amount of volume of gas that can be exhaled.		
RV (residual volume)	1.5	1.2
Amount of gas volume remaining in the lung at the end of maximal expiration.		
FRC (functional residual capacity)	2.2	2.6
Volume of gas at end expiration of normal breath.		
IRV (inspiratory reserve volume)	3.1	2.8
Inspiration in addition to normal inspiration.		
IC (inspiratory capacity)	3.6	3.1
Maximum inspiration from resting level.		
ERV (expiratory reserve volume)	1.5	1.2
Volume of air forcibly exhaled from resting position.		

*Age 40 years, weight 70 kg, height 175 cm.
†Age 40 years, weight 60 kg, height 160 cm.

completely removed from the blood. The lungs can also add substances to the blood, such as histamine and angiotensin II. The lungs can serve as a filter, trapping and dissolving small clots produced in the systemic circulation.[28]

Ventilation—Perfusion Matching

Pulmonary precapillary vasomotor and bronchiolar responses serve to match pulmonary capillary perfusion to alveolar ventilation. Unlike in the systemic circulation, where hypoxemia, decreased pH, or increased amounts of carbon dioxide cause local vasodilation in the pulmonary vascular system, any of these conditions may cause pulmonary arteriolar vasoconstriction. In well-ventilated regions, there is little vasoconstriction in response to deoxygenated blood. In poorly ventilated areas, where the amount of alveolar oxygen is less than normal, such as when a bronchus is obstructed, vasoconstriction occurs and blood is shunted to other lung areas.[17] Often this hypoxic vaso-

constriction is compounded by decreased pH, which has a similar vasoconstrictor action.[3]

Hypoxic vasoconstriction serves a useful role in diverting blood flow to areas of the lung with more abundant oxygen, thus improving pulmonary gas exchange. Hypoxic vasoconstriction occurs in conditions such as high altitude or in patients with chronic obstructive pulmonary disease.[30] When blood flow to a certain lung area is reduced, there is a subsequent decrease in the alveolar carbon dioxide concentration. The bronchial smooth muscle responds to the decreased alveolar carbon dioxide levels by constricting, thus shifting ventilation away from a poorly perfused area.[11]

Constriction of the pulmonary vessels can be induced by pharmacologic agents such as norepinephrine, serotonin, histamine, and prostaglandins.[21,24,30] Pharmacologic agents that induce vasodilation of the pulmonary vessels include isoproterenol and acetylcholine.[30]

Ventilation and perfusion must occur in equal proportion in the various regions of the lung to achieve adequate gas exchange. Gas exchange determines the levels of alveolar oxygen partial pressure (PO_2) and carbon dioxide partial pressure (PCO_2). An adequate alveolar PO_2 depends on a balance of two factors: the rate of removal of oxygen by the pulmonary arterial blood and the rate of replenishment of oxygen by alveolar ventilation. An adequate alveolar PCO_2 depends on the rate of removal of carbon dioxide by alveolar ventilation.

Impairment of gas exchange, which results in a decrease in PaO_2 and an increase in tissue PCO_2, can be caused by hypoventilation and shunt. Clinically, these conditions can result in hypoxemia.

Hypoventilation can result from trauma to the chest wall, paralysis of the respiratory muscles, and medications such as morphine sulfate and barbiturates, which depress the respiratory center. *Shunt* refers to blood that enters the arterial system without going through ventilated regions of the lung. Under normal conditions, there exists a small physiologic shunt because of the difference in PO_2 between alveolar gas and end-capillary blood. Physiologically, mixed venous blood from the pulmonary arterial bed mixes with capillary blood from pulmonary venous beds, thereby lowering the end-capillary PO_2. This difference can become larger in conditions such as ventricular septal defect, in which greater amounts of venous blood are added to arterial blood across the defect, resulting in a lower PaO_2.

An important clinical characteristic of a shunt is that the hypoxemia cannot be resolved by placing the patient on an inspired oxygen fraction (FIO_2) of 100%. Because the shunt blood bypasses the ventilated regions of the lung, it is not exposed to the higher alveolar PO_2. Another feature of a shunt results in a normal level of alveolar PCO_2 in arterial blood. Central chemoreceptors sense a rising PCO_2, thus increasing the respiratory drive. In some patients with shunt, the arterial PCO_2 may be low because of increases in respiratory drive due to hypoxemia.

A key component in pulmonary gas exchange is the ventilation—perfusion ratio ($\dot{V}/\dot{Q}$). The concentration of gases (i.e., oxygen, carbon dioxide, nitrogen) in the various regions of the lung is determined by the ratio of the rate of ventilation to the rate of perfusion (blood flow). Obstruction to ventilation or perfusion leads to alteration in this ratio and, consequently, the composition of gases. Inequality in ventilation—perfusion hinders the lung's ability to replenish oxygen and remove carbon dioxide.

STRUCTURAL CHARACTERISTICS

Pulmonary Vessels

The pulmonary trunk originates from the base of the right ventricle, extends 5 cm, and divides into the right and left pulmonary arteries. The right pulmonary artery is positioned posterior to both the aorta and superior vena cava and anterior to the right mainstem bronchus. The left pulmonary artery extends over the left main bronchus and divides into lobar branches. The pulmonary arteries and segmental and lobar branches are composed of elastic arteries to maintain low vascular resistance. These arteries contain smooth muscle with the capability of vasoconstriction and vasodilatation.

The muscular arteries have internal and external elastic laminae with a layer of smooth muscle cells. The acinour and supernumerary arteries (precapillary arteries) are muscular. Increases in pulmonary vascular resistance come from the precapillary arteries.

Arterioles are vessels with a thin intima and a single elastic lamina. These vessels make up the accessory branches of the respiratory tree and end at the alveolar capillary network.

Pulmonary Endothelium

The entire pulmonary vascular bed is lined with endothelium. The endothelium serves a number of functions, including modulating vascular smooth muscle tone, releasing relaxing and contracting mediators, and activating or deactivating circulating mediators. Angiotensin-converting enzyme, released by the pulmanary endotrelium is responsible for the conversion of angiotensin I to angiotensin II. This enzyme also deactivates the peptide bradykinin. In addition, the endothelium contains adhesion molecules that migrate to areas of inflammation when activated by local chemoattractants.

Muscles of Respiration

The inspiratory and expiratory muscles determine the rate of inspiratory and expiratory airflow and generate negative and positive intrathoracic pressures. The primary muscles of inspiration include the diaphragm and the parasternal intercartilaginous, external intercostal, and scalenus muscles. The sternocleidomastoid muscles serve as accessory muscles of inspiration. During inspiration, the diaphragm and parasternal and external intercostals contract, producing deflation of the rib cage. Abdominal muscles contribute to expiration under conditions of increased ventilatory demand such as exercise or hypercapnia.

PULMONARY VASCULAR BED

The pulmonary vascular bed provides a low-pressure and low-resistance avenue for movement of venous blood from the right heart to the left heart. It also provides a large surface area to facilitate contact between alveolar gas and blood and augment production or removal of vasoactive substances.

Pulmonary vascular resistance is seven to eight times lower than systemic resistance. No other single organ receives the entire output of one ventricle. Consequently, the pulmonary circulation has high blood flow and acts as a reservoir for the right ventricle.

The pulmonary vascular bed is regulated by passive factors such as lung volume and active factors such as alveolar gas. These mechanisms alter pulmonary vascular resistance.

BLOOD RESERVOIR

Pulmonary blood volume decreases or is diverted to the systemic circulation in conditions such as generalized systemic vasodilation, the standing position, positive end-expiratory pressure, or circulatory shock. Conditions that increase pulmonary blood volume include generalized systemic vasoconstriction,[10] the supine position, mitral stenosis, and left heart failure.

As in the systemic circulation, there is a large volume of blood sequestered in the pulmonary veins, usually 10% of the total volume, which often serves an important secondary function as a vascular volume reserve. The left heart transiently increases its output over that of the right heart to accommodate the increased volume.

EFFECTS OF LUNG PRESSURES

Because the alveolar air spaces surround collapsible capillaries, intrapleural and alveolar pressures affect pulmonary capillary pressures. Pulmonary blood flow reflects this influence during respiration in the upright and lateral recumbent positions. Both inspiration and expiration of the ventilatory cycle induce fluctuating negative intrathoracic pressures that influence the pulmonary vessels. Pulmonary capillaries are also affected by alveolar pressure to a certain degree. However, the capillary–alveolar membrane is thin and compliant enough to approximate pulmonary capillary pressure to alveolar pressure. With a change from supine to standing position, a hydrostatic pressure difference of 20 cm H_2O is created between the apex and base of the lung.

West[32–34] described the hydrostatic effect of body position on pulmonary capillary flow by dividing the lung into three regions (Fig. 3-1). The region of zone 1 is represented above the heart in an upright body position, where pulmonary alveolar pressure (PA) may exceed pulmonary arterial pressure (Pa) and pulmonary venous pressure (Pv) (PA > Pa > Pv). In a normal physiologic state, pulmonary arterial pressure is sufficient to maintain blood flow to the top of the lung. Thus, this zone does not usually develop. However, in conditions that reduce arterial pressure (e.g., hemorrhage) or increase alveolar pressure (e.g., positive end-expiratory pressure), a zone 1 region may be created. In this state, the apex of the lung continues to be ventilated yet unperfused, creating alveolar dead space that is ineffective for gas exchange.[32]

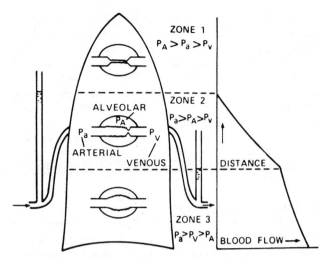

FIGURE 3-1 Model to explain the zones of the lungs. PA, alveolar pressure; Pa, pulmonary arterial pressure; Pv, pulmonary venous pressure. (From West JB: Respiratory Physiology: The Essentials, 2nd ed, p 43. Baltimore, Williams & Wilkins, 1979.)

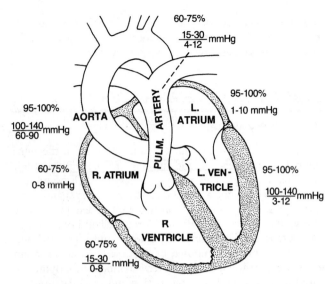

FIGURE 3-2 Heart diagram illustrating normal ranges of oxygen saturation (in percentage) and pressure (in millimeters of mercury) in heart chambers and great vessels.

The region of zone 2 is represented at the level of the left atrium of the heart, where pulmonary arterial pressure increases because of the hydrostatic effect. At this point, Pa exceeds PA, which continues to exceed venous pressures (Pa > PA > Pv). Although Pa exceeds PA, alveolar pressure is still higher than the pressure of the left atrium.

The region of zone 3, below the left atrium, is where both Pa and left atrial pressures exceed PA (Pa > Pv > PA). Blood flow, determined by the difference between arterial and venous pressures, is increased markedly in this region of the lung because of capillary distention. A zone 3 region creates a continuous column of fluid between the pulmonary artery and the left atrium. Reliable pulmonary artery pressure measurements can be obtained when the tip of the pulmonary artery catheter is located in zone 3.

ALVEOLAR—CAPILLARY TRANSFER OF OXYGEN AND CARBON DIOXIDE

Pulmonary Respiration

Each gas in a mixture of gases behaves as if it alone occupied the total volume and exerts a partial pressure independent of the other gases present. Gases equilibrate across the alveolar—capillary membranes by simple passive diffusion, moving from an area of greater partial pressure to a region of lesser partial pressure.

The partial pressure of oxygen in pulmonary arterial blood (venous blood from the body) is approximately 40 mm Hg, whereas pulmonary alveolar partial pressures of oxygen are approximately 100 mm Hg; thus, oxygen moves into the blood. The partial pressure of systemic arterial oxygen is slightly less than 100 mm Hg because of the admixture of oxygenated and deoxygenated blood. Blood from pulmonary veins is mixed with some deoxygenated blood

from bronchial veins and in the left heart is mixed with deoxygenated blood from thebesian veins draining cardiac muscle tissue. The percentage of oxygen in the different chambers of the heart is depicted in Figure 3-2.

Carbon dioxide is removed in the pulmonary capillaries. The partial pressure of carbon dioxide in pulmonary arterial blood (systemic venous blood) is 46 mm Hg and that of blood leaving the lung (which becomes systemic arterial blood) is 40 mm Hg. The release of carbon dioxide is aided by the conversion of hemoglobin to oxyhemoglobin.

Tissue Respiration

Maintenance of adequate tissue oxygenation depends on complex mechanisms, including transport of oxygen, microvascular control (systemic and local), and intact metabolic cellular function. Figure 3-3 illustrates the processes by which oxygen is transported from the atmosphere to the mitochondria.

Alveolar oxygen diffuses into the pulmonary capillaries. The amount of oxygen transferred depends on the mechanics of the ventilation—perfusion relationship of the lungs and the amount of inspired oxygen. Oxygen can be transported in two forms: dissolved in plasma (3%) or bound to hemoglobin (97%).

Oxyhemoglobin Dissociation Curve

The essential relationship between PaO_2 and arterial oxygen saturation (SaO_2) is graphically illustrated by the oxyhemoglobin dissociation curve (Fig. 4-4), originally described by Hufner in 1890. The sigmoid shape of this curve reflects the optimal conditions that facilitate oxygen loading in the lungs and oxygen release to the tissues. To describe these processes in relation to the curve, it is often divided into two segments: the association segment and the dissociation segment.

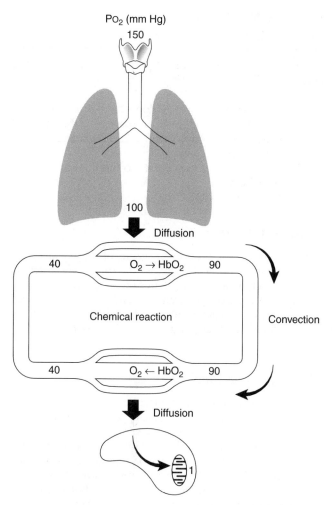

FIGURE 3-3 The processes when oxygen is transported from atmosphere to the mitochondria. (From Dantzker DR, Scharf SM: Cardiopulmonary Critical Care, 3rd ed, p 175. Philadelphia, WB Saunders, 1998.)

The upper portion of the curve, or the association segment, represents oxygen uptake, where large decreases in PaO_2 elicit only small decreases in SaO_2. The association segment also represents the body's protective mechanism to ensure that, even with a substantial decrease in PaO_2, adequate arterial oxygen content is available for transport to the cells. The lower portion of the curve, or the dissociation segment, reflects the release of oxygen to the tissues. Here, small changes in PaO_2 result in large changes in SaO_2, protecting the tissues by releasing large amounts of oxygen with minimal changes in oxygen tension.

Changes in oxyhemoglobin affinity affect the oxyhemoglobin dissociation curve and need to be considered in tissue oxygen assessment.[23] Increased affinity, caused by hypothermia, alkalosis, or decreased levels of 2,3-bisphosphoglycerate (2,3,-BPG; formerly 2,3-DPG or 2,3-diphosphoglycerate), decreases oxyhemoglobin affinity, shifting the curve to the right and thus allowing more oxygen to be released. In this way, tissue oxygenation is enhanced in the presence of decreased saturation and increased demand.

Change in the $PaCO_2$ can also cause shifts in the hemoglobin dissociation curve; this is termed the Bohr effect.[6] As blood perfuses through the lungs, carbon dioxide diffuses from the blood to the alveoli. As a result of this movement of carbon dioxide, the $PaCO_2$ is reduced, and there is a subsequent rise in pH. The hemoglobin dissociation curve shifts to the left, thus increasing the binding of hemoglobin to oxygen and allowing greater oxygen transport to the tissues.[7,21] At the tissue level, however, carbon dioxide displaces oxygen from the hemoglobin. The hemoglobin dissociation curve shifts to the right at the tissue level, facilitating higher oxygen delivery to the tissues (opposite to what occurs in the lungs). Shifts in the oxygen—hemoglobin dissociation curve have greater affects on events in the tissues than in the lungs because the relationships in the lungs are described in the flat upper position of the curve.[16]

A frequently used index of right and left shifts of the dissociation curve is the P_{50}, which is the PaO_2 at which hemoglobin is 50% saturated. A P_{50} that is higher than normal means a lower than normal affinity for oxygen. Under normal conditions (37° C, pH 7.40, PCO_2 40 mm Hg, and normal hemoglobin), the P_{50} is 27 mm Hg.

FIGURE 3-4 The oxygen–hemoglobin dissociation curve illustrates the relationship between the partial pressure of oxygen (PO_2) and the percentage of oxyhemoglobin (HbO_2) saturation. *A* indicates the situation in the lungs, and *V* indicates the situation in the venous blood returning from the tissues; see text for discussion. The small insets on the right indicate the effects of pH, PCO_2, and temperature. (From Smith JJ, Kampine JP: Circulatory Physiology: The Essentials, 2nd ed, p 9. Baltimore, Williams & Wilkins, 1980.)

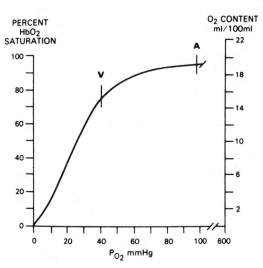
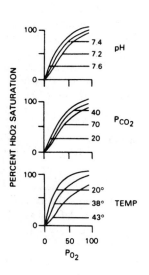

OXYGEN

The consumption of oxygen at the tissue level varies with the metabolic requirements of the individual tissues. The PaO_2 (100 mm Hg) is greater than the PO_2 of the tissues (30 mm Hg), causing oxygen to diffuse from the plasma into the tissue fluid and then into the cells. Depending on the metabolic needs of the tissues, the PO_2 of the tissues regulates the release of oxygen from the oxyhemoglobin molecule. A reduced plasma PO_2 causes the release of oxygen, which diffuses through the plasma and tissue fluid and into the cells.

The PCO_2 of the tissues (50 mm Hg) is greater than the $PaCO_2$ in systemic capillaries (46 mm Hg). Thus, carbon dioxide diffuses from the tissues into the blood. The PCO_2 in the tissues is proportional to the amount of energy expended.

The amount of oxygen released to the tissues is regulated by the PO_2 of the tissues, which is governed by the internal environment and activity of the tissues. The diffusion of carbon dioxide into the blood is determined by two factors, the PCO_2 of the tissues and the oxygen content of the blood; both factors are in turn determined by the environment of the tissues. Thus, the physiochemical system that results from this exchange of gases is controlled by the metabolic demands of the tissues.

CARBON DIOXIDE

The transport of carbon dioxide in the blood begins with the diffusion of carbon dioxide out of the tissue cells. Once carbon dioxide has diffused into the capillaries, a series of chemical reactions can occur. Carbon dioxide is carried in the blood by three mechanisms. Approximately 6% of the total is carried in the dissolved state, 20% to 25% combines with hemoglobin, and most of it combines with hydrogen to form bicarbonate. In the normal physiologic state, an average of 4 mL of carbon dioxide is transported from the tissues to the lungs in each 100 mL of blood. The amount of carbon dioxide carried in the blood can greatly alter the acid-base balance and must be carefully monitored in the critically ill patient.[22,31] Oxygen consumption ($\dot{V}O_2$) is the body's demand for oxygen and is defined as the amount of oxygen consumed at the tissue level per minute. It is derived from the difference between arterial and venous oxygen transport ($C[a–v]O_2$). $\dot{V}O_2$ can also be calculated by multiplying cardiac output (CO) by the $C(a–v)O_2$ difference times 10, which converts liters to milliliters per minute (mL/min). Normal oxygen consumption is 200 to 250 mL/min. All of the parameters that affect oxygen delivery and oxygen consumption affect the measurement of $\dot{V}O_2$.[9]

$$\dot{V}O_2 = CO\left(C[a-v]O_2\right) \times 10$$

Oxygen delivery ($\dot{D}O_2$) is the supply of oxygen to the body and is defined as the transport of oxygen to the tissues per minute. Oxygen delivery is determined by five main components: cardiac output, microvascular mechanisms, hemoglobin, PaO_2, and SaO_2.[1,8,19,29,31]

OXYGEN DELIVERY OR TRANSPORT

Oxygen transport or delivery ($\dot{D}O_2$) at the tissue level is affected by five factors:[8,9,14,15,17]

1. The effect of the rate of blood flow (cardiac output)
2. The effect of the rate of tissue metabolism and vasoregulatory mechanisms in the vascular bed (steady state, exercising, or injured)
3. The effect of hemoglobin concentration
4. The effect of the PaO_2
5. The effect of SaO_2

Cardiac Output

Cardiac output is a main determinant of oxygen delivery. Reduction in blood flow decreases the supply of oxygen to the cells, thereby initiating a series of compensatory mechanisms to increase oxygen transport and extraction. Careful monitoring of the determinants of cardiac output—heart rate, preload, afterload, and contractility—is necessary to optimize oxygen delivery.[2,20]

Microvascular Mechanisms

Pulmonary vascular tone is regulated by a number of regulatory mechanisms, including alveolar oxygen tension, the autonomic nervous system (neurogenic control), vasoactive circulatory mediators, and endothelial smooth muscle interaction.

Reduced oxygen levels in alveoli cause pulmonary vasoconstriction, diverting blood to better-ventilated regions. Hypercarbia or metabolic acidosis contributes to pulmonary vasoconstriction.

The proximal elastic arteries are innervated by the autonomic nervous system. It has been suggested that the autonomic nervous system modulates pulmonary vascular compliance rather than resistance.[11]

A number of circulating factors effect vasomotor tone. Vasoconstriction is induced by α_1 and α_2 receptors, whereas β_1 receptors mediate vasodilation. Serotonin and histamine mediate vasoconstriction in the pulmonary circulation. Angiotensin II is a potent pulmonary vasoconstrictor. Other vasodilator peptides include bradykinin, calcitonin, and substance P.

Endothelial cells act to maintain vascular tone by releasing various relaxing and constricting factors in response to physical and hormonal stimuli. The primary endothelium-relaxing factors released by the endothelial cells are nitric oxide and prostacyclin. The constricting factors include endothelin, superoxide anion, thromboxane, and prostaglandin H_2.

Hemoglobin

Hemoglobin is a protein of four subunits of porphyrin and iron. Each of the four units can bind one molecule of oxygen. Thus, four molecules of oxygen are carried by one molecule of hemoglobin when the hemoglobin is completely (100%) saturated. Oxygenation of the first heme unit in the hemoglobin molecule increases the affinity of the unit for oxygen, so that the affinity of the last heme unit for oxygen is much greater than that of the first unit. In each 100 mL of blood, there is approximately 15 g of hemoglobin. Each gram of hemoglobin binds with 1.38 mL of oxygen.

Partial Pressure of Oxygen

The remaining 3% of the oxygen content comprises oxygen dissolved in plasma. The PO_2, a well-recognized measurement of oxygen tension, is simply a reflection of the patient's plasma oxygenation. The PO_2 levels are an excellent indication of the patient's capacity for bonding oxygen to hemoglobin and the ability of oxygen to be released into the interstitial tissues. The body's plasma may carry a small percentage of the arterial oxygen, but measurement of its oxygen tension is an indirect method for determining the patient's oxygen—hemoglobin affinity.[1,2]

Arterial Oxygen Saturation

The last component involved in oxygen delivery is the SaO_2. The quantity of oxyhemoglobin, reflecting the amount of hemoglobin bound to oxygen, is measured as oxygen saturation. Saturation can be expressed as a percentage when multiplied by 100.

BLOOD OXYGEN CONTENT

The delivery of adequate oxygen for normal cellular function depends on the total amount of oxygen in the blood (oxygen content) and the ability of the heart to provide adequate blood flow (cardiac output). As discussed earlier, oxygen content reflects the amount of oxygen dissolved in plasma ($0.0031 < PO_2$) and the amount bound to hemoglobin ($1.38 <$ hemoglobin $< SaO_2$), where 1.38 is the maximum amount of oxygen carried by 1 g of hemoglobin. This expression is depicted in the following equation[1]:

$$(Hgb \times 1.38 \times SaO_2) + (0.0031 \times PaO_2)$$
$$\quad\quad 97\% \quad\quad\quad\quad\quad\quad 3\%$$

where Hgb is hemoglobin.

Assuming a normal hemoglobin of 15 g and 100% saturation, the end pulmonary capillary content is 21.2 volumes percent. The difference between arterial and venous contents is 5 volumes percent or a 25% difference, known as the $C(a–v)O_2$ difference. As tissue demands rise, for example, with exercise or febrile states, oxygen extraction increases and the $C(a–v)O_2$ difference widens. Extraction greater than 5 volumes percent occurs in reduced cardiac output states because marginal flow decreases transit time through the capillary beds and forces the body to increase extraction as a mechanism to compensate for reduced oxygen delivery. On the other hand, narrowing of the $C(a/2/v)O_2$ difference, or extraction less than 5 volumes percent, is seen in conditions related to increased oxygen supply, high-flow states, peripheral shunting, or inability of tissue to use oxygen. Therefore, a small percentage of the available oxygen is extracted from the blood.

MEASUREMENT OF OXYGEN DELIVERY OR TRANSPORT

Measurement of $\dot{D}O_2$ is calculated by multiplying total arterial oxygen content by cardiac output (CO)1[1]:

$$\dot{D}O_2 = CO \times CaO_2 \times 10^*$$
$$\text{where } CaO_2 = (Hgb \times 1.38 \times SaO_2) + (0.0031 \times PO_2)^\dagger$$
$$= CO \times Hgb \times SaO_2 \times 13.9$$

where Hgb is hemoglobin.

In patients with cardiac output of 5 L/min and a CaO_2 of 20.1 volumes percent, arterial oxygen delivery (DaO_2) is 1005 mL of oxygen/min.

Venous oxygen delivery (cardiac output < 15.5 volumes percent) is normally 775 mL/min. Again, note that a 25% difference exists between arterial and venous oxygen delivery levels. The significance of the 25% (5 volumes percent) decrease in arterial and venous content and delivery is that this difference reflects the amount of oxygen removed from the blood by the tissues. Additional oxygen remains in the venous system to be extracted by the tissues in conditions of greater oxygen demand.

Oxygen Consumption

Measurement of $\dot{V}O_2$ is derived by subtracting arterial oxygen transport (delivery) from venous oxygen transport (reserve)[27]:

$$\dot{V}O_2 = CaO_2 - CvO_2$$
$$\dot{V}O_2 = (CO \times CaO_2 \times 10) - (CO \times CvO_2 \times 10)$$

By combining the factors, the preceding can be simplified to the following equation:

$$\dot{V}O_2 = CO \times Hgb \times 13.8 \times (SaO_2 - S\bar{v}O_2)$$

where Hgb is hemoglobin and $S\bar{v}O_2$ is the mixed venous oxygen saturation.

This equation is a restatement of the Fick equation, placing $\dot{V}O_2$ on the left instead of cardiac output. This formula identifies all components of oxygen supply and demand.[5]

In a patient with normal values in a relatively steady state, normal $\dot{V}O_2$ is between 200 and 250 mL/min, as shown in the following equation[1,5]:

$$\dot{V}O_2 = 5 \text{ L/min} \times 15 \text{ g/dL} \times 13.8 \times (0.97 - 0.75)$$
$$\dot{V}O_2 = 228 \text{ mL/min}$$

Oxygen consumption is affected by several factors. Blood flow depends on the cardiac output and on the degree of constriction of the vascular bed in the tissue

---

*Correction factor for converting liters to oxygen content per 100 mL of blood.

†Amount contributed by the dissolved oxygen is minimal and not included in the equation.

(vasoregulatory mechanisms). A low hemoglobin, such as in anemia, reduces the amount of available oxygen to be delivered to the tissues. A reduced PaO_2 can affect the driving force needed to load the oxygen molecule on the hemoglobin. A decreased SaO_2 affects the affinity between oxygen and hemoglobin, enhancing the release of oxygen to the tissues. The metabolic rate of the tissues also affects the affinity of oxygen to be released.

Oxygen Consumption—Oxygen Delivery Relationship or Balance Between $\dot{V}O_2$ and DO_2

Three main compensatory mechanisms are needed to balance delivery and consumption to maintain aerobic metabolism. These mechanisms are:

1. *Cardiac output:* As oxygen demand and consumption increase, cardiac output increases to maintain adequate oxygen delivery.
2. *Vasoregulatory mechanisms (systemic vascular resistance):* The cardiac output and systemic vascular resistance actually work in conjunction with each other. Peripheral tissue beds shunt blood (vasoconstrict) to organs of greater demand.[31]
3. *Oxygen delivery-extraction (mixed venous oxygen saturation, $S\bar{v}O_2$):* Diminished oxygen delivery results in an increased oxygen extraction, reducing the amount of oxygen in venous blood returning to the heart.[12]

The balance of oxygen supply and demand can be challenged by a number of factors. An increase in $\dot{V}O_2$ is a threat to the oxygen supply—demand balance.[9] For the most part, the body consumes the oxygen it demands as long as there is adequate oxygen delivery. Once oxygen demand increases, the body's compensatory mechanisms must work to maintain oxygen delivery. If $\dot{V}O_2$ increases in a healthy person, cardiac output increases to maintain the balance between oxygen delivery and demand. If additional oxygen is required, then extraction of available oxygen increases, causing a decrease in $S\bar{v}O_2$.

A decrease in hemoglobin is another threat. As discussed previously, hemoglobin carries approximately 97% of the oxygen to the tissues. Except in certain situations, such as large volume replacements, hemoglobin is a very slowly changing value. However, frank hemorrhage or hidden intra-abdominal bleeding would result in a rapid decrease in hemoglobin. In the healthy person with mild anemia or a reduced level of hemoglobin, cardiac output usually increases as a compensatory measure to increase the delivery of oxygen.

As with other threats to the oxygen supply—demand balance, increasing oxygen extraction is a second compensatory mechanism that increases the delivery of oxygen. Failure of the ventilatory process is also a threat. In most instances, even in patients with severe pulmonary disease, the SaO_2 remains above 90% and poses little threat to the oxygen supply—demand balance. If the SaO_2 decreases to an unacceptable range, the body responds by increasing cardiac output.[3] An increase in oxygen extraction results if increases in cardiac output fail to meet oxygen demand. In the event of inadequate or nonexistent cardiac output reserve, the only remaining compensatory mechanism is to increase oxygen extraction.

A decrease in cardiac output is perhaps the most serious threat to the patient because an inadequate cardiac output eliminates one of the most important compensatory mechanisms. Therefore, a patient cannot tolerate as great a decrease in cardiac output as he or she can a decrease in SaO_2 or hemoglobin before lactic acidosis appears. Cardiac failure explains why perfusion failure, and not hypoxia or anemia, is the common cause of lactic acidosis encountered in clinical practice.[4] As cardiac function deteriorates and cardiac output decreases, the body's only remaining compensatory mechanism is to extract more available oxygen, which results in a decrease in $S\bar{v}O_2$.

MONITORING TISSUE OXYGENATION

Continuous $S\bar{v}O_2$ Interpretation

Mixed venous oxygen saturation is a parameter measured in the pulmonary arterial bed that is influenced by and dependent on the interaction between oxygen delivery and consumption.[35,36] Monitoring and trending the $S\bar{v}O_2$ provides critical information on the adequacy of the balance between oxygen delivery and consumption.[12,14,20,22,25—27,29,35,36]

Continuous $S\bar{v}O_2$ generally reflects the total body's adequacy of tissue oxygenation. The $S\bar{v}O_2$ parameter is considered a "global" indicator of the whole body's oxygen supply—demand balance. One of the only limitations of this indicator is that it is unable to specify which tissue bed or organ is suffering from an imbalance in delivery and consumption.[31]

Sampling from various venous sites in the body would give very different results. Each organ system uses oxygen in differing amounts and therefore returns blood with various $S\bar{v}O_2$ levels. For instance, the coronary circulation has the greatest need for oxygen, and $P\bar{v}O_2$ values are lowest, at 30 mm Hg (57% saturation). On the other hand, the integumentary system has a lower demand for oxygen, often returning venous blood values of 75 mm Hg (95% saturation). The $S\bar{v}O_2$ can be measured by the conventional method of sending a pulmonary arterial sample to the laboratory for interpretation or by means of a pulmonary artery catheter with a fiberoptic photometric lumen, which allows continuous monitoring of $S\bar{v}O_2$.

Pulse Oximetry

Pulse oximetry is a clinical tool that determines the percentage of hemoglobin saturation by measuring the absorbency of two wavelengths of light detected in a vascular bed. The measurement of SaO_2 is influenced by a number of clinical conditions such as elevated levels of carboxyhemoglobin, severe hypoxic states, jaundice, or shock states. In addition, the presence of nail polish on the patient's finger may invalidate the SaO_2 measurement.

Cardiac Reserve (Oxygen Extraction Ratio)

The percentage of oxygen extracted by the tissues is a useful indicator of the balance between oxygen delivery and consumption. The normal oxygen extraction ratio is 25%.[8,16,27] This ratio increases in pathologic conditions characterized by an imbalance between oxygen delivery and $\dot{V}O_2$. Thus, whenever cardiac output, hemoglobin, or PaO_2 are depressed (decreased oxygen delivery), or when excessive increases in $\dot{V}O_2$ are not met by compensatory increases in cardiac output, the oxygen extraction ratio increases. The extraction ratio is decreased in conditions where $\dot{V}O_2$ is relatively low in proportion to oxygen delivery, such as in sepsis or cirrhosis.

REFERENCES

1. Aberman A: Fundamental oxygen transport physiology in a hemodynamic monitoring context. In Schweiss JF (ed): Continuous Measurement of Blood Oxygen Saturation in the High-Risk Patient, pp 13–26. San Diego, Beach International, 1983
2. Ahrens TS: Concepts in the assessment of oxygenation. Focus in Critical Care 14: 36–44, 1987
3. Albert RK: Physiology and management of failure of arterial oxygenation. In Fallat RJ, Luce JM (eds): Clinics in Critical Care Medicine vol 14, pp 37–59. New York, Churchill Livingstone, 1988
4. Astiz ME, Rackow EC, Kaufman B et al: Relationship of oxygen delivery and mixed venous oxygenation to lactic acidosis in patients with sepsis and acute myocardial infarction. Crit Care Med 16: 655–658, 1988
5. Baele P, McMichan J, Marsh M et al: Continuous monitoring of mixed venous oxygen saturation in critically ill patients. Anesth Analg 61: 513–517, 1982
6. Bohr DF, Greenberg S, Bonaccorsi A: Mechanisms of action of vasoactive agents. In Kaley G, Altura BM (eds): Micro-circulation, Vol II, pp 311–348. Baltimore, University Park Press, 1978
7. Bone RC: Respiratory monitoring. In Fallat RJ, Luce JM (eds): Clinics in Critical Care Medicine: Cardiopulmonary Critical Care Medicine, vol 14, pp 89–111. New York, Churchill Livingstone, 1988
8. Bryan-Brown CW: Tissue blood flow and oxygen transport in critically ill patients. Crit Care Med 3(3): 103–108, 1975
9. Buran MJ: Oxygen consumption. In Snyder JV, Pinsky MR (eds): Oxygen Transport in the Critically Ill, pp 16–21. Chicago, Year Book, 1987
10. Comroe JH: Physiology of Respiration, pp 160–166. Chicago, Year Book, 1965
11. Dantzker DR, Scharf SM: Cardiopulmonary Critical Care, 3rd ed. Philadelphia, WB Saunders, 1998
12. Divertie M, McMichan J: Continuous monitoring of mixed venous oxygen saturation. Chest 85: 423–428, 1984
13. Fahey P: Continuous Measurement of Blood Oxygen Saturation in the High-Risk Patient, Vol 2. San Diego, Beach International, 1985
14. Fahey PJ, Harris K, Vanderwarf C: Clinical experience with continuous monitoring of mixed venous oxygen saturation in respiratory failure. Chest 86: 748–752, 1984
15. Fauci AS, Braunwald E, Isselbacher KJ et al: Harrison's Principles of Internal Medicine, 14th ed. New York, McGraw-Hill, 1998
16. Finch CA, Lenfant C: Oxygen transport in man. N Engl J Med 286): 407–415, 1972
17. Folkow B, Neil E: Circulation, pp 3–145. London, Oxford University Press, 1971
18. Fromm RE, Grumond J, Darley J et al: The craft of cardiopulmonary analysis. In Snyder JV, Pinsky MR (eds): Oxygen Transport in the Critically Ill, pp 249–269. Chicago, Year Book, 1987
19. Ganong WF: Review of Medical Physiology, 11th ed, pp 533–539. Los Altos, CA, Lang, 1983
20. Gardner P, Laurent-Bopp D: Continuous $S\bar{v}O_2$ monitoring: Clinical application in critical care nursing. Prog Cardiovasc Nursing 2: 9–18, 1987
21. Guyton AC: Transport of oxygen and carbon dioxide in the blood and body fluids. In Guyton AC (ed): Textbook of Medical Physiology, pp 504–515. Philadelphia, WB Saunders, 1986
22. Kandel G, Aberman A: Mixed venous oxygen saturation: Its role in the assessment of the critically ill patient. Arch Intern Med 143: 1400–1402, 1983
23. Kersten LD: Comprehensive Respiratory Nursing. Philadelphia, WB Saunders, 1989
24. Lenfant C: Pulmonary circulation. In Ruch TC, Patton HD (eds): Physiology and Biophysics II, pp 277–284. Philadelphia, WB Saunders, 1974
25. Marini JJ: Acute lung injury: Hemodynamic monitoring with the pulmonary artery catheter. Crit Care Clin 2: 551–572, 1986
26. Mims BC: Physiologic rationale of $S\bar{v}O_2$ monitoring. Critical Care Clinics of North America vol 1: 619–628, 1989
27. Nelson LD: Mixed venous oximetry. In Snyder JV, Pinsky MR (eds): Oxygen Transport in the Critically Ill, pp 235–248. Chicago, Year Book, 1987
28. Shepherd JT, Vanhoutte PM: The Human Cardiovascular System: Facts and Concepts, pp 1–106. New York, Raven Press, 1979
29. Shoemaker WC, Appel P, Bland R: Use of physiologic monitoring to predict outcome and to assist in clinical decisions in critically ill postoperative patients. Am J Surg 146: 43–150, 1983
30. Smith JJ, Kampine JP: Circulatory Physiology: The Essentials, pp 1–20, 53–72, 129–161. Baltimore, Williams & Wilkins, 1980
31. Snyder, JV: Assessment of systemic oxygen transport. In Snyder JV, Pinsky MR (eds): Oxygen Transport in the Critically Ill, pp 179–198. Chicago, Year Book, 1987
32. West JB (ed): Pulmonary Gas Exchange, Vol I. New York, Academic Press, 1980
33. West JB (ed): Pulmonary Pathophysiology: The Essentials, pp 20–41. Baltimore, Williams & Wilkins, 1977
34. West JB (ed): Respiratory Physiology: The Essentials, 2nd ed, pp 32–78. Baltimore, Williams & Wilkins, 1979
35. White KM: Continuous monitoring of mixed venous oxygen saturation ($S\bar{v}O_2$): A new assessment tool in critical care nursing: Part I. Cardiovascular Nursing 23(1): 1–6, 1987
36. White KM: Continuous monitoring of mixed venous oxygen saturation ($S\bar{v}O_2$): A new assessment tool in critical care nursing: Part II. Cardiovascular Nursing 23(2): 1–7, 1987

Control of Blood Pressure and Cardiac Output

ELIZABETH J. BRIDGES*

This chapter reviews the neurohumoral control of the cardiovascular system as it relates to both the rapid and more long-term control of cardiac output and blood pressure, and the local control of blood flow (autoregulatory, metabolic, autacoid). Several models of cardiac function are presented, including the relationship between cardiac output and central venous pressure, the Krogh model of the effect of distribution of blood volume on cardiac output, and the arterial baroreflex responses to decreased and increased blood pressure.

AFFERENT INPUT AND RECEPTORS

Arterial Baroreceptors

The arterial baroreceptors are responsible for the reflex control of blood pressure. These baroreceptors are undifferentiated nerve fibers located in the adventitia of the carotid sinus (at the bifurcation of the carotid artery) and the aortic arch (between the arch of the aorta and the bifurcation of the subclavian artery; Fig. 4-1). The receptors are mechanoreceptors that respond to distortion or a change in transmural pressure or stretch (ds/dt) of the vascular bed in which they are located. For example, the carotid baroreceptors are sensitive to external compression or massage, both of which unload them (decrease transmural pressure). Although baroreceptors are often referred to as "pressoreceptors," they in fact do not sense pressure directly, but only indirectly through change in stretch.

The baroreceptors respond to two types of input: static input (i.e., mean arterial pressure) and phasic input (i.e., pulsatile changes). Therefore, the baroreceptors are responsive to mean arterial pressure, pulse pressure, and the number of pulses per minute (e.g., heart rate).[156] The static response has a threshold effect, that is, below a certain threshold of mean arterial pressure (20 to 50 mm Hg), the receptor stops firing. Above this threshold there is an increase in rate of receptor firing in proportion to the increase in mean pressure, until a plateau of the output is reached at saturation. The phasic response increases when the rate of change of pressure rises (increasing pressure), and decreases when the rate of change in pressure decreases.

From the carotid sinus, afferent input to the nucleus tractus solitarius in the medulla is through the carotid sinus nerve (nerve of Hering), which joins the ninth cranial nerve (glossopharyngeal). The sensory input from the aortic arch is through the 10th cranial nerve (vagus). Through synaptic connections to areas located in ventrolateral medulla and *nucleus ambiguus,* sympathetic and parasympathetic output is modified by afferent feedback from the baroreceptors. The excitation or inhibition of the sympathetic and parasympathetic systems depends on the direction of the change (increase or decrease) in arterial pressure.

Cardiopulmonary Receptors

Cardiopulmonary or low-pressure baroreceptors are located in the atria, ventricles, and pulmonary arteries and veins. The properties of the cardiopulmonary baroreceptors are similar to those of the arterial baroreceptors—that is, a decrease in transmural pressure in the chamber or vessel results in a decrease in the firing rate of receptors, and vice versa. In addition, receptors located in the ventricles are sensitive to chemical stimuli. As is discussed later, in response to a decrease in atrial and, in some cases, ventricular pressure, the cardiopulmonary baroreceptors initiate reflex vasoconstriction of skeletal muscle cutaneous resistance vessels, which may be important for the rapid control of blood pressure. This reflex vasoconstriction of cutaneous resistance vessels[85,113,147] may help maintain blood pressure when the person is standing up.[145] Ironically, the cardiopulmonary baroreflex does not constrict the splanchnic vessels, which would cause the greatest transfer of blood to the heart.[47,145] Another possibility is that the vasoconstriction of

The views expressed in this chapter are those of the author and do not reflect the official policy of the Department of Defense or other departments of the United States Government.

The author thanks Dr. Loring Rowell for his expert consultation and assistance with the development of this chapter.

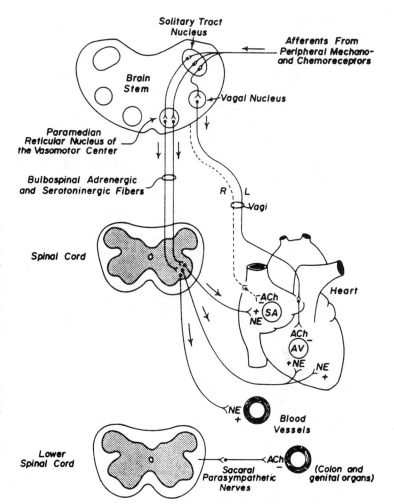

FIGURE 4-1 Origin and distribution of the adrenergic and cholinergic nerves to the cardiovascular system. The vagal fibers to the heart arise from the vagal nucleus in the brainstem. This nucleus is governed by the nucleus tractus solitarius, which is the main receiving station for afferent information from the peripheral mechanoreceptors and chemoreceptors. The mechanoreceptors are located in the carotid sinus and the receptors of the aortic arch. The carotid receptors send impulses to the central nervous system (CNS) by the carotid sinus nerve (nerve of Hering), which joins the glossopharyngeal nerve (cranial nerve IX). The aortic baroreceptors send afferent input to the CNS by the vagus nerve (cranial nerve X). The vagal nerve alters heart rate through its effect on the sinoatrial (SA) and (AV) nodes. Sympathetic fibers innervate the SA and AV nodes and the ventricular myocardium, and affect heart rate and contractility. In addition, the sympathetic fibers innervate the vasculature, and thus alter vascular tone. Ach, acetylcholine; NE, norepinephrine. (From Shepherd JT, Vanhoutte PM: The Human Cardiovascular System: Facts and Concepts, p 124. New York, Raven Press, 1979.)

cutaneous resistance vessels that has been attributed to the cardiopulmonary baroreceptors may also be a manifestation of an aortic baroreflex caused by a small change in stroke volume and the aortic pulse pressure.[47]

ATRIAL NATRIURETIC FACTOR

In response to increased atrial pressure, atrial natriuretic factor or peptide is released from the atrial tissue. In rats, atrial natriuretic factor has natriuretic and vasorelaxant properties.[37,184] However, at physiological levels in humans, the transient increase in atrial natriuretic factor in response to increased atrial pressure appears to have little acute effect on renal sodium excretion.[62] In addition, the role of atrial natriuretic factor in the long-term control of blood pressure remains unclear.[37] For example, patients with cardiomyopathy and heart failure often have an increased plasma level of atrial natriuretic factor; however, these patients demonstrate sodium retention rather than the expected increase in sodium excretion.[152] Thus, it appears that atrial natriuretic factor does not play a major role in either the rapid or slow control of blood pressure in humans.

Left Ventricular Baroreceptors

Under normal resting circumstances, control of heart rate is mediated by the sinoaortic baroreceptors. However, there are inhibitory or depressor receptors located in the inferoposterior wall of the left ventricle that modify the sinoaortic control of heart rate. In addition, under pathologic conditions, such as myocardial infarction (MI), hemorrhage, aortic stenosis or syncope, activation of these receptors has a direct inhibitory affect on heart rate.

Input to the central nervous system from the ventricular receptors, which are sensitive to both mechanical and chemical stimuli, is through nonmyelinated vagal afferents (C fibers).[18] The left ventricular end-diastolic pressure is the primary factor affecting receptor output. There is a linear relationship between receptor firing rate and left ventricular end-diastolic pressure (i.e., an increase in left ventricular end-diastolic pressure is associated with an increase in firing rate).[122] The pathophysiological effect of increased receptor firing rate is discussed later.

BEZOLD-JARISCH REFLEX

From a clinical perspective, the ventricular receptors are thought to be responsible for pathophysiological responses to several clinical conditions or situations, including MI, thrombolytic therapy, syncope, and aortic stenosis. During an acute inferoposterior MI,[18,113,181] and at the time of reperfusion of these infarctions,[183] the transient bradycardia observed is thought to be a manifestation of the depressor effect of receptors located in the inferoposterior wall of the left ventricle. During ischemia, the receptors may be distorted by bulging of the ventricular wall during systole.[177] These receptors are also thought to mediate the reflex bradycardia and hypotension that occur during coronary angiography, particularly during injection of contrast material into the arteries that supply the inferoposterior surface of the left ventricle (e.g., circumflex, right coronary artery).[132]

In severe aortic stenosis, some patients experience exertional syncope and even sudden death. The probable mechanism of the syncope is an exercise-induced increase in left ventricular pressure, which is extreme because of high aortic valve resistance, despite a decrease in aortic blood pressure. This high left ventricular pressure stimulates the ventricular baroreceptors and causes reflex vasodilation because of loss of sympathetic vasoconstriction, extreme bradycardia, and a drop in sympathetic nerve activation to zero.[112,113,122] Once these patients undergo surgical correction of the stenosis, however, the normal sympathetic vasoconstrictor response to exercise is restored.

Finally, in cases of severe hemorrhage or during head-up tilt (particularly in patients receiving a concurrent infusion of isoproterenol), the ventricular depressor reflex may be initiated in response to a forceful ventricular contraction on a relatively empty ventricle.[126,153] This forceful contraction causes distortion of the receptors, with a subsequent triggering of the cardiac depressor reflex. The reflex, which may be mediated through the release of epinephrine, results in paradoxical and unexpected bradycardia and worsening hypotension.[148] These findings remain equivocal, however.

CENTRAL NERVOUS SYSTEM REGULATION

The *nucleus tractus solitarius* is an ovoid area located in the medulla that receives efferent input from cardiovascular, respiratory, and gastrointestinal sites. The *nucleus tractus solitarius* serves as the first relay station for reflexes (e.g., baroreceptor reflex) that control circulation and respiration. From the *nucleus tractus solitarius*, there are multiple projections to areas such as (1) the ventrolateral medulla, which is responsible for sympathetic efferent activity; (2) the *nucleus ambiguus* or "cardioinhibitory center" of the medulla, which is the location of the cell bodies of the vagal parasympathetic nerves; and (3) the median preoptic nuclei, which affect the release of vasopressin. The output from the medulla depends on the perturbation of the system (i.e., an increase or decrease in blood pressure). The complete baroreflex response is discussed later. From the central nervous system, the efferent arm of the rapid control of blood pressure operates through the autonomic nervous system.

AUTONOMIC NERVOUS SYSTEM REGULATION

The autonomic nervous system, which is one branch of the peripheral nervous system, is responsible for coordination of body functions that ensure homeostasis. The autonomic nervous system is further divided into two major components: the sympathetic nervous system and the parasympathetic nervous system (Fig. 4-2).

Sympathetic Nervous System

Efferent projections from the hypothalamus and medulla terminate in the intermediolateral cells located in the gray matter of the thoracic and lumbar (thoracolumbar) sections of the spinal column (specifically, T-1 to L-2). Hence, the sympathetic nervous system is often referred to as the thoracolumbar division of the autonomic nervous system. The neuronal cell bodies, which are located in the spinal column, are generally the origin of short preganglionic efferent fibers that innervate postsynaptic sympathetic neurons located in three general groupings of ganglia (a group of nerve cell bodies). The paravertebral ganglia are located in a bilateral chain-like structure adjacent to the spinal column. This chain extends from the superior cervical ganglia, located at the level of the bifurcation of the carotid artery, to ganglia located in the sacral region. The prevertebral ganglia, which lie midline and anterior to the aorta and vertebral column, include the celiac, aorticorenal, and superior and inferior mesenteric ganglia. The third group of ganglia comprises the previsceral or terminal ganglia, which are located close to the target organs of the sympathetic nervous system. The ganglia are the site of action of ganglionic blocking agents, such as trimethaphan. These agents, which were previously used to treat hypertensive emergencies, are seldom used today because of the numerous side effects (e.g., orthostatic hypotension, inhibition of pupillary responses, paralytic ileus, circulatory collapse) associated with blocking sympathetic output at a central location.[64] The previsceral ganglia have long preganglionic fibers and short postganglionic fibers. In contrast, the paravertebral and prevertebral ganglia give rise to long postganglionic fibers, which extend to the target organs of the sympathetic nervous system (e.g., heart, lungs, vascular smooth muscle, liver, kidneys, bladder, and reproductive organs; see Fig. 4-2). Of particular importance to the control of blood pressure are the sympathetic receptors located in the heart, vasculature, kidneys, and renal medulla.

ADRENORECEPTORS

At the target organs, the postganglionic fibers terminate at the neuroeffector junction and are separated from the adrenergic receptors (adrenoreceptors) by only a small junctional gap or cleft. The adrenoreceptors have been classified into two general groups: α-adrenergic receptors and ß-adrenergic receptors. The receptor groups are further divided into subtypes, β_1 and β_2 and α_1 and α_2 (Table 4-1). The dopaminergic receptors are also characterized by subtypes: DA_1 receptors, which are located in the renal vasculature, and DA_2 receptors, which are located on the peripheral vasculature.[79,102]

Stimulation of the ß-adrenergic receptor results in activation of a cascade of events modulated by cyclic adenosine monophosphate (cAMP) that results in an influx of calcium into cell. Conversely, α-adrenergic receptor activity is modulated by inositol triphosphate and protein kinase C.[129] The

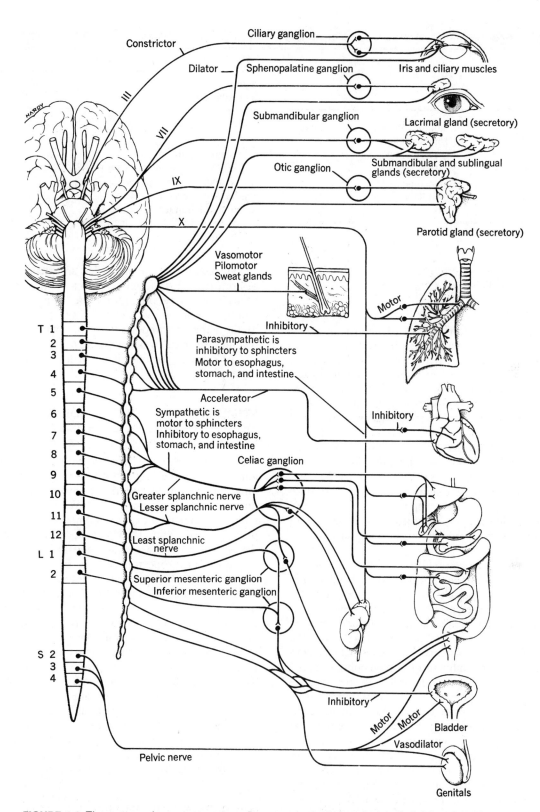

FIGURE 4-2 The autonomic nervous system. Parasymphathetic (craniosacral) divisions send long preganglionic fibers that synapse with a second nerve in ganglia located close to or within the organs that are then innervated by short postganglionic fibers. The sympathetic (thoracolumbar) division sends relatively short preganglionic fibers to the chains of paravertebral ganglia and to certain outlying ganglia. The second cell then sends relatively long postganglionic fibers to the organs they innervate. (From Rodman MJ, Smith DW: Pharmacology and Drug Therapy in Nursing, 3rd ed, p 302. Philadelphia, JB Lippincott, 1985.)

TABLE 4-1 **Cardiovascular Effects of Autonomic Nervous System Innervation**[5, 24, 41, 50, 57, 72, 127, 129]

Organ	Site	Effects Sympathetic Stimulation	Parasympathetic Stimulation
Heart	Sinoatrial/atrioventricular nodes, His-Purkinje system	+ Chronotrope (β_1,β_2)	–Chronotrope
	Myocardium	+ Inotrope (β_1, β_2, α)	–Inotrope (minor)
Systemic vasculature	Skeletal muscle	Vasodilation (β_2, presynaptic α_2)	—
	Splanchnic bed	Vasoconstriction (α_1, postsynaptic α_2)	—
	Renal flow	Vasoconstriction (β)	—
		Vasoconstriction (α)	—

end result of the receptor activation depends on the specific effector organ stimulated (see Chapter 2).

Heart. The predominant type of ß-adrenergic receptor in the heart is the $ß_1$ subtype, whereas the $ß_2$ subtype predominates in noncardiac structures (e.g., bronchi, vasculature, uterus).[23] However, approximately 20% of the ß-adrenergic receptors in the ventricle and 40% in the atria are the $ß_2$ subtype.[23,41,100,129] Stimulation of the $ß_1$ and $ß_2$ receptors in the heart increases (1) the rate of discharge of the sinoatrial node, (2) conduction across the atrioventricular node, and (3) speed of contraction in the atria and ventricles (chronotropic effect). In addition, $ß_1$ stimulation increases cardiac contractility (inotropic effect). Stimulation of the cardiac $ß_2$ receptors produces effects similar to those of $ß_1$ receptor activation, in addition to causing coronary vasodilation.[52] There are also a smaller number (approximately 14%) of α_1 receptors located in the atria and ventricles.[24] Stimulation of the α_1 receptors creates a modest inotropic response.[57]

Vasculature. Sympathetic stimulation of the arterial tree extends to the level of the terminal arterioles. Traditionally, the α_1 receptors were thought to be postsynaptic, whereas the α_2 receptors were presynaptic. The former belief is true, but the latter view has been amended to include a postsynaptic effect. Binding of norepinephrine to the vascular smooth muscle α_1 receptor initiates vasoconstriction. Conversely, α_2 presynaptic inhibition of norepinephrine release reduces vasoconstriction, a process called *passive vasodilation*. In addition to the presynaptic α_2 receptors, it has been demonstrated that there are also postsynaptic α_2 receptors located on large arterioles and, perhaps most important, on the terminal arterioles.[50,127] Stimulation of the postsynaptic α_2 receptors causes vasoconstriction of the terminal arterioles. This vasoconstriction determines the number of open capillaries, and thus capillary blood flow. This latter effect is modified by the concurrent presynaptic inhibition of norepinephrine release. The α_2-mediated vasoconstriction of the terminal arterioles can be inhibited by the presence of metabolic vasodilators (e.g., oxygen, potassium), particularly in the skeletal muscles. There are also smooth muscle $ß_2$ receptors. Stimulation of the noncardiac $ß_2$ receptors results in relaxation of smooth muscle, with subsequent bronchodilation and peripheral vasodilation.

The cutaneous circulation has an extensive distribution of both α_1 and α_2 adrenoreceptors.[20] There appears to be virtually no ß adrenoreceptors. The sympathetic cholinergic innervation of the sweat glands may be functionally linked to the large and important active cutaneous vasodilation seen in heat stress, which appears to be caused by release of an unknown cotransmitter from these cholinergic nerves.[92,139,149]

STIMULATION OF CYCLIC ADENOSINE MONOPHOSPHATE–DEPENDENT RECEPTORS

Knowledge of the steps and effects of activation of the various receptors that depend on the activation of cAMP is important to understand the mechanism of action of the numerous inotropic and vasoactive medications administered to augment cardiac function (Fig. 4-3). For example, pharmacologic stimulation of $ß_1$ adrenoreceptors with drugs such as dobutamine and dopamine results in positive inotropic and chronotropic effects. In addition, these drugs also stimulate the $ß_2$ adrenoreceptors, leading to varying degrees of peripheral vasodilation, which is both drug and dose specific. Administration of phosphodiesterase inhibitors (phosphodiesterase is the enzyme that breaks down cAMP), such as amrinone and milrinone, causes cytosolic cAMP to increase. The increased cAMP has both positive inotropic and chronotropic effects on the heart. The phosphodiesterase inhibitors also cause peripheral vasodilation in regions containing a rich supply of ß adrenoreceptors, such as the splanchnic and skeletal muscle circulations. Finally, dopamine exerts its indirect inotropic and chronotropic effects through the release of norepinephrine, and directly causes renal and peripheral vasodilation through stimulation of dopaminergic receptors.[89,111]

NEUROTRANSMITTERS

The sympathetic postganglionic fibers that innervate the arterial tree are in general noradrenergic (i.e., release norepinephrine). The one exception mentioned previously are the postganglionic fibers that innervate the sweat glands (sudomotor neurons), which have acetylcholine as their neurotransmitter.[131] Norepinephrine, which is the primary

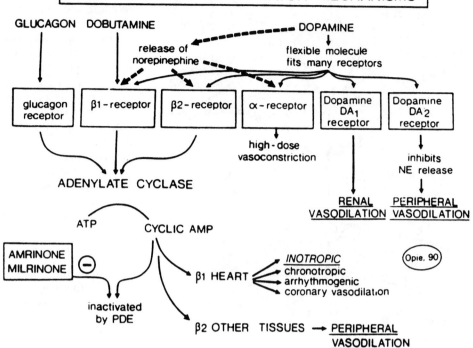

FIGURE 4-3 The basic mechanisms for combined inotropic and vasodilator effects are (1) stimulation of adenylate cyclase to elevate cyclic adenosine monophosphate (cAMP), which has positive inotropic and vasodilatory effects; (2) modulation of release of norepinephrine (NE) by dopamine receptor stimulation; and (3) inhibition of phosphodiesterase (PDE), which increases myocardial and vascular cyclic AMP. ATP, adenosine triphosphate. (From Marcus FI, Opie LH, Sonnenblick EH: Digitalis and other inotropes. In Opie LH [ed]: Drugs for the Heart, 3rd ed, p 141. Philadelphia, WB Saunders, 1991.)

noradrenergic neurotransmitter, is synthesized from tyrosine and is stored in sympathetic nerve terminals. In response to neuronal stimulation, the "packets" or quanta of norepinephrine are extruded from the axon vesicles by exocytosis.[178] The vesicular release of norepinephrine is enhanced by angiotensin II and cold, whereas the prejunctional effects of potassium, decreased PO_2, heat, autacoids (adenosine, bradykinin, serotonin, prostaglandins), nitric oxide, and acetylcholine inhibit its release[178] (Fig. 4-4). The neurotransmitters (primarily norepinephrine) diffuse over varying small distances, depending on the junctional cleft, to receptors located on effector organs.

In the heart, norepinephrine binds predominantly with ß$_1$ receptors, with a resultant increase in heart rate and cardiac contractility. The primary mechanism of action of the postsynaptic α_1 and α_2 receptors is an increase in intracellular calcium of arteries and arterioles, which initiates their vasoconstriction (see Chapter 2).

Norepinephrine is primarily (70% to 80%) deactivated by removal from the neuroeffector junction by active reuptake. A small amount is degraded in the cleft by catechol-*O*-methyl transferase, and the remainder leaks into the capillaries (spillover).[131] The spillover is usually proportional to the increase in sympathetic nervous system activation; thus, the plasma norepinephrine level can be used as a rough indicator of sympathetic nervous system activity. However, the width of the junctional cleft also affects spillover. This mechanism is particularly important in the pulmonary vasculature, where spillover is predominantly the result of the wide junctional clefts and not of a high rate of sympathetic nervous system activation or norepinephrine release.[7,8,10]

Parasympathetic Nervous System

The second branch of the autonomic nervous system is the parasympathetic nervous system. The primary parasympathetic outflow is through four cranial nerves (III, VII, IX, and X). Of importance to blood pressure and cardiac output control, the nucleus ambiguus or "cardioinhibitory center" of the medulla is the location of the cell bodies of the vagus nerve (cranial nerve X). In addition, there are cell bodies located in the spinal cord gray matter at S-2 through S-4. Hence, the parasympathetic nervous system is referred to as the craniosacral branch of the autonomic nervous system. As noted previously, the glossopharyngeal (cranial nerve IX) and the vagus nerves also carry afferent (sensory) fibers to the medulla. These afferent fibers play a critical role in the arterial baroreceptor reflex control of blood pressure. In contrast to the sympathetic nervous system, the preganglionic fibers of the parasympathetic nervous system are long, synapsing on ganglia that are close to or are directly attached to the effector organ. The postsynaptic fibers are relatively short, in contrast to the fibers of the sympathetic nervous system (see Fig. 4-2).

RECEPTORS

In the parasympathetic nervous system, the nerve fibers are cholinergic, which means they liberate acetylcholine.[131] Despite the common neurotransmitter (i.e., acetylcholine), stimulation of various receptors in the parasympathetic nervous system causes different effects. The reason for the variable response is that there are two general types of cholinergic receptors: nicotinic and muscarinic. This classification is based on responsiveness of the receptor to nicotine or muscarine.

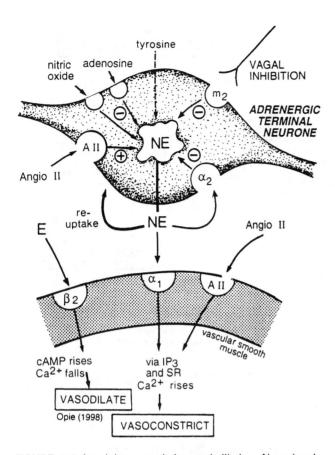

FIGURE 4-4 Arteriolar constriction and dilation. Norepinephrine (NE), released from the storage granules of the terminal neurons into the synaptic cleft, has predominantly vasoconstrictive effects acting through postsynaptic α_1 receptors. In addition, presynaptic α_2 receptors are stimulated to allow feedback inhibition of its release to modulate any excess release of NE. Parasympathetic cholinergic stimulation releases acetylcholine (Ach), which stimulates the muscarinic (m_2) receptors to inhibit the release of NE and thereby indirectly cause vasodilation. Circulating epinephrine (E) stimulates vasodilatory β_2 receptors. Angiotensin II (Angio II), formed ultimately in response to renin released from the kidneys, is also powerfully vasoconstrictive, acting both by enhancement of NE release and directly on arteriorlar receptors. cAMP, cyclic adenosine monophosphate; SR, sarcoplasmic reticulum; IP$_3$, inositol triphosphate, AII, angiotensin II. (From Opie LH: The Heart: Physiology from Cell to Circulation, 3rd ed, p 28. Philadelphia, Lippincott–Raven, 1998.)

Preganglionic cholinergic receptors, which are found in both the sympathetic and parasympathetic nervous systems, are nicotinic. The nicotinic receptors are located on autonomic ganglia and skeletal muscle end-plates. Stimulation of the nicotinic receptors is excitatory and short term (milliseconds). These receptors are blocked by curare, and in clinical practice blockade of the nicotinic receptors with various neuromuscular blocking agents (e.g., succinylcholine, pancuronium) causes musculoskeletal paralysis (blockade at the skeletal muscle end-plate) and may potentially cause hypotension because of blockade at the autonomic ganglia.[135,157]

The primary postganglionic receptor in the heart, smooth muscle, and glandular tissue is muscarinic. These receptors are stimulated by muscarine and can be antagonized by atropine and scopolamine.[131] There are subtypes of the muscarinic receptors that result in varied responses. For example, stimulation of muscarinic subtype 1 (M_1) receptors is responsible for the release of norepinephrine from the sympathetic neurons. Conversely, stimulation of muscarinic subtype 2 (M_2) receptors, which are specifically associated with vagal nerve endings in the heart, has direct and indirect negative inotropic and chronotropic effects. The direct effects are secondary to occupation of the ß-adrenergic receptors and inhibition of norepinephrine release, and the indirect effects occur through inhibition of the adrenergic second messenger cAMP.[5,72,129] Of clinical importance, the negative chronotropic and inotropic effects associated with the M_2 receptor are blocked by atropine.

Cotransmitters

At the preganglionic synapse, the primary neurotransmitter for both the sympathetic and parasympathetic nervous systems is acetylcholine. At the sympathetic nervous system neuroeffector junction, the primary neurotransmitters are norepinephrine and its precursor, dopamine, whereas the primary neurotransmitter of the postganglionic fibers of the parasympathetic nervous system is acetylcholine. However, other neurotransmitters that augment or modify the effects of the primary neurotransmitter are coreleased, and are referred to as *cotransmitters*.[28,131] For example, neuropeptide Y is the most prominent cotransmitter in the sympathetic nervous system ganglia, and vasoactive intestinal peptide is the most prominent peptide in the parasympathetic nervous system ganglia and nonadrenergic, noncholinergic nerves.[29]

Neuropeptide Y is an amino acid peptide released with norepinephrine from sympathetic nerve terminals. The primary cardiac effect of neuropeptide Y is the prejunctional modulation of the release of other neurotransmitters. For example, neuropeptide Y inhibits the release of acetylcholine from vagal nerve endings, thus attenuating the effects of the parasympathetic system on heart rate, atrioventricular conduction, and atrial contractility.[57]

SYSTEMIC HORMONES

In addition to the rapid control of arterial pressure by the autonomic nervous system, hormones such as epinephrine, arginine vasopressin, and renin–angiotensin II directly and indirectly affect the baroreceptor reflex and play an important role in the rapid control of blood pressure. Spillover of norepinephrine into the systemic circulation also affects blood pressure and cardiac output.

Epinephrine

In response to physical or emotional stressors (mental stress, exercise, hyperthermia, hypoglycemia), epinephrine is secreted into the plasma by the adrenal medulla, causing the plasma level of epinephrine to rise. Epinephrine stimulates

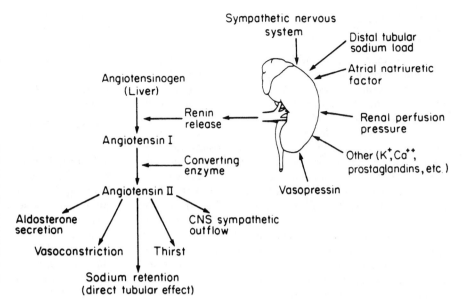

FIGURE 4-5 A schematic representation of the renin–angiotensin system showing major regulators of renin release, the biochemical cascade leading to angiotensin II release, and the major effects of angiotensin II. CNS, central nervous system. (From Dzau VJ, Orat RE: Renin–angiotensin system. In Fozzard HA, Haber E, Jennings RB et al ([eds]: The Heart and Cardiovascular System, Vol II, 2nd ed, p 1818. New York, Raven Press, 1991.)

ß$_1$ receptors in the heart and has positive chronotropic and inotropic effects. The net effect of this cardiac stimulation is an increase in cardiac output. Epinephrine also acts on the vasculature and stimulates the ß$_2$ receptors in the skeletal muscles and splanchnic arterioles, which causes vasodilation in these two large regions and potentially large decrements in the systemic vascular resistance (see Fig. 4-4). In the skin and kidneys, epinephrine stimulates the α-adrenergic receptors and causes vasoconstriction.[128,146]

Exogenously administered epinephrine has dose-specific effects. Low-dose epinephrine (0.005 to 0.02 µg/kg/min in adults) stimulates the ß adrenoreceptors and causes vasodilation and increased heart rate and contractility. Increased doses stimulate the α adrenoreceptors and increase vascular resistance and blood pressure.[186] Knowledge of these dose-specific effects is important, and although epinephrine is often administered for its vasoconstrictive effects, it may cause vasodilation if a large enough dose is not administered.

Renin–Angiotensin–Aldosterone System

The renin–angiotensin–aldosterone system plays an important role in the long-term control of arterial blood pressure, regional blood flow, and sodium balance[44] (Fig. 4-5). The renin–angiotensin–aldosterone system acts in a cascade fashion, initiated by the stimulation of renin release from the kidney. Renin is stored in and released from the juxtaglomerular cells near the renal afferent arterioles. Renin release is stimulated by three mechanisms. First, renin release occurs in response to increased sympathetic nervous system stimulation of the afferent and efferent arterioles in the renal glomeruli. The ß-adrenergic receptors in the cells of the juxtaglomerular apparatus are sensitive to neurally released and systemic catecholamines. (This effect can be blocked by ß-adrenergic blockers, e.g., propranolol.) Second, renin release is stimulated by decreased renal perfusion pressure, distending the afferent arterioles. Below a mean arterial pressure of 80 to 90 mm Hg, renin secretion is a steep and linear function of renal perfusion pressure. Finally, decreased sodium concentration in the macula densa, which is located in the early distal tubule, stimulates the juxtaglomerular apparatus to secrete renin.[44,145]

Angiotensin II is released through the proteolytic effects of renin on the plasma protein, angiotensinogen, which is synthesized and released into the plasma from the liver. Renin converts angiotensinogen to angiotensin I. Angiotensin I, which is inactive, is converted to angiotensin II by a converting enzyme located in vascular endothelium throughout the body.[151] Angiotensin-converting enzyme inhibitors exert their effect at this level of the renin–angiotensin system.

Angiotensin II has two primary actions: vasoconstriction and stimulation of aldosterone release. Angiotensin II constricts arterioles through a direct effect on the smooth muscle. The renal and splanchnic circulations are particularly sensitive to angiotensin II.[44] Angiotensin II increases vascular resistance and stimulates the heart indirectly through its potentiating actions on the sympathetic nervous system. These effects include (1) accelerating the synthesis and release of norepinephrine, (2) delaying neuronal reuptake of norepinephrine, (3) directly stimulating the sympathetic ganglia, and (4) facilitating the response to sympathetic activity and vasoconstrictor drugs.[145]

Angiotensin II also has a long-term effect on blood pressure through stimulation of aldosterone synthesis and secretion, which raises blood volume. The change in blood volume is a slow process, which is important in the long-term control of blood pressure. Aldosterone, a mineralocorticoid synthesized and secreted by the adrenal cortex, increases sodium reabsorption in the loop of Henle and decreases sodium excretion, which together lead to retention of water and expansion of blood volume.

Arginine Vasopressin (Antidiuretic Hormone)

Arginine vasopressin, or antidiuretic hormone, is a neurotransmitter synthesized in the hypothalamus and released from the neurohypophysis of the pituitary gland (posterior pituitary gland).[38] Vasopressin is primarily released in response to changes in plasma osmolality; however, vasopressin may also be released in response to a decrease in blood volume or blood pressure. As the osmolality increases the secretion of vasopressin increases. In humans, the primary effect of vasopressin is its antidiuretic effect, which is secondary to stimulation of water absorption at the distal and collecting tubules of the kidney.[39,71] The change in water absorption affects plasma osmolality. Vasopressin is exquisitely sensitive to changes in osmolality; for example, a 5- to 10-mOsm increase in osmolality causes an increase in plasma vasopressin.[13,137] The close relation between osmolality and vasopressin maintains plasma osmolality within 3% of normal in most conditions.[43] In contrast, the sensitivity of the baroreceptor system is less than that of the osmoreceptors, as demonstrated by the large (5% to 10%) iso-osmotic change in plasma volume required before vasopressin secretion is altered.

However, during hemorrhage (plasma volume decreased by > 5% to 10%), plasma levels of vasopressin are increased, in some cases 100-fold. In this case, vasopressin acts in a manner similar to renin and norepinephrine, causing vasoconstriction[156] and playing a supporting role to the sympathetic nervous system in the maintenance of blood pressure.[38] The mechanism for the hemorrhage-induced change in vasopressin secretion was previously thought to be the Henry-Gauer (cardiorenal) reflex. Identification of the Henry-Gauer reflex as the mechanism was based on the assumption that a change in atrial volume caused a change in both vasopressin secretion and activation of the renin–angiotensin–aldosterone system. Current evidence suggests that the arterial baroreceptors, and not the cardiac receptors as specified by the Henry-Gauer reflex, are the primary reflex controllers of the plasma volume–mediated release of these hormones.[145,160] In the case of hemorrhage, the change in intrathoracic volume alters the arterial pulse pressure, which decreases arterial baroreceptor stimulation and leads to increased vasopressin secretion. A similar mechanism also appears to explain the inhibition of vasopressin in response to increased thoracic volume.

Norepinephrine Spillover

Approximately 80% of the norepinephrine secreted at the neuroeffector junction is either taken up by sympathetic neurons (neuronal reuptake) or broken down by the enzymes monoamine oxidase or catechol-*O*-methyl transferase. The remaining 20% may spill into the systemic circulation, causing the plasma norepinephrine concentration to increase in proportion to sympathetic nervous system activation. Factors such as the nerve firing rate, blood flow, neuronal uptake of norepinephrine, capillary permeability, and width of the junctional cleft can also affect the level of plasma norepinephrine. Despite the effects of these factors, the plasma level of norepinephrine is considered to be a sensitive indicator of sympathetic nervous system activity.[27,48,63,145]

HEART RATE

Control of Heart Rate

The intrinsic heart rate at rest, without any neurohumoral influence, is approximately 100 to 120 beats/min. The heart rate in the intact, resting person reflects a balance between the tonically active sympathetic and parasympathetic nervous systems, with the parasympathetic nervous system predominating.[70,105,106] The predominance of the parasympathetic nervous system is manifested by a resting heart rate that is lower than the intrinsic rate. Parasympathetic predominance may also be demonstrated by abolishing the vagal influence with the administration of atropine.[6,91]

Vagal stimulation of the sinoatrial and atrioventricular nodes leads to a rapid (within one to two beats) decrease in heart rate. Conversely, when vagal stimulation is discontinued, the heart rate increases rapidly. The rapid response to vagal stimulation and the presence of a large amount of cholinesterase (the enzyme that degrades the acetylcholine that is released from the parasympathetic fibers) allows the vagus nerve to exert beat-to-beat control of heart rate. The heart rate response to sympathetic stimulation is gradual in onset, and once the sympathetic stimulation is terminated, the heart rate slowly decreases. This response is in contrast to the almost instantaneous response to vagal stimulation.[6,104,105]

As discussed later, there is an inverse relation between heart rate and arterial blood pressure. The inverse changes in heart rate are in response to baroreceptor stimulation, with the response most pronounced over a mean arterial pressure of 70 to 160 mm Hg.[34] The alterations in heart rate are achieved by a reciprocal relationship between sympathetic and parasympathetic cardiac stimulation.[95]

Changes in heart rate also occur as a result of chemosensor reflexes mediated by the carotid chemoreceptors. For example, a relatively slight excitation of the chemoreceptors leads to stimulation of the vagal center in the medulla and a decrease in heart rate. This response is considered the primary reflex effect of chemosensor stimulation.[123] With increased levels of stimulation (e.g., a marked decrease in arterial PO_2), a secondary reflex is initiated that leads to depression of the primary chemoreceptor reflex and an increase in heart rate. This reflex is caused by pulmonary hyperventilation, which leads to hypocapnia and activation of pulmonary stretch receptors. The chemosensor reflex plays only a minimal role in the control of heart rate because the primary and secondary reflexes tend to offset one another.

In patients who have received an orthotopic heart transplant, the resting heart rate is increased to approximately 100 beats/min (intrinsic rate), and the exercise-induced heart rate increase (primarily dependent on the level of circulating catecholamines) is delayed.[82,133,170]

Resting Sinus Arrhythmia

There is a direct relation between heart rate and respiration.[70] During inspiration the heart rate increases, and then falls during expiration. This respiratory-induced cyclical variation in heart rate is referred to as a *sinus arrhythmia*. The sinus arrhythmia also may occur in the absence of ventilatory movement, indicating a central control mechanism.[3]

Sinus arrhythmia is thought to be predominantly mediated by the vagus nerve. Measurement of heart rate variability is used as an indicator of the balance between parasympathetic and sympathetic nervous system input to the heart,[14,35,45,56,94,172] with decreased heart rate variability indicating an imbalance between the parasympathetic and sympathetic nervous systems. Decreased heart rate variability has been observed in patients who were post-MI, sudden cardiac arrest survivors,[30,31,35] post cardiac surgery,[80] or suffering from heart failure.[173] A decrease in heart rate variability is associated with an increase in mortality due to a sudden cardiac arrest after a MI.[15–17,36,93]

Heart Rate and Cardiac Output

The relationship between heart rate and cardiac output is defined by the equation: cardiac output = stroke volume × heart rate.

The effect of heart rate on cardiac output is not invariant (e.g., increased heart rate leads to increased cardiac output), and the effect can change over a wide range because of changes in stroke volume. As is discussed in the section on models of cardiac performance, a small increase in heart rate causes an increase in cardiac output and a decrease in stroke volume. The decrease in stroke volume is due to the effect of increased cardiac output on the peripheral volume, and a subsequent decrease in central venous pressure.[82,161] In this case, the increase in heart rate is not the direct cause of the decrease in stroke volume. It is not until the heart rate exceeds 150 beats/min that the cardiac output is decreased secondary to inadequate diastolic filling time, which decreases stroke volume.[11,70,120,150] Conversely, below a heart rate of 50 beats/min, the stroke volume is relatively fixed, and a further decrease in heart rate causes a decrease in cardiac output.[11,70,120,150]

INTRINSIC CARDIAC CONTROL

In addition to cardiac control through the autonomic nervous system and systemic hormones, cardiac output is modified by the intrinsic factors: preload, afterload, and contractility. The following discussion focuses on how these factors affect cardiac output. The specific cellular mechanisms of each of these factors are discussed in Chapter 2.

Preload

At the level of the muscle fiber, preload is defined as the force acting to stretch the ventricular fibers at end-diastole. Preload is related to cardiac output by the Frank-Starling Law of the Heart (length–tension relationship), which states that an increase in myocardial muscle fiber length is associated with an increase in the force of contraction,[166,171] and the subsequent increase in stroke volume and cardiac output.[77,154,182]

Afterload

In muscle fiber experiments, preload is the tension in the muscle before contraction and afterload is the additional tension that develops in the muscle during contraction, before shortening occurs.[77,166] At the level of the ventricle, afterload is defined as ventricular wall tension during the shortening phase of contraction, and reflects the sum of the forces against which the ventricle must act to eject blood.[82] However, given the heterogeneous direction of myocardial fibers, and the torsion or twisting of the ventricle during systole, a single measure of ventricular wall tension is inadequate to define afterload. In the intact system in vivo, afterload is defined as the pressure in the aorta during systole.[77] The aortic blood pressure is essentially equal to left ventricular pressure during the ejection phase of systole; thus, these values are interchangeable. The key factors that affect aortic blood pressure during ejection are arterial compliance, arterial resistance, and the reflection of pulse waves from the periphery.

As described by the force–velocity relation, for any given preload there is an inverse relation between afterload and muscle shortening, and thus stroke volume.[81,141,142,182] Although this relationship is observed in the isolated muscle fiber, it is not clinically apparent in people with normal cardiac function.[82] However, in people with a chronically depressed inotropic state (e.g., heart failure, cardiomyopathy), a steady state with altered ventricular dimensions (hypertrophy, dilatation) and maximal employment of the length–tension relation occurs. Therefore, in these people in the face of an increase in afterload, the reserve provided by the length–tension relationship is exhausted and stroke volume decreases acutely.[142] These findings help to explain the use of afterload-reducing agents in patients with heart failure.

In clinical practice, systemic vascular resistance, which is often considered *the* indicator of afterload, is often used interchangeably with afterload. This conceptualization is incorrect because afterload can change independently of vascular resistance. For example, in a patient who has suffered a severe hemorrhage, despite the fact that the systemic vascular resistance is increased (often to extremes), afterload is actually decreased. Recalling the original definition of afterload as the additional tension that develops in the muscle during contraction before shortening occurs helps to clarify this area of confusion. The tension or stress that develops in the ventricular wall according to the Laplace relation is:

$$\sigma = PR/2h$$

where σ is wall stress (force/cross-sectional area), P is intraventricular pressure, R is the radius of curvature of the wall, and h is wall thickness.

In hemorrhage, the radius of the ventricle is decreased, and if the compensatory actions of increased heart rate and systemic vasoconstriction are inadequate to maintain pressure, the intraventricular pressure also decreases. Thus, despite an increase in systemic vascular resistance, ventricular afterload decreases.

Contractility

Contractility refers to the intrinsic properties of cardiac myocytes that reflect the activation, formation, and cycling of cross-bridges between actin and myosin filaments. At a constant preload and afterload, an increase in contractility results in greater magnitude and velocity of shortening,[129,166] and augmented stroke volume. Contractility can be increased by an increase in circulating epinephrine and norepinephrine released from cardiac sympathetic nerves,[149] and by a decrease in the interval between beats (increasing heart rate), a phenomenon known as the treppe (staircase) effect.[81] In the intact heart, a change in contractility is defined as an alteration in cardiac performance that is independent of preload and afterload. The mechanism associated with increased contractility is an increase in the cytosolic calcium level (e.g., during ß-adrenergic stimulation) or increased sensitivity of myofibrils to calcium (e.g., use of calcium-sensitizing drug).[128–130]

The mechanism of the change in contractility differs physiologically from the change in contractile function related to a change in preload or afterload, although clinically there are no load-independent indices of contractility that are of practical utility. In the latter case, the mechanism for an increase in contractile function is known as length-dependent activation, whereby the myofilaments increase their sensitivity to cytosolic calcium as the sarcomere length increases to maximum.[2,60,76,128] This mechanism is contrary to traditional descriptions of Starling's law of the heart, which had maximal cardiac function occurring at an "optimal sarcomere length."[98] According to this conceptualization, an increase in sarcomere length was thought to give rise to optimal overlap of actin and myosin. This conceptualization has been challenged because the cardiac sarcomere normally operates at 80% to 85% of optimal length with only 10% of maximal force developed. Therefore, a mechanism other than optimal overlap, such as length-dependent calcium sensitivity, appears to be more likely.[129,140]

EXTRINSIC CONTROL: PERICARDIAL LIMITATION

In addition to the intrinsic factors that affect cardiac output, the pericardium restricts stroke volume in the face of increased filling pressures. The restrictive effects of the pericardium are particularly important in preventing excessive dilation during acute increases in cardiac volume.[169] In chronic cardiac dilation, however, there is growth of new pericardial tissue, and the pericardium actually enlarges in size and mass. As a result of this pericardial growth, there is no increase in pericardial constraint in cases of chronic cardiac dilation.[58]

After pericardiectomy, the maximal cardiac output, O_2 consumption, and left ventricular end-diastolic segment length increase.[75,176] The increase in cardiac output is related to an increase in stroke volume,[75] which is secondary to the increase in end-diastolic volume and myocardial fiber length, as described by the Frank-Starling law of the heart. Of course, the effects of pericardiectomy on stroke volume and cardiac output are apparent only during exercise.[176] In theory, a similar increase would occur in any situation that would cause an increase in venous return or end-diastolic volume, such as volume loading.

In cases in which the pericardium has been opened and reapproximated, pericardial constraint increases because of development of adhesions between the pericardium and the heart.[75] The increased constraint is manifested as an increase in intraventricular pressure for any given volume, which reflects an increase in juxtacardiac pressure.[174] This may be important in the interpretation of hemodynamic data (increased pressure for any given volume) in patients post-cardiac surgery who have had pericardial reapproximation.

VASCULAR CONTROL

Resistance and Compliance

The control of vascular resistance is crucial for the maintenance of blood pressure, as described by the equation: blood pressure = flow × resistance. The principal site for control of vascular resistance is the arterioles. More than 50% of total peripheral resistance appears across arterioles between 100 and 250 μm in diameter.[149]

Properties of Regional Circulation

There are six major organ systems. Four of these systems (i.e., muscle, brain, heart, and kidneys) are characterized as noncompliant (Δ volume/Δ pressure is small). The remaining two systems (i.e., splanchnic and skin) are compliant vascular beds ($\Delta V/\Delta P$ is large). As described later, the distribution of blood flow to the compliant versus noncompliant vascular beds determines the volume of blood available to fill the heart, and thus has a marked effect on central vascular pressure and stroke volume (Krogh model). The physical properties of the vascular system are discussed in Chapter 2.

The vascular beds with the highest conductance (lowest resistance) are the splanchnic, renal, and skeletal muscle vascular circuits. Changes in blood volume to these areas (particularly the splanchnic vascular bed) markedly affect venous return, and thus stroke volume. Of importance, the regions of high conductance have low metabolic demands at rest; thus, a large decrease in blood flow, which is needed passively to release blood volume, does not compromise the oxygen consumption of these organs. The oxygen consumption is maintained by increasing oxygen extraction, which is manifested by a widening of the arteriovenous oxygen difference.

Reflex Control of Vascular Resistance

In addition to the autonomic nervous system control of vascular resistance, other factors, such as endogenous vasoactive substances known as autacoids (histamine, serotonin, prostaglandins, bradykinin), endothelium-derived vasodilator substances (prostaglandins, endothelin, nitric oxide, and

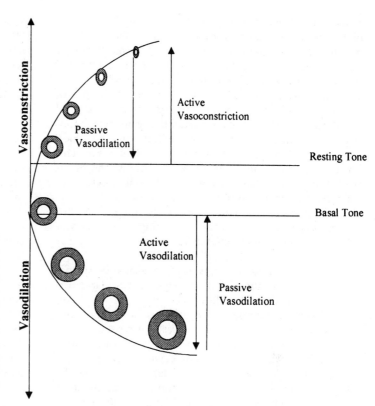

FIGURE 4-6 Schematic of active and passive changes in vascular resistance. [33,145] The vascular bed is tonically constricted (basal tone) as a result of neurohumoral and local factors (autoregulation). In addition, some vascular beds have a higher level of tone (resting tone) indicating sympathetic nervous system (SNS) stimulation. Passive vasodilation is the passive release of SNS stimulation, dilating the vessel toward basal tone. Passive vasoconstriction is the release of active vasodilatory stimuli. Active vasodilation is vascular dilation below basal tone and active vasoconstriction is constriction above basal tone. (Courtesy of Loring B. Rowell University of Washington, Seattle, WA.)

endothelium-derived hyperpolarizing factor), autoregulation, local heating, and local metabolic factors (e.g., hydrogen, potassium) all exert some local effects on vascular resistance (see Chapter 2). [146,179,180]

LONG-TERM CONTROL OF BLOOD PRESSURE

Although the sympathetic nervous system, through the sinoaortic baroreceptor reflex, plays a primary role in the rapid (minutes to hours) regulation of blood pressure, it appears to be less important in the long-term control of arterial pressure than neuroendocrine factors. [37] The probable method for the long-term control of arterial pressure is the much slower-acting fluid volume regulation, with the hypothesized mechanism being renal pressure diuresis–natriuresis. [37]

Although blood volume is not directly linked to arterial pressure, long-term arterial blood pressure control is based on the idea that arterial pressure is maintained at a level required by the kidneys to excrete a volume of urine approximately equivalent to the daily fluid intake (minus extrarenal fluid losses). [37] The kidneys sense a change in blood volume through the arterial pressure. [27,37] That arterial pressure and not fluid volume is sensed is demonstrated in disease processes associated with a combination of increased extracellular volume and decreased arterial pressure (e.g., heart failure, cirrhosis with ascites). In these cases, the kidneys retain fluid despite expanded fluid volume.

Based on this hypothesis, an increase in arterial pressure as a result of increased systemic vascular resistance would cause an increase in sodium and water excretion. As long as

sodium and water intake remained stable, the enhanced excretion would decrease extracellular volume and blood volume, and arterial pressure would decrease. According to this mechanism, an increase in systemic vascular resistance would not cause a long-term increase in arterial pressure unless renal function was impaired. [37]

Renal Excretion of Sodium Chloride and Water

Despite the putative primacy of the renal diuresis–natriuresis mechanism in the long-term control of blood pressure, a hypothesis receiving some support is that arginine vasopressin and angiotensin II provide long-term feedback to the central nervous system. In addition, neural and hormonal factors modulate the renal diuresis–natriuresis response. For example, a decrease in sodium intake stimulates renin activity, which leads to the generation of angiotensin II. An increase in angiotensin II decreases renal blood flow and the glomerular filtration rate, which indicates a shift of the pressure–natriuretic response (i.e., increased response to decreased sodium). Thus, angiotensin II appears to have an important role in the long-term modulation of renal function and the control of blood pressure. [37]

Basal Tone

All arterioles exhibit a basal level of vasoconstriction or tone. Basal tone, which is the intrinsic level of vascular tone, is independent of neural or humoral influences and serves as the baseline around which neural or humorally mediated vasoconstriction or vasodilation occurs (Fig. 4-6). Basal tone varies among organs; it is lowest in the kidneys and highest in the skeletal muscles, heart, and brain.[7,116,117] The maintenance of arteriolar tone through tonic rhythmic vasoconstriction is essential for the maintenance of blood pressure. For example, it is estimated that if this basal myogenic tone were eliminated, a minimal cardiac output of 60 to 75 L/min would be required to maintain a normal blood pressure.[116,117,146] In contrast, if the sympathetic input associated with resting tone were withdrawn, the blood pressure would decrease only from 100 to 86 mm Hg. This small decrease in blood pressure occurs because the vascular bed with the highest resting tone (skeletal muscle) normally receives only 15% of the cardiac output.

As demonstrated in Figure 4-6, active and passive vasomotion occurs around the basal and resting tone of the vascular bed. Four terms define this vasomotion:[33,146]

1. *Active vasoconstriction,* which is mediated by sympathetic stimulation, is the increase in vascular resistance above the basal level.
2. *Passive vasodilation,* in contrast to active vasoconstriction, is the reduction in vascular resistance back to the basal level due to the withdrawal of the sympathetic stimulation associated with active vasoconstriction. In some vascular beds, resistance may be increased above basal tone by tonic sympathetic stimulation. This increase in vascular tone is referred to as *resting tone.* Passive vasodilation is most easily seen in vascular beds with increased resting tone.
3. If a vascular bed has high basal tone, *active vasodilation,* which is a decrease in vascular resistance below the level maintained by basal tone, may occur (i.e., vasodilation beyond that which exists after all neural and hormonal influences are removed). In this case, the vasodilation is not merely the result of withdrawal of sympathetic tone because this action causes passive vasodilation.
4. *Passive vasoconstriction* is due to withdrawal of the stimulation causing active vasodilation.

The skeletal muscle arterioles have a high basal tone and therefore are capable of a wide range of vasoconstriction and vasodilation because there is an increased level of basal tone to be modulated. In contrast, the renal vasculature has a low basal and resting tone that can be markedly increased through sympathetic stimulation, but has little capability to undergo active vasodilation because there is so little basal tone to inhibit.

LOCAL REGULATION OF SYSTEMIC MICROVASCULAR BEDS

As noted, arteriolar resistance vessels are partially constricted under normal circumstances by a tonic rhythmic myogenic tone, and this level is modulated by neurogenic or other factors that cause active vasoconstriction or vasodilation. In the intact organism, blood flow and vascular hydrostatic pressure in the microvasculature of each organ system are controlled by complex interrelations among the effects of physical factors, locally released substances, circulating hormones, and above all by neurotransmitters secreted in response to central activation of the sympathetic nervous system. The relative predominance of local versus centrally mediated control of the microvascular bed varies among vascular beds, and it also varies among resistance, precapillary, and postcapillary blood vessels within a given vascular bed.

The large and medium-sized arterioles, which are the predominant sites of vascular resistance, are primarily under the control of the sympathetic nervous system and centrally mediated neurohumoral factors (e.g., angiotensin II). These vascular segments are influential in the control of arterial blood pressure and, by virtue of their position, they control the total amount of blood entering a specific vascular area and, therefore, the distribution of blood flow between the different vascular beds.

The terminal arterioles or precapillary vascular segments control the number of open capillaries and are under sympathetic nervous system and local control.[83] Local control mechanisms (autoregulation) that affect the terminal arterioles may have a substantial influence on exchange vessel pressures and flows and on the vascular tissue exchange of fluid and solutes.

Autoregulation

Autoregulation, which appears to occur in all organs except the lung, is the intrinsic tendency of an organ or vascular bed to maintain constant blood flow through alteration in its arteriolar tone, despite changes in arterial pressure.[86,136] Autoregulation can occur in some organs over a range of perfusion pressure of 60 to 80 mm Hg to an upper limit of 150 mm Hg (Fig. 4-7), and is independent of neural and hormonal control. There are three hypotheses to explain autoregulation: the myogenic, metabolic, and tissue pressure hypotheses.[86,136] It appears that none of these mechanisms works in isolation, and, as described later, the tissue pressure hypothesis may apply only in pathologic conditions. In addition, under certain conditions (e.g., a marked decrease in arterial perfusion with hypoxemia and decreased transmural pressure), metabolic and myogenic control promote vasodilation in an additive manner.[21,136] Conversely, with increased venous pressure, the myogenic and metabolic control systems may compete. In this case (low flow, high venous pressure), metabolically induced vasodilatation usually predominates over the myogenic response to increased vascular distention, which should stimulate vasoconstriction.[87,108,136]

MYOGENIC HYPOTHESIS

The myogenic hypothesis is based on the observation that when vascular smooth muscle is stretched, or transmural pressure increases, the smooth muscle is stimulated to contract.[84,87,136] Thus, a pressure-induced stretch in vascular smooth muscle results in vasoconstriction and subsequently decreases the flow.[51] Conversely, when the arterial pressure is decreased, the stimulus for the myogenic response is decreased, the vessel dilates, and blood flow is returned

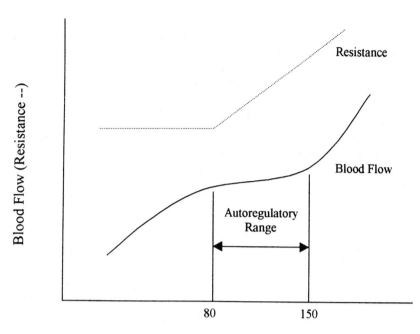

FIGURE 4-7 A schematic representation of autoregulation. The blood flow is relatively constant between an arterial pressure of 60 and 150 mm Hg because of an active increase in resistance. Below a mean pressure of 60 mm Hg and above 150 mm Hg, the flow is directly related to pressure.[51, 145]

toward control levels.[87,88] Neither the stimulus nor the mechanism for myogenic response has been clarified.[9,87,88,115]

There are two arguments against the myogenic hypothesis. First, the myogenic response senses local pressure rather than flow to control flow.[134,136,146] Autoregulation is related to the control of flow, not the control of pressure; thus, although the myogenic response may play some role in the local control of blood flow, its role in the central control of blood flow remains to be demonstrated. Second, to increase resistance and maintain a constant flow, the caliber of the arteriole must be smaller than it was before the vessel was stretched by the increased pressure. If this vasoconstriction does not occur, flow rises.[146]

METABOLIC HYPOTHESIS

The metabolic hypothesis is considered a special case of metabolic control of blood flow and is based on the idea that the concentration of a huge number of metabolites and metabolic substrates (e.g., potassium, hydrogen, O_2, CO_2, adenosine) in the interstitial space controls vascular tone. In this case, the vascular smooth muscle acts as a chemosensor. According to this hypothesis, a decrease in blood flow leads to an increase in the local concentration of a metabolite and causes vasodilation and increased blood flow.[51,136,146] The metabolic hypothesis has been suggested as a mechanism for autoregulation in organs or tissues where the primary function of blood supply is to support local metabolism. In this case, there is a close relation between blood flow and metabolic needs. However, in organ systems with high blood flow (e.g., kidney, skin), where blood flow occurs in excess of metabolic needs, there is a limited relationship between blood flow and metabolism,[146] and the metabolic hypothesis as a factor in the autoregulatory control of blood flow has not been supported.

An important point is that metabolic autoregulation is not the same as metabolically induced active and reactive hyperemia (increased blood flow), which occur in response to increased metabolic demand (e.g., intestinal vasculature during digestion or cardiac and skeletal muscle during activity) or interruption of blood flow to a vascular bed, respectively.[136]

Active hyperemia is the adaptive increase in blood flow in response to changes in the local metabolic rate due to variation in the functional activity of the surrounding cells.[136] In response to this change in functional status, the vascular resistance decreases almost immediately. In addition, there is an increase in the number of perfused capillaries (capillary recruitment) in response to metabolic stimulation.

The magnitude of the reactive hyperemia response depends on the duration of the vascular obstruction and the metabolic rate of the given vascular bed. Unlike "pure" metabolic autoregulation, this response is a combination of three components: (1) passive changes in vessel diameter due to a change in transmural pressure, (2) a myogenic response to the change in transmural pressure, and (3) a metabolic component.[87,107,136]

TISSUE PRESSURE HYPOTHESIS

The tissue pressure hypothesis states that an increase in external pressure (e.g., interstitial pressure) decreases transmural pressure (pressure inside minus pressure outside the vessel), which passively decreases the vessel diameter and decreases flow.[136] The effect of external compression on blood flow normally occurs during ventricular systole, when the coronary arteries are compressed. Clinically, the effect of transmural compression is more likely to be observed in organs constrained in a rigid container (e.g., brain, where increased cerebrospinal fluid pressure may compress cerebral vessels) or a stiff capsule (e.g., kidney).[136,146] In the lung, vascular compression due to increased external (alveolar) pressure, such as with the application of high levels of positive end-expiratory pressure, may also affect blood flow.

Tissue pressure probably does not play a major role in the control of blood flow under physiological conditions, but may be particularly important under pathologic conditions such as edema, hemorrhage into the interstitial space, or cellular swelling due to injury or hypoxemia (compartment syndrome).[136] In the latter cases, external compression may decrease blood flow below a physiologically safe level.

Endothelium-Derived Vasoactive Mediators

In vivo, in response to shear stress, pressure, and hypoxia,[32,110,121,179] and in vitro in response to numerous neurohumoral mediators (e.g., histamine, arginine vasopressin, serotonin, adenosine diphosphate, thrombin, and endothelin), endothelial cells synthesize vasoactive mediators. Perhaps the best known mediator of vasoaction is the endothelium-derived relaxing factor, nitric oxide. In addition to nitric oxide, prostaglandins and endothelium-derived hyperpolarizing factor[53] all exert vasodilatory effects that could counteract neurally and humorally mediated vasoconstriction.[179] In contrast, endothelin, which, depending on concentration, is both a vasodilator and a vasoconstrictor, is also synthesized by endothelial cells. The specifics of cellular activation and activity of these factors are described in Chapter 2.

VENOUS SYSTEM

The primary functions of the venous system are to return blood from the capillaries to the heart and to serve as a volume reservoir that counterbalances the transient imbalance between cardiac output and venous return. However, because of its capacious nature, the venous system serves not only as a reservoir (normally approximately two-thirds of total blood volume is stored in the veins, liver sinusoids, and spleen), but as a buffer against changes in cardiac output and blood pressure. The venous system can play both an active (venoconstriction) and, more important, a passive role in the maintenance of thoracic blood volume.

Neurohumoral Stimulation

The only neural control of veins is through the α-adrenergic fibers of the sympathetic nervous system.[143] Release of norepinephrine from α-adrenergic fibers causes constriction in the splanchnic and cutaneous veins, whereas withdrawal of sympathetic stimulation results in passive vasodilation. The cutaneous veins are densely innervated with α-adrenergic receptors, predominantly postsynaptic α₂ receptors.[55] There is limited ß-adrenergic stimulation in the cutaneous veins. The veins of the skeletal muscle and the small venules have virtually no innervation.

Epinephrine is the primary humoral factor that affects the veins, with actions on cutaneous vessels and, more important, splanchnic vessels. Given the preponderance of α-adrenergic receptors on the veins, stimulation by epinephrine results in venoconstriction. However, unlike the arterioles, epinephrine stimulation of ß₂-adrenergic receptors does not cause venodilation.

PASSIVE VERSUS ACTIVE EFFECTS

As noted, neurohumoral stimulation primarily affects the most capacious volume reservoirs (splanchnic and cutaneous venous bed). The question is whether translocation of blood from the venous system is primarily the consequence of active venoconstriction or of the passive effects that stem from the substantial changes in venous transmural pressure caused by arteriolar vasoconstriction or vasodilation.

Changes in upstream arteriolar tone alter downstream venous transmural pressure and the volume of blood that flows through the venous system. For example, arteriolar vasodilation increases blood flow into the highly capacious postcapillary venous beds, and the increase in their transmural venular pressure passively expands their volume. Given that total blood volume is constant, an increase in blood volume in the peripheral venous system means a decrease in the volume of the central veins that fill the heart. Conversely, vasoconstriction decreases flow into the postcapillary venous system, venous transmural pressure decreases, and the elastic recoil of the veins passively expels their volume back toward the central thoracic veins.[144]

The magnitude of passive change in venous transmural pressure depends on where the changes occur along the venous volume–pressure curve (Fig. 4-8). For example, as demonstrated in Figure 4-8, at a low venous transmural

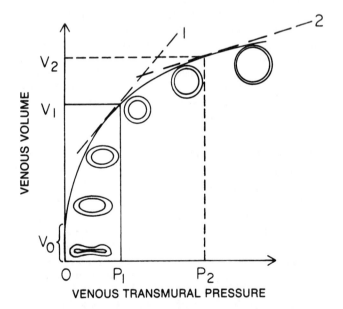

FIGURE 4-8 Typical volume–pressure curve of an isolated vein. Dashed lines (1 and 2) show the compliance (ΔV/ΔP) at two venous transmural pressures, P_1 and P_2. Note that compliance varies with pressure, being greatest at the lower pressures (line 1) and decreasing as the pressure increases (line 2). V_0 is the unstressed volume, which is the volume contained at 0 transmural pressure. The change in volume from V_2 to V_1 is the passive effect of changing pressures from P_2 to P_1. Note how changing cross–sectional geometry contributes to *passive* emptying. (From Rowell LB: Human Circulation: Regulation During Physical Stress, p 46. New York, Oxford University Press, 1986.)

pressure, the pressure–volume curve is steep and a small change in distending pressure causes a large change in volume; that is, arteriolar vasodilation, which increases venous blood flow and venous transmural pressure, causes a larger increase in venous volume expansion when the veins are not initially distended compared with the volume expansion that would occur if the veins were fully distended with decreased compliance. Conversely, passive vasoconstriction translocates a larger volume of blood to the central circulation when venular volume is normal or increased, in contrast to a situation such as hemorrhage, where the volume is already diminished (e.g., no further volume to move into the central circulation).

The passive effects of an alteration in blood flow on venous volume are exemplified in a study by Sheriff and colleagues[161] that evaluated the effect of a pacing-induced increase or decrease in cardiac output on central venous pressure. A decrease in cardiac output, which resulted in a 17 mm Hg decrease in arterial pressure, was associated with 3.9 mm Hg increase in central venous pressure. The increase in central venous pressure reflects the fall in venous flow and transmural pressure associated with the decrease in cardiac output, and the resultant passive recoil of the veins and the translocation of their blood centrally. The relation between venous volume and cardiac output is addressed further in the sections on the relation between cardiac output and central venous pressure, and the Krogh model.

The dominance of passive venous volume mobility can be altered in conditions such as hemorrhage, in which active venoconstriction of the richly innervated splanchnic veins can also play a role in the translocation of blood back to the central circulation.[71,146] In addition, vasoconstriction continues to exert its effects on venous volume, as previously described. In a study that examined the effects of a 27% decrease in cardiac output, with and without the presence of reflexes, active constriction of the splanchnic veins accounted for 21% of the translocated blood volume, whereas passive vasodilation accounted for the remaining 79%.[144] Thus, when active and passive effects are combined, the passive effects of decreased blood flow on venous volume mobility exceed the effect of simultaneous active venoconstriction.[144,145]

MODELS OF CARDIAC PERFORMANCE

Relation Between Cardiac Output and Central Venous Pressure

In the 1950s, Guyton[65,66,68] developed a model in which central venous pressure was presumed to affect cardiac output in a retrograde fashion. However, a more useful conceptualization is a model of the anterograde relationship between cardiac output and central venous pressure, that is, cardiac output affects central venous pressure.[105,145] Guyton and colleagues[67] addressed this anterograde relationship. They stated:

The normal [i.e., at rest] circulatory system operates near this limit [i.e., collapse of central veins due to increased cardiac output] so that an increase in

efficacy of the heart as a pump cannot by itself increase cardiac output more than a few percent, unless some simultaneous effect takes place in the peripheral circulatory system at the same time to translocate blood from the peripheral vessels to the heart.

The concept put forward in this statement provides answers to two questions raised by Guyton's statement: (1) Why, at rest, does an increase in cardiac output decrease the central venous pressure? Conversely, why does a decrease in cardiac output increase the central venous pressure? (2) Is it possible to correct the problem and maintain end-diastolic volume?

WHY DOES AN INCREASE IN CARDIAC OUTPUT DECREASE CENTRAL VENOUS PRESSURE?

In experiments, an increase in cardiac output secondary to an increase in heart rate was limited by a decrease in central venous pressure.[11] This inverse relationship between cardiac output and central venous pressure is demonstrated in Figure 4-9. The resistive and capacitive properties of the arteries and veins help to explain this relationship.[82,146] Of particular importance is the highly capacious nature of the postcapillary venules and small veins in most vascular beds. In response to increased blood flow (increased cardiac output), transmural pressure in the veins rises, and thus their volume rises as well. The consequent shift in blood volume from the central to the peripheral veins lowers the central venous pressure.[82,149,161] If cardiac output continues to increase, the central venous pressure approaches, and

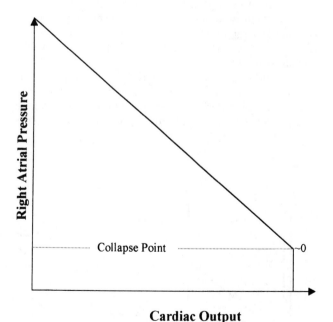

FIGURE 4-9 Schematic demonstrating the effect of raising or lowering cardiac output on right atrial pressures, which is caused in turn by the effect of blood flow on peripheral vascular volume. (Modified from Rowell LB: Human Cardiovascular Control, p 45. New York, Oxford University Press, 1993.)

eventually the central venous vasculature collapses, making it impossible to increase cardiac output further.[82] This constitutes an autolimitation on our ability to increase cardiac output when there is no extra cardiac force available to match increased venous return with cardiac output (to increase, as stated by Guyton and colleagues).

In contrast to the effects of increased cardiac output on central venous pressure, a decrease in cardiac output causes peripheral venous transmural pressure to fall. The decrease in transmural pressure allows the venous beds to collapse passively and expel their blood volume into the central circulation, thus raising end-diastolic volume, central venous pressure, and stroke volume.

Krogh Model. The ideas expressed about the inverse relationship between cardiac output and central venous pressure bring to life the importance of a simple and highly insightful model of the circulation proposed by Krogh in 1912 that helps us to understand the importance of the distribution of cardiac output on end-diastolic volume and stroke volume.[97] The Krogh model (Fig. 4-10) divides the circulation into two circuits, one compliant and the other noncompliant. In humans, the two compliant vascular beds are the splanchnic region (liver, gastrointestinal tract, pancreas) and the skin, whereas the remaining vascular beds are noncompliant.[143,145] Cardiac filling pressures depend on the ratio of flow through the noncompliant versus compliant vascular beds. For example, if, with all else constant, flow is increased to the splanchnic region relative to the skeletal muscle, cardiac filling pressures would be expected to decrease as a consequence of the distention and increased volume in the compliant splanchnic veins, whereas the volume in the noncompliant veins in the muscle would not be expected to change. This relationship can be visualized as running fluid through a piece of highly compliant tubing, such as a Penrose drain, versus running the same flow and volume through a rigid pipe. The volume in the compliant tubing increases, whereas the volume in the rigid tubing remains constant.

A clinical demonstration of the Krogh model can be achieved by administering a vasoconstricting α-adrenergic agent (e.g., phenylephrine, norepinephrine, or dopamine) to a patient who is vasodilated. Vasoconstriction of blood vessels leading into compliant vascular beds (e.g., splanchnic) results in the passive collapse of the bed, with translocation of blood into the central circulation and a subsequent increase in blood return to the heart. However, as observed in clinical practice, a decrease in blood flow to the splanchnic region is not risk free; for example, decreased gastrointestinal tract perfusion and ischemic bowel can occur if the decrease in flow is too great.

The Krogh model is also useful for understanding the potentially negative consequences of recreational hyperthermia (i.e., hot tub or sauna) on coronary blood flow and cardiac output in a person with coronary artery disease. With hyperthermia, there is vasodilation of the highly compliant cutaneous vascular bed, with a resultant large increase in cutaneous blood volume.[149] The net result is a decrease in blood volume available to the heart and a subsequent decrease in cardiac output and coronary artery perfusion. In addition, the vasodilation accelerates the rate of increase in body core temperature because of the increased cutaneous volume exposed to the hot water or air.[145,146]

The effects of environmental thermal stress plus exercise can also precipitate problems. In this case, the ability to increase cardiac output is limited by the fall in central venous pressure and stroke volume, which is caused by vasodilation of the cutaneous vascular bed and the large increase in venous volume. The body compensates (according to the Krogh model) by marked vasoconstriction in the visceral organs (including the kidneys), which can lead to ischemia and injury of these organs as well as a severe overload on the heart.[146] This finding has important implications for exercise programs that are a part of cardiac rehabilitation and highlights the need for control of ambient temperature to maximize the benefits of exercise.[145,146]

HOW IS IT POSSIBLE TO CORRECT THE PROBLEM AND MAINTAIN END-DIASTOLIC VOLUME?

The second question is, How is it possible to correct the problem of increased peripheral blood volume to maintain end-diastolic volume when cardiac output increases? For example, in response to the stress of standing, blood volume is transferred to the periphery, and a reflex increase in

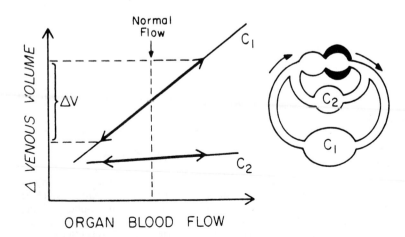

FIGURE 4-10 (Right) The Krogh model divides the circulation between two circuits, one compliant (C_1) and the other noncompliant (C_2). **(Left)** The relation between the change in organ venous volume and blood flow through a compliant organ (C_1) and a noncompliant organ (C_2). The volume of blood available to the heart is determined by the distribution of blood flow between such circuits. For example, in hyperthermia there is increased blood volume in the compliant vascular beds of the skin, and the amount of blood available to the heart is decreased. (From Rowell LB: Human Circulation: Regulation During Physical Stress, p 60. New York, Oxford University Press, 1986.)

heart rate and cardiac output is initiated to maintain blood pressure. The increase in cardiac output is maintained for only a few beats, as the left ventricular reservoir (the pulmonary veins) is rapidly depleted. As discussed, the beneficial effect of increasing cardiac output is ultimately limited by the flow-induced "relative sequestration or pooling" of blood in the periphery. Any further increase in heart rate[11,99,155] or cardiac output are met by a decrease in central venous pressure, and thus in a circular manner the cardiac output decreases. Therefore, as Guyton stated,[67] for cardiac output to be maintained it is imperative that a "simultaneous effect takes place in the peripheral circulatory system at the same time to translocate blood from the peripheral vessels to the heart." Two factors that aid in the translocation of blood from the peripheral vessels to the central circulation are the muscle pump and the respiratory pump.

Muscle Pump. During passive upright posture or tilt, blood volume in the dependent (below heart level) veins rises by 500 to 700 mL, and then slowly rises further because of filtration and slow venous expansion (i.e., creep). The central venous pressure, stroke volume, and cardiac output fall progressively to a point where the arterial blood pressure begins to fall, eventually resulting in fainting, although the increase in peripheral blood volume may be temporarily offset by the presence of intact venous valves. However, the key to surviving the stress of passive upright posture is the contraction of skeletal muscles in the legs.[61]

When the skeletal muscles in the leg relax, they do so rapidly. The sudden release of muscular compression pulls the collapsed veins open and creates negative transmural pressure (assuming the valves are competent).[101] This negative pressure occurs because the veins, which are tethered to the muscle, are pulled open as the muscle recoils.[149] This negative pressure creates an arteriovenous gradient that facilitates movement of blood into the venous beds. During muscle contraction, the muscle pump generates a gradient for flow between the venous beds and the right atrium (i.e., the muscle can increase its own blood flow by increasing the arteriovenous pressure gradient). The muscle pump, with a pumping capability *equal to that of the left ventricle,* is so important that it is often referred to as the "second heart."[149,162] Without the muscle pump, we would be unable to maintain an upright position[145,146] or to exercise.[162] As previously discussed, people with congenitally absent venous valves cannot maintain an upright position.[12]

In patients who undergo prolonged bed rest, temporary orthostatic intolerance develops. The exact mechanism of bed rest–induced orthostasis remains unclear. One factor that may contribute to orthostatic intolerance is a position-induced increase in intrathoracic blood volume, which ultimately results in a decrease in plasma volume.[19] This factor is questioned, however, because the maintenance of adequate plasma volume does not prevent bed rest–induced orthostasis. The other factor that may play a role in orthostasis is a decrease in intramuscular pressure that has been found after prolonged bed rest or surgery. A decrease in intramuscular pressure translates into an inability to compress the intramuscular veins or decrease venous transmural pressure and thus pump blood back to the heart.

Respiratory Pump. The second, but less important, mechanism that promotes blood return to the heart is the respiratory pump. The pressure difference promoting flow from the venules to the right atrium is affected by changes in intrathoracic and intra-abdominal pressures.[22] During inspiration, the diaphragm descends and intrathoracic pressure decreases and intra-abdominal pressure increases. These pressure changes create a gradient for blood flow from the point where the vena cava enters the thoracic cavity to the right atrium, and thereby increase venous return to the heart. During expiration, the diaphragm relaxes and intrathoracic pressure increases, whereas intra-abdominal pressure decreases. The increased intrathoracic pressure impedes thoracic venous flow; however, there is an increase in blood flow from the lower extremities. During mechanical ventilation, however, the relation between the respiratory cycle and venous return is reversed.[22,125,145]

Normally, the changes in venous return are not readily apparent because the liver serves as a sump to smooth out the fluctuations in venous return.[125] The liver is able to do this because it is a highly compliant vascular bed.[143] During inspiration, the diaphragm compresses the hepatic veins and essentially stops venous outflow. However, arterial inflow continues, and the liver swells with blood. During expiration, the diaphragm ascends and the compression of the hepatic veins is released. The liver discharges the increased blood volume to the right atrium, which smooths the expected respiratory oscillations.

An increase in respiratory oscillations may be observed in patients with a noncompliant liver, such as those with hepatic engorgement secondary to right heart failure or hepatic cirrhosis. In these cases, the respiration-induced fluctuations are more apparent because the liver cannot serve as a sump for blood.[124] Pericardial constriction, restrictive cardiomyopathy, and right ventricular infarction are other clinical conditions to consider when a respiration-induced increase in right atrial pressure (Kussmaul's sign) is observed.[42,167,168] In these cases, the paradoxical increase in right atrial pressure is due to the inspiration-induced increase of venous return into the nondistensible right atrium or ventricle.[167]

ADDITIONAL EFFECTS OF RESPIRATION

In addition to the effects of the respiratory pump on returning blood to the heart, respiration, or the normal rhythmic changes in intrathoracic pressure, also directly affects stroke volume, cardiac output, and blood pressure. Extreme changes in intrathoracic pressure (Valsalva maneuver) also have potentially serious consequences for patients with cardiovascular disease.

Effect of Respiration on Stroke Volume, Cardiac Output, and Blood Pressure

Venous return to the right atrium increases during inspiration, which leads to an increase in right ventricular stroke volume during inspiration. This increase in stroke volume increases the pulmonary blood volume. Conversely, the right ventricular stroke volume decreases during expiration. The exact opposite occurs on the left side of the heart, as the left ventricular stroke volume decreases during inspiration and increases during expiration.[25,69,163] The inspiratory decrease in left ventricular stroke volume occurs because the space in the pericardium is limited; that is, the right ventricular volume is increased during inspiration, thus decreasing the space available for the left ventricle. As noted, there is an increase in pulmonary blood flow due to the inspiratory increase in right ventricular stroke volume. The availability of this sump for the left ventricle helps lessen the respiratory variation in left ventricular stroke volume because the left heart can draw from the sump when right ventricular outflow decreases during expiration.[69,145]

The respiration-induced swings in stroke volume increase with increasing tidal volume and respiratory rate and decrease in patients who are status-post pericardiectomy.[69] Possible mechanisms for the decrease in left ventricular stroke volume during inspiration include decreased left ventricular compliance due to increased right ventricular volume and shifting of the interventricular septum, and increased left ventricular afterload due to the effects of the decreased intrathoracic pressure on left ventricular transmural pressure.[25,69,90,138,185] The latter concept of how respiration changes left ventricular afterload is explained by Bromberger-Barnea (1981):

If we would put a constriction on the aorta and thereby raise aortic systolic and diastolic pressure proximal to the constriction, it would be self-evident that this increase in aortic diastolic pressure represented an additional afterload to the left ventricle. . . . Lowering the pressure around the heart [due to inspiration] is analogous to raising the extra-thoracic diastolic pressure, because lowering the pressure around the heart is like lowering the whole heart and, therefore, the pressure generated by the heart to pump blood over the wall out into the periphery has to be increased (p 2173).

Normally, during inspiration there is a small decrease in systolic arterial pressure (<10 mm Hg) as a result of the decrease in stroke volume.[158] Despite its name, pulsus paradoxus, which is defined as an inspiratory decrease in systolic blood pressure of greater than 10 mm Hg, is not paradoxical, but rather is an exaggeration of the normal inspiratory decrease in systolic blood pressure.[168]

Valsalva Maneuver

The Valsalva maneuver, which is a deep breath followed by straining to expire against a closed glottis, causes an abnormal increase in intrathoracic pressures.[40,49,103,175] The hemodynamic response to the sudden increase in intrathoracic pressure associated with the Valsalva maneuver can be subdivided into four phases[73,74,103] (Fig. 4-11). During the initial phase (phase 1: strain phase), which is produced by forcefully exhaling against a closed glottis, there is a transient increase in arterial systolic and diastolic pressures due to aortic compression caused by increased intrathoracic pressure, and a marked decrease in venous return subsequent to

compression of the vena cava, as well as a decrease in pulse pressure. During the remainder of the strain phase (phase 2), there is a progressive decrease in blood pressure and cardiac output due to a decrease in venous return and left ventricular filling and stroke volume subsequent to compression of the vena cava. The decrease in cardiac output and arterial pulse pressure, which increases baroreflex-mediated sympathetic activity, is manifested as a compensatory increase in heart rate and peripheral resistance.[118,165] On release of the strain (phase 3), there is an abrupt decrease in arterial pressure (release of aortic compression) and a rapid rise in venous return (decreased caval compression with restoration of the inferior vena cava to right atrial pressure gradient) without a change in heart rate.[1] Finally, during phase 4 (overshoot), when the increased venous return reaches the left ventricle, there is a progressive increase in left ventricular stroke volume, blood pressure, and pulse pressure above baseline due to an increase in cardiac output, secondary to the increased venous return into the vasoconstricted systemic vasculature.[26,73,103,159,165] The overshoot of blood pressure, pulse pressure, and cardiac output stimulates vagal activity, leading to reflex bradycardia.[165] The autonomic nervous system plays the central role in the response to the Valsala maneuver.

The Valsalva maneuver is used to evaluate autonomic function.[59] A frequently used technique is the Valsalva ratio, which is a comparison of the heart rate response during various stages of the maneuver.[4,46,59,96,103,109,164] An example of an abnormal response to the Valsalva maneuver may be seen in patients with diabetic autonomic neuropathy.[49] In these patients, there may be a delay or absence in the tachycardia observed during the decrease in blood pressure in phase 2, and a delay or absence in the bradycardic response to the blood pressure overshoot during phase 4.[54] This latency, which is thought to reflect sympathetic and parasympathetic nervous system dysfunction,[54,164] may place these patients at increased risk for a progressive fall in blood pressure (to the point of syncope).[109]

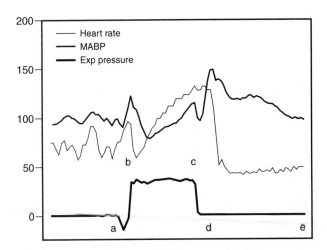

FIGURE 4-11 The normal hemodynamic response to a Valsalva maneuver. Phase 1: a–b; phase 2: b–c; phase 3: c–d; phase 4: d–e. MABP, mean arterial blood pressure; Exp pressure, expiratory pressure. (From Freeman R: Noninvasive evaluation of heart rate variability. In Low PA [ed]: Clinical Autonomic Disorders, 2nd ed, p 302. Philadelphia, Lippincott–Raven Publishers, 1997.)

In the clinical setting, the effects of the Valsalva maneuver may be observed when a patient strains during defecation or vomiting.[114] It is the reflex bradycardia and the sequelae of the Valsalva maneuver (cardiac arrhythmias, sudden cardiac arrest, cerebral and subarachnoid hemorrhage, rupture of a dissecting aortic aneurysm) that are observed clinically.[114,119] Patients who may be at increased risk for an adverse response to the Valsalva maneuver include those with cardiac disease (e.g., heart failure)[103,159] and older people, because the response to the maneuver has been shown to decrease with age.[175] Interventions to protect this high-risk group from the sequelae of the Valsalva maneuver (e.g., positioning, and avoiding straining during a bowel movement or with vomiting) need to be performed.

OVERALL CONTROL

Baroreflex Control of Blood Pressure

The arterial baroreceptor reflex is the primary mechanism for the short-term or rapid control of arterial blood pressure, whereas neurohumoral factors (predominantly the control of sodium excretion) are responsible for long-term or slower control.

ARTERIAL BARORECEPTOR RESPONSE TO DECREASED ARTERIAL PRESSURE

A decrease in blood pressure may be the result of loss of blood (hemorrhage) or a shift in blood away from the heart (standing up). In response to a decrease in arterial pressure, the baroreceptor firing rate decreases, and the firing rate through the sinus node and vagal afferents is reduced. The anatomic details of the reflex are described in Chapter 2. The response to a decrease in arterial pressure is described as follows (Fig. 4-12):

Increased Sympathetic Nervous System Activity. The primary result is an increase in total vascular resistance. This response is relatively slow (5 to 15 seconds). A small increase in stroke volume secondary to ß₁ stimulation and increased contractility also occurs. The increase in vascular resistance is the primary mechanism for restoring blood pressure because an increase in heart rate is relatively ineffective in raising cardiac output. As previously described, if the cardiac output increases without an increase in peripheral vascular tone, the central venous pressure decreases.[11,82,146,149]

The sympathetic nervous system–mediated vasoconstriction decreases blood flow to the splanchnic region, thereby causing a passive release of blood volume from its capacious veins. Visceral organs can transfer as much as 300 to 500 mL of blood into the central circulation.[144,145,147] The importance of vasoconstriction, particularly that involving the splanchnic region, is demonstrated by people with peripheral neuropathy (diabetes mellitus, Parkinson's disease) or spinal cord injury who have severe orthostatic intolerance because of an inability to constrict arterioles in the dependent regions.[145,147]

Decreased Vagal Activity Resulting in an Increase in Heart Rate. The increase in heart rate is not a primary compensatory response to a decrease in blood pressure. As described by the cardiac output–central venous pressure relation, an increase in heart rate–induced central venous pressure is of limited efficacy in increasing the cardiac output.

ARTERIAL BARORECEPTOR RESPONSE TO INCREASED ARTERIAL PRESSURE

An acute increase in blood pressure results in increased stimulation of the sinoaortic baroreceptors. The increased baroreceptor firing rate increases sinus and vagal afferent input into the nucleus tractus solitarius of the medulla. In response to the increased baroreceptor input, the following occur (Fig. 4-13):

1. A rapid (within one beat) decrease in heart rate, secondary to a sudden increase in vagal tone
2. A secondary decrease in stroke volume due to the negative inotropic effects of the increased vagal tone (minor effect)
3. A sympathetic nervous system–mediated decrease in vascular tone (minor effect)

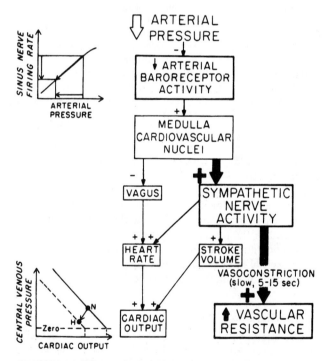

FIGURE 4-12 Summary of how the arterial baroreflex restores blood pressure back toward normal during arterial hypotension. Correction is by relatively slow (5 to 15 seconds) vasoconstriction. Increased heart rate has little or no effect if cardiac filling pressure is low and cardiac output cannot be increased, for reasons illustrated in the small graph next to "cardiac output" (central venous pressure vs. cardiac output). When normal (N) cardiac output increases, central venous pressure falls. When both cardiac output and central venous pressure are low during hemorrhage (H), output cannot rise much without collapsing central veins as central venous pressure goes to 0. (From Rowell LB: Human Cardiovascular Control, p 57. New York, Oxford University Press, 1993.)

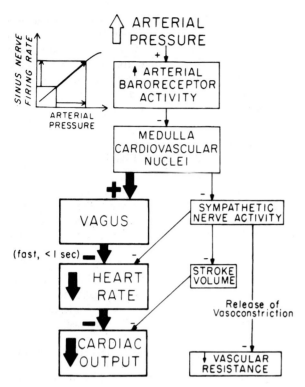

FIGURE 4-13 Summary of how the arterial baroreflex restores blood pressure back toward normal after *sudden* hypertension. Correction is *rapid* and achieved by immediate vagal activation and reduced heart rate and cardiac output. Release of tonic vasoconstriction is slow and has a minimal effect because only skeletal muscle has significant tonic vasoconstriction to be withdrawn in resting humans. (From Rowell LB: Human Cardiovascular Control, p 58. New York, Oxford University Press, 1993.)

The net result is a decrease in heart rate, with a subsequent decrease in cardiac output and blood pressure. The most important point is that the response, which occurs within one beat, is mediated by a vagally induced decrease in heart rate and cardiac output. The rapid response is extremely important in the protection of the cerebral vessels.[78] Passive vasodilation due to a decrease in sympathetic tone occurs only in the skeletal muscles, and thus cannot contribute greatly to the sudden lowering of arterial blood pressure.[145]

REFERENCES

1. Aebischer N, Malhotra R, Connors L et al: Ventricular interdependence during Valsalva maneuver as seen by two-dimensional echocardiography: New insights about an old method. J Am Soc Echocardiogr 8: 536–542, 1995
2. Allen D, Kentish J: Calcium concentration in the myoplasm of skinned ferret ventricular muscle following changes in muscle length. J Physiol (Lond) 407: 489–503, 1988
3. Anrep G, Pascual W, Rossler R: Respiratory variations in heart rate: II. The central mechanism of the respiratory arrhythmia and the inter-relations between the central and reflex mechanisms. Proc R Soc Lond 119: 218–230, 1936
4. Baldwa V, Ewing D: Heart rate response to Valsalva manoeuvre: Reproducibility in normals, and relation to variation in resting heart rate in diabetics. Br Heart J 39: 641–644, 1977
5. Bartel S, Karczewski P, Krause E: Protein phosphorylation and cardiac function: Cholinergic-adrenergic interaction. Cardiovasc Res 27: 1948–1953, 1993
6. Berne R, Levy M: Cardiovascular Physiology, 7th ed. St. Louis, Mosby, 1997
7. Bevan J: Some bases of differences in vascular response to sympathetic activity. Circ Res 45: 161–171, 1979
8. Bevan J: Some functional consequences of variation in adrenergic synaptic cleft width and in nerve density and distribution. Fed Proc 36: 2439–2443, 1977
9. Bevan J, Laher I: Pressure and flow-dependent vascular tone. FASEB J 5: 2267–2273, 1991
10. Bevan J, Su C: Variation of intra- and perisynaptic adrenergic transmitter concentration with width of synaptic cleft in vascular tissue. J Pharmacol Exp Ther 190: 30–38, 1974
11. Bevegård S, Jonsson B, Karlof I et al: Effect of changes in ventricular rate on cardiac output and central pressures at rest and during exercise in patients with artificial pacemakers. Cardiovasc Res 1: 21–33, 1967
12. Bevegård S, Lodin A: Postural circulatory changes at rest and during exercise in five patients with congenital absence of valves in the deep veins of the legs. Acta Medica Scandinavica 172: 21–29, 1962
13. Bie P: Osmoreceptors, vasopressin, and control of renal water excretion. Physiol Rev 60: 961–1048, 1980
14. Bigger JJ, Albrecht P, Steinman R et al: Comparison of time- and frequency domain-based measures of cardiac parasympathetic activity in Holter recordings after myocardial infarction. Am J Cardiol 64: 536–538, 1989
15. Bigger JJ, Fleiss J, Steinman R et al: Frequency domain measures of heart rate period variability and mortality after myocardial infarction. Circulation 85: 164–171, 1992
16. Bigger JJ, Fleiss J, Steinman R et al: RR variability in healthy, middle-aged persons compared with patients with chronic coronary heart disease or recent acute myocardial infarction. Circulation 91: 1936–1943, 1995
17. Bigger JJ, Kleiger R, Fleiss J et al: Components of heart rate variability measured during healing of acute myocardial infarction. Am J Cardiol 61: 208–215, 1988
18. Bishop V, Malliani A, Thoren P: Cardiac mechanoreceptors. In Shepherd J, Abboud F, Geiger S (eds): Handbook of Physiology, Section 2: The Cardiovascular System, Vol III: Peripheral Circulation and Organ Blood Flow (Part 2), pp 497–555. Bethesda, MD, American Physiological Society, 1983
19. Blomqvist C, Stone H: Cardiovascular adjustments to gravitational stress. In Sheperd J, Abboud F, Geiger S (eds): Handbook of Physiology, Section 2: The Cardiovascular System, Vol III: Peripheral Circulation and Organ Blood Flow (Part 2), pp 1025–1063. Bethesda, MD, American Physiological Society, 1983
20. Borbujo J, Garcia-Villalon A et al: Postjunctional α-1 and α-2 adrenoreceptors in human skin arteries: An in vitro study. J Pharmacol Exp Ther 249: 284–287, 1989
21. Borgström P, Grände P, Mellander S: An evaluation of the metabolic interaction with myogenic reactivity during blood flow autoregulation. Acta Physiol Scand 122: 275–284, 1984
22. Brecher G: Venous Return. New York, Grune & Stratton, 1956
23. Bristow M, Hershberger R, Port J et al: Beta₁ and beta₂ adrenergic receptor-mediated adenylate cyclase stimulation in nonfailing and failing human ventricular myocardium. Mol Pharmacol 35: 295–303, 1989
24. Bristow M, Monobe W, Pasmussen R et al: Alpha-1 adrenergic receptors in the nonfailing and failing human heart. J Pharmacol Exp Ther 247: 1039–1045, 1988
25. Bromberger-Barnea B: Mechanical effects of inspiration on heart functions: A review. Fed Proc 40: 2172–2177, 1981

26. Brooker J, Alderman E, Harrison D: Alterations in left ventricular volumes induced by Valsalva manoeuvre. Br Heart J 36: 713–718, 1974

27. Brooks V, Osborn J: Hormonal-sympathetic interactions in long-term regulation of arterial pressure: an hypothesis. Am J Physiol 268: R1343–R1358, 1995

28. Burnstock G: Noradrenaline and ATP: Cotransmitters and neuromodulators. J Physiol Pharmacol 46: 365–384, 1995

29. Burnstock G: Purinergic neurotransmission. In Robertson D, Low P, Polinsky R (eds): Primer on the Autonomic Nervous System, pp 99–104. San Diego, Academic Press, 1996

30. Burr R, Hamilton P, Cowan M et al: Nycthemeral profile of nonspectral heart rate variability measures in women and men: Description of a normal sample and two sudden cardiac arrest subsamples. J Electrocardiol 27(Suppl): 54–62, 1994

31. Busch S, Cowan M, Simpson T: Heart rate variability in cardiac disease. Prog Cardiovasc Nurs 7: 2–9, 1992

32. Busse R, Mülsch A, Fleming I et al: Mechanisms of nitric oxide release from the vascular endothelium. Circulation 87(Suppl V): V18–V25, 1993

33. Celander O: The range of control exercised by sympathicoadrenal system. Acta Physiol Scand 32(Suppl 116): 1–132, 1954

34. Cornish KG, Barazanji MW, Yong T et al: Volume expansion attenuates baroreflex sensitivity in the conscious nonhuman primate. Am J Physiol 257: R595–R598, 1989

35. Cowan M: Measurement of heart rate variability. West J Nurs Res 17: 32–48, 1995

36. Cowan M, Pike K, Burr R: Effects of gender and age on heart rate variability in healthy individuals and in persons after sudden cardiac arrest. J Electrocardiol 27(Suppl): 1–9, 1994

37. Cowley AJ: Long-term control of arterial blood pressure. Physiol Rev 72: 231–300, 1992

38. Cowley AJ, Liard J-F: Cardiovascular actions of vasopressin. In Gask D, Boer G (eds): Vasopressin: Principles and Properties, pp 389–433. New York, Plenum Press, 1987

39. Cunningham S: The physiology of body fluids. In Patton H, Fuchs A, Hille B et al (eds): Textbook of Physiology, Vol 2, 21st ed, pp 1098–1113. Philadelphia, WB Saunders, 1989

40. Dawson P: An historical sketch of the Valsalva experiment. Bull Hist Med 14: 295–320, 1943

41. del Monte F, Kaumann A, Poole-Wilson P: Coexistence of functioning beta-1 and beta-2 adrenoreceptors in single myocytes from human ventricle. Circulation 88: 854–863, 1993

42. Dell'Italia L, Starling M, O'Rourke R: Physical examination for exclusion of hemodynamically important right ventricular infarction. Ann Intern Med 96: 594–597, 1983

43. Dorsa D: Neurohypophyseal hormones. In Patton H, Fuchs A, Hille B et al (eds): Textbook of Physiology, Vol 2, 21st ed, pp 1173–1183. Philadelphia, WB Saunders, 1989

44. Dzau V, Pratt R: Renin-angiotensin system. In Fozzard H, Haber E, Jennings R et al (eds): The Heart and Cardiovascular System, Vol 2, pp 1817–1849. New York, Raven Press, 1991

45. Eckberg D: Human sinus arrhythmia as an index of vagal cardiac outflow. J Appl Physiol 54: 961–966, 1983

46. Eckberg D: Sympathovagal balance: A critical reappraisal. Circulation 96: 3224–3232, 1997

47. Eckberg DL: Directionally opposite left atrial and ventricular volume changes during lower body suction (Letter, Comment). J Appl Physiol 77: 1569–1570, 1994

48. Esler M, Jennings G, Lambert G et al: Overflow of catecholamine neurotransmitters to the circulation: Source, fate, and functions. Physiol Rev 70: 963–985, 1990

49. Ewing D, Burt A, Campbell I et al: Vascular reflexes in diabetic autonomic neuropathy. Lancet 2 1354–1356, 1973

50. Faber J: In situ analysis of alpha-adrenoreceptors on arteriolar and venular smooth muscle in rat skeletal muscle microcirculation. Circ Res 62: 37–50, 1988

51. Feigl E: The arterial system. In Patton H, Fuchs A, Hille B et al (eds): Textbook of Physiology, Vol 2, 21st ed, pp 849–859. Philadelphia, WB Saunders, 1989

52. Feigl E: Neural control of coronary blood flow. J Vasc Res 35: 85–92, 1998

53. Félétou M, Vanhoutte P: Endothelium-dependent hyperpolarization of canine coronary smooth muscle. Br J Pharmacol 93: 515–524, 1988

54. Ferrer M, Kennedy W, Sahinen F: Baroreflexes in patients with diabetes mellitus. Neurology 41: 1462–1466, 1991

55. Flavahan N, Linblad L, Verbeuren T et al: Cooling and alpha-1 and alpha-2 adrenergic response in cutaneous veins: Role of receptor reserve. Am J Physiol 249: H950–H955, 1985

56. Fouad F, Tazazi R, Ferrario C: Assessment of parasympathetic control of heart rate by a noninvasive method. Am J Physiol 246: H838–H842, 1984

57. Franchini K, Cowley AJ: Autonomic control of cardiac function. In Robertson D, Low P, Polinsky R (eds): Primer on the Autonomic Nervous System, pp 42–48. San Diego, Academic Press, 1996

58. Freeman G, LeWinter M: Pericardial adaptations during chronic cardiac dilation in dogs. Circ Res 54: 294–300, 1984

59. Freeman R: Noninvasive evaluation of heart rate variability. In Low P (ed): Clinical Autonomic Disorders, 2nd ed, pp 297–307. Philadelphia, Lippincott–Raven, 1997

60. Fuchs F: Mechanical modulation of the Ca^{2+} regulatory protein complex in cardiac muscle. NIPS 10: 6–12, 1995

61. Gauer O, Thron H: Postural changes in the circulation. In Hamilton W, Dow P (eds): Handbook of Physiology, Circulation, Section 2, Vol III, pp 2409–2439. Bethesda, MD, American Physiological Society, 1965

62. Goetz K: Physiology and pathophysiology of atrial peptides. Am J Physiol 254: E1–E15, 1988

63. Goldstein D: Plasma norepinephrine as an indicator of sympathetic neural activity in clinical cardiology. Am J Cardiol 48: 1147–1154, 1981

64. Grim C: Antihypertensives. In Underhill S, Woods S, Sivarajan-Froelicher E et al (eds): Cardiac Nursing, 2nd ed, pp 650–654. Philadelphia, JB Lippincott, 1990

65. Guyton A: Determination of cardiac output by equating venous return curves with cardiac response curves. Physiol Rev 35: 123–129, 1955

66. Guyton A, Abernathy B, Langston J et al: Relative importance of venous and arterial resistances in controlling venous return and cardiac output. Am J Physiol 196: 1008–1014, 1959

67. Guyton A, Douglas B, Langston J et al: Instantaneous increase in mean circulatory pressure and cardiac output at onset of muscular activity. Circ Res 11: 431–444, 1962

68. Guyton A, Lindsey A, Abernathy B et al: Venous return at various right atrial pressures and the normal venous return curve. Am J Physiol 189: 609–615, 1957

69. Guz A, Innes J, Murphy K: Respiratory modulation of left ventricular stroke volume in man measured using pulsed Doppler ultrasound. J Physiol 393: 499–512, 1987

70. Hainsworth R: The control and physiological importance of heart rate. In Malik M, Camms A (eds): Heart Rate Variability, pp 3–19. Armonk, NY, Futura, 1995

71. Hainsworth R: Vascular capacitance: Its control and importance. Rev Physiol Biochem Pharmacol 105: 101–173, 1986

72. Hamill R: Peripheral autonomic nervous system. In Robertson D, Low P, Polinsky R (eds): Primer on the Autonomic Nervous System, pp 12–25. San Diego, Academic Press, 1996

73. Hamilton W, Woodbury R, Harper H: Physiological relationships between intrathoracic, intraspinal, and arterial pressures. JAMA 107: 853–856, 1936

74. Hamilton W, Woodbury R, Harper HJ: Arterial, cerebrospinal and venous pressures in man during cough and strain. Am J Physiol 141: 42–50, 1944

75. Hammond H, White F, Bhargava V et al: Heart size and maximal cardiac output are limited by the pericardium. Am J Physiol 263: H1675–H1681, 1992

76. Hancock W, Martyn D, Huntsman L: Ca²⁺ and segment length dependence of isometric force kinetics in intact ferret cardiac muscle. Circ Res 73: 603–611, 1993

77. Hedges JR: Preload and afterload revisited. Emerg Nurs 9: 262–267, 1983

78. Heistad D, Kontos H: Cerebral circulation. In Shepherd J, Abboud F, Geiger S (eds): Handbook of Physiology, Section 2: The Cardiovascular System, Vol III: Peripheral Circulation and Organ Blood Flow (Part 2), pp 137–182. Bethesda, MD, American Physiological Society, 1983

79. Hoffman B, Lefkowitz R: Catecholamines, sympathomimetic drugs, and adrenergic receptor antagonists. In Hardman J, Goodman L, Gilman A et al (eds): Goodman and Gilman's The Pharmacological Basis of Therapeutics, 9th ed, pp 199–210. New York, McGraw-Hill, 1996

80. Hogue CJ, Stein P, Apostolidou I et al: Alterations in temporal patterns of heart rate variability after coronary artery bypass graft surgery. Anesthesiology 81: 1356–1364, 1994

81. Huntsman LL, Feigl EO: Cardiac mechanics. In Patton J, Fuchs A, Hille B et al (eds): Textbook of Physiology: Circulation, Respiration, Body Fluids, Metabolism, and Endocrinology, Vol 2, 21st ed, pp 820–833. Philadelphia, WB Saunders, 1989

82. Janicki J, Sheriff D, Robotham J et al: Cardiac output during exercise: Contributions of the cardiac, circulatory, and respiratory systems. In Rowell L, Sheperd J (eds): Handbook of Physiology. Exercise: Regulation and Integration of Multiple Systems. Vol Section 12, pp 649–704. Bethesda, MD, Oxford University Press, 1996

83. Johanson B: Myogenic responses of vascular smooth muscle. In Stevens N (ed): Smooth Muscle Contraction, pp 457–472. New York, Marcel Dekker, 1980

84. Johansson B: Myogenic tone and reactivity: Definitions based on muscle physiology. J Hypertens 7(Suppl 4): S5–S8, 1989

85. Johnson J, Rowell L, Niederberger M et al: Human splanchnic and forearm vasoconstrictor responses to reductions of right atrial and aortic pressures. Circ Res 34: 515–524, 1974

86. Johnson P: Autoregulation of blood flow. Circ Res 59: 483–495, 1986

87. Johnson P: The myogenic response. In Bohr D, Somlyo A, Sparks H (eds): Handbook of Physiology, Section 2, Vol II: Vascular Smooth Muscle, pp 409–442. Bethesda, MD, American Physiological Society, 1980

88. Johnson P: The myogenic response in the microcirculation and its interaction with other control systems. J Hypertens 7(Suppl 4): S33–S39, 1989

89. Jose P, Raymond J, Bates M et al: The renal dopamine receptors. J Am Soc Nephrol 2: 1265–1278, 1992

90. Karam M, Wise R, Natrajan T et al: Mechanism of decreased left ventricular stroke volume during inspiration in man. Circulation 69: 866–873, 1984

91. Katona P, McLean M, Dighton D et al: Sympathetic and parasympathetic cardiac control in athletes and nonathletes at rest. J Appl Physiol 52: 1652–1657, 1982

92. Kellog DJ, Pergola P, Piest K et al: Cutaneous active vasodilation is mediated by cholinergic nerve co-transmission (Abstract). FASEB J 8: A263, 1994

93. Kleiger R, Miller J, Bigger JJ et al: Decreased heart rate variability and its association with increased mortality after acute myocardial infarction. Am J Cardiol 59: 256–262, 1987

94. Kleiger R, Stein P, Bosner M et al: Time domain measurements of heart rate variability. Cardiol Clin 10: 487–498, 1992

95. Kollai M, Koizumi K: Cardiac vagal and sympathetic nerve responses to baroreceptor stimulation in the dog. Pflugers Arch 413: 365–371, 1989

96. Korner P, Tonkin A, Uther J: Reflex and mechanical circulatory effects of graded Valsalva maneuvers in normal man. J Appl Physiol 40: 434–440, 1976

97. Krogh A: The regulation of the supply of blood to the right heart. Skandinavisches Archiv fÅr Physiologie 27: 227–248, 1912

98. Lakatta E: Starling's Law of the heart is explained by an intimate interaction of muscle length and myofilament calcium activation. J Am Coll Cardiol 10: 1157–1164, 1987

99. Lancon J, Pillet M, Gabrielle F et al: Effects of atrial pacing on right ventricular contractility after coronary artery surgery. J Cardiothorac Vasc Anesth 8: 536–540, 1994

100. Lands A, Arnold A, McAuliff J: Differentiation of receptor systems activated by sympathomimetic amines. Nature 214: 597–598, 1967

101. Laughlin M: Skeletal muscle blood flow capacity: Role of muscle pump in exercise hyperemia. Am J Physiol 253: H993–H1004, 1987

102. Lefkowitz R, Hoffman B, Taylor P: Neurotransmission: The autonomic and somatic motor nervous systems. In Hardman J, Goodman L, Gilman A et al (eds): Goodman and Gilman's The Pharmacological Basis of Therapeutics, 9th ed, pp 105–139. New York, McGraw-Hill, 1996

103. Levin A: A simple test of cardiac function based upon the heart rate changes induced by the Valsalva Maneuver. Am J Cardiol 18: 90–99, 1966

104. Levy M: Neural control of cardiac function. Ballieres Clin Neurol 6: 227–244, 1997

105. Levy M, Martin P: Neural control of the heart. In Berne R (ed): Handbook of Physiology, Vol Section 2, Vol 1, pp 581–620. Bethesda, MD, American Physiological Society, 1979

106. Levy M, Zieske H: Autonomic control of cardiac pacemaker activity and atrioventricular transmission. J Appl Physiol 27: 465–470, 1969

107. Lombard J, Duling B: Multiple mechanisms of reactive hyperemia in arterioles of the hamster cheek pouch. Am J Physiol 241: H748–H755, 1981

108. Lombard J, Duling B: Relative importance of tissue oxygenation and vascular smooth muscle hypoxia in determining arteriolar response to occlusion in the hamster cheek pouch. Circ Res 41: 365–373, 1977

109. Low P: Laboratory evaluation of autonomic function. In Low P (ed): Clinical Autonomic Disorders, 2nd ed, pp 179–208. Philadelphia, Lippincott–Raven, 1997

110. Lüscher T, Vanhoutte P: The Endothelium: Modulation of Cardiovascular Function. Boca Raton, FL, CRC Press, 1990

111. Marcus F, Opie L, Sonnenblick E: Digitalis and other inotropes. In Opie L (ed): Drugs for the Heart, pp 129–154. Philadelphia, WB Saunders, 1991

112. Mark A, Abboud F, Schmid P et al: Reflex vascular response to left ventricular outflow obstruction and activation of ventricular baroreceptors in dogs. J Clin Invest 52: 1147–1153, 1973

113. Mark A, Mancia G: Cardiopulmonary baroreflexes in humans. In Shepherd J, Abboud F, Geiger S (eds): Handbook of Physiology, Section 2: The Cardiovascular System, Vol III: Peripheral Circulation and Organ Blood Flow (Part 2), pp 795–813. Bethesda, MD, American Physiological Society, 1983

114. McGuire J, Green R, Hauenstein V et al: Bed pan deaths. Am Practitioner 1: 23–28, 1950
115. Meininger G, Davis M: Cellular mechanisms involved in the vascular myogenic response. Am J Physiol 263: H647–H659, 1992
116. Mellander S: Functional aspects of myogenic vascular control. J Hypertens 7(Suppl 4): S21–S30, 1989
117. Mellander S, Johansson B: Control of resistance, exchange, and capacitance functions in the peripheral circulation. Pharmacol Rev 20: 117–196, 1968
118. Mellette H, Booth R, Ryan J et al: Hemodynamic changes associated with the Valsalva maneuver in normal adult male and female subjects (Abstract). Circulation 18: 758, 1958
119. Metzger B, Therrien B: Effect of position on cardiovascular response during the Valsalva maneuver. Nurs Res 39: 198–202, 1990
120. Miller D, Gleason W, Whalen R: Effect of ventricular rate in the cardiac output in the dog with chronic heart block. Circ Res 10: 658–663, 1962
121. Miller V, Vanhoutte P: Enhanced release of endothelium-derived factor(s) by chronic increases in blood flow. Am J Physiol 255: H446–H451, 1988
122. Minisi A, Thames M: Reflexes from ventricular receptors with vagal afferents. In Zucker I, Gilmore J (eds): Reflex Control of Circulation, pp 359–405. Boca Raton, FL, CRC Press, 1991
123. Mohrman D, Heller L: Cardiovascular Physiology, 4th ed. New York, McGraw-Hill, 1997
124. Moreno A, Burchell A: Respiratory regulation of splanchnic and systemic venous return in normal subjects and in patients with hepatic cirrhosis. Surg Gynecol Obstet 154: 257–267, 1982
125. Moreno A, Burchell A, van der Woude R et al: Respiratory regulation of splanchnic and venous return. Am J Physiol 213: 455–465, 1967
126. Oberg B, Thoren P: Increased activity in left ventricular receptors during hemorrhage or occlusion of caval veins in the cat: A possible cause of the vaso-vagal reaction. Acta Physiol Scand 85: 164–173, 1972
127. Ohyanagi M, Faber J, Nishigaki K: Differential activation of $alpha_1$- and $alpha_2$-adrenoreceptors on microvascular smooth muscle during sympathetic nerve stimulation. Circ Res 68: 232–244, 1991
128. Opie L: Heart: Physiology from Cell to Circulation. Philadelphia, Lippincott–Raven, 1998
129. Opie L: Mechanisms of cardiac contraction and relaxation. In Braunwald E (ed): Heart Disease: A Textbook of Cardiovascular Medicine, Vol 1, pp 360–393. Philadelphia, WB Saunders, 1997
130. Opie L: Regulation of myocardial contractility. J Cardiovasc Pharmacol 26(Suppl 1): S1–S9, 1995
131. Patton H: The autonomic nervous system. In Patton H, Fuchs A, Hille B et al (eds): Textbook of Physiology, Vol 1, 21st ed, pp 737–758. Philadelphia, WB Saunders, 1989
132. Perez-Gomez F, Garcia-Aguada A: Origin of ventricular reflexes caused by coronary arteriography. Br Heart J 39: 967–973, 1977
133. Perini R, Orizio C, Gamba A et al: Kinetics of heart rate and catecholamines during exercise in humans. Eur J Appl Physiol 66: 500–506, 1993
134. Price J: Influence of pressure and flow on constriction of blood vessels. J Fla Med Assoc 78: 825–827, 1991
135. Prielipp R, Coursin D: Applied pharmacology of common neuromuscular blocking agents in critical care. New Horizons 2(1): 34–47, 1994
136. Renkin E: Control of microcirculation and blood–tissue exchange. In Renkin E, Michel C (eds): Handbook of Physiology, Vol IV (Part 2), pp 627–687. Bethesda, MD, American Physiological Society, 1984
137. Robertson G: Osmoregulation of thirst and vasopressin secretion: Functional properties and their relationship to water balance. In Schrier R (ed): Vasopressin, pp 203–212. New York, Raven Press, 1985
138. Robotham J, Lixfield W, Holland L et al: Effects of respiration on cardiac performance. J Appl Physiol 44: 703–709, 1978
139. Roddie I: Circulation to skin and adipose tissue. In Shepherd J, Abboud F, Geiger S (eds): Handbook of Physiology, Section 2: The Cardiovascular System, Vol III: Peripheral Circulation and Organ Blood Flow (Part 2), pp 285–317. Bethesda, MD, American Physiological Society, 1983
140. Rodriguez E, Hunter W, Royce M et al: A method to reconstruct sarcomere lengths and orientations at transmural sites in beating canine hearts. Am J Physiol 263: H293–H306, 1992
141. Ross JJ, Covell JW, Sonnenblick EH et al: Contractile state of the heart characterized by force–velocity relations in variably afterloaded and isovolumic beats. Circ Res 18: 149–163, 1966
142. Ross JR: Afterload mismatch and preload reserve: A conceptual framework for the analysis of ventricular function. Prog Cardiovasc Dis 18: 255–264, 1976
143. Rothe C: Venous system: Physiology of the capacitance vessels. In Shepherd J, Abboud F, Geiger S (eds): Handbook of Physiology, Section 2: The Cardiovascular System, Vol III: Peripheral Circulation and Organ Blood Flow (Part 2), pp 397–452. Bethesda, MD, American Physiological Society, 1983
144. Rothe C, Gaddis M: Autoregulation of cardiac output by passive elastic characteristics of the vascular capacitance system. Circulation 81: 360–368, 1990
145. Rowell L: Human Cardiovascular Control. New York, Oxford University Press, 1993
146. Rowell L: Human Circulation: Regulation During Physical Stress. New York, Oxford University Press, 1986
147. Rowell L: Reflex control of regional circulations in humans. J Auton Nerv Syst 11: 101–114, 1984
148. Rowell L, Blackmon J: Hypotension induced by central hypovolaemia and hypoxaemia. Clin Physiol 9: 269–277, 1989
149. Rowell LB, O'Leary DS, Kellogg DLJ: Integration of cardiovascular control systems in dynamic exercise. In Rowell L, Sheperd J (eds): Handbook of Physiology, Exercise: Regulation and Integration of Multiple Systems. Vol Section 12, pp 770–838. Bethesda MD, Oxford University Press, 1996
150. Rushmer R: Constance of stroke volume in ventricular responses to exertion. Am J Physiol 196: 745–750, 1959
151. Ryan J, Stewart J, Leary W et al: Metabolism of angiotensin I in the pulmonary circulation. Biochem J 120: 221–223, 1970
152. Saito Y, Nakao H, Sugawara S et al: Atrial natriuretic polypeptide (ANP) in human ventricle increased gene expression of ANP in dilated cardiomyopathy. Biochem Biophys Res Commun 148: 211–217, 1987
153. Sander-Jensen K, Secher N, Warberg J et al: Vagal slowing of the heart during haemorrhage: Observations from 20 consecutive hypotensive patients. Br Med J 292: 364–366, 1986
154. Sarnoff SJ: Myocardial contractility as described by ventricular function curves: Observations on Starling's law of the heart. Physiol Rev 35: 107–122, 1955
155. Schaefer S, Taylor A, Lee H et al: Effect of increasing heart rate on left ventricular performance in patients with normal cardiac function. Am J Cardiol 16: 617–620, 1988
156. Scher A: Cardiovascular control. In Patton H, Fuchs A, Hille B et al (eds): Textbook of Physiology: Circulation, Respiration, Body Fluids, Metabolism, and Endocrinology, Vol 2, 21st ed, pp 972–990. Philadelphia, WB Saunders, 1989

157. Scott R: Autonomic and cardiovascular effects of neuromuscular-blocking drugs. Curr Opin Anaesth 5: 568–571, 1992

158. Shabetai R, Fowler N, Gueron M: Effects of respiration on aortic pressure and flow. Am Heart J 65: 525–533, 1963

159. Sharpey-Schafer E: Effects of Valsalva's manoeuvre on the normal and failing circulation. BMJ 1: 693–695, 1955

160. Shen Y-T, Cowley A, Vatner S: Relative roles of cardiac and arterial baroreceptors in vasopressin regulation during hemorrhage in conscious dogs. Circ Res 68: 1422–1436, 1991

161. Sheriff D, Zhou X, Scher A et al: Dependence of cardiac filling pressure on cardiac output during rest and dynamic exercise in dogs. Am J Physiol 265: H316–H322, 1993

162. Sherriff D, Rowell L, Scher A: Is the rapid rise in vascular conductance at onset of dynamic exercise due to the muscle pump? Am J Physiol 265: H1227–H1234, 1993

163. Slutsky R, Dittrich H, Peck W: Radionuclide analysis of sequential changes in central circulatory volumes: Inspiration, expiration, and the Valsalva maneuver. Crit Care Med 11: 913–917, 1983

164. Smith M, Beightol L, Fritsch et al. Valsalva's maneuver revisited: A quantitative method yielding insights into human autonomic control. Am J Physiol 271: H1240–H1249, 1996

165. Smith S, Salih M, Littler W: Assessment of beat to beat changes in cardiac output during the Valsalva manoeuvre using electrical bioimpedance. Clin Sci 72: 423–428, 1987

166. Sonnenblick EH: Force–velocity relations in mammalian heart muscle. Am J Physiol 202: 931–939, 1962

167. Spodick D: Kussmaul's sign. N Engl J Med 293: 1047–1048, 1975

168. Spodick D: The Pericardium: A Comprehensive Textbook. New York, Marcel Dekker, 1997

169. Spodick D: Threshold of pericardial constraint: The pericardial reserve and auxiliary pericardial functions (Editorial). J Am Coll Cardiol 6: 296–297, 1985

170. Squires R: Exercise training after cardiac transplantation. Med Sci Sports Exerc 23: 686–694, 1991

171. Starling E: The Linacre Lecture on the Law of the Heart, Given at Cambridge, 1915, p 147. London, Longmans, Green, 1918

172. Stein P, Bosner M, Kleiger R et al: Heart rate variability: A measure of cardiac autonomic tone. Am Heart J 127: 1376–1381, 1994

173. Stein P, Freedland K, Skala J et al: Heart rate variability is independent of age, gender, race in congestive heart failure with a recent acute exacerbation. Am J Cardiol 79: 511–512, 1997

174. Stokland O, Miller M, Lekven J et al: The significance of the intact pericardium for cardiac performance in the dog. Circ Res 47: 27–32, 1980

175. Storm D, Metzger B, Therrien B: Effects of age on autonomic cardiovascular responsiveness in healthy men and women. Nurs Res 38: 326–330, 1989

176. Stray-Gundersen J, Musch T, Haidet G et al: The effect of pericardiectomy on maximal oxygen consumption and maximal cardiac output in untrained dogs. Circ Res 58: 523–530, 1986

177. Thoren P: Left ventricular receptors activated by severe asphyxia and by coronary artery occlusion. Acta Physiol Scand 85: 455, 1972

178. Vanhoutte P, Leusen I: Vasodilatation. New York, Raven Press, 1981

179. Vanhoutte P, Mombouli J: Vascular endothelium: Vasoactive mediators. Prog Cardiovasc Dis 49: 229–238, 1996

180. Vanhoutte P, Scott-Burden T: The endothelium in health and disease. Tex Heart Inst J 21: 62–67, 1994

181. Webb S, Adgey A, Pantridge J: Autonomic disturbance at onset of acute myocardial infarction. Br Med J 3: 89–92, 1972

182. Weber K, Janicki J, Reeves R et al: Determinants of stroke volume in the isolated canine heart. J Appl Physiol 37: 742–747, 1974

183. Wei J, Markis J, Malagold M et al: Cardiovascular reflexes stimulated by reperfusion of ischemic myocardium in acute myocardial infarction. Circulation 67: 796–801, 1983

184. Wildey G, Misono K, Graham R: Atrial natriuretic factor: Biosynthesis and mechanism of action. In Fozzard H, Haber E, Jennings R et al (eds): The Heart and Cardiovascular System, Vol 2, pp 1777–1796. New York, Raven Press, 1991

185. Wise R: Effect of alterations of pleural pressure on cardiac output. South Med J 78: 423–428, 1985

186. Zaritsky A: Catecholamines, inotropic medications, and vasopressor agents. In Chernow B (ed): Essentials of Critical Care Pharmacology, 2nd ed, pp 255–272. Baltimore, Williams & Wilkins, 1994

Physiologic and Pathologic Responses

Hematopoiesis and Coagulation

HOLLY LEA
BRENDA K. ZIERLER*

The major functions of blood include nutrition, oxygenation, cleansing of wastes, and defense against microbes.[1] These functions are accomplished through the specific functions of the various components of blood. Over half of the blood volume is composed of plasma. Plasma is mainly water and serves as a transport medium for ions, proteins, hormones, and end products of cellular metabolism. The most important ions carried in the plasma are sodium, potassium, chloride, hydrogen, magnesium, and calcium. Examples of proteins transported in the plasma are immunoglobulins and the coagulation proteins. The other half of the blood volume consists of the formed elements. These include red blood cells (RBCs; erythrocytes), white blood cells (WBCs; leukocytes), and platelets. The major functions of *erythrocytes* are to carry oxygen to the tissues and carbon dioxide back to the lungs for excretion. *Leukocytes* protect against infection. *Platelets*, along with coagulation proteins, protect against blood loss through the formation of blood clots.

Because these functions are vital, a significant blood loss has devastating consequences for all body tissues. Protection against such blood losses and potential exsanguination from injuries is achieved by a complex series of events leading to hemostasis. This system is balanced by the equally complex mechanism of fibrinolysis, which dissolves clots. Knowledge of these normal processes is important as a basis for understanding the many alterations that may occur as a result of disease states or drug administration.

HEMATOPOIETIC CELLS

Hematopoiesis, or the production of blood cells, occurs primarily in the bone marrow. The liver, spleen, lymph nodes, and thymus are involved in hematopoiesis during embryonic life, but after birth *extramedullary* (outside the bone marrow) *hematopoiesis* occurs only during abnormal cir-

*The section on Hematopoiesis was written by Carina Knowlton Moravec.

cumstances. If it occurs at all after birth, extramedullary hematopoiesis occurs mainly in the liver and spleen. The pluripotent hematopoietic stem cell resides mainly in the bone marrow and in small numbers in the peripheral blood. It is the source of all the types of blood cells: erythrocytes, leukocytes, and platelets.

The *stem cell* is an immature (undifferentiated) cell that has the capacity to reproduce itself and to mature (differentiate) into any of the different types of blood cells. As the stem cell divides and matures, it differentiates into one of two committed cell lines: lymphoid or myeloid. The committed lymphoid cells eventually mature into T or B lymphocytes. The committed myeloid stem cell develops into what is called a *colony-forming unit—granulocyte, erythrocyte, macrophage, megakaryocyte* (CFU-GEMM).[22] This colony-forming unit, in turn, has the potential to develop along discrete cell lines: the erythroid line (leading to the formation of red cells), the granulocyte–monocyte line (leading to the formation of the phagocytic white cells), the megakaryocyte line (leading to the formation of platelets), the eosinophil line, and the basophil line. As the various types of blood cells mature, they are released into the peripheral circulation. Figure 5-1 shows a model for hematopoietic cell differentiation and the growth factors involved at the various stages of differentiation. Table 5-1 lists most of the known hematopoietic growth factors and the type of cell they are thought to stimulate.

The Regulation of Hematopoiesis

Because blood cells have a limited life span, they need to be replaced constantly. Usually, the amount produced is fairly constant, but depending on environmental stimuli, such as bleeding or infection, various cells may be needed in larger than normal quantities at times. Thus, each of these cell lines is regulated by cytokines that influence the rate of growth and differentiation of the stem cells in the marrow. *Cytokines* are proteins that are made by cells of the immune system and regulate the immune response. Some examples of cytokines are granulocyte–macrophage colony-stimulating factor

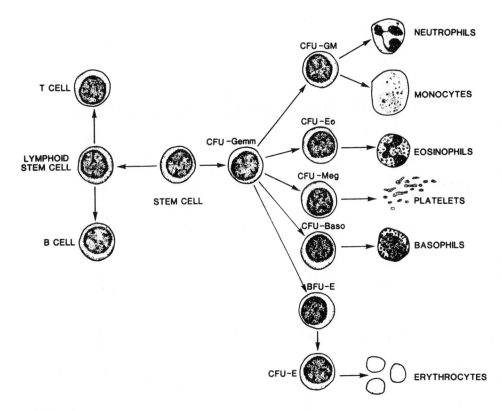

FIGURE 5-1 Diagram of hematopoiesis. The various progenitors are schematically represented. *CFU-GEMM,* multipotential progenitor for granulocytes, erythrocytes, macrophages, megakaryocytes; *CFU-GM,* progenitor for neutrophils and monocytes; *CFU-Eo,* progenitor for eosinophils; *CFU-Meg,* progenitor for megakaryocytes; *CFU-Baso,* progenitor for basophils; *BFU-E,* most primitive, committed progenitor for erythroid line; *CFU-E,* more mature progenitor for erythroid line. (From Rothstein G: Origin and development of the blood and blood-forming tissues. In Lee GR, Bithell TC, Foerster J et al [eds]: Wintrobe's Clinical Hematology, 9th ed, p 51. Philadelphia, Lea & Febiger, 1993.)

TABLE 5-1	Hematopoietic Growth Factors and Some of Their Characteristics
Factor*	**Cells Simulated**
M-CSF	Monocytes
GM-CSF	All granulocytes, megakaryocytes, erythrocytes, stem cells
G-CSF	Granulocytes, macrophages, endothelial cells
IL-3	Granulocytes, erythroid cells, multipotent progenitors
IL-4	B, T cells
IL-5	B cells, CFU-Eo
IL-6	B, T cells, CFU-GEMM, CFU-GM, BFU-E, macrophages, neural cells, hepatocytes
IL-7	B cells
IL-8	T cells, neutrophils
IL-9	BFU-E, CFU-GEMM
IL-11	B, T cells, CFU-GEMM, macrophages
Erythropoietin	CFU-E, BFU-E
c-kit ligand ("stem cell factor")	Primitive progenitors

*CSF, colony-stimulating factor; GM, granulocyte–macrophage;IL, interleukin; CFU, colony-forming unit; Eo, eosinophil; BFU, burst-forming unit; E, erythrocyte; GEMM, granulocytes, erythrocytes, macrophages, megakaryocytes.
  Adapted from Rothstein G: Origin and development of the blood and blood-forming tissues. In Lee GR, Bithell TC, Foerster J et al (eds): Wintrobe's Clinical Hematology, 9th ed, p 53. Philadelphia, Lea & Febiger, 1993.

(GM-CSF), which stimulates the growth of granulocytes and macrophages, and interleukin-3, which stimulates the stem cell. Cytokines also stimulate the function of mature immune cells.

Red Blood Cells

All tissues of the body require a steady supply of oxygen to survive. RBCs take up oxygen in the lungs, transport it, and then deliver it to the tissues. The correct number of RBCs is crucial. If the number of RBCs is too low (anemia), the oxygen-carrying capacity is compromised. Too many RBCs (polycythemia) increases the viscosity of the blood and thus slows the flow to the tissues. The rate of bone marrow stem cell differentiation into erythrocytes is primarily controlled by erythropoietin. The bulk of this hormone is produced by the kidney. The rate of RBC production is influenced by the oxygen content of the blood as sensed by the kidneys. RBC production is increased at times of blood loss, at high altitude, and in pulmonary diseases that affect the transport of oxygen from the lungs to the blood. It takes approximately 3 to 5 days for an RBC to mature in the marrow and be released into the peripheral circulation. RBCs live approximately 4 months, at which time they are disposed of by the spleen.

The mature RBC is a biconcave disc filled with hemoglobin. The heme section is the actual oxygen-transporting portion of the hemoglobin molecule. Oxygen diffuses from the lungs into the alveolar capillaries, and as the RBC passes through the lungs, the oxygen binds to each of four sites in the heme region. The remarkable oxygen-binding properties of this site allow the RBC to fill up with oxygen in the lungs and then release it at the tissue level. The characteristics of this uptake and release are demonstrated by the oxygen–hemoglobin dissociation curve (see Chapter 3). Sufficient iron is an essential factor in the normal production of heme and thus oxygen transport. In addition to its oxygen-carrying functions, hemoglobin can also bind to hydrogen, thus providing a minor means of compensating for cellular acid production (see Chapter 7).

White Blood Cells

White blood cells, all of which defend against microbes, can be divided into two major categories: phagocytes and lymphocytes. The primary role of phagocytes is to locate and kill invading microorganisms. The primary role of lymphocytes is to initiate and carry out immune responses, including the manufacture of antibodies.

Phagocytes perform their role primarily out in the tissues, where they travel toward the site of an inflammation (*chemotaxis*) and kill microbes by engulfing them (*phagocytosis*). Many substances, including complement fragments and bacterial products, stimulate this chemotactic migration. Phagocytosis is an active process that uses energy derived from anaerobic glycolysis.

Phagocytic cells are divided into two subgroups: *granulocytes* and *monocytes*. The granulocytes include neutrophils (also called "polys"), basophils, and eosinophils. *Neutrophils* are produced in huge numbers daily. Neutrophil maturation in the marrow takes 7 to 10 days. Their main function is to find and kill bacteria, especially resident microorganisms such as staphylococci and gram-negative enteric flora.[23] They also play an important role in acute inflammatory processes. Neutrophils are the first phagocytic cells to appear at the site of an acute inflammation.[9]

During severe inflammatory reactions, neutrophils can actually cause damage to surrounding tissues by releasing proteolytic enzymes and oxygen-free radicals. This process is thought to occur, for example, in the adult respiratory distress syndrome. Once in the bloodstream, a portion of the neutrophils freely circulates and another portion rolls along the blood vessel wall. This latter portion is called the *marginal pool*. Substances emanating from an injury or from an organism make the blood vessel wall sticky so that the marginated neutrophils adhere to the vessel walls. The neutrophil then releases substances that allow the endothelial cells to separate and permit the neutrophil to crawl into the connective tissue (*diapedesis*). It then migrates to the area of injury through chemotaxis. The migration of neutrophils to the tissues takes place rapidly, within 12 hours of having entered the bloodstream. An important step in making microorganisms recognizable to neutrophils is *opsonization*. Opsonization is a process in which molecules in the plasma coat the microorganism, making it more recognizable to the neutrophil.

Eosinophils develop in the marrow along the same maturation steps as neutrophils. They make up only approximately 4% of a normal WBC count. Eosinophils have been postulated to play a defensive role against parasites and in allergic reactions.[1]

Basophils account for only 0.5% to 1% of the total WBC count. The role of the basophil is not well clarified, but these cells are known to play a part in immediate hypersensitivity reactions. Basophils release histamine when stimulated, which in turn results in the signs and symptoms of allergic reaction such as rhinitis, bronchospasm, urticaria, angioedema, and anaphylaxis.[1] The relationship between basophils and mast cells, similar cells that reside in tissues, is not clearly understood.[1] However, it is thought that they are both derived from a common progenitor, the CFU-Mast.[40]

Monocytes constitute 4% to 8% of the total WBC count. Within 24 to 36 hours of entering the circulation, they migrate out to the tissues, where they undergo further maturation and are called *macrophages*.[31] There they make up the monocyte–macrophage system, which used to be called the reticuloendothelial system.[32] Hepatic Kupffer cells, alveolar macrophages, and peritoneal macrophages are examples of tissue macrophages.[22] Once lodged in their target organ, macrophages can live for up to 60 days. In the bloodstream, monocytes have similar functions to the neutrophil: to find and kill microorganisms. However, in addition, monocytes and macrophages play a crucial role in recognizing foreign invaders and presenting foreign antigens to lymphocytes, thus stimulating the immune response. They are important in killing bacteria, protozoa, cells infected with viruses, and tumor cells. In addition to their phagocytic activity, macrophages secrete biologically active products, including cytokines, that modulate the immune response (e.g., GM-CSF), enzymes that can degrade connective tissue, and chemotactic factors.[9,32]

Lymphocytes are essential components of the immune system. They recognize and are instrumental in the elimination of foreign proteins, pathogens, and tumor cells. Lymphocytes control the intensity and specificity of the immune response.[36] There are two general types of lymphocytes: *T lymphocytes* (or T cells), which provide cell-mediated immunity, and *B lymphocytes* (B cells), which produce the antibodies of humoral immunity.

As with the other cells already described, stem cell differentiation for the production of lymphocytes occurs in the bone marrow. During fetal life, lymphocytes that will become T cells migrate to the thymus gland and mature into T cells ready to participate in cell-mediated immune reactions. It is in the thymus that T cells learn to differentiate self from nonself.[37] There are four separate subsets of T cells: helper T cells, suppressor T cells, cytotoxic T cells, and memory T cells. Cell-mediated activities are of great importance in delayed hypersensitivity reactions; graft rejection; graft-versus-host disease; and in defense against fungal, protozoal, and most viral infections. Another important function of T cells is to regulate immune activities through the secretion of lymphokines.

B lymphocytes mature into cells that respond to stimulation from foreign proteins by differentiating into *memory cells* and *plasma cells*. The plasma cells in turn produce specific antibodies that inactivate or destroy foreign proteins and pathogens. These antibodies are particularly effective against bacterial infections, especially encapsulated bacteria, such as pneumococci, streptococci, meningococci, and *Hemophilus influenzae*, as well as certain viruses. One subset of T cells, the helper cells, stimulates B cells to produce antibodies. Another subset of T cells, the suppressor cells, slows the production of antibodies, preventing uncontrolled immune reactions.[1]

Memory B and T cells impart immunologic memory. These cells respond to repeated exposures to specific antigens with greater efficiency than during the first exposure. This memory provides the rationale for vaccinations.[1]

Natural killer cells, another subset of lymphocytes, kill tumor cells and cells infected by viruses by lysing them. They play an important role in tumor surveillance.

The activities of phagocytes and immune cells overlap in numerous mutually beneficial ways. For example, immune cells often participate in chronic inflammatory reactions. Conversely, engulfment of foreign protein by macrophages is a preparatory step leading to antibody production.

Platelets

Platelets are small cell fragments that are produced by the disintegration of megakaryocytes in the bone marrow.[1] It takes approximately 5 days for a stem cell to differentiate along the megakaryocyte line and produce platelets. Under normal circumstances, platelets circulate in the bloodstream for approximately 10 days. Their production is regulated by thrombopoietin, interleukin-3, and GM-CSF.[1] The primary functions of platelets include the formation of a cellular plug that temporarily arrests bleeding and the contribution of substances to the subsequent coagulation process.

HEMOSTASIS

The normal *hemostatic system* is designed to protect against bleeding from injured blood vessels.[47] Hemostasis is usually accomplished by a combination of three sequential and interrelated processes involving blood vessels, platelets, and coagulation proteins. This complex system is highly regulated to ensure that clotting occurs only at a site of injury and only as long as the integrity of the vessel is compromised. The clotting processes are balanced by the complex mechanism of *fibrinolysis,* which breaks down clots and maintains or reestablishes blood flow once the vessel leak or tear has healed. The balance between these two mechanisms and their activators and inhibitors is vital. An imbalance in one direction leads to excessive bleeding, whereas an imbalance in the other direction leads to excessive clotting. The following sections present the normal sequence of coagulation and fibrinolysis, as well as selected bleeding and clotting disorders most commonly associated with the patient experiencing cardiovascular disease.

Vascular Phase

The *vascular phase* refers to several instantaneous compensatory responses that occur when a vessel is injured. The initial vascular reaction to injury is constriction of vascular smooth muscle that limits blood loss. Thrombin is thought to play a major role in the vascular phase. In a normal vessel where the endothelial lining is intact, thrombin induces the release of nitric oxide and prostacyclin from endothelial cells, which cause vasorelaxation. During injury, the endothelial lining is disrupted, exposing smooth muscle cells. Thrombin causes these smooth muscle cells to contract and vasoconstriction occurs.[23] Capillary bleeding may be controlled by contraction of precapillary sphincters.[41] Blood loss is also reduced by the apposition of surrounding tissues and by the pressure of interstitial fluid, the increase of which is due to escape of blood from the vessel into the interstitium.

Platelet Phase

The *platelet phase* refers to the formation of a soft mass of aggregated platelets that provides a temporary patch over the injured, bleeding vessel. Almost immediately after vascular injury, platelets begin to adhere to the exposed subendothelial basement membrane and collagen fibers.[51] Adherence to the damaged vessel surface is believed to be mediated by the von Willebrand factor and a glycoprotein in the platelet membrane.[42,52] Also, loss of endothelium after injury removes factors such as prostacyclin, nitric oxide, ecto-adenosine diphosphatase, and heparan sulfate, which are important for suppression of platelet activation and for adherence to the wall.[38,60] Adherent platelets release adenosine diphosphate (ADP), which causes platelets to change from their normal shape into a spherical form with pseudopods. During activation, the platelets become sticky and adhere to each other, increasing the size of the platelet plug. ADP induces this *aggregation*.[42] ADP and collagen also trigger formation of arachidonic acid from phospholipids in the platelet membrane. This acid in turn leads to the formation of thromboxane A_2, a substance that induces further platelet aggregation.[33,42] Thromboxane A_2 causes conformational changes in glycoprotein IIb/IIIa, a receptor on the platelet surface, which expose fibrinogen binding sites. Fibrinogen then binds to adjacent platelets, advancing clot formation. Inhibition of this receptor is becoming a major target for antiplatelet therapy.[26] During activation, platelets also develop the ability to promote activation of the clotting cascade. Ultimately, aggregated platelets plug the injured vessel. The dual processes of vascular constriction and platelet plug formation are responsible for initial hemostasis in minor injuries.

Coagulation Phase

The final phase of hemostasis is the formation of a fibrin blood clot. The coagulation process is most commonly viewed as a series of enzymatic reactions in which clotting factors are sequentially activated. This process is known as the *coagulation cascade*. The clotting factors are all present in the circulating blood in their inactive form until a stimulus for clot formation occurs. Twelve different substances have been officially designated as clotting factors. These are identified in Table 5-2. All of the clotting factors except factor VIII are manufactured in the liver. Factor VIII is synthesized by endothelial cells, megakaryocytes, and many other cells in the body.[1] Four of the clotting factors require the presence of vitamin K for their production: factors II (prothrombin), VII, IX, and X. Calcium is required for most of the reactions of the clotting cascade.

TABLE 5-2 The Blood Coagulation Proteins

Factor	Synonyms
I	Fibrinogen
II	Prothrombin
III	Tissue thromboplastin, tissue factor
IV	Calcium
V	Accelerator globulin, proaccelerin, labile factor
VI*	
VII	Proconvertin, stable factor
VIII	Antihemophilic factor or globulin
IX	Christmas factor, plasma thromboplastin component
X	Stuart factor, Stuart-Prower factor
XI	Plasma thromboplastin antecedent
XII	Hageman factor
XIII	Fibrin-stabilizing factor, fibrinoligase
Prekallikrein (Fletcher factor)	
High–molecular-weight kininogen (Fitzgerald factor)	

*Factor VI was at one time used to designate activated factor V.

From Pizzo, SV: An overview of coagulation. In Koepke JA (ed): Laboratory Hematology, Vol 1, p 505. New York, Churchill Livingstone, 1984. By permission.

As studied in the laboratory, the coagulation process can be initiated by two different pathways, the *extrinsic pathway* and the *intrinsic pathway*. Although differentiating between them is helpful for understanding pathologic mechanisms, medication actions, and coagulation tests, these two pathways are functionally inseparable *in vivo*. The extrinsic pathway, whose major mediators are rapidly inactivated, is the primary initiator of the clotting cascade. The intrinsic pathway, whose major mediators are more slowly degraded, is thought to be important for maintenance and amplification of the clotting cascade.[35,38] Both extrinsic and intrinsic mechanisms eventually lead to the activation of factor X, with the remaining steps of the coagulation sequence being identical. The sequence of the coagulation process is shown in Figure 5-2.

The extrinsic pathway is initiated by the combination of tissue factor (factor III) with factor VIIa (the activated form of VII) and ionized calcium, which together convert factor X to its activated form, factor Xa. The function of the extrinsic pathway is tested in the laboratory by the prothrombin time (PT; see Chapter 11).[16] Tissue factor, also called *tissue thromboplastin*, is a membrane glycoprotein that is particularly prevalent in tissues, where it plays a vital role in the prevention of hemorrhage. It is generally found in tissues surrounding the vasculature and boundaries of vital organs.[36] Tissue factor is exposed to and binds to factor VIIa when a vascular injury occurs and allows circulating factor VIIa to come into contact with these tissues, which are normally separated from the blood.

FIGURE 5-2 Coagulation cascade and fibrin formation by the intrinsic and extrinsic pathways. The initiation of the coagulation cascade occurs after vascular injury and the exposure of tissue factor to blood. This triggers the extrinsic pathway (*right side*), shown in *heavy arrows*. The intrinsic pathway (*left side*) can be triggered when thrombin is generated, leading to the activation of factor XI. The two pathways converge by the formation of factor Xa. The activated clotting factors (except thrombin) are designated by lowercase *a* (e.g., IXa, Xa, XIa). The phospholipid (PL) bound to tissue factor apoprotein is not shown. (Reprinted with permission from *Biochemistry* 30: 10363–10370, 1991. Copyright 1991, American Chemical Society.)

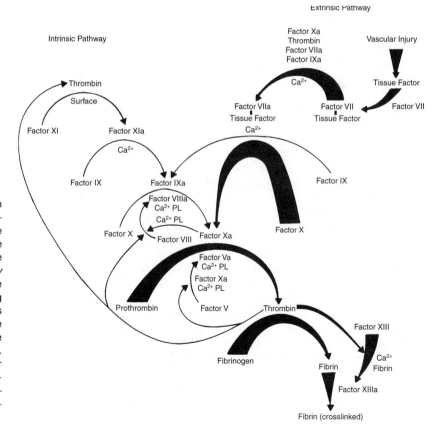

Because the intrinsic pathway is initiated by a separate set of factors that are not degraded by rapid-acting inhibitors, the process may proceed more slowly and the results may last longer and be more pronounced than those initiated by the extrinsic pathway. The function of the intrinsic pathway is commonly analyzed by the partial thromboplastin time (PTT; see Chapter 11).[17] Intrinsic activation is initiated when blood is exposed to a negatively charged surface, such as the site of blood vessel injury.[1] The negative charge, along with collagen and endotoxin, attracts factor XII, which binds to the surface and autoactivates to factor XIIa. Factor XIIa converts prekallikrein to kallikrein, which in turn converts circulating factor XII to its activated form, XIIa. Both the activated form of factor XII and kallikrein catalyze the activation of factor XI into XIa. Factor XIa, together with ionized calcium, cleaves factor IX at two sites to produce factor IXa.[39] Factor IXa, together with factor VIII, phospholipid, and ionized calcium (tenase complex), convert factor X to its activated form, factor Xa. As discussed previously, factor X can also be activated through the extrinsic pathway. From here, the coagulation process proceeds along the common pathway, regardless of whether initiation was extrinsic or intrinsic.[7,25]

The final common sequence involves the combination of factors Xa and V, phospholipid, and ionized calcium (prothrombinase complex) into a complex that converts prothrombin to thrombin. The thrombin formed subsequently cleaves the long molecule fibrinogen to fibrin. The fibrin monomer is able to polymerize spontaneously to form a loose web of fibers that is capable of stopping the bleeding in small- and medium-sized arteries and veins. The fibrin clot is eventually stabilized and thickened by the action of factor XIII, which is activated by the presence of ionized calcium and thrombin. Plasminogen and other components of the fibrinolytic mechanism are incorporated into the fibrin clot as it solidifies.[7]

Coagulation is regulated by three major mechanisms: the elimination of activated clotting factors, the protease inhibitors (inhibitors of coagulation), and the destruction of the fibrin clot.[1,46] Activated clotting factors are rapidly cleared by the liver, a protective mechanism that prevents activated clotting factors in the circulation from starting clots in inappropriate sites. They are also inactivated by antithrombin, the protein C—protein S system, and tissue factor pathway inhibitor, which is secreted in response to thrombin and works by inhibiting the tissue factor—factor VIIa—factor Xa complex. Antithrombin is the major inhibitor of thrombin, factor Xa, and factor IXa.[38] Heparin anticoagulation works through its interaction with antithrombin III and tissue factor pathway inhibitor.[1] People with an inherited deficiency of antithrombin III are prone to development of venous thromboembolism (VTE). Protein C is vitamin K dependent and neutralizes factors Va and VIIIa with the help of a cofactor, protein S. The fibrinolytic system, described in more detail in the following section, degrades the fibrin clot. Finally, endothelial cells regulate coagulation by a number of activities, including synthesis of prostaglandin I_2 and nitric oxide, which inhibit platelet aggregation and adhesion.[39]

FIBRINOLYSIS

The removal of clots when the site of vessel injury has healed is as important as the formation of the clot itself.[1] The process of fibrinolysis maintains or reestablishes blood flow. Of the numerous mechanisms known to result in fibrinolysis, most investigators consider the process mediated by plasmin to be of greatest significance.[24] Plasmin is found only in minute quantities in plasma, but its precursor, plasminogen, is normally abundant. Plasminogen is a glycoprotein with a molecular weight of approximately 90,000 that is synthesized by the liver.[16] Whether fibrinolysis occurs is controlled by the complex interplay of some substances that can activate plasminogen and others that keep it inactive. Under normal circumstances, the balance is in favor of those substances that prevent activation, thus favoring clot stability.

Activators of plasminogen are found in various tissues, blood, and urine. The best-known activator is tissue plasminogen activator (t-PA).[25] The activation process involves cleavage of a bond on the plasminogen molecule that converts it to plasmin, a proteolytic enzyme that can break down fibrin and other proteins.[42] Plasminogen inhibitors that usually prevent this activation are also present in blood and in various tissues.[42] A schematic diagram of the fibrinolytic mechanism is shown in Figure 5-3.

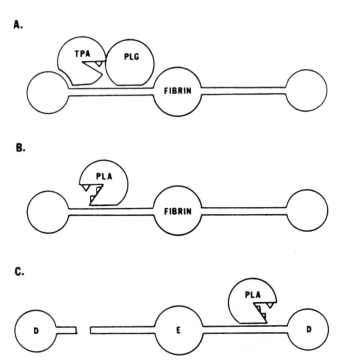

FIGURE 5-3 Schematic diagram of the fibrinolytic system. **(A)** Both tissue plasminogen activator (*TPA*), derived from endothelial cells, and plasminogen (*PLG*) are incorporated into the matrix of a fibrin clot. In the presence of fibrin, which functions as a cofactor, TPA rapidly activates plasminogen to plasmin (*PLA*). **(B, C)** Plasmin then degrades the fibrin monomer, releasing the fibrin degradation products D and E. Plasmin can be inhibited by α_2-antiplasmin, which is also present in the clot matrix, but this depends on the same binding site involved in the interaction of plasmin and fibrin. Thus, as long as the plasmin remains bound to fibrin, it remains active. (From Brandt JT: Current concepts of coagulation. Clin Obstet Gynecol 28: 13, 1985.)

DISPLAY 5-1

Bleeding Disorders

I. Vascular
  A. Autoimmune vascular purpuras (allergic, drug induced)
  B. Infections (bacterial, viral, rickettsial, protozoal)
  C. Structural malformations (hereditary or acquired)
II. Platelet
  A. Thrombocytopenia
    1. Disturbances in platelet production
      a. Megakarocytic hypoplasia (congenital or acquired)
      b. Ineffective platelet production (hereditary or acquired)
    2. Disturbances in platelet distribution
      a. Splenic pooling (splenomegaly)
      b. Vascular pooling (hypothermia)
    3. Disturbances in platelet destruction
      a. Combined consumption of disseminated intravascular coagulation (e.g., obstetric complications, neoplasms, tissue injury)
      b. Isolated platelet consumption (e.g., prosthetic valves, extracorporeal circulation, thrombotic thrombocytopenia purpura)
      c. Immune platelet destruction (e.g., idiopathic thrombocytopenia purpura, post-transfusion purpura, drugs, infections)

  B. Thrombocytosis
    1. Primary (autonomous)
      a. Essential thrombocythemia
      b. Other myeloproliferative disorders
    2. Secondary (reactive)
      a. Inflammatory disorders
      b. Blood disorders
      c. Malignancy
      d. Postoperative
      e. Response to drugs
      f. Response to exercise
III. Coagulation
  A. Congenital
    1. Hemophilia A
    2. Hemophilia B
    3. Factor XI deficiency
    4. Factor XII deficiency
    5. von Willebrand's disease
  B. Acquired
    1. Vitamin K deficiency
    2. Liver disease
    3. Nephrotic syndrome
    4. Systemic lupus erythematosus
    5. Circulating anticoagulants
    6. Disseminated intravascular coagulation

Adapted from Williams WJ: Classification and clinical manifestations of disorders of hemostasis. In Williams WJ, Beutler E, Ersley AJ et al (eds): Hematology, 4th ed, p 1338. New York, McGraw-Hill, 1990.

Fragments of the fibrin clot, known as *fibrin degradation products* (FDPs), are released into the circulation as the clot is broken down. FDPs are potent inhibitors of coagulation. They act by binding to thrombin, thus inhibiting its action, and by interfering with the binding of fibrin threads to form the fibrin clot. Except in some abnormal situations, FDPs are present in such small numbers that their anticoagulant effect is not clinically important. FDPs are measured in the clinical laboratory as a marker for disseminated intravascular coagulation (DIC).

BLEEDING DISORDERS

Bleeding can occur when the intricate relationship between the various elements in the hemostatic system is disturbed.[1] Numerous defects in the hemostatic system are possible. Furthermore, many drugs inhibit hemostasis, either as the intended drug action or as a side effect. In either event, knowledge of these pharmacologic activities is important for patient care and for patient teaching.

Bleeding disorders are usually categorized as vascular, platelet, or coagulation abnormalities. Display 5-1 lists common disorders in the three categories. In each case, bleeding is the primary manifestation. The bleeding may be minor, such as petechiae and easy bruising of the skin, or major, with massive hemorrhage. Occasionally, a defect may exist in more than one area simultaneously. DIC, for example, affects both platelets and coagulation factors. Although DIC

is actually a disorder of coagulation, it is discussed as a bleeding disorder because its major manifestation is bleeding.

Disseminated Intravascular Coagulation

DEFINITION

Disseminated intravascular coagulation is a pathologic syndrome resulting in the indiscriminate formation of fibrin clots throughout all or most of the microvasculature. Paradoxically, diffuse bleeding results and is usually the hallmark sign because clotting factors and platelets are consumed during the widespread coagulation.[1,22]

ETIOLOGY

Inappropriate coagulation results from the presence of thromboplastic substances in the bloodstream.[1] These thromboplastic substances stimulate clotting despite the lack of actual bleeding. Tissue thromboplastin is released into the circulation by damaged cells in people with massive burns, injuries, and systemic infections. DIC is a common complication of serious infections, especially gram-negative sepsis. Approximately 50% of clients with DIC have obstetric problems, whereas another 33% have cancer.[27] The fetus, placenta, and amniotic fluid contain thromboplastic substances that are released into the maternal circulation during obstetric complications such as abruptio placentae and amniotic fluid embolism. Certain malignant tumors release small amounts of thromboplastic substances into the circulation.

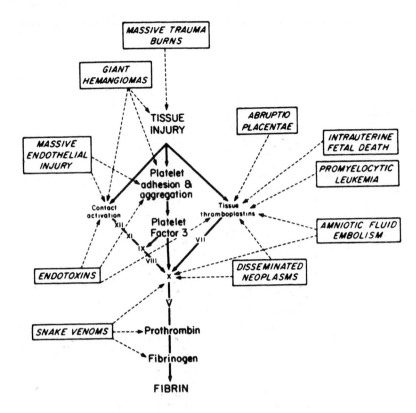

FIGURE 5-4 Factors that initiate disseminated intravascular coagulation (DIC). Normal hemostatic apparatus is within *solid arrows*. Processes that trigger DIC and the mechanisms involved are in *blocks* with *dotted arrows*. The processes illustrated are, in many cases, highly theoretic. (From Bithell TC: Acquired coagulation disorders. In Lee GR, Bithell TC, Foerster J et al [eds]: Wintrobe's Clinical Hematology, 9th ed, p 1481. Philadelphia, Lea & Febiger, 1993.)

The most critical time for the development of DIC is during chemotherapy or radiation treatment because the tumor cells are dying and releasing massive amounts of thromboplastin into the circulation. Figure 5-4 illustrates various factors that can initiate DIC. Display 5-2 lists these and other disorders associated with DIC. In the patient with cardiovascular disease, DIC is most likely to develop as a result of cardiogenic, septic, or hemorrhagic shock; acidosis; or extracorporeal circulation.

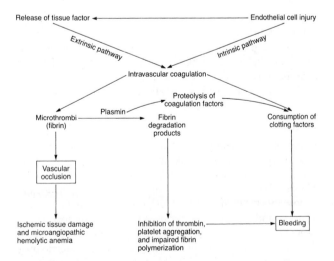

FIGURE 5-5 Schematic illustration of the major consequences of disseminated intravascular coagulation (DIC). (From Robbins SL, Angell M, Kumar V: Basic Pathology, 4th ed, p 396. Philadelphia, WB Saunders, 1987.)

PATHOLOGY

The two major consequences of DIC are bleeding and organ ischemia.[28] Widespread intravascular clotting resulting in deposition of fibrin in the microcirculation leads to ischemia in organs such as the kidney. RBCs are damaged as they pass through the fibrin strands. These damaged RBCs are called schistocytes.[23] As the disseminated clotting continues, circulating platelets and clotting factors are consumed and bleeding ensues. Fibrinolysis is activated as a result of the widespread clotting, yielding abnormally large amounts of circulating FDPs. In these large numbers, FDPs aggravate bleeding because they inhibit platelet aggregation, act as anticoagulants, and impair fibrin polymerization[28] (Fig. 5-5). FDPs are also thought to increase capillary permeability and may contribute to the development of the adult respiratory distress syndrome.[23]

CLINICAL MANIFESTATIONS

Disseminated intravascular coagulation can occur in a chronic or acute form. The chronic form is more subtle and easily goes unrecognized. The acute form tends to be more severe and sudden in onset. Clinical manifestations range in severity from prolonged bleeding from a venipuncture site to spontaneous massive hemorrhage.[28] In massive hemorrhage, bleeding occurs from mucous membranes, sites of injury (including venipuncture and injection sites, and surgical wounds), and every orifice. Deep tissue bleeding may

---

DISPLAY 5-2

Disorders Associated with Disseminated Intravascular Coagulation

Direct release of tissue thromboplastin into circulation (extrinsic pathway)

  I. Obstetric complications
     A. Abruptio placentae
     B. Abortions
        1. Septic
        2. Saline induced
     C. Retained placental tissue
     D. Amniotic fluid embolism
     E. Placenta previa
     F. Eclampsia
 II. Neoplasms
     A. Acute leukemia
     B. Lymphomas
     C. Carcinomas
     D. Others
III. Tissue injury
     A. Massive trauma
     B. Extensive burns
     C. Dissecting aneurysm of aorta
     D. Extensive surgery
     E. Fat embolism
     F. Extracorporeal circulation
     G. Head trauma
 IV. Snake bites

Pathogenesis uncertain or mixed (e.g., endothelial damage, vasculitis, stasis, hemolysis)

  I. Infections
     A. Bacterial (particularly due to gram-negative organisms)
        1. Septicemia and septic shock
        2. Meningococcemia
     B. Mycotic
        1. Histoplasmosis
        2. Aspergillosis
     C. Rickettsial
     D. Viral
        1. Herpes
        2. Rubella
        3. Smallpox
        4. Hepatitis
        5. Reyes' syndrome
 II. Autoimmune disease and hypersensitivity reactions
     A. Drug reactions
     B. Renal homograft rejection
     C. Graft-vs.-host disease
     D. Anaphylaxis
III. Miscellaneous
     A. Liver disease
     B. Heat stroke
     C. Adult respiratory distress syndrome
     D. Hypoxia and hypoperfusion

Adapted from Bitnell TC: Acquired coagulation disorders. In Lee GR, Bithell TC, Foerster J et al (eds): Wintrobe's Clinical Hematology, 9th ed, p 1481. Philadelphia, Lea & Febiger, 1993.

---

also occur. Petechiae, purpura, and ecchymosis are very common.[17] In chronic DIC, thrombosis is the most common symptom. Recurrent thrombophlebitis is the most common manifestation of chronic DIC.[1]

PHYSICAL ASSESSMENT

All patients who have undergone extracorporeal circulation or thoracic surgery or who have had septic shock, hypoxemia, or hypoperfusion are at risk for the development of DIC. Those patients who are at risk must be observed closely for signs of bleeding. Table 5-3 lists various types of bleeding that may be found on physical examination. In addition, prolonged bleeding from wounds or needle puncture sites, occult blood in body excreta or excretions (i.e., emesis, feces, urine), or bleeding from mucous membranes may signal the development of DIC. The definitive diagnosis of DIC depends on laboratory tests.[42]

MEDICAL MANAGEMENT

The *diagnosis* of DIC should be suspected whenever abnormal bleeding occurs in association with any of the disorders listed in Display 5-1. Multiple coagulation test abnormalities are found in DIC. These include prolonged PT, PTT, and thrombin time; decreased fibrinogen and platelet counts; increased FDPs; decreased levels of factors II, V, VIII, and X; and the presence of schistocytes.[12] Table 5-4 lists the laboratory abnormalities associated with DIC.[42]

The *prognosis* of DIC varies markedly depending on the underlying cause and the amount of intravascular clotting.[27] DIC may cease spontaneously, or it may respond to prompt and aggressive treatment.[28] In other cases, the organ ischemia and bleeding lead to death.

Disseminated intravascular coagulation always occurs as the result of some other underlying abnormality, and thus the treatment of DIC is directed toward improvement of the underlying disorder. For example, infection requires the use of antibiotics. Fetal death or a retained placenta requires the removal of the uterine contents. Acute promyelocytic leukemia may respond to the use of prophylactic heparin during chemotherapy.[15] General support measures, such as fluid and blood replacement and maintenance of adequate oxygenation and tissue perfusion, are also essential.[30] The bleeding may be slowed by giving the patient transfusions of platelets, fresh frozen plasma (which

TABLE 5-3	Physical Findings in Bleeding Disorders

Finding	Description	Probable Cause

Petechiae	Small capillary hemorrhages
	  Flat, 1–3 mm in diameter, do not blanch
	  with pressure, deep red or reddish-purple in color
	  Most common in dependent areas
		Vessel or platelet abnormalities, DIC

Purpura	Petechiae that have grown together to form a larger lesion	Vessel or platelet abnormalities, DIC

Ecchymoses
(bruises)
	Larger macular areas, blue-black initially, fading to
	  brownish-green, then yellow
	Due to blood in the subcutaneous tissues and skin
		Usually from veins. Common with disorders
		  of platelet and vessels as well as coagulation
		  defects, DIC

Hemarthrosis	Hemorrhage into synovial joints May have no external evidence of bleeding, only complaints of severe joint pain	Severe hereditary coagulation disorders or DIC

DIC, disseminated intravascular coagulation.
  From Bithell TC: The diagnostic approach to the bleeding disorders. In Lee GR, Bithell TC, Foerster J et al
(eds): Wintrobe's Clinical Hematology, 9th ed, p 1302. Philadelphia, Lea & Febiger, 1993.

contains all the clotting factors), and cryoprecipitate (for factor V, factor VIII, and fibrinogen replacement). The use of heparin, a potent anticoagulant, which inactivates the intravascular clotting and thus inhibits consumption of the coagulation factors, is very controversial and probably inappropriate in the face of active bleeding.[18,31,44] Heparin promotes bleeding, so platelets and clotting factors may need to be administered during heparin therapy.[31] Heparin may be used to prevent the consumption of platelets and clotting factors if laboratory tests show that DIC is beginning during chemotherapy for disorders such as acute promyelocytic leukemia.

NURSING MANAGEMENT PLAN. The nursing care of patients with cardiovascular disease in whom DIC develops is a challenge. Frequently, the bleeding is severe and associated with other problems of hypoperfusion such as brain, kidney, and liver dysfunction. In addition to managing the bleeding problem, the nurse must assist the patient and family in dealing with the possibility of death.

The primary nursing diagnoses for the patient in whom DIC has developed are the following: (1) risk for fluid volume deficit, (2) altered systemic tissue perfusion, (3) fear, and (4) anxiety. Nursing Care Plan 5-1 presents a management plan for the patient with DIC.

TABLE 5-4	Laboratory Tests in DIC

Manifestation	Acute DIC	Chronic DIC
Clinical	Usually hemorrhagic	None or thrombotic
Screening tests		
Prothrombin time, partial thromboplastin time	Usually prolonged	Normal
Platelets	Usually decreased	Normal or slightly decreased
Fibrinogen	Usually decreased, but may be normal	Usually normal
Confirmatory tests		
Fibrin monomer	Positive; can be negative, if severe	Positive
Fibrin degradation products	Strongly positive, usually >40 µg/mL	Positive, >40 µg/mL
D dimer	Positive	Positive
Other assays		
Thrombin time	Normal or abnormal	Usually normal
Factor assays	Decreased V, VIII	Normal V, VIII
Antithrombin III	May be low	Usually normal

DIC, disseminated intravascular coagulation.
  From Schmaier AH: Laboratory studies in disseminated intravascular coagulation and activated coagulation.
In Koepke J (ed): Practical Laboratory Hematology, p 480. New York, Churchill Livingstone, 1991.

NURSING CARE PLAN 5–1 ◆ The Patient with Disseminated Intravascular Coagulation

Nursing Diagnosis 1:	Potential or actual fluid volume deficit: intravascular volume deficit related to increased utilization of platelets and clotting factors and manifested by bleeding
Nursing Goal 1:	To detect early signs and symptoms of bleeding or intravascular volume deficit
Outcome Criteria:	Documentation reflects that the following were detected and reported: (1) any abnormal or excessive bleeding (on occurrence); (2) an intravascular volume deficit (within 4 hours of occurrence); (3) abnormal laboratory tests

NURSING INTERVENTIONS	RATIONALE
1. Observe for bleeding from the following sites: (1) skin—petechiae, hematoma, ecchymoses; (2) mucous membranes—epistaxis, bleeding gums, gatrointestinal (GI) bleeding; (3) wounds, incision, or puncture sites; (4) intracranial.	1.–3. Early detection of bleeding allows for prompt treatment.
2. Test all body excreta (emesis, nasogastric [NG] drainage, sputum, feces, and urine) for occult blood.	
3. Measure and record blood loss by any route: (weigh blood-soaked linen, count sanitary napkins or tampons).	3. One liter of fluid weighs approximately 1 kg.
4. Observe for signs of internal bleeding: abdominal/flank pain; pain or swollen joints; decreased level of consciousness (LOC) or headache (HA).	4. Abdominal or flank pain may indicate abdominal or retroperitoneal bleeding; swollen or painful joints may indicate bleeding into joints; HA or decreased LOC may indicate cerebral hemorrhage.
5. Monitor and record the following vital signs (VS) every 15 minutes to 1 hour during bleeding episodes and 2 to 4 hours thereafter:	5a. Inability to maintain postural adjustments in BP and pulse occurs in volume depletion before overt shock is present. Saline depletion (includes blood) should be suspected when, in response to sitting or
a. Blood pressure (BP) and pulse (postural BP and pulse if tolerated)	standing, the heart rate increases and either the diastolic BP: drops by 10 mm Hg or the systolic BP
b. Respiratory rate	decreases by
c. Central venous pressure (CVP) (if available) or neck veins	15 mm Hg (see Chapter 10).
d. Pulmonary artery wedge pressure (PAWP) (if available)	b–d. An intravascular volume deficit may be manifested by increased respiratory rate, decreased CVP and PAWP, and flat neck veins.

Nursing Goal 2:	To minimize blood loss and replace blood volume as necessary
Outcome Criteria:	Overt bleeding will cease or lessen. Intravascular volume will be maintained as evidenced by VS within the patient's normal limits.

NURSING INTERVENTIONS	RATIONALE
1. Attempt to control active bleeding by:	1. Direct pressure will stop bleeding and allow a clot to form if appropriate coagulation factors are present. Cold causes vasoconstriction, which assists in the control of bleeding.
a. Applying direct pressure where possible for 5 to 10 minutes	
b. Applying ice or cold compresses over the site of bleeding	
c. Resting the affected part and elevating above the level of the heart if possible	
d. Lavaging stomach with iced saline to control bleeding from GI tract	
2. Administer blood and blood products as ordered:	2. Whole blood may be ordered if the bleeding causes an intravascular volume deficit. Platelets, cryoprecipitate, and fresh frozen plasma may be ordered to replace platelets and clotting factors.
a. Use the appropriate administration technique for each type of transfusion	
b. Assess for adverse reactions or side effects such as chilling or anaphylaxis.	

(continued)

NURSING CARE PLAN 5–1 ◆ The Patient with Disseminated Intravascular Coagulation *(Continued)*

| **Nursing Goal 3:** | To prevent bleeding episodes. |

| **Outcome Criteria:** | Absence of active bleeding, VS within the patient's normal limits, and normal hemoglobin and hematocrit levels |

NURSING INTERVENTIONS

1. Protect the patient from injury by the following:
   a. Provide all care as gently as possible (e.g., turning, bathing).
   b. Use a soft toothbrush or cotton swabs for oral care.
   c. Use an electric rather than a safety razor.
   d. Use plastic or paper rather than adhesive tape.
   e. Assist the patient to sit or stand from a recumbent position (especially if postural hypotension is present).
2. Modify nursing interventions that may precipitate bleeding.
   a. Intramuscular and subcutaneous injections should be avoided. (If injections cannot be avoided, use a small-gauge needle.)
   b. Use central lines for fluid and medication administration.
   c. Use arterial lines for BP monitoring and blood withdrawal for laboratory tests. (If an arterial line is not available, use an intravascular line for blood withdrawal.)
   d. Apply direct pressure for 5 to 10 minutes when removing intravascular lines. Apply pressure dressing and observe frequently for bleeding.
   e. Avoid the use of NG or rectal tubes, which irritate mucous membranes.
3. Avoid the use of aspirin or aspirin-containing products.

RATIONALE

1. Patients with disseminated intravascular coagulation bleed very easily and therefore must be protected from trauma.

2. Any interruption of the skin integrity may cause excessive bleeding. Blood samples for most laboratory tests, including some coagulation tests, may be withdrawn from intravascular lines. The pressure from the BP cuff may cause ecchymoses.

3. Aspirin interferes with the function of platelets by inhibiting their release; thus, aspirin may enhance bleeding.[47]

| **Nursing Diagnosis 2:** | Potential altered systemic tissue perfusion: organ ischemica, related to deposition of fibrin or clotting within the microcirculation |

| **Nursing Goal:** | To detect decreased tissue perfusion or thrombus formation early |

| **Outcome Criteria:** | Documentation reflects that the signs of decreased tissue perfusion or thrombus formation were detected and reported within 2 hours of occurrence |

NURSING INTERVENTIONS

1. Every hour, assess and document signs of decreased tissue perfusion or thrombus formation:
   a. Cerebral—decreased LOC, restlessness, agitation, or apprehension
   b. Myocardial ischemia—chest pain, ST segment changes
   c. Renal ischemia—decreased urine output
   d. Peripheral arterial thrombus—cool, pale skin or pain in an extremity
   e. Deep vein thromosis—edema, increased skin temperature, and a reddened, tender extremity
2. Report any signs and symptoms listed above to the physician.

RATIONALE

1, 2. Early detection of organ ischemia allows for early treatment, which may prevent an infarction.

(continued)

NURSING CARE PLAN 5–1 ◆ **The Patient with Disseminated Intravascular Coagulation** *(Continued)*

Nursing Diagnosis 3:	Fear and anxiety related to hemorrhage and the possibility of death as manifested by ineffective coping
Nursing Goal:	To decrease the patient's and family's fear and anxiety
Outcome Criteria:	The patient and family demonstrate decreased anxiety and effective coping behaviors such as verbalization of their fears

NURSING INTERVENTIONS	**RATIONALE**
1. Demonstrate efficiency and competence while delivering patient care.	1. A calm competent manner increases the patient's and family's confidence and may decrease anxiety.
2. Encourage the patient and family to express their fears.	2. Unresolved anxiety increases the stress response.
3. Explain all procedures and tests to the patient and family.	3. Providing information will lessen the fear of the unknown.
4. Use flexible visiting hours and assist the family members to touch and talk to the patient (especially if the patient is intubated and there are multiple tubes and lines present).	4. The presence of a supportive family may assist in reducing both the patient's and family's anxiety.
5. Encourage the family members to eat and go home to rest if the patient is stable (reassure that you will call if there is any change in the patient's condition).	5. Adequate nutrition and rest are essential to maintain effective coping.
6. Assess the need for spiritual counseling and refer as appropriate.	6. The patient and family may find support in spiritual counseling, thereby reducing fear and anxiety.

Adapted from Wild L: Inflammatory disorders affecting vascular function. In Patrick ML, Woods SL, Cravan RF et al (eds): Medical-Surgical Nursing: Pathophysiological Concepts, 2nd ed. Philadelphia, JB Lippincott, 1991.

CLOTTING DISORDERS

Excessive or inappropriate coagulation is also of great clinical significance. Venous thrombosis involves the interacting conditions of stasis, vascular damage, and hypercoagulability. Its most common life-threatening complication, pulmonary embolism, is a major cause of mortality in hospitalized patients. Recognition of patients likely to have any of these conditions is a nursing responsibility.

Clot Formation

A *thrombus* is a clot or solid mass formed by blood components. *Thrombosis* refers to the formation or presence of blood clots in a vessel. A thrombus that breaks loose and travels in the blood vessel is termed an *embolus*—thus the term *thromboembolism*. The potential outcome from either thrombosis or embolism is ischemia, leading to infarction with cellular and tissue necrosis.[27]

A thrombus develops when the normal process of hemostasis is inappropriately activated.[28] Three factors, when all are present, predispose a patient to thrombosis. These three factors, commonly known as Virchow's triad, were first described in 1846 by Rudolf Virchow[29] (Fig. 5-6).

First, the vessel involved must have suffered some type of injury, particularly damage to the endothelial layer. *Vessel injury* may be the result of sustained pressure on the vessel or surrounding tissue, as might occur from prolonged immobility of an extremity or pressure points caused by crossed legs, elastic-topped knee socks, or a bed where the knee gatch is raised too high. Vessel wall injury can also result from direct trauma by surgery, or more commonly by intravenous (IV) or arterial catheters. Underlying vascular disease also creates vessel wall abnormalities. Chemical irritation may result from intravenous solutions and drugs. Anything that exposes collagen fibers in the vessel wall of arteries and veins may cause rapid platelet adhesion, aggregation, and thrombus formation. In addition, injury to vessels activates an inflammatory response that can be seen histologically and, in most cases, clinically.

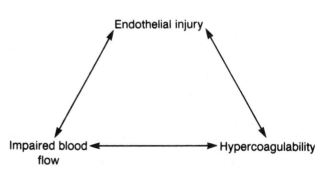

FIGURE 5-6 Virchow's triad: factors that predispose a patient to thrombosis. (From Patrick ML, Woods SL, Craven RF et al: (eds) Medical-Surgical Nursing: Pathophysiologic Concepts, 2nd ed, p 837, Philadelphia, JB Lippincott, 1991.)

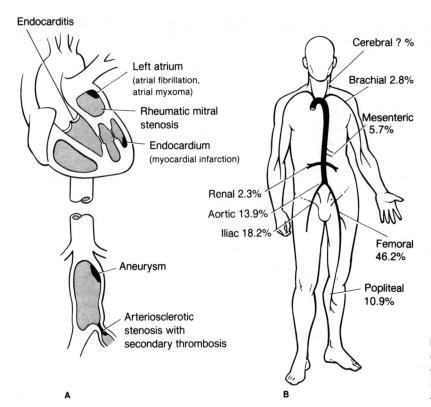

FIGURE 5-7 Sources (A) and distribution (B) of emboli. (From Patrick ML, Woods SL, Craven RF et al: [eds] Medical-Surgical Nursing: Pathophysiological Concepts, 2nd ed, p 854. Philadelphia, JB Lippincott, 1991.)

The second factor in the triad is impaired blood flow, or *stasis*, in the involved vessel. Normally the pumping action of the muscles against the venous vasculature assists venous return and is seen most vividly in the lower extremities. When an extremity is immobile for any period of time, the pumping action is lost, resulting in venous stasis. Postoperative patients have a decrease in total limb blood flow.[45] Stasis may also result from reduced cardiac output due to heart failure or shock. Alteration in blood flow leading to arterial thrombosis may be due to turbulent flow at points of arterial bifurcation or stenosis, or with aneurysms. Fortunately, the rapid blood flow in arteries tends to discourage thrombus formation. Reduced blood flow in the atria occurs with atrial fibrillation, leading to thrombus formation. When the patient's cardiac rhythm converts to a regular sinus rhythm, these thrombi can be expelled into the lungs or systemic circulation.

The final predisposing factor of Virchow's triad is *hypercoagulability* of the blood itself. Changes in blood leading to hypercoagulability may occur during pregnancy or in women taking oral contraceptive drugs in whom the changes are due to elevated levels of coagulation factors.[18] Changes in blood constituents may also occur in polycythemia, in severe anemia, or with circulating endotoxins from systemic infections.[27,39] Deficiencies in antithrombin III and reduced hepatic function may be thrombogenic factors in patients with liver disease and in premature infants.[29]

The type of thrombus formed usually differs between arteries and veins. Arterial thrombi usually begin at the site of endothelial injury or turbulence.[27] The arterial thrombus is a dry, friable, tangled mass composed of layers of platelets and coagulated fibrin. Arterial thrombi are termed "white thrombi" because they are primarily composed of platelets and fibrin, and they lack RBCs.

A venous thrombus is almost always occlusive. In the slower-moving blood of the veins, the thrombus frequently creates a long cast in the lumen of the vessel. Venous thrombi, which have a rich admixture of RBCs with tangled strands of pale gray fibrin, are termed "red thrombi."[27]

Acute Arterial Occlusion

Acute arterial occlusion is a vascular emergency. The ischemic consequences of a sudden block to arterial blood flow may be severe. Profound tissue necrosis may occur within 6 to 12 hours.[43]

ETIOLOGY AND PATHOPHYSIOLOGY

One of the most common causes of acute arterial occlusion is arterial embolism. Embolization of an arterial thrombus is usually the result of the entire thrombus detaching and ultimately lodging in a smaller arterial branch. Most arterial emboli originate in the heart. Figure 5-7 summarizes the sources of emboli as well as their eventual distribution. Most arterial emboli lodge in vessels of the lower extremities.

Acute arterial occlusion can also result from acute arterial thrombosis associated with either an existing atheromatous lesion or iatrogenic sources such as intra-arterial catheters. Arterial trauma, hematoma formation, vascular graft occlusion, and dissecting aneurysms can also lead to acute arterial occlusion.[3]

TABLE 5-5	**Acute Arterial Occlusion: Differentiation of Embolism and Thrombosis**	
	Embolism	Thrombosis
Onset	Sudden	Gradual
	May be without prior symptoms of arterial insufficiency	Usually other symptoms of arterial insufficiency
Appearance of affected limb	Yellowish, waxy, "cadaveric pallor"	Mottled, cyanotic
Pulses	Often normal in unaffected extremities	Bruits, pulse deficits in unaffected extremities
Prevalent history	Atrial fibrillation	Chronic arteriosclerosis obliterans

CLINICAL MANIFESTATIONS

Acute arterial occlusion typically presents as the "six P's": pain, pallor, paresthesias, paralysis, pulselessness, and polar (coldness).[3] Differentiation between acute arterial thrombosis and embolism can often be made from the clinical history and other assessment criteria. Table 5-5 highlights the distinguishing features of both arterial thrombosis and embolism.

MEDICAL MANAGEMENT

Arterial Doppler studies are helpful in the *diagnosis* of acute arterial occlusion. However, definitive diagnosis of arterial occlusion requires arteriography.

Surgical intervention is the treatment of choice for acute arterial occlusion due to embolization. An arterial embolectomy is performed. A small incision is made in the proximal artery, followed by the insertion of a Fogarty balloon catheter. The balloon catheter is then passed through the embolus, and the balloon is inflated and gently withdrawn to remove the embolus without incurring further damage to the vessel itself. After extraction of the embolus, the vessel is irrigated with a heparinized saline solution. An operative arteriogram is usually obtained to ensure arterial patency.[42] Regional infusions of thrombolytic agents, such as streptokinase or urokinase, are also used in conjunction with surgery to promote limb salvage. Used alone, thrombolytic agents do not usually result in limb salvage. However, they can be used alone when surgical intervention is not possible or has a poor prognosis.[6]

The effectiveness of drugs like heparin and coumarin in the treatment of arterial thrombosis appears to be in preventing extension of the thrombus and preventing VTE.[6] These drugs do not reduce the size of the thrombus. When heparin is used, a loading dose of 70 U/kg of body weight (5,000 to 10,000 U) is given intravenously, followed by a continuous infusion drip titrated to prolong PTT to 1.5 times to 3 times the baseline value.[6] Usual dosage is 10 to 15 U/kg/h.

The patient is usually maintained on postoperative intravenous heparin for 12 to 24 hours to prevent recurrent embolization. After this time, patients usually begin oral anticoagulant agents such as sodium warfarin.[2]

The *prognosis* for the patient with an acute arterial occlusion is good, provided interventions are made quickly. Limb viability is severely threatened with prolonged ischemia. Amputation of the affected extremity may be necessary if tissue necrosis ensues. The amputation rate after embolectomy is low, approximately 5% to 20%.

NURSING MANAGEMENT PLAN. Because acute arterial occlusion is medical emergency, the goals of prevention, early detection, and prompt intervention are essential to maintain limb viability. Revascularization is attempted surgically. If necrosis is severe, amputation of the extremity is necessary. Before surgery, an appropriate nursing diagnosis is anxiety related to the abrupt onset of the disorder in addition to the threat to the affected limb and the emergency surgery necessary to correct the problem. Astute assessment, explanation of procedures, and caring reassurance to the patient and family are critical nursing interventions to relieve the anxiety experienced by the patient and family.

The most common complication of fibrinolytic and anticoagulant therapies is hemorrhage. The nurse must be alert to signs and symptoms of bleeding from the surgical site, bleeding into the tissues surrounding the wound, and bleeding from other sites, such as gastrointestinal bleeding and ecchymoses at needle puncture sites. In general, all that is required to reverse the bleeding from heparin overdosage is to turn it off. However, if immediate reversal of heparin effects is needed, the patient can be given protamine. Bleeding secondary to coumarin drug administration is usually related to the time the patient has been on these drugs. The longer a patient is on coumarin drugs, the more likely bleeding complications will occur.[6] In addition, the patient may experience allergic reactions to both heparin and the thrombolytic agents.

Venous Thromboembolism

The clinical problems associated with VTE include *deep vein thrombosis* (DVT) and *pulmonary embolism* (PE). VTE is the third most common acute cardiovascular disease after cardiac ischemic syndromes and stroke. Furthermore, the incidence of VTE has not declined during a period when all other forms of cardiovascular disease are becoming less prevalent.[16] One of the most common and potentially life-threatening problems confronted by physicians is the diagnosis, prophylaxis, and treatment of PE and DVT in both medical and surgical patients. The magnitude of the problem is enormous, with a conservative estimate of 2.5 million cases of DVT and 600,000 cases of PE per year in the United States.[15] Approximately 200,000 deaths per year are related to PE. Critically ill patients typically have multiple risk factors for DVT and PE. Risk factors for VTE include age over 40 years, male sex, presence of malignancy, prior episode of VTE, major surgery (orthopedic, gynecologic, general, neurosurgical, urologic), prolonged immobilization, oral contraceptive pill, pregnancy, presence of hypercoagulable disorder, trauma, myocardial infarction, congestive heart failure, stroke, and obesity. Overall, VTE is associated with more than 300,000 hospitalizations annually. Some form of DVT develops in approximately 30% to 40% of postoperative patients, and among older patients presenting with DVT, the 1-year mortality rate exceeds 20%.[8,34]

DEEP VEIN THROMBOSIS

The major risk associated with DVT is that it can lead to PE, which kills 10% to 15% of affected patients within minutes.[6] Venous thrombosis in the lower extremity can involve superficial leg veins, the deep veins of the calf (calf vein thrombosis), and the more proximal veins, including the popliteal veins, the superficial femoral, common femoral, and iliac veins. In superficial vein thrombosis, sometimes called thrombophlebitis, the thrombosis occurs secondary to inflammation in the venous wall of the superficial venous system and is benign and self-limiting. However, the thrombi in the superficial veins can extend into the deep veins and give rise to major PE.[19]

More common is acute thrombosis of the deep venous system. This type of thrombus occurs secondary to stasis and is not associated with preexisting inflammation of the vein. Calf vein thrombosis (below-knee DVT) is thought to be less serious than proximal vein thrombosis (above-knee DVT) because thrombi in calf veins are usually small and less likely to be associated with clinical disability or major complications, such as PE. However, these thrombi can extend proximally and become dangerous. Although venous thrombi are usually attached to the vessel at the point of origin, the tail of the thrombus, which builds up behind the occluding head, may or may not be attached.[28] This tail is the part most likely to break off and create an embolus, which often lodges in a pulmonary artery, causing the signs and symptoms of a PE (see later).

Risk Factors. Certain patient populations are at high risk for the development of DVT. Several risk factors have been identified that relate to the three etiologic factors (Virchow's triad) discussed previously. The major clinical risk factor is age. The relative risk for development of DVT is increased dramatically for patients older than 40 years of age.[32] For every 20 years, the relative risk for development of DVT more than triples. For example, a 60-year-old patient is approximately 3 times more likely to have thrombosis than is a 40-year-old patient, and 10 times more likely than a 20-year-old. Changes in activity levels, decreased muscle tone, and reductions in antithrombin III levels predispose elderly patients to DVT.[45]

Patients with cardiac disease are also at risk for development of DVT. The mechanisms predisposing these patients include general cardiac insufficiency along with alterations in blood flow and hemodynamic pressures, which may decrease venous return and subsequently cause venous stasis and pooling. In addition, patients with cardiac disease may be less active and are more prone to the hazards of stasis associated with immobility (see Chapter 34).

People with a previous thrombosis are also at a higher risk for recurrent thrombosis. The risk of recurrent VTE is increased by the presence of malignancy and coagulation abnormalities and is decreased in patients who have modifiable risk factors (e.g., birth control pills, surgery, fracture, travel longer than 6 hours).[20]

Any postoperative patient is at risk for development of DVT. Patients undergoing orthopedic surgery, especially hip surgery, are at the highest risk, followed by patients undergoing general, neurosurgical, and urologic procedures. Surgery after traumatic injury is also associated with a higher incidence of thrombosis, primarily because prophylaxis is not possible, and the coagulation cascade may already be activated.[5]

Patients undergoing estrogen therapy are at risk for thrombosis. This effect is reduced with lower doses of estrogen. Estrogens are believed to induce both distention of peripheral veins and changes in the coagulation and fibrinolytic systems.[40] Because estrogen levels are elevated during pregnancy and the puerperium, these patients are also at greater risk.

The incidence of thrombosis is higher in patients with infections or malignancies.[5,45] The higher risk is suspected to be due to alterations in the coagulation system.

Clinical Manifestations. The clinical manifestations of DVT are sometimes elusive; therefore, a clinical suspicion of DVT should always be confirmed by objective diagnostic tests. The classic signs and symptoms of pain, edema, and tenderness of the leg can be caused by nonthrombotic disorders.[21] As many as 50% of patients with DVT in whom PE develops have no symptoms of deep venous disease.[40] Symptoms of DVT are pain and tenderness, mild swelling, and superficial venous dilatation in the extremity, most commonly in the calf because it is the most frequent site of the thrombosis. The classic sign of DVT is a positive Homans' sign, which can be described as pain occurring in the affected calf with forceful dorsiflexion of the foot. However, a positive Homans' sign is not specific for thrombotic disease, and therefore caution must be used when interpreting Homans' sign because any inflammation near the calf muscles may also elicit pain with dorsiflexion, and, thus, a false-positive diagnosis of thrombosis can occur.

Other signs of DVT may include warmth and redness of the affected extremity. Asymmetry between two extremities may also be present, with the affected limb being slightly larger because of the congestion and edema associated with the inflammatory process.

Medical Management. When DVT is suspected in a patient, usually by the presence of clinical signs and symptoms, further *diagnostic studies* are indicated. In addition to getting objective tests, a careful history and physical examination should be obtained. The patient's history and physical examination are important components of the diagnostic process because they may reveal an alternative cause of the patient's symptoms, and because they allow patients to be classified as having a low, intermediate, or high clinical probability for DVT. Wells and colleagues[49] have developed a simple clinical scoring system that, when combined with the results of the noninvasive tests, can be used both to simplify and reduce the costs of the diagnostic process. The scoring system includes three main components (signs and symptoms at presentation, presence or absence of risk factors, and presence or absence of possible alternative diagnosis). Using the clinical scoring system, Wells and associates[49] have shown that 80% of patients with high clinical probability have venous thrombosis, whereas only 5% of patients with low clinical probability have venous thrombosis.

The diagnostic studies include compression ultrasonography, duplex ultrasonography, venography, plethysmography, and magnetic resonance imaging.[10] Some form of ultrasound, either compression or color duplex, is usually the most common test used for diagnosing DVT.[20]

Medical *management* of acute DVT centers around prevention. The most effective way of decreasing the mortality rate from PE and morbidity from the post-thrombotic syndrome is to institute primary prophylaxis in patients at risk for VTE.[20] Patients' risk factors should be assessed and classified as low, moderate, or high risk for development of VTE based on established clinical criteria.[13] Prophylaxis is achieved by either preventing venous stasis or modulating activation of blood anticoagulation.[21] Preventive measures include mechanical methods to improve venous flow and prophylactic anticoagulation. The approach to treatment evolves from the triad of factors that predispose patients to the development of thrombosis.

Mechanical measures to deter venous stasis include intermittent pneumatic compression of the legs, graduated compression stockings, passive and active leg exercises, and early ambulation.[13]

The use of prophylactic anticoagulants has become a standard of practice for many hospitalized patients, particularly for those at highest risk for the development of DVT, as previously discussed. Prophylactic anticoagulants approved by the National Heart, Blood, and Lung Institute of the National Institutes of Health include low-dose subcutaneous heparin, low-dose warfarin, dextran,[37] and low–molecular-weight heparins (LMWHs).[21] Low-dose heparin has been shown to decrease the incidence of DVT.[5] Frequently, 5,000 U of subcutaneous heparin are given two to three times daily for the duration of bed rest and up to 1 week afterward. Larger doses do not correlate with a lowered incidence of thrombosis and tend to increase the risk of bleeding.[5,45]

Dextran may also be used as a prophylactic agent, especially with patients for whom any bleeding would be detrimental, such as neurosurgical patients. Dextran has been shown to be more effective than heparin for thromboprophylaxis in patients with hip surgery.[5]

Oral anticoagulants such as warfarin may be used. Aspirin is no longer recommended for prophylaxis of DVT.[38] LMWHs have been approved for use as prophylactic agents in North America and are proven to be safe and effective for prophylaxis in patients who are at high risk for VTE. In general surgical patients, in patients with stroke, and in patients undergoing elective hip surgery, LMWHs have been reported to be more effective than standard low-dose heparin. The LMWHs have also been shown to be more effective than warfarin in patients undergoing hip or major knee surgery.[21]

Definitive treatment for DVT centers around symptom management and prevention of embolization. PE is a serious sequel to DVT and is associated with a high mortality rate. Heparin and coumarin drugs have been the treatment of choice for DVT since the 1950s. The combination of heparin and coumarin drugs is still the most commonly used treatment for DVT. When used to treat acute DVT, heparins are usually administered based on the patient's body weight, age, and drug sensitivity. Unfractionated heparin is usually administered intravenously for 3 to 5 days, whereas LMWHs are administered subcutaneously two times daily for 5 to 7 days.[21] Patients who can be treated with LMWHs are more likely to be treated in an outpatient setting. Activated PTT is used to guide the unfractionated intravenous heparin dosage. Therapeutic range for heparin therapy is 1.5 to 2 times the baseline PTT value.[6] Coumarin drugs are administered in dosages sufficient to keep the PT at 1.3 to 2.5 times baseline. The coumarin drugs are usually started on the first or second day of heparin therapy.

Although thrombolytic therapy is more effective than heparin in producing rapid lysis of thromboemboli, it is also more expensive and is associated with a higher risk of bleeding.[29] Thrombolytic therapy usually is not recommended for patients with PE because they do well clinically with anticoagulant therapy. It is also contraindicated in postoperative patients and in situations in which there is a high risk of bleeding. Thrombolytic therapy should be considered in patients with major PE. It may also be indicated in selected patients (both young and old without risk factors for bleeding) with extensive proximal vein thrombosis (phlegmasia cerulea dolans).[30] The thrombolytic agents most often used include urokinase and t-PA. Thrombolytic therapy must be used early in the treatment of thrombi to be effective. Heparin and coumarin drugs are used after the discontinuation of thrombolytic agents.

A debate concerning the efficacy of activity limitations and elevation of the affected limb in people with documented DVT continues. Proponents suggest that the risk of embolization with activity and movement is too high, whereas opponents propose that immobility and limbs in dependent positions serve only to promote further venous stasis and its complications.

Surgical intervention for venous thrombosis is seldom necessary and is used only when other methods of treatment, as described previously, are contraindicated and the patient is at high risk for PE. In these cases, a thrombectomy or a caval interruption may be performed to prevent the passage of emboli.[5] The most common indication for venous interruption in patients with VTE is anticoagulant-induced bleeding or for those patients who are at risk for bleeding due to one of the following predisposing conditions: peptic ulcer disease, recent intracranial surgery, gastrointestinal malignancy, or an underlying hemorrhagic state.[20] Caval interruption can be accomplished by the transvenous placement of an umbrella filter into the inferior vena cava or by partial ligation of the caval segment. The umbrella filter traps emboli traveling from distal sites toward the pulmonary vasculature. Because caval interruption with an umbrella filter traps thrombi, postoperative vena caval occlusion can occur, necessitating removal of the filter.[11] Placement of an inferior vena cava filter is not considered a treatment for acute DVT, but rather a prophylactic procedure to prevent PE. Therefore, without removing the risk factors for DVT or administering anticoagulants, the patient may continue to experience acute DVT.[20]

The *prognosis* for patients with DVT is favorable. For most patients, the problem resolves quickly without complications or residual morbidity. Unfortunately, in some patients, DVT is a recurrent problem. These patients are especially at risk for PE. Recurrent DVT can also lead to the post-thrombotic syndrome. The post-thrombotic syndrome is caused by venous hypertension, which occurs as a result of recanalization of major venous thrombi leading to patent but scarred and incompetent venous valves.[20,45] Recanalization and valve destruction result in failure of the muscular pump mechanism, which leads to increased pressure in the deep veins of the calf. The high pressure can cause progressive incompetence of the valves of the perforating veins of the calf; when this happens, flow is directed from the deep vein into the superficial system during muscle contraction, which can lead to edema, impaired viability of the subcutaneous tissue (brown discoloration), and, ultimately, ulceration.[20] The post-thrombotic syndrome occurs in approximately 25% to 50% of patients with symptomatic DVT.[43] Medical management of the post-thrombotic syndrome is difficult and costly. The diagnosis of post-thrombotic syndrome should include demonstration of deep venous incompetence using Doppler ultrasonography or plethysmography.[45]

NURSING MANAGEMENT PLAN. The primary approach to nursing management of the patient at risk for DVT includes identifying the high-risk patient and implementing vigorous attempts to prevent its occurrence. Such attempts include encouraging active or passive leg exercises and early ambulation to increase muscle activity, thereby improving venous blood flow. Frequent turning, coughing, and deep breathing help reduce the risk of vessel injury and improve venous return. Other measures to promote venous return are pneumatic compression stockings, graduated compression stockings, elevating the foot of the bed 6 to 8 inches, and not raising the knee to avoid excessive popliteal pressure.

A thorough history of the patient's risk factors along with the vigilant physical assessment of extremities for any evidence of inflammation, such as redness, swelling, asymmetry, and tenderness, is critical. Any such signs and symptoms should be followed by objective diagnostic testing (see earlier).

Bleeding is the most common complication of anticoagulant and fibrinolytic therapy. The patient must be observed for sites of bleeding such as hematomas and gastrointestinal bleeding.

Because embolization is always a threat, special attention to the assessment of cardiopulmonary indicators is paramount. The signs to look for include sudden onset of dyspnea, chest pain, and tachypnea, and alterations in level of consciousness; an abnormal electrocardiogram (ECG) showing a pattern of right ventricular strain may also accompany PE (see Chapter 13).

An overview of nursing care with nursing diagnoses, goals, and outcomes appears in Nursing Care Plan 5-2 for the patient with DVT.

PULMONARY EMBOLISM

Pulmonary embolism is an acute pulmonary-vascular disorder. In the event of PE, the pulmonary vasculature may be partially or completely occluded; pulmonary infarction and necrosis may follow complete obstruction (Fig. 5-8). The incidence of symptomatic PE is estimated to be in excess of 650,000 occurrences annually and is thought to be the leading nonsurgical cause of death in hospitalized patients.[4,49] PE is fatal in approximately 38% of symptomatic patients[4]; the mortality rate is even higher in patients for whom the diagnosis was missed.

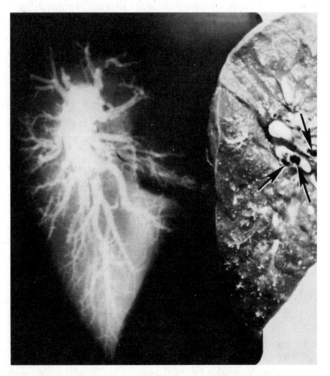

FIGURE 5-8 Multiple pulmonary emboli. The figure to the right is a lung specimen. The figure to the left shows the perfusion abnormality of this lung specimen. The *arrows* indicate large, nonocclusive thrombi in the pulmonary artery and its major branches. The perfusion defect in the apex (*top half*) of the lung indicates small emboli in at least three smaller branches of the pulmonary artery, leading to an infarct of the lung. (Courtesy of Dr. Marie Cowan, University of Washington School of Nursing, Seattle, WA.)

NURSING CARE PLAN 5–2 ◆ The Patient with Deep Vein Thrombosis

Nursing Diagnosis 1: Potential or actual altered peripheral tissue perfusion, related to the inflammatory process

Nursing Goal 1: To prevent inflammation and the formation of thrombi

Outcome Criteria: Absence of signs and symptoms of inflammation such as redness, warmth, swelling, positive Homans' sign, and tenderness or aching in affected limb

NURSING INTERVENTIONS	RATIONALE

1. Encourage movement of lower limbs:
  a. Leg exercises
  b. Early ambulation
	1. Increased muscle activity in lower extremities improves venous return by muscle pumping action, thereby reducing venous stasis.

2. Encourage turning, coughing, and deep breathing at least every 2 hours.	2. Turning helps to alleviate pressure points to tissues, thereby decreasing risk for vessel injury and venous stasis. Deep breathing increases negative intrathoracic pressure, thus promoting improved venous return.
3. Apply antiembolism stockings as ordered.	3. Antiembolism stockings improve venous flow rate in the lower limbs.
4. Administer prophylactic anticoagulants as ordered by physician.	4. Anticoagulants prevent thrombus formations. See discussions above.
5. Elevate foot of bed 6 to 8 inches.	5. Foot elevation to this level improves venous return and helps reduce venous stasis.
6. Do not elevate knee gatch of patient's bed.	6. A raised knee gatch exerts prolonged pressure on the popliteal area and vessels, which may induce vessel injury and inhibit venous return by compression.

Nursing Goal 2: To detect deep vein thrombosis early, and treat if it should occur

Outcome Criteria: Deep vein thrombosis detected within a 4-hour time span
Treatment of affected area within 1 hour of detection

NURSING INTERVENTIONS	RATIONALE
1. Assess patient every 4 to 8 hours; document and report the presence of signs and symptoms of inflammation: redness, swelling, asymmetry, tenderness and aching, shortness of breath, chest pain.	1. Presence of any signs and symptoms of inflammation may signal propagation of thrombus.

2. Implement treatment of deep vein thrombosis as ordered by physician:
  a. Administration of anticoagulants
  b. Positioning of extremity
  c. Activity restrictions
  d. Application of warm, moist heat
  e. Application of antiembolism stockings
  f. Administration of analgesics
	2. a. Anticoagulants help prevent further clot formation and may help prevent embolization.
	  b. Extremity may be elevated to promote venous return or left flat to prevent embolization of thrombi.
	  c. Some physicians require bed rest for their patients to reduce risk of embolization; others suggest moderate activity restrictions and encourage sitting for short periods to prevent further stasis and other complications of prolonged immobility.
	  d. Application of warm, moist heat increases blood flow to affected area.
	  e. Antiembolism stockings improve venous flow rate.
	  f. Analgesics help reduce discomfort experienced by patient.

(continued)

NURSING CARE PLAN 5–2 ◆ **The Patietnt with Deep Vein Thrombosis** *(Continued)*

Nursing Goal 3:	To detect potential complications of deep vein thrombosis early
Outcome Criteria:	No signs and symptoms of pulmonary embolism evident. Normal breathing patterns (no dyspnea). No complaints of chest pain. Normal heart rate and electrocardiogram. Normal mentation and awareness. Normal arterial blood gases. Signs and symptoms of pulmonary embolism detected within a 2-hour time span.

NURSING INTERVENTIONS	RATIONALE
1. Avoid rubbing or massaging the affected area.	1. Rubbing or massaging increases the danger of the thrombus breaking off and embolizing.

2. Assess, document, and report any signs and symptoms of pulmonary embolus every 2 hours and as necessary:
  a. Sudden onset of dyspnea, chest pain, tachypnea
  b. Alterations in level of consciousness
  c. Abnormal arterial blood gases
	2. Pulmonary embolism is the most common and serious sequel to thrombosis and may occur rapidly.

(Adapted from Wild L: Inflammatory disorders affecting vascular function. In Patrick ML, Woods SL, Cravan RF et al (eds): Medical-Surgical Nursing: Pathophysiological Concepts, 2nd ed. Philadelphia, JB Lippincott, 1991.)

Pulmonary embolism may be the result of either arterial or venous thrombi. Common sources of PE include deep venous thrombi from the lower legs, right atrial thrombi, septic foci (often related to intravenous drug abuse or infected vascular access sites), tumors, atheroemboli, amniotic fluid, fat, air, bone marrow, and other foreign bodies.[4]

Several factors may predispose patients to PE. These factors are similar to those risk factors for development of DVT, discussed earlier. Predisposing factors include immobility; trauma; age (the 50- to 65-year-old age bracket has the highest incidence); obesity; pregnancy and puerperium; and coexisting cardiac, neoplastic, hematologic, or metabolic disease.[4]

Pathophysiology. A PE is a mechanical obstruction to pulmonary blood flow. As a result of this obstruction, there is a local aggregation of platelets and release of vasoactive substances, which induce vasoconstriction. Histamine, serotonin, and prostaglandins are also released, causing bronchoconstriction.[15] The persistent obstruction and associated vasoconstriction and bronchoconstriction act together to produce a ventilation–perfusion (VQ) imbalance (see Chapter 3). With PE, there is adequate ventilation coupled with inadequate perfusion. Any sustained VQ mismatch results in arterial hypoxemia.

In an attempt to compensate for the VQ imbalance, the respiratory rate increases. Consequently, the partial pressure of arterial carbon dioxide ($PaCO_2$) drops as carbon dioxide is blown off. However, instead of correcting the VQ mismatch, the reduction in $PaCO_2$ induces even further bronchoconstriction and vasoconstriction, thus perpetuating the problem and its severity.[4,15]

The hemodynamic consequences of PE may be profound. Because of the decrease in arterial flow through the lungs, there is an increase in both pulmonary artery and right ventricular pressures. Cardiac output eventually decreases because of right ventricular dilatation and the lowered left ventricular preload. Systemic hypotension usually follows.[4,15]

Clinical Manifestations. Pulmonary embolism may have a sudden, abrupt onset, or it may have an insidious onset that mimics other cardiopulmonary disorders. Chest pain, the most common symptom associated with PE, has been reported by 88% of patients with angiographically documented PE. Of those patients, 74% described the chest pain as pleuritic and 14% described it as nonpleuritic.[4] Patients reported chest pain as much as 3 to 4 days before diagnosis. Dyspnea is also a common symptom associated with PE. The dyspnea experienced is usually of acute onset and is often combined with tachypnea (respiratory rate >16/min). Also, crackles can be auscultated over the affected lung.[4]

Heart rate may be elevated in patients with PE, although 44% of patients studied had heart rates within normal limits (60 to 100 beats/min). Fever, which may also be present with PE, could also account for an increase in heart rate. Other cardiac signs may include the development of a cardiac gallop or murmur located in the pulmonic valve area and an increase in the intensity of the pulmonic component of the second heart sound (S_2).

Apprehension and subtle changes in mentation or level of consciousness may also signal PE. Other symptoms of PE include coughing, diaphoresis, palpitations, hemoptysis, nausea, vomiting, chills, fever, and syncope.[4,15]

Medical Management. If a PE is suspected, immediate *diagnostic studies* are indicated because the clinical diagnosis of PE is highly nonspecific. The clinical features of PE can mimic other cardiorespiratory or musculoskeletal disorders. The diagnosis of PE should always be confirmed by objective tests. Arterial blood gas (ABG) determination, ECG, and chest roentgenography can be done quickly and are able to provide preliminary information about the patient's condition. In general, patients with PE have profound hypoxemia, with arterial oxygen (PO_2) levels ranging between 60 and 65 mm Hg.[4] Arterial $PaCO_2$ may be normal or decreased from normal as a result of tachypnea. However, if normal ABGs are found, a diagnosis of PE cannot be ruled out.

An ECG may be abnormal in patients with PE, although it is nonspecific in approximately 80% of those patients. The ECG is of greatest diagnostic value in massive PE because 87% of patients show consistent ECG changes.[4] The most common ECG finding is a pattern of right ventricular strain related to alterations in right ventricular and pulmonary artery pressures[2,15] (see Chapter 13). With PE that is not considered massive, the ECG is often normal or shows nonspecific changes.[45]

A chest roentgenogram is usually abnormal but rarely, if ever, diagnostic in PE. Most frequently, abnormalities are seen in the lower lobes. An elevated diaphragm and pleural effusions may also be evident.[4,15] Chest roentgenographic abnormalities are more common in patients who also have underlying cardiopulmonary disorders[4] (see Chapter 12).

A more definitive diagnosis can be made by means of a noninvasive lung VQ scan. In PE, a defect is evident in the perfusion portion of the scan in conjunction with a normal ventilation scan. An abnormal VQ scan suggests PE. If the VQ scan is normal, the likelihood of PE is low.[4,15] However, if the VQ scan is nondiagnostic, a pulmonary angiogram should be performed.

A definitive diagnosis of PE is best made by pulmonary angiography because a well-performed pulmonary angiogram excludes the diagnosis of PE. Although the time and costs involved with the invasive pulmonary angiography preclude its routine use in the diagnosis of PE, it remains the most reliable clinical study available.[4,12]

The first *treatment* goal for PE is to maintain cardiopulmonary function. Intensive respiratory and cardiac support may be necessary (see below).

Anticoagulation with intravenous unfractionated heparin followed by coumarin drugs is the standard treatment for PE. The aim of this therapy is to prevent local extension of the thrombus, recurrent embolization, and to accelerate fibrinolysis. Dosage is weight based and regulated to keep activated PTT between 1.5 and 2 times the baseline value. Heparin therapy is continued for 3 to 7 days, followed by warfarin therapy for at least 12 weeks.[4] The duration of the warfarin therapy depends on the patient's underlying medical condition and risk factors. If a patient has continuing risk factors, such as ongoing cancer, then the patient should remain on coumarin until the risk factor can be modified.

Thrombolysis by means of urokinase or t-PA may also be instituted. The aim of thrombolytic therapy is to accelerate the rate of dissolution of thrombi and emboli. Both regional and intravenous infusion of these drugs are effective. These drugs boost endogenous thrombolysis to dissolve the thrombus.[4,15] If infused intravenously, thrombolytic agents are infused for 2 to 72 hours. Thrombin time should be kept at one to five times baseline.[6] Regional infusions dissolve the clot directly. Thrombolytic therapy is usu-

ally followed by heparin therapy in an attempt to prevent recurrence. Thrombolysis is more expensive and is associated with a higher risk of bleeding than anticoagulant therapy and should be restricted to patients who are likely to benefit from it.[20] Patients who have the potential to benefit from thrombolytic therapy are selected patients with major venous thrombosis and those with major PE.[20]

Patients for whom anticoagulation or thrombolysis is contraindicated may be surgically treated by means of a vena caval interruption. Caval interruption, as discussed previously, helps prevent passage of emboli to the lung. In rare instances, pulmonary embolectomy may be performed in conjunction with cardiopulmonary bypass; however, mortality rates with this procedure are in excess of 50%.[15]

With prompt identification and treatment, *prognosis* is good for patients with PE. Only 10% of all PEs are considered incurable; successful treatment results in little long-term morbidity.[4] Long-term sequelae such as pulmonary hypertension and cor pulmonale may be seen in patients with underlying cardiopulmonary disease or those with massive emboli.[4,15]

NURSING MANAGEMENT PLAN. Because PE can be a life-threatening event, the emphasis of nursing management is on prevention. As discussed previously, prevention of thrombus formation and early detection of PE is essential. Fifty percent of those patients who die of PE do so within the first hour, and 75% do so within 2 hours.[4]

Analysis of Assessment Data. Any patient experiencing a sudden onset of chest pain, dyspnea, and tachypnea must be evaluated for the possibility of PE. Assessing the character of the patient's chest pain is important because most patients describe their pain as pleuritic. A 12-lead ECG and an ABG also provide useful data. Explaining all procedures and tests helps reassure the patient during a time of discomfort and anxiety about the sudden change of his or her condition.

Once the diagnosis of PE has been established, continued nursing management of the patient's cardiopulmonary function is essential. Two key nursing diagnoses include impaired gas exchange related to a VQ mismatch associated with PE and knowledge deficit regarding anticoagulant therapy.

Impaired Gas Exchange. Because profound arterial hypoxemia can accompany PE, the primary *goal* is to normalize gas exchange. By normalizing the exchange of gases and minimizing the VQ mismatch, other systemic effects of impaired gas exchange can also be ameliorated.

Interventions to support respiratory function by patient positioning and the use of supplemental oxygen may help decrease the degree of hypoxemia and the alveolar-arterial oxygen difference ($PAO_2 - PaO_2$) accompanying PE. Supplemental oxygen may be administered by face mask or, if necessary, by endotracheal intubation and mechanical ventilation. Positioning the patient with the head of the bed elevated allows for better chest expansion with respiration.

The administration of prescribed analgesics and sedatives may help relieve the patient's discomfort and anxiety.

By reducing discomfort and anxiety, respiratory rate may also decrease, thus reducing the additional vasoconstriction and bronchoconstriction caused by lower $PaCO_2$ levels.

Anticoagulants and thrombolytic agents, as described earlier, are usually ordered by the physician. These agents help decrease the recurrence of emboli and may help lyse the embolus, thus restoring normal blood flow through the pulmonary vasculature.

Frequent assessment of cardiopulmonary function is also important. Vital signs, particularly respiratory rate, heart rate, and blood pressure, should be assessed and documented hourly and as needed. Normal vital signs may indicate improved gas exchange. ABG analysis offers a quantitative assessment of gas exchange and should be obtained every 2 to 4 hours as needed.

Outcome criteria to *evaluate* normalization of gas exchange include ABG values within normal limits (see Chapter 11), heart rate between 60 and 100 beats/min, and respiratory rate less than 20/min, without dyspnea or cyanosis. In addition, the patient should be alert and oriented or at his or her baseline level of consciousness.

Knowledge Deficit. Because of the prolonged duration of anticoagulant therapy, patients require extensive teaching about the administration and follow-up schedules of oral anticoagulants, a medication identification card or band, potential hazards associated with therapy, and the signs and symptoms of bleeding and recurrent VTE.

REFERENCES

1. Babior BM, Stossel TP: Hematology: A Pathophysiological Approach, 2nd ed. New York, Churchill Livingstone, 1990
2. Bastarache MM, Giuca J, Horowitz LM et al: Assessing peripheral vascular disease: Noninvasive testing. Am J Nurs 83: 1552–1556, 1983
3. Baum PL: Heed the early warning signs of peripheral vascular disease. Nursing 15(3): 50–57, 1985
4. Bell WR, Simon TL: Current status of pulmonary thromboembolic disease: Pathophysiology, diagnosis, prevention, and treatment. Am Heart J 103: 239–261, 1982
5. Bergquist D: Postoperative Thromboembolism. New York, Springer-Verlag, 1983
6. Bithell TC: Thrombosis and antithrombotic therapy. In Lee GR, Bithell TC, Foerster J et al (eds): Wintrobe's Clinical Hematology, 9th ed, pp 1515–1551. Philadelphia, Lea & Febiger, 1992
7. Brandt JT: Current concepts of coagulation. Clin Obstet Gynecol 28: 3, 1985
8. Coccheri S, Palareti G: Prevention and treatment of deep venous thrombosis: Prevention of pulmonary embolism. Cardiologia 39(Suppl 1): 341–345, 1994
9. Cotran RS, Kumar V, Robbins SL: Robbins' Pathologic Basis of Disease, 4th ed. Philadelphia, WB Saunders, 1989
10. Davies MG, Sabiston DC: Acute deep vein thrombosis and pulmonary embolism. In Tibbs DJ, Sabiston DC, Davies MG et al (eds): Varicose Veins, Venous Disorders, and Lymphatic Problems in the Lower Limbs, pp 189–206. New York, Oxford University Press, 1998
11. Fernsebner B, Baum PL, Bartle HC: Surgical prevention of pulmonary emboli. AORN J 39: 56–64, 1984
12. Fischbach FT: A Manual of Laboratory Diagnostic Tests, 4th ed. Philadelphia, JB Lippincott, 1992
13. Gallus AS, Salzman EW, Hirsh J: Prevention of venous thromboembolism. In Colman RW, Hirsh J, Marder VJ et al (eds): Haemostasis and Thrombosis: Basic Principles and Clinical Practice, 3rd ed, pp 1331–1345. Philadelphia, JB Lippincott, 1994
14. Goldhaber SZ, Braunwald E: Pulmonary embolism. In Braunwald E (ed): Heart Disease, 4th ed, pp 1558–1580. Philadelphia, WB Saunders, 1992
15. Giuntini C, Di-Ricco G, Marini C et al: Pulmonary embolism: Epidemiology. Chest 107(Suppl 1):3S–9S, 1995
16. Handin RI: Bleeding and thrombosis. In Wilson JD, Braunwald E, Isselbacher KJ et al (eds): Harrison's Principles of Internal Medicine, 12th ed, pp 1500–1511. New York, McGraw-Hill, 1991
17. Handin RI: Disorders of coagulation and thrombosis. In Wilson JD, Braunwald E, Isselbacher KJ et al (eds): Harrison's Principles of Internal Medicine, 12th ed, pp 1505–1511. New York, McGraw-Hill, 1991
18. Harker LA: Pathogenesis of thrombosis. In Williams WJ, Beutler E, Erslev AJ et al (eds): Hematology, 4th ed, pp 1559–1568. New York, McGraw-Hill, 1990
19. Hirsh J, Hoak J: Management of deep vein thrombosis and pulmonary embolism. Circulation 93: 2212–2245, 1996
20. Hirsh J, Levine MN: Low molecular weight heparin. Blood 79: 1–77, 1992
21. Hull RD, Raskob GE, Leclerc JR et al: The diagnosis of clinically suspected venous thrombosis. Clin Chest Med 5: 439–456, 1984
22. Jandl JH: Blood: Textbook of Hematology. Boston, Little, Brown, and Company, 1987
23. Jerius H, Beall A, Woodrum D et al: Thrombin-induced vasospasm: Cellular signalling mechanisms. Surgery 123: 46–50, 1998
24. Kane KK: Fibrinolyis: A review. Ann Clin Lab Sci 14: 443, 1984
25. Kessler CM, Bell WR: Coagulation factors. In Spivak JL, Eichner ER (eds): Fundamentals of Clinical Hematology, 3rd ed, pp 367–386. Baltimore, Johns Hopkins University Press, 1993
26. Koon-Hou M, Tan ATH, Chan C et al: The clinical impact of platelet glycoprotein IIb/IIIa receptor blockade in cardiovascular medicine. Jpn Circ J 62: 233–243, 1998
27. Kumar V, Cotran RS, Robbins SL: Basic Pathology, 5th ed. Philadelphia, WB Saunders, 1992
28. Lee GR, Bithell TC, Foerster J et al: Wintrobe's Clinical Hematology, 9th ed. Philadelphia, Lea & Febiger, 1993
29. Lensing AWA, Hirsh J: Rationale and results of thrombolytic therapy for deep vein thrombosis. In Bernstein EF (ed): Vascular Diagnosis. St. Louis, Mosby-Year Book, 1993
30. Marder VJ: Consumptive thrombohemorrhagic disorders. In Williams WJ, Beutler E, Erslev AJ et al (eds): Hematology, 4th ed. New York, McGraw-Hill, 1990
31. Newcombe DS: Monocytes and macrophages. In Spivak JL, Eichner ER (eds): The Fundamentals of Clinical Hematology, 3rd ed. Baltimore, Johns Hopkins University Press, 1993
32. Nicolaides AN, Irving D: Clinical factors and the risk of deep venous thrombosis. In Nicolaides AN (ed): Thromboembolism. Baltimore, University Park Press, 1975
33. Ogston D: The Physiology of Hemostasis. Cambridge, MA, Harvard University Press, 1983
34. Olin JW, Graor RA, O'Hara P et al: The incidence of deep vein thrombosis in patients undergoing abdominal aortic aneurysm. J Vasc Surg 18: 1037–1041, 1993
35. Osterud B: Tissue factor: A complex biological role. Thromb Haemost 78: 755–758, 1997
36. Paraskevas F, Foerster J: The lymphocytes. In Lee RG, Bithell TC, Foerster J et al (eds): Wintrobe's Clinical Hematology, 9th ed, pp 354–430. Philadelphia, Lea & Febiger, 1993

37. Preventing thrombosis pulmonary embolism. Am J Nurs 86: 648, 1986

38. Rock G, Wells P: New concepts in coagulation. Crit Rev Clin Lab Sci 34: 475–501, 1997

39. Rose AG: Diseases of the veins. In Silver MD (ed): Cardiovascular Pathology, 2nd ed, pp 195–223. New York, Churchill Livingstone, 1991

40. Rothstein G: Origin and development of the blood and blood-forming tissues. In Lee GR, Bithell TC, Foerster J et al (eds): Wintrobe's Clinical Hematology, 9th ed, pp 41–78. Philadelphia, Lea & Febiger, 1993

41. Saito H: Normal hemostatic mechanisms. In Ratnoff OD, Forbes CD (eds): Disorders of Hemostasis, 2nd ed, pp 18–47. Philadelphia, WB Saunders, 1991

42. Schmaier AH: Laboratory studies in disseminated intravascular coagulation and activated coagulation. In Koepke JA (ed): Practical Laboratory Hematology, pp 395–407. New York, Churchill Livingstone, 1991

43. Shoor PM, Fogarty TJ: Acute arterial insufficiency. In Miller DC, Roon AJ (eds): Diagnosis and Management of Peripheral Vascular Disease, pp 119–134. Menlo Park, CA, Addison-Wesley, 1982

44. Strandness DE, Thiele BL: Selected Topics in Venous Disorders. Mount Kisco, NY, Futura, 1981

45. Szucs MM, Brooks HL, Grossman W et al: Diagnostic sensitivity of laboratory findings in acute pulmonary embolism. Ann Intern Med 74: 161–166, 1971

46. Thompson AR, Harker LA: Manual of Hemostasis and Thrombosis, 3rd ed. Philadelphia, FA Davis, 1983

47. Triplett DA: Hemostasis: A Case Oriented Approach. New York, Igaku-Shoin, 1985

48. Wells PS, Hirsh J, Anderson DR et al: Accuracy of clinical assessment of deep-vein thrombosis. Lancet 345: 1326–1330, 1995

49. Wenger NK: Pulmonary embolism: Recognition and management. Consultant 20: 85–96, 1980

50. Wu KK, Thiagarajan P: Role of endothelium in thrombosis and hemostasis. Annu Rev Med 47: 315–331, 1996

51. Yardumian DA, Mackie IJ, Machin SJ: Laboratory investigation of platelet function: A review of methodology. J Clin Pathol 39: 701, 1986

Fluid and Electrolyte Balance and Imbalance

LINDA FELVER

PRINCIPLES OF FLUID BALANCE

The fluid in the body serves many vital functions. In addition to being the milieu in which cellular chemistry occurs, it provides the transport medium for oxygen and other nutrients to reach the cells and for carbon dioxide and other metabolic waste products to be removed from the body. Technically, *fluid* is water plus the substances dissolved in it.

The amount of water in the body decreases as a person ages. The body ranges from 70% water by weight (newborn infant) to 60% (young or middle-aged adult) to 45% (elderly woman). Women have less water by weight than men because a higher percentage of their weight is fat. Similarly, water is a lower percentage of body weight in obese people. One liter of water weighs 1 kg (2.2 lb). Thus, a standard 70-kg (154-lb) middle-aged man (60% water) has 42 L of body water (70 kg × 0.60 = 42 kg; 42 kg = 42 L).[46]

Body Fluid Compartments

The fluid in the body lies in several compartments. The *extracellular fluid* consists primarily of vascular and interstitial fluid. Some extracellular fluid is located in bone and dense connective tissue; this fluid is not considered accessible for dynamic exchange. *Intracellular fluid,* as the name indicates, lies in the cells. *Transcellular fluid* is fluid that is secreted by epithelial cells. Examples of transcellular fluid are cerebrospinal fluid, saliva, and intestinal secretions. Many of the transcellular fluids are reabsorbed by the body after they have been secreted.

More water is located inside the cells than outside of them. Clinically, approximately two-thirds of body water in adults is considered intracellular and one-third extracellular. Thus, the 70-kg man who has 42 L of body water can be considered to have approximately 28 L of water inside the cells and 14 L of extracellular water. This extracellular water is approximately one-third vascular and two-thirds interstitial. For clinical purposes, then, the 70-kg man can be considered to have approximately 4.5 L of water in the vascular compartment and approximately 9.5 L in the interstitial compartment.

Osmolality

The relative proportion of water to particles in body fluid is measured as osmolality. Osmolality can be considered to be the degree of concentration. Technically, osmolality is defined as the number of moles of particles per kilogram of water. The normal range of osmolality of the blood is 280 to 300 mOsm/kg (lower in normal pregnancy).[10] Fluids that have osmolality within this normal range are called *isotonic*. Extracellular and intracellular fluids have the same osmolality. If the osmolality of the extracellular fluid is increased or decreased, the osmolality of the intracellular fluid changes rapidly until intracellular and extracellular fluids again have the same osmolality. This process is discussed later in the section on Fluid Distribution.

Although the osmolality of intracellular and extracellular fluids is the same, the ion composition of the two fluids differs. Thus, they have the same particle concentration, but the specific kinds of particles are different in the two fluids. Intracellular fluid has a higher concentration of protein and potassium, magnesium, and phosphate ions; extracellular fluid has a higher concentration of sodium, calcium, chloride, and bicarbonate ions.[46] Transcellular fluids are usually hypotonic; their ion composition varies widely depending on their physiologic function.

Processes Involved in Fluid Balance

Fluid balance is the net result of fluid intake, fluid distribution, fluid excretion, and fluid loss by abnormal routes. Fluid balance is maintained when fluid excretion and fluid loss through any abnormal routes are matched by fluid intake and when the fluid is distributed normally into its compartments.[46]

FLUID INTAKE

The major determinant of fluid intake in a healthy adult is habit. Thirst, another important determinant of fluid intake, can be caused by several physiologic mechanisms. These include dryness of the oral mucous membranes, increase in osmolality of the body fluids (osmoreceptor-mediated thirst), decrease in extracellular fluid volume (ECV; baroreceptor-mediated thirst), and increased renin secretion (angiotensin-mediated thirst). Osmoreceptor-mediated thirst is the most common cause of thirst in healthy adults. This mechanism becomes less effective with aging. Thus, elderly adults often have a greater need for water before they become thirsty.[6] Cultural factors have an important influence on fluid intake. For example, intake of certain herbal teas may be considered necessary by some patients when they become ill. In clinical settings, fluid intake is often regulated by health care professionals. Routes of fluid intake include oral, rectal, intravenous, and intraosseous, as well as through tubes into body cavities. Oral fluid intake includes liquids and the water contained in food, as well as water made by cellular metabolism of ingested nutrients.

FLUID DISTRIBUTION

Two types of fluid distribution operate in the body. First, fluid is distributed between the vascular and interstitial spaces, the two subcompartments of the extracellular compartment. Second, fluid is distributed between the extracellular and intracellular compartments. Different processes regulate these two types of fluid distribution.

Fluid distribution between the vascular and interstitial spaces is regulated by filtration. Filtration is the net result of four opposing forces. Two of these forces tend to move fluid out of the capillaries, whereas the other two tend to move fluid into the capillaries. Which direction the fluid moves in any one location depends on which forces are stronger. The two forces that tend to move fluid out of capillaries are the blood hydrostatic pressure (outward force against the capillary walls) and the interstitial fluid osmotic pressure (inward pulling force due to particles in interstitial fluid). The two forces that tend to move fluid into capillaries are the blood osmotic pressure (inward pulling force due to particles in blood) and the interstitial fluid hydrostatic pressure.

Usually, the blood hydrostatic pressure is highest at the arterial end of a capillary, and there is filtration from the capillary into the interstitial fluid. This flow of fluid out of the capillaries is useful in carrying oxygen, glucose, amino acids, and other nutrients to the cells that are surrounded by interstitial fluid. Most proteins are too large to cross into the interstitial fluid and remain in the capillary. At the venous end of a capillary, the blood hydrostatic pressure is usually lower and the blood osmotic pressure higher because fluid has left the capillary but the proteins have remained. These changes cause a net flow of fluid from the interstitial space back into the venous end of a capillary. The flow of fluid back into the capillaries is physiologically useful in carrying carbon dioxide, metabolic acids, and other waste products into the blood for further metabolism or excretion.

Changes in any of the four forces that determine the direction of filtration at the capillaries can cause abnormal distribution between the vascular and interstitial compartments. The most common abnormal distribution is edema, which is expansion of the interstitial space. Edema can be caused by increased blood hydrostatic pressure (e.g., venous congestion), increased interstitial fluid osmotic pressure (e.g., proteins in interstitial fluid), decreased blood osmotic pressure (e.g., hypoproteinemia), or blockage of the lymphatic system, which normally removes excess fluid from the interstitial space and returns it to the vascular compartment.

The second type of fluid distribution occurs between the extracellular and intracellular compartments. This process is regulated by osmosis. Cell membranes are freely permeable to water, but the passage of ions and other particles depends on membrane transport processes. Osmotic pressure is an inward-pulling force due to particles in a fluid. Both the extracellular and intracellular fluids exert osmotic pressure. Because the osmolality of the two compartments is normally the same, the osmotic pressures are the same. Therefore, the force pulling water into the cells is balanced by the force pulling water into the interstitial space, and the normal fluid distribution is maintained. If the osmolality of the extracellular fluid changes, however, osmosis occurs, altering the fluid distribution until the osmolality in the extracellular and intracellular compartments is again the same. For example, if the extracellular fluid becomes more concentrated (increased osmolality), then the osmotic pressure of the extracellular fluid becomes higher than the osmotic pressure of the intracellular fluid. Water leaves the intracellular compartment until the intracellular fluid becomes as concentrated as the extracellular fluid. This process decreases the amount of water that is distributed into the intracellular compartment. Similarly, if the extracellular fluid becomes more dilute (decreased osmolality), then the osmotic pressure of the extracellular fluid becomes lower than the osmotic pressure of the intracellular fluid. Water moves by osmosis into the intracellular compartment until the intracellular fluid becomes as dilute as the extracellular fluid. This process increases the amount of water that is distributed into the intracellular compartment.

In summary, fluid distribution between the vascular and interstitial compartments depends on filtration, the net result of four forces that act on fluid at the capillary level. Fluid distribution between the extracellular and intracellular compartments depends on osmosis, the movement of water across cell membranes to equilibrate particle concentrations.

FLUID EXCRETION

The normal routes of fluid excretion are respiratory tract, urine, feces, and skin (insensible perspiration and sweat). In a standard adult, approximately 400 mL of water is excreted daily through the respiratory tract, even if the person is fluid depleted. This amount increases during fever. The urine volume of a healthy adult varies according to the fluid intake, the needs of the body, and the hormonal status. It averages 1,500 mL. Major hormones that regulate urinary excretion of fluid are summarized in Table 6-1. Diuretics, ethanol, and caffeine increase urine volume. Fecal excretion of water averages 200 mL/d in healthy adults who have a normal fluid balance and a fully functioning bowel. Diarrhea causes a dramatic increase in fecal excretion of water. Insensible perspiration is fluid excretion through the skin that is not visible. It averages 500 mL/d in a healthy adult. Insensible perspiration occurs even if the person is fluid depleted. It increases during fever. Sweat is visible fluid excretion through the skin. The volume of sweat varies greatly depending primarily on thermoregulatory needs.

TABLE 6-1	Hormones That Regulate Urinary Excretion of Fluid			
Hormones	**Origin**	**Stimuli That Increase Hormone Secretion**	**Stimuli That Decrease Hormone Secretion**	**Major Physiologic Actions**
Aldosterone	Adrenal cortex (zona glomerulosa)	Angiotensin II (renin–angiotensin system is stimulated by hypovolemia or other causes of decrease blood flow through the renal artery and by stimulation of renal sympathetic nerves) Hyperkalemia	Decreased angiotensin II Hypokalemia Atrial natriuretic peptides	Kidneys retain more saline (expands extracellular fluid volume) Kidneys excrete more potassium and hydrogen ions
Atrial natriuretic peptides	Atria of heart	Increased atrial stretch (e.g., increased extracellular fluid volume)	Decreased atrial stretch	Kidneys excrete more saline (decreases extracellular fluid volume)
Antidiuretic hormone	Synthesize in preoptic and paraventricular nuclei of hypothalamus Secreted from posterior pituitary gland	Increased osmolality of body fluids Hypovolemia Physiologic and psychological stressors; surgery/anesthesia; trauma; pain; nausea	Decreased osmolality of body fluids Hypervolemia Ethanol	Kidneys retain more water (dilutes body fluids, decreasing osmolality)

From Felver L: Fluid and electrolyte balance and imbalances. In Woods SL, Froelicher ES, Halpenny CJ et al (eds): Cardiac Nursing, 3rd ed, p. 123. Philadelphia, JB Lippincott, 1995.

FLUID LOSS BY ABNORMAL ROUTES

Examples of abnormal routes of fluid loss are emesis, drains, suction, paracentesis, and hemorrhage. Third-spacing (e.g., ascites) can be considered abnormal fluid loss, even though the fluid remains in the body, because the fluid is not freely available to the normal fluid compartments.

SUMMARY OF FLUID BALANCE

In summary, the processes of fluid intake, fluid distribution, fluid excretion, and fluid loss by abnormal routes must act together to maintain fluid balance. A change in one of these processes must be matched by a change in another to maintain fluid balance. For example, if an increased urine output is matched by an increased fluid intake, fluid balance can be maintained. If changes in one or more of these processes are not matched by changes in the others, however, then a fluid imbalance occurs. Fluid imbalances may be characterized by altered *volume* of fluid (ECV imbalances), altered *concentration* of fluid (osmolality imbalances), or a combination of the two.

EXTRACELLULAR FLUID VOLUME BALANCE

The ECV is the net result of fluid intake, fluid distribution, fluid excretion, and fluid loss by abnormal routes. A normal ECV is maintained when fluid excretion and any fluid loss are balanced by fluid intake and when the fluid distribution

is normal. The body's responsiveness to administration of a fluid load has a circadian rhythm (i.e., varies in a cyclic manner over 24 hours). The kidneys can excrete an excess fluid load more efficiently if it is administered during the time that the person is normally active than if it is administered during a person's customary sleeping time.

The blood volume is an important determinant of the work of the heart and provides the medium for oxygen delivery to tissues. Therefore, ECV imbalances can interfere with cardiac function and tissue oxygenation.

Extracellular Fluid Volume Deficit

Extracellular fluid volume deficit is caused by removal of sodium-containing fluid from the vascular and interstitial spaces. Usually, the fluid is removed from the body; however, in some cases, fluid is sequestered in the peritoneal cavity, the intestinal lumen, or some other "third space." ECV deficits occur when intake of sodium-containing fluid does not keep pace with increased fluid excretion or loss of fluid through abnormal routes. Clinical causes of ECV deficit are presented in Display 6-1. ECV deficit may develop in patients with cardiac disease who take diuretics if the dosage is excessive.

The clinical manifestations of ECV deficit include sudden weight loss (unless there is third-spacing), decreased skin turgor, dryness of opposing mucous membranes, hard, dry stools, longitudinal furrows in the tongue, absence of tears and sweat, and soft, sunken eyeballs. Although weight loss occurs immediately, most of these signs appear only

---

DISPLAY 6-1

Causes of Extracellular Fluid Volume Deficit

GENERAL ETIOLOGY: LOSS OF A SODIUM-CONTAINING FLUID

Specific Examples
Renal
    Addison's disease
    Salt-wasting disorders
    Bed rest
    Excessive use of diuretics
Gastrointestinal
    Vomiting
    Diarrhea
    Fistula drainage
    Nasogastric suctioning
    Intestinal decompression
Other
    Excessive diaphoresis
    Burns
    Blood loss
    Third-space accumulation

From Felver L: Fluid and electrolyte balance and imbalances. In Patrick ML, Woods SL, Craven RF et al (eds): Medical–Surgical Nursing: Pathophysiological Concepts, 2nd ed, p. 231. Philadelphia, JB Lippincott, 1991.

DISPLAY 6-2

Causes of Extracellular Fluid Volume Excess

GENERAL ETIOLOGY: RENAL RETENTION OF SODIUM AND WATER

Specific Examples
Endocrine imbalance
    Hyperaldosteronism
    Cushing's syndrome
    Glucocorticoid therapy
Secondary to a disease process
    Chronic renal failure
    Congestive heart failure
    Cirrhosis

ADDITIONAL ETIOLOGY: EXCESS INTRAVENOUS INFUSION OF SALINE SOLUTIONS (e.g., 0.9% SALINE, RINGER'S)

From Felver L: Fluid and electrolyte balance and imbalances. In Patrick ML, Woods SL, Craven RF et al (eds): Medical–Surgical Nursing: Pathophysiological Concepts, 2nd ed, p. 233. Philadelphia, JB Lippincott, 1991.

---

after substantial fluid depletion. Cardiovascular manifestations are among the early signs; these are discussed next.

Many of the clinical manifestations of ECV deficit are evident in the cardiovascular system. Decreased volume in the vascular compartment causes postural blood pressure drop, increased small vein filling time, flat neck veins when supine (or neck veins that collapse during inspiration), and decreased central venous pressure.

A postural blood pressure drop is present if the following criteria are met in an adult: (1) blood pressure is measured with the patient supine and then standing or sitting with the legs dependent (not horizontal); (2) systolic blood pressure decreases more than 15 mm Hg; (3) diastolic blood pressure decreases 10 mm Hg or more; and (4) heart rate increases. The increase in heart rate indicates that autonomic reflexes are functioning and rules out autonomic insufficiency, which may cause the upright blood pressure to decrease when the ECV is normal. Postural blood pressure drop is not a reliable assessment for ECV deficit in patients who have transplanted hearts. The heart rate may not increase in these patients when their blood pressure drops from ECV deficit.

Small vein filling time is assessed by placing a patient's hand or foot below the level of the heart, occluding a small vein, milking it flat by stroking toward the heart, and then releasing it. If the vein takes longer than 3 to 5 seconds to refill, the patient probably has an ECV deficit (unless occlusive arterial disease is present).

The decreased preload of ECV deficit leads to decreased cardiac output, with resulting dizziness, syncope, and oliguria. If ECV deficit becomes severe, tachycardia, pallor due to cutaneous vasoconstriction, and other manifestations of hypovolemic shock occur (see Chapter 24).

Extracellular Fluid Volume Excess

Excess ECV is an overload of fluid in the vascular and interstitial compartments. It is common in patients with heart failure because their decreased cardiac output activates the renin–angiotensin–aldosterone system. Aldosterone causes renal retention of sodium and water, which expands the extracellular volume. In patients who have hypertension due to elevated renin, ECV excess also develops. Other causes of ECV excess are listed in Display 6-2. Clinical manifestations of ECV excess include sudden weight gain, peripheral edema, and the cardiovascular effects described next.

Increased vascular volume is manifested by bounding pulse, distended neck veins when upright, and elevated central venous pressure. The crackles, dyspnea, and orthopnea of pulmonary edema may be present. A sudden overload of isotonic fluid increases cardiac work and may cause heart failure, especially in an elderly person or an infant.

OSMOLALITY BALANCE

The osmolality of body fluids is determined by the relative proportion of particles and water. The serum sodium concentration usually parallels the osmolality of the blood. When the serum sodium concentration is abnormally low, the osmolality is decreased; in other words, the blood is relatively too dilute. Conversely, when the serum sodium concentration is elevated, the osmolality is increased; in that case, the blood is relatively too concentrated. Antidiuretic hormone (see Table 6-1) is the major regulator of osmolality.

Hyponatremia

Hyponatremia is a relative excess of water that causes a decreased serum sodium concentration. It is caused by a gain of water relative to salt or a loss of salt relative to water (Display 6-3). Antidiuretic hormone increases the reabsorption of water by the renal tubules and thus dilutes the body fluids. In patients who have had cardiac surgery, hyponatremia may occur in the first few days after surgery if excess free water is administered because the stressors of surgery, anesthesia, pain, and nausea increase the secretion of antidiuretic hormone.[46] Hyponatremia is common in patients with congestive heart failure.[88] Patients with chronic heart failure who have hyponatremia have a poorer prognosis than those whose serum sodium concentration is normal.[109]

Medications used by patients with cardiac disease that may cause hyponatremia include thiazide diuretics and enalapril.[20,54] Hyponatremia from thiazide diuretics occurs more frequently in women than men.[132] Although enalapril and other angiotensin-converting enzyme (ACE) inhibitors may cause hyponatremia, captopril has also been used to correct hyponatremia in selected patients.[40,145]

The hypo-osmolality of hyponatremia causes water to enter cells by osmosis. The clinical manifestations of hyponatremia are primarily nonspecific markers of cerebral dysfunction: malaise, confusion, lethargy, seizures, and coma. The extent of these manifestations depends on the speed with which hyponatremia develops as well as its severity.[133] Hyponatremia does not have significant clinical effects on cardiac electrophysiology or function.

Hypernatremia

Hypernatremia is a relative deficit of water that causes an increased serum sodium concentration. It is caused by a loss of water relative to salt or a gain of salt relative to water (Display 6-4). The hyperosmolality of hypernatremia causes water to leave cells by osmosis. The clinical manifestations are similar to those of hyponatremia: malaise, confusion,

---

DISPLAY 6-3

Causes of Hyponatremia

GENERAL ETIOLOGY: GAIN OF WATER RELATIVE TO SALT

Specific Examples
Endocrine
   Stimulation of antidiuretic hormone (stressors, postsurgical state, nausea, pain)
   Ectopic production of antidiuretic hormone
Iatrogenic Excessive tap-water enemas
   Excessive infusion of 5% dextrose in water
   Excessive use of ultrasonic nebulizer
   Hypotonic irrigating solutions
   Excessive water ingestion after poisoning
   Excessive water ingestion before ultrasound examination
Other
   Psychogenic polydipsia
   Excessive beer drinking
   Near-drowning in fresh water
   Overdose of barbiturates

GENERAL ETIOLOGY: LOSS OF SALT RELATIVE TO WATER

Specific Examples
Renal
   Salt-wasting renal disease
   Many types of diuretics, especially thiazides
Gastrointestinal
   Nasogastric suction
   Vomiting ⎫
   Diarrhea ⎬ with water but not salt replacement
   Hypotonic irrigating solutions ⎭
Other
   Burns ⎫ with water but not
   Excessive sweating ⎭ salt replacement

From Felver L: Fluid and electrolyte balance and imbalances. In Patrick ML, Woods SL, Craven RF et al (eds): Medical–Surgical Nursing: Pathophysiological Concepts, 2nd ed, p. 237. Philadelphia, JB Lippincott, 1991.

DISPLAY 6-4

Causes of Hypernatremia

GENERAL ETIOLOGY: LOSS OF WATER RELATIVE TO SALT

Specific Examples
Renal
   Diabetes insipidus
   Osmotic diuresis
   Renal concentrating disorders
Other
   Prolonged diarrhea without water replacement
   Excessive sweating without water replacement
   Dysfunctional humidifier of mechanical ventilator

GENERAL ETIOLOGY: GAIN OF SALT RELATIVE TO WATER

Specific Examples
Decreased water intake
   No access to water
   Prolonged nausea
   Difficulty swallowing fluids (e.g., advanced Parkinson's disease)
   Inability to respond to thirst (e.g., coma, paralysis, aphasia, confusion, weakness)
   Decreased thirst sensation
Increased salt intake
   Tube feedings
   Half-and-half for ulcer diet
   Excess hypertonic NaCl or $NaHCO_3$
   Near-drowning in salt water

From Felver L: Fluid and electrolyte balance and imbalances. In Patrick ML, Woods SL, Craven RF et al (eds): Medical–Surgical Nursing: Pathophysiological Concepts, 2nd ed, p. 235. Philadelphia, JB Lippincott, 1991.

lethargy, seizures, and coma.[110] Thirst (except in some elderly people) and oliguria (except in hypernatremia caused by decreased antidiuretic hormone) may also occur. As with hyponatremia, the extent of these manifestations depends on the speed with which hypernatremia develops as well as its severity. Hypernatremia also does not have significant clinical effects on cardiac electrophysiology or function.

Mixed Extracellular Fluid Volume and Osmolality Imbalances

Extracellular fluid volume and osmolality imbalances may occur at the same time in the same person. For example, in a person who has severe gastroenteritis without proper fluid replacement, concurrent ECV deficit and hypernatremia (clinical dehydration) will develop. The fluid lost in the emesis and diarrhea, plus the usual daily fluid excretion (urine, feces, respiratory, insensible through skin), is hypotonic sodium-containing fluid (analogous to isotonic saline that has extra water added). The signs and symptoms of such mixed fluid imbalances are a combination of the clinical manifestations of the two separate imbalances. In the example of clinical dehydration, the patient has the sudden weight loss, manifestations of decreased vascular volume, and signs of decreased interstitial volume that result from ECV deficit plus the thirst and nonspecific signs of cerebral dysfunction that result from hypernatremia.[46]

PRINCIPLES OF ELECTROLYTE BALANCE

Electrolyte balance is the net result of several concurrent dynamic processes. These processes are electrolyte intake, absorption, distribution, excretion, and loss through abnormal routes[45] (Table 6-2). Electrolyte intake in healthy people is primarily by the oral route; other routes of electrolyte intake include the intravenous and rectal routes, and through tubes into various body cavities. Electrolytes that are taken into the gastrointestinal tract must be absorbed into the blood. Although some electrolytes (e.g., potassium) are absorbed readily by mechanisms based on gradients, the absorption of other electrolytes (e.g., calcium and magnesium) is more complex and can be impaired by many factors.

Electrolytes are distributed into all body fluids, but their concentrations in the different body fluid compartments vary greatly. Substantial amounts of most electrolytes are located in pools outside the extracellular fluid. For example, the major pool of potassium is inside cells; the major pool of calcium is in the bones.

Electrolyte excretion occurs through the normal routes of urine, feces, and sweat. Any removal of electrolytes through other routes can be considered loss of electrolytes through an abnormal route. Examples of these abnormal routes are emesis, nasogastric suction, fistula drainage, and hemorrhage.

To maintain normal balance of any specific electrolyte, electrolyte intake and absorption must equal electrolyte excretion and electrolyte loss through abnormal routes, and the electrolyte must be distributed properly within the body. Alterations in any of these processes can cause an electrolyte imbalance.[46]

ELECTROLYTE IMBALANCES

Plasma electrolyte imbalances may have profound effects on cardiovascular function. Because cardiac function depends on ion currents across myocardial cell membranes, action potential generation, impulse conduction, and myocardial contraction are all vulnerable to alterations in electrolyte status. In addition to their effects on the myocardium itself, some electrolyte imbalances have vascular effects.

Potassium Balance

Potassium balance is the net result of potassium intake and absorption, distribution, excretion, and abnormal losses. These components are summarized in Table 6-2. Although the plasma potassium concentration describes the status of potassium in the extracellular fluid, it does not necessarily reflect the amount of potassium inside the cells. The plasma potassium concentration has a circadian rhythm, rising during the hours a person is usually active and reaching its trough when a person is usually asleep.[130] The kidneys handle an intravenous potassium load much less efficiently during the hours a person is customarily asleep.[97]

The potassium concentration of the extracellular fluid has a major influence on the function of the myocardium. Specifically, the resting membrane potential of cardiac cells is proportional to the ratio of potassium concentrations in the extracellular and intracellular fluids. The potassium concentration within cardiac cells is approximately 140 mEq/L; the normal potassium concentration of the extracellular fluid is 3.5 to 5 mEq/L. A small change in the extracellular concentration of potassium has a large effect on the extracellular/intracellular concentration ratio because the initial extracellular value is relatively small. A similar change in the intracellular potassium concentration has a lesser effect because the initial intracellular value is so large.

HYPOKALEMIA

Hypokalemia, a decrease in the plasma potassium concentration, is caused by decreased potassium intake, shift of potassium ions from the extracellular fluid into the cells, increased excretion of potassium, loss of potassium through an abnormal route, or any combination of these factors.[44] Some specific etiologic factors in these categories are listed in Display 6-5. Hypokalemia is common in patients with heart failure because of their increased secretion of aldosterone and their diuretic therapy.[29,32,88]

Catecholamines cause potassium ions to shift into cells by a ß-adrenergic mechanism. This effect may produce hypokalemia.[28,81] Plasma catecholamines increase rapidly during myocardial infarction (MI).[75] Transient hypokalemia associated with catecholamine release during a MI may cause further impairment of an already compromised myocardium[98] (see Chapter 20).

The increased potassium excretion caused by many types of diuretics is well known.[13] Many investigators believe that

TABLE 6-2	Electrolyte Homeostasis				
Electrolyte	**Sources of Intake**	**Absorption**	**Electrolyte Pool**	**Distribution**	**Excretion**

Potassium (K^+)	*Foods:*
	Almonds
	Apricots
	Bananas
	Cantaloupe
	Coffee (instant)
	Dates
	Molasses
	Oranges
	Peaches
	Potatoes
	Prunes
	Raisins
	Strawberries
	
	Intravenous:
	Packed red blood
	  cells or whole
	  blood; penicillin G
		Based on gradient
		between lumen
		and blood
		concentrations
			Inside cells	*Cause shift into cells:*
				β-adrenergic agonists
				Insulin
				Alkalosis
				Cause shift out of cells:
				Acidosis caused by
				  mineral acids
				Lack of insulin
				Cell death
					Urinary:
					Increased by in-
					  creased flow,
					  glucocorticoids
					Aldosterone
					  causes K^+
					  excretion
					Fecal:
					Increased with
					  diarrhea
					Sweat

Calcium (Ca^{2+})	*Foods:*
	Beet greens
	Broccoli
	Dairy products
	Farina
	Kale
	Milk chocolate
	Oranges
	Salmon (canned)
	Sardines
	Tofu
		Most efficient in
		duodenum;
		increased by
		vitamin D
		Decreased by
		phosphates,
		phytates,
		oxalates,
		increased
		intestinal pH,
		undigested fat,
		diarrhea,
		glucocorticoids
			Physiologically
			unavailable when
			bound in blood to
			proteins and
			small organic
			anions
			
			Bones
				Cause more binding in
				  blood:
				Alkalosis
				Citrate in blood products
				Protein plasma
				  expanders
				Increased free fatty acids
				Cause shift into bones:
				Lack of parathyroid
				  hormone
				Cause shift from bones:
				Parathyroid hormone
				High-protein diet
				Glucocorticoids
				Immobility
					Urinary:
					Decreased by
					  parathyroid
					  hormone
					Increased by
					  saline
					  diuresis, high-
					  protein diet
					Fecal:
					Increased with
					  undigested fat
					Sweat

Magnesium (Mg^{2+})	*Foods:*
	Cocoa
	Chocolate
	Dried beans and
	  peas
	Green leafy
	  vegetables
	Hard water
	Nuts
	Peanut butter
	Sea salt
	Whole grains
		Most efficient in
		terminal ileum
		Decreased by
		phosphates,
		phytates,
		undigested fat,
		alcohol, diarrhea
		Increased by
		lactose
			Physiologically
			unavailable when
			bound in blood to
			proteins and small
			organic anions
			
			Bones
			
			Inside cells
				Cause more binding in
				  blood:
				Citrate in blood products
				Increased free fatty acids
				
				Cause shift from bones:
				Parathyroid hormone
				Cause shift into cells:
				Epinephrine
				Insulin
					Urinary:
					Increased with
					  extracellular
					  fluid volume
					  expansion,
					  rising blood
					  alcohol, high-
					  protein diet,
					  acidosis
					Fecal:
					Increased with
					  undigested
					  fat, increased
					  aldosterone
					Sweat

Phosphate (P_i)	*Foods:*
	Eggs
	Meat
	Milk
	Processed foods
	Almost all foods
	  have some
	  phosphates
		Decreased by
		aluminum and
		magnesium
		antacids,
		diarrhea
			Inside cells
			
			Bones
				Cause shift into cells:
				Epinephrine
				Insulin
				Increased cellular
				  metabolism
				Cause shift out of cells:
				Ketoacidosis
				Cell death
				
				Cause shift out of bones:
				Parathyroid hormone
				Immobility
					Urinary:
					Increased by
					  parathyroid
					  hormone,
					  extracellular
					  fluid volume
					  expansion
					Fecal
					Sweat

From Felver L: Fluid and electrolyte balance and imbalances. In Woods SL, Froelicher ES, Halpenny CJ et al (eds): Cardiac Nursing, 3rd ed, p. 126. Philadelphia, JB Lippincott, 1995.

DISPLAY 6-5

Causes of Hypokalemia

GENERAL ETIOLOGY: DECREASED POTASSIUM INTAKE

Specific Examples:
Noniatrogenic
  Anorexia
  Fad diets
  Fasting
Iatrogenic
  NPO orders
  Prolonged intravenous therapy without K+

GENERAL ETIOLOGY: ENTRY OF POTASSIUM INTO CELLS

Specific Examples:
Alkalosis
Familial periodic paralysis
Hypersecretion of insulin (hyperalimentation)
Transfusion of frozen red blood cells (are low in K+)
Rapid correction of acidosis during hemodialysis
Excessive β-adrenergic stimulation

GENERAL ETIOLOGY: INCREASED POTASSIUM EXCRETION

Specific Examples:
Urinary
  Hyperaldosteronism
  Cushing's syndrome
  Glucocorticoid therapy
  Excess black licorice ingestion (aldosterone-like effect)
  Renal salt wasting
  Hypomagnesemia
  Diuretic therapy (potassium-sparing drugs excepted)
  Carbenicillin therapy
Fecal
  Diarrhea
  Laxative abuse
Other
  Excessive sweating without K+ replacement

GENERAL ETIOLOGY: POTASSIUM LOSS BY ABNORMAL ROUTE

Specific Examples:
Emesis
Nasogastric suction
Fistula drainage

From Felver L: Fluid and electrolyte balance and imbalances. In Patrick ML, Woods SL, Craven RF et al (eds): Medical–Surgical Nursing: Pathophysiological Concepts, 2nd ed, p. 245. Philadelphia, JB Lippincott, 1991.

diuretic therapy is still a matter of debate.[12,32,110,124] The necessity of monitoring the plasma potassium concentration in patients taking diuretics is clear.[146] Patients who are hypokalemic have significantly more ventricular arrhythmias after MI than do normokalemic patients.[101] The hypokalemic effect of catecholamines is stronger in patients who are taking thiazide diuretics than it is in those who are not taking diuretics. Thus, the plasma potassium concentration of patients who are taking thiazide diuretics decreases to low levels in the presence of increased catecholamines.[138] Clinical studies support the possibility that patients who have left ventricular hypertrophy, advanced atherosclerosis, chronic diuretic-induced hypokalemia, and suddenly increased circulating catecholamines are at high risk for cardiac arrhythmias and sudden death.[83]

The clinical manifestations of hypokalemia include diminished bowel sounds, abdominal distention, constipation, polyuria, skeletal muscle weakness, flaccid paralysis, cardiac arrhythmias, and postural hypotension. Cardiac and vascular effects of hypokalemia are discussed next.

Cardiac Effects of Hypokalemia. The cardiac effects of hypokalemia include changes in cell membrane resting potential. When the extracellular potassium concentration decreases, the extracellular/intracellular potassium concentration ratio decreases. This change in ratio causes cardiac muscle cells to hyperpolarize (i.e., the resting membrane potential becomes more negative). In hyperpolarized cells, the distance between resting potential and action potential is increased; hyperpolarized cells are less responsive to stimuli than are normal cells. The hyperpolarizing effect of hypokalemia on cardiac cells does not occur at all levels of hypokalemia. At low plasma potassium concentrations, a *hypopolarizing* effect may be seen and is probably due to decreased potassium conductance (analogous to decreased potassium permeability) of the cell membrane.[116] The specific alteration of cardiac cell membrane resting potential thus depends on the degree of hypokalemia. In any case, the normal resting potential is altered, which contributes to the development of arrhythmias.

In addition to its effect on cell membrane resting potential, hypokalemia increases the rate of cardiac cell diastolic depolarization. Diastolic depolarization is the normal mechanism that initiates the depolarization of pacemaker cells (see Chapter 14). Under usual circumstances, diastolic depolarization is fastest in the sinus node cells; consequently, the sinus node serves as the predominant pacemaker. During hypokalemia, however, the rate of diastolic depolarization increases in other myocardial cells, especially in diseased myocardium. Ectopic beats may arise, even from hyperpolarized cells.

Other effects of hypokalemia on the myocardium also predispose to arrhythmias. Hypokalemia decreases conduction velocity, especially in the atrioventricular node. Hypokalemia prolongs the action potential by decreasing the rate of repolarization, at least in part by decreasing cardiac cell membrane permeability to potassium efflux. The absolute refractory period is shorter than normal; the relative refractory period is prolonged. These changes in the refractory period predispose to the development of extrasystoles and reentrant arrhythmias[1,22,148,162] (see Chapter 14).

mild hypokalemia due to diuretic use is associated with an increased incidence of cardiac arrhythmias.[32,88] Another investigator, however, believes that prospective studies in hypertensive patients show that hypokalemia does not increase the incidence of ventricular arrhythmias.[110] Although the ability of hypokalemia to precipitate cardiac arrhythmias is well documented, the necessity of potassium supplementation during

The cardiac alterations of hypokalemia may cause many types of arrhythmias. Hypokalemia-induced arrhythmias include supraventricular premature depolarizations and tachycardias, atrial flutter, ventricular ectopic beats and ventricular tachycardia, torsade de pointes, and ventricular fibrillation.[25,67,85,88,114,122] Hypokalemia potentiates digitalis toxicity and may reduce the effectiveness of disopyramide.[92,146]

As might be expected from the previous discussion, electrocardiographic (ECG) changes are seen in patients with hypokalemia (see Chapter 14). The most characteristic change is the development of U waves. Other ECG changes include flattened T waves, ST segment depression, and prolonged PR interval. A prolonged QT interval may also occur in hypokalemia; the QRS complex may widen.[1,27,30,35,60,160] Figure 13-38 in Chapter 13 illustrates a typical ECG in hypokalemia.

Long-standing hypokalemia is associated with selective myocardial cell necrosis. As discussed in Chapter 25, selective myocardial cell necrosis is associated with sudden cardiac death.

Vascular Effects of Hypokalemia. In addition to the multiple cardiac effects discussed previously, hypokalemia has vascular effects. Postural hypotension often occurs in hypokalemia,[23] most likely due to impaired smooth muscle function.

Classic studies indicate that chronic potassium depletion in humans impairs vasodilation during strenuous exercise.[80] The resulting impaired muscle blood flow decreases oxygen delivery and contributes to the rhabdomyolysis that occurs with whole-body potassium depletion.[51,91,161]

HYPERKALEMIA

Hyperkalemia, an increased plasma potassium concentration, results from increased potassium intake, shift of potassium ions from the cells to the extracellular fluid, decreased potassium excretion, or any combination of these factors.[44] Examples of specific etiologic factors in each of these categories are listed in Display 6-6. Hyperkalemia may occur during hemorrhagic or hypovolemic shock and during cardiopulmonary resuscitation.[3,152]

Some medications that are commonly administered to patients with cardiac disease may cause hyperkalemia. One of the effects of *angiotensin-converting enzyme inhibitors* (ACE), such as captopril and enalapril, is decreased aldosterone release. Aldosterone normally facilitates renal excretion of potassium. When ACE inhibitors decrease the availability of aldosterone, hyperkalemia may occur.[36,146] Severe hyperkalemia from ACE inhibitors occurs more commonly in people older than 70 years of age.[119,157] *Potassium-sparing diuretics,* such as triamterene, spironolactone, and amiloride, may cause hyperkalemia, especially if given with potassium supplementation or ACE inhibitors.[2] Beta blockers (those with ß$_2$ action) promote the development of hyperkalemia by blocking catecholamine-induced potassium entry into cells. The hyperkalemic effect of beta blockade is especially pronounced during exercise, such as treadmill stress testing.[90,159] Administration of *heparin,* even in low-dose therapy, depresses the synthesis of aldosterone; hyperkalemia results in approximately 7% of

patients.[106] A massive overdose of *digitalis* causes hyperkalemia by allowing intracellular potassium to leak into the extracellular fluid.[47,146]

Another cardiovascular-related source of hyperkalemia is massive blood transfusion. While blood is stored, potassium ions leak from the erythrocytes into the plasma. The longer the storage time, the greater the potassium load contained in a unit of blood. A classic study indicates that if the blood has been in storage for more than 3 days, rewarming the blood before administration causes only minimal return of potassium to the cells.[41] Patients receiving more than 10 U of stored blood within a few hours are considered at high risk for severe hyperkalemia; however, fatal hyperkalemia has occurred with transfusion of fewer units.[100]

DISPLAY 6-6

Causes of Hyperkalemia

GENERAL ETIOLOGY: INCREASED POTASSIUM INTAKE

Specific Examples:
Excessive intravenous administration
Insufficiently mixed KCl in flexible plastic intravenous bags
Massive transfusion of blood stored longer than 3 days (K⁺ leaves red blood cells)
Large doses of intravenous potassium penicillin G (contains 1.6 mEq K⁺/million units)
Large oral intake and decreased renal excretion

GENERAL ETIOLOGY: MOVEMENT OF POTASSIUM OUT OF CELLS

Specific Examples:
Acidosis
Insulin deficiency
Massive cell death (crushing injuries, burns, cytotoxic drugs)
Arginine infusion
Large digitalis overdose
Familial periodic paralysis

GENERAL ETIOLOGY: DECREASED POTASSIUM EXCRETION

Specific Examples:
Oliguria
  Extracellular volume depletion
  Renal failure
Decreased aldosterone
  Addison's disease
  Hyporeninism
  Chronic heparin administration
  Lead poisoning
  Captopril administration
Other
  Potassium-sparing diuretics (spironolactone, triamterene, and amiloride)

From Felver L: Fluid and electrolyte balance and imbalances. In Patrick ML, Woods SL, Craven RF et al (eds): Medical–Surgical Nursing: Pathophysiological Concepts, 2nd ed, p. 248. Philadelphia, JB Lippincott, 1991.

Cardioplegic solutions used to stop the heart during cardiac surgery are often high in potassium (the cardioplegic agent). Occasionally, the use of these solutions causes hyperkalemia.[73]

Hyperkalemia may be manifested clinically by intestinal cramping and diarrhea, skeletal muscle weakness, flaccid paralysis, cardiac arrhythmias, and cardiac arrest. The cardiac effects of hyperkalemia are potentially fatal; they are discussed in the next section.

Cardiac Effects of Hyperkalemia. Hyperkalemia alters myocardial cell function in several ways. When the plasma potassium concentration increases, the extracellular/intracellular potassium concentration ratio increases. Consequently, the resting membrane potential of cardiac cells becomes partially depolarized (hypopolarized). Initially, the partial depolarization of resting cardiac cells increases their excitability because the resting potential is close to threshold potential (see Chapter 14). As the extracellular potassium concentration increases, however, the cardiac cells depolarize to the extent that they cannot repolarize. Cells in this state are nonexcitable; no further contractile activity occurs.[72]

Other effects of hyperkalemia include decreased duration of the action potential at all heart rates and increased rate of repolarization, the latter due to increased permeability of the cardiac cell membrane to potassium efflux.[155] Hyperkalemia lengthens the effective refractory period of atrial muscle[56] and slows diastolic depolarization of pacemaker cells, two antiarrhythmic effects. Cardiac cells vary in their sensitivity to the effects of hyperkalemia. Atrial cells are more sensitive than ventricular cells; the conduction system is the least affected by hyperkalemia.[56] Evidence from a patient with Wolff-Parkinson-White syndrome indicates that hyperkalemia depresses conduction in an accessory bypass tract to a greater extent than in the atrioventricular node.[135]

As the plasma potassium increases, the rate of rise of the action potential decreases. Slow upstroke velocity decreases cell-to-cell conduction velocity (see Chapter 14). Hyperkalemia decreases conduction velocity at all levels of the conduction system: atrial, atrioventricular nodal, and intraventricular.[56,61] In severe hyperkalemia, intraventricular conduction may be completely inhibited. Bundle-branch block or, less frequently, complete heart block may occur.[104]

Although some of the cellular effects of hyperkalemia are antiarrhythmogenic, cardiac arrhythmias do occur in hyperkalemia. The differential effects of hyperkalemia on different cell types cause slow and nonhomogeneous conduction to cells with variable degrees of excitability.

When intra-atrial conduction is depressed, sinus node impulses may be delayed in exit or may fail to propagate. This situation gives rise to Wenckebach (type I) or Mobitz (type II) sinoatrial block (see Chapter 14). Reentrant ventricular arrhythmias may arise from nonhomogeneous increases in the rate of repolarization.[144] A unidirectional conduction block in the ventricular myocardium may result in reentry ventricular tachycardia. Ventricular tachycardia may terminate in ventricular fibrillation.[4,89] Asystolic cardiac arrest is also a potentially fatal event.[37,71,117,137] Hyperkalemia enhances the slowing of cardiac conduction by pro-

cainamide.[149] It also may cause heart block with digitalis and serious arrhythmias with concurrent use of disopyramide.[146]

The characteristic ECG changes of hyperkalemia arise from the electrophysiologic changes previously described. The T waves become peaked (tented) with a narrow base and symmetric shape (see Fig. 13-39 in Chapter 13). The QRS complex widens; ST depression may occur. Hyperkalemia also causes decreased amplitude and prolongation of P waves and PR prolongation. As the plasma potassium concentration increases to high levels, the P waves disappear. A sine-wave pattern appears in severe, often terminal, hyperkalemia.[24,27,30,60,96,158]

The ECG changes of hyperkalemia are not well correlated with plasma potassium levels.[57] Although the ECG is usually abnormal with severe hyperkalemia (serum potassium greater than 8 mEq/L), minimal ECG changes have been observed in patients with serum potassium concentrations greater than 9 mEq/L.[140,165] The rate of rise of the plasma potassium concentration may contribute more to the ECG changes in hyperkalemia than does the absolute plasma potassium level. In patients with ventricular pacing and atrial fibrillation, the development of hyperkalemia may be recognized by loss of atrial activity and widened QRS complex.[69] Occasionally, the ECG in hyperkalemia mimics MI.[79]

During myocardial ischemia, potassium concentration rises quickly in the extracellular spaces of the myocardium.[107] The clinical effect of these localized areas of high potassium concentration is not yet understood. During exercise, elevated catecholamines counteract the negative cardiac effects of hyperkalemia in normal hearts; this protective effect is diminished in ischemic hearts.[105,112]

Hyperkalemia also has an indirect cardiac effect in that it stimulates aldosterone secretion. Through its saline-retaining action on the kidneys, aldosterone expands the ECV, which may have a detrimental effect on patients in heart failure.

Vascular Effects of Hyperkalemia. In high concentrations, potassium ions cause contraction of smooth muscle of coronary arteries.[48,113] Both animal and human research using coronary arteries indicates that hyperkalemia reduces the smooth muscle relaxation normally mediated by endothelium-derived hyperpolarizing factor.[64,65] Clinically, the constricting effect of hyperkalemia has been observed as coronary artery spasm arising from intracoronary injection of a glyceryl trinitrate solution containing 40 mEq/L potassium.[156]

Calcium Balance

Calcium balance is the net result of calcium intake and absorption, distribution, excretion, and abnormal losses. These components are summarized in Table 6-2. Calcium in the plasma exists in three forms: protein bound, complexed, and ionized (free). The calcium that is bound to plasma proteins and complexed with small anions (e.g., citrate) is physiologically inactive. Only the ionized calcium is physiologically active. The commonly used laboratory measure for extracellular calcium is the total calcium concentration (bound, complexed, and ionized), although ionized calcium measurements are available clinically in many locations.

Calcium ions play crucial roles in the automaticity of the sinus and atrioventricular nodes, in the plateau phase of the Purkinje and ventricular cell action potentials, in excitation–contraction coupling, and in cardiac and vascular muscle contraction (see Chapters 1 and 14). Not unexpectedly, one of the cardiac effects of an abnormal extracellular calcium concentration is altered duration of the plateau phase. Extracellular fluid calcium imbalances are less likely to cause cardiac arrhythmias than are potassium imbalances, but arrhythmias associated with hypercalcemia have been fatal. In addition to their cardiac effects, acute calcium imbalances also affect the vasculature.

HYPOCALCEMIA

Hypocalcemia may be defined as a decreased extracellular *total* calcium concentration or as a decreased extracellular *ionized* calcium concentration. The first definition refers to the commonly measured total calcium value. The second definition of hypocalcemia, however, is used in this chapter because decreases in ionized calcium concentration cause physiologic effects even if the total plasma concentration is within normal limits.

Hypocalcemia results from decreased calcium intake or absorption, decreased physiologic availability of calcium, increased calcium excretion, loss of calcium by an abnormal route, or any combination of these factors.[44] Display 6-7 lists specific etiologic factors for hypocalcemia. Several of these specific factors may cause hypocalcemia in patients with cardiac disease. The preservative used in storage of blood contains citrate, which complexes with calcium ions. Large or rapid transfusions of citrated blood cause transient hypocalcemia by decreasing the physiologic availability of calcium in the blood.[31] Similarly, rapid administration of proteinaceous plasma expanders such as albumin also decreases the physiologic availability of plasma calcium and may cause symptomatic hypocalcemia.[82]

Hypocalcemia increases neuromuscular excitability. The clinical manifestations of hypocalcemia may include digital and perioral paresthesias, positive Chvostek's sign, positive Trousseau's sign, muscle twitching and cramping, grimacing, hyperactive reflexes, tetany, carpopedal spasm, laryngospasm, seizures, cardiac arrhythmias, cardiac arrest, and hypotension (with acute hypocalcemia).

Cardiac Effects of Hypocalcemia. Hypocalcemia prolongs the plateau phase, thereby increasing the duration of the cardiac action potential. In addition, hypocalcemia slows atrioventricular and intraventricular conduction to a moderate degree.[30]

These hypocalcemia-related changes in the myocardium usually are not great enough to give rise to significant cardiac arrhythmias in clinical settings, although they may occasionally predispose to ventricular fibrillation or ventricular tachycardia.[27,78] Although hypocalcemia does not usually cause major clinical arrhythmias, it does cause characteristic alterations in the ECG (see Fig. 13-40 in Chapter 13). Hypocalcemia prolongs the ST segment. This finding is not unexpected because hypocalcemia prolongs the plateau phase of the action potential. The prolongation of the ST segment is the cause of the prolonged QT interval that is

---

---

observed in hypocalcemia.[27] T-wave duration is unchanged. The degree of prolongation of the QT interval is not a reliable indicator of the degree of hypocalcemia or of the decrease in ionized calcium concentration, but it is influenced by the rate of decrease of the ionized calcium.[31]

Hypocalcemia impairs myocardial contractility and thus may cause heart failure.[52,74,139] Patients who already have heart failure may decompensate if they become hypocalcemic. Hypocalcemia-associated heart failure may be unresponsive to digitalis until the hypocalcemia is corrected.[146] Although the role of calcium ions in the regulation of myocardial contraction is clear (see Chapter 14), the mechanism by which hypocalcemia interferes with this process is not fully understood. Because most of the calcium ions that initiate myocardial contraction come from the sarcoplasmic reticulum rather than directly from the extracellular fluid, the major effect of hypocalcemia on myocardial contractility is probably indirect. In a normal heart, hypocalcemia reduces stroke work at any particular left ventricular end-diastolic pressure. This impairment is even greater in an ischemic heart. In hypocalcemic critically ill patients, stroke work increases when the hypocalcemia is corrected.[150]

Patients who are given albumin during resuscitation from hypovolemic shock may also exhibit impaired myocardial contractility when the ionized calcium binds to the albumin and becomes physiologically unavailable.[82] During left coronary angiography, the blood in the coronary sinus has a reduced level of ionized calcium within 5 seconds of injection of iodinated contrast media.[62] This may depress left ventricular function.

Vascular Effects of Hypocalcemia. Calcium ions play several important roles in contraction of vascular smooth muscle. They are involved in the action potential, in the regulation of cell membrane permeability, and in excitation–contraction coupling. In smooth muscle, as well as in cardiac muscle, contraction is initiated by an increase in cytoplasmic calcium. Most of the calcium ions that initiate the contraction come from the sarcoplasmic reticulum rather than from the extracellular fluid. For this reason, it is possible for vascular smooth muscle to contract in a calcium-free extracellular medium in laboratory experiments.[131] Therefore, any short-term effects of hypocalcemia on the vasculature are more likely to arise from alterations in cell membrane permeability than from alteration in the contractile mechanisms.

Acute (but not chronic) hypocalcemia causes hypotension.[52,59] The mechanisms involved are not completely understood but include both decreased peripheral vascular resistance and impaired cardiac function. The systemic vascular resistance of patients undergoing coronary artery bypass grafting in whom ionized hypocalcemia develops at the end of surgery can be increased significantly with intravenous calcium gluconate.[53] Correction of ionized hypocalcemia in critically ill patients increases mean arterial blood pressure.[150] In laboratory preparations, reduction of the extracellular calcium concentration well below physiologic levels reduces both isometric force and maximal shortening velocity of portal vein smooth muscle.[5] The vasodilator action of acute hypocalcemia also occurs in renal blood vessels.[18]

HYPERCALCEMIA

Hypercalcemia is caused by increased intake or absorption of calcium, shift of calcium from the bones into the extracellular fluid, decreased calcium excretion, or any combination of these factors.[44] Specific etiologic factors are listed under these categories in Display 6-8. Note that thiazide diuretics, often administered to patients with cardiac disease, decrease the urinary excretion of calcium.[146] Another type of diuretic should be substituted if hypercalcemia develops.

The clinical manifestations of hypercalcemia include anorexia, nausea, vomiting, constipation, abdominal pain, polyuria, renal calculi, skeletal muscle weakness, diminished reflexes, confusion, lethargy, possible personality change,

---

DISPLAY 6-8

Causes of Hypercalcemia

GENERAL ETIOLOGY: INCREASED CALCIUM INTAKE OR ABSORPTION

Specific Examples:
Milk–alkali syndrome
Excessive intake of vitamin D
Sarcoidosis

GENERAL ETIOLOGY: RELEASE OF CALCIUM FROM BONE

Specific Examples:
Hyperparathyroidism
Prolonged immobilization
Multiple myeloma
Leukemia
Bone tumors (primary or metastatic)
Many other malignancies (e.g., breast cancer) that produce bone-resorbing substances

GENERAL ETIOLOGY: DECREASED CALCIUM EXCRETION

Specific Examples:
Thiazide diuretics
Familial hypocalciuric hypercalcemia

From Felver L: Fluid and electrolyte balance and imbalances. In Patrick ML, Woods SL, Craven RF et al (eds): Medical–Surgical Nursing: Pathophysiological Concepts, 2nd ed, p. 254. Philadelphia, JB Lippincott, 1991.

---

frank psychosis, cardiac arrhythmias, and hypertension (with acute hypercalcemia).

Cardiac Effects of Hypercalcemia. Hypercalcemia shortens the plateau phase of the cardiac action potential, thereby decreasing the duration of the action potential. In addition, it increases the rate of diastolic depolarization of sinus node cells and may increase the initial rate of rise and amplitude of the action potential. It may also delay atrioventricular conduction. Acute hypercalcemia increases myocardial contractility.[147]

Cardiac arrhythmias may arise from hypercalcemia. First-degree atrioventricular block, second-degree heart block, complete heart block, paroxysmal atrial fibrillation, severe bradycardia, and tachy-brady syndrome have been reported.[7,16,27] Hypercalcemia potentiates digitalis toxicity. Patients taking digitalis may acquire heart block if they become hypercalcemic.[146] Sudden death has occurred in severe hypercalcemia, possibly due to ventricular fibrillation.

The ECG in hypercalcemia reflects the short plateau phase in a shortened ST segment (see Fig. 13-41 in Chapter 13). The QT interval is decreased as a result and may be so short that it is difficult to see. The length of the QT interval is a clinically unreliable index of the extent of hypercalcemia.[31,163] Severe hypercalcemia has been accompanied by lengthening of the QRS complex, increased QRS voltage, and diffuse flattening and localized biphasic changes of T waves.[16,30,39] Another ECG abnormality that may be observed during severe hypercalcemia is a J wave at the junction between the QRS and ST segments.[136]

Vascular Effects of Hypercalcemia. Acute hypercalcemia causes vasoconstriction, a response present in normotensive and intensified in hypertensive laboratory rats.[111] The vasoconstrictive response is abolished in the presence of calcium channel blocker agents. Clinically, this acute vasoconstriction may manifest as vasospasm. Spasm of the coronary arteries due to excess extracellular calcium can produce myocardial ischemia and its related problems. Vasospasm of cerebral arteries followed by infarction has also occurred in a hypercalcemic patient.[153]

Increased *intracellular* calcium in vascular smooth muscle causes increased vascular resistance. In many people with essential hypertension, increased intracellular calcium occurs with normal plasma calcium levels. Parathyroid hormone and parathyroid hormone-related factor are implicated in transepithelial calcium transport.[42,115] This physiologic process explains why acute hypercalcemia causes hypertension in people with intact parathyroid glands, but not in people who do not have parathyroid function.[9,50] This hypercalcemic hypertension is likely caused by increased peripheral vascular resistance,[18] although some researchers believe that the effect of elevated calcium concentration on blood pressure is due only to increased myocardial contractility.[147] Acute hypercalcemia stimulates the adrenal glands to release catecholamines, which contributes to the hypertensive effect.[94] In laboratory studies, the combination of catecholamines and acute hypercalcemia raises renal vascular resistance by more than twice the increase produced by hypercalcemia alone.[77] This could be clinically important in patients already at high risk for renal dysfunction.

Magnesium Balance

Magnesium balance is the net result of magnesium intake and absorption, distribution, excretion, and abnormal losses. These components are summarized in Table 6-2. Similar to calcium, magnesium in the plasma exists in three forms: protein bound, complexed, and ionized (free). Only the ionized magnesium is physiologically active; however, the only widely available clinical laboratory measure for magnesium is the total serum magnesium concentration (bound, complexed, and ionized).

Magnesium, like potassium, is primarily an intracellular ion. For this reason, plasma levels of magnesium do not necessarily reflect the intracellular magnesium content. Total-body magnesium depletion may be present even when the plasma magnesium is normal. Intracellular magnesium is a cofactor for many enzymes, including Na^+-K^+ adenosine triphosphatase (ATPase). Changes in magnesium balance, especially hypomagnesemia, cause alterations in ion transport across membranes. Because the function of both cardiac and smooth muscle depends on ion fluxes, magnesium imbalances have both myocardial and vascular effects.

HYPOMAGNESEMIA AND TOTAL-BODY MAGNESIUM DEPLETION

Hypomagnesemia and total-body magnesium depletion are caused by decreased magnesium intake or absorption, decreased physiologic availability of magnesium, increased magnesium excretion, loss of magnesium by an abnormal route, or any combination of these factors.[44] Specific etiologic factors for hypomagnesemia are listed in Display 6-9. Hypomagnesemia and total-body magnesium depletion are common in chronic alcoholism; therefore, patients who are diagnosed with alcoholic cardiomyopathy need assessment for hypomagnesemia. Both serum and skeletal muscle magnesium decrease significantly after open heart surgery with a prime that is low in magnesium.[127]

Diuretics (except for spironolactone, triamterene, and amiloride) and digitalis both cause increased renal excretion of magnesium and can lead to hypomagnesemia. Patients with heart failure are at high risk for hypomagnesemia or

---

DISPLAY 6-9

Causes of Hypomagnesemia

GENERAL ETIOLOGY: DECREASED MAGNESIUM INTAKE OR ABSORPTION

Specific Examples:
Chronic malnutrition
Prolonged intravenous therapy without Mg^{2+}
Malabsorption syndromes
Chronic diarrhea
Steatorrhea
Pancreatitis
Resection of ileum
Chronic alcoholism

GENERAL ETIOLOGY: INCREASED MAGNESIUM EXCRETION

Specific Examples:
Urinary
    Diabetic ketoacidosis
    Chronic alcoholism
    Diuretic therapy
    Hyperaldosteronism
    Gentamicin toxicity
    Diuretic phase of acute renal failure
Fecal
    Steatorrhea
    Pancreatitis

GENERAL ETIOLOGY: MAGNESIUM LOSS BY ABNORMAL ROUTE

Specific Examples:
Emesis
Nasogastric suction
Fistula drainage

From Felver L: Fluid and electrolyte balance and imbalances. In Patrick ML, Woods SL, Craven RF et al (eds): Medical–Surgical Nursing: Pathophysiological Concepts, 2nd ed, p. 261. Philadelphia, JB Lippincott, 1991.

total-body magnesium depletion.[26,29,38] In addition to diuretic and digitalis therapy, they often have congestion of the splanchnic vessels, which decreases magnesium absorption. Also, the secondary hyperaldosteronism and elevated catecholamines of heart failure increase urinary excretion of magnesium.

Patients with ischemic heart disease, with or without acute MI, often have magnesium depletion. Patients admitted to a coronary care unit after acute MI are frequently hypomagnesemic and their red blood cell (RBC) magnesium is decreased as well.[143] Normomagnesemic patients with ischemic heart disease and low RBC magnesium have more cardiac events and a more unfavorable outcome than patients with normal RBC magnesium.[87] Hypomagnesemia may be an etiologic factor for MI as well as a result of pathophysiologic changes immediately after MI.

Hypomagnesemia causes increased neuromuscular excitability. The signs and symptoms of hypomagnesemia include hyperactive reflexes, positive Chvostek's sign, positive Trousseau's sign, leg and foot cramps, muscle twitching, grimacing, tremors, dysphagia, nystagmus, ataxia, tetany, seizures, extreme confusion, cardiac arrhythmias, and hypertension. Patients with total-body magnesium depletion but normal or near-normal plasma magnesium concentrations may not display the neuromuscular effects but still may have significant cardiovascular effects.[38]

Cardiac Effects of Hypomagnesemia and Total-Body Magnesium Depletion.

Magnesium is a cofactor for Na^+-K^+ ATPase, the enzyme that plays a major role in the regulation of intracellular potassium concentration in the myocardium. When magnesium is deficient, the decreased intracellular magnesium leads to decreased activity of this enzyme. As a result, the intracellular potassium ion concentration decreases and intracellular sodium concentration increases in myocardial cells. Decreased activity of Na^+-K^+ ATPase interferes with the reentry of potassium ions into depolarized cells and promotes diastolic leak of potassium from cells that are already depolarized. In addition, hypomagnesemia causes increased membrane permeability to potassium, an effect that also tends to decrease intracellular potassium concentration in the myocardium.

In hypomagnesemia, the sinus node has an increased spontaneous firing rate, and there is a rate-dependent decrease in the duration of the cardiac action potential.[17] The absolute refractory period is shortened, and the relative refractory period is lengthened. Hypomagnesemia thus predisposes to arrhythmias, especially tachyarrhythmias. The imbalance is associated with supraventricular tachycardia, ventricular ectopic beats, ventricular tachycardia, ventricular fibrillation, and torsade de pointes.[141,142] Whether these arrhythmias are due directly to the hypomagnesemia itself or to hypomagnesemia-induced changes in potassium transport across myocardial membranes is uncertain. What is clear, however, is that both hypomagnesemia and total-body magnesium depletion lead to cardiac arrhythmias that can be corrected only by the administration of magnesium. In patients who are not hypomagnesemic, magnesium has been used pharmacologically to treat arrhythmias, including

atrial fibrillation, ventricular tachycardia, and torsade de pointes, and to reduce arrhythmias after coronary artery bypass graft surgery, in acute MI, and in heart failure.[19,63,84,95] Using a special technique to measure free ionized magnesium in the blood, researchers have found that most of the patients who responded well to magnesium treatment of their arrhythmias had preexisting low ionized magnesium.[55,68]

Heart muscle magnesium content decreases after acute MI.[134] This post-MI magnesium decrease may be due to leakage of magnesium from necrotic cells and interference with ion transport in hypoxic cells. Another mechanism for the cardiac muscle magnesium decrease after MI may be the action of catecholamines, which cause loss of cardiac muscle magnesium in animal experiments.[128] It is likely that localized decreases of myocardial magnesium after acute MI predispose to the development of cardiac arrhythmias. Intravenous magnesium reduces the frequency of arrhythmias and mortality in patients with acute MI, regardless of whether they have preexisting hypomagnesemia.[66,68,76]

Hypomagnesemia potentiates digitalis toxicity.[146] Hypomagnesemia-related digitalis toxicity arises in part from the intracellular potassium deficiency caused by the magnesium imbalance. In addition, hypomagnesemia increases the uptake of digitalis by myocardial cells.[70] Digitalis toxicity arrhythmias have been observed in patients with therapeutic digitalis levels and either decreased serum magnesium levels or normal serum levels with total-body magnesium depletion.

The ECG changes in hypomagnesemia are not easily characterized; rather, they are somewhat nonspecific. Prolongation of the QT interval is frequently observed in hypomagnesemia. This ECG change is probably due to the altered potassium transport caused by hypomagnesemia. Other ECG changes seen with hypomagnesemia are ST segment depression, prolonged PR interval, wide QRS complex, and T-wave abnormalities, such as flattening, inversion, peaking, or bifid T wave.[27,154]

Total-body magnesium depletion is associated with cardiomyopathy and may be a contributing factor to its development.[38] Hypomagnesemia increases the secretion of catecholamines from the adrenal medulla and causes an increase in aldosterone.[99,128] These hormonal changes affect cardiovascular function by their usual actions.

Vascular Effects of Hypomagnesemia and Total-Body Magnesium Depletion.

Hypomagnesemia has important effects on vascular smooth muscle. A decrease in the extracellular magnesium concentration causes arteriolar vasoconstriction, in part by increasing the intracellular calcium concentration in vascular smooth muscle. The resulting increased peripheral vascular resistance causes the hypertension that often accompanies acute or chronic hypomagnesemia. In addition to this direct vasoconstrictive effect, hypomagnesemia also increases the vascular response to the vasoconstrictors acetylcholine, angiotensin, and norepinephrine.[43]

The vascular actions of hypomagnesemia promote the occurrence of vasospasm. The coronary arteries are extremely sensitive to the effects of hypomagnesemia. ECG evidence of acute myocardial ischemia due to coronary artery spasm has been observed in clinical hypomagnesemia.[21] Sudden death ischemic heart disease, associated with a reduced dietary intake of magnesium, may be the result of coronary vasospasm. Plasma free fatty acids bind ionized magnesium, rendering it physiologically inactive. An increase in plasma free fatty acids thus causes a decrease in the amount of ionized magnesium. In patients who have total-body magnesium depletion, it is possible that epinephrine-induced increases in plasma free fatty acids are a triggering factor for coronary vasospasm (and subsequent sudden death).

Total-body magnesium depletion (with or without hypomagnesemia) appears to play an important role in the development of atherosclerosis and ischemic heart disease. Epidemiologic studies show an association between low magnesium content of drinking water and increased incidence of MI.[123] Clinical studies demonstrate increased frequency of episodes of variant angina in men with total-body magnesium depletion.[126] Patients with low total-body magnesium also have decreased serum high-density lipoprotein cholesterol and apolipoprotein A-I.[102] Laboratory studies using cultured human endothelial cells demonstrate increased transport of low-density lipoprotein during magnesium deficiency.[164] Animal studies demonstrate plasma elevation of inflammatory cytokines that stimulate oxygen free radical formation and increased sensitivity of tissues to lipid peroxidation.[58,93,120] Thus, magnesium deficiency causes changes that are part of the atherosclerotic process. In addition, studies with magnesium-deficient animals and humans demonstrate significant increases in platelet aggregation, thromboxane, and endothelin-1 and significant decreases in plasma antithrombin III.[99,129] These changes may contribute to clot formation in coronary arteries.

As mentioned previously, it is well established that hypomagnesemia produces hypertension. In addition, total-body magnesium depletion, without hypomagnesemia, is associated with essential hypertension. Magnesium-deficient animals produce inflammatory cytokines that are potent vasodilators.[93] Clinical studies in hypertensive patients show total-body magnesium depletion, elevated RBC free calcium, and decreased RBC free magnesium compared with normotensive people.[8,108] These results are consistent with a role for total-body magnesium depletion in essential hypertension.

In summary, the vascular effects of hypomagnesemia include vasoconstriction, increased peripheral resistance, hypertension, increased vasoconstrictive response to humoral vasoactive agents, and a tendency to vasospasm. Current evidence relates total-body magnesium depletion, with or without hypomagnesemia, to both ischemic heart disease and essential hypertension.

HYPERMAGNESEMIA

Hypermagnesemia is caused by increased magnesium intake or absorption, increased physiologic availability of magnesium, decreased magnesium excretion, or any combination of these factors.[44] Specific etiologic factors for hypermagnesemia are listed in Display 6-10. Elderly people who use

---

DISPLAY 6-10

Causes of Hypermagnesemia

GENERAL ETIOLOGY: INCREASED MAGNESIUM INTAKE OR ABSORPTION

Specific Examples:
Aspiration of sea water
Excessive use of Mg^{2+}-containing cathartics
Excessive use of Mg^{2+}-containing urologic irrigating solutions
Excessive magnesium in dialysis fluid
Excessive intravenous infusion of Mg^{2+}

GENERAL ETIOLOGY: DECREASED MAGNESIUM EXCRETION

Specific Examples:
Oliguric renal failure
Adrenal insufficiency

From Felver L: Fluid and electrolyte balance and imbalances. In Patrick ML, Woods SL, Craven RF et al (eds): Medical–Surgical Nursing: Pathophysiological Concepts, 2nd ed, p. 262. Philadelphia, JB Lippincott, 1991.

---

magnesium-containing antacids and cathartics are at especially high risk for development of hypermagnesemia.[49]

The cardiac effects (bradycardia, arrhythmias, cardiac arrest) and vascular effects (flushing, hypotension) of hypermagnesemia are discussed next. In addition to these effects, hypermagnesemia may cause a subjective sensation of warmth, diaphoresis, drowsiness, lethargy, coma, diminished deep tendon reflexes, flaccid skeletal muscle paralysis, and respiratory depression.

Cardiac Effects of Hypermagnesemia. A plasma excess of magnesium interferes with cardiac conduction throughout the heart. Complete heart block may occur at high plasma levels of magnesium. Hypermagnesemia inhibits myocardial contraction and depresses membrane excitability, although intracellular contractile mechanisms remain intact.[34,121,146]

Hypermagnesemia causes clinically significant supraventricular bradycardia. Cardiac arrest in asystole may be fatal in severe hypermagnesemia.[118,151] The ECG changes associated with hypermagnesemia include prolonged PR interval and increased duration of the QRS complex.[30,118,142] These changes are somewhat variable and do not present a classic, easily recognizable picture.

Vascular Effects of Hypermagnesemia. Hypermagnesemia causes peripheral vasodilation, which leads to hypotension. Vasodilation of cutaneous vessels in hypermagnesemia causes flushing. Hypermagnesemia reduces peripheral vascular resistance by inhibiting calcium movement into vascular smooth muscle cells, inhibiting calcium release from intracellular storage, and depressing contractile responses to vasoactive substances such as epinephrine and angiotensin II.[38,142,146]

Phosphate Balance

Phosphate balance is the net result of phosphate intake and absorption, distribution, excretion, and abnormal losses. These components are summarized in Table 6-2.

The normal range of serum phosphate concentration is 2.5 to 4.5 mg/dL. A moderate hypophosphatemia (1 to 2.4 mg/dL) may be asymptomatic. A serum phosphate below 1 mg/dL, however, usually has dramatic effects. For this reason, it is termed *severe symptomatic hypophosphatemia*. Severe symptomatic hypophosphatemia is caused by decreased intake or absorption of phosphate, shift of phosphate into cells, or increased phosphate excretion.[44] Specific etiologic factors included in these categories are presented in Display 6-11.

Of importance to patients with cardiac disease is the decrease in plasma phosphate concentration that occurs with intravenous glucose administration. Glucose infusion by itself does not usually cause severe symptomatic hypophosphatemia; however, if glucose infusion is combined with other factors, such as diuretics that increase phosphate excretion, severe symptomatic hypophosphatemia may result. Insulin, as well as glucose, promotes the movement of phosphate into cells. Glucose–insulin–potassium solution administered intravenously to increase myocardial performance can decrease plasma phosphate for up to 18 hours. Catecholamines and ß-adrenergic agonist drugs also shift phosphate into cells and predispose to hypophosphatemia.[14]

Hypophosphatemia is common in chronic alcoholism. Patients newly diagnosed with alcoholic cardiomyopathy need to have their phosphate levels checked; if they undergo alcohol withdrawal, the phosphate levels need monitoring for at least 4 days.[33,45]

The signs and symptoms of severe symptomatic hypophosphatemia include anorexia, nausea, malaise, diminished reflexes, paresthesias, muscle aching, muscle weakness, severe debility, acute respiratory failure, hemolysis, confusion, stupor, seizures, coma, and impaired cardiac function. These effects of hypophosphatemia are primarily due to decreased intracellular ATP and to decreased 2,3-diphosphoglycerate in the RBCs. Decreased erythrocyte 2,3-diphosphoglycerate causes tissue hypoxia by increasing hemoglobin–oxygen affinity, which reduces oxygen release.[86]

CARDIAC EFFECTS OF SEVERE SYMPTOMATIC HYPOPHOSPHATEMIA

Severe hypophosphatemia impairs myocardial function by decreasing cardiac contractility and stroke work.[11] This cardiac impairment may progress to severe congestive cardiomyopathy. The decreased cardiac performance of hypophosphatemia is reversed by the administration of phosphate; in one study of patients in the surgical ICU, the cardiac index increased 18% after correction of hypophosphatemia.[166]

The role of hypophosphatemia in cardiac arrhythmias is not well understood. A study of patients with MI showed that hypophosphatemia was a significant predictor of ventricular tachycardia during the first 24 hours of hospitalization.[103] Cardiorespiratory arrest has also been attributed to severe hypophosphatemia.[15]

DISPLAY 6-11

Factors That Decrease Plasma Phosphate

GENERAL ETIOLOGY: DECREASED PHOSPHATE INTAKE OR ABSORPTION

Specific Examples:
PROLONGED OR EXCESSIVE ANTACID USE*
Malabsorption syndrome
Chronic diarrhea
Chronic alcoholism

GENERAL ETIOLOGY: MOVEMENT OF PHOSPHATE INTO CELLS

Specific Examples:
HYPERALIMENTATION
REFEEDING AFTER STARVATION
RESPIRATORY ALKALOSIS (HYPERVENTILATION)
Intravenous glucose, fructose, lactate, or bicarbonate
Insulin
Epinephrine
Androgen therapy

GENERAL ETIOLOGY: INCREASED PHOSPHATE EXCRETION

Specific Examples:
DIABETIC KETOACIDOSIS
ALCOHOL WITHDRAWAL
DIURETIC PHASE AFTER SEVERE BURNS
Diuretic therapy
Corticosteroid therapy
Early chronic renal failure
Renal tubular acidosis
Hyperparathyroidism
Osteoporosis, osteomalacia
Multiple myeloma
Gout

GENERAL ETIOLOGY: PHOSPHATE LOSS BY ABNORMAL ROUTE

Specific Examples:
Emesis
Hemodialysis

*Capitalized type denotes single causes of severe symptomatic hypophosphatemia.
From Felver L: Fluid and electrolyte balance and imbalances. In Patrick ML, Woods SL, Craven RF et al (eds): Medical–Surgical Nursing: Pathophysiological Concepts, 2nd ed, p. 257. Philadelphia, JB Lippincott, 1991.

VASCULAR EFFECTS OF SEVERE SYMPTOMATIC HYPOPHOSPHATEMIA

Long-term phosphate depletion in rats causes decreased mean arterial pressure, decreased arteriolar responsiveness to norepinephrine and angiotensin II, increased systemic vascular resistance, increased plasma renin activity, increased plasma norepinephrine, and no change in plasma epinephrine.[125] The clinical significance of these findings is not yet fully understood. Mean arterial pressure in hypophosphatemic patients increases after phosphate repletion.[11] It is likely that this effect is due to a vascular as well as a myocardial action.

SUMMARY

Fluid balance is determined by the interplay of fluid intake, distribution, excretion, and fluid loss through abnormal routes. The two types of fluid imbalances are ECV imbalances and osmolality imbalances. ECV imbalances are increases or decreases in the amount of fluid in the vascular and interstitial compartments. Osmolality imbalances are alterations in the concentration of body fluids and result in movement of water into or out of cells due to osmosis. Extracellular volume and osmolality imbalances may occur concurrently or separately in patients with cardiac disease.

A normal plasma electrolyte concentration is necessary for optimal cardiovascular function. Because electrolytes play important roles in the generation of action potentials and the contraction of both cardiac and smooth muscle, electrolyte imbalances exert both cardiac and vascular effects. The effects of a specific electrolyte imbalance depend on the specific role of that electrolyte in normal cardiovascular function.

People who do not have cardiovascular disease may acquire an electrolyte imbalance that subsequently causes cardiovascular impairment. In addition, patients who have preexisting cardiovascular disease have specific risk factors for electrolyte imbalances. If imbalances develop in these patients, the cardiovascular effects of the electrolyte imbalances may cause severe disturbance to an already compromised cardiovascular system. Successful nursing management of these patients involves careful assessment of risk factors, elimination of those risk factors where possible, surveillance for the manifestations of fluid and electrolyte imbalances, and nursing interventions to protect and support function during the correction of fluid and electrolyte imbalances.[44-46]

REFERENCES

1. Akita M, Kuwahara M, Tsubone H et al: ECG changes during furosemide-induced hypokalemia in the rat. J Electrocardiol 31: 45–49, 1998
2. Anonymous: Effectiveness of spironolactone added to an angiotensin-converting enzyme inhibitor and loop diuretic for severe chronic congestive heart failure. Am J Cardiol 78: 902–907, 1996
3. Antognini JF, Mark K: Hyperkalemia associated with haemorrhagic shock in rabbits: Modification by succinylcholine, vecuronium and blood transfusion. Acta Anaesthesiol Scand 39: 1125–1127, 1995
4. Appleby M, Fischer M, Martin M: Myocardial infarction, hyperkalemia and ventricular tachycardia in a young male body-builder. Int J Cardiol 44: 171–174, 1994
5. Arner A, Malmqvist U, Uvelius B: Effects of Ca^{2+} on force–velocity characteristics of normal and hypertrophic smooth muscle of the rat portal vein. Acta Physiol Scand 124: 525–533, 1985
6. Ayus JC, Arieff A: Abnormalities of water metabolism in the elderly. Semin Nephrol 16: 277–288, 1996
7. Badertscher E, Warnica JW, Ernst DS: Acute hypercalcemia and severe bradycardia in a patient with breast cancer. CMAJ 148: 1506–1508, 1993
8. Barbagallo M, Gupta RK, Bardicef O et al: Altered ionic effects of insulin in hypertension: Role of basal ion levels in determining cellular responsiveness. J Clin Endocrinol Metab 82: 1761–1765, 1997
9. Bedani PL, Gilli P: Hypertensive emergency due to acute renal failure secondary to rhabdomyolysis (Letter). Nephron 69: 120–121, 1995
10. Blackburn ST, Loper DL: Maternal, Fetal, and Neonatal Physiology. Philadelphia, WB Saunders, 1992
11. Bollaert PE, Levy B, Nace L et al: Hemodynamic and metabolic effects of rapid correction of hypophosphatemia in patients with septic shock. Chest 107: 1698–1701, 1995
12. Bourke E, Delaney V: Prevention of hypokalemia caused by diuretics. Heart Disease and Stroke 3(2): 63–67, 1994
13. Braxmeyer DL, Keyes JL: The pathophysiology of potassium balance. Crit Care Nurs 16(5): 59–71, 1996
14. Brown GR, Greenwood JK: Drug- and nutrition-induced hypophosphatemia: Mechanisms and relevance in the critically ill. Ann Pharmacother 28: 626–632, 1994
15. Cariem AK, Lemmer ER, Adams MG et al: Severe hypophosphatemia in anorexia nervosa. Postgrad Med J 70: 825–827, 1994
16. Carpenter C, May ME: Case report: Cardiotoxic calcemia. Am J Med Sci 307: 43–44, 1994
17. Carpentier RG, Posner P, Bloom S: Sinoatrial automaticity and transmembrane potentials in hamsters on a magnesium-deficient diet. J Cardiovasc Pharmacol 7: 919–923, 1985
18. Castelli I, Steiner LA, Kaufmann MA et al: Renovascular responses to high and low perfusate calcium steady-state experiments in the isolated perfused rat kidney with baseline vascular tone. J Surg Res 61: 51–57, 1996
19. Casthely PA, Yoganathan T, Komer C et al: Magnesium and arrhythmias after coronary artery bypass surgery. J Cardiothorac Vasc Anesth 8: 188–191, 1994
20. Castrillon JL, Mediavilla A, Mendez MA et al: Syndrome of inappropriate antidiuretic hormone secretion and enalapril. J Intern Med 233: 89–91, 1993
21. Chadda KD: Clinical hypomagnesemia, coronary spasm and cardiac arrhythmia. Magnesium 5: 47–52, 1986
22. Chah Q, Braly G, Bouzita K et al: Effects of hypokalemia on the various parts of the conduction of the dog heart in situ. Naunyn Schmiedebergs Arch Pharmacol 319: 178–183, 1982
23. Chan TY: Indapamide-induced severe hyponatremia and hypokalemia. Ann Pharmacother 29: 1124–1128, 1995
24. Chava NR: Tall T waves: Electrocardiographic differential diagnosis. Heart Lung 13: 168–172, 1984
25. Chvilicek JP, Hurlbert BJ, Hill GE: Diuretic-induced hypokalemia inducing torsades de pointes. Can J Anaesth 42: 1137–1139, 1995
26. Costello RB, Moser-Veillon PB, DiBlanco R: Magnesium supplementation in patients with congestive heart failure. J Am Coll Nutr 16: 22–31, 1997
27. Cummins RO, Graves JR: ACLS Scenarios: Core Concepts for Case-Based Learning. St Louis, Mosby, 1996
28. Darbar D, Smith M, Morike K et al: Epinephrine-induced changes in serum potassium and cardiac repolarization and effects of pretreatment with propranolol and diltiazem. Am J Cardiol 77: 1351–1355, 1996
29. Dargie HJ: Interrelation of electrolytes and renin–angiotensin system in congestive heart failure. Am J Cardiol 65: 29E–32E, 1990

30. Davenport J, Morton PG: Identifying nonischemic causes of life-threatening arrhythmias. Am J Nurs 97(11): 50–55, 1997

31. Davis TM, Singh B, Choo KE et al: Dynamic assessment of the electrocardiographic QT interval during citrate infusion in healthy volunteers. Br Heart J 76: 523–526, 1995

32. Dei Cas L, Metra M, Leier CV: Electrolyte disturbances in chronic heart failure: Metabolic and clinical aspects. Clin Cardiol 18: 370–376, 1995

33. De Marchi S, Cecchin E, Basile A et al: Renal tubular dysfunction in chronic alcohol abuse: Effects of abstinence. N Engl J Med 329: 1927–1934, 1993

34. Dichtl A, Vierling W: Inhibition by magnesium of calcium inward current in heart ventricular muscle. Eur J Pharmacol 204: 243–248, 1991

35. Dietz T, Bissett JK, Talley JD: The effects of hypokalemia on the heart. J Ark Med Soc 94: 79–81, 1997

36. Doman K, Perlmutter JA, Muhammedi M et al: Life-threatening hyperkalemia associated with captopril administration. South Med J 86: 1269–1272, 1993

37. Dornan RI, Royston D: Suxamethonium-related hyperkalemic cardiac arrest in intensive care (Letter). Anaesthesia 50: 1006, 1995

38. Douban S, Brodsky MA, Whang DD et al: Significance of magnesium in congestive heart failure. Am Heart J 132: 664–671, 1996

39. Douglas PS, Carmichael KA, Palevsky PM: Extreme hypercalcemia and electrocardiographic changes. Am J Cardiol 54: 674, 1984

40. Elisef M, Theodorou J, Pappas C et al: Successful treatment of hyponatremia with angiotensin-converting enzyme inhibitors in patients with congestive heart failure. Cardiology 86: 477–480, 1995

41. Eurenius S, Smith RM: The effect of warming on the serum potassium content of stored blood. Anesthesiology 38: 482–484, 1973

42. Fardella C, Rodriguez-Portales JA: Intracellular calcium and blood pressure: comparison between primary hyperparathyroidism and essential hypertension. J Endocrinol Invest 18: 827–832, 1995

43. Farago M, Szabo C, Dora E et al: Contractile and endothelium-dependent dilatory responses of cerebral arteries at various extracellular magnesium concentrations. J Cerebral Blood Flow Metab 11: 161–164, 1991

44. Felver L: Caring for people with fluid, electrolyte, and acid-base imbalances. In Luckmann J (ed): Saunders Manual of Nursing Care, pp. 235–290. Philadelphia, WB Saunders, 1997

45. Felver L: Fluid and electrolyte balance and imbalances. In Patrick ML, Woods SL, Craven RF et al (eds): Medical-Surgical Nursing: Pathophysiological Concepts, 2nd ed., pp. 228–270. Philadelphia, JB Lippincott, 1991

46. Felver L: Fluid and electrolyte homeostasis and imbalances. In Copstead L (ed): Perspectives on Pathophysiology, pp. 538–545. Philadelphia, WB Saunders, 1995

47. Fenton F, Smally AJ, Laut J: Hyperkalemia and digoxin toxicity in a patient with kidney failure. Ann Emerg Med 28: 440–441, 1996

48. Flores NA, Davies AL, Sheridan DJ: Microangiographic investigation of the effects of radiographic contrast media and hyperkalemia on coronary artery calibre in the rabbit. Q J Exp Physiol 74: 181–195, 1989

49. Fung MC, Weintraub M, Brown DL: Hypermagnesemia: Elderly over-the-counter drug users at risk. Arch Fam Med 4: 718–723, 1995

50. Gennari C, Nami R, Bianchini C et al: Blood pressure effects of acute hypercalcemia in normal subjects and thyroparathy-roidectomized patients. Miner Electrolyte Metab 11: 369–373, 1985

51. Genovese A, Spadaro G, Santoro L et al: Giardiasis as a cause of hypokalemic myopathy in congenital immunodeficiency. Int J Clin Lab Res 26: 132–135, 1996

52. Ghent S, Judson MA, Rosansky SJ: Refractory hypotension associated with hypocalcemia and renal disease. Am J Kidney Dis 23: 430–432, 1994

53. Goertz AW, Lass M, Schutz W et al: Influence of intravenous calcium gluconate on saphenous vein graft flow in closed-chest patients. J Cardiothorac Vasc Anesth 8: 541–544, 1994

54. Gonzalez-Martinez H, Gaspard JJ, Espino DV: Hyponatremia due to enalapril in an elderly patient. Arch Fam Med 2: 791–793, 1993

55. Gottlieb SS: Effects of intravenous magnesium sulphate on arrhythmias in patients with congestive heart failure. Am Heart J 125: 1645–1650, 1993

56. Gould L, Reddy CVR, Becker WH et al: Effect of potassium infusion on the human conduction system. Angiology 31: 666–676, 1980

57. Greenberg A: Hyperkalemia: Treatment options. Semin Nephrol 18: 46–57, 1998

58. Gueux E, Azais-Braesco V, Bussiere L et al: Effect of magnesium deficiency on triacylglycerol-rich lipoprotein and tissue susceptibility to peroxidation in relation to vitamin E content. Br J Nutr 74: 849–856, 1995

59. Gurtoo A, Goswami R, Dingh B et al: Hypocalcemia-induced reversible hemodynamic dysfunction. Int J Cardiol 43: 91–93, 1994

60. Halperin ML, Goldstein MB: Fluid, Electrolyte, and Acid-Base Physiology, 2nd ed. Philadelphia, WB Saunders, 1994

61. Hariman RJ, Chen CM: Effects of hyperkalemia on sinus nodal function in dogs: Sino-ventricular conduction. Cardiovasc Res 17: 509–517, 1983

62. Hayakawa K, Mitsumori M, Uwatoko H: Acute electrolyte disturbances in coronary sinus during left coronary arteriography in man. Acta Radiol 34: 230–236, 1993

63. Hays JV, Gilman JK, Rubal BJ: Effect of magnesium sulfate on ventricular rate control in atrial fibrillation. Ann Emerg Med 24: 61–64, 1994

64. He GW: Hyperkalemia exposure impairs EDHF-mediated endothelial function in the human coronary artery. Ann Thorac Surg 63: 84–87, 1997

65. He GW, Yang CQ, Yang JA: Depolarizing cardiac arrest and endothelium-derived hyperpolarizing factor-mediated hyperpolarization and relaxation in coronary arteries: The effect and mechanism. J Thorac Cardiovasc Surg 113: 932–941, 1997

66. Heesch CM, Eichhorn EJ: Magnesium in acute myocardial infarction. Ann Emerg Med 24: 1154–1160, 1994

67. Higham PD, Adams PC, Murray A et al: Plasma potassium, serum magnesium and ventricular fibrillation: A prospective study. QJM 86: 609–617, 1993

68. Horner SM: Efficacy of intravenous magnesium in acute myocardial infarction in reducing arrhythmias and mortality. Circulation 86: 774–779, 1992

69. Howard JA, Kosowsky BD: Electrocardiographic diagnosis of hyperkalemia in the presence of ventricular pacing and atrial fibrillation. Chest 78: 491–492, 1980

70. Iseri LT: Potassium, magnesium, and digitalis toxicity. In Whang R (ed): Potassium: Its Biologic Significance, pp. 125–136. Boca Raton, FL, CRC Press, 1982

71. Jackson MA, Lodwick R, Hutchinson SG: Hyperkalemic cardiac arrest successfully treated with peritoneal dialysis. BMJ 312: 1289–1290, 1996

72. Jovanovic A, Alekseev AE, Lopez JR et al: Adenosine prevents hyperkalemia-induced calcium loading in cardiac cells:

Relevance for cardioplegia. Ann Thorac Surg 63: 153–161, 1997

73. Kao YJ, Mian T, Kleinman S: Hyperkalaemia: A complication of warm heart surgery. Can J Anaesth 40: 67–70, 1993

74. Karademir S, Altuntas B, Tezic T et al: Left ventricular dysfunction due to hypocalcemia in a neonate. Jpn Heart J 34: 355–359, 1993

75. Karlsberg RP, Cryer PE, Roberts S: Serial plasma catecholamine response early in the course of clinical acute myocardial infarction: Relationship to infarct extent and mortality. Am Heart J 102: 24–29, 1981

76. Kasaoka S, Tsuruta R, Nakashima K et al: Effect of intravenous magnesium sulfate on cardiac arrhythmias in critically ill patients with low serum ionized magnesium. Jpn Circ J 60: 871–875, 1996

77. Kaufmann MA, Pargger H, Castelli I et al: Renal vascular responses to high and low ionized calcium: Influence of norepinephrine in the isolated perfused rat kidney. J Trauma 41: 110–115, 1996

78. Klasaer AE, Scalzo AJ, Blume C et al: Marked hypocalcemia and ventricular fibrillation in two pediatric patients exposed to a fluoride-containing wheel cleaner. Ann Emerg Med 28:713–718, 1996

79. Klein LW, Meller J: Hyperkalemia-induced pseudoinfarction pattern. Mt Sinai J Med 50: 428–431, 1983

80. Knochel J, Schlein E: On the mechanism of rhabdomyolysis in potassium depletion. J Clin Invest 51: 1750–1758, 1972

81. Kolloch RE, Kruse HJ, Friedrich R et al: Role of epinephrine-induced hypokalemia in the regulation of renin and aldosterone in humans. J Lab Clin Med 127: 50–56, 1996

82. Kovalik SG, Ledgerwood AM, Lucas CE et al: The cardiac effect of altered calcium homeostasis after albumin resuscitation. J Trauma 21: 275–279, 1981

83. Kuller JH, Hulley SB, Cohen JD et al: Unexpected effects of treating hypertension in men with electrocardiographic abnormalities: A critical analysis. Circulation 73: 114–123, 1986

84. Kurita T: Antiarrhythmic effect of parenteral magnesium on ventricular tachycardia associated with long QT syndrome. Magnes Res 7: 155–157, 1994

85. Kurita T, Ohe T, Maed, K et al: QRS alteration-induced torsade de pointes in a patient with an artificial pacemaker and hypokalemia. Jpn Circ J 60: 189–191, 1996

86. Larsen VH, Waldau T, Gravesen H et al: Erythrocyte 2, 3-diphosphoglycerate depletion associated with hypophosphatemia detected by routine arterial blood gas analysis. Scand J Clin Lab Invest 224: 83–87, 1996

87. Lasserre B, Spoerri M, Moullet V et al: Should magnesium therapy be considered for the treatment of coronary heart disease? II. Epidemiological evidence in outpatients with and without coronary heart disease. Magnes Res 7: 45–53, 1994

88. Leier CV, Dei Cas L, Metra M: Clinical relevance and management of the major electrolyte abnormalities in congestive heart failure: Hyponatremia, hypokalemia, and hypomagnesemia. Am Heart J 128: 564–574, 1994

89. Lin JL, Lim PS, Leu ML et al: Outcomes of severe hyperkalemia in cardiopulmonary resuscitation with concomitant hemodialysis. Intensive Care Med 20: 287–290, 1994

90. Lindinger MI: Potassium regulation during exercise and recovery in humans: Implications for skeletal and cardiac muscle. J Mol Cell Cardiol 27: 1011–1022, 1995

91. Lucatello A, Sturani A, DiNardo A et al: Acute renal failure in rhabdomyolysis associated with hypokalemia. Nephron 67: 115–116, 1994

92. McDonough AA, Wang J, Farley RA: Significance of sodium pump isoforms in digitalis therapy. J Mol Cell Cardiol 27: 1001–1009, 1995

93. Mak IT, Komarov AM, Wagner TL et al: Enhanced NO production during Mg deficiency and its role in mediating red blood cell glutathione loss. Am J Physiol 271: C385–C390, 1996

94. Marone C, Beretta-Piccoli C, Weidmann P: Acute hypercalcemic hypertension in man: Role of hemodynamics, catecholamines, and renin. Kidney Int 20: 92–96, 1980

95. Merrill JJ, DeWeese G, Wharton JM: Magnesium reversal of digoxin-facilitated ventricular rate during atrial fibrillation in the Wolff-Parkinson-White syndrome. Am J Med 97: 25–28, 1994

96. Metcalfe MJ, Seidelin PH: Images in cardiology: ECG changes of severe hyperkalemia. Br Heart J 72: 260, 1994

97. Moore-Ede MC, Meguid M, Fitzpatrick G et al: Circadian variation in response to potassium infusion. Clin Pharmacol Ther 23: 218–227, 1978

98. Morgan DB, Young RM: Acute transient hypokalemia: New interpretation of a common event. Lancet 2: 751–752, 1982

99. Nadler JL, Buchanan T, Natarajan R et al: Magnesium deficiency produces insulin resistance and increased thromboxane synthesis. Hypertension 21: 1024–1029, 1993

100. Narins R (ed): Clinical Disorders of Fluid and Electrolyte Metabolism, 5th ed. New York, McGraw-Hill, 1994

101. Nordrehaug JE: Malignant arrhythmia in relation to serum potassium in acute myocardial infarction. Am J Cardiol 56: 20D–23D, 1985

102. Nozue T, Kobayashi A, Uemasu F et al: Magnesium status, serum HDL cholesterol, and apolipoprotein A-1 levels. J Pediatr Gastroenterol Nutr 20: 316–318, 1995

103. Ognibene A, Ciniglio R, Greifenstein A et al: Ventricular tachycardia in acute myocardial infarction: The role of hypophosphatemia. South Med J 87: 65–69, 1994

104. Ohmae M, Rabkin SW: Hyperkalemia-induced bundle branch block and complete heart block. Clin Cardiol 4: 43–46, 1981

105. O'Neill M, Sears CE, Paterson DJ: Interactive effects of K⁺, acid, norepinephrine and ischemia on the heart: Implications of exercise. J Appl Physiol 82: 1046–1052, 1997

106. Oster JR, Singer I, Fishman LM: Heparin-induced aldosterone suppression and hyperkalemia. Am J Med 98: 575–586, 1995

107. Owens LM, Fralix TA, Murphy E et al: Correlation of ischemia-induced extracellular and intracellular ion changes to cell-to-cell electrical uncoupling in isolated blood-perfused rabbit hearts. Circulation 94: 10–13, 1996

108. Ozono R, Oshima T, Matsura H et al: Systemic magnesium deficiency disclosed by magnesium loading test in patients with essential hypertension. Hypertens Res 18: 39–42, 1995

109. Panciroli C, Galioni G, Oddone A et al: Prognostic value of hyponatremia in patients with severe chronic heart failure. Angiology 41: 631–638, 1990

110. Papademetriou V: Effect of diuretics on cardiac arrhythmias and left ventricular hypertrophy in hypertension. Cardiology 84(Suppl 2): 43–47, 1994

111. Pargger H, Kaufmann MA, Drop LJ: Renal vascular hyperresponsiveness to elevated ionized calcium in spontaneous hypertensive rat kidneys. Intensive Care Med 24: 61–70, 1998

112. Paterson DJ: Antiarrhythmic mechanisms during exercise. J Appl Physiol 80: 1853–1862, 1996

113. Pérez JE, Saffitz JE, Gutiérrez FA et al: Coronary artery spasm in intact dogs induced by potassium and serotonin. Circ Res 52: 423–431, 1983

114. Peterson EW, Chen KG, Elkins N et al: NMR spectroscopy studies of severe hypokalemia in isolated rat hearts. Am J Physiol 269: H1981–H1987, 1995

115. Philbrick WM, Wysolmerski JJ, Galbraith S et al: Defining the roles of parathyroid hormone-related protein in normal physiology. Physiol Rev 76: 127–173, 1996

116. Pitts BJR, Entman ML: The heart and cellular potassium fluxes. In Whang R (ed): Potassium: Its Biologic Significance, pp. 110–118. Boca Raton, FL, CRC Press, 1982

117. Quick G, Bastani B: Prolonged asystolic hyperkalemic cardiac arrest with no neurologic sequelae. Ann Emerg Med 24: 305–311, 1994

118. Qureshi T, Malonakos TK: Acute hypermagnesemia after laxative use. Ann Emerg Med 28: 552–555, 1996

119. Reardon LC, Macpherson DS: Hyperkalemia in patients using angiotensin-converting enzyme inhibitors: How much should we worry? Arch Intern Med 158: 26–32, 1998

120. Rayssiguier Y, Gueux E, Bussiere L et al: Dietary magnesium affects susceptibility of lipoproteins and tissues to peroxidation in rats. J Am Coll Nutr 12: 133–137, 1993

121. Reinhart RA: Clinical correlates of the molecular and cellular actions of magnesium on the cardiovascular system. Am Heart J 121: 1513–1521, 1991

122. Roden DM: A practical approach to torsades de pointes. Clin Cardiol 20: 285–290, 1997

123. Rylander R: Environmental magnesium deficiency as a cardiovascular risk factor. J Cardiovasc Risk 3: 4–10, 1996

124. Saggar-Malik AK, Cappuccio FP: Potassium supplements and potassium-sparing diuretics: A review and guide to appropriate use. Drugs 46: 986–1008, 1993

125. Saglikes Y, Massry SG, Iseki K et al: Effect of phosphate depletion on blood pressure and vascular reactivity to norepinephrine and angiotensin II in the rat. Am J Physiol 248: F93–F99, 1985

126. Satake K, Lee JD, Shimuzu H et al: Relation between severity of magnesium deficiency and frequency of anginal attacks in men with variant angina. J Am Coll Cardiol 28: 897–902, 1996

127. Satur AMR, Stubington SR, Jennings A et al: Magnesium flux during and after open heart operations in children. Ann Thorac Surg 59: 921–927, 1995

128. Seelig M: Consequences of magnesium deficiency on the enhancement of stress reactions: Preventive and therapeutic implications. J Am Coll Nutr 13: 429–446, 1994

129. Serebruany VL, Herzog WR, Edenbaum LR et al: Changes in the haemostatic profile during magnesium deficiency in swine. Magnes Res 9: 155–163, 1996

130. Solomon R, Weinberg MS, Dubey A: The diurnal rhythm of plasma potassium: Relationship to diuretic therapy. J Cardiovasc Pharmacol 17: 854–859, 1991

131. Somlyo AP: Excitation-contraction coupling and the ultrastructure of smooth muscle. Circ Res 57: 497–507, 1985

132. Sonnenblick M, Friedlander Y, Rosin AJ: Diuretic-induced severe hyponatremia: Review and analysis of 129 reported patients. Chest 103: 601–606, 1993

133. Soupart A, Decaux G: Therapeutic recommendations for management of severe hyponatremia: Current concepts on pathogenesis and prevention of neurologic complications. Clin Nephrol 46: 149–169, 1996

134. Speich M, Bousquet B, Nicolas G: Concentrations of magnesium, calcium, potassium, and sodium in human heart muscle after acute myocardial infarction. Clin Chem 26: 1662–1665, 1980

135. Sridharan MR, Flowers NC: Hyperkalemia and Wolff-Parkinson-White type preexcitation syndrome. J Electrocardiol 19: 183–188, 1986

136. Sridharan MR, Horan LG: Electrocardiographic J wave of hypercalcemia. Am J Cardiol 54: 672–673, 1984

137. Strivens E, Siddiqi A, Fluck, R et al: Hyperkalemic cardiac arrest: may occur secondary to misuse of diuretics and potassium supplements (Letter). BMJ 313: 693, 1996

138. Struthers AD, Whitesmith R, Reid JL: Prior thiazide diuretic treatment increases adrenaline-induced hypokalemia. Lancet 1: 1358–1360, 1983

139. Suzuki T, Ikeda U, Fujikawa H et al: Hypocalcemic heart failure: A reversible form of heart muscle disease. Clin Cardiol 21: 227–228, 1998

140. Szerlip HM, Weiss J, Singer I: Profound hyperkalemia without electrocardiographic manifestations. Am J Kidney Dis 7: 461–465, 1986

141. Topol EJ, Lerman BB: Hypomagnesemic torsades de pointes. Am J Cardiol 52: 1367–1368, 1983

142. Toto KH, Yucha CB: Magnesium: Homeostasis, imbalances, and therapeutic uses. Crit Care Nurs Clin North Am 6: 767–783, 1994

143. Tsutsui M, Shimokawa H, Yoshihara S et al: Intracellular magnesium deficiency in acute myocardial infarction. Jpn Heart J 34: 391–401, 1993

144. Tsutsumi T, Wyatt RF, Abildskov JA: Effects of hyperkalemia on local changes of repolarization duration in canine left ventricle. J Electrocardiol 16: 1–6, 1983

145. Tueth MJ, Broderick-Cantwell J: Successful treatment with captopril of an elderly man with polydipsia and hyponatremia. J Geriatr Psychiatry Neurol 6: 112–114, 1993

146. United States Pharmacopeial Convention: USP DI (Vol I): Drug Information for the Health Care Professional, 18th ed. Rockville, MD, USP, 1998

147. Van Kuijk WH, Mulder AW, Peels CH et al: Influence of changes in ionized calcium on cardiovascular reactivity during hemodialysis. Clin Nephrol 47: 190–196, 1997

148. Veress G: Hypokalemia associated with infra-His Mobitz type second degree A-V block. Chest 105: 1616–1617, 1994

149. Villemaire C, Nattel S: Modulation of procainamide's effect on cardiac conduction in dogs by extracellular potassium concentration: A quantitative analysis. Circulation 89: 2870–2878, 1994

150. Vincent JL, Bredas P, Jankowski S et al: Correction of hypocalcemia in the critically ill: What is the hemodynamic benefit? Intensive Care Med 21: 838–841, 1995

151. Vissers RJ, Purssell R: Iatrogenic magnesium overdose: Two cases. J Emerg Med 14: 187–191, 1996

152. Voelckel W, Kroesen, G: Unexpected return of cardiac action after termination of cardiopulmonary resuscitation. Resuscitation 32: 27–29, 1996

153. Walker GL, Williamson PM, Ravich RBM et al: Hypercalcemia associated with cerebral vasospasm causing infarction. J Neurol Neurosurg Psychiatry 43: 464–467, 1980

154. Wan-chun C, Xin-xiang F, Zhen-jia P et al: ECG changes in early stage of magnesium deficiency. Am Heart J 104: 1115–1116, 1982

155. Watanabe I, Kanda A, Engle CL et al: Comparison of effects of regional ischemia and hyperkalemia on the membrane action potentials of the in situ pig heart. J Cardiovasc Electrophysiol 8: 1229–1236, 1997

156. Webb SC, Canepa-Anson R, Rickards AF et al: High potassium concentration in a parenteral preparation of glyceryl trinitrite. Br Heart J 50: 395–396, 1983

157. Weir MR: Non-diuretic-based antihypertensive therapy and potassium homeostasis in elderly patients. Coron Artery Dis 8: 499–504, 1997

158. Weizenberg A, Class RN, Surawicz B: Effects of hyperkalemia on the electrocardiogram of patients receiving digitalis. Am J Cardiol 55: 968–973, 1985

159. Wheeldon M, McDevitt DG, Lipworth BJ: The effects of lower than conventional doses of oral nadolol on relative beta 1/beta 2-adrenoceptor blockade. Br J Clin Pharmacol 38: 103–108, 1994

160. Williams MJ, Hammond-Tooke GD, Restieaux NJ: Hypokalemic periodic paralysis with cardiac arrhythmia and prolonged QT interval (Letter). Aust N Z J Med 25: 549, 1995

161. Williams SG, Davison AG, Glynn MJ: Hypokalaemic rhabdomyolysis: An unusual presentation of coeliac disease. Eur J Gastroenterol Hepatol 7: 183–184, 1995

162. Wong KC, Schafer PG, Schultz JR: Hypokalemia and anesthetic implications. Anesth Analg 77: 1238–1260, 1993

163. Wortsman J, Frank S: The QT interval in clinical hypercalcemia. Clin Cardiol 4: 87–90, 1981

164. Yokoyama S, Su J, Kashima K et al: Combined effects of magnesium deficiency and an atherogenic level of low density lipoprotein on uptake and metabolism of low density lipoprotein by cultured human endothelial cells: II. electron microscopic data. Magnes Res 7: 97–105, 1994

165. Yu AS: Atypical electrocardiographic changes in severe hyperkalemia. Am J Cardiol 77: 906–908, 1996

166. Zazzo JF, Troche G, Ruel P et al: High incidence of hypophosphatemia in surgical intensive care patients: efficacy of phosphorus therapy on myocardial function. Intensive Care Med 21: 826–831, 1995

Acid-Base Balance and Imbalances

LINDA FELVER

PRINCIPLES OF ACID-BASE BALANCE

The degree of acidity of the body fluids plays an important role in physiology. It influences the structure and function of many enzymes and also modifies the affinity between oxygen and hemoglobin. Deviations of acid-base balance from normal can affect cellular function and tissue oxygenation. In the extreme, they can be fatal.

Terminology Review

An *acid* is a substance that donates hydrogen ions (H⁺) in solution. A *base* is a substance that accepts hydrogen ions. The more hydrogen ions a solution contains, the more acidic it is. The actual number of hydrogen ions in extracellular fluid is small and unwieldy to write (0.00004 mmol/L).[25] Therefore, the degree of acidity of body fluids is reported as the pH. The pH is the negative logarithm of the hydrogen ion concentration. It ranges from 1 (very acidic) to 14 (very alkaline). A pH of 7 is neutral. The blood is normally slightly alkaline. The normal pH range of the blood is 7.35 to 7.45.

If the pH of the blood falls below the normal range (i.e., becomes more acidic), a patient has *acidemia*. The process that tends to decrease the pH is called *acidosis*. Similarly, if the pH of the blood rises above the normal range (i.e., becomes more alkaline), a patient has *alkalemia*. The process that tends to decrease the pH is called *alkalosis*.

Processes Involved in Acid-Base Balance

Normal cellular metabolism continually produces acids, which can cause dangerous acidemia without the closely regulated processes by which the body maintains pH within the normal range. After acid production, these processes of acid buffering and acid excretion work to maintain or reestablish a normal pH.

ACID PRODUCTION

Cellular metabolism produces two types of acids: carbonic acid and metabolic acids. Carbonic acid (H_2CO_3) is produced as carbon dioxide (CO_2); the enzyme carbonic anhydrase combines the CO_2 with water (H_2O) to produce carbonic acid. In a standard adult, approximately 15,000 mmol of carbonic acid are generated per day from metabolism of carbohydrates and fats.[25]

Metabolic acids are produced primarily from the metabolism of phosphate-containing compounds and amino acids that contain sulfur. These metabolic acids include sulfuric and phosphoric acids. Metabolic acids are handled differently by the body than carbonic acid. For this reason, they are sometimes called *noncarbonic acids*.

Cellular metabolism also produces small amounts of base (bicarbonate ions; HCO_3^-) as a result of oxidation of small organic anions such as citrate. Much more metabolic acid is produced than base. In a standard adult, a net 50 to 100 mEq of hydrogen ions is generated per day from metabolism.[11,25]

ACID BUFFERING

Buffers in the body act to minimize changes in pH due to gain of acid or base. They neutralize acids by taking up excess hydrogen ions and neutralize bases by releasing hydrogen ions. Buffers are located in all body fluids; however, the most important roles are played by the buffers in the extracellular fluid, intracellular fluid, bone, and urine. Different body fluids contain different buffers, which meet specific needs (Table 7-1).

The major extracellular buffer is the carbonic acid-bicarbonate-carbon dioxide buffer system (commonly termed the *bicarbonate buffer system*). Carbonic acid is a weak acid, which means that it dissociates partially when in solution so that it is in equilibrium with bicarbonate and hydrogen ions. The carbonic acid concentration can be altered by variations in alveolar ventilation (variations in

TABLE 7-1	The Major Buffers		
Extracellular Fluid	**Intracellular Fluid**	**Bone**	**Urine**
Bicarbonate	Proteins	Carbonates	Inorganic phosphates
Inorganic phosphates	Organic and inorganic phosphates	Phosphates	
Plasma proteins	Hemoglobin (erythrocytes)		

CO_2 excretion). The chemical equation for the bicarbonate buffer system is written as follows:

$$CO_2 + H_2O \rightleftharpoons H_2CO_3 \rightleftharpoons H^+ + HCO_3^-$$

carbon   water   carbonic   hydrogen   bicarbonate
dioxide   acid   ion   ion

To maintain the pH of the blood within the normal range, there must be 20 bicarbonate ions for every carbonic acid molecule. The Henderson-Hasselbalch equation, a mathematical description of the pH of a buffered solution, shows how this 20:1 ratio is necessary:

$$pH = pKa + \log \frac{[A^-]}{[HA]} \quad \text{(general equation)}$$

$$pH = 6.1 + \log \frac{[HCO_3^-]}{[H_2CO_3]} \quad \text{(substituting values for bicarbonate buffer system)}$$

$$pH = 6.1 + \log \frac{20}{1}$$

$$pH = 6.1 + 1.3$$

$$pH = 7.4$$

A buffer system cannot buffer its own acid. Thus, the bicarbonate buffer system cannot buffer carbonic acid. The carbonic acid that is produced by cells (as CO_2 and H_2O) is buffered primarily by intracellular buffers. The bicarbonate buffer system is a major buffer for metabolic acids. Table 7-2 summarizes the role of buffers with respect to acid or base loads.

ACID EXCRETION

Even though the buffers minimize pH changes as acid is produced, they have a limited capacity. Therefore, acid excretion mechanisms are necessary to maintain acid-base balance. The body has two acid excretion mechanisms: carbonic acid is excreted by the lungs, and metabolic acids are excreted by the kidneys.

Role of the Lungs. The lungs excrete carbonic acid in the form of carbon dioxide and water. They cannot excrete metabolic acids. When alveolar ventilation increases (increased rate and depth of ventilation), more carbonic acid is excreted. Conversely, when alveolar ventilation decreases, less carbonic acid is excreted. Because carbonic acid is essentially carbon dioxide and water, the body actually senses and regulates the partial pressure of carbon dioxide ($PaCO_2$).

If carbonic acid begins to accumulate (increased $PaCO_2$), chemoreceptors in the medulla and carotid and aortic bodies are stimulated by the increased $PaCO_2$ and decreased pH.[10] The resulting increase in alveolar ventilation causes the excretion of the excess carbonic acid. Similarly, if too little carbonic acid is present (decreased $PaCO_2$), the chemoreceptors are less stimulated, and alveolar ventilation decreases somewhat to retain carbonic acid in the body. Hypoxia, sensed by the carotid chemoreceptors, stimulates alveolar ventilation and may override the suppression of ventilation from decreased $PaCO_2$. In a healthy person, alveolar ventilation changes rapidly in response to changes in $PaCO_2$, and thus carbonic acid is excreted at a rate effective in maintaining acid-base balance.

Role of the Kidneys. The kidneys excrete metabolic acids. They cannot excrete carbonic acid.

The renal epithelial cells that line the proximal tubules secrete hydrogen ions into the renal tubular fluid and reabsorb bicarbonate ions in the process. Bicarbonate is the major extracellular buffer of metabolic acids. Therefore, the bicarbonate ion concentration indicates how much metabolic acid is present. A decreased serum bicarbonate concentration indicates increased amounts of metabolic acid. When the proximal tubular cells secrete hydrogen ions that are eventually excreted in the urine, they replenish the bicarbonate ions that were used in buffering. Hydrogen ions are also secreted into the renal tubular fluid by cells that line the distal tubules and collecting ducts. The distal tubular cells can also secrete bicarbonate into the tubular fluid or reabsorb it into the blood.

If the urine were to become too acidic, it could damage the cells that line the urinary tract. Fortunately, the urine does not become dangerously acidic because the hydrogen ions in the renal tubules are buffered by the urine buffers or combine chemically with ammonia. Ammonia (NH_3) is produced by renal tubular cells and then diffuses into the tubular fluid.[8] Hydrogen ions combine with ammonia in the tubular fluid to produce ammonium ions (NH_4^+). Because ammonium ions are charged particles, they cannot cross the cell membranes to enter the blood; thus, they are "trapped" in the renal tubular fluid and excreted in the urine. An increase in acid in the body (decreased pH) causes the production of more ammonia, which facilitates renal excretion of acid. This process begins within 2 hours but takes several days to be maximally effective.[25]

Thus, the kidneys have several mechanisms that result in the excretion of metabolic acids that are produced by cellular metabolism. These mechanisms can be adjusted to excrete more acid or less acid, thereby maintaining the bicarbonate ion concentration within normal limits. Changes in renal function with normal aging cause elderly people to excrete acid loads more slowly than younger adults.

TABLE 7-2	Role of Buffers with Respect to an Acid or Base Load		
Buffers	**Carbonic Acid Load**	**Metabolic Acid Load**	**Base (Bicarbonate) Load**
Extracellular			
Bicarbonate	Not effective	Major role (immediate action)	Not effective
Others	Minor role (immediate action)	Minor role (immediate action)	Minor role (immediate action)
Intracellular	Major role (10–30 minutes)	Important role (2–4 hours)	Important role (hours)
Bone	Probably unimportant	Important role (2–4 hours)	Important role (hours)

Summary of Acid-Base Balance

Cellular metabolism produces carbonic acid and metabolic acids. These acids must be excreted to maintain normal acid-base balance. Buffers in all body fluids act to minimize changes in pH due to an acid load or a bicarbonate (base) load. Carbonic acid is excreted by the lungs; increases or decreases in alveolar ventilation regulate the amount of carbonic acid excretion. The $PaCO_2$ is the clinical indicator of carbonic acid. Metabolic acids are excreted by the kidneys, which can excrete more or less acid as needed. The plasma bicarbonate ion concentration is the clinical indicator of the amount of metabolic acid. Table 7-3 summarizes the physiologic responses that maintain acid-base balance.

ACID-BASE IMBALANCES

Acid-base imbalances occur when the capacity of the buffers to modulate pH changes is exceeded. Two terms are important in understanding the physiologic responses to acid-base imbalances. *Correction* of the imbalance occurs when the original problem is fixed so that the pH, $PaCO_2$, and plasma bicarbonate ion concentration can return to normal. *Compensation* for an acid-base imbalance restores the pH toward normal but does not correct the problem that originally caused the imbalance. In many cases, an acid-base imbalance persists long enough that compensatory physiologic processes occur. A partially compensated acid-base imbalance is characterized by abnormal pH,

$PaCO_2$, and plasma bicarbonate ion concentration. However, the pH is not as abnormal as it was before the partial compensation. When an acid-base imbalance is fully compensated, the pH is in the normal range, but the $PaCO_2$ and plasma bicarbonate ion concentration are both abnormal. By moving the pH toward normal, compensation for an acid-base imbalance helps to protect cells from death.

Acidosis

A patient who has acidosis has processes that tend to decrease the pH of the blood below normal by creating a relative excess of acid. The resulting acidemia may persist or may be lessened by the body's compensatory response. A pH below 6.9 is usually fatal. Acidosis is classified as respiratory or metabolic, depending on what type of acid is initially in relative excess.

RESPIRATORY ACIDOSIS

Respiratory acidosis occurs when too much carbonic acid accumulates in the blood. Clinically, the increase of carbonic acid is measured as an increased $PaCO_2$. Carbonic acid is normally excreted by the lungs. Thus, any factor that decreases respiration or ventilation can cause respiratory acidosis (Display 7-1). Patients in whom cor pulmonale develops because of chronic lung disease commonly have chronic respiratory acidosis.

Carbon dioxide diffuses readily through membranes. Thus, the pH of cerebrospinal fluid (CSF) decreases when

TABLE 7-3	Summary of Physiologic Responses that Maintain Acid-Base Balance	
Mechanism	**Response to Decreasing pH (Blood too Acidic)**	**Response to Increasing pH (Blood too Alkaline)**
Buffers	Basic portion of buffer pair (e.g., Pr⁻ for protein buffer system) accepts H⁺	Acidic portion of buffer pair (e.g., HPr for protein buffer system) releases H⁺
Respiratory system	Increasing rate and depth of respiration removes carbonic acid from the body	Decreasing rate and depth of respiration retains carbonic acid in the body
Renal system	Increased secretion of H⁺ from extracellular fluid into renal tubular fluid	Decreased secretion of H⁺
	Increased reabsorption of HCO_3^- from renal tubular fluid into extracellular fluid	Decreased reabsorption of HCO_3^-
	Increased production of NH_3	Decreased production of NH_3

Adapted from Felver L: Acid-base balance and imbalances. In Patrick M, Bruno P, Woods S et al (eds). Medical–Surgical Nursing: Pathophysiological Concepts. 2nd ed, p 273. Philadelphia, JB Lippincott, 1991.

DISPLAY 7–1

Causes of Respiratory Acidosis

GENERAL ETIOLOGY: DECREASED GASEOUS EXCHANGE

Specific Examples
Decreased alveolar ventilation
Chronic obstructive pulmonary disease
Emphysema
Severe asthma
Sleep apnea (obstructive type)
Atelectasis
Pneumonia
Adult respiratory distress syndrome
Pulmonary edema
Hypoventilation by way of mechanical ventilator

GENERAL ETIOLOGY: IMPAIRED NEUROMUSCULAR FUNCTION OF CHEST

Specific Examples
Chest injury
Surgical incision (pain limits respirations)
Poliomyelitis
Guillain-Barré syndrome
Respiratory muscle fatigue
Myasthenia gravis
Hypokalemia
Kyphoscoliosis
Pickwickian syndrome (obesity limits chest expansion)

GENERAL ETIOLOGY: SUPPRESSION OF NEURAL VENTILATORY MECHANISMS IN BRAIN STEM (MEDULLA)

Specific Examples
Narcotics
Barbiturates
Sleep apnea (central type)

From Felver L: Acid-base balance and imbalances. In Patrick M, Bruno P, Woods S et al (eds): Medical–Surgical Nursing: Pathophysiological Concepts, 2nd ed, p 275. Philadelphia, JB Lippincott, 1991.

---

respiratory acidosis occurs. As excess CO_2 enters the brain cells, intracellular acidosis alters enzyme activity and central nervous system (CNS) depression results. The clinical manifestations of respiratory acidosis are CNS depression (disorientation, lethargy, somnolence), headache, blurred vision, tachycardia, and cardiac arrhythmias.

Respiratory acidosis can be corrected only by restoring lung function because the lungs are the only route of excretion of carbonic acid. If the kidneys compensate by excreting more than the usual amount of metabolic acids, the pH moves back toward normal, even though the blood chemistry remains abnormal. Excretion of more metabolic acids raises the bicarbonate ion concentration because fewer bicarbonate ions are used in buffering. Thus, renal compensation for respiratory acidosis restores the 20:1 ratio of bicarbonate to carbonic acid, even though the absolute values of both are elevated. Restoring the 20:1 ratio normalizes the pH. Renal compensation for respiratory acidosis takes 3 to 5 days to be fully effective. A compensated respiratory acidosis is characterized by an elevated $PaCO_2$ (the sign of the primary problem), an elevated bicarbonate ion concentration (the sign of the renal compensation), and a pH that is decreased (partially compensated) or normal (fully compensated).

In respiratory acidosis, excess CO_2 diffuses into cardiac cells. Although intracellular buffering of carbonic acid may protect intracellular pH in cardiac cells more effectively than in many other types of cells, the intracellular pH in cardiac cells does decrease.[12,28] Respiratory acidosis depresses cardiac contractility.[12,27] The negative effects of decreased myocardial cell contractility in respiratory acidosis are partially offset by increased sympathetic neural discharge and increased catecholamine levels. Tachycardia and cardiac arrhythmias in patients with respiratory acidosis may be due to the increased circulating catecholamines. Clinical evidence indicates that cardiac arrhythmias in asthma patients with respiratory arrest and respiratory acidosis are due to hypoxia rather than to the acidosis.[19]

Respiratory acidosis also affects blood vessels, altering both peripheral vascular resistance and distribution of blood flow. Peripheral vascular resistance decreases[2] owing to peripheral vasodilation. Coronary vasodilation also occurs.[9] The peripheral vasculature becomes less sensitive to α- and β-adrenergic stimulation. Baroreflex sensitivity also decreases.[29] Decreased peripheral vascular resistance and decreased cardiac contractility cause hypotension. The hypotension may be diminished by vasoconstriction in splanchnic[21] and peripheral venous beds (the venous capacitance beds). This response increases central arterial blood volume.

The decreased pH in the CSF causes cerebral vasodilation,[1,24] increasing cerebral blood flow. This is the cause of the headache that is experienced by many patients with respiratory acidosis. Increased cerebral blood flow from cerebral vasodilation may also raise CSF pressure and cause papilledema. In contrast to its effect on other vascular beds, respiratory acidosis causes vasoconstriction in the pulmonary vasculature.[20,30] The resulting increase in pulmonary vascular resistance may worsen the clinical status of patients with preexisting right heart failure.

In summary, the major cardiovascular effects of respiratory acidosis are tachycardia, cardiac arrhythmias, decreased cardiac contractility, decreased peripheral vascular resistance, increased pulmonary vascular resistance, and shift of blood flow from the venous capacitance beds into the central and cerebral arterial beds.

METABOLIC ACIDOSIS

Metabolic acidosis is caused by relatively too much metabolic acid. It can be due to a gain of acid or a loss of base. Acid can be gained from intake of acids or substances that are converted to acid in the body, from an increased rate of normal metabolism, from production of unusual acids due to altered metabolic processes, or from factors that decrease renal excretion of acid. Bicarbonate ions (base) can be lost in the urine or through the gastrointestinal tract. Display 7-2

DISPLAY 7–2

Causes of Metabolic Acidosis

GENERAL ETIOLOGY: ACID ACCUMULATION BY INGESTION OF ACID OR ACID PRECURSORS
Specific Examples
Aspirin (acetylsalicylic acid)
Methanol (converted to formic acid)
Ethylene glycol (converted to oxalic acid)
Paraldehyde (converted to acetic and chloroacetic acids)
Boric acid
Elemental sulfur (sulfuric acid)
Ammonium chloride (releases H⁺)

GENERAL ETIOLOGY: ACID ACCUMULATION BY INCREASED PRODUCTION OF METABOLIC ACIDS
Specific Examples
Hyperthyroidism
Hypermetabolic state after burns, trauma, or sepsis
Lactic acidosis
Shock

GENERAL ETIOLOGY: ACID ACCUMULATION BY UTILIZATION OF ABNORMAL OR INCOMPLETE METABOLIC PATHWAYS
Specific Examples
Diabetic ketoacidosis
Alcoholic ketoacidosis
Starvation ketoacidosis

GENERAL ETIOLOGY: ACID ACCUMULATION BY IMPAIRED ACID EXCRETION
Specific Examples
Oliguric renal failure
Severe hypovolemia
Shock
Renal tubular acidosis (type 1)
Hypoaldosteronism

GENERAL ETIOLOGY: PRIMARY DECREASE OF BICARBONATE
Specific Examples
Urinary route. Renal tubular acidosis (type 2)
Gastrointestinal route
    Severe diarrhea
    Intestinal decompression
    Ureterosigmoidostomy
    Fistula drainage
    Vomiting of intestinal contents
    Cholestyramine therapy

Adapted from Felver L: Acid-base balance and imbalances. In Patrick M, Bruno P, Woods S et al (eds): Medical–Surgical Nursing: Pathophysiological Concepts, 2nd ed, p 277. Philadelphia, JB Lippincott, 1991.

---

lists clinical conditions that cause metabolic acidosis by each of these mechanisms. Cardiogenic shock causes metabolic acidosis by accumulation of lactic acid from anaerobic metabolism and through failure of the decreased circulation to deliver metabolic acids to the kidneys for excretion. No matter what its cause, metabolic acidosis is characterized by a decreased plasma bicarbonate ion concentration. The bicarbonate is either depleted by being used to buffer excess metabolic acids or is lost directly from the body.

Metabolic acidosis can be corrected physiologically only by the kidneys, which are the sole excretory route for metabolic acids. Renal correction of metabolic acidosis may take several days. Meanwhile, respiratory compensation occurs within hours. The respiratory compensation for metabolic acidosis is hyperventilation. By increasing the excretion of carbonic acid, hyperventilation makes the blood less acid. This makes the blood chemistry more abnormal (decreased $PaCO_2$) but tends to restore the 20:1 ratio of bicarbonate to carbonic acid and move the pH toward the normal range, thus helping to preserve cellular function. Compensated metabolic acidosis is characterized by a decreased $PaCO_2$ (the sign of the respiratory compensation), a decreased bicarbonate ion concentration (the sign of the primary problem), and a pH that is decreased (partially compensated) or normal (fully compensated).

The clinical manifestations of metabolic acidosis include headache, abdominal pain, cardiac arrhythmias, and CNS depression (confusion, drowsiness, lethargy, stupor, coma). The CNS depression arises from decreased pH of the CSF and resultant intracellular acidosis of brain cells. The exact cause of the abdominal pain is not clearly understood. Patients are tachypneic from the compensatory hyperventilation.

Metabolic acidosis depresses cardiac contractility by causing intracellular acidosis, which alters delivery of calcium ions to the myofilaments and inhibits myofilament responsiveness to calcium.[17,23,26] Cardiac arrhythmias may be related to an increase in circulating catecholamine levels caused by metabolic acidosis. This catecholamine increase helps preserve cardiac output during mild metabolic acidosis.[15] However, acidosis decreases the affinity of β-adrenergic receptors.[18] Thus, in more severe metabolic acidosis, the catecholamine effect on cardiac output is less pronounced and the decreased myocardial contractility becomes predominant. Coronary artery occlusion causes myocardial acidosis, so that these cardiac effects occur in patients with myocardial infarction without the systemic effects of metabolic acidosis.

Increased circulating catecholamines also protect the arterial blood pressure from the peripheral vasodilation caused by acidosis. Coronary vasodilation[14] and pulmonary vasoconstriction[16] occur. Mild cerebral vasodilation[1,24] is probably responsible for the headache experienced by some patients. Constriction of the venous capacitance vessels increases central blood volume. The vascular effects of acid-base imbalances are summarized in Table 7-4.

Alkalosis

A patient who has alkalosis has processes that tend to increase the pH of the blood above normal by creating a relative excess of base (a relative deficit of acid). The resulting alkalemia may persist or may be modulated by a compensatory response. A pH above 7.8 is usually fatal. Alkalosis is classified as respiratory or metabolic, depending on what type of acid is initially in relative deficit.

TABLE 7-4	Vascular Effects of Acid-Base Imbalances			
Vascular Bed	**Respiratory Acidosis**	**Metabolic Acidosis**	**Respiratory Alkalosis**	**Metabolic Alkalosis**
Peripheral	Vasodilation	Vasodilation	Vasoconstriction (debatable)	Vasoconstriction (likely)
Coronary	Vasodilation	Vasodilation	Vasoconstriction	Vasoconstriction
Cerebral	Vasodilation	Vasodilation	Vasoconstriction	Vasoconstriction
Pulmonary	Vasoconstriction	Vasoconstriction	Vasodilation	Vasodilation

RESPIRATORY ALKALOSIS

Respiratory alkalosis occurs when there is too little carbonic acid in the blood. Clinically, the decreased carbonic acid is measured as a decreased $PaCO_2$. Any factor that causes hyperventilation can cause excretion of too much carbonic acid, leading to respiratory alkalosis (Display 7-3).

Note that hypoxia, as from pulmonary embolism or severe anemia, causes appropriate hyperventilation with resultant respiratory alkalosis. In such cases, the cause of the hypoxia should be the primary focus of treatment rather than the respiratory alkalosis.

Patients who have respiratory alkalosis may evidence light-headedness, diaphoresis, paresthesias (digital and circumoral), muscle cramps, carpal and pedal spasms, tetany, syncope, and cardiac arrhythmias. Most of these manifestations are the result of increased neuromuscular excitability. The CSF becomes alkalotic. Chvostek's and Trousseau's signs (nonspecific signs of increased neuromuscular excitability) are positive in many of these patients.

Respiratory alkalosis can be corrected only by the lungs. If any compensation occurs, it is performed by the kidneys, which increase the urinary excretion of bicarbonate ions to restore the 20:1 ratio of bicarbonate ion to carbonic acid. Renal compensation for a respiratory acid-base imbalance requires several days. Most cases of respiratory alkalosis have a short duration; therefore, the disorder is often uncompensated or partially compensated. Compensated respiratory alkalosis is characterized by a decreased $PaCO_2$ (the sign of the primary problem), a decreased bicarbonate ion concentration (the sign of the renal compensation), and a pH that is increased (partially compensated) or normal (fully compensated).

Respiratory alkalosis causes increased pH inside myocardial cells[13] and increases cardiac contractility by increasing the calcium sensitivity of myofibrils.[3,22] The imbalance increases sympathetic nervous system activity and circulating catecholamine levels. Cardiac arrhythmias may result. Although respiratory alkalosis may cause peripheral vasodilation, which decreases peripheral vascular resistance, it is likely to cause peripheral vasoconstriction and increased peripheral vascular resistance.[5] Respiratory alkalosis also causes pulmonary vasodilation,[7,30] coronary vasoconstriction, and cerebral vasoconstriction.[4] This latter effect reduces intracranial pressure and cerebral blood flow and may be the reason for the light-headedness and syncope experienced by some patients with respiratory alkalosis.

METABOLIC ALKALOSIS

Metabolic alkalosis is caused by relatively too little metabolic acid. It can be due to a loss of acid or a gain of base. Acid can be lost through the gastrointestinal tract or in the urine. Acid may also be shifted into cells and thus "lost" from the blood. Base (bicarbonate ions) may be gained from intake of bicarbonate or of substances that are converted to bicarbonate in the body. Patients receiving the combination of loop diuretics and thiazide diuretics for treatment of severe congestive heart failure may develop metabolic alkalosis associated with extracellular volume contraction.[6] A patient with hypovolemic shock from hemorrhage may develop a metabolic alkalosis if 8 or more units of packed red cells or other forms of blood are infused in a short time because the liver metabolizes the citrate in the blood into bicarbonate. Additional causes of metabolic alkalosis are listed in Display 7-4.

The initial clinical manifestations of metabolic alkalosis are often milder than those of respiratory alkalosis because bicarbonate ions cross membranes (and thus alter CSF and intracellular pH) less rapidly than does carbon dioxide. These clinical manifestations may include light-headedness, paresthesias, muscle cramps, carpal and pedal spasms, and cardiac arrhythmias. An initial CNS excitation is followed by the CNS depression of severe

---

DISPLAY 7–3

Causes of Respiratory Alkalosis

GENERAL ETIOLOGY: HYPERVENTILATION

Specific Examples
Anxiety or fear
Pain
Prolonged crying and gasping
Hypoxemia (high altitudes, pulmonary disease, or
  pulmonary embolism)
Some brain injuries
Hyperventilation by means of mechanical ventilator
Stimulation of neural ventilatory mechanisms in brain stem
  (medulla)
  High fever
  Meningitis
  Encephalitis
  Salicylates (overdose)
  Progesterone (high levels)
  Gram-negative septicemia

Adapted from Felver L: Acid-base balance and imbalances. In
  Patrick M, Bruno P, Woods S et al (eds): Medical–Surgical
  Nursing: Pathophysiological Concepts, 2nd ed, p 281.
  Philadelphia, JB Lippincott, 1991.

DISPLAY 7-4

Causes of Metabolic Alkalosis

GENERAL ETIOLOGY: DECREASE OF ACID

Specific Examples
Gastrointestinal
    Emesis
    Gastric suction
Urinary route
    Hyperaldosteronism
    Glucocorticoid excess
    Chronic excessive ingestion of black licorice (contains aldosterone-like compounds)
    Diuretic therapy
Acid movement into cells
    Hypokalemia

GENERAL ETIOLOGY: INCREASE OF BASE (BICARBONATE IONS)

Specific Examples
Excess infusion or ingestion of $NaHCO_3$
Excess administration of lactate or acetate (bicarbonate precursors)
Massive blood transfusion (citrate is a bicarbonate precursor)
Extracellular fluid volume deficit (contraction alkalosis)

Adapted from Felver L: Acid-base balance and imbalances. In Patrick M, Bruno P, Woods S et al (eds). Medical–Surgical Nursing: Pathophysiological Concepts, 2nd ed, p 283. Philadelphia, JB Lippincott, 1991.

---

metabolic alkalosis: confusion, lethargy, and coma. The plasma bicarbonate ion concentration is elevated.

Correction of metabolic alkalosis must be accomplished by the kidneys because they are the excretory organs for bicarbonate ions. Compensation for the disorder, therefore, is the role of the lungs. Because the bicarbonate ion concentration is increased in metabolic alkalosis, the 20:1 ratio of bicarbonate ion to carbonic acid that creates a normal pH can be restored by increasing the amount of carbonic acid in the blood. Thus, the respiratory compensation for metabolic alkalosis is decreased rate and depth of respiration. This compensatory hypoventilation retains carbonic acid (carbon dioxide and water) in the body, which tends to normalize the pH. Compensatory hypoventilation, however, is limited by the body's need for oxygen, so full compensation for metabolic alkalosis is not common. Compensated metabolic alkalosis is characterized by an increased $PaCO_2$ (the sign of the respiratory compensation), an increased bicarbonate ion concentration (the sign of the primary problem), and a pH that is somewhat increased (partially compensated).

Metabolic alkalosis causes increased cardiac contractility by increasing calcium sensitivity,[17] although intracellular pH does not increase in myocardial cells as it does in respiratory alkalosis.[13] Cardiac arrhythmias may occur. Vascular effects are likely to include peripheral vasoconstriction. Other vascular effects of metabolic alkalosis are coronary vasocon-striction, pulmonary vasodilation, and cerebral vasoconstriction with resulting decreased cerebral blood flow and light-headedness.

Principles of Interpreting Arterial Blood Gas Reports

Arterial blood gases are used to assess a patient's acid-base status. The material presented earlier in this chapter provides the basis for understanding and interpreting acid-base aspects of arterial blood gases. The principles are summarized in this section. The PaO_2, a measure of oxygenation, is not discussed here.

The first laboratory value to consider is the pH. If it is below the normal range (less than 7.35 or the reported laboratory normal), then the patient has acidosis. If it is above the normal range (greater than 7.45 or the reported laboratory normal), then the patient has alkalosis. If the pH is within the normal range, there may be no acid-base imbalance, or the patient may have a fully compensated imbalance. For purposes of interpretation, then, if the pH is less than 7.40, the patient is tentatively considered to have acidosis; if the pH is greater than 7.40, the patient is tentatively considered to have alkalosis.

The next value to consider is the $PaCO_2$. If the $PaCO_2$ is above the normal range, then the patient has respiratory acidosis. This respiratory acidosis may be the primary problem, or it may be compensatory. On the other hand, if the $PaCO_2$ is below the normal range, then the patient has respiratory alkalosis. This respiratory alkalosis may be the primary problem or it may be compensatory. If the $PaCO_2$ is within the normal range, then the patient does not have a respiratory acid-base disorder.

A basic understanding of acid-base imbalances facilitates differentiating between primary and compensatory respiratory imbalances. If the patient has *primary respiratory acidosis*, then the pH would be expected to be below 7.40. A *compensatory respiratory acidosis* would occur in response to a metabolic alkalosis, so the pH would be above 7.40.

The third laboratory value to consider is the bicarbonate ion concentration. If it is above the normal range, the patient has metabolic alkalosis, which may be the primary problem or may be compensatory. If the bicarbonate ion concentration is below the normal range, then the patient has primary or compensatory metabolic acidosis. A bicarbonate ion concentration within the normal range indicates no metabolic acid-base disorder. The differentiation between primary and compensatory imbalances is made by considering the pH. A patient who has a *primary metabolic acidosis* would be expected to have a pH below 7.40. A *compensatory metabolic acidosis* would be a response to a primary respiratory alkalosis, so the pH would be above 7.40. Following similar logic, with a *primary metabolic alkalosis*, the pH would be above 7.40; with a *compensatory metabolic alkalosis*, the pH would be below that value.

Once the three values have been examined, the final step in interpreting arterial blood gas values is to compare the interpretation with the patient's history and condition to verify that it makes sense. The principles of laboratory value interpretation presented in this section apply to

TABLE 7-5	Mixed Acid-Base Imbalances		
Concurrent Primary Acid-Base Imbalances	**Example of Etiology**	**Blood Gas Values**
Respiratory acidosis and metabolic alkalosis	COPD and emesis	pH possibly near normal $PaCO_2$ increased HCO_3^- increased
Respiratory alkalosis and metabolic acidosis	Salicylate poisoning	pH possibly near normal $PaCO_2$ decreased HCO_3^- decreased
Respiratory acidosis and metabolic acidosis	COPD and diarrhea	pH greatly decreased $PaCO_2$ increased HCO_3^- increased
Respiratory alkalosis and metabolic alkalosis	Hyperventilation from pain or sepsis and massive blood transfusion	pH greatly increased $PaCO_2$ decreased HCO_3^- increased
Metabolic acidosis and metabolic alkalosis	Renal failure and emesis	Values depend on severity and duration of the two imbalances
Two different kinds of metabolic acidosis	Diabetic ketoacidosis and lactic acidosis	pH greatly decreased $PaCO_2$ normal or decreased (compensation) HCO_3^- decreased

COPD, chronic obstructive pulmonary disease.
From Felver L: Acid-base balance and imbalances. In Patrick M, Bruno P, Woods S et al (eds): Medical–Surgical Nursing: Pathophysiological Concepts, 2nd ed, p 287. Philadelphia, JB Lippincott, 1991.

patients who have only one primary acid-base imbalance. Mixed acid-base imbalances (more than one concurrent primary imbalance) are presented in the next section.

Mixed Acid–Base Imbalances

Occasionally, a patient may have more than one primary acid-base imbalance at the same time. In this circumstance, coexisting primary acidosis and alkalosis may somewhat neutralize each other so that the pH is near normal while the $PaCO_2$ and bicarbonate ion concentration are grossly abnormal. Alternatively, two primary disorders that cause the same pH alteration (e.g., types of coexisting alkalosis) can create a pH that rapidly approaches the fatal limit. Examples of mixed acid-base imbalances are presented in Table 7-5.

SUMMARY

This chapter describes the mechanisms by which the body maintains acid-base balance and explains acid-base imbalances. Respiratory acid-base imbalances are disorders of too much or too little carbonic acid (carbon dioxide and water). Their laboratory marker is an altered $PaCO_2$. The body compensates for an ongoing respiratory acid-base disorder by excreting more or fewer metabolic acids in the urine to normalize the pH.

Metabolic acid-base imbalances are disorders of too many or too few metabolic acids. Their laboratory marker is an altered bicarbonate ion concentration. The body compensates for metabolic acid-base disorders by adjusting alveolar ventilation to excrete more or less carbonic acid to normalize the pH.

In addition to their other effects, acid-base imbalances alter cardiac contractility and may cause cardiac arrhythmias. They influence the degree of vasoconstriction in various vascular beds. Thus, an understanding of acid-base balance and imbalances is important in the care of cardiac patients.

REFERENCES

1. Aalkajaer C, Peng HL: pH and smooth muscle. Acta Physiol Scand 161: 557–566, 1997
2. Carvalho CR, Barbas CS, Medeiros DM et al: Temporal hemodynamic effects of permissive hypercapnia associated with ideal PEEP in ARDS. Am J Respir Crit Care Med 156: 1458–1466, 1997
3. Churcott CS, Moyes CD, Bressler BH et al: Temperature and pH effects on Ca+ sensitivity of cardiac myofibrils: A comparison of trout with mammals. Am J Physiol 267: R62–R70, 1994
4. Combes P, Durand M: Combined effects of nicardipine and hypocapnic alkalosis on cerebral vasomotor activity and intracranial pressure in man. Eur J Clin Pharmacol 41: 207–210, 1991
5. Combes P, Fauvage B: Systemic vasomotor interaction between nicardipine and hypocapnic alkalosis in man. Intensive Care Med 18: 89–92, 1992
6. Dormans TF, Gerlag PG, Russel FG et al: Combination diuretic therapy in severe congestive heart failure. Drugs 55: 165–172, 1998
7. Fineman JA, Wong J, Solfer SJ: Hyperoxia and alkalosis produce pulmonary vasodilation independent of endothelium-derived nitric oxide in newborn lambs. Pediatr Res 33: 341–346, 1993
8. Good DW: Ammonium transport by the thick ascending limb of Henle's loop. Annu Rev Physiol 56: 623–654, 1994
9. Gurivicius J, Salem MR, Metwally AA et al: Contribution of nitric oxide to coronary vasodilation during hypercapnic acidosis. Am J Physiol 268: H39–H47, 1995

10. Guyton AC, Hall JE: Textbook of Medical Physiology, 9th ed. Philadelphia, WB Saunders, 1996

11. Halperin ML, Goldstein MB: Fluid, Electrolyte, and Acid-Base Physiology, 2nd ed. Philadelphia, WB Saunders, 1994

12. Harrison SM, Frampton JE, McCall E et al: Contraction and intracellular Ca^{2+}, Na^+, and H^+ during acidosis in rat ventricular myocytes. Am J Physiol 262: C348–C357, 1992

13. Hunjan S, Mason RP, Mehta VD et al: Simultaneous intracellular and extracellular pH measurement in the heart by 19F NMR of 6-fluoropyridoxol. Magn Reson Med 39: 551–556, 1998

14. Ishizaka H, Kuo L: Acidosis-induced coronary arteriolar dilation is mediated by ATP-sensitive potassium channels in vascular smooth muscle. Circ Res 78: 50–57, 1996

15. Leitch SP, Patterson DJ: Interactive effects of K^+, acidosis, and catecholamines on isolated rabbit heart: Implications for exercise. J Appl Physiol 77: 1164–1171, 1994

16. Lejeune P, Brimioulle S, Leeman M et al: Enhancement of hypoxic pulmonary vasoconstriction by metabolic acidosis in dog. Anesthesiology 73: 256–264, 1990

17. Mayoux E, Coutry N, Lechene P et al: Effects of acidosis and alkalosis on mechanical properties of hypertrophied rat heart fiber bundles. Am J Physiol 266: H2052–H2060, 1994

18. Modest VE, Butterworth JF IV: Effect of pH and lidocaine on beta-adrenergic receptor binding: Interaction during resuscitation? Chest 108: 1373–1379, 1995

19. Molfino NA, Nannini LJ, Martelli AN et al: Respiratory arrest in near-fatal asthma. N Engl J Med 324: 285–288, 1991

20. Mora GA, Pizarro C, Jacobs MJ et al: Experimental model of single ventricle: Influence of carbon dioxide on pulmonary vascular dynamics. Circulation 90(5): II43–II46, 1994

21. Nakanishi T, Su H, Momma K: Developmental changes in the effect of acidosis on contraction, intracellular pH, and calcium in the rabbit mesenteric small artery. Pediatr Res 42: 750–757, 1997

22. Onishi K, Sekioka K, Ishisu R et al: Decrease in oxygen cost of contractility during hypocapnic alkalosis in canine hearts. Am J Physiol 270: H1905–H1913, 1996

23. Orchard CH, Kentish JC: Effects of changes of pH on the contractile function of cardiac muscle. Am J Physiol 258: C967–C981, 1990

24. Peng HL, Jensen PE, Nilsson H et al: Effect of acidosis on tension and $[Ca^{2+}]i$ in rat cerebral arteries: Is there a role for membrane potential? Am J Physiol 274: H655–H662, 1998

25. Rose BD: Clinical Physiology of Acid-Base and Electrolyte Disorders, 4th ed. New York, McGraw-Hill, 1994

26. Serieix D, Delayance S, Paris M et al: Tris-hydroxymethyl aminomethane and sodium bicarbonate to buffer metabolic acidosis in an isolated heart model. Am J Respir Crit Care Med 155: 957–963, 1997

27. Tang WC, Weil MH, Gazmuri RJ et al: Reversible impairment of myocardial contractility due to hypercarbic acidosis in the isolated perfused rat heart. Crit Care Med 19: 218–224, 1991

28. Vandenberg JI, Metcalfe JC, Grace AA: Intracellular pH recovery during respiratory acidosis in perfused hearts. Am J Physiol 266: C489–C497, 1994

29. Watanabe Y, Dohi S, Iida H et al: The effects of bupivacaine and ropivacaine on baroreflex sensitivity with or without respiratory acidosis and alkalosis in rats. Anesth Analg 84: 398–404, 1997

30. Yamaguchi K, Takasugi T, Fujita H et al: Endothelial modulation of pH-dependent pressor response in isolated perfused rat lungs. Am J Physiol 270: H252–H258, 1996

8

Sleep

KATHRYN A. LEE

*The sleeping patient is still a patient, his disease goes on not only while he sleeps but may indeed progress in an entirely different fashion from its progression during the waking state.**

Disrupted sleep and sleep-related changes in physiologic function have a significant impact on patients with cardiovascular disease. This chapter examines normal sleep patterns, changes in cardiorespiratory and other physiologic functions during sleep, interactions between sleep and cardiovascular disease, and nursing management to promote adequate restful sleep.

NATURE OF SLEEP

Approximately one-third of life is spent asleep, and the recurring cycle of sleep and wakefulness is the most noticeable human circadian (daily) rhythm. Sleep can be defined behaviorally as a spontaneous, reversible, recurring state of reduced awareness of and responsiveness to the environment, usually accompanied by a recumbent posture, relative motor inactivity, and closed eyes.[35] Sleep is also an active physiologic process that alternates between two different states, non—rapid-eye-movement (NREM) sleep and rapid-eye-movement (REM) sleep, with a total of five stages. Sleep stages and wakefulness are identified by *polysomnography,* the application of a set of pattern recognition rules to a recording of three electrophysiologic signals. Brain waves are recorded using the electroencephalogram (EEG), eye movements using the electro-oculogram, and muscle tone using the chin electromyogram (EMG; Fig. 8-1). At the usual recording speed of 1 cm/s, a standard 30-cm page represents a 30-second period, or *epoch.* Each epoch is assigned a single sleep stage score based primarily on changes in EEG frequency (in cycles/second, or hertz [Hz]) and amplitude (in microvolts [μV]), with confirmation by the electro-oculogram and EMG patterns.[36,180] In addition to the sleep staging signals, polysomnography often includes other physiologic variables, such as respiratory movements of the chest and abdomen, airflow at the nose and mouth, arterial oxygen saturation, electrocardiogram (ECG), and leg movements (anterior tibialis EMG)[142] (Fig. 8–2).

*From Eugene D. Robin: Some interrelationships between sleep and disease. Arch Intern Med 102: 674, 1958.

States of Wakefulness and Sleep

Typical EEG patterns during wakefulness and sleep are shown in Figure 8-3. During relaxed wakefulness with the eyes closed, the EEG consists mostly of α waves, which have a frequency of 8 to 13 Hz, on a background of faster, mixed-frequency, low-amplitude activity. REMs and blinks may occur, and muscle tone is usually at its highest level.[36,66,180]

Non—rapid-eye-movement sleep is divided somewhat arbitrarily into four stages based on the EEG pattern. Sleep depth increases from stage 1 to 4 in that the sleeper becomes harder to awaken.[19,35] In stages 1 and 2, or light sleep, the EEG consists of relatively low-amplitude waves with a predominant frequency of 2 to 7 Hz. High, narrow-vertex sharp waves may appear late in stage 1. Stage 2 is identified by two sporadic waveforms that stand out from the background EEG, sleep spindles and K complexes. Sleep spindles are waxing—waning bursts of waves in the 12- to 14-Hz range. They originate in the thalamus and are thought to reflect impulses that inhibit the relay of sensory information to the cerebral cortex.[213] K complexes consist of a sharp negative wave (upward deflection by EEG recording convention) followed by a slower positive wave (downward deflection). They occur spontaneously and in response to mild external stimuli, such as sounds.[66] Stages 3 and 4, also called slow-wave or deep sleep, are differentiated by the percentage of slow (2 Hz or less), high-amplitude (>75 μV) EEG waves. They account for 20% to 50% of the epoch in stage 3 and over 50% in stage 4. The eyes are relatively quiet during NREM sleep, except for slow rolling movements that usually occur at the beginning of stage 1. Muscle tone is moderately reduced from the waking level.[36,66,180]

Rapid-eye-movement sleep is a different neurophysiologic state. It is considered a single stage, although two types of REM events have been identified, tonic and phasic. Tonic events occur throughout a period of REM sleep. They include intense brain activity with a mixed-frequency, relatively low-amplitude EEG similar to stage 1 and complete loss of postural muscle tone due to hyperpolarization of spinal motoneurons. The sleeper has an active brain in a paralyzed body, with only the diaphragm and extraocular

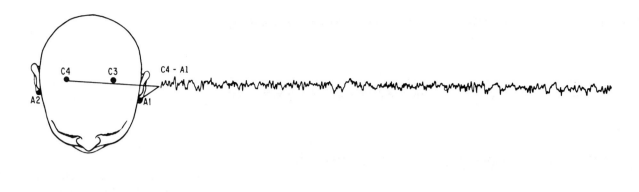

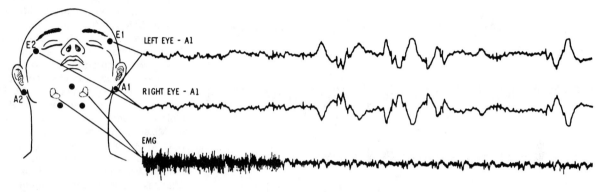

FIGURE 8-1 Placement of electrodes for **(top)** electroencephalogram and **(bottom)** electro-oculogram and electromyogram in polygraphic sleep recordings. (From Rechtschaffen A, Kales A [eds]): A Manual of Standardized Terminology, Techniques and Scoring System for Sleep Stages of Human Subjects, p 15. Los Angeles, Brain Information Service/Brain Research Institute, University of California, 1968.)

FIGURE 8-2 Recording of multiple physiologic signals in a formal polysomnographic sleep evaluation. In this example, the patient has an obstructive apnea with cessation of oral and nasal airflow despite effort to breathe. The interrupted breathing is accompanied by a decrease in oxygen saturation and slowing of the heart rate and is followed by an arousal. ECG, electrocardiogram; EEG, electroencephalogram; EMG, electromyogram: EOG, electro-oculogram. (From White D: Obstructive sleep apnea. Hosp Pract 27(5A): 68, 1992.)

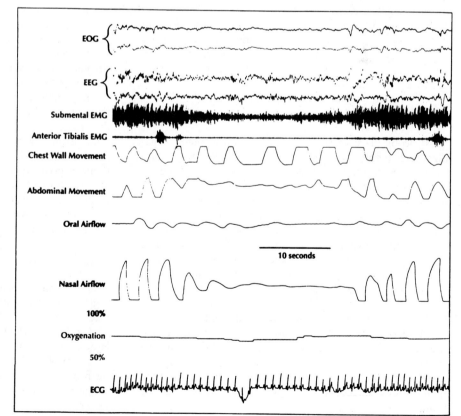

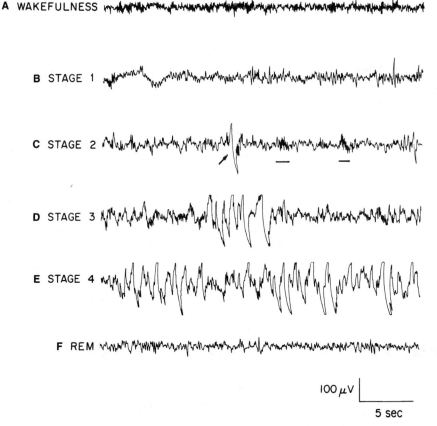

FIGURE 8-3 Electroencephalogram patterns in wakefulness and sleep in a young adult. **(A)** Rhythmic α-wave activity at 8 to 10 Hz in relaxed wakefulness with the eyes closed. **(B)** Mixed-frequency, relatively low-amplitude waves in non–rapid-eye-movement stage 1, with a vertex sharp wave toward the end of the tracing. **(C)** K complex *(arrow)* and sleep spindles *(underscored)* begin in stage 2. **(D, E)** Progressively greater percentages of slow, high-amplitude waves in stages 3 and 4. **(F)** Mixed-frequency, relatively low-amplitude waves in rapid-eye-movement sleep, similar to the pattern in stage 1. (From Dement W, Richardson G. Prinz P et al: Changes of sleep and wakefulness with age. In Finch CE, Schneider EL (eds): Handbook of the Biology of Aging, 2nd ed, p 694. New York, Van Nostrand Reinhold, 1985.)

muscles retaining substantial tone. Phasic events occur intermittently in REM sleep, including bursts of REMs for which the stage is named, muscle twitches in the face and distal extremities (potent motor excitation briefly overrides the paralysis), and fluctuations in blood pressure, heart rate, and breathing.[36,39,66] The depth of REM sleep is usually similar to that found in NREM stage 2.[19]

Sleep Cycle

Most people have their major sleep period at night, organized in a rhythmic sequence of sleep stages (Fig. 8-4). After a short period of relaxed wakefulness, a young adult enters sleep with a few minutes of stage 1, followed by a descent into stage 2 for 10 to 25 minutes, a few minutes of stage 3, and about 20 to 40 minutes of stage 4. The sleeper then reascends through stages 3 and 2 and has a first brief REM period approximately 90 minutes after sleep onset. The cycle begins again with stage 2 and repeats another three to five times during the night. Slow-wave sleep occupies less of the second cycle and may then disappear, whereas REM periods lengthen across the night. Therefore, most slow-wave sleep occurs in the first third of the night, and most REM occurs in the last third. If an awakening occurs, the sleep cycle starts again with stage 1. Thus, frequent disruptions of sleep interfere with advancing far enough into the cycle to reach slow-wave and REM sleep, and the time spent in these stages is reduced, whereas the time in stage 1 is increased.[35]

Adults sleep on their sides for approximately two-thirds of the night. Position changes occur two or three times per hour, with major body shifts at changes from stage 4 to lighter NREM stages or from REM to NREM sleep.[52,125] A sudden muscle contraction involving all or part of the body (hypnic jerk) occasionally accompanies sleep onset, often in association with stress or irregular sleep schedules.[35,81]

Approximately 90% of people awakened from REM sleep and 60% awakened from NREM sleep report having dreams. In NREM sleep, this involuntary mental activity tends to have a dull, sketchy, thought-like quality without much real thinking or involvement toward any particular point or goal. In contrast, dreams recalled from REM sleep are usually vivid, well-formed, story-like narratives. Dreams include more visual imagery and emotional tone as the night progresses in relation to longer REM periods and greater intensity of phasic events.[38,73,224]

Sleep Time

Healthy, young adults sleep approximately 7.5 to 8.5 hours nightly. Approximately 5% of the sleep period is spent in stage 1, 45% to 55% in stage 2, 20% in stages 3 and 4, and 20% to 25% in REM sleep, with little or no time awake.[35] In large survey studies, unusually short or long sleep lengths (less than 4 to 6 hours or more than 9 to 10 hours) have been associated with increased rates of illness and death, suggesting that common factors may affect both sleep and general health status.[122,241]

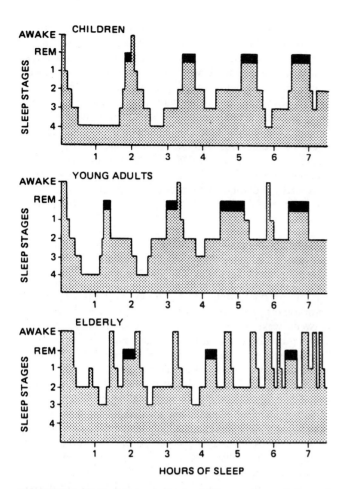

FIGURE 8-4 Normal sleep cycles in children, young adults, and the elderly. Rapid-eye-movement (REM) sleep (*darkened area*) occurs cyclically throughout the night at intervals of approximately 90 minutes in all age groups and shows little variation in the different age groups, whereas stage 4 non-REM (NREM) sleep decreases with age. In addition, the elderly have frequent awakenings and a marked increase in total wake time. (From Kales A, Kales JD: Sleep disorder. N Engl J Med 290: 488, 1974.)

Sleepiness

A continuum between being very alert and very sleepy provides a background for all waking endeavors and is a far more important dimension of human function than commonly recognized. Physiologic sleepiness, defined as the tendency to fall asleep, may go unnoticed subjectively when masked by stimulating factors such as movement, excitement, high motivation, or hunger. As personal experience attests, however, a sleep tendency can be unmasked by situational factors such as boredom, a warm, dark room, or a prolonged, dull task. Sleepiness has a biphasic circadian rhythm, with an increased sleep tendency in the mid-afternoon and—as is well known to night-shift workers—in the early morning hours[2,34,192] (Fig. 8-5). Many adults are chronically sleepy in the daytime because of insufficient or disrupted nighttime sleep. For example, people often voluntarily shorten their weekday sleep periods because of perceived social or job constraints.[181,188] Sleepy people experience fatigue, difficulty concentrating, and memory lapses and may unintentionally fall asleep at inopportune times. Sleepiness has serious consequences for public safety, with numerous examples of transportation and industrial accidents in which sleepiness was a contributing factor.[141,148]

Effect of Aging

With increasing age, particularly in men, sleep becomes lighter and more fragmented (see Fig. 8-4). In contrast to young adults, older people usually spend more time in bed but less time asleep (reduced sleep efficiency) and are more easily awakened from sleep. The time needed to fall asleep (sleep latency) shows little change with aging, but more nighttime awakenings, brief arousals, and stage changes occur. There is a striking reduction in slow-wave sleep (stages 3 and 4) and an increase in stage 1 sleep, with little change in the percentages of stage 2 and REM sleep. Bedtime and wakeup time come earlier (circadian phase advance), the daytime sleep tendency may be increased,

FIGURE 8-5 Mean sleep latency in minutes in young adults (*open circles*) and old adults (*solid circles*) at different times of day. The shaded area represents the nighttime sleep period. A biphasic rhythm exists with maximal sleepiness in the mid-afternoon and early morning, as indicated by shorter latencies. (From Richardson GS, Carskadon MA, Orav EF et al: Circadian variation of sleep tendency in elderly and young adult subjects. Sleep 5(Suppl 2): S87, 1982.)

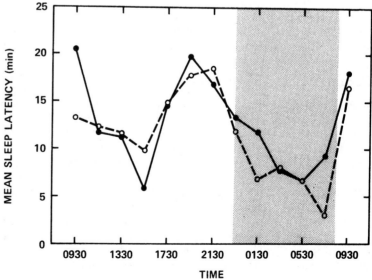

daytime napping is more common, and tolerance for changes in the sleep—wake schedule is reduced. These age-related sleep patterns occur independently of illness and may be related to changes in the body's circadian pacemaker, probably located in the suprachiasmatic nucleus of the anterior hypothalamus.[16,29,34] Sleep apnea (discussed later) and periodic leg movements (involuntary repetitive jerks) are more common in older adults and can contribute to sleep disruption.[3,4] Other factors may include poor sleep habits, a reduced activity level, psychological concerns, physical illness, and medications.[16,138,183] Not surprisingly, older people often complain about their sleep and use sleeping pills more often than other age groups.[247]

Function of Sleep

Despite intense scientific study and general consensus that sleep is a physiologic necessity, its function remains speculative. Sleep is clearly needed for alert waking function, and continued wakefulness leads predictably to sleepiness and reduced mental performance. After several weeks of sleep deprivation, rats manifest a syndrome of debilitation and impaired thermoregulation, and eventually die.[179] Horne[99] makes a distinction between *core* and *optional* sleep. He argues that core sleep, including most of slow-wave sleep and part of REM sleep, is essential to repair waking wear and tear on the brain. The longer a person is awake before sleeping, the longer is the period of core sleep. The remaining, optional sleep is under the behavioral drive to sleep associated with the sleep—wake rhythm and can be modified somewhat to suit individual circumstances.[99]

PHYSIOLOGIC RESPONSES DURING SLEEP

The physiologic basis of nursing care has rested almost entirely on studies of responses during wakefulness. The notion that regulatory processes may be different during sleep is relatively recent. Sleep has been found, however, to affect the regulation of virtually every physiologic process that has been studied, with most major functions differing between the NREM and REM states. Findings related to cardiovascular and respiratory function have particular importance for cardiovascular nursing care.

Cardiovascular Responses

Sleep is accompanied by changes in blood pressure and heart rate, both major determinants of myocardial oxygen demand. NREM sleep appears to be a relatively protected state because blood pressure and heart rate decrease and become more stable as sleep progresses to deeper stages. During slow-wave sleep, blood pressure is approximately 10% to 20% lower than in quiet wakefulness, whereas the heart rate is decreased by approximately 5% to 10%.[26,41,116,206,209] Brief surges in blood pressure and heart rate occur with K complexes, arousals, and large body movements.[100,206,209] Sharp increases occur with morning awakening and beginning the day's activities,[72,130,155] as well

as after other periods of sleep, such as afternoon naps.[155] The decreased blood pressure in NREM sleep is related to reduced sympathetic vasomotor tone in skeletal muscle vessels, whereas the decrease in heart rate reflects enhanced vagal parasympathetic input to the heart.[100,137,166,209]

Rapid-eye-movement sleep brings an increase in cardiovascular demands. Although blood pressure and heart rate have average levels near those observed in light NREM sleep or quiet wakefulness, their variability increases markedly during phasic REM sleep, with wide, erratic fluctuations.[41,116,206,209,250] These changes are related to bursts of increased sympathetic activity and to reduced vagal input to the heart.[100,137,166,209,250]

Respiratory Responses

Sleep alters breathing patterns, ventilation, and arterial blood gas values. Periodic breathing, a cyclic waxing and waning of tidal volume, sometimes with brief apnea, is common at sleep onset in association with fluctuations between wakefulness and light sleep. Breathing is remarkably regular, however, in stable stage 2 and slow-wave sleep. The pattern becomes faster and more erratic during phasic REM sleep, and brief apnea is common.[121,233]

Minute ventilation falls during NREM sleep, mainly because of reduced tidal volume, with an average decrease of approximately 13% in stage 2 and 15% in stage 4 compared with quiet wakefulness. This hypoventilation leads to small changes in arterial blood gases, including a mild hypercapnia, with rises of 2 to 7 mm Hg in carbon dioxide tension and decreases of 0.01 to 0.06 units in pH, and a mild hypoxemia, with decreases of 3 to 10 mm Hg in oxygen tension and 2% or less in oxygen saturation.[121,233] Data about REM sleep are somewhat contradictory but suggest that minute ventilation, tidal volume, and respiratory frequency are similar to those in NREM sleep, with comparable or greater changes in blood gas values.[121,233]

Factors that contribute to hypoventilation in NREM sleep include reduced central drive to breathe due to loss of the wakefulness stimulus and increased upper airway resistance to airflow due to reduced pharyngeal muscle tone. Tone in the intercostal muscles and diaphragm, however, is maintained or increased.[103,121] In REM sleep, tone is lost in both the intercostal and upper airway muscles, reducing the rib cage contribution to breathing and increasing upper airway resistance; the diaphragm, however, is relatively spared from REM-related paralysis. Phasic REM sleep also includes dysrhythmic changes in stimulation of brainstem respiratory neurons, resulting in the erratic breathing pattern.[121,233]

The arterial blood gas changes stimulate an adaptive increase in ventilation, although the response is less effective in sleep than in wakefulness. In men, the ventilatory responses to both hypercapnia and hypoxemia decrease by approximately half from wakefulness to NREM sleep, with a further reduction in REM sleep. Women respond similarly to hypercapnia but somewhat differently to hypoxemia—women have a lower ventilatory response than men when awake and little change in NREM sleep, but a similar fall in REM sleep.[58,233] Prior sleep deprivation impairs the ventilatory responses during wakefulness.[42,198,235]

Waking up is a second adaptive response to blood gas changes during sleep because the change stimulates ventilation and permits voluntary action to cope with the situation, such as moving a pillow that interferes with breathing. Hypercapnia is a relatively effective arousal stimulus, awakening most healthy subjects before carbon dioxide tension rises 15 mm Hg; concurrent hypoxemia enhances the response. Hypoxemia alone, however, is a poor arousal stimulus; study subjects often fail to awaken despite an oxygen saturation as low as 70%.[58,233]

Adaptive responses that protect the airways also are less effective during sleep. Respiratory secretions are cleared less readily owing to diminished mucociliary clearance,[10] and the tendency to aspirate increases.[102] In addition, sleep suppresses the protective cough response to irritating substances in the airways. Coughing during sleep is rare and has not been documented during slow-wave sleep.[58,105,175]

Aging also affects breathing during sleep. Research suggests that approximately one-fourth to one-third of elderly people,[12] and perhaps far more,[4] have a significant number of periods during sleep when breathing is reduced (hypopnea) or absent (apnea) for 10 seconds or longer. The arousals that terminate apneas, although adaptive responses, may account for some of the sleep fragmentation found in the elderly. The long-term effect of sleep-disordered breathing is uncertain, but some evidence suggests that it may insidiously contribute to development of hypertension, arrhythmias, and reduced pulmonary function.[13,14]

Other Responses

Body temperature is regulated at a lower set-point in NREM sleep than in wakefulness. In combination with reduced motor activity, this results in a decrease in temperature at sleep onset.[9] The normal regulating mechanisms are markedly inhibited during REM sleep, however, and during this stage of sleep, body temperature is influenced more by the environment than the hypothalamus.[78] Body temperature also has an independent circadian rhythm that, in day-active people, peaks in the late afternoon and reaches a minimum in the early morning hours of sleep.[147,151] Body temperature rhythms become altered when patients are receiving hemodialysis, and this alteration can adversely affect sleep.[171]

Sleep length depends on the phase of the circadian temperature rhythm at bedtime because the rising phase triggers awakening from sleep. A sleep period that begins when body temperature is low—for example, going to bed at 3 AM—is relatively short because temperature soon rises. In contrast, a sleep period that begins when temperature is high is relatively long because a rise in temperature does not occur for some time.[47,75] The body temperature rhythm shifts a little earlier (phase advance) with aging, which may partly explain why many older people have an earlier wakeup time than younger adults.[31]

Neurologic changes in sleep include higher brain blood flow than when awake. A small to moderate rise in brain blood flow occurs in NREM sleep that can be explained by the mild hypercapnia associated with reduced ventilation. The marked rise in brain blood flow in REM sleep, however, cannot be explained by hypercapnia alone.[58,80] Brain imaging techniques show that metabolic activity in the brain in NREM sleep is approximately one-fourth to one-third lower than in quiet wakefulness, whereas in REM sleep it is similar to the waking level. Areas with higher metabolic activity in REM sleep include the left side of the brain (right side when awake), limbic system (involved in emotions), and visual association areas.[76] Poor performance on tasks after sleep deprivation is associated with reduced metabolic activity in the frontal lobes, thalamus, and midbrain, which may be associated with the state of reduced alertness.[246] Intracranial pressure has been observed to increase at sleep onset and during light sleep, decrease variably during slow-wave sleep, and rise significantly during REM sleep, perhaps in relation to increased brain blood flow.[161]

Urine flow is reduced and more concentrated during sleep, particularly during the REM state, with a diminished excretion of sodium, chloride, potassium, and calcium. The mechanisms involved in these changes in urine flow and electrolyte excretion are complex and include changes in renal blood flow, glomerular filtration, hormone secretion (vasopressin, aldosterone, prolactin, parathormone), and sympathetic neural stimulation.[194] Because nighttime potassium excretion is reduced, potassium infusions given at that time may lead to higher serum levels than daytime infusions.[150]

From infancy to old age, males have penile erections (nocturnal penile tumescence) during REM sleep. Total tumescence time is greatest just before and during puberty and then may gradually decline. Sleep-related erectile activity can be monitored to aid in differentiating physical and psychological components of impotence.[113]

Endocrine hormone secretion is influenced by sleep. For example, growth hormone secretion is highly dependent on sleep. Most secretion occurs during the first few hours after sleep onset in association with slow-wave sleep. If sleep is advanced or delayed, growth hormone secretion shifts accordingly. In contrast, thyroid hormone and cortisol secretion are suppressed by sleep but also have independent circadian rhythms. Thyroid hormone secretion rises to a late evening peak, whereas cortisol concentration increases in the latter half of the night and peaks toward the end of the normal sleep period or soon after awakening in the morning.[146]

The hormone melatonin, which is secreted by the pineal gland, induces sleepiness and is under study as a therapeutic agent. Melatonin has a marked circadian rhythm that is closely linked to the light—dark cycle and to the sleep—wake, temperature, and cortisol rhythms. A late evening surge in melatonin begins at darkness, approximately 2 hours before bedtime, and is considered a marker of the body's circadian timing system. Secretion peaks at approximately 3 AM, then is suppressed by daylight to levels that are barely detectable. Bright light exposure suppresses melatonin secretion and can be used to reset a person's circadian clock.[46,128,201]

SLEEP AND CARDIOVASCULAR DISEASE

Altered sleep patterns are a common human response to illness. In addition, physiologic changes during sleep sometimes accentuate the underlying health problem. The sleeping hours merit special attention in patients with cardiovascular disease because both poor sleep and adverse physiologic changes can occur.

Sleep in Coronary Heart Disease

Although more than 13 million Americans are estimated to have coronary heart disease,[163] research about their sleep patterns remains relatively limited. Available information is often based on small numbers of subjects and is complicated by variations in age, sex, type and severity of cardiovascular impairment, medications, and study methods that make comparison of findings difficult. Despite these limitations, however, the research conveys a consistent theme that patients with coronary heart disease often have disturbed sleep.

Impaired cardiac function from any cause can produce symptoms such as chest pain and dyspnea that interfere with sleep. Even when patients with a variety of diseases are considered, cardiovascular symptoms are a major factor associated with complaints of reduced total sleep and increased nighttime wakefulness.[106] The psychological impact of heart disease also has a major impact on sleep. A myocardial infarction (MI), for example, not only affects physical health and comfort, but influences social relationships, living patterns, work options and income, and sense of personal vulnerability. Fears of death, reinfarction, or inability to resume former living patterns are common.[44,88,156] It is not surprising that anxiety and depression, typically accompanied by poor sleep, are common after an MI, and many patients report troublesome insomnia that lasts for months and sometimes years.[199,205,214,215,243]

Poor sleep also appears to be a precursor to MI. Complaints of insomnia, habitual short sleep, waking up exhausted, daytime sleepiness, and frequent napping are common in the preceding months.[5,32,223] A common link with the period of depression that often precedes an MI is a possible explanation for these symptoms.[5,32]

Sleep in the Coronary Care Unit

Specialized coronary care units (CCUs) convincingly reduce hospital deaths after MI,[163] but they can be far from optimal environments for sleep. The setting is unfamiliar and perhaps frightening to patients, the schedule and bedtime routine differ from those at home, noise and lighting may never be completely suppressed, interruptions for patient care procedures are frequent, and personnel may lack awareness that patients have a problem sleeping. In addition, some medications may result in the appearance of "sleep" when in fact the patient is merely experiencing the sedating side effect of the medication and is not truly asleep or perceiving that sleep occurred.

In polysomnographic studies, CCU patients typically have a pattern of light, fragmented sleep with reduced slow-wave and REM sleep, frequent stage changes, and considerable nighttime wakefulness.[37,55,114,183] Although total sleep time is not necessarily reduced, the normal circadian sleep—wake rhythm is disrupted, with sleep occurring off and on during the 24 hours.[114] Sleep is more disturbed as illness severity increases,[55] with an MI compared with angina,[114]

and during hemodynamic monitoring.[37] Sleep patterns usually improve over time,[205] probably in relation to such factors as improved health status, fewer interruptions for care, and increased familiarity with the CCU environment.

Sleep After Cardiac Surgery

Sleep disruption after surgery is related to the magnitude of procedure and associated postoperative care. Patients who undergo cardiac surgery experience dramatic sleep pattern disturbances. Severe sleep deprivation is common in the early postoperative period, with only a few hours of fragmented sleep each 24 hours and virtual absence of slow-wave and REM sleep.[64,107,168] Contributing factors may include persistent interruptions and activity, high noise and lighting levels, anxiety, pain, and medications.[107,110,143,168,229,244] Sleep deprivation often is implicated as a risk factor for the postoperative delirium that develops in some cardiac surgical patients. Severity of sleep loss, however, does not differentiate patients with delirium from those who recover uneventfully.[107,168]

Although sleep patterns gradually improve after cardiac surgery, slow-wave and REM sleep may be suppressed for several weeks after the patient returns home,[168] with many patients reporting continuing sleep disturbances.[117] A contributing factor for some patients with heart valve replacements is noise generated by the mechanical valve prosthesis, including audible high-frequency closing clicks and low-frequency sounds conducted by body tissues.[152]

CARDIAC EVENTS DURING SLEEP

For many years, there has been speculation that sleep is a time of increased physiologic risk for patients with cardiovascular disease, particularly the early morning hours when sleep is primarily REM with its bursts of sympathetic activity, or when medications are discontinued and REM rebound occurs. A growing database suggests that patients can experience both beneficial and potentially harmful physiologic changes during sleep.

Angina

Anginal chest pain results from myocardial ischemia, an imbalance between coronary blood flow and myocardial requirements (see Chapter 20). In its classic form, angina is precipitated by physical exertion or other situations that increase myocardial oxygen demand.[109] Blood pressure and heart rate characteristically increase before appearance of ischemic changes in the ECG in both daytime and sleep-related anginal episodes (see Chapter 15).[131,177,178]

Classic (effort) angina occurs more often in the morning hours after awakening than at night.[162,186] Sleep is generally a time of reduced myocardial demand because of decreased blood pressure and heart rate. Patients with known daytime ischemia report relatively few nighttime anginal episodes and usually have reduced or unchanged ECG evidence of ischemia.[115,131] When greater ischemic changes occur at night, they are often asymptomatic (silent ischemia).[136,162,178,216] Nighttime chest pain is more likely to occur in patients with other symptoms of cardiac impairment, such as congestive failure.[129] Anginal episodes have a variable relation to sleep stage. Two early reports linked angina to REM sleep,[165,237] but most studies found no particular sleep stage predominance.[136,216]

Variant (Prinzmetal) angina is a less common form of ischemic chest pain. It is caused by coronary artery spasm and is characterized by angina at rest and ST segment elevation. Variant angina has a clear circadian rhythm, with episodes clustering in the early morning hours of sleep.[6,7,162,227,232] At one time, increased sympathetic activity during REM sleep was the proposed mechanism for coronary spasm. Except for an anecdotal report,[118] however, no consistent association between REM sleep and variant angina has been found. In addition, variant angina is not preceded by a rise in heart rate[177,227] and seldom occurs near the noontime peak of plasma norepinephrine,[176] which are other manifestations of sympathetic activity. The mechanism that underlies coronary artery spasm remains unclear.

Arrhythmias

Sinus bradycardia and sinus arrhythmia are the most frequent changes in heart rhythm during sleep in healthy people, consistent with the dominance of parasympathetic activity. Bradycardia during sleep is more common in men than in women, and the difference between daytime and nighttime heart rates decreases with age.[111] Heart rates less than 40 beats/min and sinus pauses longer than 2 seconds are rare,[27,69,111,207] except in highly trained athletes.[225,226] Although heart rate usually is lowest in slow-wave sleep, little information is available about sleep stage relations of bradyarrhythmias. A few instances of unusually long episodes of sinus arrest during REM sleep were reported and probably are related to abnormal vagal parasympathetic activity.[84]

Premature ventricular contractions (PVCs) are common after an MI and, when frequent or complex, carry a higher mortality risk[15,154] (see Chapter 14). Sleep usually suppresses the frequency of PVCs in both healthy people[27,69,207,219] and those with heart disease.[132,133,174] Nighttime PVCs have no consistent relation to sleep stage.[65,149,191] The mechanism of PVC reduction during sleep is probably a decrease in cardiac sympathetic activity with an increase in vagal parasympathetic activity.[153] PVC frequency, however, also may be independently related to heart rate[174,242] and is increased by hypoxemia.[95,204] The latter mechanism is especially important in patients with sleep apnea and chronic obstructive pulmonary disease (COPD), in whom PVCs are clearly more common during sleep than wakefulness (see discussion later).

In evaluating the evidence about sleep-related arrhythmias, Motta and Guilleminault[153] concluded that fewer arrhythmias occur during sleep than during wakefulness, although a subset of patients experience an increase in arrhythmias. They stated that concern about dangerous arrhythmias being precipitated by REM sleep remains speculative and probably is true in only a small number of patients.[153]

Timing of Cardiovascular Events

The timing of MIs has a marked circadian pattern, with the highest frequency of onset in the period between 6 AM and 12 noon. A major peak occurs at approximately 8 to 10 AM, with a three– to fourfold increase compared with the minimum at approximately 11 PM to 1 AM.[97,159,240] The morning peak is absent or reduced in groups receiving β-adrenergic blocking agents[97,159,172,240] or aspirin.[185] The morning rise in MI onset probably is related to increased sympathetic activity on awakening and assuming an upright posture, which leads to increased blood pressure, heart rate, coronary vascular tone, and platelet aggregation.[25,160] The timing of cardioprotective medication to cover the period of increased morning risk is a promising preventive approach.[74,157,240] Like MI, sudden cardiac death,[158,239] transient myocardial ischemia,[162,186] and stroke[8,139,140] occur more often in the morning than at other times of day and probably are triggered by similar underlying physiologic processes.

CARDIOVASCULAR CONSEQUENCES OF BREATHING DISORDERS IN SLEEP

Sleep-related changes in breathing and oxygenation have important cardiovascular consequences. This section focuses on the cardiovascular impact of sleep in COPD, sleep apnea, and snoring.

Chronic Obstructive Pulmonary Disease

During REM sleep, patients with COPD can have repeated episodes of hypoventilation, with large decreases in oxygen saturation and a mild hypercapnia, as REM-related changes in breathing interact with disease-related alterations in pulmonary function. For example, both REM sleep and COPD are associated with reduced ventilation and with diminished ventilatory and arousal responses to arterial blood gas changes. In addition, patients with COPD increasingly depend on the intercostal and accessory muscles of breathing, yet their activity is inhibited during REM sleep.[57,59,173] Alcohol consumed before bedtime may aggravate the nighttime hypoxemia.[23,62] Sleeping pills in general have not worsened breathing, but adverse effects in some people suggest caution.[17,45,212]

Cardiovascular consequences of sleep-related hypoxemia in COPD included marked elevations in pulmonary artery pressure,[22,40] daytime pulmonary hypertension,[126] increased frequency of PVCs,[71,203] and an increase in myocardial oxygen demand to a level much like that in maximal exercise at the time when the arterial oxygen supply is low.[127,204] Not surprisingly, patients with COPD often sleep badly, with light sleep that is fragmented by arousals.[24,43,68] Use of low-flow nocturnal oxygen to relieve nocturnal hypoxemia reduces cardiovascular complications,[22,70] probably improves sleep,[30,57] and may prolong survival.[144,164]

Obstructive Sleep Apnea

Patients with sleep apnea repeatedly stop breathing during sleep for periods of 10 seconds or longer. Apnea can be obstructive (a collapsed upper airway blocks airflow despite effort to breathe), central (no respiratory effort), or mixed (central, then obstructive component). A predominance of obstructive apnea is the most common pattern and can lead to repetitive episodes of hypoxemia that are terminated by brief arousals. Typical patients are middle-aged men who are overweight, snore loudly during sleep, and experience daytime sleepiness that interferes with normal activities; women with sleep apnea are usually postmenopausal.[85,112,234] Sleep apnea is likely to be worsened by sleep deprivation,[86,217] alcohol ingestion,[18,86,104,200] and sedative or hypnotic use.[56]

Obstructive sleep apnea has significant cardiovascular consequences. Systemic and pulmonary arterial pressures rise and increase in a stepwise fashion with repeated apnea. Daytime systemic hypertension occurs in 40% to 60% of patients and, conversely, approximately 20% to 30% of hypertensive patients have sleep apnea.[87,202] Whether the hypertension is caused directly by sleep apnea or a related common factor, such as obesity, is unclear.[98] Cardiac arrhythmias are relatively common and include PVCs, atrioventricular block, and bradycardia. Virtually every apnea is associated with a progressive sinus bradycardia, sometimes with a prolonged sinus pause, followed by an abrupt tachycardia when breathing resumes. A fall and subsequent rise in cardiac output parallel the heart rate changes.[83] Obstructive sleep apnea predominates in the same group at highest risk for coronary heart disease (middle-aged and older men), but little data are available on the extent to which one condition may influence the other.[54,65,101,195]

To minimize possible complications, early diagnosis and treatment are critical.[28] The treatment of choice for obstructive sleep apnea is nasally applied continuous positive airway pressure (CPAP). A soft, firmly fitting nasal mask is held in place by straps and attached to a bedside blower that provides continuous pressure (usually 5 to 15 cm H_2O) to prevent collapse of the upper airway. Recent improvements in CPAP devices include gradual onset of pressure and separate control of inspiratory and expiratory pressures.[197] Conservative treatment strategies include weight loss, learning to sleep in a side-lying position (as by putting a ball in a pouch on the pajama back), and avoidance of alcohol and sedatives. Pharmacologic approaches with purported respiratory stimulants (e.g., acetazolamide, methylprogesterone, protriptyline) have had variable effectiveness, and supplemental nighttime oxygen often worsens the apnea. Occasionally, surgery is done to enlarge the upper airway (uvulopalatopharyngoplasty) or to bypass it (tracheostomy) when other measures do not alleviate the apnea.[112,196,234] If the patient has been receiving antihypertensive medication, the dosage may need adjustment when the sleep apnea is effectively managed.

Central Sleep Apnea

Patients with severe congestive heart failure often have a pattern of periodic (Cheyne-Stokes) breathing during light sleep in which periods of central apnea alternate with hyper-

pnea. This breathing pattern causes recurrent episodes of hypoxemia that can further impair the failing heart and frequent arousals during the hyperpneic phase that disrupt sleep and impair subsequent daytime alertness.[50,67,90,248] One mechanism for the abnormal breathing pattern is prolonged circulation time that delays the ventilatory responses to blood gas changes. The resulting hypoxemia sets up a vicious cycle whereby increased ventilation improves oxygenation but lowers carbon dioxide tension below the apneic threshold; the resulting apnea then leads to hypoxemia, which perpetuates the cycle. In addition, cardiac enlargement and pulmonary congestion reduce gas stores in the lungs, which allows wider swings in blood gas values with changes in ventilation.[90,248] Effective treatment of the heart failure[11,50] and low-flow oxygen therapy during sleep[89] help to correct the hypoxemia and stabilize the breathing pattern. Use of nasal CPAP has variable results.[82,218]

Snoring

Epidemiologic studies indicate that habitual snoring is associated with a greater prevalence of coronary heart disease,[48,119,120] hypertension,[77,119] and stroke.[120,169,170,211] Snoring is more common and becomes habitual earlier in men than in women. By 60 to 65 years of age, more than 60% of men and 40% of women are chronic snorers.[134] Snoring is a primarily inspiratory noise during sleep caused by partial upper airway obstruction and vibration of the soft tissues during breathing. Snoring intensifies as NREM sleep deepens and diminishes in REM sleep to a level comparable with NREM stage 2. Heavy snoring is associated with reduced ventilation, obstructive apnea during light sleep and especially REM sleep, transient falls in arterial oxygen, and elevated systemic and pulmonary arterial pressures. Factors that worsen snoring include obesity, supine position, sleep deprivation, use of alcohol or sedatives, and smoking.[135]

NURSING MANAGEMENT PLAN

Assessment

A sleep assessment (Table 8-1) is a systematic collection of data that includes information about a patient's usual sleep patterns, sleep effectiveness, bedtime routines, and sleep environment. Because sleep-related breathing disorders predominate in the same group at highest risk for cardiovascular disease, the patient (or bed partner) should be asked about two cardinal symptoms of sleep apnea: snoring and daytime sleepiness.[91,236] The patient's physical appearance provides additional data. A variety of factors related to the patient's pathophysiologic disorder, treatments, environment, personal habits or concerns, and maturational status can contribute to sleep problems, and these should be explored. If the patient can be observed during sleep, a variety of physiologic variables can be monitored. Objective data from a polysomnographic sleep study may be available for occasional patients, but for most, a sleep history and direct observation are the primary assessment methods. Observational judgments that patients are asleep or awake are correct approximately 75% of the time.[63] When

TABLE 8-1 | Sleep Assessment

Sleep Patterns	**Current and Potential Related Factors**
Bedtime/wakeup time	*PATHOPHYSIOLOGY AND SYMPTOMS*
Time to fall asleep	Pain
Mid-sleep awakenings	Dyspnea
Time of final awakening	Nausea
Total sleep time	Mobility restriction
Movement during sleep	Others
Snoring	*TREATMENT*
Morning/afternoon/evening naps	Medications
Sleep Effectiveness	Monitoring/treatment devices
Rest/refreshment on awakening	*ENVIRONMENT*
Subjective sleep quality	Bed/bedding
Daytime alertness	Lighting
Ability to perform daytime activities	Sound (including conversation)
Bedtime Routines	Temperature
Bedtime rituals	Odors
Use of sleep medication	Activities
Use of other sleep aids	Interruptions by caregivers
Sleeping positions	*PERSONAL BEHAVIORS AND CONCERNS*
Sleep Environment	Sleep–wake schedule changes
Bed/bedding	Worry about illness
Lighting	Concerns about family/work
Sound	Depression
Temperature	*MATURATIONAL STATUS*
Bed/room partner (including pets)	Age
Physical Observations	Menopausal status
Yawning	**Physiologic Alterations in Sleep**
Dozing	Heart rate/rhythm
Drawn appearance	Hemodynamic monitoring
Decreased attention span	Respiratory pattern
Irritability	Respiratory pauses
Obesity	Snoring
	Oxygen saturation
	Movement in sleep

disturbed sleep is a significant ongoing problem, a sleep diary is an excellent way to document frequency and severity of symptoms and their effect on daily activities, evaluate progress of treatment, and promote self-management.[60,189]

In hospital settings, nurses are the only group of health care providers with bedside responsibility for patients throughout the 24 hours and with a regular opportunity to observe patients while they sleep. Symptoms such as snoring, respiratory pauses, and restless movements are important clues of sleep apnea. Monitoring devices provide a wealth of information about the sleep-related occurrence of myocardial ischemia, cardiac arrhythmias, systemic and pulmonary arterial pressure changes, drops in oxygen saturation, and other physiologic events. Periods of REM sleep predominate in the early morning hours and can be identified with reasonable certainty by the presence of easily observed REMs and muscle twitches in the face. Assessment during this time is particularly important for patients with respiratory disorders and for some patients with cardiovascular disease.

Nursing Diagnosis

A nursing diagnosis of sleep pattern disturbance is made when patients experience or are at risk of experiencing a change in the quantity or quality of sleep that causes discomfort or interferes with daily life.[33] The typical presenting complaint is either insomnia (difficulty falling asleep or staying asleep) or excessive sleepiness.[220] The diagnostic statement should include the related factors that contribute to the problem to provide specificity and suggest direction for intervention. The statement may also include the signs and symptoms that indicate sleep is disturbed. For example, a patient with a recent MI may have a nursing diagnosis of "sleep pattern disturbance related to intermittent chest pain, anxiety, and disruptions of care as evidenced by difficulty falling asleep and frequent nighttime awakenings." A patient with COPD complicated by heart failure may have a diagnosis of "sleep pattern disturbance related to recurrent nighttime hypoxemia evidenced by frequent nighttime awakenings and excessive daytime sleepiness."

Nursing Goals

The general nursing management plan focuses on promoting adequate, restful sleep for patients with cardiovascular disorders. One nursing goal is to prevent or reduce the factors that are disturbing the patient's sleep or that have potential to do so. A second goal is to provide bedtime routines, comfort measures, and a setting conducive to sleep. A third goal is to detect alterations in physiologic function that are caused by or may accentuate the underlying health problem. A fourth goal is to assist patients to learn behavioral patterns to enhance the quality of their sleep.

Outcome Criteria

Ideally, patients should be able to fall asleep easily at bedtime and sustain sleep for an adequate period. They should awaken feeling rested and refreshed and remain alert during normal daily activities. They should be able to describe and carry out practices of daily living that promote good sleep quality and daytime alertness.

Interventions

SLEEP HYGIENE

Sleep hygiene refers to practices of daily living that promote good sleep.[210,220] These behaviors reinforce the time and place for sleep and control factors that interfere with sleep. Sleep hygiene is an effective, low-technology approach that fits with common sense and principles of sleep regulation. It is the foundation for intervention when sleep is disturbed and is an important component of patient teaching for health maintenance.[93,94,210]

To reinforce the time for sleep, patients should be advised to go to bed and get up at approximately the same times each day, carry out a regular bedtime routine, and limit napping. Exposure to outdoor morning light helps to maintain the setting of the circadian timing system. To the extent possible in hospital settings, patients should have the opportunity to sleep during their accustomed hours and to maintain familiar routines. This is particularly important for elderly patients who already experience less deep, restorative sleep because of their age.[183] Increased napping commonly occurs during illness and may be particularly important during recovery from cardiac surgery or other cardiac events,[205] but the effect on nighttime sleep and physical recovery has not been studied.

The place for sleep should be physically comfortable and psychologically conducive to sleep. To keep the bed associated with sleep, it should be reserved for that purpose rather than serving as a hub for other activities. When lying in bed does not lead to sleep, the patient should be advised to get up, engage in quiet activity until drowsy, and then return to bed. Trying too hard to sleep is counterproductive; it is bet-

ter to engage in some distraction and let sleep come naturally. The psychological associations that are established when patients must spend considerable waking time in bed have not been studied.

Strenuous physical activity, worry, and anxiety lead to physiologic arousal that interferes with sleep. Moderate exercise usually is perceived as more beneficial to sleep when performed early in the day rather than late in the evening.[92,228] If patients tend to dwell on their concerns after going to bed, setting aside planned "worry time" an hour or two before bedtime may be helpful. Consumption of stimulants such as caffeine containing beverages should be restricted to the early part of the day[220,231]; nicotine in tobacco products is also a mild stimulant that interferes with falling sleep.[208] Although alcohol in moderate doses helps some people fall asleep, their sleep will likely be fragmented by brief, frequent arousals, and their total sleep time will be reduced.[187] Massage and other relaxation measures have been shown to be beneficial in reducing anxiety and inducing sleep in critically ill patients.

ENVIRONMENTAL MANAGEMENT

Nurses have considerable control over the hospital patient's physical environment, particularly lighting and sound levels. Most people prefer a darkened, quiet room for sleep. The level of noise (or sound unwanted by the listener)[167] tends to be particularly high in intensive care units—and a major source of that noise is the staff.[205,221] Noise can be reduced by conscious effort to avoid unnecessary or loud conversation, close doors to patients' rooms, use equipment quietly, turn off unnecessary equipment or alarms, consider sound level when deciding on equipment purchases, and give attention to acoustic features when participating in design of hospital units.[96,222,245,249] Some patients may find that soothing background sounds, such as provided by audiotapes of ocean surf or patter of rain, aid their sleep.[238]

A major challenge to nurses working in hospital settings, especially intensive care units, is limiting disruptions of patients' sleep while still providing the care necessary in cardiovascular disorders and surgery. Nursing care should be planned to protect, or at least minimally disrupt, the hours patients spend in sleep. Most patients' daily life schedules include the major sleep period at night, and routine procedures should be avoided during that time. Although protecting the entire sleep period may not be possible, the nursing plan should reflect awareness of the typical 90-minute sleep cycle and should cluster nursing care to provide opportunities for full cycles to occur. Research is needed to determine the success of these sleep opportunities and possible adverse effects of grouping patient care procedures.

Nurses must be assertive in alerting other health care providers to the patient's need for sleep and in identifying untimely disruptions. Skills of diplomacy, coordination, and priority setting are needed to get important procedures done without fragmenting either the patient's sleep or the health care provider's routine. Sophisticated monitoring equipment permits assessment of many physiologic parameters without disturbing the patient. Necessary interruptions should, when possible, be done at times when otherwise unavoidable activities occur.

Drawing morning blood specimens for laboratory tests is routine in many hospital settings, and in intensive care units, morning care also may occur at times when patients would otherwise be asleep. Although this helps to distribute workload across the 24 hours and to prepare patients and their laboratory data for the day shift and morning physicians' rounds, it shortens the total sleep period and particularly interferes with REM sleep. Health care providers should reevaluate these traditional practices.

COMFORT AND RELAXATION

Patients with pain, dyspnea, or simply wrinkled bedding can find it difficult to sleep or even rest at ease. Analgesics should be administered when indicated to alleviate pain. Careful positioning and dry, wrinkle-free beds enhance patient comfort. Various kinds of relaxation techniques may be used to produce a calm inner state through reduction of arousal. They have the advantages of helping to promote sleep and providing a general coping skill to deal with daily life stresses.[21,108] Traditional presleep back rubs are assumed to promote relaxation, although their actual effect on sleep has not been studied.

SLEEP MEDICATION

In general, sleep hygiene and other nonpharmacologic strategies should be used before sleep-promoting medications are considered in managing insomnia. In 1983, a national consensus conference recommended that use of hypnotics be limited to temporary insomnia. What can make insomnia serious is not sleep loss *per se* but resulting daytime sleepiness and inattentiveness that interfere with work, driving, and other activities. When hypnotics are used, patients should receive the lowest effective dose for the shortest clinically necessary period—a few days or, at most, a few weeks. There is no indication for the chronic use of sleep medication for persistent insomnia.[53]

In the United States, benzodiazepines are the hypnotics of choice. Short-acting agents such as triazolam (Halcion; Upjohn, Kalamazoo, MI) and a sedative—hypnotic drug such as zolpidem (Ambien) are preferred to avoid a daytime carryover effect. If daytime sedation is desired, a long-acting agent such as flurazepam (Dalmane; Roche Laboratories, Nutley, NJ) can be used. If hypnotics are abruptly discontinued, sleep is likely to worsen (rebound insomnia). This effect can be reduced by tapering the dose. Patients with sleep apnea or heavy snoring are not good candidates for hypnotic medications because they may worsen hypoxemia and the related sleep disturbance.[145,230]

THE HEALTH CARE PROVIDERS' SLEEP

Hospital nurses, physicians, and others who work night shift or rotating schedules often experience irregular sleep—wake schedules and inferior sleep, causing reduced alertness and general fatigue. This is accentuated by the pronounced circadian alertness—sleepiness rhythm, with maximal sleepiness and lowest performance at approximately 4 to 5 AM, at the low point of the body temperature rhythm.[34,123,184,192] Mental tasks that require sustained visual attention, such as monitoring an ECG oscilloscope or driving home from work, are more affected than are physical tasks.[49,79,124,193] Suggested coping strategies include staying on a night schedule on nonwork days (often socially unattractive), using rotation schedules that move forward around the clock rather than backward, and taking a nap before going to work.[182,190] Use of melatonin in the evening to help reset the circadian timing system, or bright light therapy to suppress natural melatonin secretion from the pineal gland, also appear to be promising strategies.[46,51]

SUMMARY

Patients with cardiovascular disease often have disturbed sleep, especially in intensive cardiac care settings, and may be at risk for physiologic changes during sleep that adversely affect their health status. Despite the widely held belief that sleep promotes well-being, hospital practices are rarely designed to encourage optimal sleep. Research is needed to clarify the role of both nighttime sleep and daytime naps in recovery from cardiovascular disease and surgery (what are optimal sleep patterns?) and to identify nursing interventions that prevent sleep deprivation, minimize adverse sleep-related physiologic changes, and promote good sleep.

REFERENCES

1. Åkerstedt T: Shifted sleep hours. Ann Clin Res 17: 273–279, 1985
2. Åkerstedt T: Sleepiness as a consequence of shift work. Sleep 11: 17–34, 1988
3. Ancoli-Israel S, Kripke DF, Klauber MR et al: Periodic limb movements in sleep in community-dwelling elderly. Sleep 14: 496–500, 1991
4. Ancoli-Israel S, Kripke DF, Klauber MR et al: Sleep-disordered breathing in community-dwelling elderly. Sleep 14: 486–495, 1991
5. Appels A, Schouten E: Waking up exhausted as risk indicator of myocardial infarction. Am J Cardiol 68: 395–398, 1991
6. Araki H, Koiwaya Y, Nakagaki O et al: Diurnal distribution of ST-segment elevation and related arrhythmias in patients with variant angina: A study by ambulatory ECG monitoring. Circulation 67: 995–1000, 1983
7. Araki H, Nakamura M: Diurnal variation of variant angina. Int J Cardiol 5: 402–405, 1984
8. Argentino C, Toni D, Rasura M et al: Circadian variation in the frequency of ischemic stroke. Stroke 21: 387–389, 1990
9. Barrett J, Lack L, Morris M: The sleep-evoked decrease of body temperature. Sleep 16: 93–99, 1993
10. Bateman JRM, Pavia D, Clarke SW: The retention of lung secretions during the night in normal subjects. Clinical Science and Molecular Medicine 55: 523–527, 1978
11. Baylor P, Tayloe D, Owen D et al: Cardiac failure presenting as sleep apnea: Elimination of apnea following medical management of cardiac failure. Chest 94: 1298–1300, 1988
12. Berry DTR, Phillips BA: Sleep-disordered breathing in the elderly: Review and methodological comment. Clin Psychol Rev 8: 101–120, 1988

13. Berry DTR, Phillips BA, Cook YR et al: Sleep-disordered breathing in healthy aged persons: Possible daytime sequelae. J Gerontol 42: 620–626, 1987

14. Berry DTR, Phillips BA, Cook YR et al: Sleep-disordered breathing in healthy aged persons: One-year follow-up of daytime sequelae. Sleep 12: 211–215, 1989

15. Bigger JT, Fleiss JL, Kleiger K et al: The relationship between ventricular arrhythmias, left ventricular dysfunction and mortality in the 2 years after myocardial infarction. Circulation 69: 250–258, 1984

16. Bliwise DL: Sleep in normal aging and dementia (review). Sleep 16: 40–81, 1993

17. Block AJ, Dolly FR, Slayton PC: Does flurazepam ingestion affect breathing and oxygenation during sleep in patients with chronic obstructive lung disease. Am Rev Respir Dis 129: 230–233, 1984

18. Block AJ, Hellard DW, Slayton PC: Effect of alcohol ingestion on breathing and oxygenation during sleep. Am J Med 80: 595–600, 1986

19. Bonnet MH: Depth of sleep. In Carskadon MA (ed): Encyclopedia of Sleep and Dreaming, pp 186–188. New York, Macmillan, 1993

20. Bonnet MH, Arand DL: Caffeine use as a model of acute and chronic insomnia. Sleep 15: 526–536, 1992

21. Bootzin RR, Perlis ME: Nonpharmacologic treatments of insomnia. J Clin Psychiatry 53(Suppl): 37–41, 1992

22. Boysen PG, Block AJ, Wynne JW et al: Nocturnal pulmonary hypertension in patients with chronic obstructive pulmonary disease. Chest 76: 536–542, 1979

23. Brander PE, Kuitunen T, Salmi T et al: Nocturnal oxygen saturation in advanced chronic obstructive pulmonary disease after a moderate dose of ethanol. Eur Respir J 5: 308–312, 1992

24. Brezinova V, Catterall JR, Douglas NJ et al: Night sleep of patients with chronic ventilatory failure and age matched controls: Number and duration of the EEG episodes on intervening wakefulness and drowsiness. Sleep 5: 123–130, 1982

25. Brezinski DA, Tofler GH, Muller JE et al: Morning increase in platelet aggregability: Association with assumption of the upright posture. Circulation 78: 35–40, 1988

26. Bristow JD, Honour AJ, Pickering TG et al: Cardiovascular and respiratory changes during sleep in normal and hypertensive subjects. Cardiovasc Res 3: 476–485, 1969

27. Brodsky M, Wu D, Denes P et al: Arrhythmias documented by 24 hour continuous electrocardiographic monitoring in 50 male medical students without apparent heart disease. Am J Cardiol 30: 390–395, 1977

28. Buckle P, Pouliot Z, Millar T et al: Polysomnography in acutely ill intensive care unit patients. Chest 102: 288–291, 1992

29. Buysse DJ, Browman KE, Monk TH et al: Napping and 24-hour sleep/wake patterns in health elderly and young adults. J Am Geriatr Soc 40: 779–786, 1992

30. Calverly PMA, Brezinova V, Douglas NJ et al: The effect of oxygenation on sleep quality in chronic bronchitis and emphysema. Am Rev Respir Dis 126: 206–210, 1982

31. Campbell SS, Gillin JC, Kripke DF et al: Gender differences in the circadian temperature rhythms of healthy elderly subjects: Relationships to sleep quality. Sleep 12: 529–536, 1989

32. Carney RM, Freedland KE, Jaffe AS: Insomnia and depression prior to myocardial infarction. Psychosom Med 52: 603–609, 1990

33. Carpenito LJ: Sleep pattern disturbance. In Nursing Diagnosis: Application to Clinical Practice, 5th ed, pp 723–730. Philadelphia, JB Lippincott, 1993

34. Carskadon MA: Ontogeny of human sleepiness as measured by sleep latency. In Dinges DF, Broughton RJ (eds): Sleep and Alertness: Chronobiological, Behavioral, and Medical Aspects of Napping, pp 53–69. New York, Raven Press, 1989

35. Carskadon MA, Dement WC: Normal human sleep: An overview. In Kryger MH, Roth T, Dement WC (eds): Principles and Practice of Sleep Medicine, 2nd ed, pp 16–25. Philadelphia, WB Saunders, 1994

36. Carskadon MA, Rechtschaffen A: Monitoring and staging human sleep. In Kryger MH, Roth R, Dement WC (eds): Principles and Practice of Sleep Medicine, 2nd ed, pp 943–960. Philadelphia, WB Saunders, 1994

37. Cassano GB, Maggini C, Guazzelli M: Nocturnal angina and sleep. Prog Neuropsychopharmacol Biol Psychiatry 5: 99–104, 1981

38. Cavallero C, Cicogna P, Natale V et al: Slow wave sleep dreaming. Sleep 15: 562–566, 1992

39. Chase MH, Morales FR: Motor control. In Carskadon MA (ed): Encyclopedia of Sleep and Dreaming, pp 383–384. New York, Macmillan, 1993

40. Coccagna G, Lugaresi E: Arterial blood gases and pulmonary and systemic arterial pressure during sleep in chronic obstructive pulmonary disease. Sleep 1: 117–124, 1978

41. Coccagna G, Mantovani M, Brignani F et al: Arterial pressure changes during spontaneous sleep in man. Electroencephalogr Clin Neurophysiol 31: 277–281, 1971

42. Cooper KR, Phillips BA: Effect of short-term sleep loss on breathing. J Appl Physiol 53: 855–858, 1982

43. Cormick W, Olson LG, Hensley MJ et al: Nocturnal hypoxaemia and quality of sleep in patients with chronic obstructive lung disease. Thorax 41: 846–854, 1986

44. Croog SH: Recovery and rehabilitation of heart patients: Psychosocial aspects. In Krantz DS, Baum A, Singer JE (eds): Handbook of Psychology and Health, Vol 1: Cardiovascular Disorders and Behavior, pp 295–334. Hillsdale, NJ, Lawrence Erlbaum Associates, 1983

45. Cummiskey J, Guilleminault C, Del Rio G et al: The effects of flurazepam on sleep studies in patients with chronic obstructive pulmonary disease. Chest 84: 143–147, 1983

46. Czeisler CA, Johnson MP, Duffy JF et al: Exposure to bright light and darkness to treat physiologic maladaptation to night work. N Engl J Med 322: 1253–1259, 1990

47. Czeisler CA, Weitzman ED, Moore-Ede MC et al: Human sleep: Its duration and organization depend on its circadian phase. Science 210: 1264–1267, 1980

48. D'Alessandro R, Magelli C, Gamberini G et al: Snoring every night as a risk factor for myocardial infarction: A case-control study. Br Med J 300: 1557–1558, 1990

49. Daly BJ, Wilson CA: The effect of fatigue on the vigilance of nurses monitoring electrocardiograms. Heart Lung 12: 384–388, 1983

50. Dark DS, Pingleton SK, Kerby GR et al: Breathing pattern abnormalities and arterial oxygen desaturation during sleep in the congestive heart failure syndrome: Improvement following medical therapy. Chest 91: 833–836, 1987

51. Dawson D, Campbell SS: Timed exposure to bright light improves sleep and alertness during simulated night shifts. Sleep 14: 511–516, 1991

52. DeKoninck JD, Lorrain D, Gagnon P: Sleep positions and position shifts in five age groups: An ontogenetic picture. Sleep 15: 143–149, 1992

53. Dement WC: The proper use of sleeping pills in the primary care setting. J Clin Psychiatry 53(Suppl): 50–56, 1992

54. De Olazabal JR, Miller MJ, Cook WR et al: Disordered breathing and hypoxia during sleep in coronary artery disease. Chest 82: 548–552, 1982

55. Dohno S, Paskewitz DA, Lynch JJ et al: Some aspects of sleep disturbance in coronary care patients. Percep Mot Skills 48: 199–205, 1979

56. Dolly FR, Block AJ: Effect of flurazepam on sleep-disordered breathing and nocturnal oxygen desaturation in asymptomatic subjects. Am J Med 73: 239–243, 1982

57. Douglas NJ: Nocturnal hypoxemia in patients with chronic obstructive pulmonary disease. Clin Chest Med 13: 523–532, 1992

58. Douglas NJ: Control of ventilation during sleep. In Kryger MH, Roth T, Dement WC (eds): Principles and Practice of Sleep Medicine, 2nd ed, pp 204–211. Philadelphia, WB Saunders, 1994

59. Douglas NJ, Flenley DC: Breathing during sleep in patients with obstructive lung disease. Am Rev Respir Dis 141: 1055–1070, 1990

60. Douglass AB, Carskadon MA, Houser R: Historical data base, questionnaires, sleep and life cycle diaries. In Miles LE, Broughton RJ (eds): Medical Monitoring in the Home and Work Environment, pp 17–28. New York, Raven Press, 1990

61. Dunn C, Sleep J, Collett, D: Sensing and improvement: An experimental study to evaluate the use of aromatherapy, massage and periods of rest in an intensive care unit. J Adv Nurs 21(1): 34–40, 1995

62. Easton PA, West P, Meatherall RC et al: The effect of excessive ethanol ingestion on sleep in severe chronic obstructive pulmonary disease. Sleep 10: 224–233, 1987

63. Edwards GB, Schuring LM: Pilot study: Validating staff nurses' observations of sleep and wake states among critically ill patients, using polysomnography. Am J Crit Care 2: 125–131, 1993

64. Elwell EL, Frankel BL, Snyder F: A polygraphic sleep study of five cardiotomy patients (Abstract). Sleep Res 3: 133, 1974

65. Erickson RS: Nighttime Sleep and Cardiopulmonary Function During Recovery from Myocardial Infarction. Unpublished doctoral dissertation. Seattle, University of Washington, 1987

66. Erwin CW, Somerville ER, Radtke RA: A review of electroencephalographic features of normal sleep. J Clin Neurophysiol 1: 253–274, 1984

67. Findley LJ, Zwillich CW, Ancoli-Israel S et al: Cheyne-Stokes breathing during sleep in patients with left ventricular heart failure. South Med J 78: 11–15, 1985

68. Fleetham J, West P, Mezon B et al: Sleep, arousals, and oxygen desaturation in chronic obstructive pulmonary disease: The effect of oxygen therapy. Am Rev Respir Dis 126: 429–433, 1982

69. Fleg JL, Kennedy HL: Cardiac arrhythmias in a healthy elderly population. Chest 81: 302–307, 1982

70. Fletcher EC, Levin DC: Cardiopulmonary dynamics during sleep in subjects with chronic obstructive pulmonary disease: Effect of short and long term oxygen. Chest 86: 6–14, 1984

71. Flick MB, Block AJ: Nocturnal vs. diurnal cardiac arrhythmias in hospitalized patients with chronic obstructive pulmonary disease. Chest 75: 8–11, 1979

72. Floras JS, Jones JV, Johnston JA et al: Arousal and the circadian rhythm of blood pressure. Clini Science Mol Med 55(Suppl A): 395S–397S, 1978

73. Foulkes D: Dreaming: A Cognitive–Psychological Analysis. Hillsdale, NJ, Lawrence Erlbaum Associates, 1985

74. George CFP: Cardiovascular disease and sleep. In Kryger MH, Roth T, Dement WC (eds): Principles and Practice of Sleep Medicine, 2nd ed, pp 835–846. Philadelphia, WB Saunders, 1994

75. Gillberg M, Akerstedt T: Body temperature and sleep at different times of day. Sleep 5: 378–388, 1982

76. Gillin JC, Buchsbaum MS, Wu JC: Cerebral metabolism. In Carskadon MA (ed): Encyclopedia of Sleep and Dreaming, pp 96–98. New York, Macmillan, 1993

77. Gislason T, Aberg H, Taube A: Snoring and systemic hypertension: An epidemiological study. Acta Medica Scandinavica 222: 415–421, 1987

78. Glotzbach SF, Heller HC: Temperature regulation. In Kryger MH, Roth T, Dement WC (eds): Principles and Practice of Sleep Medicine, 2nd ed, pp 201–275. Philadelphia, WB Saunders, 1994

79. Gold DR, Rogacz S, Bock N et al: Rotating shift work, sleep, and accidents related to sleepiness in hospital nurses. Am J Public Health 82: 1011–1014, 1992

80. Greenberg JH: Sleep and cerebral circulation. In Orem J, Barnes CD (eds): Physiology in Sleep, pp 57–95. New York, Academic Press, 1980

81. Guilleminault C: Hypnic jerks. In Carskadon MA (ed): Encyclopedia of Sleep and Dreaming, p 290. New York, Macmillan, 1993

82. Guilleminault C, Clerk A, Labanowski M et al: Cardiac failure and benzodiazepines. Sleep 16: 524–528, 1993

83. Guilleminault C, Motta J, Mihm F et al: Obstructive sleep apnea and cardiac index. Chest 89: 331–334, 1986

84. Guilleminault C, Pool P, Motta J et al: Sinus arrest during REM sleep in young adults. N Engl J Med 311: 1006–1010, 1984

85. Guilleminault C, Quera-Salva MA, Partinen M et al: Women and the obstructive sleep apnea syndrome. Chest 93: 104–109, 1988

86. Guilleminault C, Rosekind M: The arousal threshold: Sleep deprivation, sleep fragmentation, and obstructive sleep apnea syndrome. Bulletin Europeen de Physiophathologie Respiratoire 17: 341–349, 1981

87. Guilleminault C, Suzuki M: Sleep-related hemodynamics and hypertension with partial or complete upper airway obstruction during sleep. Sleep 15(Suppl): S20–S24, 1992

88. Hackett TP, Rosenbaum JF, Tesar GE: Emotion, psychiatric disorders, and the heart. In Braunwald E (ed): Heart Disease: A Textbook of Cardiovascular Medicine, 3rd ed, pp 1883–1900. Philadelphia, WB Saunders, 1988

89. Hanley PJ, Millar TW, Steljes DG et al: The effect of oxygen on respiration and sleep in patients with congestive heart failure. Ann Intern Med 111: 777–782, 1989

90. Hanley PJ, Millar TW, Steljes DG et al: Respiration and abnormal sleep in patients with congestive heart failure. Chest 96: 480–488, 1989

91. Haraldsson P-O, Carenfelt C, Knutsson E et al: Preliminary report: Validity of symptom analysis and daytime polysomnography in diagnosis of sleep apnea. Sleep 15: 261–263, 1992

92. Hasan J, Urponen H, Vuori I et al: Exercise habits and sleep in a middle-aged Finnish population. Acta Physiol Scand 133(Suppl 574): 33–35, 1988

93. Hauri PJ: Sleep hygiene, relaxation therapy, and cognitive interventions. In Hauri PJ (ed): Case Studies in Insomnia, pp 65–84. New York, Plenum, 1991

94. Hauri P, Linde S: No More Sleepless Nights. New York, John Wiley & Sons, 1991

95. Heistad DD, Abboud FM: Circulatory adjustments to hypoxia. Circulation 61: 463–470, 1980

96. Hilton BA: Noise in acute patient care areas. Res Nurs Health 8: 283–291, 1985

97. Hjalmarson Å, Gilpin EA, Nicod P et al: Differing circadian patterns of symptom onset in subgroups of patients with acute myocardial infarction. Circulation 80: 267–275, 1989

98. Hoffstein V, Chan CK, Slutsky AS: Sleep apnea and systemic hypertension: A causal association review. Am J Med 91: 190–196, 1991

99. Horne J: Why We Sleep: The Functions of Sleep in Humans and Other Mammals. Oxford, Oxford University Press, 1988

100. Hornyak M, Cejnar M, Elam M et al: Sympathetic muscle nerve activity during sleep in man. Brain 114: 1281–1295, 1991

101. Hung J, Whitford EG, Parsons RW et al: Association of sleep apnoea with myocardial infarction in men. Lancet 336: 261–264, 1990

102. Huxley EJ, Viroslav J, Gray WR et al: Pharyngeal aspiration in normal adults and patients with depressed consciousness. Am J Med 64: 564–568, 1978

103. Ingrassia TS, Nelson SB, Harris CD et al: Influence of sleep state on CO_2 responsiveness. Am Rev Respir Dis 144: 1125–1129, 1991

104. Issa FG, Sullivan CE: Alcohol, snoring and sleep apnoea. J Neurol Neurosurg Psychiatry 45: 353–359, 1982

105. Jamal K, McMahon G, Edgell G et al: Cough and arousal to inhaled citric acid in sleeping humans (Abstract). Am Rev Respir Dis 127: 237, 1983

106. Johns MW, Egan P, Gay TJA et al: Sleep habits and symptoms in male medical and surgical patients. Br Med J 2: 509–512, 1970

107. Johns MW, Large AA, Masterton JP et al: Sleep and delirium after open heart surgery. Br J Surg 61: 377–381, 1974

108. Johnson JE: Progressive relaxation and the sleep of older non-institutionalized women. Appl Nurs Res 4: 165–170, 1991

109. Joint International Society and Federation of Cardiology/World Health Organization Task Force on Standardization of Clinical Nomenclature: Nomenclature and criteria for diagnosis of ischemic heart disease. Circulation 59: 607–609, 1979

110. Jones J, Hoggart B, Withey J et al: What the patients say: A study of reactions to an intensive care unit. Intensive Care Med 5: 89–92, 1979

111. Kantelip J-P, Sage E, Duchene-Marullaz P: Findings on ambulatory electrocardiographic monitoring in subects older than 80 years. Am J Cardiol 57: 398–401, 1986

112. Kaplan J, Staats BA: Obstructive sleep apnea syndrome. Mayo Clin Proc 65: 1087–1094, 1990

113. Karacan I: Evaluation of nocturnal penile tumescence and impotence. In Guilleminault C (ed): Sleeping and Waking Disorders: Indications and Techniques, pp 343–371. Boston, Butterworth, 1982

114. Karacan I, Green JR, Taylor WJ et al: Sleep in post–myocardial infarction patients. In Eliot RS (ed): Contemporary Problems in Cardiology, Vol 1: Stress and the Heart, pp 163–195. Mount Kisco, NY, Futura, 1974

115. Karacan I, Williams RL, Taylor WJ: Sleep characteristics of patients with angina pectoris. Psychosomatics 10: 280–284, 1969

116. Khatri IM, Freis ED: Hemodynamic changes during sleep. J Appl Physiol 22: 867–873, 1967

117. King KB, Parrinello KA: Patient perceptions of recovery from coronary artery bypass grafting after discharge from the hospital. Heart Lung 17: 708–715, 1988

118. King MJ, Zir LM, Kaltman AJ et al: Variant angina associated with angiographically demonstrated coronary artery spasm and REM sleep. Am J Med Sci 265: 419–422, 1973

119. Koskenvuo M, Kaprio J, Partinen M et al: Snoring as a risk factor for hypertension and angina pectoris. Lancet 1: 893–896, 1985

120. Koskenvuo M, Kaprio J, Telakivi T et al: Snoring as a risk factor for ischaemic heart disease and stroke in men. Br Med J 294: 16–19, 1987

121. Krieger J: Breathing during sleep in normal subjects. In Kryger MH, Roth T, Dement WC (eds): Principles and Practice of Sleep Medicine, 2nd ed, pp 212–223. Philadelphia, WB Saunders, 1994

122. Kripke DF, Simons RN, Garfinkel L et al: Short and long sleep and sleeping pills: Is increased mortality associated? Arch Gen Psychiatry 36: 103–116, 1979

123. Lee KA: Circadian temperature rhythms in relation to menstrual cycle phase. J Biol Rhythms 3: 255–263, 1988

124. Lee KA: Self-reported sleep disturbances in employed women. Sleep 15: 493–498, 1992

125. Lee R: Sleep positions. In Carskadon MA (ed): Encyclopedia of Sleep and Dreaming, pp 570–572. New York, Macmillan, 1993

126. Levi-Valensi P, Weitzenblum E, Rida Z et al: Sleep-related oxygen desaturation and daytime pulmonary haemodynamics in COPD patients. Eur Respir J 5: 301–307, 1991

127. Levy PA, Guilleminault C, Fagret D et al: Changes in left ventricular ejection fraction during REM sleep and exercise in chronic obstructive pulmonary disease and sleep apnoea syndrome. Eur Respir J 4: 347–352, 1991

128. Lewy AJ, Sack RL: The dim light melatonin onset as a marker for circadian phase position. Chronobiol Int 62: 93–102, 1989

129. Lichstein E, Alosilla C, Chadda KD et al: Significance and treatment of nocturnal angina preceding myocardial infarction. Am Heart J 93: 723–726, 1977

130. Littler WA: Sleep and blood pressure: Further observations. Am Heart J 97: 35–37, 1979

131. Littler WA, Honour AJ, Sleight P et al: Direct arterial pressure and the electrocardiogram in unrestricted patients with angina pectoris. Circulation 48: 125–133, 1973

132. Lopes MG, Runge P, Harrison DC et al: Comparison of 24 versus 12 hours of ambulatory monitoring. Chest 67: 269–273, 1975

133. Lown B, Tykocinski M, Gargein A et al: Sleep and ventricular premature beats. Circulation 48: 691–701, 1973

134. Lugaresi E, Cirignotta F, Coccagna G et al: Some epidemiological data on snoring and cardiocirculatory disturbances. Sleep 3: 221–224, 1980

135. Lugaresi E, Cirignotta F, Montagna P et al: Snoring: Pathogenic, clinical, and therapeutic aspects. In Kryger MH, Roth T, Dement WC (eds): Principles and Practice of Sleep Medicine, 2nd ed, pp 621–629. Philadelphia, WB Saunders, 1994

136. Maggini C, Guazzelli M, Mauri M et al: Relation of transient myocardial ischemia to the sleep pattern in patients with "primary" angina. In Maseri A, Klassen GA, Lesch M (eds): Primary and Secondary Angina Pectoris, pp 157–167. New York, Grune & Stratton, 1978

137. Mancia G: Autonomic modulation of the cardiovascular system during sleep (Editorial). N Engl J Med 328: 347–349, 1993

138. Mant A, Eyland EA, Hewitt H et al: Sleep-disordered breathing in elderly people and subjective sleep–wake disturbance. Age Ageing 21: 262–268, 1992

139. Marler JR, Price TR, Clark GL et al: Morning increase in onset of ischemic stroke. Stroke 20: 473–476, 1989

140. Marsh EE, Biller J, Adams HP et al: Circadian variation in onset of acute ischemic stroke. Arch Neurol 47: 1178–1180, 1990

141. Martikainen K, Urponen H, Partinen M et al: Daytime sleepiness: A risk factor in community life. Acta Neurol Scand 86: 337–341, 1992

142. Martin RJ, Block AJ, Cohn MA et al: Indications and standards for cardiopulmonary sleep studies. Sleep 8: 371–379, 1985

143. McFadden EH, Giblin EC: Sleep deprivation in patients having open–heart surgery. Nurs Res 20: 249–254, 1971

144. Medical Research Council Working Party: Long term domiciliary oxygen therapy in chronic hypoxic cor pulmonale complicating chronic bronchitis and emphysema. Lancet 1: 681–686, 1981

145. Mendels J: Criteria for selection of appropriate benzodiazepine hypnotic therapy. J Clin Psychiatry 52(Suppl): 42–46, 1991

146. Mendelson WB: Neuroendocrinology and sleep. In Human Sleep: Research and Clinical Care, pp 129–179. New York, Plenum, 1987

147. Minors DS, Waterhouse JM: The circadian rhythm of deep body temperature. In Circadian Rhythms and the Human, pp 24–40. Bristol, United Kingdom, Wright PSG, 1981

148. Mitler MM, Carskadon MA, Czeisler et al: Catastrophes, sleep, and public policy: Consensus report. Sleep 11: 100–109, 1988

149. Monti JM, Folle LE, Lepuffo C et al: The incidence of premature contractions in coronary patients during the sleep–wake cycle. Cardiology 60: 257–264, 1975

150. Moore-Ede MC, Meguid MM, Fitzpatrick GF et al: Circadian variation in response to potassium infusion. Clin Pharmacol Ther 23: 218–227, 1978

151. Moore-Ede MC, Sulzman FM, Fuller CA: The Clocks that Time Us. Cambridge, Harvard University Press, 1982

152. Moritz A, Steinseifer U, Kobinia G et al: Closing sounds and related complaints after heart valve replacement with St Jude Medical, Duromedics Edwards, Bjårk-Shiley Monostrut, and Carbomedics prostheses. Br Heart J 67: 460–465, 1992

153. Motta J, Guilleminault C: Cardiac dysfunction during sleep. Ann Clin Res 17: 190–198, 1985

154. Mukharji J, Rude RE, Poole WK et al: Risk factors for sudden death after acute myocardial infarction: Two-year follow-up. Am J Cardiol 54: 31–36, 1984

155. Mulcahy D, Wright C, Sparrow J et al: Heart rate and blood pressure consequences of an afternoon SIESTA (Snooze-induced excitation of sympathetic triggered activity). Am J Cardiol 71: 611–614, 1993

156. Mullan PD: Cutting back after a heart attack: An overview. Health Education Monographs 6: 295–311, 1978

157. Muller JE: Morning increase of onset of myocardial infarction: Implications concerning triggering events. Cardiology 76: 96–104, 1989

158. Muller JE, Ludmer PL, Willich SN et al: Circadian variation in the frequency of sudden cardiac death. Circulation 75: 131–138, 1987

159. Muller JE, Stone PH, Turi ZG et al: Circadian variation in the frequency of onset of acute myocardial infarction. N Engl J Med 313: 1315–1322, 1985

160. Muller JE, Tofler GH, Stone PH: Circadian variation and triggers of onset of acute cardiovascular disease. Circulation 79: 733–743, 1989

161. Munari C, Calbucci F: Correlations between intracranial pressure and EEG during coma and sleep. Electroencephalogr Clin Neurophysiol 51: 170–176, 1981

162. Nademanee K, Intarachot V, Josephson MA et al: Circadian variation in occurrence of transient overt and silent myocardial ischemia in chronic stable angina and comparison with Prinzmetal angina in men. Am J Cardiol 60: 494–498, 1987

163. 1998 Cardiovascular Diseases: American Heart Association Web Page (1998). Available: http://www.amhrt.org/Scientific/HSstats98/03cardio.html

164. Nocturnal Oxygen Therapy Trial Group: Continuous or nocturnal oxygen therapy in hypoxemic chronic obstructive lung disease: A clinical trial. Ann Intern Med 93: 391–398, 1980

165. Nowlin JB, Troyer WG, Collins WS et al: The association of nocturnal angina pectoris with dreaming. Ann Intern Med 63: 1040–1046, 1965

166. Okada H, Iwase S, Mano T et al: Changes in muscle sympathetic nerve activity during sleep in humans. Neurology 41: 1961–1966, 1991

167. Olishifski JB, Standard JJ: Industrial noise. In Plog BA (ed): Fundamentals of Industrial Hygiene, 3rd ed, pp 163–189. Chicago, National Safety Council, 1988

168. Orr WC, Stahl ML: Sleep disturbances after open heart surgery. Am J Cardiol 39: 196–201, 1977

169. Palomäki H: Snoring and the risk of ischemic brain infarction. Stroke 22: 1021–1025, 1991

170. Palomäki H, Partinen M, Erkinjuntti T et al: Snoring, sleep apnea syndrome, and stroke. Neurology 42(Suppl 6): 75–82, 1992

171. Parker KP, Bliwise DL: Timing of hemodialysis affects the rhythm of oral body temperature (Abstract). Sleep 21(Suppl 3): 210, 1998

172. Peters RW, Muller JE, Goldstein S et al: Propranolol and the morning increase in the frequency of sudden cardiac death (BHAT study). Am J Cardiol 63: 1518–1520, 1989

173. Phillipson EA, Goldstein RS: Breathing during sleep in chronic obstructive pulmonary disease: State of the art. Chest 85(Suppl): 24S–30S, 1984

174. Pickering TG, Johnson J, Houour AM: Comparison of the effects of sleep, exercise and autonomic drugs on ventricular extrasystoles, using ambulatory monitoring of electrocardiogram and electroencephalogram. Am J Med 65: 575–583, 1978

175. Power JT, Stewart IC, Connaughton JJ et al: Nocturnal cough in patients with chronic bronchitis and emphysema. Am Rev Respir Dis 130: 999–1001, 1984

176. Prinz PN, Vitiello MV, Smallwood RG et al: Plasma norepinephrine in normal young and aged men: Relationship with sleep. J Gerontol 39: 561–567, 1984

177. Quyyumi AA, Efthimiou J, Quyyumi A et al: Nocturnal angina: Precipitating factors in patients with coronary artery disease and those with variant angina. Br Heart J 56: 346–352, 1986

178. Quyyumi AA, Wright CA, Mockus LJ et al: Mechanisms of nocturnal angina pectoris: Importance of increased myocardial oxygen demand in patients with severe coronary artery disease. Lancet 1: 1207–1209, 1984

179. Rechtschaffen A, Bergmann BM, Everson CA et al: Sleep deprivation in the rat: X. Integration and discussion of the findings. Sleep 12: 68–87, 1989

180. Rechtschaffen A, Kales A (eds): A Manual of Standardized Terminology, Techniques and Scoring System for Sleep Stages of Human Subjects. Los Angeles, Brain Information Service/Brain Research Institute, University of California, 1968

181. Reynolds CF, Jennings R, Hoch CC et al: Daytime sleepiness in the healthy "old old": A comparison with young adults. J Am Geriatr Assoc 39: 957–962, 1991

182. Rezents KJ, Lee KA: Shiftwork and health: Rationale for occupational health nurse management. AAOHN Update Series 5(18): 2–7, 1994

183. Richards KC: Sleep promotion. Critical Care Nursing Clinics of North America 8(1): 39–52, 1996

184. Richardson GS, Carskadon MA, Orav EJ et al: Circadian variation of sleep tendency in elderly and young adult subjects. Sleep 5(Suppl 2): S82–S94, 1982

185. Ridker PM, Manson JE, Buring JE et al: Circadian variation of acute myocardial infarction and the effect of low-dose

aspirin in a randomized trial of physicians. Circulation 82: 897–902, 1990

186. Rocco MB, Barry J, Campbell S et al: Circadian variation of transient myocardial ischemia in patients with coronary artery disease. Circulation 75: 395–400, 1987

187. Roehrs TA: Alcohol. In Carskadon MA (ed): Encyclopedia of Sleep and Dreaming, pp 21–23. New York, Macmillan, 1993

188. Roehrs T, Zorick F, Sicklesteel J et al: Excessive daytime sleepiness associated with insufficient sleep. Sleep 6: 319–325, 1983

189. Rogers AE, Caruso CC, Aldrich MS: Reliability of sleep diaries for assessment of sleep/wake patterns. Nurs Res 42: 368–372, 1993

190. Rosa RR: Intervention factors for promoting adjustment to nightwork and shiftwork. Occup Med 5: 391–415, 1990

191. Rosenblatt G, Hartmann E, Zwilling GR: Cardiac irritability during sleep and dreaming. J Psychosom Res 17: 129–134, 1973

192. Roth T, Roehrs TA, Carskadon MA et al: Daytime sleepiness and alertness. In Kryger MH, Roth T, Dement WC (eds): Principles and Practice of Sleep Medicine, 2nd ed, pp 40–49. Philadelphia, WB Saunders, 1994

193. Rubin R, Orris P, Lau SL et al: Neurobehavioral effects of the on-call experience in housestaff physicians. J Occup Med 33: 13–18, 1991

194. Rubin RT: Hormonal regulation of renal function during sleep. In Orem J, Barnes CD (eds): Physiology in Sleep, pp 181–201. New York, Academic Press, 1980

195. Saito T, Yoshikawa T, Sakamoto Y et al: Sleep apnea in patients with acute myocardial infarction. Crit Care Med 19: 938–941, 1991

196. Sanders MH: The management of sleep-disordered breathing. In Martin RJ (ed): Cardiorespiratory Disorders During Sleep, 2nd ed, pp 141–187. Mount Kisco, NY, Futura, 1990

197. Sanders MH, Stiller RA. Positive airway pressure in the treatment of sleep-related breathing disorders. In Chokroverty S (ed): Sleep Disorders Medicine: Basic Science, Technical Considerations, and Clinical Aspects, pp 455–471. Boston, Butterworth-Heinemann, 1994

198. Schiffman PL, Trontell MC, Mazar MF et al: Sleep deprivation decreases ventilatory response to CO_2 but not load compensation. Chest 84: 695–698, 198

199. Schleifer SJ, Macari-Hinson MM, Coyle DA et al: The nature and course of depression following myocardial infarction. Arch Intern Med 149: 1785–1789, 1989

200. Scrima L, Broudy M, Nay K et al: Increased severity of obstructive sleep apnea after bedtime alcohol ingestion: Diagnostic potential and proposed mechanism of action. Sleep 5: 318–328, 1982

201. Shanahan TL: Melatonin. In Carskadon MA (ed): Encyclopedia of Sleep and Dreaming, pp 359–360. New York, Macmillan, 1993

202. Shepard JW: Hypertension, cardiac arrhythmias, myocardial infarction, and stroke in relation to obstructive sleep apnea. Clin Chest Med 13: 437–457, 1992

203. Shepard JW, Garrison MW, Grither DA et al: Relationship of ventricular ectopy to nocturnal oxygen desaturation in patients with chronic obstructive pulmonary disease. Am J Med 78: 28–34, 1985

204. Shepard JW, Schweitzer PK, Keller CA et al: Myocardial stress: Exercise versus sleep in patients with COPD. Chest 86: 366–374, 1984

205. Simpson T, Lee R, Cameron C: Relationship among dimensions and factors that impair sleep after cardiac surgery. Res Nurs Health 19: 213–223, 1996

206. Snyder F, Hobson JA, Morrison DF et al: Changes in respiration, heart rate, and systolic blood pressure in human sleep. J Appl Physiol 19: 417–422, 1964

207. Sobotka PA, Mayer JH, Bauernfeind RA et al: Arrhythmias documented by 24-hour continuous ambulatory electrocardiographic monitoring in young women without apparent heart disease. Am Heart J 101: 753–759, 1981

208. Soldatos CR, Kales JD, Scharf MB et al: Cigarette smoking associated with sleep difficulty. Science 207: 551–553, 1980

209. Sommers VK, Dyken ME, Mark AI et al: Sympathetic-nerve activity during sleep in normal subjects. N Engl J Med 328: 303–307, 1993

210. Spielman AJ, Glovinsky PB: Sleep hygiene. In Carskadon MA (ed): Encyclopedia of Sleep and Dreaming, pp 550–553. New York: Macmillan, 1993

211. Spriggs DA, French JM, Murdy JM et al: Snoring increases the risk of stroke and adversely affects prognosis. Q J Med 84: 555–562, 1992

212. Steens RD, Pouliot Z, Millar TW et al: Effects of zolpedem and triazolam on sleep and respiration in mild to moderate chronic obstructive pulmonary disease. Sleep 14: 318–326, 1993

213. Steriade M: Sleep spindles. In Carskadon MA (ed): Encyclopedia of Sleep and Dreaming, pp 573–576. New York, Macmillan, 1993

214. Stern MJ, Pascale L, Ackerman A: Life adjustment post-myocardial infarction. Ann Intern Med 137: 1680–1685, 1977

215. Stern M, Pascale L, McLoone JB: Psychosocial adaptation following an acute myocardial infarction. Chronic Dis 29: 513–526, 1976

216. Stern S, Tzivoni D: Dynamic changes in the ST-T segment during sleep in ischemic heart disease. Am J Cardiol 32: 17–20, 1973

217. Stoohs RA, Itoi A, Hyde P et al: The effect of partial, prolonged sleep deprivation on snoring and obstructive sleep apnea (Abstract). Sleep Res 22: 349, 1993

218. Takasaki Y, Orr D, Popkin J: Effect of nasal continuous positive airway pressure of sleep apnea in congestive heart failure. American Review of Respiratory Disease 140: 140–157, 1989

219. Tammaro AE, Casale G, de Nicola P: Circadian rhythms of heart rate and premature ventricular beats in the aged. Age Ageing 15: 93–98, 1986

220. Thorpy MJ (Chairman): International Classification of Sleep Disorders: Diagnostic and Coding Manual. Lawrence KS, Allen Press, 1990

221. Topf M, Bookman M, Arand D: Effects of critical care unit noise on the subjective quality of sleep. J Adv Nurs 24: 545–551, 1996

222. Topf M, Davis JE: Critical care unit noise and rapid eye movement (REM) sleep. Heart Lung 22: 252–258, 1993

223. van Diest R: Subjective sleep characteristics as coronary risk factors, their association with type A behavior and vital exhaustion. J Psychosom Res 34: 415–426, 1990

224. Verdone P: Psychophysiology of dreaming. In Carskadon MA (ed): Encyclopedia of Sleep and Dreaming, pp 479–483. New York, Macmillan, 1993

225. Viitasalo M, Halonen L, Partinen M et al: Sleep and cardiac rhythm in healthy men. Ann Med 23: 135–139, 1991

226. Viitasalo MT, Kala R, Eisalo A: Ambulatory electrocardiographic recordings in endurance athletes. Br Heart J 47: 213–220, 1982

227. von Arnim T, Höfling B, Schreiber M: Characteristics of episodes of ST elevation or ST depression during ambulatory monitoring in patients subsequently undergoing coronary angiography. Br Heart J 54: 484–488, 1985

228. Vuori I, Urponen H, Hasan J et al: Epidemiology of exercise effects on sleep. Acta Physiol Scand 133(Suppl 574): 3–7, 1988

229. Walker BB: The postsurgery heart patient: Amount of uninterrupted time for sleep and rest during the first, second, and third postoperative days in a teaching hospital. Nurs Res 21: 164–169, 1972

230. Walsh JK, Fillingim JM: Role of hypnotic drugs in general practice. Am J Med 88(Suppl 3A): 34S–38S, 1990

231. Walsh JK, Muehlbach MJ, Humm TM et al: Effect of caffeine on physiological sleep tendency and ability to sustain wakefulness at night. Psychopharmacology 101: 271–273, 1990

232. Waters DD, Miller DD, Bouchard A et al: Circadian variation in variant angina. Am J Cardiol 54: 61–64, 1984

233. White DP: Ventilation and the control of respiration during sleep: Normal mechanisms, pathologic nocturnal hypoventilation, and central sleep apnea. In Martin RJ (ed): Cardiorespiratory Disorders During Sleep, 2nd ed, pp 53–108. Mount Kisco, NY, Futura, 1990

234. White DP: Obstructive sleep apnea. Hosp Pract 27: 57–84, 1992

235. White DP, Douglas NJ, Pickett CK et al: Sleep deprivation and the control of ventilation. Am Rev Respir Dis 128: 984–986, 1983

236. Wiggins CL, Schmidt-Nowara WW, Coultas DB et al: Comparison of self- and spouse reports of snoring and other symptoms associated with sleep apnea syndrome. Sleep 13: 245–252, 1990

237. Williams JC, Dace MC, Karacan I et al: The risk of sleep in the cardiac patient (Abstract). Clin Res 17: 64, 1969

238. Williamson JW: The effects of ocean sounds on sleep after coronary artery bypass graft surgery. Am J Crit Care 1: 91–97, 1992

239. Willich SN, Levy D, Rocco MB et al: Circadian variation in the incidence of sudden cardiac death in the Framingham Heart Study population. Am J Cardiol 60: 801–806, 1987

240. Willich SN, Linderer T, Wegscheider K et al: Increased morning incidence of myocardial infarction in the ISAM study: Absence with prior β-adrenergic blockade. Circulation 80: 853–858, 1989

241. Wingard DL, Berkman LF: Mortality risk associated with sleep patterns among adults. Sleep 6: 102–107, 1983

242. Winkle RA: The relationship between ventricular ectopic beat frequency and heart rate. Circulation 66: 439–446, 1982

243. Wishnie HA, Hackett TP, Cassem NH: Psychological hazards of convalescence following myocardial infarction. JAMA 215: 1292–1296, 1971

244. Woods NF: Patterns of sleep in postcardiotomy patients. Nurs Res 21: 347–352, 1972

245. Woods NF, Falk SA: Noise stimuli in the acute care area. Nurs Res 23: 144–150, 1974

246. Wu JC, Gillin JC, Buschsbaum MS et al: The effect of sleep deprivation on cerebral glucose metabolic rate in normal humans assessed with positron emission tomography. Sleep 14: 155–162, 1991

247. Wysowski DK, Baum C: Outpatient use of prescription sedative-hypnotic drugs in the United States, 1970 through 1989. Arch Intern Med 151: 1779–1783, 1991

248. Yamashiro Y, Kryger MH: Sleep in heart failure. Sleep 16: 513–523, 1993

249. Yinnon AM, Ilan Y, Tadmor B et al: Quality of sleep in the medical department. Br J Clin Pract 46: 88–91, 1992

250. Zemaityte D, Varoneckas G, Sokolov E: Heart rhythm control during sleep. Psychophysiology 21: 279–289, 1984

Physiologic Adaptations With Aging

RUTH F. CRAVEN

Aging is a normal developmental process during which physiologic and psychosocial changes occur. Wide variation in the aging process exists among individuals as a result of varied environmental exposures, social relationships, genetic endowment, and health status. Whereas maximum life span (the age reached by the longest-lived survivors) for humans is 114 to 120 years, the average human life span is approximately 75 years. Developmental changes and adaptations continue throughout aging until death.

The life span is divided into phases, with the commonly used periods for these phases being infancy (birth to 1 year), early childhood (1 to 6 years), late childhood (7 to 10 years), adolescence (11 to 18 years), young adulthood (19 to 35 years), early middle age (36 to 49 years), late middle age (50 to 64 years), young-old (65 to 74 years), old (75 to 85 years), and old-old (86 years and older). The group of elderly who are aged 85 years or older is the most rapidly growing segment of the elderly population (Fig. 9-1). The elderly in this age group typically have a noticeable decline in functional ability and have one or more chronic disorders.

Aging is a multifactorial process with both genetic and environmental components. Each system in an organism, each tissue in a system, and each cell type in a tissue appears to have its own trajectory of aging.[4] Theories of the biologic aspects of aging have been developed and studied.[8,9] The theories can be divided into three groups: organ theories, physiologic theories, and genome-based theories. The organ theories examine age changes in the body brought about by the possible initiation from a "master" organ system, such as the immune or neurologic system. The physiologic theories analyze cell functioning as related to waste product accumulation or molecular changes. The genome-based theories attribute age changes to the individual's genetic endowment and suggest that a predetermined series of events programmed into cells or random mutations or cell errors are responsible for the process of aging. Probably no one theory can totally explain the aging process, but rather some or all of these theories may be involved in the complete explanation.

The nurse needs to be aware of several concepts in addressing the health care needs of the elderly:

1. Age-related changes are gradual and individual, and different systems age at different rates within an individual.
2. Complex functions that require multisystem coordination show the most obvious decline and require the greatest compensation and support.
3. Vulnerability to disease increases with age.
4. Stressful situations (physiologic or psychosocial) produce a more pronounced reaction in the elderly and require a longer period of time for readjustment.[1]

Although Americans are living longer, they are not necessarily healthier and, with increasing age, are at increased risk of becoming ill. Chronic illnesses, such as arthritis, cardiac and vascular problems, and diabetes are the major health problems of the elderly (Fig. 9-2). Because of the lifestyle changes in young and middle-aged adults, particularly in the areas of diet and exercise, the elderly in the near future may be sufficiently healthier that definitions and expectations of the aging process may need to be revised. At present, however, heart disease is the leading health problem for the elderly (Fig. 9-3).

When the elderly become ill, there is frequently an atypical presentation, such as missing or altered symptoms. Confusion is often one of the earliest indications of a change in health status. Restlessness, confusion, or altered mentation often occur in the presence of illness and should not be confused with dementia, providing that dementia was not present before the illness. Acute onset or unexplained deterioration of health should be carefully evaluated and not accepted as a normal concomitant of aging.

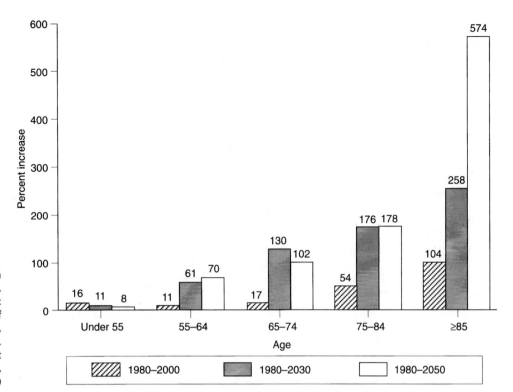

FIGURE 9-1 Projected growth in population by age group, 1980–2050. (From Spencer G: Projections of the population of the United States, by age, sex, and race: 1988–2080. U.S. Bureau of the Census, Current Population Reports Series P-25, No. 1018, Hyattsville, MD, 1989.)

The older person who is ill has many adjustments and adaptations to make. The social supports (family and friends) available to that person may be fewer in number or less able to be supportive because of their own debilities, such as a spouse who is also ill or an adult child who has other responsibilities, such as being in the work force.

Apprehension, worry, and fear of becoming dependent and helpless may add to the emotional burden of the current illness. Of those older adults between 80 and 84 years of age, 30% require assistance with daily activities, and of those adults who are 85 years and older, 50% require assistance.

The elderly require careful, thorough nursing management during an acute illness and afterward. Discharge planning that begins with the admission process and includes consideration of living arrangements, care providers, and support services is especially important for the elderly, who are often most adversely affected by the shorter hospitalizations and nursing care visits that accompany managed care.

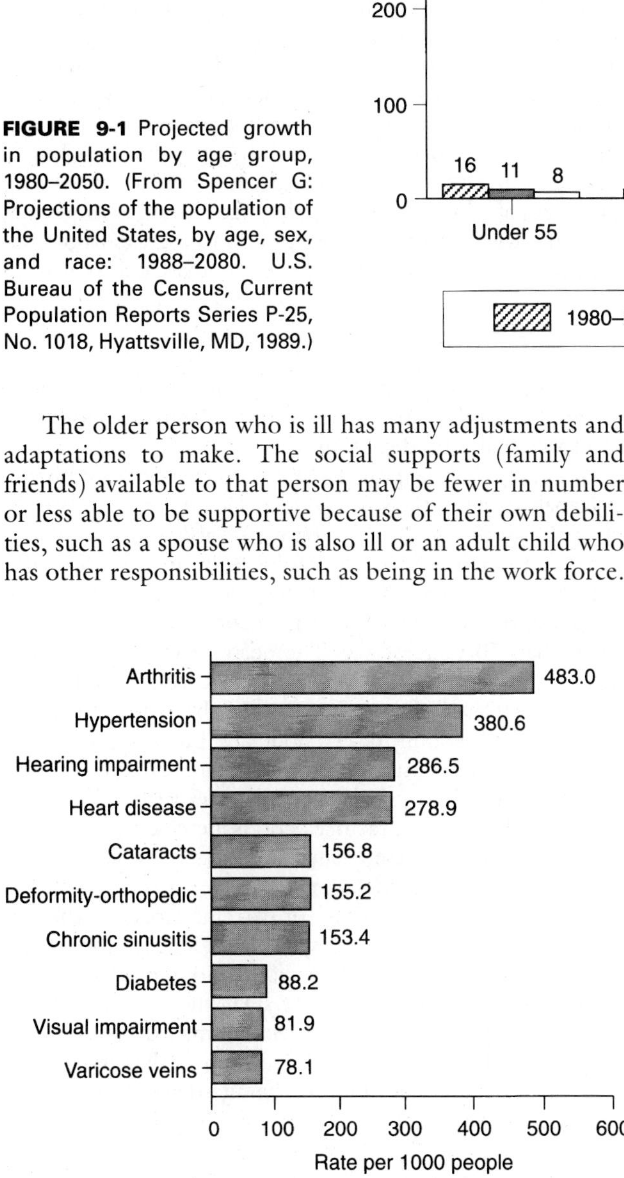

FIGURE 9-2 The top 10 chronic conditions for people older than 65 years of age, 1989. (From National Center for Health Statistics: Current estimates from the National Health Interview Survey, 1989. Vital and Health Statistics Series 10, No. 176, Washington, DC, 1990.)

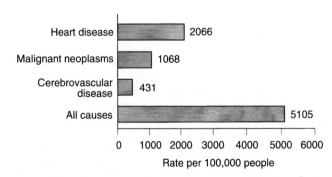

FIGURE 9-3 The top causes of death among older people, 1988. (From National Center for Health Statistics: Advance report of final mortality statistics, 1988. Monthly Vital Statistics Report Vol. 39, No. 7, Supplement, Washington, DC, November 1990.)

GENERAL PHYSIOLOGIC CHANGES

Aging is an integral part of the continuum that begins at conception and ends at death. As contrasted with the developmental growth and maturation of childhood and adolescence, aging is characterized by a decline in function and by changes that are decremental in nature. The inability to maintain homeostasis in a broad range of environments and with a variety of physiologic challenges is central to the decline in function.

Changes related to aging may be classified or categorized in several ways. Kenny[11] suggests the following scheme:

1. Change in which the function is totally lost (e.g., female reproductive ability)
2. Changes in or loss of function related to loss of structure (e.g., altered kidney function related to loss of nephrons)
3. Changes in efficiency without structural loss (e.g., reduction in conduction velocity in aging nerve fibers)
4. Changes resulting from interruptions in a control system (e.g., the rise in gonadotropins in women with the reduction in feedback control of sex hormones)
5. Rarely, increased function (e.g., secretion of antidiuretic hormone in response to osmotic challenge)

In reviewing the age-related changes in selected systems, the changes in structure and function of each system are discussed along with the changes appropriate to the system.

CARDIOVASCULAR CHANGES

One of the challenges in discussing aging changes in any system is that of separating changes that can be attributed only to age from changes related to disease. This is particularly true in the cardiovascular system. This discussion attempts to identify what is known about changes in cardiovascular structure and function that result from aging changes and, subsequently, increase vulnerability to disease.

Cardiac Structural Changes

Although there are some differences in findings, it is now agreed that there is myocardial hypertrophy from aging alone. Structural changes during aging are dominated by some left ventricular wall and septal hypertrophy and by left atrial and ventricular widening.[17] The left ventricular wall may be 25% thicker at age 80 than at age 30 years.[8]

Changes in the myocardial cells include the accumulation of lipofuscin (a lipid-containing material), which is thought to be a consequence of biologic aging; deposits of amyloid; and an increase in myocardial collagen and connective tissues.[8,9] The effects of these changes on function are unclear.

Aging changes in the valves are characterized by increases in fibrosis, collagen degeneration, lipid accumulation, and calcification. Calcifications of the aortic valve ring can contribute to stenosis and valvular incompetency in aging.[8,9]

Cardiac Functional Changes

In the absence of disease or preexisting dysfunction, resting heart rate is relatively unchanged with age. For the elderly who are free of coronary disease and maintain normal, active lives, cardiac output (i.e., heart rate, stroke volume, and diastolic volume) is not markedly affected by age.[16] However, some studies report a decrease in cardiac output in adult men of approximately 0.7% per year; for example, the cardiac output is approximately 5.0 L/min at age 20 and may fall to approximately 3.5 L/min by age 75 years. Conflicting findings add to the problem of separating normal aging from cardiac disease. From a clinical viewpoint, the agreement that is important is that there is an age-related decline in maximum heart rate with stress from exercise, illness, or other sources. In normal living, activity is adjusted according to the accompanying decline in heart rate. In the presence of illness or stress, this age-related change may combine with cardiac disease, leading to a greater potential for cardiac failure and for decreased functional capacity.

Electrical System

Because research on the cardiac electrical system cannot be rigidly controlled in humans, data presented should be interpreted and used cautiously.

In aging there appears to be a decrease in the number of pacemaker cells in the sinus node and a greater irregularity in their shape. By age 75 years, only 10% of original nodal cells remain, although this is compatible with normal pacemaker activity. The number of conducting cells in the atrioventricular (AV) node and the left bundle branch decreases in people older than 70 years of age. The decrease in the number of cells in the bundle of His begins over age 40 and in the right bundle over age 50 years. Some studies have noted increases in fat and collagen in the AV node and bundle.[12] Idiopathic bundle-branch fibrosis is a common cause of chronic atrioventricular block in people older than 65 years of age. The atrial and AV nodal refractory periods increase with age. It is not clear whether these changes are caused by altered catecholamine or vagal stimulation with age.

In the absence of disease or extreme stress on the cardiac function, the electrical system is adequate for normal conductivity. The normal electrocardiogram shows little change with age. There may be small increases in the PR, QRS, and QT intervals along with a small decrease in the amplitude of the QRS complex. When challenged by disease or adverse circumstances, the age-dependent changes increase the potential for conduction difficulties.

Vascular System

STRUCTURAL CHANGES

With advancing age, a series of structural changes take place in the vascular system. The vessel diameter tends to increase and the intimal and medial layers tend to thicken.[2] In the arterial intima, the endothelial cells become irregular in size and shape with an increase in connective tissue. Calcification and lipid deposition also occur. In the media, roughening of the surface of the muscle cells combines with calcification, increased collagen content, and elastin disorganization and fragmentation. Changes in the adventitia solely related to aging are not well documented.

FUNCTIONAL CHANGES

As a result of less elasticity and increased connective tissue, the arterial walls are less distensible and less compliant with aging. There also appears to be diminished responsiveness to β-adrenergic stimulation.[8] A question exists regarding a change in distensibility of baroreceptors or in the central response to them, but no clear data are available.

Elevation of the blood pressure usually is not considered a normal age change; however, it is a change that frequently occurs with the process of aging. Systolic hypertension in the elderly, in particular, is a distinct pathologic process and accounts for more than 50% of cases of hypertension. It is defined as a systolic pressure greater than 160 mm Hg and diastolic pressure below 95 mm Hg and is probably the result of arterial stiffening and loss of arterial compliance that occur with aging.[3] Treatment of systolic hypertension presents a dilemma because it is frequently labile with wide variance in the systolic readings, and the medications available for treatment primarily affect the diastolic pressure. Although there is a significant correlation between morbidity and mortality and the presence of systolic hypertension, there is very little agreement regarding treatment of systolic hypertension (see Chapter 32).

In summary, cardiovascular changes related to aging begin in the middle adult years and progress during the later years. When stressed by exercise or illness, the aged heart may exhibit decreased cardiac output, which, when combined with vascular changes, leads to the alterations in overall performance associated with aging.

RESPIRATORY CHANGES

In the absence of disease, the changes that occur in the lungs from maturity through the aging process are so gradual that the lungs are capable of providing normal gas exchange throughout life. However, the lungs are continuously exposed to the external environment and to various internal assaults; hence, it is difficult to separate changes due solely to aging from those related to injury or disease processes.

Structural Changes

The aging lung undergoes gradual, subtle changes. There is a gradual reduction in weight over the life span (approximately 20%).[13] Decreased elasticity in the lung tissue combines with increased stiffness and calcification of thoracic joints and intercostal muscles to produce a decrease in chest wall compliance with aging and an increased anteroposterior diameter of the chest. The resulting reduced mobility of the thorax leads to increased residual air volume and to a breathing pattern that is augmented by the increased use of diaphragmatic and abdominal muscles in breathing. The activity of the cilia is decreased, producing less ciliary clearance.

Functional Changes

The typical changes in lung function with age include decreased lung recoil, increased closing volume, altered lung volumes, and decreased maximum expiratory flow volume.[13] Nonemphysematous enlargement of the alveoli resulting from loss of lung elastic recoil is accepted as a normal change of aging. The effect of this change is decreased efficiency of gas-diffusing capacity and increased residual volume.

During expiration, airways in the dependent lung regions close and no longer participate in respiration. With aging, the lung volume at which these airways close (closing volume) may exceed the functional residual capacity, leading to closure of distal airways before the end of a normal breath and while still in a sitting position.[13] Loss of lung recoil and the effects of gravity on the dependent areas of lungs allow the airways to close at a higher lung volume and lead to nonuniformity of ventilation (Fig. 9-4).

The total lung capacity changes very little with age. There is an increase, however, in residual volume for reasons previously discussed and in the ratio of residual volume to total lung capacity. When increased closing capacity closes terminal airways, these airways no longer actively participate in ventilation, resulting in reduced maximal expiratory flow (V_{max}) and in decreased forced expiratory volume (FEV_1), which is measured in the first second of forced expiration.

As a result of changes in airway closure, diffusing capacity, lung volumes, and lung structure, a lower arterial oxygen tension is seen in the elderly. The arterial oxygen

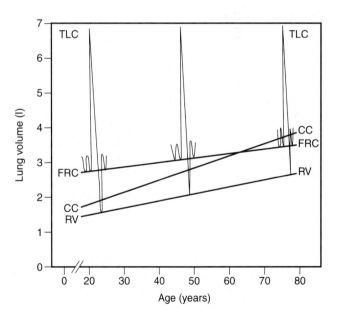

FIGURE 9-4 Changes in lung volumes with age. CC, closing capacity; FRC, functional residual capacity; RV, residual volume; TLC, total lung capacity. (Peterson DD, Fishman AP: The lungs in later life. In Fishman AP (ed): Update: Pulmonary Diseases and Disorders, pp 123–136. New York, McGraw-Hill, 1982.)

(PaO_2) decreases approximately 4 mm Hg per decade, whereas arterial carbon dioxide ($PaCO_2$) and pH remain unchanged.

Host defense mechanisms of airway clearance and immune system functions located in the airway and lung tissue respond less vigorously with age.[16] When combined with the decreased cough reflex resulting from decreased cilia activity, the consequence is that the elderly person is more vulnerable to infections (e.g., pneumonia, tuberculosis), mechanical irritation, and, possibly, tumor formation.

In summary, although the lung undergoes some structural and functional changes, the nondiseased respiratory system continues to be capable of supporting physical challenges throughout life.

RENAL CHANGES

The kidney is an organ with complex functions that are intimately related with other organ systems, such as the cardiovascular, endocrine, and neurologic systems. In discussing the aging kidney, changes are discussed as they relate to intrinsic changes in the kidney as well as those adaptive changes that result from the effects of other systems.

Structural Changes

The volume and weight of the kidney decline during the aging process. By the ninth decade, renal mass declines up to 25%,[10] with cortical mass lost to a greater extent than medullary mass. As a consequence, the number of nephrons declines with age by 30% to 40% compared with the number present at 20 years of age.

Functional Changes

As an accompaniment to the structural changes, the effective renal plasma flow and the glomerular filtration rate (GFR) progressively decline in the elderly.[9] The reduced renal perfusion and reduction in number of nephrons contribute to the reduction of GFR by 30% to 50% between 30 and 80 years of age. Because of the decrease in muscle mass with aging, there is not a corresponding rise in serum creatinine to go along with the reduced GFR.[10] Creatinine clearance, not serum creatinine, should be the criterion for renal clearance. The formula for predicting creatinine clearance is[14]

$$\text{Creatinine clearance} = \frac{(140 - \text{age}) \times \text{body weight in kg}}{72 \times \text{serum creatinine in mg} / \text{dL}}$$

$$\times 0.85 \text{ for women}$$

The clinical importance of this formula is apparent when determinations about kidney function and appropriate drug dosage need to be made. The decline in GFR reduces the renal clearance of those medications normally removed by the kidney.[14]

The aging kidney's tendency to lose salt is related to nephron loss, with increased osmotic load per nephron leading to mild osmotic diuresis and the age-related changes in the renin-aldosterone system. Lower levels of renin (decreased by 30% to 50% in older adults) are related to 30% to 50% reductions in plasma concentration of aldosterone. When this is combined with the decreased GFR, elderly people are therefore at risk for expansion of extracellular fluid volume when faced with an acute salt load (from diet, drugs, or intravenous fluids).

The limited ability of the kidney to regulate salt balance is compounded by diminished ability to concentrate urine maximally. The elderly also cannot maximally suppress antidiuretic hormone secretion in the presence of reduced serum osmolality.[10] Therefore, the elderly person has more difficulty retaining fluid when it is necessary, as in situations of decreased circulating fluid volume (e.g., dehydration), and in excreting fluid, as in situations of excess circulating fluid volume (e.g., congestive heart failure). The ability to concentrate urine declines moderately, with the usual value (specific gravity) of 1.032 decreasing to 1.024 at age 80 years.[5] Vitamin D hydroxylation in the kidney is reduced and may contribute to a decreased intestinal absorption of calcium.

There are many functions of the kidney (e.g., erythropoietin production, hormone metabolism) that have yet to be thoroughly studied. Of those changes that have been described, the clinical effects on drugs and their excretion and on fluid balance are of primary importance.

HEPATIC CHANGES

Structural Changes

The liver declines in weight after 50 years of age. This reduction in weight (18% to 24% between age 30 and 80 years) is accompanied by a gradual increase in collagen. The liver also undergoes a decrease in blood flow (approximately 35%); hepatocyte size is altered; and the liver takes on a darker brown color because of pigmented lipofuscin granules.

Functional Changes

Studies of hepatic function in the elderly are of particular interest because of the liver's role in metabolism of drugs, as well as other metabolic activities.[6] With aging, there is a decrease in hepatic size and in regional blood flow to the liver and in the response of enzymes in the liver.[18] Hepatic flow in people older than 65 years of age may be only 40% to 60% of that of people in their fourth decade. Although it is not clear that the reduced size, decreased enzyme response, and decreased blood flow affect the general function of the liver, they do alter the hepatic clearance for drugs whose metabolism and excretion depend on the liver. There is a broad decline in drug clearance of 10% to 30% between young adulthood and old age.

DRUGS AND THE ELDERLY

Drug Absorption

Little is known about absorption of oral drugs from the intestines, but it seems to be mildly decreased or unchanged with age. The observation of a 40% to 50% reduction in splanchnic blood flow would support the concept of reduced intestinal absorption in the elderly.[10]

Drug Distribution

Decreased serum albumin concentration is linked to decreased binding capacity of drugs. Drugs that are bound are inactive in terms of therapeutic effect. Unbound, or free, drug is free to exert therapeutic effects. This is one reason why a smaller dosage of drug may exert the same therapeutic effect in an older person as a regular dosage in a younger person.

With aging, lean body mass decreases by approximately 10% and body fat increases by the same amount. This, along with decreased total body water, may also contribute to the retention of fat-soluble drugs, so that they exert effects over a longer period of time because of depot action.

Drug Metabolism and Excretion

The regional blood flow to the liver decreases by as much as 1.5% per year, and thus the blood flow in a 65-year-old man is 55% to 60% that of a 20-year-old. Diminished blood flow to the liver results in less drug passing through the liver to be available for metabolism.

Reduction in liver mass and in blood flow lead to less effective activity of the hepatic enzymes involved in drug metabolism. The decreased activity of drug-metabolizing enzymes contributes to the decreased metabolism of drugs in the elderly.

The other route of drug excretion is the kidney. As was previously described, changes in the kidney may lead to decreased excretion of active drug with consequent prolonged half-lives of drugs and sustained or increased levels of free drug in the serum.

As a result of these changes in absorption, distribution, metabolism, and excretion, greater care must be exercised with drug administration to the elderly. Giving drugs in smaller doses and less frequently may accomplish an adequate therapeutic effect. If adverse reactions or side effects occur, it may be more prudent to discontinue a suspected drug rather than add another drug to counteract the effects. The elderly are vulnerable to adverse effects from drugs for many reasons (e.g., age changes, chronic conditions, polypharmacy). Consequently, clinical professionals must exercise caution and responsibility where drugs and the elderly are concerned.[7,15]

SUMMARY

In summary, cardiovascular function declines progressively with age, and because of the interrelatedness of the major systems, it is affected by and affects the other systems as well. Respiratory, renal, and heptic functions are independent and interconnected with cardiovascular function so that normal age-related changes in any or all of these systems exacerbates changes in other systems. One significant area where this interconnectedness is exemplified is in drug therapy. The ongoing question and dilemma for the health care provider is differentiating between decline in function that occurs with age and problems resulting from specific cardiovascular diseases.

REFERENCES

1. Berry AL, Davignon D: Changes with aging. In Patrick M et al (eds): Medical–Surgical Nursing, 2nd ed, pp 55–70. Philadelphia, JB Lippincott, 1991
2. Bilato C, Crow MT: Atherosclerosis and vascular biology of aging. Aging 8: 221–234, 1996
3. Black HR: New concepts in hypertension: Focus on the elderly. Am Heart J 135: S2–S7, 1998
4. Cristofalo VJ, Gerhard GS, Pignolo RJ: Molecular biology of aging. Surg Clin North Am 74: 1–21, 1994
5. Davies I, O'Neill PA, McLean KA et al: Age-associated alterations in thirst and arginine vasopressin in response to a water or sodium load. Age Ageing 24: 151–159, 1995
6. Geokas M, Conteas C, Majumdar A: The aging gastrointestinal tract, liver, and pancreas. Clin Geriatr Med 1: 177–206, 1985
7. Gurwitz JH, Avorn J: The ambiguous relation between aging and adverse drug reactions. Ann Intern Med 114: 956–966, 1991
8. Hazzard WR, Andres R, Bierman EL et al: Principles of Geriatric Medicine and Gerontology, 2nd ed. New York, McGraw-Hill, 1990
9. Kane RL, Ouslander JG, Abrass IB: Essentials of Clinical Geriatrics, 2nd ed. New York, McGraw-Hill, 1989
10. Kaysen G, Myers B: The aging kidney. Clin Geriatr Med 1: 207–222, 1985
11. Kenny RA: Physiology of aging. Clin Geriatr Med 1: 37–60, 1985
12. Klausner S, Schwartz A: The aging heart. Clin Geriatr Med 1: 119–142, 1985
13. Krumpe P, Knudson R, Parsons G et al: The aging respiratory system. Clin Geriatr Med 1: 143–176, 1985
14. Malmrose LC, Gray SL, Pieper CF et al: Measured vs estimated creatinine clearance in a high-functioning elderly sample: MacArthur Foundation Study of Successful Aging. J Am Geriatr Soc 41: 715–721, 1993
15. Montamat SC, Cusack B: Overcoming problems with polypharmacy and drug misuse in the elderly. Clin Geriatr Med 8: 143–158, 1992
16. Schneider EL, Rowe JW, Johnson TG et al (eds): Handbook of the Biology of Aging, 4th ed. New York, Academic Press, 1996
17. Svanborg A: Age-related changes in cardiac physiology: Can they be postponed or treated by drugs? Drugs Aging 11: 253, 1997
18. Vogt BL, Richie JP: Fasting-induced depletion of glutathione in the aging mouse. Biochem Pharmacol 46: 257–263, 1993

Assessment of Heart Disease

10

History Taking and Physical Examination

BARBARA S. LEVINE
SANDRA UNDERHILL MOTZER

Assessment data, which are obtained from the patient's history, physical examination, and diagnostic tests, are used to formulate clinical diagnoses, establish patient goals, plan care, and evaluate patient outcomes. A complete history and physical examination includes the same content areas, whether elicited by nurses or physicians. A complete history and physical examination is impractical in most clinical situations. The inclusion of appropriate content areas is determined by the patient's clinical condition and the purpose and context of the clinical encounter. Specific content areas may be investigated in greater detail by clinicians from different disciplines, and the data may be used in different ways. Nurses must be able to incorporate historical data into the nursing assessment so that the interdependent nursing and medical responsibilities are completed in the correct priority sequence. Conversely, physicians need to be aware of the data elicited by nurses so that the complete database is the foundation for the total plan of care.

This chapter focuses on history taking and physical examination of the patient with heart disease. Emphasis is placed on those sections of the health history and physical examination that are affected by heart disease. General assessment techniques, with their rationale, are described. Competence in obtaining a history and in performing a physical examination cannot be achieved simply by reading the material presented. It is vitally important to become actively involved in clinical assessment, ideally with a qualified preceptor. Many hours of practice are required before the beginning student becomes skilled in assessment techniques.

CARDIOVASCULAR HISTORY

Cardiac patients who are acutely ill require a different initial history than do cardiac patients with stable or chronic conditions. A patient experiencing a myocardial infarction requires immediate, and possibly life-saving, medical and nursing interventions (e.g., relief of chest discomfort and treatment of arrhythmia) rather than an extensive inter-

view. For this patient, a few-well chosen questions regarding chest discomfort using the patient's descriptors is important. In addition, associated symptoms (such as shortness of breath or palpitations), drug allergies and reactions, current medications, history of cardiac and other major illnesses, and smoking history should be determined while assessing vital signs (heart rate and rhythm and blood pressure) and starting an intravenous line. As the patient's condition stabilizes, a more extensive history should be obtained. Cardiac patients who are not acutely ill benefit from a more detailed history and physical examination.

A comprehensive history includes the following areas:

- Identifying information
- Chief complaint or presenting problem
- History of the present illness
- Past history
- Review of systems
- Family history
- Personal and social history
- Perceived health status
- Functional patterns

The responsibility for obtaining particular portions of the health history varies with practice model and setting. In traditional, hospital-based practice models, the first six areas of the history are usually obtained by a physician, some data related to personal and social history are obtained by a physician and some by a nurse, and data related to perceived health status and functional patterns are obtained by a nurse. In collaborative practice models, all data may be obtained by an advanced-practice nurse or responsibility for all areas of data collection may be shared by the physician, advanced-practice nurse, nurse, and other members of the health care team. The cardiac nurse uses the data to make informed clinical judgments, to monitor change over time, to identify patient and family learning needs, and to coordinate care across settings.

TABLE 10-1	Differential Diagnosis of Episodic Chest Pain Resembling Angina Pectoris					
Diagnosis	**Duration**	**Quality**	**Provocation**	**Relief**	**Location**	**Comment**
Effort angina	5–15 min	Visceral (pressure)	During effort or motion	Rest, nitroglycerin	Substernal radiates	First episode vivid
Rest angina	5–15 min	Visceral (pressure)	Spontaneous	Nitroglycerin	Substernal radiates	Often nocturnal
Mitral prolapse	Minutes to hours	Superficial (rarely visceral)	Spontaneous (no pattern)	Time	Left anterior	No pattern, variable character
Esophageal reflux	10–60 min	Visceral	Recumbency, lack of food	Food, antacid	Substernal epigastric	Rarely radiates
Esophageal spasm	5–60 min	Visceral	Spontaneous, cold liquids, exercise	Nitroglycerin	Substernal radiates	Mimics angina
Peptic ulcer	Hours	Visceral (burning)	Lack of food, "acid" foods	Food, antacids	Epigastric substernal	
Biliary disease	Hours	Visceral (wax and wane)	Spontaneous, food	Time, analgesia	Epigastric radiates	Colic
Cervical disc	Variable (gradually subsides)	Superficial	Head and neck movement, palpation	Time, analgesia	Arm, neck	Not relieved by rest
Hyperventilation	2–3 min	Visceral	Emotion tachypnea	Stimulus removal	Substernal	Facial paresthesia
Musculoskeletal	Variable	Superficial	Movement, palpation	Time, analgesia	Multiple	Tenderness
Pulmonary	30 minutes+	Visceral (pressure)	Often spontaneous	Rest, time, bronchodilator	Substernal	Dyspneic

From Christie LG Jr, Conti CR: Systematic approach to the evaluation of angina-like chest pain. Am Heart J 102: 899, 1981.

HEALTH HISTORY

The health history is the patient's story of his or her diseases, symptoms, illness experiences, and responses to actual and potential health problems. The history-taking process may be the first phase in establishing a therapeutic relationship. The history is a precise, concise, chronologic description of the patient's current health status. The patient is the primary source of historical data; however, questioning of family members or close friends may provide essential information about symptoms and the impact of heart disease on family members. For example, the bed partner is more likely than the patient to provide a history of periodic respiration or sleep apnea.

The primary symptoms of heart disease include chest discomfort, dyspnea, syncope, palpitations, edema, cough, hemoptysis, and excess fatigue. Heart disease develops slowly and the patient may have a long period of asymptomatic disease and may present initially with acute collapse. To describe the health history, a sample symptom, chest discomfort, is used throughout. Guidelines are useful in differentiating chest discomfort due to serious, life-threatening conditions from those conditions that are less serious or would be treated in a different manner.[10] Table 10-1 summarizes conditions associated with chest discomfort.

IDENTIFYING INFORMATION

The patient's name, the name by which he or she prefers to be called, his or her age and birth date, and date and time of the interview are all recorded under identification of the patient. It is assumed that all data in the history are obtained from the patient; when this is not the case, secondary data sources (e.g., family member, clinical records) should be identified. The use of an interpreter should also be recorded.

CHIEF COMPLAINT OR PRESENTING PROBLEM

The chief complaint or presenting problem is the reason the person has sought health care and represents his or her priority for treatment. It should be recorded within quotation marks exactly as stated. The chief complaint also should indicate duration, such as "chest discomfort for 2 hours." An asymptomatic patient may present because of a community screening activity—for example, "high blood cholesterol discovered on finger-stick last month."

A patient may have more than one chief complaint. Some complaints are closely related and may be listed together, such as "chest discomfort and weakness for 2 hours." If complaints are unrelated, they should be listed separately in the order of importance to the patient. In general, "the greater the number of symptoms, the less the significance of each."[32]

There are four important points to remember when evaluating chest discomfort:[46]

1. For a patient who has a history of or who is at risk for development of coronary heart disease, always assume that the chest discomfort is secondary to ischemia until proven otherwise. This practice is important because unrelieved myocardial ischemia is immediately life threatening and can extend infarct size, resulting in serious complications such as lethal arrhythmia or cardiogenic shock. Chest discomfort related to other conditions, such as pulmonary emboli, usually is not as immediately life threatening.

2. There may be little correlation between the severity of the chest discomfort and the gravity of its cause. That is, pain is a subjective experience and depends in part on a lifetime of learned reactions to it. A stoic person may not admit to having much discomfort and yet may be having a large myocardial infarction. Another person may express extreme pain and yet may be experiencing stable angina rather than an acute myocardial infarction. Stress can increase pain. Taking into account the patient's usual response to pain (often obtained from a family member) may assist the nurse to interpret the patient's pain response better. In addition, older adults or people with diabetes may have altered sensory perception and little or no discomfort in the presence of severe disease.[8] When present, positive objective signs, such as ST segment shifts on the electrocardiogram, are clear indicators of the significance of the subjective symptom. It is important to realize that the absence of electrocardiographic criteria for ischemia or infarction does not eliminate the clinical significance of the chest pain.

3. There is a poor correlation between the location of chest discomfort and its source because of the concept of "referred pain," which is pain originating in one location but being interpreted by the patient as occurring in another location. Commonly, cardiac discomfort is perceived as being in the arm, jaw, neck, or epigastric area rather than in the chest (see Fig. 20-13).

4. The patient may have more than one clinical problem occurring simultaneously, particularly if he or she has delayed seeking medical assistance.

HISTORY OF THE PRESENT ILLNESS

For the symptomatic patient, obtaining the history of the present illness starts with a more detailed discussion of the chief complaint. Begin with an open-ended question, such as "Tell me more about your chest discomfort." There is a wide range in patients' abilities to express thoughts accurately, chronologically, and succinctly. Some patients need guidance more than others. Listen to the patient. It is best to let patients tell their stories in a comfortable manner. However, patients who appear to be rambling need to be redirected by clarifying or leading questions. The information that must be obtained when describing any symptom is the time and manner of onset, frequency and duration, location, quality, quantity, setting, associated symptoms, alleviating or aggravating factors, pertinent negative responses, impact of the symptom on usual or desired activities, and the meaning attributed to the symptom by the patient.

The *time of onset* should be recorded when possible with both the date and time, for example, "9 PM on December 22nd." When the patient presents with chest discomfort it is essential to know how long the discomfort has been present and if it has been present continuously since onset. The *manner of onset* is the way in which the symptom began. For example, discomfort may begin suddenly and reach maximum intensity immediately, or there may be a growing awareness of the discomfort over time. *Frequency and duration* should be stated specifically rather than generally—for example, "once a week," "once a day," or "more than three times a day." Likewise, patients should be assisted to express the duration of the discomfort, as in "2 minutes," "15 minutes," or "1 hour." For patients with a history of angina, it is also important to determine if there has been any change in frequency or duration of chest discomfort, which suggests worsening of the underlying disease.

Ask the patient to describe the exact *location* of the symptom by pointing to it. Cardiac pain is diffuse and the patient often rubs a hand over the sternum and precordium. Chest pain that can be precisely located with a fingertip is usually related to chest wall abnormalities.[5] If the pain radiates, the patient should trace its path with a fingertip. The *quality* of a symptom refers to its unique characteristics, such as color, appearance, and texture. Chest discomfort is so subjective that its quality is particularly difficult to describe. Thus, whenever possible, it is important to use the patient's own words (in quotation marks). Words that patients often use to describe chest discomfort include constriction, aching, pressure, squeezing, heaviness, indigestion, burning, strangling, choking in throat, and expansion.[8] The patient's response to the symptom also should be recorded; for example, "It makes me stop what I'm doing and sit down," or "I can continue my activities without stopping."

Quantity refers to the size, extent, or amount of the symptom. The quantity of the chest discomfort is described in terms of its severity. Again, quantity is extremely subjective and might be rated best on a 10-point scale, ranging from "barely noticeable" (1) to "the worst pain ever" (10). The severity of pain should be recorded as a fraction (e.g., 2/10 or 10/10).

Ask patients to describe the *setting* and if they were alone or with someone when the symptom occurred. If the symptom has occurred before, ascertain if the setting, circumstances, or the presence of another person is consistent during symptom onset. This information may be useful later in counseling or helping a patient gain insight into the development of his or her symptoms. Chest discomfort that is reliably associated with activity (e.g., walking up hill) is a specific indicator of cardiac ischemia.

The patient should be asked to describe any *associated symptoms* that always accompany the chief complaint. For example, palpitations and dizziness might always precede the chest discomfort. If the patient mentions associated symptoms, these should be described in the same manner as the chief complaint (i.e., quality, quantity, onset, duration). It is important to note whether these associated symptoms occur consistently with the chief complaint or occur independently at other times.

Alleviating factors, such as resting, changing position, or taking medication, should be noted. Change in the time it takes for alleviating factors to be effective should be identified. For example, if in the past the chest discomfort resolved with 5 minutes of rest and now requires 10 minutes, worsening or a new pathologic process is suggested. *Aggravating factors,* such as eating, exercising, or being in a cold climate, also must be recorded. These factors can provide helpful diagnostic information. To complete the present illness history, it is also important to record any *pertinent negative responses* to the interviewer's questions, such as "The chest discomfort is not made worse by strenuous exercise." The patient should be specifically asked about palpitations, dizziness, syncope, dyspnea, orthopnea, and paroxysmal nocturnal dyspnea, if these symptoms have not already been described.

Impact of the symptom on usual or desired activities should be explored. Some people with recurrent chest discomfort reduce their activity over time to try and prevent chest discomfort. It is essential that clinicians understand how the symptom or disease has affected the patient's activity and perceived quality of life.

Throughout the interview, the nurse observes the patient carefully and may begin to understand the meaning the illness has for the patient. The personal meaning of the illness can amplify or reduce the symptom experience and course of action. For example, a 38-year-old, female cardiac nurse who experiences chest discomfort may attend to the symptom and seek assistance urgently, or she may ignore the symptom and dismiss it as indigestion.

The results of diagnostic or laboratory testing specifically related to heart disease are included in the *history of present illness.* Prior cardiac events (e.g., coronary artery bypass surgery or myocardial infarction) are included also.

We recommend that cardiovascular risk factors and current activity be added in a separate paragraph to the conventional content of the history of present illness. Risk factors for coronary heart disease are discussed in Chapter 29.

Sample questions that may be used in assessing the patient with acute or recurrent chest discomfort follow. Similar questions may be generated to assess patients with other symptoms. However, it is important to phrase the questions according to the appropriateness of the situation and logically to pursue areas where further clarification is necessary.

- When exactly do you get the discomfort?
- What were you doing when the chest discomfort occurred?
- Exactly how often does the chest discomfort occur?
- How many minutes does it usually last?
- Can you point to the exact location where it starts?
- Does the discomfort move anywhere else?

- If so, can you trace its path with your fingertip?
- What words would you use to describe how the discomfort feels?
- What do you do when you have the chest discomfort?
- Quantify your discomfort on a 1-to-10 scale.
- Where were you when the discomfort occurred?
- If the chest discomfort has occurred before, have you always been in the same place?
- Were you alone at the time or with someone?
- Did you notice any other symptoms that occurred at the same time?
- If yes, does this other symptom ever occur by itself?
- What can you do to make the chest discomfort better?
- What can you do to make it worse?
- Are you taking any medication to improve your chest discomfort?
- If yes, what is the medication?
- Does any medication you are taking affect your chest discomfort?
- If yes, what is the medication?
- What time of day do you prefer to take your medication?
- What activities have you given up because of your chest discomfort?
- What do you think this chest discomfort means?

PAST HISTORY

The past history includes past illnesses and interventions not directly related to the present illness. For a patient with chest discomfort, the history of a previous myocardial infarction, coronary artery bypass surgery, or cholecystectomy belongs in the *history of present illness,* whereas a remote appendectomy does not. Major elements of the *past history* include childhood and adult illnesses, accidents and injuries, current health status, current medications, allergies, and health maintenance. Always ask about major illnesses such as chronic obstructive airway disease, diabetes mellitus, bleeding disorders, and acquired immunodeficiency syndrome.

Allergic reactions (e.g., to drugs, food, environmental agents, or animals) also should be noted. Always ask if the patient has an allergy to penicillin or to commonly used emergency drugs, such as lidocaine hydrochloride and morphine sulfate. Allergy to shellfish suggests iodine sensitivity and is important because agents used in cardiac diagnostic tests may contain iodine. Both the allergen and the reaction should always be noted, because some patients confuse an allergic reaction with a drug's side effect.

Medication history includes all prescription and over-the-counter drugs and home remedies. Over-the-counter preparations that increase heart rate or afterload may precipitate or worsen symptoms. If the patient has brought medications with him or her, these should be reviewed by the nurse and then sent home or to the appropriate area for safekeeping.

FAMILY HISTORY

The major purpose of the family history is to assess risk factors affecting the patient's current or future health. Notations regarding the age and health status of each first degree family member are made: living and well, deceased, and the possible or confirmed diagnosis now or at death. Family occurrences of diabetes, kidney disease, tuberculosis, cancer, arthritis, asthma, allergies, mental illness, alcoholism, and drug addiction are included. A family history of coronary heart disease, myocardial infarction, or sudden death would be included in the history of present illness for a patient presenting with chest discomfort.

PERSONAL AND SOCIAL HISTORY

The personal and social history includes important and relevant information about the patient as a person. An individual's response to illness is determined in part by his or her cultural background, socioeconomic standing, education, and beliefs about the illness. Major elements include health habits, home situation, and supports and resources. Occupational history may be included here or in the past history. *Health habits* include alcohol, drug, or tobacco use, nutrition, sleep, and physical activity. Use of alcohol and the amount per time period (day, week, year) should be recorded. The use of recreational drugs, especially cocaine, should also be assessed. The cigarette smoking history should be recorded as the number of pack-years (packs per day multiplied by the number of years) the patient has smoked. Other tobacco use, such as pipe or cigar smoking or chewing tobacco, should be recorded. Special diets, such as low-sodium or low-fat diets, should be identified and the patient's usual eating pattern described. The usual number of hours the patient sleeps and circumstances that impair or facilitate sleep should be assessed.

Current Living Circumstances. These include marital status, number of children, occupation, financial resources, and hobbies.

Perceived Health and Coping Challenges. The patient's perception of his or her current health status as either good or bad is helpful in assessing how he or she views its effect on daily living. For example, a 42-year-old man with an old anterior myocardial infarction is seen in the clinic. His chief complaint is extreme fatigue that prevents him from working a full 8-hour day at the office. Initial investigation focuses on ruling out any new process affecting the adequacy of cardiac output, such as a left ventricular aneurysm. Nonpathophysiologic causes for fatigue must be considered also, such as fear of overstressing his heart and sudden death, changes in the work situation, family difficulties, or depression.

Being aware of patients' goals in terms of health and lifestyle are important in determining whether their expectations are realistic. "What do you see yourself doing 3 months from now?" is a good way to ask the patient to define the goal. Another approach is ascertaining what changes the patient would be willing to make in life if the goal could not be achieved.

Assessing the patient's and family's expectations of health care has implications for teaching. For example, is the patient with unstable angina pectoris who has been admitted after "cardiac catheterization" able to explain what the test was and why it resulted in admission? Communication among the health care team members is essential before planning any teaching.

Resources and Support System. It is important to consider the patient's strengths and support system when planning care across the continuum: environmental resources, such as the proximity to the hospital; personal-social support, such as a spouse to provide home care; and economic support, such as adequate insurance, are all examples. Needed resources that are not readily available also must be considered. Knowledge of the patient's health benefits and financial status assists the health care team in designing an affordable therapeutic regimen: for example, the avoidance of expensive combination or sustained-release medications when other drugs and dosage forms that are as effective and less costly are available.

REVIEW OF SYSTEMS

To ensure that all important areas have been considered, a systematic review of all body systems is conducted. Lists of major symptoms associated with each body system are included in health assessment textbooks.[2,26] Some clinicians prefer to conduct the review of systems simultaneously with the physical examination. For the patient with chest discomfort, the review of the cardiac, pulmonary, and gastrointestinal system is logically included in the history of present illness.

FUNCTIONAL PATTERNS

Clinical information related to function is collected in the following areas:[20]

- ◆ Health perception—health management
- ◆ Nutrition—metabolism
- ◆ Elimination
- ◆ Activity—exercise
- ◆ Cognitive—perceptual
- ◆ Sleep—rest
- ◆ Self-perception, self-concept
- ◆ Roles and relationships
- ◆ Sexuality
- ◆ Coping—stress
- ◆ Values—beliefs

Information collected within these functional patterns does not duplicate information collected within other areas of the health history. The sequence of data gathered in the functional assessment is determined by the patient's clinical condition and the purpose of the encounter. Relevant data obtained earlier in the history should not be repeated.

For the acutely ill cardiac patient who is admitted to the hospital, areas that affect the hospital experience are assessed first. As the patient is able, all functional patterns are assessed. To facilitate the gathering of subjective information for the functional assessment, examples of questions, using the sample symptom of chest discomfort, follow. Functional assessment is an ongoing process that evaluates the effect of intervention on patient outcome.

Health Perception—Health Management. Collect the following information:

- What concerns do you have about your health or hospitalization?
- What things are important to you while you are hospitalized? How can we make this experience as easy as possible for you?
- What do you think caused this illness (symptom)?
- Compared with others your age, how would you rate your general health?
- What things do you believe are important to maintain your health?

Nutrition—Metabolism. Collect the following information:

- What do you like to eat (including cultural or ethnic favorites)?
- How are your foods prepared (canned or commercially prepared foods versus fresh foods)?
- Do you usually eat in a restaurant, fast-food outlet, or at home?
- Who shops for groceries?
- Who prepares the meals?
- Are you on a special diet?

Elimination. Collect the following information:

- Is the amount that you urinate normal for you?
- Do you ever get up at night to use the bathroom? If so, how many times?
- If there was a change in elimination pattern, when did you notice it?
- Do you sometimes lose urine or find that you cannot quite make it to the bathroom?
- Do you take a diuretic? If so, when do you take it?
- What is your usual frequency of bowel movements? When was your last movement?
- Are there things you do to maintain that pattern?

Activity—Exercise. Collect the following information:

- Have you noticed a change in your usual or desired activity level?
- Do you have sufficient energy for your desired activities?
- What is the most strenuous activity you perform on a regular basis? How often and how long?
- What leisure or recreational activities do you enjoy? Are you currently able to participate in these activities?
- Are you satisfied with your current level of activity?

Cognitive—Perceptual. Collect the following information:

- Do you have any difficulty with seeing or hearing? Glasses or hearing aid?
- Do you think as fast as you used to? As clearly?
- In general, what is the easiest way for you to learn new material? Any learning difficulties?
- Do you understand why you are in the hospital?
- What does your diagnosis mean to you?

- What is your understanding of the treatment plan?
- Do you understand the risk factors for heart disease and how to modify them?
- Do you understand how long you will be in the hospital and when you can return to your usual activities of daily living?

Sleep—Rest. Collect the following information:

- How many hours do you usually sleep? What hours?
- Do you have difficulty falling asleep or staying asleep? Has this been a change for you or have you always had this difficulty?
- Do you follow a specific bedtime routine or ritual?

Self-Perception, Self-Concept. Collect the following information:

- How would you describe yourself? Your personality? Your approach to life?
- Most of the time, do you feel good about yourself?
- Have you noticed changes in yourself or your body? Do these changes concern you?

Roles and Relationships. Collect the following information:

- Do you live alone? With whom do you live?
- Do you have a close friend or confidant?
- How do you and those close to you feel about your illness?
- Do you often feel lonely? Do you feel part of the neighborhood in which you live?

Sexuality. Collect the following information:

- Have you experienced any changes in your sexuality? Problems in sexual relationships?
- For women: are you still menstruating? Are you taking hormone replacements?

Coping—Stress. Collect the following information:

- Do you feel tense or anxious much of the time? What helps? Do you use medicines for this?
- When you feel stressed, who is most helpful to you?
- When you have big problems in your life, how do you handle them? Does that usually work for you?

Values—Beliefs. Collect the following information:

- Are you generally satisfied with your life?
- Is religion important to you?
- Do you hold religious or other beliefs that you wish to observe here?

Functional and Therapeutic Classification

After the history is completed, it may be possible to categorize the patient according to the New York Heart Association's Functional and Therapeutic Classification[35] (Table 10-2). This classification may be helpful in assessing

TABLE 10-2	Functional and Therapeutic Classification of Patients with Diseases of the Heart

Functional Classification		**Therapeutic Classification**	
Class I	Patients with cardiac disease but without resulting limitations of physical activity. Ordinary physical activity does not cause undue fatigue, palpitation, dyspnea, or anginal pain.	Class A	Patients with cardiac disease whose physical activity need not be restricted in any way.
Class II	Patients with cardiac disease resulting in slight limitation of physical activity. They are comfortable at rest. Ordinary physical activity results in fatigue, palpitation, dyspnea, or anginal pain.	Class B	Patients with cardiac disease whose ordinary physical activity need not be restricted, but who should be advised against severe or competitive efforts.
Class III	Patients with cardiac disease resulting in marked limitation of physical activity. They are comfortable at rest. Less than ordinary physical activity causes fatigue, palpitation, dyspnea, or anginal pain.	Class C	Patients with cardiac disease whose ordinary physical activity should be moderately restricted and whose more strenuous efforts should be discontinued.
Class IV	Patients with cardiac disease resulting in inability to carry on any physical activity without discomfort. Symptoms of cardiac insufficiency or of the anginal syndrome may be present even at rest. If any physical activity is undertaken, discomfort is increased.	Class D	Patients with cardiac disease whose ordinary physical activity should be markedly restricted.
		Class E	Patients with cardiac disease who should be at complete rest, confined to bed or chair.

From New York Heart Association Criteria Committee: Diseases of the Heart and Blood Vessels: Nomenclature and Criteria for Diagnosis, 6th ed. Boston, Little, Brown, 1964.

symptom severity and monitoring effects of treatment over time. The patient's functional classification may improve as recovery from an acute event, such as myocardial infarction, occurs or as intervention is optimized. Conversely, it may decline with worsening or additional disease.

PHYSICAL ASSESSMENT

Assessment of physical findings confirms or expands data obtained in the health history. Baseline information is obtained at the initial encounter and frequency of subsequent assessments is based on the clinical encounter. Change in the data over time documents progression of, or recovery from acute disease; new disease; the effectiveness of current interventions; and the patient's current functional status. The type, degree, and rate of change assist the nurse in identifying or predicting immediate or long-term problems, formulating nursing diagnoses, planning care, and establishing individual patient outcome criteria.

In the acutely ill cardiac patient, segments of the physical examination are performed every 2 to 4 hours or more frequently if indicated. Although some data may be available from monitoring devices, physical examination assists in evaluating the accuracy of those data. As the acutely ill patient improves, assessments are routinely done once per shift or more frequently if indicated. If a rapid change in patient condition occurs, the initial assessment is problem focused and the complete assessment is done at a later time. Because nurses spend 24 hours per day with the hospitalized patient, they are in the best position to identify any changes that occur. It is to the patient's benefit for changes to be detected early, before serious complications develop. The cardiac nurse who telephones the physician to report

that the patient "just does not look good" lacks the credibility of the nurse who identifies "a new S_3 gallop, bilateral crackles halfway up the posterior lung fields, and jugular venous pressure of 14 cm H_2O." Any changes observed in the examination should be documented in the patient's record and reported to the physician. To collect, correlate, and interpret the data accurately, a thorough understanding of the cardiac cycle (see Chapter 1) is essential. A cardiac physical assessment should include an evaluation of:

♦ The heart as a pump—reduced pulse pressure, cardiac enlargement, and presence of murmurs and gallop rhythms
♦ Filling volumes and pressures—the degree of jugular venous pressure and the presence or absence of crackles, peripheral edema, and postural changes in blood pressure
♦ Cardiac output—heart rate, blood pressure, pulse pressure, systemic vascular resistance, urine output, and central nervous system manifestations
♦ Compensatory mechanisms—increased filling volumes, peripheral vasoconstriction, and elevated heart rate

The order and techniques of examination proceed logically. The precise order may vary with the setting and the condition of the patient. With practice, the focused cardiovascular examination can be done in approximately 10 minutes:

♦ General appearance
♦ Head
♦ Arterial pulse
♦ Jugular venous pressure
♦ Blood pressure

- ◆ Peripheral vasculature
- ◆ Heart
- ◆ Lungs
- ◆ Abdomen

General Appearance

Observe the general appearance of the patient while the history is being obtained. The patient's appearance and responses provide cues to the cardiovascular status. Note general build, skin color, presence of shortness of breath, and distention of neck veins. Assess the patient's level of distress. If he or she is in pain, the patient's response to it may assist in the differential diagnosis. For example, moving about is a characteristic response to the pain of myocardial infarction, whereas sitting quietly is more characteristic of angina, and leaning forward is more characteristic of pericarditis.[38] Some abnormalities of the arterial pulses may be observed unobtrusively. For example, patients with severe aortic insufficiency may have bounding pulses that cause the head to bob.[38] Note appropriateness of weight; malnutrition and cachexia are associated with chronic, severe heart failure.[36] Skeletal manifestations of Marfan's syndrome, tall stature and arachnodactyly, may be observed. Level of consciousness should be described. Appropriateness of thought content, reflecting the adequacy of cerebral perfusion, is particularly important to evaluate. Family members who are most familiar with the patient can be of help in alerting the examiner to subtle behavior changes. The nurse also should be aware of the patient's anxiety level, not only to attempt to put the patient more at ease, but to realize its effects on the cardiovascular system.

Head

The examination of the head includes assessment of facial characteristics, color, temperature, and eyes. For advanced-practice nurses, a funduscopic examination also may be performed.

FACIAL CHARACTERISTICS

Examination of the facial characteristics may aid in the recognition of disorders affecting the cardiovascular system. *Coronary heart disease* is suggested by the presence of an earlobe crease in a person younger than 45 years of age. *Rheumatic heart disease* with severe mitral stenosis is associated with a malar flush, cyanotic lips, and slight jaundice from hepatic congestion. With severe aortic regurgitation, head bobbing with each heartbeat (de Musset's sign) may be present. Infective endocarditis is associated with a "café au lait" complexion. *Constrictive pericarditis* and *tricuspid valve disease* tend to cause facial edema. *Pheochromocytoma* is associated with episodic facial flushing, as well as severe hypertension and tachyarrhythmia.[5,9,37]

Systemic lupus erythematosus may present with a butterfly rash on the face and may suggest inflammatory heart disease. A systemic lupus erythematosus-like syndrome frequently occurs with procainamide administration but disappears after discontinuation of the drug. *Myxedema* is characterized by dry, sparse hair; loss of lateral eyebrows; a dull, expressionless face; and periorbital puffiness. Because a myocardial effect of hypothyroidism is reduced cardiac output, heart failure may develop in these patients. *Cushing's syndrome* is characterized by moon facies, hirsutism, acne, and centripetal obesity with thin extremities. High blood pressure frequently occurs with Cushing's syndrome.[5,9,36]

COLOR

Cyanosis is the bluish discoloration seen through the skin and mucous membranes when the concentration of reduced hemoglobin exceeds 5 g/100 mL of blood. *Peripheral cyanosis* implies reduced blood flow to the periphery. Because more time is available for the tissues to extract oxygen from the hemoglobin molecule, the arteriovenous oxygen difference widens. Cyanosis of the nose, lips, and earlobes is considered peripheral. Peripheral cyanosis may occur physiologically with the vasoconstriction associated with anxiety or a cold environment, or pathologically in conditions that reduce blood flow to the periphery, such as cardiogenic shock.

Central cyanosis, as observed in the buccal mucosa, implies serious heart or lung disease and is accompanied by peripheral cyanosis. In severe heart disease, a right-to-left shunt exists in which blood passes through the lungs without being fully oxygenated, as happens in severe heart failure with interstitial pulmonary edema. In severe lung disease, changes produced by chronic obstructive airway disease or fibrosis impede oxygenation.

Pallor can denote anemia (with concomitant decreased oxygen-carrying capacity) or an increased systemic vascular resistance. *Jaundice* can be associated with hepatic engorgement from right ventricular failure.

TEMPERATURE

Temperature reflects the balance of heat production and dissipation in the body. Normal oral temperature is considered to be 37° C (98.6° F). However, there is a diurnal pattern of temperature fluctuation, with temperatures as low as 35.8° C (96.4° F) orally in the early morning to as high as 37.3° C (99.1° F) orally in the late afternoon or evening. Oral temperatures average 0.6° C (1.0° F) lower than rectal temperatures.[30] Normal body temperature may be less than 37° C in older adults because of reduced heat production (lower metabolic activity, less muscle mass and activity) and conservation (less insulation).[28]

In hospitalized patients, body temperature usually is measured on admission and then every 4 hours or more often if indicated. After cardiac surgery, temperature is measured every 15 to 30 minutes until rewarming is complete, and every 1 to 4 hours until normothermia is achieved. Measure the temperature orally unless the patient is unconscious or unable to close his or her mouth. Body temperatures also may be measured rectally, by means of a pulmonary artery catheter equipped with a thermistor, by means of a thermistor-equipped urinary bladder catheter, or with a device that measures temperature in the insulated auditory meatus close to the tympanic membrane.

Pulmonary artery, urinary bladder, tympanic, and rectal temperatures are all considered to be core temperatures;

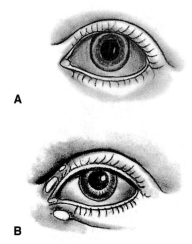

A

B

FIGURE 10-1 Eye changes suggestive of hyperlipoproteinemia. **(A)** Corneal arcus. **(B)** Xanthelasmas. (From Bates B: A Guide to Physical Examination 5th ed, pp 202, 200. Philadelphia, JB Lippincott, 1991.)

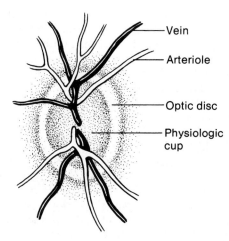

Vein

Arteriole

Optic disc

Physiologic cup

FIGURE 10-2 Funduscopic examination of retinal structures. (From Bates B: A Guide to Physical Examination, 3rd ed, p 79. Philadelphia, JB Lippincott, 1983.)

however, they actually measure somewhat different things, and simultaneous measurements may not agree, especially during hypothermia. Pulmonary artery temperature measures the mean blood temperature that results from core thermogenesis and peripheral heat loss or gain. Because urine is a filtrate of blood, urinary bladder temperature also reflects mean blood temperature, but may be falsely low in the setting of low-output renal failure. During hypothermia after cardiac surgery, rectal temperatures reflect peripheral, rather than core, temperatures.[40]

EYES

The eyes are examined for vision and appearance. A funduscopic examination may be performed.

Vision. Vision is assessed to determine if defects exist that may affect activities of daily living. The examination is as simple as having the patient read a name tag or identify an object.

Appearance. Corneal arcus, a thin, grayish-white circle around the iris, may occur normally with aging (Fig. 10-1*A*). When seen in white people younger than age 40 years, corneal arcus suggests hyperlipidemia. *Xanthelasmas* are slightly raised, yellowish plaques of cholesterol in the skin that appear along the nasal side of one or both eyelids (see Fig. 10-1*B*). They are associated with hyperlipidemia but also may occur normally. *Ophthalmitis* and *petechial* and *subconjunctival hemorrhages* of the upper and lower eyelids are seen with bacterial endocarditis.

Fundi. Examination of the ocular fundi provides the only opportunity for direct visualization of blood vessels. Vascular changes from high blood pressure and diabetes mellitus can be detected in the arteries and small veins of the retina. In general health care, funduscopic examination is conducted without pharmacologic dilation of the pupils. Phys-

iologic dilation may be maximized by darkening the room and asking the patient to gaze off in the distance. Photographs printed in books are taken through a maximally dilated pupil with a special camera. The view through the ophthalmoscope is only a small portion of the retina. It is necessary to direct the ophthalmoscope in varying directions, following blood vessels and observing the retinal structures and background.

The *funduscopic examination technique* is as follows[2]:

- ◆ Darken the room.
- ◆ Turn on the ophthalmoscope light; select the large round beam of white light.
- ◆ Adjust the lens disc to 0 diopters, keeping your index finger on the ophthalmoscope throughout the examination.
- ◆ Use your right hand and right eye to examine the patient's right eye; use your left hand and left eye to examine the patient's left eye.
- ◆ Place your opposite thumb over the patient's eyebrow to gain proprioceptive guidance as you move closer to the patient.
- ◆ Ask the patient to look straight ahead and to fix his or her gaze on a distant point.
- ◆ Brace the ophthalmoscope firmly against your face, with your eye directly behind the sight hole.
- ◆ Position yourself 6 inches (15 cm) away from the patient and 15 degrees lateral to his or her line of vision. Shine the light beam on the patient's pupil and note the *red reflex*. Absence of a *red reflex* suggests a lens opacity, such as a cataract.
- ◆ With both of your eyes open and keeping the light beam focused on the red reflex, move horizontally at a 15–degree angle slowly toward the patient. When you are approximately 1.5 to 2 inches (3 to 5 cm) from the patient, the optic disc or blood vessels should come into view (Fig. 10-2). Rotate lenses with your index finger until fundic structures are as clearly visible as possible.

◆ To overcome corneal reflection (light reflected back into the examiner's eye), direct the light beam toward the edge of the pupil rather than through its center.

◆ Examine the *optic disc,* a yellowish-orange to creamy pink oval or round structure. If you do not see the disc, follow a blood vessel centrally (by noting the angles of vessel branching and the progressive enlargement of vessel size toward the disc) until it is visible. Assess disc border clarity (nasal margin may be normally somewhat blurred) and color.

◆ Identify the *retinal arteries* and *veins* using the differential criteria of color, size, and light reflex (or reflection; Fig. 10-3*A*). Arteries and veins appear to originate from the *physiologic cup,* a small, white depression in the optic disc. Arteries are light red, two-thirds to four-fifths the diameter of veins, and have a bright light reflex. Veins are dark red, larger than arteries, and have an inconspicuous or absent light reflex. Follow the vessels peripherally in all directions, noting the character of the arteriovenous crossings. To examine the extreme periphery, instruct the patient to look up, down, temporally, and nasally.

◆ Assess the retina for any *lesions,* noting size, shape, color, and distribution.

Optic disc edema (swollen optic disc with blurred margins) is present in patients with increased intracranial pressure, retinal venous outflow obstruction, inflammation, or ischemia[1,3] (Fig. 10-4). *Beading* (abnormal constriction) of a retinal vein is common in diabetic retinopathy. With high blood pressure, thickening of the walls and narrowing of the lumen of retinal arteries develop. These changes are observed as *focal narrowing,* a *narrowed column of blood,* and a *narrowed light reflex* (see Fig. 10-3*B*). If opacity is such that no blood column is visible, the artery appears as a *silver wire artery* (see Fig. 10-3*C*). With increased filling and tortuosity, arteries closest to the optic disc manifest an increased light reflex and are known as *copper wire arteries* (see Fig. 10-3*D*). Arteriovenous crossings also are affected by thickening of the artery walls, demonstrated by *tapering* of the vein on either side of the artery (see Fig. 10-3*E*), *arteriovenous nicking* (abrupt cessation of the vein on either side of the artery; see Fig. 10-3*F*), or *banking* of the vein (venous twisting distal to the artery, forming a dark, wide buckle; see Fig. 10-3*G*).[1,3]

Red spots in the retina may be due to hemorrhage or microaneurysms, which can be associated with hypertension, diabetes, or a number of other conditions.[1,2] *Roth's spots,* hemorrhages with white centers, occur with subacute bacterial endocarditis and leukemia.[1,37] *Cotton wool patches* are white or gray and have large irregular shapes and fuzzy borders (Fig. 10-5*A*). They occur with hypertension and are seen frequently in patients with acquired immunodeficiency syndrome. *Hard exudates* are small, creamy white or yellow lesions with well-defined borders (see Fig. 10-5*B*). They occur frequently in clusters and are indicative of diabetes, hypertension, and other conditions.[2] Abnormalities of the fundi are difficult to see and require much practice.

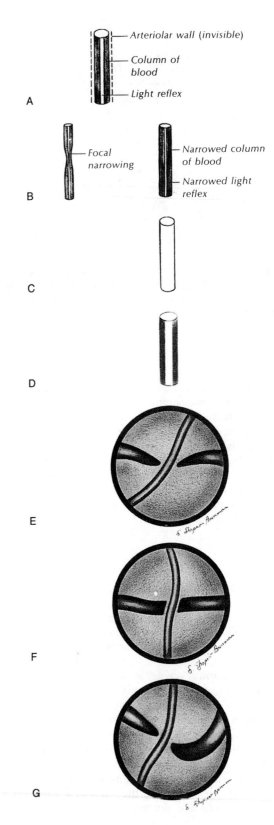

FIGURE 10-3 Vascular changes associated with high blood pressure. **(A)** Normal. **(B)** Spasm and thickening of arteriolar walls. **(C)** Silver wire arterioles. **(D)** Copper wire arterioles. **(E)** Venous tapering. **(F)** Arteriovenous nicking. **(G)** Venous banking. (From Bates B: A Guide to Physical Examination, 5th ed, p 208. Philadelphia, JB Lippincott, 1991.)

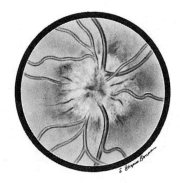

FIGURE 10-4 Papilledema. The optic disc is swollen, its margins are blurred, and the physiologic cup is not visible. (From Bates B: A Guide to Physical Examination, 5th ed, p 207. Philadelphia, JB Lippincott, 1991.)

Arterial Pulse

Information about pulse rate, rhythm, amplitude and contour, and obstruction to blood flow is obtained from palpation of the arterial pulse. Pulses should be evaluated at baseline, before and after vascular procedures that might impair blood flow, and with the onset of any symptom associated with reduced peripheral flow or ischemia. On initial examination, both carotid, both radial, both femoral, both tibial, and both dorsal pulses should be assessed.

PULSE RATE AND RHYTHM

Pulse rate and rhythm commonly are assessed in the radial artery. However, in certain clinical situations, such as shock

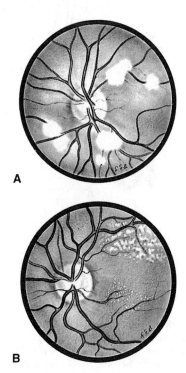

FIGURE 10-5 Light-colored spots in the retina. **(A)** Cotton wool patches. **(B)** Hard exudates. (From Bates B: A Guide to Physical Examination, 5th ed, p 210. Philadelphia, JB Lippincott, 1991.)

(with very low-amplitude or absent peripheral pulses) or during cardiac arrest (when information about central blood flow is essential), pulses should be assessed in the more centrally located carotid artery.

Pulse Rate. The pulse rate at rest usually is between 60 and 100 (average of approximately 70) pulsations per minute. A lower resting heart rate is common in athletes. Conditions or activities such as exercise, fever, and stress increase the pulse rate. Hypothermia, certain drugs, and heart blocks, for example, decrease the pulse rate. Each pulse wave is indicative of a cardiac contraction. However, each cardiac contraction does not necessarily result in a peripheral pulse. In patients with heart disease, pulse rate may be slower than heart rate because not all cardiac contractions are perfused peripherally. Extremely fast heart rates, such as atrial fibrillation with an uncontrolled ventricular response or premature supraventricular or ventricular contractions, have shortened diastolic filling times, resulting in reduced stroke volume and, therefore, diminished or absent pulses. For this reason, pulse rate should not be recorded from the heart rate display on the cardiac monitor or counted from an electrocardiographic strip.

Using the pads of the index and middle fingers, compress the artery until maximum pulsation is detected. Count the rate. If regular, count for 15 seconds and multiply by 4; if irregular, count for a full minute, noting the variations in rhythm.

In all cardiac patients and in any patient with an irregular heart rate, simultaneously auscultate the apical rate and palpate the peripheral rate (*apical-radial rate*); record both rates. It is important that the apical-radial rates be counted during the *same* minute. If the apical-radial difference is very large, if the rate is very fast, or if the examiner is not yet skilled, it may be helpful to have two people count for the same minute.

Pulse Rhythm. Pulse rhythm is normally regular. Physiologic variation can occur with respiration. During inspiration, blood flow to the right heart is increased, right ventricular output is enhanced, and pulmonary venous capacitance is increased. Consequently, blood flow to the left heart is reduced, causing a drop in left ventricular stroke volume. Cardiac output is maintained by a compensatory increase in heart rate (mediated by the baroreceptors). During expiration, the large amount of blood residing in the pulmonary vascular bed during inspiration reaches the left heart. Left ventricular contractility is enhanced by means of the Frank-Starling mechanism, increasing left ventricular stroke volume. Because an increased heart rate is no longer needed to maintain cardiac output, the heart rate returns to baseline. This physiologically irregular rhythm is termed *sinus arrhythmia.* It is common in people younger than 40 years of age.

Other irregular rhythms are not normal. The irregularity should be described as regularly irregular (e.g., every other pulse wave is early) or irregularly irregular (e.g., atrial fibrillation). Occasional, early pulsations that are perceived as transient skips or breaks in an otherwise regular rhythm are common and are not necessarily abnormal.

PULSE AMPLITUDE AND CONTOUR

Pulses are described in a variety of ways. The simplest classification is absent, present, and bounding. A 0-to-4 scale is often used, and pulses are graded as follows: absent (0), diminished (1+), normal (2+), moderately increased (3+), and markedly increased (4+).[36] This scale is fairly subjective and, although an individual tends to be internally consistent over time, different people may grade the same pulse differently. There are also other scales in which the numbers are defined differently.

The amplitude of an arterial pulse is a function of the pulse pressure, which is related to stroke volume, elasticity of the arterial tree, and velocity of left ventricular ejection. Increased stroke volume, as occurs with exercise or excitement, results in increased amplitude and a bounding arterial pulse.

Small, weak pulses (Fig. 10-6*B*) have a diminished pulse pressure, which is indicative of a reduced stroke volume and ejection fraction and of increased systemic vascular resistance.

Large, bounding pulses result from an increased pulse pressure (see Fig. 10-6*C*). Increased pulse pressure is caused by increased stroke volume and ejection velocity and by diminished peripheral vasoconstriction. *Corrigan's pulse* is a bounding pulse visible in the carotid artery. It occurs with aortic regurgitation.

The amplitude of a pulse contributes to its contour, but contour refers to the rate of rise and the shape of the arterial pulse. Because of the distortion that occurs when the pulse wave is transmitted peripherally, pulse contour is best assessed in the carotid arteries. The *normal pulse contour* has a rapid and smooth upstroke. The dicrotic notch is not palpable (see Fig. 10-6*A*), although the dicrotic wave (see Fig. 10-6*I*) may be palpable in heart failure and in febrile states.[23] Usually it is palpable only in the peripheral arteries.

Pulsus bisferiens (see Fig. 10-6*D*) is characterized by a rapid upstroke and double systolic peak. This pulse may be present in idiopathic hypertrophic subaortic stenosis, aortic stenosis with regurgitation, and pure aortic insufficiency.

Pulsus alternans (see Fig. 10-6*E*) is a regular rhythm in which strong pulse waves alternate with weak ones. It is an ominous sign when it occurs at normal heart rates and suggests serious heart disease. The difference in amplitude may be slight and difficult to palpate. The presence of pulsus alternans can be confirmed with a sphygmomanometer. The cuff is inflated above systolic pressure and slowly released until the first heart sound is audible. Cuff pressure is held at this point and the pulse palpated to determine if every pulse is audible.

Bigeminal pulses (see Fig. 10-6*F*), which should not be confused with pulsus alternans, are caused by a bigeminal, premature ectopic rhythm. Note that every other pulse wave is not only diminished but is early.

Pulsus paradoxus (see Fig. 10-6*G*) is the reduction in strength of the arterial pulse that can be felt during abnormal inspiratory decline of left ventricular filling. However, it is more apparent and can be quantified if sphygmomanometry is used. (Refer to the discussion of the determination of paradoxical blood pressure, later.)

Pulsus parvus et tardus (see Fig. 10-6*H*) is found in severe aortic stenosis. It resembles the double systolic beat

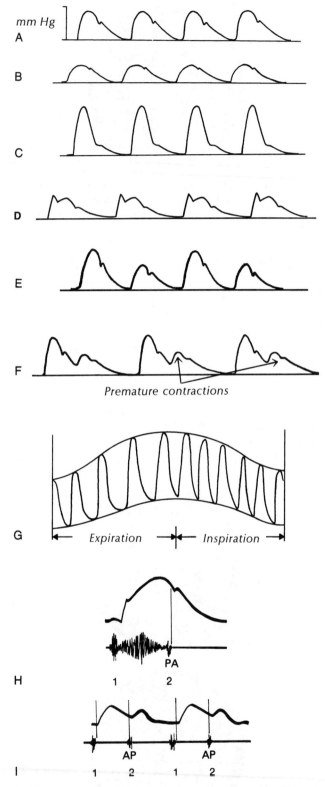

FIGURE 10-6 Normal and abnormal pulses. **(A)** Normal. **(B)** Small and weak. **(C)** Large and bounding. **(D)** Bisferiens. **(E)** Pulsus alternans. **(F)** Bigeminal. **(G)** Pulsus paradoxus. **(H)** Parvus et tardus. **(I)** Dicrotic. (A–G from Bates B: A Guide to Physical Examination, 5th ed, p 308. Philadelphia, JB Lippincott, 1991; **H,I** adapted from Hurst JW, Schlant, RC: Examination of the arteries and their pulsation. In Hurst JW, Logue RB, Schlant RC et al [eds]: The Heart, 4th ed, pp 186–187. New York, McGraw-Hill, 1978.)

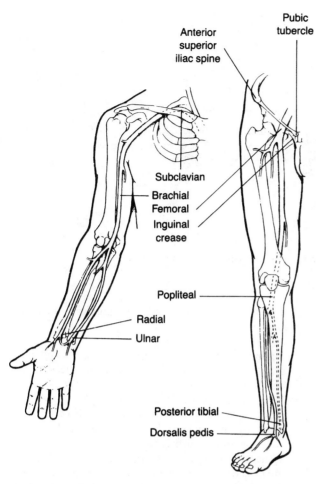

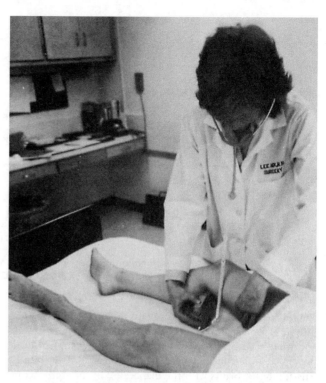

FIGURE 10-8 Use of Doppler probe. (From Greenfield LJ: Acute venous thrombosis and pulmonary embolism. In Hardy JD [ed]: Hardy's Textbook of Surgery, p 973. Philadelphia, JB Lippincott, 1983.)

FIGURE 10-7 Peripheral arteries and their landmarks. (From Boozer M, Craven RF: Assessment of vascular function. In Patrick ML, Woods SL, Craven RF et al [eds]: Medical–Surgical Nursing: Pathophysiological Concepts, p 595. Philadelphia, JB Lippincott, 1986.)

in pulsus bisferiens, but its upstroke is more gradual and the pulse pressure is smaller. Usually it is palpable only in the carotid artery.

Carotid Pulse. The carotid artery is best for assessing pulse-wave amplitude and contour. Observe the neck for pulsations. Carotid pulsations are visible bilaterally just medial to the sternocleidomastoid muscle. Place your fingertips along the medial border of the sternocleidomastoid muscle in the lower half of the neck. Press posteriorly to feel the artery. Palpate well below the upper border of the thyroid cartilage to avoid compressing the carotid sinus, which might result in a reflex drop in heart rate or blood pressure. Compare one side with the other, but do not palpate both sides simultaneously because brain blood flow might be interrupted. Using the side with the strongest pulsations, assess the amplitude and contour of the pulse wave and determine whether it occurs in early systole or has a delayed upstroke.

Peripheral Circulation. In the legs, assess femoral, popliteal, dorsalis pedis, and posterior tibial pulses (Fig. 10-7). The popliteal pulse is never directly palpable; only the transmitted pulsations can be detected.[12] In the arms, assess brachial, radial, and ulnar pulses. When assessing peripheral circulation, always compare one side with the other. An *Allen test* should be performed before radial arterial cannulation to evaluate radial and ulnar arterial patency. Simultaneously compress the radial and ulnar arteries and ask the patient to make a fist. The hand blanches. Ask the patient to open his or her fist. Release the pressure from the ulnar artery while maintaining pressure on the radial artery. The hand color returns to normal if the ulnar artery is patent. Repeat the process releasing pressure from the radial artery. If dual circulation to the hand is not present, do not attempt radial arterial puncture or cannulation.

In shock states associated with reduced cardiac output and elevated systemic vascular resistance, or with arterial insufficiency, pulses may not be palpable in the periphery. In this case, *Doppler ultrasound* should be used to evaluate arterial flow. Using light pressure so that the artery is not occluded, place the Doppler probe (with conducting gel) over the general area of the artery to be assessed. Move the probe until the arterial signal is audible. Mark the location of the pulse with indelible ink (Fig. 10-8).

BRUITS

Bruits are arterial sounds, similar to cardiac murmurs, that occur with turbulence of blood flow. Bruits in the carotid arteries may indicate a partial obstruction to cerebral blood flow, whereas bruits in the femoral arteries

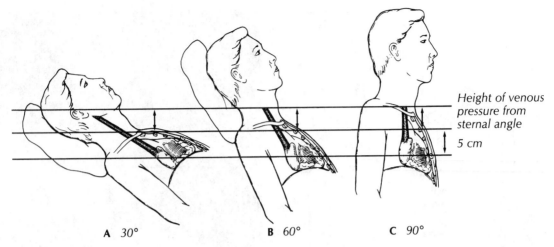

Height of venous
pressure from
sternal angle

5 cm

A 30°   B 60°   C 90°

FIGURE 10-9 Assessment of jugular venous pressure. (From Bates B: A Guide to Physical Examination, 5th ed, p 276. Philadelphia, JB Lippincott, 1991.)

suggest partial obstruction to blood flow to the legs. When listening for carotid bruits, instruct the patient to exhale and then hold his or her breath during the examination to prevent bruits from being obscured by respiratory sounds. Auscultate for bruits with the diaphragm of the stethoscope over the carotid, renal, iliac, and femoral arteries.

Jugular Venous Pulse

Inspection of the jugular venous pulse can reveal important information about right heart hemodynamics. The level of the jugular venous pressure reflects the right atrial pressure and, in most instances, reflects the right ventricular diastolic pressure (filling pressure). The pattern of the jugular venous pulse can reveal abnormalities of conduction and abnormal function of the tricuspid valve.[5] Assess the right side of the neck because right heart hemodynamics are transmitted more directly to the right, rather than to the left, jugular vein. It is important to inspect the skin for evidence of previous cannulation of the vessel that may result in thrombosis and affect the accuracy of pressure measurement. Oblique light may assist in visualizing the jugular veins.

JUGULAR VENOUS PRESSURE

Jugular venous pressure reflects filling volume and pressure on the right side of the heart. Jugular veins act like manometers; blood in the jugular veins assumes the level that corresponds to the right atrial (central venous) pressure. The normal jugular venous pressure is less than 9 cm H_2O.[5] The right internal jugular vein provides the most accurate reflection of right heart hemodynamics because it is in an almost straight line with the innominate vein and the superior vena cava.[36] It lies deep to the sternocleidomastoid muscle; however, the pulsations are usually transmitted to the skin. The top level of skin pulsation is recorded as the jugular venous pressure. If the right internal jugular vein is not visible, the right external jugular vein may be used to measure jugular venous pressure,[37] although it is more subject to thrombosis or compression, and the presence of venous valves may make

the data less reliable. To measure the jugular venous pressure, follow these steps (Fig. 10-9):

◆ Begin with the patient supine; the head and trunk should be in a straight line without significant flexion of the neck.
◆ Position the patient's backrest so that the jugular meniscus can be seen in the lower half of the neck. Elevating the backrest 15 to 30 degrees above horizontal is usually sufficient.
◆ Visualize the right internal jugular vein and identify the level of peak excursion. If the external jugular vein is used, identify the level at which it appears collapsed.
◆ Place a ruler vertically on the sternal angle (angle of Lewis). Position a straight edge (e.g., tongue blade) horizontally at the highest point of the jugular vein so that it intersects the ruler at a right angle and measure the vertical distance above the sternal angle.

If the top of the neck veins is more than 3 cm above the sternal angle, venous pressure is abnormally elevated.[33] Elevated venous pressure reflects right ventricular failure (and is a late finding in left ventricular failure), reduced right ventricular compliance, pericardial disease, hypervolemia, tricuspid valve stenosis, and obstruction of the superior vena cava.[36] During inspiration, the jugular venous pressure normally declines, although the amplitude of the a wave may increase.[5] With the patient in the horizontal position, if the neck veins collapse on deep inspiration (intrathoracic pressure of –5 cm H_2O), the central venous pressure is less than 5 cm H_2O.

Abdominojugular reflux occurs in right ventricular failure. It can be demonstrated by pressing the periumbilical area firmly for 30 to 60 seconds and observing the jugular venous pressure. If there is a rise in the jugular venous pressure by 1 cm or more that is sustained throughout pressure application, abdominojugular reflux is present.[16,32] *Kussmaul's sign* is a paradoxical elevation of jugular venous pressure during inspiration and may occur in patients with chronic constrictive pericarditis, heart failure, or tricuspid stenosis.

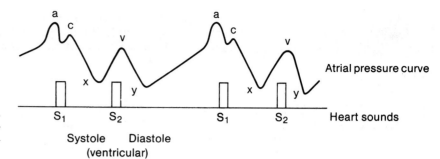

FIGURE 10-10 Patterns of the venous pulse. (From Bates B: A Guide to Physical Examination, 3rd ed, p 169. Philadelphia, JB Lippincott, 1983.)

PATTERNS OF THE VENOUS PULSE

Before evaluating the venous pulse, it is important to discriminate between venous and carotid pulsations. Venous pulse waves are observed more readily than they are palpated. The descents are often more easily seen than the peaks and are inward movements.[5] The carotid pulsation is a brisk, outward movement. Palpation of the jugular vein obliterates the pulsations except in extreme venous hypertension.[36] Palpation of the carotid does not obliterate the observable pulsation in the neck.

Right atrial systole increases right atrial pressure and causes venous distention and the resulting a wave (Fig. 10-10). Atrial emptying and relaxation, and descent of the atrial floor during ventricular systole, results in the x descent. The c wave occurs simultaneously with the carotid arterial pulse, interrupting the x descent. The c wave may be related to tricuspid valve closure and bulging into the right atrium, or it may be an artifact from the adjacent carotid pulse. The v wave reflects the rise in right atrial pressure from atrial filling during ventricular contraction while the tricuspid valve is closed. The y descent results from reduction in right atrial volume and pressure when the tricuspid valve opens.[36]

Timing of the venous pulse can be appreciated by auscultating the heart or palpating the carotid artery on the opposite side of the neck. The a wave occurs just before the first heart sound or carotid pulse and has a sharp rise followed by the rapid x descent. The v wave occurs immediately after the arterial pulse and has a slower, undulating pattern. The y descent is less steep than the x descent. Consistently large a waves are seen in tricuspid stenosis, pulmonary hypertension, and right ventricular failure. *Cannon a waves* are seen in patients with atrioventricular dissociation as the right atrium contracts against the closed tricuspid valve.[37] The a wave is absent in atrial fibrillation because of the absence of coordinated atrial contraction. Elevated v waves and rapid y descents suggest tricuspid regurgitation or increased intravascular volume. Blunting of the y descent suggests impaired atrial emptying in early ventricular diastole, such as occurs in tricuspid stenosis, pericardial disease, or cardiac tamponade.

Blood Pressure

Systemic arterial blood pressure can be measured indirectly or directly. Indirect measurement of blood pressure is most common and is described in this section. Direct measurement of blood pressure, an invasive technique requiring placement of an arterial catheter, may be necessary in certain conditions, such as clinical shock. Direct measurement of blood pressure is discussed in Chapter 19 (Hemodynamic Monitoring).

Blood pressure should be measured at each health encounter. Measurements should be taken in a quiet room at a comfortable temperature. Exertion, exposure to cold, eating, and smoking should be avoided for 30 minutes before measurement; postural change should be avoided for 5 minutes before measurement.[25,37]

Evaluate the patient's current blood pressure. If it differs greatly from the usual, immediate intervention may be required. Optimal blood pressure in people 18 years of age or older is defined as less than 120/80 mm Hg and normal pressure is defined as less than 130/85 mm Hg.[25] Hypertension is defined as systolic blood pressure of 140 mm Hg or greater, diastolic blood pressure of 90 mm Hg or greater, or taking antihypertensive medication.[25] Results from the recent Hypertension Optimal Treatment trial indicate that lowering blood pressure below this "normal" level in people with hypertension significantly reduced cardiovascular mortality.[22] (See Chapter 32 for treatment of hypertension.) In western societies, blood pressure tends to increase with increasing age. This is not biologic and there is clear evidence that lowering blood pressure in older adults reduces the risk of stroke, cardiac disease, and all-cause mortality.[24] The higher the blood pressure, the greater the increase in the heart's work and oxygen consumption. Blood pressures less than 90/60 mm Hg may decrease blood and oxygen delivery to an already compromised myocardium. Taking into account symptoms of myocardial ischemia and adequacy of cerebral and peripheral perfusion may enable the examiner to judge more accurately the clinical significance of blood pressure changes in the cardiac patient.

SPHYGMOMANOMETER

Blood pressure is measured indirectly using a sphygmomanometer (inflatable bladder inside a pressure cuff, a manometer, and an inflation system) and stethoscope. Stethoscopes are described later in this chapter.

Bladder and Cuff. The inflatable bladder fits inside a nondistensible covering, termed the *cuff*. Size and placement of the bladder (rather than the cuff) are crucial in obtaining accurate blood pressure measurements. The

TABLE 10-3	Recommended Ideal Arm Circumference, Arm Circumference Ranges, and Correction of Systolic and Diastolic Readings for Adult Blood Pressure Cuffs of Different Bladder Widths at Various Arm Circumferences					

Cuff width (cm)	12		15		18	
Ideal arm circumference (cm)	30.0		37.5		45.0	
Arm circumference range (cm)	26–33		33–41		>41	
Arm Circumference (CM)	**SBP**	**DBP**	**SBP**	**DBP**	**SBP**	**DBP**
26	+5	+3	+7	+5	+9	+5
28	+3	+2	+5	+4	+8	+5
30	0	0	+4	+3	+7	+4
32	−2	−1	+3	+2	+6	+4
34	−4	−3	+2	+1	+5	+3
36	−6	−4	0	+1	+5	+3
38	−8	−6	−1	0	+4	+2
40	−10	−7	−2	−1	+3	+1
42	−12	−9	−4	−2	+2	+1
44	−14	−10	−5	−3	+1	0
46	−16	−11	−6	−3	0	0
48	−18	−13	−7	−4	−1	−1
50	−21	−14	−9	−5	−1	−1

SBP, systolic correction in millimeters of mercury; DBP, diastolic correction in millimeters of mercury.

For correction of blood pressure readings in individual patients, positive numbers should be added to and negative numbers subtracted from the readings obtained.

From Frohlich ED, Grim C, Labarthe DR et al (eds): Recommendations for Human Blood Pressure Determination by Sphygmomanometers, p. 10. Dallas, American Heart Association, 1987. By permission of the American Heart Association, Inc.

bladder width should be 40% of the circumference of the limb (usually the arm) to be used. Bladders that are too narrow for the size of the limb reflect a falsely elevated blood pressure, whereas bladders that are too wide reflect an erroneously low blood pressure. Bladder length, which also affects accuracy of measurement, should be approximately twice that of width, or 80% of the limb circumference. Inflatable bladders and cuffs are available in various sizes. Table 10-3 summarizes recommended bladder dimensions for blood pressure cuffs. It is important to remember that cuff size is determined by patient size, not patient age.[18,37]

Manometers. There are two types of manometers: mercury and aneroid. *Mercury manometers,* which are the most reliable, can be mounted either on a portable stand or on the wall above the bed or table. A reservoir of mercury (Hg) is attached to the bottom of the manometer, which is calibrated in millimeters (mm). In response to pressure exerted on the bulb, mercury rises vertically in the manometer. As pressure is released from the bag, the column of mercury falls, and blood pressure can be measured in millimeters of mercury. It is important that the meniscus of the mercury be at eye level when the blood pressure is measured. The blood pressure reading should be taken at the top of the meniscus. If the wall mounting is too high or the portable stand too low, errors in blood pressure determinations will be made.

Inspect the tube of mercury for dirt and signs of oxidation and observe that the level of the meniscus is at zero when no pressure is applied. A clogged air vent or filter at the top of the manometer results in a sluggish response to declining pressure and an erroneous measurement. The filter and vent should be serviced annually.

Aneroid manometers have round gauges calibrated in millimeters of mercury, or torr (1 torr = 1 mm Hg), and affixed to the blood pressure cuff. Advantages of the aneroid manometer are that it is easily seen, conveniently portable, and, with the cuff, composes one unit. Unfortunately, the calibration of the dial frequently becomes inaccurate. It is important before each use to check that the indicator needle is pointing to the zero mark on the dial. If the needle is either below or above this mark, the blood pressure reading will be incorrect and the scale may no longer be linear.

Calibration of an aneroid manometer is performed using a mercury manometer as the reference manometer (Fig. 10-11). The mercury manometer must be functioning correctly to obtain reliable results.[36] These sphygmomanometers should be recalibrated by qualified personnel at least yearly or whenever the needle does not point to zero.

The inflation system of aneroid manometers consists of the bulb, exhaust valve, and tubing. The bladder should be able to be inflated and deflated gradually or rapidly. Check frequently for pressure leaks greater than 1 mm Hg per second and for smooth, efficient functioning of the apparatus.[36]

Electronic devices can be used for measuring blood pressure, but the reading should be validated with a mercury manometer. Electronic devices are more sensitive to artifact

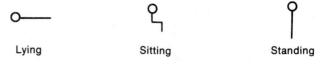

Lying   Sitting   Standing

FIGURE 10-12 Symbols used to record a patient's position during blood pressure determination.

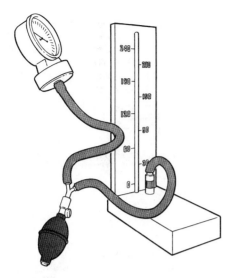

FIGURE 10-11 Calibration of an aneroid manometer. Disconnect the cuffs from both the aneroid and reference manometers. Attach a bulb to a Y connector and the Y connector to the tubes to each of the manometers. Inflate the bulb and observe the pressure at several points over the entire range on both manometers. The pressures should be equal on both manometers. (From Cunningham SL: Hypertension. In Patrick ML, Woods SL, Craven RF et al [eds]: Medical–Surgical Nursing: Pathophysiological Concepts, p 609. Philadelphia, JB Lippincott, 1986.)

such as patient movement or muscle contraction. These devices do not require use of a stethoscope and may be used by patients for self-monitoring of blood pressure.

TECHNIQUE

On initial examination, blood pressure should be recorded in both arms and, in infants, in one leg as well. Subsequently, the arm with the higher blood pressure should be used. Indicate whether the blood pressure was taken on the right arm or left arm. Avoid possible development of lymphedema after mastectomy by always taking the patient's blood pressures on the arm *opposite* the affected side. Avoid taking blood pressure on an arm with an arteriovenous shunt or fistula, as well as those with subclavian stenosis.[37]

Differences in blood pressure between the arms or between the arms and the legs have important diagnostic implications. In patients with occlusive arterial disease of the subclavian artery, the blood pressure is lower in the affected arm. In patients with coarctation of the aorta or dissecting aortic aneurysm, depending on the location of the lesion, the blood pressure may be higher in one arm than the other, or in both arms (proximal) compared with the legs (distal).

Bladder and Cuff Position. The deflated cuff is placed snugly around the arm, with the bladder covering the inner aspect of the arm and the brachial artery. The lower margin of the cuff should be 2.5 cm above the antecubital space.

Arm Position. As long as the patient's arm is at heart level, the blood pressure can be determined with the patient in any position. Errors up to 10 mm Hg, both systolic and diastolic, can be made if the arm is not at the correct level. Falsely elevated pressures are obtained if the arm is lower than the heart; falsely low pressures are measured if the arm is higher than the heart. The arm must be supported during pressure determination.

Patient Position. The patient's position during blood pressure measurement always should be recorded. Use the symbols or drawings shown in Figure 10-12.

Palpation. After the cuff is in place, the brachial artery is palpated continuously. Once the brachial or radial pulse is obtained, the cuff is inflated rapidly. The pressure at which the pulse disappears should be noted, but the cuff inflation should continue for another 30 mm Hg before the actual measurement of the blood pressure begins. For example, if the brachial pulse disappears when the cuff pressure is 110 mm Hg, the cuff should be pumped to 140 mm Hg before starting. The cuff should not be inflated further than necessary, because high cuff pressures are uncomfortable, create undue anxiety in the patient, and tend to raise the patient's blood pressure. The pressure in the cuff should be reduced gradually by 2 to 3 mm Hg per second. The point at which the brachial pulse is first detected on expiration is the systolic blood pressure. Diastolic blood pressure cannot be determined accurately by this method.[19] Once measurement is made, the cuff should be deflated rapidly. If possible, allow a minimum of 1 to 2 minutes before the blood pressure is measured again to release venous blood.

Systolic blood pressure is measured by palpation in patients whose blood pressures cannot be heard, for example, patients in shock. It is also useful when checking blood pressures frequently (e.g., every 1 to 2 minutes). Palpated blood pressures are charted using "P" as diastolic pressure (e.g., 90/P).

Auscultation. Preparation of the patient and use of the blood pressure equipment are identical in the auscultatory method. After the brachial pulse has been located, the stethoscope is applied over the artery using light pressure. Heavy pressure might partially occlude the artery, creating turbulence in the blood flow, prolonging phase IV (see later), and falsely lowering the diastolic blood pressure. Care must be taken to avoid causing extraneous noise, such as from the stethoscope touching the cuff or any other material.

Korotkoff sounds are the sounds created by turbulence of blood flow within the vessel caused by constriction of the blood pressure cuff (Fig. 10-13). The five Korotkoff sounds are summarized in Table 10-4.

Systolic blood pressure is the highest point at which initial tapping (phase I) is heard in two consecutive beats (to

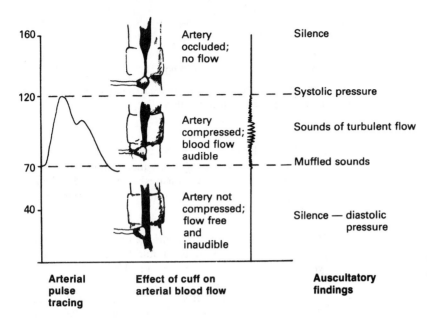

FIGURE 10-13 Auscultation of the blood pressure. (Adapted from Bates B: A Guide to Physical Examination, 5th ed, p 284. Philadelphia, JB Lippincott, 1991.)

ascertain that the sound is not extraneous) during expiration. Systolic blood pressure is higher in the expiratory phase compared to the inspiratory phase of the respiratory cycle (see section on Measurement of Paradoxical Blood Pressure, later). Systolic blood pressure should be read to the nearest 2 mm Hg mark on the manometer.

Diastolic blood pressure is equated with disappearance of Korotkoff sounds (phase V) in adults. Phase V most closely approximates intra-arterial diastolic pressure. Muffling of sounds (phase IV) usually occurs at pressures 5 to 10 mm Hg higher than intra-arterial diastolic pressures and, therefore, is not a good indicator of diastolic blood pressure in adults. However, muffling, rather than disappearance of sounds, is a better index of intra-arterial diastolic pressure in children and in adults with hyperkinetic states. Hyperkinetic

conditions, including hyperthyroidism, aortic insufficiency, and exercise, increase the rate of blood flow, resulting in disappearance of sounds (absence of turbulence) far below intra-arterial diastolic pressure. In children and adults with hyperkinetic states, sounds can be detected below muffling for much longer than normal.[29] As with systolic blood pressure, read diastolic pressure to the nearest 2 mm Hg mark on the manometer. If there is a difference of 10 mm Hg or more between disappearance and muffling of sounds, record both diastolic pressures (e.g., 140/56/20 mm Hg).[6]

In some patients, Korotkoff sounds may be soft and could result in falsely low blood pressure values. To augment the loudness of Korotkoff sounds, increase brachial flow by having the patient open and clench a fist; quickly inflate cuff to a value 30 mm above the palpable systolic blood pressure. If necessary, sounds can be further augmented by elevating the arm before inflating the cuff.[12]

Auscultatory gap is a temporary disappearance of sound that occurs during the latter part of phase I and phase II (Fig. 10-14). It is particularly common in patients with

TABLE 10-4	**Phases of Korotkoff Sounds**	
Phase	Sound	Recorded as
I	First appearance of faint, clear tapping sounds that gradually increase in intensity.	Systolic blood pressure.
II	Sounds assume a swishing or murmur-like quality.	
III	Sounds become crisper and increase in intensity.	
IV	Distinct muffling abruptly occurs, and the sounds become soft and blowing.	Diastolic blood pressure in **children** <13 years of age.
V	Disappearance of sounds.	Diastolic blood pressure in most* **adults.**

*Note: In pregnant women and in persons with high cardiac output or peripheral vasodilation, use Phase IV muffling.

Perloff D, Grim C, Flack J et al: Human blood pressure determination by sphygmomanometry. Circulation 88: 2460–2470, 1993.

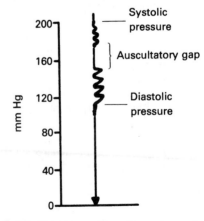

FIGURE 10-14 Auscultatory gap. (From Bates B: A Guide to Physical Examination, 5th ed, p 283. Philadelphia, JB Lippincott, 1991.)

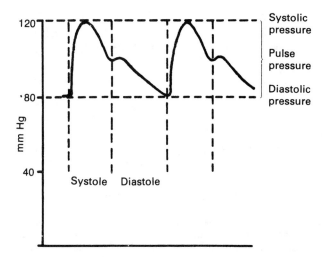

FIGURE 10-15 Measurement of pulse pressure. (From Bates B: A Guide to Physical Examination, 5th ed, p 274. Philadelphia, JB Lippincott, 1991.)

high blood pressure,[29] venous distention, or reduced velocity of arterial flow (e.g., severe aortic stenosis).[36] The auscultatory gap can be as wide as 40 mm Hg. Serious errors in blood pressure measurement can be made if the cuff is not inflated high enough to exceed true systolic pressure. Systolic blood pressure would be underestimated if the second appearance of the Korotkoff sounds were recorded as phase I. Diastolic blood pressure would be overestimated if the first muffling of sounds was considered to be phase IV. The auscultatory gap can be avoided if a preliminary palpable blood pressure is obtained before auscultation.

MEASUREMENT OF PULSE PRESSURE

Pulse pressure is the difference between the systolic and diastolic blood pressures, expressed in millimeters of mercury. For example, if the blood pressure is 120/80 mm Hg, the pulse pressure is 40 mm Hg (Fig. 10-15). Pulse pressure reflects stroke volume, ejection velocity, and systemic vascular resistance. Use pulse pressure as a noninvasive indicator of the patient's ability to maintain cardiac output.

Pulse pressure is increased in many situations. A widened pulse pressure is seen in sinus bradycardia, complete heart block, aortic regurgitation, anxiety, exercise, and catecholamine infusion, which are examples of situations characterized by increased stroke volume. Examples of conditions that increase pulse pressure by reducing systemic vascular resistance are fever, hot environment, and exercise. Conditions such as atherosclerosis, aging, and high blood pressure widen the pulse pressure because of decreased distensibility of the aorta, arteries, and arterioles. A narrowed pulse pressure also can be caused by many factors: reduced ejection velocity in heart failure, shock, and hypovolemia; mechanical obstruction to systolic outflow in aortic stenosis, mitral stenosis, and mitral insufficiency; peripheral vasoconstriction in shock and with certain drugs; and artifactually from an auscultatory gap.[36,38] If the pulse pressure in the cardiac patient falls below 30 mm Hg, further assessment of the patient's cardiovascular status may be indicated.

MEASUREMENT OF POSTURAL BLOOD PRESSURE

Postural (orthostatic) hypotension occurs when the blood pressure drops after an upright posture is assumed. It usually is accompanied by dizziness, lightheadedness, or syncope. Although there are many causes of postural hypotension, the three most commonly seen in the cardiac patient are (1) intravascular volume depletion, which often results from aggressive diuretic therapy, inadequate intake, or intravascular to extravascular fluid shift; (2) inadequate vasoconstrictor mechanisms, which may be a primary pathologic process but also result from immobility; and (3) autonomic insufficiency, which is often related to the sympathetic blocking drugs used in the cardiac patient. Postural changes in blood pressure, along with the appropriate history, can help the clinician differentiate between them.[27,34] Postural changes in blood pressure and pulse should be measured in patients who are older than age 65 years, diabetic, receiving antihypertensive therapy, or who complain of dizziness or syncope. Important points to remember are the following:

- Position the patient supine and as flat as symptoms permit for 10 minutes before the initial measurement of blood pressure and heart rate.
- Always check supine measurements before upright measurements.
- Always record both heart rate and blood pressure at each postural change.
- Do not remove the blood pressure cuff between position changes, but do check to see that it remains placed correctly.
- Safety considerations may require assessment of blood pressure and pulse with the patient seated with legs in the dependent position before standing. Measurement of blood pressure and pulse in this position is not sufficient to rule out orthostasis.[27,38]
- Have the patient assume a standing position. Measure the blood pressure and pulse immediately and after 2 minutes. If orthostasis is strongly suspected and not apparent after 2 minutes, continue to monitor blood pressure and pulse every 2 minutes for 10 minutes. If the purpose of collecting the data is to assess falls risk, another approach is to ask the patient to get out of bed as he or she normally does and evaluate the change in pulse rate and blood pressure and associated symptoms at the patient's rate of position change.
- Be alert for any signs or symptoms of patient distress, including dizziness, weakness, blurring of vision, and syncope. When the patient returns to a recumbent position, these symptoms should reverse and the blood pressure and pulse return to normal.
- Record any signs or symptoms that accompany the postural change.

Normal postural responses are a transient increased heart rate of 5 to 20 beats per minute (to offset reduced stroke volume and to maintain cardiac output), a drop in systolic pressure of less than 10 mm Hg, and an increase in diastolic pressure of approximately 5 mm Hg. *Orthostasis* is defined as a drop in systolic pressure of 20 mm Hg or greater or a drop in diastolic pressure of at least 10 mm Hg within 3 minutes of standing,[11] although any drop in diastolic pressure is cause for concern.[5,34] The change from lying to sitting position is not sufficient to make a diagnosis of orthostasis; it may be used as a screening test because decreased blood pressure, increased pulse, or symptoms in the sitting position presage similar events in the erect position. Often, the change in blood pressure does not meet the criteria for orthostasis, but it is accompanied by a significant change in heart rate or associated symptoms, or both. These circumstances identify people at risk and should prompt further investigation by the cardiac nurse of the patient's present volume status and vasodilatory or cardioinhibitory drug regimen.

The presence of intravascular volume depletion (such as with diuretic therapy) should be suspected when, in response to sitting or standing, the heart rate increases and the systolic pressure decreases by 15 mm Hg and the diastolic blood pressure drops by 10 mm Hg.[34] It is difficult to differentiate intravascular volume loss from inadequate vasoconstrictor mechanisms solely by changes in vital signs accompanying postural changes. With intravascular volume depletion, reflexes to maintain cardiac output (increased heart rate and peripheral vasoconstriction) function correctly, but because of reduced intravascular fluid volume, these reflexes are not adequate to maintain systemic arterial pressure and the blood pressure falls. With inadequate vasoconstrictor mechanisms, the heart rate responds appropriately also, but blood pressure drops because of diminished peripheral vasoconstriction. Differentiation, therefore, depends in part on the patient's history. However, intravascular depletion and inadequate vasoconstrictor mechanisms are not mutually exclusive. The following is an example of a postural blood pressure recording showing either saline depletion or inadequate vasoconstrictor mechanisms.

Blood Pressure	Heart Rate	Patient Position
120/70 mm Hg	70 bpm	
100/55 mm Hg	90 bpm	
98/52 mm Hg	94 bpm	
150/90 mm Hg	60 bpm	
100/60 mm Hg	60 bpm	

MEASUREMENT OF PARADOXICAL BLOOD PRESSURE

Paradoxical blood pressure is an exaggerated decrease in the systolic blood pressure during inspiration. The mechanism is complex and controversial. Normally, during inspiration, blood flow into the right heart is increased, right ventricular output is enhanced, and pulmonary venous capacitance is increased. Consequently, less blood reaches the left ventricle, which reduces left ventricular stroke volume by approximately 7% and arterial pressure by approximately 3%.[44]

During cardiac tamponade, effects of respiration on both right and left ventricular filling appear to be greater than normal, causing a reduction of 10 mm Hg or more in

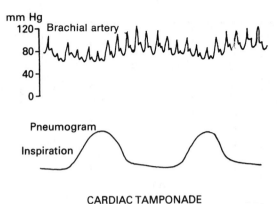

CARDIAC TAMPONADE

FIGURE 10-16 Paradoxical blood pressure in cardiac tamponade. The paradox is greater than 20 mm Hg. (Adapted from Fowler NO: Examination of the Heart, Part 2: Inspection and Palpation of Arterial and Venous Pulses, p 33. New York, American Heart Association, 1972. By permission of the American Heart Association, Inc.)

systolic pressure during inspiration[15,17] (Fig. 10–16). In addition, echocardiography has demonstrated a shift of the intraventricular septum to the left, further impairing left ventricular filling and stroke volume. With high intrapericardial pressures, the thin-walled right ventricle may collapse during diastole, further impairing venous return and cardiac output.[5,15] Chronic obstructive airway disease, constrictive pericarditis, pulmonary emboli, restrictive cardiomyopathy, and cardiogenic shock have also been associated with an abnormal inspiratory decline of blood pressure. Echocardiographic studies of patients with emphysema demonstrate both an augmented inspiratory filling of the right ventricle and an exaggerated inspiratory decline of left ventricular filling.[9]

The patient should breathe normally and must not exaggerate respiratory effort during an examination for a paradoxical blood pressure. As before, the nurse should inflate and gradually deflate the cuff until the first systolic sound is heard on expiration and continue slowly releasing the cuff pressure until sounds are heard both on inspiration and expiration. The difference between the two is termed the *paradox,* and it normally is less than 10 mm Hg.[5] For example, if the first systolic sound occurs at 140 mm Hg during expiration and Korotkoff sounds begin appearing with both inspiration and expiration at 120 mm Hg, the paradox is 20 mm Hg. Paradoxical blood pressures should be determined as a baseline in all patients on the cardiac care unit and routinely in all patients with pericarditis or with heart catheters, such as a temporary pacing wire.

BLOOD PRESSURE MEASUREMENT UNDER SPECIAL CONDITIONS

Arrhythmia. With very irregular rhythms, accurate assessment of blood pressure is difficult because of the beat-to-beat variation in both stroke volume and blood pressure. Systolic blood pressure is related directly to the stroke volume and duration of the preceding cycle. Pulse pressure is related inversely to pulse cycle duration. A short cycle (reduced ventricular filling time) increases the diastolic blood pressure of that cycle and reduces systolic blood pressure during the next cycle. A long pulse cycle (increased ventricular filling time) causes a decreased diastolic blood pressure in that cycle but an increased systolic blood pressure in the next cycle.[32]

Any arrhythmia that alters stroke volume and cardiac output can be detected during blood pressure measurement. Always record the presence of an irregular cardiac rhythm along with the blood pressure.

Premature ectopic beats (either ventricular or supraventricular) have a short cycle followed by a long cycle (postextrasystolic beat). If they occur only occasionally, they have minimal effects on blood pressure. In *bigeminal rhythms,* as the blood pressure cuff is deflated, Korotkoff sounds of the alternate strong beats are heard first and are half as fast as the heart rate. Further reduction in cuff pressure enables the listener to hear the alternating weaker sounds produced by the ectopic impulses as well.

Pulsus alternans, indicative of severe organic heart disease and left heart failure, also is manifested by alternating strong and weak pulses but with a regular cadence. Pulsus alternans can occur with ectopic bigeminal rhythms that are interpolated rather than premature, but in this instance it does not necessarily indicate severe organic heart disease.

Because pulse cycle length changes constantly in *atrial fibrillation,* both systolic and diastolic blood pressures must be approximated.[5,37] For systolic blood pressure, average a series of readings (three to five) of phase I pressures. For diastolic blood pressure, average the pressure readings obtained in phases IV and V.

Atrioventricular dissociation can be detected during auscultation of blood pressure. Examples of rhythms with atrioventricular dissociation include *ventricular tachycardia, high-grade* or *complete atrioventricular block,* and *asynchronous ventricular pacing.* In atrioventricular dissociation, an occasional, well-timed atrial contraction contributes to diastolic ventricular filling. This "atrial kick" augments the stroke volume for that beat. As the cuff bladder is deflated, phase I sounds periodically are increased.

Clinical Shock. In shock states associated with reduced cardiac output and elevated systemic vascular resistance, Korotkoff sounds may not be generated in the periphery. Direct measurement of blood pressure may be required to manage these critically ill patients. When indirect cuff measurements are compared with direct (femoral arterial) pressure measurements, direct pressures are higher than auscultated pressures. In hypotensive states, when direct measurement of blood pressure is not feasible, *Doppler ultrasound* may provide a more reliable indirect measurement of systolic blood pressure than the auscultatory method. Place the Doppler probe (with conducting gel) over the patient's artery. As in auscultatory measurement, inflate the cuff and listen for the arterial signal as the bladder is deflated. Cuff widths of 50% of the arm circumference have been recommended for the Doppler technique.[29]

Obesity. Cuff size and bladder size frequently are too small for use in the obese patient. If a proper-sized cuff can-

not be used, apply a standard cuff to the forearm 13 cm from the elbow and auscultate the radial artery to obtain the blood pressure measurement.

Thigh Blood Pressure Measurement. Blood pressures are measured in the thigh if the arms cannot be used or to confirm or rule out certain conditions that alter circulation, such as coarctation of the aorta or dissecting aortic aneurysm.

For thigh blood pressure measurement, use a cuff and bladder that are both longer and wider than an arm cuff. Recommendations for the exact sizes of the thigh cuff and bladder have not been made. With the patient in the prone position, apply the compression bladder over the posterior aspect of the mid-thigh. Place the stethoscope over the artery in the popliteal fossa and auscultate in the same manner as described previously. If the patient is unable to tolerate the prone position, have the patient remain supine with the knee slightly flexed. Apply the stethoscope over the popliteal artery. When cuffs of the correct size are used for both arms and legs, pressures should vary by only a few millimeters of mercury. (The arm cuff, incorrectly used on the thigh, produces a falsely high value.)

Community Blood Pressure Readings. Blood pressures taken in the patient's home may provide a better indication of basal blood pressure than those obtained in an office or clinic setting. However, if the patient takes his or her own blood pressure, readings may be elevated because of the isometric exercise required to inflate the cuff and because of the concentration necessary. Many fire stations and hospital auxiliaries provide blood pressure measurement as a community service. Alternately, a fully automated system that measures blood pressure at preset intervals over the 24-hour period may be used.

Pseudohypertension. Misleadingly high blood pressure values may be obtained in older adults because of excessive vascular stiffness.[25] Pseudohypertension should be suspected in the presence of high blood pressure values and the absence of target organ damage. To confirm suspected pseudohypertension, inflate the cuff above systolic pressure and palpate the radial artery. Presence of a palpable, pulseless radial artery provides additional evidence of pseudohypertension.

Peripheral Vascular System

Adequacy of both arterial and venous circulation is assessed when examining the extremities. Always make arm-to-arm and leg-to-leg comparisons. Careful examination of the lower extremities is impossible without removing shoes and stockings.

INSPECTION AND PALPATION

Inspection and palpation are the primary techniques used in examining the peripheral vasculature (see section on Bruits, earlier). Observe and compare (right to left) size, temperature, symmetry, swelling, venous pattern, pigmentation, scars, and ulcers. Palpate the superficial lymph nodes, noting their size, consistency, discreteness, and any tenderness.

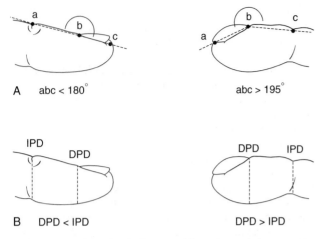

FIGURE 10-17 Clubbing is diagnosed from the angle between the base of the nail and the skin next to the cuticle and by phalangeal depth. **(A)** In healthy adults, the hyponychial angle is 180 degrees (*left*); with clubbing, the angle increases above 195 degrees (*right*). **(B)** The ratio of distal phalangeal depth (DPD) to interphalangeal depth (IPD) is normally less then 1 (*left*). In clubbing, it exceeds 1.0 (*right*). (After Hansen-Flaschen, Nordberg; Clubbing and hypertrophic osteoarthropathy. Clin Chest Med 8: 291, 1987.)

CLUBBING

Clubbing is a pathologic sign that is defined as focal enlargement of the terminal phalanges. Two diagnostic findings are present in clubbing: change in the angle between the base of the nail and the phalangeal skin, and "floating" nails. When viewed from the side, the base angle normally is less than 180 degrees and the distal phalangeal diameter is less than the interphalangeal diameter. In clubbing, the base angle becomes 195 degrees or greater and the distal phalangeal diameter becomes greater than the interphalangeal diameter[7] (Fig. 10-17). Floating nails can be detected by palpating the base of the nail while moving the tip of the nail. Rather than a firm anchor, the base of the nail appears to float or move under the palpating finger. Clubbing may develop in a variety of conditions, including congenital heart disease and lung abscess; its cause is unknown.

ARTERIAL CIRCULATION

Adequacy of peripheral arterial circulation is assessed by arterial pulse; skin color, temperature, and moistness; and capillary refill time. Pulse-wave analysis and skin color are described earlier in this chapter in the sections on Arterial Pulse and Head, respectively.

Temperature and Moistness. Temperature and moistness are controlled by the autonomic nervous system. Normally, hands and feet are warm and dry. Under stress, the periphery may be cool and moist. In cardiogenic shock, skin becomes cold and clammy.

Capillary Refill Time. Capillary refill time provides an estimate of the rate of peripheral blood flow. When the tip of the fingernail is depressed, the nail bed blanches. When the pressure is released quickly, the area is reperfused and

becomes pink. Normally, reperfusion occurs almost instantaneously. More sluggish reperfusion indicates a slower peripheral circulation, such as in heart failure.

Peripheral Atherosclerosis. Risk factors for peripheral atherosclerosis include advancing age, diabetes mellitus, hyperlipidemia, and tobacco use. Peripheral atherosclerosis may present with pain or fatigue in the muscles (intermittent claudication) that occurs with exercise and resolves with rest. Physical findings of chronic arterial insufficiency include decreased or absent pulses, reduced skin temperature, hair loss, thickened nails, smooth shiny skin, and pallor or cyanosis. Elevation of the feet and repeated flexing of the calf muscles may produce pallor of the soles of the feet. Returning the feet to a dependent position may produce rubor secondary to reactive hyperemia. If the ankle—brachial systolic pressure index (calculated by dividing the ankle systolic pressure by the brachial systolic pressure) is less than 0.8, it is highly probable (>95%) that arterial insufficiency is present. When vascular ulcers associated with arterial insufficiency occur, they are more commonly located near the lateral malleolus. Acute arterial occlusion produces sudden cessation of blood flow to an extremity. Severe pain, numbness, and coldness develop in the affected extremity quickly (within 1 hour). Physical findings include loss of pulse distal to the occlusion, decreased skin temperature, loss of sensation, weakness, and absent deep tendon reflexes.[13]

VENOUS CIRCULATION

Edema. Edema is an abnormal accumulation of fluid in the interstitium. Causes include right-sided heart failure, hypoalbuminemia, excessive renal retention of sodium and water, venous stasis from obstruction or insufficiency, lymphedema, orthostatic edema, or increased capillary permeability.[2] In the cardiac patient, peripheral edema frequently occurs because of sodium and water retention and right-sided heart failure. Bilateral edema of the lower extremities suggests a systemic etiology; unilateral edema is usually the result of a local etiology. A weight gain of 10 pounds (indicative of 5 L of extracellular fluid volume) precedes visible edema in most patients.

Interstitial edema occurs in the most dependent part of the body, its location varying with the patient's posture. With sitting or standing, edema develops in the lower extremities. With bed rest, edema forms in the sacrum. Because the distribution of edema fluid varies with position, daily weights provide the best serial assessment of edema. *Pitting edema* is a depression in the skin from pressure. To demonstrate the presence of pitting edema, the nurse presses firmly with his or her thumb over a bony surface such as the sacrum, medial malleolus, the dorsum of each foot, and the shins. When the thumb is withdrawn, an indentation persists for a short time. The severity of edema is described on a five-point scale, from none (0) to very marked (4). *Pigmentation, reddening, induration,* and *fibrosis* of the skin and subcutaneous tissues of the lower extremities may result from long-standing edema.[13] *Skin mobility* is decreased by edema.

Thrombophlebitis. Thrombophlebitis is inflammation of the vein associated with a clot. Diagnosis is made using subjective and objective data.

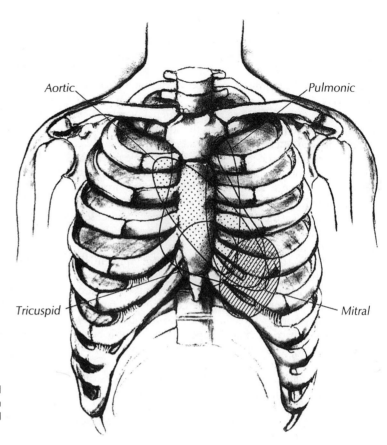

FIGURE 10-18 Areas to be assessed in the precordial examination. (Drawn from Leatham A: An Introduction to the Examination of the Cardiovascular System, 2nd ed, p 20. Oxford, Oxford University Press, 1979.)

In *superficial thrombophlebitis,* the affected vein is hard, red, sensitive to pressure, warm to touch, and engorged. *Deep vein thrombosis* may be asymptomatic or associated with pain, warmth, and mottling of the leg. With severe edema, the leg may be cool and cyanotic. Deep vein thrombosis can cause thromboembolism, resulting in a pulmonary embolus.[13,21] Among hospitalized patients, hip surgery is the most common precipitant of deep venous thrombosis.[43] Elicitation of pain with dorsiflexion of the foot (*Homans' sign*) is an unreliable diagnostic sign. Noninvasive imaging with duplex venous ultrasonography or plethysmography is required for diagnosis.[13]

Varicose Veins. Varicose veins are tortuous dilations of the superficial veins that result from defective venous valves, intrinsic weakness of the vein wall, high intraluminal pressure, or arteriovenous fistulas. Patients may be concerned about the appearance of their legs or may complain of a dull ache that is present with standing and relieved by elevation. Visual inspection of the legs with the patient in the standing position confirms the presence of varicose veins.

Chronic Venous Insufficiency. Chronic venous insufficiency (incompetence of venous valves) may follow deep venous thrombosis or may occur without previous thrombosis. It may be unilateral, but more commonly is bilateral. Patients complain of a dull ache in the legs that is present with standing and relieved by elevation. Physical examination reveals increased leg circumference, edema, and superficial varicose veins. Erythema, dermatitis, and hyperpigmentation may

develop in the distal lower extremity.[13] When venous ulcers occur, they are more common near the medial malleolus.

Heart

The precordium should be assessed in an orderly fashion using the techniques of inspection, palpation, and auscultation. Careful inspection and palpation provide better information on heart size than does percussion. Percussion is most useful in the rare instance where dextrocardia is suspected.[37] The room should be quiet and permit privacy. Both the patient and the examiner should be in comfortable positions before beginning the examination.

Topographic Anatomy

Knowledge of the topographic anatomy of the cardiac and vascular structures is essential to understanding the clinical findings. The *left ventricle* is primarily a posterior structure and is evaluated on the anterior chest wall at the cardiac apex, which is normally in the fifth intercostal space (ICS) at, or slightly medial to, the mid-clavicular line (MCL). The *right ventricle* is anterior to the left ventricle and underlies the sternum and the lower left sternal border at the fourth and fifth ICS. The *right atrium* is just lateral to the lower right sternal border. The outflow tracts of both ventricles underlie the third left ICS (Erb's point). The main *pulmonary artery* underlies the second left ICS, and the *ascending aorta* underlies the second right ICS[31,32,45] (Fig. 10-18).

INSPECTION

Inspect the precordium with the patient supine, the chest exposed, and the backrest slightly elevated. Stand at the foot or right side of the bed or examining table. Tangential lighting allows the examiner to detect chest wall movements more easily.

Note any *pulsations* (outward movement) or *retractions* (inward movement) and describe the location by ICS and distance in centimeters from the sternum or the MCL. Determine whether it occurs in systole or diastole by timing it with the carotid pulse or the heart sounds. In general, retractions are more easily seen, and pulsations are more easily palpated.

When visible, the normal *apex impulse* can be seen within the fifth ICS at or just medial to the MCL. It is an early systolic pulsation with a rapid upstroke and downstroke. A late systolic retraction, 1 to 2 cm long, in the fourth or fifth ICS may also be normally seen and is produced by ventricular emptying. The apex impulse cannot be seen in every patient. It is easily detected in thin patients, whereas it may not be visible in those who are obese or have large breasts or barrel chests. An apex impulse that is below the fifth ICS, lateral to the MCL, or seen in more than one ICS represents left ventricular enlargement.

Slight movement over the sternum or the epigastrium can be normal in thin people and in those with fever or anemia who may have hyperdynamic heartbeats. A *sternal rise* that is sustained after systole begins usually indicates right ventricular enlargement. Pulsations in other areas are abnormal. For example, pulsation over the second right ICS may represent an aortic aneurysm, and pulsation over the second left ICS can represent increased filling pressure or flow in the pulmonary artery.

Paradoxical movement of the left anterior precordium is suggestive of a left ventricular aneurysm. With paradoxical movement, as the apex contracts, the aneurysmic area bulges. This ectopic impulse usually is seen above the apex impulse. The visibility of abnormal pulsations can be enhanced by balancing a tongue depressor on the chest over the pulsation.

PALPATION

Movement that was not visible on inspection may be detected by palpation. All areas should be palpated using either the ball of the palm (at the base of the fingers) or the fingertips. In general, the palm surface is more sensitive to *thrills* (vibrations), whereas fingertips are more sensitive to *pulsations*. Thrills indicate turbulence of blood flow and are associated with murmurs. Impulses are described in terms of *location, size, amplitude, duration,* and *time in the cardiac cycle* (systole or diastole). To facilitate measurement of the horizontal location in centimeters from the MCL, or the size of the impulse, it is helpful for the examiner to measure his or her hand and use it as a "ruler." For example, the distance from the tip of the finger to the first joint, the second joint, and the third joint can be used.

Assess the apex impulse for location, size, amplitude, and duration. The apex impulse is, by definition, the furthest point leftward and downward at which a cardiac pulsation can be seen or felt.[32] The normal apex impulse is felt as a light tap, extending over 3 cm or less. The apex impulse is felt immediately after the first heart sound and lasts halfway through systole. An impulse that is diffuse (felt over two ICSs), increased in amplitude, or laterally or inferiorly displaced suggests increased volume load and left ventricular dilatation, such as occurs in mitral insufficiency or left ventricular failure. An impulse that is sustained, enlarged, and, sometimes, laterally displaced suggests obstruction to outflow with increased ventricular pressure load and concentric hypertrophy of the muscle, such as occurs in aortic stenosis or systemic hypertension.[5,38] If the apex impulse cannot be felt with the patient lying supine, examine the patient in the left lateral position, which brings the apex of the heart against the chest wall; the quality of the apex beat still can be determined even though its size and position may be slightly altered. A diastolic outward pulsation indicates impaired ventricular filling and corresponds to an S_3 (early to mid-diastole) or S_4 (late diastole) heard on auscultation.

Next, palpate the right ventricular area. The presence of a pulsation suggests right ventricular enlargement. Palpation of the epigastrium, by placing the palmar surface of the hand over the area and sliding the fingers toward the xiphoid, can also detect right ventricular enlargement. Pulsations beating down on the fingertips indicate right ventricular movement. Pulsations pushing upward against the hand originate in the aorta. An increased aortic pulse could indicate abdominal aortic aneurysm or aortic regurgitation. Hepatic pulsations may be felt in the epigastrium but also over the right upper abdomen. The liver may pulsate with tricuspid valve disease, severe right ventricular failure, or pulmonary hypertension.[32] A thrill at the lower left sternal border suggests tricuspid valve disease.

Then, palpate the third left ICS and the second left and right ICSs. Systolic pulsations in the second left or right ICS suggest increased pressure or enlargement of the pulmonary artery or the aorta, respectively; thrills suggest pulmonary or aortic valve abnormalities.

AUSCULTATION

Stethoscope. A good-quality stethoscope is required for cardiac auscultation. Although the human ear is able to hear sounds ranging in frequency from 20 cycles per second, or Hertz (Hz), to 20,000 Hz, it is most sensitive to 1,000 to 5,000 Hz. The frequency of most heart sounds is less than 1,000 Hz. The stethoscope must transmit these low-frequency sounds to the ear.

The parts of the stethoscope are the ear pieces, tubing, and chest pieces. The ear pieces should fit comfortably into the ear canal and be snug enough so that extraneous sound cannot enter. They also must be kept free of ear wax. Double tubing with a small internal diameter (3 mm) should extend from the ear pieces to the chest pieces. In addition, the tubing should be reasonably short (25 to 30 cm) so that the sound is not diluted and should be thick to minimize room noise.[44]

There are two basic types of chest pieces, the diaphragm and the bell. The *diaphragm,* which brings out higher frequencies and filters out the lower ones, is useful for listening to the first and second heart sounds (S_1 and S_2), high-frequency murmurs, and lung sounds. The diaphragm should be pressed firmly against the chest wall. The *bell* filters out high-frequency sounds and accentuates the low-frequency ones. Diastolic filling sounds and the low-frequency murmurs of mitral and tricuspid stenosis are heard best with the bell.[45] The bell should rest lightly on the chest; if firm pressure is applied, the skin becomes taut and acts like a diaphragm. When auscultating heart sounds, the nurse stands on the patient's right side so that as he or she places the bell of the stethoscope on the patient's chest, the chest piece is balanced. Because the bell does not have to be held in place, the possibilities of creating extraneous sounds and filtering out low frequencies are reduced.

As part of a cardiac examination, all areas identified in Figure 10-18 should be auscultated except the epigastrium. The listener's goals when auscultating the precordium are to identify normal heart sounds, the heart rate, and rhythm; extra diastolic and systolic sounds; murmurs; and pericardial friction rubs.

Technique. The stethoscope is placed directly on the chest wall; adequate auscultation of the heart and lungs through clothing is impossible. The room should be quiet; the patient and examiner should be comfortable. Cardiac auscultation should be performed with the patient in three positions: supine, lying partially on the left side, and sitting up, leaning forward. The examiner can begin listening either at the cardiac apex or at the base. Beginning at the apex allows the examiner to focus initially on the first heart sound, clearly identify systole and diastole, and think through the cardiac cycle while listening at each site. The apex is the location of the apex impulse identified by palpation. Remember that left ventricular enlargement shifts the apex from the normal location. The timing of extra sounds in the cardiac cycle, the location in which they are best heard, and the quality of the sound are used to differentiate one from another.

It is important to proceed in a systematic manner. Inching the stethoscope up and down the chest wall is a useful technique and allows the examiner to focus on specific events in the cardiac cycle (Table 10-5). At each location, listen sequentially to four events: S_1, systole (interval between S_1 and S_2), S_2, and diastole (interval between S_2 and S_1). For example, begin at the apical area with the diaphragm of the stethoscope and focus on S_1 and S_2. Normally, S_1 is louder than or equal to S_2 at the apex. Listen carefully during systole and during diastole for clicks, murmurs, or other extra sounds. Inch the stethoscope toward the sternum to the right ventricular area and listen for a split S_1. Continue to move the stethoscope up the left sternal border to the second left ICS and note the change in relative intensity of the heart sounds. Normally, S_2 is louder than S_1 at the base. Continue to listen for splitting of the second heart sound and, if present, determine whether it is physiologic or abnormal. Move the stethoscope to the second right ICS and listen for an ejection sound in early systole after S_1. Listen with the bell along the lower sternal border for right ventricular S_3 and S_4. Move the bell to the apical area and listen for left ventricular S_3 and S_4. An opening sound of the mitral valve (high frequency) can be dis-

TABLE 10-5	Auscultatory Technique	
Location	**Chest Piece**	**Sounds**
Apex	Diaphragm	S_1 intensity; opening sounds; murmurs from aortic and mitral valve
	Bell	Left S_3, S_4; murmurs
Left sternal border	Diaphragm	S_2 intensity; split S_1; murmurs from tricuspid and pulmonic valves and from atrial septal defects
	Bell	Right S_3, S_4
Base	Diaphragm	Split S_2; ejection sounds; murmurs from aortic vale
	Bell	Murmurs from aortic valve or dilated aorta

tinguished from an S_3 by pressing firmly with the bell to stretch the skin. Stretching the skin causes it to act as a diaphragm and filters out low-frequency sounds.

Normal Heart Sounds. Normal heart sounds consist of the first and second heart sounds, S_1 and S_2. Both are of relatively high frequency and can therefore be heard clearly with the diaphragm of the stethoscope. Systole is normally shorter than diastole; with slow heart rates (100 beats/min), the two sounds are easily distinguished by the cadence of the rhythm (Fig. 10-19). However, in more rapid rhythms, diastole shortens so that systole and diastole are of equal duration or, as the rate increases further, diastole becomes shorter than systole. To identify systole and diastole properly in this instance, the examiner should palpate the carotid artery while listening to the heart; the carotid upstroke immediately follows S_1.

Phonocardiograms or echocardiograms can be used to validate the auscultatory findings. In a phonocardiogram, heart sounds, electrocardiogram, and carotid pulse tracings are recorded simultaneously. Phonocardiograms are most often used for research or teaching. Echocardiograms are used clinically to demonstrate abnormalities of valve structure and cardiac function.[36]

The *first heart sound* is due primarily to closure of the mitral and tricuspid valves and is therefore heard loudest at the apex of the heart. Phonetically, if the heart sounds are "lub-dup," S_1 is the "lub." Mitral and tricuspid closure usually is heard as a single sound.

The intensity of the S_1 depends on leaflet mobility, position of the atrioventricular valves at the onset of systole, and

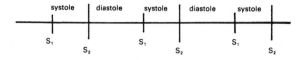

FIGURE 10-19 Normal heart sounds.

the rate of ventricular upstroke. A loud S_1 is noted clinically in mitral stenosis when the cusps are mobile; with a short PR interval (0.08 to 0.13 second) because the leaflets are wide open when systolic contraction begins; in tachycardia, hyperthyroidism, or exercise because of an increased rate of pressure rise in the ventricle; and in the presence of a mechanical prosthetic mitral valve. Most commonly, a soft S_1 is due to poor conduction of sound through the chest wall, but other causes include a fixed or immobile valve; a long PR interval (0.20 to 0.26 second) or a slow heart rate, which allows the atrioventricular valves to float back into position before the onset of ventricular systole; low flow at the end of diastole; and β-adrenergic or calcium channel blockers that reduce the rate of rise of ventricular pressure. The intensity of S_1 varies from beat to beat in atrial fibrillation because diastolic filling time is not constant. In a regular rhythm with a variable S_1 intensity, complete heart block should be suspected.[42] Variation in the intensity of S_1 can be evaluated by listening carefully to the relative intensity of S_1 and S_2 at the apex and the base. For example, when the intensity of S_1 is increased, it may be equal to or louder than S_2 at the base.[5] When assessing variation in S_1, it is helpful to have the patient hold his or her breath because respiratory movements may cause variation in the intensity of heart sounds.

Splitting of the first heart sound occurs when tricuspid closure is delayed and is best heard at the lower left sternal border. Pathologic splitting of S_1 results from right bundle-branch block, tricuspid stenosis, and atrial septal defect.[45] Splitting of S_1 helps to differentiate supraventricular from ventricular tachycardia. In supraventricular rhythms, S_1 is normal; in ventricular rhythms it is split.[32] Unfortunately, when supraventricular rhythms are conducted aberrantly, S_1 is split.

The *second heart sound* results primarily from closure of the aortic and pulmonic valves and is loudest at the base of the heart. Phonetically, the "dup" of the "lub-dup" is the S_2. The intensity of S_2 is determined by the pressure in the receiving vessels, the mobility of the valve leaflets, the degree of apposition of the leaflets, and the size of the aortic root. Intensity is increased with systemic or pulmonary hypertension, ascending aortic aneurysm, and in the presence of a mechanical prosthetic aortic valve. Intensity may be diminished in heart failure, myocardial infarction, pulmonary embolism, clinical shock, and stenosis of the aortic or pulmonic valve.[32]

Physiologic (normal) *splitting* of S_2 occurs during inspiration. During inspiration, an increased amount of blood is returned to the right side of the heart and a decreased amount of blood is returned to the left side of the heart due to trapping in the expanded lung. Pulmonic valve closure (P_2) is delayed because of the extra time needed for the increased blood volume to pass through the pulmonic valve, and aortic valve closure (A_2) occurs slightly early because of the relatively smaller amount of blood ejected from the left ventricle. In addition, the time of closure of P_2 is affected by the "hang out" interval, which is inversely related to pulmonary vascular impedance. During inspiration, the pulmonary vascular impedance decreases and P_2 is delayed; on expiration the opposite occurs.[41] If the two

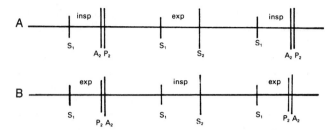

FIGURE 10-20 Splitting of the S_2. **(A)** Physiologic splitting. During inspiration (*insp*), the P_2 sound is delayed. **(B)** Paradoxical splitting. During expiration (*exp*), A_2 is delayed.

components are fairly close together, it is difficult to appreciate two distinct and separate sounds. A physiologic split S_2 may seem muffled or sound like a short drum roll on inspiration compared with expiration. On expiration, the split sounds merge (Fig. 10-20A). Normal splitting should be evaluated during quiet respiration and may be better heard with the patient sitting.[32] In pathologic splitting of S_2 (wide or fixed splits), the second sound is split during both inspiration and expiration, although there may be some respiratory variation in the amount of the split.

Paradoxical (abnormal) *splitting* of S_2 also can occur. Paradoxical splitting is due to any mechanism that causes late aortic valve closure (A_2), such as electrical delay (left bundle-branch block, right ventricular pacing, or right ventricular ectopy), mechanical obstruction (aortic stenosis or systolic hypertension), or impaired left ventricular contractile function (left ventricular failure or left ventricular ischemia; see Fig. 10-20B). Because P_2 is soft and A_2 is comparably loud and easily transmitted, a split S_2 is heard best in the second left ICS (pulmonary outflow tract). In paradoxical splitting, the second component (aortic closure) is louder than the first component (pulmonic closure).

Normally, A_2 is louder than P_2, even in the pulmonic area, and P_2 is not well heard, if at all, in other areas of the precordium. In pulmonary hypertension, the intensity of P_2 increases so that A_2 is less than or equal to P_2. The loud P_2 can the be heard in other areas of the precordium, particularly the lower left sternal border and the cardiac apex.[5]

Extra Diastolic Sounds. Extra diastolic sounds consist of diastolic filling sounds and opening snaps. *Diastolic filling sounds* (S_3 and S_4) occur as blood enters a noncompliant ventricle during the two phases of rapid ventricular filling: the end of the early rapid filling phase, as active ventricular relaxation ceases (S_3); and, with atrial contraction, the active, rapid filling phase (S_4). Three theories have been proposed to explain the generation of the third and fourth heart sounds: the mitral valve theory, the chest wall theory, and the ventricular wall vibration theory. The last is the most widely accepted theory. Sound is produced within the ventricle by the abrupt decrease in wall motion (S_3) or with rapid filling of a noncompliant ventricle that causes a rapid deceleration of blood flow.[41] Diastolic filling sounds can arise from either or both ventricles. The cadence suggests the sound of a galloping horse, and these sounds are sometimes called diastolic gallops.

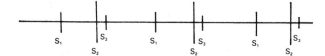

FIGURE 10-21 An S_3 gallop immediately follows the S_2.

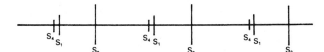

FIGURE 10-22 An S_4 gallop immediately precedes the S_1.

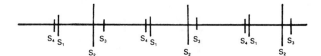

FIGURE 10-23 Quadruple rhythm.

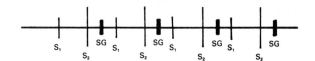

FIGURE 10-24 Summation gallop.

A *physiologic* S_3 can be heard in healthy children or young adults but usually disappears by 40 years of age. Its disappearance with advancing age has been attributed to decreased ventricular wall compliance with reduced early ventricular filling.[32] An S_3 in people older than age 40 years is usually pathologic and signals impaired systolic function.[42] It is one of the first clinical findings associated with cardiac decompensation, such as left ventricular heart failure (left ventricular S_3), primary pulmonary hypertension and cor pulmonale (right ventricular S_3), or insufficiency of the mitral, aortic, or tricuspid valves. An S_3 follows the S_2 in a "lub-dup-*ta*" cadence (Fig. 10-21). Using the bell of the stethoscope, listen for a left ventricular S_3 over the apex of the heart; for a right ventricular S_3, listen over the lower left sternal border. By having the patient in the left lateral position, the apex is brought forward against the chest wall, making the left ventricular S_3 louder and, therefore, easier to hear.

The S_4 occurs after atrial contraction as the blood is ejected into a noncompliant ventricle, producing a rapid elevation of ventricular pressure, and signals diastolic dysfunction.[42] Even though it is the fourth heart sound, because the S_4 occurs at the end of ventricular diastole, it is heard immediately before S_1 and sounds like "*ta*-lub-dup" (Fig. 10-22). The S_4 is heard in most patients who have had a myocardial infarction, in a large number of patients experiencing angina pectoris, and in patients with coronary heart disease. It is also heard in patients with left ventricular hypertrophy due to hypertension, hypertrophic cardiomyopathy, or aortic stenosis. It is common in the elderly because of the decreased compliance of the ventricle that occurs with age and the prevalence of hypertension and aortic stenosis in this population. An S_4 does not necessarily imply cardiac failure in people with ventricular hypertrophy. Because atrial contraction is necessary to produce an S_4, it is not heard in patients with atrial fibrillation. As with the S_3, listen for an S_4 using the bell of the stethoscope. A left ventricular S_4 is heard best at the apex, with the patient lying in the left lateral position; right ventricular S_4 is loudest over the lower left sternal border. Inching the stethoscope from the apex to the lower left sternal border can be helpful in differentiating right- and left-sided sounds. Left-sided sounds fade and right-sided sounds get louder as the stethoscope approaches the sternum.

A *quadruple rhythm* may be heard in patients with severe cardiac failure and both systolic and diastolic dysfunction. If the heart rate is slow enough, four distinct heart sounds (S_1, S_2, and both S_3 and S_4) can be heard (Fig. 10-23). However, if a patient is ill enough to have a quadruple rhythm, tachycardia also usually is present. In this case, a *summation gallop* is heard, in which the S_3 and S_4 gallops fuse in mid-diastole to one loud diastolic sound. The summation gallop resembles the sound of a galloping horse (Fig. 10-24).

It stands to reason that in a noncompliant ventricle there should be more resistance to active ventricular filling than to passive ventricular filling; therefore, an S_4 gallop should be generated more easily than an S_3 gallop. Therefore, one would expect all patients with normal sinus rhythm who have an S_3 gallop to have an S_4 gallop as well. However, patients with normal sinus rhythm frequently have only an S_3. The cause for this finding is unknown, although one possibility may be an absence of actual mechanical atrial contraction in spite of electrical atrial activity.

Opening snaps are associated with the opening of a stenotic mitral valve. Opening sounds are not heard with normal valves. The sound is heard in very early diastole, medial to the cardiac apex. The sound can be loud and transmitted throughout the precordium (Fig. 10-25). Unlike an S_3, an opening snap has a high-pitched, snapping quality and is heard best with the diaphragm of the stethoscope.[2,45]

Extra Systolic Sounds. Extra systolic sounds consist of early systolic ejection sounds and systolic clicks. *Early ejection sounds* (Fig. 10-26) coincide with the opening of the

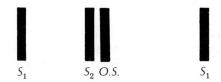

FIGURE 10-25 Opening snap (OS). (From Bates B: A Guide to Physical Examination, 5th ed, p 313. Philadelphia, JB Lippincott, 1991.)

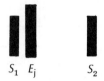

FIGURE 10-26 Early systolic ejection sound. (From Bates B: A Guide to Physical Examination, 5th ed, p 312. Philadelphia, JB Lippincott, 1991.)

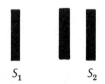

FIGURE 10-27 Mid- to late systolic click. (From Bates B: A Guide to Physical Examination, 4th ed, p 301. Philadelphia, JB Lippincott, 1987.)

aortic and pulmonic valves. They are heard shortly after S_1 and are high-pitched and clicking in quality. An *aortic ejection sound* is heard at the base or apex and accompanies a dilated aorta or aortic stenosis. *Pulmonic ejection sounds* are heard loudest in the second or third left ICSs and occur with pulmonary artery dilatation, pulmonary hypertension, and pulmonary stenosis.[38] *Mid- to late systolic clicks* are associated with mitral valve prolapse; they occur from tensing of the leaflet or chordae when the limit of excursion is reached, and frequently they are followed by a murmur (Fig. 10-27).

Murmurs. Heart murmurs are sounds produced in the heart or great vessels by turbulent blood flow. Turbulent blood flow can be produced by[2]:

♦ Increased rate of flow across a normal valve (exercise, pregnancy, anemia)
♦ Flow across a partial obstruction (valvular stenosis, pulmonary or systemic hypertension)
♦ Flow across an irregularity without obstruction (bicuspid aortic valve, thickening of aortic cusps with aging)
♦ Flow into a dilated vessel (dilation of the aortic root)
♦ Backward flow across an incompetent valve or through a ventricular septal defect

Murmurs are classified according to systolic or diastolic *timing* (Fig. 10-28); *intensity* (Table 10-6); *location* (where the murmur is heard loudest); *radiation,* such as to the back, neck, or axilla; *configuration* (Fig. 10-29); *quality,* such as harsh, rough, rumbling, blowing, squeaking, or musical; and *duration* (see Fig. 10-28).[39,45] Murmurs may be organic (due to intrinsic cardiovascular disease), functional (produced by circulatory disturbances such as anemia, pregnancy), or innocent (occur in the absence of disease).[32]

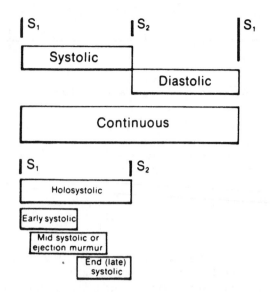

FIGURE 10-28 Classification of murmurs by timing. (From Tilkian A, Conover M: Understanding Heart Sounds and Murmurs, 3rd ed, p 99. Philadelphia, WB Saunders, 1993.)

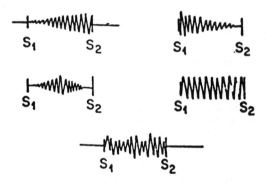

FIGURE 10-29 Configuration of murmurs. **(A)** Crescendo. **(B)** Decrescendo. **(C)** Crescendo–decrescendo (diamond). **(D)** Plateau: (even). **(E)** Variable (uneven). (From Perloff JK: Physical Examination of the Heart and Circulation, p 208. Philadelphia, WB Saunders, 1990.)

TABLE 10-6	Grading the Intensity of a Murmur
Grade	**Clinical Findings**
I/VI	Very faint; heard only after listener "tuned in"; may not be heard in all positions
II/VI	Quiet, but heard immediately after placing the stethoscope on the chest
III/VI	Moderately loud
IV/VI	Loud
V/VI	Very loud; may be heard with stethoscope partly off the chest; associated with a thrill
VI/VI	May be heard with stethoscope entirely off chest; associated with a thrill

Adapted from Bates B: A Guide to Physical Examination, 5th ed, p 301. Philadelphia, JB Lippincott, 1991.

In adults, the most common systolic murmurs are produced by semilunar valve stenosis (ejection murmurs), atrioventricular valve insufficiency (regurgitant or holosystolic murmurs), and ventricular septal defect (early systolic murmurs) secondary to myocardial infarction. In older adults, the murmur of aortic sclerosis (thickening of aortic valve leaflets) is common. The most common diastolic murmurs are produced by the reverse set of circumstances: insufficiency of semilunar valves (early regurgitant murmurs) and stenosis of the atrioventricular valves (mid- to late diastolic rumbles). The loudness of the murmur may not correlate with the severity of the valvular lesion; for example, a patient with a grade V to VI murmur in whom cardiogenic shock develops actually may have reduced intensity of the murmur because of diminished cardiac blood flow. Refer to Chapter 27 for descriptions of the murmurs of aortic and mitral stenosis and regurgitation.

Recognizing an innocent murmur is an important and difficult skill. The innocent murmur can often be diagnosed by its clinical features and the absence of other clinical abnormalities. Clinical features of innocent murmurs include the following: always systolic, soft, short, modified by change in posture, normal S_2, and most common at left sternal border.[32] Echocardiography may be needed to confirm its innocence, and follow-up is essential. The precordial "whoop" or "honk" may be an innocent finding in patients without organic heart disease or may represent an exaggerated phase of an organic murmur.[32,45]

In the cardiac care unit, nurses are most often concerned with changes in murmurs rather than in their diagnosis. However, it is important accurately to diagnose the onset of murmurs of papillary muscle dysfunction and aortic insufficiency.

Normally, papillary muscle contraction allows for complete closure of the atrioventricular valves. However, when the papillary muscles are ischemic (most often in the left ventricle), they are unable to contract properly, preventing the chordae tendineae from being held tautly and, in turn, from holding the mitral valve leaflets closed during left ventricular contraction. Blood is therefore allowed to flow backward through the mitral valve (mitral regurgitation) during systole. The murmur of mitral regurgitation secondary to papillary muscle dysfunction is systolic (occurring in early to mid-systole) and usually soft, high pitched, and crescendo—decrescendo in configuration. In the presence of heart failure or angina, the murmur may become holosystolic.

A new murmur of *papillary muscle dysfunction* in the patient with acute myocardial infarction must be recognized immediately because interventions must be instituted to relieve the papillary muscle ischemia and prevent progression to papillary muscle infarction. Should the papillary muscles infarct, they also may rupture; there is a high mortality rate associated with papillary muscle rupture because of the development of sudden and profound heart failure.

In the setting of acute aortic dissection, coronary artery bypass grafting with a friable aorta, or aortic valve replacement, *new-onset aortic insufficiency* indicates retro-

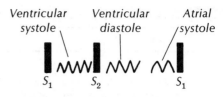

FIGURE 10-30 Pericardial friction rub. (From Bates B: A Guide to Physical Examination, 5th ed, p 320. Philadelphia, JB Lippincott, 1991.)

grade dissection of the aorta, or valve dehiscence. The murmur of aortic insufficiency is an early diastolic, decrescendo murmur, heard at the second right or third left ICS that radiates toward the apex. In acute aortic insufficiency, the intensity of S_1 is frequently diminished because of the increase in ventricular volume, and P_2 may be accentuated because of the rapid rise in pulmonary vascular pressure.[5] Acute left ventricular failure may result from volume overload alone or, in the case of continued retrograde dissection, from myocardial infarction secondary to dissection of the coronary arteries.

Pericardial Friction Rubs. Pericardial friction rubs are characteristic of pericarditis, which occurs in more than 15% of patients with acute myocardial infarction. A pericardial friction rub develops in approximately 7% of patients with myocardial infarction, commonly by the fourth day after myocardial infarction. Rubs may be transient, lasting only several hours. The rub occurs with heart movement; each movement creates its own short, scratchy sound (Fig. 10-30). Pericardial friction rubs are classified as three-component (atrial systole, ventricular systole, and ventricular diastole), two-component (ventricular systole and diastole), or one-component (ventricular systole) rubs. One-component rubs may be difficult to differentiate from a murmur. Rubs are best heard either with the patient sitting upright and leaning forward with the breath expelled (most appropriate for the patient with an acute myocardial infarction) or with the patient on his or her hands and knees in bed or on the examination table (useful in a nonacute situation). A pericardial friction rub can be heard with or without a pericardial effusion. Pericardial friction rubs can be differentiated from pleural friction rubs by having the patient hold his or her breath.

Pericardial friction rubs are common in postoperative cardiac patients. Also, a respirophasic squeak may be heard that is related to mediastinal or pleural tubes. Air in the mediastinum produces a crunching sound (Hamman's sign) during auscultation of the precordium.

Dynamic Auscultation. Dynamic auscultation can be used to aid in the interpretation of heart sounds and murmurs. A variety of physiologic or pharmacologic maneuvers can be used to alter circulatory dynamics: respiration, postural changes, the Valsalva maneuver, postextrasystolic beats, isometric exercise, and vasoactive agents.[5,32] Table 10-7 summarizes the auscultatory effects of these maneuvers.

TABLE 10-7	**Auscultatory Effects of Physiologic and Pharmacologic Maneuvers**		
Maneuver	**Effect**	**Maneuver**	**Effect**
Inspiration	Physiologically splits S_2	Valsalva maneuver	
	Attenuates left ventricular S_3 and S_4, mitral opening snap, and pulmonic ejection sound	Phase II	Attenuates S_3 and S_4 Narrows A_2–P_2 interval
	Accentuates right ventricular S_3 and S_4, tricuspid opening snap, and right heart murmurs	Phase III Phase IV	Widens A_2–P_2 interval Returns to baseline or transiently accentuates S_3 and S_4
	Hastens and accentuates click-murmur of mitral valve prolapse	Postextrasystolic beats	Augments murmurs of aortic and pulmonic stenosis, tricuspid and aortic regurgitation, and hypertrophic obstructive cardiomyopathy
Expiration	Paradoxically splits S_2		Delays click, murmur of mitral valve prolapse
	Accentuates left ventricular S_3 and S_4, mitral opening snap, and left heart murmurs		
	Attenuates right ventricular S_3 and S_4 and tricuspid opening snap	Isometric exercise	Accentuates left ventricular S_3 and S_4 and murmurs of aortic regurgitation, rheumatic mitral regurgitation, ventricular septal defect, mitral stenosis
Lying down	Widens split S_2 in all respiratory phases Augments first right, then left, ventricular S_3 and S_4 Augments most systolic murmurs		Attenuates murmur of aortic stenosis Delays click, murmur of mitral valve prolapse
	Diminishes systolic murmur of hypertrophic obstructive cardiomyopathy	Amyl nitrate	Augments opening snaps; S_3; and murmurs of aortic, pulmonic, mitral, and tricuspid stenosis, and tricuspid regurgitation
	Delays and attenuates click, murmur of mitral valve prolapse		
Sudden standing	Narrows split S_2 in all respiratory phases Diminishes first right, then left, ventricular S_3 and S_4 Diminishes most systolic murmurs Accentuates systolic murmur of hypertrophic obstructive cardiomyopathy		Diminishes murmurs of mitral and aortic regurgitation, ventricular septal defect, and Austin Flint Hastens click, murmur of mitral valve prolapse
	Hastens and accentuates click, murmur of mitral valve prolapse	Methoxamine and phenylephrine	Accentuates murmurs of aortic and mitral regurgitation, and ventricular septal defect
Squatting	Augments right and left ventricular S_3 and S_4, and most murmurs		Diminishes murmurs of hypertrophic obstructive cardiomyopathy and aortic stenosis
	Delays click and murmur of mitral valve prolapse		Delays click, murmur of mitral valve prolapse

Adapted from Braunwald E: The physical examination. In Braunwald E (ed): Heart Disease: A Textbook of Cardiovascular Medicine, 2nd ed, pp 35–38. Philadelphia, WB Saunders, 1984.

Respiration affects blood flow. *Inspiration* increases venous return to the right heart, increasing right ventricular diastolic pressure, stroke volume, and ejection time. Pulmonary vascular impedance is reduced, with increases in pulmonary vascular capacitance. With a normal respiratory rate, blood return to the left ventricle is reduced, resulting in decreased left ventricular diastolic pressure, stroke volume, and ejection time. Transmission of the augmented right ventricular volume to the left ventricle is delayed by three to four cardiac cycles in the pulmonary vasculature. All of the auscultatory events generated by the right heart are augmented during inspiration.[45] The use of the Müller maneuver (sustained inspiratory effort against a closed glottis) further augments the auscultatory effects of inspiration. *Expiration* increases venous return to the left heart, increasing left ventricular diastolic pressure, stroke volume, and ejection time.[38]

The *Valsalva maneuver* (forced expiration against a closed glottis) has variable effects associated with each of its four phases. In *phase I,* the *initial* phase, intrathoracic pressure increases, causing a transient elevation in left ventricular output. In *phase II,* the *straining* phase, venous return is decreased; first right, then left ventricular filling is reduced; stroke volume, mean arterial pressure, and pulse pressure are reduced; and heart rate is increased. In *phase III,* the *release* phase, venous return is increased, with subsequent increases in right, then left, ventricular filling. In *phase IV,* the *overshoot* phase, right ventricular filling and stroke volume return to baseline or may be elevated briefly. The return to baseline of left ventricular hemodynamics is delayed for six to eight beats and also may be elevated briefly.[38,45] During phase II, all murmurs diminish except those of hypertrophic cardiomyopathy and mitral valve prolapse. The Valsalva maneuver should not be held for more than 10 seconds because it reduces cardiac output.

Postural change from sitting or standing to lying down increases venous return first to the right and then to the left ventricle. Recumbence and passive leg raising cause most auscultatory cardiac events to increase except the murmurs of idiopathic hypertrophic subaortic stenosis and mitral valve prolapse. Sudden standing has the opposite effect; it reduces venous return and causes most murmurs, except hypertrophic cardiomyopathy and mitral valve prolapse, to decrease. Squatting simultaneously increases venous return and systemic vascular resistance.[38]

Postextrasystolic beats, if followed by a pause, increase ventricular filling and cardiac contractility. Similar hemodynamic changes occur with diastolic pauses in atrial fibrillation and sinus arrhythmia.[5]

Isometric exercise increases systemic vascular resistance, arterial pressure, heart rate, cardiac output, left ventricular filling pressure, and heart size. Using a calibrated handgrip device, the patient sustains the handgrip for 20 to 30 seconds. The handgrip enhances S_3 and S_4 and aortic regurgitant murmurs. Avoid isometric exercise in patients with myocardial ischemia or ventricular arrhythmia. The patient should never perform the Valsalva maneuver simultaneously with isometric exercise.[5,44]

Pharmacologic agents used in dynamic auscultation are amyl nitrate, methoxamine, and phenylephrine. Inhalation of *amyl nitrate* for 10 to 15 seconds causes marked vasodilatation, reducing systemic arterial pressure and producing a reflex tachycardia, followed by an increase in stroke volume and venous return. *Methoxamine* and *phenylephrine* increase systemic vascular resistance. Both cause a reflex drop in heart rate and decrease contractility and cardiac output. Methoxamine, 3 to 5 mg intravenously, results in blood pressure changes of 20 to 40 mm Hg, lasting 10 to 20 minutes. Phenylephrine, 0.5 mg intravenously, elevates blood pressure 30 mm Hg for 3 to 5 minutes.[5]

Lungs

The respiratory assessment described in this chapter is elementary and is designed to assist the cardiac nurse in identifying respiratory manifestations seen in patients with heart disease. The room should be quiet and the patient's chest exposed. Proceed in a systematic manner: inspect, palpate, percuss, and auscultate. Always compare one side with the other; always place the stethoscope in direct contact with the chest wall. Begin with examination of the posterior chest, if possible, with the patient sitting upright and arms folded across the chest. Follow with assessment of the anterior chest with the patient lying down. Only the upper and lower lobes of the lung are accessible by posterior chest examination; to assess the right middle lobe, the lateral and anterior chest must be examined[2] (Fig. 10-31).

INSPECTION

Respiratory Rate, Depth, Rhythm, and Effort. Normally, the respiratory rate is less than 16 breaths/min and the rhythm is regular (Fig. 10-32*A*). *Tachypnea,* rapid, shallow breathing, may be noted in patients who have heart failure, pain, or anxiety (see Fig. 10-32*B*). *Bradypnea,* slow breathing, can be noted during sleep or after administration of respiratory depressant agents, such as morphine sulfate or anesthesia (see Fig. 10-32*C*). *Cheyne-Stokes respirations,* characterized by periods of alternating depth and apnea, occur in patients with severe left ventricular failure (see Fig. 10-32*D*). Of particular concern is the duration of the apneic period. Use of accessory muscles of respiration, an upright, forward-leaning position, and pursed-lip breathing are visible signs of increased respiratory effort. Retraction of the ICSs is seen in severe asthma or upper airway obstruction.[2] A prolonged expiratory phase is associated with early airway obstruction.

Cough and Sputum. A dry, hacking *cough* from irritation of small airways is common in patients with pulmonary congestion from heart failure or patients taking angiotensin-converting enzyme inhibitors. *Pink, frothy sputum* is indicative of pulmonary edema. Although an occasional cough may be normal, sputum production is always abnormal.

Chest Configuration. With *normal* chest configuration, the anteroposterior to lateral diameter ratio ranges from 1 : 2 to 5 : 7 (Fig. 10-33*A*). With a *barrel chest,* associated with pulmonary emphysema and aging, the anteroposterior to lateral diameter ratio increases to 1 : 1 or more (see Fig. 10-33*B*). *Kyphoscoliosis,* an abnormal spinal curvature, may prevent the patient from fully expanding his or her lungs (see Fig. 10-33*C*).

POSTERIOR CHEST

Palpation. Palpation is performed to identify areas of tenderness, respiratory excursion, and any observed abnormality and to elicit tactile fremitus. To assess *respiratory excursion,*

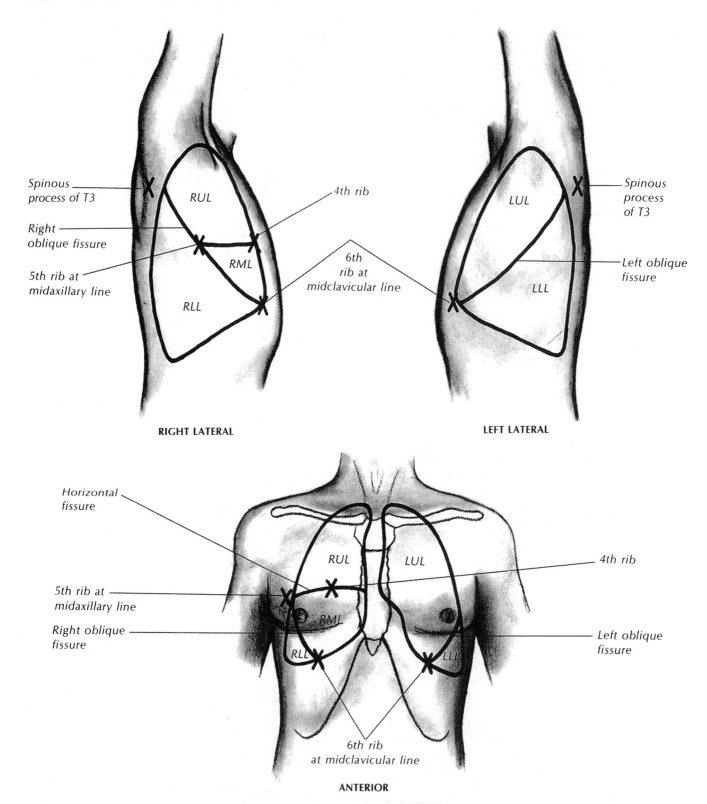

FIGURE 10-31 Lobar localization. (From Bates B: A Guide to Physical Examination, 5th ed, p 237. Philadelphia, JB Lippincott, 1991.)

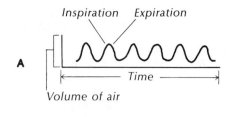

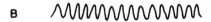

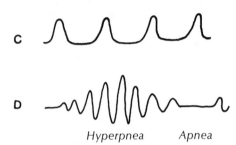

FIGURE 10-32 Respiratory rate and rhythm. **(A)** Normal. **(B)** Tachypnea. **(C)** Bradypnea. **(D)** Cheyne-Stokes. (From Bates B: A Guide to Physical Examination, 5th ed, p 256. Philadelphia, JB Lippincott, 1991.)

the examiner places his or her thumbs slightly to either side of the spine and parallel to the 10th ribs (Fig. 10-34). As the patient inhales deeply, the examiner evaluates the depth and symmetry of the patient's breath by the movement of his or her thumbs.

Fremitus is the palpable vibration transmitted to the chest wall through the bronchopulmonary system when the patient speaks. The patient is asked to repeat the word "ninety-nine," and the nurse uses the ball of his or her hand to palpate and compare areas over the posterior chest. Fremitus is decreased with air or fluid in the pleural space and by an obstructed bronchus; it is increased by lung consolidation. To estimate the level of the diaphragm bilaterally, the examiner places the ulnar surface of his or her hand parallel to its expected level and progressively moves the hand downward until fremitus is no longer felt. Posteriorly, the diaphragm is located between the 10th and 12th (with deep inspiration) ribs. An abnormally high diaphragm suggests a pleural effusion or atelectasis.

Percussion. Percussion causes vibrations in the underlying tissues, resulting in sounds that indicate if the tissues are solid or filled with fluid or air (Table 10-8). The technique of percussion involves the examiner placing the passive finger firmly over the area to be percussed and striking the distal interphalangeal joint of the middle finger of that hand with the middle finger of the opposite hand (Fig. 10-35). Percuss across both shoulders and then at 5-cm intervals down the back (Fig. 10-36), making side-to-side comparisons. Normal lung tissue (air-filled) produces *resonance.* *Dullness* replaces resonance when fluid or solid tissue replaces air-filled tissue. In patients with emphysema and air trapping, *hyper-resonance* replaces resonance. *Diaphragmatic excursion* can be ascertained by percussion of the border between resonance (lung tissue) and dullness (muscle) in expiration and inspiration. Normal excursion is 5 to 6 cm.

Auscultation. Airflow, obstruction, and the condition of the lungs and pleural space can be assessed with auscultation. Use the diaphragm of the stethoscope pressed firmly on the skin in the sequence illustrated in Figure 10-36. Ask the patient to breathe slowly and deeply through his or her mouth because nose breathing changes the pitch of the sounds. Listen through one full breath in each location for pitch, intensity, and duration of inspiration and expiration.

Normal breath sounds (vesicular) are heard in peripheral lung tissue away from large airways. They are soft, low-pitched, blowing sounds. The inspiratory—expiratory time ratio is 5 : 2. Normal breath sounds are diminished at the

TABLE 10-8	Sounds Produced by Percussion			
Percussion Sound	Relative Intensity	Relative Pitch	Relative Duration	Example Location
Flatness	Soft	High	Short	Thigh
Dullness	Medium	Medium	Medium	Liver
Resonance	Loud	Low	Long	Normal lung
Hyper-resonance	Very loud	Lower	Longer	Emphysematous lung
Tympany	Loud	*	*	Gastric air bubble or puffed-out cheek

*Distinguished mainly by its musical timbre.
From Bates B: A Guide to Physical Examination, 5th ed, p 247. Philadelphia, JB Lippincott, 1991.

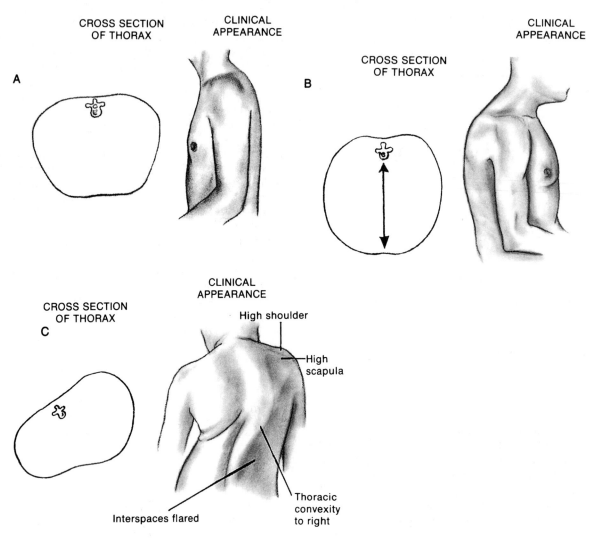

CROSS SECTION OF THORAX | CLINICAL APPEARANCE

A

B

CROSS SECTION OF THORAX | CLINICAL APPEARANCE

C

CROSS SECTION OF THORAX | CLINICAL APPEARANCE

High shoulder

High scapula

Thoracic convexity to right

Interspaces flared

FIGURE 10-33 Chest wall configurations. **(A)** Normal. **(B)** Barrel chest. **(C)** Kyphoscoliosis. (From Bates B: A Guide to Physical Examination, 5th ed, p 257. Philadelphia, JB Lippincott, 1991.)

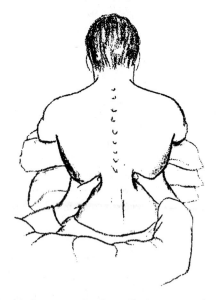

FIGURE 10-34 Assessment of respiratory excursion. (From Bates B: A Guide to Physical Examination, 4th ed, p 246. Philadelphia, JB Lippincott, 1987.)

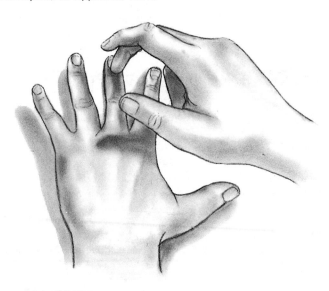

FIGURE 10-35 The technique of percussion. (From Bates B: A Guide to Physical Examination, 5th ed, p 246. Philadelphia, JB Lippincott, 1991.)

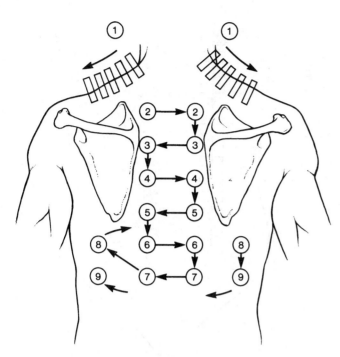

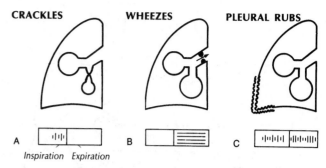

FIGURE 10-37 Adventitious breath sounds. **(A)** Crackles. **(B)** Wheezes. **(C)** Pleural friction rubs. (From Bates B: A Guide to Physical Examination, 4th ed, pp 248–249. Philadelphia, JB Lippincott, 1987.)

FIGURE 10-36 Sequence of posterior percussion and auscultation. (From Bates B: A Guide to Physical Examination, 3rd ed, p 142, Philadelphia, JB Lippincott, 1983.)

bases. The sounds are decreased in obese patients and with shallow breathing or pleural effusion, and they are increased with exercise.

Bronchovesicular sounds are heard normally in the areas around the mainstem bronchi (below the clavicles and between the scapulae). They have moderate pitch and intensity, with an inspiratory—expiratory time ratio of 1 : 1. These sounds are abnormal if heard in the lung periphery.

Bronchial sounds, heard normally over the bronchial areas, are loud and high pitched. Expiratory time is greater than inspiratory time. If heard in the lung periphery, bronchial sounds are abnormal.

Adventitious breath sounds are superimposed over normal breath sounds. There are two categories of adventitious sounds: discontinuous (crackles) and continuous (wheezes and pleural friction rubs). When adventitious breath sounds are heard, note loudness, pitch, duration, number, timing (phase of respiratory cycle), location on the chest wall, and persistence from breath to breath. Have the patient cough and note any change in adventitious sounds.[2]

Crackles are discrete, discontinuous sounds that are similar to the sound generated by rubbing hairs together in front of the ears (Fig. 10-37A). Crackles are attributed to fluid in the alveoli or to explosive reopening of alveoli. Heart failure or atelectasis associated with bed rest, splinting from ischemic or incisional pain, or the effects of pain medication and sedatives often result in development of crackles. Typically, crackles are noted first at the bases (because of gravity's effect on fluid accumulation and decreased ventilation of basilar tissue), but may progress to all portions of the lung fields.

Wheezes are continuous, musical sounds from rapid air movement through constricted airways. They are heard

most often on expiration but can be heard during both inspiration and expiration (see Fig. 10-37B). Although wheezes are characteristic of obstructive lung disease, they can be caused by interstitial pulmonary edema compressing small airways. β-adrenergic blocking agents, such as propranolol, may precipitate airway narrowing, especially in patients with underlying pulmonary disease. A fixed wheeze is characteristic of an endobronchial mass or tumor.

Transmitted voice sounds may be louder and clearer than normal (bronchophony, whispered pectroliloquy) when heard through the chest wall. The quality of voice sounds may have a nasal or bleating character (egophony). Transmitted voice sounds suggest consolidation of lung tissue.

Pleural friction rubs result from inflamed pleura rubbing together. A pleural friction rub, characteristic of pleuritis, is a coarse, grating sound that can be heard on inspiration and expiration (see Fig. 10-37C).

ANTERIOR CHEST

Palpation. Tenderness of the pectoral muscles or costal cartilage suggests a musculoskeletal origin of chest pain. Respiratory excursion is assessed in the same manner as on the posterior chest, except that the examiner's thumbs are placed along each costal margin. Assess vocal or tactile fremitus. Fremitus normally is diminished over the precordium.[2]

Percussion. The pattern for percussion of the anterior chest is diagrammed in Figure 10-38. Gently displace a female patient's breast before percussion. Dullness is produced by the heart between the third and fifth ICSs. Note and mark the upper border of liver dullness.

Auscultation. Listen for breath sounds over the patient's anterior and lateral chest. Place the stethoscope in the sequence illustrated in Figure 10-8. If indicated, assess for transmitted voice sounds.[2]

Abdomen

The abdominal examination presented here has a narrow focus. Purposes include evaluation of bowel tones, determination of liver size, assessment of bladder distention, and auscultation for bruits. After anesthesia, resumption of

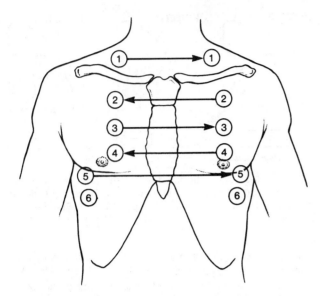

FIGURE 10-38 Sequence of anterior percussion and auscultation. (From Bates B: A Guide to Physical Examination, 3rd ed, p 146. Philadelphia, JB Lippincott, 1983.)

bowel tones must be confirmed before initiating a diet. Liver engorgement occurs because of decreased venous return secondary to right ventricular failure. Urine output is an important indicator of cardiac output. In a patient who is unable to void (e.g., secondary to strict bed rest or after atropine sulfate administration) or who has not voided despite adequate fluid intake, always assess for bladder distention before initiating other measures.

INSPECTION

Observe the abdomen for symmetry and visible peristalsis. Note the presence of abdominal distention. Abdominally localized obesity (waist-to-hip ratio >0.85) is associated with coronary artery disease and with adult-onset diabetes mellitus.

AUSCULTATION

Auscultate the abdomen after observation because palpation and percussion can either increase or diminish bowel sounds. Gently place the diaphragm of the stethoscope on the abdomen. Listen over all quadrants. Normal bowel sounds consist of clicks and gurgles, at a frequency of 5 to 34 per minute. It is necessary to listen for 2 minutes or more to determine that bowel sounds are absent. Borborygmi (prolonged gurgles of hyperperistalsis) also may be heard. Bowel sounds are increased with diarrhea and early intestinal obstruction, and they are decreased or absent with paralytic ileus and peritonitis.[2] Listen for bruits over the renal, ischial, and femoral arteries.

PERCUSSION

Determination of Liver Size. Percussion of the liver (Fig. 10-39) should start in the right MCL, at or below the umbilicus, and proceed upward from an area of tympany (intestine) to an area of dullness (liver). Identify the lower edge of the liver in the MCL. Next, percuss downward at

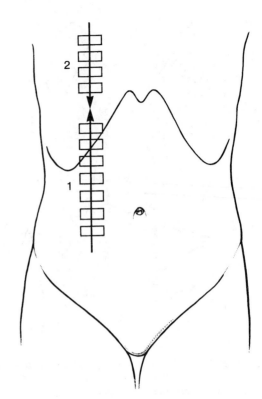

FIGURE 10-39 Percussion of the liver. (From Bates B: A Guide to Physical Examination, 3rd ed, p 236. Philadelphia, JB Lippincott, 1983.)

the MCL from resonance (lung) to dullness (liver). Measure the distance from the upper to the lower liver edge at the MCL; the normal liver span is 6 to 12 cm (Fig. 10-40). A right pleural effusion or lung consolidation (dullness) may obscure the upper border. Gas in the colon (tympany) may obscure the lower edge.

Assessment of Bladder Distention. Percuss downward from the umbilicus to the symphysis pubis. Suprapubic dullness may indicate a distended urinary bladder. If percussion

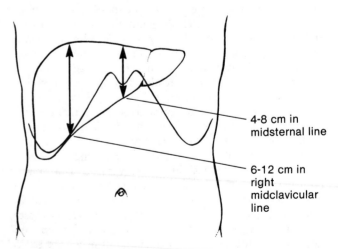

4-8 cm in midsternal line

6-12 cm in right midclavicular line

FIGURE 10-40 Measurement of liver span. (From Bates B: A Guide to Physical Examination, 3rd ed, p 236. Philadelphia, JB Lippincott, 1983.)

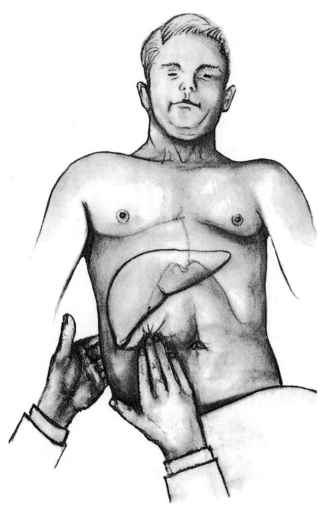

FIGURE 10-41 Palpation of the liver. (From Bates B: A Guide to Physical Examination, 4th ed. Philadelphia, JB Lippincott, 1987.)

does not confirm suspicions of a distended urinary bladder, palpate gently above the symphysis pubis. If ascites is present, neither abdominal percussion nor palpation may reveal bladder distention.

PALPATION

Determination of Liver Size. Deep palpation is necessary to feel the liver. It is imperative that the patient is relaxed. Place the left hand under the patient's 11th and 12th ribs for support. The liver is easier to palpate if the examiner pushes up with this hand. Place the right hand on the abdomen below the lower edge of dullness, with the fingers pointing toward the right costal margin. As the patient takes a deep abdominal breath and then exhales, gently but firmly push in and up with the fingers (Fig. 10-41). With each exhalation, move the hand further toward the liver. The liver edge should come down to meet the fingers. Normally, it feels firm with a smooth edge. It should not be tender. With venous engorgement from right heart failure, the liver is enlarged, firm, tender, and smooth.

REFERENCES

1. Anderson WB: Examination of the retina. In Schlant RC, Alexander RW (eds): Hurst's The Heart Arteries and Veins, 8th ed, pp 315–320. New York, McGraw-Hill, 1994
2. Bates B: A Guide to Physical Examination, 6th ed. Philadelphia, JB Lippincott, 1995
3. Bates B: A Guide to Physical Examination, 5th ed, p 208. Philadelphia, JB Lippincott, 1991
4. Bates B: A Guide to Physical Examination, 3rd ed, p 79. Philadelphia, JB Lippincott, 1983
5. Braunwald E: The physical examination. In Braunwald E (ed): Heart Disease: A Textbook of Cardiovascular Medicine, 2nd ed, pp 35–38. Philadelphia, WB Saunders, 1984
6. Boozer M, Craven RF: Assessment of vascular function. In Patrick ML, Woods SL, Craven RF et al (eds): Medical–Surgical Nursing: Pathophysiological Concepts, p 593–599. Philadelphia, JB Lippincott, 1986
7. Charan NB, Carvalho P: Cardinal symptoms and signs in respiratory disease. In Pierson DJ, Kacmarek RM (eds): Foundations of Respiratory Care, pp 672–674. New York, Churchill Livingston, 1992
8. Chatterjee K: The history. In Parmley W, Chatterjee K (eds): Cardiology, 2nd ed, Vol 1, pp 3.2–3.10. Philadelphia, JB Lippincott, 1991
9. Chatterjee K: Bedside evaluation of the heart: The physical examination. In Parmley W, Chatterjee K (eds): Cardiology, 2nd ed, Vol 1, pp 3.11–3.53. Philadelphia, JB Lippincott, 1991
10. Christie LG Jr, Conti CR: Systematic approach to the evaluation of angina-like chest pain. Am Heart J 102: 897–912, 1981
11. Consensus Committee of the American Autonomic Society and the American Academy of Neurology: Consensus statement on the definition of orthostatic hypotension, pure autonomic failure, and multiple system atrophy. Neurology 46: 1470, 1996
12. Constant J: Essentials of Bedside Cardiology. Boston, Little, Brown, 1989
13. Creager MA, Dzau VJ: Vascular diseases of the extremities. In Isselbacher KJ, Braunwald E, Wilson JD et al (eds): Harrison's Principles of Internal Medicine, 13th ed, pp 1135–1143. New York, McGraw-Hill, 1994
14. Cunningham SL: Hypertension. In Patrick ML, Woods SL, Craven RF et al (eds): Medical–Surgical Nursing: Pathophysiological Concepts, pp. 603–621. Philadelphia, JB Lippincott, 1986
15. Dornhorst AC, Howard R, Leathart GL: Pulsus paradoxus. Lancet 1: 746–748, 1952
16. Ewy GA: The abdominojugular test: Technique and hemodynamic correlates. Ann Intern Med 109: pp. 456–460, 1988
17. Fowler NO: Examination of the Heart, Part 2: Inspection and Palpation of Arterial and Venous Pulses, p 33. New York, American Heart Association, 1972
18. Frolich ED, Grim, C, Labarthe DR et al (eds): Recommendations for Human Blood Pressure Determination by Sphygmomanometers, p 10. Dallas, American Heart Association, 1987
19. Geddes LA: The Direct and Indirect Measurement of Blood Pressure. Chicago, Year Book, 1973
20. Gordon M: Nursing Diagnosis Process and Application. New York, McGraw-Hill, 1982.
21. Greenfield LJ: Acute venous thrombosis and pulmonary embolism. In Hardy JD (ed): Hardy's Textbook of Surgery, p 973. Philadelphia, JB Lippincott, 1983
22. Hansson L, Zanchetti A, Carruthers SG et al: Effects of intensive blood-pressure lowering and low-dose aspirin in patients with hypertension: Principal results of the Hypertension Optimal Treatment (HOT) randomised trial. Lancet 351: 1755–1762, 1998

23. Hurst JW, Schlant RC: Examination of the arteries and their pulsation. In Hurst, JW, Logue RB, Schlant RC et al (eds): The Heart, 4th ed, pp 186–187. New York, McGraw-Hill, 1978

24. Insuna JT, Sacks HS, Lau TS, et al: Drug treatment of hypertension in the elderly: A meta-analysis. Ann Intern Med 121: 355–362, 1994

25. Joint National Committee on Detection, Evaluation, and Treatment of High Blood Pressure: The Sixth Report of the Joint National Committee on Detection, Evaluation, and Treatment of High Blood Pressure. Bethesda, MD, The National Heart, Blood, and Lung Institute, National Institutes of Health, 1997

26. Judge RD, Zuidema GD, Fitzgerald FT (eds): Clinical Diagnosis, 5th ed. Boston, Little, Brown, 1989

27. Kapoor WN: Syncope and hypotension. In Braunwald E (ed): Heart Disease: A Textbook of Cardiovascular Medicine, 5th ed, pp 863–875. Philadelphia, WB Saunders, 1997

28. Kenney RA: Physiology of aging. Clin Geriatr Med 1: 37–59, 1988

29. Kirkendall WM, Feinleib MD, Freis ED et al (eds): Recommendations for Human Blood Pressure Determination by Sphygmomanometers. Dallas, American Heart Association, 1980

30. Laurent DJ: A Comparison of Axillary, Oral, and Rectal Temperatures to Pulmonary Artery Blood Temperature in Acutely Ill Patients. Unpublished Master's Thesis, Seattle, University of Washington, 1979

31. Leatham A: An Introduction to the Examination of the Cardiovascular System, 2nd ed, p 20. Oxford, Oxford University Press, 1979

32. Marriott HJL: Bedside Cardiac Diagnosis. Philadelphia, JB Lippincott, 1993

33. McGee SR: Physical examination of venous pressure: A critical review. Am Heart J 136: 10–18, 1998

34. Memmer M: Acute orthostatic hypotension. Heart Lung 17: 134–140, 1988

35. New York Heart Association Criteria Committee: Diseases of the Heart and Blood Vessels: Nomenclature and Criteria for Diagnosis, 6th ed. Boston, Little, Brown, 1964

36. O'Rourke RA, Silverman ME, Schlant RC: General examination of the patient. In Schlant RC, Alexander RW (eds): Hurst's The Heart, Arteries, and Veins, 8th ed, pp 217–251. New York, McGraw-Hill, 1994

37. Perloff D, Grim C, Flack J et al: Human blood pressure determination by sphygmomanometry. Circulation 88: 2460–2470, 1993

38. Perloff, JK, Braunwald E: Physical examination of the heart and circulation. In Braunwald E (ed): Heart Disease: A Textbook of Cardiovascular Medicine, 5th ed, pp 15–52. Philadelphia, WB Saunders, 1997

39. Perloff JK: Physical Examination of the Heart and Circulation, p 208. Philadelphia, WB Saunders, 1990

40. Phillips R, Skov P: Rewarming and cardiac surgery: A review. Heart Lung 17: 511–519, 1988

41. Ronan J: Cardiac auscultation: The first and second heart sounds. Heart Disease and Stroke 1: 113–116, 1992

42. Ronan J: Cardiac auscultation: The third and fourth heart sounds. Heart Disease and Stroke 1: 267–270, 1992

43. Runge MS and Harker LA: Thrombus formation and dissolution. In Schlant RC, Alexander RW (eds): Hurst's The Heart, Arteries, and Veins, 8th ed, pp 173–183. New York, McGraw-Hill, 1994

44. Ruskin J, Bache RJ, Rembert JC et al: Pressure-flow studies in man: Effect of respiration on left ventricular stroke volume. Circulation 48: 79–85, 1973

45. Tilkian A, Conover M: Understanding Heart Sounds and Murmurs with an Introduction to Lung Sounds, 3rd ed. Philadelphia, WB Saunders, 1993

46. Underhill SL: Assessment of cardiovascular function. In Brunner LS, Suddarth DS (eds): Textbook of Medical–Surgical Nursing, 5th ed, pp 457–563. Philadelphia, JB Lippincott, 1984

Laboratory Tests Using Blood

MARGARET WOODING BAKER

Diagnosis, treatment, and management of patients requires a multimodal, multidisciplinary approach. Along with an in-depth history and physical, the clinician frequently depends on test results to complete the assessment picture. One of the most frequently used testing modalities is laboratory tests of blood specimens. A host of variables can affect interpretation of blood specimen results. Accurate interpretation starts with proper specimen collection. The nurse has a key role in maximizing the conditions under which specimens are collected,[67,90] thereby controlling for as many variables as possible.

BLOOD SPECIMEN COLLECTION

Collection of blood specimens is a process that involves three phases: patient preparation, collection of the blood sample, and interpretation of results. As mentioned earlier, the nurse plays an important role during this process.

Patient Preparation

Adequate preparation of the patient and their family involves education. Frequently, proper specimen collection and interpretation requires compliance with instructions about food or fluid restrictions, taking or withholding medications, and meeting criteria for proper timing of the blood sample.[90] When the blood sample is taken, patients should receive an explanation about what tests are being drawn, why they have been ordered, and when results will be available. If the sample is being obtained by venipuncture, arterial puncture, or vascular port access, preparation of the patient includes a reminder about pain during the procedure and the importance of complying with instructions to maintain a certain position.

Universal Precautions

All blood is considered a source of potential infection. Universal precautions, as well as organizational policies and procedures, should be followed when collecting and transporting specimens. Universal precautions include the use of gloves during phlebotomy (or at any time there is risk of exposure to blood or body fluids), complete avoidance of recapping needles, proper disposal of sharps, and proper handwashing. When there is the potential that blood or body fluids will splash, protective clothing and eyewear should be worn. Spills should be cleaned with an Environmental Protection Agency (EPA)-approved germicide or a 1:100 solution of household bleach, and soiled linen should be bagged at the location where it was used. Last, institutional policies should be followed with regard to isolation or transport of patients who have highly transmittable organisms, as well as disposal of infective waste.[22,90,99]

Blood Sample Collection

General guidelines for blood sample collection have been developed that help to ensure patient and clinician safety and maximize interpretation of results. The clinician should consider the policies and procedures of his or her organization with regard to blood specimen collection, as well as the standards for professional, national, and international organizations.

Control of variability can be enhanced by use of proper technique during collection and processing of the specimen. The practice of having patients clench and unclench their fist in preparation for specimen collection from the arm should be avoided. This maneuver causes an increase in the metabolic activity of muscle tissue, thereby affecting certain laboratory results. With just 1 minute of fist-clenching, plasma potassium can increase by as much as 1.0 to 1.5 mmol/L. The possibility for hemolysis is enhanced by repeatedly clenching the fist during specimen withdrawal.[57]

The use of a tourniquet produces changes as well. Once a tourniquet is placed on the arm, veins dilate because of their inability to drain. Under these conditions, return of fluid and electrolytes to the vein is decreased or prohibited, resulting in a hemoconcentrated specimen.[67] In addition, despite decreased circulation of fresh blood to the tissues, cells continue their metabolic processes, leading to an increased concentration in metabolic waste products, such as lactate. In this more acidic environment, potassium leaks out of cells.[32] In general, the tourniquet should not be left on more than 1 or 2 minutes. Cellular injury and hemolysis can be caused by the prolonged use of a tourniquet, described as 3 minutes or longer.[123] Longer use may be unavoidable during a difficult venipuncture. In such cases, information about a difficult venipuncture should be noted on the laboratory slip to assist with interpretation of results.[90]

Blood specimens can be contaminated in several ways. During collection, contamination may occur from intravenous (IV) fluids. Blood draws should not be done on the same arm as an infusion. If the infusion arm cannot be avoided, a tourniquet may be placed between the IV site and the phlebotomy site. Slowing the IV to a keep-open rate (if not contraindicated) for 3 to 5 minutes before the draw may help to reduce contamination of the blood sample.[90] In any event, it should be noted on the laboratory slip that the sample was obtained under these conditions.

Contamination may also be introduced by improper use of blood tubes. Most specimen collection tubes contain some form of anticoagulant. If blood has been mistakenly collected in one tube containing anticoagulant, it should never be poured into a different tube. Also, blood entering one tube should never be allowed to contaminate remaining blood that will be introduced into another tube.

Another source of contamination is introduced when routine samples are drawn from arterial lines, vascular catheters, or ports. The use of an indwelling intravascular catheter allows access to the patient's blood supply without further invasive procedure. Comfort for the patient and ease and speed of periodic specimen collection are some of the benefits of using an intravascular line for blood sampling.[20,72,100,104] Intravascular catheters may be kept patent by continuous or intermittent infusion, or by instilling saline or heparin solutions. Sometimes, solutions delivered through the catheter may contain medications. The infusate or any additives may dilute blood constituents. This dilution would have the effect of lowering the concentration of the desired sample.

The diameter and length of the catheter are important determinants when considering this hemodilution. Several studies have been successful in establishing accuracy for specific laboratory tests after a minimal blood discard volume. Research has explored the use of central venous, intra-arterial, and pulmonary artery catheters, including both the right atrial (RA) port and vascular infusion port (VIP). Certain precisely controlled studies have quantified a discard volume for specific blood tests. Research has demonstrated that a 1- to 6-mL discard volume is sufficient for most intravascular catheters.[18,21,27,47,48,72,110,123,137] At the very minimum, the initial discard needs to equal the dead space of the device or tubing. The institution's policy and procedure manual should be consulted for recommended withdrawal and discard from vascular devices. Additional sources, such as professional nursing society standards, may assist in making decisions about recommended discard volumes.

Whether sampling from a pulmonary artery catheter, central venous line, arterial catheter, or other intravascular

catheter, attention should be paid to the feasibility of interruption of the system. The pulmonary artery catheter presents particular problems. Both the RA port and VIP are useful for the administration of drugs and fluids. Although the RA port allows access to the central circulation, use of this port for cardiac output calculations makes it difficult to infuse drugs or fluids (a large amount of the infusate might be delivered during delivery of the cardiac output injectate). Consequently, the VIP is chosen for fluid and drug infusion. In this situation, the use of the RA port may be preferable for blood withdrawal. If vasoactive drugs are not infusing through the VIP, it may also be used for blood sampling; the proximal opening into the RA is upstream of any drugs or fluids infusing through the RA port and the possibility of contamination of the blood sample by infusates is minimized.

Questions persist about appropriate discard from vascular catheters (instilled with heparin) when drawing blood for coagulation studies. Inconsistent results may increase the cost to the patient through repeated testing, wasted blood, or erroneous treatment decisions.[20,72] Various studies indicate that accurate results for activated partial thromboplastin time (aPTT) can be obtained if a minimal amount is withdrawn and discarded prior to filling blood specimen tubes. However, recommendations differ with respect to how much should be withdrawn and discarded.[55,74,75,128] Reliable results have been established for the partial thromboplastin time (PTT) drawn from a heparinized catheter.[47] However, sampling for thrombin time and prothrombin time (PT) has been shown to produce inaccurate results, particularly when a heparinized catheter is used.[12,47,120] Heparin adhering to a catheter can alter the test results.[30,60] Again, the nurse may refer to policy and procedure manuals or professional organization standards for guidance. In any event, coordination in obtaining multiple blood specimens decreases the amount of blood that is eventually discarded and the number of times that the sterile system is invaded, thus reducing risk of introducing infection.

Early investigations of sepsis associated with intravascular monitoring equipment discouraged frequent blood sampling from the system.[122] These reports identified stopcocks and pressure transducers as the most frequent reservoirs for endemic contamination.[139,141] The incidence of local infection and bacteremia has been reduced by the use of disposable transducers and the percutaneous sheath systems used to introduce pulmonary artery catheters.[145] The withdrawal of blood from an intravascular catheter should be considered a sterile procedure. Once removed, caps used to cover stopcock openings should always be replaced with a sterile cap. The person performing the procedure should be gloved. Syringes, used once, should be discarded.

Types of Specimens

When blood is withdrawn from the body, it eventually clots. The fluid that separates from the clot is called *serum*. Plasma, from unclotted blood, contains fibrinogen, which is eventually converted to fibrin. Most blood tests are done on serum, and therefore require use of a tube that allows blood to clot. Red-top tubes contain no additives; they are used for chemistries, drug monitoring, radioimmunoassays, serology, and blood typing. Lavender-top tubes, which contain ethylenediaminetetraacetic acid (EDTA), are usually used for hematology and certain chemistries. Green-top tubes contain heparin as the anticoagulant and can be used for chemistries, arterial blood gases and hormone levels. Blue-top tubes, used for coagulation studies, contain citrate. Sodium fluoride, found in gray-top tubes, prevents glycolysis and may be used to test blood glucose in its *in vivo* state.[67]

When multiple blood samples are drawn at the same collection time, the preferred order is as follows: tubes with no preservative (red-top); tubes with mild anticoagulants (green, gray, blue, black); lavender-top tubes should be collected last. Blood for coagulation studies should never be drawn first because tissue injury can initiate the clotting process and result in falsely low levels of coagulation factors.[32] Specimens in tubes with additives should be rotated gently to mix the anticoagulant with the blood. They should never be shaken.[67]

Hemolysis refers to the lysis of red blood cells. When extracellular fluid (plasma) is used for analysis, inaccurate results are produced if the specimen is hemolyzed. Hemolysis may occur *in vivo,* as in hemolytic disease states such as transfusion reactions. Hemolysis may also occur in some infections and with the use of some drugs.[33] A deficiency of the enzyme glucose-6-phosphate dehydrogenase, responsible for generating chemicals needed for maintenance of normal red cell fragility, contributes to hemolysis.

Hemolysis may also occur as a result of improper collection technique or specimen transport. Specimens may be hemolyzed if they are collected from a poorly flowing venipuncture. Greater hemolysis occurs with the use of a large-bore needle than with a small-bore needle.[19,32] Failure to dry alcohol from the venipuncture site also results in hemolysis.[124] Blood should never be forcibly withdrawn from the venipuncture, nor should it be forcibly entered into the collection tube by pushing on the syringe barrel to fill faster.[32]

Specimens should be handled carefully when placed in collection tubes and when transported to the laboratory; rough handling may lead to hemolysis. Hemolysis increases the laboratory values of lactate dehydrogenase (LDH), aspartate aminotransferase (AST or SGOT), and phosphorus, as well as potassium, magnesium, and calcium.[138]

Proper specimen collection includes accurate identification of the patient and accurate labeling of the specimen at the site of collection.[90] It also includes rapid transport to the laboratory, because cells remain viable after collection and continue their metabolic processes. Specimens that are left to stand unprocessed often yield inaccurate results.[32]

Interpretation of Results

Inherent physiologic variability exists based on patient age, sex, ethnicity, and health status (such as pregnancy or post-myocardial infarction [MI]). These physiologic differences affect interpretation of results. Physiologic changes associated with the aging process bring concomitant changes in some expected laboratory results. Because men usually have more muscle mass than women, sex differences are seen in substances related to muscle function or metabolism, such as creatinine. According to Dufour,[32] numerous studies have documented significant differences among European, African, and Asian populations in testing for cholesterol, enzymes, and hormones. Various physiologic states, such as pregnancy, stress, and endurance exercise, also introduce situational changes in expected results.

Cyclic variability produces daily, monthly, or yearly patterns in physiologic states. These cycles are often taken into consideration in the collection or interpretation of laboratory results. As a result, most routine specimens, at least in the hospital setting, are drawn in the early morning to control for any circadian variability.

Blood tests are sometimes affected by the ingestion of food or fluids. Not only are results affected by the absorption of dietary components into the blood after a meal, but hormonal and metabolic changes occur as well. Partial control for the variability introduced by food or fluid ingestion can be achieved either by drawing early morning, premeal specimens, or by having the patient fast for 8 to 12 hours. The latter is especially important in lipid testing.[32]

The timing of blood sampling should include consideration of the effect of medications on the interpretation of results. Medications affect results of many specimens drawn for chemistry, hematology, coagulation, and hormonal and enzyme studies. Knowledge of the effect of the drug assists in proper timing or subsequent interpretation of the results. Consideration should also be given to the effects of other influences, including over-the-counter medications, caffeine, nicotine and ethanol,[32] home remedies, and herbal therapies.

In therapeutic drug monitoring, blood drug levels are monitored to evaluate the effects of drug therapy, make decisions regarding dosage, prevent toxicity, and monitor patient adherence. Timing of the blood sample usually depends on the half-life of the drug; samples drawn at projected peak level assist in monitoring for toxicity, whereas levels drawn at trough help to verify the minimum satisfactory therapeutic level for that patient.[23,129,132] Regardless of the purpose of the blood sample, drugs that may affect interpretation of results should be noted on the laboratory slip. For therapeutic drug monitoring, it is important to note the date and time of the last dose as well.[90]

Sometimes, differences based on position are negligible. In other cases, they are significant. Patient position during (and before) sampling can affect results. In the upright position, there may be a shift in extracellular fluid volume into the tissues. With the resulting increased concentration of proteins and protein-bound substances in the vascular space, samples for proteins, enzymes, hematocrit (Hct), calcium, iron, hormones, and several drugs may show an average 5% to 8% increase. Redistribution of extracellular fluid volume and electrolytes within the vascular space does not stabilize until a patient has assumed the sitting position for at least 15 minutes (from a standing position)[32], and in some cases 20 to 30 minutes.[67] In some settings, such as the hospital, it is not difficult to stabilize the patient's position and thus reduce variability.[90] In other settings, such as ambulatory care, significant variability is introduced if the patient is not made to sit for at least 15 minutes before the blood draw. Because control over sitting time is not usually feasible or practical, care should be taken in the interpretation of results. Exercising immediately before blood sample collection frequently produces significantly erroneous results, especially with enzyme evaluation. Forearm exercises before blood withdrawal may lead to hemolysis.[67,108]

Different laboratories use different equipment and methods by which to test specimens. Specific reference ranges are usually reported alongside the patient's results on the laboratory report. In an effort to establish a standard for communicating laboratory results, the World Health Organization has recommended that the medical and scientific community throughout the world adopt the use of the International System of Units (ISU).[67] An international unit is defined as the number of moles of substrate converted per second under defined conditions.[131] Thus, many laboratories may report results in different ways, depending on their accepted standard of practice.[71] Most laboratories also report critical (or panic) values. These values should be reported promptly to the provider so that results may be evaluated (and decisions made) in light of patient condition.

Except for arterial blood gases, most reference ranges have been established for venous blood samples. Because arterial blood has higher concentrations of glucose and oxygen and lower concentrations of waste products (ammonia, potassium, lactate), an arterial source (instead of venous) should be noted on the laboratory slip. Capillary samples yield results that are closer to arterial blood than venous.

Critical evaluation of laboratory results should take into account how the reference, or "normal" values, were determined. Patients who have been seen for a long time by the same provider, or those who have been seen within the same health care organization, sometimes establish their own reference range. Reference ranges for a specific disease are sometimes established through large-scale clinical trials.

In most circumstances, each laboratory establishes its own reference values by testing a group that is easy to recruit. It is possible, however, that this technique may not reflect the usual values or range of values of the group that the organization serves. When samples are taken from volunteers, such as those who agree to give a blood sample for reference testing in exchange for a free cholesterol screening, bias may be introduced because those who are likely to volunteer may be those who have or suspect they have illness already. When reference samples are taken from patients who are undergoing routine physical examinations or elective surgery, results may reflect a mix of the surrounding population. Again, these reference values need to be considered in light of who was included or excluded from testing. Usually, those who drink alcohol, smoke, or take certain medications are excluded from reference range testing. However, this is likely to establish a narrow range of "normal" values, thereby increasing the number of people in the served population who fall outside the established range. Additional care should be taken in interpreting results if the laboratory reports only one set of reference values.[32]

Clinicians who are aware of how reference ranges are obtained are in a better position to interpret laboratory results accurately for their patients. In all situations, interpretation of results should be done in light of all factors that introduce variability, and in light of the clinical condition, remembering that "normal" values do not necessarily indicate absence of disease, just as "abnormal" values do not necessarily establish a pathologic state.[32]

CARDIAC MARKERS

The internal environment of the healthy person is in a state of balance with respect to water, electrolytes, energy storage and use, and metabolic end products. Stability is maintained through homeostatic mechanisms that regulate the activities of cells and organs. During periods of critical illness, a disruption in cell membrane stability may cause chemical substances that are responsible for intracellular homeostatic mechanisms to appear in the blood. Frequent evaluation of blood results is a means by which the status of the internal environment and the extent and nature of tissue damage can be monitored.

Certain intracellular enzymes and proteins are rarely found in measurable amounts in the blood of healthy people. However, after an event leading to cellular injury, these substances may leak into the blood. In irreversible cellular damage, smaller intracellular components are released earlier than larger ones, accounting for differences in timing in the appearance of these substances in the blood after damage has occurred.[32] Because of the importance of the timing of the appearance (and disappearance) of enzymes in the blood, it is crucial that ordered enzyme tests are drawn on time. It is equally important that the date and time of the blood draw are noted on the laboratory slip so that the temporal sequence of the rise and fall can be established by those interpreting the results.[68,99]

Diagnosis of MI, reinfarction, or other types of myocardial damage is made through evaluation of 12-lead electrocardiograms (ECGs), clinical signs and symptoms, and evaluation of enzymes: creatine kinase ([CK] and its isoenzymes, isoforms, and mass activity), LDH, and AST. Newer tests available to clinicians include measurement of troponins and myoglobin. Investigators are studying additional markers for utility in assisting with diagnosis of MI, including glycogen phosphorylase, fatty-acid–binding proteins, myosin light chains, and inflammatory markers, such as C-reactive protein and serum amyloid A.[14,151]

Myocardial Proteins

TROPONINS

Troponins are a protein complex that regulate actin–myosin interaction in striated muscle. They are found in both cardiac and skeletal muscle. Three isotypes have been identified: troponin-T (cTnT), troponin-I (cTnI), and troponin-C (cTnC).[99] Isotypes T and I are both found in the myocardium. The normal range for cTnI is 0 to 2 ng/mL, and the normal range for cTnT is 0 to 3.1 ng/mL. Both are elevated in MI.[32] A cTnI level greater than 1.5 ng/mL is consistent with acute MI.[71]

Troponin-I is actually found exclusively in the myocardium and has 100% sensitivity for MI. It is not elevated in patients with either acute or chronic severe skeletal muscle injury, despite elevation in CK-MB.[4] Given the high rate of false-positive and false-negative CK-MB results in diagnosing blunt cardiac trauma,[93] cTnI is emerging as an accurate test for confirming presence of myocardial damage during cardiac contusion.[3] Unlike CK-MB or cTnT, cTnI elevations are not found in the blood of marathon runners or patients with muscle disease (acute or chronic) unless there has been injury to the myocardium.[83] Unlike cTnT, cTnI is not elevated in patients with renal insufficiency or failure.[14]

Troponin-T is also elevated in muscle damage and renal failure.[23,32] Despite its high sensitivity for MI, its specificity has not yet been defined.[4] It has been suggested that cTnT concentrations may be of use in diagnosing perioperative MI after coronary artery bypass grafting. cTnT may also be a strong predictor of significant complication after MI, helping to identify those who require bypass surgery. In addition, release of cTnT in donor hearts correlates with the need for inotropic support after cardiac transplantation, and may be of some use in evaluating high-risk donor hearts.[14] It has not been found useful as a predictor of cardiac allograft rejection.[140]

With such high sensitivity, the troponins may be enormously useful markers in the early diagnosis of MI because they are either low or undetectable in healthy people, but in the event of an MI, are detectable as early as 3 to 4 hours after injury.[23,32] Then, a second, slower release occurs. Because most troponin is so tightly bound to muscle, it is released slowly and may remain detectable for 1 to 2 weeks post-MI.[4,32] This late-phase presence of troponins may represent death of the contractile apparatus.[83] Testing for troponins requires a 5-mL specimen in a red-top tube.

MYOGLOBIN

Myoglobin is a low–molecular-weight oxygen-binding protein. Found in the myocardium and skeletal muscle, it is similar to hemoglobin (Hgb).[14] Myoglobin is released into the circulation after damage to the heart or skeletal muscle. Compared with CK levels in evaluation of myocardial damage, myoglobin is more sensitive (serial measurements taken in the first 6 hours after the onset of pain are nearly 100%), but not as specific because of its release after skeletal muscle injury as well. False-positive rates range anywhere from 0% to 22%.[99,129] Levels increase in 2 to 4 hours, peak 8 to 12 hours after MI, and return to normal (undetectable) as early as 12 hours, but usually after 24 to 30 hours. Because of the rapid increase in myoglobin levels after myocardial injury, it is useful as a basis for making decisions about thrombolytic therapy or emergency angioplasty within 6 hours of MI.[99,121]

Elevated myoglobin levels are seen after MI, reinfarction, skeletal muscle injury, trauma, severe burns, electrical shock, polymyositis, alcoholic myopathy, delirium tremens, metabolic disorders (e.g., myxedema), malignant hyperthermia, systemic lupus erythematosus, muscular dystrophy, rhabdomyolysis, and seizures.[67,99] Very high levels of myoglobin are toxic to the kidneys, and careful monitoring of renal function is warranted.[99,132] False-positive results occur in renal failure, when myoglobin is not excreted.[90] Myoglobin levels are usually evaluated along with serial determinations of CK, LDH, and AST, serial ECGs, and assessment of patient signs and symptoms. Tests for myoglobin require 5 mL of venous blood in a red-top tube.[67]

Cardiac Enzymes

Enzymes are protein substances that catalyze chemical reactions in cells but do not themselves enter into the reaction. Substrates in the cells bind to the enzymes and form products. After the reaction, the enzyme molecule is free to undergo the same reaction with other substrate molecules. Specific enzymes are responsible for nearly every chemical reaction in the body. Some enzymes are present in almost all cells; others are specific to cells of certain organs.

CREATINE KINASE

Creatine kinase is an enzyme specific to cells of the brain, myocardium, and skeletal muscle, but it also is found in minimal amounts in other tissues such as smooth muscle. In these organ systems, the function of CK is primarily that of energy production, where it serves as a catalyst in the phosphorylation of adenosine diphosphate (ADP) to creatine and adenosine triphosphate (ATP). In this manner, CK is responsible for the transfer of an energy-rich bond to ADP. This reaction provides a rapid means of forming ATP for contractile activity in muscle as well as for energy requirements in nonmuscle tissue. The reaction is reversible, and ATP can phosphorylate creatine to form creatine phosphate and ADP during periods of rest.[91,92,132]

In an acute MI, inadequate oxygen delivery to the myocardium causes cell injury. An acidic environment promotes the activity of lysosomal enzymes, which are responsible for cell membrane damage or destruction. CK is among the cellular enzymes that diffuse from the damaged cell into the blood. It is released after irreversible injury.[132] The appearance of CK in the blood indicates cardiac, cerebral, or skeletal muscle necrosis or injury and follows a predictable rise and fall over a specified time (Fig. 11-1). Its presence may also indicate a neurologic pathologic process.[99]

The average peak CK level after MI is approximately 1,200 U/L. The MB fraction averages 11%, with a relative index of 6%.[32] Total CK increases are seen in acute MI,[67,90,99] unstable angina,[68,99,132] shock, malignant hyperthermia, myopathies, myocarditis,[67,99] cardiac aneurysm surgery, cardiac defibrillation,[68,99] and sustained ventricular arrhythmias. Less frequent causes are electrical cardioversion, cardiac catheterization, and stroke.[90] Rises in total CK are also seen with major surgery, vigorous exercise, and alcoholic myopathy, and after intramuscular (IM) injections;[67,90] just one IM injection 24 to 48 hours before measurement may increase CK by over 1,000 U/L.[32,68,90,99] CK levels as high as 5,000 to 10,000 U/L can be seen after cardiopulmonary resuscitation.[32] It is thought that CK-MB levels rise only slightly after cardiac pacemaker implantation and therefore should not interfere with attempts to evaluate such patients for MI.[46]

Specimens for CK are collected on admission, 12 hours later, and then every day for 3 days.[68,99] CK and CK isoenzyme results should be evaluated along with AST and LDH, ECG results, and clinical signs and symptoms. Laboratory

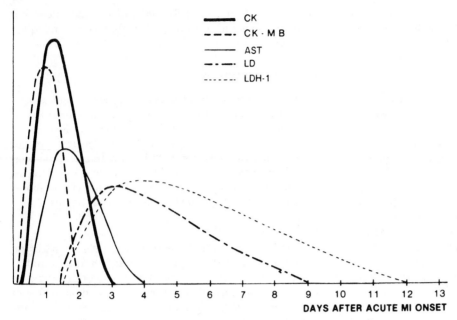

FIGURE 11-1 Patterns and timing of elevation for creatine kinase (CK), creatine kinase-MB (CK-MB), lactate dehydrogenase (LDH), lactate dehydrogenase-1 (LDH-1), and aspartate aminotransferase (AST). MI, myocardial infarction. (Adapted and reproduced with permission from Ravel R: Clinical Laboratory Medicine: Clinical Application of Laboratory Data, 4th ed. Copyright © 1984 by Year Book Medical Publishers, Inc., Chicago.)

slips should be marked with the date and time of any IM injections given to the patient in the prior 24 to 48 hours. Caution should be exercised in interpretation of CKs drawn in the emergency department. Only 25% to 40% of patients who are having an MI have an abnormal CK at that point. An initial normal CK level should *never* be used to make a decision about discharge from the emergency department, or to withhold thrombolytic therapy.[32,121]

The importance of monitoring the concentration of serum CK is related to its specificity in the organ in which it functions. Slightly different molecular forms (isoenzymes, or *isozymes*) of CK have different tissues of origin (Table 11-1). The three CK isoenzymes are combinations of the protein subunits, M and B, named for their primary sites of isolation, the muscle (M) and brain (B).[38] CK-MM is the predominant muscle isoenzyme, found in cardiac and skeletal muscle. It also can be detected in normal serum. The myocardium is primarily responsible for the CK-MB form.

CK-BB is present in the brain, lung, stomach, prostate, and smooth muscle of the gastrointestinal tract and bladder.[38,133] Diagnostic precision depends on laboratory analysis of CK isoenzymes and may well be imperative in critically ill patients with multiple organ system involvement.

Because of the wide range in baseline values among "healthy" people, and various enzyme assay techniques, there are no uniform reference values for CK and CK isoenzymes.[32] Consequently, the practice of reporting the isoenzyme as a percentage of the total CK, as well as in units per liter of blood (U/L), has been encouraged.[80] A nationwide survey of the analyses for CK and its isoenzymes revealed that 99% of 300 participating laboratories reported CK isoenzyme results in units per liter, and 69% of the laboratories also reported isoenzymes as a percentage of the total CK activity.[16] The reference values reported by laboratories may vary, suggesting possible regional variations in normal serum levels for CK and its isoenzymes.

TABLE 11-1 **Distribution of Total Creatine Kinase and Creatine Kinase Isoenzymes in Human Tissue**

Tissue	Total CK*	CK-MM†	CK-BB†	CK-MB†
Normal serum	Trace	97%–100%	0%	0%–3%
Skeletal muscle	1,894–3,281	99%–100%	<1%	<1%
Heart	356–402	76%–78%	0%–2%	22%
Bladder	162	2%	92%	6%
Bowel	125–160	3%–4%	96%	0%–1%
Brain	157	0	100%	0%
Lung	8.7–14	16%–35%	64%–84%	0%–1%

CK, creatine kinase.
*Expressed in units per liter (U/L)
†Expressed as percentage of total CK.
Data from Galen RS: Myocardial infarction: A clinician's guide to the isoenzymes. Resident and Staff Physician 23: 67–75, 1977; Lott JA, Stang JM: Serum enzymes and isoenzymes in the diagnosis and differential diagnosis of myocardial ischemia and necrosis. Clin Chem 26: 1241–1250, 1980; and Tsung SM; Creatine kinase isoenzyme patterns in human tissue obtained at surgery. Clin Chem 22: 173–175, 1976.

Age, sex, race, physical activity, lean body mass, medications, and other unidentified factors are known to affect total CK. A patient's baseline CK level is related to his or her overall muscle mass.[99] Adults have lower values than children. Serum CK declines with age; the elderly have very low values, sometimes making the diagnosis of MI difficult. CK values measured in women are lower than those of men; European Americans have lower values than African Americans. Chronic exercise raises serum CK levels; however, there is a training effect, and well-trained athletes have smaller increases in CK after physical exertion.[81] Medications that may increase CK include anticoagulants, aspirin, furosemide, captopril, lovastatin, lidocaine, propranolol, and morphine.[99]

Creatine Kinase-BB.

The brain fraction CK-BB (CK-1) is seen infrequently in serum. Its rare appearance has been associated with Reye's syndrome, brain trauma, cerebral contusions, and cerebrovascular accidents.[53,90,97,102,111,118] The presence of CK-BB in association with cancer has been reported.[26] Other causes of serum CK-BB activity include malignant hyperpyrexia, bowel infarctions, renal failure, and after central nervous system surgery.[37,38] More recently, however, serum CK-BB has been reported after cardiac arrest.[77,78,88] The presence of CK-BB after cardiac arrest has implications in the care of postarrest survivors. Investigators have been able to show that the maximum cerebrospinal fluid CK-BB concentration is related to neurologic outcome, Glasgow Coma Scale scores, the presence of intracranial pressure plateau waves, and histologic brain damage on death.[11,53,69,78,138] Results of studies are now emerging that have attempted to correlate serum CK-BB levels with neurologic outcome.[77,88] Some researchers have suggested that a more favorable outcome is associated with a return to normal of serum CK-BB within 36 hours of a cerebral injury. Longstreth and coworkers[77] suggested that persistence or reappearance of serum CK-BB more than 6 hours after cardiac arrest was associated with poor outcome. In a study by Massey and Goe,[88] however, no relationship was shown.

Creatine Kinase-MM.

Creatine kinase-MM constitutes almost all of the CK total in healthy people. Skeletal muscle injury or severe muscle exertion is the most frequent source of high serum CK-MM (CK-3) levels. Specific examples include myopathy, vigorous exercise, multiple intramuscular injections, electroconvulsive therapy, cardioversion, surgery,[99] muscular dystrophy, convulsions, and delirium tremens. Elevations in CK-MM fractions have also been noted in conditions producing less obvious effects on muscle, such as hypokalemia and hypothyroidism. Alcohol has a direct toxic effect on muscle, and elevations of CK-MM can be detected in alcoholic patients.[105]

Some controversy continues as to whether skeletal muscle also contains CK-MB. One investigator reported that type I muscle fibers contain CK-MM, and that type II muscle fibers contain both CK-MM and CK-MB.[105] However, tissue studies done by Tsung[133] determined that CK-MB in skeletal muscle is responsible for less than 1% of the total CK activity in skeletal muscle, and that CK-MM is the primary muscle isoenzyme.

The analysis of blood for CK-MM can be a useful tool for differential diagnosis in complex situations. The normal range of CK-MM in the blood is 94% to 100%.[67] Isoforms MM1 and MM3 are the most useful for evaluation of cardiac disease. A ratio of MM3:MM1 greater than 1 is suggestive of acute myocardial injury. The presence of CK-MM, rather than CK-MB, in the serum of patients who experienced electric countershock accounted for a total CK elevation in 30 patients studied by Ehsani and coworkers.[33] This finding supported the belief that myocardial injury in such situations was minimal and that CK-MB was likely to appear in the serum only after abnormally vigorous and repetitive countershock. It is now accepted that total CK elevation after electric countershock, formerly thought to be of myocardial origin, is of skeletal muscle origin (CK-MM).

Exercise stress testing may negligibly elevate the total serum CK.[80] A study of the sera of 62 subjects after performance of stress exercise to a symptom-tolerated maximum revealed that CK elevations, if present, were of the CK-MM fraction and were associated with the amount of work performed.[125] Of marathon participants, 14% to 100% have elevated CK-MB.[81]

A study of 210 patients after cardiac catheterization demonstrated that an increase in the serum activity of total CK activity was also of the CK-MM fraction. This issue was first examined by Roberts and coworkers,[107] who showed similar results in 42 patients. After balloon angioplasty of the coronary arteries, subtle myocardial injury may be reflected by increased CK-MB.[81] If CK-MB is seen after cardiac catheterization without balloon angioplasty, injury to the myocardium should be considered.[80]

At one time, it was thought that victims of primary cardiac arrest had experienced an MI, based on the case history and total CK elevation. In 1975, Cobb and coworkers[25] reported that the CK elevation was not of myocardial origin (CK-MB) but probably due to cardiopulmonary resuscitation (CK-MM). This information has become an important determinant in the implication of several other cardiovascular diseases or processes that are now known to lead to primary cardiac arrest.

Creatine Kinase-MB.

Since 1975, CK-MB (CK-2) isoenzyme analysis has been an accepted means for diagnosis of an acute MI. Roberts and associates[105] examined tissue extracts obtained during surgery and demonstrated that the myocardium was the only tissue containing sufficient CK-MB to account for plasma increases. The same studies revealed that the sera of 300 hospitalized patients showed elevated CK-MB plasma levels after an MI (0.089 international units per mL [IU/mL]), but low levels after cardiac catheterization and noncardiac surgery (0.004 IU/mL).[107] This study was followed by others that determined that CK-MB isoenzyme activity was most specific in differentiating an MI from other myocardial events and could be defined by a predictable rise and fall over a period of 3 days.[119]

When CK-MB is released from myocardial tissue, it has a biologic half-life in blood of hours to days (see Fig. 11-1). Total CK and CK-MB rise within 4 to 6 hours after an acute MI. Peak levels are seen within 12 to 24 hours and are more than six times their normal value. If no additional myocyte necrosis occurs, levels return to normal within 3 to 4 days.[68] Elevated CK-MB levels have also been reported after myocardial damage from unstable angina,[132] in cardiac surgery or coronary angioplasty, after defibrillation, in vigorous exercise, and after intramuscular injections, trauma, and surgery.[90] Early and abnormally high increases in CK are sometimes seen after reperfusion by percutaneous transluminal coronary angioplasty (PTCA) or thrombolytic agents.[103] By 6 to 8 hours postangioplasty, 20% of patients have a mild increase in CK-MB. Elevations are occasionally seen in pericarditis, myocarditis, viral myositis, and sustained tachyarrhythmias.[129] An increase in CK-MB may occur after cardioversion, but only with the use of 400 J or more. The time course for increase is different for that of MI, with the mild increase of CK-MB peaking within 4 hours of cardioversion.

Although not very specific, CK-MB increases are seen after blunt cardiac trauma, as happens in steering wheel injuries. However, they are so nonspecific that much doubt has been shed on the utility of CK and CK-MB levels in ruling out myocardial contusion. These tests may be abandoned in favor of the high specificity of cTnI.[3,51,54,101] Noncardiac increases in CK-MB are seen with trauma, skeletal muscle disease, Reye's syndrome, hypothyroidism, labor, and the peripartum period.[42]

Since 1975, studies have attempted to quantify the rise in CK-MB with such factors as ejection fraction and infarct size. Dyskinesis and akinesis have been associated with a higher CK level than hypokinesis ($r = 0.68$, $P < 0.01$) in 21 patients studied by Hori and coworkers.[58] They also found that the ejection fraction in patients with anterior wall MI was lower than that in those with inferior wall MI with the same CK-MB values.[58] However, neither the ejection fraction values nor the clinical importance of the values was discussed.

Elevated CK-MB levels occur after PTCA and IV or intracoronary thrombolysis. Normally there is no elevation of CK-MB with PTCA unless the procedure is performed early in an evolving MI in an effort to limit the infarct size. Monitoring of CK-MB after elective PTCA, however, has been suggested as important in ruling out myocardial damage. After successful elective PTCA, an elevation of CK-MB of 2% to 21% was found in 20% of 128 patients studied by Oh and colleagues.[98] A mild myocardial necrosis was suspected in these patients. Length of hospital stay was twice that of patients without an elevated CK-MB. A high CK-MB is anticipated after fibrinolytic therapy, which takes place during the first few hours of symptoms suggestive of an acute MI. Early high CK-MB activity is considered to indicate successful reperfusion of the coronary artery. This "washout" of CK-MB, indicating revascularization, can be differentiated from the elevated CK-MB occurring after myocardial injury by its peak at approximately 12 to 14 hours after symptom onset[89] (Fig. 11-2).

Other clinical situations may lead to a rise in serum CK-MB and are associated with myocardial cell injury or selected necrosis. Creatine kinase may be elevated with heart failure (without MI) and is usually attributed to circulatory failure secondary to heart failure or myocardial injury. In the presence of coronary heart disease (CHD), tachyarrhythmias compromise diastolic filling time and may

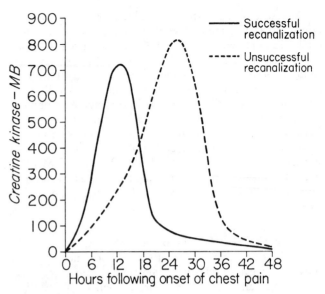

FIGURE 11-2 The pattern of total creatine kinase-MB (CK-MB) activity after successful emergency percutaneous transluminal coronary angioplasty (PTCA) or thrombolytic therapy (*solid line*) and unsuccessful PTCA or thrombolytic therapy (*dashed line*). Successful recanalization results in a "washout" of CK-MB (units/liter) at approximately 13 hours after onset of symptoms; an appearance of CK-MB at 22 to 30 hours indicates unsuccessful recanalization.[89] (From Goe MR: Creatine kinase enzyme determination: Implications for cardiovascular nursing. Prog Cardiovasc Nurs 2 [2]: 48, 1987.)

lead to focal cell injury. The CK-MB in this situation is abnormal. Arrhythmias without CHD do not lead to the release of CK-MB.[79,80]

Just as the ECG may show changes with brain injury, such as subdural hematoma, CK-MB levels may be elevated. Although the exact mechanism is not known, it is believed that a selected myocardial cell necrosis accompanies some head injuries. Subendocardial hemorrhage has been shown at autopsy of patients with CK-MB elevations after head injury.[67] Finally, the appearance of CK-MM and CK-MB after extreme hypothermia reflects severe skeletal and cardiac muscle damage.[80]

The patient in the critical care unit may have been admitted to rule out MI or for recovery after aortocoronary bypass surgery. In addition, patients admitted with other diagnoses, including primary cardiac arrest, metabolic disorders, trauma, or respiratory disorders, can be found in these units. Each of these patients is at risk for myocardial injury and presents a complex diagnostic picture if acute MI develops. Assay of CK-MB may be the only way to make a differential diagnosis.

Serum CK-MB greater than 5% of the total CK indicates myocardial injury. Some laboratories, however, continue to report isoenzyme results only in units per liter. In the interlaboratory survey performed by Boone and coworkers,[16] a wide range for normal levels of CK-MB was reported: 0 to 24 U/L. In this case, a CK-MB in excess of the reference value (independent of total CK elevation) would indicate an MI, a possible erroneous interpretation.

| TABLE 11-2 | Comparison of Sensitivity and Specificity of Various Tests for Myocardial Infarction* |

Test	Sensitivity (%)	Specificity (%)
Electrocardiogram	63–84	100
Aspartate aminotransferase increased	89–97	48–88
CK increased	93–100	57–88
CK-MB increased	94–100	93–100
LDH increased	87	88
LDH–1 > LDH–2 (on third day after chest pain)	61–90	94–99

CK, creatine kinase; LDH, lactate dehydrogenase.

*Range of values provided because different studies used various methods, periods after onset of symptoms, benchmarks for establishing the diagnosis, and so forth. Refers to levels in serum.
High sensitivity of CK-MB is combined with the high specificity of LDH isozymes by ordering both performed on same specimen where the diagnosis is uncertain.
From Wallach J: Interpretation of Diagnostic Tests: A Synopsis of Laboratory Medicine, 5th ed. Boston, Little, Brown, 1992.

| TABLE 11-3 | Noncardiac Disorders Resulting in Elevation of Creatine Kinase-MB and Lactate Dehydrogenase-1 |

Elevated Creatine Kinase-MB
Muscular dystrophies[38,79]
Hypothermia, hyperthermia[79,80]
Hypothyroidism[138]
Acute cholecystitis[138]
Duchenne's muscular dystrophy[38,79,80]
Alcohol overdose[79,80,138]
Delirium tremens[79]
Polymyositis[38,81]
Carcinomas (e.g., prostate, breast)[117]
Dermatomyositis[38,79]
Viral myositis[38]
Extreme exercise[81]
Peripartum period[138]
Severe skeletal muscle trauma (rhabdomyolysis due to crush injury or viral infection)[38,79,80,138]
Reye's syndrome[38,79,80,138]
Poisoning[80]

Elevated Lactate Dehydrogenase-1
Pulmonary embolism[80]
Acute renal infarction[38]
Hemolytic anemia[38,138]
Pernicious anemia[38,138]
Hemolysis associated with prosthetic heart valves[38]
Pregnancy[138]

The same survey determined that 66% of the laboratories reported a CK-MB fraction of 0% to 5% of the total CK as the upper limit of normal.[16] Comparison of total CK to CK-MB can be diagnostic, with a relative index greater than 2.5 highly suggestive of an acute MI.[99]

Although CK-MB is an accurate indicator of myocardial damage and is considered to be 96% to 99% sensitive for MI (Table 11-2), it is not 100% specific for MI.[80] CK-MB can also be found in other cardiac and noncardiac disorders (Table 11-3), which can usually be distinguished clinically from an MI and present no diagnostic problem.

Creatine Kinase Activity After Cardiac Surgery. Until recently, the enzymatic criteria for diagnosis of a perioperative MI during aortocoronary bypass surgery remained a problem because of the myocardial cellular injury produced during surgery.[38] Elevations in CK-MB have been associated with aortic cross-clamp time and duration of extracorporeal circulation.[133] At one time, it was thought that only a total CK level of 1200 U/L or greater could be diagnostic of perioperative infarct.[15] However, studies have revealed that a small peak of CK-MB, having a shorter peak time and a rapid disappearance, was present after aortocoronary bypass surgery, whereas a peak CK-MB occurred later and lasted longer after an acute MI.[34,45,70] A peak activity seen 4 to 7 hours after coronary artery bypass grafting reflects reversible myocardial ischemia, whereas a peak of more than 50 U/L occurring at 21 hours may indicate MI.[34] Because perioperative MI has an influence on surgical prognosis, it has been suggested that multiple determinants of CK-MB be performed beyond 48 hours after cardiac surgery to rule out the occurrence of perioperative MI. Mass concentration of CK-MB and determination of the CK-MB time–activity curve are also sensitive diagnostic aids.[50] With multiple determinations, the finding

of a delayed peak or reappearance of CK-MB would be indicative of myocardial cell necrosis, a meaningful event in terms of length of hospitalization, treatment decisions, and rehabilitation. Figure 11-3 illustrates the typical patterns after aortocoronary bypass surgery and an acute MI.

The techniques used during valve replacement and atriotomy cause a postoperative elevation of CK-MB that is greater than that in patients who have had a coronary bypass procedure.[40,61] This pattern of CK-MB activity led one group of investigators to suggest that the appearance of mean CK-MB levels of 93 to 103 U/L at 18 hours after aortic or mitral valve replacement precluded the diagnosis of perioperative MI (percentage of total CK was not discussed).[61] However, it has been suggested that the diagnosis of perioperative MI is possible if two determinations of CK-MB are made between 18 and 30 hours after surgery, by which time CK-MB activity from other tissues (skeletal muscle or atrial myocardium) has disappeared. Sensitivity and specificity for MI were said to approach 99% if the two CK-MB determinations taken between 18 and 30 hours were 5% or more of the total CK.[45] Autotransfusion of shed mediastinal blood may complicate the assessment of perioperative MI after cardiac surgery. Reinfusion of autotransfused blood after internal mammary artery dissection is associated with high levels of total CK (MB fraction is normal) and LDH. Care should be taken when interpreting serial enzyme results in such a situation.[96]

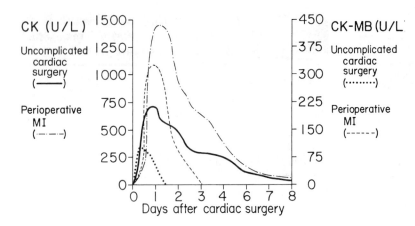

FIGURE 11-3 The pattern of total creatine kinase (CK) and creatine kinase-MB (CK-MB) activity after uncomplicated cardiac surgery (*dark lines*) and cardiac surgery with perioperative myocardial infarction (MI; *lighter lines*). After surgery, peak CK activity occurs at 22 hours and returns to normal after 5 days. The CK-MB activity appears approximately 4 hours after surgery and disappears within 48 hours. With an acute MI, CK-MB activity is considerably higher, occuring at approximately 21 to 24 hours after the onset of symptoms (the same time as total CK).[34,45,94] (From Goe MR: Creatine kinase enzyme determination: Implications for cardiovascular nursing. Prog Cardiovasc Nurs 2[2]: 47, 1987.)

It is clear that whenever the question of myocardial damage arises, the analysis of CK isoenzymes is of diagnostic value. Identification of the isoenzyme responsible for total CK elevation in complex clinical situations could eliminate or confirm cardiac disease as a consideration in further treatment.

Creatine Kinase-MB Mass Concentration. Analysis of CK isoenzyme types depends on assessing functional "activity." An alternate approach has been developed that directly measures the mass concentration of CK (in micrograms per liter). Techniques to measure mass concentration allow CK to be determined more quickly. Rapid determination is of value in the emergency room when treatment decisions are being made, when coronary patency is evaluated after thrombolysis,[24] after cardiac surgery when perioperative MI is evaluated,[50] and to select high-risk patients with unstable angina.[84] Collinson and coworkers[29] looked at 73 patients who had a diagnostic rise in CK; they measured CK-MB concentration and determined the slope in the rise of CK. They reported that 100% sensitivity and specificity for MI was shown within 4 hours of admission.[29,81] A bedside test of cardiac markers is being evaluated, using newer monoclonal immunoassay techniques.[17] These findings have cost and comfort implications for patients with an uncertain admission diagnosis.

Creatine Kinase Isoforms. Serum isoforms similar to CK-MM and CK-MB are part of the normal clearance process for CK and are present in all human sera. After release from injured myocardium, isoforms of CK-MM and CK-MB are converted in the circulation into three CK-MM isoforms and two CK-MB isoforms.[106] Studies have now shown that CK-MM isoform patterns provide a means of assessing the time of necrosis.[62] Similar results have been demonstrated for isoforms of CK-MB. Normally, MB-1 and MB-2 isoforms are found in a 1:1 ratio. However, when infarction occurs, the total CK-MB level may be normal, but a change in the ratio of MB-2 to MB-1 of 1.5 or greater is diagnostic of an MI.[106] These isoforms have appeared in sera early after MI (1 to 4 hours), while total CK and CK-MB are still within normal limits.[62] The significance of these findings is that isoforms have become potential early indicators of MI capable of facilitating rapid diagnosis and intervention.[6,63,113,150]

Laboratory Measurement of Creatine Kinase. Plasma CK sampling is among the most common laboratory assays. It is particularly useful in the cardiac care unit, where the presence of CK isoenzymes has many important and life-threatening implications. The determination of an accurate serum CK level depends on several variables in measurement and procedural techniques. Table 11-4 describes typical serum CK values found in patients with MI and in healthy people.

The collection of plasma for CK interpretation presents some problems in methodology. Dilution of the CK specimen with either distilled water or saline may lead to changes in enzyme kinetic activity (an indicator of enzyme concentration) when certain assay techniques are used.[57] The test requires 1 to 3 mL of blood. CK must be collected in a timely manner because the half-life of the isoenzyme in the body may be as short as 2 to 5 hours. Any delay in collection of blood for CK-BB activity should be particularly avoided. The CK-BB isoenzyme is unstable in blood already collected, and serum should be frozen as soon as possible

TABLE 11-4	**Reference Values for Creatine Kinase and Creatine Kinase-MB***		
Population	**Total CK (U/L)**	**CK-MB (U/L)**	**CK-MB (%)**
Ranges reported as normal	95–100	0–5	0–5
Healthy laboratory controls	42–123	0–1.4	0–2
Hospitalized patients	217–1140	0–8	0–1.1
Acute myocardial infarction patients	144–4125	6.8–336	4–19

CK, creatine kinase.

*U/L = international units per liter of blood

$$\% = \frac{CK - MB}{Total\ CK} \times 100$$

Results are usually reported in units per liter or percentage at either 30° C or 37° C.

Data from Boone DJ, Duncan PH, MacNeil ML et al: Results of a nationwide survey of analyses for creatine kinase and creatine kinase isoenzymes. Clin Chem 30: 33–37, 1984; and Varat MA, Mercer DW: Cardiac specific creatine phosphokinase isoenzyme in the diagnosis of acute myocardial infarction. Circulation 51: 855–859, 1975.

after the blood is drawn to minimize inactivation in the tube. Methods to reactivate this isoenzyme in serum may make this test less sensitive to time delay.[2,78] A baseline CK-MB, drawn during the first 4 hours after a suspected MI, may be of value in identifying atypical, chronically elevated CK (the immunoglobulin complex of CK-BB or CK of mitochondrial, rather than cytoplasmic, origin) when certain assay techniques are used.[87]

Serum or plasma should be separated from the erythrocytes immediately after clotting is completed. Assays for CK-MB or CK-BB require that the serum be frozen until assayed. Results are reported in units per liter. However, measurement of CK-MM is not sensitive to storage. Isoenzyme results are also described as a percentage of the total CK. The assay is performed at either 30° C (room temperature) or 37° C.[10] The assay temperature should be reported with the results.

Slight hemolysis can be tolerated for CK assay because red blood cells do not contain CK. However, specimens with a visible degree of hemolysis may contain adenylate kinase, which may falsely increase CK-MB results.[105] Assay mixtures for total CK used by many clinical laboratories now contain specific inhibitors of adenylate kinase, preventing falsely elevated total CK results.

Creatine kinase isoenzymes can be analyzed using several techniques, which accounts for the wide diversity in normal ranges (reference intervals) as well as diagnostic values. Immunoassay is simple, relatively speedy, and precise. Because of this, it is the most widely used technique for measuring CK. Electrophoresis is less sensitive and less accurate. Immunoinhibition is not widely used because false-positive results are relatively common.[32] The range of reference values for upper limits of normal for the CK isoenzymes is given in Table 11-5.

LACTATE DEHYDROGENASE

Lactate dehydrogenase is an enzyme that catalyzes the reversible conversion of lactate to pyruvate, providing ATP for energy during periods of anaerobic metabolism.[105,132] LDH is present in nearly all metabolizing cells and is released during tissue injury.[90] LDH is widely distributed in the body. It can be found in skeletal muscle, red blood cells, kidney, liver, pancreas, lungs, and brain.[38,99,105] Because of its presence in multiple organs throughout the body, evaluation of LDH is used to establish many diagnoses, including MI. Drugs that may cause an elevated LDH include clofibrate, codeine, meperidine, morphine, and procainamide.[90]

During the early stages of an MI, the myocardial cell, in the absence of oxygen, is unable to use its usual source of energy, free fatty acids. However, anaerobic metabolism of pyruvate to form lactate can take place without oxygen and can sustain the cell for several minutes after occlusion of the coronary artery. LDH facilitates this alternate energy pathway. Eventually, on cell death and subsequent lysis of the plasma membrane, the LDH is among the substances released into the serum. The serum LDH is thought to rise by two mechanisms: (1) the release of LDH from red blood cells in the infarction zone, and (2) the release of LDH from necrosing myocytes.[121]

Measurement of the total LDH is often used to confirm the diagnosis of acute MI established by CK-MB assay. LDH activity starts within 12 to 48 hours after the MI, reaches a peak between 48 and 72 hours, and returns to normal in approximately 7 to 14 days (Fig. 11-4). The prolonged time course of detection makes evaluation of MI possible when patients present late after the onset of symptoms. It has a predictive value ranging from 90% to 95% when used to diagnose MI.[90,129,132]

Lactate dehydrogenase is actually a group of isoenzymes with variable molecular forms.[38] These isoenzymes have different concentrations in different tissues and therefore may be identified by separation. It is the isoenzyme identification and the pattern of elevation that make confirmation of myocardial cell injury possible. This pattern has added value in that the abnormal elevation of one isoenzyme may not lead to elevation of the total LDH level; in this case, the identification of an elevated LDH isoenzyme may be the only evidence of myocardial cell injury.[105]

Lactate Dehydrogenase Isoenzymes. Five main fractions (isoenzymes) of LDH are assayed. LDH-1 is found in the heart, kidney, and red blood cells and is the fraction observed after MI. Post-MI, LDH-1 may remain elevated after total LDH returns to normal.[138] LDH-2 is the most plentiful of the isoenzymes and found mainly in the heart and kidney. LDH-1 and LDH-2 are known as the cardiac fractions. LDH-3, the pulmonary fraction, is prominent in the lungs, with lesser amounts found in the adrenal glands, spleen, pancreas, thyroid, and lymph nodes. LDH-4 and LDH-5 are the hepatic fractions. Both are also found in the skeletal muscle and kidneys. LDH-4 is also found in the brain.[67]

With such an array of forms, it becomes necessary to analyze the distribution pattern of LDH isoenzymes to diagnose MI. Electrophoretic analysis can show the relative contribution of all five isoenzymes. Figure 11-4 illustrates the normal pattern and the pattern demonstrated with acute MI. Normally, LDH-1 is less prevalent than LDH-2; the ratio of LDH-1 to LDH-2 is less than 1. In an acute MI, the ratio is reversed and greater than 1.[79] This finding

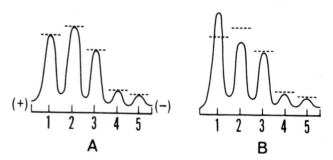

FIGURE 11-4 Lactate dephydrogenase (LDH) isoenzyme patterns. **(A)** Normal. **(B)** Fraction 1 increased with LDH-1 greater than LDH-2; "flipped" pattern of acute myocardial infarction. (Adapted and reproduced with permission from Ravel R: Clinical Laboratory Medicine. Clinical Application of Laboratory Data, 4th ed. Copyright © 1984 by Year Book Medical Publishers, Inc., Chicago.)

TABLE 11-5	Normal Reference Ranges for Laboratory Blood Tests

Blood Test	Reference Range	Blood Test	Reference Range
Hematologic Studies		**Blood Chemistries–(cont.)**	
Red blood cell count[130]		Base excess, deficit	0 ± 2.3 mEq/L[148]
Men	$4.6–6.2 \times 10^6$	SaO_2	98%[148]
Women	$4.2–5.4 \times 10^6$	$S\bar{v}CO_2$	75%[148]
Hematocrit[130]		Bilirubin	
Men	40%–50%	Total	0.2–1.3 mg/dL[148]
Women	38%–47%	Direct	0–20 mg/dL[148]
Hemoglobin[130]		Calcium	
Men	13.5–18.0 g/100 mL	Total	8.9–10.3 mg/dL[148]
Women	12.0–16.0 g/100 mL	Free (ionized)	4.6–5.1 mg/dL[148]
Corpuscle indices[130]		Creatinine[148]	
Mean corpuscular volume	82–98 fl	Men	0.9–1.4 mg/dL
Mean corpuscular hemoglobin	27–31 pg	Women	0.8–1.3 mg/dL
Mean corpuscular hemoglobin concentration	32%–36%	Glucose (fasting)	65–110 mg/dL[148]
		Magnesium	1.3–2.2 mEq/L[148]
White blood cell count[130]		Phosphorus	2.5–4.5 mg/dL[148]
Total	4,500–11,000/mm³	Phosphatase, alkaline	35–148 U[148]
Differential (in number of cells/mm³ blood)		Protein (total)	6.5–8.5 g/dL[148]
		Urea nitrogen	8–26 mg/dL[148]
Total leukocytes	5,000–10,000 (100%)	Uric acid[148]	65–110 mg/dL[148]
Total neutrophils	3,000–7,000 (60%–70%)	Men	4.0–8.5 mg/dL
Lymphocytes	1,500–3,000 (20%–30%)	Women	2.8–7.5 mg/dL
Monocytes	375–500 (2%–6%)	**Serum Enzymes***	
Eosinophils	50–400 (1%–4%)	CK-MM	95%–100%[16]
Basophils	0–50 (0.1%)	CK-MB	0%–5%[16]
Sedimentation rate	0–30 mm/hr[148]	CK-BB	0%[16]
Coagulation Studies*		LDH-1	Dependent on assay technique ratio
Platelet count	250,000–500,000/mm³ [132]	LDH-1: LDH-2 ratio	<1.0[80]
Prothrombin time	12–15 sec[130]	Aspartate aminotransferase	<50 U/L[38]
Partial thromboplastin time	60–70 sec[130]	**Myocardial Proteins**	
Activated partial thromboplastin time	35–45 sec[132]	Troponin-I[35]	0–2 ng/mL
		Troponin-T[35]	0–3.1 ng/mL
Activated clotting time	75–105 sec[132]	Myoglobin[35]	20–90 ng/mL
Fibrinogen level	160–300 mg/dL[132]	Men:	10–75 ng/mL
Thrombin time	11.3–18.5 sec[148]	Women:	
Blood Chemistries		**Cholesterol**	
Serum electrolytes[148]		Total blood cholesterol[95]	
Sodium	135–145 mEq/L	Desirable	<200 mg/dL
Potassium	3.3–4.9 mEq/L	Borderline high	200–239 mg/dL
Chloride	97–110 mEq/L	High	≥240 mg/dL
Carbon dioxide	22–31 mEq/L	LDL-cholesterol[95]	
Blood gases		Desirable	<130 mg/dL
pH	7.35–7.45[148]	Borderline high	130–159 mg/dL
PaO_2	80–105 mm Hg[148]	High	≥160 mg/dL
$PaCO_2$	35–45 mm Hg[148]	HDL-cholesterol	>35 mg/dL[109]
Bicarbonate	22–29 mEq/L[132]	Apolipoprotein A	120 mg/dL[112]
		Apolipoprotein B	134 mg/dL[95]

CK, creatine kinase; LDH, lactate dehydrogenase; LDL, low-density lipoprotein; HDL, high-density lipoprotein.
*Examples: regional laboratory techniques and methods may result in variations.

is known as a "flipped" LDH pattern (see Table 11-3). The flipped pattern usually occurs within 12 to 24 hours of acute MI, and by 48 hours has occurred in 80% of patients with MI.[99]

Lactate Dehydrogenase Activity After Cardiac Surgery.
A flipped LDH-1 to LDH-2 ratio is shown by 100% of patients with a perioperative MI. However, approximately 25% of surgical patients without MI also exhibit this pattern because of hemolysis from the extracorporeal circulation.[38] The analysis of α-hydroxybutyrate dehydrogenase (represents LDH-1 intermixed with small amounts of other isoenzymes) is thought by some to be more specific for myocardial damage. An enzyme found primarily in heart muscle, α-hydroxybutyrate dehydrogenase is similar to LDH-1 and rises 8 to 10 hours post-MI.[67] The activity of this enzyme subunit peaks later and at higher levels after an acute MI than after aortocoronary bypass surgery.[94] The finding of LDH-1 on days 2 to 4 after cardiac surgery appears to be a good discriminator of perioperative MI.[50] In addition, LDH isoenzyme analysis may be of help in evaluating postsurgical chest pain when the response to surgical intervention has started to normalize.

Laboratory Measurement of Lactate Dehydrogenase.
Lactate dehydrogenase isoenzymes are best analyzed by electrophoresis. The quality of the enzyme samples and the handling in the laboratory determines whether valid results are obtained. Because of the amount of LDH in red blood cells, hemolyzed specimens may not be used for analysis.[32,67,90] A minimum of 2 mL of blood is required for assay.[52] The serum can be stored at room temperature for up to 48 hours if it cannot be analyzed for LDH immediately. However, if LDH isoenzyme analysis is desired, the sample should be stored at 25° C and analyzed within 24 hours. The normal reference ranges for LDH isoenzyme activity are listed in Table 11-5.

ASPARTATE AMINOTRANSFERASE

Aspartate aminotransferase, formerly known as serum glutamic-oxaloacetic transaminase (SGOT or GOT), is located in the cell cytoplasm and in the mitochondria, where it catalyzes amino acid activity.[52] This enzyme, although not specific to myocardial tissue, was the first to be used extensively to confirm an MI.[73] The enzyme is widely distributed, with high concentrations in the liver, skeletal muscle, kidney, red blood cells, and myocardium.[52] It is found in lesser amounts in the lungs, pancreas, and brain.[68,90,132] The presence of AST in so many organ systems reduces its specificity for MI.[81] Therefore, it is used in concert with CK and LDH. AST usually is evaluated to rule out MI or to diagnose and monitor hepatocellular diseases.

After an acute MI, AST rises sharply within the first 8 to 12 hours, peaks in 24 to 48 hours, and returns to normal by the fifth or sixth day[68,90] (see Fig. 11-2). AST levels are said to relate roughly to the extent of the MI and are elevated in 90% to 95% of patients with acute MI.[90,105] However, because it is found in quantity in other tissues, care must be taken in interpretation of AST levels. If there is only cardiac injury, the AST usually is not over

500 U/L. Levels over 1,000 U/L in patients with heart failure are probably due to concomitant hepatic congestion or necrosis.[132]

Aspartate aminotransferase is also elevated with cardiac surgery, cardiac catheterization and angioplasty,[99] severe angina, acute pulmonary embolus,[68] renal infarction,[23] acute pancreatitis, musculoskeletal diseases, trauma, and strenuous exercise. Drugs that may increase AST levels include antihypertensives, coumarin, digitalis preparations, salicylates, verapamil,[68,99] and theophylline.[90] False elevations are seen in pyridoxine deficiency (beriberi, pregnancy), uremia, or diabetic ketoacidosis. Levels are slightly increased in the elderly.[67] In chronic conditions, such as severe, longstanding liver disease, the elevation is usually persistent.[99]

Laboratory Measurement of Aspartate Aminotransferase.
The analysis of AST requires a minimum of 1 mL of blood. Because AST is found in red blood cells, hemolyzed specimens should not be used to test AST. The assay is performed spectrophotometrically.[52] The specimen may be stored after collection if immediate analysis is not possible. The reference range for normal AST is listed in Table 11-5.

HEMATOLOGIC STUDIES

Cells in the circulating blood are responsible for oxygen and carbon dioxide transport and the body's immune response. Erythrocytes (red blood cells), leukocytes (white blood cells [WBCs]), and platelets are formed in the bone marrow and are suspended in the plasma (see Chapter 5). Blood is also the transport system for electrolytes, products of metabolism, hormones, and plasma proteins. The blood volume in a normal adult is approximately 8% of the body weight.[40] An appreciation of the roles of erythrocytes, leukocytes, and other hematologic parameters is an important prerequisite to understanding deviations from normal. This approach is helpful in planning care based on an assessment of the demands of daily living. Each of the aspects of a hematologic study has meaning for patients in terms of their ability to withstand the effects of a cardiac event.

Complete Blood Cell Count

A complete blood cell count (CBC) is important for evaluating the oxygen-carrying capacity of the blood and the response of the body to invasion by foreign cells such as bacteria. Excessive bleeding, bone marrow disease, hemolytic disorders, some drugs, and infections can alter the number of leukocytes, erythrocytes, or platelets in the blood. Because of this, the CBC of the patient with cardiac disease is closely monitored. A baseline study can be compared with subsequent studies to evaluate bleeding, the effects of treatment, or the presence of infection (see Table 11-5).

RED BLOOD CELL COUNT

Red blood cells (RBCs; erythrocytes) are formed in the bone marrow and constitute the majority of peripheral cells. They contain Hgb and are responsible for transporting oxygen to the tissues (and carbon dioxide from tissues).

The average life span of an RBC is 120 days, after which it is removed from the blood by the liver, spleen, or bone marrow.

When the RBC count is more than 10% below the expected normal value, the patient is said to be anemic. Conditions under which there are a decreased number of RBCs include cirrhosis, hemorrhage, presence of prosthetic valves, renal disease, chronic illnesses, and various malignancies of the bone marrow.[23,99] Anemia from any cause must be looked for in the patient with cardiac disease because it may precipitate angina, aggravate heart failure, or contribute to a diagnosis of subacute bacterial endocarditis.[130] An Hgb reduced to 5 g/dL manifests clinically as cyanosis.

An RBC increase is seen in congenital heart disease, severe chronic obstructive pulmonary disease, and polycythemia vera. It is falsely high in extracellular fluid deficit (volume contraction) and falsely low with extracellular fluid excess.[99] The production of RBCs is inhibited by a rise in circulating RBC levels and stimulated by anemia and hypoxemia. The RBC count represents the number of RBCs in 1 μL of whole blood.

HEMATOCRIT

The Hct is the volume of packed RBCs found in 100 mL of blood. As an indirect measure of the RBC count, Hct increases and decreases with the RBC count. Normal ranges for Hct differ by sex and age group.[99] Physical training is known to decrease the Hct level. Findings suggests that physical training may be of value in lowering blood viscosity in patients post-MI.[126]

HEMOGLOBIN

The RBCs contain a complex protein compound called *hemoglobin*. Hgb is the oxygen-carrying protein of the RBC and is an important component of the acid-base buffer system. Insufficient amounts of Hgb place a strain on the cardiovascular system, and may cause MI, angina, congestive heart failure (CHF) or stroke. There is a diurnal variation in Hgb, which varies by as much as 1 g/dL between its peak at 8 AM and its nadir at 8 PM.[99]

CORPUSCULAR INDICES

With the RBC count, the quantity of Hgb, and the Hct, the characteristics of individual RBCs can be described in terms of cell size (mean corpuscular volume [MCV]), amount of Hgb present in a single cell (mean corpuscular Hgb [MCH]), and the proportion of each cell occupied by Hgb (mean corpuscular Hgb concentration [MCHC]). The indices are calculated by these formulas:[144]

$$MCV = \frac{Hematocrit\ (as\ \%) \times 10}{RBC\ count\ (millions\ per\ mm^3)}$$

$$MCH = \frac{Hemoglobin\ (as\ g/100\ mL) \times 10}{RBC\ count}$$

$$MCHC = \frac{Hemoglobin}{Hematocrit}$$

WHITE BLOOD CELL COUNT

The WBCs, or leukocytes, work to defend against foreign matter and cells in the body. There are five types of WBCs: neutrophils, eosinophils, basophils, monocytes, and lymphocytes. Neutrophils, the most numerous circulating WBCs, are responsible for phagocytosis and are stimulated by acute bacterial infections or trauma. When their production is significantly increased, immature forms (bands or stab cells) are released in the blood. Eosinophils are able to phagocytize antigen—antibody complexes and are increased during allergic and parasitic conditions. Basophils (mast cells) are increased during the healing phase of infection or inflammation. Monocytes are capable of fighting bacteria in a way similar to neutrophils, as well as removing debris and microorganisms from the blood. Lymphocytes play a role in chronic or viral infections. T lymphocytes, which mature in the thymus, are responsible for cellular-type immune reactions. B lymphocytes, which mature in the bone marrow, play a major role in humoral immunity (antibody production).[67,68,99]

Elevated WBC counts in the patient with cardiac disease may be due to MI, bacterial endocarditis, or Dressler's syndrome. After MI, the elevation may be a result of the body's normal response to stress. On approximately the fourth day after an acute MI, WBCs may be elevated. Leukocytosis occurs as the infarcted site is invaded by leukocytes and macrophages that engulf and phagocytose necrotic tissue.

Although an elevated temperature after MI may be expected, an elevated WBC count should always suggest the possibility of concomitant infection. A urinary or respiratory tract infection or an infection secondary to an invasive procedure is a possibility during an extended illness. In this case, the presence of band cells (immature neutrophils), coupled with leukocytosis, suggests the bone marrow is putting out more cells in response to stress or infection. An elevated WBC count has also been associated with CHD. WBC counts were obtained from participants in the Framingham, Massachusetts, offspring study. An increase in WBC count in men was related to the development of cardiovascular disease.[65]

Drugs that may cause an increase in WBCs include aspirin, procainamide, allopurinol, heparin, digoxin, and epinephrine. WBCs have a diurnal variation, with counts generally lower in the morning than in the afternoon.[67]

WHITE CELL DIFFERENTIAL

The differential count is a descriptive list of the types of WBCs. The differential for each of the five leukocyte types is usually expressed as a percentage of the total leukocyte count; the total should add up to 100 (see Table 11-5).

CELL MORPHOLOGY

Occasionally, a CBC includes a description of any abnormal cell types. Immature RBCs (reticulocytes) may be noted. The presence of these cells is a clue that there may be increased demands on RBC production or that cell function may be impaired. Normoblasts appear in blood after severe stress, such as massive hemorrhage or hemolysis, or cardiac arrest. Megaloblasts can be seen in a severe vitamin B_{12} or folate deficiency. Fragmented RBCs may suggest disseminated intravascular coagulopathy (DIC)[1] and are also seen in people with prosthetic valves. Microcytes may indicate a nutritional iron-deficiency anemia. Target cells are seen in liver disease. The appearance of nucleated RBCs and immature WBCs (myelocytes) may indicate severely depressed bone marrow activity, requiring measures to protect the patient from infection. If the neutrophil count is less than 1,000 cells/mm[3], there is a slight risk of infection; if the count is less than 500 cells/mm[3], infection is frequent.[35]

ERYTHROCYTE SEDIMENTATION RATE

The erythrocyte sedimentation rate (ESR) measures the speed at which anticoagulated erythrocytes settle in a long, narrow tube. The speed depends on the size of the clumps into which the cells aggregate in the presence of blood fibrinogen. The ESR is a nonspecific indicator of inflammatory disease. It may be elevated in MI and bacterial endocarditis; it is usually low in CHF.[67,90] Although many factors affect the ESR and it is considered a test with neither disease nor organ specificity, it is a useful test in differentiating the pain of pericarditis and Dressler's syndrome from anginal pain. The degree of increase of the ESR does not correlate with severity or prognosis.[138]

BLOOD CULTURES

Blood cultures are indicated when a fever of unknown origin is present. Blood cultures identify pathogenic organisms in the blood (bacteremia). The blood is drawn and placed into specialized culture media. Policies differ with regard to the number and timing of cultures considered adequate for diagnosis; the policy and procedure of the institution should be followed. Regardless of the number of cultures recommended and the timing between them, collection of blood cultures requires meticulous technique to protect the specimen from contamination. Sampling should be done while the temperature is still elevated and before treatment with antibiotics. The blood samples are cultured in the laboratory at 37° C. Preliminary results should be available within 24 hours, but final results may not be available for a week or more.

COMPLETE BLOOD COUNT AFTER CARDIAC SURGERY

The Hgb and Hct levels are monitored after cardiac surgery to evaluate blood loss. Immediately after cardiac surgery, there are rapid shifts in extracellular fluid volume status because of the hemodilutional effects of cardiopulmonary bypass and the rewarming that follows induced hypothermia. This fluid shift may be reflected in a reduced Hgb or Hct level. Frequent monitoring of the WBC count helps identify any leukocytosis and infection. Cardiopulmonary bypass results in a period of reduced phagocytic activity that renders the patient more at risk for infection.[116]

LABORATORY MEASUREMENT OF COMPLETE BLOOD CELL VALUES

The RBC and WBC counts are done by an automated counter that directly measures all parameters, including Hct, corpuscular indices, and platelets. The precision of the Hct analysis is ±2 points. Consequently, a change in measurement by as much as 4 points may not indicate a change in the true Hct.

Activity and change in position may raise Hct and Hgb levels; Hgb may be higher by 8% in the morning than in the evening.[31] A minimum of 2 mL of blood is required for assay. The usual precautions should be taken to avoid hemolysis and ensure accuracy. The specimen should be rapidly transported to the laboratory to avoid changes in distribution of the cells within the plasma. Red blood cell tests can be done using capillary blood, but massage of the fingertip or earlobe can lead to cell destruction and alter the sample. If difficulty is encountered in locating a vein, the tourniquet should be removed long enough to allow restoration of circulation to avoid a hemoconcentrated sample.[132] In one study, application of a tourniquet for 3 minutes led to a rise of 3.9 points in Hct; hemolysis was avoided when the tourniquet was applied for less than 1 minute.[86] A blood smear should also be examined if there is an abnormality in one or more of the CBC parameters (to evaluate the size, shape, and color of the RBCs, WBCs, and platelets).

Coagulation Studies

Drug-induced anticoagulation is a routine procedure in the cardiac care unit and requires close monitoring of blood coagulation mechanisms. Anticoagulation is used after thrombolytic therapy, during cardiac surgery, to prevent formation of venous thrombus associated with prolonged bed rest and hemostasis, to prevent formation of intracardiac thrombus, and in treatment for established thrombus and embolus (see Chapter 5 for a discussion of coagulation).

The prevention and treatment of blood coagulation are complex and involve a number of hemostatic functions that play roles in the body's homeostasis. Therapy involves interference with this homeostatic mechanism. An understanding of the laboratory tests used to evaluate the effectiveness of treatment is vital to prevent undesired outcomes of anticoagulation therapy. The normal ranges for the coagulation factors and the methods used depend on the laboratory. Typical reference ranges, however, are listed in Table 11-5.

PLATELET COUNT

Platelets are elements of the blood that promote coagulation and are produced by the bone marrow. They contribute to blood clotting by clumping or sticking to rough surfaces and injured sites.[67] The average life span of a platelet is 7 to 9 days.

Platelet counts are useful for monitoring the course of a disease or treatment. Thrombocytopenia (low platelet count) is a common cause of abnormal bleeding.[1] There is a serious risk of hemorrhage when the platelet count is less than 50,000/mm,[3] and a spontaneous bleed may occur when platelets are less than 20,000/mm.[3] Bleeding due to thrombocytopenia is characterized by petechiae, bleeding from the gums or tongue, or epistaxis.[142]

Thrombocytopenia may occur by several mechanisms: reduced platelet production, sequestration of platelets, accelerated platelet destruction, loss from hemorrhage, and dilution from massive blood transfusions that contain few platelets.

Specific conditions that cause a decrease in platelets include hemorrhage, hypersplenism, leukemia, prosthetic heart valves, DIC, lupus, hemolytic anemia, and infection. Medications that decrease the platelet count include acetaminophen, aspirin, chemotherapy, histamine blocking agents, hydralazine, indomethacin, quinidine, and thiazide diuretics.[99] The concurrent use of heparin with antiplatelet agents increases the risk of bleeding. After a large number of blood transfusions (14 units or more), and occasionally after extracorporeal circulation, the platelet count is low.[86]

Increased amounts may be seen in malignant disorders, polycythemia vera, postsplenectomy syndrome, and rheumatoid arthritis.[99] Platelet counts may also be increased in those who live at high altitude, or in strenuous exercise. Other situations may give rise to thrombocytopenia, including idiopathic thrombocytopenic purpura, systemic lupus erythematosus, chronic lymphocytic leukemia, and lymphoma.[1] Platelets are activated by thrombolytic agents.[36] Aspirin has been incorporated into the treatment plan after MI to prevent hypercoagulability due to platelet aggregation.

PROTHROMBIN TIME

The PT is used to evaluate the extrinsic system and common pathway in the clotting mechanism. Specifically, it measures the activity of prothrombin, fibrinogen, and factors V, VII, and X. Prothrombin is synthesized by the liver. PT may be prolonged in heart failure, vitamin K deficiency, liver disease, bile duct obstruction, coumarin ingestion, DIC, massive blood transfusion, salicylate intoxication, and alcohol use.[67,68,99] Severe liver damage may prolong PT. Drugs that may prolong PT include some antibiotics, allopurinol, cimetidine, warfarin, heparin, quinidine, and aspirin.[67]

Decreased PT is seen in thrombophlebitis, MI, and pulmonary embolus. Medications that may decrease PT include digitalis preparations, diuretics, diphenhydramine, and metaproterenol.[67]

The PT is used mainly for monitoring patients on warfarin (Coumadin). Warfarin inhibits vitamin K-dependent synthesis of clotting factors II, VII, IX, and X. Therapeutic PTs are considered to be 1.5 to 2 times normal, or a 15% to 50% change in the normal value. If the PT is allowed to prolong greater than 2.5 times the control value, there is a risk of bleeding.[68] The World Health Organization has recommended the use of an international standardized ratio (INR) for reporting PTs. With the INR, standardized PT results are available for physicians in different parts of the country and the world. These standardized results are independent of the reagents used and adjust for the type of instrument used. The therapeutic INR in most situations ranges from 2.0 to 3.5. However, different ranges have been established for deep vein thrombosis prophylaxis (1.5 to 2.0), deep vein thrombosis (2.0 to 3.0), prevention of embolus in atrial fibrillation (2.0 to 3.0), pulmonary embolism (3.0 to 4.0), and prosthetic valve prophylaxis (2.5 to 3.5). The INR should not be used to initiate warfarin therapy; it should be used only once the patient is thought to be on a stable dose.[67,99,115]

PARTIAL THROMBOPLASTIN TIME AND ACTIVATED PARTIAL THROMBOPLASTIN TIME

The PTT and aPTT measure the intrinsic coagulation system and are used in assessing patients receiving unfractionated heparin. With the newer low–molecular-weight heparin, neither PTT nor aPTT changes, so laboratory monitoring is not required.[59,134] The PTT measures deficiencies in all factors except factors VII and XIII, whereas the aPTT measures all coagulation factors except platelet factor III, factor XIII, and factor VII.[1] The aPTT is measured by adding test reagents to PTT to shorten clotting time. When clotting time is shortened, minor clotting defects can be detected.[67,99]

The therapeutic range for both PTT and aPTT is maintained at 1.5 to 2.5 times the patient's baseline value. The aPTT is usually drawn 30 to 60 minutes before the patient's next dose of heparin. For results less than 50 seconds, an increase in the heparin dose should be considered. Conversely, a decrease in dose should be considered for values greater than 100 seconds.[99]

The PTT and aPTT are prolonged in heparin administration, congenital clotting factor deficiencies, cirrhosis of the liver, vitamin K deficiency, and DIC. Antihistamines, ascorbic acid, chlorpromazine, and salicylates may also cause an increase.

ACTIVATED CLOTTING TIME

The activated clotting time (ACT) is used during cardiac surgery to monitor heparinization. The time it takes whole blood to clot reflects the activity of the intrinsic clotting mechanism.[132] During extracorporeal heparin therapy, the ACT is kept at four to six times the baseline value.

Tests to measure ACT are simple and easy to use at the bedside. The use of ACT rather than aPTT to monitor heparin therapy in patients with unstable angina or acute MI may result in much steadier levels of anticoagulation and prevent ischemic recurrences.[92]

FIBRINOGEN LEVEL

Fibrinogen is a plasma protein synthesized by the liver.[68] This test measures the conversion of fibrinogen to fibrin by thrombin.[132] Fibrinogen levels are elevated in acute infections, collagen disease, inflammatory diseases, and hepatitis. Decreased levels are seen in severe liver disease, DIC, leukemia, and obstetric complications. Thrombolytic therapy may also affect fibrinogen levels. Intracoronary and IV streptokinase therapies lower fibrinogen levels to below 100 mg/dL. Urokinase therapy, however, minimally decreases fibrinogen, whereas tissue plasminogen activator therapy does not reduce fibrinogen.[117] Low fibrinogen levels (<100 mg/dL) may occur as a result of cardiac surgery, DIC, or other fibrinolytic disorders.[1] The most common use of the test is in differentiating these clinical conditions from liver disease, in which the fibrinogen level is rarely less than 100 mg/dL.

THROMBIN TIME

The time required for a thrombin solution to clot plasma is measured with the thrombin time.[1] Thrombin is the factor that directly converts fibrinogen to fibrin, and the formation of thrombin is the common pathway for both the intrinsic and extrinsic coagulation systems. The thrombin time moderates the thrombin–fibrinogen reaction and adequate formation of a fibrin clot.[132] Thrombin time is elevated by liver disorders, systemic lupus erythematosus, uremia, and DIC. The thrombin time may be used after fibrinolytic enzyme therapy (streptokinase) to assess the extent of hypofibrinogenemia. The thrombin time is prolonged after streptokinase therapy if antibody has not combined with the streptokinase antigen. In the rare event that thrombin time is not elevated after streptokinase infusion, the patient is presumed to have a large amount of streptococcal antibody, which renders streptokinase therapy ineffective. The thrombin time is prolonged with the use of urokinase and heparin and is too sensitive to heparin to monitor heparin therapy. Heparin contamination of specimens is common. The PTT, PT, and thrombin time should be measured concurrently because the thrombin time is too nonspecific to be used alone to assess antico-agulation therapy.

COAGULATION STUDIES AFTER CARDIAC SURGERY

The nature of cardiac surgery calls for close attention to coagulation factors. Prolonged cardiopulmonary bypass, heparinization during surgery, and coagulopathies can contribute to bleeding after surgery. Tests commonly followed immediately after surgery are ACT, platelet count, fibrinogen level, PT, and PTT.[85] After valve replacement or revascularization, heparin therapy, oral anticoagulant therapy, and antiplatelet agents (low-dose salicylates and dipyridamole) are commonly administered. Heparin is given either through infusion or subcutaneously during the early postoperative period; the PTT is considered the best index of unfractionated heparin activity. A risk for bleeding accompanies long-term anticoagulation therapy, and the PT is monitored for patients receiving warfarin during and after hospital discharge.[146]

LABORATORY MEASUREMENT OF COAGULATION STUDIES

Blood specimens for coagulation studies should be placed in collection tubes prepared specifically for this purpose. The laboratory should be contacted for specifics such as type of collection tube and amount of blood required. For most studies, an exact amount of blood is required: exactly 1 mL for ACT, and 4.5 mL for thrombin, PT, and PTT. Care must be taken after the specimen is withdrawn to prevent bleeding from a venipuncture site; pressure should be maintained over the site for a minimum of 3 to 5 minutes.[19] Rapid transportation of the specimen to the laboratory is essential because analysis should be done immediately.

A number of factors may contribute to the variability of coagulation studies. The timing of the determination of the test is critical, and the maximum effect of the anticoagulant must be considered. Results of coagulation studies require careful assessment because they are influenced by diet, med-ications (including over-the-counter medications), alcohol consumption, and physical activity. Circadian variations in the response of the coagulation may influence therapeutic response to anticoagulants.[13] Other, unknown factors affect laboratory coagulation studies. Consequently, dose adjustments of anticoagulants should be followed by repeated testing.

Nursing Considerations After Hematologic Studies

Abnormal bleeding, anemias, the inflammatory response, and infection indicate several nursing diagnoses, including decreased cardiac output, fluid volume deficit, altered tissue perfusion, and impaired tissue integrity. The cardiac nurse should be aware of any actual or potential problems related to hematologic abnormalities. Knowledge of normal values, as well as those factors that alter function of the cells or homeostatic mechanisms, is required for recognition of deviations from normal. Attention to the results is important; communication to the physician, if necessary, should be based on an understanding of the ramifications of an altered value. Intervention should be based on a physiologic conceptualization of the mechanisms involved in altered hematologic values. Attention to the hematologic values alone, however, should never become the focus of nursing intervention. The ability of the patient to tolerate the condition should be assessed from a daily living status that incorporates resources as well as the demands of the illness.[22]

ARTERIAL BLOOD GASES

Arterial blood gases are frequently assessed in the patient with cardiac disease. Tissue oxygenation, carbon dioxide removal, and acid–base status are analyzed through the assay of arterial blood gases. Arterial blood gas results guide treatment decisions in ventilated patients and critically ill, nonventilated patients. They are also drawn to establish a preoperative baseline.[99] Complete discussions of these parameters can be found in Chapter 7. A knowledge of the normal blood gas values and the meaning of deviation from normal is essential to treatment decisions.

The arterial oxygen saturation (SaO_2) and the mixed venous saturation ($S\bar{v}O_2$) reflect the relationship between oxygen supply and demand and the extent of overall tissue utilization of O_2. Continuous monitoring of SaO_2 (oxygen supply) can be achieved through pulse oximetry; laboratory analysis, however, is useful in distinguishing the SaO_2 at PaO_2 levels above 65 mm Hg.[82] A fiberoptic pulmonary artery catheter is capable of evaluating $S\bar{v}O_2$ levels continuously. This information is useful in determining the ideal mode of respiratory intervention, the effect of nursing care on tissue O_2 demands, physiologic alterations requiring increased supply of O_2, and the reflection of physiologic changes on cardiac output.[143] Calibration of the $S\bar{v}O_2$ catheter oximeter should be performed every 24 hours by laboratory O_2 saturation analysis. Table 11-5 provides normal values for SaO_2 and $S\bar{v}O_2$.

BLOOD CHEMISTRIES

The body's homeostatic mechanisms are responsible for a stable internal environment. The chemical regulation of cellular and plasma metabolites is among the most precise mechanisms in the body. During periods of critical illness, these mechanisms may be inadequate or dramatically altered. The functional alterations that result from altered values are sometimes life threatening. An awareness of the factors affecting blood chemistry homeostasis, as well as the consequences of elevated or decreased levels, aids the nurse in making appropriate patient care decisions.

Some blood chemistry tests are drawn routinely on admission to the hospital to establish the patient's baseline. Other tests are performed frequently over a day and may indicate the need for intervention in the form of altered therapy and treatment modalities. "Normal" or reference values may differ between laboratories or among populations. Typical reference ranges for selected blood chemistry values can be found in Table 11-5.

Serum Electrolytes

SODIUM

Sodium is the major cation in the extracellular space. It has several major functions: maintenance of osmotic pressure, regulation of acid–base balance (by combining with chloride or bicarbonate ions), and transmission of nerve impulses by the sodium pump.[23,99,132] Sodium balance is regulated by aldosterone, atrial natriuretic hormone, and antidiuretic hormone (ADH). Aldosterone causes sodium conservation (and water retention) by stimulating the kidneys to reabsorb sodium. It is secreted in response to low extracellular sodium levels, an increase in intracellular potassium, low blood volume or cardiac output, and physical or emotional stress.[90,99] When serum sodium levels are too high, atrial natriuretic hormone is secreted from the atrium and acts as an antagonist to renin and aldosterone.[67] ADH, secreted by the posterior pituitary gland, controls serum sodium by regulation of the amount of intracellular fluid reabsorbed at the distal tubules.[90,99]

POTASSIUM

Potassium is the major intracellular cation, in concentrations of approximately 150 mEq/L. It is regulated in a very tight range in the extracellular fluid. Potassium plays a crucial role in initiating and sustaining cardiac and skeletal muscle contraction. It is also important for acid–base balance and maintenance of oncotic pressure.

Maintenance of potassium within the normal range is crucial in the care of a patient with cardiac disease. Failure to do so results in dangerous sequelae for the patient. In general, potassium levels in patients with cardiac disease are maintained above 4.0 mEq/L. Special care should be taken in patients with cardiac disease receiving potassium-sparing diuretics or angiotensin-converting enzyme inhibitors, especially in light of decreased renal blood flow. Potassium levels are falsely elevated by analysis of hemolyzed specimens. Prolonged use of a tourniquet, having the patient clench and unclench a fist before blood draw, or delayed processing of the specimen all may cause hemolysis.[109,138]

CHLORIDE

Chloride is the major extracellular anion. It helps to maintain electrical neutrality and acts as an acid–base buffer. The rise and fall of chloride levels follows sodium and bicarbonate shifts. When carbon dioxide increases, chloride shifts to the intracellular space as bicarbonate goes extracellular. Along with sodium, chloride also helps to maintain osmotic pressure. Found primarily in hydrochloric acid in stomach secretions, chloride also provides the acid medium for digestion and enzyme activation.[67,90,99]

CALCIUM

Calcium is found mainly in the bones and teeth, with only approximately 10% found in the blood.[90] Calcium is essential for the formation of bones and for blood coagulation. Calcium ions affect neuromuscular excitability and cellular and capillary permeability.[144] It is essential for nerve transmission and cardiac and skeletal muscle contraction. Calcium also contributes to anion–cation balance. Calcium can be found ionized (free) in the serum or bound to serum albumin. The ionized calcium, which is approximately one-half of the total calcium, is the fraction important to cardiac and neuromuscular excitability.[99] In acidosis, more calcium appears in the ionized form; in alkalotic environments, most of the calcium remains protein bound.[67]

Calcium levels in the blood follow a diurnal variation, with the lowest values occurring in the early morning, and highest values occurring at mid-evening.[23] Ionized calcium is difficult to measure, so total calcium is reported in most hospitals. In some situations, the measured calcium level may be low, but by estimating the amount bound to protein, the ionized calcium may be found to be normal. The formula for the computation of ionized calcium is shown in Table 11-6. Decreased serum sodium (<120 mEq/L) increases protein-bound calcium and consequently increases the total calcium; the opposite is true of increased serum sodium.[138]

MAGNESIUM

Magnesium is essential in many enzymatic activities involving lipid, carbohydrate, and protein metabolism. It is predominantly an intracellular ion. Most of the body's magnesium is stored in the bones in an insoluble state; one-third is bound to protein, and approximately 1% is found in the serum. Because of its importance in phosphorylation of ATP, magnesium is seen as a critical component of almost all metabolic processes.[99] Its importance in the care of patients with cardiac disease stems from its role in neuromuscular regulation. Low levels of magnesium precipitate cardiac arrhythmias because of increased cardiac irritability. Hypermagnesemia results in depressed neuromuscular conduction, and consequent slowing of conduction in the heart. Ventricular arrhythmias after MI have been associated with magnesium deficiency. A 24-hour magnesium infusion has been recommended for patients suspected of having

TABLE 11-6	Computation Formulas

Computation of Ionized Calcium

Serum calcium can be presumed to be normal if:

(4.5 − albumin level) × (0.8) + lab value for total calcium = 8.8 to 11.0 mEq/L

1. Obtain total calcium level (normal = 8.8–10.5 mEq/L). If it is less than normal (e.g., <8.8 mEq/L), follow the steps below.
2. Obtain serum albumin level (normal = 4.5 g/dL).
3. If serum albumin level is decreased, subtract the decreased level from normal value for albumin (e.g., albumin level is measured at 3.0; 4.5 [normal] − 3.0 [measured] = 1.5).
4. For every 1.0 decrease in albumin, add 0.8 to calcium level (e.g., for above example, 1.5 × 0.8 = 1.2).
5. Add the calculated figure to the total calcium level (e.g., 7.8 + 1.2 = 9 mEq/L, calcium is within normal range).
6. One-half of this level (9/2) is 4.5, within the normal range for ionized calcium (normal ionized calcium = 4.5–5.0).

Computation of Anion Gap

Anion gap = [sodium (140) + potassium (4.0)] − bicarbonate (24) + chloride (110)] = 10 − 12 mEq/L

Computation of Serum Osmolality

Two times the serum sodium + serum glucose (Glu) divided by 18 + blood urea nitrogen (BUN) divided by 1.8 = serum osmolality ([2 × Sodium] + [Glucose/18] + [BUN/1.8]) = 280 − 300, mOsm/kg

(e.g., 2 × 122 + 198/2 + 18/1.8 = 265 mOsm (water or intracellular fluid excess); 2 × 155 + 108/2 + 5.4/1.8 = 318 mOsm [water or intracellular fluid deficit])

MI.[5,149] Magnesium levels should be monitored carefully in patients on digitalis preparations. Low magnesium levels are known to enhance the effect of digitalis, leading to toxicity.[67,68,90,99,129]

CARBON DIOXIDE

Measurement of carbon dioxide assists the clinician in evaluation of electrolyte status and acid–base balance. Because approximately 80% of carbon dioxide is found as bicarbonate, it is a good reflection of the bicarbonate level. The carbon dioxide level should not be confused with the PCO_2 obtained from blood gas readings.

ANION GAP

The anion gap measures the normal balance between positive and negative electrolytes in the serum. It describes the relationship between serum sodium (a cation) and bicarbonate and chloride (anions). A normal anion gap is 12 mEq/L. A value greater than this is considered abnormal. This test is useful in determining whether an acid–base imbalance is due to an increase in organic acid (increased lactic acid or ketoacids, or ingestion of acid such as salicylic acid). In this case, the anion gap increases. With mineral acid problems (decreased bicarbonate or increased hydrochloric acid), the anion gap is normal. A formula for computation of the anion gap is given in Table 11-6.

SERUM OSMOLALITY

Serum osmolality reflects the osmotic property of the blood. It is an important parameter in determining whether water excess or deficit exists. Either of these problems can present in the cardiac care unit, where fluid management is often a problem. The most dramatic alterations in osmolality can be seen with inappropriate ADH secretion or failure of ADH secretion in conditions characterized by low blood volume (see Chapter 6). Normal serum osmolality is 280 to 300 mOsm/kg. The osmolality can be measured in the laboratory or calculated with a simple formula (see Table 11-6).

SERUM ELECTROLYTES AFTER CARDIAC SURGERY

Fluid volume shifts and changes in electrolytes and serum osmolality are common after cardiac surgery. The examination of serum electrolytes at least every 3 to 4 hours during the first 24 hours after surgery has been recommended. Changes in potassium may be rapid; sodium may be increased; total calcium may be decreased; and total circulating volume may be increased. The hemodilutional effects of cardiopulmonary bypass are responsible for these changes as well as changes in renal function that, in turn, may affect fluid volume and electrolyte status.[85] During and after cardiac surgery, changes in plasma potassium concentration may develop.[76,114] There appears to be a decrease in potassium during hypothermia and an increase during rewarming, which has been attributed to washout of ischemic areas or to a direct effect of temperature on the transmembrane distribution of potassium.[76] Sodium, chloride, calcium, and magnesium have not shown changes. However, serum sodium does fall after surgery if large amounts of glucose-containing fluids have been infused. In this situation, glucose is metabolized slowly and draws fluid from the cells by its osmotic effect. Consequently, the sodium is diluted.[94]

Errors in measurement can be costly to the patient in terms of safety, health status, and cost-effective practice. Because changes in potassium are closely watched and treatment is initiated when the level falls within a very narrow range, the chances for error are great. It has been suggested that potassium replacement during rewarming be handled cautiously.[76]

Selected Chemistries

ALKALINE PHOSPHATASE

Alkaline phosphatase is an enzyme released in liver and bone disease. An increased serum level suggests an abnormality in the liver or bones, but can be associated with chronic therapeutic use of anticonvulsant drugs such as phenobarbital or phenytoin.[138]

BILIRUBIN

Bilirubin is a product of Hgb breakdown and is removed from the body by the liver. Elevated direct bilirubin is the result of obstructive jaundice due to extrahepatic (stones or tumor) or intrahepatic (damaged liver cells) causes.

Increases in indirect bilirubin occur with hepatocellular dysfunction or an increase in RBC destruction (e.g., transfusion reaction or hemolytic anemia). Care should be taken not to hemolyze the sample. The sample should also be protected from bright light because bilirubin levels are reduced after 1 hour of such exposure.[23,67,68,99]

CATECHOLAMINES

Epinephrine and norepinephrine are elevated in pheochromocytoma, a tumor of the adrenal medulla. Pheochromocytoma is a cause of high blood pressure.

CREATININE

Creatinine is a waste product formed during muscle protein metabolism. Serum creatinine is a reflection of the excretory function of the kidney. It is evaluated in conjunction with blood urea nitrogen (BUN), but is a more sensitive indicator of renal function. People with large muscle mass have higher serum creatinine levels than do those with less muscle, such as the elderly, amputees, and patients with muscle disease.[67,68,90,99,132]

GLUCOSE

Glucose is elevated whenever endogenous epinephrine is mobilized. Conditions in which this would be expected include chronic renal failure, acute pancreatitis, acute MI, CHF, extensive surgery, and infections. Mild hyperglycemia can be expected whenever the patient is under stress. Diabetes mellitus is frequently the cause of marked hyperglycemia. MI may precipitate diabetes in a person with latent diabetes.[138] Ideally, blood specimens for glucose determination should be drawn when the patient is fasting.

PROTEIN

Total protein measurement includes albumin (53%) and globulin (15% α, 12% ß, and 20% γ). These protein components can be quantified with the use of protein electrophoresis. Albumin (4 to 5.5 g/dL) contributes to the balance of osmotic pressure between blood and tissues. Globulins (2 to 3 g/dL) influence osmotic pressure and include the immunoglobulins (antibodies). Because albumin is produced in the liver, a low serum albumin level is seen in liver disease. Low serum albumin also reflects poor nutritional status, and the finding should prompt a complete nutritional assessment. The half-life of albumin is 18 days. If albumin is reduced, edema results because albumin accounts for 90% of the serum colloid osmotic pressure. Albumin is reduced in heart failure because of hypervolemic dilution.[138] The α- and ß-globulins tend to decrease with abnormal liver function. The γ-globulins, the body's antibodies, increase with chronic disease.[144]

UREA NITROGEN

Urea nitrogen is the end product of protein metabolism. It is produced by the liver and excreted by the kidney. Increases in BUN are referred to as *azotemia*. Prerenal azotemia occurs whenever a disease or condition affects urea nitrogen before the kidneys are actually damaged or diseased. Postrenal azotemia is the result of any condition that affects BUN after it has cleared the kidney, such as in ureteral and urethral obstruction. BUN levels in the elderly may be slightly higher because the number of nephrons tends to decrease in the aging process. The BUN may be higher in hospitalized patients because of their increased catabolic state.[23,68,90,99,132]

URIC ACID

Uric acid is the end product of purine metabolism; it is increased in gout. Severe renal disease results in a high level of serum uric acid because excretion is reduced. Large doses of salicylates may interfere with accurate test results.[144]

SELECTED CHEMISTRIES AFTER CARDIAC SURGERY

Blood test results related to renal function are of particular importance after cardiac surgery. Anesthesia and the length of time associated with cardiopulmonary circulatory bypass present potential hazards to the surgical patient. The anesthetic agent may produce hypotension and subsequent reduced renal perfusion and injury to the glomeruli. Cardiopulmonary bypass may damage cellular elements, which must be cleared from the system. Observation of the renal system parameters (BUN and creatinine) gives clues to kidney function.

Laboratory Blood Chemistry Analysis

The sampling of serum for chemistry measurement requires 1 mL of blood for most tests. If a multichannel, random-access analyzer is used for a defined battery of tests, 2.5 mL of serum is required. Hemolysis should be avoided for most tests. Delays before analysis lead to prolonged contact of cells with serum and should be avoided for most samples because some products can shift from the cells into the serum. Preservatives may allow for increased stability of samples for some laboratory values, which can increase the storage time up to 48 hours. Once the laboratory work is completed, the results should be communicated rapidly to a health team member if intervention is indicated.

Nursing Considerations After Blood Chemistry Measurement

Variations in blood chemistry can substantiate nursing diagnoses of intracellular fluid volume excess or deficit, altered (decreased) cardiac output related to volume deficit or electromechanical conduction disturbances, impaired gas exchange, impaired physical mobility, altered patterns of urinary elimination, activity intolerance, and altered tissue perfusion.

Blood Lipids

Alterations of blood lipid levels have been identified as a CHD risk factor.[64] Certain lipoproteinemias have been identified as contributing to total plasma cholesterol levels.

TABLE 11-7 Factors That Influence Low-Density Lipoprotein (LDL) and High-Density Lipoprotein (HDL) Levels

LDL Levels

Increased with
  Diets high in cholesterol[28,112]
  Diets high in saturated fat[28,112]
  Alcohol[44]
  Strict vegetarian diet[28]
  Hypothyroidism[44,112]
  Obesity[28]
  Obstructive liver disease[94,112]
  Nephrosis[94,112]
  Thiazide diuretics[49]
  β-Adrenergic blocking agents[94]
  Progestin and anabolic steroids[94]
Decreased with
  Low-cholesterol diet[112]
  Low-fat diet[112]
  Alcohol restriction[147]
  Regular strenuous exercise[28]

HDL Levels

Increased with
  Not smoking[56]
  Lean body mass[56]
  Estrogen[56]
  Vigorous exercise[28,43]
  Diet low in sucrose and starch[56]
  Increased clearance of very–low-density lipoprotein
    (triglyceride)[43]
  Alcohol[28]
Decreased with
  Cigarette smoking[28,56,94]
  Obesity[28,43,56,94]
  Progesterone[43,94]
  Male gender[112]
  Sedentary lifestyle[112]
  Hypertriglyceridemia[43,94,112]
  Non–insulin-dependent diabetes mellitus[43]
  Strict vegetarian diet[28]
  Hypertriglyceridemia[43,94,112]
  Anabolic steroids[94]
  Starvation[43]
  β-Adrenergic blocking agents[94]
  Infectious illness[28]

Plasma normally contains insoluble lipid elements: free fatty acids; exogenous triglycerides; endogenous triglycerides, which are manufactured in the liver; cholesterol; and phospholipids. To be transported, each is attached to a protein. Distinguishing lipoprotein abnormalities is useful because therapy is based on an understanding of the origin of the problem (see Chapter 33).

BLOOD LIPID LABORATORY MEASUREMENT

Elevated lipid levels are considered a risk factor for cardiovascular disease. Cholesterol and the protein components of high-density lipoproteins (HDL-C) and low-density lipoproteins (LDL-C) are evaluated by electrophoresis when hyperlipoproteinemia is suspected. In most people, the cholesterol values remain constant over 24 hours; a nonfasting blood sample for measurement of total blood cholesterol is acceptable. However, a nonfasting sample for triglyceride, HDL-C, and LDL-C levels is of less value. Consequently, if triglyceride and lipoprotein analysis is indicated, measurements should be obtained after a 12- to 14-hour fast.[28] Lipoprotein electrophoresis is necessary to evaluate serum for hyperlipoproteinemia. The major apolipoproteins of HDL (apolipoprotein A-I) and LDL (apolipoprotein B) have been described as good predictors of CHD.[112,138] Measurement of these apolipoproteins may replace lipoprotein assay in assessing the risk of CHD.[41,112] A low ratio of apolipoprotein A-I to apolipoprotein B may be a highly accurate predictor of CHD.[41,138] Because lipids may be abnormal if drawn while the patient is having an acute MI or is otherwise undergoing considerable acute

stress, it is recommended that lipid studies be done at another time. A number of factors are known to influence LDL and HDL levels (Table 11-7). Table 11-5 lists plasma lipid reference values.

SERUM CONCENTRATION OF SELECTED DRUGS

Serum levels of cardiac drugs are frequently obtained to determine the effectiveness of drug therapy. Usual ranges of therapeutic and toxic serum concentrations of selected drugs are given in Table 11-8.

The serum concentrations must always be interpreted in the context of all the clinical data. For example, digitalis intoxication can occur within the usual range of therapeutic serum concentrations if the patient has hypokalemia, hypercalcemia, hypomagnesemia, acid-base imbalances, increased adrenergic tone, hypothyroidism, hypoxemia, or myocardial ischemia.[70]

Digitoxin, phenytoin, and quinidine are chiefly bound to serum albumin. Bound fractions have no pharmacologic effect. The determination of a drug in the serum is usually the total amount bound and unbound. Usually, the amount of unbound drug is a fairly constant percentage of the total. In situations where there is less albumin or when the drug-binding ability of the albumin is depressed (such as in uremia), or where other drugs that are highly bound to protein are also given, the amount of drug bound is less. Thus, serious toxicity can result even within the normal therapeutic range because of an increase in non–protein-bound drug.[8,70]

TABLE 11-8	Therapeutic Reference Ranges and Toxic Levels of Common Drugs	
Drug	**Therapeutic Range**	**Toxic Level**
Amiodarone	1.0–3.4 µg/mL[127,130]	
Bretylium	0.8–2.4 µg/mL[130]	
Digitoxin	15 ng/mL[127]	>40 ng/mL[127]
Digoxin	0.5–2.0 µg/mL[148]	>4.0 ng/mL[130]
Diltiazem	100–200 ng/mL[127]	
Disopyramide	1.5–5.0 µg/mL[127,130]	>9.0 µg/mL[127]
Encainide	10.0–135 µg/mL[127]	
Flecainide	0.2–1.0 µg/mL[127,130]	
Lidocaine	1.5–5.0 µg/mL[127,130]	>6.0 µg/mL[130]
Lorcainide	200–500 ng/mL[127]	
Metoprolol	120–200 ng/mL[130]	
Mexiletine	0.5–2.0 µg/mL[127,130]	>3.0 µg/mL[130]
N-Acetylprocainamide (NAPA)	2.0–22.0 µg/mL[130]	
Nifedipine	50–100 ng/mL[130]	
Phenytoin	10–20 µg/mL[127,130,148]	>18 µg/mL[130]
Procainamide	4.0–8.0 µg/mL[127,130]	>10 µg/mL[130]
Propafenone	64–1044 ng/mL[127]	
Propranolol	30–50 ng/mL[127]	
Quinidine	2.5–5.0 µg/mL[127,130]	>6.0 µg/mL[130]
Theophylline	10–20 µg/mL[127,130,148]	>20 µg/mL[130]
Tocainide	4.0–10.0 µg/mL[127]	>10 µg/mL[127]
Verapamil	50–400 ng/mL[127]	

Serum concentrations of drugs can be altered by many mechanisms. A number of factors are known to alter digoxin concentration when the dosage is kept constant, including altered absorption, impaired renal excretion, drug interaction, and impaired metabolism.[7] Theophylline concentration is increased in neonates, in the elderly, with obesity, with high carbohydrate diets, and with some comorbid conditions. Theophylline concentration is reduced in children, with a low carbohydrate diet, with eating charcoal-cooked meats, and with some drugs.[9] There is as much as a 50-fold difference in plasma concentration of phenytoin among patients taking the same dosage; altered metabolism and altered protein binding account for the large individual variation in the disposition of phenytoin.[8]

The blood specimen to determine serum concentration of a drug usually is drawn 1 to 2 hours after an oral drug is given because absorption and distribution are usually complete by this time.[70] However, peak and trough times are frequently defined for individual drugs; these times should be considered in the timing of specimens for therapeutic drug level monitoring.

REFERENCES

1. Abbey EE: Bleeding disorders. In Campbell JW, Frisse M (eds): Manual of Medical Therapeutics, 24th ed, pp 285–288. Boston, Little, Brown, 1983
2. Abbott LB, Lott JA: Reactivation of serum creatine kinase isoenzyme BB inpatients with malignancies. Clin Chem 30: 1861–1863, 1984
3. Adams JE, Dávila-Román VG, Bessey PQ, et al: Improved detection of cardiac contusion with cardiac troponin I. Am Heart J 131: 308–312, 1996
4. Adams JE, Bodor GS, Dávila-Román VG, et al: Cardiac troponin I: A marker with high specificity for cardiac injury. Circulation 88: 101–106, 1993
5. Adult advanced cardiac life support, part III. JAMA 268: 2199–2241, 1992
6. Apple FS: Diagnostic use of CK-MM and CK-MB isoforms for detecting myocardial infarction. Clin Lab Med 9: 643–655, 1989
7. Aronson JK, Hardman M, Reynolds DJM: ABC of monitoring drug therapy: Digoxin. BMJ 305: 1149–1152, 1992
8. Aronson JK, Hardman M, Reynolds DJM: ABC of monitoring drug therapy: Phenytoin. BMJ 305: 1215–1218, 1992
9. Aronson JK, Hardman M, Reynolds DJM: ABC of monitoring drug therapy: Theophylline. BMJ 305: 1355–1358, 1992
10. Baer DM, Dito WR (eds): Interpretations in Therapeutic Drug Monitoring, p 90. Chicago, ASCP, 1981
11. Bakay RAE, Ward AA: Enzymatic changes in serum and cerebrospinal fluid in neurological injury. J Neurosurg 58: 27–37, 1983
12. Baranowski L: Central venous access devices: Current technologies, uses, and management strategies. J Intravenous Nursing 16: 167–191, 1993
13. Becker RC, Corrao JM: Circadian variations in cardiovascular disease. Cleve Clinic J Med 56: 676–679, 1989
14. Birdi I, Angelini GD, Bryan AJ: Biochemical markers of myocardial injury during cardiac operations. Ann Thorac Surg 63: 879–874, 1997
15. Bolooki H: The significance of serum enzyme studies in patients undergoing direct coronary artery surgery. J Thorac Cardiovasc Surg 65: 863, 1973
16. Boone DJ, Duncan PH, MacNeil ML et al: Results of a nationwide survey of analyses for creatine kinase and creatine kinase isoenzymes. Clin Chem 30: 33–37, 1984
17. Brogan GX, Bock JL, McCuskey CF et al: Evaluation of cardiac status CK-MB/myoglobin device for rapidly ruling out acute myocardial infarction. Clin Lab Med 17: 655–658, 1997
18. Burns PK, Gregersen RA, Underhill SL: Adequate discard volume determinations to obtain accurate coagulation studies from heparinized arterial lines (Abstract). Circulation 72: II-96, 1985
19. Calam RR: Reviewing the importance of specimen collection. J Am Med Technology 39: 297–301, 1977
20. Cannon K, Mitchell KA, Fabian TC: Prospective randomized evaluation of two methods of drawing coagulation studies from heparinized arterial lines. Heart Lung 14: 392–395, 1985
21. Carlson KK, Snyder ML, Wallace HH: Obtaining reliable plasma sodium and glucose determinations from pulmonary artery catheters (Abstract). Heart Lung 15: 307–308, 1985
22. Carnevali D: Nursing Care Planning: Diagnosis and Management, 3rd ed. Philadelphia, JB Lippincott, 1983
23. Chernecky CC, Berger BJ: Laboratory Tests and Diagnostic Procedures, 2nd ed. Philadelphia, WB Saunders, 1997
24. Christenson RH, Clemmensen P, Ohman EM et al: Relative increase in creatine kinase MB isoenzyme during reperfusion after myocardial infarction is method dependent. Clin Chem 36: 1444–1449, 1990
25. Cobb LA, Baum RS, Alvarez H et al: Resuscitation from out-of-hospital ventricular fibrillation: Four years follow-up. Circulation 52(Suppl 3): 223–235, 1975

26. Coolen RB, Pragay DA, Nosanchuk JS et al: Elevation of brain-type creatine kinase in serum from patients with carcinoma. Cancer 44: 1414–1418, 1979

27. Coombs DL, Russo LE, Underhill SL et al: Withdrawal of blood specimens from radial artery catheters for serum sodium and hematocrit studies (Abstract). Circulation 70: II-288, 1984

28. Cooper GR, Myers GL, Smith SJ, Schlant RC: Blood lipid measurements: Variations and practical utility. JAMA 267: 1652–1660, 1992

29. Collinson PO, Rasalki SB, Kuwana T et al: Early diagnosis of acute myocardial infarction by CK-MB mass measurements. Ann Clin Biochem 29: 43–47, 1992

30. Costentino F: Central venous catheters. In Plumer A: Principles and Practices of Intravenous Therapy, pp 323–369. Boston, Little, Brown, 1987

31. Dacie JV, Lewis SM (eds): Practical Hematology, 6th ed, pp 7–12. Edinburgh, Churchill Livingstone, 1984

32. Dufour DR: Clinical Use of Laboratory Data: A Practical Guide. Baltimore, Williams & Wilkins, 1998

33. Ehsani A, Ewy GA, Sobel BE: Effects of electrical countershock on serum creatine phosphokinase (CPK) isoenzyme activity. Am J Cardiol 37: 12–18, 1976

34. Farah SY, Moss DW, Ribeiro P et al: Interpretation of changes in the activity of creatine kinase MB isoenzyme in serum after coronary artery bypass grafting. Clin Chim Acta 141: 219–225, 1984

35. Finch SC: Neutropenia. In Williams WJ, Buetler B, Erslev AJ et al (eds): Hematology, 3rd ed, pp 773–793. New York, McGraw-Hill, 1983

36. Fitzgerald DJ, Catella R, Roy L, Fitzgerald GA: Market platelet activation in vivo after intravenous streptokinase in patients with acute myocardial infarction. Circulation 77: 142–150, 1988

37. Fried MW, Murthy UK, Hassig SR et al: Creatine kinase isoenzymes in the diagnosis of intestinal infarction. Dig Dis Sci 36: 1589–1593, 1991

38. Galen RS: Isoenzymes in cardiac and noncardiac disorders. In Galen RS, Brennan L (eds): Laboratory Diagnosis and Patient Monitoring: Clinical Chemistry, pp 113–136. Oradell, NJ, Medical Economics, 1981

39. Galen RS: Myocardial infarction: A clinician's guide to the isoenzymes. Resident and Staff Physician 23: 67–75, 1977

40. Ganong WF: Circulating body fluids. In Ganong WF (ed): Review of Medical Physiology, 13th ed, pp 429–449. Los Altos, CA, Lange Medical, 1987

41. Genest J, McNamara JR, Ordovas JM et al: Lipoprotein cholesterol, apolipoprotein A-1 and B and lipoprotein (a) abnormalities in men with premature coronary artery disease. J Am Coll Cardiol 19: 792–802, 1992

42. Gersh BJ, Clements IP: Acute myocardial infarction. In Giuliani E, Gersh BJ, McGoon MD et al (eds): Mayo Clinic Practice of Cardiology, 3rd ed, pp 1226–1229. St. Louis, Mosby, 1996

43. Glatter TR: Hyperlipidemia. Postgrad Med 76: 49–59, 1984

44. Gotto AM: Clinical diagnosis of hyperlipoproteinemia. Am J Med 74(5A): 5–9, 1983

45. Graeber GM: Creatine kinase (CK): Its use in the evaluation of perioperative MI. Surg Clin North Am 65: 539–551, 1985

46. Gram-Hansen P, Nielsen FE, Kalusen IC. Creatine kinase-MB activity after implantation of a cardiac pacemaker. Am J Cardiol 66: 862–863, 1990

47. Gregersen RA, Underhill SL, Detter JC et al: Accurate coagulation studies from heparinized radial artery catheters. Heart Lung 16: 686–693, 1987

48. Gregersen RA, Underhill SL, Detter JC: Withdrawal of blood specimens from heparinized radial artery catheters for coagulation studies (Abstract). Circulation 68: III-23, 1983

49. Grundy SM: Can modification of risk factors reduce coronary heart disease? In SM Rahimtoola (ed): Controversies in Coronary Artery Disease, pp 283–296. Philadelphia, FA Davis, 1983

50. Gulbis B, Unger P, Lenaers A et al: Mass concentration of creatine kinase MB isoenzyme and lactate dehydrogenase isoenzyme 1 in diagnosis of perioperative myocardial infarction after coronary bypass surgery. Clin Chem 36: 1784–1788, 1990

51. Gunnar WP, Martin M, Smith RF et al: The utility of cardiac evaluation in the hemodynamically stable patient with suspected myocardial contusion. Am Surg 57: 373–377, 1991

52. Halsted JA: Diagnostic procedures and tests. In Halsted JA (ed): The Laboratory in Clinical Medicine, pp 530–535. Philadelphia, WB Saunders, 1976

53. Hans P, Born JD, Chapelle J-P et al: Creatine kinase isoenzymes in severe head injury. J Neurosurg 58: 689–692, 1983

54. Healey MA, Brown R, Fleiszer D: Blunt cardiac injury: Is this diagnosis necessary? J Trauma 30: 137–146, 1990

55. Heap MJ, Ridley SA, Hodson K et al: Are coagulation studies on blood sampled from arterial lines valid? Anaesthesia 52: 640–645, 1997

56. Heiss G, Hohnson NJ, Reiland S et al: The epidemiology of plasma high-density lipoprotein cholesterol levels: The Lipid Research Clinics Program Prevalence Study. Circulation 62(Suppl IV): IV-116–IV-136, 1980

57. Henry RJ, Cannon DC, Winkelman JW: Enzymes. In Henry RJ, Cannon DC, Winkelman JW (eds): Clinical Chemistry: Principles and Techniques, pp 818–904. Hagerstown, MD, Harper & Row, 1974

58. Hori M, Inoue M, Fukui S et al: Correlation of infarct size estimated from the total CK released in patients with acute myocardial infarction. Br Heart J 41: 433–440, 1979

59. Huang JN, Shimamura A: Low-molecular-weight heparins. Hematol Oncol Clin North Am 12, 1251–1281, 1998

60. Intravenous Nursing Standards of Practice. J Intravenous Nurs 13(Suppl): S1–S98, 1990

61. Jarvinen A, Mattila T, Kyosola K: Serum CK-MB isoenzyme after aortic and mitral valve replacements. Ann Clin Res 15: 189–193, 1983

62. Kanemitsu F, Okigake T: Creatine kinase MB isoforms for early diagnosis and monitoring of acute myocardial infarction. Clin Chim Acta 206: 191–199, 1992

63. Johnston JB, Messina M: Erroneous laboratory values obtained from central catheters. J Intravenous Nurs 14: 13–15, 1991

64. Kannel WB: Recent findings of the Framingham Study. Resident and Staff Physician 24: 56–71, 1978

65. Kannel WB, Anderson K, Wilson PF: White blood cell count and cardiovascular disease: Insights from the Framingham Study. JAMA 267: 1253–1256, 1992

66. Kaste M, Somer H, Konttinen A: Brain-type creatine kinase isoenzyme: Occurrence in serum in acute cerebral disorders. Arch Neurol 34: 142–144, 1977

67. Kee JL: Laboratory and Diagnostic Tests With Nursing Implications, 5th ed. Stamford, CT, Appleton & Lange, 1999

68. Kee JL: Handbook of Laboratory Diagnostic Tests with Nursing Implications, 3rd ed. Stamford, CT, Appleton & Lange, 1998

69. Kjekshus JK, Vaagenes P, Hetland O: Assessment of cerebral injury with spinal fluid creatine kinase (CSF-CK) in patients after cardiac resuscitation. Scand J Clin Lab Invest 40: 437–444, 1980

70. Koch-Weser J: Serum drug concentrations as therapeutic guides. N Engl J Med 287: 227–231, 1972

71. Kratz AK, Lewandrowski KB: Normal reference laboratory values. N Engl J Med 339: 1063–1072, 1998

72. Krueger K, Carrico CJ, Detter JC et al: The reliability of laboratory data from blood samples collected through pulmonary artery catheters. Arch Pathol Lab Med 105: 343–344, 1980

73. LaDue JS, Wroblewski F, Karmen A: Serum glutamic oxaloacetic transaminase activity in human acute transmural myocardial infarction. Science 120: 497–499, 1954

74. Laxson CJ, Titler MG: Drawing coagulation studies from arterial lines: An integrative literature review. Am J Crit Care 3: 16–22, 1994

75. Lew JKL, Hutchinson R, Lin ES: Intra-arterial blood sampling for clotting studies: Effects of heparin contamination. Anaesthesia 46: 719–721, 1991

76. Lim M, Linton AF, Band DM: Rise in plasma potassium during rewarming in open-heart surgery. Lancet 1: 241–242, 1983

77. Longstreth WT, Clayson KJ, Sumi SM: Cerebrospinal fluid and serum creatine kinase BB activity after out-of-hospital cardiac arrest. Neurology 31: 455–458, 1981

78. Longstreth WT, Clayson KJ, Chandler WL et al: Cerebrospinal fluid creatine kinase activity and neurologic recovery after cardiac arrest. Neurology 34: 834–837, 1984

79. Lott JA: Serum enzyme determinations in the diagnosis of acute myocardial infarction: An update. Hum Pathol 15: 706–716, 1984

80. Lott JA, Stang JM: Serum enzymes and isoenzymes in the diagnosis and differential diagnosis of myocardial ischemia and necrosis. Clin Chem 26: 1241–1250, 1980

81. Lott JA, Stang JM: Differential diagnosis of patients with abnormal serum creatine kinase isoenzymes. Clin Lab Med 9: 627–642, 1989

82. Luce JM, Tyler ML, Pierson DJ (eds): Intensive Respiratory Care. Philadelphia, WB Saunders, 1984

83. Mangano DT: Beyond CK-MB: Biochemical markers for perioperative myocardial infarction. Anesthesiology 81: 1317–1320, 1994

84. Markenvard J, Dellborg M, Jagenberg R et al: The predictive value of CK-MB mass concentration in unstable angina pectoris: Preliminary report. J Intern Med 231: 433–436, 1992

85. Markmann PJ, Wallace P: Nursing care in the intensive care unit. In McCauley KM, Brest AN, McGoon DW (eds): McGoon's Cardiac Surgery: An Interprofessional Approach to Patient Care, pp 319–354. Philadelphia, FA Davis, 1985

86. Masouredes SP: Preservation and clinical use of erythrocytes and whole blood. In Williams WJ, Buetler E, Erslev AJ et al (eds): Hematology, 4th ed, pp 1628–1646. New York, McGraw-Hill, 1990

87. Massey TH, Butts WC: Development and clinical evaluation of a microcentrifugal analyzer method for determining creatine kinase MB isoenzyme. Clin Chem 29: 533–538, 1983

88. Massey TH, Goe MR: Transient creatine kinase-BB activity in serum or plasma after cardiac or respiratory arrest. Clin Chem 30: 50–55, 1984

89. Mathey DG, Kuck K H, Tilsner V et al: Nonsurgical coronary recanalization in acute transmural myocardial infarction. Circulation 63: 481–497, 1981

90. McFarland MB, Grant MM: Nursing Implications of Laboratory Tests, 3rd ed. Albany, NY, Delmar, 1994

91. McFarland MB, Grant MM: Nursing Implications of Laboratory Tests, pp 89–107. New York, Wiley Medical, 1988

92. Melandri G, Branze A, Traini AM et al: On the value of the activated clotting time for monitoring heparin therapy in acute coronary syndromes. Am J Cardiol 71: 469–470, 1993

93. Miller FA: Cardiac trauma. In Giuliani E, Gersh BJ, McGoon MD et al (eds): Mayo Clinic Practice of Cardiology, 3rd ed, pp 1706–1707. St. Louis, Mosby, 1996

94. Miyazawa K, Fukuyama H, Yamaguchi I et al: Serial determinations of serum enzymes following aorta-coronary bypass surgery and acute myocardial infarction. Jpn Heart J 26: 45–52, 1985

95. National Cholesterol Education Program Expert Panel on Detection, Evaluation, and Treatment of High Blood Cholesterol in Adults. Arch Intern Med 148: 36–69, 1988

96. Nguyen DM, Gilfix BM, Dennis F et al: Impact of transfusion of mediastinal shed blood on serum levels of cardiac enzymes. Ann Thorac Surg 62: 109–114, 1996

97. Nordby HK, Urdal P: Creatine kinase BB in blood as index or prognosis and effect of treatment after severe head injury. Acta Neurochir 76: 131–136, 1985

98. Oh JK, Shub C, Ilstrup DM et al: Creatine kinase release after successful percutaneous transluminal coronary angioplasty. Am Heart J 109: 1225–1231, 1985

99. Pagana KD, Pagana TJ: Mosby's Manual of Diagnostic and Laboratory Tests. St. Louis, Mosby, 1998

100. Palermo LM, Andrews RV, Ellison N: Avoidance of heparin contamination in coagulation studies drawn from indwelling lines. Anesth Analg 59: 222–224, 1980

101. Paone RF, Peacock JB, Smith DLT: Diagnosis of myocardial contusion. South Med J 86: 867–870, 1993

102. Phillips JP, Jones HM, Hitchcock R et al: Radioimmunoassay of serum creatine kinase BB as index of brain damage after head injury. BMJ 281: 777–779, 1980

103. Prinkey LA: Diagnostic testing. In Guzzetta CE, Dossey BM (eds): Cardiovascular Nursing: Holistic Practice, pp 128–130. St. Louis, Mosby, 1992

104. Pryor AC: The intra-arterial line: A site for obtaining coagulation studies. Heart Lung 12: 586–590, 1983

105. Ravel R: Cardiac, pulmonary, and miscellaneous diagnostic procedures. In Ravel R (ed): Clinical Laboratory Medicine: Clinical Application of Laboratory Data, 4th ed, pp 227–441. Chicago, Year Book, 1984

106. Roberts R, Morris D, Pratt CM et al: Pathophysiology, recognition and treatment of acute myocardial infarction and its complications. In Schlant RC, Alexander RW (eds): Hurst's The Heart: Arteries and Veins, 8th ed, pp 1117–1122. New York, McGraw-Hill, 1994

107. Roberts R, Gowda KS, Ludbrook PA et al: Specificity of elevated serum MB creatine phosphokinase activity in the diagnosis of acute myocardial infarction. Am J Cardiol 36: 433–437, 1975

108. Romano AT, Yourn GW: Mild forearm exercise during exercise and its effect on potassium determinations. Clin Chem 23: 303–304, 1977

109. Rose BD: Clinical Physiology of Acid-Base and Electrolyte Disorders, 2nd ed, pp 275–276. New York, McGraw-Hill, 1984

110. Russo LE, Coombs DL, Underhill SL et al: Reliable measurements of serum potassium and glucose from radial artery lines (Abstract). Heart Lung 13: 310, 1984

111. Ruzak-Skocir B: Cerebrospinal fluid CK enzyme and CK isoenzymes in the outcome prognosis of cerebrovascular disease. Neurologia/Croatica 40: 247–256, 1991

112. Schaefer ER, Levy RL: Pathogenesis and management of lipoprotein disorders. N Engl J Med 312: 1300–1310, 1985

113. Schofer J, Ress-Grigolo G, Voigt KD et al: Early detection of coronary artery patency after thrombolysis by determination of the MM creatine kinase isoforms in patients with acute myocardial infarction. Am Heart J 123: 846–853, 1992

114. Schwartz AJ, Geer RT: Cardiac anesthesia. In McCauley KM, Brest AM, McGoon DC (eds): McGoon's Cardiac Surgery:

An Interprofessional Approach to Care, pp 289–315. Philadelphia, FA Davis, 1985

115. Severson AL, Baldwin LR, DeLoughery TG: International normalized ratio in anticoagulant therapy: Understanding the issues. Am J Crit Care 6: 88–94, 1997

116. Silva J, Hoekesma H, FeKety FR: Transient defects in phagocytic functions during cardiopulmonary bypass. J Thorac Cardiovasc Surg 67: 175–183, 1974

117. Sipperly ME: Thrombolytic therapy update. Crit Care Nurse 5(6): 30–34, 1985

118. Skogseid LM, Nordby HK, Urdal P et al: Increased serum creatine kinase BB and neuron specific enolase following head injury indicates brain damage. Acta Neurochir (Wien) 115: 106–111, 1992

119. Smith AF, Radford D, Wong CP et al: Creatine kinase MB isoenzyme studies in diagnosis of myocardial infarction. Br Heart J 38: 225–232, 1976

120. Snyder M, Gregersen R, Underhill SL et al: Partial thromboplastin and thrombin time blood specimens collection through pulmonary artery catheters (Abstract). Heart Lung 15: 315, 1986

121. Sobel BE, Jaffe AS: The value and limitations of cardiac enzymes in the recognition of acute myocardial infarction. Heart Disease and Stroke 2(1): 26–32, 1993

122. Spaccavento LJ, Hawley H: Infections associated with intraarterial lines. Heart Lung 11: 118–122, 1982

123. Statland BE, Bokelund H, Winkel P: Factors contributing to intra–individual variations of serum constituents: Effects of posture and tourniquet application on variation of serum constituents in healthy subjects. Clin Chem 20: 1513–1519, 1974

124. Statland BE, Winkel P: Sources of variation in laboratory measurements. In Henry JB (ed): Clinical Diagnosis and Management by Laboratory Methods, pp 3–28. Philadelphia, WB Saunders, 1979

125. Steele BW, Gobel FL, Nelson RR et al: Creatine kinase isoenzyme activity following cardiac catheterization and exercise stress testing. Chest 73: 489–496, 1978

126. Suzuki T, Yamauchi K, Yamada Y et al: Blood coagulability and fibrolytic activity before and after physical training during the recovery phase of acute myocardial infarction. Clin Cardiol 15: 358–364, 1992

127. Taylor WJ, Caviness MHD: A Textbook for the Clinical Application of Therapeutic Drug Monitoring. Irving, TX, Abbott Laboratories, 1986

128. Templin K, Shively M, Riley J: Accuracy of drawing coagulation samples from heparinized arterial lines. Am J Crit Care 2: 88–95, 1993

129. Tilkian SM, Conover MB, Tilkian AG: Clinical and Nursing Implications of Laboratory Tests, 5th ed. St. Louis, Mosby, 1995

130. Tilkian SM, Conover MB, Tilkian A: Clinical Implications of Laboratory Tests, 4th ed. St. Louis, CV Mosby, 1987

131. Treseler KM: Clinical Laboratory and Diagnostic Tests: Significance and Nursing Implications, 3rd ed. Norwalk, CT, Appleton & Lange, 1995

132. Treseler KM: Clinical Laboratory Tests: Significance and Implications for Nursing, 2nd ed. Englewood Cliffs, NJ, Prentice–Hall, 1988

133. Tsung SM: Creatine kinase isoenzyme patterns in human tissue obtained at surgery. Clin Chem 22: 173–175, 1976

134. Turpie AGG: Antithrombotic therapy in coronary ischaemia: The expanding role of low-molecular-weight heparin. Haemostasis 28(Suppl 3): 35–42, 1998

135. Vaagenes P, Kjekshus J, Torvik A: The relationship between cerebrospinal fluid creatine kinase and morphologic changes in the brain after transient cardiac arrest. Circulation 61: 1194–1199, 1980

136. Varat MA, Mercer DW: Cardiac specific creatine phosphokinase isoenzyme in the diagnosis of acute myocardial infarction. Circulation 51: 855–859, 1975

137. Wallace HH, Carlson KK, Snyder ML et al: Obtaining reliable plasma glucose and potassium values from intraarterial catheters (Abstract). Heart Lung 15: 317, 1986

138. Wallach J: Interpretation of Diagnostic Tests: A Synopsis of Laboratory Medicine, 5th ed. Boston, Little, Brown, 1992

139. Walrath JM, Abbott NK, Caplan E et al: Stopcocks: Bacterial contamination in invasive monitoring systems. Heart Lung 8: 100–104, 1979

140. Wang CW, Steinhubl SR, Castellani WJ et al: Inability of serum myocyte death markers to predict acute cardiac allograft rejection. Transplantation 62: 1938–1941, 1996

141. Weinstein RA, Emori TG, Anderson RL et al: Pressure transducers as a source of bacteremia after open heart surgery. Chest 69: 338–344, 1976

142. Weiss HJ: Platelet physiology and abnormalities of platelet function. N Engl J Med 293: 531–540, 1977

143. White KM: Completing the hemodynamic picture: SvO_2. Heart Lung 14: 272–280, 1985

144. Widmann FK: Goodale's Clinical Interpretation of Laboratory Tests, 9th ed. Philadelphia, FA Davis, 1983

145. Wiedemann HP, Matthay MA, Matthay RA: Cardiovascular-pulmonary monitoring in the intensive care unit, part 2. Chest 85: 656–668, 1984

146. Wilson H: Perioperative use of cardiac drugs. In McCauley KM, Brest AN, McGoon DC (eds): McGoon's Cardiac Surgery: An Interprofessional Approach to Patient Care. Philadelphia, FA Davis, 1985

147. Witztum JL: Diagnosis and treatment of hyperlipidemia. Hospital Medicine 14(6): 60–63, 65, 67, 71–80, 1978

148. Woodley M, Whelan A (eds): Manual of Medical Therapeutics, 27th ed, pp 517–523. Boston, Little, Brown, 1992

149. Woods KL, Fletcher S, Roffe C, Haider Y: Intravenous magnesium sulphate in suspected acute myocardial infarction: Results of the second Leicester Intravenous Magnesium Intervention Trial (LIMIT-2). Lancet 339: 1553–1558, 1992

150. Wu AH: Creatine kinase isoforms in ischemic heart disease. Clin Chem 35: 7–13, 1989

151. Yamada T, Matsumori A, Tamaki S et al: Myosin light chain I grade: A simple marker for the severity and prognosis of patients with acute myocardial infarction. Am Heart J 135: 329–334, 1998

Radiologic Examination of the Chest

JON S. HUSEBY

A cardiac care nurse may be the first health care professional to see the chest radiograph of a patient in acute distress. Valuable time may be saved if the nurse is able to recognize the presence of an abnormality. Knowledge of chest radiograph interpretation and the disease processes that an abnormal film indicates can help in the nurse's understanding of disease pathophysiology, thereby allowing for better patient care; dual reading of radiographs significantly increases diagnostic accuracy and decreases the incidence of missed abnormalities. This chapter is divided into five sections:

1. How x-rays work
2. Interpretation of chest radiographs
3. Chest film findings in myocardial infarction (MI) and conditions that may mimic an acute MI
4. Chest film findings in complications of acute MI
5. Miscellaneous uses of the chest radiograph

HOW X-RAYS WORK

X-rays are radiant energy, like light, except that these waves are shorter and can pass through opaque objects. They are produced by bombarding a tungsten target with an electron beam and are channeled so that a narrow but diverging beam is emitted from the tube. When an x-ray exposure is taken, the tube is usually aimed so that the rays pass through the subject to the x-ray film in either a posterior to anterior (posteroanterior) or anterior to posterior (anteroposterior) direction (Figs. 12-1 and 12-2). Because the x-rays are diverging and subject to reflection (scatter), structures more distant from the film are magnified and less distinctly outlined. In general, chest radiographs are taken in the posteroanterior direction because this places the heart, an anterior structure, closer to the film, resulting in less magnification and allowing the cardiac outline to be seen clearly.

Anteroposterior chest radiographs are often taken in cardiac care units (CCUs) because it is difficult to put the x-ray tube behind the patient. The x-ray film is therefore placed behind the patient. Because the heart is relatively far away from the x-ray film, its outline is somewhat less distinct and the heart size is magnified. Moreover, the distance between the tube and the patient in CCUs is shorter than usual to cut down x-ray scatter. This also results in greater magnification.

The degree of darkness of the x-ray film depends on how much x-ray energy traverses the patient and exposes the film. This depends on the density of the material through which the x-ray beam passes. The chest has four major types of tissue densities through which rays must pass: bone, water, fat, and air. Because bone is the densest of these, fewer and less energetic x-rays pass through this substance. Thus, the shadow on the x-ray film cast by bone is light. (An x-ray picture is like a photographic negative, with white color indicating lack of exposure and black color indicating intense exposure.) The lung, which is largely air, is least dense; therefore it appears black on a chest radiograph. Soft tissues and blood are largely water, with similar densities, between those of bone and air. Fat is usually visibly less dense than other soft tissues. Thus, a chest radiograph is actually a shadowgraph.

The reason a structure can be outlined is that the shadow of one density contrasts with that of an adjacent density. If two structures are of equal density and adjacent to each other, a single combined shadow results. If two structures of similar density are in different planes or are separated by a structure of a different density, then the two structures are seen on x-ray film as separate. This property of the x-ray shadowgraph is helpful in determining where a certain density lies. For example, if a density on a posteroanterior chest radiograph is inseparable from and therefore adjacent to the descending thoracic aorta, then the observer knows that this abnormal density is in the posterior chest; if the density is inseparable from the right heart border, then the density is in an anterior position, because the heart is an anterior structure.

INTERPRETATION OF CHEST RADIOGRAPHS

A chest radiograph is usually read as though the reader were looking at the patient. The x-ray film is placed on a

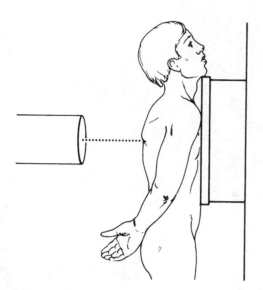

FIGURE 12-1 Positioning a patient for a posteroanterior (PA) frontal chest radiograph. The x-ray tube is behind the patient, and the x-ray film is close to his anterior chest.

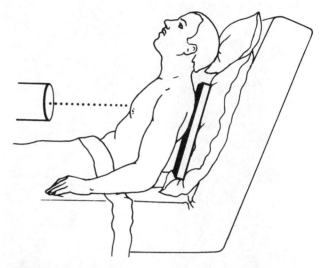

FIGURE 12-2 Typical cardiac care unit (CCU) patient positioned for an anteroposterior (AP) chest radiograph. Note that, as often occurs in the CCU, the patient's chest is not perfectly perpendicular to the x-ray tube. This placement is called a *lordotic position* and causes the heart to appear large and indistinct.

viewbox so that the patient's right side is to the viewer's left and the patient's left side is to the viewer's right. To ensure that all anatomic structures are seen, radiographs are read according to a certain pattern. This method is called the directed-search method. It is common practice to look at soft tissues, bones, and diaphragms first, then at the lungs from apex to base, and finally at the outline of the

heart and the aorta. Most structures in the chest, except the heart, are bilateral. Thus, if an abnormality is found on one side of the chest, the other side should be observed to ensure that this abnormality is not present there also. Even if an obvious abnormality is present, a directed search should be completed so that additional disease is not missed. Figure 12-3*A* is a normal posteroanterior chest

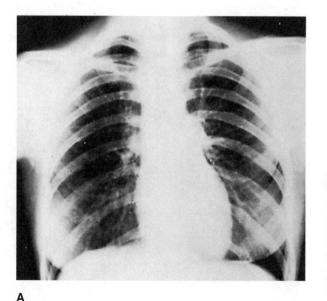

A

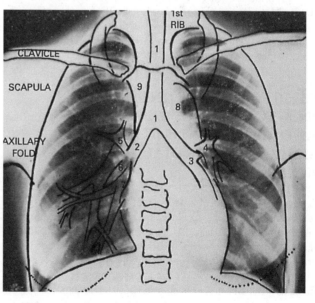

B

FIGURE 12-3 (**A**) Normal posteroanterior chest radiograph. (**B**) Outline of structures visible on normal posteroanterior chest radiograph. The diagrammatic overlay shows the normal anatomic structures: (*1*) trachea, (*2*) right main bronchus, (*3*) left main bronchus, (*4*) left pulmonary artery, (*5*) right upper lobe pulmonary artery, (*6*) right interlobar artery, (*7*) right lower and middle lobe vein, (*8*) aortic knob, (*9*) superior vena cava. (Adapted from Fraser RG, Pare JAP, Pare PD et al: Diagnosis of Disease of the Chest, pp 288–290. Philadelphia, WB Saunders, 1988.)

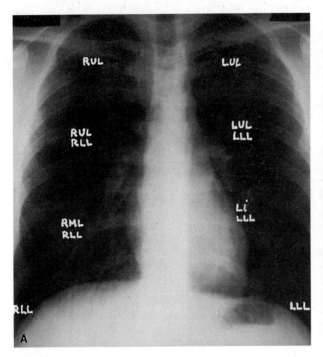

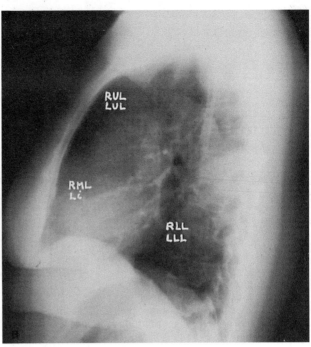

FIGURE 12-4 **(A)** Location of the lung lobes on the frontal chest radiograph. Because some lobes are anterior and some posterior, an abnormality in a certain area on a frontal chest radiograph can be in one of two lobes. Obtaining a lateral film or noticing whether an anterior or posterior structure is obliterated by an abnormal density can help with localization. RUL, right upper lobe; RLL, right lower lobe; LLL, left lower lobe; RML, right middle lobe; LUL, left upper lobe; Li, lingula. **(B)** Location of lung lobes in a lateral radiograph. Abnormalities of the right middle lobe and lingula would go undetected with posterior chest auscultation.

radiograph and Figure 12-3*B* indicates what structures the shadows represent. Figure 12-4*A* shows the location of various lung lobes on a frontal projection and Figure 12-4*B*, a lateral film, shows the location of these lobes when the chest is viewed from the side.

CHEST FILM FINDINGS IN MYOCARDIAL INFARCTION AND CONDITIONS THAT MAY MIMIC MYOCARDIAL INFARCTION

A bedside chest film of a patient with an uncomplicated MI is shown in Figure 12-5. Note that this is basically a normal chest film except that, possibly because of pain, the patient has failed to take a deep breath and thus the lung fields are not as large as they would normally appear. This is a lordotic view, which decreases the apparent height of the lung fields as well. Because it is an anteroposterior exposure, the patient's heart appears enlarged, although in reality it may not be. Patients with MI or pulmonary thromboembolism may have normal chest radiographs. A ventilation-perfusion lung scan or pulmonary angiogram is necessary to diagnose the latter. Table 12-1 includes conditions that may mimic an acute MI. Figures 12-6 through 12-14 are radiographs

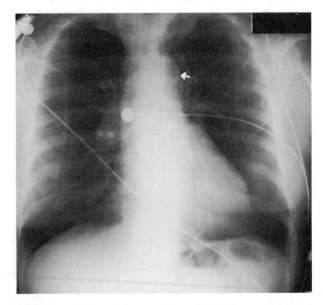

FIGURE 12-5 Normal chest radiograph. This is an anteroposterior lordotic radiograph of a patient admitted to rule out myocardial infarction. The lung fields are clear. Because this is an anteroposterior film, heart size cannot be accurately assessed (see text). Monitoring leads are visible, and calcium is present in the aortic knob (*arrow*).

(*Text continues on page 258*)

TABLE 12-1	**Differential Diagnosis of Acute Myocardial Infarction (MI)**

Pericarditis

Pulmonary embolus

Dissecting thoracic aortic aneurysm

Pleurisy

Pneumonia

Pancoast tumor

Abdominal problem (ruptured viscus, esophageal spasm, cholelithiasis)

Herpes zoster

Thoracic musculoskeletal pain

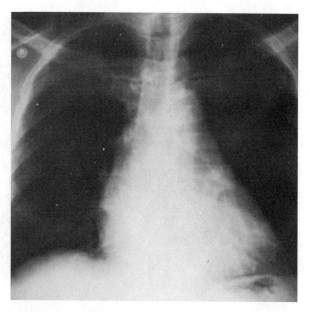

FIGURE 12-6 Pericardial effusion. This patient was admitted to rule out myocardial infarction. A pericardial friction rub was present. ST segments were elevated across the precordium, consistent with pericarditis. However, pericarditis was not diagnosed, and the patient was heparinized. Subsequently, he bled into the pericardium and cardiac tamponade developed. Cardiomegaly may be difficult to distinguish from a pericardial effusion. An echocardiogram can differentiate between the two.

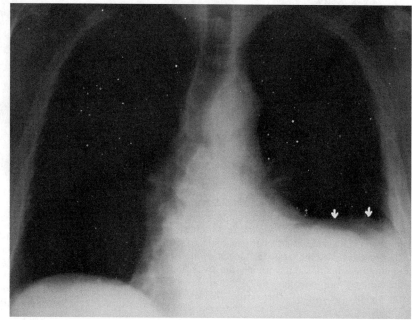

FIGURE 12-7 Left pleural effusion. Some common causes of pleural effusion are pulmonary embolus, heart failure, and neoplasm. Pulmonary embolus, an infection in the pleural space, or a neoplasm may cause acute chest pain. Physical findings of pleural effusion include absent breath sounds, dullness on percussion, and possibly (if massive) shift of the trachea to the side away from the pleural effusion. The presence of free pleural fluid can be documented by filming the patient with left side down and noting that the fluid shifts with gravity. An x-ray film taken in this position is known as a *left lateral decubitus radiograph.*

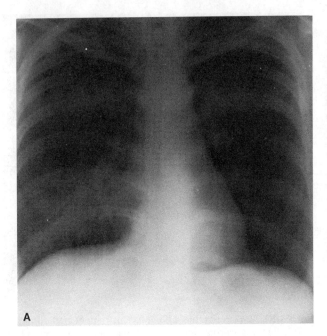

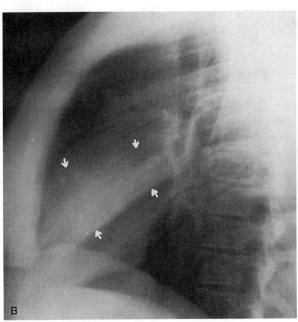

FIGURE 12-8 (A) Right middle lobe pneumonia. The patient usually has cough, sputum, fever, chills, and possible chest pain. Physical findings include bronchial breathing, crackles, and dullness over the right anterior chest. The infiltrate obscures the right heart border, indicating that the infiltrate is in an anterior position. (B) The middle lobe location is confirmed on the lateral chest radiograph (*arrows*).

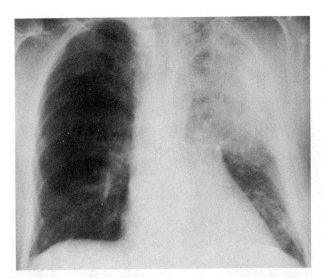

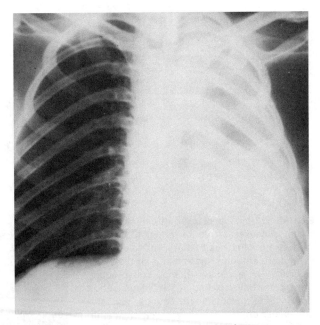

FIGURE 12-9 Left upper lobe pneumonia. Symptoms and signs are as in right middle lobe pneumonia, although the signs of consolidation (bronchial breathing, crackles, and dullness to percussion) are heard over the left upper chest. In pneumonia, egophony is heard over areas of consolidated lung. The patient is instructed to say the letter "e," and the lung is auscultated to demonstrate this finding. Normally the "e" sound is heard, but consolidated lung changes the "e" to an "a" that sounds like the "bleating of a goat." This sign is also known as "an e-to-a change."

FIGURE 12-10 Massive atelectasis of the left lung. The patient may have acute shortness of breath. Volume loss in the left chest is indicated by the shift of the heart to the left (right heart border over the spine), tracheal shift (noted by a shift of the tracheostomy tube), and by elevation of the left hemidiaphragm. Physical findings of atelectasis include absent breath sounds, dullness on percussion, and evidence of tracheal shift.

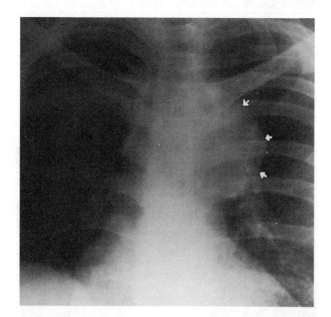

FIGURE 12-11 Dissecting aortic aneurysm. The mediastinum is widened (*arrows*). The patient may have chest pain radiating to the neck or through to the back. Blood pressure may be higher in the right arm than in the left. A murmur of aortic insufficiency may be present.

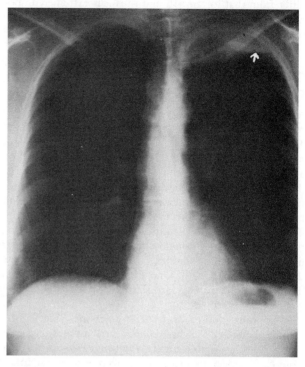

FIGURE 12-13 Pancoast tumor, a bronchogenic carcinoma in the apex of the left lung. In this location, it invades the brachial plexus and pleura. Patients may have left-sided chest pain that radiates into the neck and down the left arm, and thus may stimulate a myocardial infarction. They frequently have neurologic abnormalities in the involved arm.

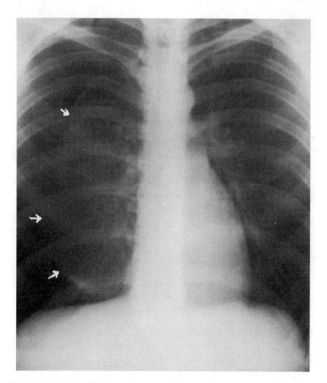

FIGURE 12-12 Pneumothorax. The patient may have acute chest pain and shortness of breath. Physical findings include absent or reduced breath sounds on the side of the pneumothorax and tympany or a hollow sound on chest percussion, with possibly a shift of the trachea to the side away from the pneumothorax. The *arrows* indicate the outer border of the right lung. The remainder of the right chest cavity is filled with air in the pleural space.

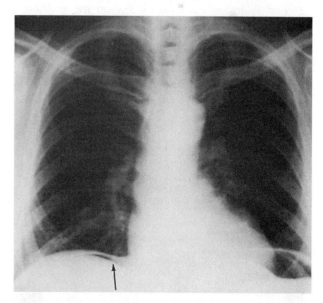

FIGURE 12-14 Free air under the diaphragm (*arrow*). This patient had epigastric pain and diaphoresis. The admission radiograph showed free air under the diaphragm consistent with a perforated viscus. At operation, a perforated peptic ulcer was found. The patient must be upright for the air to be seen under the diaphragm.

of some conditions encountered in the differential diagnosis of an acute MI. The treatment for these conditions may differ from that for an MI, and thus it is extremely important to obtain a chest film early in a patient's course to help rule out these conditions.

CHEST FILM FINDINGS IN COMPLICATIONS OF ACUTE MYOCARDIAL INFARCTION

Table 12-2 lists some of the complications of MI. *Acute pulmonary edema* (Figs. 12-15 and 12-16) may result from a wide variety of causes, including myocardial dysfunction due to ischemia, fluid overload, arrhythmias, papillary muscle rupture, ruptured interventricular septum, and development of a ventricular aneurysm. *Pericarditis* is usually manifested by a new and pleuritic type of pain different from that of an infarct, although it may seem similar. If pericardial fluid is absent or minimal, a pericardial rub is heard, and the cardiac outline may be normal. If a *pericardial effusion* develops, the rub may disappear and the chest film looks like that in Figure 12-6 or 12-17.

Symptoms due to *ventricular aneurysms* (Fig. 12-18) include congestive heart failure, arrhythmias, systemic emboli, and intractable angina. *Pulmonary emboli* may arise from clots within the heart or the deep venous system and may show *pleural effusion* (see Fig. 12-7), atelectasis, or consolidation on the radiograph, but commonly the chest radiograph is normal.

MISCELLANEOUS USES OF THE CHEST RADIOGRAPH

Figures 12-19 through 12-26 are examples of how the chest radiograph is used to confirm the position of

TABLE 12-2	Complications of Acute Myocardial Infarction (MI)

Congestive heart failure
Arrhythmias
Pericarditis, Dressler's syndrome
Pulmonary or systemic emboli
Ventricular aneurysm
Rupture of ventricular septum, papillary muscle, or ventricle

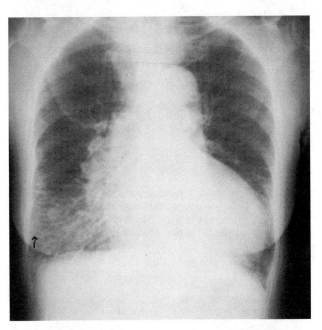

FIGURE 12-16 Cardiogenic pulmonary edema with cardiomegaly. In this radiograph, Kerley B lines are seen (*arrow*). These represent dilated pulmonary lymph vessels, which facilitate pulmonary edema removal from the alveolar spaces.

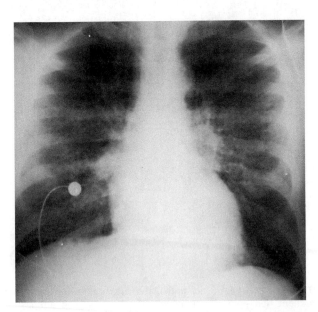

FIGURE 12-15 Cardiogenic pulmonary edema. This radiograph shows bilateral fluffy densities. The fact that right and left sides are equally involved somewhat contradicts a diagnosis of pneumonia. Physical findings would include an S₃ gallop, distended neck veins, and bilateral crackles. In myocardial infarction, pulmonary edema may occur without cardiac enlargement (cardiomegaly).

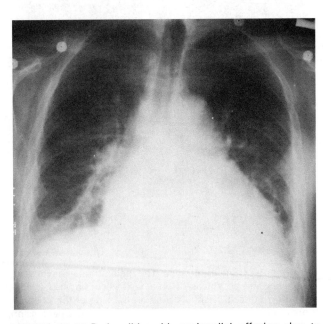

FIGURE 12-17 Pericarditis with pericardial effusion due to myocardial infarction. A pericardial friction rub may be present, and the electrocardiogram may show generalized ST segment elevation and PR segment depression. Neck veins are elevated and pulmonary artery catheterization may show equal elevation of right- and left-sided pressures. The diagnosis is confirmed by echocardiography.

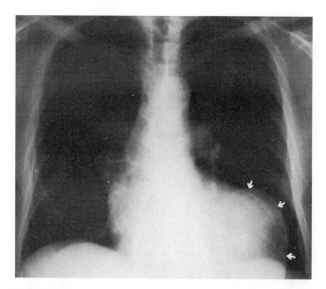

FIGURE 12-18 Left ventricular aneurysm. The heart is enlarged. This long-standing aneurysm is outlined by calcium (*arrows*); acutely, the patient may have arrhythmias, intractable angina, left ventricular failure, or systemic emboli. The electrocardiogram shows persistent elevation of the ST segment, and physical examination may reveal a rocking or abnormally pulsating precordium.

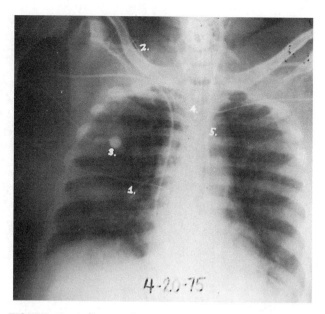

FIGURE 12-19 Chest radiograph of a patient with pulmonary edema, showing the position of (*1*) pulmonary artery (Swan-Ganz) catheter; (*2*) incorrect position of central venous pressure catheter ending in neck, not thorax; (*3*) cardiac monitoring leads; (*4*) tracheostomy tube; and (*5*) nasogastric tube.

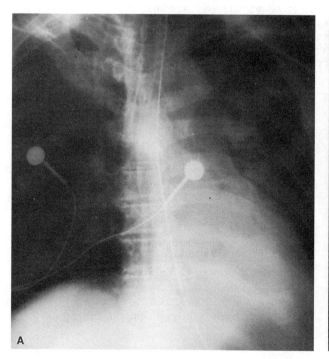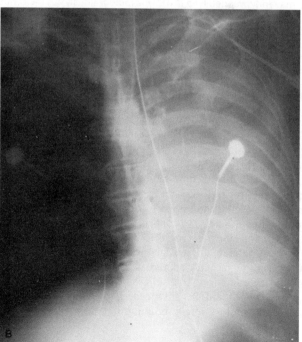

FIGURE 12-20 (**A**) Endotracheal tube positioned in right main stem bronchus. (**B**) If tube is left in this position, atelectasis of the left lung would result. The tube should be positioned several centimeters above the carina.

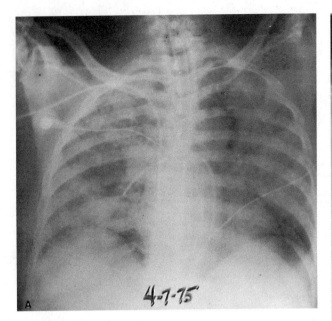

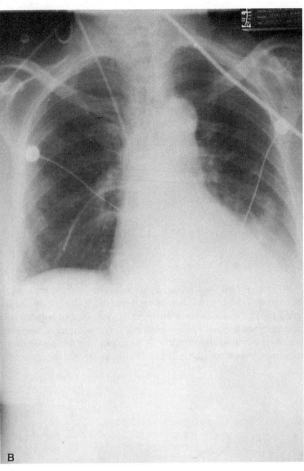

FIGURE 12-21 (**A**) Proper position of a pulmonary artery catheter. However, waveform analysis is essential to confirm accurate placement because even in this position the catheter would be permanently wedged (see text). This radiograph shows the diffuse pulmonary edema seen in a patient with the adult respiratory distress syndrome (ARDS). ARDS is noncardiogenic pulmonary edema; the wedge pressure is low or normal, and edema forms because the pulmonary capillaries are injured or "leaky." ARDS may occur in some cases of myocardial infarction. (**B**) Improper position of pulmonary artery line (too far out into the right lower lobe pulmonary artery). If the catheter is left in this position, pulmonary infarction can occur.

invasively placed lines, tubes, and wires. Figure 12-19 is a radiograph of a patient in cardiogenic shock. All tubes are in correct position except the central venous pressure line (see legend).

Figure 12-20 indicates the results of an improperly positioned endotracheal tube, and Figure 12-21*A* indicates the proper position of a pulmonary artery catheter. Whereas the chest radiograph helps to confirm its position, careful analysis of the waveform is crucial to the prevention of complications. A permanently wedged tracing (Fig. 12-21*B*) indicates that the catheter should be pulled back to prevent pulmonary infarction. If a right ventricular tracing is seen, the catheter should be advanced, if possible, to prevent arrhythmias and to obtain meaningful data.

Figure 12-22 shows a chest tube in the right pleural space placed to correct a right pneumothorax, and Figure 12-23 shows correct placement of an intra-aortic balloon pump catheter placed to improve the cardiac output in a patient with cardiogenic shock.

Figures 12-24, 12-25, and 12-26 show proper placement of unipolar, dual-chamber, and epicardial pacemaker electrodes.

The chest radiograph provides useful data that aid in the total assessment of the patient in the CCU. Early diagnosis of complications and improperly placed invasive lines improves patient care, and knowledge of the radiographic findings in disease processes augments the nurse's understanding of cardiopulmonary pathophysiology.

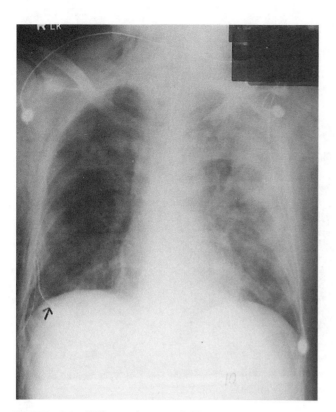

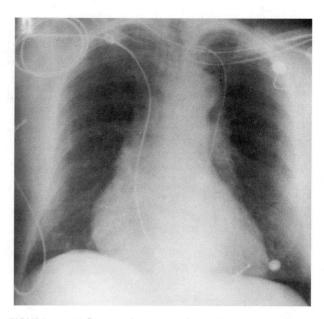

FIGURE 12-24 Proper placement of a right ventricular pace-maker electrode.

FIGURE 12-22 Diffuse pulmonary infiltrates due to adult respiratory distress syndrome. A right-sided pneumothorax has been treated with a chest tube (*arrow*). Air has also dissected up the tracheobronchial tree and into the neck. Air is seen in the soft tissues of the neck and thorax (*right side*). Air under the skin is known as subcutaneous emphysema and may occur without a pneumothorax if alveoli rupture deep in the lung, away from the pleural surface. Crackles are felt when the skin is palpated, and these may be mistaken for rales.

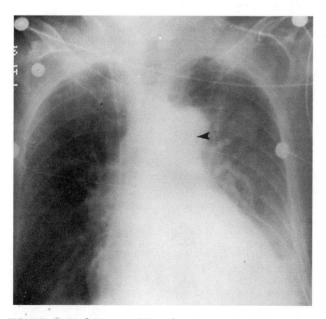

FIGURE 12-23 Correct position of an intra-aortic balloon pump catheter just below the arch of the aorta. *Arrow* indicates position of the catheter tip.

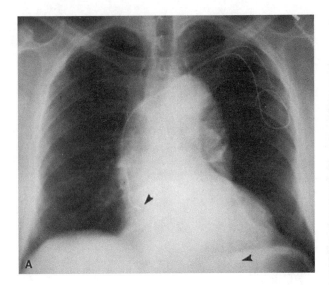

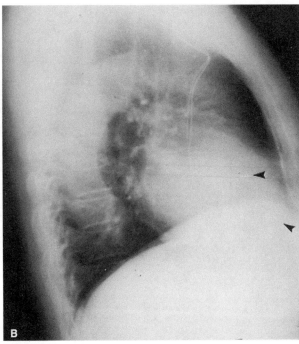

FIGURE 12-25 Proper position of a dual-chamber pacing electrodes in the right atrium and right ventricle. **(A)** posteroanterior view. **(B)** Lateral view. Dual-chamber pacing may improve cardiac output in some patients.

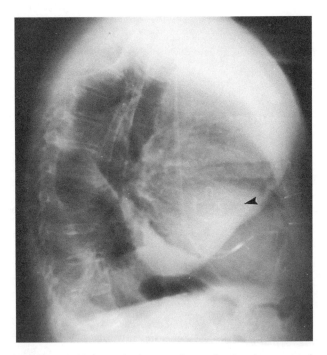

FIGURE 12-26 Lateral chest radiograph showing properly placed epicardial pacing wires placed during cardiac surgery. *Arrow* indicates tip of one wire. These are usually removed several days after surgery. A dual-chamber pacemaker is also in place. A correctly positioned aortic porcine valve is shown (*arrow*).

BIBLIOGRAPHY

Fraser RG, Pare JAP, Pare PD et al: Diagnosis of Diseases of the Chest, pp 1–295. Philadelphia, WB Saunders, 1988

George RB, Light RW, Matthay MA et al: Chest Medicine: Essentials of Pulmonary and Critical Care Medicine, pp 81–92. Baltimore, Williams & Wilkins, 1995

Lillington GA: A Diagnostic Approach to Chest Diseases, pp 23–27. Baltimore, Williams & Wilkins, 1987

13

Electrocardiography

CAROL JACOBSON

ELECTRICAL CONDUCTION THROUGH THE HEART

The electrical impulse of the heart is the stimulus for cardiac contraction. The conduction system (Fig. 13-1) is responsible for the initiation of the electrical impulse and its sequential spread through the atria, atrioventricular (AV) junction, and ventricles.

The Cardiac Conduction System

The conduction system of the heart consists of the following structures.

SINUS NODE

The sinus or sinoatrial (SA) node is a small group of cells in the high right atrium that functions as the normal pacemaker of the heart because it has the fastest rate of automaticity. The SA node normally depolarizes between 60 to 100 times per minute.

ATRIOVENTRICULAR NODE

The AV node is a small group of cells in the low right atrium near the tricuspid valve. The AV node has three main functions:

1. Its major job is to slow conduction of the impulse from the atria to the ventricles to allow time for the atria to contract and empty their blood into the ventricles.
2. It has automaticity at a rate of 40 to 60 beats/min and can function as a backup pacemaker if the SA node fails.
3. It screens out rapid atrial impulses to protect the ventricles from dangerously fast rates when the atrial rate is very rapid.

BUNDLE OF HIS

The bundle of His is a short bundle of fibers at the bottom of the AV node leading to the bundle branches. Conduction velocity accelerates in the bundle of His and the impulse is transmitted to both bundle branches.

BUNDLE BRANCHES

The bundle branches are bundles of fibers that rapidly conduct the impulse into the right and left ventricles. The *right bundle* branch travels along the right side of the interventricular septum and carries the impulse into the right ventricle. The *left bundle branch* has two main divisions, the anterior fascicle and the posterior fascicle, which carry the impulse into the left ventricle.

PURKINJE FIBERS

The Purkinje fibers are hair-like fibers that spread out from the bundle branches along the endocardial surface of both ventricles and rapidly conduct the impulse to the ventricular muscle cells. Cells in the Purkinje system have automaticity at a rate of 20 to 40 beats/min and can function as a backup pacemaker if all other pacemakers fail.

Origin and Spread of the Electrical Impulse Through the Heart

The impulse normally begins in the SA node, located in the high right atrium, because the SA node has the fastest rate of automaticity of all potential pacemaker cells in the heart. The impulse spreads from the SA node through both atria in an inferior and leftward direction, resulting in depolarization of the atrial muscle. When the impulse reaches the AV node, its conduction velocity is slowed before it continues into the ventricles. The slowing in the AV node is necessary to allow time for the atria to contract and empty their blood into the ventricles before the ventricles contract. When the impulse emerges from the AV node, it travels rapidly through the bundle of His and down the right and left bundle branches

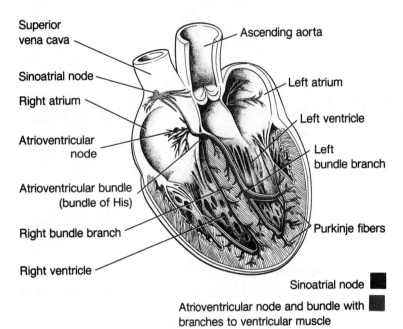

Superior
vena cava

Ascending aorta

Sinoatrial node

Left atrium

Right atrium

Left ventricle

Atrioventricular
node

Left
bundle branch

Atrioventricular bundle
(bundle of His)

Right bundle branch

Purkinje fibers

Right ventricle

Sinoatrial node ■

Atrioventricular node and bundle with ■
branches to ventricular muscle

FIGURE 13-1 Cardiac conduction system. (From Jacobson C: Cardiac arrhythmias and conduction abnormalities. In Patrick ML, Woods SL, Craven RF et al [eds]: Medical–Surgical Nursing, 2nd ed, p 649. Philadelphia, JB Lippincott, 1991.)

into the Purkinje network of both ventricles, and results in depolarization of the ventricular muscle. The spread of this wave of depolarization through the heart produces the classic surface electrocardiogram (ECG), which can be recorded by an electrocardiograph (ECG machine) or monitored continuously on a bedside cardiac monitor.

Waves, Complexes, and Intervals of the Cardiac Cycle

The ECG waves, complexes, and intervals are illustrated in Figure 13-2. Table 13-1 summarizes normal waveform configurations in each of the 12 ECG leads.

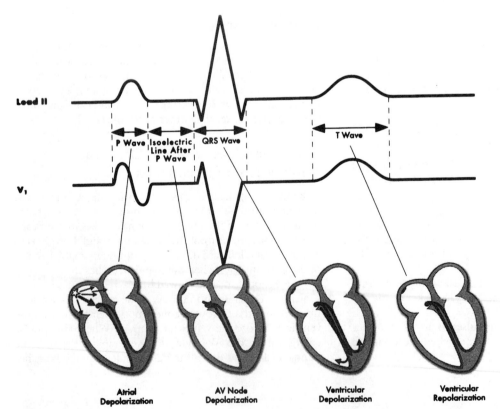

Lead II

V₁

P Wave | Isoelectric Line After P Wave | QRS Wave

T Wave

Atrial
Depolarization

AV Node
Depolarization

Ventricular
Depolarization

Ventricular
Repolarization

FIGURE 13-2 Waves, complexes, and intervals of the cardiac cycle in leads II and V₁.

TABLE 13-1	Normal Electrocardiogram Waveform Configuration in Each of the 12 Leads					
Lead	P Wave	Q Wave	R Wave	S Wave	T Wave	ST Segment
I	Upright	Small	Largest wave of complex	Small (less than R or none)	Upright	May vary from +1 to –0.5 mm
II	Upright	Small or none	Large (vertical heart)	Small (less than R or none)	Upright	May vary from +1 to –0.5 mm
III	Upright, diphasic, or inverted	Usually small or none (for large Q to be diagnostic, a Q must also be present in a VF)	None to large	None to large (horizontal heart)	Upright, diphasic, or inverted	May vary from +1 to –0.5 mm
aVR	Inverted	Small, none, or large	Small or none	Large (may be QS complex)	Inverted	May vary from +1 to –0.5 mm
aVL	Upright, diphasic, or inverted	Small, none, or large (to be diagnostic, Q must also be present in I or precordial leads)	Small, none, or large (horizontal heart)	None to large (vertical heart)	Upright, diphasic, or inverted	May vary from +1 to –0.5 mm
aVF	Upright	Small or none	Small, none, or large (vertical heart)	None to large (horizontal heart)	Upright, diphasic, or inverted	May vary from +1 to –0.5 mm
V_1	Upright, diphasic, or inverted	None or QS complex	Less than S wave or none	Large (may be QS)	Upright, diphasic, or inverted	May vary from 0 to +3 mm
V_2	Upright	None (rare QS)	Less than S wave, or none (larger than V_1)	Large (may be QS)	Upright	May vary from 0 to +3 mm
V_3	Upright	Small or none	Less, greater, or equal to S wave; (larger than V_2)	Large (greater, less, or equal to R wave)	Upright	May vary from 0 to +3 mm
V_4	Upright	Small or none	Greater than S (larger than V_3)	Smaller than R (smaller than V_3)	Upright	May vary from +1 to –0.5 mm
V_5	Upright	Small	Larger than R in V_4; less than 26 mm	Smaller than S in V_4	Upright	May vary from +1 to –0.5 mm
V_6	Upright	Small	Large; less than 26 mm	Smaller than S in V_5	Upright	May vary from +1 to –0.5 mm

U waves may follow T waves, particularly in leads V_2 to V_4, are upright; and are of lower amplitude than T waves.

Adapted from Goldschlager N, Goldman MJ: Principles of Clinical Electrocardiography, 13th ed. Norwalk, CT, Appleton & Lange, 1989.

P WAVE

The P wave represents atrial muscle depolarization. It is normally small, smoothly rounded, and no taller than 2.5 mm or wider than 0.11 second.

QRS COMPLEX

The QRS complex represents ventricular muscle depolarization. The shape of the QRS complex depends on the lead being recorded and the ventricular activation sequence; not all leads record all waves of the QRS complex. A Q wave is an initial negative deflection from baseline and should be less than 0.03 second in duration and less than 25% of the R-wave amplitude. An R wave is the first positive deflection from baseline. An S wave is a negative deflection that follows an R wave. When a complex is all positive, it is just an R wave; when it is all negative, it is called a QS. Regardless of the shape of the complex, ventricular depolarization waves are called QRS complexes (Fig. 13-3). The width of the QRS complex represents intraventricular conduction time and is measured from the point at which it first leaves the baseline to the end of the last appearing wave. Normal QRS width is 0.04 to 0.10 second.

T WAVE

The T wave represents ventricular muscle repolarization. It follows the QRS complex and is normally in the same direction as the QRS complex. The T wave is usually rounded and slightly asymmetric, rising more slowly than it descends. T waves are not normally taller than 5 mm in any limb lead or 10 mm in any precordial lead.

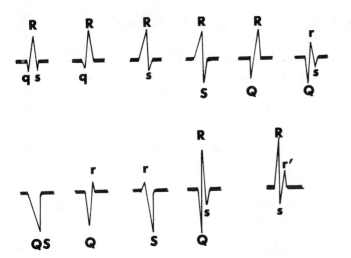

FIGURE 13-3 Examples of various QRS complexes.

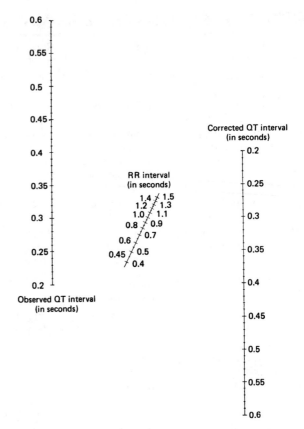

FIGURE 13-4 Nomogram for rate correction of QT interval. Measure the observed QT interval and the RR interval. Mark these values in the respective columns of the chart (left and middle). Place a ruler across these two points. The point at which the extension of this line crosses the third column is the corrected QT interval (QTc). (From Kissin M, Schwarzschild MM, Bakst H: A nomogram for rate correction of the QT interval in the electrocardiogram. Am Heart J 35: 991, 1948.)

U WAVE

The U wave is a small, rounded wave that sometimes follows the T wave and is most prominent in leads V_2 or V_3. The U wave is normally in the same direction as the T wave but is only approximately 10% of its amplitude. The U wave is thought to be part of the ventricular repolarization process and may represent repolarization of the Purkinje network or certain endocardial cells in the ventricle, or summation of ventricular afterdepolarizations.

PR INTERVAL

The PR interval is measured from the beginning of the P wave to the beginning of the QRS complex and represents the time required for the impulse to travel through the atria, AV junction, and Purkinje system. The normal PR interval is 0.12 to 0.20 second.

ST SEGMENT

The ST segment represents the period of time when the ventricle is still depolarized. It begins at the end of the QRS complex (J point) and extends to the beginning of the T wave. The ST segment should be at the isoelectric line and gently curve up into the T wave.

QT INTERVAL

The QT interval measures the duration of ventricular activation and recovery and is measured from the beginning of the QRS complex to the end of the T wave. The QT interval varies inversely with the heart rate and must be corrected to a heart rate of 60 after measurement (QTc interval). Because the QT interval adjusts gradually to a change in heart rate, accurate measurement of the QTc can be done only after several regular and equal cardiac cycles. The normal QTc is usually less than half the preceding RR interval at normal heart rates, but a more accurate evaluation can be done using the nomogram for rate correction of the QT interval (Fig. 13-4). The upper limit of normal QTc has been stated as 0.42 second for men and 0.43 second for women,[4] but may be as long as 0.44 second for men and 0.47 second for women.

BASIC ELECTROCARDIOGRAPHY

The ECG is the graphic record of the electrical activity of the heart. The spread of the electrical impulse through the heart produces weak electrical currents through the entire body, which can be detected and amplified by the ECG machine and recorded on calibrated graph paper. These amplified signals form the ECG tracing, consisting of the waveforms and intervals described previously, and is inscribed onto grid paper that moves beneath the recording stylus (pen) at standard speed of 25 mm/s. The grid on the paper consists of a series of small and large boxes, both horizontally and vertically; horizontal boxes measure time, and vertical boxes measure voltage (Fig. 13-5). Each small box horizontally is equal to 0.04 second, and each large box horizontally is equal to 0.20 second. On the vertical axis, each small box measures 1 mm and is equal to 0.1 mV; each large box measures 5 mm and is equal to 0.5 mV. In addition to the grid, most ECG paper places a vertical line in the top margin at 3-second intervals or places a mark at 1-second intervals.

The waveforms of the cardiac cycle can be recorded by a bedside cardiac monitor and displayed continuously on an oscilloscope or recorded on a rhythm strip, which consists of the same grid as described previously. The standard 12-lead ECG simultaneously records 12 different views of

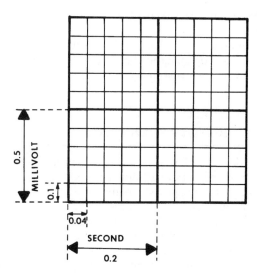

FIGURE 13-5 Time and voltage lines on electrocardiogram paper at standard paper speed of 25 mm/s. Horizontal axis measures time: each small box = 0.04 second, one large box = 0.20 second. Vertical axis measures voltage: each small box = 1 mm or 0.1 mV, one large box = 5 mm or 0.5 mV.

electrical activity as it travels through the heart and displays all 12 views on a full-page layout, which consists of the same grid. The 12 leads of the ECG are described in detail in following sections.

Determining Heart Rate on the Electrocardiogram

Heart rate can be determined from the ECG strip by several methods. An easy method that can be used for both regular and irregular rhythms is to count the number of RR intervals (not R waves) in a 6-second strip and multiply that number by 10, because there are 10 6-second intervals in 1 minute (Fig. 13-6*A*).

Another method that can be used only if the rhythm is regular is to count the number of large boxes between two R waves and divide that number into 300, because there are 300 large boxes in a 1-minute strip. The most accurate method to use for a regular rhythm is to count the number of small boxes between two R waves and divide that number into 1,500, because there are 1,500 small boxes in a 1-minute strip. The easiest way to do either of these methods is to use the rate ruler in Figure 13-6*B*.

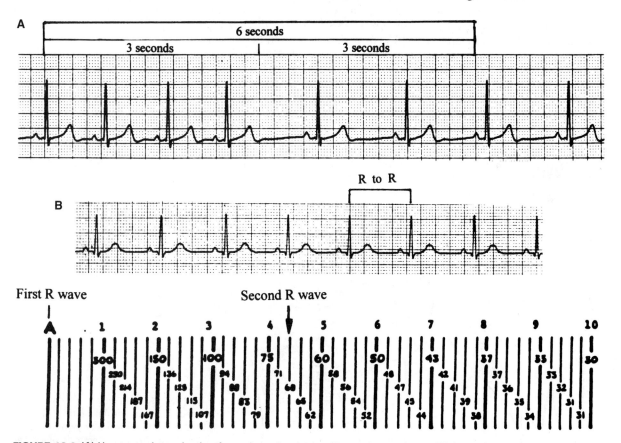

FIGURE 13-6 **(A)** Heart rate determination for an irregular rhythm. Count the number or RR intervals in a 6-second strip and multiply by 10. In **(A)**, there are almost six complete RR intervals in a 6-second strip; the heart rate is 60 beats/min. **(B)** Heart rate determination for a regular rhythm using the rate ruler. Count the number of large and small boxes between R waves on the rhythm strip. In **(B)**, there are four large boxes and two small boxes between the R waves marked on the strip. On the rate ruler, the first R wave is represented by the thick line marked "A." Each large box on the electrocardiogram paper is represented by a thick line on the rate ruler and is numbered at the top; each small box on the strip is represented by a thin line on the ruler. The number on the line on the ruler that corresponds to the second R wave on the strip represents the heart rate. In **(B)**, count four large boxes at the top of the ruler and then two small boxes; the heart rate is 68 beats/min (represented by the arrow). (Rate ruler in **B** from Marriott HJL: Practical Electrocardiography, 8th ed, p 15. Baltimore, Williams & Wilkins, 1988.)

Determining the Cardiac Rhythm on the Electrocardiogram

The first step in interpreting a 12-lead ECG is to determine the cardiac rhythm. A rhythm strip should be analyzed in a systematic manner to aid in rhythm interpretation until the learner is able to identify arrhythmias by scanning the strip. See Chapter 14 for detailed information on the normal cardiac rhythm and both basic and advanced arrhythmias. The following steps provide a systematic approach to rhythm interpretation.

Regularity: First determine if the rhythm is regular or irregular because this information determines the method of heart rate calculation. If the rhythm is irregular, determine if the irregularity is random or if it occurs in a pattern (i.e., repetitive groups of beats separated by a pause).

Rate: Determine the heart rate as described previously. Determine both atrial and ventricular rates if they are not the same.

P waves: Locate P waves and note their shape and relationship to QRS complexes. Determine if all P waves look alike and if they have a consistent relationship to QRS complexes (i.e., one P wave before every QRS, two or more P waves before each QRS) or if they occur randomly and are unrelated to QRS complexes.

PR interval: Measure the PR interval of several complexes in a row to determine if it is of normal duration and consistent for all complexes.

QRS width: Measure the QRS complex and determine if it is normal or wide.

Determine the rhythm based on an analysis of the information obtained in these steps. See Chapter 14 for details on arrhythmia analysis.

THE 12-LEAD ELECTROCARDIOGRAM

The 12-lead ECG records electrical activity as it spreads through the heart from 12 different leads that are recorded through electrodes placed on the arms, legs, and specific spots on the chest. Each lead represents a different view of the heart and consists of two electrodes with opposite polarity (bipolar) or one electrode and a reference point (unipolar). A *bipolar* lead has a positive pole and a negative pole, with each contributing equally to the recording. A *unipolar* lead has one positive pole and a reference pole in the center of the chest that is algebraically determined by the ECG machine. The reference pole represents the center of the electrical field of the heart and has a zero potential, so only the positive pole of a unipolar lead contributes to the tracing.

The standard 12-lead ECG consists of 6 limb leads that record electrical activity in the frontal plane–traveling up/down and right/left in the heart; and 6 precordial leads that record electrical activity in the horizontal plane–traveling anterior/posterior and right/left. Limb leads are recorded by electrodes placed on the arms and legs, whereas precordial leads are recorded by electrodes placed on the chest (Fig. 13-7). For convenience in contin-

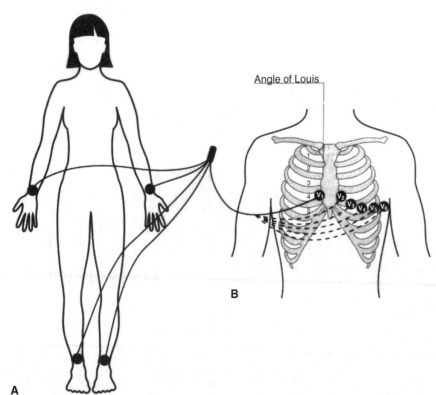

Angle of Louis

A

B

FIGURE 13-7 Electrode placement for limb leads and precordial leads. **(A)** Limb electrodes can be placed anywhere on the arms and legs. **(B)** Chest electrode placement. V_1 = fourth intercostal space at right sternal border; V_2 = fourth intercostal space at left sternal border; V_3 = halfway between V_2 and V_4 in a straight line; V_4 = fifth intercostal space at mid-clavicular line; V_5 = same level as V_4 at anterior axillary line; V_6 = same level as V_4 at mid-axillary line.

uous bedside monitoring, arm electrodes can be placed on the shoulders and leg electrodes on the lower part of the rib cage rather than on the limbs without significantly altering the signals recorded.

A camera analogy makes the 12-lead ECG easier to understand. Each lead of the ECG represents a picture of the electrical activity in the heart taken by the camera. In any lead, the positive electrode is the recording electrode or the camera lens. The negative electrode tells the camera which way to "shoot" its picture and determines the direction in which the positive electrode records. When the positive electrode sees electrical activity traveling toward it, it records an upright deflection on the ECG. When the positive electrode sees electrical activity traveling away from it, it records a negative deflection (Fig. 13-8). If the electrical activity travels perpendicular to a positive electrode, either a diphasic deflection or no activity is recorded. The ECG records three bipolar frontal plane leads—lead I, lead II, and lead III—and three unipolar frontal plane leads: aVR, aVL, and aVF. In addition, there are six unipolar precordial leads: V_1, V_2, V_3, V_4, V_5, and V_6.

Bipolar Leads

Figure 13-9*A* illustrates the three bipolar frontal plane leads. In each lead, the camera represents the positive pole of the lead. In lead I, the positive electrode is on the left arm and the negative on the right arm. Any electrical activity in the heart that travels toward the positive electrode (camera lens) on the left arm is recorded as an upright deflection and any traveling away from it is recorded as a negative deflection. In lead II, the positive electrode is on the left leg and the negative electrode is on the right arm. Any electrical activity traveling toward the left leg electrode (camera lens) is recorded as an upright deflection and any traveling away from it toward the right arm electrode is recorded as a negative deflection. In lead III, the positive electrode is on the left leg and the negative electrode is on the left arm. Any electrical activity coming toward the left leg electrode (camera lens) is recorded upright and any traveling away from it toward the left arm is recorded negative. The right leg electrode serves as a ground and does not contribute to the signals recorded. The electrical sum

of the voltages in the three bipolar frontal plane leads equals zero potential and forms a virtual ground in the center of the triangle used by the unipolar leads as their reference point.

Unipolar Leads

Figure 13-9*B* illustrates the three unipolar frontal plane leads, aVR, aVL, and aVF. The camera represents the location of the positive electrode: on the right shoulder for aVR, on the left shoulder for aVL, and at the foot (left leg) for aVF. The "negative end" of the unipolar lead is the reference point in the center of the chest that is obtained as described previously. The same principles apply to unipolar leads: any electrical activity traveling toward the positive electrode is recorded as an upright deflection and any traveling away from it is recorded as a negative deflection. Figure 13-9*C* shows the six unipolar precordial leads recording from their locations on the chest and "shooting" toward the reference point in the center of the heart.

Right Chest and Posterior Leads

Additional leads can be recorded on the right chest or posterior thorax to gain additional information about right ventricular or posterior infarction or right ventricular hypertrophy (RVH). Figure 13-10 shows lead placement for obtaining right chest leads and posterior leads.

The Hexaxial Reference System

Figure 13-11*A* shows the *hexaxial reference system* that is formed when the six frontal plane leads are moved together in such a way that they bisect each other in the center. Each lead is labeled at its positive end to make it easy to remember where the positive electrode is. In Figure 13-11*B*, the hexaxial reference system is superimposed over a drawing of the heart to illustrate how each lead views the heart. The reference system forms a 360-degree circle surrounding the heart with 180 positive degrees and 180 negative degrees. By convention, the positive end of lead I is designated 0 degrees and the six leads divide the circle into 30-degree segments, as labeled in the figure.

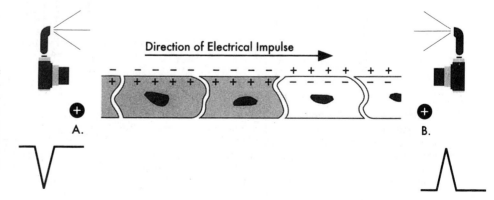

FIGURE 13-8 A strip of cardiac muscle depolarizing in the direction of the arrow. A positive electrode at *B* sees depolarization coming toward it and records an upright deflection. A positive electrode at *A* sees depolarization going away from it and records a negative deflection.

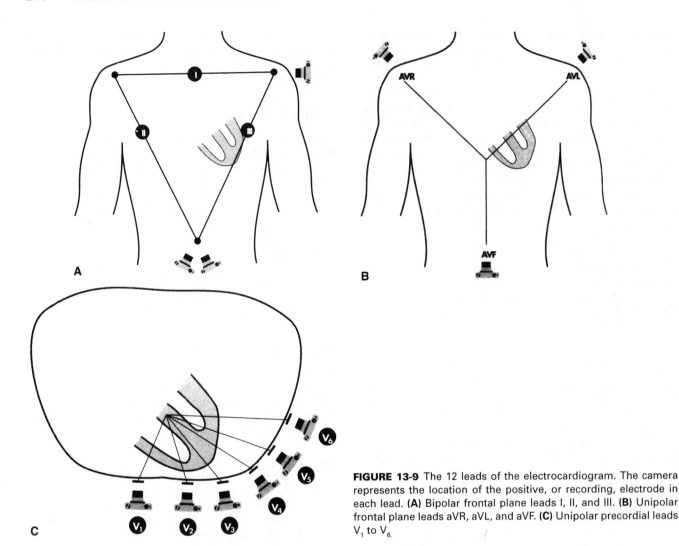

FIGURE 13-9 The 12 leads of the electrocardiogram. The camera represents the location of the positive, or recording, electrode in each lead. **(A)** Bipolar frontal plane leads I, II, and III. **(B)** Unipolar frontal plane leads aVR, aVL, and aVF. **(C)** Unipolar precordial leads V_1 to V_6.

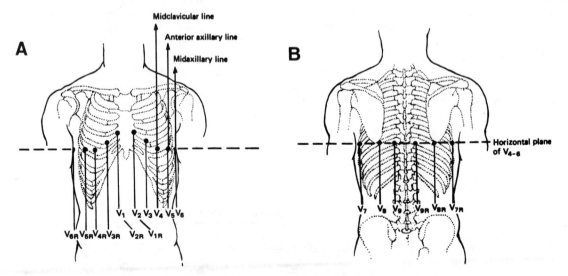

FIGURE 13-10 (A) Electrode placement for the six standard precordial leads and for right precordial leads. Right chest leads are a mirror image of left chest leads: V_{1R} is the same as standard V_2, V_{2R} is the same as standard V_1, V_{3R} is halfway between V_{2R} and V_{4R}, V_{4R} is the fifth intercostal space at the right mid-clavicular line, V_{5R} is the same level as V_{4R} in the right anterior axillary line, and V_{6R} is same level in right mid-axillary line. **(B)** Electrode placement for left posterior leads: V_7, posterior axillary line; V_8, posterior scapular line; V_9, left border of spine. All three are in the same horizontal plane of V_4 to V_6. (From Goldman MJ: Principles of Clinical Electrocardiography, 12th ed. Los Altos, CA, Lange Medical Publications, 1986.)

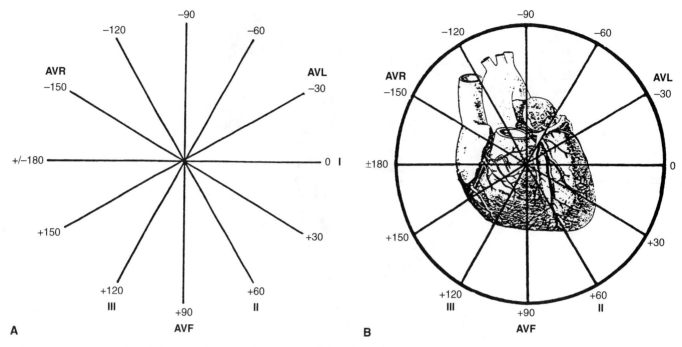

FIGURE 13-11 Hexaxial reference system (or axis wheel). Each lead is labeled at its positive end in both examples. **(A)** All six frontal plane leads bisect each other. The degrees of the axis wheel are shown. **(B)** The axis wheel superimposed on the heart to demonstrate each lead's view of the heart. Leads I and aVL face the left lateral wall, and leads II, III, and aVF face the inferior surface.

The 12 Views of the Heart

The normal sequence of depolarization through the heart and the resulting P, QRS, and T waves for each frontal plane lead are illustrated in Figure 13-12A. The impulse normally originates in the SA node high in the right atrium and spreads leftward through the left atrium and downward toward the AV node low in the right atrium. Leads I and aVL, with their positive electrode (camera lens) on the left side of the body, record this leftward electrical activity as an upright P wave because the positive electrode sees atrial depolarization coming toward it. Leads II, III, and aVF, with their positive electrode at the bottom of the heart, record the downward spread of atrial activity as upright P waves for the same reason. Lead aVR, with its positive electrode on the right shoulder, sees the electrical activity moving away from it and records a negative P wave.

As the impulse spreads through the AV node, no electrical activity is recorded because the AV node is too small to be recorded by surface leads. As the impulse exits the AV node, it moves through the bundle of His and enters the right and left bundle branches. The left bundle branch sprouts some Purkinje fibers high on the left side of the septum that carry the impulse into the septum and cause it to depolarize first in a left-to-right direction. The electrical impulse then enters the Purkinje system of both ventricular free walls simultaneously and depolarizes them from endocardium to epicardium (indicated by the small arrows through the ventricles in Fig. 13-12A). Millions of electrical impulses travel through the ventricles in three dimensions simultaneously, but if averaged together they move downward, leftward, and posterior toward the large left ventricle, as indicated by the large arrow in the same figure. This large arrow represents the *mean axis,* which is the net

direction of electrical depolarization through the ventricles when all the smaller arrows are averaged together.

The QRS complex is recorded as the ventricles depolarize. Leads I and aVL, with their positive electrodes on the left side of the body, see the septum depolarizing away from them and record a small negative deflection (Q wave). They then see the large left ventricular free wall depolarizing toward them and record an upright deflection (R wave). Leads II, III, and aVF, with their positive electrodes at the bottom of the heart, may not see septal activity at all and not record any deflection. If these leads see septal activity coming slightly toward them, they record a positive deflection. They all then see the forces moving downward toward them and record an upright deflection (R wave). Lead aVR, positive on the right shoulder, sees all activity moving away from it and records a negative deflection (QS complex).

The six precordial leads record electrical activity traveling in the horizontal plane. Figure 13-12B illustrates the position of the precordial leads and how they record electrical activity as it spreads through the ventricles in the horizontal plane. Lead V_1 is located on the front of the chest and records a small R wave as the septum depolarizes toward it from left to right. It then records a deep S wave as depolarization spreads away from it through the thick left ventricle. As the positive electrode is moved across the precordium from the V_1 to the V_6 position, it records progressively more left ventricular forces and the R wave gets progressively larger. Lead V_6 is located on the left side of the chest and usually records a small Q wave as the septum depolarizes from left to right away from the positive electrode, and a large R wave as electrical activity spreads toward the positive electrode through the thick left ventricle. Normal R-wave progression means that the R wave gets

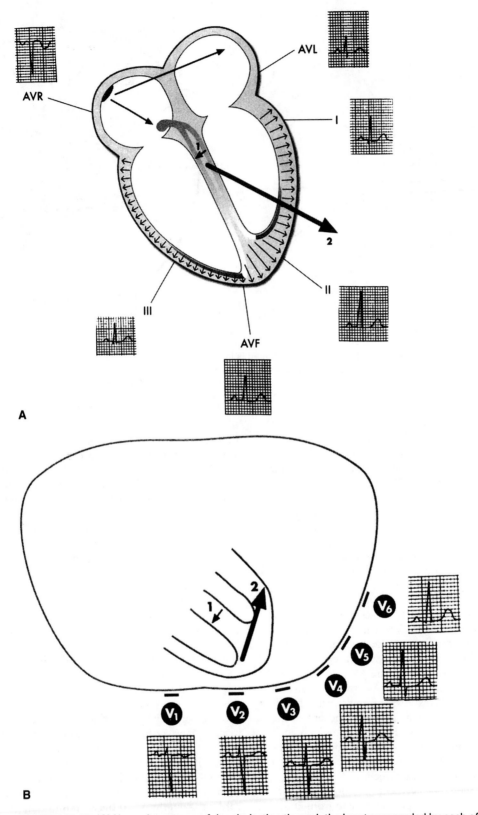

FIGURE 13-12 (A) Normal sequence of depolarization through the heart as recorded by each of the frontal plane leads. **(B)** Cross-section of the thorax illustrating how the six precordial leads record normal electrical activity in the ventricles. In both examples, the *small arrow* (*1*) shows the initial direction of depolarization through the septum, followed by the mean direction of ventricular free wall depolarization (*larger arrow* [*2*]).

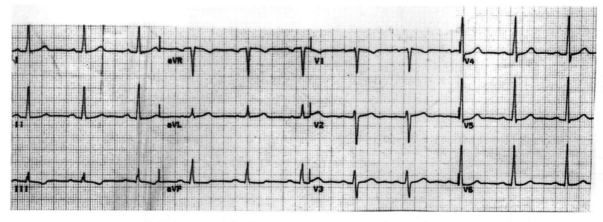

FIGURE 13-13 Normal 12-lead electrocardiogram.

progressively larger from V_1 to V_6, or that V_6 is predominantly an R wave compared with V_1, which is predominantly an S wave. Sometimes the largest precordial R wave is recorded in lead V_4 or V_5, which is a normal variant.

The Normal Adult 12-Lead Electrocardiogram

Table 13-1 lists normal waveform configurations for each of the 12 leads and Figure 13-13 shows a normal 12-lead ECG. Normal sinus rhythm is present, and the axis is +45 degrees. P waves are normal (they are flat in V_2, but this is not necessarily abnormal) and T waves are normal (inverted in lead III is a normal variant). The QRS complex is normal (0.08 second wide), there are no abnormal Q waves, and R-wave progression is normal across the precordium. The ST segment is at baseline in all leads. This ECG can be used for comparison as abnormalities are discussed throughout this chapter.

AXIS DETERMINATION

Conduction of a wave of depolarization through the myocardium results in propagation of thousands of electrical potentials in multiple directions. Over 80% of these potentials are balanced by similar instantaneous charges moving in opposite directions. Balanced alterations in electrical potentials result in an algebraic "canceling out" of these instantaneous vectors. What remains as the detected and amplified ECG tracing is the net vector, which reveals the magnitude, direction, and polarity of the mean electrical force as it courses through the myocardium. Frontal plane axis can be determined for P waves, QRS complexes, and T waves. This section deals only with QRS axis determination.

The normal QRS axis is defined as –30 to +110 degrees because most of the electrical forces in a normal heart are directed downward and leftward toward the large left ventricle. Left axis deviation is defined as –31 to –90 degrees and occurs when most of the forces move in a leftward and superior direction, as can happen in left ventricular hyper-

trophy, left anterior fascicular block (LAFB), inferior myocardial infarction (MI), left bundle-branch block (LBBB), several congenital defects, and some arrhythmias, especially ventricular tachycardia and Wolff-Parkinson-White syndrome. Right axis deviation is defined as +110 to +180 degrees and occurs when most of the forces move rightward, as can happen in RVH, left posterior fascicular block (LPFB), right bundle-branch block (RBBB), dextrocardia, ventricular tachycardia, and Wolff-Parkinson-White syndrome. When most of the forces are directed superior and rightward between –90 and –180 degrees, the term *indeterminate axis* is used. This axis can occur with ventricular tachycardia and occasionally with bifascicular block. Figure 13-14 shows the axis wheel divided into its normal, left deviation, right deviation, and indeterminate sections.

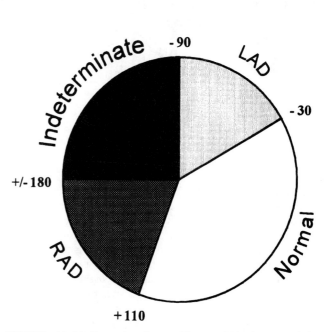

FIGURE 13-14 Normal axis = –30 to +110 degrees; left axis deviation (LAD) = –30 degrees to –90 degrees; right axis deviation (RAD) = +110 to 180 degrees; indeterminate axis = –90 to –180 degrees.

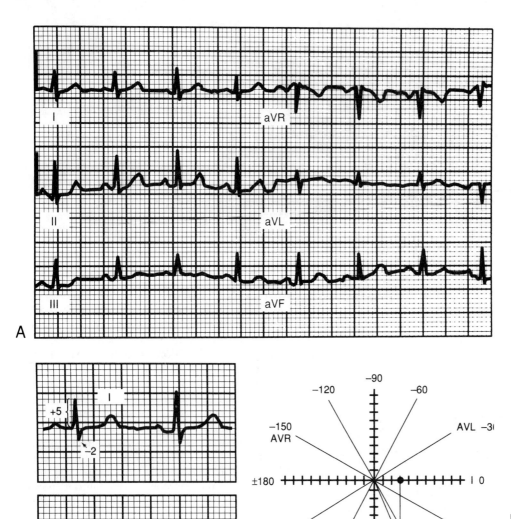

FIGURE 13-15 Calculating the mean QRS axis. **(A)** The six frontal plane leads of an electrocardiogram. **(B)** Lead I and lead aVF enlarged. See text for instructions on calculating the axis using leads I and aVF on the axis wheel.

The mean frontal plane QRS axis can be determined in a number of ways. The most accurate method is to average the forces moving right and left with those moving up and down because this represents the frontal plane. Because lead I is the most direct right/left lead and lead aVF is the most direct up/down lead, it is easiest to use these two perpendicular leads to calculate the mean axis. Figure 13-15*A* shows the frontal plane leads of a 12-lead ECG. In Figure 13-15*B*, leads I and aVF are shown enlarged along with the axis wheel with small hash marks along the axes of lead I and lead aVF. These hash marks represent the small 1-mV boxes on the ECG paper. To determine the mean QRS axis, follow these steps:

1. Look at the QRS complex in lead I and count the number of positive and negative boxes. Mark the net vector along the appropriate end of lead I on the axis wheel. In Figure 13-15*B*, the QRS complex in lead I is five boxes positive and two boxes negative, resulting in a net three boxes positive, or +3. Count three hash marks toward the positive end of lead I and put a mark on the axis wheel at that spot.
2. Look at the QRS complex in aVF and follow the same procedure as before. In this example, the QRS complex in aVF is eight boxes positive and has two very small negative deflections that equal approximately one box when added together, resulting in a

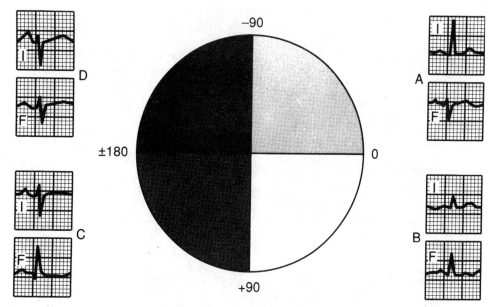

FIGURE 13-16 The four quadrants of the axis wheel. **(A)** Left quadrant, lead I is positive and lead aVF is negative. **(B)** Normal quadrant, both leads I and aVF are positive. **(C)** Right quadrant, lead I is negative and lead aVF is positive. **(D)** Indeterminate quadrant, both leads I and aVF are negative. (From Marriott HJL: Practical Electrocardiography, 8th ed. Baltimore, Williams & Wilkins, 1988.)

net +7. Count seven hash marks along the positive end of the aVF axis and place a mark at that spot.

3. Draw a perpendicular line down from the mark on the lead I axis and a perpendicular line across from the mark on the aVF axis.

4. Draw a line from the center of the axis wheel to the spot where these two perpendicular lines meet. This line is the mean QRS axis—approximately +65 degrees.

A quick but less accurate method of axis determination is to place the axis in its proper quadrant of the axis wheel by looking at lead I and aVF, because these leads divide the wheel into four quadrants. As illustrated in Figure 13-16, if both of these leads are positive, the axis falls in the normal quadrant, 0 to +90 degrees. If lead I is positive and aVF is negative, the axis falls in the left quadrant, 0 to –90 degrees. If lead I is negative and aVF is positive, the axis falls in the right quadrant, +90 to +180 degrees. If both leads are negative, the axis falls in the indeterminate quadrant or "no-man's-land," –90 to –180 degrees. Locating the correct quadrant is often adequate, but because the portion of the left quadrant for 0 to –30 degrees is considered normal, it is necessary to be more precise in describing the axis when it falls in the left quadrant. To fine-tune the axis quickly, find the limb lead with the smallest or most equiphasic QRS complex. This lead is not seeing much electrical force if it is equiphasic or very small, and therefore its perpendicular lead must be seeing most of the forces. Locate the perpendicular lead (lead I and aVF are perpendicular, lead II and aVL are perpendicular, lead III and aVR are perpendicular) and see if the QRS is positive or negative in that lead. If it is positive, the axis is directed toward the positive end of the lead, and if it is negative, the axis is directed toward the negative end of the lead. Using the ECG in Figure 13-15A, do the following:

1. Place the axis in its correct quadrant by looking at lead I and aVF. Because both leads are positive, the axis is in the normal quadrant.

2. Find the smallest or most equiphasic limb lead. Lead aVL is the most equiphasic lead in this example.

3. Find the lead that is perpendicular to the equiphasic lead and note if it is positive or negative. Lead II is perpendicular to aVL and lead II is positive in this example. Therefore the axis is directed toward the positive end of lead II, which is +60 degrees.

Using the ECG in Figure 13-17A, first place the axis in the appropriate quadrant by using lead I and aVF. Lead I is upright and aVF is negative, placing the axis in the left quadrant. However, because 30 degrees of the left quadrant is considered normal, we need to fine-tune the axis to determine where in the left quadrant it actually falls. Lead aVR is the most equiphasic lead in this ECG, which means that most of the electrical force is moving perpendicular to aVR. Lead III is perpendicular to aVR, and lead III is negative in this ECG, indicating that the axis is directed toward the negative pole of lead III. The axis is –60 degrees. The axis wheel shows how to count boxes in this example.

Using the ECG in Figure 13-17B, place the axis in the appropriate quadrant. Because lead I is negative and aVF is positive, the axis is in the right quadrant. The most equiphasic lead is aVR, and lead III is perpendicular to aVR. Because lead III is positive, the axis is directed toward the positive pole of lead III, or +150 degrees. The axis wheel shows how boxes are counted in this example.

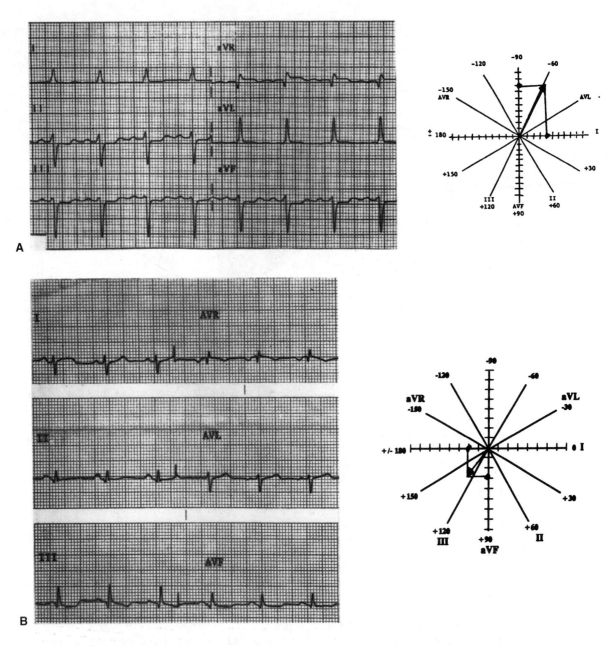

FIGURE 13-17 (A) Frontal plane leads demonstrating left axis deviation. Lead I is 5 boxes positive, and aVF is 2 boxes positive and 10 boxes negative, for a net of –8. The axis is –60 degrees. This is an example of left anterior fascicular block. **(B)** Frontal plane leads demonstrating right axis deviation. Lead I is two boxes positive and five boxes negative, for a net –3. Lead aVF is two boxes positive. The axis is +150 degrees. This is an example of left posterior fascicular block.

INTRAVENTRICULAR CONDUCTION ABNORMALITIES

The intraventricular conduction system consists of the right bundle branch and the left main bundle branch, which fans out into septal fascicles, an anterior fascicle, and a posterior fascicle. There are numerous individual anatomic variations, but the intraventricular conduction system is generally regarded to consist of three major fascicles that diverge from the bundle of His: (1) the right bundle branch, (2) the anterior division of the left bundle branch (left anterior fascicle), and (3) the posterior division of the left bundle branch (left

posterior fascicle; Fig. 13-18). Block may occur in any part of this conduction system. Monofascicular block is block in only one of the three major fascicles. Bifascicular block can mean block in both divisions of the left bundle branch, but it is more commonly used to describe the combination of RBBB and either LAFB or LPFB. Trifascicular block means block in all three major divisions.

Bundle-Branch Block

When one of the bundle branches is blocked, the ventricles depolarize asynchronously. Bundle-branch block is charac-

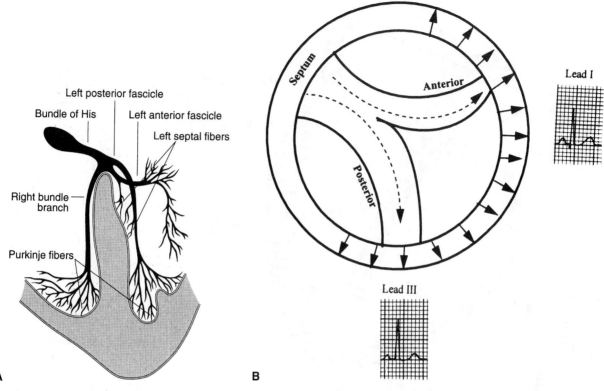

FIGURE 13-18 (A) Intraventricular conduction system. Right bundle branch carries impulse into right ventricle. Left main bundle branch divides into anterior and posterior fascicles which carry impulse into left ventricle. **(B)** Diagram of left ventricle as seen looking up from apex toward base. Anterior fascicle carries impulse upward and leftward, whereas posterior fascicle carries impulse downward and rightward in left ventricle. QRS complexes in leads I and III are shown.

terized by a delay of excitation to one ventricle and abnormal spread of electrical activity through the ventricle whose bundle is blocked. This delayed conduction results in widening of the QRS complex to 0.12 second or greater and a characteristic pattern best recognized in precordial leads V_1 and V_6 and limb leads I and aVL.

Normal ventricular depolarization as recorded by leads V_1 and V_6 is illustrated in Figure 13-19. The positive electrode for V_1 is located on the front of the chest at the fourth intercostal space to the right of the sternum, close to the right ventricle. The positive electrode for V_6 is located in the left mid-axillary line at the fifth intercostal space, close to the left ventricle. Lead V_1 records a small R wave as the septum depolarizes from left to right toward the positive electrode. It then records a negative deflection (S wave) as the main forces travel away from the positive electrode toward the left ventricle, resulting in the normal rS complex in V_1. Lead V_6 records a small Q wave as the septum depolarizes left to right away from the positive electrode. It then records a tall R wave as the main forces travel toward the left ventricle, resulting in the normal qR complex in V_6. When both ventricles depolarize together, the QRS width is less than 0.12 second.

RIGHT BUNDLE-BRANCH BLOCK

Figure 13-20*A* illustrates the spread of electrical forces in the ventricles when the right bundle branch is blocked. Three separate forces occur:

1. Septal activation occurs first from left to right, resulting in the normal small R wave in V_1 and small Q wave in V_6.
2. The left ventricle is activated next through the normally functioning left bundle branch. Depolarization spreads normally through the Purkinje fibers in the left ventricle, causing an S wave in V_1 as the impulse travels away from its positive electrode and an R wave in V_6 as the impulse travels toward the positive electrode in V_6.
3. The right ventricle depolarizes late and abnormally as the impulse spreads by cell-to-cell conduction through the right ventricle. This abnormal activation causes a wide second R wave (called R') in V_1 as it travels toward the positive electrode in V_1, and a wide S wave in V_6 as it travels away from the positive electrode in V_6. Because muscle cell-to-cell conduction is much slower than conduction through the Purkinje system, the QRS complex widens to 0.12 second or greater.

Typical uncomplicated RBBB can be recognized by a wide rSR' pattern in V_1 and a wide qRs pattern in V_6 and in leads I and aVL, because the positive electrode in these two limb leads is located on the left side of the body. Figure 13-20*B* illustrates three variations of the RBBB pattern most commonly seen. If a patient with RBBB has a septal MI, the initial small R wave usually seen in lead V_1 in

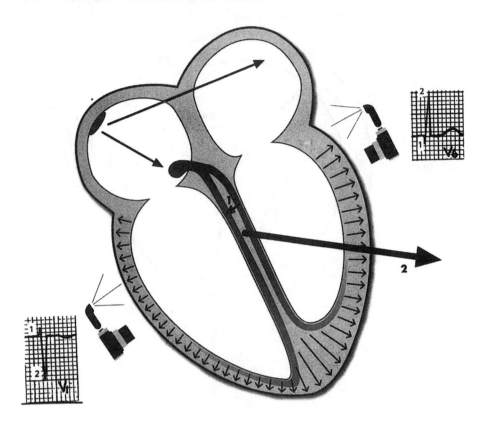

FIGURE 13-19 Normal ventricular activation as recorded by leads V_1 and V_6.

RBBB disappears because the septum no longer depolarizes normally from left to right, resulting in a qR pattern as seen in the second example in Figure 13-20*B*. Sometimes RBBB presents as a wide R wave in lead V_1 that may or may not be notched, as shown in the third example of Figure 13-20*B*. The ECG in Figure 13-20*C* is an example of typical RBBB.

LEFT BUNDLE-BRANCH BLOCK

Figure 13-21*A* illustrates the spread of electrical forces through the ventricles when the left bundle branch is blocked. In LBBB, the septum does not depolarize in its normal left-to-right direction because the block occurs above the Purkinje fibers that normally activate the left side of the septum. This causes the loss of the normal small R wave in V_1 and loss of the Q wave in V_6, lead I, and aVL. The loss of normal initial QRS forces in LBBB makes identification of MI more difficult. Two main forces occur in LBBB:

1. The right ventricle is activated first through the Purkinje fibers. Because the right ventricular free wall is so much thinner than the left ventricle, forces traveling through it are often not recorded in V_1. Sometimes a small, narrow R wave is recorded in V_1 during LBBB, and this is most likely the result of forces traveling through the right ventricular free wall.

2. The left ventricle depolarizes late and abnormally as the impulse spreads by cell-to-cell conduction through the thick left ventricle. This causes V_1 to record a wide negative QS complex as the impulse travels away from its positive electrode. The lateral leads V_6, I, and aVL record a wide R wave as the impulse travels through the large left ventricle toward their positive electrodes. The QRS widens to 0.12 second or greater due to the slow cell-to-cell conduction in the left ventricle.

Left bundle-branch block is recognized by a wide QS complex in V_1 and wide R waves with no Q waves in V_6, lead I, or aVL. Figure 13-21*B* shows two commonly seen LBBB patterns, the most common being the QS in lead V_1; the rS pattern is seen in approximately 30% of LBBB.[5] The ECG in Figure 13-21*C* illustrates LBBB.

Fascicular Blocks

The term *fascicular block* or *hemiblock* is used to describe block in either division of the left bundle branch. In fascicular block, both ventricles depolarize simultaneously so the QRS remains narrow, but the direction of left ventricular depolarization is altered. The most useful ECG leads for recognizing fascicular block are leads I and aVF for the axis, and leads I and III for the typical pattern of fascicular block.

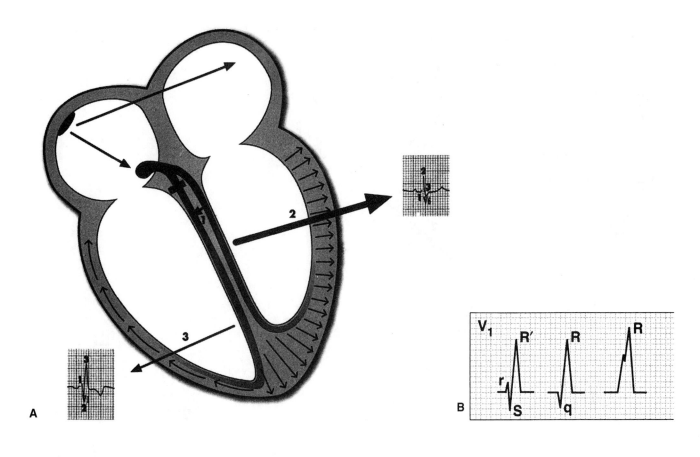

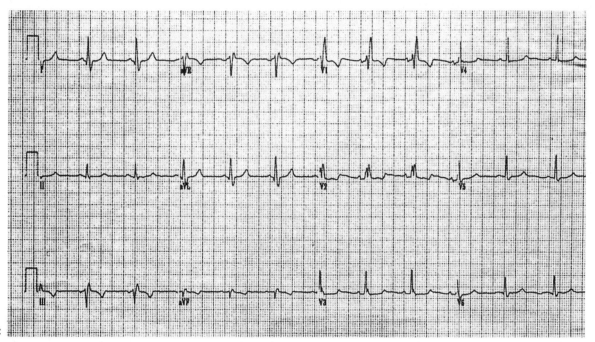

FIGURE 13-20 **(A)** Ventricular depolarization with right bundle-branch block (RBBB) as recorded by leads V_1 and V_6. **(B)** Three commonly seen variations of the RBBB pattern. **(C)** Twelve-lead electrocardiogram illustrating RBBB.

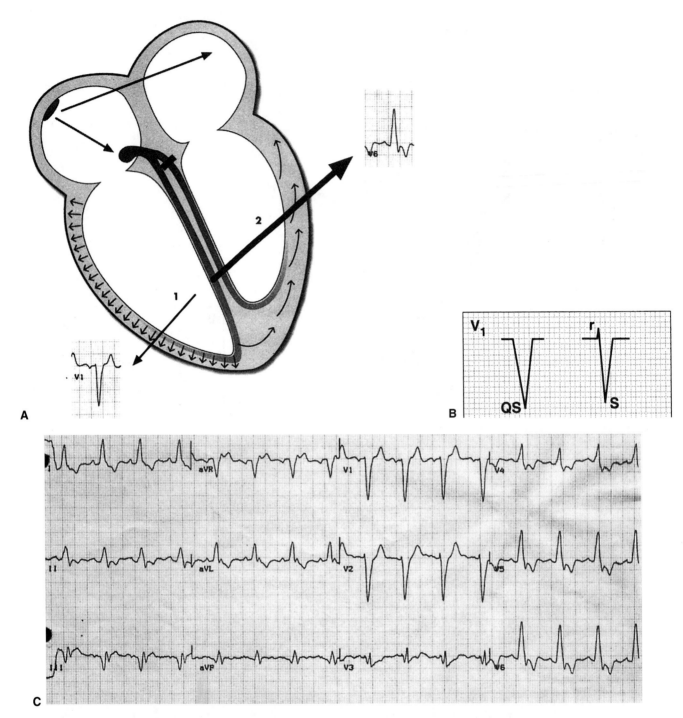

FIGURE 13-21 (A) Ventricular depolarization with left bundle-branch block (LBBB) as recorded by leads V₁ and V₆. **(B)** Two commonly seen patterns of LBBB. **(C)** Twelve-lead electrocardiogram illustrating LBBB.

Figure 13-18*A* illustrates the normal intraventricular conduction system and the relationship between the anterior and posterior divisions of the left bundle. In Figure 13-18*B*, imagine the apex of the left ventricle cut away and tipped toward you as you look up the barrel of the left ventricle. The main left bundle is seen coming from the septum into the left ventricle and dividing into the anterior and posterior fascicles, which course toward the anterior and posterior papillary muscles, respectively. When the left ventricular free wall is activated normally, the anterior fascicle carries the electrical

impulse in a superior and leftward direction and the posterior fascicle carries it downward and rightward. Because free wall activation proceeds in both directions simultaneously, most of the forces cancel each other and result in the normal QRS shape seen in leads I and III and a normal QRS axis as the combined forces proceed downward and leftward through the left ventricle. When fascicular block occurs, left ventricular activation proceeds from one site instead of both simultaneously, removing the cancellation and altering the shape of the QRS in leads I and III. Because the left ventricle is depo-

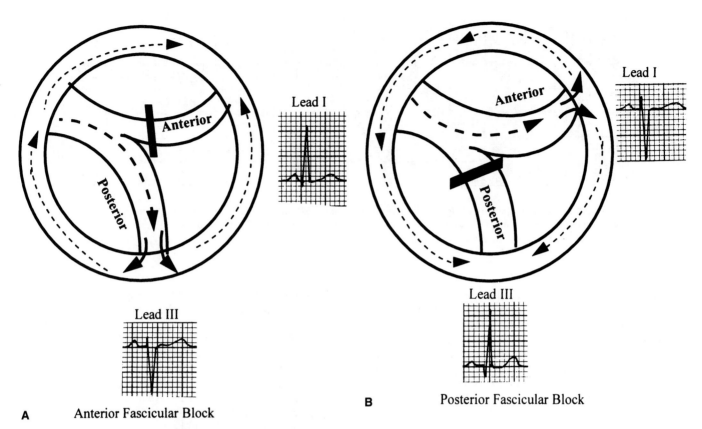

FIGURE 13-22 (A) Anterior fascicular block. Impulse depolarizes left ventricle in downward and rightward direction first through posterior fascicle, then travels upward and to the left, resulting in left axis deviation, Q wave in lead I, S wave in lead III. **(B)** Posterior fascicular block. Impulse depolarizes left ventricle in upward and leftward direction first through anterior fascicle, then travels downward and rightward, resulting in right axis deviation, S wave in lead I, Q wave in lead III.

larized in an abnormal direction, an axis deviation always results from fascicular block.

LEFT ANTERIOR FASCICULAR BLOCK

In LAFB (also called *anterior hemiblock*), the impulse conducts through the posterior fascicle and begins depolarizing the ventricle in an inferior and rightward direction. It then travels through the left ventricular free wall in a superior and leftward direction, resulting in a left axis deviation. The degree of left axis deviation required to diagnose LAFB is controversial, with some experts stating –45 to –90 degrees, and others at least –60 degrees. The initial forces are directed inferiorly and rightward, causing a small Q wave in lead I and a small R wave in lead III. The forces then travel superiorly and leftward, causing a normal R wave in lead I and an abnormally deep S wave in lead III. There may or may not be a Q wave in lead I, depending on whether initial septal activation is directed to the left or to the right.[3] Figure 13-22*A* is an example of LAFB. The ECG characteristics of LAFB are:

1. Left axis deviation (–45 degrees or more)
2. Small Q in lead I, large S in lead III (QI, SIII), or an rS pattern in II, III, aVF
3. QRS duration not prolonged more than 0.11 second
4. Increased QRS voltage in limb leads due to loss of cancellation of forces in left ventricle

LEFT POSTERIOR FASCICULAR BLOCK

In LPFB (also called *posterior hemiblock*), the impulse conducts through the anterior fascicle and begins depolarizing the ventricle in a superior and leftward direction. It then travels through the left ventricular free wall in an inferior and rightward direction, resulting in a right axis deviation. The initial forces are directed superiorly and leftward, causing a small R wave in lead I and a small Q wave in lead III. The forces then travel inferiorly and rightward, causing a deep S wave in lead I and a tall R wave in lead III. Before diagnosing LPFB, the clinician must rule out RVH because RVH can cause the identical frontal plane picture. Figure 13-22*B* is an example of LPFB. The ECG characteristics of LPFB are:

1. Right axis deviation (>110 degrees)
2. Small R in lead I and aVL, small Q in II, III, aVF (SI, QIII), or an rS pattern in leads I and aVL
3. Normal QRS duration (not >0.11 second)
4. Increased QRS voltage due to loss of cancellation of QRS forces
5. No evidence of RVH

Bifascicular Block

Bifascicular block means that two of the three major fascicles are blocked. Because block in both divisions of the left bundle branch presents as complete LBBB, the term

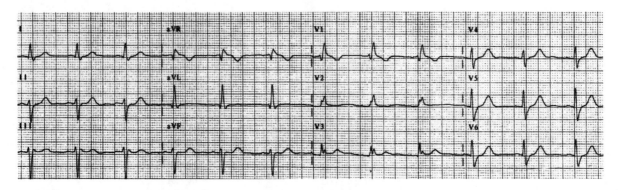

FIGURE 13-23 Electrocardiogram of right bundle-branch block (RBBB) and left anterior fascicular block (LAFB). Rhythm is sinus, QRS width is 0.12 second, there is left axis deviation (–60 degrees) due to LAFB, and V₁ shows the typical rsR' pattern of RBBB.

bifascicular block is usually used to refer to block in the right bundle branch along with block in either the anterior or posterior divisions of the left bundle branch. The ECG displays the typical RBBB morphology (wide QRS and rsR' pattern, or one of its variants) along with an axis deviation consistent with the fascicular block. Figure 13-23 is an example of RBBB and LAFB. Figure 13-24 shows RBBB and LPFB.

ISCHEMIA, INJURY, AND INFARCTION

Myocardial ischemia is the result of an imbalance between myocardial O_2 supply and demand and is a reversible process if blood flow is restored before cellular damage occurs. Ischemia can result from increased myocardial O_2 demands or from decreased myocardial O_2 supply. If ischemia is severe and blood flow is not restored relatively soon, cellular injury and eventually necrosis (infarction) result. Myocardial infarction can occur because of blockage of a coronary artery with

thrombus or from severe and prolonged ischemia due to coronary artery spasm or unrelieved obstruction of a coronary artery. When infarction does occur, there are three "zones" of tissue involvement, each of which produces characteristic changes on the ECG (Fig. 13-25).

Myocardial ischemia can result in several changes on the ECG (Fig. 13-26). The most familiar pattern of ischemia is T-wave inversion, although T-wave inversion is often a nonspecific finding and can be due to a variety of causes other than ischemia.[3,5,6] Other indicators of ischemia include ST segment depression of 0.5 mm or more, an ST segment that remains on the baseline longer than 0.12 second; an ST segment that forms a sharp angle with the upright T wave; tall, wide-based T waves; and inverted U waves.[6] Display 13-1 lists several causes of ST segment and T-wave changes.

Myocardial injury is most often indicated by ST segment elevation of 1 mm or more above the baseline. Other signs of acute injury include a straightening of the ST segment that slopes up to the peak of the T wave without spending any time on the baseline; tall, peaked T waves; and symmetric T-wave inversion[3,6] (Fig. 13-27).

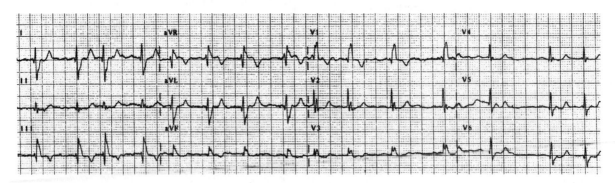

FIGURE 13-24 Electrocardiogram of right bundle-branch block (RBBB) and left posterior fascicular block (LPFB). Rhythm is atrial fibrillation, QRS width is 0.12 second, there is right axis deviation (approximately +150 degrees) due to LPFB, and V₁ shows the typical rsR' pattern of RBBB.

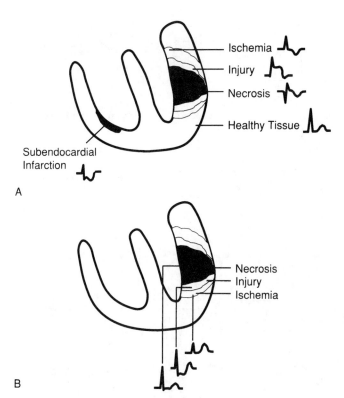

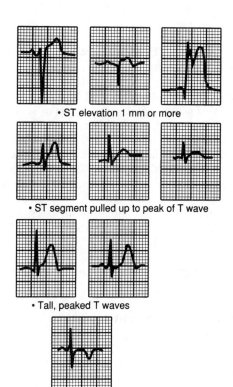

FIGURE 13-25 Zones of ischemia, injury, and infarction with associated electrocardiogram changes. **(A)** Indicative changes of ischemia, injury, and necrosis seen in leads facing the injured area. **(B)** Reciprocal changes often seen in leads not directly facing the involved area.

• ST elevation 1 mm or more

• ST segment pulled up to peak of T wave

• Tall, peaked T waves

• Symmetrical T inversion

FIGURE 13-27 Electrocardiographic patterns associated with acute myocardial injury.

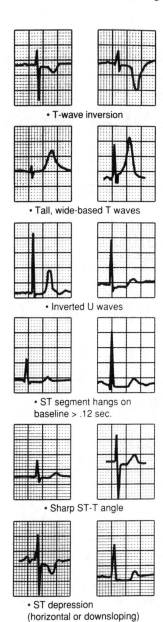

• T-wave inversion

• Tall, wide-based T waves

• Inverted U waves

• ST segment hangs on baseline > .12 sec.

• Sharp ST-T angle

• ST depression (horizontal or downsloping)

FIGURE 13-26 Electrocardiographic patterns associated with myocardial ischemia.

DISPLAY 13-1

Causes of ST Segment and T-Wave Changes

Aberrant conduction	Intracranial hemorrhage
Amyloidosis	Myocardial metastases
Bundle-branch block	Myocarditis
Cardiomyopathy	Paced rhythm
Cocaine vasospasm	Pancreatitis or acute abdomen
Drugs	Pericarditis
Early repolarization	Physical training
Hemiblock	Printzmetal's angina
Hypercalcemia	Pulmonary embolism
Hyperkalemia	Tachycardia
Hyperventilation	Ventricular aneurysm
Hypocalcemia	Ventricular hypertrophy
Hypoglycemia	Ventricular rhythms
Hypokalemia	Wolff-Parkinson-White syndrome
Hypothermia	

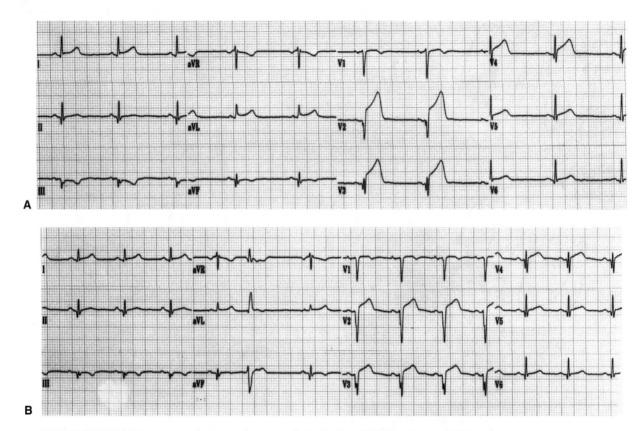

FIGURE 13-28 (A) Early acute anterior wall myocardial infarction (MI). Note abnormal R-wave progression in V$_{1-3}$ and ST segment elevation with tall, wide-based T waves in V$_{2-4}$. Q waves are present in inferior leads, indicating prior inferior wall MI. **(B)** Same patient 9 hours later. Q waves have developed in V$_{1-4}$ and ST segments are still elevated.

Necrosis or death of myocardial tissue is indicated on the ECG by development of new Q waves or deepening of preexisting Q waves. Abnormal Q waves are greater than 0.03 second wide or 25% of the ensuing R-wave amplitude. (See Figs. 13-12 and 13-13 for examples of normal Q waves; Figs. 13-28, 13-29, and 13-30 show examples of abnormal Q waves.) Display 13-2 lists conditions other than infarction that can result in development of Q waves.[6,7,10] Traditionally, it was taught that the presence of Q waves indicates transmural MI extending through the entire thickness of the muscle, and that subendocardial infarction involving less than the entire thickness of the muscle does not produce Q waves. It is now thought that Q waves can develop transiently with severe ischemia and that infarction can occur without the development of Q waves. Subendocardial infarction is recognized by decreased amplitude of R waves, ST segment depression, and T-wave inversion. The newer terms *Q wave* and *non-Q wave* MI are replacing the older terms of *transmural* and *subendocardial* infarction. In any case, the presence of abnormal Q waves is still considered indicative of myocardial necrosis.

The ECG reflects the progression of the infarction from the acute stage through the fully evolved stage. Very early MI often causes peaking and widening of the T waves followed within minutes by ST segment elevation. ST segment elevation can persist for hours to several days but resolves more quickly with successful reperfusion. Once the ST segment has returned to baseline, ECG evidence of the acute stage is lost. Q waves appear within hours of pain onset and usually remain forever, although sometimes Q waves disappear over the years after infarction. T-wave inversion occurs within hours after infarction and can last for months. T waves often return to their previous upright position within a few months after acute MI. Thus, an *evolving infarct* is one in which serial ECGs show ST segments returning toward baseline, the development of Q waves, and T-wave inversion. The term *old infarction* or *infarct of undetermined age* is used when the first ECG recorded shows Q waves, ST segment at baseline, and T waves either inverted or upright, indicating that an MI occurred at some point in the past.

Locating the Infarction From the Electrocardiogram

ST segment elevation, Q waves, and T-wave inversion are recorded in leads facing the damaged myocardium and are called the *indicative changes* of infarction. Other leads not facing the involved tissue are often affected by the loss of

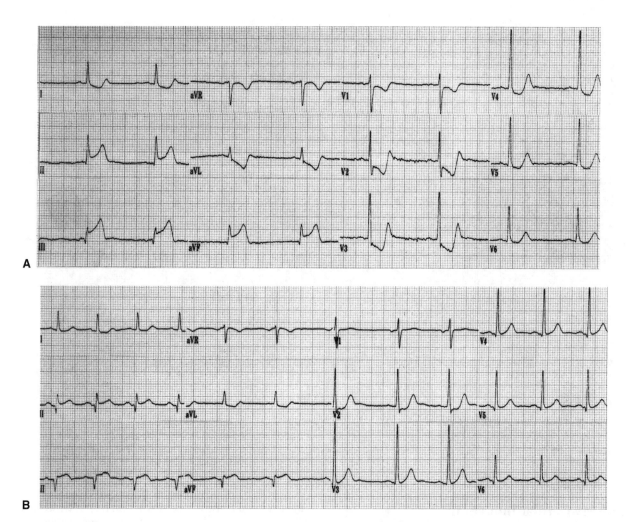

FIGURE 13-29 (A) Early acute inferior wall myocardial infarction. Note ST segment elevation in leads II, III, and aVF and reciprocal ST depression in V_{1-6}, I, and aVL. **(B)** Same patient next day. Q waves have developed and ST segments are coming down in inferior leads, and most of the reciprocal ST segment depression has resolved.

electrical forces in damaged tissue and record mirror-image changes called *reciprocal changes*. Figure 13-25 illustrates indicative and reciprocal changes associated with MI and Table 13-2 lists leads in which indicative and reciprocal changes are found in each of the major types of MI. Figure 13-31 illustrates how to localize ischemia, injury, and infarction using the 12–lead ECG.

Anterior Myocardial Infarction

Anterior wall MI (see Fig. 13-28) is due to occlusion of the left anterior descending coronary artery and is recognized by indicative changes in leads facing the anterior wall (V_{1-4}). Reciprocal changes are often recorded in the lateral leads I and aVL and the inferior leads II, III, and aVF. Loss of normal R-wave progression or development of Q waves and ST elevation in V_{1-4} are seen in anterior infarction. If only the septum is infarcted, changes occur only in leads V_{1-2}, but if

the entire anterior wall is involved, changes are seen in V_{1-4}. Anterior wall infarction that extends laterally and involves leads I and aVL is often referred to as extensive anterior or anterolateral infarction (Fig. 13-32).

Inferior Myocardial Infarction

Inferior wall MI (see Fig. 13-30) is usually due to occlusion of the right coronary artery and is diagnosed by indicative changes in leads II, III, and aVF. Reciprocal changes are often seen in leads I, aVL, or the V leads. In people with left dominant coronary circulation, the circumflex artery supplies the inferior surface of the heart and circumflex occlusion is the cause of inferior MI. Lead III can have a Q wave normally, but if the Q wave is large and accompanied by Q waves in leads II or aVF, it is considered indicative of inferior MI. Approximately 40% of inferior MIs involve the right ventricle (Fig. 13-33).

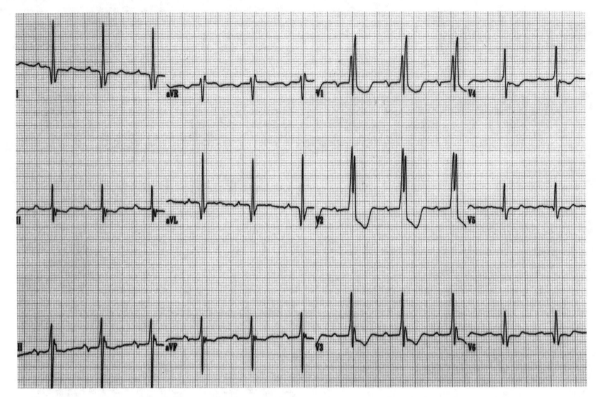

FIGURE 13-30 Lateral wall myocardial infarction (MI). Note deep Q waves in leads I, aVL, and V$_6$. ST segments are at baseline, indicating that this is an old MI. Right bundle-branch block is also present.

Lateral Myocardial Infarction

Lateral wall MI is due to circumflex artery occlusion and presents with indicative changes in leads I, aVL, and sometimes V$_{5-6}$, with reciprocal changes in inferior or anterior leads (see Fig. 13-30). Lateral wall MI does not often occur alone but commonly accompanies anterior MI, as it does in Figure 13-32.

Posterior Myocardial Infarction

Posterior wall MI (Fig. 13-34) is due to right coronary artery occlusion or to circumflex occlusion in left-dominant circulation, and usually occurs in conjunction with inferior MI. ECG changes of posterior MI are less obvious because in the standard 12-lead ECG there are no leads that face the posterior wall, and therefore there are no indicative changes recorded. The diagnosis is made by observing reciprocal changes in the anterior leads, especially V$_1$ and V$_2$, but often all the way to V$_4$. Reciprocal changes seen in these leads include a taller R wave than normal (mirror image of the Q wave that would be recorded over the posterior wall), ST segment depression (mirror image of the ST segment elevation from the posterior wall), and upright, tall T waves (mirror image of the T-wave inversion from the posterior wall).

DISPLAY 13-2

Causes of Noninfarction Q Waves

Ventricular hypertrophy
Anterior and posterior hemiblock
Hypertrophic cardiomyopathy
Ventricular preexcitation (Wolff-Parkinson-White syndrome)
Pulmonary embolism
Incomplete left bundle-branch block
Cardiac amyloidosis

TABLE 13-2 **Electrocardiographic Changes Associated with Myocardial Infarction (MI)**

Location of MI	Indicative Changes	Reciprocal Changes
Anterior	V$_1$ to V$_4$	I, aVL, II, III, aVF
Septal	V$_1$, V$_2$	I, aVL
Inferior	II, III, aVF	I, aVL, V$_1$ to V$_4$
Posterior	None	V$_1$ to V$_4$
Lateral	I, aVL, V$_5$, V$_6$	II, III, aVF, V$_1$, V$_2$
Right ventricle	V$_3$R to V$_6$R	

From Chuley, p 430.

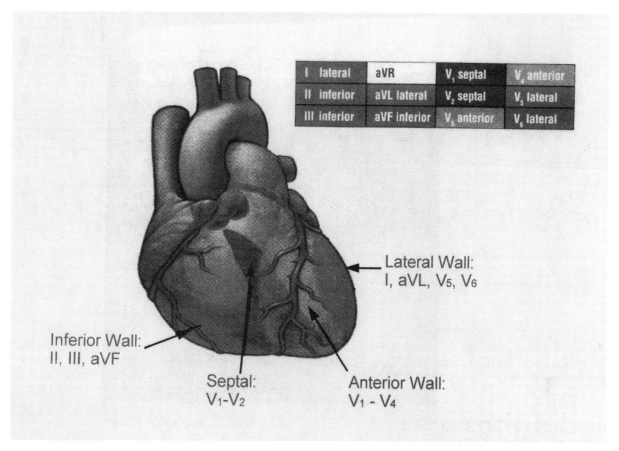

I	lateral	aVR		V₁ septal		V₄ anterior
II	inferior	aVL lateral		V₂ septal		V₅ lateral
III	inferior	aVF inferior		V₃ anterior		V₆ lateral

Lateral Wall:
I, aVL, V5, V6

Inferior Wall:
II, III, aVF

Septal:
V1-V2

Anterior Wall:
V1 - V4

FIGURE 13-31 Localizing myocardial ischemia, injury, or infarction using the 12-lead electrocardiogram (ECG). Standard 12-lead ECG format is illustrated at upper right, with leads color-coded to area of heart each lead faces. (From Cummins RO [ed]: Advanced Cardiac Life Support, p 9-27. Dallas, American Heart Association, 1997.)

Right Ventricular Myocardial Infarction

Right ventricular MI (RVMI; see Fig. 13-33) occurs in up to 45% of inferior MIs, and therefore it usually is associated with indicative changes in the inferior leads II, III, and aVF. In addition, it is not uncommon to see ST segment elevation in V_1 as well, because V_1 is the chest lead that is closest to the right ventricle. ST segment elevation in V_1 together with ST segment elevation in the inferior leads is suspect for

RVMI. Another clue is discordance between the ST segment in V_1 and the ST segment in V_2. Usually, when the ST segment in V_1 is elevated, it is related to anterior or septal MI, in which case the ST segment in V_2 is also elevated. Discordance means that the ST segments do not point in the same direction—V_1 shows ST segment elevation, whereas V_2 is either normal or shows ST segment depression. This finding is suspect for RVMI. When RVMI is suspected, right-sided chest leads should be obtained (see

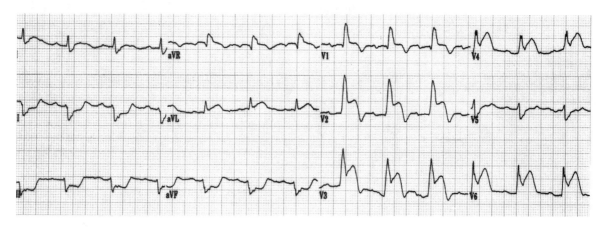

FIGURE 13-32 Acute anterolateral wall myocardial infarction. ST segment elevation is present in leads I, aVL, and V_{2-6}. Reciprocal ST segment depression is present in III, aVF, and aVR.

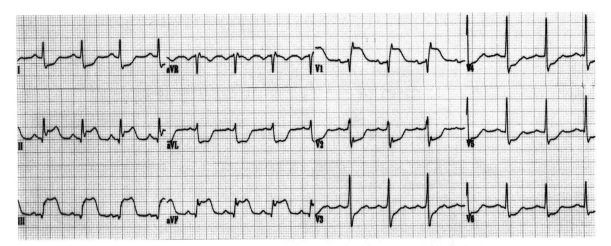

FIGURE 13-33 Acute right ventricular myocardial infarction. ST segment elevation is present in leads II, III, aVF, and V_1; reciprocal ST segment depression in all other leads. Note the discordant ST segment elevation in V_1 and depression in V_2.

Fig. 13-10). Leads V_{3R} through V_{6R} develop ST segment elevation when acute RVMI is present. Lead V_{4R} is the most sensitive and specific lead for recognition of RVMI.

ATRIAL AND VENTRICULAR ENLARGEMENT (HYPERTROPHY)

Each of the four heart chambers can enlarge because of hypertrophy or dilation. Each chamber is discussed separately.

Atrial Enlargement

Atrial enlargement due to hypertrophy or dilation may be determined from the ECG. Normal P waves are no wider than 0.11 second or taller than 2.5 mm. They are usually upright in leads I, II, and V_{4-6}, and diphasic with the initial portion upright and the terminal portion negative in V_1. Right atrial depolarization forms the first half of the P wave and left atrial depolarization forms the second half.

LEFT ATRIAL ENLARGEMENT

Left atrial enlargement is caused by conditions that increase pressure or volume in the left atrium, such as mitral stenosis, mitral regurgitation, systemic hypertension, and left heart failure. Left atrial enlargement can be manifested on the ECG in the following ways (see Fig. 13-35):

1. The P wave is wider than 0.11 second and often notched in leads I, II, aVL, and V_{4-6} (termed *P mitrale*).
2. The terminal negative component of the P wave in lead V_1 or V_2 is 1 mm or more in depth, greater than

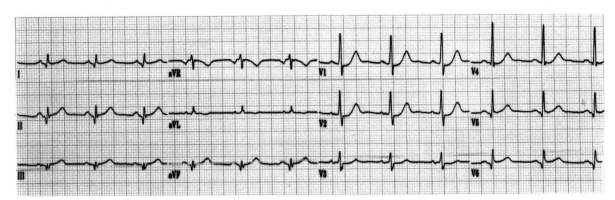

FIGURE 13-34 Posterior wall myocardial infarction (MI). Large R waves and ST segment depression are present in V_1 and V_2. Q waves and wide-based T waves in II, III, and aVF indicate probable inferior MI as well.

Normal   LAE   RAE

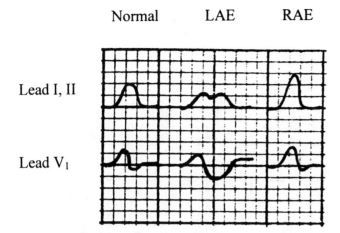

Lead I, II

Lead V₁

FIGURE 13-35 Normal P waves compared with those of left atrial enlargement (LAE) and right atrial enlargement (RAE). LAE causes widening and notching of P waves in many leads and enlargement of the terminal negative portion of the P wave in V₁. RAE causes tall, peaked P waves in many leads and enlargement of the initial upright portion of the P wave in V₁.

0.04 second in duration, and directed toward the left and posterior.

RIGHT ATRIAL ENLARGEMENT

Right atrial enlargement is commonly caused by conditions that increase the work of the right atrium, such as pulmonary hypertension, pulmonary or tricuspid stenosis or regurgitation, and congenital heart disease. Right atrial enlargement can be manifested on the ECG in the following ways (see Fig. 13-35):

1. The P waves are tall and peaked (>2.5 mm) in leads II, III, and aVF and inverted in lead aVL. The P waves in leads V_{1-3} are sharp and pointed.
2. The positive component of the P wave in leads V_1 and V_2 is greater than 1 mm in height and width.

BIATRIAL ENLARGEMENT

Biatrial enlargement occurs when both atria become enlarged. It is sometimes seen in mitral valve disease, atrial septal defect, multiple valvular defects, and biventricular failure. Biatrial enlargement is manifested on the ECG in the following ways:

1. The P wave is greater than 2.5 mm in lead II.
2. The P wave is longer than 0.11 second in lead II.
3. The P wave is notched.

Ventricular Enlargement

The ventricles can enlarge because of increased pressure or volume in the chamber. Enlargement of the right and left ventricles is discussed separately.

Left Ventricular Enlargement

Left ventricular enlargement (LVE) caused by increased volume (diastolic overload or increased preload) or increased pressure (systolic overload or increased afterload) can be expressed on the ECG (Fig. 13-36). Both QRS and ST-T-wave changes can be seen with LVE. The most characteristic effect of LVE is increased amplitude of the R wave in leads facing the left ventricle (leads I, aVL, V_5, and V_6) as more forces travel through the enlarged left ventricle. There is a concurrent decrease in R-wave amplitude and increase in S-wave amplitude in leads facing the right ventricle (leads V_1 and V_2). The intrinsicoid deflection (the time from the beginning of the QRS complex to the peak of the R wave) is slightly delayed in leads facing the left ventricle, and the QRS width approaches the upper limit of normal because of the increased time required for electrical forces to travel through the thick left ventricular muscle.[1,5]

The ST-T-wave changes that occur reflect repolarization abnormalities and may be due to hypertrophy or may be secondary consequences of dilation or ischemia. The term *strain* is often used to describe the ST-T-wave changes that commonly occur with LVE. ST segment depression, often downsloping, with T-wave inversion commonly develops in left chest leads. Increased T-wave amplitude may be found in leads that show large R waves, and ST segments may be elevated in leads that show deep S waves. ST segment depression and T-wave inversion accompany more severe hypertrophy and ventricular dysfunction.[8]

A variety of methods have been proposed to help diagnose LVE on the ECG, and Table 13-3 lists several of these methods. The ECG changes seen with hypertrophy or dilation of the left ventricle lack sensitivity but have high specificity.[3,6,8] There are more false-positive than true-positive diagnoses, and autopsy data show that voltage changes consistent with LVE can be present in the absence of LVE.[3]

RIGHT VENTRICULAR ENLARGEMENT

Right ventricular enlargement (RVE) may be caused by any condition that produces a sufficient load on the right ventricle, such as pulmonary disease or congenital or acquired heart disease, particularly mitral valve disease. The electrical events of the right ventricle are normally masked by the events taking place nearly simultaneously in the dominant left ventricle. As the right ventricle enlarges, these right-sided (or anterior) forces are revealed and may become the dominant forces if the right ventricle becomes as large or larger than the left. The normal sequence of depolarization is altered, resulting in ECG changes in axis, QRS morphology and voltage, and ST-T waves (Fig. 13-37).

The most obvious ECG change with RVE is a reversal of normal R-wave progression in precordial leads. R waves become dominant and the S wave shrinks in right chest leads, whereas R waves shrink and S waves dominate in left-sided leads. The same "strain" pattern described previously

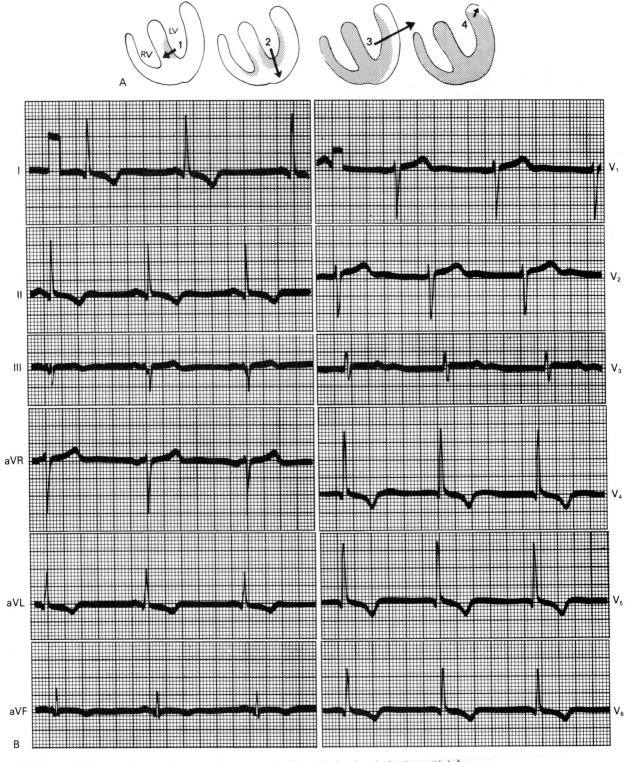

FIGURE 13-36 **(A)** Shaded area represents the sequence of ventricular depolarization with left ventricular enlargement (LVE). **(B)** Electrocardiographic changes with LVE. Deep S wave (or Q wave) in leads V_1 and V_2; tall R wave in leads V_5, V_6, and I. (Note that leads V_1 through V_6 are recorded at half the standard voltage.) (From Bernreiter M: Electrocardiography, p 97. Philadelphia, JB Lippincott, 1963.)

TABLE 13-3	Methods to Diagnose Left Ventricular Enlargement on the Electrocardiogram (ECG)
Author/Method	**ECG Criteria Favoring LVE**

Author/Method	ECG Criteria Favoring LVE	
Dubin[2]	R wave in lead I + S wave in lead III >26 mm	
	S wave in lead V_1 + R wave in lead V_5 or V_6 >35 mm	
Sokolow and Lyon[10, 11]	R wave in VL ≥11 mm	
	S wave in lead V_1 + R wave in lead V_5 or V_6 >35 mm	
	R wave in V_5 or V_6 >26 mm	
Estes' Scorecard[6]	*Criteria*	*Points**
	1. R or S wave in limb lead 20 mm or more	
	S wave in lead V_1, V_2, or V_3 25 mm or more ⎫	
	R wave in lead V_4, V_5, or V_6 25 mm or more ⎭	3
	2. Any ST shift (without digitalis)	3
	Typical ST strain (with digitalis)	1
	3. Left axis deviation −30 degrees or more	2
	4. QRS interval 0.09 second or more	1
	5. Intrinsicoid deflection in V_5 and V_6 0.05 second or more	1
	6. P-wave terminal force in V_1 >0.04 second	3
	Total possible	14
Scotts Criteria[6]	Limb leads	
	R in 1 + S in 3 >25 mm	
	R in aVL >7.5 mm	
	R in aVF >20 mm	
	S in aVR >14 mm	
	Chest leads	
	S in V_1 or V_2 + R in V_5 or V_6 >35 mm	
	R in V_5 or V_6 >26 mm	
	R + S in any V lead >45 mm	
Cornell Index[11]	Women: R in aVL + S in V_3 >20 mm	
	Men: R in aVL + S in V_3 >28 mm	

LVE, left ventricular enlargement.
  *5 = LVE; 4 = probable LVE.

with ST segment depression and T-wave inversion occurs in right chest leads and in leads II, III, and aVF. Ten ECG features commonly seen with RVE are listed in Display 13-3. The presence of one of the criteria listed is highly indicative of RVE. These features seen with RVE are highly specific but lack sensitivity[8]—that is, when a named feature is evident, the diagnosis of RVE is certain, but there may be considerable enlargement present before this feature becomes evident.

ELECTROLYTE IMBALANCES

Hypokalemia (serum potassium <3 mEq/L) may produce a number of ECG changes (Fig. 13-38). Prominent U waves develop and as serum potassium levels drop, the T and U waves may merge together and the U wave may become larger than the T wave. ST segment depression and T-wave flattening occur, P waves widen, and the PR interval may prolong. Arrhythmias, especially premature ventricular contractions, are common with hypokalemia. These ST-T- and U-wave changes correlate fairly well with serum potassium levels but are not specific for hypokalemia because they can also result from administration of certain drugs and from ventricular hypertrophy.

Hyperkalemia (serum potassium >5 mEq/L) may produce tall, narrow-based, peaked T waves and QT interval shortening (Fig. 13-39). As the potassium level rises, QRS complexes widen and ST segment elevation may occur. First-degree AV block often occurs. P waves flatten and eventually may disappear. With severe hyperkalemia the QRS complex becomes broad and bizarre with a sine wave formation, and ventricular fibrillation may ensue. These ECG changes are typical of hyperkalemia but do

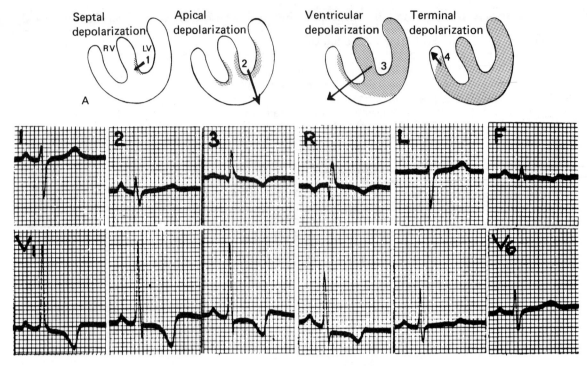

FIGURE 13-37 (A) Shaded area represents the sequence of ventricular depolarization with right ventricular enlargement. **(B)** Right ventricular hypertrophy. Note marked right axis deviation and reversal of normal R-wave progression across the precordium, with large R waves in V_{1-3} and S wave in V_6. (From Marriott HJL: Marriott's Manual of Electrocardiography, p 84. Orlando, FL, Trinity Press, 1995.)

DISPLAY 13-3

Diagnostic Criteria for Right Ventricular Enlargement

R/S radio in V_5 or V_6 ≤1
S wave in V_5 or V_6 ≥7 mm
S_1, S_2, S_3 pattern
S_1, Q_3 pattern
Right axis deviation +110 degrees[9] (≥ +90 degrees[8])
R/S ratio in V_1 >1 (with R wave >5 mm)
R wave in V_1 ≥7 mm
P pulmonale
QR in V_1
R wave in V_5 or V_6 ≤4 mm (with S in V_1 ≤2 mm)

Presence of one criterion indicates right ventricular enlargement with 95% specificity; two criteria indicate 99% specificity or higher.[8]
Data from Mirvis DM: Electrocardiography: A Physiologic Approach. St. Louis, CV Mosby, 1993; and Murphy MI, Thenabadu PN, Blue LR et al: Descriptive characteristics of the electrocardiogram from autopsied men free of cardiopulmonary disease: A basis for evaluating criteria for ventricular hypertrophy. Am J Cardiol 52: 1275–1280, 1983.

---

not correlate well with the actual serum potassium level. Some people do not show ECG changes until serum levels are quite high, whereas others show changes at lower potassium levels.

Hypocalcemia (serum calcium <6.1 mg/dL) prolongs the ST segment and the QT interval (Fig. 13-40). The prolonged QT interval is due to the abnormally long ST segment rather than to abnormal repolarization, as can occur with quinidine or other drugs (see Chapter 14). T waves are usually unchanged, but terminal T-wave inversion may occur.

Hypercalcemia (serum calcium >12 mg/dL) shortens the QT interval, especially the distance from the beginning of the QRS to the peak of the T wave (Fig. 13-41). The ST segment practically disappears and the proximal limb of the T wave takes off from the end of the QRS complex. Arrhythmias are uncommon in states of calcium imbalance.

Hypomagnesemia can produce arrhythmias and predispose to digitalis toxicity. ECG effects of hypomagnesemia resemble those of hypokalemia—most notably, QT interval prolongation. These deficits in magnesium and potassium levels frequently occur concurrently; it has not been determined what independent effects result from hypomagnesemia.

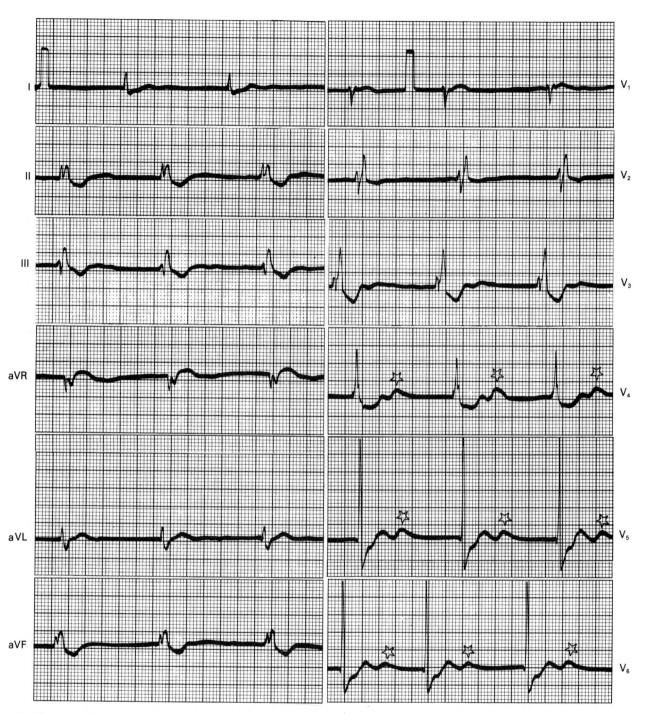

FIGURE 13-38 Electrocardiographic effects of hypokalemia. (From Bernreiter M: Electrocardiography, p 158. Philadelphia, JB Lippincott, 1963.)

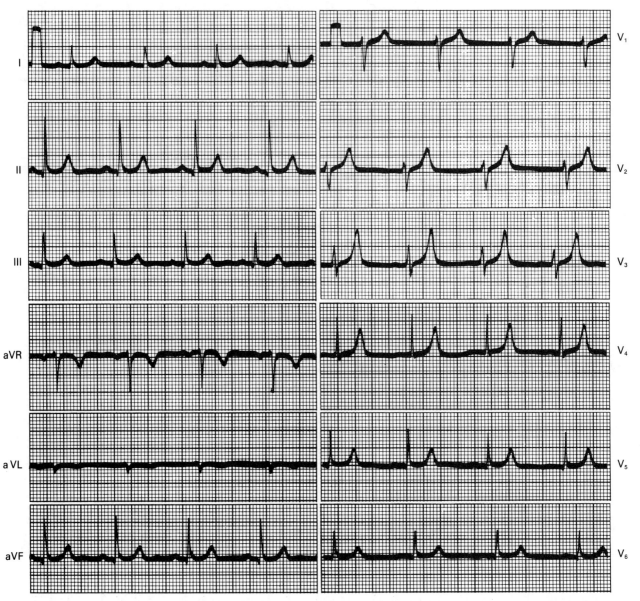

FIGURE 13-39 Electrocardiographic effects of hyperkalemia. (Note that all V leads are shown at half the standard voltage). (From Bernreiter M: Electrocardiography, p 155. Philadelphia, JB Lippincott, 1963.)

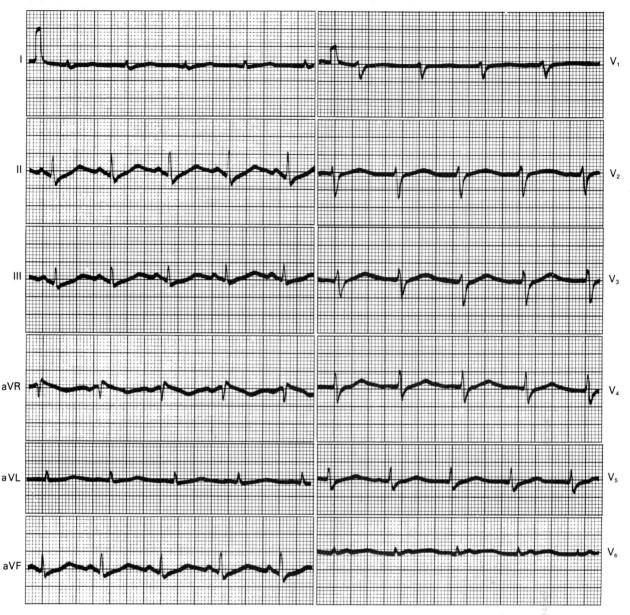

FIGURE 13-40 Electrocardiographic effects of hypocalcemia. (Note that all V leads are shown at half the standard voltage.) (From Bernreiter M: Electrocardiography, p 162. Philadelphia, JB Lippincott, 1963.)

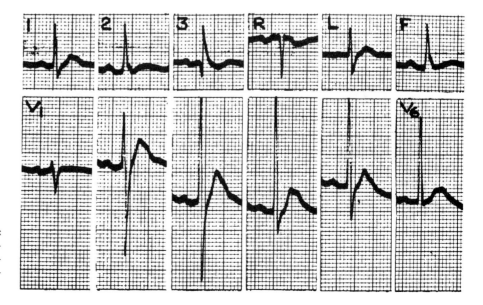

FIGURE 13-41 Electrocardiographic effects of hypercalcemia. (From Marriott HJL: Marriott's Manual of Electrocardiography, p 142. Orlando, FL, Trinity Press, 1995.)

REFERENCES

1. Conover MB: Understanding Electrocardiography, 7th ed. St. Louis, Mosby, 1996
2. Dubin D: Rapid Interpretation of EKGs, 3rd ed. Tampa, FL, Cover, 1988
3. Fisch C: Electrocardiography. In Braunwald E (ed): Heart Disease, 5th ed, pp 108–152. Philadelphia, WB Saunders, 1997
4. Goldschlager N, Goldman MJ: Principles of Clinical Electrocardiography, 13th ed. Norwalk, CT, Appleton & Lange, 1989
5. Marriott HJL: Marriott's Manual of Electrocardiography. Orlando, FL, Trinity Press, 1995
6. Marriott HJL: Practical Electrocardiography, 8th ed. Baltimore, Williams & Wilkins, 1988
7. Marriott HJL: Emergency Electrocardiography. Naples FL, Trinity Press, 1997
8. Mirvis DM: Electrocardiography: A Physiologic Approach. St. Louis, CV Mosby, 1993
9. Murphy MI, Thenabadu PN, Blue LR et al: Descriptive characteristics of the electrocardiogram from autopsied men free of cardiopulmonary disease: A basis for evaluating criteria for ventricular hypertrophy. Am J Cardiol 52: 1275–1280, 1983
10. Sokolow M, Lyon TP: The ventricular complex in left ventricular hypertrophy as obtained by unipolar precordial and limb leads. Am Heart J 37: 161–186, 1949
11. Wagner GS: Marriott's Practical Electrocardiography, 9th ed. Baltimore, Williams & Wilkins, 1994
12. Zipes DP: Specific arrhythmias: Diagnosis and treatment. In Braunwald E (ed): Heart Disease, 5th ed, pp 604–702. Philadelphia, WB Saunders, 1997.

Arrhythmias and Conduction Disturbances

CAROL JACOBSON

MECHANISMS OF ARRHYTHMIAS

Cardiac arrhythmias result from abnormal impulse initiation, abnormal impulse conduction, or both mechanisms together. The major mechanisms of arrhythmias are enhanced normal automaticity, abnormal automaticity, triggered activity resulting from afterdepolarizations, conduction blocks, and reentry. Although all of these mechanisms have been shown to cause arrhythmias in the laboratory, it is not possible to prove which mechanism is responsible for a particular arrhythmia using currently available diagnostic tools in the clinical setting. However, it is possible to postulate the mechanism of many clinical arrhythmias based on their characteristics and behavior and to list rhythms most consistent with known electrophysiologic mechanisms.[3,32,70,92,93,109] Some arrhythmias, such as atrioventricular (AV) nodal reentry tachycardia, atrial flutter, some ventricular tachycardias (VTs), and reentry tachycardias involving accessory pathways, have been proven to be caused by reentry. This section describes the major mechanisms of arrhythmias and lists arrhythmias suggested or proven to be caused by each mechanism whenever possible.

Abnormal Impulse Initiation

Abnormal impulse initiation can be due to enhanced normal automaticity, abnormal automaticity, or afterdepolarizations. It is important to understand the normal property of automaticity before considering these mechanisms.

AUTOMATICITY

The sinus node (or sinoatrial node) is the normal pacemaker of the heart because it has the fastest rate of automaticity. Other cells in the heart also have the property of automaticity, including cells in the atria, coronary sinus, AV junction, AV valves, and Purkinje system. The rates of these other pacemakers are slower than the rate of the sinus node; therefore, they are suppressed by the sinus node under normal conditions, a phenomenon known as *overdrive suppres-*

sion. The site of fastest impulse initiation is referred to as the *dominant pacemaker,* whereas sites of impulse formation that are suppressed by the dominant site are called *subsidiary* or *latent pacemakers.*

ENHANCED NORMAL AUTOMATICITY

Impulse initiation can be shifted from the sinus node to other parts of the heart if the rate of the sinus node drops below that of a subsidiary pacemaker or if the automatic rate of a subsidiary pacemaker rises above that of the sinus node. Increased vagal tone, drugs, or disease of the sinus node can decrease its rate of automaticity or can cause exit block of its impulse, thus allowing subsidiary pacemakers to assume control of the heart. Examples of clinical arrhythmias due to shifting of the pacemaker from the sinus node include atrial, junctional, or ventricular escape rhythms that occur due to sinus bradycardia or AV block. Such "escape" pacemaker activity cannot be considered abnormal because it is a manifestation of the normal automaticity of these cells.

Subsidiary pacemaker activity can be enhanced by factors that decrease the transmembrane resting potential (TRP), decrease the threshold potential, or increase the rate of diastolic phase 4 depolarization of the subsidiary pacemaker cells. Figure 14-1 illustrates how these mechanisms can change the rate of firing of pacemaker cells.

Enhanced normal automaticity can occur with sympathetic stimulation, drugs such as digitalis and sympathomimetic agents, or with disease states such as coronary artery disease or chronic pulmonary disease.[37] Clinical arrhythmias that may be due to enhanced normal automaticity include sinus tachycardia, wandering atrial pacemaker (WAP), some atrial tachycardias, junctional tachycardia, some accelerated ventricular rhythms, and ventricular parasystole.[36,60]

ABNORMAL AUTOMATICITY

Atrial and ventricular myocardial cells that do not normally show automaticity can develop abnormal automaticity

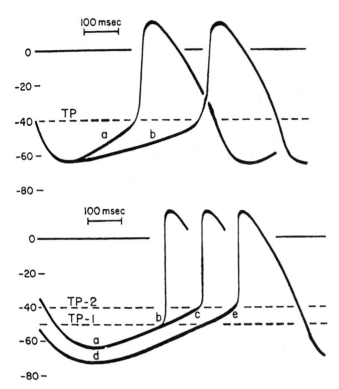

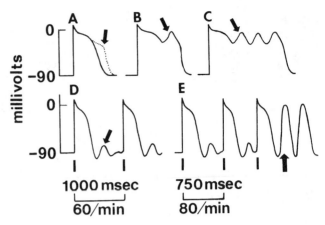

FIGURE 14-2 **(A)** An early afterdepolarization (*arrow*). **(B)** A single triggered action potential caused by this afterdepolarization (*arrow*). **(C)** A train of triggered action potentials (*arrow*). **(D,E)** Action potentials caused by propagating impulses (indicated by vertical lines), followed by delayed afterdepolarization (*arrow* in **D**). **(E)** Triggered activity caused by the afterdepolarization (*arrow*). (From Wit A, Rosen M: Cellular electrophysiology of cardiac arrhythmias: I. Arrhythmias caused by abnormal impulse generation. Modern Concepts in Cardiovascular Disease 50: 5, 1981. By permission of the American Heart Association, Inc.)

FIGURE 14-1 Diagram illustrating the principal mechanisms underlying changes in the frequency of discharge of a pacemaker fiber. The *upper diagram* shows a reduction in rate caused by a decrease in the slope of diastolic, or pacemaker, depolarization from a to b, and thus an increase in the time required for the membrane potential to decline to the threshold potential (TP) level. The *lower diagram* shows the reduction in the rate associated with a shift in the level of the threshold potential from TP-1 to TP-2, and a corresponding increase in cycle length (b to c); also illustrated is a further reduction in rate due to an increase in the maximal diastolic potential level (compare a with c and d with e). (From Hoffman BF, Cranefield PF: Electrophysiology of the Heart. New York, McGraw-Hill, 1960. Used with permission of the McGraw-Hill Book Company.)

when their TRP is reduced.[34,36,92,93,102,104,105,108,109] Abnormal automaticity that occurs in either atrial or ventricular cells, or in otherwise normal pacemaker cells at reduced membrane potentials, is thought to depend on the slow inward current carried mainly by calcium (*slow channels*) because the normal fast sodium channels are at least partially inactivated at reduced membrane potentials.[34,36,71,92,93,102,104,109] These arrhythmias are not always controlled with calcium channel blockers, which may indicate that abnormalities of sodium conduction also play an important role in abnormal automaticity.

The resting potential of a cell can be reduced (e.g., from –90 to –70 mV) and the cell partially depolarized by anything that increases the extracellular potassium concentration, decreases the intracellular potassium concentration, increases the permeability of the membrane to sodium, or decreases the membrane permeability to potassium.[34,92,102,105,109] Ischemia, hypoxia, acidosis, hyperkalemia, digitalis toxicity, chamber enlargement or dilation, stretch, and other metabolic abnormalities or drugs can reduce the

resting potential and result in abnormal automaticity.[34,66,104] Hypoxia and ischemia affect the TRP by decreasing the amount of oxygen available to supply adenosine triphosphate in amounts sufficient to operate the sodium–potassium pump efficiently. Anything that interferes with proper operation of this pump, like digitalis, reduces normal resting ionic gradients across the cell membrane and results in reduction of the resting potential. When the TRP is reduced at rest, the cell is partially depolarized and the time required for spontaneous diastolic depolarization to reach threshold is reduced, thus increasing pacemaker activity (see Fig. 14-1). For the same reason, automaticity is increased when the threshold potential is reduced (e.g., from –40 to –50 mV) by ischemia or drug effects because less time is required for phase 4 depolarization to reach the lower threshold. The rate of phase 4 depolarization can be increased by several factors, including local norepinephrine release at ischemic sites, systemic catecholamine release, reduced vagal tone, and drugs.

Clinical arrhythmias that may be due to abnormal automaticity include some atrial tachycardias, accelerated ventricular rhythm, and some VTs associated with acute myocardial infarction (MI).[60,93,108,109]

TRIGGERED ACTIVITY DUE TO AFTERDEPOLARIZATIONS

Afterdepolarization is a transient depolarization that occurs at some time during or right after repolarization of an action potential. Early afterdepolarizations occur during the repolarization of an action potential. Delayed afterdepolarizations occur after repolarization is complete but before the next action potential is due to occur. Figure 14-2 shows both early and delayed afterdepolarizations.

Early Afterdepolarizations. Early afterdepolarizations occur during phase 2 or 3 of an action potential that was initiated from a high resting membrane potential (−75 to −90 mV). Early afterdepolarizations occur when repolarization is delayed and are thought to result from activation of the slow channels because they arise during repolarization at a time when the fast channels are largely inactivated.[34,70,93,102,104–106] If this afterdepolarization is large enough to reach threshold, a second upstroke occurs, causing an "early" beat. This second upstroke is called a *triggered beat* because it depends on and arises as a result of the preceding action potential. The triggered beat may be followed by its own afterdepolarization, which initiates yet another upstroke. This activity may be sustained for several beats and may terminate only when the membrane finally repolarizes to a high enough level to extinguish the rhythmic activity. This mechanism of abnormal impulse formation differs from abnormal automaticity in that automatic beats result from spontaneous initiation of each impulse, whereas beats due to afterdepolarizations depend on a preceding impulse.

Early afterdepolarizations have been shown to occur in the presence of hypoxia, acidosis, hypokalemia, hypomagnesemia, hypothermia, high PCO_2, and high concentrations of catecholamines, and in areas of stretch or mechanical injury.[104,106] These findings suggest that certain arrhythmias seen soon after MI, in patients with enlarged hearts from heart failure, or in patients with ventricular aneurysms may be due to early afterdepolarizations.[102,105,106] Triggered activity due to early afterdepolarizations is enhanced by slow heart rates and is usually associated with prolongation of the repolarization phase of the action potential.[6,93,106] The proarrhythmic effects of many drugs, especially class IA and III antiarrhythmics, are thought to be due to their ability to prolong repolarization in cardiac cells and cause early afterdepolarizations.[106] Clinical arrhythmias thought to be due to early afterdepolarizations include drug-induced torsades de pointes, torsades de pointes (TdP) due to electrolyte imbalances, and ventricular arrhythmias in patients with congenital long QT syndrome.[6,93,106,109]

Studies[85,86] have demonstrated cells in the deep subepicardial region of the canine ventricle that have electrophysiologic characteristics intermediate between those of muscle cells and Purkinje cells. These cells are called *M cells* and have been shown to prolong their action potentials and induce early afterdepolarizations in response to slowing of the heart rate and in the presence of quinidine. There is some evidence that M cells are also present in the human ventricle[25] and that repolarization of M cells contributes to the genesis of the U wave on the electrocardiogram (ECG).[6,7] Others believe that U waves may represent a summation of early afterdepolarizations occurring throughout the heart.[41] Research continues into the possible relationship between M cells and certain clinical arrhythmias, especially reperfusion arrhythmias after myocardial ischemia, TdP, right ventricular outflow tract (RVOT) tachycardia, and reentrant arrhythmias.

Delayed Afterdepolarizations. Delayed afterdepolarizations occur after the membrane has repolarized to its original level after an action potential. Subthreshold afterdepolarizations do not result in triggered activity, but if the delayed afterdepolarization is large enough to reach threshold, a triggered impulse arises. This triggered impulse may also be followed by its own afterdepolarization, leading to trains of triggered beats. Again, the mechanism differs from automaticity in that afterdepolarizations depend on and arise as a result of preceding action potentials.

Delayed afterdepolarizations occur in association with increased intracellular calcium levels, which commonly occur with digitalis toxicity.[6,102,104,106] There is a direct relation between amplitude of delayed afterdepolarizations and heart rate: as the heart rate increases, so does afterdepolarization amplitude. Thus, triggered activity tends to occur after premature beats or at rapid heart rates. Factors that increase delayed afterdepolarization amplitude and contribute to triggered arrhythmias include high concentrations of catecholamines and digitalis, and hypokalemia.[3,6,34,72,102,104–106,109] Delayed afterdepolarizations can also occur in the presence of rheumatic heart disease and cardiomyopathy.[6,104,106] Clinical arrhythmias that may be due to delayed afterdepolarizations include digitalis toxic rhythms like accelerated junctional rhythm and atrial tachycardia, idiopathic VT originating in the RVOT, and accelerated idioventricular rhythm after MI.[6,93,106,109]

Abnormal Impulse Conduction

Abnormal impulse conduction can occur as a result of conduction blocks or reentry.

CONDUCTION BLOCK

The electrical impulse can be prevented from propagating through the heart for a variety of reasons. If the propagating impulse is not strong enough to excite the tissue ahead of it, conduction will fail (see following section on Decremental Conduction). If an impulse arrives at an area where the tissue is still refractory after a previous depolarization it will not be able to conduct further (see section on Phase 3 Block, later). If an impulse reaches tissue that is abnormally depolarized due to ischemia, disease, or drugs, it may not be able to conduct at all or will conduct with delay (see section on Phase 4 Block, later). Scar tissue from previous MI, surgery, or catheter ablation also prevents conduction.

Decremental Conduction. Decremental conduction is the progressive decrease in conduction velocity of an impulse as it travels through a region of myocardium. Decremental conduction is a normal function of the AV node, delaying the impulse in the AV node long enough for atrial contraction to contribute to ventricular filling. Decremental conduction normally occurs in areas of the heart where resting potentials are low and action potentials depend on slow channels, such as the AV and sinus nodes. It can also occur in areas where resting potentials are low due to ischemia, disease, or drugs. Under such circumstances, conduction velocity is slow because of the slower rate of rise of the action potential that occurs when cells are stimulated at reduced resting potentials. At times, decremental conduction can be so pronounced that the impulse fails to conduct,

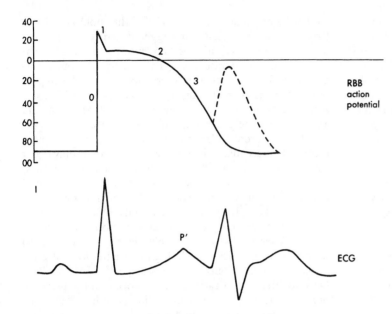

FIGURE 14-3 Phase 3 block. The electrocardiogram on the bottom shows a normal beat followed by a premature atrial beat that conducts with right bundle-branch block. The action potentials on top illustrate that the early beat entered the right bundle during phase 3, when the membrane potential was still reduced. The resulting action potential is a slow channel response, and conduction fails. (From Marriott HJL, Conover M: Advanced Concepts in Arrhythmias, 3rd ed, p 217. St. Louis, CV Mosby, 1998.)

thus leading to block. This failure of conduction can occur in the sinus node, leading to sinus exit block; in the AV node, leading to AV block; or in the bundle-branch system, causing bundle-branch block.

Phase 3 Block. When a cell is stimulated during phase 3 of the action potential, conduction is impaired because the membrane has not yet returned to its resting level. Whenever a cell is stimulated at a less negative membrane potential, the rate of rise of the action potential, and thus conduction velocity, is slow because only part of the fast sodium channels is available. Figure 14-3 illustrates phase 3 block occurring in the right bundle branch, resulting in aberrant conduction of the impulse with a right bundle-branch block (RBBB) pattern.

Phase 3 block (also called short-cycle aberrancy[84]) can occur in normal hearts if impulses are premature enough to reach fibers during their normal refractory period, resulting in aberrant conduction of premature beats. It is also responsible for rate-dependent bundle-branch blocks and for the

aberration that commonly occurs when cycle lengths are very irregular, as in atrial fibrillation. Phase 3 block can occur pathologically if the refractory period is abnormally prolonged by drugs or disease.

Phase 4 Block. Phase 4 block (also called long-cycle aberrancy[84]) occurs late in diastole when fibers are stimulated at reduced membrane potentials secondary to spontaneous phase 4 depolarization. In this case, the membrane has begun to depolarize spontaneously during its normal phase 4. By the time a stimulus arrives, the resting potential has been reduced enough to cause slow conduction. Again, whenever a cell is stimulated at a reduced membrane potential, only some of the sodium channels are available, and slow conduction results. Figure 14-4 shows a normal right bundle-branch action potential followed by spontaneous phase 4 depolarization. By the time the second impulse arrives in that bundle, membrane potential has been reduced enough to cause slow conduction and RBBB.

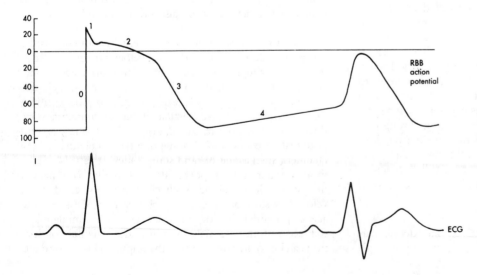

FIGURE 14-4 Phase 4 block. The electrocardiogram on the bottom shows a normal beat followed by a pause and a second beat that conducts with right bundle-branch (RBB) block. The action potential on top illustrates that the pause after the first normal action potential allowed sufficient time for spontaneous phase 4 depolarization to occur in the RBB. The impulse after the pause enters the RBB at a time when its membrane potential is reduced, resulting in conduction failure. (From Marriott HJL, Conover M: Advanced Concepts in Arrhythmias, 3rd ed, p 219. St. Louis, CV Mosby, 1989.)

Phase 4 block is responsible for abnormal conduction that occurs only at the end of long cycles or for so-called "bradycardia-dependent bundle-branch block." Phase 4 block is uncommon and is considered pathologic when it occurs.

REENTRY

Reentry is a type of conduction abnormality that leads to the occurrence of premature beats or sustained tachycardias rather than to block and is thought to be responsible for more clinically important arrhythmias than any other mechanism.[75] Reentry can occur in areas of the heart where conduction velocity is abnormally slow because of ischemia, electrolyte abnormalities, drugs, or disease. *Reentry* means that an impulse can travel through an area of myocardium, depolarize it, and then reenter that same area to depolarize it again. For reentry to occur, there must be an area of unidirectional block in which an impulse can conduct in one direction but not in the opposite direction. In addition, conduction velocity must be slow enough relative to tissue refractoriness and circuit length to allow the impulse to continue propagating in a circular manner.[75,103] Figure 14-5*A* illustrates normal conduction of an impulse through an area of myocardium, and Figure 14-5*B* shows reentry occurring as a result of an area of unidirectional block and slow conduction.

For reentry to occur, an area of unidirectional block is necessary to allow an impulse to conduct in one direction and to provide a return pathway by which the original stimulus can reenter a previously depolarized area. Conduction velocity must be slow enough and the refractory period short enough to allow time for the previously stimulated area to recover its ability to conduct. If the refractory period of the previously stimulated tissue is long or conduction velocity is fast, the impulse dies out because it encounters tissue that is unable to conduct.

Based on these general concepts, three main types of reentry have been described.[34,60,75] *Anatomic reentry* (see Fig. 14-5) involves an anatomic obstacle around which the circulating wave of depolarization can travel. *Functional reentry* does not require an anatomic obstacle but depends on local differences in conduction velocity and refractoriness among neighboring fibers that allow an impulse to circulate repeatedly around the area. *Anisotropic reentry* is caused by structural differences among adjacent fibers that cause variations in conduction velocity and repolarization between these fibers. An impulse conducts more rapidly when it travels along the length of fibers than it does when it travels in the transverse direction across fibers. These differences in conduction velocity can result in unidirectional block and slow conduction, leading to reentry.

When an impulse travels the reentry loop only once, a single premature beat results. If conduction velocity is slow enough and the refractory period of normal tissue is short enough, a single impulse could travel the loop numerous times, resulting in a run of premature beats or in a sustained tachycardia. Reentry that occurs in small loops of tissue, such as the AV node or Purkinje tissue, is called *microreentry*. If the reentry loop involves large tracts of tissue, such as AV bypass tracts or the bundle-branch system in the ventricles, it is called *macroreentry*.

Many clinical dysrhythmias are thought to be due to reentry, including most VTs, atrial fibrillation, atrial flutter, and some atrial tachycardias.[34,55,75,93,109] Arrhythmias that are known to involve discrete reentry circuits are atrial flutter, AV nodal reentry tachycardia (AVNRT), AV reentrant tachycardia using an accessory pathway in Wolff-Parkinson-White syndrome, and bundle-branch reentry VT.

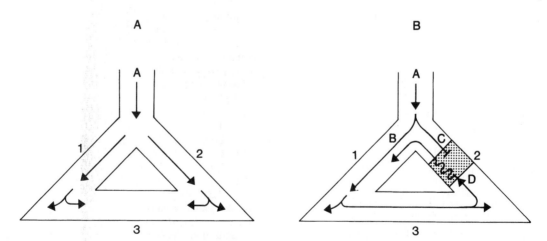

FIGURE 14-5 (A) Normal conduction of an impulse through cardiac muscle. **(B)** Area of unidirectional block and reentry (*shaded area*). The impulse enters at point A and depolarizes limb 1 normally but is blocked from stimulating limb 2 at point C. It continues around from limb 1 to depolarize limb 3 and enters limb 2 from below the are of unidirectional block. At point D, the impulse is able to conduct backward through the depressed segment and reenter limb 1 at point B. (Adapted from Rosen MR, Danilo P: Electrophysiological basis for cardiac arrhythmias. In Narula OS (ed): Cardiac Arrhythmias: Electrophysiology, Diagnosis, Management, p 9. Baltimore, Williams & Wilkins, 1979.)

BASIC ARRHYTHMIAS AND CONDUCTION DISTURBANCES

An *arrhythmia* is any cardiac rhythm that is not normal sinus rhythm at a normal rate. Arrhythmias can be due to abnormal impulse initiation, either at an abnormal rate or from a site other than the sinus node, or abnormal impulse conduction through any part of the heart. This section focuses on arrhythmias that originate in the sinus node, atria, AV node, and ventricles, as well as basic AV conduction disturbances. Refer to Tables 14-1 through 14-4 for information related to antiarrhythmic drug therapy. The advanced cardiac life support (ACLS) algorithms for current recommendations for the acute treatment of arrhythmias can be found in Chapter 25.

Rhythms Originating in the Sinus Node

The sinus node is the normal pacemaker of the heart because it has the highest rate of automaticity of all potential pacemaker sites. The arrhythmias that originate in the sinus node are sinus bradycardia, sinus tachycardia, sinus arrhythmia, sinus arrest, sinus exit block, and sick sinus syndrome.

NORMAL SINUS RHYTHM

The sinus node normally fires at a regular rate of 60 to 100 beats/min. The impulse spreads from the sinus node through the atria and to the AV node, where it encounters a slight delay before it travels through the bundle of His, right and left bundle branches, and Purkinje fibers into the ventricles. The spread of this wave of depolarization through the

(text continued on page 14)

TABLE 14-1   **Classification of Antiarrhythmic Drugs**

Class	Action	Electrocardiographic Effect	Examples	Potential for Left Ventricular Depression	Proarrhythmic Potential
IA	Sodium channel blockade Prolong repolarization time Slow conduction velocity Suppress automaticity	↑ QRS, ↑ QT	Quinidine, procainamide, disopyramide	+ + +++	+++ ++ ++
IB	Sodium channel blockade Accelerate repolarization	↓ QT	Lidocaine, tocainide, mexiletine	+ ++ ++	+ + +
IC	Sodium channel blockade Marked slowing of conduction No effect on repolarization	↑↑ QRS	Flecainide, propafenone, moricizine (also has IA and IB effects)	+++ ++ ++	+++ ++ ++
II	Beta blockade	↓ HR, ↑ PR	Acebutolol, atenolol, esmolol, metoprolol, propranolol, timolol, sotalol (other blockers are available but not usually used as antiarrhythmics)	+++ ++	0 ++
III	Potassium channel blockade Prolong repolarization time	↑ QT	Amiodarone, sotalol, bretylium, ibutilide	+ ++ 0 +	+ ++ + +++
IV	Calcium channel blockade	↓ HR, ↑ PR	Verapamil, diltiazem, (other calcium channel blockers are available but not usually used as antiarrhythmics)	+++ ++	+ +

+++, greatest; ++, moderate; +, least; ↑, increased; ↓, decreased; HR, heart rate; PR, PR interval; QRS, QRS width; QT, QT interval.

TABLE 14-2   Antiarrhythmic Drugs

Drug (Class)	Indication	Dose/Administration/ Therapeutic Level/Half-Life	Side Effects	Comments
Adenosine (unclassified) *Adenocard*	First-line therapy to terminate AV nodal active SVTs (AVNRT, CMT). Can be diagnostic in AV nodal passive rhythms by causing AV block and revealing atrial mechanism. VT arising in the right ventricular outflow tract and those due to afterdepolarizations may respond to adenosine.	6 mg given very rapidly IV followed by rapid saline flush. May follow with 12 mg if needed and repeat 12 mg if no effect. Half life = 9s	Acute onset of AV block usually lasting a few seconds. May result in brief period of asystole or bradycardia that is not responsive to atropine. Torsades de pointes can occur in patients who are susceptible to bradycardia-dependent arrhythmias. Flushing, hot flash, acute dyspnea lasting a few seconds, chest pressure.	Very short half-life so side effects are transient. Warn patients about side effects before giving drug—especially dyspnea. It may be helpful to have patients take a deep breath while injecting drug to lessen dyspneic sensation. Should not be used when arrhythmia is known to be atrial fibrillation or flutter. Monitor ECG during administration and be prepared for cardioversion. May accelerate accessory pathway conduction and should not be used when antegrade conduction is occurring over accessory pathway. May rarely accelerate ventricular rate in atrial flutter. **Drug interactions:** Theophylline (and related drugs) and caffeine antagonize effects of adenosine and make it ineffective. Dipyridamole and carbamazepine potential effects of adenosine.
Amiodarone (III) *Cordarone*	Life-threatening ventricular arrhythmias: recurrent VF, recurrent hemodynamically unstable VT. Also used for conversion of the atrial fibrillation to sinus and maintenance of NSR; treatment of atrial tachycardia, CMT. Slow conduction through accessory pathways in atrial fibrillation or CMT.	**PO:** 800–1,600 mg qd for 1–3 w, then 600–800 mg qd for 4 w. Maintenance: 100–400 mg/d. May be given as single daily dose or bid if GI intolerance occurs. **IV:** 1,000 mg over first 24 h given as follows: **First rapid infusion:** 150 mg over first 10 min (15 mg/min; add 3 mL [150 mg] to 100 mL D$_5$W). Infuse 100 mL over 10 min.	Bradycardia, heart block. Proarrhythmia (VF, incessant VT, torsades de pointes). Hypotension with IV form. Pulmonary fibrosis, corneal microdeposits, photosensitivity, blue skin, thyroid dysfunction (hypo and hyper), liver dysfunction. Tremor, malaise, fatigue, GI upsets, dizziness, poor coordination, peripheral neuropathy, involuntary movements.	Give with meals to ↓ GI intolerance. Baseline chest radiograph, renal, liver, thyroid function tests. Takes several weeks to achieve therapeutic blood levels and for side effects to decrease after stopping drug. Is not dialyzable. Monitor K$^+$ and Mg^{2+} levels. Monitor QTc interval.

(continued)

TABLE 14-2   Antiarrhythmic Drugs (Continued)

Drug (Class)	Indication	Dose/Administration/ Therapeutic Level/Half-Life	Side Effects	Comments
		Followed by slow infusion: 360 mg over next 6 h (1 mg/min; add 18 mL [900 mg] to 500 mL D$_5$W). Infuse at 33.6 mL/h. **Maintenance infusion:** 540 mg over next 18 h (0.5 mg/min; decrease rate of slow loading infusion to 0.5 mg/min). Infuse at 16.8 mL/h. May continue with 0.5 mg/min for 2–3 w if needed. Central line recommended for long-term infusions. If breakthrough VT occurs, may give supplemental doses of 150 mg over 10 min (150 mg added to 100 mL D$_5$W). **IV to PO transition** *Duration of IV PO dose* <1 w 800–1,600 mg qd 1–3 w 600–800 mg qd >3 w 400 mg qd Therapeutic level = 1–2.5 µg/mL Very long half-life (26–107 d, average 53 d)	Liver enzyme elevations are common but occur in patients with MI, CHF, shock, multiple defibrillations, and so forth. It is unknown if elevations in liver enzymes are due to amiodarone or to associated conditions commonly present in these patients. Hepatocellular necrosis has occurred in patients who received IV amiodarone at rates higher than recommended.	**Drug interactions:** ↑ Protime with coumarin drugs. ↑ Serum levels of digoxin, quinidine, procainamide, cyclosporine. May double flecainide level. Cimetidine ↑ serum amiodarone levels. Cholestyramine and phenytoin ↓ serum amiodarone levels. Additive effects on ↓ HR and ↓ AV conduction with beta blockers and Ca^{2+} blockers. **Special precautions with IV form:** Physically incompatible with aminophylline, heparin, cefamandole, cefazolin, mezlocillin, sodium bicarbonate. Must be delivered using a *volumetric pump* (not drop counter) because drop size is altered by drug.
Atenolol (beta blocker) *Tenormin*	Ventricular rate control in atrial fibrillation/flutter. Slow conduction through AV node in AVNRT and CMT.	**Initial dose:** 12.5–25 mg PO qd **Maintenance dose:** 50–100 mg PO qd Beta blocking plasma concentration = 0.2–5 µg/mL Half-life = 6–9 h	Hypotension, bradycardia, AV block, diarrhea, wheezing, CHF.	Cardioselective beta blocker used primarily for hypertension. **Drug interactions:** Additive effects on HR, AV conduction, BP, and ↑ potential for CHF when given with negative inotropic drugs, Ca^{2+} blockers, digoxin.
Atropine (anticholinergic, parasympatholytic)	Treatment of symptomatic bradycardia (sinus, junctional, AV block) and asystole.	**Symptomatic bradycardia:** 0.5–1 mg IV. May repeat q 3–5 min to total of 0.04 mg/kg. **Asystole:** 1 mg IV, repeat q 3–5 min to total vagolytic dose of 0.04 mg/kg. May be given down endotracheal tube during cardiac arrest if no IV available: use 2–2.5 mg. Half-life = 2–5 h	CV: tachycardia, chest pain, ventricular tachycardia/fibrillation (rare). CNS: drowsiness, confusion, dizziness, insomnia, nervousness. GI: dry mouth, ↓ GI motility, constipation, nausea. Other: urinary retention, hot flushed skin, rash.	Doses <0.5 mg may cause paradoxical bradycardia. Causes pupils to dilate (significant when checking pupils during cardiac arrest situation). **Drug interactions:** Incompatible with aminophylline, metaraminol, norepinephrine, pentobarbital, sodium bicarbonate.

Drug	Indications	Dosing	Adverse Effects	Contraindications / Drug Interactions
Bretylium (III)	IV treatment of VF and pulseless VT. Treatment of sustained VT.	**VF and pulseless VT:** 5 mg/kg rapid IV bolus. May repeat with 10 mg/kg bolus if needed. **Hemodynamically stable VT:** 5–10 mg/kg IV over 8–10 min. If successful, follow with IV infusion at 1–2 mg/min. Therapeutic level = 0.5–3 μg/mL (not well established, limited clinical use) Half-life = 13 h	CV: hypotension (due to peripheral vasodilation). GI: May cause projectile vomiting.	Causes an initial catecholamine release with tachycardia, hypertension, anxiety, flushing, headache. No known drug interactions.
Digoxin (unclassified)	Ventricular rate control in atrial fibrillation/flutter. Also used as an inotropic agent in CHF.	**PO loading dose:** 0.5–1 mg divided into 3 or 4 doses at 6- to 8-h intervals. **PO maintenance dose:** 0.125–0.5 mg qd. **IV loading dose:** 0.5–1 mg divided into 3 or 4 doses given at 4- to 8-h intervals. Therapeutic level = 0.8–2 ng/mL. Half-life = 36–48 h	CV: bradycardia, AV block. Digoxin toxicity: sinus exit block, AV block, atrial tachycardia with block, bidirectional tachycardia, fascicular tachycardia, accelerated junctional rhythm, regularization of the ventricular response to atrial fibrillation. Visual disturbances (halo vision), anorexia, nausea, vomiting, malaise, headache, weakness, disorientation, seizures.	Contraindicated in patients with WPW. Digoxin toxicity is more common in the presence of hypokalemia, renal failure, pulmonary or thyroid disease and in older people. **Drug interactions:** The following drugs ↓ digoxin levels: cholestyramine, antacids, kaopectate, neomycin, sulfasalazine, para-aminosalicylic acid. The following drugs ↑ digoxin levels: Erythromycin, tetracycline, quinidine, amiodarone, verapamil, spironolactone, nicardipine, indomethacin.
Diltiazem (Ca²⁺ blocker) *Cardizem*	Ventricular rate control in atrial fibrillation/flutter. Slow conduction through AV node in AVNRT and CMT.	180–360 mg/d in divided doses. **IV:** 0.25 mg/kg bolus over 2 min. If needed, repeat with 0.35 mg/kg over 2 min. **IV infusion:** 10–15 mg/h. Therapeutic level = 50–200 ng/mL Half-life = 4–56 h	Bradycardia, heart block, CHF, hypotension, flushing, angina, syncope, insomnia, ringing ears, edema, headache, nausea. Less depression of contractility than with verapamil, but watch for CHF.	Contraindicated in patients with accessory pathways (WPW, short PR syndrome) **Drug interactions:** Additive effects on HR, AV conduction, BP, and ↑ potential for CHF when given with negative inotropic drugs, Ca²⁺ blockers, digoxin.
Disopyramide (IA) *Norpace*	Effective in treating PVCs but not recommended because of proarrhythmic effects. Suppresses sustained VT. Effective in preventing atrial fibrillation and flutter. Slows conduction through accessory pathways.	Total daily dose = 400–800 mg in divided doses, usually 150 mg q6h. Sustained-release form = 300 mg q12h. Therapeutic level = 3–6 μg/mL Half-life = 4–10 h	Anticholinergic effects: dry mouth, urinary retention, constipation, precipitation or exacerbation of glaucoma. CV: marked negative inotropic effects, CHF, prolongs QT interval, proarrhythmic (less than quinidine or procainamide), ↑ SVR.	Monitor QT interval. **Drug interactions:** May potentiate effect of coumarin drugs. Additive negative inotropic effects with beta blockers or Ca²⁺ blockers. Phenobarbital, dilantin, rifampin, ↓ disopyramide levels. Quinidine ↑ disopyramide level.

(continued)

TABLE 14-2   **Antiarrhythmic Drugs** *(Continued)*

Drug (Class)	Indication	Dose/Administration/ Therapeutic Level/Half-Life	Side Effects	Comments
Epinephrine *Adrenalin*	Treatment of any cardiac arrest situation requiring cardiopulmonary resuscitation: VF, pulseless VT, asystole, Pulseless Electrical Activity.	1 mg IV bolus every 3–5 min during resuscitation efforts. May be given by endotracheal tube if IV access not available: use 2 to 2.5 mg. Alternative dosing can be used for cardiac arrest but has not been shown to improve outcomes. **Intermediate dose:** 2–5 mg IV every 3–5 min. **Escalating dose:** 1 mg, 3 mg, 5 mg, 3 min apart. **High dose:** 0.1 mg/kg q 3–5 min. May be infused at 2–10 µg/min to maintain BP during symptomatic bradycardia.	CV: tachycardia, hypertension, arrhythmias, angina. CNS: restlessness, headache, tremor stroke. Other: nausea, ↓ urine output, transient tachypnea.	**Drug interactions:** Has potential to cause arrhythmias when given with bretylium, digoxin, other sympathomimetic agents. Physically incompatible with aminophylline, ampicillin, cephapirin, sodium bicarbonate, and other alkaline solutions.
Esmolol (beta blocker) *Brevebloc*	Rapid control of ventricular rate in atrial fibrillation/flutter.	**Loading infusion:** 500 µg/kg/min for 1 min. **Maintenance infusion:** 50–100 µg/kg/min. Use dosing chart that comes with drug. Beta blocking plasma concentration = 0.15–1 µg/mL. Half-life = 9 min.	Hypotension, dizziness, diaphoresis, nausea.	Cardioselective beta blocker. Short half-life so effects reversed within 10–20 min after stopping drug. **Drug interactions:** May increase digoxin level. Additive effects on HR, AV conduction, BP, and ↑ potential for CHF when given with negative inotropic drugs, Ca²⁺ blockers, digoxin. Incompatible with sodium bicarbonate, furosemide, diazepam, thiopental.
Flecainide (IC) *Tambocor*	In absence of structural heart disease: Conversion of atrial fibrillation to sinus and maintenance of NSR. Treatment of SVTs: AVNRT, CMT. Slow conduction through accessory pathways in atrial fibrillation or CMT.	100–200 mg PO q12h. Therapeutic level = 0.2–1 µg/mL. (Plasma levels do not correlate with efficacy but incidence of CV toxicity greater when levels >1 µg/mL.) Half-life = 12–27 h.	CV: marked proarrhythmia, marked negative inotropic effects (CHF), bradycardia, heart block. CNS: blurred vision, dizziness, flushing, ringing ears, drowsiness, headache. Other: bad taste, constipation, edema, abdomina pain.	Higher mortality rate in patients post-MI when studied in CAST. Safest in patients with normal left ventricular function. Should not be used in patients with recent MI. Prolongs QT interval, potential for proarrhythmia. Monitor for CHF. Full therapeutic effect may take up to 5 days.

Drug	Use	Dose	Side effects	Drug interactions
	Life-threatening ventricular arrhythmias (sustained VT).			**Drug interactions:** ↑ digoxin levels. Cimetidine, amiodarone, propranolol increase flecainide levels. Additive negative inotropic effects with beta blockers, Ca²⁺ blockers, disopyramide.
Ibutilide (III) *Corvert*	Conversion of atrial fibrillation or flutter to sinus. First drug approved by Food and Drug Administration specifically for this indication.	IV infusion of 1 mg over 10 min. May repeat same dose in 10 min if needed. In patients <60 kg: 0.01 mg/kg. Half-life = 6 h	Hypotension, VT, bundle-branch block, AV block, nausea, headache.	Prolongs QT interval and may be proarrhythmic. Proarrhythmia usually occurs within 40 min. Monitor ECG continuously during administration and at least 4 h after. Conversion to NSR usually occurs within 20–30 min of infusion. **Drug interactions:** Do not give other class I or class III agents within 4 h.
Lidocaine (IB)	Treatment of ventricular arrhythmias: VT, VF. Effective for PVC suppression, but PVC suppression not usually recommended.	**For VT:** 1 mg/kg IV bolus over 3 min followed by infusion at 2–4 mg/min. Repeat bolus of 0.5 mg/kg in 10 min to maintain therapeutic level. May repeat to total of 3 mg/kg. **For VF pulseless VT:** 1.5 mg/kg IV bolus. May repeat with same amount and follow with infusion at 2–4 mg/min. May be given by endotracheal tube during cardiac arrest if no IV available. Therapeutic level = 1.4–5 µg/mL Half-life of bolus = 10 min Half-life once therapeutic level reached = 1.5–2 h	Side effects relatively rare. CNS: lightheadedness, dizziness, tremor, agitation, tinnitus, blurred vision, convulsions, respiratory depression and arrest. CV: bradycardia, asystole, hypotension, shock.	Decrease dose to half if liver disease or low liver blood flow (shock). **Drug interactions:** Beta blockers and cimetidine increase lidocaine levels. Glucagon and isoproterenol may increase liver blood flow and ↓ lidocaine levels.
Magnesium	May be useful for treatment or prevention of both supraventricular and ventricular arrhythmias after MI or cardiac surgery. Treatment of choice for torsades de pointes and VF or pulseless VT refractory to other drugs.	1–2 g diluted in 10 mL D$_5$W over 1–2 min. May be given IV push for VF or torsades de pointes. Infusion of 0.5–1 g/h for up to 24 h.	CV: hypotension, bradycardia, heart block, cardiac arrest. CNS: weakness, drowsiness, peripheral neuromuscular blockade, absent deep tendon reflexes. Other: ↓ respiratory rate, respiratory paralysis.	**Drug interactions:** CNS depression when used with general anesthetics, barbiturates, opiate analgesics. Additive effects with neuromuscular blocking agents. Incompatible with calcium, sodium bicarbonate, ciprofloxacin.

(continued)

TABLE 14-2 Antiarrhythmic Drugs *(Continued)*

Drug (Class)	Indication	Dose/Administration/Therapeutic Level/Half-Life	Side Effects	Comments
Metoprolol (beta blocker) *Lopressor*	Ventricular rate control in atrial fibrillation/flutter. Slow conduction through AV note in AVNRT and CMT.	PO: 100–450 mg qd. IV: 5 mg q 2–5 min for three doses (used in acute MI). Beta blocking plasma concentration = 50–100 ng/mL. Half-life = 3–4 h.	Hypotension, bradycardia, AV block.	Cardioselective beta blocker. **Drug interactions:** Additive effects on HR, AV conduction, BP, and ↑ potential for CHF when given with negative inotropic drugs, Ca²⁺ blockers, digoxin.
Mexiletine (IB) *Mexitil*	Acute and chronic treatment of symptomatic VT.	PO loading dose: 400 mg. **Maintenance dose:** 200–400 mg q8h. Therapeutic level = 0.5–2 µg/mL. Half-life = 10–17 h.	GI: nausea, vomiting, heartburn, anorexia, diarrhea. CNS: tremor, dizziness, ataxia, slurred speech, paresthesias, seizures, hallucinations, emotional instability, insomnia, memory impairment. CV: bradycardia, hypotension, CHF, proarrhythmia (rare compared with other agents). Other: thrombocytopenia, fever, rash, positive antinuclear antibody.	Often given in combination with other antiarrhythmics with increased effectiveness (quinidine, disopyramide, propafenone, amiodarone). **Drug interactions:** Phenobarbital, dilantin, rifampin ↓ mexiletine levels. Cimetidine ↑ mexiletine levels. Mexiletine ↑ theophylline levels.
Procainamide (IA) *Pronestyl*	Conversion of atrial fibrillation to sinus and maintenance of NSR. Suppresses premature atrial complexes, atrial tachycardia, atrial flutter and fibrillation. Slows conduction through accessory pathways. Effective in terminating and preventing VT. Effective in treating PVCs, but not recommended because of proarrhythmic effects.	**PO dose:** 3–7.5 g qd in divided doses 3–4 times a day (never more than 6 h between doses). Sustained-release forms q6h. **IV loading dose:** 17 mg/kg at 20 mg/min. If rapid loading is needed, give 100 mg doses over 5 min to total of 1–1.5 g. IV drip 2–4 mg/min. Therapeutic level = 4–10 µg/mL (may be as high as 5–32 mg/L to prevent sustained VT) Half-life = 3–4 h. Active metabolite is NAPA: therapeutic level = 9–12 mg/L	GI: nausea, vomiting, anorexia. CV: bradycardia, heart block, proarrhythmia (less than with quinidine). Prolongs QT interval. Hypotension with IV use. CNS: headache, insomnia, dizziness, psychosis, hallucinations, depression. Lupus-like syndrome with long-term use (15%–25% of patients who take drug >1 y). Other: rash, fever, swollen joints, agranulocytosis, pancytopenia.	Monitor QT intervals, QRS width, PR. Monitor NAPA level (active metabolite). Watch for hypotension with IV use. **Drug interactions:** Amiodarone, cimetidine, ranitidine, ↑ procainamide levels. Alcohol ↓ procainamide levels. Additive effects on conduction system disease when given with other class IA, class IC, tricyclic antidepressants, or Ca²⁺ blockers.
Propafenone (IC) *Rhythmol* Also has beta blocker effects	Conversion of atrial fibrillation to sinus and maintenance of NSR. Slow conduction through accessory pathways. Life-threatening ventricular arrhythmias (sustained VT).	150–300 mg tid. Therapeutic level = 0.2–3 µg/mL. Half-life = 2–10 h in normal metabolizers, up to 32 h in slow metabolizers.	GI: nausea, anorexia, constipation, metallic taste. CNS: dizziness, headache, blurred vision. CV: CHF, bradycardia, AV block, bundle-branch block, proarrhythmia.	Was not included in CAST but is same class as drugs shown to cause higher mortality post-MI. Watch for proarrhythmia.

Drug	Indications	Dosage	Side effects	Drug interactions / Monitoring
Propranolol (beta blocker) *Inderal*	Ventricular rate control in atrial fibrillation/flutter. Treatment of SVTs (slow AVT node conduction): AVNRT, CMT. Effective in some types of VT: exercise induced, digitalis induced. Effective in reducing incidence of VF and sudden death post-MI.	**PO:** 10–30 mg 3–4 times a day. **IV:** 1–3 mg at rate of 1 mg/min. Beta blocking plasma concentration = 50–100 ng/mL. Half-life = 3–5 h.	CV: bradycardia, heart block, hypotension, CHF. GI: nausea, vomiting, stomach discomfort, constipation, diarrhea. CNS: dreams, hallucinations, insomnia, depression. Other: bronchospasm, exacerbation of peripheral vascular disease, fatigue, hypoglycemia, impotence.	**Drug interactions:** ↑ Digoxin levels. Potentiates coumarin drugs. Has mild beta blocker and Ca²⁺ blocker effects. ↑ Cyclosporin levels. Quinidine and cimetidine ↑ propafenone levels. Noncardioselective beta blocker.
Quinidine (IA)	Conversion of atrial fibrillation to sinus and maintenance of NSR. May be used for other SVTs: atrial tachycardia, AVNRT, accessory pathways. Effective in treating PVCs and VT, but not recommended because of proarrhythmic effects.	**Sulfate:** 200–400 mg q6–8h. **Gluconate:** 324-mg sustained-release tabs, 1–2 q8–12h. Therapeutic level = 2–5 µg/mL Half-life = 7–9 h.	GI: nausea, diarrhea, abdominal pain. CV: hypotension, bradycardia, tachycardia, torsades de pointes, CHF. Prolongs QTc interval, proarrhythmia. CNS: cinchonism (tinnitus, hearing loss, confusion, delirium, visual disturbances, psychosis). Other: fever, headache, rashes, leukopenia, thrombocytopenia.	**Drug interactions:** Additive effects on HR, AV conduction, BP, and ↑ potential for CHF when given with negative inotropic drugs, Ca²⁺ blockers, digoxin. Give with food. Monitor QT interval, QRS width, PR. Watch for proarrhythmia (torsades de pointes). IV use rare (hypotension). **Drug interactions:** ↑ Digoxin levels. Increased bleeding when used with coumarin drugs. Dilantin, phenobarbital, rifampin, nifedipine, sodium bicarbonate, thiazide diuretics all ↓ quinidine levels. Cimetidine, amiodarone, verapamil all ↑ quinidine levels.
Sotalol (III) *Betapace* Has beta blocker effects	Conversion of atrial fibrillation to sinus and maintenance of NSR. Treatment of SVT. Slow conduction through accessory pathways. Life-threatening VT, VF.	80 mg bid × 3 d, then 160 mg bid × 3 d. 240–320 mg bid if necessary. Therapeutic level = 1–4 µg/mL (not clinically useful). Half-life = 10–20 h.	CV: bradycardia, heart block, CHF, proarrhythmia. Other: bronchospasm, fatigue, weakness, GI symptoms, dizziness, dyspnea, hypotension.	Prolongs QT interval, potential for proarrhythmia. Watch for bradycardia, AV block, and new or worsening CHF. No known drug interactions.
Tocainide (IB) *Tonocard*	Acute and chronic treatment of symptomatic VT.	400–600 mg q8h PO. Therapeutic level = 4–10 µg/mL Half-life = 11–15 h.	GI: nausea, vomiting, heartburn, anorexia, diarrhea. CNS: tremor, dizziness, ataxia, slurred speech, paresthesias, seizures, hallucinations, emotional instability, insomnia, memory impairment.	Give with food to ↓ GI effects. Can cause blood dyscrasias: monitor blood counts weekly for first 12 wk of therapy and frequently thereafter. No known drug interactions.

(continued)

TABLE 14-2 Antiarrhythmic Drugs *(Continued)*

Drug (Class)	Indication	Dose/Administration/ Therapeutic Level/Half-Life	Side Effects	Comments
			CV: bradycardia, hypotension, CHF, proarrhythmia (rare compared with other agents). Other: agranulocytosis, fever, rash, positive antinuclear antibody, pulmonary fibrosis.	
Verapamil (Ca²⁺ blocker) *Calan*	Ventricular rate control in atrial fibrillation/flutter. Slow conduction through AV note in AVNRT and CMT.	**PO:** 80–120 mg tid or qid. **IV:** 2.5–5 mg over 2 min. May repeat with 5–10 mg if needed. Therapeutic level = 80–400 ng/mL Half-life = 3–7 h.	Bradycardia, heart block, CHF, hypotension, fatigue, headache, edema, constipation.	Contraindicated in patients with accessory pathways (WPW, short PR syndrome) **Drug interactions:** Additive effects on HR, AV conduction, BP, and ↑ potential for CHF when given with negative inotropic drugs, Ca²⁺ blockers, digoxin.

AV, atrioventricular; AVNRT, atrioventricular nodal reentry tachycardia; BP, blood pressure; CAST, Cardiac Arrhythmia Suppression Trial; CHF, congestive heart failure; CMT, circus movement tachycardia; CNS, central nervous system; CV, cardiovascular; ECG, electrocardiogram; GI, gastrointestinal; HR, heart rate; IV, intravenous; MI, myocardial infarction; NAPA, *N*-acetyl procainamide; NSR, normal sinus rhythm; PO, oral; PVC, premature ventricular complex; SVT, supraventricular tachycardia; VF, ventricular fibrillation; VT, ventricular tachycardia; WPW, Wolff-Parkinson-White syndrome.

TABLE 14-3	Common Therapies for Tachyarrhythmias

Treatment	Atrial Fibrillation or Flutter, Atrial Tachycardia	AVNRT	CMT	VT
Adenosine 6 mg very rapidly IV. May repeat with 12 mg very rapidly IV if no effect within 2–3 min. May repeat 12-mg dose once more.	Slows AV conduction and unmasks atrial mechanism. (If atrial rate <250 = atrial tachycardia. If atrial rate >250 = atrial flutter. If atrial rhythm very rapid and chaotic with no formed P waves = atrial fibrillation.) Temporary slowing of ventricular rate only. Does not terminate atrial arrhythmia. Should not be used when mechanism is known to be atrial flutter, atrial fibrillation, or ectopic atrial tachycardia, or if atrial fibrillation with accessory pathway conduction is suspected.	**Drug of choice for treatment of PSVT when mechanism is unknown or if known AVNRT.** Terminates rhythm by blocking conduction through AV node. Does not prevent recurrence.	**Drug of choice for treatment of PSVT if mechanism unknown or if known CMT.** Terminates rhythm by blocking conduction through AV node. Does not prevent recurrence.	No effect but also no harm.
Beta blockers Esmolol (Brevebloc) Atenolol (Tenormin) Metoprolol (Lopressor)	Slow AV conduction and provide long-term control of ventricular rate. Usually do not convert atrial arrhythmias to sinus rhythm.	May terminate AVNRT by blocking conduction through slow pathway in AV node. Do not prevent recurrence unless they suppress initiating PACs.	May terminate CMT by blocking conduction through AV node. Do not prevent recurrence unless they suppress initiating PACs or PVCs.	Not indicated for acute treatment of VT episode. May be used for prevention of some types of VT.
Calcium channel blockers Diltiazem (Cardizem) Verapamil (Calan)	Slow Av conduction and provide long-term control of ventricular rate. Usually do not convert atrial arrhythmias to sinus rhythm. **Do not use in atrial fibrillation with accessory pathway conduction.**	May terminate AVNRT by blocking conduction through slow or fast pathway in AV node. Do not prevent recurrence unless they suppress initiating PACs.	May terminate CMT by blocking conduction through AV node. Do not prevent recurrence unless suppress initiating PACs or PVCs.	**Do not use for wide QRS tachycardia of uncertain type.** Generally not indicated for VT (except for "verapamil-sensitive" type of VT).
Cardioversion First choice for hemodynamically unstable tachycardias.	If rapid ventricular response results in hemodynamic instability. Terminates individual episode but does not prevent recurrence.	If rapid rate results in hemodynamic instability. Terminates individual episode but does not prevent recurrence.	If rapid rate results in hemodynamic instability. Terminates individual episode but does not prevent recurrence.	If rapid rate results in hemodynamic instability. Terminates individual episode but does not prevent recurrence.

(continued)

| TABLE 14-3 | Common Therapies for Tachyarrhythmias *(Continued)* |

Treatment	Atrial Fibrillation or Flutter, Atrial Tachycardia	AVNRT	CMT	VT
Ibutilide (Corvert) 1 mg over 10 min. May repeat same dose in 10 min if needed.	**Becoming drug of choice to convert atrial fibrillation or flutter to normal sinus rhythm.** Usually converts within 20 min. Causes prolonged QT interval and may cause torsades de pointes.	Not indicated.	Not indicated.	Not indicated.
Procainamide IV loading dose 17 mg/kg at 20 mg/min. Oral sustained release up to 1,000–1,300 mg/d.	**Drug of choice for atrial fibrillation with accessory pathway conduction** because it prolongs refractory period of pathway and slows ventricular rate. May also convert atrial arrhythmias to sinus rhythm.	May terminate AVNRT by slowing conduction through fast pathways in AV node. May prevent recurrence by suppressing initiating PACs.	May terminate CMT by slowing conduction through accessory pathway. May prevent recurrence by suppressing initiating PACs or PVCs.	May terminate VT or slow its rate. **Good choice for treating wide QRS tachycardias of unknown type or known VT.**
Radiofrequency catheter ablation	Atrial flutter focus can sometimes be ablated. Ablation of AV node in drug-refractory atrial fibrillation sometimes done, and pacemaker inserted when ventricular rate control not possible with drugs.	Ablation of slow pathway in AV node prevents recurrence of AVNRT.	Ablation of accessory pathway prevents recurrence of CMT.	Ablation of VT focus may be helpful in VT originating in right ventricular outflow tract. Ablation of right bundle-branch sometimes successful in bundle-branch reentry VT.

AV, atrioventricular; AVNRT, atrioventricular nodal reentry tachycardia; CMT, circus movement tachycardia using accessory pathway; IV, intravenous; PAC, premature atrial complex; PSVT, paroxysmal supraventricular tachycardia; PVC, premature ventricular complex; VT, ventricular tachycardia.

TABLE 14-4   **Common Therapies for Bradyarrhythmias**

Treatment	Sinus Bradycardia, Junctional Bradycardia	Second-Degree AV Block—Type I Wenckebach	Second-Degree AV Block—Type II	Third-Degree AV Block	Asystole
Atropine (0.5–1 mg IV)	↑ Sinus rate, may ↑ rate of junctional pacemaker. May stimulate sinus rhythm when junctional pacemaker in control of ventricles. Usually very effective, especially for sinus bradycardia.	↑ Sinus rate and ↑ AV nodal conduction. Usually very effective.	Should be used with caution in type II block—may cause slowing of ventricular rate. Type II block is due to disease below the AV node where atropine has no effect. Atropine ↑ sinus rate and AV conduction, thus increasing number of impulses reaching diseased bundle branches.	Usually has no effect on complete AV block. If junctional rhythm is controlling ventricles, atropine may increase rate of junctional focus.	Given in addition to epinephrine to treat asystole. Give 1 mg IV every 3 min to total vagolytic dose of 0.04 mg/kg.
Epinephrine	May be infused at 2–10 µg/min to maintain BP while waiting for pacing to be instituted.	May be infused at 2–10 µg/min to maintain BP while waiting for pacing to be instituted.	May be infused at 2–10 µg/min to maintain BP while waiting for pacing to be instituted.	May be infused at 2–10 µg/min to maintain BP while waiting for pacing to be instituted.	IV bolus of 1 mg every 3–5 min during resuscitation efforts.
Transcutaneous pacing	Not usually needed but may be used for severe bradycardia until transvenous pacing wire can be placed.	Not usually needed. May be used temporarily until transvenous pacing can be instituted if symptomatic bradycardia is unresponsive to atropine.	May be used temporarily until transvenous pacing can be instituted if symptomatic bradycardia.	May be required in symptomatic patients until transvenous pacing wire can be placed.	May be helpful if instituted early in resuscitation efforts.
Temporary transvenous pacing	May be necessary on short-term basis if symptomatic bradycardia is unresponsive to atropine, especially in presence of inferior MI. Usually not needed for more than a few days, because sinus node function usually improves.	May be necessary on short-term basis if symptomatic bradycardia is unresponsive to atropine, especially in presence of inferior MI. Usually not needed for more than a few days, because block usually resolves.	May be necessary to stabilize patient with symptomatic bradycardia, especially in anterior MI. Often used as bridge to permanent pacemaker insertion if block does not resolve.	May be necessary to stabilize patient with symptomatic third-degree block regardless of cause. Often used as bridge to permanent pacemaker insertion if block does not resolve.	Not usually attempted during resuscitation because of difficulties placing wire during resuscitation, unless transcutaneous pacing not available. If used, success rate better if instituted early in resuscitation attempt.

AV, atrioventricular; BP, blood pressure; IV, intravenous; MI, myocardial infarction.

heart gives rise to the classic surface ECG, which can be monitored at the bedside. Chapter 13 presents information on the origin of the waves and intervals of the cardiac cycle.

The characteristics of normal sinus rhythm include the following:

Rate: 60 to 100 beats/min

Rhythm: Regular

P waves: Precede every QRS complex and are consistent in shape

PR interval: 0.12 to 0.20 second

QRS complex: 0.04 to 0.10 second

Example: Normal sinus rhythm—rate, 65 beats/min; PR interval, 0.14 second; QRS interval, 0.06 second

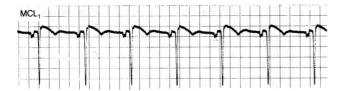

SINUS BRADYCARDIA

Sinus bradycardia is discharge of the sinus node at a rate slower than 60 beats/min. It can be a normal variant, especially in athletes and during sleep. Sinus bradycardia may be a response to vagal stimulation, such as carotid sinus massage (CSM), ocular pressure, or vomiting. Disease processes that can cause sinus bradycardia include inferior wall MI, myxedema, obstructive jaundice, uremia, increased intracranial pressure, glaucoma, anorexia nervosa, and sick sinus syndrome.[20,59,110] Sinus bradycardia can be a response to several medications, including digitalis, beta blockers, and calcium channel blockers.

The following are ECG characteristics of sinus bradycardia:

Rate: Less than 60 beats/min

Rhythm: Regular

P waves: Precede every QRS, consistent shape

PR interval: Usually normal (0.12 to 0.20 second)

QRS complex: Usually normal (0.04 to 0.10 second)

Conduction: Normal through atria, AV node, bundle branches, and ventricles

Example: Sinus bradycardia—rate, 40 beats/min

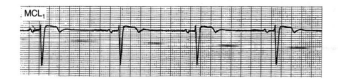

Sinus bradycardia does not require treatment unless the patient is symptomatic. If the arrhythmia is accompanied by hypotension, restlessness, diaphoresis, chest pain, or other signs of hemodynamic compromise or by ventricular ectopy, atropine, 0.5 to 1 mg intravenously (IV) is the treatment of choice. Attempts should be made to decrease vagal stimulation, and if bradycardia is due to medications, they should be held until their need has been reevaluated. See Chapter 25 for the ACLS algorithm for treatment of symptomatic bradycardia.

SINUS TACHYCARDIA

Sinus tachycardia is sinus rhythm at a rate faster than 100 beats/min. It is a normal response to anything that stimulates the sympathetic nervous system, including sympathomimetic drugs, exercise, and emotion. Sinus tachycardia that persists at rest usually indicates some underlying problem, such as fever, blood loss, anxiety, heart failure, hypermetabolic states, or anemia.[59,110] Sinus tachycardia is a normal physiologic response to a decrease in cardiac output. Drugs that can cause sinus tachycardia include atropine, isoproterenol, epinephrine, dopamine, dobutamine, norepinephrine, nitroprusside, and caffeine.

The ECG characteristics of sinus tachycardia include the following:

Rate: Greater than 100 beats/min

Rhythm: Regular

P waves: Precede every QRS; have consistent shape; may be buried in the preceding T wave

PR interval: Usually normal; may be difficult to measure if P waves are buried in T waves

QRS complex: Usually normal

Conduction: Normal through atria, AV node, bundle branches, and ventricles

Example: Sinus tachycardia—rate, 125 beats/min

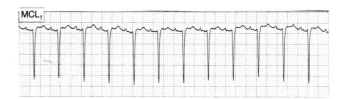

Treatment of sinus tachycardia is directed at the cause. Because this arrhythmia is a physiologic response to a decrease in cardiac output, it should never be ignored, especially in the cardiac patient. Because the ventricles fill with blood and the coronary arteries perfuse during diastole, persistent tachycardia can cause decreased stroke volume, decreased cardiac output, and decreased coronary perfusion secondary to the decreased diastolic time that occurs with rapid heart rates. Carotid sinus pressure may slow the heart rate temporarily and thereby help in ruling out other arrhythmias. Beta blockers are used to treat tachycardia in patients with acute MI without signs of heart failure or contraindications to beta blocker therapy.

SINUS ARRHYTHMIA

Sinus arrhythmia occurs when the sinus node discharges irregularly. It occurs as a normal phenomenon and is commonly associated with the phases of respiration. During inspiration, the sinus node fires faster; during expiration, it slows. Other than this phasic increase and decrease in rate, sinus arrhythmia looks like normal sinus rhythm. The following characteristics are typical of sinus arrhythmia:

Rate: 60 to 100 beats/min

Rhythm: Irregular; phasic increase and decrease in rate, which may be related to respiration

P waves: Precede every QRS; have consistent shape

PR interval: Usually normal

QRS complex: Usually normal

Conduction: Normal through atria, AV node, bundle branches, ventricles

Example: Sinus arrhythmia

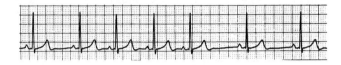

Treatment of sinus arrhythmia is usually not necessary, but the administration of atropine may increase the rate or abolish the irregularity.

SINUS ARREST

Sinus arrest occurs when sinus node automaticity is depressed and impulses are not formed when expected. This results in the absence of a P wave at the time it is expected to occur, and unless there is escape of a junctional or ventricular pacemaker, the QRS complex is also missing. If only one sinus impulse fails to form, the term *sinus pause* is usually used, whereas if more than one sinus impulse in a row fails to form, sinus arrest has occurred. Because the sinus node has depressed automaticity and does not form impulses regularly as expected, the P-P interval in sinus arrest is not an exact multiple of the sinus cycle. Causes of sinus arrest include vagal stimulation, carotid sinus sensi-

tivity, MI interrupting the blood supply to the sinus node, and drugs such as digitalis, beta blockers, and calcium channel blockers. Sinus arrest is characterized by the following ECG changes.

Rate: Atrial—usually within normal range but may be in bradycardic range if several sinus impulses fail to form. Ventricular—usually within normal range but may be in bradycardic range if several sinus impulses fail to form and there are no junctional or ventricular escape beats. Occasionally, the ventricular rate may be faster than the atrial rate because of junctional or ventricular escape beats that occur during the period of sinus arrest.

Rhythm: Irregular due to absence of sinus node discharge

P waves: Present when sinus node is firing and absent during periods of sinus arrest. When present, they precede every QRS complex and are consistent in shape. If junctional escape beats occur, P waves may be inverted either before or after the junctional QRS.

PR interval: Usually normal when P waves are present. If junctional escape beats occur, the PR interval is short when the P wave precedes the junctional QRS.

QRS complex: Usually normal when sinus node is functioning and absent during periods of sinus arrest unless escape beats occur. If ventricular escape beats occur, QRS complex is wide.

Conduction: Normal through atria, AV node, bundle branches, and ventricles when sinus node is firing. When the sinus node fails to form impulses, there is no conduction through the atria. If a junctional escape beat occurs, ventricular conduction is usually normal, whereas if a ventricular escape beat occurs, conduction through the ventricles is abnormally slow.

Examples: (A) Sinus pause. (B) Sinus pause and sinus arrest with a junctional escape beat

Treatment of sinus arrest is aimed at the cause and at increasing ventricular rate if the patient is symptomatic. Any offending drugs should be discontinued, and vagal stimulation should be minimized. If periods of sinus arrest are frequent and causing hemodynamic compromise, atropine, 0.5 to 1 mg IV, may increase the rate. Pacemaker therapy may be necessary if all other forms of management fail.

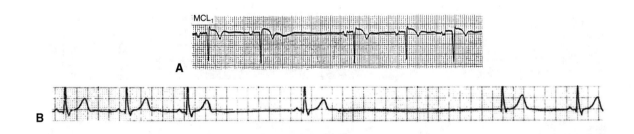

SINUS EXIT BLOCK

Sinus exit block occurs when the impulse is formed in the sinus node normally but fails to exit the node to excite atrial tissue. Sinus exit block can be type I, type II, or complete. The section of this chapter on Complex Arrhythmias and Conduction Disturbances contains a discussion of sinus Wenckebach, which is type I sinus exit block. Type II sinus exit block looks exactly like sinus arrest except for the P-P intervals, which are multiples of the basic sinus cycle length. Complete sinus exit block exists when no impulses reach the atria from the sinus node and no P waves occur. In this case, either a junctional or ventricular pacemaker emerges to take over pacing duties, or asystole occurs.

Rate: Atrial—usually within normal range but may be in bradycardic range if several sinus impulses fail to exit the sinus node. Ventricular—usually in normal range but may be in bradycardic range if no junctional or ventricular escape beats occur during periods of sinus exit block.

Rhythm: Irregular due to pauses caused by sinus exit block

P waves: Present except when impulse fails to exit sinus node. When present, they precede every QRS and are consistent in shape. The P-P interval is an exact multiple of the sinus cycle because impulses are formed regularly but occasionally fail to exit the sinus node.

PR interval: Usually normal when P waves are present

QRS complexes: Usually normal when sinus impulse conducts and absent when exit block occurs. If ventricular escape beats occur, QRS is wide.

Conduction: Normal through atria, AV node, bundle branches, and ventricles when impulse exits sinus node normally

Example: Sinus exit block. The length of the pause is exactly double the sinus rate. (From Huff J, Doernbach DP, White RD: ECG Workout, 2nd ed, p 53. Philadelphia, JB Lippincott, 1993.)

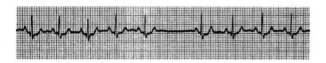

Treatment of sinus exit block depends on the resulting ventricular rate and its hemodynamic significance. Atropine may cause an increase in rate if bradycardia is symptomatic. Pacing may be necessary, especially with complete sinus exit block. Otherwise, the treatment is similar to that of sinus arrest.

SICK SINUS SYNDROME

The term *sick sinus syndrome* is used to describe rhythms in which there is marked sinus bradycardia, sinus pauses, or periods of sinus arrest alternating with paroxysms of rapid atrial arrhythmias, especially atrial flutter or atrial fibrillation. The term *brady-tachy syndrome* is commonly used to describe the same arrhythmias.[59,110] During periods of sinus bradycardia or arrest, junctional escape rhythms commonly occur, and AV block is also often associated with sick sinus syndrome. Causes of sick sinus syndrome include inflammatory cardiac disease, cardiomyopathy, sclerodegenerative processes involving both the sinus and AV nodes, and drugs such as beta blockers, calcium channel blockers, digitalis, amiodarone, propafenone, and adenosine.[42,59,110] ECG characteristics of sick sinus syndrome include:

Rate: Varies from bradycardic to tachycardic rates depending on sinus node function, rate of escape pacemakers, and presence of atrial tachyarrhythmias

Rhythm: Irregular. Pauses of 3 seconds or more can occur during periods of sinus arrest. Regularity of rhythm depends on reliability of sinus node and escape pacemakers, and on type of tachyarrhythmia present (e.g., atrial fibrillation is very irregular).

P waves: Usually normal during periods of sinus rhythm. Absent during periods of sinus arrest or atrial fibrillation, inverted with junctional rhythms. Flutter waves are present during periods of atrial flutter.

PR interval: May be normal or prolonged depending on state of AV conduction

QRS complex: Usually normal unless there is associated bundle-branch block or ventricular escape rhythms

Conduction: Normal through the atria when the sinus node is in control, abnormal through atria during periods of atrial tachyarrhythmias. AV conduction may be normal or abnormal depending on degree of AV node disease. Conduction through ventricles normal unless bundle-branch block is present or a ventricular escape rhythm occurs.

Example: Sick sinus syndrome. Intermittent sinus arrest with junctional escape beats (filled circles in top strip), then a short episode of atrial flutter followed by almost 5 seconds of asystole before a junctional escape rhythm resumes. (From Zipes DP: Specific arrhythmias: Diagnosis and treatment. In Braunwald E (ed): Heart Disease, 4th ed, p 677. Philadelphia, WB Saunders, 1992.)

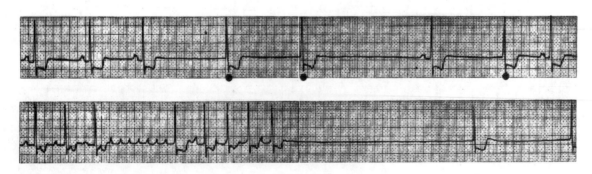

Treatment of sick sinus syndrome may include atropine for bradyarrhythmias and antiarrhythmics such as quinidine, procainamide, or others for tachyarrhythmias. Permanent pacing is usually necessary because drugs used to treat the tachyarrhythmias aggravate bradycardia and often further depress sinus node function.

Rhythms Originating in the Atria

Ectopic impulses or reentry circuits can occur in the atrial myocardium, resulting in several atrial arrhythmias: premature atrial complex (PAC), WAP, atrial tachycardia, multifocal atrial tachycardia (MAT), atrial flutter, and atrial fibrillation. See Chapter 25 for the ACLS algorithm for treatment of tachycardias.

PREMATURE ATRIAL COMPLEXES

A PAC occurs when an irritable focus in the atria fires before the next sinus impulse is due. PACs can be caused by caffeine, alcohol, nicotine, stretch on the atria (as in congestive heart failure [CHF] or pulmonary disease), interruption of atrial blood supply by myocardial ischemia or MI, anxiety, and hypermetabolic states. PACs can also occur in normal hearts.

The ECG characteristics of PACs include the following:

Rate: Usually within normal range

Rhythm: Usually regular except when PACs occur, resulting in early beats. PACs often have a noncompensatory pause (interval between the complex before and that after the PAC is less than two normal R-R intervals) because premature depolarization of the atria by the PAC usually causes premature depolarization of the sinus node, thus causing the sinus node to "reset" itself.

P waves: Precede every QRS. The configuration of the premature P wave differs from that of the sinus P waves because the premature impulse originates in a different part of the atria and depolarizes them in a different way. Very early P waves may be buried in the preceding T wave.

PR interval: May be normal or long depending on the prematurity of the beat. Very early PACs may find the AV junction still partially refractory and unable to conduct at a normal rate, resulting in a prolonged PR interval.

QRS complex: May be normal, aberrant (wide), or absent, depending on the prematurity of the beat. If the ventricles have repolarized completely, they are able to conduct the early impulse normally, resulting in a normal QRS. If the PAC occurs during the relative refractory period of the bundle branches or ventricles, the impulse conducts aberrantly and the QRS is wide. If the PAC occurs very early during the complete refractory period of the bundle branches or ventricles, the impulse does not conduct to the ventricles and the QRS is absent.

Conduction: PACs travel through the atria differently from sinus impulses because they originate from a different spot. Conduction through the AV node, bundle branches, and ventricles is usually normal unless the PAC is very early (see previous discussion of PR interval and QRS complex).

Examples: (A) Sinus rhythm with PACs. (B) Sinus rhythm with a nonconducted PAC.

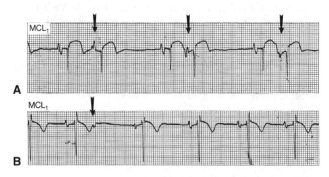

Treatment of PACs usually is unnecessary because they do not cause hemodynamic compromise. Frequent PACs may precede more serious arrhythmias such as atrial fibrillation. Drugs such as quinidine, disopyramide, and procainamide can be used to suppress atrial activity if necessary.

WANDERING ATRIAL PACEMAKER

Wandering atrial pacemaker refers to rhythms that exhibit varying P-wave morphology as the site of impulse formation shifts from the sinus node to the atria to the AV junction.[110] This occurs when two (usually sinus and junctional) or more supraventricular pacemakers compete with each other for control of the heart. Because the rates of these competing pacemakers are almost identical, it is common to have atrial fusion occur as the atria are activated by more than one wave of depolarization at a time, resulting in varying P-wave morphology. WAP can be due to increased vagal tone that slows the sinus pacemaker or to enhanced automaticity in atrial or junctional pacemaker cells, causing them to compete with the sinus node for control.

Wandering atrial pacemaker is characterized as follows:

Rate: 60 to 100 beats/min

Rhythm: May be slightly irregular

P waves: Exhibit varying shapes (upright, flat, inverted, notched) as impulses originate in different parts of the atria or junction and as atrial fusion occurs. At least three different P-wave configurations should be seen.

PR interval: May vary depending on proximity of the pacemaker to the AV node

QRS complex: Usually normal

Conduction: Conduction through the atria varies as it is depolarized from different spots. Conduction through the bundle branches and ventricles is usually normal.

Example: WAP

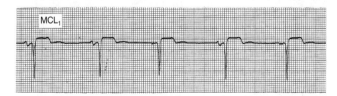

Treatment of WAP is not usually necessary. If heart rate is slow enough to be symptomatic, atropine can be given.

MULTIFOCAL ATRIAL TACHYCARDIA

Multifocal atrial tachycardia is rapid firing of several ectopic atrial foci at a rate faster than 100 beats/min. MAT is most commonly associated with chronic pulmonary disease, CHF, hypokalemia, hypomagnesemia, acute MI, and theophylline toxicity.[37,83,110]

The ECG characteristics of MAT include the following:

Rate: Usually 100 to 130 beats/min

Rhythm: Usually irregular

P waves: Vary in shape because they originate in different spots in the atria. At least three different P waves are seen. They usually precede each QRS complex, but some may be blocked in the AV node.

PR interval: May vary depending on proximity of each ectopic atrial focus to the AV node and the prematurity of atrial impulses

QRS complex: Usually normal

Conduction: Usually normal through the AV node and ventricles. Aberrant ventricular conduction may occur if an impulse is conducted into the ventricles while they are partially refractory.

Example: MAT

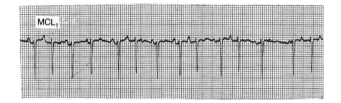

Treatment of MAT is directed toward eliminating the cause, including hypoxia and electrolyte imbalances. Antiarrhythmic therapy is often ineffective. Beta blockers, verapamil, flecainide, and amiodarone have been reported to be successful.[37,83] Beta blockers seem to work best but must be used with caution because pulmonary disease is usually associated with MAT. Theophylline may need to be discontinued. If MAT is chronic and unresponsive to drug therapy, radiofrequency ablation of the AV node and insertion of a permanent pacemaker may be necessary to control the ventricular rate.[83]

ATRIAL TACHYCARDIA AND PAROXYSMAL ATRIAL TACHYCARDIA

Atrial tachycardia is a rapid atrial rhythm at a rate of 120 to 250 beats/min. This rhythm may be due to rapid firing of an ectopic atrial focus or to an atrial reentry circuit that allows an impulse to travel rapidly and repeatedly around a pathway in the atria.[83,110] When the arrhythmia abruptly starts and terminates, the term *paroxysmal atrial tachycardia* is used. Atrial tachycardia has been associated with caffeine, tobacco, alcohol, mitral valve disease, rheumatic heart disease, chronic obstructive pulmonary disease, acute MI, and digitalis toxicity.

If the atrial rate is very rapid, the AV node begins to block some of the impulses attempting to travel through it

to protect the ventricles from excessively rapid rates. In normal, healthy hearts, the AV node can usually conduct each atrial impulse up to rates of approximately 180 beats/min. In patients with cardiac disease or in those who take drugs that slow AV conduction, the AV node cannot conduct each impulse, and atrial tachycardia with block occurs.

The ECG characteristics of atrial tachycardia include the following:

Rate: Atrial rate is 120 to 250 beats/min. The ventricular rate depends on the amount of block at the AV node and may be the same as the atrial rate or slower.

Rhythm: Regular unless there is variable block at the AV node

P waves: Differ in configuration from sinus P waves because they are ectopic. Precede each QRS complex but may be hidden in preceding T wave. When block is present, more than one P wave appears before each QRS complex.

PR interval: May be shorter or longer than normal but often difficult to measure because of hidden P waves

QRS complex: Usually normal but may be wide if aberrant conduction is present

Conduction: Usually normal through the AV node and into the ventricles. In atrial tachycardia with block, some atrial impulses do not conduct into the ventricles. Aberrant ventricular conduction may occur if atrial impulses are conducted into the ventricles while the bundle branches are still partially refractory.

Examples: Atrial tachycardia. Both strips are from the same patient. (A) Atrial tachycardia at a rate of 187 beats/min. (B) Atrial tachycardia with block, occurring after administration of propranolol.

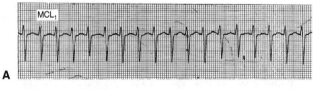

A

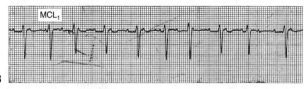

B

Treatment of atrial tachycardia is directed toward eliminating the cause and decreasing the ventricular rate. Sedation alone may terminate the rhythm or slow the rate. If the patient is severely symptomatic, cardioversion may be necessary to terminate the episode. Vagal stimulation, either through CSM or Valsalva maneuver, or adenosine may terminate some episodes of atrial tachycardia. Beta blockers, verapamil, and diltiazem increase block at the AV node and may slow ventricular response or terminate the tachycardia. Digitalis slows ventricular rate by increasing block at the AV node, but it can also be the cause of atrial tachycardia with block and should be discontinued if that is the case. Type IA, IC, and III antiarrhythmics may be effective in reducing the number of tachycardia episodes. Radiofrequency catheter ablation of the ectopic focus or reentry circuit is successful in many cases.

ATRIAL FLUTTER

In atrial flutter, the atria are depolarized at rates of 250 to 450 times per minute. A reentry circuit in the right atrium is responsible for type I (classic) atrial flutter and usually results in an atrial rate of 300 beats/min.[83,94,95] Type II flutter is more rapid, with atrial rates in the 400 to 450 beats/min range, and less is known about the mechanism of this type of flutter. At such rapid atrial rates, the AV node usually blocks at least half of the impulses to protect the ventricles from excessive rates. Because atrial flutter most often occurs at a rate of 300 beats/min, and because the AV node usually blocks half of those impulses, a ventricular rate of 150 beats/min is common. Therefore, whenever a ventricular rate of 150 beats/min is seen, the diagnosis of atrial flutter with 2 : 1 conduction should be suspected until proved otherwise. Causes of atrial flutter include rheumatic heart disease, atherosclerotic heart disease, thyrotoxicosis, CHF, cardiac surgery, and myocardial ischemia or MI.

Atrial flutter is characterized as follows:

Rate: Atrial rate varies between 250 to 450 beats/min, most commonly 300 beats/min. Ventricular rate varies depending on the amount of block at the AV node, most commonly 150 beats/min and rarely 300 beats/min. Ventricular rates can be within the normal range when atrial flutter is treated with appropriate drugs. Rarely, 1 : 1 conduction results in a ventricular rate of 300 beats/min.

Rhythm: Atrial rhythm is regular. Ventricular rhythm may be regular or irregular because of varying AV block.

P waves: F waves (flutter waves) are seen, characterized by a regular, sawtooth pattern thought to be composed of the atrial depolarization wave followed by the atrial repolarization, or atrial T wave. One F wave is usually hidden in the QRS complex, and when 2 : 1 conduction occurs, F waves may not be readily apparent. Flutter waves are best seen in the inferior leads (II, III, and avF) and may appear more like individual P waves in lead V$_1$.

PR interval: May be consistent or may vary in a Wenckebach-type pattern (see section on Multilevel Atrioventricular Block, under Complex Arrhythmias and Conduction Disturbances)

QRS complex: Usually normal; aberration can occur

Conduction: Usually normal through the AV node and ventricles. Multilevel AV block commonly occurs (see section Complex Arrhythmias and Conduction Disturbances).

Examples: Atrial flutter. All strips are from the same patient. (A) Atrial flutter with 2 : 1 conduction. (B) Ventricular rate slows momentarily and flutter waves are clearly visible at a rate of 300 beats/min. (C) Atrial flutter with variable conduction.

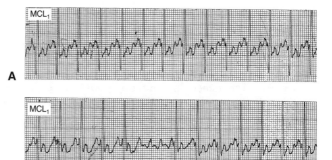

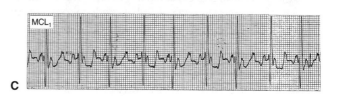

Because the ventricular rate in atrial flutter can be rapid, symptoms associated with decreased cardiac output can occur. Mural thrombi may form in the atria because there is no strong atrial contraction and blood stasis occurs, leading to a risk of systemic or pulmonary emboli. Persistent atrial flutter is uncommon; it usually converts to either sinus rhythm or atrial fibrillation spontaneously or as a result of drug therapy.

The immediate goal of treatment depends on the hemodynamic consequences of the arrhythmia. Excessively rapid ventricular rates need to be controlled immediately if cardiac output is significantly compromised. Cardioversion may be necessary as an immediate treatment, especially if 1 : 1 conduction occurs. Verapamil, diltiazem, beta blockers, or digitalis can be used to slow ventricular rate. Type IA (quinidine and procainamide), type IC (flecainide, propafenone), or type III antiarrhythmics (sotalol, amiodarone) may convert flutter to sinus rhythm. These agents are also useful in maintaining sinus rhythm after conversion. Drugs that slow the atrial rate, like quinidine, should never be given without prior treatment to ensure adequate AV block if the ventricular response to flutter is rapid. The danger of giving quinidine alone is that as atrial rate slows from 300 to 200 beats/min, for example, it is possible for the AV node to conduct each impulse rather than block impulses, thus leading to even faster ventricular rates.

A new type III antiarrhythmic agent, ibutilide (Corvert), can be given IV and is often successful in converting atrial flutter to sinus rhythm if flutter is recent in onset. Rapid atrial pacing can also be used to terminate atrial flutter, especially when it occurs after cardiac surgery. Radiofrequency catheter ablation of the flutter reentry circuit is becoming the treatment of choice for chronic or recurrent atrial flutter.

ATRIAL FIBRILLATION

Atrial fibrillation is an extremely rapid and disorganized pattern of depolarization in the atria. The mechanism of this arrhythmia is most likely multiple reentry circuits in the atria.[29] Atrial fibrillation is the most common rhythm seen (next to sinus rhythm) and can be chronic or occur in paroxysms. Atrial fibrillation commonly occurs in the presence of atherosclerotic or rheumatic heart disease, thyrotoxicosis,

CHF, valve disease, pulmonary disease, MI, and congenital heart disease, and after cardiac surgery.

Atrial fibrillation is characterized as follows:

Rate: Atrial rate is 400 to 600 beats/min or faster. Ventricular rate varies depending on the amount of block at the AV node. In new-onset atrial fibrillation, the ventricular response is usually rapid, 110 to 160 beats/min; in treated atrial fibrillation, the ventricular rate is controlled in the normal range of 60 to 100 beats/min.

Rhythm: Irregular. One of the distinguishing features of atrial fibrillation is the marked irregularity of the ventricular response because of concealed conduction in the AV junction (see section on Complex Arrhythmias and Conduction Disturbances). If the ventricular response is ever regular in the presence of atrial fibrillation, AV dissociation should be suspected.

P waves: Not present. Atrial activity is chaotic, with no formed atrial impulses visible. Irregular F waves are often seen and vary in size from coarse to very fine.

PR interval: Not measurable because there are no P waves

QRS complex: Usually normal; aberration is common

Conduction: Intra-atrial conduction is disorganized and irregular. Most of the atrial impulses are blocked in the AV junction; those impulses that are conducted through the AV junction are usually conducted normally through the ventricles. If an atrial impulse reaches the bundle-branch system during its refractory period, aberrant intraventricular conduction can occur.

Examples: (A) Atrial fibrillation. (B) Alternating coarse and fine atrial fibrillation (sometimes called *atrial fib-flutter*). (C) Fine atrial fibrillation. (D) Atrial fibrillation with a slow and regular ventricular response, most likely due to complete AV block.

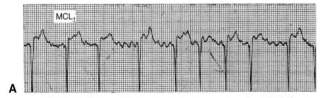

A

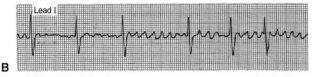

B

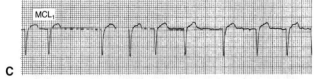

C

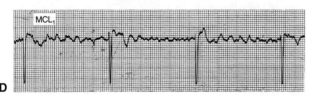

D

If the ventricular response to atrial fibrillation is rapid, cardiac output can be reduced secondary to decreased diastolic filling time in the ventricles. Because the atria quiver rather than contract, atrial kick is lost, which can also reduce cardiac output. Another possible complication is mural thrombus formation in the atria due to stasis of blood. This can lead to pulmonary or systemic embolization if clots dislodge spontaneously or with conversion to sinus rhythm.

Treatment of atrial fibrillation is directed toward eliminating the cause, controlling ventricular rate, restoring and maintaining sinus rhythm, and preventing thromboembolism. Cardioversion may be necessary if the patient is hemodynamically unstable because of rapid ventricular rates. Diltiazem, verapamil, beta blockers, and digitalis are commonly used to reduce ventricular rate by increasing block at the AV node. Atrial antiarrhythmic drugs used to convert atrial fibrillation to sinus rhythm and to maintain sinus rhythm include type IA agents (quinidine, procainamide, disopyramide), type IC agents (flecainide, propafenone), and type III agents (amiodarone, sotalol). Ibutilide is a new type III antiarrhythmic used for rapid conversion of atrial fibrillation to sinus rhythm and works best in new-onset atrial fibrillation. Anticoagulation with a coumarin drug is necessary if atrial fibrillation is chronic.

SUPRAVENTRICULAR TACHYCARDIA

The term *supraventricular tachycardia* (SVT) is used for tachycardias that originate above the ventricles for which the exact mechanism cannot be determined from the ECG. Atrial tachycardia, atrial flutter, and junctional tachycardia can all cause SVT. AVNRT and circus movement tachycardia (CMT) using an accessory pathway are the two most common mechanisms of SVT. (See section on Complex Arrhythmias and Conduction Disturbances for discussion of these two causes of SVT). SVT is characterized by the following:

Rate: Greater than 100 beats/min, can be as fast as 280 beats/min

Rhythm: Regular

P waves: Usually not visible, making the exact mechanism of the tachycardia uncertain

PR interval: Not measurable if P waves cannot be seen

QRS complex: Usually narrow; may be wide if aberrant ventricular conduction occurs

Conduction: Conduction through the atria varies depending on the mechanism of tachycardia. Atria may depolarize in a retrograde direction when the mechanism is AVNRT or CMT. Conduction through ventricles is normal unless bundle-branch block is present or there is anterograde conduction through an accessory pathway.

Example: SVT with a narrow QRS and no identifiable P waves

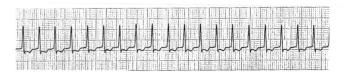

Treatment of SVT depends on the patient's tolerance of the arrhythmia. If the ventricular rate is fast enough to cause hemodynamic instability, cardioversion is the treatment of choice. Drugs such as adenosine, beta blockers, calcium channel blockers, and digitalis can slow ventricular rate or terminate many SVTs. (See section on Complex Arrhythmias and Conduction Disturbances for more detailed information on treating SVTs.)

Rhythms Originating in the Atrioventricular Junction

Cells surrounding the AV node in the AV junctional area have automaticity and are capable of initiating impulses and controlling the heart rhythm. Junctional arrhythmias include premature junctional complex (PJC), junctional rhythm, and junctional tachycardia.

Junctional beats and junctional rhythms can appear any of three ways on the ECG depending on the location of the junctional pacemaker and the speed of conduction of the impulse into the atria and ventricles:

1. When a junctional focus fires, the wave of depolarization spreads backward (retrograde) into the atria as well as forward (anterograde) into the ventricles. If the impulse arrives in the atria before it arrives in the ventricles, the ECG shows a P wave (usually inverted because the atria are depolarized from bottom to top) followed immediately by a QRS complex as the impulse reaches the ventricles. In this case, the PR interval is short, usually 0.10 second or less.
2. If the junctional impulse reaches both the atria and the ventricles at the same time, only a QRS is seen on the ECG because the ventricles are much larger than the atria, and only ventricular depolarization is seen, even though the atria are also depolarizing.
3. If the junctional impulse reaches the ventricles before it reaches the atria, the QRS precedes the P wave on the ECG. Again, the P wave usually is inverted because of retrograde atrial depolarization, and the RP interval (distance from the beginning of the QRS to the beginning of the following P wave) is short, usually 0.10 second or less.

PREMATURE JUNCTIONAL COMPLEXES

Premature junctional complexes are due to an irritable focus in the AV junction. Irritability can be due to coronary heart disease (CHD) or MI disrupting blood flow to the AV junction, nicotine, caffeine, catecholamines, or drugs such as digitalis.

Premature junctional complexes have the following ECG characteristics:

Rate: 60 to 100 beats/min or the rate of the basic rhythm

Rhythm: Irregular because of the early beats

P waves: May occur before, during, or after the QRS complex and are inverted in the inferior leads (II, III, aVF)

PR interval: Short, usually 0.10 second or less when P waves precede the QRS

QRS complex: Usually normal but may be aberrant if the PJC occurs very early and conducts into the ventricles during the refractory period of a bundle branch

Conduction: Retrograde through the atria, usually normal through the ventricles

Example: Sinus rhythm with two PJCs

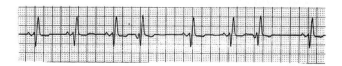

No treatment is necessary for PJCs.

JUNCTIONAL RHYTHM AND JUNCTIONAL TACHYCARDIA

Junctional rhythm can occur if the sinus node rate falls below the automatic rate of an AV junctional pacemaker, or in the presence of digitalis toxicity. Junctional rhythms commonly occur after inferior wall MI because the blood supply to the sinus node and the AV junction is disrupted. The rhythms are classified according to their rate; junctional rhythm usually occurs at a rate of 40 to 60 beats/min, accelerated junctional rhythm occurs at a rate of 60 to 100 beats/min, and junctional tachycardia occurs at a rate of 100 to 250 beats/min.

Junctional rhythm has the following ECG characteristics:

Rate: Usually 40 to 60 beats/min; accelerated junctional rhythm, 60 to 100 beats/min; junctional tachycardia, 100 to 250 beats/min

Rhythm: Regular

P waves: May precede or follow QRS

PR interval: Short, 0.10 second or less

QRS complex: Usually normal

Conduction: Retrograde through the atria, normal through the ventricles

Examples: (A) Junctional rhythm (rate, 43 beats/min). (B) Accelerated junctional rhythm (rate, 84 beats/min).

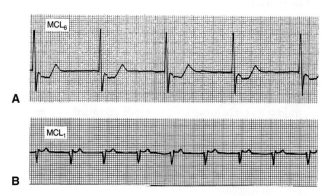

Junctional rhythm rarely requires treatment unless the rate is too slow or too fast to maintain cardiac output. If the rate is slow, atropine can be given to increase the sinus rate and override the junctional focus or increase the rate

of firing of the junctional pacemaker. If the rate is fast, drugs such as verapamil, beta blockers, quinidine, or digitalis may be effective in slowing the rate or terminating the arrhythmia. Cardioversion may be necessary if the rate is so rapid that cardiac output is severely limited. Because digitalis toxicity is a common cause of junctional rhythms, the drug should be held until serum levels return to normal and the arrhythmia stops.

Rhythms Originating in the Ventricles

Ventricular arrhythmias originate in the ventricular muscle or Purkinje system and are considered to be more dangerous than other arrhythmias because of their potential to limit cardiac output severely. However, as with any arrhythmia, ventricular rate is a key determinant of how well a patient can tolerate a ventricular rhythm. Ventricular arrhythmias include premature ventricular complex (PVC), accelerated ventricular rhythm, VT, ventricular flutter, ventricular fibrillation, and ventricular asystole. See Chapter 25 for the ACLS algorithm for treatment of ventricular fibrillation and pulseless VT.

PREMATURE VENTRICULAR COMPLEXES

Premature ventricular complexes are caused by premature depolarization of cells in the ventricular myocardium or Purkinje system due to enhanced normal automaticity or abnormal automaticity, reentry in the ventricles, or afterdepolarizations. PVCs can be caused by hypoxia, myocardial ischemia, hypokalemia, acidosis, exercise, increased levels of circulating catecholamines, digitalis toxicity, and other causes. PVCs increase with aging and are more common in people with CHD and other forms of heart disease. PVCs are not dangerous in people with normal hearts but are associated with higher mortality rates in patients with structural heart disease or acute MI, especially if left ventricular function is reduced. PVCs are considered potentially malignant when they occur more frequently than 10 per hour or are repetitive (i.e., occur in pairs, triplets, or more than three in a row) in patients with coronary disease, previous MI, or cardiomyopathy.[10,73]

Premature ventricular complexes have the following ECG characteristics:

Rate: 60 to 100 beats/min or the rate of the basic rhythm

Rhythm: Irregular because of the early beats

P waves: Not related to the PVCs. Sinus rhythm is often not interrupted, so sinus P waves can frequently be seen occurring regularly throughout the rhythm. P waves may follow PVCs because of retrograde conduction from the ventricle backward through the atria; these P waves are inverted in the inferior leads (II, III, aVF).

PR interval: Not present before most PVCs. If a P wave happens, by coincidence, to precede a PVC, the PR interval is short.

QRS complex: Wide and bizarre, usually greater than 0.12 second in duration. May vary in morphology if

PVCs originate from more than one focus in the ventricles. T waves are usually in the opposite direction from the QRS complex.

Conduction: Impulses originating in the ventricles conduct through the ventricular myocardium from muscle cell to muscle cell rather than through Purkinje fibers, resulting in wide QRS complexes. Some PVCs may conduct retrograde into the atria, resulting in inverted P waves that follow the PVC. When the sinus rhythm is undisturbed by PVCs, the atria depolarize normally.

Examples: (A) Normal sinus rhythm with PVCs. (B) Sinus rhythm with multifocal PVCs. (C) Paired PVCs. (D) R-on-T PVCs resulting in short runs of VT.

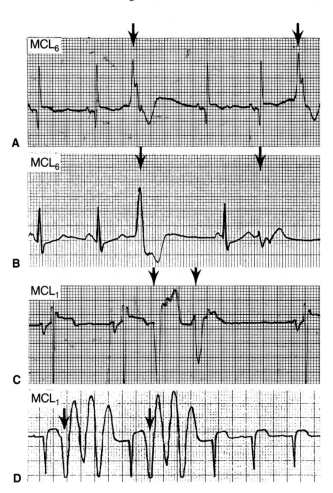

The significance of PVCs depends on the clinical setting in which they occur. Many people have chronic PVCs that do not need to be treated, and most of these people are asymptomatic. In the setting of an acute MI or myocardial ischemia, PVCs may be precursors of more dangerous ventricular arrhythmias. Unless PVCs result in hemodynamic instability or symptomatic VT, most physicians elect not to treat them, although some prefer to treat PVCs that occur in the first 24 to 48 hours after acute MI or after cardiac surgery.

There is no evidence that suppression of PVCs reduces mortality, especially in patients with no structural heart disease. The Cardiac Arrhythmia Suppression Trial (CAST)[14] was terminated early after demonstrating a 2.4 times higher risk of death and a 3.6 times greater risk of nonfatal cardiac arrest and arrhythmic death in patients post-MI taking encainide or flecainide to suppress ventricular ectopy. These results have led physicians to avoid administration of class I antiarrhythmic agents to suppress PVCs and has made them wary of using other antiarrhythmic agents for that purpose as well.

If PVCs are to be treated, intravenous lidocaine is recommended as the first drug. Other antiarrhythmic agents such as procainamide or bretylium can be used IV for acute control. Oral maintenance therapy with class I antiarrhythmics is becoming less common, and the use of class III antiarrhythmics such as amiodarone and sotalol is gaining favor in the treatment of ventricular arrhythmias.[8,54,87]

ACCELERATED IDIOVENTRICULAR RHYTHM

Accelerated idioventricular ventricular rhythm occurs when an ectopic focus in the ventricles fires at a rate of 50 to 100 beats/min. Accelerated idioventricular ventricular rhythm commonly occurs in the presence of inferior MI and during reperfusion with thrombolytic therapy, when the rate of the sinus node slows below the rate of the latent ventricular pacemaker. (See section on Complex Arrhythmias and Conduction Disturbances for a discussion of AV dissociation.) The ECG characteristics of accelerated ventricular rhythm include the following:

Rate: 50 to 100 beats/min

Rhythm: Usually regular

P waves: May be seen but are dissociated from the QRS. If retrograde conduction from the ventricle to the atria occurs, P waves follow the QRS complex.

PR interval: Not present

QRS complex: Wide and bizarre

Conduction: If sinus rhythm is the basic rhythm, atrial conduction is normal. Impulses originating in the ventricles conduct through the ventricular myocardium by cell-to-cell conduction, resulting in the wide QRS complex.

Example: Sinus rhythm with accelerated ventricular rhythm at a rate of 58 beats/min

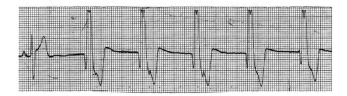

The treatment of accelerated ventricular rhythm depends on its cause and how well it is tolerated by the patient. This arrhythmia alone is usually not harmful because the ventricular rate is within normal limits and usually adequate to maintain cardiac output. If the patient is symptomatic because of the loss of atrial kick, atropine can be used to increase the rate of the sinus node and overdrive the ventricular rhythm. Suppressive therapy is rarely used because abolishing the ventricular rhythm may leave an even less desirable heart rate. Usually, accelerated ventricular rhythm is transient and benign and does not require treatment.

VENTRICULAR TACHYCARDIA

Ventricular tachycardia is a rapid ventricular rhythm most likely due to reentry in the ventricles, although automaticity of an ectopic focus and afterdepolarizations may also be mechanisms of VT. The causes of VT are the same as those of PVCs, but VT is considerably more dangerous than PVCs because of its effect of decreasing cardiac output and its tendency to degenerate into ventricular fibrillation. When VT lasts for less than 30 seconds, it is called *nonsustained* VT. If it lasts longer than 30 seconds or requires immediate treatment because of hemodynamic compromise, it is called *sustained* VT.[57] ECG characteristics of VT include the following:

Rate: Ventricular rate is usually 100 to 220 beats/min

Rhythm: Usually regular but may be slightly irregular

P waves: Often dissociated from QRS complexes. If sinus rhythm is the underlying basic rhythm, regular P waves may be seen but are not related to QRS complexes. P waves are often buried in QRS complexes or T waves. VT may conduct retrograde to the atria and P waves can be seen after each QRS.

PR interval: Not measurable because of dissociation of P waves from QRS complexes

QRS complex: Wide and bizarre, greater than 0.12 second in duration. When QRS complexes are the same morphology, the term *monomorphic VT* is used. When QRS complexes are different morphologies, the term *polymorphic VT* is used (see section on Complex Arrhythmias and Conduction Disturbances).

Conduction: Impulse originates in one ventricle and spreads by muscle cell-to-cell conduction through both ventricles. There may be retrograde conduction through the atria, but often the sinus node continues to fire regularly and depolarizes the atria normally. Rarely, one of these sinus impulses may conduct normally through the AV node and into the ventricle before the next ectopic ventricular impulse fires, resulting in a normal QRS complex, called a *capture beat*. Occasionally, a *fusion beat* may occur as the ventricles are depolarized by a descending sinus impulse and the ventricular ectopic impulse simultaneously, resulting in a QRS complex that looks different from both the normal beats and the ventricular beats.

Examples: (A) Sinus rhythm with a PVC and a run of VT. (B) VT. AV dissociation is evidenced by independently occurring P waves. (C) VT with a fusion beat (fourth complex).

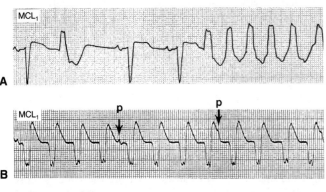

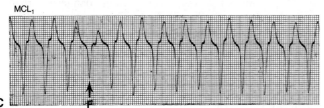

Immediate treatment of VT depends on how well the rhythm is tolerated by the patient. The two main determinants of patient tolerance of any tachycardia are ventricular rate and underlying left ventricular function. VT can be an emergency if cardiac output is severely decreased because of a very rapid rate or poor left ventricular function. The preferred immediate treatment for severely symptomatic VT is cardioversion, but defibrillation can be performed if there is not time to synchronize the shock. If the patient is not severely symptomatic, lidocaine is the drug of first choice for acute treatment of VT. IV procainamide, bretylium, amiodarone, or magnesium sulfate can also be used for acute treatment. Maintenance therapy may be prescribed with the same drugs used for PVCs, with increasing emphasis on class III agents with beta blocker effects, like amiodarone and sotalol. See Chapter 25 for the ACLS algorithm for treatment of VT.

VENTRICULAR FLUTTER

Ventricular flutter is similar to VT, but the rate is faster. Hemodynamically, ventricular flutter is more dangerous because there is virtually no cardiac output. ECG characteristics of ventricular flutter are as follows:

Rate: Ventricular rate is usually 220 to 400 beats/min

Rhythm: Usually regular

P waves: None seen

PR interval: None measurable

QRS complex: Very wide, regular, sine-wave type of pattern

Conduction: Originates in the ventricle and spreads through muscle cell-to-cell conduction, resulting in very wide, bizarre complexes

Example: Ventricular flutter

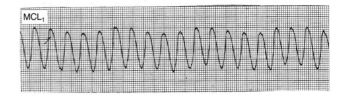

Ventricular flutter is fatal unless treated immediately by defibrillation. If a defibrillator is not immediately available, cardiopulmonary resuscitation (CPR) should be started. After the rhythm is converted, antiarrhythmic drug therapy should be initiated to prevent recurrence. Drug therapy is similar to that used for VT.

VENTRICULAR FIBRILLATION

Ventricular fibrillation is rapid, ineffective quivering of the ventricles and is fatal without immediate treatment. Electrical activity originates in the ventricles and spreads in a chaotic, irregular pattern throughout both ventricles. There is no cardiac output or palpable pulse with ventricular fibrillation. ECG characteristics of ventricular fibrillation include the following:

Rate: Rapid, uncoordinated, ineffective

Rhythm: Chaotic, irregular

P waves: None seen

PR interval: None

QRS complex: No formed QRS complexes seen; rapid, irregular undulations without any specific pattern. This erratic electrical activity can be coarse or fine.

Conduction: Multiple ectopic foci firing simultaneously in ventricles and depolarizing them irregularly and without any organized pattern. Ventricles are not contracting.

Examples: (A) Coarse ventricular fibrillation. (B) Fine ventricular fibrillation.

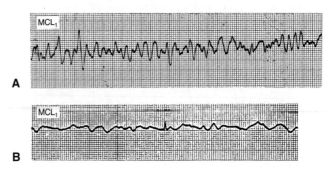

Ventricular fibrillation requires immediate defibrillation. Synchronized cardioversion is not possible because there are

no formed QRS complexes on which to synchronize the shock. CPR must be performed if a defibrillator is not immediately available. The American Heart Association guidelines for ventricular fibrillation and pulseless VT call for CPR until a defibrillator is available, then defibrillation at 200 J.[22] If ventricular fibrillation continues, an immediate second shock at 300 J and a third shock at 360 J, if necessary, are recommended. If ventricular fibrillation does not convert after three shocks, CPR needs to be continued and drug therapy initiated. Antiarrhythmic agents such as lidocaine, procainamide, magnesium, and bretylium are commonly used in an effort to convert ventricular fibrillation. Once the rhythm has converted, maintenance therapy with intravenous antiarrhythmic agents is continued. Drugs with beta blocker effects plus the ability to prolong repolarization (class III effects), like amiodarone and sotalol, are preferred agents for maintenance therapy of lethal ventricular arrhythmias.[8,54,87]

VENTRICULAR ASYSTOLE

Ventricular asystole is the absence of any ventricular rhythm; there is no QRS complex, no pulse, and no cardiac output. This is always fatal unless treated immediately. Ventricular asystole has the following characteristics:

Rate: None

Rhythm: None

P waves: May be present if the sinus node is functioning

PR interval: None

QRS complex: None

Conduction: Atrial conduction may be normal if the sinus node is functioning. There is no conduction into the ventricles.

Example: Ventricular asystole. Two P waves are seen at the beginning of the strip.

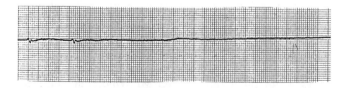

Cardiopulmonary resuscitation must be initiated immediately if the patient is to survive. IV epinephrine and atropine may be given in an effort to stimulate a rhythm. If pacing is to be used, external pacing should be instituted early in the resuscitation attempt. Asystole has a very poor prognosis despite the best resuscitation efforts because it usually represents extensive myocardial ischemia or severe underlying metabolic problems. See Chapter 25 for the ACLS algorithm for treatment of asystole.

Conduction Abnormalities

The term *AV block* is used to describe arrhythmias in which there is delayed or failed conduction of supraventricular impulses into the ventricles. AV blocks have been classified according to location of the block and severity of the conduction abnormality. The following classification of AV blocks is discussed in this section:

First-degree AV block
Second-degree AV block
Type I
Type II
High-grade AV block
Type I
Type II
Third-degree AV block

FIRST-DEGREE ATRIOVENTRICULAR BLOCK

First-degree AV block is defined as prolonged AV conduction time of supraventricular impulses into the ventricles. This delay usually occurs in the AV node, and all impulses conduct to the ventricles, but with delayed conduction times. First-degree AV block can be due to CHD, rheumatic heart disease, increased vagal tone, inflammatory diseases, collagen disease, or administration of digitalis, beta blockers, or calcium channel blockers. First-degree AV block can be recognized by the following ECG characteristics:

Rate: Can occur at any sinus rate, usually 60 to 100 beats/min

Rhythm: Regular

P waves: Normal, precede every QRS

PR interval: Greater than 0.20 second. PR intervals as long as 1 second or more have been reported.[74]

QRS complex: Usually normal unless bundle-branch block exists

Conduction: Normal through the atria, delayed through the AV node, normal through the ventricles

Example: First-degree AV block (PR interval, 0.44 second)

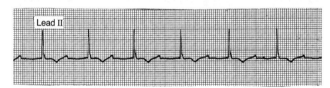

First-degree AV block does not require any specific treatment, but it should be observed for progression to more serious block.

SECOND-DEGREE ATRIOVENTRICULAR BLOCK

Second-degree AV block occurs when one atrial impulse at a time fails to be conducted to the ventricles. Second-degree AV block can be divided into two distinct categories: type I block, occurring in the AV node, and type II block, occurring below the AV node in the bundle of His or bundle-branch system.

Type I (Wenckebach). Type I second-degree AV block, often referred to as *Wenckebach or Mobitz I,* is a progressive increase in conduction times of consecutive atrial impulses into the ventricles until one impulse fails to conduct, or is "dropped." This appears on the ECG as gradually lengthening PR intervals until one P wave fails to conduct and is not followed by a QRS complex, resulting in a pause, after which the cycle repeats itself. This type of block is commonly associated with inferior wall MI, chronic CHD, aortic valve disease, mitral valve prolapse, atrial septal defects, and administration of digitalis, beta blockers, or calcium channel blockers. (See section on Complex Arrhythmias and Conduction Disturbances for a more detailed discussion of Wenckebach conduction.)

Type I second-degree AV block can be recognized by the following ECG characteristics:

Rate: Can occur at any sinus or atrial rate

Rhythm: Irregular unless 2 : 1 conduction is present. Overall appearance of the rhythm demonstrates group beating (i.e., groups of beats separated by pauses).

P waves: Normal. Some P waves are not conducted to the ventricles, but only one at a time fails to conduct.

PR interval: Gradually lengthens in consecutive beats. The PR interval preceding the pause is longer than that following the pause. When 2 : 1 conduction is present, PR intervals are constant.

QRS complex: Usually normal unless there is associated bundle-branch block

Conduction: Normal through the atria, progressively delayed through the AV node until an impulse fails to conduct. Ventricular conduction is normal. Wenckebach conduction ratios describe the number of P waves to QRS complexes: 6 : 5 conduction means six P waves resulted in five QRS complexes, or every sixth P wave is blocked. Conduction ratios can vary from low (e.g., 2 : 1, 3 : 2) to high (e.g., 12 : 11, 15 : 14).

Examples: (A) Second-degree AV block, type I (Wenckebach) with 3 : 2 conduction. (B) Second-degree AV block, type I. Note that the PR interval preceding the pause is longer than the PR interval after the pause.

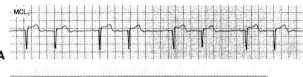

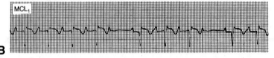

The treatment of type I second-degree AV block depends on the conduction ratio, the resulting ventricular rate, and, most important, the patient's tolerance for the rhythm. If ventricular rates are slow enough to decrease cardiac output, the treatment is atropine to increase the sinus

rate and speed conduction through the AV node. At higher conduction ratios, where the ventricular rate is within a normal range, no treatment is necessary. If the block is due to digitalis or beta blockers, those drugs should be held. This type of block is usually temporary and benign and seldom requires pacing, although temporary pacing may be needed when the ventricular rate is slow.

Type II. Type II second-degree AV block, also called *Mobitz II,* is sudden failure of conduction of an atrial impulse to the ventricles without progressive increases in conduction time of consecutive P waves. Type II block occurs below the AV node and is usually associated with bundle-branch block; therefore, the dropped beats are usually a manifestation of bilateral bundle-branch block. This form of block appears on the ECG much the same as type I block, except that there is no progressive increase in PR intervals before the blocked beats. Type II block is less common but more serious than type I block. It occurs in rheumatic heart disease, CHD, and primary disease of the conduction system, and in the presence of acute anterior wall MI.

Type II second-degree AV block can be recognized by the following ECG characteristics:

Rate: Can occur at any basic rate

Rhythm: Irregular due to blocked beats unless 2 : 1 conduction is present

P waves: Usually regular and precede each QRS. Periodically, a P wave is not followed by a QRS complex.

PR interval: Constant before all conducted beats. The PR interval preceding the pause is the same as that after the pause.

QRS complex: Almost always wide because of associated bundle-branch block

Conduction: Normal through the atria and through the AV node but intermittently blocked in the bundle-branch system and fails to reach the ventricles. Conduction through the ventricles is abnormally slow because of associated bundle-branch block. Conduction ratios can vary from 2 : 1 to only occasional blocked beats.

Example: Second-degree AV block, type II. All PR intervals are constant. (From Conover MB: *Understanding Electrocardiography,* 7th ed. St. Louis, CV Mosby, 1996.)

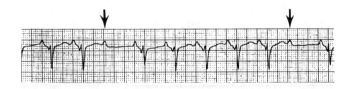

Type II block is more dangerous than type I because of a higher incidence of associated symptoms and progression to complete AV block. When it occurs in the presence of anterior wall MI, it is associated with a high mortality rate because of the extent of muscle damage necessary to produce this degree of block below the AV node.

Treatment usually includes pacemaker therapy because this type of block is often permanent and progresses to complete block. External pacing can be used for treatment of symptomatic type II block until transvenous pacing can be initiated. Atropine is not recommended because it may result in further slowing of ventricular rate by increasing the number of impulses conducting through the AV node and bombarding the diseased bundles with more impulses than they can handle, resulting in further conduction failure.

2 : 1 Conduction. The 2 : 1 conduction ratio deserves special mention because it continues to be the source of much confusion and disagreement among arrhythmia experts. The 2 : 1 block is failure of conduction of every other atrial impulse. Because only one P wave at a time is blocked, it is by definition a second-degree block. If the lesion causing conduction failure is in the AV node, it is type I block; if it is below the AV node, it is type II block. One source of confusion is the lack of progressive prolongation in PR intervals in type I block with 2 : 1 conduction, which has led educators for years to teach that all 2 : 1 block was "Mobitz II" block. Type I block with 2 : 1 conduction does not present with progressively prolonging PR intervals because there are no *consecutively conducted* beats in 2 : 1 block. The progressive prolongation of PR interval that characterizes Wenckebach behavior occurs on consecutively conducted P waves in type I block, so when there is block of every other P wave, this typical behavior is not seen. However, the location of the lesion does not change, so if the lesion is in the AV node, it is type I block regardless of the conduction ratio.

When a patient presents with a 2 : 1 conduction ratio, it is sometimes impossible to determine whether the block is type I or II without intracardiac recordings. However, an educated guess can be made depending on the length of the PR interval, the QRS width, and the clinical situation. The following ECG findings can be very helpful in determining the type of block in 2 : 1 conduction in the absence of intracardiac recordings:

PR interval: Often longer than normal (more than 0.20 second) in type I and normal in type II. Sometimes the PR in type I is normal on conducted beats because the blocked P wave allows enough time for the AV node to recover so that it is able to conduct every other P wave with a normal PR interval. If there are any periods of typical Wenckebach conduction with progressive lengthening of the PR interval on consecutively conducted P waves (even if it only happens once), it is type I block.

QRS complex: Usually narrow in type I and almost always wide in type II. Exceptions can occur in type I when there is a coincidental bundle-branch block that widens the QRS, and in type II when the block is in the His bundle (still below the AV node, thus type II), resulting in a narrow QRS. Type II block is rare compared with type I, and intra-His type II block is even rarer, so the odds are greatly in favor of type I block when the QRS is narrow.

Example: (A) Top strip shows 2 : 1 conduction that can be assumed to be type I because of the narrow QRS complex. Second strip proves that it is type I when consecutive P waves conduct with increasing PR intervals. (B) Top strip shows 2 : 1 conduction that can be assumed to be type II because of wide QRS. Second strip proves that it is type II when consecutively conducted PR intervals remain constant.

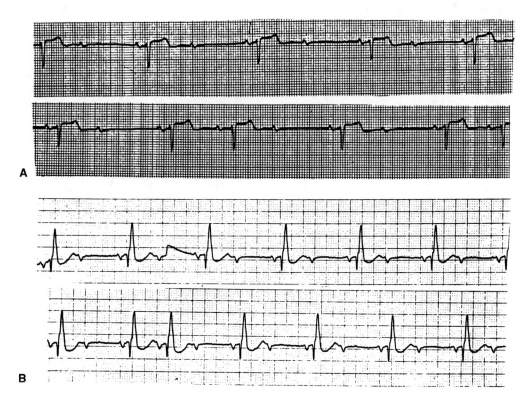

HIGH-GRADE ATRIOVENTRICULAR BLOCK

High-grade AV block (also called advanced AV block) is present when two or more consecutive atrial impulses are blocked, the atrial rate is reasonable (less than 135 beats/min), and conduction fails because of the block itself and not because of interference from an escape pacemaker.[59] If the atrial rate is very fast, as in atrial flutter with rates of 300 beats/min, physiologic AV block occurs as a normal function of the AV node and therefore cannot be called high-grade block—hence the arbitrary atrial rate limit of 135 beats/min. If a junctional or ventricular escape beat or rhythm occurs as a result of failed conduction of impulses into the ventricles and interferes with the ability of atrial impulses to conduct by causing refractoriness in the AV node or ventricles, high-grade block cannot be diagnosed; the mere presence of the escape beat or rhythm may be the cause of failed conduction, rather than a true block in the AV node or bundle-branch system.

High-grade AV block may be type I, occurring in the AV node, or type II, occurring below the AV node. High-grade block can be recognized by these ECG characteristics:

Rate: Atrial rate less than 135 beats/min

Rhythm: Regular or irregular, depending on conduction pattern

P waves: Normal, present before every conducted QRS, but several P waves may not be followed by QRS complexes

PR interval: Constant before conducted beats; may be normal or prolonged

QRS complex: Usually normal in type I block and wide in type II block

Conduction: Normal through the atria. Two or more consecutive atrial impulses fail to conduct to the ventricles. Ventricular conduction is normal in type I and abnormally slow in type II block.

Example: High-grade (advanced) AV block

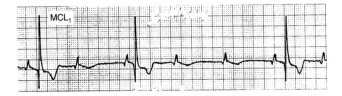

The significance of high-grade block depends on the conduction ratio and the resulting ventricular rate. Because ventricular rates tend to be slow, this arrhythmia is frequently symptomatic and requires treatment. Atropine can be given and is usually more effective in type I block. External cardiac pacing may be necessary until a temporary transvenous pacemaker can be inserted, and permanent pacing is usually necessary in type II high-grade block.

THIRD-DEGREE ATRIOVENTRICULAR BLOCK (COMPLETE BLOCK)

Third-degree AV block is complete failure of conduction of all atrial impulses to the ventricles. In third-degree AV block, there is complete AV dissociation; the atria are usually under the control of the sinus node, and either a junctional or ventricular pacemaker controls the ventricles. This arrhythmia can be diagnosed only when the opportunity for conduction is optimal and still does not occur.[19] The ventricular rate is usually less than 45 beats/min[59]; a faster rate could indicate an accelerated junctional or ventricular rhythm that is interfering with conduction from the atria into the ventricles by causing physiologic refractoriness in the conduction system, thus causing a physiologic block that must be differentiated from the abnormal conduction system function of complete AV block.

Causes of complete AV block include CHD, MI, Lev's or Lenegre's disease, cardiac surgery, congenital heart disease, and digitalis toxicity. Third-degree AV block can be recognized from the following ECG criteria:

Rate: Atrial rate is usually normal; ventricular rate is less than 45 beats/min

Rhythm: Regular

P waves: Normal but dissociated from QRS complexes

PR interval: No consistent PR intervals because there is no relation between P waves and QRS complexes

QRS complex: Normal if ventricles controlled by a junctional pacemaker, wide if controlled by a ventricular pacemaker

Conduction: Normal through the atria. All impulses are blocked at the AV node or in the bundle branches, so there is no conduction to the ventricles. Conduction through the ventricles is normal if a junctional escape rhythm occurs and is abnormally slow if a ventricular escape rhythm occurs.

Examples: (A) Third-degree AV block with a junctional pacemaker at a rate of 37 beats/min. (B) Third-degree AV block with a ventricular pacemaker at a rate of 30 beats/min.

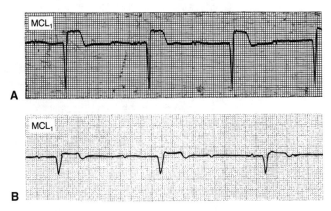

Third-degree AV block can occur without significant symptoms if it is of gradual onset and the heart has time to compensate for the slow ventricular rate. If it occurs suddenly in the presence of acute MI, its significance depends on the resulting ventricular rate and the patient's tolerance. If symptoms of decreased cardiac output occur, external cardiac pacing can be used to maintain a ventricular rate until transvenous pacing can be initiated. Dopamine or epinephrine infusions can be used to maintain blood pressure and CPR should be performed until a pacemaker can be inserted if cardiac output is severely decreased.

COMPLEX ARRHYTHMIAS AND CONDUCTION DISTURBANCES

Abnormalities of cardiac rhythm can range from simple to advanced to complex. Disorders of the heart beat provide a constant challenge to those interested in the study of arrhythmias. This section discusses advanced concepts in arrhythmia interpretation and provides clues to aid in the recognition of selected advanced arrhythmias.

Preexcitation Syndromes

Preexcitation refers to early activation of the ventricular myocardium by supraventricular impulses entering the ventricles through accessory pathways. These pathways are capable of carrying the impulse directly into the ventricle, bypassing all or part of the normal AV conduction system. The most common accessory pathway is an AV bypass tract, the bundle of Kent, which originates in the atrium and inserts in the ventricle, bypassing the entire conduction system. Other accessory pathways include AV nodal bypass tracts, which carry the impulse from the sinus node or atrium into the conduction system below the AV node (sometimes called *James fibers* or *atriohisian fibers*), and nodoventricular or fasciculoventricular connections, which originate in or below the AV node and carry the impulse directly into the ventricular myocardium (*Mahaim fibers*).[35,58,101]

The most common type of preexcitation syndrome is Wolff-Parkinson-White (WPW) syndrome, in which the impulse is transmitted down the bundle of Kent directly into the ventricles, bypassing the AV node. In Lown-Ganong-Levine (LGL) syndrome, the impulse bypasses the AV node but enters the normal conduction system at some point below the node or in the His bundle.

WOLFF-PARKINSON-WHITE SYNDROME

In WPW syndrome, the ventricle is stimulated prematurely through the Kent bundle while the impulse is simultaneously conducted through the normal AV junctional conduction system. Impulses travel faster down the accessory pathway because they bypass the normal AV node delay. Part of the ventricle receives the impulse early through the accessory pathway and begins to depolarize before the rest of the ventricle is activated through the His-Purkinje system. Early stimulation of the ventricle results in a short PR interval and a widened QRS complex as the impulse begins to depolarize the ventricle through muscle cell-to-cell conduction. Premature ventricular stimulation forms a characteristic slurring of the initial portion of the QRS complex, called a *delta wave*. The remainder of the QRS complex is normal because the rest of the ventricle is then activated normally through the Purkinje system. This type of preexcitation results in fusion beats in the ventricles as they are depolarized simultaneously by the impulse coming through the accessory pathway and through the AV node.

The degree of preexcitation can vary depending on the relative rates of conduction through the bypass connection and the AV node, and it determines the length of the PR interval and the size of the delta wave (Fig. 14-6). Maximal preexcitation occurs when the ventricles are activated totally by the accessory pathway, resulting in an extremely short PR interval and uniformly wide QRS complex. Less than

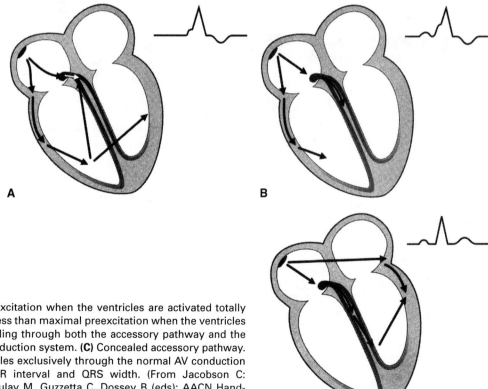

A   **B**

FIGURE 14-6 (A) Maximal preexcitation when the ventricles are activated totally by the accessory pathway. **(B)** Less than maximal preexcitation when the ventricles are activated by impulses traveling through both the accessory pathway and the normal atrioventricular (AV) conduction system. **(C)** Concealed accessory pathway. The impulse reaches the ventricles exclusively through the normal AV conduction system, resulting in normal PR interval and QRS width. (From Jacobson C: Advanced ECG concepts. In Chulay M, Guzzetta C, Dossey B (eds): AACN Handbook of Critical Care Nursing, p 434. Stamford, CT, Appleton & Lange, 1997.)

C

maximal preexcitation occurs when the impulse enters the ventricle through both pathways simultaneously, and the length of the PR interval and size of delta wave depend on how much of the ventricle is depolarized through the bypass connection. A concealed pathway is present when the ventricles are depolarized exclusively through the normal conduction system even though a bypass tract exists. In this case, the PR interval and QRS complex are normal because the accessory pathway is not being used for anterograde conduction.

Accessory pathways can be located in multiple places around the valve rings, the septum, and the free walls of both ventricles (Fig. 14-7). The ECG can be helpful in identifying location of accessory pathways: atrial origin can be deduced from polarity of the P waves during orthodromic tachycardia, and the ventricular insertion site can be inferred from the polarity of delta waves during sinus rhythm.[20,35,58-60,98] Approximately 46% to 60% are in left lateral, 25% posterolateral, 2% anteroseptal, and 13% to 21% in right lateral locations.[58] Figure 14-8 illustrates two examples of preexcitation during sinus rhythm.

Preexcitation syndromes are clinically significant because the presence of two pathways provides the opportunity for reentry of the impulse and may result in rapid reentrant tachycardias. Atrial fibrillation can become life threatening when conducted to the ventricle through an accessory pathway. The incidence of tachycardias in WPW syndrome is estimated to be from 40% to 80%,[19,101] with reentrant tachycardia accounting for 75% to 80% and atrial flutter or fibrillation for 20% to 25% of all tachycardias.[19] (See section on Supraventricular Tachycardia, later, for information on reentrant arrhythmias associated with accessory pathways.)

Atrial fibrillation and atrial flutter that occur in the presence of an accessory pathway are particularly dangerous because of the extremely rapid ventricular rate that can result from conduction of the atrial impulses directly into the ventricle through the bypass track. The ventricular rate can be as fast as 250 to 300 beats/min and can deteriorate into ventricular fibrillation, resulting in sudden death. Atrial fibrillation with anterograde conduction over an accessory pathway presents on the ECG as a very rapid, irregular, wide QRS rhythm. The irregularity of the ventricular response helps to differentiate this rhythm from other wide QRS tachycardias.

The ECG characteristics of atrial fibrillation with anterograde conduction through an accessory pathway are as follows (Fig. 14-9):

Rate: Ventricular rates up to 300 beats/min

Rhythm: Irregular. Often appears as groups of very short R-R intervals alternating with groups of longer R-R intervals. The longest R-R intervals are often more than twice the shortest R-R intervals.

P waves: None, because atria are fibrillating

PR interval: None

QRS complex: Wide, bizarre due to abnormal depolarization of ventricles through accessory pathway

Conduction: Disorganized and chaotic through atria. Atrial impulses conduct into ventricles through accessory pathway, resulting in muscle cell-to-cell conduction through ventricles.

Immediate treatment of atrial fibrillation with anterograde conduction through an accessory pathway depends on ventricular rate and the patient's tolerance of the dysrhythmia. Cardioversion is the treatment of choice when severe hemodynamic impairment occurs. Drug treatment is directed at slowing conduction through the accessory pathway and restoring and maintaining sinus rhythm. Drugs that increase the refractory period and depress conduction in the bypass tract include quinidine, procainamide,

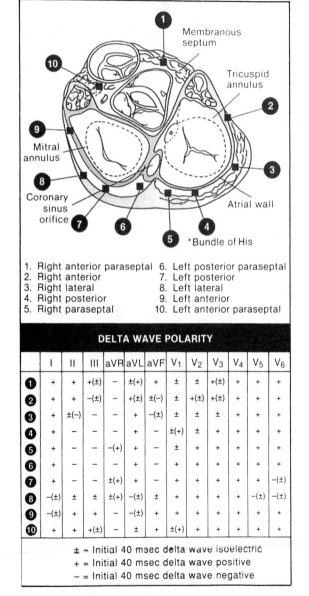

1. Right anterior paraseptal
2. Right anterior
3. Right lateral
4. Right posterior
5. Right paraseptal
6. Left posterior paraseptal
7. Left posterior
8. Left lateral
9. Left anterior
10. Left anterior paraseptal

	I	II	III	aVR	aVL	aVF	V₁	V₂	V₃	V₄	V₅	V₆
1	+	+	+(±)	−	±(+)	+	±	±	+(±)	+	+	+
2	+	+	−(±)	−	+(±)	±(−)	±	+(±)	+(±)	+	+	+
3	+	±(−)	−	−	+	−(±)	±	±	±	+	+	+
4	+	−	−	−	+	−	±(+)	±	+	+	+	+
5	+	−	−	−(+)	+	−	±	+	+	+	+	+
6	+	−	−	−	+	−	+	+	+	+	+	+
7	+	−	−	±(+)	+	−	+	+	+	+	+	−(±)
8	−(±)	±	±	±(+)	−(±)	±	+	+	+	+	−(±)	−(±)
9	−(±)	+	+	−	−(±)	+	+	+	+	+	+	+
10	+	+	+(±)	−	±	+	±(+)	+	+	+	+	+

DELTA WAVE POLARITY

± = Initial 40 msec delta wave isoelectric
+ = Initial 40 msec delta wave positive
− = Initial 40 msec delta wave negative

FIGURE 14-7 Sites of the potential position of accessory pathways. Delta-wave polarity in the 12-lead electrocardiogram is shown in the table at the bottom. (From Gallagher JJ, Pritchell EL, Sealy WC, et al: The preexcitation syndromes. Prog Cardiovasc Dis 20: 285, 1978, and adapted from Zipes DP: Specific arrhythmias: Diagnosis and treatment. In Braunwald E (ed): Heart Disease, 4th ed, p 697. Philadephia, WB Saunders, 1992.)

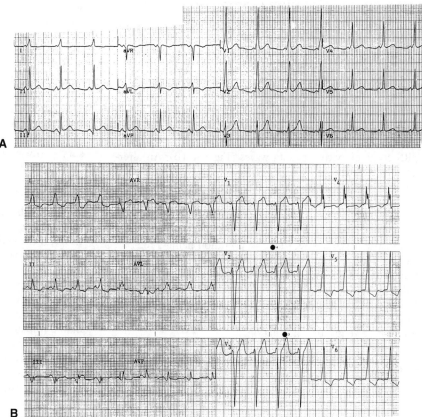

FIGURE 14-8 (A) Wolff-Parkinson-White (WPW) pattern of short PR interval and delta waves. Lead V₁ is positive (formerly referred to as *type A* pattern). **(B)** WPW pattern with short PR, delta waves, and a negative V₁ (formerly referred to as *type B* pattern).

flecainide, propafenone, amiodarone, and sotalol.[67] Many of these drugs are also effective in preventing recurrences of atrial fibrillation. Digoxin and calcium channel blockers are contraindicated whenever the tachycardia is due to anterograde conduction through an accessory pathway because they shorten the refractory period and accelerate conduction through the bypass tract.[20,62,67]

Wolff-Parkinson-White syndrome can resemble other conditions usually diagnosed by ECG. The presence of anteriorly directed delta waves can simulate RBBB, posterior or inferior MI, right ventricular hypertrophy, or posterior fascicular block. Posteriorly directed delta waves can simulate left bundle-branch block (LBBB), anterior MI, anterior fascicular block, and left ventricular hypertrophy.[18,35,59]

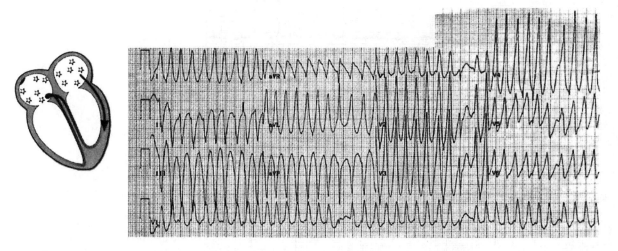

FIGURE 14-9 Atrial fibrillation conducting anterograde through an accessory pathway. Note the extremely short R-R intervals in the V leads. QRS is fast, wide, and irregular. (From Jacobson C: Advanced ECG concepts. In Chulay M, Guzzetta C, Dossey B (eds): AACN Handbook of Critical Care Nursing, p 440. Stamford, CT, Appleton & Lange, 1997.)

LOWN-GANONG-LEVINE SYNDROME

Lown-Ganong-Levine syndrome describes the combination of a short PR interval, normal QRS complex, and recurrent palpitations. The mechanism may involve an accessory pathway that originates in the atrium and terminates below the area of physiologic delay in the AV node or in the bundle of His.[59,107] A supraventricular impulse travels down the accessory pathway faster than through the AV node, causing a short PR interval, but the ventricles depolarize normally through the His-Purkinje system, resulting in a normal QRS complex without delta waves (Fig. 14-10). An alternative mechanism may be enhanced AV node conduction that allows a supraventricular impulse to conduct more rapidly than usual through an intranodal bypass tract, thus avoiding the usual AV conduction delay.[59,107] LGL syndrome is associated with the same types of tachyarrhythmias seen in WPW syndrome, the most common being a regular, narrow QRS tachycardia due to reentry of the impulse using one of the two pathways in an anterograde direction and the other in a retrograde direction. Atrial flutter and fibrillation that occurs in the presence of LGL syndrome can result in extremely rapid ventricular rates that can deteriorate into ventricular fibrillation.

TREATMENT

The WPW and LGL syndromes do not require treatment unless they are associated with symptomatic tachyarrhythmias. Ideally, specific therapy should be based on a known mechanism of the arrhythmia and knowledge of a drug's effect on that mechanism in both conduction pathways. This knowledge is best gained through electrophysiologic study, which is done to (1) confirm the presence of preexcitation, (2) identify the mechanism of the associated tachyarrhythmia, (3) localize the site of the accessory pathway, (4) confirm participation of the accessory pathway in maintenance of the tachycardia, (5) determine the functional behavior of the accessory pathway, and (6) determine the effects of different drugs on conduction velocity and refractoriness in both pathways.[35] If the arrhythmia is due to reentry, therapy is directed toward changing the conduction time or the refractory period in the AV node or in the accessory pathway, or both, so that reentry is abolished. Prolonging the refractory period in the AV node or in the bypass tract or inducing block in either of these pathways can interrupt reentry and stop the tachycardia. If atrial fibrillation is the mechanism, treatment is aimed at preventing the occurrence of the arrhythmia and slowing conduction through the accessory pathway.

Medical treatment of tachyarrhythmias associated with preexcitation syndromes depends on the degree of hemodynamic compromise caused by the arrhythmia and on the mechanism of the arrhythmia. Cardioversion is the treatment of choice for any tachycardia causing severe hemodynamic impairment. If the patient is not seriously symptomatic and has a regular, narrow QRS tachycardia, indicating conduction down the AV node, vagal maneuvers such as CSM or Valsalva maneuver, or the administration of adenosine, may terminate the arrhythmia by causing conduction delay in the AV node. Adenosine is the drug of choice in this situation because of its immediate and short-term effect of slowing conduction in the AV node. Beta blockers and calcium channel blockers, especially verapamil, can be used to slow AV node conduction, but they also have a depres-

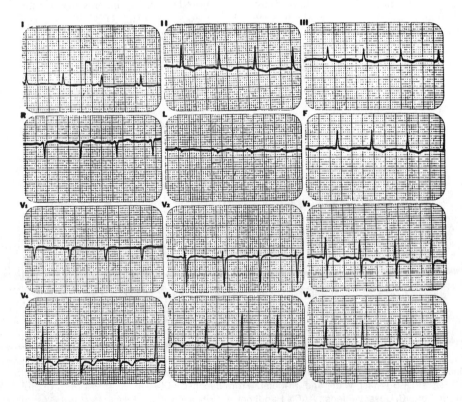

FIGURE 14-10 Lown-Ganong-Levine syndrome. Note short PR interval and normal QRS.

sant effect on myocardial contractility. IV procainamide is an alternative choice for acute therapy because it prolongs the refractory period in all parts of the circuit (atrium, AV node, ventricle, and accessory pathway). Class IC drugs (flecainide, propafenone) are most effective as chronic therapy.[107] Amiodarone and sotalol are also effective but have several side effects to be considered.

Tachycardias with wide QRS complexes, indicating conduction down the accessory pathway, are best treated with IV procainamide, which increases the refractory period and depresses conduction in the bypass tract.[107] Propranolol has no effect on the accessory pathway; digitalis and verapamil are contraindicated in this setting because they may shorten the refractory period in the accessory pathway and facilitate conduction through it.[20,62,107] Chronic therapy with class IC drugs is most effective, and class IA drugs or amiodarone may also be useful.[107]

Radiofrequency catheter ablation of the bypass tract offers a cure for tachycardias associated with accessory pathways. The reported success rate for controlling tachycardias using radiofrequency ablation without medications ranges from 88% to 99%.[77,107] (See Chapter 15 for more information about electrophysiology studies and ablation in management of arrhythmias.)

Supraventricular Tachycardia

The term *supraventricular tachycardia* is used to denote a rhythm originating above the ventricles but whose exact mechanism cannot be determined from the surface ECG. Usually, SVT is used to describe narrow QRS tachycardias because the narrow QRS denotes normal intraventricular conduction through the His-Purkinje system from a supraventricular focus. It is possible for an SVT to conduct with bundle-branch block, which would result in a wide QRS but would not change the fact that the rhythm is supraventricular. Thus, SVT can be used for wide QRS rhythms that are known to be coming from above the ventricles.

Supraventricular tachycardias can be classified into those that are AV nodal passive and those that are AV nodal active. AV nodal passive SVTs are those in which the AV node does not play a part in the maintenance of the tachycardia but serves only to conduct passively the supraventricular rhythm into the ventricles. AV nodal passive SVTs include atrial tachycardia, atrial flutter, and atrial fibrillation, all of which arise from within the atria and do not need the AV node's participation to sustain the atrial arrhythmia. AV nodal active tachycardias require participation of the AV node in the maintenance of the tachycardia. The two most common causes of a regular, narrow QRS tachycardia are AVNRT and CMT using an accessory pathway, both of which require the AV node as part of the reentry circuit that sustains the tachycardia.

Atrial fibrillation is usually easily recognized owing to its irregularity, but atrial tachycardia, atrial flutter, junctional tachycardia, AVNRT, and CMT can all present as a regular, narrow QRS tachycardia whose mechanism often cannot be determined from the ECG. Because AVNRT and CMT are responsible for most regular, narrow QRS tachycardias, these two are discussed in detail here.

ATRIOVENTRICULAR NODAL REENTRY TACHYCARDIA

Atrioventricular nodal reentry tachycardia is the most common mechanism of SVT and is responsible for up to 60% of regular, narrow QRS tachycardias.[2,20,33] This rhythm involves dual AV nodal pathways: a fast-conducting pathway with a long refractory period and a slow-conducting pathway with a short refractory period.[2,20,33,43,59] In AVNRT, a reentry circuit is set up in the AV node, using one pathway (usually the slow pathway) for the anterograde limb and the other pathway (usually the fast pathway) as the retrograde limb (Fig. 14-11).

Normally, the sinus impulse conducts down the fast pathway into the ventricles, resulting in a normal PR interval of 0.12 to 0.20 second. If a PAC occurs before the fast pathway with its long refractory period has recovered, the impulse conducts down the slow pathway because of its shorter refractory period, resulting in a PAC with a long PR interval. The long conduction time through the slow pathway allows the fast pathway time to recover, making it possible for the impulse to conduct backward into the fast pathway. The returning impulse can then reenter the slow pathway and initiate a circuit in the AV node, resulting in AVNRT. Figure 14-11 illustrates the most common mechanism of AVNRT. The resulting rhythm is usually a narrow QRS tachycardia because the ventricles are activated through the normal His-Purkinje system. P waves are either not visible at all or are seen peeking out at the end of the QRS complex because the atria are activated in a retrograde direction at the same time as the ventricles are being depolarized in an anterograde direction[9,20,33,43,44,59,64,99] (Fig. 14-12). In the presence of preexisting bundle-branch block or rate-dependent bundle-branch block, the QRS in AVNRT is wide.

In approximately 4% of cases of AVNRT, the fast pathway is used as the anterograde limb and the slow pathway as the retrograde limb of the circuit.[59,60] This results in a long R-P tachycardia in which the P wave appears in front of the QRS because atrial activation is delayed owing to slow conduction backward through the slow pathway. These P waves are inverted in inferior leads because the atria are depolarized in a retrograde direction.

Atrioventricular nodal reentry tachycardia is an AV nodal active SVT because the AV node's participation is required to maintain the tachycardia. Therefore, anything that blocks the AV node, such as vagal stimulation or drugs like adenosine, beta blockers, or calcium channel blockers, can terminate the rhythm. AVNRT is usually well tolerated unless the rate is extremely rapid. Many people with this arrhythmia learn to stop it by coughing or breath holding, which stimulates the vagus nerve. Acute medical treatment involves administering any of the previously mentioned drugs, but adenosine is the first-line drug recommended in ACLS guidelines.[22] Radiofrequency ablation offers a cure for the arrhythmia by destroying the slow pathway.[38,52,77]

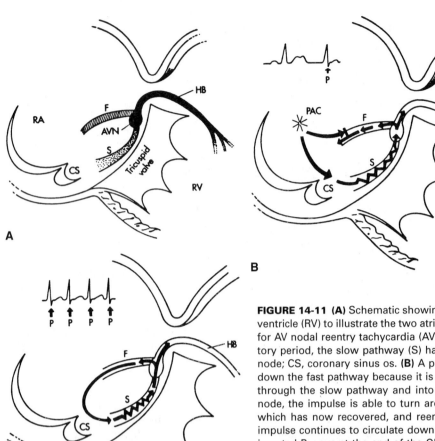

A

B

C

FIGURE 14-11 (A) Schematic showing cutaway view of right atrium (RA) and right ventricle (RV) to illustrate the two atrioventricular (AV) nodal pathways responsible for AV nodal reentry tachycardia (AVNRT). The fast pathway (F) has a long refractory period, the slow pathway (S) has a short refractory period. AVN, body of AV node; CS, coronary sinus os. **(B)** A premature atrial complex is unable to conduct down the fast pathway because it is still refractory, so it conducts to the AV node through the slow pathway and into the ventricle with a long PR interval. In the node, the impulse is able to turn around and conduct back up the fast pathway, which has now recovered, and reenter the atrium. **(C)** AVNRT results when the impulse continues to circulate down the slow and up the fast pathways. Note the inverted P wave at the end of the QRS complex as the atria and ventricles depolarize simultaneously. (From Conover MB: Understanding Electrocardiography, 7th ed. St. Louis, Mosby, 1996, and adapted from Keim S, Werner P: Jazayeri M, et al: Localization of the fast and slow pathways in antrioventricular nodal reentrant tachycardia by intraoperative ice mapping. Circulation 86(3): 919-925, 1992.)

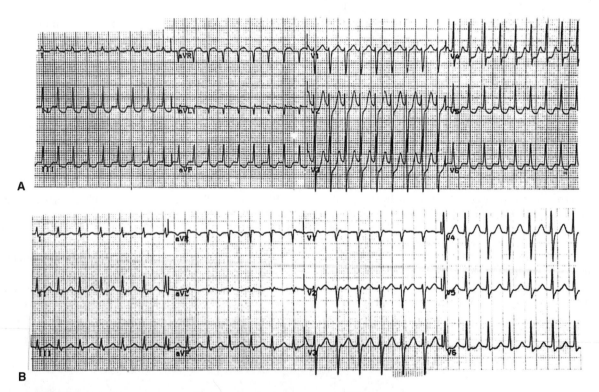

A

B

FIGURE 14-12 (A) Atrioventricular nodal reentry tachycardia (AVNRT); rate —214 beats/min. No P waves are visible. **(B)** AVNRT; rate—150 beats/min. P waves distort the end of the QRS complex in leads II, III, aVF, and V_{1-3}.

CIRCUS MOVEMENT TACHYCARDIA

Circus movement tachycardia is an SVT that occurs in people who have accessory pathways, also called *bypass tracts,* that allow impulses to conduct directly from atria to ventricles (see section on Preexcitation Syndromes, earlier). The term *AV reciprocating tachycardia* is also used to describe this arrhythmia, but to avoid confusion between AV reciprocating tachycardia and AVNRT, the term CMT is used here. Approximately 40% of regular, narrow QRS tachycardias are due to CMT using an accessory pathway.[43]

In CMT, the reentry circuit involves the atria, AV node, ventricle, and accessory pathway. The term *orthodromic* is used to describe the most common type of CMT, in which the AV node is used as the anterograde limb and the accessory pathway as the retrograde limb of the circuit. This results in a narrow QRS tachycardia because the ventricles are depolarized through the His-Purkinje system. If bundle-branch block is present, the QRS is wide. Because the atria and ventricles depolarize separately, the P waves in CMT, if visible, are often seen in the ST segment or between the QRS complexes, usually closer to the preceding QRS than the following QRS[9,20,43,44,59,64] (Fig 14-13*A*).

The term *antidromic* is used to describe a rare form of CMT in which the accessory pathway is used as the anterograde limb of the circuit and the AV node as the retrograde limb. This results in a wide QRS tachycardia because the ventricles are depolarized abnormally through the accessory pathway, and it is often indistinguishable from VT (see Fig. 14-13*B*).

Like AVNRT, CMT is an AV nodal active tachycardia because the AV node is necessary for maintenance of the tachycardia. Vagal maneuvers or any drug that blocks the AV node can terminate the tachycardia. Treatment of an acute episode is aimed at slowing conduction through the AV node with adenosine, beta blockers, or calcium channel blockers, or at slowing conduction through the accessory pathway with IV procainamide. Radiofrequency ablation offers a cure by destroying the accessory pathway.[38]

Ventricular Tachycardia

Ventricular tachycardia can be one of the most serious arrhythmias encountered in cardiac patients and often requires immediate treatment to prevent hemodynamic collapse and possible deterioration into ventricular fibrillation. Three types of VT are commonly seen in patients with cardiac disease: (1) monomorphic VT, (2) polymorphic VT, and (3) TdP.

MONOMORPHIC VENTRICULAR TACHYCARDIA

Monomorphic VT, the most common type, refers to a VT in which all of the QRS complexes are of the same morphology, indicating that they originate from the same spot in the ventricles (Fig. 14-14). Monomorphic VT often occurs in patients with dilated cardiomyopathy or a history of MI, especially in those with an ejection fraction of less than 40%. Most of these VTs occur within 1 year of the infarct, but many patients present with their first episode 5 or more years after MI.[57] This type of VT is treated acutely with the usual antiarrhythmic therapy used for ventricular arrhythmias: lidocaine, procainamide, bretylium, and IV amiodarone. Amiodarone and sotalol are more effective than other types of antiarrhythmics for chronic therapy. An implantable cardioverter-defibrillator is often required in patients with recurrent VT that is resistant to drug therapy.

Another type of monomorphic VT arises in the RVOT, occurs in patients with no structural heart disease, and is often induced by exercise. RVOT tachycardia presents with an LBBB morphology and inferior or rightward axis. RVOT tachycardia may respond to vagal maneuvers or adenosine. Beta blockers seem to work best for chronic therapy and

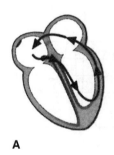
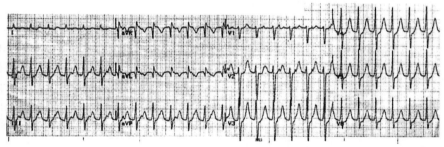

A

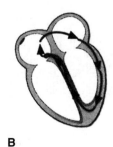

B

FIGURE 14-13 (A) Orthodromic circus movement tachycardia using the atrioventricular (AV) node as anterograde limb and accessory pathway as retrograde limb of the reentry circuit. P waves are visible on the upstroke of the T wave in most leads. **(B)** Antidromic circus movement tachycardia using the accessory pathway as the anterograde limb and the AV node as the retrograde limb of the reentry circuit. (From Jacobson C: Advanced ECG concepts. In Chulay M, Guzzetta C, Dossey B (eds): AACN Handbook of Critical Care Nursing, p 439. Stamford, CT, Appleton & Lange, 1997.)

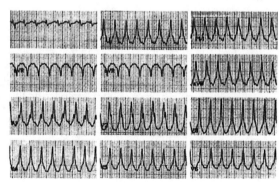

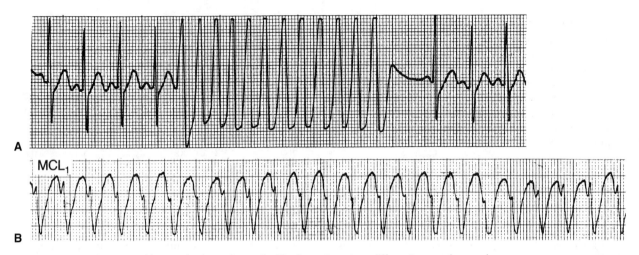

FIGURE 14-14 Monomorphic ventricular tachycardia. Tracings show two different examples, each with QRS complexes of one morphology.

calcium channel blockers have been successful in some patients. Radiofrequency catheter ablation is often successful in destroying the focus in this type of VT.[57,78]

Monomorphic VT arising in the left ventricle in young people with no structural heart disease presents with an RBBB morphology and superior axis. This VT is often sensitive to verapamil or other calcium channel blockers but not to beta blockers.[57] Radiofrequency catheter ablation is difficult because of the left ventricular location of the tachycardia and has only been done in a few patients.

POLYMORPHIC VENTRICULAR TACHYCARDIA

Polymorphic VT refers to VT with unstable, continuously varying QRS morphology often occurring at rates of approximately 200 beats/min[28,51,81] (Fig. 14-15). Polymorphic VT is classified based on whether it is associated with normal or pro-

longed QT or QTU intervals. If a long QT interval is present, it is called TdP (see later). Polymorphic VT with a normal QT or QTU interval is thought to be due to reentry, especially in the ischemic heart. The varying QRS morphologies can be explained by beat-to-beat variations in ventricular activation pattern due to changing sites and configuration of reentry circuits.[28] Polymorphic VT may respond to the same antiarrhythmic drugs used to treat monomorphic VT, especially beta blockers and amiodarone, or to revascularization by surgery or angioplasty when associated with ongoing ischemia.

TORSADES DE POINTES

Torsades de pointes means "twisting of the points" and describes a special type of VT in which the QRS complexes display continuously changing morphologies and seem to twist around an imaginary line, often resembling ventricular fibrillation (Figs. 14-16 and 14-17). The underlying

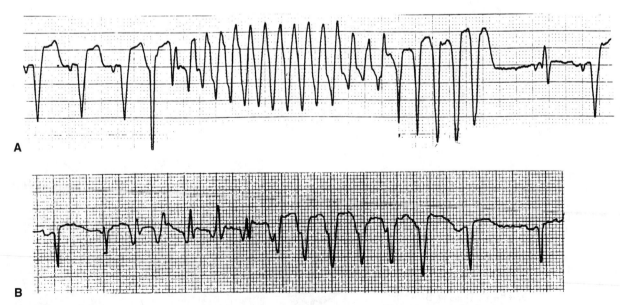

FIGURE 14-15 Polymorphic ventricular tachycardia. Two examples with varying QRS morphologies.

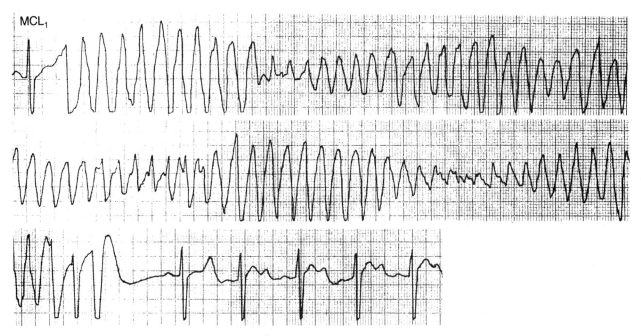

FIGURE 14-16 Torsades de pointes. Note characteristic features: **(1)** multiform RS complexes that twist around the baseline, **(2)** initiation by a premature ventricular complex with a long coupling interval, **(3)** associated long QT interval and wide TU waves during sinus rhythm.

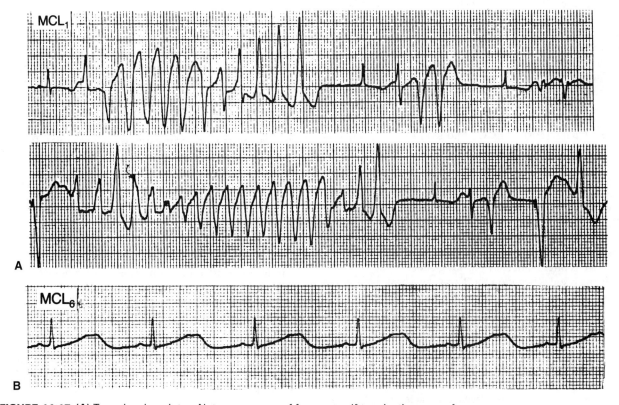

FIGURE 14-17 (A) Torsades de pointes. Note occurrence of frequent self-terminating runs of ventricular tachycardia initiated by premature ventricular complexes with long coupling intervals. QT is difficult to measure because of frequency of ventricular beats, but it appears long. **(B)** Sinus rhythm with very long QT interval and TU waves typical of abnormal repolarization. Torsades de pointes developed in the patient shortly after this strip was taken.

cause of this type of VT is delayed ventricular repolarization, which is manifested on the ECG as a prolonged QT or QTU interval. The differentiation of TdP from polymorphic VT and ventricular fibrillation is extremely important because TdP does not respond to conventional antiarrhythmic therapy and is usually made worse by the drugs used to treat ordinary VT.

The main differentiating factor between TdP and other types of VT is its association with a long QT or QTU interval, indicating repolarization abnormalities not seen in ordinary VT.[1,28,40,65,69,91] The QT interval is a rough estimate of ventricular repolarization time, although the end of the T wave may not indicate the end of repolarization because some areas of the ventricle may continue to repolarize with potentials too small to be detected on the surface ECG.[31] Prolongation of ventricular repolarization is reflected in a prolonged QT interval, and a U wave is frequently seen after the T wave or merging with the T wave in patients with long QT intervals associated with ventricular dysrhythmias. QT prolongation can occur in certain inherited congenital conditions (e.g., Jervell and Lange-Nielsen syndromes associated with deafness, and Romano-Ward syndrome without deafness). QT prolongation can occur secondary to administration of certain drugs, most notably quinidine and other class IA antiarrhythmic agents, as well as class III antiarrhythmic agents. Phenothiazines, tricyclic antidepressants, certain antibiotics, antihistamines, and other drugs have also been implicated as causing TdP.[46,69,88] Other factors that can lead to delayed repolarization include electrolyte imbalances, especially hypokalemia and hypomagnesemia; cerebral events such as cerebral vascular accidents and subarachnoid hemorrhage; CHD; right radical neck dissection; and liquid protein weight-loss diets.[46,47,69,88,91]

The underlying electrophysiology of TdP appears to be prolonged and uneven refractory periods in the ventricles, leading to longer repolarization times during which reentry[28,46,47,69,88] or early afterdepolarizations[11,21,27,28,69] can occur. Characteristic ECG findings of TdP include (1) markedly prolonged QT intervals with wide TU waves; (2) initiation of the arrhythmia by an R-on-T PVC with a long coupling interval; and (3) wide, bizarre, multiform QRS complexes that change direction frequently, appearing to twist around the isoelectric line (see Figs. 14-16 and 14-17). TdP is usually associated with bradycardia and is "pause dependent," meaning that it tends to occur after pauses produced by PVCs or sudden slowing of the heart rate. TdP is often initiated by a "long-short" cycle sequence in which episodes begin on the T wave of a beat that follows a long cycle. Ventricular rate during TdP is commonly 200 to 250 beats/min. TdP is usually self-terminating and occurs in repeated episodes, but it can deteriorate into ventricular fibrillation, requiring countershock.

Treatment of TdP is aimed at shortening the refractory period and unifying repolarization by increasing the heart rate and correcting any contributing causes, such as electrolyte imbalances. Cardiac pacing at rates of 100 to 110 beats/min can be instituted until the underlying cause is corrected. Magnesium can suppress the arrhythmia in both the acquired and congenital forms by reducing the amplitude of afterdepolarizations thought to cause TdP.[45,46,90]

Drugs such as quinidine, procainamide, disopyramide, sotalol, and amiodarone are contraindicated because they prolong the refractory period.

Aberrancy Versus Ventricular Ectopy

One of the most frequently encountered problems in working with cardiac patients is differentiating ventricular ectopy from aberrantly conducted supraventricular beats, both of which can cause a wide QRS complex. The term *aberrant* refers to the temporary abnormal intraventricular conduction of supraventricular impulses. *Ectopy* refers to impulse initiation anywhere other than the sinus node. Because an aberrantly conducted supraventricular beat can look almost identical to a ventricular ectopic beat, it is sometimes impossible to tell them apart. The problem with aberration is that it can mimic ventricular ectopy, which requires specific treatment and carries a different prognosis than aberrancy. Aberrancy is always secondary to some other primary disturbance and does not itself require treatment; therefore, nurses must be able to make the distinction and accurately identify which mechanism is responsible for the arrhythmia being observed whenever possible. Although many criteria have been proposed to aid in differentiating these two causes of wide QRS rhythms, this section concentrates only on selected criteria that seem to be the most helpful in the everyday clinical situation. Table 14-5 lists the ECG clues most helpful for differentiating wide QRS rhythms.

MECHANISMS OF ABERRATION

Aberrancy can occur whenever the His-Purkinje system is still partly or completely refractory when a supraventricular impulse attempts to traverse it. The refractory period of the conduction system is directly proportional to preceding cycle length. Long cycles (slow heart rates) are followed by long refractory periods, whereas short cycles (fast heart rates) are followed by short refractory periods. Supraventricular beats that occur early in the cycle, like PACs, may enter the conduction system during its refractory period and be conducted aberrantly. Similarly, beats that follow a sudden lengthening of the cycle may be conducted aberrantly because of the increased length of the refractory period that occurs when the cycle lengthens. There are three situations in which aberration is likely to occur[84]: (1) early supraventricular beats (e.g., PACs), (2) rapid heart rates where the supraventricular focus conducts into the intraventricular conduction system so rapidly that the bundles do not have time to repolarize completely, and (3) irregular rhythms where cycle lengths are constantly changing (e.g., atrial fibrillation). In addition, the right bundle branch has a longer refractory period than the left; therefore, aberrant beats tend to be conducted most often with an RBBB pattern. Figures 14-18 and 14-19 illustrate these principles of refractory periods and cycle lengths.

ELECTROCARDIOGRAPHIC CRITERIA

P Waves. When trying to make the distinction between aberrancy and ventricular ectopy, a helpful first step is to search for P waves and note their relation to QRS

TABLE 14-5	Electrocardiographic Clues for Differentiating Wide QRS Rhythms	
Electrocardiogram Feature	**Aberrancy**	**Ventricular Ectopy**
P waves	Precede QRS complexes (may be hidden in T waves)	Dissociated from QRS or occur at rate slower than QRS. If 1 : 1 ventriculoatrial conduction is present, retrograde P waves follow every QRS.
Right bundle-branch block QRS morphology	Triphasic rsR' in V_1 Triphasic qRs in V_6	Monophasic R wave or diphasic qR complex in V_1 Left "rabbit ear" taller in V_1 Monophasic QS or diphasic rS in V_6
Left bundle-branch block QRS morphology	Narrow R wave (<0.04 s) in V_1 Straight downstroke of S wave in V_1 (often slurs or notches on upstroke) Usually no Q wave in V_6	Wide R wave (>0.03 s) in V_1 Slurring or notching on downstroke of S wave in V_1 Delay of >0.06 s to nadir of S wave in V_1 Any Q wave in V_6
Precordial QRS concordance	Positive concordance may occur with WPW	Negative concordance favors VT Positive concordance favors VT if WPW ruled out
Fusion or capture beats		Strong evidence in favor of VT
QRS axis	Often normal May be deviated to right or left	Indeterminate axis favors VT Often deviated to left or right
QRS width	Usually <0.14 s unless preexisting bundle-branch block	QRS >0.16 s favors VT

VT, ventricular tachycardia; WPW, Wolff-Parkinson-White syndrome.

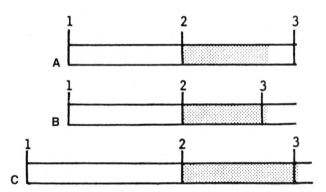

FIGURE 14-18 In the diagrams, 1, 2, and 3 are consecutive beats, and the shaded area represents the refractory period of some part of the conducting system after the second beat. **(A)** There are two regular cycles with normal conduction. The length of the refractory period is directly proportional to preceding cycle length. **(B)** Beat 3 occurs early and enters part of the conduction system during its refractory period, thus conducting aberrantly. **(C)** The first cycle is lengthened, resulting in a longer refractory period after beat 2. Beat 3 occurs no earlier than it did in **(A)**, but conducts aberrantly because the refractory period is prolonged. (From Marriott HJL: Practical Electrocardiography, 8th ed, p 236. Baltimore, Williams & Wilkins, 1988.)

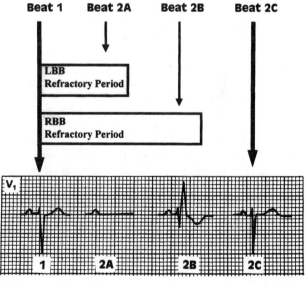

FIGURE 14-19 Diagram of refractory periods in the bundle branches and the effect of cycle length on conduction. The right bundle has a longer refractory period than the left. Beat 2A occurs so early that it cannot conduct through either bundle branch. Beat 2B encounters a refractory right bundle and conducts with right bundle-branch block. Beat 2C falls outside the refractory period of both bundles and is able to conduct normally. (From Jacobson C: Advanced ECG concepts. In Chulay M, Guzzetta C, Dossey B (eds): AACN Handbook of Critical Care Nursing, p 440. Stamford, CT, Appleton & Lange, 1997.)

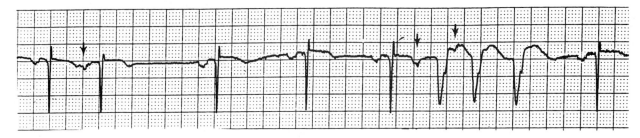

FIGURE 14-20 Sinus rhythm with premature atrial complexes (PACs) and three wide QRS beats that could be mistaken for ventricular tachycardia. The second beat in the strip is a PAC that conducts normally. Note the P waves preceding the wide QRS complexes, indicating aberrant conduction.

complexes. Atrial activity (represented by a P wave) preceding a wide beat or a run of tachycardia strongly favors a supraventricular origin of that beat or tachycardia. Figure 14-20 illustrates an early ectopic P wave initiating three beats of a wide QRS rhythm that could easily be mistaken for PVCs.

An exception to the preceding P wave rule is the case of end-diastolic PVCs that occur after the sinus P wave has occurred. Figure 14-21 shows sinus rhythm with an end-diastolic PVC occurring immediately after the sinus P wave. In this case, the P wave preceding the wide QRS is merely a coincidence and does not represent aberrant conduction; the PR interval is much too short to have conducted that beat. In addition, the P wave preceding the wide QRS is not early; it is the regularly scheduled sinus beat coming on time. Thus, early P waves that precede early wide QRS complexes are usually related to those QRSs, whereas "on time" P waves in front of end-diastolic PVCs are not early and do not cause the wide QRS, although they may result in ventricular fusion beats.

P waves seen during a wide-complex tachycardia can be very helpful in making the differential diagnosis between SVT with aberration and VT. It is common for the sinus node to continue to fire regularly and independently of the ventricular focus when VT occurs. By noting the relationship between P waves and QRS complexes, it is sometimes possible to demonstrate AV dissociation, which means that the atria and ventricles are under the control of separate pacemakers (Fig. 14-22). Therefore, the presence of independent P waves in a wide QRS tachycardia indicates AV dissociation and is diagnostic of VT, whereas P waves seen before each QRS complex indicate a supraventricular origin of the rhythm. Figure 14-23 illustrates how P waves can be useful in differentiating two similar wide QRS tachycardias due to two different mechanisms.

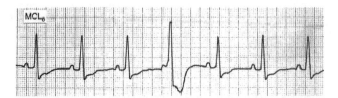

FIGURE 14-21 Sinus rhythm with one end-diastolic premature ventricular complex (PVC). The P wave preceding the PVC is the sinus P wave that coincidentally occurred just before the PVC.

QRS Morphology. The shape of the QRS complexes in a wide QRS tachycardia can be helpful in determining the mechanism of the arrhythmia. The following sections discuss the morphologic clues for wide-complex tachycardias with RBBB and LBBB morphologies.

RIGHT BUNDLE-BRANCH BLOCK PATTERN (QRS UPRIGHT IN V_1). Because the right bundle has a longer refractory period than the left, an impulse entering the conduction system early or at very rapid rates is more likely to encounter a still-refractory right bundle branch; therefore, most (80% to 85%) aberrantly conducted beats conduct with RBBB. However, approximately 60% of ventricular ectopic beats simulate an RBBB pattern.[61,76] Studies have shown that of those beats presenting with an RBBB pattern in lead V_1, most aberrantly conducted supraventricular beats (70%) show a triphasic rsR' pattern, whereas almost all ectopic ventricular beats (92%) show a monophasic (R) or biphasic (qR) pattern.[30,61,76,99,100] Therefore, a wide QRS complex with a triphasic pattern of RBBB in lead V_1 strongly favors aberrancy, whereas a monophasic or biphasic complex of RBBB type favors ventricular ectopy.

Other morphologic clues are presented in Figure 14-24. A monophasic or biphasic complex of RBBB type in lead V_1 with a taller left "rabbit ear" favors ectopy, whereas a taller right "rabbit ear" favors neither. Often V_6 is as helpful as V_1; a triphasic qRs complex in V_6 favors RBBB aberrancy, whereas a monophasic QS complex or a biphasic rS complex favors ventricular ectopy. Figure 14-25A shows VT with RBBB morphology.

LEFT BUNDLE-BRANCH BLOCK PATTERN (QRS NEGATIVE IN V_1). Leads V_1 or V_2 and V_6 also offer morphologic clues for tachycardias with LBBB morphology[48] (see Fig. 14-24). Three characteristics of the QRS complex in V_1 or V_2 favor a ventricular origin: a wide initial r wave of greater than 0.03 second, slurring or notching on the downstroke of the S wave, and a delay of 0.06 second or more from the beginning of the QRS to the nadir (deepest part) of the S wave. In addition, any q wave (qR or QS) in V_6 favors a ventricular origin. Figure 14-25B shows VT with LBBB morphology.

Brugada and colleagues[12] suggest that additional morphologic clues in the precordial leads V_1 through V_6 can also be helpful. They suggest that a helpful first step in diagnosing a wide QRS rhythm is to scan the precordial

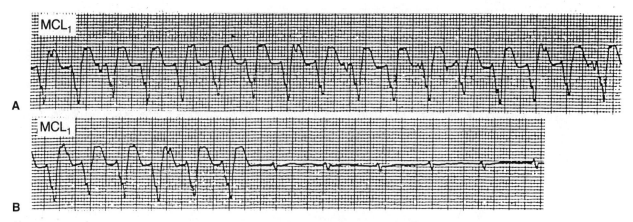

FIGURE 14-22 **(A)** Ventricular tachycardia (VT) at a rate of 136 beats/min. Independent P waves can be seen throughout the strip. **(B)** Sudden termination of VT, revealing the underlying sinus rhythm at a rate of 94 beats/min.

leads to see if any lead shows an rS complex. If no precordial lead shows an rS pattern, VT is the likely diagnosis. If any precordial lead displays an rS pattern in which the measurement from onset of the r wave to nadir of the S wave exceeds 100 milliseconds (0.10 second), it favors the diagnosis of VT. They also emphasize that the presence of AV dissociation or any of the morphologic clues found in leads V_1, V_2, or V_6 discussed previously favor the diagnosis of VT[5], (Fig. 14-26).

Lead V_6 or MCL_6 can be useful in differentiating supraventricular rhythms with aberrancy from ventricular ectopy.[23,24] In wide QRS rhythms of either RBBB or LBBB pattern, an interval of 50 milliseconds (0.05 second) or less from the onset of the QRS to the tallest peak of the R wave or nadir of the S wave favors a supraventricular origin, whereas an interval of 70 milliseconds (0.07 second) or more favors a ventricular origin (Fig. 14-27).

Fusion and Capture Beats. Ventricular fusion beats are produced when a supraventricular impulse and an ectopic ventricular impulse both contribute to ventricular depolarization. The resulting QRS complex does not look like a normally conducted beat or like the pure ventricular ectopic

beat because it is formed by a combination of both depolarization waves. The shape and width of fusion beats vary depending on the relative contributions of both the supraventricular and the ventricular impulses. The presence of fusion beats indicates AV dissociation; the atria and the

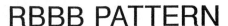

RBBB PATTERN

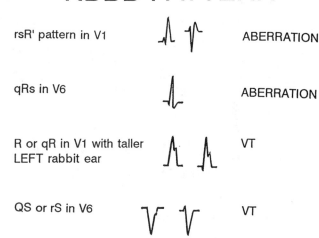

LBBB PATTERN

In Leads V1 or V2:

Wide R,
Slurred downstroke,
>.06 sec to nadir of S ⩔ VT

Any Q (qR or QS) in V6 ⩔ VT

FIGURE 14-24 Morphology clues for wide QRS beats and rhythms with right bundle-branch block (RBBB) pattern and left bundle-branch block (LBBB) pattern.

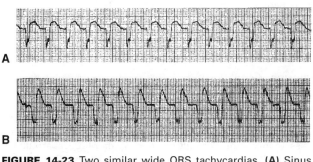

FIGURE 14-23 Two similar wide QRS tachycardias. **(A)** Sinus tachycardia; rate-115 beats/min. P waves can be seen preceding each QRS, indicating a supraventricular origin of the tachycardia. **(B)** P waves are independent of QRS complexes, indicating atrioventricular dissociation that favors ventricular tachycardia.

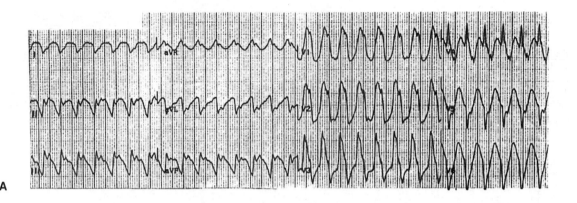

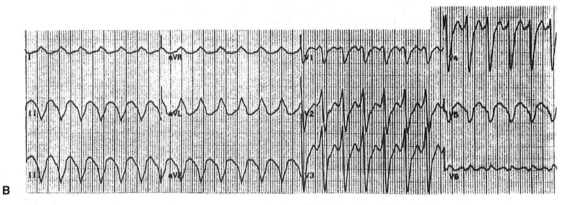

FIGURE 14-25 (A) Twelve-lead electrocardiogram (ECG) of ventricular tachycardia (VT) with right bundle-branch block morphology. Note monophasic R wave with taller left rabbit ear in V_1 and QS complex in V_6. The indeterminate QRS axis also favors VT. **(B)** Twelve-lead ECG of VT with left bundle-branch block morphology. Note wide R waves in V_1 and V_2, and qR pattern in V_6. (From Jacobson C: Advanced ECG concepts. In Chulay M, Guzzetta C, Dossey B (eds): AACN Handbook of Critical Care Nursing, p 444. Stamford, CT, Appleton & Lange, 1997.)

THE NETHERLANDS CLUES
Any of the following = VT

No RS in any precordial lead

R to S interval > 100ms
in any precordial lead

AV dissociation

Morphology criteria for VT present in V1-2 and V6

FIGURE 14-26 The Netherlands clues (so named because these clues originated in The Netherlands from research done by Brugada and colleagues[13]). In a wide QRS tachycardia, if no precordial lead displays an RS complex, or if any precordial lead displays an RS complex that measures greater than 100 milliseconds from onset to nadir, ventricular tachycardia (VT) is the favored diagnosis. Atrioventricular dissociation and the morphology clues favoring VT in V_{1-2} and V_6 are also helpful.

THE SAN FRANCISCO CLUE
In either RBBB or LBBB morphologies

In V6 or MCL6:

Onset of QRS to tallest peak
or to nadir < 50 ms   ABERRATION

Onset of QRS to tallest peak
or to nadir > 70ms   VT

FIGURE 14-27 The San Francisco clue (so named because these clues originated from research done in San Francisco by Drew and Scheinman[24]). In wide QRS tachycardias of either right or left bundle-branch block morphology, if measurement from beginning of QRS to tallest peak or to nadir of S wave is less than 50 milliseconds (ms) in V_6 or MCL_6, aberration is favored. If the measurement is more than 70 ms, VT is favored.

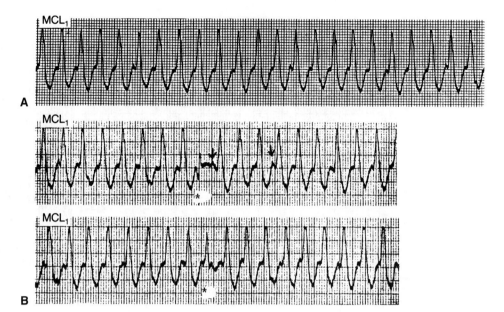

FIGURE 14-28 (A) Wide QRS tachycardia at a rate of approximately 200 beats/min. P waves are not easily recognizable, but the monophasic upright QRS morphology in V_1 favors ventricular tachycardia (VT). **(B)** Same patient with fusion beats among the wide QRS complexes (*asterisks*). *Arrows* point to P waves occurring independently of QRS complexes. Fusion beats and independent P waves are diagnostic of VT.

ventricles are under the control of separate pacemakers. Capture beats occur when, in the presence of AV dissociation, a supraventricular impulse manages to conduct into the ventricles and "capture" them, resulting in a normally conducted QRS complex. Thus, the presence of fusion or capture beats in a run of wide QRS tachycardia is diagnostic of VT, but unfortunately capture beats are rare and cannot be counted on to make the diagnosis[30] (Fig. 14-28).

Cycle Length Variations. Ashman's phenomenon states that a beat that terminates a short cycle after a long cycle tends to be aberrantly conducted.[20,59] Because the refractory period of the conduction system varies with preceding cycle length, a beat that terminates a long cycle has a long refractory period, causing the next beat to conduct aberrantly if it occurs early (i.e., terminates a short cycle). This aberrant conduction usually occurs with RBBB because the right bundle branch has a longer refractory period than the left. Thus, aberration tends to occur in early beats that cause a shortening of the cycle, such as PACs, or only in the first beat of a run of SVT. Ashman's phenomenon does not prove aberration, it merely explains it if it occurs. Therefore, the presence of a beat that meets Ashman criteria (i.e., terminates a short cycle after a long cycle) does not prove that the wide beat is aberrant, because a PVC could just as easily have occurred in the same spot.

Depending only on cycle lengths to aid in the differentiation of aberration from ectopy is unreliable for another reason as well. By the "rule of bigeminy," a long cycle can also precipitate a PVC.[53,60] The mechanism responsible for this seems to be that the area of unidirectional block that allows the reentry of the impulse in the ventricular myocardium is able to conduct the impulse in a retrograde direction only after a certain rest period (i.e., a long cycle). Once a PVC has occurred, the pause that follows results in another long cycle, which allows another VPB; thus, ventricular bigeminy tends to perpetuate itself. Because a long preceding cycle can occur in both aberration and ectopy, it

alone cannot be used with certainty in differentiating the two mechanisms. However, the absence of a long preceding cycle favors ectopy and is evidence against aberration.[59]

Atrial fibrillation presents special difficulties in the differentiation of wide QRS complexes. The absence of P waves prevents the use of P-wave clues, and the variations in cycle length that are common in atrial fibrillation or atrial flutter provide a perfect set-up for both aberrant conduction and ventricular reentry. It is necessary to rely heavily on QRS morphology and it is helpful to compare cycle lengths. When comparing cycle sequences in atrial fibrillation or flutter, it is important to look at several sequences and not only at the sequence containing the beat with the wide QRS. Figure 14-29A shows atrial flutter with an aberrantly conducted beat that terminates a short cycle after a long cycle (i.e., Ashman's phenomenon). In Figure 14-29B, beat 5 terminates a cycle that is shorter than the preceding cycle, but in comparing other cycle sequences in the same strip, note that beat 21 terminates an even shorter cycle that follows the longest cycle in the strip and still conducts normally. The absence of aberration in beat 21 where it would be expected because of cycle lengths helps to identify beat 5 as a PVC.

It is common in the presence of atrial fibrillation to see both RBBB and LBBB aberration in the same patient. An interesting finding in many cases is that the two forms of aberration are often separated from one another by one normally conducted beat.[59,60] The mechanism of this phenomenon is not understood, but it occurs often enough to make it a useful clue in differentiating aberration from bifocal ventricular ectopy (Fig. 14-30).

Whenever possible, it is useful to compare conduction during atrial fibrillation with conduction that occurs in the same patient during sinus rhythm. Figure 14-31A is from a patient in atrial fibrillation with many episodes of LBBB aberration resembling VT. Note that whenever the ventricular response to atrial fibrillation slows even slightly, normal conduction resumes. Also note that the aberrantly conducted

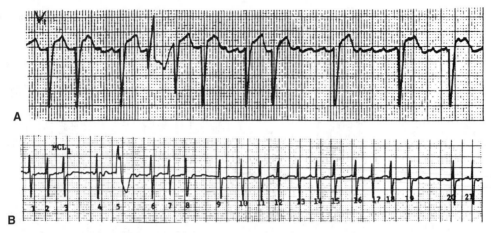

FIGURE 14-29 (A) Atrial flutter with one aberrantly conducted beat. Note the triphasic rSR' complex of right bundle-branch block in V₁. **(B)** Atrial fibrillation with a premature ventricular complex (beat no. 5). The monophasic QRS with taller left "rabbit ear" favors a ventricular origin. Comparison of cycle lengths indicates that if any beat in this strip should be conducted aberrantly, it is beat no. 21, which terminates a short cycle after the longest cycle in the strip. If the heart can conduct beat 21 normally, there is no reason why it would conduct beat no. 5 aberrantly.

beats occur in an irregular pattern, just as the ventricular response to atrial fibrillation typically occurs, and that the morphology favors LBBB rather than VT. The irregularity is a helpful observation because VT, although it does not have to be perfectly regular, is seldom as irregular as the ventricular response to atrial fibrillation. Figure 14-31*B* is from the same patient during one of his frequent episodes of sinus rhythm. Note that during the sinus rhythm, there are no aberrantly conducted beats. When sinus rhythm is restored, the ventricular rate slows and the cycle lengths become reg-

ular, both of which remove the opportunity for aberration to occur. If the wide beats that occur during atrial fibrillation were ventricular ectopic beats, they would be just as likely to occur during sinus rhythm. The disappearance of the wide QRS complexes every time sinus rhythm is restored helps make the diagnosis of aberration in Figure 14-31*A*.

Intra-atrial Electrograms and Esophageal Leads. Recording the electrogram from a lead in or on the right atrium or from a lead positioned behind the atria in the

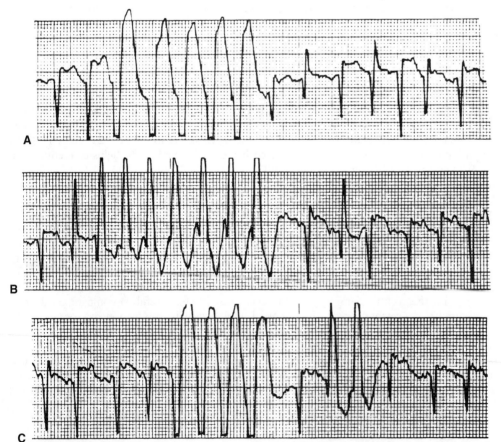

FIGURE 14-30 Atrial fibrillation with both left **(A)** and right **(B)** bundle-branch block aberration. **(C)** Left bundle-branch block aberration and right bundle-branch block aberration are separated by a single normal beat.

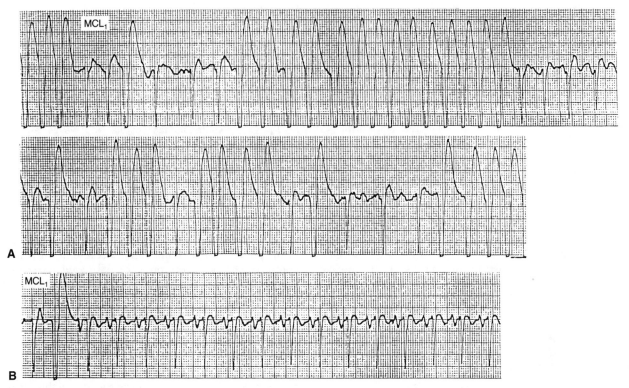

FIGURE 14-31 (A) Atrial fibrillation with frequent left bundle-branch block aberration resembling ventricular tachycardia. Normal conduction resumes whenever the ventricular rate slows even slightly. **(B)** Same patient during one of his frequent episodes of sinus tachycardia, restored after the second beat. During sinus tachycardia, no aberration occurs because the rate is slower and cycle lengths are regular, removing the opportunity for aberration.

esophagus is a useful technique for demonstrating the relationship between atrial and ventricular electrical activity. When the lead is positioned in or very near the atria, atrial activity records as a large deflection and ventricular activity records as a smaller deflection, making it easier to see if P waves are associated with or dissociated from the QRS complexes. Figure 14-32 shows an intra-atrial recording from a patient with a wide QRS tachycardia in whom the diagnosis was uncertain. AV dissociation is clearly present, as demonstrated by very large "P" waves and smaller QRS

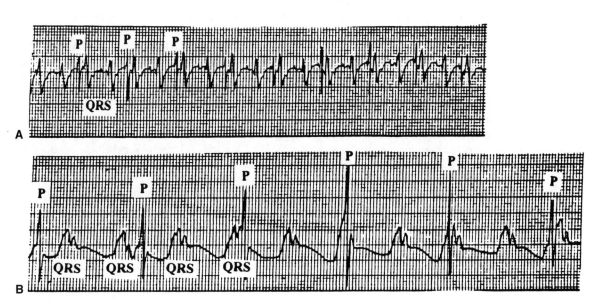

FIGURE 14-32 Intra-atrial recording of a wide QRS tachycardia at regular paper speed **(A)** and double paper speed **(B)** Atrioventricular dissociation is apparent and is diagnostic of ventricular tachycardia.

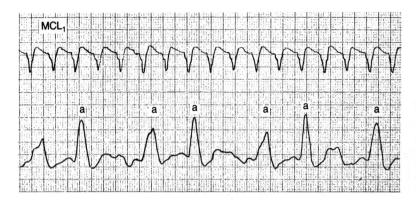

FIGURE 14-33 Electrocardiogram (ECG) and a central venous pressure (CVP) tracing of a patient in ventricular tachycardia. No P waves can be seen for certain in the ECG, but the CVP shows exaggerated a waves when the right atrium contracts against the closed tricuspid valve during atrioventricular dissociation.

deflections. When recording an atrial electrogram, the recorder should be run at double the normal paper speed (i.e., at 50 mm/sec instead of the usual 25 mm/sec) to make it easier to differentiate atrial and ventricular activity.

CLINICAL CRITERIA

Several clinical criteria can be used to aid in the differentiation of aberration from ectopy.

Heart Sounds. Varying intensity of the S_1 heart sound occurs whenever the atrial activity is dissociated from ventricular activity, as frequently occurs in VT. The S_1 sound is produced by the closure of the AV valves, and its intensity depends on the proximity of the valve leaflets to one another at the time of ventricular systole. When atrial activity and ventricular activity are dissociated, the atria contract in variable relationship to the ventricles and the valve leaflets are at times wide open when ventricular systole occurs, causing a loud sound when they close. At other times, the leaflets have drifted closer together before ventricular systole and the resulting sound is softer. When there is a 1 : 1 relation between atrial and ventricular contraction, as occurs in a supraventricular rhythm, the intensity of S_1 is constant because the valve leaflets are in the same position every time they close. Thus, variable intensity of S_1 favors VT when AV dissociation is present.

Neck Veins. When AV dissociation is present, atrial and ventricular contraction is asynchronous and the atria and the ventricles occasionally contract simultaneously. When this occurs, the atria contract against closed AV valves, and blood from the right atrium has no place to go except back up into the neck veins. Observation of the patient's neck veins during AV dissociation reveals irregularly occurring "cannon a waves," which are large pulsations seen in the neck veins as blood is forced backward during atrial contraction. When atrial activity precedes ventricular activity, as it does in some SVTs (e.g., sinus or atrial tachycardia), cannon a waves are not seen. When atrial activity occurs simultaneously with or after ventricular activity in a 1 : 1 relationship (as it may in junctional tachycardia or VT with retrograde conduction, AVNRT, or in SVT due to an accessory pathway), cannon a waves are often seen with each beat. No a waves at all occur in the presence of atrial fibrillation because the atria do not contract. Therefore, the presence of *irregularly occurring* cannon a waves in the jugular pulse or in the central venous pressure or pulmonary wedge pressure tracing in the presence of a wide QRS tachycardia favors VT (Fig. 14-33).

Response to Vagal Maneuvers. Carotid sinus massage or other vagal-stimulating maneuvers, such as the Valsalva maneuver, are often used in the presence of a rapid heart rate either to terminate a supraventricular rhythm or diagnose the mechanism of the tachycardia. A sinus tachycardia usually responds to CSM by slowing its rate, whereas some SVTs (especially AVNRT or CMT) may convert to sinus rhythm. Atrial rhythms, such as atrial tachycardia, flutter, or fibrillation, usually respond with a slowing of the ventricular response but not by conversion to sinus rhythm. VT typically does not respond to CSM, and occasionally there is no response from a supraventricular rhythm. Therefore, if the rate of the tachycardia slows in response to CSM or the rhythm converts to sinus rhythm, a supraventricular origin of the tachycardia is favored; if there is no response, neither aberration nor ectopy is favored.

Wenckebach Conduction

Wenckebach conduction is a progressive increase in conduction time of an impulse from its site of origin to its site of termination. AV Wenckebach is a common clinical occurrence and is easily recognized. It is known that Wenckebach conduction can occur in other areas of the heart, including the sinus node,[82] various levels of the AV node,[39,50] the bundle branches,[72] and reentry loops in the ventricles,[15] as well as from ectopic foci.[20,63] Recognition of Wenckebach conduction from these other sites is not as easy as recognizing AV Wenckebach, although Wenckebach conduction occurring anywhere in the heart follows the same rules as AV Wenckebach conduction. Therefore, a thorough understanding of typical AV Wenckebach conduction is necessary as a basis for recognizing Wenckebach conduction in other areas of the heart. This section describes the characteristics of typical AV Wenckebach conduction, the most commonly occurring atypical types of AV Wenckebach conduction, and Wenckebach conduction in other areas of the heart.

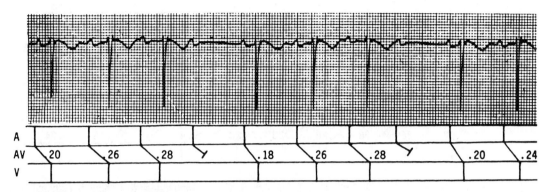

FIGURE 14-34 Typical atrioventricular (AV) Wenckebach conduction: The PR intervals gradually increase before the pause; R-R intervals shorten before the pause; the pause measures less than twice any R-R interval; the overall appearance is one of group beating. (In this and all other ladder diagrams, A, atria; AV, AV junction; V, ventricles. The slant of the line through the AV area represents conduction time through the AV junction. PR intervals are measured in seconds.) (From Jacobson C: Interpretation of complex arrhythmias. In Woods SL (ed): Cardiovascular Critical Care Nursing, p 194. New York, Churchill Livingstone, 1983. By permission.)

ATRIOVENTRICULAR WENCKEBACH

Wenckebach (type I) AV block is a progressive increase in conduction time of consecutive impulses from atria to ventricles until an impulse fails to be conducted, or is "blocked." It is characterized by progressive lengthening of the PR interval on consecutively conducted beats until the final P wave of the sequence is followed by a pause rather than by a QRS; then the cycle repeats itself (Fig. 14-34). The following are characteristics of typical AV Wenckebach conduction:

1. The PR interval progressively increases with each consecutively conducted beat.
2. The largest increment in PR interval usually occurs between the first and second beats in the cycle.
3. R-R intervals gradually shorten before the pause.
4. The pause is less than twice the length of any other cycle.
5. The overall appearance of the rhythm demonstrates group beating.

Typical AV Wenckebach conduction occurs most often at lower conduction ratios, such as 4 : 3 (four P waves to three QRS complexes), whereas atypical forms tend to be more common at higher conduction ratios, such as 8 : 7 conduction.[13,26,97]

The gradual shortening of R-R intervals before the pause occurs because even though PR intervals gradually increase, they increase by decreasing amounts each time. Figure 14-35 illustrates this concept with a ladder diagram showing each beat of a Wenckebach cycle as a solid line compared with the previous beat as a dotted line. It can be readily seen that the AV conduction time progressively increases from 0.18 second to 0.30, 0.36, and 0.38 second, but the amount of increase decreases from 0.12 to 0.06 to 0.02 second, which causes the R-R intervals to shorten. Note also that the length of the pause is less than twice the length of any other cycle in the sequence. Figure 14-34 illustrates these common characteristics of typical AV Wenckebach conduction.

Atypical AV Wenckebach conduction occurs when the conduction delay is inconsistent and not all the usual features

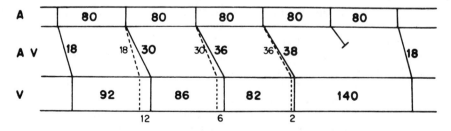

FIGURE 14-35 Diagram of typical Wenckebach cycle. Numbers are hundredths of a second. Solid lines represent the current cycle, compared with dotted lines representing the previous cycle. Note that atrioventricular conduction time gets longer with each cycle, but each increase is smaller than the preceding increase, causing R-R intervals to shorten. (From Watanabe Y, Driefus L: Atrioventricular block: Basic concepts. In Mandel WJ (ed): Cardiac Arrhythmias: Their Mechanisms, Diagnosis, and Management, p 420. Philadelphia, JB Lippincott, 1995.)

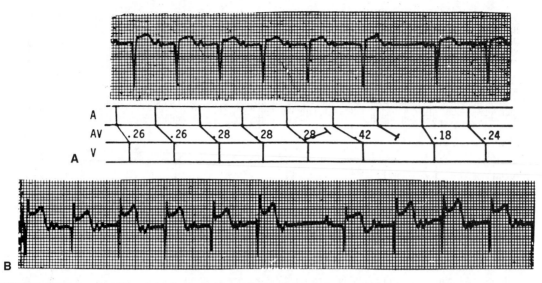

FIGURE 14-36 Atypical Wenckebach conduction. **(A)** Gradual lengthening of PR intervals until the sixth beat of the cycle, when the PR interval is suddenly longer than expected. The ladder diagram illustrates a possible explanation for the suddenly prolonged PR interval: reentry of the impulse back into the atrioventricular node causes it to be more refractory than expected to the next sinus impulse. PR intervals are shown in seconds. **(B)** Very gradual increases in PR intervals from 0.28 second in the first beat to 0.30 second in the last beat of the cycle. Note that the PR interval that follows the pause is 0.24 second. (From Jacobson C: Interpretation of complex arrhythmias. In Woods SL (ed): Cardiovascular Critical Care Nursing, p 196. New York, Churchill Livingstone, 1983. By permission.)

of typical Wenckebach conduction are present.[13,97] The following are some commonly occurring atypical patterns:

1. The last PR interval of the cycle increases in length more than expected (Fig. 14-36*A*). A possible explanation for this unexpected lengthening of the last PR interval is that prolonged conduction time of the next-to-last beat in the cycle allows the AV node to recover some of its conductivity, thus enabling the impulse to reenter the AV node and propagate back toward the atria at the same time as it proceeds into the ventricles. This retrograde conduction through the AV node causes the node to be more refractory when the next sinus impulse arrives, thus prolonging conduction time of the last impulse in the cycle more than would normally be expected, resulting in the excessive length of the last PR interval.[26]

2. Conduction times can increase so gradually that the changes in PR intervals are not easily seen on the ECG (see Fig. 14-36*B*). For this reason, it is important to compare the PR interval preceding the pause with the PR interval after the pause. When Wenckebach conduction is present, the PR interval preceding the pause is longer than the PR interval after the pause.

3. Conduction times can remain the same for several beats within a cycle or can vary within a cycle. In these cases, PR intervals may remain constant for several beats or may actually get smaller at one point in the cycle. Again, it is important to compare the PR interval preceding the pause with the PR interval after the pause to help establish the presence of Wenckebach conduction.

Wenckebach conduction can occur through the AV node in rhythms other than normal sinus rhythm. Figure 14-37*A* shows atrial tachycardia with a gradual Wenckebach conduction pattern. Figure 14-37*B* shows a rhythm that could be mistaken for atrial fibrillation with a rapid ventricular response. The overall appearance of the rhythm reveals group beating, and P waves occurring at a rate of 214 beats/min can be seen in the pauses. Once P waves have been identified, it is easy to see that PR intervals progressively increase until a P wave fails to conduct to the ventricles, resulting in the pause.

WENCKEBACH CONDUCTION IN THE SINUS NODE

Sinus Wenckebach conduction is a form of sinus exit block in which sinus impulses are formed normally in the sinus node but take progressively longer to exit from the sinus node into the atria, until finally one impulse is completely blocked and fails to reach the atria. It is impossible to see this progressive prolongation of sinoatrial conduction time directly because the ECG does not show sinus node activity. What is seen on the ECG is the P wave as the atria depolarize in response to the sinus impulse. Therefore, sinus Wenckebach conduction appears on the ECG as progressive shortening of the P-P intervals until a P wave fails to appear. The length of the P-P interval that includes the pause is less than twice the length of any other P-P interval in the sequence. After the pause, the cycle repeats itself, thus giving the appearance of group beating (Fig. 14-38).

Sinus Wenckebach conduction is more easily understood if compared with typical AV Wenckebach conduction. In AV Wenckebach conduction, the progressive con-

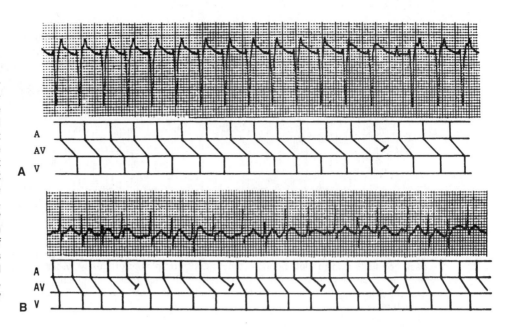

FIGURE 14-37 Atrial tachycardia with Wenckebach conduction. **(A)** P waves visible at a rate of 167 beats/min. The PR interval increases gradually from the first beat to the beat preceding the pause, and the PR interval that follows the pause is the shortest one in the strip. **(B)** P waves are visible at a rate of 214 beats/min, and PR intervals gradually increase before the pause. (From Jacobson C: Interpretation of complex arrhythmias. In Woods SL (ed): Cardiovascular Critical Care Nursing. New York, Churchill Livingstone, 1983. By permission.)

duction delay takes place across the AV node and can be measured in the PR interval. In sinus Wenckebach conduction, the progressive conduction delay takes place across the sinoatrial junction and cannot be directly measured. AV Wenckebach conduction displays progressive shortening of R-R intervals until a P wave fails to conduct to the ventricles, resulting in a pause. This cycle then repeats itself, giving the appearance of group beating. Sinus Wenckebach conduction displays progressive shortening of the P-P intervals until an impulse fails to reach the atria, resulting in a pause and the absence of the next expected P wave. The cycle then repeats itself, giving the appearance of group beating. The P-P intervals shorten in sinus Wenckebach conduction for the same reason the R-R intervals shorten in AV Wenckebach conduction; even though the impulse takes progressively longer to exit from the sinus node, it takes longer by a smaller amount each time (see Fig. 14-35). The PR intervals remain constant in sinus

Wenckebach conduction because the conduction delay is from sinus node to atria, not through the AV node.

WENCKEBACH CONDUCTION IN THE BUNDLE BRANCHES

Wenckebach conduction in the bundle-branch system is a progressive delay in conduction of the impulse down a bundle branch into its ventricle until an impulse is totally blocked in that bundle branch. The ECG demonstrates progressive widening of the QRS complex in successive beats until the last beat in the Wenckebach cycle shows complete bundle-branch block. Figure 14-39 shows Wenckebach conduction in the left and right bundle branches. The QRS complex gradually widens as the impulse is conducted progressively more slowly through the involved bundle branch. The first beat in the sequence is conducted normally because the impulse in the preceding beat is completely blocked in

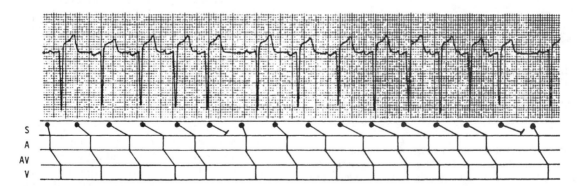

FIGURE 14-38 Sinus Wenckebach conduction. S indicates the sinus node, which is not visible on the electrocardiogram. The slant of the line through the S level indicates conduction time from sinus node to the atria. Note that sinoatrial conduction times progressively increase until a sinus impulse is completely blocked. PR intervals are constant, and P-P intervals gradually shorten before each pause. (From Jacobson C: Interpretation of complex arrhythmias. In Woods SL (ed): Cardiovascular Critical Care Nursing, p 199. New York, Churchill Livingstone, 1983. By permission.)

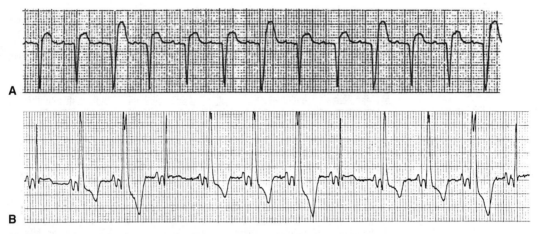

FIGURE 14-39 Wenckebach conduction in the bundle branches. **(A)** Sinus rhythm with Wenckebach conduction in the left bundle branch. QRS complexes gradually widen until complete left bundle-branch block occurs. **(B)** Sinus rhythm with Wenckebach conduction in the right bundle branch. QRS complexes gradually develop a wider terminal R wave until complete right bundle-branch block occurs.

the affected bundle, allowing a prolonged recovery time in that bundle branch. This prolonged recovery time allows the next beat to travel without delay through the affected bundle branch, resulting in a normal QRS complex.

Figure 14-40 shows Wenckebach conduction in the left anterior fascicle of the left bundle branch. The ECG shows progressive left axis deviation as the impulse is conducted progressively more slowly through the anterior fascicle.

WENCKEBACH CONDUCTION IN REENTRANT PATHWAYS

Ectopic beats can be caused by reentry of an original stimulus into previously depolarized areas of the heart through reentry pathways. Reentry can occur in various parts of the heart and is postulated to be a common cause of PVCs when it occurs in the ventricles. One of the hallmarks of reentry in the ventricles is the presence of constant coupling intervals between the normal beat and the PVC.[15] The coupling interval represents conduction time through the ventricular reen-

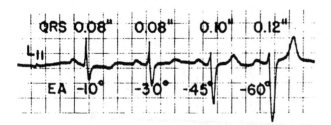

FIGURE 14-40 Wenckebach conduction in the left anterior fascicle of the left bundle branch. Lead II shows progressive left axis deviation from −10 to −60 degrees as conduction is progressively delayed through the left anterior fascicle. EA, electrical axis. The QRS gradually widens, possibly because of progressive right bundle-branch block. (From Sclarovsky S, Strasberg B, Agmon J: Coexistent Wenckebach phenomenon in the distal branches of the specialized conduction system. Chest 73: 534, 1978.)

try pathway and is usually fixed or constant, indicating that reentering impulses take the same amount of time to travel the reentry loop each time they occur. Fixed coupling has been one of the main criteria used in differentiating randomly occurring PVCs from ventricular parasystole.

Wenckebach conduction through the reentry pathway has been postulated as being responsible for variable coupling intervals in the absence of parasystole.[15] Figure 14-41 shows sinus rhythm with ventricular bigeminy. The coupling intervals gradually increase until finally a PVC fails to appear. The ladder diagram illustrates progressively prolonged conduction times through the reentry loop until the fifth reentering impulse fails to travel through the loop, resulting in the absence of a PVC. Typically, conduction times through the reentry pathway increase by decreasing increments, just as PR intervals do in AV Wenckebach, and interectopic intervals decrease before the blocked impulse, just as R-R intervals do in AV Wenckebach conduction. Figure 14-41 illustrates an atypical case of Wenckebach conduction because the last conduction time through the reentry pathway is longer than would be expected; conduction times increase by decreasing amounts during the first three trips around the loop, then increase by a longer amount for the final circuit.

WENCKEBACH EXIT BLOCK FROM AN ECTOPIC FOCUS

Wenckebach exit block can occur from an ectopic atrial, junctional, or ventricular focus just as it can from the sinus node. Wenckebach conduction from an ectopic focus is a progressive increase in conduction time of an impulse from its site of origin into surrounding tissue. Figure 14-42*A* shows atrial fibrillation with a regular junctional rhythm controlling the ventricles, a sign of digitalis toxicity. In Figure 14-42*B*, note the group beating and gradually shortening R-R intervals typical of Wenckebach conduction. The ladder diagram illustrates that the ectopic junctional focus is firing regularly, but the impulse takes progressively longer to exit into the AV junctional tissue until finally an impulse

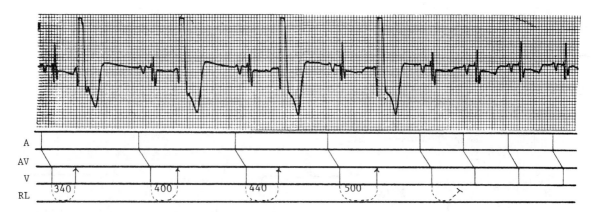

FIGURE 14-41 Wenckebach conduction through the reentry loop. Coupling intervals gradually increase from 340 to 500 milliseconds until the fifth reentering impulse is blocked in the loop. Interectopic intervals decrease slightly before the blocked impulse. Coupling intervals are shown in milliseconds. RL, reentry loop.

fails to exit from its site of origin, resulting in a pause. The sequence repeats itself, giving the appearance of group beating. In Figure 14-42*C*, the conduction ratio changes to 3 : 2, resulting in groups of two beats.

Figure 14-43*A* is a 12-lead ECG tracing showing multiple runs of VT. Note that in each lead, the R-R intervals gradually decrease during the runs of tachycardia, as happens in typical Wenckebach conduction. Figure 14-43*B* shows an enlarged lead II with a ladder diagram illustrating that the ectopic ventricular focus fires regularly, but conduction times from the ectopic focus into the ventricle gradually increase until an impulse finally fails to exit from its site of origin, resulting in the termination of the tachycardia.

Multilevel Atrioventricular Block

A block in impulse conduction can exist at more than one level in the AV conduction system, including multiple levels in the AV node (upper, middle, or lower parts of the AV node), His-Purkinje system, and AV bypass tracts.[4,17,39,50,97] *Alternating Wenckebach* is a term used to describe rhythms that demonstrate Wenckebach conduction of alternate atrial impulses (i.e., sinus or atrial rhythms with 2 : 1 conduction, in which the PR intervals of conducted beats progressively increase until two or more P waves are blocked). Alternating Wenckebach conduction can occur in the presence of sinus rhythm, atrial tachycardia, or atrial flutter and can be explained by postulating block

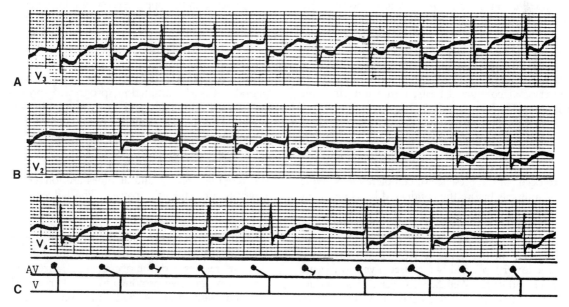

FIGURE 14-42 Wenckebach exit block from an atrioventricular junctional focus. **(A)** Atrial fibrillation with an accelerated junctional rhythm controlling the ventricles. **(B)** A 5 : 4 Wenckebach exit block from the junctional focus. Note group beating and gradual shortening of R-R intervals. **(C)** A 3 : 2 Wenckebach exit block from the junctional focus. (From Marriott HJL, Conover M: Advanced Concepts in Arrhythmias, 2nd ed, p 79. St. Louis, CV Mosby, 1989.)

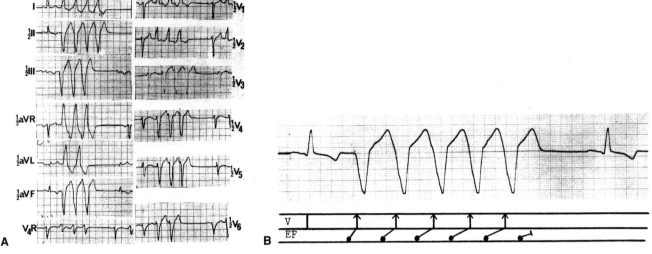

FIGURE 14-43 Ventricular tachycardia (VT) with Wenckebach exit block. **(A)** A 12-lead electrocardiogram (ECG) showing runs of VT. Note that R-R intervals decrease progressively in each lead. **(B)** Enlarged lead II from ECG in **(A)**. Ladder diagram illustrates a VT Wenckebach conduction from the ventricular focus. EF, ectopic focus. (From Peter T, Harper RW, Vohra JK et al: The electrocardiographic recognition of Wenckebach phenomenon in sites other than the atrioventricular junction. Heart Lung 5: 747, 1976.)

at two or more levels in the AV conduction system. For the purposes of this discussion, the term *multilevel block* refers to two levels of block in the AV node.

In multilevel AV block, conduction in the upper level of the AV node can be either Wenckebach or 2 : 1 block, as can conduction in the lower level. Rhythms in which Wenckebach conduction is present in the upper level display a variety of patterns depending on the length of the Wenckebach cycle and the type of block in the lower level. These rhythms may contain one, two, or more consecutively blocked P waves. Rhythms in which there is 2 : 1 conduction in the upper level and Wenckebach conduction in the lower level demonstrate the group beating of typical Wenckebach conduction and progressive prolongation in the PR interval of conducted beats, terminating in three blocked P waves.

Figure 14-44*A* illustrates sinus tachycardia with 2 : 1 and 3 : 1 conduction and could be mistaken for complete AV block because PR intervals are so inconsistent, except that the ventricular response is not regular, as would be expected to occur in the presence of complete block. Note that the PR intervals before the conducted beats gradually increase until two P waves are completely blocked after the third QRS complex. The ladder diagram below illustrates two levels of block in the AV node; 7 : 6 Wenckebach conduction is present in the upper level, 2 : 1 conduction is present in the lower level, and two consecutive P waves are blocked at the end of the Wenckebach cycle. This conduction pattern, ending with two blocked P waves, occurs when there is an odd number of P waves in the Wenckebach cycle in the upper level.[4,50]

The strip in Figure 14-44*B* shows sinus tachycardia with varying PR intervals and frequent nonconducted P waves. Note that the PR intervals of alternate beats are progressively prolonged and that only one P wave at a time is blocked. The ladder diagram shows two levels of block in the AV node, with Wenckebach conduction in the upper level, an even number of atrial complexes in each Wenckebach cycle, and 2 : 1 conduction in the lower level. When there are even numbers of atrial beats in the Wenckebach cycle, the P wave blocked in the upper level follows a beat that has been conducted in the lower level; therefore, the beat blocked in the upper level would have been blocked in the lower level if it had been conducted that far.[50] Thus, P waves 5, 9, and 15 are conducted through the lower level of 2 : 1 block even though the previous P wave was not blocked on that level.

Figure 14-44*C* demonstrates sinus tachycardia with periods of 1 : 1 conduction, progressive prolongation of successive PR intervals, and a varying number of blocked P waves. This pattern could be mistaken for typical AV Wenckebach conduction except that there are times when more than one P wave in a row is blocked. In addition, the PR intervals that follow the pauses are not necessarily the shortest PR intervals and at times are longer than the PR intervals preceding the pauses. The ladder diagram illustrates two levels of AV block with Wenckebach conduction in both levels.

When 2 : 1 conduction is present in the upper level and Wenckebach conduction occurs in the lower level, the rhythm presents with the overall appearance of group beating and progressive prolongation of alternate PR intervals and ends with three blocked atrial impulses. Figure 14-45 shows atrial flutter with a ventricular response that occurs in groups of two. Note that the FR intervals (the distance from the beginning of a flutter wave to the beginning of the QRS complex) of alternate atrial beats gradually prolong and that the cycle ends with three blocked atrial impulses.

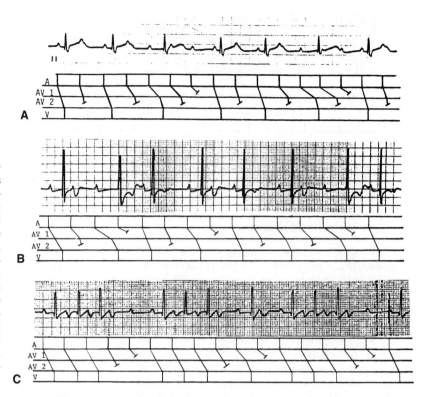

FIGURE 14-44 Multilevel atrioventricular (AV) block. The AV area in the ladder diagrams is divided into two levels to show conduction patterns in each level. **(A)** Sinus tachycardia with 7:6 Wenckebach conduction in the upper level of the AV junction and 2:1 conduction in the lower level. **(B)** Wenckebach conduction, 4:3 and 6:5, in the upper level and 2:1 conduction below. **(C)** Wenckebach conduction in both levels. (**A** adapted from Halpern MS, Nau GJ, Levi RJ et al: Wenckebach periods of alternate beats: Clinical and experimental observations. Circulation 48: 42, 1973; **B** and **C** adapted from Kosowsky B, Latif P, Radoff AM: Multilevel atrioventricular block. Circulation 54: 918, 1976. By permission of the American Heart Association, Inc.)

The ladder diagram illustrates two levels of AV block with 2:1 conduction in the upper level and Wenckebach with 3:2 conduction in the lower level.

Figure 14-46 shows atrial flutter with a variable ventricular response. Note that the QRS complexes occur in groups, the FR interval of alternate beats is gradually prolonged, and the cycle ends with three blocked atrial impulses. These are all signs of multilevel block with 2:1 conduction in the upper level and Wenckebach conduction in the lower level. Note also that the flutter waves occur in groups of two with alternately longer and shorter F-F intervals, a sign of Wenckebach conduction. The ladder diagram illustrates Wenckebach exit block from the flutter focus in the atrium, leading to the grouping of flutter waves. There are two levels of block in the AV node, with 2:1 conduction in the upper level and Wenckebach with 5:4 conduction in the lower level, causing the grouping of QRS complexes.

The mechanism of multilevel AV block is not known but is thought to involve concealed conduction of impulses to various depths in the AV node or His-Purkinje system, affecting the conduction of subsequent impulses through those regions.[50] This type of block has been shown to be a common response to rapid atrial pacing, atrial tachycardia or flutter, and administration of digitalis for treatment of atrial flutter.[16,17,50] It has also been shown to be a sign of advanced digitalis toxicity[16] and to occur in patients with primary disease of the conduction system or with inferior MI.[16,79] The clinical significance of multilevel AV block appears to depend on whether the sites of block are in the AV node, considered to be common and benign, or below the AV node in the His-Purkinje system, thought to be more dangerous; or whether the block is tachycardia dependent, thus benign, or associated with MI and possibly more dangerous.[16,17,50,79]

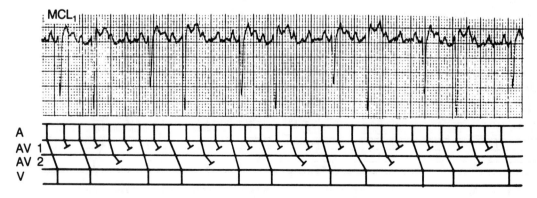

FIGURE 14-45 Atrial flutter and multilevel AV block with 2:1 conduction in the upper level and 3:2 Wenckebach conduction in the lower level. Note group beating and progressive increase in alternate FR intervals.

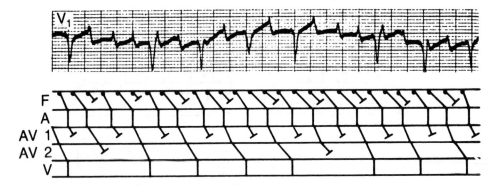

FIGURE 14-46 Atrial flutter with 3 : 2 Wenckebach exit block out of the flutter focus. In the atrioventricular junction, there are two levels of block: 2 : 1 conduction in the upper level and 5 : 4 Wenckebach conduction in the lower level. (Adapted from Marriott HJL, Conover M: Advanced Concepts in Arrhythmias, 2nd ed, p 344. St. Louis, CV Mosby, 1989.)

Atrioventricular Dissociation

Atrioventricular dissociation means that the atria and ventricles are under the control of separate pacemakers and are beating independently of each other. Usually the atria are controlled by the sinus node, but they can also be under the control of an atrial focus, as in atrial tachycardia, flutter, or fibrillation. The ventricles can be under the control of a junctional pacemaker or a ventricular pacemaker. AV dissociation is not a primary arrhythmia but is always secondary to some other disturbance that results in dissociation. Complete AV dissociation means that the atria and ventricles are always controlled by separate pacemakers and that the two different pacemakers never conduct into the other chamber to "capture" it. Incomplete dissociation occurs when one chamber is occasionally depolarized by the other chamber's pacemaker.

Atrioventricular dissociation can be secondary to (1) slowing of the primary pacemaker (sinus node), (2) acceleration of a subsidiary pacemaker (AV junction or ventricle), (3) AV block, or (4) interference, or can result from a combination of these causes.[20,59,109]

If the rate of the sinus node slows below the rate of a subsidiary pacemaker in the AV junction or in the ventricles, the subsidiary pacemaker assumes control of the ventricles while the atria are still under the control of the sinus node. This dissociation, sometimes called *dissociation by default,* lasts until a sinus impulse occurs at a time when it can be conducted into the ventricles and regain control of them or until it speeds up enough to override the subsidiary pacemaker (Fig. 14-47).

Atrioventricular dissociation can result from the acceleration of a subsidiary pacemaker, either junctional or ventricular, that fires faster than the sinus node and thus assumes control of the ventricles (*dissociation by usurpation*). Dissociation lasts until the rate of the subsidiary pacemaker slows below the rate of the sinus node or the sinus accelerates to a rate faster than that of the subsidiary pacemaker (Fig. 14-48). VT is an example of AV dissociation due to acceleration of a ventricular pacemaker; VT can be diagnosed by demonstrating independently occurring P waves, thus proving AV dissociation (see Fig. 14-22).

Complete AV block is a form of AV dissociation because none of the atrial impulses conducts to the ventricles and the atria and ventricles are under the control of separate pacemakers (Fig. 14-49). Remember: every complete AV block is AV dissociation, but not every AV dissociation is complete AV block!

Atrioventricular dissociation can result when an ectopic impulse, usually junctional or ventricular, makes the AV node refractory to the next sinus impulse, interfering with the conduction of the sinus impulse and allowing another pacemaker to control the ventricles (Fig. 14-50). Anything that causes a pause in the rhythm, like a premature beat, a blocked P wave, or sudden termination of a tachycardia can allow the escape of a subsidiary pacemaker and result in AV dissociation.

The term *isorhythmic dissociation* refers to AV dissociation with the atrial focus and the focus that controls the ventricles firing at almost identical rates. It is characterized by P waves that move into and out of the QRS complex, always staying close on either side or in the middle of the QRS (Fig. 14-51).

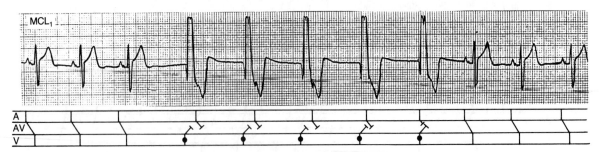

FIGURE 14-47 Atrioventricular (AV) dissociation due to slowing of the primary pacemaker. Sinus arrhythmia is present; the sinus rate slows after the third beat, allowing a ventricular escape pacemaker to take control of the ventricles at a rate of 60 beats/min. AV dissociation lasts until the rate of the sinus node becomes faster than the rate of the ventricular pacemaker.

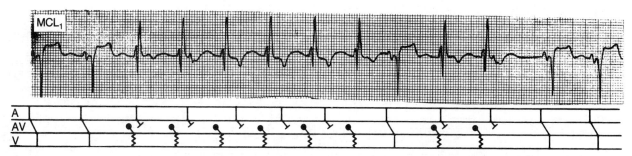

FIGURE 14-48 Atrioventricular dissociation due to acceleration of a subsidiary pacemaker. An accelerated junctional pacemaker assumes control of the ventricles and conducts aberrantly (right bundle-branch block) at a rate of 88 beats/min. Sinus arrhythmia is present at a rate in the 70s. Vertical wavy line indicates aberrant conduction.

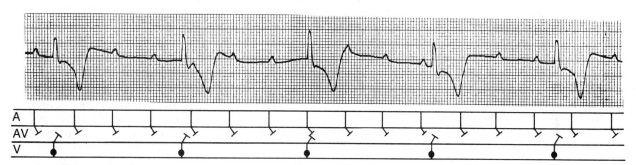

FIGURE 14-49 Atrioventricular (AV) dissociation due to complete AV block. Sinus tachycardia at a rate of 115 beats/min with third-degree AV block and a ventricular pacemaker controlling the ventricles at a rate of 34 beats/min. (From Jacobson C: Interpretation of complex arrhythmias. In Woods SL (ed): Cardiovascular Critical Care Nursing, p 216. New York, Churchill Livingstone, 1983. By permission.)

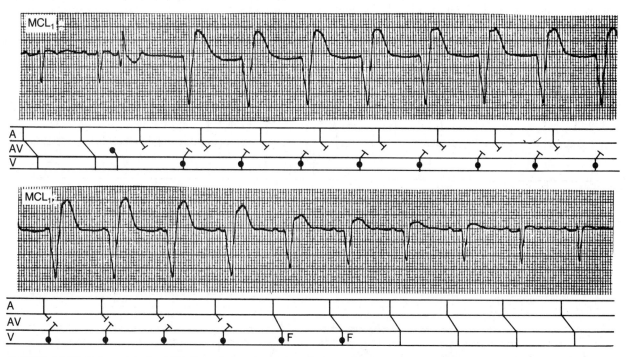

FIGURE 14-50 Atrioventricular (AV) dissociation due to interference. Strips are continuous. Sinus rhythm is present at a rate of 68 beats/min. The third beat in the top strip is a premature junctional beat that interferes with conduction of the next sinus impulse, which in turn is not conducted through the AV node. The resulting pause allows a ventricular rhythm to emerge at a rate of 65 beats/min. The bottom strip shows the slightly faster sinus P waves emerging in front of the QRS until ventricular capture occurs in the seventh beat. F, fusion beats. (From Jacobson C: Interpretation of complex arrhythmias. In Woods SL (ed): Cardiovascular Critical Care Nursing. New York, Churchill Livingstone, 1983. By permission.)

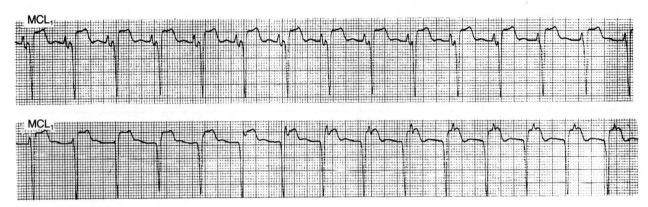

FIGURE 14-51 Isorhythmic dissociation. There is dissociation between a sinus rhythm and a junctional rhythm, both at a rate of approximately 88 beats/min. P waves disappear into the QRS complex toward the end of the top strip and emerge on the other side of the QRS in the bottom strip, always staying close to the QRS or in the middle of it.

Parasystole

Parasystole is an ectopic focus that fires regularly and independently of the dominant cardiac rhythm and is protected from being depolarized by impulses from the dominant pacemaker. Parasystole can occur in the atria, AV junction, or ventricles, but it occurs most often in the ventricles, where it is most easily recognized. The parasystolic focus is an automatic focus that spontaneously depolarizes but is surrounded by tissue with low excitability, causing decremental conduction of impulses coming from the dominant pacemaker and entrance block of outside stimuli. This same tissue may prevent conduction of the parasystolic impulse into surrounding tissue, causing exit block from the parasystolic focus.[20,49,59]

Parasystole is diagnosed from the ECG by the following criteria: (1) marked variation in coupling intervals of ectopic beats; (2) presence of interectopic intervals (the distance from one ectopic beat to the next) that are multiples of a common denominator; and (3) the presence of fusion beats resulting from the simultaneous depolarization of a chamber, either atria or ventricles, by the dominant rhythm and the parasystolic focus. A simple ventricular parasystole appears on the ECG as PVCs occurring at a regular rate, or a multiple of the rate, whenever the ventricular focus fires at a time when the ventricle is not refractory as a result of depolarization by the dominant pacemaker (Fig. 14-52). When the parasystolic focus fires during the refractory period of the ventricle, its impulse is unable to excite surrounding refractory tissue and it cannot be seen on the ECG. Coupling intervals vary because the parasystolic focus is an independently firing automatic focus that is not related to the sinus rhythm and therefore does not depend on the sinus rhythm for its existence. PVCs due to reentry have

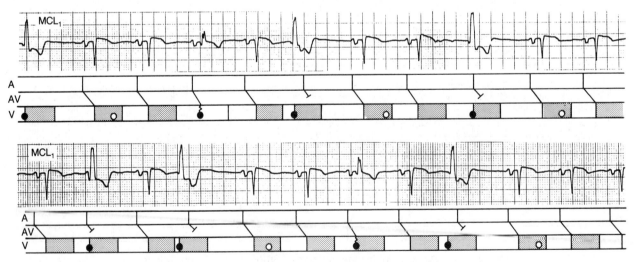

FIGURE 14-52 Ventricular parasystole. Sinus arrhythmia is present at a rate in the 60s with multiple premature ventricular complexes. Note the following characteristics of ventricular parasystole: (1) marked variation in coupling intervals, (2) presence of fusion beats, and (3) interectopic intervals that are a multiple of the basic parasystolic rate of 38 beats/min. The ladder diagram illustrates the parasystolic focus firing regularly at a rate of 38 beats/min. Solid circles indicate the parasystolic focus that is seen on the electrocardiogram (ECG); open circles indicate the focus firing but not seen on the ECG; the shaded area represents ventricular refractory period.

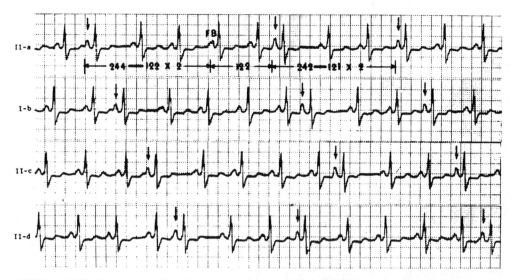

FIGURE 14-53 Sinus rhythm at a rate of 75 beats/min with atrial parasystole at a rate of 50 beats/min. Strips are continuous. *Arrows* indicate the atrial parasystolic P waves. Note an atrial fusion beat (FB). The numbers represent hundredths of a second. (From Chung EK: Electrocardiography: Practical Applications With Vectorial Principles, 2nd ed, p 552. Hagerstown, MD, Harper & Row, 1980.)

fixed coupling intervals because they depend on the preceding impulse for their existence. Ventricular fusion beats occur whenever the parasystolic focus fires at the same time that the dominant focus enters the ventricles and begins to depolarize them. Atrial or junctional parasystole behaves the same way, with coupling intervals measured from normal P wave to ectopic P wave and fusion beats occurring in the atria (Fig. 14-53).

A parasystolic focus usually fires at rates between 38 to 60 beats/min but has been reported to occur at rates up to 300 beats/min. The focus may fire regularly, exhibiting regular interectopic intervals or intervals that are exact multiples of its basic interval (a variation of 0.10 second is allowed before intervals are considered irregular); it may fire irregularly, resulting in irregular interectopic intervals. Several factors responsible for variance in parasystolic firing rate have been identified:[20,49,56,68]

- ◆ Intermittent firing of the parasystolic focus.
- ◆ Change in the firing rate of the parasystolic focus secondary to ischemia, drug effects, electrolyte imbalances, autonomic influences, or any factor known to influence phase 4 depolarization of automatic cells.
- ◆ Varying degrees of exit block from the parasystolic focus. Block can be type I (Wenckebach exit block), with impulses taking progressively longer to exit from the parasystolic focus into surrounding tissue, or type II, with sudden absence of an impulse where it would otherwise be expected. Exit block from a parasystolic focus is presumed to be present whenever the focus fires but fails to appear on the ECG when the refractory period of the ventricles is over.
- ◆ Varying degrees of entrance block of the dominant impulse into the parasystolic focus. Although entrance block is the protective mechanism that

allows the parasystolic focus to continue firing regularly without interference from the dominant pacemaker, a temporary loss of this protection can occur, and the dominant impulses can enter and reset the parasystolic focus.

Although simple parasystole can be recognized by the usual ECG criteria, more complicated forms of parasystole can occur when entrance or exit block is present, fixed coupling occurs, or more than one parasystolic focus fires at the same time.

Concealed Conduction

Concealed conduction is conduction of an impulse into a part of the conduction system but not completely through it, causing refractoriness that affects conduction or formation of subsequent impulses. Concealed conduction can occur in an anterograde direction from supraventricular impulses into the AV junction or His-Purkinje system, or in a retrograde direction from the ventricles backward into the AV junction. Because the original impulse never reaches its final destination, there is no evidence on the ECG that concealed conduction has occurred other than its influence on the conduction or formation of subsequent impulses.

Three types of concealed conduction are discussed next: (1) concealed conduction affecting subsequent impulse conduction, (2) concealed conduction affecting subsequent impulse formation, and (3) concealed impulse formation affecting subsequent impulse conduction.[20,96]

CONCEALED CONDUCTION AFFECTING SUBSEQUENT IMPULSE CONDUCTION

The most common example of concealed conduction occurs in atrial fibrillation, when the AV node is bombarded with

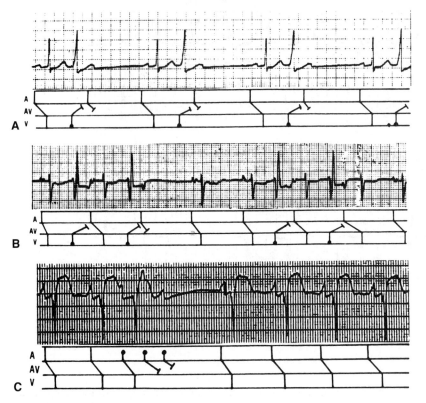

FIGURE 14-54 Concealed conduction affecting conduction of subsequent impulses. **(A)** Concealed conduction of premature ventricular complexes (PVCs) into the atrioventricular (AV) node, causing block of subsequent P waves. **(B)** Concealed conduction of PVCs into the AV node, causing varying degrees of conduction delay of subsequent sinus beats with a pseudo-Wenckebach pattern. **(C)** Sinus rhythm with three premature atrial complexes (PACs). The first is conducted with delay; the second is not conducted completely through to the ventricles but is conducted far enough into the AV node to cause complete block of the third PAC. (From Jacobson C: Interpretation of complex arrhythmias. In Woods SL (ed): Cardiovascular Critical Care Nursing, p 207. New York Churchill Livingstone, 1983. By permission.)

hundreds of impulses each minute, most of which are blocked in the AV node. Many of these impulses are conducted to various depths in the AV node, leaving it refractory to following impulses and causing the characteristic irregular ventricular response in atrial fibrillation. Because the impulses that incompletely penetrate the AV node never reach the ventricles, there is no evidence on the ECG that they conducted at all, other than their effect on preventing conduction of following impulses.

Another common example of concealed conduction is illustrated in Figure 14-54. Figure 14-54*A* shows sinus tachycardia with ventricular bigeminy. The sinus beat that follows each PVC is not conducted, presumably because of concealed conduction of the PVC backward into the AV node, causing it to be refractory and preventing the conduction of the next sinus impulse. Figure 14-54*B* shows sinus rhythm with frequent PVCs that conduct retrograde into the AV node, causing varying degrees of refractoriness that impede conduction of following sinus beats. Some

PVCs are followed by sinus beats with prolonged PR intervals and others by beats that are completely blocked; both situations are due to retrograde concealed conduction of the ventricular impulse into the AV node.

Figure 14-54*C* shows sinus rhythm with three PACs. The first PAC conducts with delay; the second is not conducted completely into the ventricle but is conducted far enough into the AV node to prevent the conduction of the third PAC.

CONCEALED CONDUCTION AFFECTING SUBSEQUENT IMPULSE FORMATION

In the presence of AV dissociation between a sinus pacemaker and an AV junctional pacemaker controlling the ventricles, the sinus impulse may occasionally conduct far enough into the AV junction to reset the junctional pacemaker and prevent the formation of the next expected junctional impulse. Figure 14-55 shows AV dissociation

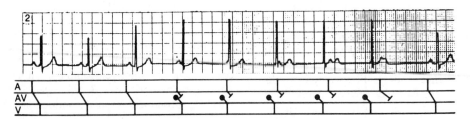

FIGURE 14-55 Concealed conduction affecting subsequent impulse formation. Atrioventricular (AV) dissociation between a junctional rhythm at a rate of 64 beats/min and a slightly slower sinus rhythm. The sinus P wave that follows the eighth QRS complex conducts far enough into the AV node to depolarize the junctional focus before it is due to fire again, causing the pause after the eighth beat. (Adapted from Marriott HJL, Conover M: Advanced Concepts in Arrhythmias, 2nd ed, p 321. St. Louis, CV Mosby, 1989.)

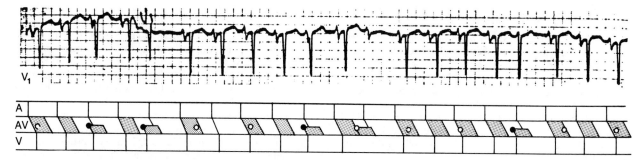

FIGURE 14-56 Concealed impulse formation affecting subsequent conduction. Sinus rhythm is present at a rate of 84 beats/min; an atrioventricular (AV) junctional parasystolic focus is firing at a rate of 48 beats/min. Concealed formation of the junctional focus after the 11th beat prevents conduction of the next sinus impulse, simulating type II second-degree AV block. Solid circles indicate the junctional parasystolic focus seen on the electrocardiogram (ECG); open circles indicate the focus firing but not seen on the ECG; the shaded area indicates the refractory period in the AV junction. (Adapted from Watanabe Y: Terminology and electrophysiologic concepts in cardiac arrhythmias: II. Concealed conduction. Pacing Clin Electrophysiol 1: 354, 1978.)

between a junctional rhythm at a rate of 64 beats/min and a slightly slower sinus rhythm. The pause that occurs near the end of the strip is due to concealed conduction of the sinus impulse into the AV junctional focus, preventing the formation of the next expected junctional beat.

CONCEALED IMPULSE FORMATION AFFECTING SUBSEQUENT IMPULSE CONDUCTION

If an impulse is formed in the AV junction but is blocked in both the anterograde and retrograde directions, there is no evidence on the ECG that the impulse ever existed unless it interferes with conduction of a following impulse. Such concealed junctional beats can imitate type I and II AV block, and their recognition may prevent misdiagnosis of a nonexistent conduction disturbance.[20,96] Figure 14-56 illustrates sinus rhythm with junctional parasystole at a rate of approximately 50 beats/min. The sinus impulse that follows beat 11 is blocked, simulating type II second-degree AV block, but this can be explained by concealed formation of the junctional parasystolic focus that fails to reach the ventricles but causes refractoriness in the AV node, preventing conduction of the next sinus impulse.

REFERENCES

1. Abildskov JA, Green LS: Long QT syndromes. In Fisch C, Surawicz B (eds): Cardiac Electrophysiology and Arrhythmias, pp 223–230. New York, Elsevier, 1991
2. Akhtar M: Atrioventricular nodal reentrant tachycardia. Med Clin North Am 68: 819, 1984
3. Akhtar M, Tchou PJ, Jazayeri M: Mechanisms of clinical tachycardias. Am J Cardiol 61: 9A–91A, 1988
4. Amat Y, Leon F, Chuquimia R et al: Alternating Wenckebach periodicity: A common electrophysiologic response. Am J Cardiol 36: 757, 1975
5. Andries E, Brugada P, Brugada J et al: A practical approach to the diagnosis of a tachycardia with a wide QRS complex. In Podrid PJ, Kowey PR (eds): Cardiac Arrhythmia: Mechanisms, Diagnosis, and Management, pp 1022–1038. Baltimore, Williams & Wilkins, 1995
6. Antzelevitch C, Sicouri S: Clinical relevance of cardiac arrhythmias generated by afterdepolarizations. J Am Coll Cardiol 23: 259–277, 1994
7. Antzelevitch C, Sicouri S, Lukas A et al: Clinical implications of electrical heterogeneity in the heart: The electrophysiology and pharmacology of epicardial, M, and endocardial cells. In Podrid PJ, Kowey PR (eds): Cardiac Arrhythmia: Mechanisms, Diagnosis, and Management, pp 88–107. Baltimore, Williams & Wilkins, 1995
8. Banerji S, Kayser SR: Antiarrhythmic drug therapy: Part IV. Ventricular arrhythmias. Prog Cardiovasc Nurs 12: 32–36, 1997
9. Bar FW, Brugada P, Willem RM et al: Differential diagnosis of tachycardia with narrow QRS complex (shorter than 0.12 second). Am J Cardiol 54: 555, 1984
10. Bigger TJ: Definition of benign versus malignant ventricular arrhythmias: Targets for treatment. Am J Cardiol 52: 47C–54C, 1983
11. Birnbaum Y, Sclarovsky S, Ronen B et al: Polymorphous ventricular tachycardia early after acute myocardial infarction. Am J Cardiol 71: 745, 1993
12. Brugada P, Brugada J, Mont L et al: A new approach to the differential diagnosis of a regular tachycardia with a wide QRS complex. Circulation 83: 1649–1659, 1991
13. Cabeen WR, Roberts NK, Child JS: Recognition of Wenckebach phenomenon. West J Med 129: 521, 1978
14. Cardiac Arrhythmia Suppression Trial Investigators: Preliminary report: Effect of encainide and flecainide on mortality in a randomized trial of arrhythmia suppression after myocardial infarction. N Engl J Med 321: 406–411, 1989
15. Carleton RA: Wenckebach (type I) behavior of ventricular reentry. Chest 71: 740, 1977
16. Castellanos A, Sung RJ, Aldrich JL et al: Electrocardiographic manifestations and clinical significance of atrioventricular nodal alternating Wenckebach periods. Chest 73: 69, 1978
17. Castellanos A, Sung RJ, Aldrich JL et al: Alternating Wenckebach periods occurring in the atria, His-Purkinje system, ventricles and Kent bundle. Am J Cardiol 40: 853, 1977
18. Chung EK: Electrocardiography: Practical Applications With Vectorial Principles, 2nd ed. Hagerstown, MD, Harper & Row, 1980
19. Chung EK: Tachyarrhythmias related to Wolff-Parkinson-White syndrome. Heart Lung 6: 262, 1977

20. Conover MB: Understanding Electrocardiography, 7th ed. St Louis, CV Mosby, 1996

21. Cranefield PF, Aronson RS: Torsade de pointes and other pause-induced ventricular tachycardias: The short-long-short sequence and early afterdepolarizations. Pacing Clin Electrophysiol 11: 670, 1988

22. Cummins RO (ed): Advanced Cardiac Life Support. American Heart Association, Dallas TX, 1997

23. Drew BJ, Scheinman MM: Value of electrocardiographic leads MCL$_1$, MCL$_6$ and other selected leads in the diagnosis of wide QRS complex tachycardia. J Am Coll Cardiol 18: 1025, 1991

24. Drew BJ, Scheinman M, Dracup K: MCL1 and MCL6 compared to V1 and V6 in distinguishing aberrant supraventricular from ventricular ectopic beats. Pacing Clin Electrophysiol 14: 1375, 1991

25. Drouin E, Charpentier F, Gauthier C et al: Evidence for the presence of M cells in the human ventricle. (Abstract) Pacing Clin Electrophysiol 16(Suppl II): 876, 1993

26. El-Sherif N, Aranda J, Befeler B et al: Atypical Wenckebach periodicity simulating Mobitz II AV block. Br Heart J 40: 1376, 1978

27. El-Sherif N, Zeiler RH, Craelius W et al: QTU prolongation and polymorphic tachyarrhythmias due to bradycardia-dependent early afterdepolarizations: Afterdepolarizations and ventricular arrhythmias. Circ Res 63(2), 286–305, 1988

28. El-Sherif N: Polymorphic ventricular tachycardia. In Podrid PJ, Kowey PR (eds): Cardiac Arrhythmia: Mechanisms, Diagnosis, and Management, pp 936–950. Baltimore, Williams & Wilkins, 1995

29. Falk RH: Atrial fibrillation. In Podrid PJ, Kowey PR (eds): Cardiac Arrhythmia: Mechanisms, Diagnosis, and Management, pp 803–827. Baltimore, Williams & Wilkins, 1995

30. Fisch C: Differential diagnosis of wide QRS tachycardia. In Fisch C, Surawicz B (eds): Cardiac Electrophysiology and Arrhythmias, pp 199–209. New York, Elsevier, 1991.

31. Fisch C: Electrocardiography. In Braunwald E (ed): Heart Disease, 5th ed., Vol. I, pp 108–152. Philadelphia, WB Saunders, 1997

32. Fisch C: Electrocardiogram and mechanisms of arrhythmias. In Podrid PJ, Kowey PR (eds): Cardiac Arrhythmia: Mechanisms, Diagnosis, and Management, pp 211–218. Baltimore, Williams & Wilkins, 1995

33. Fogel RI, Prystowsky EN: Atrioventricular nodal reentry. In Podrid PJ, Kowey PR (eds): Cardiac Arrhythmia: Mechanisms, Diagnosis, and Management, pp 828–846. Baltimore, Williams & Wilkins, 1995

34. Gadsby DC, Karagueuzian HS, Wit AL: Normal and abnormal electrical activity in cardiac cells. In Mandel WJ (ed): Cardiac Arrhythmias: Their Mechanisms, Diagnosis, and Management, 3rd ed., pp 55–82. Philadelphia, JB Lippincott, 1995

35. Gallagher JJ, Pritchett EL, Sealy WC et al: The preexcitation syndromes. Prog Cardiovasc Dis 20: 279, 1978

36. Gilmour R: Enhanced automaticity. In Podrid PJ, Kowey PR (eds): Cardiac Arrhythmia Mechanisms Diagnosis, and Management, pp 78–87. Baltimore, Williams & Wilkins, 1995.

37. Goldberger JJ, Kadish AH: Atrial premature depolarizations, junctional premature depolarizations, multifocal atrial tachycardia, and atrial tachycardia. In Podrid PJ, Kowey PR (eds): Cardiac Arrhythmia: Mechanisms, Diagnosis, and Management, pp 768–789. Baltimore, Williams & Wilkins, 1995

38. Haissaguerre M, Fischer FM, Clementy J: Role of catheter ablation for treatment of supraventricular tachyarrhythmias. In Mandel WJ (ed): Cardiac Arrhythmias: Their Mechanisms, Diagnosis, and Management, 3rd ed. Philadelphia, JB Lippincott, 1995.

39. Halpern MS, Nau GJ, Levi RJ et al: Wenckebach periods of alternate beats: Clinical and experimental observations. Circulation 48: 41, 1973

40. Jackman WM, Clark M, Friday KJ et al: Ventricular tachyarrhythmias in the long QT syndromes. Med Clin North Am 68: 1079, 1984

41. Jackman WM, Szabo B, Friday KJ et al: Ventricular tachyarrhythmias related to early afterdepolarizations and triggered firing: Relationship to QT interval prolongation and potential therapeutic role of calcium channel blocking agents. J Cardiovasc Electrophysiol 1: 170–195, 1990

42. Jordan JL, Mandel WJ: Disorders of sinus function. In Mandel WJ (ed): Cardiac Arrhythmias: Their Mechanisms, Diagnosis, and Management, 3rd ed., pp 245–295. Philadelphia, JB Lippincott, 1995

43. Josephson ME, Wellens HJJ: Differential diagnosis of supraventricular tachycardia. Cardiol Clin 8: 411, 1990

44. Kay NG, Pressley JC, Packer DL et al: Value of the 12-lead electrocardiogram in discriminating atrioventricular nodal reciprocating tachycardia from circus movement atrioventricular tachycardia utilizing a retrograde accessory pathway. Am J Cardiol 59: 296, 1987

45. Keren A, Tzivoni D: Magnesium therapy in ventricular arrhythmias. Pacing Clin Electrophysiol 13: 937, 1990

46. Khan MM, Logan KR, McComb JM et al: Management of recurrent ventricular tachyarrhythmias associated with Q-T prolongation. Am J Cardiol 47: 1301, 1981

47. Kim HS, Chung EK: Torsade de pointes: Polymorphous ventricular tachycardia. Heart Lung 12: 269, 1983

48. Kindwall KE, Brown J, Josephson ME: Electrocardiographic criteria for ventricular tachycardia in wide complex left bundle branch block morphology tachycardia. Am J Cardiol 61: 1279, 1988

49. Kinoshita S: Mechanisms of ventricular parasystole. Circulation 58: 715, 1978

50. Kosowsky BD, Latif P, Radoff AM: Multilevel atrioventricular block. Circulation 54: 914, 1976

51. Krikler DM, Parelman M, Rowland E et al: Ventricular tachycardia and ventricular fibrillation. In Mandel WJ (ed): Cardiac Arrhythmias: Their Mechanisms, Diagnosis, and Management, 3rd ed., pp 649–691. Philadelphia, JB Lippincott, 1995

52. Kuck K, Schluter M, Cappato R: Catheter ablation for supraventricular tachycardia. In Podrid PJ, Kowey PR (eds): Cardiac Arrhythmia: Mechanisms, Diagnosis, and Management, pp 666–678. Baltimore, Williams & Wilkins, 1995

53. Langendorf R, Pick A, Winternitz M: Mechanisms of intermittent ventricular bigeminy: I. Appearance of ectopic beats dependent upon length of the ventricular cycle, the "rule of bigeminy." Circulation 11: 422, 1955

54. Lazarra R: From first class to third class: Recent upheaval in antiarrhythmic therapy—lessons from clinical trials. Am J Cardiol 78(Suppl 4A): 28–33, 1996

55. Lesh MD, Van Hare GF, Epstein LM et al: Radiofrequency catheter ablation of atrial arrhythmias: Results and mechanisms. Circulation 89: 1074, 1994

56. Lightfoot PR: Parasystole simulating ventricular bigeminy with Wenckebach type coupling prolongation. J Electrocardiol 11: 385, 1978

57. Mandel WJ: Sustained monomorphic ventricular tachycardia. In Podrid PJ, Kowey PR (eds): Cardiac Arrhythmia: Mechanisms, Diagnosis, and Management, pp 919–935. Baltimore, Williams & Wilkins, 1995

58. Marinchak RA, Rials SJ: Tachycardias in Wolff-Parkinson-White syndrome including atrioventricular reciprocating tachycardia, atrial flutter, and atrial fibrillation. In Podrid PJ, Kowey PR (eds): Cardiac Arrhythmia: Mechanisms, Diagnosis, and Management, pp 847–874. Baltimore, Williams & Wilkins, 1995

59. Marriott HJL: Practical Electrocardiography, 8th ed. Baltimore, Williams & Wilkins, 1988

60. Marriott HJL, Conover M: Advanced Concepts in Arrhythmias, 3rd ed. St. Louis, CV Mosby, 1998

61. Marriott HJL, Sandler A: Criteria, old and new for differentiating between ectopic ventricular beats and aberrant ventricular conduction in the presence of atrial fibrillation. Prog Cardiovasc Dis 9: 18, 1966

62. McGovern G, Garan H, Ruskin JN: Precipitation of cardiac arrest by verapamil in patients with Wolff-Parkinson-White syndrome. Ann Intern Med 104: 791, 1986

63. Mirvis DM, Bandura JP, Brody DA: Wenckebach-type exit block from an ectopic focus as a cause of variable coupling. J Electrocardiol 9: 365, 1976

64. Morady F, Scheinman MM: Paroxysmal supraventricular tachycardia: Part I. Diagnosis. Modern Concepts in Cardiovascular Disease 51: 107, 1982

65. Moss AJ, Robinson J: Clinical features of the idiopathic long QT syndrome. Circulation 85(Suppl I):I-140, 1992

66. Norris JF, Zipes DP,: Electrophysiology of the slow channel. In Podrid PJ, Kowey PR (eds): Cardiac Arrhythmia: Mechanisms, Diagnosis, and Management, pp 33–40. Baltimore, Williams & Wilkins, 1995

67. Opie LH: Drugs for the Heart, 4th ed. Philadelphia, WB Saunders, 1995

68. Pick A, Langendorf R: Parasystole and its variants. Med Clin North Am 60: 125, 1976

69. Priori SG, Diehi L, Schwartz PJ: Torsade de pointes. In Podrid PJ, Kowey PR (eds): Cardiac Arrhythmia: Mechanisms, Diagnosis, and Management, pp 957–963. Baltimore, Williams & Wilkins, 1995.

70. Rosen MR: Mechanisms for arrhythmias. Am J Cardiol 61: 2A–8A, 1988

71. Rosen MR: Fast response action potential. In Podrid PJ, Kowey PR (eds): Cardiac Arrhythmia: Mechanisms, Diagnosis, and Management, pp 41–47. Baltimore, Williams & Wilkins, 1995

72. Rosenbaum MB, Nau GJ, Levi RJ et al: Wenckebach periods in the bundle branches. Circulation 40: 79, 1969

73. Rubin AM, Morganroth J, Kowey PB: Ventricular premature depolarizations. In Podrid PJ, Kowey PR (eds): Cardiac Arrhythmia: Mechanisms, Diagnosis, and Management, pp 891–906. Baltimore, Williams & Wilkins, 1995

74. Rusterholz AP, Marriott HJL: How long can the P-R interval be? Am J Noninvasive Cardiol 8: 11–13, 1994

75. Samuels F, Hessen SE, Dreifus LS: Reentry and development of arrhythmias: Preclinical and clinical data. In Podrid PJ, Kowey PR (eds): Cardiac Arrhythmia: Mechanisms, Diagnosis, and Management, pp 60–69. Baltimore, Williams & Wilkins, 1995

76. Sandler IA, Marriott HJL: The differential morphology of anomalous ventricular complexes of RBBB-type in lead V$_1$: Ventricular ectopy versus aberration. Circulation 31: 551, 1965

77. Scheinman M: Catheter ablation for cardiac arrhythmias: Personnel and facilities. Pacing Clin Electrophysiol 15: 715, 1992

78. Scheinman MM: The role of catheter ablation in the management of patients with ventricular tachycardia. In Podrid PJ, Kowey PR (eds): Cardiac Arrhythmia: Mechanisms, Diagnosis, and Management, pp 660–666. Baltimore, Williams & Wilkins, 1995

79. Sclarovsky S, Lervin R, Strasberg B et al: Dissociation of the atrioventricular node in acute inferior wall infarction: Transverse dissociation (alternate Wenckebach periods). Chest 73: 634, 1978

80. Sclarovsky S, Strasberg B, Agmon J: Coexistent Wenckebach phenomenon in the distal branches of the specialized conduction system. Chest 73: 534, 1978

81. Sclarovsky S, Strasberg B, Lewin RF et al: Polymorphous ventricular tachycardia: Clinical features and treatment. Am J Cardiol 44: 339, 1979

82. Shamroth L, Dove E: The Wenckebach phenomenon in sinoatrial block. Br Heart J 28: 350, 1966

83. Shenasa H, Curry P, Shenasa M: Atrial arrhythmias: Clinical concepts and advances in mechanism and management. In Mandel WJ (ed): Cardiac Arrhythmias: Their Mechanisms, Diagnosis, and Management, 3rd ed., pp 327–367. Philadelphia, JB Lippincott, 1995

84. Singer DH, Cohen HC: Aberrancy: electrophysiologic mechanisms and electrocardiographic correlates. In Mandel WJ (ed): Cardiac Arrhythmias: Their Mechanisms, Diagnosis, and Management, 3rd ed., pp 461–511. Philadelphia, JB Lippincott, 1995

85. Sicouri S, Antzelevitch C: A subpopulation of cells with unique electrophysiological properties in the deep subepicardium of the canine ventricle: The M cell. Circ Res 68(6): 1729–1741, 1991

86. Sicouri S, Antzelevitch C: Drug-induced afterdepolarizations and triggered activity occur in a discrete subpopulation of ventricular muscle cell (M cells) in the canine heart: Quinidine and digitalis. J Cardiovasc Electrophysiol 4: 48, 1993.

87. Singh BN: The coming of age of the class III antiarrhythmic principle: Retrospective and future trends. Am J Cardiol 78(Suppl 4A): 17–27, 1996

88. Smith WM, Gallagher JJ: "Les torsades de pointes": An unusual ventricular arrhythmia. Ann Intern Med 93: 578, 1980

89. Stewart RB, Bardy GH, Greene HL: Wide complex tachycardia: Misdiagnosis and outcome after emergent therapy. Ann Intern Med 104: 766, 1986

90. Tzivoni D, Banai S, Schuger C et al: Treatment of torsades de pointes with magnesium sulfate. Circulation 77: 392, 1988

91. Tzivoni D, Keren A, Stern S: Torsades de pointes versus polymorphous ventricular tachycardia. Am J Cardiol 52: 639, 1983

92. Waldo AL, Wit AL: Mechanism of cardiac arrhythmias and conduction disturbances. In Schlant RC, Alexander RW (eds): Hurst's The Heart, 8th ed., pp 659–704. New York, McGraw-Hill, 1994

93. Waldo AL, Wit AL: Mechanisms of cardiac arrhythmias. Lancet 341: 1989, 1993

94. Waldo AL: Atrial flutter. In Podrid PJ, Kowey PR (eds): Cardiac Arrhythmia: Mechanisms, Diagnosis, and Management, pp 790–802. Baltimore, Williams & Wilkins, 1995

95. Waldo AL, Henthorn RW, Plumb VJ: Atrial flutter: Recent observations in man. In Josephson ME, Wellens HJJ (eds): Tachycardias: Mechanisms, Diagnosis, Treatment, pp 113–135. Philadelphia, Lea & Febiger, 1984

96. Watanabe Y: Terminology and electrophysiologic concepts in cardiac arrhythmias: II. Concealed conduction. Pacing Clin Electrophysiol 1: 345, 1978

97. Watanabe Y, Dreifus LS, Mazgalev T: Atrioventricular block: Basic concepts. In Mandel WJ (ed): Cardiac Arrhythmias: Their Mechanisms, Diagnosis, and Management, 3rd ed., pp 417–434 Philadelphia, JB Lippincott, 1995

98. Wellens HJJ: Differential diagnosis of narrow QRS tachycardia. In Fisch C, Surawicz B (eds): Cardiac Electrophysiology and Arrhythmias, pp 164–175. New York, Elsevier, 1991

99. Wellens HJJ, Conover M: The ECG in Emergency Decision Making. Philadelphia, WB Saunders, 1991

100. Wellens HJ, Frits WH, Lie KI: The value of the electrocardiogram in the differential diagnosis of a tachycardia with a widened QRS complex. Am J Med 64: 27, 1978

101. Wellens HJJ, Smeets J, Gorgels A et al: Wolff-Parkinson-White syndrome. In Mandel WJ (ed): Cardiac Arrhythmias: Their Mechanisms, Diagnosis, and Management, 3rd ed, pp 389–413. Philadelphia, JB Lippincott, 1995

102. Wit AL, Rosen MR: Pathophysiologic mechanisms of cardiac arrhythmias. Am Heart J 106: 798, 1983

103. Wit AL, Rosen MR: Cellular electrophysiology of cardiac arrhythmias: Part II. Arrhythmias caused by abnormal impulse conduction. Modern Concepts in Cardiovascular Disease 50: 7, 1981

104. Wit AL, Rosen MR: Cellular electrophysiology of cardiac arrhythmias: Part I: Arrhythmias caused by abnormal impulse generation. Modern Concepts in Cardiovascular Disease 50: 1, 1981

105. Wit AL, Rosen MR: Cellular electrophysiology of cardiac arrhythmias. In Josephson ME, Wellens HJJ (eds): Tachycardias: Mechanisms, Diagnosis, Treatment, pp 1–27. Philadelphia, Lea & Febiger, 1984

106. Wit A: Triggered activity. In Podrid PJ, Kowey PR (eds): Cardiac Arrhythmia: Mechanisms, Diagnosis, and Management, pp 70–77. Baltimore, Williams & Wilkins, 1995

107. Young GD, Kerr CR, Yeung-Lai-Wah JA: Preexcitation other than Wolff-Parkinson-White syndrome. In Podrid PJ, Kowey PR (eds): Cardiac Arrhythmia: Mechanisms, Diagnosis, and Management, pp 875–890. Baltimore, Williams & Wilkins, 1995

108. Zipes DP, Heger JJ, Prystowsky EN: Pathophysiology of arrhythmias: Clinical electrophysiology. Am Heart J 106: 812, 1983

109. Zipes DP: Genesis of cardiac arrhythmias: Electrophysiological considerations. In Braunwald E (ed): Heart Disease, 5th ed, Vol I, pp 548–592. Philadelphia, WB Saunders, 1997

110. Zipes DP: Specific arrhythmias: Diagnosis and treatment. In Braunwald E (ed): Heart Disease: A Textbook of Cardiovascular Medicine, 5th ed., Vol I, pp 640–704. Philadelphia, WB Saunders, 1997

DRUG TABLES AND DRUG THERAPY REFERENCES

Anderson JL: Sotalol, bretylium, and other class 3 antiarrhythmic agents. In Podrid PJ, Kowey PR (eds): Cardiac Arrhythmia: Mechanisms, Diagnosis, and Management, pp 450–466. Baltimore, Williams & Wilkins, 1995

Campbell RWF: Class 1B antiarrhythmic agents. In Podrid PJ, Kowey PR (eds): Cardiac Arrhythmia: Mechanisms, Diagnosis, and Management, pp 391–404. Baltimore, Williams & Wilkins, 1995

Bond EF: Antiarrhythmic drugs. In Underhill SL, Woods SL, Sivarajan Froelicher E et al (eds): Cardiovascular Medications for Cardiac Nursing, pp 73–121. Philadelphia, JB Lippincott, 1990

DiMarco JP: Adenosine. In Podrid PJ, Kowey PR (eds): Cardiac Arrhythmia: Mechanisms, Diagnosis, and Management, pp 488–498. Baltimore, Williams & Wilkins, 1995

Frishman WH, Cavusoglu E: β-Adrenergic blockers and their role in the therapy of arrhythmias. In Podrid PJ, Kowey PR (eds): Cardiac Arrhythmia: Mechanisms, Diagnosis, and Management, pp 421–434. Baltimore, Williams & Wilkins, 1995

Giardina EV, Lipka LJ: Class 1A antiarrhythmic agents: Quinidine, procainamide, disopyramide. In Podrid PJ, Kowey PR (eds): Cardiac Arrhythmia: Mechanisms, Diagnosis, and Management, pp 396–391. Baltimore, Williams & Wilkins, 1995

Hondeghem LM: Receptor physiology and its relationship to antiarrhythmic drugs. In Podrid PJ, Kowey PR (eds): Cardiac Arrhythmia: Mechanisms, Diagnosis, and Management, pp 347–354. Baltimore, Williams & Wilkins, 1995

Johnson JH, Jadonath RL, Marchlinski FE: Digoxin. In Podrid PJ, Kowey PR (eds): Cardiac Arrhythmia: Mechanisms, Diagnosis, and Management, pp 478–488. Baltimore, Williams & Wilkins, 1995

Kayser SR: Antiarrhythmic drug therapy: Part I. General principles of drug selection. Prog Cardiovasc Nurs 11(2): 33–37, 1996

Kayser SR: Antiarrhythmic drug therapy: Part II. Specific drugs. Prog Cardiovasc Nurs 11(3): 33–38, 1996

Kayser SR: Antiarrhythmic drug therapy: Part III. Atrial fibrillation. Prog Cardiovasc Nurs 11(4): 35–43, 1996

Kayser SR: Antiarrhythmic drug therapy: Part III. Ventricular arrhythmias. Prog Cardiovasc Nurs 12(3): 32–36, 1997

Kayser SR: Ibutilide: A new drug for the rapid termination of atrial fibrillation and atrial flutter. Prog Cardiovasc Nurs 12(1): 39–43, 1997

Keen JH, Baird MS, Allen JH: Critical Care and Emergency Drug Reference, 2nd ed. St. Louis, Mosby, 1996

Kowey PR, Marinchak RA, Rials SJ et al: Acute treatment of atrial fibrillation. Am J Cardiol 81(5A): 16C–22C, 1998

Lauer MS, Eagle KA: Arrhythmias following cardiac surgery. In Podrid PJ, Kowey PR (eds): Cardiac Arrhythmia: Mechanisms, Diagnosis, and Management, pp 1206–1218. Baltimore, Williams & Wilkins, 1995

Naccarelli GV, Dougherty AH: Amiodarone: A review of its pharmacologic, antiarrhythmic, and adverse effects. In Podrid PJ, Kowey PR (eds): Cardiac Arrhythmia: Mechanisms, Diagnosis, and Management, pp 434–449. Baltimore, Williams & Wilkins, 1995

Naccarelli GV, Lee KS, Gibson JK et al: Electrophysiology and pharmacology of ibutilide. Am J Cardiol 78(Suppl 8A): 12–16, 1996

Opie LH: Drugs for the Heart, 4th ed. Philadelphia, WB Saunders, 1995

Pill MW: Ibutilide: A new antiarrhythmic agent for the critical care environment. Critical Care Nurse 17: 19–22, 1997

Podrid PJ: Aggravation of arrhythmia by antiarrhythmic drugs. In Podrid PJ, Kowey PR (eds): Cardiac Arrhythmia: Mechanisms, Diagnosis, and Management, pp 507–522. Baltimore, Williams & Wilkins, 1995

Pratt CM: Class 1C antiarrhythmic agents: Propafenone, flecainide, and ethmozine. In Podrid PJ, Kowey PR (eds): Cardiac Arrhythmia: Mechanisms, Diagnosis, and Management, pp 404–421. Baltimore, Williams & Wilkins, 1995

Siddoway LA: Pharmacologic principles of antiarrhythmic drugs. In Podrid PJ, Kowey PR (eds): Cardiac Arrhythmia: Mechanisms, Diagnosis, and Management, pp 355–368. Baltimore, Williams & Wilkins, 1995

Singh BN: Controlling cardiac arrhythmias with calcium channel blockers. In Podrid PJ, Kowey PR (eds): Cardiac Arrhythmia: Mechanisms, Diagnosis, and Management, pp 466–478. Baltimore, Williams & Wilkins, 1995

Stambler BS, Wood MA, Ellenbogen KA et al: Efficacy and safety of repeated intravenous doses of ibutilide for rapid conversion of atrial flutter or fibrillation. Circulation 94: 1613, 1996

15

Cardiac Electrophysiology Procedures

SUSAN BLANCHER
CAROLYN CHANDLER MAIN

The use of cardiac electrophysiology (EP) procedures has expanded in recent years to include both diagnostic testing and interventional treatment procedures. In general, diagnostic EP studies are performed to determine an arrhythmia diagnosis or EP mechanism of a known arrhythmia. Interventional or therapeutic EP studies include endocardial catheter ablation and surgical procedures for both supraventricular and ventricular arrhythmias. The placement of implantable cardioverter-defibrillators for management of ventricular tachycardia (VT) and ventricular fibrillation (VF) is also an interventional EP procedure and is discussed in Chapter 25. A knowledge of electrocardiography (see Chapter 13), normal cardiac activation (see Chapter 1), and cardiac activation during arrhythmias (see Chapter 14) is needed to understand EP studies.

DIAGNOSTIC ELECTROPHYSIOLOGY STUDIES

Before an EP study, a patient needs to be prepared for the procedure. This preparation and the techniques, complications, and indications of EP studies are presented here.

Patient Preparation

Preparation for EP procedures is similar to that for cardiac catheterization (see Chapter 18). Patients are fasting and usually sedated during EP studies. The degree of sedation depends on the type of study being performed and the preferences of the center performing the procedures. A peripheral intravenous line is required for medication administration. Systemic anticoagulation may be used during EP studies to decrease the incidence of thromboembolic complications.[33,46] Appropriate emergency and resuscitation equipment is required for all EP procedures.

Techniques

During invasive EP testing, spontaneous and pacing-induced intracardiac and surface electrical signals are recorded. The normal timing and sequence of electrical activation can be observed and measured during a normal or baseline rhythm. Abnormal timing and electrical activation sequences are recorded and studied during tachyarrhythmias. Programmed electrical stimulation may also be used to induce and analyze paroxysmal arrhythmias that are the same as or similar to a patient's clinical arrhythmia.[39]

Flexible catheters with at least 2 and up to 10 electrodes are introduced percutaneously. The catheters are advanced using fluoroscopy into the heart. The right and left femoral, subclavian, internal jugular, and median cephalic veins are the most commonly used venous access sites. One to several catheters may be placed depending on the type of study to be performed (Fig. 15-1). The usual intracardiac recording sites include the high right atrium, right ventricular apex, right ventricular outflow tract, coronary sinus, and the His bundle region. Occasionally, the left ventricle is used during a diagnostic study for programmed electrical stimulation if VT cannot be induced from the right ventricle.

After the catheters are in place and connected to the physiologic recording equipment, intervals are measured from both the 12-lead electrocardiogram (ECG) and the intracardiac electrograms in the baseline state (Fig. 15-2). The AH interval is a measurement of conduction time from the low right atrium through the atrioventricular (AV) node to the His bundle and is an approximation of AV node conduction time. The AH interval can vary a great deal depending on the patient's autonomic state.[39] The HV interval represents conduction time from the onset of His bundle depolarization to the onset of ventricular activity. The normal HV interval measurement is 35 to 55 milliseconds.[29] After baseline recordings, various pacing techniques may be performed to assess the patient's electrical conduction system. Refractory periods for the atrium, AV node, and ventricle are recorded. Attempts to induce and document the arrhythmia

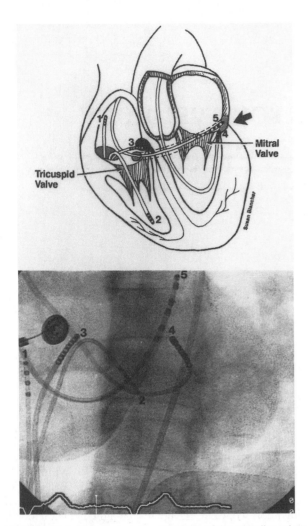

FIGURE 15-1 Diagram and radiograph of intracardiac placement of catheters. The radiograph shows the left anterior oblique view. 1, right atrial recording catheter; 2, right ventricular recording; catheter 3, His recording catheter; 4, ablating catheter; 5, mapping catheter. (From Fellows CL, Brett C, Main CC: Radio-frequency catheter ablation of Wolff-Parkinson-White syndrome. Virginia Mason Clinic Bulletin 46:45–51, 1992.)

and to relate the clinical symptoms are then made. The patient must be adequately prepared before the study and should understand that arrhythmia induction is one of the primary goals of the study. The cardiologist attempts to gather as much information as possible depending on the type of arrhythmia induced and how well it is hemodynamically tolerated. If the patient is hemodynamically unstable, such as during VF or rapid VT, documentation of the arrhythmia with a 12-lead ECG is almost always obtained before attempting to terminate it. It is important to note the method of arrhythmia termination. Tachycardias may be self-terminating or require antitachycardia pacing to stop them. Occasionally, it is necessary to cardiovert or defibrillate the patient to stop the arrhythmia.

If the patient is hemodynamically stable during a ventricular arrhythmia, attempts to map its origin can be performed. Recordings are made at various locations in the heart and compared with a reference signal, usually a surface ECG lead. The site of earliest activation is closest to the site where the arrhythmia originates.

Complications

Horowitz[33] reviewed the experience of his EP laboratory and the laboratories of five others. During a 4-year period, 8,545 EP studies were performed on 4,015 patients. Five deaths (0.12%) occurred, all due to intractable VF. The complications that occurred most frequently after EP studies were cardiac perforation (0.5%) and major venous thrombosis (0.5%). Cardiac perforation and pericardial effusion resolved without treatment in most patients; five patients required pericardial drainage or open repair. The femoral catheter site was the location of thrombosis for 95% of the 20 patients with venous thrombosis. Pulmonary emboli followed venous thrombosis in nine patients (0.2%). A slightly higher incidence of venous thrombosis (1.1%) and pulmonary emboli (1.6%) was found in a study by DiMarco and others[14] of 359 patients during 1,062 EP studies. They reported a 10% incidence of the use of countershock to terminate unstable VT; all patients returned to their original rhythm without complications. Systemic or catheter site infections were reported in 1.7% of patients in the study by DiMarco and colleagues[14] but were not reported in Horowitz's study.[33] Major hemorrhage and arterial injury are uncommon complications of EP studies.[33]

Indications

A list of indications for EP testing is provided in Display 15-1. Specific clinical indications are discussed in the subsequent sections. Indications for testing narrow-complex, supraventricular tachyarrhythmias are discussed in the section on Interventional Electrophysiology and Catheter Ablation.

CARDIAC ARREST SURVIVORS

People who survive a cardiac arrest not associated with an acute transmural myocardial infarction are at high risk for recurrence. The 2-year recurrence rate has been reported at 47%.[65] VF was the rhythm most commonly found at the time of cardiac arrest.[4,10,25,26,55] VT and VF were induced during EP testing in a baseline, antiarrhythmic drug-free state in 70% to 80% of patients resuscitated from cardiac arrest.[53,62,63,68,76]

The goal of EP-guided, serial, antiarrhythmic drug testing is to identify a drug that is effective in suppressing inducible VT or VF and subsequent recurrent cardiac arrest. After a drug has been given, EP testing is repeated. If an antiarrhythmic drug prevents VT or VF induction, then a prediction of drug efficacy is made.[63,71] VT or VF suppression has been reported in 26% to 80% of cardiac arrest survivors.[53,62,63,68,76] Wilber and colleagues[76] estimated the risk for recurrent cardiac arrest to be 6% at 1 year and 15% at 3 years for patients whose arrhythmias were noninducible during EP testing. Antiarrhythmic medications may also provoke or exacerbate arrhythmias; this situation is referred to as a *proarrhythmic effect.*[1]

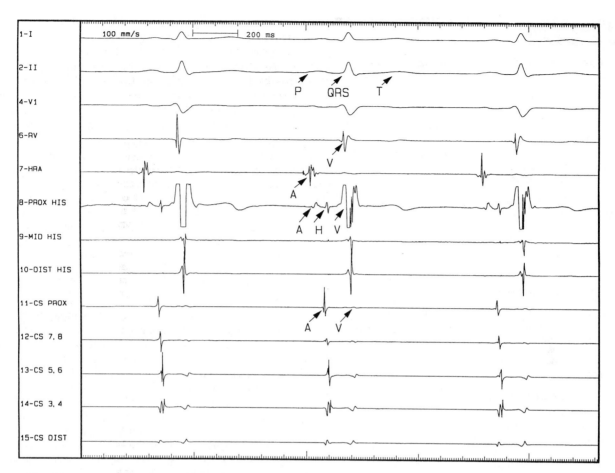

FIGURE 15-2 Basic intervals. Channel 1-I is lead I; channel 2-II is lead II; channel 4-V1 is lead V_1; channel 6-RV is a right ventricular tracing (V); channel 7-RA is a right atrial tracing (A); channel 8-HIS PROX is a tracing from the proximal portion of the His bundle; channel 9-HIS MID is a tracing from the middle portion of the His bundle; channel 10-HIS DIST is a tracing from the distal portion of the His bundle. On channel 8-HIS PROX, the first waveform represents atrial depolarization (A) and occurs slightly later than the P wave on lead II. The next waveform is the His bundle deflection (H). The last waveform represents ventricular depolarization (V), corresponding to the QRS complex. Atrial and ventricular tracings are also recorded on channels 11–15-CS and reflect proximal to distal coronary sinus electrograms.

Electrophysiology testing is recommended for patients who receive nonpharmacologic drug therapy. Implantation of combination antitachycardia pacemakers and implantable cardioverter-defibrillators usually requires a baseline EP test and may require postimplantation testing to allow for correct programming of the device. Knowledge of baseline conduction and the presence of concurrent atrial arrhythmias is also helpful for appropriate device selection (see Chapter 26).

WIDE-COMPLEX TACHYCARDIAS

Wide-complex tachycardias can be caused by VT, supraventricular tachycardia with aberration, or preexcitation syndromes such as antidromic reciprocating tachycardia, in which an accessory bypass tract is the antegrade limb and the AV node is the retrograde limb of the tachycardia. Although guidelines and criteria[16,43,74,75] have been established to help practitioners diagnose wide-complex tachycardias using the 12-lead ECG, necessary criteria may

be difficult to identify, and the diagnosis may not be certain. In these cases, EP studies are necessary to confirm or establish a diagnosis so that proper, safe treatment can be initiated.[1]

During invasive EP testing for wide-complex arrhythmias, the timing and sequence of atrial activation in relation to ventricular activation are recorded. Although it may be difficult to distinguish the various preexcitation syndromes from VT, the presence of AV dissociation favors a diagnosis of VT.

SYNCOPE

Syncope is defined as a sudden, transient loss of consciousness accompanied by loss of postural tone.[52] Syncope is a common medical problem, with many potential causes (Display 15-2). The etiology is unclear in approximately half of patients who present with syncope.[40] Some cases may be benign and self-limiting. The 1-year mortality rate for presumed cardiac causes of syncope has been reported at

---

DISPLAY 15-1

Indications for Electrophysiology Study

DEFINITE INDICATIONS

Sustained ventricular tachycardia or cardiac arrest occurring in the absence of acute myocardial infarction, antiarrhythmic drug toxicity, or electrolyte imbalance, particularly when baseline ventricular ectopic frequency is too low to permit assessment of antiarrhythmic drug efficacy by electrocardiographic monitoring

Syncope of uncertain etiology in which noncardiac causes have been ruled unlikely

Wide QRS tachycardia of uncertain etiology

Evaluation of a device for the detection and electrical termination of tachycardias

Symptomatic Wolff-Parkinson-White syndrome

Frequent symptomatic regular supraventricular tachycardia, particularly when this is unresponsive to medical therapy

Second-degree atrioventricular block in which the level of block is uncertain

INDICATION NOT ESTABLISHED

Asymptomatic Wolff-Parkinson-White syndrome
Postmyocardial infarction
Nonsustained ventricular tachycardia
Cardiomyopathy
Frequent ventricular ectopy
Any supraventricular tachycardia

NONINDICATIONS

Asymptomatic sinus bradycardia
Asymptomatic bundle-branch block
Palpitations
Atrial fibrillation or flutter
Third-degree atrioventricular block or type II second-degree atrioventricular block

From Cooper MJ, Anderson KP, Mason JW: Invasive electrophysiological studies. In Zipes DP, Jalife J (eds): Cardiac Electrophysiology From Cell to Bedside, pp 837–849. Philadelphia, WB Saunders, 1990.

20% to 30%.[17,40,41] Even though patients are routinely referred to EP centers for syncope evaluation, invasive EP testing is not always indicated. A thorough history, physical examination, and noninvasive testing can frequently uncover the mechanism and direct treatment.

The history, including observers' statements, is extremely important to assist in directing the syncope evaluation. A description of onset and recovery can provide clues for the cause. For example, a sudden onset without any warning signs or symptoms suggests a cardiac arrhythmia. Recovery from syncope due to cardiac causes is usually rapid, without neurologic sequelae, while recovery from a seizure is usually associated with a period of drowsiness and confusion.

The physical examination should include orthostatic vital signs and carotid sinus pressure in patients who do not have cerebrovascular disease or carotid bruits.[57] A positive carotid sinus test is documented by recording a pause of 3 seconds or longer or a blood pressure decrease of greater than 50 mm Hg without symptoms. A 30 mm Hg blood pressure decrease with symptoms is also considered an abnormal test result.[70] Reproduction of symptoms may suggest the cause of syncope, especially if other causes are ruled out.

Once the practitioner determines that a cardiac cause is most likely, a series of noninvasive tests may be indicated. The 12-lead ECG should be evaluated for arrhythmias, long QT syndrome, left ventricular hypertrophy, preexcitation, conduction abnormalities, and ischemia or infarction. An echocardiogram helps to rule out or confirm the presence of structural heart disease and to evaluate left ventricular function. EP study results suggest that an arrhythmia is more likely to be the cause of syncope in patients who have structural heart disease, such as a prior myocardial infarction. Ambulatory monitoring for 24 to 48 hours may be helpful if the patient is having frequent symptoms. If symptoms are not frequent enough, patient-activated transtelephonic event recorders[50] or a subcutaneously implanted loop recorder system (Medtronic, Inc. Bedford, NH) may be helpful in documenting an arrhythmia.[44]

The signal-averaged ECG has been reported as useful in screening patients at risk for VT-induced syncope.[24,45,56,77] This technique involves recording, amplifying, and filtering the surface ECG. Low-amplitude, high-frequency signals, called *late potentials,* are detected at the terminal portion of the QRS.[5,28] Delayed myocardial activation in areas of scar tissue represented by late potentials is thought to be the cause of ventricular arrhythmias. Prediction of VT by signal-averaged ECG is more accurate in patients with coronary artery disease.[45] A positive test in a patient with known heart disease is an indication for invasive EP testing.[56]

The head-upright tilt test is a noninvasive, provocative test used to try to reproduce and diagnose neurally mediated syncope (NMS). NMS is manifested by a combination of vasodilation and bradycardia, which occurs when the feedback mechanisms between the parasympathetic nervous system and sympathetic nervous system break down. Both systems are thought to activate alternately or simultaneously. Normal circulatory function is interrupted when both systems discharge rapidly. Vagal stimulation becomes exaggerated, causing bradycardia and hypotension in the presence of sympathetic nervous system stimulation.[9,60] During the head-upright tilt test, the patient is placed on a tilt table with a foot board. There are various protocols for inducing NMS. Basically, an upright tilt at 60 to 80 degrees for 10 to 60 minutes is performed. Isoproterenol is administered in increasing doses until a positive result or until the end of the protocol is reached without documentation of syncope. A positive response reproduces the patient's symptoms along with documentation of bradycardia, hypotension, or both.[2,21,27,67,69]

Invasive EP studies are indicated when a noninvasive evaluation for syncope is negative and the suspicion for a cardiac cause remains high.[3,12,13,22,32,53,58,61,72] Sinus node function is evaluated by measuring the sinus node recovery time. Overdrive pacing is performed in the high right

DISPLAY 15-2

Classification of Syncope

CARDIOVASCULAR

Reflex
Vasovagal
Vagovagal (situational)
  Micturition
  Deglutition
  Defecation
  Glossopharyngeal neuralgia
  Postprandial
  Tussive
  Supine hypotensive syndrome of near-term pregnancy
  Valsalva
  Oculovagal
  Sneeze
  Instrumentation
  Diving
  Jacuzzi
  Weight lifting
  Trumpet playing
Orthostatic
  Hyperadrenergic (e.g., volume depletion)
  Hypoadrenergic
    Primary autonomic insufficiency
    Secondary autonomic insufficiency (e.g., neurologic disorders or drugs)
Carotid sinus syncope
  Cardioinhibitory
  Vasodepressor
  Mixed
  Central

Cardiac
Mechanical (obstructive)
  Aortic stenosis
  Hypertrophic cardiomyopathy
  Pulmonary embolism
  Aortic dissection
  Myocardial infarction
  Mitral stenosis
  Left atrial myxoma
  Pulmonic stenosis
  Cardiac tamponade
  Prosthetic valve malfunction
  Global myocardial ischemia
  Tetralogy of Fallot
  Pulmonary hypertension
Electrical (dysrhythmic)
  Atrioventricular block
  Sick sinus syndrome
  Supraventricular or ventricular arrhythmias
  Long QT syndrome
  Pacemaker related

NONCARDIOVASCULAR

Neurologic
Vertebrobasilar transient ischemic attack
  Atherosclerosis
  Mechanical
Subclavian steal syndrome
Takayasu disease
Normal pressure hydrocephalus
Unwitnessed seizure
Orthostatic syncope

Metabolic
Hypoxia
Hypoglycemia
Hyperventilation

Psychiatric
Panic disorders
Major depression
Hysteria

UNEXPLAINED

From Manolis, AS, Linzer M, Salem D et al: Syncope: Current diagnostic evaluation and management. Ann Intern Med 112: 850–863, 1990.

atrium for 30 to 60 seconds.[51,79] A prolonged sinus node recovery time may be an indication of sick sinus syndrome. The His-Purkinje system is evaluated by measuring the HV interval during sinus rhythm and during incremental atrial pacing and atrial refractory period determinations. A prolonged HV interval is an indication of infrahisian disease.[1] AV node function is also evaluated by incremental atrial pacing and refractory period determinations. The Wenckebach point is recorded during incremental pacing, whereas the effective refractory periods of the atrium and AV node are recorded with the introduction of atrial extrastimuli. The atrium is refractory when the atrial extrastimuli fail to capture the atrium. The AV node is refractory when the atrial extrastimuli capture the atrium but fail to result in a His bundle depolarization (AV block). Permanent pacing may be indicated if abnormalities are found. Attempts are also made to induce ventricular and supraventricular tachycardia during EP testing for syncope.

In all cases, the findings of the EP study along with reproduction of the patient's symptoms and other findings in the work-up must be evaluated carefully to determine the appropriate course of therapy. Syncope remains unexplained in approximately half of cases.[40] The prognosis for this latter group of patients is good.[15]

INTERVENTIONAL ELECTROPHYSIOLOGY AND CATHETER ABLATION

This interventional procedure includes both a diagnostic EP study and catheter ablation. The mechanism of the arrhythmia is confirmed during the first part of the procedure, and the ablation takes place during the second part. Most centers combine the diagnostic and therapeutic segments of the study into one procedure.[8,59]

Radiofrequency Catheter Ablation

Catheter ablation techniques have been in use for over 10 years. High-energy, direct-current shocks were delivered through catheters, using a standard defibrillator, to the endocardial ablation site.[23,66] The technique was not widely used, however, because of the high complication rate, including cardiac tamponade and immediate and late sudden death.[18,19,30,42] As a result, efforts to find a safer energy source were pursued. In 1986, radiofrequency (RF) energy was applied through catheters to create endocardial lesions.[34,47] RF energy is a form of electrical energy that is produced by high-frequency alternating current. As the current passes through tissue, heat is created.[34] RF current is used in the operating room to coagulate blood vessels and to ablate abnormal tissue during neurosurgery. RF current used during endocardial catheter ablation is alternating current with a 500,000- to 750,000-Hz frequency range. The current passes from the electrode tip to a large–surface-area skin patch. The current is typically applied for 10 to 60 seconds at a time using 45 to 55 V. Catheter delivery of RF energy causes tissue heating in a small area around the electrode. The typical lesion is $3 \times 4 \times 5$ mm.[35]

Techniques

The first part of the procedure, the diagnostic phase, was described previously. After a diagnosis is made, an ablating catheter is positioned at the target area. The ablating catheter can be steered and has four to six electrodes 2 to 5 mm apart. The catheter tip is 4 or 5 mm long and serves as the electrode through which RF current is applied. The target area is located using fluoroscopy and by observing the electrogram patterns recorded by the distal mapping electrode pair.

Indications

Combination EP study and catheter ablation procedures are indicated for patients with supraventricular tachycardias due to accessory pathways (APs), AV nodal reentry tachycardia, intra-atrial tachycardias due to either an automatic or reentrant mechanism, atrial fibrillation, and atrial flutter. These procedures are also indicated for some patients with certain types of VT.[31,36-38,47,48]

ATRIOVENTRICULAR NODAL REENTRANT TACHYCARDIA

Dual AV nodal pathways are the substrate for AV nodal reentrant tachycardia (AVNRT). This arrhythmia is responsible for 60% to 70% of paroxysmal supraventricular tachycardias (PSVTs).[8] The fast pathway has a longer effective refractory period and the slow pathway has a shorter refractory period. The typical form of AVNRT is initiated when a premature beat from the atrium is blocked in the fast pathway. The early beat conducts down the slow pathway and then reenters back into the atrium through the fast pathway. This impulse continues to conduct down the slow pathway and up the fast pathway, thus perpetuating the reentry circuit and the tachycardia. Slow pathway ablation is accomplished by mapping the slow pathway region, which extends from the posterior interatrial septum near the coronary sinus ostium to the anterior interatrial septum. After characteristic electrograms are recorded, RF energy is applied through the distal mapping and ablating electrode (Fig. 15-3). Repeat programmed stimulation is performed after the ablation in an attempt to induce the tachycardia. The procedure is considered successful when AVNRT cannot be induced. Complete heart block is a potential serious complication because of the close proximity of the slow pathway to the compact AV node and has been reported to occur 1.3% to 3% of the time. The success rate is nearly 100%.[36,78]

ATRIOVENTRICULAR REENTRANT TACHYCARDIA

Both Wolff-Parkinson-White (WPW) syndrome and concealed AV bypass tracts are responsible for 30% to 40% of PSVTs.[8] The anatomy is basically the same. The AP is a small bundle of muscle fibers that cross the AV groove on either the right or left side of the heart, creating an extra electrical connection that can conduct in one or both directions. When the AP conducts in an anterograde direction, a delta wave can be observed on the ECG and is characteris-

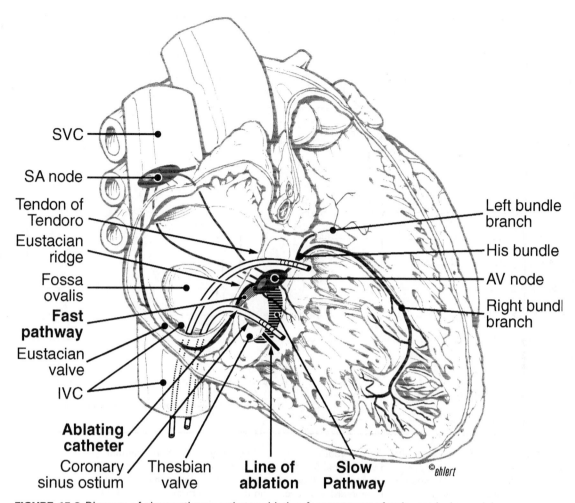

SVC

SA node

Tendon of
Tendoro

Eustacian
ridge

Fossa
ovalis

**Fast
pathway**

Eustacian
valve

IVC

**Ablating
catheter**

Coronary
sinus ostium

Thesbian
valve

**Line of
ablation**

**Slow
Pathway**

Left bundle
branch

His bundle

AV node

Right bundl
branch

©*ehlert*

FIGURE 15-3 Diagram of slow pathway catheter ablation for treatment of atrioventricular nodal reentrant tachycardia (AVNRT).

tic of WPW syndrome. PSVT is initiated in the same manner as described for AVNRT. The AV node serves as the antegrade limb of the tachycardia and the AP serves as the retrograde limb of the tachycardia. If atrial fibrillation occurs in a patient with WPW syndrome, a life-threatening situation may develop if conduction over the AP is rapid enough to induce VF.

Catheter ablation of AV bypass tracts on the left side of the heart involves one of two techniques. The mapping and ablating catheter can be advanced from the femoral artery retrograde across the aortic valve. The catheter is then positioned either under or on the mitral valve annulus. When the catheter is positioned properly, the AP activation can be recorded.[7,38] RF current is then applied. If the patient has WPW syndrome, the delta wave on the ECG disappears during RF energy application (Fig. 15-4). It is necessary to ablate so that both antegrade and retrograde conduction over the bypass tract are abolished. Testing is performed after ablating to assess for retrograde conduction and to try to induce tachycardia. Another approach to the mitral annulus is by means of transseptal catheterization. In this approach, the ablating and mapping catheter is advanced to the left atrium through the right heart using a special sheath

assembly to cross the interatrial septum. Both approaches have an 85% success rate.[48]

ATRIAL FIBRILLATION OR FLUTTER

Complete AV node ablation is indicated for patients who have chronic or paroxysmal atrial fibrillation or flutter with a rapid ventricular response. This procedure should be performed only in patients for whom conventional antiarrhythmic drug therapy has failed or for whom the side effects from effective doses of medication are intolerable. This procedure is performed by advancing the ablating catheter from the right femoral vein to the area of the AV node. Complete heart block or a junctional escape rhythm is the result. Permanent, rate-responsive pacing is indicated after AV node ablation, and the patient may discontinue all antiarrhythmic medications.[37,47] Continuous anticoagulation is recommended because the underlying arrhythmia is still present. Left ventricular dysfunction due to chronic, rapid heart rates in atrial fibrillation has been reported to improve after AV node ablation.[30] In addition, over 80% of patients report improved quality of life with increased exercise tolerance after this procedure.[20]

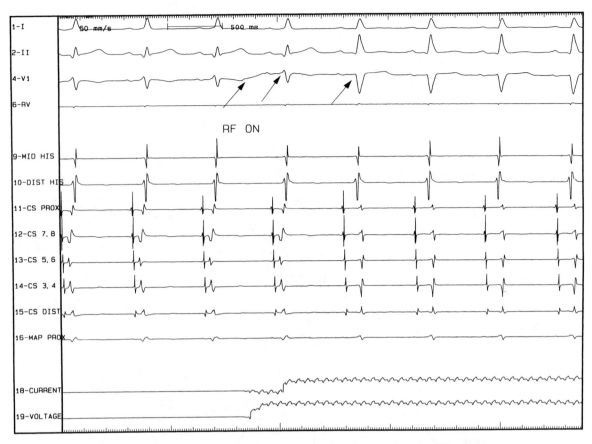

FIGURE 15-4 Loss of delta wave after onset of radiofrequency (RF) energy application. Channel 1, lead I; channel 2, lead II; channel 4, lead V_1; channel 6, right ventricular tracing; channels 9 and 10, His bundle electrograms ; channels 11–15, coronary sinus (CS) electrograms. Notice that before RF energy is applied, the earliest ventricular depolarization occurs on the CS electrogram labeld CS 5, 6, corresponding to the left posterior septal position. This location is where the mapping and ablating catheter was positioned under the mitral valve anulus. After RF energy (see current and voltage channels) application, the delta wave disappears (leads I, II_1, V_1), and the ventricular activation sequence changes to normal on all coronary sinus electrograms.

Primary ablation of typical or type 1 atrial flutter is being performed in some centers. This procedure involves ablation of a discrete anatomic region thought to be responsible for the arrhythmia. Ablation in the lower right atrium within a zone of critical slow conduction creates a *line of block* that prevents perpetuation of the arrhythmia. Success rates in an experienced center were reported to be 88% (n = 51). Although the procedure was safe with an extremely low complication rate, the recurrence of atrial flutter or the development of new-onset or recurrent atrial fibrillation was not uncommon. Repeat ablation was successful in most cases.[64]

ATRIAL ARRHYTHMIAS

Arrhythmias that originate in the atria and arise from either reentrant circuits or abnormal foci can often be treated with catheter ablation. Patients who have undergone atrial surgery for congenital heart disease may have fixed anatomic barriers within scar tissue, which facilitate a reentrant tachycardia. Arrhythmias that arise from abnormal atrial foci have increased automaticity because of their mechanism and can

be found in either the left or right atrium. The effective site for ablation in both cases is determined by methodically mapping the appropriate atrium during tachycardia. The earliest atrial endocardial electrogram marks the origin of the tachycardia.[49]

VENTRICULAR TACHYCARDIA

Ablation of paroxysmal VT is a new and challenging therapy for patients whose tachycardia is suited to study and ablation. For a VT focus to be ablated, the tachycardia must be inducible, monomorphic, and tolerated for long enough periods to enable accurate mapping. For a successful ablation, the type of VT must be determined.

Bundle-branch reentrant tachycardia conducts antegrade over the right bundle and retrograde over the left bundle. This type of VT occurs in patients who have severe ischemic or idiopathic cardiomyopathy. The VT is rapid because it uses the His-Purkinje system. Ablation of the right bundle usually abolishes this VT.

Benign monomorphic VT (idiopathic VT) usually occurs in young people with no structural heart disease. The VT can arise from the right ventricular outflow tract or from the inferior left ventricular septum. Various EP techniques are used to map the presumed site of origin before ablating. RF ablation is successful in this group of patients.

VT associated with coronary artery disease is usually due to a reentrant mechanism. One of the problems encountered with ablating in this situation is that these patients may have many tachycardia circuits.[48] Ablation can be attempted if a single monomorphic VT is identified. Techniques to identify the best ablation site are still under development.

NURSING CARE OF THE PATIENT UNDERGOING ELECTROPHYSIOLOGY PROCEDURES

Health care professionals caring for EP patients must recognize that the procedure the patient is undergoing plays a relatively small, though pivotal, part in the entire arrhythmia experience. The need for patient education throughout all phases of the experience has been well documented.[6,11,54,73] Teaching before the study must include discussions about the nature of the test, a description of the procedure, procedure length, success rates, and complication rates. Nurses must also include postprocedure instructions and discharge instructions. After the procedure, the patient must keep the affected leg straight for 3 to 4 hours to allow the venous puncture site to heal and for 4 to 6 hours if the femoral artery was punctured. The preliminary results of the procedure should be shared immediately with the patient and family. Frequent explanations may be required at first if the patient is recovering from heavy sedation. After a successful ablation, patients have no restrictions.

Most of the intraprocedure and postprocedure nursing care is centered around monitoring the patient for potential complications related to the procedure.[54] In most instances, patients are anxious before and during EP procedures. Adequate sedation to allow for patient comfort should be provided. Oversedation must be prevented. Nurses must be alert for major complications directly related to placement of catheters inside the heart. Bleeding from catheter insertion sites, tamponade from perforation, and tachyarrhythmias and bradyarrhythmias can all occur both during and after the EP procedure. Nurses who care for patients with arrhythmia in any setting should be prepared to handle any emergency that may arise. Other potential problems to monitor for include thrombophlebitis, thromboembolism, and infection.

REFERENCES

1. ACC/AHA Task Force Report: Guidelines for Clinical Intracardiac Electrophysiologic Studies: A report of the American College of Cardiology/American Heart Association Task Force on Assessment of Diagnostic and Therapeutic Cardiovascular Procedures. Circulation 80: 1925–1939, 1989
2. Almquist A, Goldenberg IF, Milstein S et al: Provocation of bradycardia and hypotension by isoproterenol and upright posture in patients with unexplained syncope. N Engl J Med 320: 346–351, 1989
3. Bass EB, Elson JJ, Fogoros RN et al: Long-term prognosis of patients undergoing electrophysiology studies for syncope of unknown origin. Am J Cardiol 62: 1186–1191, 1988
4. Bayes de Luna A, Coumel P, Leclercq JF: Ambulatory sudden cardiac death: Mechanisms of production of fatal arrhythmia on the basis of data from 157 cases. Am Heart J 117: 151–159, 1989
5. Berbari EJ, Lazzara R: An introduction to high resolution ECG recordings of cardiac late potentials. Arch Intern Med 148: 1859–1863, 1988
6. Berry VA. Wolff-Parkinson-White syndrome and the use of radiofrequency catheter ablation. Heart Lung 22: 15–25, 1993
7. Calkins H, Kim YN, Schmaltz S et al: Electrogram criteria for identification of appropriate target sites for radiofrequency catheter ablation of accessory connections. Circulation 85: 565–573, 1992
8. Calkins H, Sousa J, El-Atassi R et al: Diagnosis and cure of the Wolff-Parkinson-White syndrome or paroxysmal supraventricular tachycardias during a single electrophysiologic test. N Engl J Med 324: 1612–1618, 1991
9. Clutter C: Neurally mediated syncope. J Cardiovasc Nurs 5: 65–73, 1991
10. Cobb L, Hallstrom AP: Clinical predictors and characteristics of the sudden cardiac death syndrome. In Proceedings USA-USSR First Joint Symposium on Sudden Death. DHEW Publication no. Washington, DC: (NIH) 78-1470, 1977
11. Connelly AG: An examination of stressors in the patient undergoing cardiac electrophysiologic studies. Heart Lung 21: 335–342, 1992
12. Denes P, Uretz E, Ezri MD et al: Clinical predictors of electrophysiologic testing in patients with syncope of unknown origin. Arch Intern Med 148: 1922–1928, 1988
13. DiMarco JP, Garan H, Harthorne JW et al: Intracardiac electrophysiologic techniques in recurrent syncope of unknown cause. Ann Intern Med 95: 542–548, 1981
14. DiMarco JP, Garan H, Ruskin JN: Complications in patients undergoing electrophysiologic procedures. Ann Intern Med 97: 490–493, 1982
15. Doherty JU, Pembrook-Rogers D, Grogan E et al: Electrophysiologic evaluation and follow-up characteristics of patients with recurrent unexplained syncope and pre-syncope. Am J Cardiol 55: 703–708, 1985
16. Dongas J, Lehman MH, Mahmud R et al: Value of preexisting bundle branch block in the ECG differentiation of supraventricular from ventricular origin of wide QRS tachycardia. Am J Cardiol 55: 717–721, 1985
17. Eagle KA, Black HR, Cook EF et al: Evaluation of prognostic classifications for patients with syncope. Ann Intern Med 100: 755–757, 1984
18. Evans GJ, Scheinman MM, Bardy G et al: Predictors of in-hospital mortality after DC catheter ablation of atrioventricular junction: Results of a prospective, international, multicenter study. Circulation 84: 1924–1937, 1991
19. Evans GJ, Scheinman MM, Zipes DP et al: The percutaneous cardiac mapping and ablation registry: Final summary of results. Pacing Clin Electrophysiol 11: 1621–1626, 1989
20. Fitzpatrick AP, Kourouyan HD, Siu A et al: Quality of life and outcomes after radiofrequency His-bundle ablation and permanent pacemaker implantation: Impact of treatment in paroxysmal and established atrial fibrillation. Am Heart J 121: 499–507, 1996
21. Fitzpatrick AP, Theodorakis G, Vardas P et al: Methodology of head-up tilt testing in patients with unexplained syncope. J Am Coll Cardiol 17: 125–130, 1991

22. Fujimura O, Yee R, Klein GJ et al: The diagnostic sensitivity of electrophysiologic testing in patients with syncope caused by transient bradycardia. N Engl J Med 321: 1703–1707, 1989

23. Gallagher JJ, Svenson RH, Kasell JH et al: Catheter technique for closed-chest ablation of the atrioventricular conduction system. N Engl J Med 306: 194–200, 1982

24. Gang ES, Peter T, Rosenthal ME et al: Detection of late potentials on the surface electrocardiogram in unexplained syncope. Am J Cardiol 58: 1014–1020, 1986

25. Gradman AH, Bell PA, DeBusk RF: Sudden death during ambulatory monitoring. Circulation 55: 210–211, 1977

26. Greene HL: Sudden arrhythmic cardiac death: Mechanisms, resuscitation, and classification. Am J Cardiol 65: 4B–12B, 1990

27. Grubb BP, Temesy-Armos P, Moore J et al: Head-upright tilt table testing in evaluation and management of the malignant vasovagal syndrome. Am J Cardiol 69: 904–908, 1992

28. Hall PA, Atwood JE, Myers J et al: The signal averaged surface electrocardiogram and the identification of late potentials. Prog Cardiovasc Dis 31: 295–317, 1989

29. Hammill SC, Sugrue DD, Gersh BJ et al: Clinical intracardiac electrophysiologic testing: Technique, diagnostic indications, and therapeutic uses. Mayo Clin Proc 61: 478–503, 1986

30. Hauer R, Straks W, Borst C et al: Electrical catheter ablation in the left and right ventricular wall in dogs: Relation between delivered energy and histopathologic changes. J Am Coll Cardiol 8: 637–643, 1988

31. Heinz G, Siostrzonek P, Kreiner G et al: Improvement in left ventricular systolic function after successful radiofrequency His bundle ablation for drug refractory, chronic atrial fibrillation and recurrent atrial flutter. Am J Cardiol 69: 489–492, 1992

32. Hess DS, Morady F, Scheinman MM: Electrophysiologic testing in the evaluation of patients with syncope of undetermined origin. Am J Cardiol 50: 1309–1315, 1982

33. Horowitz LH: Safety of electrophysiologic studies. Circulation 73: II-28–II-30, 1986

34. Huang S, Bharati S, Graham A et al: Closed chest catheter desiccation of the atrioventricular junction using radiofrequency energy: A new method of catheter ablation. J Am Coll Cardiol 9: 349–358, 1987

35. Huang SKS, Graham AR, Bharati S et al: Short- and long-term effects of transcatheter ablation of the coronary sinus by radiofrequency energy. Circulation 78: 416–427, 1988

36. Jackman WM, Beckman KJ, McClelland JH et al: Treatment of supraventricular tachycardia due to atrioventricular nodal reentry, by radiofrequency catheter ablation of slow-pathway conduction. N Engl J Med 327: 313–318, 1992

37. Jackman WM, Wang X, Friday KJ et al: Catheter ablation of atrioventricular junction using radiofrequency current in 17 patients. Circulation 83: 1562–1576, 1991

38. Jackman WM, Wang X, Friday KJ et al: Catheter ablation of atrioventricular pathways (Wolff-Parkinson-White syndrome) by radiofrequency current. N Engl J Med 324: 1605–1611, 1991

39. Josephson ME: Electrophysiologic investigation: General concepts. In Josephson ME (ed): Clinical Cardiac Electrophysiology Techniques and Interpretations, 2nd ed, pp 22–70. Philadelphia, Lea & Febiger, 1993

40. Kapoor WN, Karpf M, Wieand S et al: A prospective evaluation and followup of patients with syncope. N Engl J Med 309: 197–204, 1983

41. Kapoor WN, Snustad D, Peterson J et al: Syncope in the elderly. Am J Med 80: 419–428, 1986

42. Kempf FJ, Falcone R, Iozzo R et al: Anatomic and hemodynamic effects of catheter-delivered ablation energies in the ventricle. Am J Cardiol 56: 373–377, 1985

43. Kindwall KE, Brown B, Josephson ME: ECG criteria for ventricular tachycardia in wide complex left bundle branch block morphology tachycardias secondary to coronary artery disease. Am J Cardiol 61: 1279–1283, 1988

44. Krahn AD, Klein GJ, Norris C, Yee R: The etiology of syncope in patients with negative tilt table and electrophysiology testing. Circulation 92: 1819–1824, 1995

45. Kuchar DL, Thorburn CW, Sammel NL: Signal-averaged electrocardiogram for evaluation of recurrent syncope. Am J Cardiol 58: 949–953, 1986

46. Kutcher KL: Cardiac electrophysiologic mapping techniques. Focus on Critical Care 12(4): 26–30, 1985

47. Langberg JJ, Chin MC, Rosenqvist M et al: Catheter ablation of the atrioventricular junction with radiofrequency energy. Circulation 80: 1527–1535, 1989

48. Lesh MD: Interventional electrophysiology: State-of-the-art 1993. Am Heart J 126: 686–698, 1993

49. Lesh MD, Van Hare GF, Epstein LM et al: Radiofrequency catheter ablation of atrial arrhythmias results and mechanisms. Circulation 89: 1074–1089, 1994

50. Linzer M, Prystowsky EN, Brunetti LL et al: Recurrent syncope of unknown origin diagnosed by ambulatory continuous loop ECG recording. Am Heart J 116: 1632–1634, 1988

51. Mandel WH, Hayakawa H, Danzig R et al: Evaluation of sinoatrial node function in man by overdrive suppression. Circulation 44: 59–66, 1971

52. Manolis AS, Linzer M, Salem D et al: Syncope: Current diagnostic evaluation and management. Ann Intern Med 112: 850–863, 1990

53. Morady F, Scheinman MM, Hess DS et al: Electrophysiologic testing in the management of survivors of out-of-hospital cardiac arrest. Am J Cardiol 51: 85–89, 1983

54. Moulton L, Grant J, Miller B et al: Radiofrequency catheter ablation for supraventricular tachycardia. Heart Lung 22: 3–14, 1993

55. Myerburg RJ, Conde CA, Sung RJ et al: Clinical, electrophysiologic, and hemodynamic profile of patients resuscitated from prehospital cardiac arrest. Am J Med 68: 568–576, 1980

56. Nalos PC, Gang ES, Mandel WJ et al: The signal averaged electrocardiogram as a screening test for inducibility of sustained ventricular tachycardia in high risk patients: A prospective study. J Am Coll Cardiol 9: 539–548, 1987

57. Nelson SD, Kou WH, De Buitleir M et al: Value of programmed ventricular stimulation in presumed carotid sinus syndrome. Am J Cardiol 60: 1073–1077, 1987

58. Olshansky B, Mazuz M, Martins JB: Significance of inducible tachycardia in patients with recurrent syncope of unknown origin: A long term followup. J Am Coll Cardiol 5: 216–223, 1985

59. Prystowsky EN, Noble RJ: Electrophysiologic studies: Who to refer. Heart Disease and Stroke 1: 188–194, 1992

60. Purcell JA: Provoking vasodepressor syncope with head-up tilt-table testing. Prog Cardiovasc Nurs 7: 15–18, 1992

61. Reiffel JA, Wang P, Bower R et al: Electrophysiologic testing in patients with recurrent syncope: Are results predicted by prior ambulatory monitoring? Am Heart J 110: 1146–1153, 1985

62. Roy D, Waxman HL, Kienzle MG et al: Clinical characteristics and long-term follow-up in 119 survivors of cardiac arrest: Relation to inducibility at electrophysiologic testing. Am J Cardiol 52: 969–974, 1983

63. Ruskin JN, DiMarco JP, Garan H: Electrophysiologic observations and selection of long-term antiarrhythmic therapy. N Engl J Med 303: 607–613, 1980

64. Saxon LA, Kalman JM, Olgin JE et al: Results of radiofrequency catheter ablation for atrial flutter. Am J Cardiol 77: 1014–1016, 1996

65. Schaffer WA, Cobb LA: Recurrent ventricular fibrillation and modes of death in survivors of out-of-hospital ventricular fibrillation. N Engl J Med 293: 259–262, 1975

66. Scheinman MM, Morady F, Hess D et al: Catheter induced ablation of the atrioventricular junction to control refractory supraventricular arrhythmias. JAMA 248: 851–855, 1982
67. Sheldon R, Killam S: Methodology of isoproterenol-tilt table testing in patients with syncope. J Am Coll Cardiol 19: 773–779, 1992
68. Skale BT, Miles WM, Heger JJ et al: Survivors of cardiac arrest: Prevention of recurrence by drug therapy as predicted by electrophysiologic testing or electrocardiographic monitoring. Am J Cardiol 57: 113–119, 1986
69. Sra JS, Anderson AJ, Sheikh SH et al: Unexplained syncope evaluated by electrophysiologic studies and head-up tilt testing. Ann Intern Med 114: 1013–1019, 1991
70. Sugrue DD, Wood DL, McGoon MD: Carotid sinus hypersensitivity and syncope. Mayo Clin Proc 59: 637–640, 1984
71. Swerdlow CD, Winkle RA, Mason JW: Determinants of survival with ventricular tachyarrhythmias. N Engl J Med 308: 1436–1442, 1983
72. Teichman SL, Felder SD, Matos JA et al: The value of electrophysiologic studies in syncope of undetermined origin: Report of 150 cases. Am Heart J 110: 469–479, 1985
73. Tyndall A: A nursing perspective of the invasive electrophysiologic approach to treatment of ventricular arrhythmias. Heart Lung 12: 620–630, 1983
74. Wellens HJJ, Bar FW, Lie KI: The value of the ECG in the differential diagnosis of a tachycardia with a widened QRS complex. Am J Med 64: 27–33, 1978
75. Wellens HJJ, Brugada P, Heddle WF: The value of the 12 lead ECG in diagnosis type and mechanism of a tachycardia: A survey among 22 cardiologists. J Am Coll Cardiol 4: 176–179, 1984
76. Wilber DJ, Garan H, Finkelstein D et al: Use of electrophysiologic testing in the prediction of long-term outcome. N Engl J Med 318: 19–24, 1988
77. Winters SL, Stewart D, Gomes JA: Signal averaging of the surface QRS complex predicts inducibility of ventricular tachycardia in patients with syncope of unknown origin: A prospective study. J Am Coll Cardiol 10: 775–781, 1987
78. Wu D, Yeh S, Wang C et al: A simple technique for selective radiofrequency ablation of the slow pathway in atrioventricular node reentrant tachycardia. J Am Coll Cardiol 21: 1612–1621, 1993
79. Yee R, Strauss HC: Electrophysiologic mechanisms: Sinus node dysfunction. Circulation 75(Suppl III): 12–18, 1987

16

Echocardiography, Radioisotope Studies, Electron Beam Computed Tomography, Magnetic Resonance Imaging, and Phonocardiography

MARGARET L. HALL

Over the years, there has been a great interest in developing reliable and simple tests of the heart and blood vessels that, in contrast to cardiac catheterization, do not present a risk of morbidity or mortality to the patient. Less invasive tests are even more important for critically ill patients, who may tolerate complications of invasive studies less well than those who are not ill. In addition, tests are needed that can supply accurate, reproducible diagnostic information quickly with minimal moving of the patient and reduced overall cost.

Several indirect, noninvasive measures of cardiovascular function are in common use, including the electrocardiogram (ECG) and the indirect auscultatory method of blood pressure measurement. A number of ingenious low-technology tests have been developed but abandoned, such as ballistocardiography (a test developed to assess cardiac output using the body's recoil from the ejection of blood as measured on a low-friction, moving table) and apexcardiography (a graphic display of the left ventricular [LV] impulse as evaluated by palpation). Other tests, such as the calculation of systolic time intervals and phonocardiography, continue to be used for research or educational purposes. In the last third of the century, the rapid advancement in computer science and technology has allowed us to organize and format information obtained from a variety of physical phenomena. This has greatly increased our understanding of cardiac anatomy, physiology, and metabolism both in health and disease.

Echocardiography and Doppler echocardiography have developed from rudimentary research tools into major components in the diagnostic evaluation of heart disease. The bulk of this chapter is devoted to the discussion of this modality because of its widespread use and availability in evaluating heart disease. Almost all hospitals and many large or specialized clinics are now capable of performing a wide variety of cardiac and vascular ultrasound examinations. Radioisotope studies for evaluation of coronary artery disease of global quantitative myocardial function are widely available. Standard computed tomography, electron beam computed tomography (EBCT), and magnetic resonance imaging (MRI) are all used in a more limited fashion, but continue to grow in utility for the cardiac patient. Phonocardiography is available primarily as a teaching tool in academic centers.

The cardiac nurse can participate in the successful completion of these examinations by educating and orienting patients (How is the test done? Why is the test being done? Is the test uncomfortable?) and by providing reassurance and occasional assistance during the procedure. Achieving these goals rests on an understanding of the patient's condition, the specific clinical questions that may be answered by the test, and the general principles of the examination.

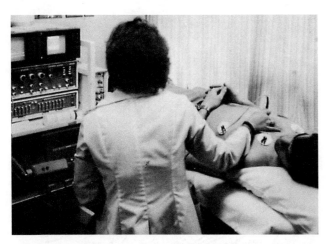

FIGURE 16-1 Position of patient and examiner for echocardiogram. Portable machinery permits the examination at bedside with no loss in quality. (From Chang S: M-Mode Echocardiographic Techniques and Pattern Recognition. Philadelphia, Lea & Febiger, 1976.)

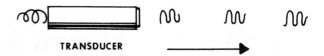

FIGURE 16-2 Transducer emits short bursts of sound.

The importance of sonographers, nuclear technologists, and radiology technicians cannot be overestimated in the successful completion of these examinations. These specialists must possess a sophisticated knowledge of cardiac anatomy, physiology, and pathophysiology and must understand the physics and mechanics that govern examination equipment and techniques.

Particularly in echocardiography, the sonographer's ability to vary the testing routine intelligently based on preliminary findings is so important that some centers perform echocardiography with a physician in attendance solely to guide the information collection. Other centers devote long training periods to sonographers so that they may perform examinations independently for subsequent physician interpretation. Whenever possible, it is helpful for nurses to observe the examinations in progress on their patients. This observation gives nurses an opportunity to discuss structure identification with the sonographer or physician and can contribute much to their understanding of anatomy, physiology, and pathophysiology (Fig. 16-1).

ECHOCARDIOGRAPHY

The study of ultrasound, the designation given to sound waves of frequencies higher than the human ear can detect, began nearly a century ago. The development of sonar (from *so*und *na*vigation *r*anging) probably represents the first widespread use of pulsed ultrasound for remote object detection and localization. Today, ultrasound technology is used extensively for anatomic evaluation of abdominal structures and fetal development and is therefore frequently familiar to patients and their families.

Technical Aspects

Echocardiography and Doppler imaging operate much like sonar; this analogy is often useful in explaining the test to patients. The ultrasound transducer serves both as a sender and a detector of sound waves. These high-frequency (2.5 to 5 MHz) waves are generated by the application of changing voltage to a substance called a *piezoelectric crystal*. This crystal deforms slightly under the influence of the voltage, and a sound wave is generated. The waves are generated in short bursts (e.g., 1 microsecond), after which the transducer operates as a receiver for the remainder of 1 millisecond, then another short burst of sound is generated and received (Fig. 16-2). These sound waves cannot be heard or felt by the patient and produce no known damaging effect on tissues.

The speed of sound through any medium is determined by the density of the medium; denser media transmit sound faster than less dense media. Whenever the ultrasound wave strikes a change in tissue density (such as that between blood and muscle or between soft tissue and bone), a portion of the wave is reflected back to the transducer. The density differences within the body are relatively minor. This means that the speed of the sound wave can be assumed to be nearly constant, and therefore the time between sound emission and sound detection can be used to calculate the distance between the transducer and the reflected tissue interface. The intensity of returning sound is greatest when the tissue interface is perpendicular to the sound beam and least when parallel to the sound beam.

When the ultrasound signal returns to the crystal, it once again deforms it and thereby generates a voltage. This voltage is detected by the echocardiograph, processed by a computer, and displayed on an oscilloscope or on recording paper.

The transducer sound beam is like a flashlight beam shined into a darkened room. Changes in the angulation of the transducer demonstrate different structures or parts of structures. If the objects in the room are stationary, then moving the flashlight through several degrees of arc illuminates each of the objects in the room.

For moving structures like the heart, such a system would result in an unclear sound signal because, over a period of time, the distance from transducer to tissue density interface would change continuously. This problem was first solved by the development of what is called *M-mode* (*M* for *motion*) *echocardiography*. A schematic representation of an M-mode scan is shown in Figure 16-3. In this figure, the transducer is slowly rotated on the chest wall, as shown in Figure 16-4. The contours in the M-mode tracing are caused by cardiac motion relative to the transducer and thus bear little resemblance to our usual visual image of the heart. On an M-mode scan, time is on the horizontal axis,

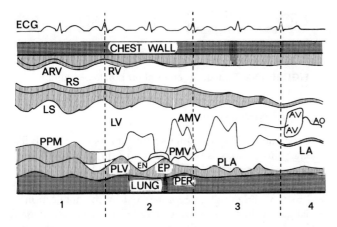

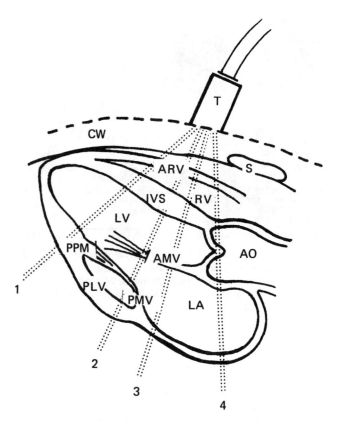

FIGURE 16-3 Schematic representation of an echocardiogram from the four transducer positions, illustrated in Figure 16-4. *ARV*, anterior right ventricular wall; *RS*, right side of interventricular septum; *LS*, left side of ventricular septum; *PPM*, posterior papillary muscle; *RV*, right ventricle; *LV*, left ventricle; *PLV*, posterior left ventricular wall; *EN*, endocardium; *EP*, epicardium; *PER*, pericardium; *AMV*, anterior mitral valve leaflet; *PMV*, posterior mitral valve leaflet; *PLA*, posterior left atrial wall; *AV*, aortic valve cusps; *AO*, aorta; *LA*, left atrium. (Adapted from Feigenbaum H: Clinical application of echocardiography. Prog Cardiovasc Dis 14: 531, 1972.)

and the distance from the tissue density interface to the transducer is on the vertical axis.

Two-dimensional (2-D) echocardiography is a further refinement on this technique. In 2-D echocardiography, the transducer sender-detector rotates mechanically or electrically through several degrees of arc. The resulting image, which is displayed on a video screen and recorded on videotape, represents a tomographic "slice" of cardiac structures, more closely resembling actual cardiac anatomy. Incorrect positioning or beam angulation, however, can significantly alter the appearance in 2-D echocardiography and obscure diagnostic information. Just as the body can be examined from several different views, so the cardiac anatomy can be viewed from several acoustic "windows." Because sound waves are diffused by air (lung) and totally reflected by bone (ribs), only a few surface locations on the chest and abdomen can be used for examination of the heart. The most common of these are shown in Figures 16-5 through 16-10, with the usual images they produce. Many modifications of these views are routinely used by experienced sonographers.

Echocardiographic measurements are frequently obtained from the M-mode images because the resolution is usually better than that on the corresponding 2-D study. The exact methods of measuring the dimensions or motion of each structure are standardized by convention. Because of anatomic variation, all such measurements cannot be obtained in all patients, so some parameters may be evaluated by general appearance rather than by exact measurement.

DOPPLER ECHOCARDIOGRAPHY

The *Doppler principle* states that the frequency of sound emitted or reflected from the moving object is changed in a

FIGURE 16-4 Schematic representation of the course of the ultrasonic beam to achieve the echo represented in Figure 16-3. *CW*, chest wall; *T*, transducer; *S*, sternum. Other abbreviations are defined in the legend to Figure 16-3. (Adapted from Feigenbaum H: Clinical application of echocardiography. Prog Cardiovasc Dis 14: 531, 1972.)

predictable way by the motion of the object. When the object moves toward the detector, the frequency increases; when the object moves away from the detector, the frequency decreases. This principle is best illustrated by the change in pitch (sound frequency) detected as a whistling train approaches and then recedes. In clinical Doppler, sound waves are reflected off moving red blood cells. The Doppler frequency shift is in the audible range and can be displayed as an audible signal or as a spectral image graphed with frequency on the vertical axis and time on the horizontal axis (Fig. 16-11). The Doppler waveform is recorded with the same transducer used for 2-D and M-mode echocardiography (in most instances). It can be adjusted to "listen" at a certain point in the 2-D image so as to "hear" blood flow velocity at that point in a process known as *pulsed Doppler.* Alternatively, the transducer may "listen" for all the velocities generated along the line of the sound beam. Technical aspects govern the choice between these two modes. Doppler shift is greatest when flow is exactly parallel to the sound beam (in contrast to M-mode or 2-D echocardiography). The magnitude of the frequency shift is related to the flow velocity increase across the area (valve orifice, outflow tract) by the formula: $P = 4V^2$, where P is the peak pressure gradient across the orifice and V is the velocity (in meters per second) of the sampled red blood cells. The timing of the waveform (systolic versus diastolic)

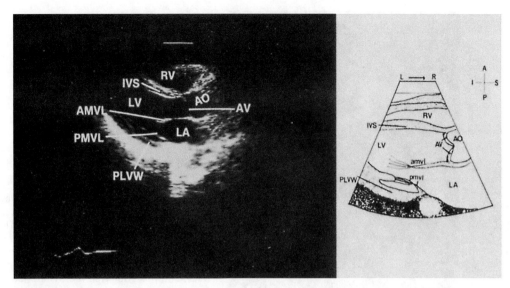

FIGURE 16-5 Parasternal long-axis view of the left ventricle. Still frame **(left)** with schematic drawing **(right)** of the long-axis left ventricular view. The aorta (*AO*) and aortic valve (*AV*) are seen at the right of the screen, and the left ventricle (*LV*) is at the left. The interventricular septum (*IVS*) is relatively horizontal and continuous with the anterior wall of the aorta. The right ventricle (*RV*) is anterior, and the posterior left ventricular wall (*PLVW*) and the left atrium (*LA*) are posterior. The anterior mitral valve leaflet (*AMVL*) and the posterior mitral valve leaflet (*PMVL*) are seen in the center of the picture. (From Levine RB, Brown SA, Janko C et al: Two-Dimensional and Doppler Echocardiographic Technique, p 8. Seattle, University of Washington, 1984.)

is determined from the superimposed ECG. By convention, flow toward the transducer is indicated as a positive waveform and flow away from the transducer as a negative waveform. Thus, Doppler can record the location, timing, direction, and magnitude of blood flow velocity.

Color Doppler transforms sectors of recorded flow signals into different colors that are then superimposed on the real-time 2-D image. By convention, red is used for signals moving toward the transducer and blue is used for signals moving away from the transducer. The intensity of the color

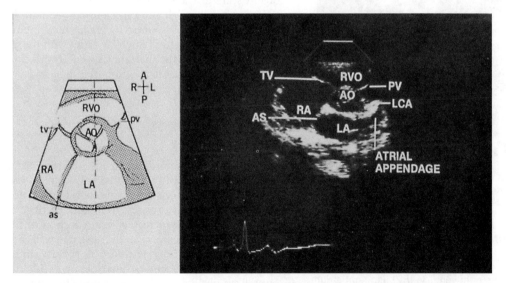

FIGURE 16-6 Parasternal short-axis view at level of great vessels. Still frame **(right)** with schematic drawing **(left)** of the short-axis great vessels view. The right ventricular outflow tract (*RVO*) is seen anteriorly, and the aorta (*AO*) with the three aortic valve leaflets is noted in the center of the picture. The left atrium (*LA*) is beneath the aorta, with the interatrial septum (*AS*) usually identifiable. The tricuspid valve (*TV*) is noted to the left of the screen, and the pulmonic valve (*PV*) is frequently seen to the right. *LCA*, left coronary artery. (From Levine RB, Brown SA, Janko C et al: Two-Dimensional and Doppler Echocardiographic Technique, p 21. Seattle, University of Washington, 1984.)

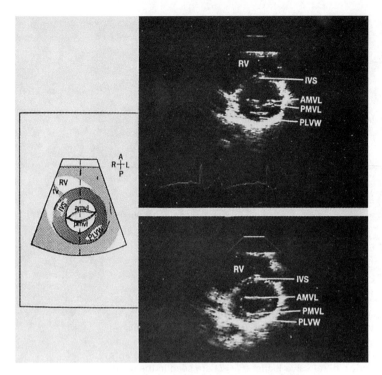

FIGURE 16-7 Parasternal short-axis view at level of mitral valve. Still frames **(right)** with schematic drawing **(left)** of the short-axis mitral valve view. The anterior and posterior mitral valve leaflets (*AMVL* and *PMVL*) are seen with the left ventricle posterior to the right ventricle (*RV*). The left ventricular walls, interventricular septum (*IVS*), and posterior wall (*PLVW*) are identified. The still frame on the top shows the mitral valve leaflets closed in systole. The still frame on the bottom shows the mitral valve leaflets open in diastole. (From Levine RB, Brown SA, Janko C et al: Two-Dimensional and Doppler Echocardiographic Technique, p 15. Seattle, University of Washington, 1984.)

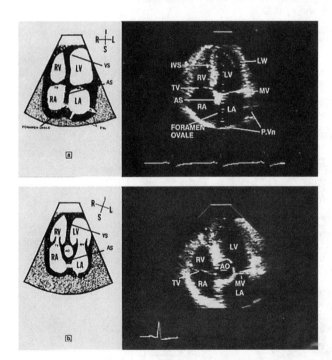

FIGURE 16-8 Apical four-chamber view. Still frames **(right)** with schematic drawings **(left)** of the apical views. The upper panel shows the four-chamber view. The left ventricle (*LV*) and left atrium (*LA*) appear on the right of the screen, with the mitral valve (*MV*) between the two. The right ventricle (*RV*) and right atrium (*RA*) are on the left, with the tricuspid valve (*TV*) between them. The interventricular septum (*IVS*) is seen at the top center of the screen, extending inferiorly and continuous with the interatrial septum (*AS*). Note the clear space at the level of the foramen ovale and the pulmonary veins (*P.Vn*) entering the left atrium. *AO*, aorta; *LW*, left ventricular wall. (From Levine RB, Brown SA, Janko C et al: Two-Dimensional and Doppler Echocardiographic Technique, p 27. Seattle, University of Washington, 1984.)

indicates velocity, with faster signals appearing lighter and slower signals appearing darker. Turbulence is indicated by a mosaic color pattern or by color mixture (e.g., green, yellow). Because an entire sector is imaged, color Doppler is much less tedious than pulsed Doppler mapping and is useful as a screening tool for valvular regurgitation. Good-quality scans give a sense of the pattern of blood flow within the chamber through the cardiac cycle. A high degree of sonographer skill is required to obtain meaningful images because the color pattern intensity varies with the gain (sensitivity) settings on the machine as well as with the severity of the lesion. Standardization of recording and interpretation is still evolving.

Diagnostic Aspects

LEFT VENTRICLE

In high-quality echocardiograms, the endocardial and epicardial surfaces of both the posterior LV wall and the interventricular septum can be measured. The thickness measured in diastole correlates well with actual anatomic thickness and, when increased, is a reflection of LV hypertrophy. The distance between the posterior wall and septum in the parasternal long-axis view is the LV intracavitary dimension. This dimension increases with LV dilatation. Overall systolic function can be assessed from the difference between end-diastolic and end-systolic dimensions as seen from several 2-D views; segmental wall motion abnormalities, as may occur in coronary heart disease (CHD), and myocardial thinning, as may occur after myocardial infarction (MI), may be evident. Differences in myocardial function before and after exercise can increase the diagnostic accuracy of exercise testing (discussed later).

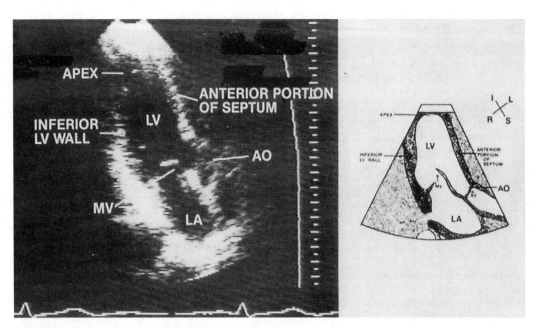

FIGURE 16-9 Apical long-axis view. Still frame **(left)** with schematic drawing **(right)** of the apical long-axis view of the left ventricle. The apex of the left ventricle is seen at the top of the screen with the left atrium (*LA*) at the bottom. The anterior portion of the septum is on the right, and the inferior left ventricular wall is on the left. The anterior mitral valve leaflet and posterior mitral valve leaflet are clearly demonstrated. The aortic root (*AR*) and aortic valve (*AV*) are seen on the right and inferiorly. *MV*, mitral valve. (From Levine RB, Brown SA, Janko C et al: Two-Dimensional and Doppler Echocardiographic Technique, p 30. Seattle, University of Washington, 1984.)

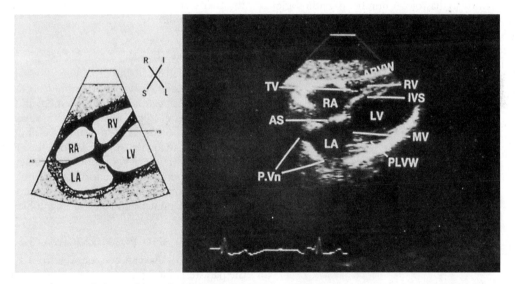

FIGURE 16-10 Subcostal four-chamber view. Still frame **(right)** with schematic drawing **(left)** of the subcostal four-chamber view. The right ventricle (*RV*) is seen at the top of the screen, with the left ventricle (*LV*) at the bottom toward the right. The ventricles are slightly foreshortened in this view. The interventricular septum (*IVS*), atrial septum (*AS*), mitral valve (*MV*), and tricuspid valve (*TV*) are readily apparent. The right atrium (*RA*) is seen at the left, with the left atrium (*LA*) below it. *ARVW*, anterior right ventricular wall; *PLVW*, posterior left ventricular wall; *P.Vn*, pulmonary veins. (From Levine RB, Brown SA, Janko C et al: Two-Dimensional and Doppler Echocardiographic Technique, p 33. Seattle, University of Washington, 1984.)

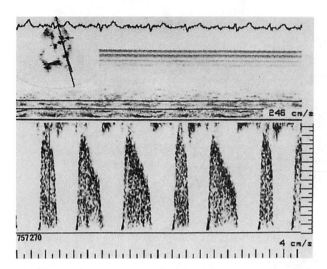

FIGURE 16-11 Doppler spectral display taken from the area of the mitral orifice, apical four-chamber view, in a patient with mitral stenosis. (From Feigenbaum H: Echocardiography, 4th ed. Philadelphia, Lea & Febiger, 1986.)

INTERVENTRICULAR SEPTUM

The interventricular septum should be assessed for both thickness (particularly as related to LV posterior wall thickness) and motion. Because the septum is normally functionally part of the left ventricle, it should move posteriorly in systole and anteriorly in diastole. A number of pathologic conditions can alter septal motion, including right ventricular (RV) volume or pressure overload and intraventricular conduction defects (left bundle-branch block). Interventricular septal motion is also altered after any sort of cardiac surgery involving opening of the pericardium.

In the absence of aortic insufficiency or outflow tract obstruction, the Doppler velocity of blood flow in the LV outflow tract can be a rough guide to cardiac output. Because the dimensions of the LV outflow tract change minimally throughout systole, the time—velocity integral in this area is primarily a reflection of the volume of blood ejected.

RIGHT VENTRICLE

As with the left ventricle, the right ventricle can be assessed for wall thickness, systolic function, and intracavitary dimension.

LEFT ATRIUM

Left atrial (LA) dimension is assessed from the parasternal long-axis view, but it is also seen well on the apical four-chamber view. Increases in LA dimension usually reflect increases in LA pressure or volume, as may occur with mitral valve disease (either stenosis or regurgitation), increased LV pressure, or normally with advancing age. Rarely, echo-producing structures, such as clot or tumor, can be seen in the left atrium. In the apical four-chamber view, LA size can be used as a general guide to right atrial size.

MITRAL VALVE

The mitral valve is usually the most vigorously moving structure on both the 2-D and M-mode echocardiogram and can serve as a marker for orienting the observer. The motion of the mitral valve is determined by the difference in pressure between the left atrium and the left ventricle over the course of the cardiac cycle. In the case of a pliable valve, Doppler LV inflow velocity as recorded at the mitral orifice parallels the motion of the mitral valve. Abnormal motion is seen in some forms of mitral valve disease, with decreased or increased cardiac output, with LV diastolic noncompliance (a normal finding in the very elderly), and with cardiac rhythm disturbance such as atrial fibrillation. Multiple dense echoes may be recorded in the region of the mitral valve, corresponding to mitral annular or valvular calcification.

AORTIC ROOT

Measurements of the diameter of the aortic root are made from the parasternal long-axis view. Aortic root dilatation occurs to some extent with aging and in some pathologic conditions such as Marfan's syndrome. It can also occur in conjunction with aortic stenosis or insufficiency. The amplitude of the aortic root excursion is a reflection of the force and volume of LV systolic ejection. Aortic root dissection can be diagnosed from the presence of an additional linear structure moving parallel to the anterior and posterior aortic walls.[1] The abnormal anatomic relation of the aortic root to other cardiac structures helps define some forms of congenital heart disease.

AORTIC VALVE

The aortic valve can be visually assessed from parasternal long- and short-axis views. It should be thin, pliable, and trileaflet. Calcification, valve thickening, and mild limitation in mobility are commonly seen with advancing age. The presence of a bicuspid aortic valve is well demonstrated on a technically adequate study. Diastolic flow disturbance may be recorded in the LV outflow tract when aortic insufficiency is present; aortic stenosis can be quantitated and an accurate estimate of aortic valve area obtained from a combination of Doppler and echocardiographic techniques.

TRICUSPID AND PULMONIC VALVES

The tricuspid valve can be seen well from a modification of the parasternal long-axis view and also from the apical four-chamber view. It should be thin and pliable. Tricuspid regurgitation can be imaged by Doppler sampling in the right atrium. The velocity of tricuspid regurgitation increases with increasing pulmonary pressure. The pulmonic valve can often be imaged from a modification of the parasternal short-axis view. Its motion resembles that of the aortic valve. The Doppler waveform is characteristically more symmetric (i.e., rate of rise approximately equal to rate of decline). When pulmonary hypertension is present, the waveform looks more like an aortic or arterial waveform, which has a more rapid rate of rise than rate of decline.

PERICARDIUM

The posterior parietal pericardial echo is a thin line behind the epicardial LV posterior wall and is often the brightest interface seen on the echocardiogram. Multiple dense echoes arising from this structure can be seen with pericardial thickening; however, echocardiography is usually somewhat insensitive to this unless it is severe. An echolucent space between the epicardium and pericardium anteriorly, inferiorly, or posteriorly can be seen with a pericardial effusion. A pericardial fat pad may be indistinguishable from a small anterior effusion. Tiny pericardial effusions without tamponade are frequent in congestive heart failure, renal failure, and reduced serum proteins of any cause (severe generalized volume excess, malnutrition).

STRESS ECHOCARDIOGRAPHY

The two techniques of exercise (bicycle or treadmill) testing and echocardiography can be used together to increase the diagnostic accuracy of standard exercise testing. In this technique, four standard echocardiographic views (parasternal long axis, parasternal short axis, apical four chamber, apical two chamber) are obtained with ECG gating before exercise testing and displayed on a single screen image as a "cine loop" or single recurring cardiac cycle. Stress testing is performed in the standard fashion, and the four views are obtained rapidly during the first 90 seconds of recovery. The images can then be shuffled or reformatted with computer-assisted techniques to juxtapose the pre-exercise and postexercise images from each view. The normal response to exercise is an increase in contractility. Areas of hypoperfusion appear normal on the rest images and become relatively hypokinetic with exercise. Areas of infarction show hypokinesis or akinesis at rest and with exercise. In stress echocardiography, it is extremely important to obtain all the images within the shortest possible period of time after exercise. Patients must be carefully coached to assist the sonographer by breathing properly during this image acquisition sequence.

In patients who are unable to perform exercise, progressively increasing doses of dobutamine can be infused, beginning at 5 μg/kg/min and increasing to as much as 40 μg/kg/min in stepwise fashion. The same echocardiographic views are serially recorded. Atropine can be used in small doses for heart rate augmentation in patients who fail to achieve an adequate heart rate response with dobutamine alone. Cardiac response to dobutamine closely approximates that which would be expected from exercise. Exercise echocardiography and dobutamine stress echocardiography are extremely sensitive for two- and three-vessel disease and somewhat more sensitive than standard exercise testing for single-vessel disease.

TRANSESOPHAGEAL ECHOCARDIOGRAPHY

A piezoelectric crystal can be mounted on an endoscope, replacing the fiberoptics used by the gastroenterologist to view the upper gastrointestinal tract. Echocardiographic images are obtained from within the esophagus or stomach and are often of much higher quality than transthoracic images because of elimination of acoustic impedance from ribs, sternum, and air-filled lungs. Obviously, this procedure is somewhat more invasive than standard transthoracic echocardiography. The complications relate primarily to the esophageal intubation and include trauma to the oropharynx, esophagus, or stomach; hypoxemia; aspiration; and rare vagal reaction. It is essential to have one practitioner, often a cardiac or gastroenterology nurse, devoted to monitoring the patient. Most complications can be prevented by careful manipulation of the scope by experienced operators, meticulous attention to airway management, appropriate sedation of the patient, and continuous oxygen and ECG monitoring.

Technique

The oropharynx is anesthetized, and the patient is given sufficient sedation to be relaxed but not asleep because patient cooperation to swallow the endoscope is necessary. The operator may prefer the sitting or the left lateral decubitus position for scope introduction. The scope is advanced to the stomach, where flexion of the tip allows imaging of the heart through the stomach wall and diaphragm. The endoscope is then slowly withdrawn and views of cardiac structures are obtained at several levels in the esophagus in various 2-D planes. The endoscope can be rotated on withdrawal to survey the ascending aorta. The entire procedure usually takes approximately 15 to 20 minutes.

Indications

Transesophageal echocardiography is indicated when views obtained from transthoracic windows are of inadequate diagnostic quality. It is also indicated for several specific conditions in which the transesophageal approach has been shown to be more sensitive or to provide information that would not be shown on a transesophageal study. These include bacterial endocarditis, aortic dissection, regurgitation through or around a prosthetic mitral or tricuspid valve, LA thrombus (particularly involving the LA appendage), intracardiac source of embolus in stroke or systemic embolization, interatrial septal defect, and in some forms of congenital heart disease.

Transesophageal echocardiography is used for continuous monitoring of myocardial function during cardiac surgery and noncardiac surgery in patients with heart disease. During cardiac surgery, transesophageal echocardiography is routinely used to confirm the adequacy and competence of mitral valve repair before the chest is closed. In coronary artery bypass surgery, the left ventricle can be surveyed before and after revascularization for segmental wall function. During noncardiac surgery in patients with known CHD, transesophageal echocardiography can be used to survey for wall motion abnormalities that may indicate the presence of myocardial ischemia.

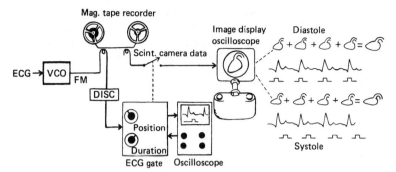

FIGURE 16-12 Diagrammatic representation of computer-assisted radioisotope ventriculography. ECG, electrocardiograph. (Adapted from Kostuk WJ, Ehsani AA, Karliner JS et al: Left ventricular performance after myocardial infarction assessed by radioisotope angiocardiography. Circulation 47: 242, 1973. By permission of the American Heart Association, Inc.)

RADIOISOTOPE EVALUATION OF THE HEART

Radionuclides, substances that emit radioactivity, have been used as tracers in the body for more than 60 years. Over the past 30 years, since the development of the gamma (γ)-ray camera by Anger, the use of radionuclides to study the heart has been the subject of much research. The great interest in these techniques has been stimulated by scientific advances in the fields of nuclear engineering, computer technology, and radiopharmaceuticals.

Technical Aspects

Radionuclides are atoms in an unstable form. They have a finite probability of spontaneously converting to a more stable configuration. When they do so, small amounts of energy in the form of γ-rays are emitted. The rate at which atoms in a given sample undergo this conversion is denoted by the half-life, the time required for one-half of the sample to undergo the conversion. Half-lives of radioactive substances may vary from a fraction of a second to millennia; the half-life for any given radionuclide is always the same. In nuclear studies of the heart, certain radionuclides have gained popularity primarily because their half-lives are appropriate for study, because of their ability to be combined with biologic substances, and because of the ease with which they can be acquired and stored. Two common radionuclides used in cardiac examination are thallium-201 and technetium-99m methoxyisobutyl isonitrile (sestamibi).

The radioactive decay is detected outside the body as a scintillation (flash of light); the detector is a γ-scintillation camera. The camera can function as a scanning device to detect the distribution of radioactivity in relatively stationary structures (as in the lung scan) or, when used with cardiac rhythm gating, can be adjusted to examine cardiac function and structure. Most examinations of the heart are now done as single-photon emission computed tomography, which yields imaging information in a format somewhat similar to radiographic computed tomography.

Clinical Applications

MYOCARDIAL FUNCTION

The changing intracardiac blood pool through the cardiac cycle (Fig. 16-12) can be imaged to obtain information about myocardial global and regional function. The computer uses the ECG signal for timing (*gating*) and divides the cardiac cycle into many small segments. Each of these segments is surveyed individually for radioactivity, and then radioactive scintillation counts from corresponding time segments are summed to augment image clarity. In this way, the manner in which the radioactivity (and hence the blood pool) changes over the cardiac cycle is demonstrated.[3] This summed cardiac cycle can be played back as a cine loop video display of a normally recurring cardiac cycle. LV and RV ejection fraction and segmental wall performance are obtained (Fig. 16-13). The video display resembles a contrast LV or RV angiogram. Variation in radioactive counts over time is analyzed to provide information about diastolic as well as systolic function. Valvular regurgitation and its severity, quantification of intracardiac shunts, and distinction of pericardial constriction from restrictive cardiomy-

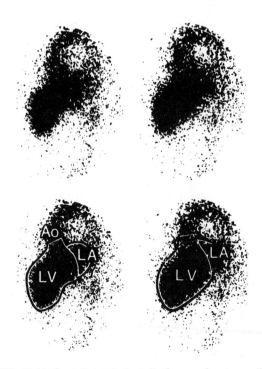

FIGURE 16-13 Systolic and diastolic frames from a radioisotope angiogram. AO, aorta; LA, left atrium; LV, left ventricle. (Adapted from Kostuk WJ, Ehsani AA, Karliner JS et al: Left ventricular performance after myocardial infarction assessed by radioisotope angiocardiography. Circulation 47: 244, 1973. By permission of the American Heart Association, Inc.)

opathy are all obtainable from blood pool studies. Rhythm disturbances such as atrial fibrillation or frequent premature contractions alter beat-to-beat filling and cycle length and may decrease quantitative accuracy.

MYOCARDIAL PERFUSION IMAGING

Thallium-201 is a radionuclide that behaves like potassium in the body. Because there is a dynamic equilibrium for potassium between cells and the blood pool, potassium and therefore thallium-201 distribute in myocardium in proportion to blood flow. "Cold" spots on resting images correspond to areas of reduced blood flow that occur in MI or severe resting ischemia. Technetium-99m can be complexed with a variety of ligands and used for similar imaging. Technetium has a shorter half-life and yields higher counts per unit time. This makes multiple injections on the same day possible. Paired rest—exercise studies are performed to evaluate transient ischemia. In this method, patients are exercised to a maximal level, which induces a relative (expected physiologic) hyperemia through normal, patent coronary arteries. At this point, the radioisotope is injected and initial scanning shows a discrepancy between these hyperemic areas served by normal vessels and areas with relatively less radioactivity fed by partially obstructed vessels. After recovery from exercise, the patients are rescanned. At this point, the radionuclide has redistributed proportional to the blood flow, which is similar at rest in all areas served by patent (even though stenotic) coronary arteries. Because there is no exercise-induced hyperemia, the heart once again shows a relatively homogeneous uptake of radioactivity.

Dual isotope protocols using thallium-201 for the rest images and technetium-99m sestamibi for the exercise images are used routinely. In addition to increasing greatly the clinical identification and quantification of coronary artery disease, these examinations predict the probability of serious cardiac events occurring within the ensuing year.[2] Radionuclide exercise testing is particularly helpful when ECG criteria for ischemia are unreliable or not applicable (e.g., in left bundle-branch block, LV hypertrophy, digitalis therapy).

POSITRON EMISSION TOMOGRAPHY

Myocardial Metabolism Scanning

Some radionuclides emit positrons rather than γ-rays. In the body, the positron travels a short distance after emission and interacts with an electron. This interaction causes annihilation of both particles, which are converted to high-energy photons that depart at an angle of 180 degrees from each other. Scintillation detectors are complexed with a computer and require the simultaneous detection of both photons, thus giving high-resolution planar images or even three-dimensional images. A positron-emitting carbon can be complexed to palmitic acid to image free fatty acid metabolism in the heart (fatty acids are the heart's primary fuel; thus, areas of transient ischemia show reduced uptake during ischemia and augmented accumulation with reper-

fusion, and areas of infarct show decreased uptake chronically). These positron emitters can be complexed to glucose to measure myocardial uptake of exogenous glucose, which appears to increase during ischemia. This technology requires a cyclotron to generate the tracers, which usually are short-lived; thus, widespread application of the technique is limited by the cost of the required generating and detection equipment. Positron emitters will, no doubt, contribute to our understanding of myocardial metabolism in various normal and pathologic states.

Risks of Radionuclides

In contrast to radioactive substances used for therapeutic (tissue ablation) purposes, radiopharmaceuticals used for imaging have short half-lives (minutes to several hours), contributing to their decay in the body and are used in small amounts. Thus, there is no need to isolate patients who have had these studies, and no particular precautions are needed for disposal of body substances (urine, stool). The risk to a fetus is likely to be small, but pregnant personnel should remember that radioactivity decreases dramatically with distance from the source and that prolonged close-range contact with patients soon after a study should be avoided. Radiopharmaceuticals are always protected in lead containers or handled with lead protection. Personnel who work in nuclear medicine departments wear detecting badges like those worn by radiology personnel to monitor their exposure.

ELECTRON BEAM COMPUTED TOMOGRAPHY

Electron beam computed tomography, also referred to as *ultrafast computed tomography,* uses a much larger generator of x-rays than is used in the standard radiograph or computed tomography scan. This results in much faster image acquisition with a higher degree of resolution. EBCT technology has been used to detect microcalcifications in the coronary arteries. This presence and magnitude of coronary calcification correlate strongly with the presence of hemodynamically significant coronary stenosis. This modality appears most useful for identifying early coronary artery disease at a time when clinically significant stenosis has not yet occurred. Such patients would have negative exercise tests but probably should be targeted for aggressive risk factor control.

Electron beam computed tomography is not yet widely used, but it has great potential to improve rapid and exact diagnostic imaging in a variety of suspected conditions such as pulmonary embolus, diseases of the great vessels, pericardial disease, and congenital heart disease.

MAGNETIC RESONANCE IMAGING

Magnetic resonance imaging is one of the newer techniques for anatomic imaging. It is based on the observation that atoms (usually those with odd numbers of protons and neutrons) have a net nuclear spin. This spin can be disturbed by the application of radiofrequency pulses from a large and powerful magnet. When the magnet is turned off, the nuclei return to their initial spin state in a process known as *relaxation*. This relaxation generates a small amount of energy, which can be detected and evaluated mathematically from two different planes (T1, T2). The spectroscopic imaging of the relaxation of various molecules can be used with computer signal processing and ECG gating to produce high-resolution images of the heart that reflect local metabolism as well as anatomic structures. Because the magnet is extremely powerful, patients with any metal implanted prostheses (joints, plates) may be at risk for dislodgment of these devices. In addition, pacemaker reed switches may be moved from demand to fixed-rate mode when the patient is near the magnet. MRI is an attractive modality because of the potential for examining physiology (metabolism) as well as anatomy and because of its totally noninvasive nature. Its place in the armamentarium of cardiac tests remains undetermined, although vigorous research in this area is underway and should result in some unique applications of this technology. MRI is somewhat limited by long data acquisition times, but newer system advances will most likely overcome this limitation.

PHONOCARDIOGRAPHY

In phonocardiography, one or more sound-sensitive transducers are placed on the chest so that they can detect the externally audible heart sounds. The impulses thus obtained are recorded on graph paper along with the ECG. Because heart sounds come in a variety of frequencies, from 20 to 400 cycles/s, microphones of different sensitivities can be used so that all audible events may be recorded.

Phonocardiography has been used with various other external recording methods, such as apexcardiography, echocardiography, and carotid pulse recordings. This is done to obtain objective documentation and graphic display of the various physical findings that the experienced examiner may observe (Fig. 16-14).

Phonocardiography has been used as a research tool with intracardiac pressure monitoring and other simultaneously recorded data in deducing the exact origins of normal and abnormal heart sounds. It is also occasionally used to document auscultatory findings.

Phonocardiography is probably most useful as an education tool. The phonocardiogram offers a graphic display of the relative timing and duration of cardiac sounds and assists the student in developing the ability to discriminate not only the presence or absence of sounds, but also the relative intensities, duration, and timing within the cardiac cycle. Because the exact nature of the heart sounds as recorded by the phonocardiogram rarely has clinical importance over the observations that can be made by the experienced clinician, and because the instrumentation requires a certain degree of technical expertise, phonocardiography remains a technique primarily of research and education.

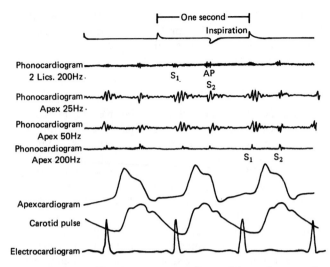

FIGURE 16-14 Simultaneous recordings of four phonocardiograms, with apex and carotid impulses and electrocardiogram simultaneously recorded. AP, apical pulse. (Adapted from Seigel W: In Hurst JW, Logue RB, Schlant RC et al (eds): The Heart. New York, McGraw-Hill, 1978.)

IMAGING IN CARDIAC PATHOLOGY

Cardiomyopathy

Cardiomyopathy is a general term that indicates pathologic changes involving the heart muscle. These changes are almost always associated with systolic dysfunction, occasionally with diastolic dysfunction, and at times with massive LV or RV dilatation. These abnormalities are usually easily appreciated on standard echocardiography but can also be demonstrated by EBCT and MRI.

CONGESTIVE CARDIOMYOPATHY

Congestive cardiomyopathy can occur in diffuse CHD, in response to alcohol or other toxins such as anthracycline drugs used in cancer chemotherapy, or in a variety of degenerative, metabolic, nutritional, infectious, and genetic disorders involving the myocardial cells. Most patients with congestive cardiomyopathy that is not due to CHD or valvular disease have no specific etiology identified. The diagnosis of congestive cardiomyopathy is supported by an echocardiogram that shows increased LV intracavitary dimensions with a decrease in ventricular wall motion. Global systolic dysfunction can be seen with CHD and, conversely, segmental wall motion abnormalities are occasionally seen when cardiomyopathy is of a non-CHD etiology. The mitral valve shows decreased opening amplitude due to reduced rate and volume of flow, reflecting the small difference in pressure between left atrium and left ventricle during diastole; the left atrium is often dilated; LV outflow tract velocity on Doppler imaging may be reduced, reflecting decreased cardiac output; and Doppler assay of the atrium may show mitral or tricuspid regurgitation. Small pericardial effusions are occasionally seen. The presence of poor LV function with good RV function usually indicates a CHD etiology.

HYPERTROPHIC CARDIOMYOPATHY

Hypertrophic cardiomyopathy occurs in conditions of increased LV afterload (aortic stenosis or systemic hypertension) but may also occur as an idiopathic or genetic disorder or in conjunction with rare diseases such as progressive systemic sclerosis. The echocardiographic findings are increased wall thickness, usually with normal or reduced intracavitary dimensions. Diastolic flow velocity across the mitral valve may be low in early diastole and high with atrial systole (the opposite of that normally seen). LA enlargement is usually present. A subtype of hypertrophic cardiomyopathy is idiopathic hypertrophic subaortic stenosis. In this disorder, the ventricular septum is disproportionately thick and may cause obstruction of the LV outflow tract during systole. Echocardiographic findings include disproportionate septal thickening, narrowing of the outflow tract, abnormal motion of the anterior mitral leaflet during systole, and mid-systolic closure of the aortic valve as the obstruction begins. There may be an acceleration in Doppler velocity between the LV cavity and outflow tract, reflecting the pressure gradient across the obstruction.

INFILTRATIVE CARDIOMYOPATHY

Infiltrative cardiomyopathy is characterized by abnormal echocardiographic texture of the LV muscle, normal or increased LV wall thickness, normal or reduced LV intracavitary dimension, often LA enlargement, and correlative findings of the infiltrative substance (e.g., amyloid, iron) on biopsy of heart or other tissues.

Valvular Heart Disease

All four cardiac valves may display congenital or acquired abnormalities that can be assessed by a combination of echocardiography and Doppler imaging.

MITRAL STENOSIS

Mitral stenosis almost always occurs secondary to rheumatic disease and is characterized by calcification of the leaflet tips, variable mobility of the leaflet bellies, thickening and fusion of the chordae tendineae, and LA enlargement due to chronic LA pressure overload. The LV cavity is often small, and measurements reflective of cardiac output (LV outflow velocity) may be reduced. Doppler shows increased velocity through the mitral orifice. The mitral valve area, as would be measured at cardiac catheterization, can be estimated from the time required for the velocity of this signal to diminish by half. This measurement is termed the *mitral pressure half-time*. Calculation of valve area using this measurement correlates well with invasive assessment and is independent of flow across the valve. Patients with mitral stenosis often have associated mitral regurgitation. They may also have pulmonary hypertension (discussed later).

MITRAL REGURGITATION

Mitral regurgitation occurs in a variety of pathologic conditions that involve the mitral valve, its annulus, or its support apparatus. No 2-D or M-mode findings are pathognomonic for mitral regurgitation unless it is the result of chordal rupture and flail mitral leaflet. In this instance, the mitral leaflet may be seen flickering into the left atrium during ventricular systole. The degree of LA enlargement is a function of the chronicity and severity of mitral regurgitation as well as the presence of associated conditions (LV diastolic dysfunction, mitral stenosis). Mitral regurgitation can be roughly quantified by the area of the left atrium over which the mitral regurgitation Doppler signal can be recorded. Because this represents a chronic volume overload for the left ventricle, LV dilatation with increased LV wall motion may be found with moderate or severe mitral regurgitation. Tiny amounts of mitral regurgitation are often seen in normal people. Mitral regurgitation can be detected with first-pass radionuclide studies.

MITRAL VALVE PROLAPSE

Mitral valve prolapse is a condition in which diagnosis depends primarily on physical examination findings but in which the echocardiographic findings provide strong supportive data. The 2-D images are characterized by prolapse of the mitral leaflets into the left atrium during ventricular systole. The leaflets may be large, thickened, or redundant; mitral regurgitation of variable degree may be present. Abnormal valve motion with minimal or no structural change may be seen in otherwise normal young adults; the distinction between this relatively benign condition and true myxomatous degeneration of the valve should be made when possible.

AORTIC STENOSIS

The diagnosis of aortic stenosis can be suspected, but not confirmed, on M-mode and 2-D studies by the presence of a thickened, immobile aortic valve. The Doppler velocity in the LV outflow tract compared with that in the ascending aorta can be used in a formula to estimate the aortic valve area. In many cases, this correlates closely with invasively determined valve area. Associated findings may include aortic insufficiency, LV hypertrophy, and a bicuspid rather than tricuspid valve.

AORTIC INSUFFICIENCY

Aortic insufficiency can be determined from the presence of characteristic diastolic flow disturbance in the LV outflow tract during diastole. Associated findings include signs of LV volume overload (chamber dilatation with increased wall motion). Fluttering of the anterior mitral leaflet on 2-D and M-mode studies occurs in cases in which the regurgitant jet strikes the leaflet during diastole (Fig. 16-15). When aortic regurgitation occurs acutely, as in aortic dissection or endocarditis, the left ventricle may not be dilated, the regurgitant jet may be recorded in early diastole only, and the mitral valve may close prematurely owing to the rapid rise in LV end-diastolic pressure in the noncompliant left ventricle.

PULMONIC INSUFFICIENCY

Pulmonic valvular insufficiency of a minor degree is observed frequently when pulsed Doppler imaging of the RV outflow tract is carefully performed. Pathologically, it

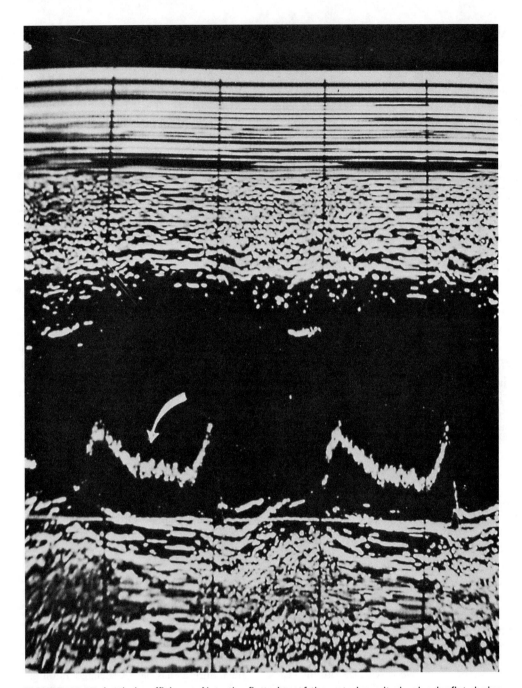

FIGURE 16-15 Aortic insufficiency. Note the fluttering of the anterior mitral valve leaflet during diastole due to the regurgitant jet of blood (*arrow*).

may occur in conjunction with congenital pulmonary valve abnormalities, pulmonary hypertension, and, rarely, endocarditis.

TRICUSPID REGURGITATION

Tricuspid regurgitation is imaged by Doppler in a fashion similar to mitral regurgitation. Because the amplitude of a Doppler waveform is a function of the pressure difference across the orifice, the velocity of the tricuspid regurgitation jet can be converted to a pressure gradient (see Doppler equation given previously). This value can be added to the clinically estimated right atrial pressure (central or jugular venous pressure) to estimate pulmonary artery systolic pressure. Pulmonary artery hypertension occurs in chronic left-sided pressure or volume overload, pulmonary disease (cor pulmonale), pulmonary embolus, and, rarely, as an idiopathic disorder.

PROSTHETIC CARDIAC VALVES

All prosthetic heart valves can be imaged using transthoracic echocardiography. The movement of mechanical parts or the leaflets of tissue valves can frequently but not always be imaged. Metal valve parts reflect back nearly 100% of the echo pulses, thus causing "shadows" or acoustic impedance preventing evaluation of structures or Doppler flow immediately behind the valve. Prosthetic valves are often better evaluated using transesophageal echocardiography. Transesophageal Doppler evaluation gives the best quantification of prosthetic or periprosthetic mitral insufficiency.

BACTERIAL ENDOCARDITIS

Bacterial endocarditis can be strongly suspected from a transthoracic echocardiogram showing highly mobile echogenic structures moving with the valve, particularly when associated with valvular incompetence. Transesophageal echocardiography has a higher diagnostic yield in identifying vegetations. The absence of vegetations, however, does not exclude the diagnosis.

PERICARDIAL DISEASE

As mentioned previously, pericardial disease can be suspected from a thickened pericardium, but detection and quantification are difficult with echocardiography and better appreciated with standard computed tomography, EBCT, or MRI. Pericardial effusion (with or without tamponade) is a diagnosis best made by 2-D echocardiography showing the echolucent space in the area of the effusion. Abnormalities in RV and right atrial motion indicating chamber collapse occur when tamponade is present, but clinical correlation is always needed. The echocardiogram can be used to direct pericardiocentesis.

Intracardiac Masses and Foreign Bodies

Intracardiac tumors and masses, LA myxomas, intraventricular or intra-atrial thrombi, intracavitary catheters, electrodes or other foreign bodies, and intramyocardial or intrapericardial tumors can be imaged with 2-D and M-mode echocardiography.

INTRACARDIAC SOURCE OF EMBOLUS

The heart is a prime suspect for origin of embolus in embolic stroke. Many such strokes arise in the left atrium in the presence of atrial fibrillation without other cardiac abnormalities. Unsuspected endocarditis or mural thrombi may be seen from a transthoracic echocardiogram. Diagnostic yield, however, is much higher with transesophageal echocardiography, which may identify LA appendage clot, interatrial septal aneurysm with or without atrial septal defect, or unidentified vegetations of endocarditis.

Echocardiographic contrast using a 10-mL bolus of agitated saline improves the possibility of identifying intracardiac shunts compared with Doppler interrogation alone. A patent foramen ovale or small atrial septal defect with right-to-left shunt can be the cause of a "paradoxical" cerebral or systemic embolus.

CORONARY HEART DISEASE WITH SEGMENTAL WALL MOTION ABNORMALITIES

Coronary disease is well evaluated with radionuclide studies, and coronary calcifications can be shown with EBCT. Segmental wall motion abnormalities (either transient or permanent) involving the left ventricle are easily appreciated on 2-D echocardiography as well. With good images, the origins of the right and left coronary ostia can be seen at the level of the aortic valve on parasternal short-axis views. Myocardial thinning from old MIs, as well as LV aneurysms or pseudoaneurysms, can be imaged.

CONCLUSION

Cardiac imaging is a rapidly expanding field of both clinical and research endeavor. Advances will continue to make the rapid, safe, and accurate identification of cardiac lesions easier. The clinician will ultimately have many testing modalities available, and intelligent use of the potential of these examinations, as well as the need for overall cost containment in the current health care milieu, will guide practice into the new century.

REFERENCES

1. Clark RD: Case Studies in Echocardiography. Philadelphia, WB Saunders, 1977
2. Hachamovitch R, Berman DS, Kiat H et al: Exercise myocardial perfusion SPECT in patients without known coronary artery disease. Circulation 93: 905—914, 1996
3. Kostuk WJ, Ehsani AA, Karliner JS et al: Left ventricular performance after myocardial infarction assessed by radioisotope angiocardiography. Circulation 47: 242—248, 1973

BIBLIOGRAPHY

Ashburn WL, Schelbert HR, Verba JW: Left ventricular ejection fraction: A review of several radionuclide angiographic approaches using the scintillation camera. Prog Cardiovasc Dis 20:267–284, 1978

Skorton DJ, Schelbert HR, Wolf GL, Brundage BH (eds). Marcus Cardiac Imaging, 2nd ed. Philadelphia, WB Saunders, 1996

Woods SL, Sivarajan Froelicher E, Halpenny CJ, Underhill Motzer S, (eds). Cardiac Nursing, 3rd ed. Philadelphia, JB Lippincott Company, 1995

Exercise Testing

JONATHAN MYERS

Exercise testing is a widely used, noninvasive procedure that provides diagnostic, prognostic, and functional information for a wide spectrum of patients with cardiovascular, pulmonary, and other disorders. Graded exercise tests are used to assess a patient's ability to tolerate increased physical activity while electrocardiographic, hemodynamic, and symptomatic responses are monitored in a controlled environment. Graded, progressive exercise can produce abnormalities that are not present at rest, the most important of which are manifestations of myocardial ischemia, including ST segment changes on the electrocardiogram, symptoms, and electrical instability. The test is also commonly used to evaluate other system disorders, such as gas exchange abnormalities in patients with pulmonary disease or chronic heart failure, symptoms associated with peripheral vascular disease, and even neurologic diseases.

In cardiovascular medicine, the exercise test is commonly used for evaluating the efficacy of medical therapy, for the assessment of interventions, and as a first-choice diagnostic tool in patients with suspected coronary artery disease (CAD), a role in which it functions as a "gatekeeper" to more expensive and invasive procedures.[50] In the latter role, the test has become even more important in the current era of health care cost containment. Although originally developed as a diagnostic tool, recent studies have established the role of the exercise test in the selection of patients for cardiac transplantation, risk stratification after a myocardial infarction (MI), and the assessment of disability.[17,22,65]

Because of the need to standardize the implementation and interpretation of the exercise test, professional organizations such as the American Heart Association (AHA), the American College of Cardiology (ACC),[22,83] the American College of Sports Medicine (ACSM),[2] and the American Association of Cardiovascular and Pulmonary Rehabilitation[1] have developed guidelines designed to optimize the test's safety, methodology, and objectives. The ACSM has developed certification programs for professional competency in exercise testing.[2,3] ACSM certification has been strongly recommended for nurses, technicians, or physiologists who oversee exercise testing in clinical settings.[3,36] This chapter describes the applications, methodology, and principles of exercise testing for the cardiovascular nurse and the professional standards for exercise testing described in the aforementioned guidelines.

INDICATIONS AND OBJECTIVES

The exercise test has numerous indications. Surveys have shown that the most common reason patients are referred for exercise testing is for the evaluation of chest pain[56] or, more generally, to assess signs and symptoms of coronary disease. Other common clinical objectives include the following to evaluate:

- Physiologic response of post-MI and postrevascularization patients to exercise
- Functional capacity for the purpose of exercise prescription
- Exercise capacity for the purpose of work classification (disability evaluation) and risk stratification (prognosis)
- The efficacy of medical, surgical, or pharmacologic treatment
- The presence and severity of arrhythmias
- Preoperative physiologic status
- Intermittent claudication

SAFETY AND PERSONNEL

Provided that contraindications to exercise testing are considered and patients who undergo exercise testing are appropriate, the test has been shown to be extremely safe. Widely cited data from the Cooper Clinic in Dallas[30] suggest that an event serious enough to require hospitalization (e.g., sustained arrhythmia, heart attack, or death) occurs at a rate of 0.8 per 10,000 tests. Earlier surveys conducted in the 1970s suggested a somewhat higher event rate, ranging in the order of 1 to 4 per 10,000.[24,26,80,90] It has been suggested that the apparent improvement in the safety of the test reflected in the more recent surveys is due to a significantly better understanding of when and when not to perform the test and when to terminate the test, and better preparation for any emergency that may arise.[22,24]

DISPLAY 17-1

Contraindications to Exercise Testing

ABSOLUTE

1. A recent change in the resting electrocardiogram suggesting infarction or other acute cardiac event
2. Recent complicated myocardial infarction
3. Unstable angina
4. Uncontrolled ventricular arrhythmia
5. Uncontrolled atrial arrhythmia that compromises cardiac function
6. Third-degree atrioventricular heart block without pacemaker
7. Acute congestive heart failure
8. Severe aortic stenosis
9. Suspected or known dissecting aneurysm
10. Active or suspected myocarditis or pericarditis
11. Thrombophlebitis or intracardiac thrombi
12. Recent systemic or pulmonary embolus
13. Acute infections
14. Significant emotional distress (psychosis)

RELATIVE

1. Resting diastolic blood pressure >115 mm Hg or resting systolic blood pressure >200 mm Hg
2. Moderate valvular heart disease
3. Known electrolyte abnormalities (hypokalemia, hypomagnesemia)
4. Fixed-rate pacemaker
5. Frequent or complex ectopy
6. Ventricular aneurysm
7. Uncontrolled metabolic disease (e.g.,diabetes, thyrotoxicosis, or myxedema)
8. Chronic infectious disease (e.g., mononucleosis or myxedema)
9. Neuromuscular, musculoskeletal, or rheumatoid disorders that are exacerbated by exercise
10. Advanced or complicated pregnancy

From American College of Sports Medicine: Guidelines for Exercise Testing and Prescription, 5th ed., p. 42. Philadelphia, Williams & Wilkins, 1998.

Clinical judgment is the most important consideration when deciding which patients should undergo exercise testing. Contraindications to testing usually describe conditions of cardiovascular instability, such as unstable angina, uncontrolled heart failure, and arrhythmias. A listing of the absolute and relative contraindications to testing is provided in Display 17-1.

Historically, professional guidelines have suggested that physician supervision was necessary for all exercise testing in the clinical setting. Given the remarkable safety record of exercise testing, particularly in recent years,[90] there is now some debate over the need for physician supervision for all exercise testing.[24] This has important implications for nursing because the nurse is frequently the person who prepares the patient and serves as the technician conducting the test, and in many centers may supervise the test as a surrogate for the physician. Although the recent AHA/ACC guidelines[22]

continue to recommend physician supervision when testing patients with heart disease in a clinical setting, the guidelines also state that ". . . exercise testing in selected patients can be safely performed by properly trained nurses, exercise physiologists, physical therapists, or medical technicians working directly under the supervision of a physician, who should be in the immediate vicinity and available for emergencies." The ACSM has outlined general guidelines for conditions in which physician supervision is recommended.[2] The nurse, physiologist, or technician conducting the test should have a comprehensive knowledge of the indications, contraindications, equipment, physiologic responses to exercise, and clinical condition of the patient to optimize the information yield and conduct the test safely.

A joint statement by the American College of Chest Physicians, the ACC, and the AHA regarding physician competence in exercise testing outlined the cognitive skills needed to perform exercise testing.[83] These included knowledge of indications and contraindications to testing, basic exercise physiology, principles of interpretation, and emergency procedures. The committee suggested that at least 50 procedures were required during training to achieve these skills. ACSM certification[2,3] is widely used to establish competency for technicians, nurses, or physiologists who oversee exercise testing and training.

PRETEST CONSIDERATIONS

Before an exercise test, all patients should undergo a complete medical history and a physical examination to identify contraindications to exercise testing.[22,26] If the reason the patient was referred for the test in unclear, it should be postponed until this is clarified. The medical history should include any remote or recent medical problems, symptoms, medication use, and findings from previous examinations and tests. Major CAD risk factors and signs and symptoms suggesting cardiopulmonary disease should be identified. Physical activity patterns, vocational requirements, and family history of cardiopulmonary and metabolic disorders should also be assessed. Identification of absolute contraindications (see Display 17-1) should result in cancellation of the test and referral of the patient to the primary physician for further medical management. Patients with relative contraindications may be tested only after careful evaluation of the risk–benefit ratio.

Detailed verbal and written instructions, provided to the patient in advance, should include a request that the patient refrain from ingesting food, alcohol, and caffeine or using tobacco products within 3 hours of testing. Patients should be well rested and avoid vigorous activity the day of the test. Clothing should be comfortable and provide freedom of movement as well as allow access for electrode and blood pressure cuff placement. Properly fitting shoes with rubber soles should be worn to ensure good traction, particularly if a treadmill is the mode of testing. A thorough explanation of the potential risks and discomforts associated with exercise testing should be provided. Written informed consent has important ethical and legal implications and ensures the patient knows and understands the purposes

TABLE 17-1	Common Drugs and Their Impact on Exercise Testing				
Drug	**Indications**	**Heart Rate**	**Blood Pressure**	**Electrocardiogram**	**Exercise Capacity**
Beta blockers	Angina, hypertension, myocardial infarction, arrhythmias, tremors, migraine headaches	Rest: ↓ Exercise: ↓	Rest: ↓ Exercise: ↓	↓ Signs of ischemia	↑ In those with angina ↓ In those without angina
Calcium channel blockers	Angina, coronary artery spasm, hypertension	Rest: ↓ Exercise: ↓	Rest: ↓ Exercise: ↓	↓ Signs of ischemia	↑ In those with angina
Digoxin	CHF, arrhythmias	No change	Rest: ↓ Exercise: ↓	Delayed signs of ischemia	↑ In those with angina (and CHF)
Nitrates	Angina	No change	Rest: ↓ Exercise: ↓	Delayed signs of ischemia	↑ In those with angina (and CHF)

CHF, congestive heart failure.

and risks associated with the exercise test. There is sufficient case law to suggest that informed consent should always be obtained before beginning a test, although this issue has also been debated.[36] Last, a demonstration of how to get on and off the testing apparatus should be given, what is expected of the patient should be described (reporting of symptoms, level of exertion, testing end points), and any questions the patient has should be answered.

Whether patients should remain on all cardiovascular medicines has been the source of some debate. Many commonly used drugs can influence hemodynamic and electrocardiographic responses to exercise[2,22,26] (Table 17-1), but removing patients from their medicines they usually take can cause instability of symptoms, rhythm, blood pressure, and other problems. Recent versions of the aforementioned exercise testing guidelines[1,2,22,83] suggest that most patients can remain on their medical regimen for testing without greatly compromising the diagnostic performance of the test. Tapering beta blockers or discontinuing antianginal medications for several days before testing should be reserved for particular patients in whom diagnostic sensitivity is paramount, and the tapering process should be carefully supervised by a physician.

Preparation for Electrocardiogram

Diagnostically, the electrocardiographic response is the cornerstone of the clinical exercise test. Thus, reliable test interpretation and patient safety mandate a high-quality exercise electrocardiogram. Critical to obtaining a high-quality electrocardiogram tracing are proper skin preparation and precise electrode placement. The goal of skin preparation is to decrease the resistance at the skin–electrode interface and thus improve the signal-to-noise ratio. After removing hair from the general areas of placement, each site should be vigorously rubbed with an alcohol pad to remove skin oil. The skin should be abraded using a product designed further to reduce resistance by removing the superficial layers of skin (e.g., abrasive pads, gels). Finally, each electrode should be carefully placed in the proper location to ensure good skin contact with both the conducting gel and adhesive surfaces of the electrode.

The Mason-Likar limb lead placement[54] (Fig. 17-1) is the standard configuration clinically because it provides a 12-lead electrocardiogram with less artifact and less restriction to movement than the standard limb placement. However, the Mason-Likar placement can result in differences in electrocardiographic amplitude and axis compared with the standard limb placement.[28,44,76] Because these shifts may be

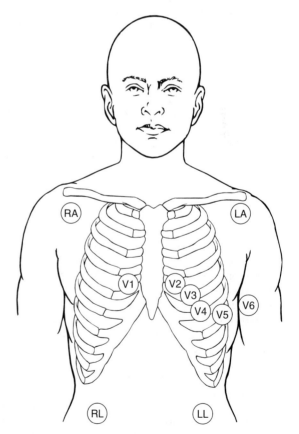

FIGURE 17-1 The Mason-Likar simulated 12-lead electrocardiogram electrode placement for exercise testing. (From Froelicher VF Myers J, Follansbee WP et al: Exercise and the Heart. St. Louis, Mosby-Yearbook, 1993, with permission.)

misinterpreted as diagnostic changes, it is often recommended that a resting supine electrocardiogram be recorded using the standard limb lead placement. It is also important to note that position changes may alter the interpretation of the electrocardiogram. For this reason, diagnostic ST segment changes should always be made relative to the resting exercise baseline position (i.e., upright rather than supine for treadmill and cycle ergometry).

EXERCISE TEST SELECTION

The purpose of the test, the health and fitness of the patient, the exercise modality, and the exercise protocol are fundamental considerations when selecting the appropriate test for a given patient. In many exercise laboratories, these issues are determined by custom and the availability of equipment, but each can have a profound effect on the response to the exercise test. For example, a treadmill test may be inappropriate for a patient who has difficulty with balance or gait, such as someone who has had a stroke or is otherwise neurologically impaired, or someone who has severe peripheral vascular disease that prevents him or her from walking. A bicycle ergometer would be a more appropriate choice for such patients. Test specificity should also be considered. For example, it would be more appropriate to use a cycle ergometer to assess physiologic responses to a cycling program. Likewise, if a person is being assessed for readiness for return to work that requires arm strength, an arm ergometer test may give more appropriate information than a treadmill test.

Modalities

An ideal exercise mode increases total body and myocardial oxygen demand to its highest level safely and in moderate, continuous, and equal increments. This requires a *dynamic* exercise device that uses major muscle groups, permitting large increases in cardiac output, oxygen delivery, and gas exchange. Many modalities have been used for diagnostic testing, including cycle ergometers, treadmills, arm ergometers, steps, and, more recently, pharmacologic agents. *Isometric*, or *static* exercise, which involves muscle contraction without movement of the corresponding joint, causes a greater increase in systolic blood pressure and heart rate in relation to total body oxygen uptake, and therefore a greater pressure load on the heart compared with dynamic exercise. Thus, it is not preferred for diagnostic exercise testing. However, isometric exercise has been used to provide occupation-specific information for a patient whose job requires an extensive amount of isometric activity.

The bicycle ergometer and the treadmill are the most commonly used dynamic exercise devices. Bicycle ergometer testing is more commonly used in Europe, whereas the treadmill is more often used in the United States. The bicycle is usually less expensive, occupies less space, and is quieter. Upper body motion is decreased, making blood pressure and electrocardiographic recordings easier. The workload administered by simple, mechanically braked bicycle ergometers is not always accurate and depends on ped-

aling speed, causing variations in the work performed. More expensive, electronically braked bicycle ergometers maintain the workload at a specified level over a wide range of pedaling speeds, and these have become the standard in most exercise laboratories. Bicycle ergometer work is commonly expressed in kilogram-meters per minute (kgm/min) or watts. The treadmill is usually more expensive than the cycle ergometer, is relatively immobile, and makes more noise. Researchers comparing treadmill and bicycle ergometer exercise tests have reported maximal oxygen uptake to be roughly 10% to 20% higher and maximal heart rate 5% to 20% higher on the treadmill.[15,34,37,63,95] Significant ST segment changes are reported more frequently and angina is elicited more frequently during treadmill testing compared with the cycle ergometer.[63,95] In addition, exercise-induced myocardial ischemia by thallium scintigraphy was reported to be greater after treadmill testing than cycle ergometry.[34] Although most of these differences are minor, if assessing the functional limits of the patient and eliciting subjective or objective signs of ischemia are important goals of the test, the treadmill may be preferable.

Protocols

The purpose of the test and the person tested are important considerations in selecting the protocol. Exercise testing may be performed for diagnostic purposes, for functional assessment, or for risk stratification. An often ignored but nevertheless consistent recommendation in the recent exercise testing guidelines is that the protocol be individualized for the patient being tested.[2,22,64,91] For example, a maximal, symptom-limited test on a relatively demanding protocol would not be appropriate (or very informative) for a severely limited patient. Likewise, a very gradual protocol might not be useful for an apparently healthy, active person. Use of submaximal testing, gas exchange techniques, the presence of a physician, and the exercise mode and protocol should be determined by considering the person being tested and the goals of the test.

The most commonly used exercise protocols, their stages, and the MET level (metabolic equivalents; an estimated value representing a multiple of the resting metabolic rate) for each stage are outlined in Figure 17-2. The most suitable protocols for clinical testing should include a low-intensity warm-up phase followed by progressive, continuous exercise in which the demand is elevated to a patient's maximal level within a total duration of 8 to 12 minutes.[2,22,15,63] In the absence of gas exchange techniques, it is important to report exercise capacity in METs rather than exercise time, so that exercise capacity can be compared uniformly between protocols. METs can be estimated from any protocol using standardized equations that have been put into tabular form.[2,22,61] In general, 1 MET represents an increment on the treadmill of approximately 1 mph or 2.5% grade. On a cycle ergometer, 1 MET represents an increment of roughly 20 W (120 kg·m/min) for a 70-kg person. The assumptions necessary for predicting MET levels from treadmill or cycle ergometer work rates (including not holding the handrails, that oxygen uptake is constant [i.e., steady-state exercise is performed], that the subject is healthy, and that all people are

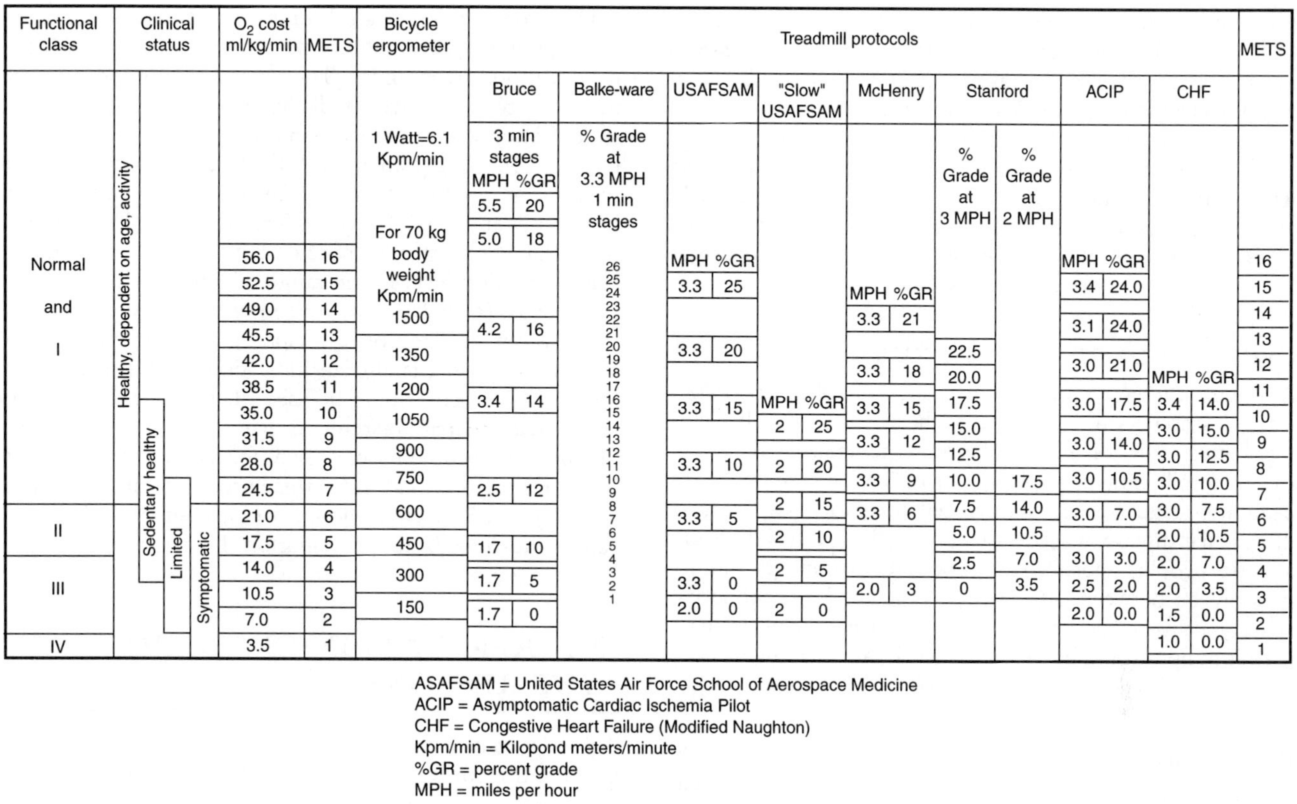

FIGURE 17-2 presents stages, workloads, and oxygen cost per stage of some commonly used protocols.

Functional class	Clinical status	O₂ cost ml/kg/min	METS	Bicycle ergometer	Bruce (3 min stages) MPH	%GR	Balke-ware %Grade at 3.3 MPH (1 min stages)	USAFSAM MPH	%GR	"Slow" USAFSAM MPH	%GR	McHenry MPH	%GR	Stanford %Grade at 3 MPH	Stanford %Grade at 2 MPH	ACIP MPH	%GR	CHF MPH	%GR	METS
				1 Watt = 6.1 Kpm/min	5.5	20														
					5.0	18														
Normal and I	Healthy, dependent on age, activity	56.0	16				26													16
		52.5	15				25	3.3	25							3.4	24.0			15
		49.0	14	For 70 kg body weight Kpm/min 1500			24 / 23					3.3	21			3.1	24.0			14
		45.5	13		4.2	16	22 / 21													13
	Sedentary healthy	42.0	12	1350			20 / 19	3.3	20					22.5		3.0	21.0			12
		38.5	11	1200	3.4	14	18 / 17					3.3	18	20.0						11
		35.0	10	1050			16 / 15	3.3	15	2	25	3.3	15	17.5		3.0	17.5	3.4	14.0	10
		31.5	9	900			14 / 13					3.3	12	15.0		3.0	14.0	3.0	15.0	9
		28.0	8	750			12 / 11	3.3	10	2	20	3.3	9	12.5		3.0	10.5	3.0	12.5	8
		24.5	7		2.5	12	10 / 9			2	15			10.0	17.5			3.0	10.0	7
II	Limited	21.0	6	600			8 / 7	3.3	5	2	10	3.3	6	7.5	14.0	3.0	7.0	3.0	7.5	6
		17.5	5	450	1.7	10	6 / 5							5.0	10.5	3.0	3.0	2.0	10.5	5
III	Symptomatic	14.0	4	300	1.7	5	4 / 3			2	5			2.5	7.0	2.5	2.0	2.0	7.0	4
		10.5	3	150			2 / 1	3.3	0	2	0	2.0	3	0	3.5	2.0	0.0	2.0	3.5	3
		7.0	2		1.7	0		2.0	0									1.5	0.0	2
IV		3.5	1															1.0	0.0	1

ASAFSAM = United States Air Force School of Aerospace Medicine
ACIP = Asymptomatic Cardiac Ischemia Pilot
CHF = Congestive Heart Failure (Modified Naughton)
Kpm/min = Kilopond meters/minute
%GR = percent grade
MPH = miles per hour

FIGURE 17-2 Stages, workloads, and oxygen cost per stage of some commonly used protocols.

similar in their walking efficiency) raise uncertainties as to the accuracy of estimating the work performed for an individual patient. For example, the steady-state requirement is rarely met for most patients on most exercise protocols; most clinical testing is performed among patients with varying degrees of cardiovascular or pulmonary disease; and people vary widely in their walking efficiency.[61] It has therefore been recommended that a patient be ascribed a MET level only for stages in which all or most of a given stage duration has been completed.

BRUCE TREADMILL PROTOCOL

Surveys have shown that the Bruce protocol is the most widely used in North America.[89] An advantage of using this test is that a great deal of functional and prognostic data have been generated over several decades using the Bruce protocol, and many published normative values have been derived from this protocol. For example, the most robust databases on the use of the exercise test for assessing prognosis, such as those from the Coronary Artery Surgery Study (CASS)[93] and the Duke Treadmill Score,[51] were generated from patients who underwent exercise testing using the Bruce test. Numerous studies have shown that patients who are unable to complete the first stage of this protocol (approximately 5 METs) have an extremely poor prognosis.[60,65,93] However, the disadvantages of the Bruce protocol include its large and unequal increments in work, which have been shown to result in less accurate estimates of exercise capacity, particularly for patients with cardiac disease. Investigations have demonstrated that work rate increments that are too large or rapid result in a tendency to overestimate exercise capacity, less reliability for studying the effects of therapy, and possibly even lowered sensitivity for detecting coronary disease.[15,63,64,73,77]

BALKE TREADMILLL PROTOCOL

The Balke protocol, and modifications of it, have been widely used for clinical exercise testing. It uses constant walking speeds (2.0 or 3.0 mph) and modest increments in grade (2.5% or 5.0%), and it has been used particularly often in studies assessing angina responses. Modifications of the original Balke treadmill protocol have become widespread. One modification, developed by the United States School of Aerospace Medicine (Balke-Ware),[96] consists of 5% grade increases every 2 minutes and a constant brisk walking speed of 3.3 mph (after an initial warm-up of 2.0 mph), which has been considered the most efficient speed for walking. The constant speed is advantageous in that it requires only an initial adaptation in stride.

NAUGHTON TREADMILL PROTOCOL

The Naughton treadmill protocol[69] is a low-level test that has become common for multicenter trials in patients with chronic heart failure. The test begins with 2-minute stages at 1 and 2 mph and 0% grade, then continually increases grade in approximately 1-MET increments at a constant speed of 2 mph for the next 8 minutes. Speed then increases to 3 mph with a slight drop in grade, followed by increases in grade equivalent to approximately 1 MET. The Naughton protocol provides reasonable and gradual work rate increases for patients with more advanced heart disease. Because this protocol has been used extensively in patients with congestive heart failure, it provides a substantial amount of functional and prognostic comparative data. The Naughton test, however, can result in tests of excessive duration among more fit subjects.

CYCLE ERGOMETER PROTOCOLS

Although there are specific bicycle protocols named for early researchers in Europe, such as Astrand,[6] bicycle ergometer protocols tend to be more generalized than for the treadmill. For example, 15- to 25-W increments per 2-minute stage are commonly used for patients with cardiovascular disease, whereas for apparently healthy adults or athletic people, appropriate work rate increments might typically be between 40 and 50 W/stage. Most modern, electronically braked cycle ergometers have controllers that permit ramp testing, in which the work rate increments can be individualized in continuous fashion (see next section).

RAMP TESTING

An approach to exercise testing that has gained interest in recent years is the ramp protocol, in which work increases constantly and continuously. In 1981, Whipp and colleagues[94] first described cardiopulmonary responses to a ramp test on a cycle ergometer, and many of the gas exchange equipment manufacturers now include ramp software. Treadmills have also been adapted to conduct ramp tests.[62,63] The ramp protocol uses a constant and continuous increase in metabolic demand that replaces the "staging" used in conventional exercise tests. The uniform increase in work allows for a steady rise in cardiopulmonary responses and permits a more accurate estimation of oxygen uptake.[63] The recent call for "optimizing" exercise testing[15,22,64,91] would appear to be facilitated by the ramp approach, because large work increments are avoided and increases in work are individualized, permitting test duration to be targeted. Because there are no stages *per se*, the errors associated with predicting exercise capacity alluded to previously are lessened.[22,63]

SUBMAXIMAL TESTING

In general, maximal, symptom-limited tests are not considered appropriate until patients are more than 1 month post-MI or postsurgery. Thus, submaximal exercise testing has an important role clinically for predischarge, post-MI or postbypass surgery evaluations. Submaximal tests have been shown to be important in risk stratification,[17,27,72] for making appropriate activity recommendations, or for recognizing the need for modification of the medical regimen or for further interventions in patients who have sustained a cardiac event. A submaximal, predischarge test appears to be as predictive for future events as a symptom-limited test

among patients less than 1 month post-MI. Submaximal testing is also appropriate for patients with a high probability of serious arrhythmias. The testing end points for submaximal testing have traditionally been arbitrary, but should always be based on clinical judgment. A heart rate limit of 140 beats/min and a MET level of 7 are often used for patients younger than 40 years of age, and limits of 130 beats/min and a MET level of 5 are often used for patients older than 40 years. For those on beta blockers, a Borg perceived exertion level in the range of 7 to 8 (1 to 10 scale) or 15 to 16 (6 to 20 scale) are conservative end points. The initial onset of symptoms, including fatigue, shortness of breath, or angina, is also an indication to stop the test. A low-level protocol should be used, that is, one that uses no more than 1-MET increments per stage. The Naughton protocol[69,70] is commonly used for submaximal testing. Ramp testing is also ideal for this purpose because the ramp rate (such as 5 METs achieved over a 10-minute duration) can be individualized depending on the patient tested.[63]

INTERPRETATION OF EXERCISE TEST RESPONSES

The important exercise test responses that should be monitored and recorded are heart rate, blood pressure, electrocardiographic changes, exercise capacity, and subjective responses, including chest discomfort, undue fatigue, shortness of breath, leg pain, and rating of perceived exertion. Each of these responses should be described in a comprehensive test report. Useful programs have been developed that automatically summarize the test responses and use regression equations that report pretest and post-test risks of coronary disease, and some provide mortality estimates.[25] An example of one such report is presented in Display 17-2.

Heart Rate

Heart rate increases linearly with oxygen uptake during exercise. Of the two major components of cardiac output, heart rate and stroke volume, heart rate is responsible for most of the increase in cardiac output during exercise, particularly at higher levels. Thus, maximal heart rate achieved is a major determinant of exercise capacity.[26,35] The inability to appropriately increase heart rate during exercise (chronotropic incompetence) has been associated with the presence of heart disease and a worse prognosis.[35,47] Although maximal heart rate has been difficult to explain physiologically,[33] it is affected by age, gender, health, type of exercise, body position, blood volume, and environment. Of these factors, age is the most important. There is an inverse relationship between maximal heart rate and age, with correlation coefficients typically in the order of –0.40. However, the scatter around the regression line is quite large, with standard deviations ranging from 10 to 15 beats/min (Fig. 17-3). Thus, age-predicted "target" maximal heart rate is a limited measurement for clinical purposes and should not be used as an end point for exercise testing.[2,22,35]

DISPLAY 17-2

Example of an Automated Exercise Test Summary Report with Diagnostic and Prognostic Probabilities Generated From a Computer Program[25]

PRETEST INFORMATION

This patient is a 74-year-old active white male outpatient 70 inches tall, weighing 180 lbs, who underwent a treadmill test on June 25, 1997. This exercise test was performed to evaluate symptoms/signs of possible heart disease or elevated risk factors.

Current Cardiac Medications:
The patient is not taking any cardiac medications.

Medical History:
The patient has the following symptoms: uncertain chest pain. The patient has no history of dysrhythmias.

Risk Factors:
The patient is currently not smoking but has 15 pack-years of smoking. The patient is 8 lbs over the average appropriate body mass index. Other risk factors include low high-density lipoprotein level (31 mg/dL) and non–insulin-dependent diabetes mellitus.

History of Cardiac Events:
No previous myocardial infarction. No bypass surgery performed. No percutaneous transluminal coronary angioplasty performed. No catheterization performed.

Resting ECG:
The resting ECG is abnormal because of the following: left ventricular hypertrophy. The ejection fraction is approximately 45% based on the resting ECG.

Pulmonary Function:
Forced vital capacity was 3.4 L (90.4% of expected), and the forced expiratory volume was 76.2% (normal is >75%).

EXERCISE TEST INFORMATION

Exercise Capacity
The patient achieved 4.3 estimated METs and 4.1 measured METs at a perceived exertion level of 18 of 20 on the Borg scale. The test was terminated because of ST changes.

Hemodynamic Data	Heart Rate	Blood Pressure	Double Product (×1,000)
Resting:	65 bpm	146/70 mm Hg	9.5
At max. exercise:	116 bpm	122/70 mm Hg	14.1

Chest Pain
Typical angina occurred during exercise.

Exercise ECG Response
The resting ECG shows no ST depression in V_5.
At maximal exercise, the ST segments showed 4 mm of downsloping depression in the lateral and inferior leads. In recovery, the ST segments showed 3 mm of downsloping depression in the lateral and inferior leads. No significant dysrhythmias occurred in response to exercise. No bundle-branch blocks or conduction defects were present at rest or developed during exercise.

CONCLUSIONS

ST segments exhibited abnormal depression during exercise and abnormal depression in recovery (abnormal ST response).
Exertional hypotension occurred (systolic blood pressure dropped below pretest standing SBP).
The exertional hypotension could be due to ischemia (ST depression).
The patient achieved 66% of normal exercise capacity for age, and 90% of normal maximal heart rate for age.
The patient has a high probability of having severe coronary artery disease.
Estimated prognosis from treadmill scores may be worse than expected for age, sex, and race.

(continued)

DISPLAY 17-2 *(CONTINUED)*

Example of an Automated Exercise Test Summary Report with Diagnostic and Prognostic Probabilities Generated From a Computer Program[25]

PROGNOSTIC ADDENDUM

Cardiovascular Mortality Prediction

The Framingham score (age, sex, cholesterol, diabetes, smoking, left ventricular hypertrophy, SBP) estimates a 5-year incidence of cardiovascular events (angina, myocardial infarction, or death) of 11% (as expected for age and gender). For comparison with the treadmill scores, the age-expected annual mortality rate from any cause is 5.1% (National Center for Health Statistics, 1990).

The Duke Score (METs, ST depression, and angina) estimates an annual cardiovascular mortality of 9.5% (not greater than two times the age-expected mortality). The Froelicher score (METs, congestive heart failure, SBP rise, and ST depression) estimates an annual cardiovascular mortality of 15.7% (three times the age-expected mortality).

Angiographic Coronary Artery Disease Prediction

The patient has no recorded history of coronary disease. Pretest probabilities for any significant coronary disease are 50% (CASS, 1981 [chest pain, age, gender]), 71% (Morise, 1992), and 51% (Do/Froelicher, 1995). Pretest probabilities for severe coronary disease are 22% (Duke, 1993), 52% (Morise, 1992), and 17% (Do/Froelicher, 1995).

The post-test probabilities for any clinically significant coronary artery disease are 99% (Detrano, 1992) due to age, 98% (Morise, 1992) due to age and diabetes mellitus, and 94% (Do/Froelicher, 1995) due to abnormal ST depression.

The probabilities of having severe coronary artery disease are 75% (Detrano, 1992) due to abnormal ST depression, 91% (Morise, 1992) due to age abnormal ST depression, and 74% (Do/Froelicher, 1995) due to abnormal ST depression.

Operative Mortality Prediction

If the patient would be selected for nonemergent bypass surgery and no renal dysfunction was present, the estimated operative morality rates are 9% (Parsonnet, 1989), 2% (NY State Dept. of Health, 1992), and 3% (VA, 1993). This is partially based on an estimated EF of 45%, so compare to measured EF.

Treadmill Report: Department of Cardiology

Disclaimer: This report was computer generated and the results are dependent on rules and correct data entry. It must be overread by a physician.

EF, ejection fraction; ECG, electrocardiographic; METs, metabolic equivalents; SBP, systolic blood pressure.

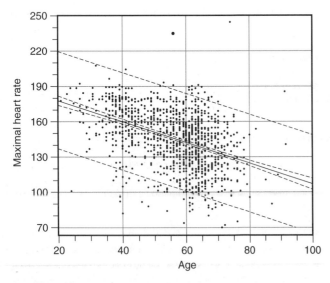

FIGURE 17-3 The relationship between maximal heart rate and age among patients referred for exercise testing. *Inner lines* represent the standard error; *outer lines* represent 95% confidence limits. (From Morris et al; J. Am Coll Cardiol 22:175–182, 1994, with permission.)

Blood Pressure

Assessment of systolic and diastolic blood pressure at rest and during the exercise test is important for patient safety and can provide important diagnostic and prognostic information. Properly trained personnel can obtain accurate and reliable blood pressures using noninvasive auscultory techniques, and guidelines have been developed for this purpose.[7,41] Blood pressure should be measured at rest before the test in both the supine and standing positions. Resting blood pressure, when measured before an exercise test, may be elevated compared with normal resting conditions because of pretest anxiety. Uncontrolled hypertension is a relative contraindication to exercise testing.[22] However, if blood pressure is elevated due to anxiety, it is not uncommon or of concern to observe a slight drop in blood pressure during the initial stage of an exercise test when the workloads are light.

The increase in systolic blood pressure during exercise reflects the inotropic reserve of the left ventricle. Systolic and diastolic blood pressure should be assessed during the last minute of each exercise stage and more frequently if hypotensive or hypertensive responses are observed. Normally, systolic blood pressure increases in parallel with an increase in work rate, and it is not uncommon in healthy people to exceed 200 mm Hg. In general, a value above 250 mm Hg is an indication to terminate the exercise test.[2,22] Diastolic pressure normally stays the same or increases slightly during exercise. The fifth Korotkov sound, however, can frequently be heard all the way to zero in a young, healthy person. A diastolic blood pressure exceeding 115 mm Hg is an indication to terminate the exercise test.[2,22] A decrease in systolic blood pressure with progressive exercise suggests that cardiac output is unable to increase in accordance with the work rate and is usually a reflection of severe ischemia. If systolic blood pressure appears to drop, it should be remeasured immediately, and if the drop is confirmed, the test should be terminated. The clinical consequences of abnormal blood pressure responses to exercise range from modest[27,55] to severe, in which decreases in systolic blood pressure have been associated with ventricular fibrillation in the laboratory.[39] Dubach and colleagues[20] have observed that systolic blood pressure must drop below the standing resting value to be prognostically valuable, whereas others have suggested that more modest decreases, in the order of 10 to 20 mm Hg, are associated with severe ischemia, left ventricular impairment, a high incidence of future cardiac events, or all three.[81,92]

Exercise Capacity

Exercise capacity can be an extremely important test response to document because it has important implications concerning the efficacy of current therapies, the assessment of disability, and risk stratification. A patient's exercise capacity says a great deal about overall cardiovascular health. The most accurate method of measuring exercise capacity is with the use of ventilatory gas exchange techniques, but this requires specialized equipment and is not available in many clinical laboratories. Exercise capacity is therefore usually expressed as exercise duration, watts achieved (on a bicycle ergometer), maximal exercise stage, or METs. In the absence of gas exchange techniques, it is preferable to express exercise capacity in METs rather than exercise time. This is because a MET value can be ascribed to any speed and grade on a treadmill or workload achieved on a cycle ergometer; therefore, exercise capacity can be compared uniformly between protocols.

As mentioned previously in the discussion on protocols, there can be a great deal of uncertainly in predicting a person's energy cost from the treadmill or cycle ergometer workload. How accurately a MET level predicts a person's true oxygen uptake depends on several factors. For most patients with cardiovascular or pulmonary disease, there is a substantial overprediction of the MET level.[2,23,61,63] The error associated with this prediction is accentuated when rapidly incremented protocols are used, when patients are unaccustomed to walking on a treadmill or pedaling a cycle ergometer, and when patients are allowed to use handrail support.[2,34,61]

Exercise capacity should be expressed as both an absolute value and as a relative percentage of normal for age and gender. The latter can be important because exercise capacity declines with increasing age and higher values are observed in men. Thus, when measuring or estimating oxygen uptake or MET levels, it is useful to have reference val-

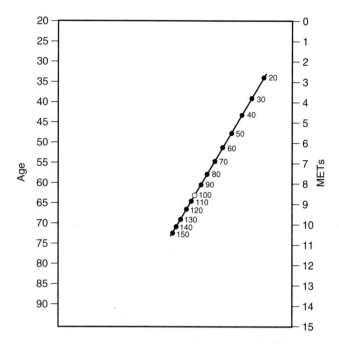

FIGURE 17-4 Nomograms of percentage normal exercise capacity for age in 1,388 male veterans referred for exercise testing (based on metabolic task equivalents [METs]). (From Morris CK et al: J Am Coll Cardiol 22: 175–182, 1994, with permission.)

ues for comparison. Normal reference values can facilitate communication with patients and between physicians regarding levels of exercise capacity in relation to a given patient's peers. Figures 17-4 and 17-5 are illustrations of nomograms for male patients referred for exercise testing. Expressing relative exercise capacity using a nomogram is

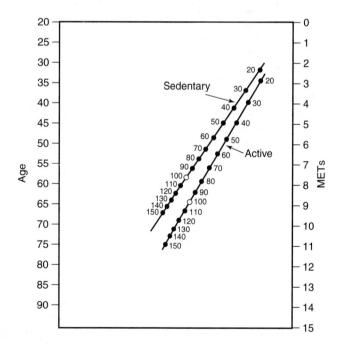

FIGURE 17-5 Nomogram of percentage normal exercise capacity for age among active and sedentary men referred for exercise testing (based on metabolic equivalents [METs]). (From Morris CK et al: J Am Coll Cardiol 22: 175–182, 1994, with permission.

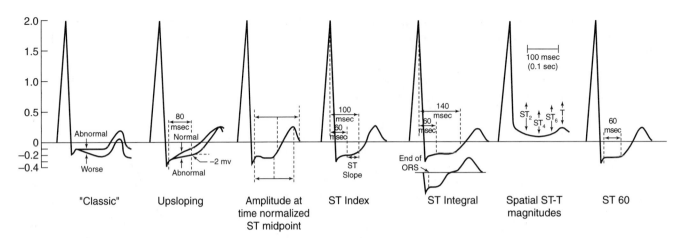

FIGURE 17-6 Normal and abnormal ST segment responses to exercise and the various criteria for ST segment depression.

advantageous because it offers a simple visual method of classifying a patient's response, without having to make cumbersome calculations from a particular regression equation. However, there are numerous available regression equations for "normal," all are population specific, and numerous factors affect a person's exercise tolerances beside age and gender, including height, weight, body composition, activity status, and exercise test mode used, in addition to many clinical factors such as smoking history, heart disease, and medications.[3,61]

Electrocardiographic Responses

In patients with CAD, exercise can cause an imbalance between myocardial oxygen supply and demand (ischemia), which can result in an alteration (depression or elevation relative to the baseline) in the ST segment of the electrocardiogram. These changes are the foundation of the exercise test clinically. Normal and abnormal ST segment responses to exercise are illustrated in Figure 17-6. Ever since electrocardiographic changes were first associated with myocardial ischemia in the 1920s, the diagnostic electrocardiographic criteria and leads that exhibit abnormalities during exercise have been the source of significant debate. Numerous electrocardiographic criteria, including complex mathematical constructs, combined scores, and ST areas during exercise and recovery, have been proposed to diagnose optimally the presence of CAD. Few of these studies however, have fol-

lowed accepted rules for evaluating a diagnostic test.[74] Virtually every edition of exercise testing guidelines that has been published suggests the application of a traditional diagnostic criterion: 1 mm or greater ST segment depression that is horizontal or downsloping 60 to 80 milliseconds after the J-point (a "positive" response). ST segment depression greater than 1 mm that is downsloping is in general indicative of more severe CAD. Most (probably >90%) ST changes occur in the lateral precordial leads.[22] Although it has historically been thought that the diagnostic performance of the test was incomplete without all 12 leads, more recent studies suggest that ST segment changes isolated to the inferior leads are frequently false positive responses.[57]

The significance of ST segment elevation depends on the presence or absence of Q waves. When ST elevation occurs in the presence of a normal resting electrocardiogram, it is usually indicative of severe transmural ischemia, it can be arrhythmogenic, and it localizes the ischemia. Conversely, exercise-induced ST segment elevation occurring in leads *with* Q waves is more common and is related to the presence of dyskinetic areas. This response is relatively common in patients after an MI and is of much less concern. Examples of these two responses are illustrated in Figure 17-7.

There are several important nuances concerning the proper measurement of exercise-induced ST segment changes. ST segment depression is measured as a change from the isoelectric line (PR segment) and is considered abnormal if the

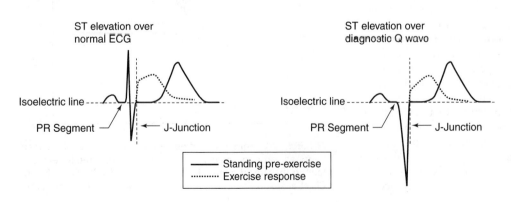

FIGURE 17-7 Example of exercise-induced ST segment elevation when the resting electrocardiogram is normal (*left*) and when the resting ECG has a diagnostic Q wave (*right*).

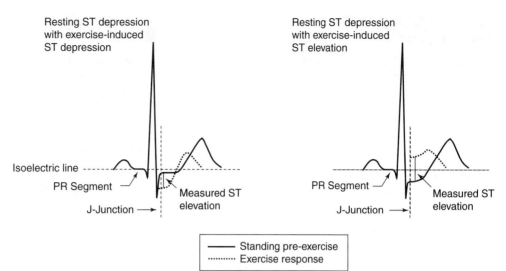

FIGURE 17-8 Example of how exercise-induced ST segment depression (*left*) and elevation (*right*) are measured when the electrocardiogram shows ST depression at rest.

next 60 to 80 milliseconds after the J-point is flat or downsloping (see Fig. 17-6). However, in patients who exhibit ST segment depression at rest, exercise-induced ST depression is measured from the baseline (resting) level (Fig. 17-8). In contrast, ST segment elevation is measured from the level at which the ST segment starts, and slope is not considered. The significance of upsloping or horizontal ST segment depression with T-wave inversion has been debated. Infarction, ventricular aneurysm, bundle-branch block, hypokalemia, ventricular hypertrophy, abnormal oxygen-carrying capacity of blood due to anemia, pulmonary disease, and drugs such as digoxin and quinidine may all influence the ST segment response; these and other conditions may cause exercise-induced ST segment depression that is not due to CAD (see section on False-Positive and False-Negative Responses).

Arrhythmias During Exercise Testing

Arrhythmias can occur during the exercise test or recovery period and can range in severity from life threatening to benign. There has been a great deal of debate about the importance of arrhythmias during exercise. The occurrence of "serious" arrhythmias during exercise, although rare, is an indication to terminate the exercise test. Arrhythmias may be overt, such as ventricular tachycardia, or more subtle, such as unifocal premature ventricular complexes (PVCs) increasing in frequency, or a period of supraventricular tachycardia. Arrhythmias for which there should be no debate about stopping the test include second- or third-degree heart block and ventricular tachycardia of any duration. Other arrhythmias that have been generally classified as "significant" or "complex" include R-on-T PVCs, frequent unifocal or multifocal PVCs (constituting 30% or more of the beats per minute), and coupling of PVCs (two in succession).[2,22] Any of these complex arrhythmias can be a precursor to sudden cardiac death. Electrophysiologic testing is commonly used to evaluate more fully complex arrhythmias and direct appropriate treatment. When there is doubt as to the nature or origin of the arrhythmia, the test should be stopped. However, isolated PVCs, even when they occur frequently, are not as ominous as previously thought. Recent studies have demonstrated that the occurrence of PVCs during an exercise test has minimal prognostic impact.[22,97] PVCs should be interpreted in the context of "the company they keep," such that the decision to terminate the test should be made based on the patient's history and whether the patient remains hemodynamically stable or the arrhythmias are accompanied by symptoms.

Subjective Responses

Assessment of symptoms and perception of effort during the exercise test are not only important to maximize safety; these subjective measures yield valuable diagnostic information. Obtaining careful assessments of subjective measures during the exercise test requires thorough explanations to ensure the patient understands what is expected of him or her and how to communicate these responses to those conducting the test. Angina and dyspnea are the most common cardiopulmonary symptoms elicited during exercise and each is typically evaluated using a four-point scale[2] (Display 17-3). These scales should be carefully explained to patients before the exercise test. Patients should be encouraged to report any and all symptoms during exercise.

It is important to distinguish between typical and atypical angina because they have quite different diagnostic implications. Typical angina tends to be consistent in its presentation and location, is brought on by physical or emotional stress, and is relieved by rest or nitroglycerin. Atypical angina refers to pain that has an unusual location, prolonged duration, or inconsistent precipitating factors that are unresponsive to nitroglycerin. Exercise-induced chest discomfort that has the characteristics of stable, typical angina provides better confirmation of the presence of significant CAD than any other test response. A patient exhibiting the combination of typical angina and an abnormal ST response has a 98% probability of having significant CAD. An important indication to stop the exercise test is moderately severe angina (level 3 on a scale of 1 to 4; see Display 17-3), which should correspond with pain that would normally cause the patient to stop daily activities or take a sublingual nitroglycerin pill.[64,68]

DISPLAY 17-3

Angina and Dyspnea Scales

ANGINA SCALE

1+	Onset of discomfort
2+	Moderate, bothersome
3+	Moderately severe
4+	Severe; most pain ever experienced

DYSPNEA SCALE

1+	Mild, noticeable to patient but not observer
2+	Mild, some difficulty, noticeable to observer
3+	Moderate difficulty, but can continue
4+	Severe difficulty, patient cannot continue

DISPLAY 17-4

Indications for Stopping an Exercise Test

ABSOLUTE

- Drop in systolic blood pressure of >10 mm Hg from baseline despite an increase in workload, when accompanied by other evidence of ischemia
- Moderate to severe angina
- Increasing nervous system symptoms (e.g., ataxia, dizziness, or syncope)
- Signs of poor perfusion (cyanosis or pallor)
- Technical difficulties in monitoring electrocardiogram or systolic blood pressure
- Subject's desire to stop
- Sustained ventricular tachycardia
- ST elevation (≥1.0 mm) in leads without diagnostic Q waves (other than V_1 or aVR)

RELATIVE

- Drop in systolic blood pressure of ≥10 mm Hg from baseline blood pressure despite an increase in workload, in the absence of other evidence of ischemia
- ST or QRS changes such as excessive ST depression (>2 mm of horizontal or downsloping ST segment depression) or marked axis shift
- Arrhythmias other than sustained ventricular tachycardia, including multifocal PVCs, triplets of PVCs, supraventricular tachycardia, heart block, or bradyarrhythmias
- Fatigue, shortness of breath, wheezing, leg cramps, or claudication
- Development of bundle-branch block or intraventricular conduction delay that cannot be distinguished from ventricular tachycardia
- Increasing chest pain
- Hypertensive response*

PVC, premature ventricular complex.
*In the absence of definitive evidence, the Committee suggests systolic blood pressure of >250 mm Hg or a diastolic blood pressure of 115 mm Hg.
From Fletcher GF, Froelicher VF, Hartley LH et al: Exercise standards: A statement for health professionals from the American Heart Association. Circulation 91: 580–615, 1995.

Dyspnea may be the predominant symptom in some patients with CAD, but it is more often associated with reduced left ventricular function or chronic obstructive pulmonary disease. In the former, it is usually accompanied by a poor exercise capacity and can occur with impaired systolic function. Dyspnea is also commonly quantified using a scale of 1 to 4 (see Display 17-3). *Claudication* is indicative of peripheral vascular disease. If peripheral vascular disease is known or suspected, pretest determination of the presence and strength of peripheral pulses should be made so that post-test comparisons are possible. Leg fatigue not related to claudication is often experienced at maximum exercise; a careful distinction should be made between these two symptoms.

Dizziness and lightheadedness may reflect cerebral hypoxia and may coincide with a feeling of exhaustion at maximum exercise. Lightheadedness can also be a sign of left ventricular dysfunction or hypotension. Dizziness may be accompanied by signs of gray or ashen pallor, diaphoresis, ataxic gait, dyspnea, and strained appearance as blood is maximally shunted to the exercising muscles. Trained observers should be able to recognize these responses and make a determination as to when the test should be stopped.

TEST TERMINATION

The usual goal of the exercise test in patients with known or suspected disease is to achieve a maximal level of exertion. This permits the greatest information yield from the test. However, achieving a maximal effort should be superseded by any of the clinical indications to stop the test (Display 17-4), by clinical judgment, or by the patient's request to stop. The reason for stopping the test should be carefully recorded because the symptoms or signs manifested by exercise often relate to the mechanism of impairment.

Determining the end point of an exercise test can be problematic. It requires integration of objective physiologic data and termination criteria with subjective judgment based on clinical experience. Some patients may be unable or unwilling to exercise to an adequate level. In patients with suspected coronary disease, a symptom-limited, maximal test is usually more diagnostic. Thus, patients should be instructed to exercise to the point at which they can no longer continue because of fatigue, dyspnea, or other symptoms. They should be informed that the test will be terminated if abnormal responses are observed by the operators. Although patients should be encouraged to exercise as long as possible, they should not be pushed beyond their capacity and any request to stop the test should be honored. Inability to fully monitor the patient's responses because of technical difficulties should result in immediate termination of the test. Most problems can be avoided by having an experienced physician, nurse, or exercise physiologist standing

DISPLAY 17-5

Borg Rating of Perceived Exertion Scale

6	
7	Very, very light
8	
9	Very light
10	
11	Fairly light
12	
13	Somewhat hard
14	
15	Hard
16	
17	Very hard
18	
19	Very, very hard
20	

From Borg GAV: An Introduction to Borg's RPE Scale. Ithaca, NY, Movement Publications, 1985.

next to the patient, measuring blood pressure and assessing patient appearance during the test. The exercise technician should operate the recorder and treadmill, take appropriate tracings, enter data on a form, and alert the physician to any abnormalities that may appear on the monitor.

Although many efforts have been made to objectify maximal effort, such as age-predicted maximal heart rate, a plateau in oxygen uptake, exceeding the ventilatory threshold, or a respiratory exchange ratio greater than unity, all have considerable measurement error and intersubject variability.[35,66,67,71,87] These problems are true regardless of the population tested. The 95% confidence limits for maximal heart rate based on age, for example, range considerably (see Fig. 17-2); therefore, this end point is maximal for some and submaximal for others.[25] The classic index of cardiopulmonary limits, a plateau in oxygen uptake, is not observed in many patients, is poorly reproducible, and has been confused by the many different criteria applied.[66,67,71,87] Although subjective, the Borg perceived exertion scale is helpful for assessing exercise effort[10] (Display 17-5). Good judgment on the part of the physician remains the most effective criterion for terminating exercise.

RECOVERY PERIOD

Some debate exists as to whether the postexercise recovery period should be an active or passive process. This decision should be made based on the purpose of the exercise test. If the test is performed for diagnostic purposes, it appears to be of value to place the patient in the supine position immediately after stopping exercise. The increase in venous return to the heart observed in the supine position results in increases in ventricular volume, wall stress, and, consequently, myocardial oxygen demand. Several studies have shown that ST segment abnormalities are enhanced in the supine position and that an active recovery may attenuate

the magnitude of these changes.[22,46] Once thought to be false-positive responses, ST segment changes 2 to 4 minutes into recovery are now known to be particularly important for the detection of ischemia. Patients with symptom-limiting angina or dyspnea may become more uncomfortable in the supine position and should recover in a seated upright or semirecumbent position. If the test is performed for nondiagnostic purposes such as for a fitness evaluation in a healthy or athletic person, an active recovery may be safer and more comfortable.

Typically, an active recovery consists of walking on the treadmill at a speed of 1.5 to 2.0 mph or continuing to pedal the cycle ergometer slowly at a work rate ranging from 0 to 25 W. An active recovery decreases the risk of hypotension and may minimize the risk of dysrhythmias secondary to elevated catecholamines in the postexercise period. A passive, standing recovery should be avoided because of potential complications associated with venous pooling. Regardless of the method of recovery, patients should be monitored for at least 6 to 8 minutes into the postexercise period. Blood pressure, the electrocardiogram, and symptoms should be monitored and recorded at 2-minute intervals for the duration of the recovery period. The recovery period should be extended as long as necessary to resolve symptoms or abnormal hemodynamic or electrocardiographic responses. After completion of the recovery portion of the test, patients should be given post-test instructions that include avoidance of long, hot showers or baths. In addition, patients should be told they may experience fatigue and muscle soreness and to avoid any heavy exertion that day. Any pain or discomfort during the day after the test should be reported to their physician immediately.

ASSESSING TEST ACCURACY

All diagnostic tests misclassify patients a certain percentage of the time. In the context of the exercise test, this is not a trivial issue, because people who are inaccurately identified as having disease may be subjected unnecessarily to additional, more invasive, and costly procedures. When the test is performed properly, it commonly serves the very important purpose of screening those who should or should not undergo these additional procedures. On the other hand, a patient with significant CAD who is incorrectly classified as normal may not receive needed medical therapy and thus be at high risk for a coronary event. How accurately the exercise test distinguishes people with disease from those without disease depends on the population tested, the definition of disease, and the criteria used for an abnormal test.

The most common terms used to describe test accuracy are *sensitivity* and *specificity*. Sensitivity is the percentage of times a test correctly identifies those with CAD. Specificity is the percentage of times a test correctly identifies those without cardiovascular disease. Sensitivity and specificity are inversely related and are affected by the choice of discriminant value for abnormal, the definition of disease, and, most important, by the prevalence of disease in the population tested. For example, if the population has a greater severity of disease (such as triple-vessel or left main coronary disease), the test will have a higher sensitivity. Alternatively, the test will have a higher specificity (and low sensitivity) when performed in a group of younger, healthier subjects.

Meta-analysis of the exercise testing literature indicates that the exercise test has, on the average, a sensitivity of approximately 68% and a specificity of approximately 77%.[29] However, these values range widely in the various studies; sensitivity can be as low as 40% among patients with single-vessel disease, but greater than 90% among those with triple-vessel disease. Conversely, the specificity of the test is usually quite low (i.e., < 50% to 60%) in patients who have more severe CAD, but is quite high in populations that are relatively healthy. These values reported in the literature and the inverse relationship between sensitivity and specificity underscore the importance of considering the patient's pretest characteristics (chest pain and CAD risk factors) before beginning the test. No test result can be interpreted accurately without considering the patient in the context of his or her pretest characteristics.

Another important term that helps define the diagnostic value of a test is the *predictive value*. The predictive value of an abnormal test (positive predictive value) is the percentage of people with an abnormal test result who have disease. Conversely, the predictive value of a normal test (negative predictive value) is the percentage of people with a normal test result who do not have disease. The predictive value of a test cannot be determined directly from the sensitivity and specificity but are strongly associated with the prevalence of disease in the population tested. The calculations used to determine sensitivity, specificity, and predictive value are presented in Display 17-6.

False-Positive and False-Negative Responses

The factors associated with a false-positive or false-negative response should also be considered before the test. A *false-positive* response is defined as an abnormal exercise test response in a person without significant heart disease and causes the specificity to be decreased. A *false-negative* response occurs when the test is normal in a person with disease and causes the sensitivity of the test to be reduced. Factors associated with false-positive and false-negative responses are listed in Display 17-7. In people whom the probability of a false-positive or false-negative test is high, an alternative procedure (exercise or pharmacologic echocardiogram or radionuclide test) may be appropriate.

ANCILLARY METHODS FOR THE DETECTION OF CORONARY ARTERY DISEASE

Several ancillary imaging techniques have been shown to provide a valuable complement to exercise electrocardiography for the evaluation of patients with known or suspected CAD. These techniques are particularly helpful among patients with equivocal exercise electrocardiograms or those likely to exhibit false-positive or false-negative responses. They are frequently used to clarify abnormal ST segment responses in asymptomatic people or those in whom the cause of chest discomfort remains uncertain. When exercise electrocardiography and an imaging technique are combined, the diagnostic and prognostic accuracy is enhanced.[12] For example, patients exhibiting both a positive exercise electrocardiogram and a positive radionuclide scan have been shown to have a 2.6-fold increased risk for subsequent coronary events.[45]

The major imaging procedures are myocardial perfusion and ventricular function studies using radionuclide techniques, exercise echocardiography, and pharmacologic stress testing. Because these techniques are often used in conjunction with or as a surrogate for standard exercise testing, they are briefly discussed here. Detailed reviews of these topics are available elsewhere.[26,78]

Myocardial Perfusion Imaging

The most commonly used technique to evaluate myocardial perfusion is the application of the radionuclide thallium-201.[8,26] When thallium-201 is injected intravenously at maximal exercise, it is rapidly extracted from the blood by living cells in the myocardium. Uptake of thallium-201 is similar to that of potassium in living cells. Radiologic images are then taken, which reveal areas of absent, poor, or moderately poor uptake of thallium-201. When exercise images are compared with rest images, the differences in uptake of thallium-201 indicate areas of decreased blood flow. At the same time, if areas absent of thallium-201 uptake occur at rest, it can be assumed that this represents areas of myocardial scarring and not ischemia with exercise. This information, along with the exercise test, can be more definitive in the evaluation of the extent and localization of ischemia.

Perfusion imaging with technetium-99m sestamibi has become common. This imaging agent permits higher dosing with less radiation exposure than thallium, resulting in improved images that are sharper and have less artifact and attenuation. Sestamibi is the preferred imaging agent for obtaining tomographic images of the heart using single-photon emission computed tomography (SPECT). SPECT images are obtained with a gamma camera, which rotates 180 degrees around the patient, stopping at preset angles to record the image. Cardiac images are then displayed in slices from three different axes to allow visualization of the heart in three dimensions. Thus, multiple myocardial segments can be viewed individually, without the overlap of segments that occurs with planar imaging.[8] As in thallium-201 imaging, perfusion defects that are present during exercise but not seen at rest suggest ischemia. Perfusion defects that are present during exercise and persist at rest suggest previous MI or scar. In this manner, the extent and distribution of ischemic myocardium can be identified.

Perfusion imaging of the coronary anatomy has been shown to be somewhat more sensitive and specific than the exercise electrocardiogram for detecting CAD. An extensive review of the literature suggested the sensitivity and specificity of exercise thallium scintigraphy for detecting coronary disease were in the order of 84% and 87%, respectively.[45] This modality also permits the localization of ischemia, which is not possible with ST segment depression on the electrocardiogram. This technique is especially helpful in patients with equivocal exercise electrocardiograms, those taking digoxin, or those with left bundle-branch block, in whom the interpretation of electrocardiographic changes is more problematic.[22,26]

Ventricular Function Studies

Ventricular function is commonly evaluated with the use of the radioisotope technetium-99m. This radioisotope is administered as an intravenous bolus, and its transit through the ventricles is measured by special cameras. Technetium-99m is also used to label red blood cells for equilibrium blood pool studies. Both of these methods have been used extensively in the evaluation of left and right ventricular function after acute MI and other cardiac events. This technique can be performed at rest as well as at maximal exercise. When performed at maximal exercise, it has the capability of determining decreased ventricular function compared with rest measures. This can help in the diagnosis of ischemic abnormalities as well as exercise-induced ventricular dysfunction. In addition to measures of ejection fraction, measures of specific regional wall motion can also be taken.[11,31,32]

The limitations of thallium, sestamibi SPECT, and technetium imaging include their higher cost and exposure of the patient to ionizing radiation. Additional equipment and personnel are also required for image acquisition and interpretation, including a nuclear technician to administer the radioactive isotope and acquire the images, and a physician trained in nuclear medicine to reconstruct and interpret the images.

Exercise Echocardiographic Imaging

Echocardiographic imaging of the heart is being increasingly used during exercise and pharmacologic stress testing. This technique is frequently combined with an exercise electrocardiogram to increase the sensitivity and specificity of exercise testing. Typically, a resting two-dimensional image is taken, and repeat images are obtained at peak exercise or immediately afterward. If images are taken after exercise, they must be obtained within 1 to 2 minutes because abnormal wall motion begins to normalize after this point. Rest and stress images are compared side by side in a cine-loop display that is gated during systole from the QRS complex. Myocardial contractility normally increases with exercise, whereas ischemia causes hypokinesis, akinesis, and dyskinesis of the affected segments. Therefore, a test is considered positive if wall motion abnormalities develop in previously normal territories with exercise or worsen in an already abnormal segment.[4,26]

Some advantages of exercise echocardiography over nuclear imaging include the absence of exposure to ionizing radiation and a shorter amount of time required for testing. Like standard exercise testing and radionuclide techniques, the diagnostic accuracy of echocardiography depends primarily on the specific methodology used and the pretest probability of CAD in the subjects tested. The accuracy of echocardiographic testing also depends on observer experience. Reviews of studies published since the advent of exercise echocardiography in the early 1980s suggest that the average sensitivity and specificity of this technique for detecting coronary disease are both approximately 85%.[5,26] The limitations of exercise echocardiography include dependence on the operator for obtaining adequate, timely images, and some variation exists in image interpretation. In addition, as much as 20% of patients have inadequate echocardiographic windows secondary to body habitus or lung interference.[84]

Pharmacologic Stress Techniques

It is advantageous to use pharmacologic stress techniques for patients who are unable to exercise on a treadmill or cycle ergometer to an adequate level. These include patients who have orthopedic limitations, peripheral vascular disease, and chronic obstructive pulmonary disease or other limiting pulmonary diseases; elderly patients with low functional capacity; diabetic patients with severe neuropathy; and patients with neuromuscular conditions. For these patients, pharmacologic methods can be extremely useful for evaluating coronary blood flow and myocardial function. Pharmacologic stress is a relatively new area with important applications for echocardiographic and nuclear techniques, but only limited data are available directly comparing pharmacologic stress testing with standard exercise testing.

Two types of pharmacologic stress agents have been used: those that increase coronary blood flow through coronary vasodilation, and those that increase myocardial oxygen demand by increasing heart rate. The commonly used coronary vasodilators are adenosine and dipyridamole (Persantine), whereas dobutamine is used to increase myocardial oxygen demand. The vasodilators cause greatly increased endocardial and epicardial blood flow in normal coronary arteries but not in stenotic segments, whereas dobutamine can create an imbalance between myocardial oxygen supply and demand by increasing heart rate and contractility. These drugs are given intravenously and, when associated with an imaging technique such as thallium-201 scintigraphy, sestamibi, or echocardiography, can provide important information about coronary artery stenosis. Comparisons between dipyridamole and standard exercise testing have demonstrated dipyridamole to have a diagnostic accuracy similar to or slightly better than that of standard exercise testing.[9,86] The disadvantages of dipyridamole and adenosine stress testing include side effects (40% to 50% of patients have minor side effects) and lack of cardiovascular response (approximately 10% of patients).[26,40,75]

GAS EXCHANGE TECHNIQUES

Because of the inaccuracies associated with estimating oxygen uptake and METs from work rate (i.e., treadmill speed and grade), many laboratories directly measure expired gases. The measurement of gas exchange and ventilatory variables provides an added dimension to the exercise test by increasing the information obtained concerning a patient's cardiopulmonary function. The direct measurement of VO_2 has been shown to be more reliable and reproducible than estimated values from treadmill or cycle ergometer work rate.[61] Peak VO_2 is the most accurate measurement of functional capacity and is a useful reflection of overall cardiopulmonary health. Measurement of expired gases is not considered necessary for all clinical exercise testing, but the additional information provides important physiologic data. Heart and lung diseases frequently manifest themselves through gas exchange abnormalities during exercise, and the information obtained is increasingly used in clinical trials to assess objectively the response to interventions. Moreover, a growing body of literature suggests that exercise capacity measured directly by gas exchange techniques provides superior prognostic information relative to exercise time or estimated METs.[49,61,65] Situations in which gas exchange measurements are appropriate include the following[22]:

- When a precise response to a specific therapeutic intervention is needed for a particular patient
- When a research question is being addressed
- When the etiology of exercise limitation or dyspnea is uncertain
- To evaluate exercise capacity in patients with heart failure to assist in the estimation of prognosis and assess the need for transplantation
- To assist in the development of an appropriate exercise prescription for cardiac rehabilitation

The use of these techniques, however, requires added attention to detail and a working knowledge of the equipment and basic physiology. This is particularly important given advances in automation for the collection and calculation of expired gasses.

PROGNOSIS

The exercise test has been shown to be of value for estimating prognosis in patients with a wide range of severity of cardiovascular diseases.[22,26,51,60,65,93] One of the most important clinical applications of the exercise test is the identification of low-risk patients in whom catheterization (and revascularization) can be safely deferred. There are several reasons why accurately establishing prognosis is important. An estimate of prognosis provides answers to patients' questions regarding the probable outcome of their illness, which may be useful to the patients in planning return to work and making decisions regarding disability, recreational activities, and finances. A second reason to estimate prognosis is to identify patients for whom interventions might improve outcome. Combining clinical and exercise test information into scores has been shown to improve the estimation risk among men and women undergoing exercise testing.[17,51]

EXERCISE TESTING IN SPECIAL POPULATIONS

Women

The interpretation of exercise testing results in women is more challenging than that in men.[14,22] Exercise-induced ST segment depression is less sensitive among women compared with men.[38,58] Test specificity is also thought to be lower among women, but there is a wide variation in the reported studies.[22] Some of these differences may be explained by differences in the meaning of chest pain presentation between men and women; although typical angina is as meaningful in women older than 60 years of age as it is in men, nearly half the women with anginal symptoms in the CASS study (who were younger than 65 years of age) had normal coronary arteries.[43] Other possible explanations for the lower test accuracy in women include lower disease prevalence, higher incidence of mitral valve prolapse and syndrome X (chest pain without coronary disease), differences in microvascular function, and possibly hormonal differences.[16,22]

The accuracy for diagnosing CAD in women has been shown to be better with the use of multivariate methods[79] and by the addition of nuclear or echocardiographic imaging techniques.[16,52,59] Thus, when exercise testing is performed in women, factors that may affect test accuracy should be carefully considered; when appropriate or if the exercise testing results are uncertain, a radionuclide imaging procedure should be considered. The optimal strategy for circumventing false-positive test results in women remains to be defined. Nevertheless, the current AHA/ACC guidelines suggest that there are insufficient data to justify routine radionuclide imaging procedures as the initial test for CAD in women.[22]

The Elderly

The prevalence of CAD increases with increasing age, and the exercise test can be an extremely useful tool for diagnosing CAD in the elderly. However, exercise testing in the elderly can be difficult given their frequently compromised ability to exercise in the context of an increased prevalence of CAD. The occurrence of fatigue and lightheadedness due to muscle weakness and deconditioning, vasoregulatory abnormalities, and difficulties with gait are important concerns in these patients. Thus, a test modality and protocol should be chosen that provides the highest degree of safety. For instance, cycle ergometry may be more appropriate for elderly patients who have a residual deficit from a cerebral vascular accident. In addition, the testing protocol should be modified considering the expected levels of exercise tolerance. More gradually incremented protocols, such as the Balke, ramp, or Naughton, are usually more suitable in the elderly population. The elderly are more likely to present with more complex medication regimens, more comorbidity, and increased prevalence of aortic stenosis and other valvular diseases, in addition to more severe CAD. For these reasons, the elderly require particularly close evaluation before clearance for exercise testing, a modified testing protocol, and particular attention to appropriate end points.[14,22]

Interpretation of the exercise test in the elderly can also differ significantly from that in younger people. Resting electrocardiographic abnormalities, including prior MI, left ventricular hypertrophy, and intraventricular conduction delays, may compromise the diagnostic accuracy of the exercise test. Nevertheless, the application of standard ST segment criteria among elderly subjects has been shown to have similar diagnostic characteristics as in younger subjects.[38] No doubt because of the higher prevalence of CAD in the elderly, test sensitivity has even been shown to be relatively higher among the elderly (84%), although specificity is somewhat lower (70%).[42] Thus, despite several problems posed by elderly subjects that require additional attention, exercise testing is not contraindicated in this group.[22]

Patients Postcardiac Transplantation

Over the last two decades, transplantation has become a widely used and successful treatment option for patients with end-stage heart failure. The 1-year survival rate for patients who undergo this procedure is now approximately 90%, compared with only 50% to 60% in patients with severe heart failure who receive medical treatment.[18] The hemodynamic response to exercise in patients who have undergone cardiac transplantation has been characterized since the early 1970s.[82,85,88] Because the heart is denervated, some intriguing hemodynamic responses are observed. Orthotopic transplantation removes the nervous system connections to the heart. Thus, the heart is not responsive to the normal actions of the parasympathetic and sympathetic systems. The absence of vagal tone explains the high resting heart rates in these patients (100 to 110 beats/min) and the relatively slow adaptation of the heart to a given amount of submaximal work.[88] This slows the delivery of oxygen to the working tissue, contributing to an earlier-than-normal metabolic acidosis and hyperventilation during exercise.[13,19,53,82,85] Although transplantation significantly improves the hemodynamic and ventilatory response to exercise, the transplanted patient still exhibits many of the responses typical of the patient with chronic heart failure.[53] These include heightened ventilatory responses attributable to uneven matching of ventilation to perfusion and an increase in physiologic dead space. Maximal heart rate is lower in transplant recipients compared with normal subjects, which contributes to a reduction in cardiac output and peak VO_2; the a-VO_2 arteriovenous oxygen difference widens as a compensatory mechanism.

The exercise test in patients who have undergone cardiac transplantation is less a diagnostic and more a functional tool. In the latter role, it is useful for assessing and modifying therapy in these patients, in addition to evaluating the appropriateness of daily activities and return to work. Although rare cases of chest pain associated with accelerated graft atherosclerosis have been reported in transplant recipients, decentralization of the myocardium usually eliminates anginal symptoms. Exercise electrocardiography is also inadequate in terms of assessing ischemia, as evidenced by its low sensitivity (21% or less).[21] Thus, radionuclide testing may be more useful for assessing ischemia in these patients.

SUMMARY

Although there have been advances in technologies related to the diagnosis of CAD, the numerous applications and widespread availability of the exercise test continue to make it one of the more important tools in cardiovascular medicine. The test is increasingly being supervised by nonphysicians,[24] and the cardiovascular nurse's role has expanded in many centers to include exercise test supervision. Thus, an understanding of proper methodology, conduct, indications, and the physiology related to exercise testing are increasingly recognized skills. A good understanding of these principles can also assist the nurse in applying the information gained from the exercise test to patients with various cardiovascular diseases. In addition to diagnostic and prognostic information, these applications include the assessment of therapy, exercise prescription, and helping to guide medical/surgical management decisions for the patient.

REFERENCES

1. American Association of Cardiovascular and Pulmonary Rehabilitation: Guidelines for Cardiac Rehabilitation Programs. Champaign, IL, Human Kinetics, 1991
2. American College of Sports Medicine: Guidelines for Exercise Testing and Exercise Prescription, 5th ed. Philadelphia, Williams & Wilkins, 1995
3. American College of Sports Medicine: Resource Manual for Guidelines for Exercise Testing and Prescription, 5th ed. Philadelphia, Williams & Wilkins, 1998
4. Armstrong W, Marcovitz PA: In Braunwald E (ed): Stress Echocardiography: Heart Disease Updates, pp 1–10. Philadelphia, WB Saunders, 1993
5. Armstrong WF, Pellikka PA, Ryan T et al: Stress echocardiography: Recommendations for performance and interpretation of stress echocardiography. J Am Soc Echocardiogr 11: 97–104, 1998
6. Åstrand P-O, Rodahl K: Textbook of Work Physiology, 3rd ed. New York, McGraw-Hill, 1986
7. Bailey RH, Bauer JH: A review of common errors in the indirect measurement of blood pressure. Arch Intern Med 153: 2741–2748, 1993
8. Berger BC, Watson DD, Taylor GJ et al: Quantitative thallium-201 exercise scintigraphy for detection of coronary artery disease. J Nucl Med 22: 585–593, 1981
9. Bolognese L, Sarasso G, Aralda D et al: High dose dipyridamole echocardiography early after uncomplicated acute myocardial infarction: Correlation with exercise testing and coronary angiography. J Am Coll Cardiol 14: 357–363, 1989
10. Borg GAV: Psychophysical bases of perceived exertion. Med Sci Sports Exerc 14: 377–381, 1982
11. Borges-Neto S: Perfusion and function assessment by nuclear cardiology techniques. Curr Opin Cardiol 12: 581–586, 1997
12. Borges-Neto S, Shaw LJ, Kesler KL et al: Prediction of severe coronary artery disease by combined rest and exercise radionuclide angiocardiography and tomographic perfusion imaging with technetium 99m-labeled sestamibi: A comparison with clinical and electrocardiographic data. J Nucl Cardiol 4: 189–194, 1997
13. Brubaker PH, Berry MJ, Brozena SC et al: Relationship of lactate and ventilatory thresholds in cardiac transplant patients. Med Sci Sports Exerc 25: 191–196, 1993
14. Bryant BA, Limacher MC: Exercise testing in selected patient groups: Women, the elderly, and the asymptomatic. Primary Care 21: 517–534, 1994
15. Buchfuhrer MJ, Hansen JE, Robinson TE et al: Optimizing the exercise protocol for cardiopulmonary assessment. J Appl Physiol 55: 1558–1564, 1983
16. Cerqueira MD: Diagnostic testing strategies for coronary artery disease: Special issues related to gender. Am J Cardiol 75: 52D–60D, 1995
17. Chang JA, Froelicher VF: Clinical and exercise test markers of prognosis in patients with stable coronary artery disease. Curr Probl Cardiol 19: 533–538, 1994
18. Costanzo MR, Augustine S, Bourge R et al: Selection and treatment of candidates for heart transplantation: A statement for health professionals from the Committee on Heart Failure and Cardiac Transplantation of the Council on Clinical Cardiology, American Heart Association. Circulation 92: 3593–3612, 1995
19. Degre SGL, Niset GL, DeSmet JM et al: Cardiorespiratory response to early exercise testing after orthotopic cardiac transplantation. Am J Cardiol 60: 926–928, 1987
20. Dubach P, Froelicher VF, Klein J et al: Exercise induced hypotension in a male population: Criteria, causes, and prognosis. Circulation 78: 1380–1387, 1988
21. Ehrman JK, Keteyian SJ, Levine AB et al: Exercise stress tests after cardiac transplantation. Am J Cardiol 71: 1372–1373, 1993
22. Fletcher GF, Froelicher VF, Hartley LH et al: Exercise standards: A statement for health professionals from the American Heart Association. Circulation 91: 580–615, 1995
23. Foster C, Crowe AJ, Danies E et al: Predicting functional capacity during treadmill testing independent of exercise protocol. Med Sci Sports Exerc 28: 752–756, 1996
24. Franklin BA, Gordon S, Timmis GC et al: Is direct physician supervision of exercise stress testing routinely necessary? Chest 111: 262–264, 1997
25. Froelicher VF: Exercise Test Reporting Aid (EXTRA) Software. St. Louis, Mosby-Year Book, 1996
26. Froelicher VF, Myers J, Follansbee WP et al: Exercise and the Heart, 3rd ed. St. Louis, CV Mosby, 1993
27. Sivarajan Froelicher E: Usefulness of exercise testing shortly after acute myocardial infarction for predicting 10-year mortality. Am J Cardio 74:318-323, 1994
28. Gamble P, McManus H, Jensen D et al: A comparison of the standard 12 lead electrocardiogram to exercise electrode placement. Chest 85: 616–622, 1984
29. Gianrossi R, Detrano R, Mulvihill D et al: Exercise-induced ST depression in the diagnosis of coronary artery disease: A meta analysis. Circulation 80: 87–98, 1989
30. Gibbons L, Blair SN, Kohl HW et al: The safety of maximal exercise testing. Circulation 80: 846–852, 1989
31. Gibbons RJ: Nuclear cardiology. In Guiliani ER, Fyster V, Gersh BJ et al (eds): Cardiology: Fundamentals and Practice, 2nd ed., pp 161–180. St. Louis, CV Mosby, 1991
32. Gibbons RJ: Rest and exercise radionuclide angiography for diagnosis in chronic ischemic heart disease. Circulation 84(Suppl 1): I-93–I-99, 1991
33. Graettinger W, Smith D, Neutel J et al: Relationship of left ventricular structure to maximal heart rate during exercise. Chest 107: 341–345, 1995
34. Hambrecht R, Schuler GC, Muth T et al: Greater diagnostic sensitivity of treadmill versus cycle exercise testing of asymptomatic men with coronary artery disease. Am J Cardiol 70: 141–146, 1992
35. Hammond K, Froelicher VF: Normal and abnormal heart rate responses to exercise. Prog Cardiovasc Dis 27: 271–296, 1985
36. Herbert DL, Herbert WG: Legal Aspects of Preventive, Rehabilitative, and Recreational Exercise Programs, 3rd ed. Canton, PRC, 1993
37. Hermansen L, Saltin B: Oxygen uptake during maximal treadmill and bicycle exercise. J Appl Physiol 26: 31–37, 1969
38. Hlatky MA, Pryor DB, Harrell FE Jr et al: Factors affecting sensitivity and specificity of exercise electrocardiography: Multivariable analysis. Am J Med 77: 64–71, 1984

39. Irving JB, Bruce RA: Exertional hypotension and postexertional ventricular fibrillation in stress testing. Am J Cardiol 39: 849–851, 1977

40. Iskandrian AS: Single-photon emission computed tomographic thallium imaging with adenosine, dipyridamole, and exercise. Am Heart J 122: 279–284, 1991

41. Iyriboz Y, Hearon CM: Blood pressure measurement at rest and during exercise: Controversies, guidelines, and procedures. J Cardiopulm Rehabil 12: 277–287, 1992

42. Kasser IS, Bruce RA: Comparative effects of aging and coronary heart disease on submaximal and maximal exercise. Circulation 39: 759–774, 1969;

43. Kennedy H, Killip T, Fischer L et al: The clinical spectrum of coronary artery disease and its surgical and medical management: 1974–1979, the Coronary Artery Surgery Study. Circulation 56: 756–761, 1977

44. Kleiner JP, Nelson WP, Boland MJ: The 12 lead electrocardiogram in exercise testing. Arch Intern Med 138: 1572–1573, 1978

45. Kotler TS, Diamond GA: Exercise thallium-201 scintigraphy in the diagnosis and prognosis of coronary artery disease. Ann Intern Med 113: 684–702, 1990

46. Lachterman B, Lehmann KG, Abrahamson D et al: "Recovery only" ST segment depression and the predictive accuracy of the exercise test. Ann Intern Med 112: 11–16, 1990

47. Lauer MS, Okin PM, Larson MG et al: Impaired heart rate response to graded exercise: Prognostic implications of chronotropic incompetence in the Framingham Heart Study. Circulation 93: 1520–1526, 1996

48. Levites R, Baker T, Anderson GJ: The significance of hypotension developing during treadmill exercise testing. Am Heart J 95: 747–753, 1978

49. Mancini DM, Eisen H, Kussmaul W et al: Value of peak oxygen consumption for optimal timing of cardiac transplantation in ambulatory patients with heart failure. Circulation 83: 778–786, 1991

50. Marcus R, Lowe R, Froelicher VF et al: The exercise test as gatekeeper: Limiting access or appropriately directing resources? Chest 107: 1442–1446, 1995

51. Mark DB, Hlatky MA, Harell FE et al: Exercise treadmill score for predicting prognosis in coronary artery disease. Ann Intern Med 106: 793–800, 1987

52. Marwick TH, Anderson T, Williams MJ et al: Exercise echocardiography is an accurate and cost-efficient technique for detection of coronary artery disease in women. J Am Coll Cardiol 26: 335–341, 1995

53. Marzo KP, Wilson JR, Mancini DM: Effects of cardiac transplantation on ventilatory response to exercise. Am J Cardiol 69: 547–553, 1992

54. Mason RE, Likar I: A new system of multiple-lead exercise electrocardiography. Am Heart J 71: 196–205, 1966

55. Mazzotta G, Scopinaro G, Falcidieno M et al: Significance of abnormal blood pressure response during exercise-induced myocardial dysfunction after recent acute myocardial infarction. Am J Cardiol 59: 1256–1260, 1987

56. Miranda CP, Lehmann KG, Froelicher VF: Indications, criteria for interpretation, and utilization of exercise testing in patients with coronary disease: Results of a survey. J Cardiopulm Rehabil 9: 479–484, 1989

57. Miranda CP, Liu J, Kadar A et al: Usefulness of exercise induced ST segment depression in the inferior leads during exercise testing as a marker for coronary artery disease. Am J Cardiol 69: 303–307, 1992

58. Morise AP, Diamond GA: Comparison of the sensitivity and specificity of exercise electrocardiography in biased and unbiased populations of men and women. Am Heart J 130: 741–747, 1995

59. Morise AP, Diamond GA, Detrano R et al: Incremental value of exercise electrocardiography and thallium-201 testing in men and women for the presence and extent of coronary artery disease. Am Heart J 130: 267–276, 1995

60. Morris CK, Ueshima K, Kawaguchi T et al: The prognostic value of exercise capacity: A review of the literature. Am Heart J 122: 1423–1431, 1991

61. Myers J: Essentials of Cardiopulmonary Exercise Testing. Champaign, IL, Human Kinetics, 1996

62. Myers J, Buchanan N, Smith D et al: Individualized ramp treadmill: Observations on a new protocol. Chest 101: 2305–2415, 1992

63. Myers J, Buchanan N, Walsh D et al: Comparison of the ramp versus standard exercise protocols. J Am Coll Cardiol 17: 1334–1342, 1991

64. Myers J, Froelicher VF: Optimizing the exercise test for pharmacologic studies in patients with angina pectoris. In Ardissino D, Savonitto S, Opie LH (eds): Drug Evaluation in Angina Pectoris. pp 41–52. Pavia, Italy, Kluwer Academic, 1994

65. Myers J, Gullestad L: The role of exercise testing and gas-exchange measurement in the prognostic assessment of patients with heart failure. Curr Opin Cardiol 13: 145–155, 1998

66. Myers J, Walsh D, Buchanan N et al: Can maximal cardiopulmonary capacity be recognized by a plateau in oxygen uptake? Chest 96: 1312–1316, 1989

67. Myers J, Walsh D, Sullivan M et al: Effect of sampling on variability and plateau in oxygen uptake. J Appl Physiol 68: 404–410, 1990

68. Myers JN: Perception of chest pain during exercise testing in patients with coronary artery disease. Med Sci Sports Exerc 26: 1082–1086, 1994

69. Naughton J, Balke B, Nagle F: Refinements in methods of evaluation and physical conditioning before and after myocardial infarction. Am J Cardiol 14: 837–843, 1964

70. Naughton JP, Haiden R: Methods of exercise testing. In Naughton JP, Hellerstien HK, Mohler LC (eds): Exercise Testing and Exercise Training in Coronary Heart Disease, pp 79–91. New York, Academic Press, 1973

71. Noakes T: Implications of exercise testing for prediction of athletic performance: A contemporary perspective. Med Sci Sports Exerc 20: 319–330, 1988

72. Olona M, Candell-Riera J, Permanyer-Miralda G et al: Strategies for prognostic assessment of uncomplicated first myocardial infarction: 5-year follow-up study. J Am Coll Cardiol 25: 815–822, 1995

73. Panza J, Quyyumi AA, Diodati JG et al: prediction of the frequency and duration of ambulatory myocardial ischemia in patients with stable coronary artery disease by determination of the ischemia threshold from exercise testing: Importance of the exercise protocol. J Am Coll Cardiol 17: 657–663, 1991

74. Philbrick JT, Horowitz, Feinstein AR: Methodological problems of exercise testing for coronary artery disease: Groups, analysis and bias. Am J Cardiol 64: 1117–1122, 1989

75. Ranhosky A, Kempthorne-Rawson J, and the Intravenous Dipyridamole Thallium Imaging Study Group: The safety of intravenous dipyridamole thallium myocardial perfusion imaging. Circulation 81: 1205–1209, 1990

76. Rautaharju PM, Prineas RJ, Crow RS et al: The effect of modified limb positions on electrocardiographic wave amplitudes. J. Electrocardiol 13: 109–114, 1980

77. Redwood DR, Rosing DR, Goldstein RE et al: Importance of the design of an exercise protocol in the evaluation of patients with angina pectoris. Circulation 43: 618–628, 1971

78. Ritchie JL, Bateman TM, Bonow RO et al: Guidelines for clinical use of cardiac radionuclide imaging: Report of the American College of Cardiology/American Heart Association Task Force on Assessment of Diagnostic and Therapeutic Cardiovascular Procedures (Subcommittee on Coronary Artery Bypass Graft Surgery). J Am Coll Cardiol 17: 543–589, 1991

79. Robert AR, Melin JA, Detry JM: Logistic discriminant analysis improves diagnostic accuracy of exercise testing for coronary artery disease in women. Circulation 83: 1202–1209, 1991

80. Rochmis P, Blackburn H: Exercise tests: A survey of procedures, safety, and litigation experience in approximately 170,000 tests. JAMA 217: 1061–1066, 1971

81. San Marco M, Pontius S, Selvester R: Abnormal blood pressure response and marked ischemia ST segment depression as predictors of severe coronary artery disease. Circulation 61: 572–578, 1980

82. Savin W, Haskell WL, Schroeder JS et al: Cardiorespiratory responses of cardiac transplant patients to graded, symptom-limited exercise. Circulation 62: 55–60, 1980

83. Schlant R, Friesinger GC, Leonard JJ: Clinical competence in exercise testing: A statement for physicians from the ACP/ACC/AHA Task Force on Clinical Privileges in Cardiology. Circulation 82: 1884–1888, 1990

84. Schmidt DH, Port SC, Gal RA: Nuclear cardiology and echocardiography: Noninvasive tests for diagnosing patients with coronary artery disease. In Pollack M, Schmidt DH (eds): Heart Disease and Rehabilitation, 3rd ed., pp 81–94. Champaign, IL, Human Kinetics, 1995

85. Schroeder JS: Hemodynamic performance of the human transplanted heart. Transplant Proc 11: 304–308, 1979

86. Severi S, Picano E, Michelassi C et al: Diagnostic and prognostic value of dipyridamole echocardiography in patients with suspected coronary artery disease: Comparison with exercise electrocardiography. Circulation 89: 1160–1173, 1994

87. Stachenfeld NS, Eskenazi M, Gleim GW et al: Predictive accuracy of criteria used to assess maximal oxygen consumption. Am Heart J 123: 922–926, 1992

88. Stinson EB, Griepp RL, Schroeder JS et al: Hemodynamic observations one and two years after cardiac transplantation in man. Circulation 14: 1181–1193, 1972

89. Stuart RJ, Ellestad MH: National survey of exercise stress testing facilities. Chest 77: 94–97, 1980

90. Thompson P: The Safety of Exercise Testing and Participation. In Durstine JL, King AC, Painter PL, Roitman JL, Zwirin LD, Kenney WL (eds): Resource Manual for Guidelines for Exercise Resting and Prescription, 2nd ed, pp 359–363. Philadelphia, Lea & Febiger, 1993

91. Webster MWI, Sharpe DN: Exercise testing in angina pectoris: The importance of protocol design in clinical trials. Am Heart J 117: 505–508, 1989

92. Weiner DA, McCabe CH, Cutler SS, et al: Decrease in systolic blood pressure during exercise testing: Reproducibility, response to coronary artery bypass surgery and prognostic significance. Am J Cardiol 49: 1627–1632, 1982

93. Weiner DA, Ryan TJ, McCabe CH et al: Value of exercise testing in determining the risk classification and the response to coronary artery bypass grafting in three-vessel coronary artery disease: A report from the Coronary Artery Surgery Study (CASS) registry. Am J Cardiol 60: 262–266, 1987

94. Whipp BJ, Davis JA, Torres F et al: A test to determine parameters of aerobic function during exercise. J Appl Physiol 50: 217–221, 1981

95. Wicks JR, Sutton JR, Oldridge NB et al: Comparison of the electrocardiographic changes induced by maximum exercise testing with treadmill and cycle ergometer. Circulation 57: 1066–1069, 1978

96. Wolthius RA, Froelicher VF, Fischer J et al: New practical treadmill protocol for clinical use. Am J Cardiol 39: 697–700, 1977

97. Yang JC, Wesley RC, Froelicher VF: Ventricular tachycardia during routine treadmill testing: Risk and prognosis. Arch Intern Med 151: 349–353, 1991

18

Cardiac Catheterization

MARY McMAHON BUSCH
ROXANNE JUEL
KATHERINE M. NEWTON

Cardiac catheterization is widely used for diagnostic evaluation and therapeutic intervention in the management of patients with cardiac disease. The nurse's role in pre-catheterization teaching and intracatheterization and post-catheterization care is well recognized.[1,6] The many nursing responsibilities related to cardiac catheterization are outlined in the *Guidelines for Cardiac Catheterization and Cardiac Catheterization Laboratories* of the American College of Cardiology/American Heart Association (ACC/AHA) Ad Hoc Task Force on Cardiac Catheterization.[1]

Cardiac catheterization developed as a result of 50 years of clinical effort. The first documented cardiac catheterization was performed by Werner Forssman in 1929.[24] Guided by fluoroscopy, Forssman passed a catheter into his own right heart through an antecubital vein. He then walked upstairs to the radiology department and confirmed the catheter position by radiograph. The techniques of right and left heart catheterization were developed during the 1940s and 1950s.[14,15,55] In 1953, the percutaneous techniques of arterial catheterization were introduced by Seldinger,[62] and in 1959, selective coronary arteriography was introduced by Sones and colleagues.[64,65]

Important advances related to cardiac catheterization included the development of quantitative angiography for determination of cardiac output (CO) and ejection fraction; therapeutic interventions, including percutaneous transluminal coronary angioplasty (PTCA), laser therapy, atherectomy, stent placement, electrophysiologic mapping, and catheter ablation for the management of arrhythmias; and valvuloplasty.[25,50]

Although noninvasive diagnostic techniques have an important role, cardiac catheterization remains the most definitive procedure for the diagnosis and evaluation of coronary disease.[25] This chapter describes cardiac catheterization procedures and their possible complications. It also describes the nursing care given before and after catheterization and the interpretation of data as they relate to coronary heart disease (CHD).

INDICATIONS

Cardiac catheterization is indicated in a wide variety of circumstances. It is essential in evaluating patients with con-

genital or valvular heart disease for surgery (see Chapter 27), and the catheterization laboratory is also the site for interventional cardiology techniques (see Chapter 21). The most frequent use of cardiac catheterization is to confirm or define the extent of suspected CHD. Anatomic and physiologic severity of disease are determined, and the presence or absence of related conditions is explored.[6]

The ACC/AHA Task Force has published indications for cardiac catheterization.[1] Indications for coronary angiography are classified for specific clinical presentations, including asymptomatic patients, symptomatic patients, atypical chest pain of uncertain origin, and acute myocardial infarction (MI). Class I indications are those for which there is general agreement that coronary angiography is indicated. Class II indications are "conditions for which coronary angiography is frequently performed, but there is a divergence of opinion with respect to its justification in terms of value and appropriateness."[51] Class I indications are summarized here. The reader is referred to the ACC/AHA guidelines for a more complete discussion.[1]

Asymptomatic patients may have known or suspected CHD, such as patients without symptoms after MI or those with exercise-induced electrocardiogram (ECG) abnormalities without accompanying angina pectoris. In asymptomatic patients, class I indications include the following[1]:

1. Evidence of high risk on noninvasive testing, including exercise ECG, thallium scintigraphy, radionuclide ventriculography, and quantitative two-dimensional echocardiography
2. High-risk occupations that involve the safety of others, including airline pilots, bus drivers, truck drivers, and air traffic controllers, or occupations that require sudden vigorous activity, such as firefighters or police officers
3. Successful resuscitation from cardiac arrest that occurred without obvious precipitating cause

In patients with symptoms thought to be due to CHD, class I indications include the following[1]:

1. Angina pectoris inadequately responsive to medical therapy, thrombolysis, PTCA, or coronary bypass surgery
2. Unstable angina pectoris

3. Prinzmetal or variant angina pectoris
4. Angina pectoris in association with high-risk results on noninvasive tests, history of MI or hypertension with ST segment depression, intolerance to medical therapy, occupation or lifestyle that necessitates diagnosis, or episodic pulmonary edema or symptoms of left ventricular failure without obvious cause
5. Before major vascular surgery
6. After resuscitation from cardiac arrest or from sustained ventricular tachycardia in the absence of acute MI

Class I indications after MI include the following[1]:

1. Within 6 hours of onset of symptoms in patients who are candidates for PTCA and in whom intravenous (IV) thrombolysis is contraindicated
2. After 6 hours of onset of symptoms but before hospital discharge in patients with recurrent chest pain, suspected mitral regurgitation, or ruptured interventricular septum causing heart failure or shock or suspected subacute cardiac rupture
3. During convalescence in patients who have angina at rest or with minimal activity, congestive heart failure, left ventricular ejection fraction less than 45%, evidence of myocardial ischemia, on laboratory testing, or non–Q-wave MI

CONTRAINDICATIONS

Cardiac catheterization has relatively few contraindications. Any correctable illness or condition that, if corrected, would improve the safety of the procedure should be managed before catheterization. These conditions include uncontrolled ventricular irritability, uncorrected electrolyte hypokalemia or digitalis toxicity, decompensated congestive heart failure, and severe renal insufficiency or anuria unless dialysis is planned after the procedure.[4] Other relative contraindications are recent stroke (within 1 month), active gastrointestinal bleeding, active infection, severe, uncontrolled hypertension, lack of appropriate emergency surgical backup, and the patient's refusal of the therapeutic procedures to be directed by the catheterization results.[51] The following are conditions for which the ACC/AHA Task Force agrees that coronary angiography is generally not indicated:[1]

1. Patients asymptomatic after coronary artery bypass surgery or PTCA and with no evidence of ischemia, unless they provide informed consent for institutionally approved research purposes
2. Symptomatic patients with mild, clinically stable angina pectoris who do not have impaired ventricular function or exercise studies suggesting high risk
3. Symptomatic patients with well controlled angina pectoris or patients after MI who are not candidates for either coronary artery bypass surgery or angioplasty because of advanced age or a life expectancy limited by other illness
4. Completed MI with uncomplicated infarction without prior thrombolytic therapy
5. Patients with severe left ventricular dysfunction in the absence of angina pectoris or evidence of ischemia

Anticoagulation as a contraindication is debated. Grossman[25] suggested that oral anticoagulants should be withheld for 48 hours before catheterization. In patients who must remain on anticoagulants, the use of heparin is favored because its effects may be quickly reversed with protamine sulfate if cardiac perforation or hemorrhage occurs.[18,25]

PATIENT PREPARATION

Patients are usually admitted for cardiac catheterization the day of the procedure. The physician performing the catheterization explains the procedure and obtains informed consent before procedure admission.

Precatheterization orders usually include the following:

1. Chest radiograph
2. Hematocrit, hemoglobin, complete blood count, differential
3. Urinalysis
4. Standard 12-lead ECG
5. Nothing by mouth after midnight (or after a light breakfast if the catheterization is to take place in the afternoon)
6. Preparation of catheterization site (antibacterial scrub of both groin or antecubital areas)
7. Patient to void before going to catheterization laboratory
8. Premedication

Various premedications may be prescribed. A sedative or sedative hypnotic is frequently ordered.[50] When coronary arteriography is planned, atropine sulfate may be ordered to help prevent the bradycardia and vasovagal reactions that often occur with contrast injections into the coronary arteries. Patients with a history of allergy to iodine-containing substances, such as seafood or contrast agents, should be given an antihistamine such as diphenhydramine hydrochloride and treated with glucocorticosteroids before the procedure.[52] For these patients, the use of nonionic contrast agents is recommended.[52] The use of prophylactic antibiotics is not recommended.[25]

Patients who wear artificial dentures, glasses, or hearing aids should be sent to the laboratory wearing them.[47,48] The patient is better able to communicate when dentures and hearing aids are in place. Glasses allow the patient to view the videotape playback and help keep the patient better oriented to the surroundings.

Nursing Assessment and Patient Teaching

Nursing assessment and teaching are an important part of patient preparation.[48,53]

The nursing assessment includes the patient's heart rate and rhythm, blood pressure, evaluation of the peripheral pulses of the arms and legs, and assessment of heart and lung sounds. The sites for best palpation of the patient's dorsalis pedis and posterior tibial pulses are marked on the skin. This information will be used for comparison in evaluating peripheral pulses after the catheterization procedure. A conscious sedation assessment is performed, including assessment of the patient's cardiovascular, respiratory, and renal systems. Care is taken to identify characteristics or conditions that may cause the patient to be at greater risk for complications associated with conscious sedation. Characteristics associated with greater conscious sedation risk include history of difficult intubation; history of difficulty with sedation; morbid obesity; sleep apnea; extremes of age; severe cardiac, respiratory, renal, hepatic, or central nervous system disease; and history of substance abuse.[42] Patients with diabetes are questioned about the type of insulin they use. Those who take NPH insulin may be sensitized to protamine and are at increased risk for severe protamine reactions if it is used to reverse the effects of heparin.[66] The nursing assessment also includes an evaluation of the patient's emotional status and attitude toward catheterization.

- ◆ Is this the patient's first cardiac catheterization?
- ◆ What are the patient's apprehensions about the procedure?
- ◆ What has the patient heard about cardiac catheterization? (Patients have sometimes heard "horror stories" from friends or acquaintances about catheterization experiences and may therefore need reassurance about the safety of the procedure.)
- ◆ What decisions are being faced? (Patients may be facing good or bad news about the absence or presence and extent of disease. Thus, the period before catheterization most likely is a time of anxiety and fear for a variety of reasons. Discussion and reassurance may help to relieve some of these feelings.)

The catheterization laboratory confronts the patient with new sights, sounds, and experiences that may be intimidating and frightening. Teaching is aimed at preparing the patient for this experience. In some institutions, patients are given a tour of the laboratory before the procedure.[48] A printed booklet to which the patient can refer is also helpful. The following points should be covered in patient teaching:

1. The patient will be given nothing by mouth for 6 to 12 hours before the catheterization and will be asked to void before leaving the unit.
2. Medication will be given before or during the procedure, if prescribed, but the patient will be awake during the procedure.
3. The patient should be instructed in deep breathing or stopping the breath without bearing down and in coughing on request. With deep inspiration, the diaphragm descends, preventing it from obstructing the view of the coronary arteries in some radiographic projections. Bearing down (Valsalva maneuver) increases intra-abdominal pressure and may raise the diaphragm, obstructing the view. After the injection of contrast medium, coughing will be requested to help clear the material from the coronary arteries. The rapid movement of the diaphragm also acts as a mechanical stimulant to the heart and helps prevent the bradycardia that may accompany the injection of contrast medium.[61]
4. The appearance of the laboratory should be explained to the patient, including the general function of the equipment.

5. The patient will wear a gown to the laboratory; both arms may be slipped out of the gown for ECG electrode placement in the laboratory.
6. The patient will lie on a table that tends to be hard.
7. The catheter insertion site will be washed, and hair will be removed with a razor or other depilatory.[32]
8. The expected length of the procedure should be explained to the patient.
9. The patient will be given a local anesthetic at the catheter entry site, but the procedure is rarely totally pain free. The patient should let the staff know if the anesthetic begins to wear off so that more may be given.
10. The patient may have hot flashes or experience nausea during injection of the coronary arteries with contrast medium.
11. The patient should report angina or other chest pain to the staff.
12. The patient should be told the expected length of bed rest after the catheterization.

Outpatient Cardiac Catheterization

In this cost-driven health care environment, an estimated 80% of diagnostic cardiac catheterizations are outpatient procedures.[22,30,56] Advantages include decreased costs and avoidance of an unnecessary overnight hospital stay.[47] Patients considered for outpatient cardiac catheterization are those with stable coronary symptoms. Patients in whom the outpatient procedure is contraindicated include those with unstable, accelerated, crescendo, or preinfarction angina pectoris; uncompensated congestive heart failure; severe aortic stenosis; suspected left main coronary disease; known bleeding disorders; and metabolically unstable patients with intercurrent disease or uncontrolled arrhythmias.

Additional considerations include the distance the patient lives from the hospital and the availability of someone to drive the patient home.

Preprocedure teaching is best done before hospital admission. The content is similar to that for patients undergoing an inpatient procedure. Patients who have significant left main coronary disease or complications during the procedure are usually admitted to the hospital for overnight observation.

After the procedure, the patient spends 3 to 6 hours in a short-stay unit, ambulatory recovery, or similar setting. Postprocedure orders are the same for inpatient and outpatient cardiac catheterization. After the required period of bed rest, the patient is observed for 30 to 60 minutes while sitting, standing, and walking. During this time, discharge instructions are reviewed. The patient is then allowed to leave. Results of the catheterization are reviewed with the patient by the cardiologist before discharge.

PROCEDURE

Cardiac Catheterization Laboratory

The cardiac catheterization laboratory is a specially equipped radiologic laboratory for the study of children and adults with known or suspected heart disease. The laboratory usually has the following equipment:[6]

1. A fluoroscope with image intensifier. Fluoroscopy is the continuous presentation of an x-ray image on a fluorescent screen. This allows the viewing of structures in motion. Traditional fluoroscopy presents a dim image that cannot be filmed and must be viewed in a darkened room. The image intensifier receives the fluoroscopic image and increases its brightness, permitting filming (cinefluoroscopy) or digital acquisition of motion pictures and viewing of the image with a television camera, television screen, and videotape recorder.
2. A video tape recorder for filming the fluoroscopic image for instant replay and for transmitting the image to a monitor, so that catheter progression, contrast medium test doses, and so forth, can be monitored.
3. Single or biplane cameras linked to the image intensifier for filming of cine or digital angiograms.
4. An x-ray table. The image intensifiers are mounted on a C-arm that rotates around the patient.
5. Pressure transducers and a multichannel physiologic recorder.
6. Equipment for CO determination.
7. Advanced cardiac life support drugs and equipment.
8. A cardioverter–defibrillator.
9. An ECG with continuous monitor display.
10. A standby pacemaker, either a temporary transvenous electrode and pulse generator system or an external transthoracic pacemaker.

Catheterization Approach

Cardiac catheterization is usually accomplished by percutaneous methods (the Seldinger technique). Direct exposure of the vein and artery (Sones technique) may also be used.[62] The percutaneous method is used for the femoral artery and vein[27]; direct exposure is used for the brachial artery and basilic vein.[4] All chambers and vessels may be cannulated using either approach, and both approaches have high degrees of safety. Although physician preference often dictates which approach is used, specific factors may favor the use of one approach over the other.

The *percutaneous femoral approach* is preferred because of its speed and repeatability and because arteriotomy and arterial repair are not required. Its use is indicated in cases of decreased or absent radial or brachial pulse. When tight aortic stenosis makes retrograde catheterization difficult or impossible, the percutaneous transseptal approach is used for left heart catheterization.[25]

The *direct brachial approach* is indicated in cases of known vascular disease of the abdominal aorta or iliac or femoral arteries, or thrombotic disease of the femoral veins or inferior vena cava.[25] Severe hypertension, a wide pulse pressure due to aortic regurgitation, and anticoagulant therapy are associated with an increased risk of bleeding when the percutaneous approach is used.[25] In cases of severe obesity, the direct approach is used for better visu-

alization and control of bleeding.[25] A disadvantage of the direct approach is that it can be repeated only once or twice. Arterial thrombosis occurs more frequently with this approach, and the patient must return for removal of the sutures.

PERCUTANEOUS CATHETERIZATION

Percutaneous catheterization is accomplished using the technique described by Seldinger or a modified Seldinger technique[62] (Fig. 18-1). The same technique is used for both arterial and venous entry. The vessels are located, and local anesthetic is given. The percutaneous needle has a sharp inner obturator. A small incision is made in the skin over the vein or artery, and the needle is passed through both walls of the vessel. The needle and obturator are pulled back into the vessel lumen and the obturator is removed. A guide wire is passed through the needle, into the vessel. The needle is removed and a hemostatic introducer sheath is advanced over the guide wire and placed within the vessel. The modified Seldinger technique is commonly used. This technique uses a single-wall needle puncture without an inner obturator. Catheters are exchanged by inserting a guide wire into the catheter and inserting the catheter with the guide wire through the introducer sheath, into the vessel. Four to 6 cm of the guide wire is advanced past the distal end of the catheter, so that the wire leads as the catheter and wire are advanced to the aortic arch. The

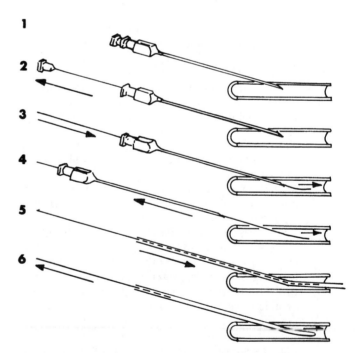

FIGURE 18-1 Catheterization by the Seldinger technique. **(1)** Arterial puncture; **(2)** removal of stylet; **(3)** insertion of guide wire through needle; **(4)** withdrawal of needle, leaving guide wire in artery; **(5)** introduction of catheter into artery over guide wire; **(6)** withdrawal of guide wire. (Reproduced by permission from Daily EK, Schroeder JS: Techniques in Bedside Hemodynamic Monitoring, 3rd ed, p 110. St. Louis, CV Mosby, 1985.)

guide wire is removed from the catheter completely before catheter placement. This procedure can be repeated several times during the catheterization.[3]

DIRECT BRACHIAL APPROACH

Local anesthesia is used and the brachial pulse is identified. An incision is made over the medial vein for right heart catheterization or over both the vein and the brachial artery if right and left heart catheterization is planned. The vein and artery are approached by blunt dissection and are brought to the surface and tagged with surgical tape. Venotomy and arteriotomy are performed using scissors or a scalpel. The distal segment of the artery is flushed with heparinized saline to prevent clotting from distal arterial stasis. The catheterization is performed. After catheterization, the distal brachial artery is aspirated until a forceful backflow is achieved, and heparinized saline is injected. The arterial incision is then sutured. Some laboratories also recommend the routine use of a Fogarty catheter for removal of clots in the distal segment as protection against thrombosis. The vein may be tied off, sutured, or used for an IV line.[27]

Right Heart Catheterization

Right heart catheterization (Fig. 18-2) is used to obtain right heart pressures, to evaluate the pulmonic and tricuspid valves, to sample blood oxygen content of right heart chambers for detection of left-to-right shunt, to determine CO, and to evaluate mitral valve stenosis or mitral valve insufficiency by the transseptal approach.[20]

The right heart can be approached through the femoral vein and the inferior vena cava or through the basilic vein and superior vena cava.[3,27] Once the inferior vena cava or superior vena cava is reached, the catheter is advanced through the right atrium, right ventricle, and pulmonary artery to a distal pulmonary vessel. Right ventricular irritability may be noted when the catheter tip passes through

the right ventricle. The course of the catheter is followed with pressure monitoring through the catheter and with fluoroscopy. When indicated, blood samples are taken, and pressures are recorded as the catheter is advanced. If left heart catheterization is planned, the catheter may be left in the distal pulmonary vessel, so that simultaneous left ventricular and pulmonary artery wedge pressure waveforms can be recorded. As the catheter is removed, pull-back pressures can be recorded from the pulmonary artery to the right ventricle and from the right ventricle to the right atrium. These pressures are used to determine valve gradients and evaluate pulmonic and tricuspid valve function. Blood samples can also be taken as the catheter is withdrawn for detection of left-to-right shunts.[29] If pulmonic or tricuspid valve disease is suspected, contrast can be injected for digital imaging of the right atrium, right ventricle, or pulmonary artery.

Left Heart Catheterization

Left heart catheterization (Fig. 18-3) is used to obtain pressure measurements to evaluate mitral and aortic valve and left ventricular function, to use angiography to evaluate mitral and aortic valve disease, and to perform left ventriculography.[20]

The two main approaches into the left heart are retrograde entry, through the aortic valve by either the percutaneous femoral or direct brachial approach, and transseptal entry, from the right atrium.[3,27] The progress of the catheter in both approaches is followed by fluoroscopy and pressure measurement. In the retrograde approach, the catheter is threaded along the aorta and across the aortic valve to the left ventricle. For mitral valve studies, simultaneous pulmonary

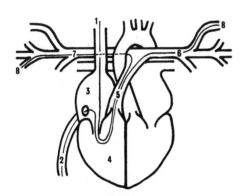

FIGURE 18-2 Right heart catheterization through the superior and inferior venae cavae. Catheters are in the wedge position. Chambers and vessels that may be catheterized are numbered: **(1)** superior vena cava; **(2)** inferior vena cava: **(3)** right atrium; **(4)** right ventricle; **(5)** main pulmonary artery; **(6)** left pulmonary artery; **(7)** right pulmonary artery; **(8)** pulmonary artery wedge. (From Directions in Cardiovascular Medicine 4: Cardiac Catheterization, p 25. Somerville, NJ, Hoechst Pharmaceuticals, 1972.)

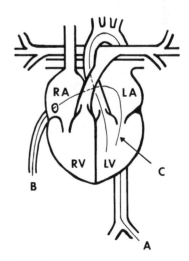

FIGURE 18-3 Left heart catheterization, showing the three approaches for catheterizing the left heart. **(A)** Retrograde approach across the aortic valve by way of the femoral or brachial artery; **(B)** transseptal approach through the right femoral vein and inferior vena cava across the atrial septum; **(C)** direct transthoracic puncture. (From Directions in Cardiovascular Medicine 4: Cardiac Catheterization, p 26. Somerville, NJ, Hoechst Pharmaceuticals, 1972.)

artery wedge and left ventricular pressures or simultaneous left atrial and left ventricular pressures are recorded to evaluate pressure differences across the valve. To evaluate the aortic valve function, pull-back pressure is recorded as the catheter is withdrawn from the left ventricle to the aorta. Digital or cineangiography may be performed during contrast injection of the left atrium, left ventricle, or aortic root to evaluate valve function further.

A third, rarely used, approach to left ventricular catheterization is direct left ventricular puncture (see Fig. 18-3). This technique is used only when the other techniques of entering the left ventricle are unsuccessful, most frequently in cases of severe aortic stenosis.[3,35] Complications occur in approximately 3% of these procedures and include chest pain, cardiac tamponade, pneumothorax, hemothorax, pleural effusion, ventricular arrhythmias, vasovagal responses, and intramyocardial injection of contrast medium.[3]

TRANSSEPTAL LEFT HEART CATHETERIZATION

The transseptal approach to left heart catheterization is indicated in the following situations[3,35]:

◆ When left heart catheterization has not been possible by the retrograde approach owing to severe aortic stenosis or a prosthetic valve

◆ To obtain left atrial angiograms to study mitral valve motion in mitral stenosis
◆ To rule out pulmonary venous obstruction through simultaneous left atrial and pulmonary artery wedge pressures
◆ When pulmonary artery wedge tracings are inaccurate because of pulmonary hypertension or other pulmonary disease

This approach is contraindicated for patients on anticoagulant therapy because of the danger of hemorrhage and tamponade if myocardial puncture occurs. When location of the necessary anatomic landmarks is impossible, as in patients who have severe chest deformities, abnormal heart position, or a huge right atrium, or in those who cannot lie flat, the transseptal approach is also inadvisable.[3,35]

Transseptal catheterization is done only through the right femoral vein and inferior vena cava, using percutaneous techniques and the needle described by Brockenbrough and Braunwald[11] (Fig. 18-4). The transseptal catheter is threaded into the right atrium over a guide wire, which is then removed. The transseptal needle, with a blunt stylet extending beyond its tip to prevent the needle from puncturing the catheter, is threaded up the catheter, the stylet is withdrawn, and the needle is connected to a pressure transducer. The catheter and needle are guided together to the fossa ovalis, where the needle is advanced to

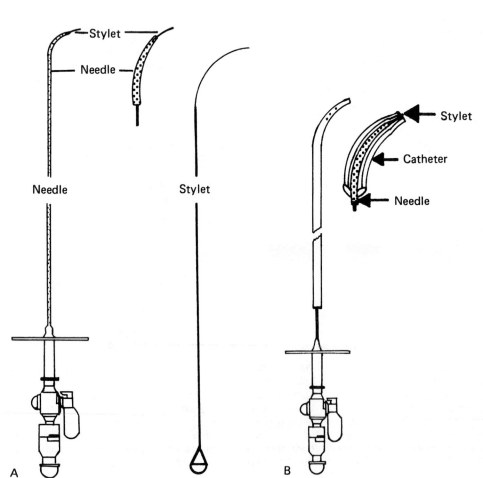

FIGURE 18-4 Transseptal needle, stylet, and catheter. **(A)** Brockenbrough transseptal needle and Bing stylet; **(B)** transseptal needle, catheter, and stylet matched before insertion. (From Conti CR: Percutaneous approach and transseptal catheterization. In Grossman W [ed]: Cardiac Catheterization and Angiography, pp 35–36. Philadelphia, Lea & Febiger, 1976.)

perforate the atrial septum. After perforation of the septum, left atrial pressure is recorded and a blood sample is drawn to confirm the catheter location. The catheter and needle are advanced well into the left atrium, the needle is withdrawn, and the desired studies are performed. The catheter may also be advanced to enter the left ventricle.[3,35]

Ventriculography

Ventriculography is performed to evaluate valve structure or function, to define ventricular anatomy, and to evaluate ventricular function.[37,41] Ventriculography is accomplished by opacifying the ventricular cavity with contrast medium and filming ventricular motion (Fig. 18-5). Digital or cineangiography is single- or biplane filming of the image on an image intensifier by a motion picture camera during cardiac catheterization. Single- or biplane 35-mm movie films are taken at rates of 30, 50, 60, or 90 frames/s. This technique provides a clear sense of movement and the dynamic events of the cardiac cycle, television visualization, instant replay capability, and low x-ray exposure.[6,41] More recently, digital image acquisition is taking the place of cineangiography.

The catheter used for contrast injection during ventriculography must be capable of delivering a large amount of contrast medium (30 to 50 mL) in a short period (10 to 20 mL/s).[41] Many types of catheters are available for ventricular injections. Catheters with side holes, with or without an end hole, are preferred to end-hole catheters because they have less tendency to recoil. Catheter stability is also important to minimize the risk of ventricular arrhythmias during injection.[37] Arrhythmias change the quality of contraction and thus make it impossible to use ventriculography for studies of ventricular function.[41]

Contrast injection is accomplished by power injection. A test dose is first delivered by low-pressure injection to ensure proper catheter placement. The power injection is then made. Patients often feel a hot flash, experience nausea with the injection, and occasionally vomit.[37] The principal complications of injection are arrhythmias, intramyocardial or pericardial injection of contrast medium, and embolism from injection of air or thrombi.

Coronary Arteriography

Coronary arteriography can be performed using either the percutaneous femoral approach of Judkins[39] or the direct brachial approach described by Sones and Shirey.[64]

With the *Judkins technique* (Fig. 18-6), two preformed polyurethane catheters are used for catheterization of the right and left coronary arteries. The catheters are guided over a guide wire through the distal aortic arch to the coronary ostia, the guide is withdrawn, and the catheter is filled with contrast medium.

With the *direct approach* (Fig. 18-7), a single catheter is manipulated for selective catheterization of both the right and left coronary arteries. During passage of the catheter from the subclavian artery to the aortic arch, the patient may be asked to shrug the shoulders, turn the head to the left, or take a deep breath to assist passage of the catheter.

Certain principles apply to both techniques. The ventriculogram may be performed before the coronary arteriogram because intracoronary contrast medium may have a depressant effect on ventricular function.[49] In very sick

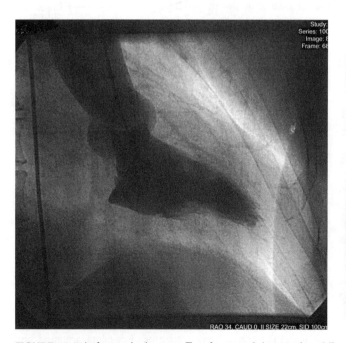
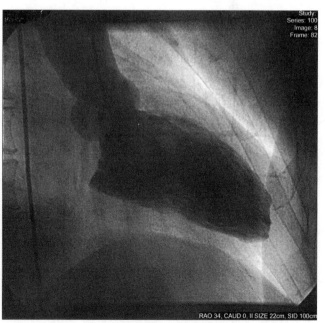

FIGURE 18-5 Left ventriculogram. Two frames, right anterior oblique of projection, demonstrating left ventricle in systole **(A)** and diastole **(B)**. (Courtesy of Virginia Mason Medical Center, Seattle, Washington.)

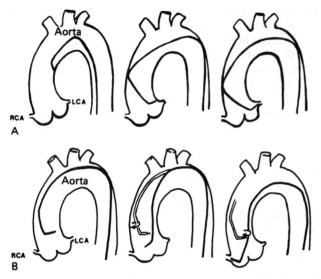

FIGURE 18-6 Coronary artery catheterization by the Sones technique (anterior view). **(A)** Catheter is introduced through the brachial artery to the aortic root and into the right coronary artery (*RCA*). **(B)** After right coronary catheterization, catheter is rotated, and left coronary artery (*LCA*) is catheterized. (From Conti CR: Coronary arteriography. In Grossman W [ed]: Cardiac Catheterization and Angiography, pp 126–127. Philadelphia, Lea & Febiger, 1976.)

patients, coronary angiography may be performed first because it is usually better tolerated than the ventriculogram.[52] Anticoagulant therapy (heparin) is administered intravenously before coronary arteriography to prevent complications from thrombus formation. The ECG and arterial pressure must be closely monitored. Images of both the right

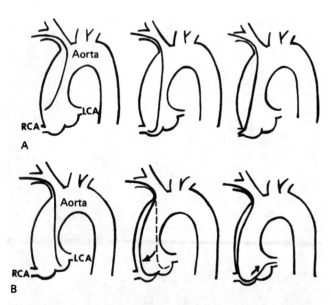

FIGURE 18-7 Coronary artery catheterization by the Judkins technique. **(A)** Catheterization of left coronary artery (*LCA*); **(B)** catheterization of right coronary artery (*RCA*). (From Judkins MP: Percutaneous transfemoral selective coronary arteriography. Radiol Clin North Am 6: 471, 1968.)

and left coronary arteries are recorded in the left anterior oblique (LAO) and right anterior oblique (RAO) views[52] (Fig. 18-8). Frontal, LAO, and RAO films from axial or lordotic angles may also be taken to view specific lesions more clearly. The patient is asked to take a deep breath and hold it without bearing down, just before the injection, to clear the diaphragm from the field. After the injection, the patient is told to breathe and cough, which helps clear the contrast medium from the coronary arteries. Imaging of the coronary arteries may also be performed after the administration of nitroglycerin or other vasodilators to evaluate the effects on the coronary circulation, including the collateral vessels.[52]

Cardiac Output Studies

The most commonly used methods of CO determination are quantitative angiography and the dilution method. Of these, the first is most frequently used for CO determination when coronary arteriography and ventriculography are performed.[28]

An older technique, the direct Fick method, may still be used to a limited extent at some institutions.

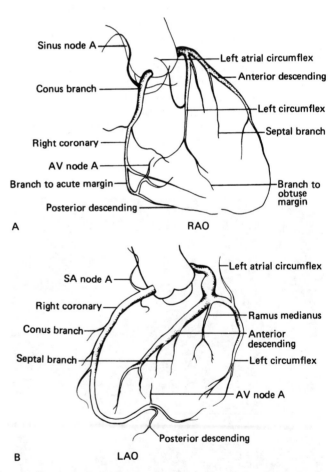

FIGURE 18-8 Spatial appearance of the coronary anatomy in the right anterior oblique (*RAO*) view **(A)** and in the left anterior oblique (*LAO*) view **(B)**. (From Abrams HL, Abrams DF: Coronary arteriography: I. Principles, procedures, interpretation, and applications. In Abrams [ed]: Angiography, 2nd ed, p 402. Boston, Little, Brown, 1971.)

QUANTITATIVE ANGIOGRAPHY

In quantitative angiography, ventricular end-systolic and end-diastolic volumes are determined from the ventriculogram.[63] Single- or biplane films can be used. This method assumes that the left ventricle is of a given shape, most commonly ellipsoid.[19,58,59] The ventricular cavity is outlined at end-systole and end-diastole from the ventriculogram (Fig. 18-9). Correction factors are applied to compensate for the magnification and distortion that occur with filming, and the true dimensions of the ventricle at end-systole and end-diastole are determined. From these dimensions, the left ventricular end-systolic and end-diastolic volumes are calculated. Stroke volume is then obtained by subtracting the end-systolic volume from the end-diastolic volume.[63] Computer software that performs these computations is available.

The advantages and uses of quantitative angiography include eliminating the need for right heart catheterization (which is required for other methods), thus shortening the catheterization time. Because this method reveals the actual ventricular volumes, the left ventricular ejection fraction can be obtained:

$$\text{Ejection Fraction} = \frac{\text{Stroke volume}}{\text{End = diastolic volume}}$$

This parameter, not obtainable with other CO methods, is important in evaluating left ventricular function. The CO obtained by quantitative angiography represents the total CO.[63] In aortic or mitral insufficiency, some of this volume is regurgitant and does not take part in effective circulation.

THERMODILUTION AND INDICATOR DILUTION METHODS

Thermodilution and indicator dilution methods are based on the principle that if a known amount of an indicator is added to an unknown quantity of flowing liquid, and the concentration of the indicator is then measured downstream, the time course of its concentration gives a quantitative index of the flow.[28] Applied to the circulatory system, the amount of indicator, its dilution within the circulation, and the time during which the first circulation of the substance occurs can be used to compute CO.

The thermodilution technique using cold or room-temperature dextrose or saline injectate solution is the most frequently used CO method in cardiac catheterization laboratories. Before the thermodilution method, other dye indicator dilution methods were used. The benefits of the thermodilution technique are that (1) it is performed over a short period, and is therefore more likely to be recorded during a period of steady state; (2) it is most accurate in patients with normal or high CO; (3) the indicator used is inert and inexpensive; (4) it does not require an arterial puncture; and (5) the computer analysis or thermopalpation curve is reasonably simple to interpret.[28] Drawbacks of this method include its unreliability in the presence of significant tricuspid regurgitation and its tendency to overestimate CO in patients with low CO.[28] (See Chapter 19 for further discussion of this technique.)

DIRECT FICK METHOD

The direct Fick method has largely been replaced by the thermodilution method for CO determination. The Fick method, although scientifically superior, requires equipment and processes that are not considered standard in modern cardiac catheterization laboratories. This method is based on the Fick principle, which states that the amount of substance taken up or released by an organ is equal to the product of the organ's blood flow rate and its arterial–mixed venous oxygen difference.[21] The direct Fick

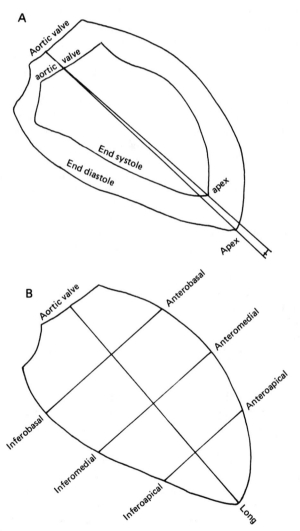

FIGURE 18-9 **(A)** End-systolic and end-diastolic endocardiac silhouettes are superimposed with correction for apical rotation. **(B)** This reference system for ventricular wall motion analysis consists of a long axis and six transverse hemiaxes that quadrisect it at right angles. (From Yang SS, Bentivoglio LG, Maranhao V et al: From Cardiac Catheterization Data to Hemodynamic Parameters, 2nd ed, pp 376–377. Philadelphia, FA Davis, 1978.)

method for CO determination uses the lungs as the organ, oxygen (O_2) as the substance, and CO as the organ's flow. Thus, the formula for CO becomes:

$$CO(L/min) = \frac{O_2 \text{ consumption (mL/min)}}{\left[\begin{array}{c}\text{Pulmonary venous } O_2 \\ \text{content (mL/L)}\end{array}\right] - \left[\begin{array}{c}\text{Pulmonary arterial} \\ O_2 \text{ content (mL/L)}\end{array}\right]}$$

Oxygen consumption is usually measured by one of two methods. In the *polarographic oxygen method,* room air enters at a constant rate through a hood or mask around the patient's head and is carried past a polarographic sensor, which determines the oxygen content of the mixed air (room air plus expired air). Oxygen consumption is calculated from the fractional contents of oxygen in the room air, the oxygen content of the mixed air, and the rate of air flow through the hood. In the *Douglas bag method,* the patient breathes through a mouthpiece that allows inhalation of room air and expiration into a collecting bag (Douglas bag). The mouthpiece must be tightly sealed, the nose clamped, and the collection period carefully timed.[28] Expired air is collected during a measured period of at least 3 minutes. The volume of expired air and its oxygen content are measured. Oxygen consumption is computed from the volume and oxygen content of expired air, the oxygen content of the room air, and the time over which the sample was collected.[28]

Pulmonary venous oxygen content can be measured from any systemic artery. Pulmonary arterial oxygen content is measured directly because the most complete mixing of venous blood occurs in the pulmonary artery. The blood samples are drawn simultaneously during the period of expired air collection. A steady state must exist during the period of air collection because arterial oxygen and venous oxygen are sampled at only one point during the collection period.[28]

Radiographic Angiographic Contrast Agents

The two types of contrast agents are the widely used high- and low-osmolar ionic agents and nonionic low-osmolar agents. Both types of agents contain iodine, which absorbs x-rays and thus provides their imaging properties.[6,36] The hemodynamic and other side effects of contrast agents are related to their osmolality and their chemical and pharmacologic differences.[10,38] Ionic agents have osmolalities as high as six to seven times that of blood, whereas the nonionic agents have an osmolality approximately three times that of blood.[6,36] Nonionic agents are associated with fewer side effects and less dramatic hemodynamic reactions than ionic agents, particularly in high-risk patients. Nonionic agents are significantly more costly than ionic agents.[6,10,36]

Most catheterization laboratories continue to use both ionic and nonionic agents, with many following specific guidelines for agent choice.[12] Indications for use of nonionic agents include unstable ischemic syndromes including acute MI, congestive heart failure, diabetes mellitus, ejection fraction less than 30%, acute or chronic renal insuffi-

ciency, hypotension, severe bradycardia, history of contrast allergy, severe valvular heart disease, internal mammary artery injection, history of transient ischemic attack or recent stroke, and PTCA.[10,33,36]

The hemodynamic effects of contrast agents are well documented. These effects vary with the site and volume of the injection as well as with the osmolality, sodium content, and calcium concentration of the agent used.[38] Immediate effects (10 to 120 seconds) are seen with both ventriculography and coronary angiography, whereas long-term effects are seen primarily with ventriculography or other injections that require large amounts of contrast medium.[38]

After left ventricular injection, there is depression of left ventricular contractility and an increase in intravascular volume, and left ventricular end-diastolic pressure rises.[38] As contrast reaches the systemic arterial system, there is arteriolar vasodilation; this response increases with the osmolality of the agent used. There is a corresponding decrease in arterial pressure.[37,38] These effects peak within 2 to 3 minutes, and values return to normal within 5 minutes.[38]

With coronary arteriography, immediate effects of contrast may include sinus bradycardia, systemic arterial hypotension, an increase in left ventricular end-diastolic pressure, arrhythmias, myocardial ischemia, and T-wave changes on the ECG.[37,38] Usually, these changes revert quickly to normal when the catheter is withdrawn from the coronary ostia and the patient coughs, clearing the contrast medium from the coronary arteries.[37]

The high osmolarity of contrast medium raises serum osmolality. In response, plasma volume increases when water moves from the extravascular to the intravascular space. Both hematocrit and hemoglobin levels fall, whereas left atrial and left ventricular end-diastolic pressures increase in response to the increased intravascular volume.[38] CO and stroke volume increase as a secondary response to the reduced systemic vascular resistance (afterload) and increased filling volume and pressures (preload).[38]

Contrast agents act as an osmotic diuretic.[38] The diuresis that occurs after catheterization may result in water and saline deficits, which precipitate hypotension. For this reason, patients should be given IV replacement or be encouraged to drink liquids on returning from the laboratory.

THE NURSE IN THE CARDIAC CATHETERIZATION LABORATORY

Nurses working in cardiac catheterization laboratories fill many roles. In some laboratories, the nurses scrub and assist in the procedure; in others, they are responsible for monitoring pressure and cardiac rhythm, assisting with hemodynamic studies such as CO determination, and administering IV conscious sedation.[42,46] The nurse may visit the patient before the procedure to teach and help in preparing the patient.[48] The nurse ideally has a background in intensive or coronary care and a thorough knowledge of cardiovascular drugs, arrhythmias, the principles of IV conscious sedation, sterile technique, cardiac anatomy and physiology, pacemakers, and the concepts of catheter flushing and clot and embolus formation and prevention.[46] Changes in the patient's emotional status, alertness, vocal responses, and facial expressions are important indices of the patient's tolerance of the procedure. The nurse's alertness to these clues and early intervention with reassurance or appropriate medication may help to prevent more serious events, such as vasovagal reactions and coronary artery spasm.[43]

Complications and Nursing Care After Cardiac Catheterization

The nursing care of patients after cardiac catheterization is directed toward the prevention and detection of complications. Although complications are infrequent, they do occur and may be life threatening (Table 18-1). Early detection and intervention are essential in preventing permanent disability and death.

The most frequent complication during catheterization is arrhythmia. Ventricular arrhythmias often occur in response to catheter manipulation or contrast medium injection and tend not to recur after the predisposing stimulus is removed. Atrial and junctional arrhythmias and varying degrees of blocks also occur in response to these stimuli, and bradycardia is common in response to injection of the coronary arteries with contrast.[26,33]

Allergic reactions to the contrast medium may occur. Sneezing, itching of the eyes or skin, urticaria, bronchospasm, or other beginning signs of allergy are treated with antihistamines and corticosteroids. Patients with known or suspected allergies to iodine-containing substances such as seafood or with a prior allergic reaction to radiographic contrast may be treated with antihistamines or methylprednisolone before the procedure, and nonionic contrast may be used.[33,36]

POSTPROCEDURE CARE

After the procedure, the femoral arterial or venous introducer sheaths are removed and manual or mechanical pressure is applied to the sheath entry site until hemostasis is achieved. Nurses caring for patients after cardiac catheterization must be prepared to perform sheath removal according to institutional policies and guidelines, and must be able to recognize complications associated with this procedure.[7,45,60]

After returning from the laboratory, the patient must be thoroughly assessed. Information about the approach used, the procedures performed, and any complications experienced during the catheterization should be obtained from the physician, nurse, or technician. Table 18-2 lists typical postcatheterization protocols. These vary among institutions. The elements of the nursing assessment and intervention and potential findings are listed and explained in the following sections.

Psychological Assessment and Patient Teaching. Patients are often tired, hungry, and uncomfortable when they return from the laboratory. They are usually relieved that the procedure is over and may already know the preliminary findings of their study. This news may be good or bad, and it is important to find out what the patient has been told and what this means. The patient may have questions about surgery or about what to expect next. Some patients are anxious or depressed. Giving patients the opportunity to express their feelings about the procedure helps to calm and relax them. Reassure the patient by describing the sensations that can be expected, such as thirst and the frequent

TABLE 18-2	Postcatheterization Protocols

1. Assess vital signs, function every 15 min for 1 h, every 30 min for 1 h, and hourly for 4 h or until discharge.
2. Assess catheterization site for bleeding, hematoma formation, and swelling. Assess peripheral pulses and neurovascular status every 15 min for 1 h, every 30 min for 1 h, and hourly for 4 h or until discharge.
3. Resume precatheterization diet and medications.
4. Administer analgesic agents as needed.
5. Notify physician if any of the following occur:
   a. Decrease in peripheral pulses
   b. New hematoma or increase in size of existing hematoma
   c. Unusually severe catheter insertion site pain or affected extremity pain
   d. Onset of chest discomfort or shortness of breath

Femoral Approach

6. Place patient on bed rest for 6 h. The head of the bed may be raised to 30 degrees.
7. Apply sandbag or ice pack to catheter insertion site.
8. Instruct patient not to flex or hyperextend the hip joint of the affected leg for 12 h, and to use the bed controls to elevate the head of the bed.

Brachial Approach

6. Place patient on bed rest for 2–3 h. The head of the bed may be raised to 30 degrees.
7. Release pressure dressing 30 min after return from the catheterization laboratory and reapply pressure dressing or Ace bandage to affected arm.
8. Instruct patient not to flex or hyperextend or lie on the affected arm for 24 h.
   Instruct the patient regarding dressing changes and when to return for suture removal.

TABLE 18-1	Complications of Cardiac Catheterization	

	Incidence (%)	
Complication	Brachial	Femoral
Arrhythmias	0.45 (54)	0.45 (54)
Vascular emboli, thrombosis	0.91–2.79 (17, 54)	0.22–0.36 (17, 54)
Stroke	0.06 (54)	0.06 (54)
Myocardial infarction	0.06–0.42 (17, 54)	0.07–0.22 (17, 54)
Death	0.09–0.51 (41, 54)	0.11–0.14 (41, 54)
Hemorrhage	0.01 (54)	0.12 (54)
Contrast reactions	0.22 (54)	0.28 (54)

need to urinate even though the patient has had nothing to eat or drink for several hours. Reemphasize the need for bed rest and the need to keep the catheterized limb immobile. Let the patient know that frequent checking of vital signs is routine and not a cause for alarm. Before hospital discharge, the patient should be instructed regarding symptoms for which to call the physician and site care (Table 18-3).

Circulatory Integrity of Entry Site. The most frequent complication of cardiac catheterization is arterial thrombosis.[33,40,54] Thus, careful assessments of the entry site and limb are important elements of postcatheterization nursing care. The site should be checked for visible bleeding, swelling, or tenderness. The arterial pulse at the site and at points distal to it should be compared with pulses on the opposite limb and those recorded before the procedure. Capillary filling and the warmth of the limb should also be evaluated. Blanching, cramping, coolness, pain, numbness, or tingling may indicate reduced perfusion and must be carefully evaluated. A diminished or absent pulse is a sign of serious arterial occlusion. The first step, if any of these signs occur, is to check the dressing. A dressing applied too tightly may result in arterial compression if swelling or

hematoma occurs. If this is not the case, the physician should be notified immediately, and steps should be taken to preserve the limb, as indicated. Bleeding and hematoma are other complications at the entry site.[33] These may occur when a patient moves the limb too vigorously, when the dressing is not sufficiently tight, or because of inadequate suturing at a brachial site. Pressure should be applied, the dressing reapplied, if appropriate, and the physician notified. When pressure is applied at an arterial site, the pulse distal to the site should remain palpable.

Blood Pressure Findings. Evaluation of the blood pressure should include checking for orthostatic hypotension and paradoxical pulse as well as comparing the precatheterization and postcatheterization values. Mild systolic hypotension frequently occurs after cardiac catheterization and is usually not of concern.[26] Angiographic contrast medium acts as an osmotic diuretic, and patients frequently return with signs of volume depletion, including orthostatic hypotension. Patients are thus kept on bed rest until fluid balance is restored with oral liquids or by intravenous replacement. *Hypotension* may also be a response to the drugs given during the procedure. Vasodilators are often administered during coronary arteriography or ventriculography. Protamine sulfate, which may be given to reverse the effects of heparin after coronary arteriography, has direct effects on the myocardium and vascular smooth muscle, resulting in vasodilatation, bradycardia, and hypotension.[26] If the blood pressure is less than 75% to 80% of baseline, other causes such as blood loss or arrhythmias must be considered and assessed, and the physician notified. *Paradoxical pulse* suggests pericardial tamponade, which may occur as a result of perforation of the myocardium. In patients with known perforation, this sign should be specifically assessed with each blood pressure measurement, and if it occurs, the physician should be notified.

Heart Rate and Rhythm. A mild sinus tachycardia (100 to 120 beats/min) is not unusual after catheterization and may be a sign of anxiety, an indication of saline and water loss due to diuresis, or a reaction to medication such as atropine. Fluids, time, and reassurance often bring the heart rate down to more normal levels. Heart rates above 120 beats/min should be evaluated for other causes such as hemorrhage, more severe fluid imbalance, fever, or arrhythmias. Bradycardia may indicate vasovagal responses, arrhythmias, or infarction and should be assessed by ECG and correlated with other clinical signs such as pain and blood pressure.

Temperature. Early increases in temperature may occur because of the fluid loss that occurs with catheterization. More persistent elevations may indicate infection or pyrogenic reactions.

Urinary Output. Because angiographic contrast medium acts as an osmotic diuretic, patients have an increase in urine output for a short time after catheterization.

TABLE 18-3	**Patient Discharge Instructions for Inpatient and Outpatient Catheterization**

1. Report the following symptoms to your physician if they occur:
   a. New bleeding or swelling at the catheterization site
   b. Increased tenderness, redness, drainage, or pain at the catheterization site
   c. Fever
   d. Change in color (pallor), temperature (coolness), or sensation (numbness) in the leg or arm used for catheterization
2. Acetaminophen or other non–aspirin-containing analgesic may be taken every 3 to 4 h as needed for pain.
3. If stitches are present, wear an adhesive bandage until they are removed. Otherwise, cover site with an adhesive bandage for 24 h.
4. Patient may shower the day after the procedure. Tub bath should be avoided for 48 h after the procedure.
5. Patient to see physician for follow-up appointment ____ .
6. Continue prescribed medications as before unless otherwise indicated by your physician.
7. Avoid strenuous activity for 24 h.
8. Patient must be driven home and be accompanied by a responsible adult until the following morning.

Adapted from Preparing You for Cardiac Catheterization, and Ambulatory Recovery Facility Post Cardiac Catheterization Instructions. University Hospital, University of Washington, Seattle, Washington

OTHER POSSIBLE PROBLEMS

Myocardial infarction, stroke, and congestive heart failure are all potential complications after cardiac catheterization. The nurse caring for patients after cardiac catheterization should be aware of the signs and symptoms of these complications. (See Chapters 19 and 21 for more complete discussion of these specific problems.)

INTERPRETATION OF DATA

Table 18-4 lists normal ranges for some of the data gathered during cardiac catheterization. The assessment of coronary artery disease involves evaluation of the coronary vasculature and left ventricular function.

The first step in evaluating the coronary arteriogram is to determine whether the coronaries are unobstructed and free of lesions. Each major artery is traced along its entire length, and branches and collaterals are noted and evaluated for irregularities or narrowing.[52] When occlusion is present, the degree of disease and the suitability of the artery for revascularization are of primary concern. The American Heart Association Ad Hoc Committee for Grading of Coronary Artery Disease has recommended the following system for grading occlusions:[2]

1. Normal: No decrease in lumen diameter
2. 25%: Decrease in lumen diameter up to 25%
3. 50%: Decrease in lumen diameter of 26% to 50%
4. 75%: Decrease in lumen diameter of 51% to 75%
5. 90%: Decrease in lumen diameter of 76% to 90%
6. 99%: Hair-width lumen with greater than 90% narrowing
7. 100%: Total occlusion

In addition to grading the occlusion, the condition of the distal artery must be evaluated. The distal artery may be identified by antegrade or collateral flow, and its caliber and suitability as a recipient for bypass grafting is evaluated. Arteries with high degrees of peripheral involvement are less suitable for bypass grafting. The proximity of the occlusion determines the amount of myocardium in jeopardy. A subjective evaluation of the degree of arterial flow is made by observing the time required for perfused arteries to fill and clear. Contrast medium clears faster with higher flow rates. Intermittent luminal obstruction due to systolic constriction from encircling muscle bands or to coronary artery spasm is also observed, and its degree, distribution, and pattern are evaluated.[6] If bypass grafts have been injected, they are evaluated in the same manner for patency, flow indices, and the condition of the perfused artery. Figures 18-10 and 18-11 show normal and abnormal angiograms of the right and left coronary arteries.

Evaluation of myocardial function is an important part of the evaluation of coronary artery disease. Patterns of ventricular contraction are evaluated by superimposing the

TABLE 18-4	Normal Adult Values for Data Collected During Cardiac Catheterization
Pressures	(mm Hg)[43]
Systemic arterial	
Peak-systolic	100–140
End-diastolic	60–90
Mean	70–105
Left ventricular	
Peak-systolic	100–140
End-diastolic	3–12
Left atrial	
Left atrial mean (or PAWP)	1–10
a wave	3–15
v wave	3–12
Pulmonary artery	
Peak-systolic	15–30
End-diastolic	3–12
Systolic mean	9–16
Right ventricular	
Peak-systolic	15–30
End-diastolic	0–8
Right atrial	
Mean	0–8
a wave	2–10
v wave	2–10
Left Ventricular Volumes[23]	
End-systolic volume (mL/m²)	20–30
End-diastolic volume (mL/m²)	70–79
Ejection fraction (%)	58–72
Resistance (dynes/s/cm⁻⁵)[43]	
Total systemic resistance	900–1440
Pulmonary arteriolar (vascular) resistance	37–97
Flow[16]	
Cardiac output (L/min)	4.0–8.0
Cardiac index (L/min/m²)	2.5–4.0
Stroke index (mL/beat/m²)	35–70
Stroke volume (mL/beat)	60–130
Oxygen consumption (mL/min/m²)	125
Oxygen Saturation (%)[16]	
Right atrium	60–75
Right ventricle	60–75
Pulmonary artery	60–75
Left atrium	95–99
Left ventricle	95–99
Aorta	95–99

PAWP, pulmonary artery wedge pressure.

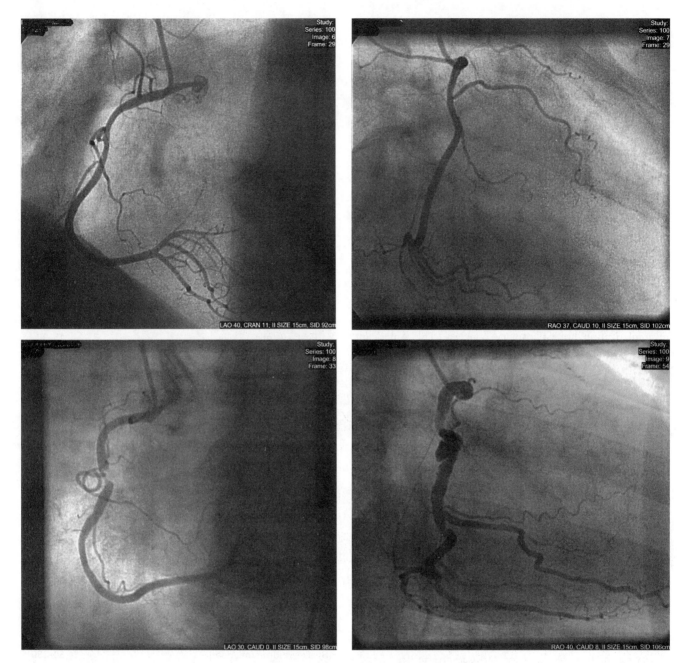

FIGURE 18-10 Right coronary artery (RCA). **(A and B)** Normal right coronary artery in the left anterior oblique (*LAO*) and right anterior oblique (*RAO*) projections. **(C)** RCA, LAO projection with 90% narrowing of the proximal portion of the vessel. **(D)** RCA, RAO projection with multiple obstructions. (Courtesy of Virginia Mason Medical Center, Seattle, Washington.)

systolic and diastolic outlines of the left ventricular chamber in the RAO and LAO projections.[41] In the RAO projection, a long axis is drawn from the apex to the aortic valve commissure aligned at the aortic valve or the midpoint of the long axis (see Fig. 18-9*A*). The anterior, inferior, and apical regions of the left ventricle can be examined in the RAO projection. In the LAO projection, septal and inferior wall motion abnormalities may be seen.[41] Many methods are used to subdivide the areas of the ventricular wall by region[8,39,67]

(see Fig. 18-9*B*). The ventricular contractile state of each region may then be qualitatively classified (Fig. 18-12). Regional contraction may be classified as follows:[39]

1. Normal
2. Mild hypokinesia—a mild reduction in myocardial contraction
3. Severe hypokinesia—a more severe reduction in myocardial contraction

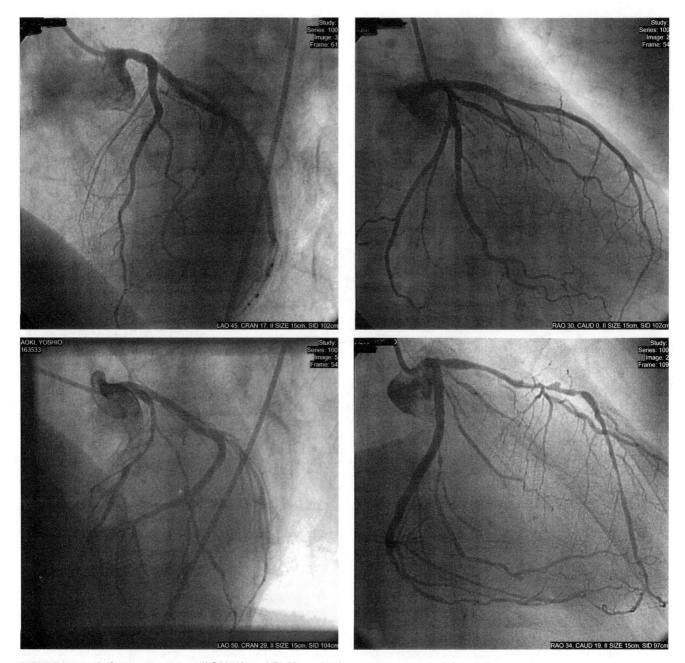

FIGURE 18-11 Left coronary artery (LCA). **(A** and **B)** Normal left coronary artery in left anterior oblique (*LAO*) and right anterior oblique (*RAO*) projections. **(C** and **D)** LCA. Severe left main lesion shown in LAO and RAO projections with multiple obstructions in the left anterior descending and the obtuse marginal branches of the left circumflex. (Courtesy of Virginia Mason Medical Center, Seattle, Washington.)

4. Akinesia—the total absence of wall motion in a discrete area
5. Dyskinesia—a disturbance in the temporal sequence of left ventricular wall contraction
6. Aneurysm—paradoxical systolic expansion of a portion of the left ventricular wall

The reversibility of myocardial contraction abnormalities is an important consideration in the decision for sur-

gery. Reversibility of abnormal contractility can be evaluated with ventriculography after administration of nitroglycerin or catecholamines or by observing postextrasystolic potentiation after premature contractions.[49,52] If these maneuvers or events result in improved contractility, revascularization may also improve contractility. Improved function is more common with hypokinesis than with akinesis or dyskinesis.[6,9,57] The presence of collateral vessels and the lack of Q waves favor the reversibility of hypokinesis.[9]

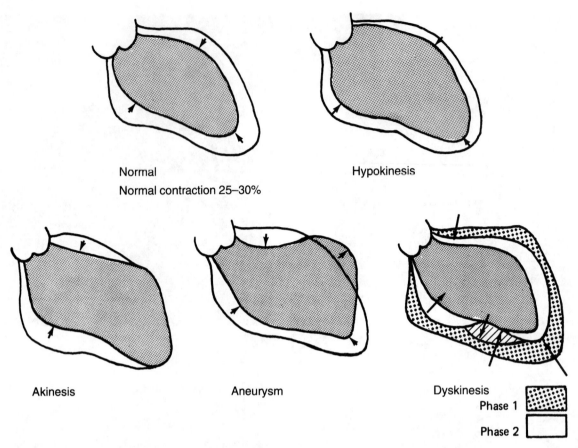

FIGURE 18-12 Normal contraction and contraction abnormalities viewed in the right anterior oblique projection. *Arrows* illustrate motion from end-diastole to end-systole. (Adapted from Herman MV, Heinle RA, Klein MD et al: Localized disorders in myocardial contraction, asynergy and its role in congestive heart failure. N Engl J Med 277: 225, 1967.)

REFERENCES

1. American College of Cardiology/American Heart Association: Cardiac catheterization and guidelines for cardiac catheterization laboratories. Circulation 84: 2213–2247, 1991
2. Austen WB, Edwards RL, Frye RL et al: A reporting system on patients evaluated for coronary artery disease: Report of the ad hoc committee for grading of coronary artery disease, Council on Cardiovascular Surgery, American Heart Association. Circulation 51: 7–40, 1975
3. Baim DS, Grossman W: Percutaneous approach, including transseptal catheterization and apical left ventricular puncture. In Grossman W, Baim DS (eds): Cardiac Catheterization and Angiography, pp 62–81. Philadelphia, Lea & Febiger, 1991
4. Baim DS, Grossman W: Coronary angiography. In Grossman W, Baim DS (eds): Cardiac Catheterization and Angiography, pp 185–214. Philadelphia, Lea & Febiger, 1991
5. Baim DS, Paulin S: Angiography: Principles underlying proper utilization of cineangiographic equipment and contrast agents. In Grossman W, Baim DS (eds): Cardiac Catheterization and Angiography, pp 15–27. Philadelphia, Lea & Febiger, 1991
6. Banka VS, Bodenheimer MM, Helfant RH: Determinants of reversible asynergy, the native coronary circulation. Circulation 52: 810–816, 1975
7. Bogart MA: Time to hemostasis: A comparison of manual versus mechanical compression of the femoral artery. Am J Crit Care 4: 149–156, 1995
8. Bolson EL, Kliman S, Sheehan F et al: Left ventricular segmental wall motion: A new method using local direction information. Computers in Cardiology 245, 248, 1980
9. Bourassa MB, Lisperance J, Campeau L et al: Fate of left ventricular contraction following aortocoronary venous grafts: Early and late postoperative modifications. Circulation 46: 724–730, 1972
10. Brinker JA: Selection of a contrast agent in the cardiac catheterization laboratory. Am J Cardiol 66: 26F–33F, 1990
11. Brockenbrough EC, Braunwald E: A new technique for left ventricular angiography and transseptal left heart catheterization. Am J Cardiol 6: 1062–1064, 1960
12. Cameron A, Sheldon WC, Balter S: Cardiac catheterization laboratory survey: 1990 Society for Cardiac Angiography and Interventions Laboratory Performance Standards Committee. Cathet Cardiovasc Diagn 27: 267–275, 1992
13. Clark DA, Moscovich MD, Vetrovec GW, Wexler L: Guidelines for the performance of outpatients catheterization and angiographic procedures. Cathet Cardiovasc Diagn 27: 5–7, 1992
14. Cournand AF, Ranges CS: Catheterization of the right auricle in man. Proc Soc Exp Biol Med 46: 462, 1941
15. Cournand AF, Riley RL, Breed ES et al: Measurement of cardiac output in man using the technique of catheterization of the right auricle or ventricle. J Clin Invest 24: 106–116, 1945
16. Daily EK, Schroeder JS: Techniques in Bedside Hemodynamic Monitoring, 3rd ed. St. Louis, CV Mosby, 1985

17. Davis K, Kennedy JW, Kemp HG et al: Complications of coronary arteriography for the collaborative study of coronary artery surgery (CASS). Circulation 59: 1105–1112, 1979

18. Dehmer GJ, Haagen D, Malloy CR, Schmitz JM: Anticoagulation with heparin during cardiac catheterization and its reversal by protamine. Cathet Cardiovasc Diagn 13: 16–21, 1987

19. Dodge HT, Hay RE, Sandler H: An angiographic method for directly determining left ventricular stroke volume in man. Circ Res 11: 739–745, 1962

20. Edwards M, Payton V: Cardiac catheterization, teaching and technique. Nurs Clin North Am 11: 271–281, 1976

21. Fick A: Uber die Messung des Blutquantums in den Herzventrikeln, p 16. Wurzburg, Germany, SB Physmed, 1870

22. Fierens E: Outpatient coronary arteriography. Cathet Cardiovasc Diagn 10: 27–32, 1984

23. Fifer MA, Grossman W: Measurement of ventricular volumes, ejection fraction, mass, wall stress, and regional wall motion. In Grossman W, Baim DS (eds): Cardiac Catheterization and Angiography, pp 300–318. Philadelphia, Lea & Febiger, 1991

24. Forssman W: Die Sondierung des rechter Herzens. Klin Wochenschr 8: 2085, 1929

25. Grossman W: Cardiac catheterization: Historical perspective and present practice. In Grossman W, Baim DS (eds): Cardiac Catheterization and Angiography, pp 3–14. Philadelphia, Lea & Febiger, 1991

26. Grossman W: Complication of cardiac catheterization: Incidence, causes, and prevention. In Grossman W, Baim DS (eds): Cardiac Catheterization and Angiography, pp 28–43. Philadelphia, Lea & Febiger, 1991

27. Grossman W: Cardiac catheterization by direct exposure of artery and vein. In Grossman W, Baim DS (eds): Cardiac Catheterization and Angiography, pp 47–61. Philadelphia, Lea & Febiger, 1991

28. Grossman W: Blood flow measurement: The cardiac output. In Grossman W, Baim DS (eds): Cardiac Catheterization and Angiography, pp 105–122. Philadelphia, Lea & Febiger, 1991

29. Grossman W: Shunt detection and measurement. In Grossman W, Baim DS (eds): Cardiac Catheterization and Angiography, pp 166–181. Philadelphia, Lea & Febiger, 1991

30. Health and Public Policy Committee, American College of Physicians: The safety and efficacy of ambulatory cardiac catheterization in the hospital and freestanding setting. Ann Intern Med 103: 294–298, 1985

31. Herman MV, Heinle RA, Klein MD et al: Localized disorders in myocardial contraction, asynergy and its role in congestive heart failure. N Engl J Med 277: 222–232, 1967

32. Heupler FA, Heisler M, Keys TF et al: Infection prevention guidelines for cardiac catheterization laboratories. Cathet Cardiovasc Diagn 25: 260–263, 1992

33. Hildner FJ: Risks of cardiac catheterization. In Pepine CJ, Hill JA, Lambert CR (eds): Diagnostic and Therapeutic Cardiac Catheterization, pp 22–37. Baltimore, Williams & Wilkins, 1989

34. Hill JA, Grabowski EF: Relationship of anticoagulation and radiographic contrast agents to thrombosis during coronary angiography and angioplasty: Are there real concerns? Cathet Cardiovasc Diagn 25: 200–208, 1992

35. Hill JA, Lamber DR, Pepine CJ: Review of techniques. In Pepine CJ, Hill JA, Lambert CR (eds): Diagnostic and Therapeutic Cardiac Catheterization, pp 71–91. Baltimore, Williams & Wilkins, 1989

36. Hill JA, Lambert CR, Pepine CJ: Radiographic contrast agents. In Pepine CJ, Hill JA, Lambert CR (eds): Diagnostic and Therapeutic Cardiac Catheterization, pp 140–150. Baltimore, Williams & Wilkins, 1989

37. Hillis LD, Grossman W. Cardiac ventriculography. In Grossman W, Baim DS (eds): Cardiac Catheterization and Angiography, pp 215–228. Philadelphia, Lea & Febiger, 1991

38. Hirshfeld JW: Cardiovascular effects of iodinated contrast agents. Am J Cardiol 66: 9F–17F, 1990

39. Judkins MP: Percutaneous transfemoral selective coronary arteriography. Radiol Clin North Am 6: 467–492, 1968

40. Kennedy JW: Registry Committee of the Society for Cardiac Angiography: Mortality related to cardiac catheterization and angiography. Cathet Cardiovasc Diagn 8: 323–340, 1982

41. Kennedy JW, Sheehan FH: Ventriculography. In Pepine CJ, Hill JA, Lambert CR (eds): Diagnostic and Therapeutic Cardiac Catheterization, pp 161–175. Baltimore, Williams & Wilkins, 1989

42. Kixmiller JM, Schick L: Conscious sedation in cardiovascular procedures. Critical Care Nursing Clinics of North America 9: 301–312, 1997

43. Lambert CR, Pepine CJ, Nichols WW: Pressure measurement. In Pepine CJ, Hill JA, Lambert CR (eds): Diagnostic and Therapeutic Cardiac Catheterization, pp 283–297. Baltimore, Williams & Wilkins, 1989

44. Lange RA, Hillis LD: Assessment of cardiovascular function. In Pepine CJ, Hill JA, Lambert CR (eds): Diagnostic and Therapeutic Cardiac Catheterization, pp 346–378. Baltimore, Williams & Wilkins, 1989

45. Lazzara D, Pfersdorf P, Sedlacek M: Femoral compression. Nursing 97 27(12): 54–57, 1997

46. McCracken MJ, Chapman MJ: The cardiac catheterization suite. In Bashore TM (ed): Invasive Cardiology Principles and Techniques, pp 5–17. Toronto, BC Decker, 1990

47. Montes P: Managing Outpatient Catheterization. Am J Nurs 97: 34–37, 1997

48. Owens P, Bashore TM: The preparation and care of the patient and the laboratory. In Bashore TM (ed): Invasive Cardiology Principles and Techniques, pp 19–39. Toronto, BC Decker, 1990

49. Pasternak RD, Reis GJ: Profiles in coronary artery disease. In Grossman W, Baim DS (eds): Cardiac Catheterization and Angiography, pp 582–607. Philadelphia, Lea & Febiger, 1991

50. Pepine CJ, Hill JA, Lambert CR: History of the development and application of cardiac catheterization. In Pepine CJ, Hill JA, Lambert CR (eds): Diagnostic and Therapeutic Cardiac Catheterization, pp 3–10. Baltimore, Williams & Wilkins, 1989

51. Pepine CJ, Hill JA, Lambert CR: Indication and contraindications. In Pepine CJ, Hill JA, Lambert CR (eds): Diagnostic and Therapeutic Cardiac Catheterization, pp 13–21. Baltimore, Williams & Wilkins, 1989

52. Pepine CJ, Lambert DR, Hill JA: Coronary angiography. In Pepine CJ, Hill JA, Lambert CR (eds): Diagnostic and Therapeutic Cardiac Catheterization, pp 176–201. Baltimore, Williams & Wilkins, 1989

53. Piazzo D, Jackson BS: Nursing decisions, experiences in clinical problem solving: Sara N., an anxious patient undergoing cardiac catheterization. RN 39: 41–47, 1976

54. Society for Cardiac Angiography: Registry Committee Annual Report. New York: Society for Cardiac Angiography, December 1987

55. Richards DW: Cardiac output by catheterization technique in various clinical conditions. Fed Proc 4: 215–220, 1945

56. Rogers WF, Moothart RW: Outpatient arteriography and cardiac catheterization: Effective alternatives to inpatient procedures. AJR Am J Roentgenol 144: 233–234, 1985

57. Saltiel J, Lesperanel J, Bourassa MG et al: Reversibility of left ventricular dysfunction following aorto-coronary bypass grafts. AJR Am J Roentgenol 110: 739–746, 1970

58. Sandler H, Dodge HT: The use of single plane angiocardiograms for the calculation of left ventricular volume in man. Am Heart J 75: 325–334, 1968

59. Sandler H, Dodge HT: Quantitation of valvular insufficiency by angiocardiography in man. Clin Res 8: 191, 1960

60. Schickel S, Cronin SN, Mize A et al: Removal of femoral sheaths by registered nurses: Issues and outcomes. Critical Care Nursing 16: 32–36, 1996

61. Schultz DD, Olivas GS: The use of cough cardiopulmonary resuscitation in clinical practice. Heart Lung 15: 273–280, 1986

62. Seldinger SI: Catheter replacement of the needle in percutaneous arteriography. Acta Radiol 29: 368–376, 1953

63. Skelton TN: Angiographic techniques and data analysis. In Bashore TM (ed): Invasive Cardiology Principles and Techniques, pp 199–238. Toronto, BC Decker, 1990

64. Sones FM, Shirey EK: Cine coronary arteriography. Modern Concepts in Cardiovascular Disease 31: 735–738, 1962

65. Sones FM, Shirey EK, Prondfit WL et al: Cine-coronary arteriography. Circulation 20: 773, 1959

66. Stewart WJ, McSweeney SM, Kellet MA et al: Increased risk of severe protamine reactions in NPH insulin-dependent diabetics undergoing cardiac catheterization. Circulation 5: 788–792, 1984

67. Yang SS, Bentivoglio LG, Maranhao V et al: From Cardiac Catheterization Data to Hemodynamic Parameters, 2nd ed. Philadelphia, FA Davis, 1978

Hemodynamic Monitoring

ELIZABETH J. BRIDGES

Invasive catheters (arterial catheters, central venous catheters, pulmonary artery [PA] catheters) are placed in critically ill patients when acute changes in cardiopulmonary function occur that require more extensive assessment than the standard clinical measurement of vital signs (heart rate [HR], blood pressure, respiratory rate). Physiologic measures are obtained to assess preload, afterload, contractility, and the components of oxygen delivery. Information about the factors that affect cardiac output (CO) and oxygen supply and demand are used to guide and evaluate the effectiveness of therapy.

TECHNICAL ASPECTS OF INVASIVE PRESSURE MONITORING

Invasive measurement of intravascular (blood pressure) and intracardiac (right atrial [RA] and PA) pressures involves gaining access into an artery or vein. The catheter is connected to fluid-filled tubing and a pressure transducer that communicates with the bedside monitor. The components of the pressure monitoring system are illustrated in Figure 19-1.

Pressure monitoring systems are divided into two components: the components of the electrical system and the components of the fluid or "plumbing" system.[150,151] The electrical system consists of the amplifier, the oscilloscope, the processor or display, and the analog recorder. The amplifier increases or amplifies the signal from the transducer, and the signal is displayed on the oscilloscope as a pressure waveform, and numerically as a digital display. The analog recorder records the pressure waveform on pressure graph paper.

The components of the fluid or plumbing system are in direct contact with the patient's vascular system and carry the mechanical signal to the transducer. These components consist of the vascular catheter, the noncompliant pressure tubing, a continuous-flush device that allows continuous and manual flushing of the catheter tubing system, two or three stopcocks, pressure transducer, an infusion pressure bag, and flush solution of normal saline. The flush solution usually contains heparin to maintain catheter patency. The amount of heparin added to the solution varies among institutions. The infusion pressure bag must be maintained at

300 mm Hg to allow the continuous-flush device to deliver a rate of 1 to 3 mL/h.[143,335] The plumbing system components are disposable items and should be replaced in accordance with the information in Table 19-1.

Reference Level

Correct referencing is crucial to ensure the accuracy of pressure measurements. In 1945, Winsor and Burch[504] conducted studies to determine a reference for the measurement of venous pressure, which they defined as the phlebostatic axis and phlebostatic level. The *phlebostatic axis* is the intersection of two reference lines: first, an imaginary line from the fourth intercostal space (ICS) at the point where it joins the sternum, drawn out to the side of the body; second, a line drawn *midway* between the anterior and posterior surfaces of the chest. The *phlebostatic level* is a horizontal line through the phlebostatic axis. As the patient moves from the flat to the upright position, the phlebostatic level rotates on the axis and remains horizontal (Fig. 19-2). The phlebostatic axis should be marked on the patient's chest to ensure consistent pressure readings.[509]

Although Winsor and Burch identified the phlebostatic axis as the reference level for venous (RA) pressures, it has also been identified as the reference for the left atrium (LA).[237,349,471] It is important to note that the PA catheter is referenced to the *mid-LA*, not to the PA catheter tip.[84] In subjects with normal chest wall configuration, the mid-axillary line (MAL) has also been identified as a valid reference level for the RA and LA.[236] However, use of the MAL in patients with varied chest configuration may result in a potential pressure difference of up to 6 mm Hg.[20] Therefore, use of the MAL as a reference is not recommended.

Even though patients are frequently placed in a lateral position, hemodynamic monitoring in this position has been complicated by the need to identify angle-specific LA references. Attainment of valid and reliable PA pressures was not possible because the use of a reference point above or below the LA resulted in the inclusion of hydrostatic pressure component; thus, the measured pressures were underestimated or overestimated.[46,54,180,233,236,237,499] The effect of varying reference levels on pressures recorded

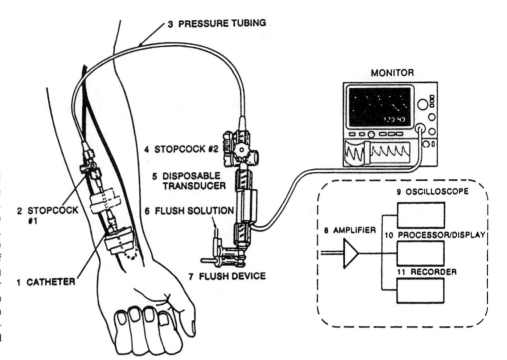

FIGURE 19-1 Components used to monitor blood pressure directly are nearly the same, independent of whether the catheter is in an artery (radial, brachial, or femoral) or in the pulmonary artery. The size of the transducer and plumbing components were enlarged for the illustration. (Adapted from Gardner RM, Hollingsworth KW: Optimizing ECG and pressure monitoring. Crit Care Med 14: 651, 1986.)

was demonstrated by Ross,[383] who placed patients in the 30-degree right and left lateral positions, and then used various reference points. As demonstrated in Figure 19-3, for every 1 cm the reference point is above the LA, the measured pressure decreases by 0.73 mm Hg. Conversely, for every 1 cm the reference point is below the LA, the measured pressure increases by 0.73 mm Hg.

Using chest radiography, Kennedy and colleagues[242] identified the fourth ICS mid-sternal line as the LA reference in the 90-degree lateral decubitus position. Using computed tomography, Paolella and colleagues[349] identified the fourth ICS left parasternal border in the left-lateral decubitus position and the fourth ICS at the mid-sternum in the right-lateral decubitus position as the reference for

TABLE 19-1	Summary of Recommended Frequency for Replacement of Intravascular Devices and Catheter Site Dressings[212,300,354]	
Device	**Replacement and Relocation of Device**	**Dressing Change**
Peripheral arterial line	Replace/relocate catheter and insertion site *no more* frequently than every 4 days for infection control purposes. Replace disposable transducer, continuous-flush device, flush solution every 96 hours.	Replace dressing when the catheter is replaced or when the dressing becomes damp, loosened, or soiled, or when inspection of the site is necessary.
Central venous line	Do not routinely replace percutaneously inserted catheters by either rotating the insertion site or by guide wire exchange. No recommendation for hang time of intravenous fluids.	No recommendation. Replace when the catheter is replaced or when the dressing becomes damp, loosened, or soiled, or when inspection of the site is necessary.
PA catheter	Replace at least every 5 days. If feasible, replace the sheath (introducer) every 5 days even if the PA catheter has already been removed. No recommendation for hang time of intravenous fluids. No recommendation for replacement of transducer, flush solution, tubing.	No recommendation. Replace when the catheter is replaced or when the dressing becomes damp, loosened, or soiled, or when inspection of the site is necessary.

PA, pulmonary artery.

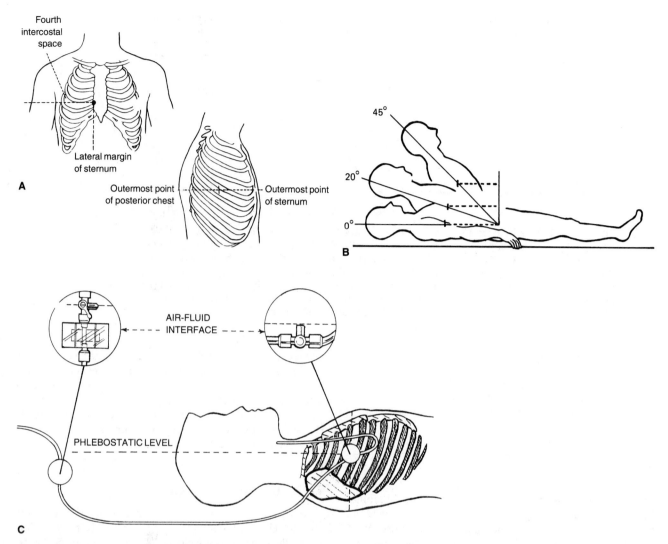

FIGURE 19-2 The phlebostatic axis and the phlebostatic level. **(A)** The phlebostatic axis is the crossing of two reference lines: (1) a line from the fourth intercostal space at the point where it joins the sternum, drawn out to the side of the body beneath the axilla; and (2) a line midway between the anterior and posterior surfaces of the chest. **(B)** The phlebostatic level is a horizontal line through the phlebostatic axis. The air–fluid interface of the stopcock of the transducer or the zero mark on the manometer must be level with this axis for accurate measurements. Moving from the flat to erect positions, the patient moves the chest and therefore the reference level; the phlebostatic level stays horizontal through the same reference point. (Adapted from Shinn JA, Woods SL, Huseby JS: Effect of intermittent positive pressure ventilation upon pulmonary capillary wedge pressures in acutely ill patients. Heart Lung 8: 324: 1979.) **(C)** Two methods for referencing the pressure system to the phlebostatic axis. The system can be referenced by placing the air–fluid interface of either the in-line stopcock or the stopcock on top of the transducer at the phlebostatic level. (From Bridges EJ, Woods SL: Pulmonary artery pressure measurement: State of the art. Heart Lung 22: 101, 1993.)

the LA. The difference between these two measurements is clinically insignificant.

In the 30-degree lateral recumbent position, the reference level for the mid-LA is approximately one-half the vertical distance from the surface of the bed to the left-sternal border in the right and left 30-degree lateral positions[471,472] (Fig. 19-4). Using this reference level, there were statistically ($P < 0.05$), but not clinically, significant pressure changes in the 30-degree right and left lateral positions (0-degree backrest elevation) in hemodynami-

cally stable postcardiac surgery patients during the first 24 postoperative hours. However, individual response to position needs to be assessed.[41] In addition, use of the reference point identified in the supine, 0-degree backrest position (phlebostatic axis) would on average introduce a maximal error of 1 mm Hg; therefore, from a pragmatic perspective, when the patient is placed in the 30-degree lateral position, the transducer does not need to be moved from the position that was level with the supine phlebostatic axis.

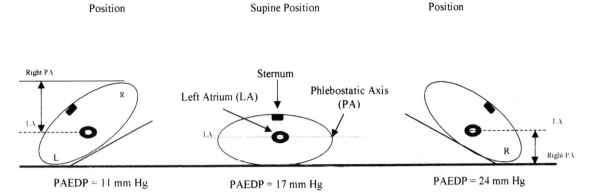

Left 30°-Lateral Position

Supine Position

Right 30°Lateral Position

PAEDP = 11 mm Hg

PAEDP = 17 mm Hg

PAEDP = 24 mm Hg

FIGURE 19-3 Work by Ross and Jones[383] demonstrates the effect of varying references on measured pressures. The pulmonary artery end-diastolic (PAED) pressure in the supine position using the phlebostatic axis as the reference was 17 mm Hg. When the phlebostatic axis was used with the patient in the 30-degree left lateral position, the PAED pressure was 11 mm Hg because the reference was above the left atrium. With the patient in the right 30-degree lateral position, using the PA, the PAED pressure was 24 mm Hg, reflecting the inclusion of hydrostatic pressure from a reference point below the left atrium. PA, phlebostatic axis; LA, left atrium.

Zeroing and Referencing

Zeroing is performed by opening the system to air to establish atmospheric pressure as zero and to compensate for offset caused by hydrostatic pressure or offset in the pressure transducer, amplifier, oscilloscope, recorder, or digital delays.[151] The disposable transducer-catheter systems currently in use demonstrate minimal zero drift.[3] Zero drift is related to the offset in the electrical and plumbing components of the system; thus, zeroing is primarily performed to correct for the offset caused by hydrostatic pressure. In addition, calibrating disposable pressure transducers and fixed-calibration bedside pressure monitoring systems is no longer recommended.[147]

Referencing is accomplished by placing the air–fluid interface (stopcock) of the catheter system at a specified reference point to negate the weight effect of the catheter tubing (see Fig. 19-2). The act of simultaneously zeroing and referencing ensures that the pressures being measured are intracardiac. The procedure for referencing and zeroing is outlined in Display 19-1. When the air–fluid interface on the stopcock is placed above the phlebostatic level, the pressure measurement is lower as a result of decreased hydrostatic pressure. When the air–fluid interface is positioned below the phlebostatic level, the pressure measurement is falsely increased. For every 1.36 cm of discrepancy, the measured pressure is altered by 1 mm Hg, a potentially treatable difference.[150,152,153,319]

Dynamic Response Characteristics

The dynamic response characteristics of the catheter-transducer system reflect the system's ability to reproduce faithfully a pressure waveform. The dynamic response can be determined by evaluating the system's natural (resonant) frequency and damping coefficient (Fig. 19-5). The damping coefficient is a measure of how quickly the system dampens and eventually arrests the oscillations.[149,152] A certain degree of damping is desirable for optimal fidelity and suppression of unwanted high-frequency vibration or noise.

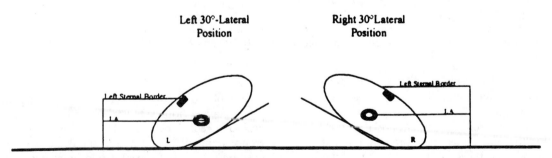

Left 30°-Lateral Position

Right 30°Lateral Position

FIGURE 19-4 Left atrial reference point in 30-degree lateral position. The reference point is located one-half the vertical distance between the surface of the bed and the left sternal border in both right and left 30-degree lateral positions. PA, phlebostatic axis; LA, left atrium. (From VanEtta DJ: Location of the Left Atrium in Thirty-Degree Right and Thirty-Degree Left Lateral Recumbency in Adults. Unpublished master's thesis. University of Washington, Seattle. Adapted with permission.)

DISPLAY 19-1

Protocol for Obtaining Pulmonary Artery and Pulmonary Artery Wedge Pressures Using Digital and Analog Recordings

1. Explain procedure to patient
2. Position patient in
   a. Supine position with backrest up to 60 degrees
   b. Lateral position at 30 or 90 degrees
3. Allow 5 minutes for pressure stabilization after position change
4. Reference and zero the pressure-transducer system
   a. Locate the reference point
      (1) Supine: line bisecting fourth ICS at the sternum and one-half anteroposterior diameter
      (2) 30-degree lateral (right and left): one-half distance from left sternal border to surface of bed
      (3) 90-degree lateral (right): fourth ICS at the mid-sternum
      (4) 90-degree lateral (left): fourth ICS left parasternal border
   b. Level the air–fluid interface (not the transducer) with the reference level (use either the in-line stopcock or the stopcock on the top of the transducer)

   (1) Spontaneous: Immediately before inspiratory trough

   c. Remove the cap from the stopcock using aseptic technique
      (1) Spontaneous: Immediately before inspiratory trough
   d. Turn stopcock "off" to the patient and "open" to air
   e. Activate the "Zero" button on the monitor
   f. Close stopcock and replace cap
   g. Reference and zero the system anytime the patient's position changes
5. Check and troubleshoot the dynamic response characteristics of the system every shift, if the waveform characteristics change, or if the system has been disturbed (blood draw, tubing change; (see Figure 19-5)
6. Identify end-expiratory waveform
   a. Determine pressures using analog (graphic) tracing (analog pressure method recommended over "freeze screen" or digital methods)
   b. Record end-expiratory pressures

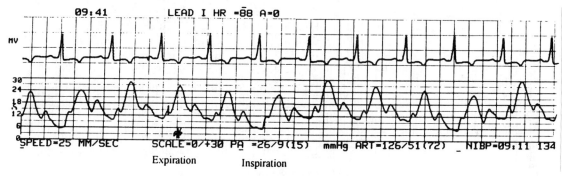

Figure PA Systolic = 27 mm Hg; PAEDP = 13 mm Hg; PA mean = 19 mm Hg

(2) Mechanical ventilation: Immediately before inspiratory rise

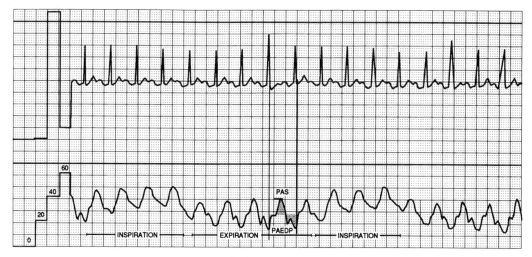

Figure: PA systolic = 44 mm Hg; PAEDP = 22 mm Hg; PA mean = 33 mm Hg

(continued)

Protocol for Obtaining Pulmonary Artery and Pulmonary Artery Wedge Pressures Using Digital and Analog Recordings

(3) Intermittent mechanical ventilation: Determine from analog display only

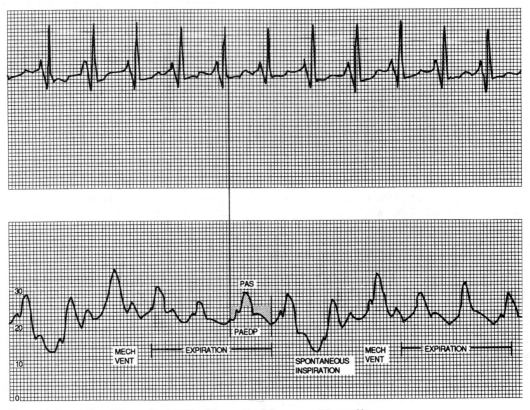

Figure: PA systolic = 28 mm Hg; PAED = 21 mm Hg; PA mean = 23 mm Hg

7. If digital data are the only available method, record the PAW pressure using the following:
   a. Controlled mechanical ventilation: diastolic mode (lowest pressure)
   b. Assisted ventilation: digital mean
   c. Spontaneous ventilation: systolic mode (highest pressure)

8. Evaluate pressures for normal fluctuation and trends (amount of fluctuation may be patient populations specific)[41, 44, 54, 315, 328]
   a. PA systolic: 4–7 mm Hg
   b. PA mean: 4–5 mm Hg
   c. PAED: 4–7 mm Hg
   d. PAW: 4 mm Hg

ICS, intercostal space; PA, pulmonary artery; PAEDP, pulmonary artery end-diastolic pressure; PAW, pulmonary artery wedge.

An underdamped system is characterized by too many frequency components, without a reduction in amplitude,[336] resulting in falsely high systolic (15 to 30 mm Hg) and low diastolic pressures. An overdamped system loses its characteristic landmarks, and the waveform appears unnaturally smooth with a diminished or absent dicrotic notch.[149] Falsely low systolic and high diastolic pressure readings are the result of an overdamped system. Studies of PA catheters have demonstrated a decreased natural frequency[395]; thus, the performance of the steps for assessing the dynamic response characteristics and troubleshooting the system as outlined in Figure 19-5 are imperative to optimize the systems. The key to optimizing the system is that the simpler the system (shorter tubing, fewer stopcocks), the better its ability to reproduce faithfully the pressure waveforms.[43,149,152,161]

Decision Making Algorithm

How to Assess Dynamic Response Characteristics

1. Determine Natural Frequency of System (Fn)
   a. Fast Flush System and Record Strip
   b. Measure period (t) of once cycle
   c. Fn=Paper speed (mm/sec)/one cycle (mm)
2. Determine Amplitude Ratio
   Compare the amplitude of two successive peaks (A2/A1)
3. Plot Amplitude Ratio Against Natural Frequency
   -Apply algorithm if system other than OPTIMAL or ADEQUATE

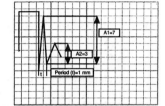

Example:
1) Determine Fn
   Paper Speed=25 mm/sec
   t=1 mm
   Fn=25/1=25 cycles/sec
2) Determine Amplitude
   A2/A1=3/7=0.43
3) Plot on graph=ADEQUATE

Frequency versus Amplitude Ratio Plot

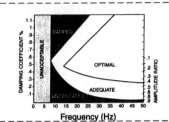

Frequency versus damping coefficient plot that illustrates the five areas into which the catheter, tubing, and transducer systems fall. Systems in the optimal area reproduce even the most demanding (fast heart rate and rapid systolic upstroke) waveforms without distortion. Systems in the adequate area reproduce the most typical waveforms with little or no distortion. All other areas cause serious wave distortion. (Gardner, RM Hollingsworth, KW: Optimizing the electrocardiogram and pressure monitoring. Crit Care Med 14: 651-658m 1986. With permission).

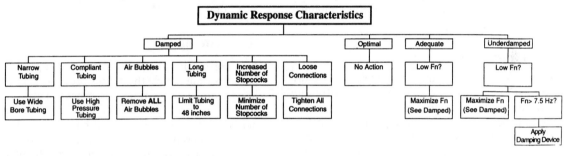

FIGURE 19-5 Dynamic response characteristics. From Bridges EJ, Middleton R. Direct arterial vs. oscillometric monitoring of blood pressure: Stop comparing and pick one (A decision making algorithm) Critical Care Nurse, 17(3):58–72, 1997. With permission.

DIRECT ARTERIAL PRESSURE MONITORING

Indications

Intra-arterial monitoring is indicated when precise and continuous monitoring is required. Examples of clinical conditions warranting direct arterial monitoring include acute hypertensive crises, hypotension, any shock state, frequent drawing of arterial blood samples, monitoring of vasoactive pharmacologic support, and during aggressive respiratory support (high positive end-expiratory pressures [PEEP]).[175,473]

Catheter Placement

Sites for intra-arterial catheterization include the radial, brachial, femoral, dorsalis pedis, and axillary arteries.[72,217,406] Important considerations in site selection include adequate collateral circulation, patient comfort, and avoidance of areas at increased risk for infection (e.g., groin), if possible. The most common insertion site is the radial artery because of the presence of collateral circulation, which decreases the risk of vascular complications. The radial and ulnar

artery/superficial palmar arteries provide a dual blood supply to the hand. This dual blood supply is important if radial artery perfusion becomes temporarily or permanently compromised as a result of catheter placement. Before radial artery cannulation is attempted, collateral circulation to the hand must be assessed. Tests used to determine collateral circulation include the Allen test, plethysmography, and pulse oximetry.[96,175,217]

The brachial artery is used less frequently because it does not have good collateral circulation, which in theory increases the risk for diffuse distal ischemia. However, in facilities that routinely perform brachial cannulation, the complication rate is not increased.[283] Regardless of the insertion site, ongoing assessment of collateral circulation must be made while the catheter is in place.

Complications Related to Arterial Catheterization

INFECTION

Infection is the most clinically important complication of vascular cannulation.[406] Conditions that place a patient at risk include immunosuppression, arterial insufficiency

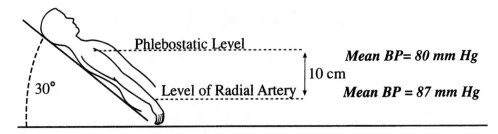

FIGURE 19-6 Effect of two reference points on the measured mean arterial pressure (MAP) in a patient in the 30-degree supine position. If the distance between the phlebostatic level and the radial insertion site is 10 cm, the MAP measured by the arterial line referenced to the radial insertion site will be 7.3 mm Hg than the pressure measured in the arterial line referenced to the phlebostatic level (1 cm = 0.73 mm Hg). (From Bridges EJ, Middleton R: Direct arterial vs oscillometric monitoring of blood pressure: Stop comparing and pick one [a decision making algorithm]. Critical Care Nurse 17(3): 66, 1997.)

states, and catheters placed by surgical cutdown or left in place longer than 4 days.[175,231] Careful hand washing and changing the equipment set-up down to the arterial catheter hub every 96 hours are recommended to minimize contamination and bacterial growth.[354]

ARTERIAL THROMBOSIS

Arterial thrombosis is an uncommon complication of vascular cannulation since the advent of continuous heparinized flush systems. There remains a risk of arterial thrombosis in patients with catheters larger than 20 gauge; with tapered, polypropylene catheters; and with catheters in place more than 4 days.[231] Aspiration of the clot or removal of the catheter is recommended if thrombosis is suspected.

A large clinical study was undertaken to evaluate the effects of heparinized and nonheparinized flush solutions on the patency of arterial pressure lines.[335] Results indicated that heparinized flush solution was associated with increased arterial line patency rates. Variables affecting patency included insertion site (femoral sites have greater patency rate), anticoagulants and antithrombotics (these agents increase chance of patency), catheter length (arterial catheters or sheaths longer than 2 inches were more likely to remain patent), and sex (men have higher patency rates than women).

DISTAL ISCHEMIA

Distal ischemia may be due to thrombosis (distal embolization) or local occlusion.[292] Risk factors for ischemia include severe peripheral vascular disease, hypotension, and the use of vasopressor drugs. Assessment of distal perfusion (skin color/temperature, capillary refill) should be performed daily and after any manipulation of the catheter.[367] In addition, the use of heparinized continuous-flush solutions decreases the incidence of thrombus formation,[335] and thus the risk for distal embolization.

AIR EMBOLIZATION

Air can enter at several areas (connections, stopcocks) in the intra-arterial catheter and tubing system. Air that enters the arterial system rapidly passes through the heart into the aorta. Depending on the position of the patient, an air embolus can enter the cerebral or coronary arteries and potentially obstruct flow of blood to the tissue of the brain or heart. Maintaining the integrity of the system and using a continuous-flush device are essential for preventing air entry into the system.

Referencing

Pressure in blood vessels has three components: dynamic blood pressure (i.e., the blood pressure generated by the heart, equal to flow times resistance), hydrostatic pressure (related to fluid density, gravitational acceleration, and height of the column of blood between the heart and the vessels), and static pressure (related to the volume of blood in the vascular system at zero flow).[388] The blood pressure is the same at all points along a vertical level. However, pressure at different vertical levels reflects not only the dynamic pressure, but the hydrostatic pressure.

Referencing is performed to correct for the change in hydrostatic pressure in vessels above and below the heart. If the patient is in a supine position and then is placed into a semi-Fowler's position without the catheter system being re-referenced, the patient will seem to have an increase in pressure when, in fact, his or her aortic blood pressure may be unchanged or even decreased.[158] However, if the catheter is referenced to the LA, there is minimal position-related pressure difference[82,84,245] (Fig. 19-6). Therefore, it is recommended that the arterial pressure monitoring system be referenced at the level of the heart.[42,43,402]

Interpretation of Arterial Pressure Data

The arterial pressure can be described by a mean arterial pressure (MAP) and fluctuations about the mean.[140,341] The systolic and diastolic pressures describe the fluctuation about the mean. The MAP, which represents the average pressure through a cardiac cycle, is affected by the CO and systemic vascular resistance (SVR) as described by the following equation[140]:

$$\text{Mean arterial pressure} = \text{CO} \times \text{SVR}$$

The factors that affect the mean, systolic, and diastolic arterial pressures are described in Chapter 2. Recall of these factors is important when assessing changes in blood pressure. The systolic pressure is affected by left ventricular

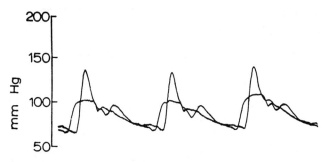

FIGURE 19-7 Simultaneous recordings of aortic and radial arterial pressure waves. (From Rowell LD, Brengelmann GL, Blackmon RJ et al: Disparities between aortic and peripheral pulse pressures induced by upright exercise and vasomotor changes in man. Circulation 37: 954–964, 1968.)

(LV) stroke volume (SV), peak rate of ejection, and distensibility of the vessel walls. Diastolic pressure is primarily affected by arterial peripheral resistance. The pulse pressure, which is the difference between systolic and diastolic pressures, is determined by SV and elasticity of the arteries.

The important point with regard to hemodynamic monitoring is that the peripheral systolic pressure may be as much as 5 to 20 mm Hg higher than the central aortic pressure as a result of reflection of the arterial pulse wave back from the periphery and the end-pressure product[210,342–344,389] (Fig. 19-7). Both peripheral wave reflection and the end-pressure product, which is the result of the conversion of kinetic energy from flowing blood into pressure as the blood strikes the upstream-looking arterial catheter, result in the augmentation of the systolic blood pressure.[43,183] However, the MAP and the diastolic pressure are relatively unchanged in the periphery. The MAP provides a more consistent value to evaluate and guide therapy.[288,290]

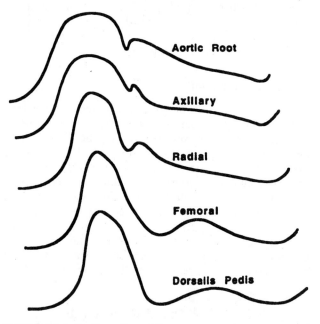

FIGURE 19-8 Configuration of the pressure-pulse wave at various sites in the arterial tree. (From Varon AJ: Arterial, central venous, and pulmonary artery catheters. In Taylor RW, Kirby RR (eds): Critical Care, 3rd ed, pp 847–865. Philadelphia, Lippincott–Raven, 1997.)

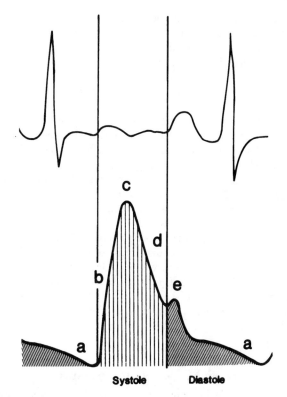

FIGURE 19-9 Components of arterial waveform during cardiac cycle. The pulse wave a to c waveform occurs as blood is ejected into the aorta from the ventricle during systole. Volume displacement occurs at point c. Segment d occurs during late systole as the ventricles empty and forward movement slows. Closure of the aortic valve is reflected as the dicrotic notch, point e. At point e, the pulmonic valve is also closed and the atrioventricular valves are opening. Upstroke of the arterial waveform begins approximately 0.2 seconds after the QRS complex. (From Campbell B: Arterial waveforms: Monitoring changes in figuration. Heart Lung 26: 204–214, 1997.)

Of clinical interest, vasodilator drugs (e.g., nitroglycerin, nitroprusside) can substantially decrease aortic pressure without a clinically measurable change in brachial pressure.[240,338,339,341,491,512] This variable effect is the result of the reduction in pulse-wave reflection. These findings may explain why a patient may "look better" after the initiation of vasodilator therapy even though there has been no marked decrease in blood pressure or preload.

Arterial Waveform Analysis

The arterial pressure waveform changes its contour when recorded at different sites along the arterial circuit[290,342,389] (Fig. 19-8). The pulse pressure and the systolic pressure increase and the ascending limb of the waveform becomes steeper. In addition, the incisura is gradually replaced by a later diastolic wave (dicrotic notch) that is the result of peripheral pressure pulse reflection.[340,342,473]

The arterial pressure waveform is characterized by a steep upstroke caused by ventricular systole, which is followed by a brief, peaked, sustained pressure (anacrotic shoulder). At the end of systole, pressure falls in the aorta and LV, resulting in a downward deflection (Fig. 19-9).

When LV pressure falls below aortic pressure, the aortic valve closes (incisura). Pressure in the aorta continues to decrease and is reflected on the arterial pressure waveform as a gradual downslope until the next ventricular systole. Systolic pressure is recorded at the peak of the waveform, and diastolic pressure is read at end-diastole just before the rapid rise in the waveform.

Examples of the effect of cardiovascular disease on arterial waveforms include atherosclerosis, dilated cardiomyopathy, valvular disorders, and cardiac arrhythmias.[52,344] With atherosclerosis, there is a change in the elasticity of the arteries. This change results in an increase in the systolic waveform and a decrease in the size of the diastolic wave and dicrotic notch.[52,256,330,337] These changes, which are the result of pulse-wave reflection from the periphery, are also observed with systemic vasoconstriction. As discussed, the use of vasodilator agents may decrease peripheral reflection and decrease the systolic pressure in the aorta. However, the changes in the waveform may not be noticeable at the level of the brachial or radial artery.[240,338,339,341,427,512] With dilated cardiomyopathy, the SV and MAP are decreased and the arterial waveform is characterized by a late, secondary systolic peak.

Direct Arterial Versus Cuff Pressure

The intra-arterial blood pressure is often compared with the auscultatory or oscillometric blood pressure to assess if the systolic and diastolic pressures are similar. There is no basis for this practice.[210]

The direct method using the intra-arterial system is based on pressure, whereas the oscillometric methods depends on flow-induced oscillations in the arterial wall.[43,175,371] An erroneous assumption is that pressure equals flow. As described by a derivation of Ohm's law (pressure = flow × resistance), if resistance remains constant, there is a direct relationship between pressure and flow. However, in clinical practice, resistance is seldom constant.[210] Thus, blood pressure may appear adequate while flow is decreased, or pressure may be low although perfusion remains adequate. Although the systolic pressure may vary depending on the measurement method used, the mean pressure is a relatively stable value across a wide variety of patients and may provide a better means of monitoring the patient.[277,352,477]

In addition to the physical factors that cause the differences in arterial pressure measured in various locations in the body, there are also technical factors that affect measurement accuracy. For example, the accuracy of direct arterial pressure may be affected by excessive tubing length (>4 feet), air bubbles in the tubing, and incorrect referencing. Oscillometric measurement is affected by factors such as cuff size, loose cuff application, the presence of intrinsic (shivering, arm motion) and extrinsic movement (external compression of the cuff, passive arm motion), and variations in anatomy and physiology (respiratory variation, arrhythmias, patient talking, conically shaped arms).[42,43] Several algorithms have been developed to guide assessment of the physiologic and technical factors that affect direct and oscillometric arterial pressure measurements, and to aid in answering the question, "Which do you believe, the arterial line or the cuff?"[43,174,196,235,253]

Blood-Drawing Procedure from an Arterial Line

1. Turn off monitor alarm.
2. Aseptically remove cap from distal stopcock.
3. Insert syringe into stopcock and turn stopcock away from patient.
4. Draw six times dead space of a-line (see manufacturer specifications).
5. Turn stopcock off.
6. Insert syringe and turn stopcock away from patient.
7. Draw specimen.
8. Flush system/stopcock.
9. Return stopcock to original position and aseptically cap.
10. Turn on monitor alarm

Blood Drawing

Blood samples can be withdrawn for laboratory determination. The procedure for manual withdrawal is outlined in Display 19-2. In-line blood drawing systems are now being used to eliminate potential contact with contaminated blood and to decrease blood loss.[358,425]

Prothrombin time and partial thromboplastin time can be drawn from an arterial line. The prothrombin and partial thromboplastin time measurements obtained from an arterial line are similar to those obtained by venous stick from a patient not receiving additional systemic heparin. However, there is a potential for heparin contamination in the arterial line; thus, the catheter must be adequately cleared before obtaining the specimen. The current recommendation is that the dead space (see manufacturer information) plus 2 mL[458] or six times the dead space[258] (which is approximately equal to the dead space plus 2 mL) should be withdrawn before obtaining the specimen.

Catheter Removal

When the need for continuous intra-arterial monitoring ends, the physician or the nurse should remove the catheter. The procedure is first explained to the patient. To remove the catheter, the tape or sutures are removed. The catheter is removed quickly, and the site is immediately compressed for 5 to 10 minutes, or longer if the patient is receiving anticoagulants or has a coagulopathy. At the end of the 5 to 10 minutes, the site is checked for bleeding, hematoma, and distal circulatory impairment. Direct compression is held until there are no signs of bleeding. If the patient is thought to have an infection, the enterocutaneous portion (distal tip) of the catheter may be sent to the laboratory for culturing.

CENTRAL VENOUS PRESSURE MONITORING

The central venous pressure (CVP) directly reflects RA pressure (RAP) and indirectly reflects the preload of the right ventricle (RV) or RV end-diastolic pressure. The CVP is determined by vascular tone, the volume of blood returning to the heart, the pumping ability of the heart, and patient position (supine, standing).

The CVP is measured in the superior vena cava or the RA by a water manometer in centimeters of water (cm H_2O) or by a pressure transducer (the recommended method) in millimeters or mercury (mm Hg).[473] Normally, the CVP ranges from 3 to 8 cm H_2O or 2 to 6 mm Hg (1 mm Hg = 1.36 cm H_2O). In the supine position, a CVP of less than 2 mm Hg may indicate hypovolemia, vasodilation, or increased myocardial contractility. An increased CVP may indicate increased circulatory blood volume, vasoconstriction, or decreased contractility of the myocardium. An increased CVP is also observed in clinical states such as RV failure, tricuspid insufficiency, positive-pressure breathing, pericardial tamponade, pulmonary embolus, and obstructive pulmonary disease.

Indications

The measurement of CVP or RAP is indicated to secure venous access, to administer vasoactive drugs and parenteral nutrition, and to monitoring of right heart preload. Hemodynamic monitoring using a CVP is most often performed when cardiopulmonary function is relatively normal.[447,473]

Catheter Placement

Insertion of a CVP catheter is achieved percutaneously or by venous cutdown through a central or peripheral vein. Acceptable insertion sites include the medial basilica, lateral cephalic, internal or external jugular, and subclavian veins.[231] Selection of the appropriate site depends on the skill of the clinician inserting the catheter, physical structure and age of the patient, thoracic deformities, and clinical circumstances.

Limitations

The CVP is not an accurate indicator of LV function or left heart preload.[23,69,135] In the presence of normal right heart function, severe deterioration of LV function may not be reflected by a change in RAP or CVP. For example, in an acute myocardial infarction (MI), the CVP may remain unchanged in the presence of acute LV dysfunction. An increased CVP is usually an indication of later stages of LV failure, although the CVP may remain normal even in the presence of high PA pressures and pulmonary edema.

Complications

Complications associated with CVP monitoring include localized infection, atrial or ventricular arrhythmias, vessel laceration, RV perforation, thrombophlebitis, hematoma formation at the insertion site, and pneumothorax.[429,451] Percutaneous insertion into the internal jugular vein or the subclavian vein may potentially result in a pneumothorax.

Measurement Technique

The CVP system is referenced by placing the air–fluid interface of the stopcock at the level of the phlebostatic axis. The hemodynamically stable patient can be positioned up to 45 degrees when the CVP is measured, provided that the air–fluid interface of the stopcock is repositioned to the phlebostatic axis.[363]

An area of confusion is related to which port to transduce when measuring the CVP with a triple-lumen catheter. There are no research-based, standardized recommendations regarding port selection. There is some evidence that the pressures measured from the various ports may be different; however, in general, the differences are not large.[393,405] Because of the potential for a clinically significant change in pressure depending on the port transduced, it seems prudent to transduce consistently one port, and if a change in the site of monitoring is necessary, to annotate the change on the flowsheet.

Interpretation of Data

Useful clinical information can be obtained by examining the pressure waves that are developed in the atria and great veins

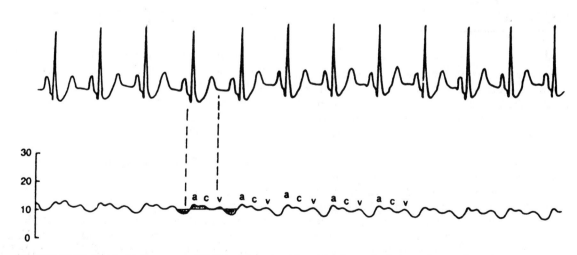

FIGURE 19-10 Right atrial pressure (RAP) is determined by obtaining a dual-channel recording of the electrocardiographic and RAP waveforms. The a and v waves are identified and the mean RAP determined by bisecting these waves. (From Gardner PE: Pulmonary artery pressure monitoring. AACN Clinical Issues in Critical Care Nursing 4: 103, 1993.)

TABLE 19-2	Relation of Right Atrial and Pulmonary Artery Pressures to Electrocardiographic Findings	
Waveform	**Mechanical Activity**	**Electrocardiographic Findings**
RA Pressure (2–6 mm Hg)		
a wave	RA contraction	PR interval
x descent	RA relaxation	
c wave	Tricuspid valve closure	QRS
v wave	Venous inflow into right atrium against closed tricuspid valve	T wave
y descent	Passive RA filling	
PA Pressure		
PA systolic (15–25 mm Hg)	Right ventricular systole into PA	After QRS, near T wave
PA end-diastolic (8–12 mm Hg)	Left ventricular end-diastole	0.08 after onset of QRS (does not apply for bundle-branch block)
PA Wedge Pressure (6–12 mm Hg)		
a wave	LA contraction	After PR interval
x descent	LA relaxation	
c wave (not usually seen)	Mitral valve closure	QRS
v wave	Venous inflow into left atrium against closed mitral valve	TP interval
y descent	Passive LA filling	

LA, left atrial; PA, pulmonary artery; RA, right atrial.

during the cardiac cycle (Fig. 19-10). There are five mechanical components of the RAP waveform. The mean RAP is determined by bisecting the a, c, and v waves so that there are equal areas above and below the bisection. A dual-channel strip chart recorder should be used to identify the corresponding venous pressure waves (a, c, and v waves) with the electrical events on the electrocardiogram (ECG)[404,408] (Table 19-2). The RAP tracing may be useful in the diagnosis of wide-complex tachyarrhythmias of unknown origin, tricuspid insufficiency, pericardial tamponade, and constrictive pericarditis.[473]

PULMONARY ARTERY PRESSURE MONITORING

Indications

Since its introduction in 1970,[450] invasive hemodynamic monitoring with a PA catheter has become one of the most commonly used diagnostic tools in critical care.[166] Despite the widespread use and reports of improved diagnostic accuracy,[123] there has been a recent call for a reduction or restriction of use of the PA catheter.[76,77,86] In response to this call, a national conference developed a consensus statement based on the current state of knowledge regarding PA catheter use in specific patient populations, and made recommendations for use of the PA catheter in clinical practice.[351] The recommendations addressed the question of whether management with PA catheters improves patient outcome. Some of the general recommendations from the conference include (1) there is no basis for a U.S. Food and Drug Administration moratorium on PA catheters; (2) clinicians should care-

fully consider the risks and benefits of PA catheter use, and patients or their surrogates should be fully informed before use; (3) clinician knowledge about the use of the PA catheter and its complications should be improved; and (4) current training, credentialing, and continuing quality improvement issues related to the PA catheter should be reevaluated.[351]

In addition to the potential for improvement of diagnostic accuracy and outcomes in certain patient populations, analysis of waveform morphology may be useful in the differential diagnosis and evaluation of conditions such as cardiogenic shock, cardiac tamponade, pulmonary hypertension, and valvular dysfunction.[123,306,441]

Description of the Pulmonary Artery Catheter

The PA catheter is a multilumen, polyvinylchloride catheter with a variable external diameter. Many models of PA catheters are available (Fig. 19-11). The standard thermodilution catheter is 7.5 French in diameter and 110 cm long and is marked in 10-cm increments. The balloon is inflated with a maximum of 1.5 mL of air.

Insertion of the Pulmonary Artery Catheter

The catheter is inserted percutaneously, with or without the use of fluoroscopy. Once the RA is reached, the balloon, located on the distal end of the catheter, is inflated and the catheter is "floated" through the RA and RV and out into the PA, where it wedges in a branch of the PA.[449,498] Once the characteristic PA wedge pressure (PAWP) tracing has been obtained, the balloon

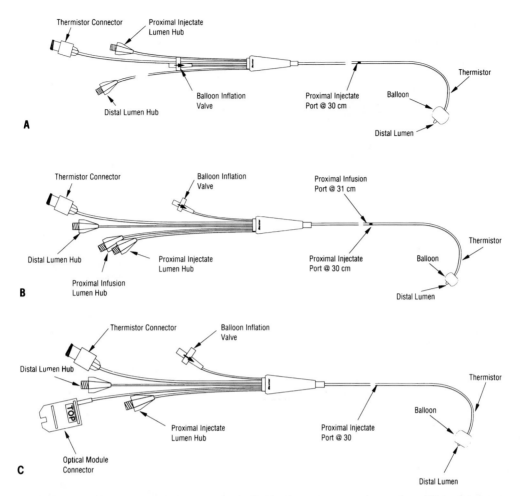

FIGURE 19-11 Catheter model examples. **(A)** Traditional pulmonary artery (PA) catheter. **(B)** Venous infusion port PA catheter. **(C)** Oximetry PA catheter. *(continued)*

is deflated, allowing the catheter to recoil slightly into the PA. The catheter is left in the balloon-down position to prevent pulmonary infarction. Table 19-6 outlines the nursing responsibilities during insertion of the PA catheter.

Pulmonary Artery Waveform Characteristics

As the catheter passes through the heart, three pressure waveforms can be visualized using a PA catheter: RA, PA, and PAWP (Fig 19-12).

PULMONARY ARTERY PRESSURE

Pulmonary artery pressures provide an index of the pressure within the pulmonary vasculature and are affected by compliance of the LV, pulmonary vascular pressure, CO (blood flow to the lungs), and the state of the lung tissue. The PA pressure increases slightly with age. For example, in healthy people older than 60 years of age, the mean PA pressure was 16 ± 3 mm Hg and the pulmonary vascular resistance (PVR) was 124 ± 32 dynes/s/cm^{-5}. In contrast, people younger than 60 years of age had a mean PA pressure and PVR of $12 \pm$ mm Hg and $70 \pm$ dynes/s/cm^{-5}, respectively.[93]

Three PA pressures are measured: systolic, diastolic, and mean. The PA systolic pressure reflects the flow of blood into the PA from the RV. In the absence of elevated pulmonary vascular pressure or RV outflow obstruction, PA systolic pressure is equal to RV systolic pressure.[143] During diastole, the mitral valve is open, and a continuous column of blood from the PA to the LA and LV exists; therefore, the pressure just before contraction (end-diastole) is approximately equal in the PA, LA, and LV. As a result of the diastolic equalization, the PA end-diastolic pressure (PAEDP) is often used as an indirect indicator of PAWP and LV end-diastolic pressure (LVEDP).[36,39,126,130,372,401] The difference between the RV diastolic pressure and PAEDP (an increase in the diastolic pressure as the catheter passes across the pulmonic valve) is an important characteristic in determining whether the catheter tip is correctly positioned in the PA or has flipped back into the right ventricle (see Fig. 19-12).

PULMONARY ARTERY WEDGE PRESSURE

The PAWP is obtained by inflation of the balloon on the distal end of the PA catheter, which allows the catheter to float forward to wedge in a segment of the PA. The wedged catheter creates a static column of blood through the

(text continues on page 441)

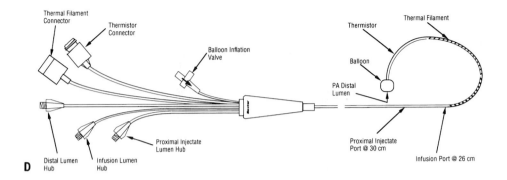

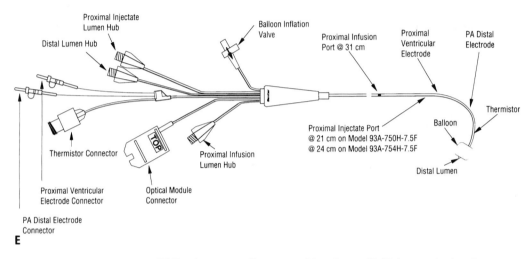

FIGURE 19-11 *(CONTINUED)* **(D)** Continuous cardiac output PA catheter. **(E)** Right ventricular ejection fraction oximetry PA catheter. (Courtesy of Baxter Healthcare Corporation, Edwards Critical-Care Division, Santa Ana, CA.)

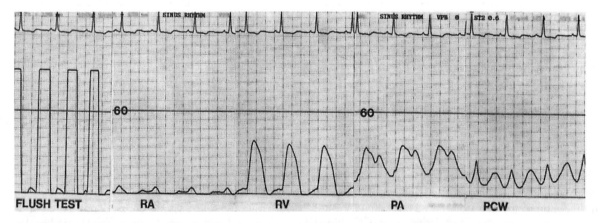

FIGURE 19-12 Characteristic waveforms observed as the pulmonary artery (PA) catheter is "floated" from the right atrium through the right ventricle and into the PA, where it finally wedges. Note that the mean right atrial pressure (RAP) is similar to the right ventricular end-diastolic pressure (RVEDP), the RV systolic and PA systolic pressures are similar, and there is a step-up in pressure as the catheter crosses the pulmonic valve and enters the PA. In a correctly positioned catheter, the PA wedge pressure is lower than the mean PA pressure and has a waveform that is relatively similar to the RAP (although slightly delayed relative to the electrocardiogram). (From Sharkey S: A Guide to Interpretation of Hemodynamic Data in the Coronary Care Unit. Philadelphia, Lippincott–Raven, 1997.)

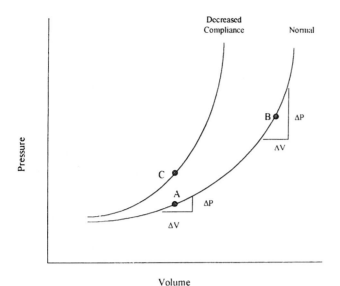

FIGURE 19-13 Pressure–volume curves. The result of the curvilinear pressure–volume relationship is that compliance is greater at a lower filling volume (point A) compared with a higher volume (point B). In addition, a decrease in compliance without a change in filling volume is manifested by a left shift of the curve. Thus, for any given filling volume, the measured pressure is increased (point A to point C). Therefore, a change in the measured pressure may indicate an increase in filling volume or an alteration in compliance.[262]

pulmonary vasculature, which acts as an extension of the fluid within the catheter system and allows retrograde transmission of left heart pressures to the distal port of the catheter. There is in general a good relationship between the mean PAWP and mean LA pressure.[21,252] However, as demonstrated by the pressure—volume curve (Fig. 19-13), any alteration in myocardial compliance may affect the pressure–volume relation and limit the usefulness of the PAWP as an indicator of left heart preload. Absolute PAWP values should be used with caution in any situation that alters myocardial compliance, such as LV dysfunction or MI (particularly involving the posteroinferior surface of the heart).[397]

In addition to being an indirect indicator of LVEDP (preload), the PAWP is also an indicator of the capillary pressure (P_{cap}) and the risk for the development of pulmonary edema. In patients with MI, an increase in PAWP above 18 mm Hg is associated with the onset of pulmonary congestion.[136] However, as demonstrated in Figure 19-14, the PAWP underestimates the P_{cap} when there is increased resistance in the postcapillary vessels.[79,80,261,336]

Pulmonary Artery Waveform Interpretation

Pulmonary artery waveform interpretation can be simplified by remembering that electrical activity, as indicated by the ECG, precedes mechanical activity (pressure waveforms).[45] The relation of ECG to waveform characteristics is outlined in Table 19-2.

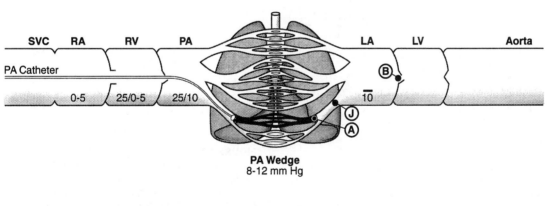

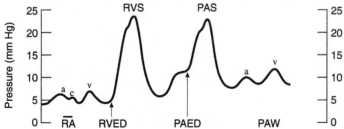

FIGURE 19-14 Schema of the principle underlying the use of the pulmonary artery wedge pressure (PAWP) as an indicator of left ventricular (LV) preload and characteristic waveforms. When the inflated balloon on the catheter obstructs arterial flow, the catheter records the pressure at the junction of the static column of fluid and flowing venous channels (J-point). The PAWP underestimates the pulmonary capillary pressure (P_{cap}) when there is increased resistance in the postcapillary vessels proximal to the J-point (point A). The PAWP overestimates LV end-diastolic pressure (LVEDP) in the presence of obstruction distal to the J-point (point B; e.g., mitral stenosis, left atrial myxoma), whereas the PAWP underestimates the LVEDP in the presence of premature closure of the mitral valve as a result of aortic insufficiency.[261, 336]

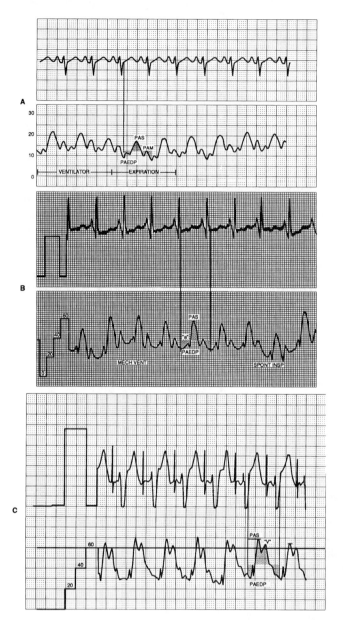

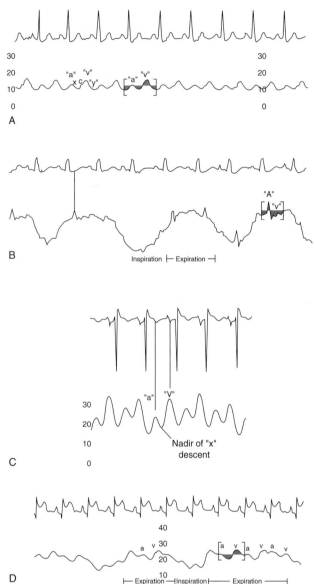

FIGURE 19-15 Pulmonary artery (PA) pressure determination. **(A)** Normal PA pressure waveform. Pulmonary artery systolic (PAS) pressure = 18 mm Hg, pulmonary artery end-diastolic pressure (PAEDP) = 10 mm Hg; PA mean pressure = 12 mm Hg. **(B)** Elevated PA pressure related to left ventricular failure and acute respiratory distress syndrome (ARDS). Patient is on intermittent mandatory ventilation. PAS = 58 mm Hg; PAEDP = 30 mm Hg; PA mean = 38 mm Hg. **(C)** Patient with vegetation on mitral valve resulting in acute mitral insufficiency. Note the v wave on the downstroke of the PA waveform (bifid waveform). PAS = 68 mm Hg; PAEDP = 32 mm Hg; PAM = 48 mm Hg.

FIGURE 19-16 Pulmonary artery (PA) wedge pressure determination. **(A)** Normal PA wedge pressure tracing. The mean PA wedge pressure is read on an end-expiratory waveform and is determined by bisecting the a and v waves so there is an equal area above and below the bisection. PA wedge pressure = 12 mm Hg. **(B)** PA wedge pressure in spontaneously breathing patient. Note the sharp a wave associated with acute congestive heart failure. PA wedge pressure = 22 mm Hg. Pressure is read immediately before the inspiratory trough. **(C)** PA wedge pressure with elevated v wave in a spontaneously breathing patient who was complaining of chest pain. The PA wedge pressure is read at the nadir of the x descent. Note the relation of the v wave to the TP interval of the electrocardiogram. PA wedge pressure = 17 mm Hg. **(D)** Elevated a and v waves. Patient with a history of an inferolateral myocardial infarction with signs and symptoms of congestive heart failure. The increased a and v waves are consistent with left ventricular failure. PA wedge pressure = 24 mm Hg.

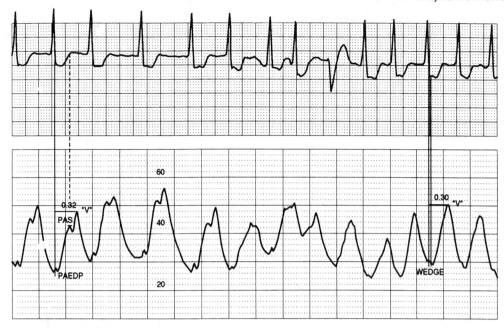

FIGURE 19-17 Pulmonary artery (PA) pressure or PA wedge pressure. In the presence of a large v wave, the PA wedge pressure tracing may mimic a PA tracing. Comparison of the PA and PA wedge pressure relative to the electrocardiogram reveals the following: (1) the v wave of the PA wedge pressure occurs during the TP interval, whereas the initial systolic upstroke of PA waveform is closely related to the end of the QRS complex; and (2) the PA v wave is a sharp upward deflection on the descending limb of the PA pressure curve, having the same temporal relation as the v wave in the PA wedge pressure tracing. PA wedge pressure = 30 mm Hg.

PULMONARY ARTERY PRESSURE

The PA systolic pressure is represented by a steep rise during RV ejection and usually occurs after the QRS complex or near the T wave of the ECG. The PAEDP is measured 0.08 second after the onset of the QRS,[274] and the PA mean is determined by bisecting the end-expiratory waveform so there is an equal area above and below the bisection (Fig. 19-15A). In the presence of LV dysfunction, the presystolic a wave may provide a more consistent index of LVEDP than PAEDP and PAWP; however, the presence of this wave is variable.[369]

Elevated PA pressures occur with:

1. Increased PVR (see Fig. 19-15B)
   a. Pulmonary hypertension
   b. Chronic obstructive pulmonary disease
   c. Acute respiratory distress syndrome (ARDS)
   d. Hypoxia
   e. Pulmonary embolus
2. Increased pulmonary venous pressure
   a. LV failure
   b. Mitral stenosis
3. Increased pulmonary blood flow
   a. Hypervolemia
   b. Atrial and ventricular septal defects
4. Mitral insufficiency (see Fig. 19-15C).

PULMONARY ARTERY WEDGE PRESSURE

The PAWP waveform is similar to the LA pressure waveform but is slightly damped and phase delayed (50 to 70 milliseconds) because of pulmonary vascular transmission.[252] The PAWP is a mean pressure and is determined by bisecting the a and v waves, so there is an equal area above and below the bisection (Fig. 19-16A).

Pulmonary artery wedge pressure waveforms are useful in the diagnosis of various cardiac lesions:

1. Elevated a wave: conditions that increase resistance to LV filling
   a. Mitral stenosis
   b. LV failure (see Fig. 19-16B)
   c. Acutely ischemic LV
2. Elevated v wave: conditions that cause increased LA filling during ventricular systole (see Fig. 19-16C)
   a. Acute mitral insufficiency (Fig. 19-17)
   b. Ventricular septal defect
   c. Aortic regurgitation

The giant V wave in acute mitral regurgitation and ventricular septal defect is the result of augmented LA filling. The height of the V wave is determined by LA loading volume and compliance and LV afterload, and is not a consistent indicator of disease severity.[110,202] In the presence of a large V wave (V wave 10 mm Hg greater than a wave) associated with mitral regurgitation, LVEDP is best correlated ($r = 0.89$) with the trough or nadir of the x descent[202] (see Fig. 19-16C). The PAWP and peak of the a wave overestimate the LVEDP. The clinical importance of the giant V wave, regardless of etiology, is the marked increase in P_{cap}, with the potential development of pulmonary edema. The ECG is useful in differentiating a bifid PA waveform from a PA wedge with a large V wave (see Fig. 19-17).

3. Elevated a and v waves
   a. Cardiac tamponade (Fig. 19-18)
   b. Hypervolemia

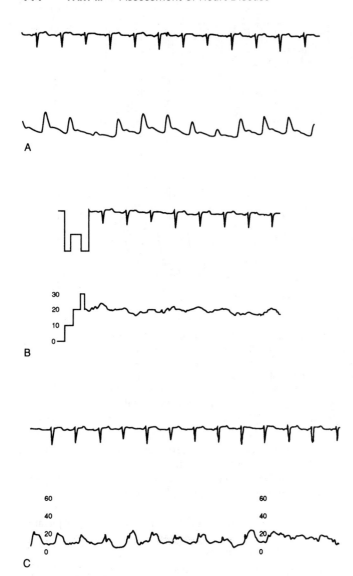

FIGURE 19-18 Pericardial tamponade in a spontaneously breathing patient. **(A)** Arterial waveform. Note the electrical alternans, alternating height or duration of the QRS complex, and pulsus paradoxus on the arterial waveform. **(B)** Right atrial pressure (RAP) = 20 mm Hg. **(C)** Pulmonary artery (PA) to PA wedge pressure. Pulmonary artery systolic (PAS) pressure = 26 mm Hg; pulmonary artery end-diastolic pressure (PAEDP) = 17 mm Hg; PA mean pressure = 19 mm Hg; PA wedge pressure = 20 mm Hg. Equalization of the diastolic pressures is the result of circumferential compression of all cardiac chambers.

c. Constrictive pericarditis
d. LV failure (see Fig. 19-16D)
e. Mitral stenosis (Fig. 19-19)

In mitral stenosis, a pressure gradient develops between the LA and LV; therefore, the PA and PAWP are not accurate indices of LV pressure.[252]

Technical Aspects of Pulmonary Artery Pressure Monitoring

Numerous research studies have evaluated the technical aspects of PA pressure measurement.[45,234] The use of incor-

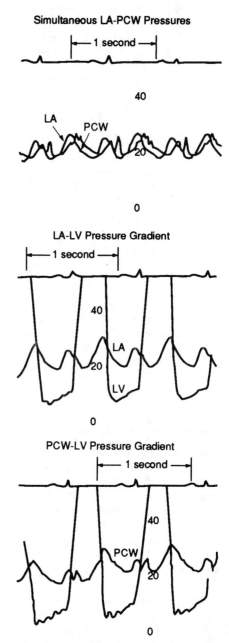

FIGURE 19-19 Hemodynamic recordings from patient with mitral stenosis. **(Top)** Simultaneous left atrial (LA) and pulmonary capillary wedge (PCW) pressure recordings. There is a time delay of 80 milliseconds, and the *y* descent of the PCW tracing is slightly delayed. **(Middle)** Simultaneous LA and left ventricular (LV) pressure recordings. **(Bottom)** Simultaneous PCW and LV pressure recordings. The PCW is an accurate indicator of LA **(Top)**, but there is a marked pressure gradient between the PCW and LV pressure **(Middle)**, and LA and LV pressure **(Bottom)**. (From Lange RA, Moore DM, Cigarroa RG et al: Use of pulmonary capillary wedge pressure to assess severity of mitral stenosis: Is true left atrial pressure needed in this condition? J Am Coll Cardiol 13: 825–829, 1989.)

rect technique may result in the introduction of error into pressure measurements and potentiate therapeutic mismanagement of critically ill patients.[312] Nursing responsibilities during PA catheter insertion are summarized in Display 19-3.

Nursing Responsibilities During Pulmonary Artery Catheter Insertion

1. Prepare equipment
   a. Flush solution: 1–4 U heparin/mL of 5% dextrose in water or normal saline; remove all air from bag.
   b. Attach to pressure tubing with macrodrip chamber.
   c. Place flush solution in pressure bag (300 mm Hg delivers solution at 3 mL/h)
   d. Flush transducer/pressure tubing/stopcocks using aseptic technique. Ensure *all* air bubbles are removed.
   e. Attach pressure tubing to transducer system or cable, and reference system to patient's phlebostatic axis and zero system.
2. Assist during insertion
   a. Attach pressure tubing to proximal and distal ports—flush system.
   b. Determine integrity of balloon—provider inserting PA catheter places catheter tip in sterile water and inflates the balloon; the balloon should be symmetric and not cover the tip.
   c. Transduce distal lumen on oscilloscope
   d. Inflate balloon at physician's direction (generally after catheter reaches right atrium).
   e. Monitor oscilloscope for characteristic waveform changes (see Fig. 19-12) and ectopy.
   f. Record waveforms and pressures as catheter passes from right atrium to PAW position.
   g. Deflate balloon once PAW has been obtained, and note return of characteristic PA waveform.
   h. Secure catheter and note insertion distance.
   i. Apply sterile occlusive dressing.
   j. Obtain chest radiograph to confirm catheter placement.

PA, pulmonary artery; PAW, pulmonary artery wedge.

POSITIONING

Supine With Backrest Elevation. Traditionally, PA and PAWP measurements have been obtained with the patient *supine* and flat; however, this position may be poorly tolerated by patients with increased intracranial pressure or pulmonary dysfunction. Research has shown that in a wide variety of critically ill patients, accurate PA pressure and PAWP can be obtained in the supine position with legs extended and a backrest elevation up to 60 degrees.[50,66,73,102,167,257,305,365,507–509] LA pressure can be measured with a backrest elevation up to 30 degrees as long as the phlebostatic axis is used as the reference level.[379] Measurement of PA pressures in the sitting position (legs dependent) is not recommended.[138,509]

Because some patients vary in response to position change, pressure measurements obtained in the flat, supine position should be compared with those measurements obtained with backrest elevation before assuming no difference. An algorithm developed by Gawlinski[157] for evaluating a patient's response to position change is outlined in Figure 19-20.

Lateral Position. In studies with a wide variety of patient populations, PA pressures obtained in the 90-degree lateral position were similar to those obtained in the supine position with the backrest flat.[48,185,242] In this position, an angle-specific reference point (mid-sternum at the fourth ICS) was used. In studies by Whitman[494] and Ross and Jones[383] using the supine phlebostatic axis as the reference, there were no clinically or statistically significant differences in the 20- or 30-degree lateral positions, respectively. However, in seven other studies regarding the effect of 30- to 60-degree lateral positions on PA pressures, statistically and clinically significant pressure changes relative to the supine position were found.[4,46,54,180,233,500] In the latter studies, the *mid-sternum* was used as the reference, potentially introducing measurement error related to placement of the reference level above or below the LA (see Fig. 19-3).

Research has demonstrated that the level of the LA in the 30-degree lateral position is a point one-half the distance from the surface of the bed to the left sternal border at the fourth ICS[471] (see Fig. 19-4). Using this reference point, there were no clinically significant pressure changes in most of the trauma patients[113] and postcardiac surgery patients studied in the supine and 30-degree right and left lateral positions.[41] These research studies demonstrate the importance of accurate referencing. However, as with supine backrest elevation, individual response to position should be assessed.

Three studies evaluated the effect of lateral position with backrest elevation and found clinically and statistically significant pressure changes relative to the flat, supine position.[54,180,346] However, in a study by Ross and Jones,[383] where the reference point was not moved from the supine reference, there were no significant ($P > 0.05$) pressure changes. If the potential error related to not moving the reference point is corrected, the results are similar to those of Bridges.[41] This finding reinforces the importance of correct referencing. Further research related to the effect of lateral position with backrest elevation using an angle-specific LA reference is needed.

PULMONARY EFFECTS

Correct function of the PA catheter requires a continuous column of fluid between the catheter tip and the LA. There are three physiologic zones in the lung, which depend on the interaction of alveolar, arterial, and venous pressures.[490] Alteration in any of these pressures may affect the fluid column between the catheter tip and the LA and alter the accuracy of PA pressure measurements. The delineation of the various lung zones is not as clearcut as initially thought, and within any given level of the lung, all three zone conditions may coexist.[168,169,170,171] Presence of catheter tip outside of zone 3 is one of the most common causes of inaccurate PAWP measurements.[312] Because the presence of a zone 3 vascular bed is crucial for accurate PA pressure measurements, assessment of this factor should be performed routinely.

There are three general methods that are useful in assessing for a zone 3 catheter placement.[41] First, anatomically, approximately 50% of the lung volume is below the LA,[139] and vascular beds below the level of the LA have an increased propensity for zone 3 characteristics.[168,169,172,173,484]

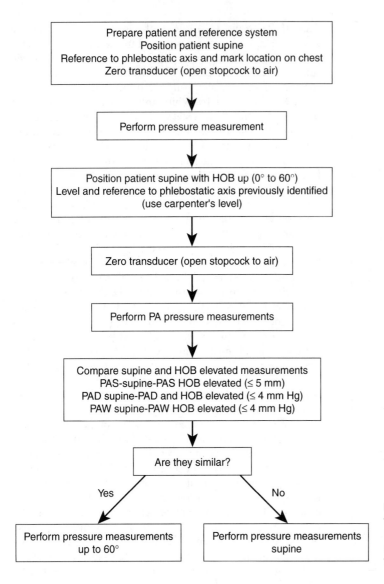

FIGURE 19-20 Algorithm for research-based practices for backrest position and pulmonary artery (PA) pressure measurement. (Gawlinski, A: Facts and fallacies of patient positioning and hemodynamic measurement. J Cardiovasc Nurs 12: 1–15, 1997. Adapted with permission.)

In the anteroposterior chest radiograph, the level of the LA is located approximately 3 cm below the carina, and the carina is vertically close to the bifurcation of the PA.[22] Therefore, the patient's anteroposterior chest radiograph can be reviewed to determine if the PA catheter is correctly placed[200,229,282,409,463] (Fig. 19-21).

Second, during wedging, the PA should be analyzed for the following changes. First, the PA waveform should flatten into a characteristic atrial waveform, although in some cases distinct a and v waves may not be discernible. Second, the waveform should immediately return to a PA configuration with deflation of the balloon. A partial wedge pressure is characterized as a waveform different from the phasic PA waveform, but intermediate between the phasic PA waveform and the atrial waveform. Partial PAW pressures do not accurately reflect left heart pressures and should not be used.[311,313] Finally, the PAWP should be lower than the mean PA pressure in the absence of a large V wave.[261]

The third method involves evaluating respiratory artifact induced by mechanical ventilation (inspiratory peak value minus expiratory peak value) on the PA pressure and PAWP tracings.[456] In patients with zone 2 placement, where there is increased respiratory artifact reflecting changes in alveolar pressure, the change in the ratio of the PAWP changes relative to changes in the PA pressure (ΔPAWP/ΔPA pressure) is greater than 2 at all levels of PEEP. A value of 1 for the ratio indicates no respiratory artifact due to zone 2 compression.

In addition, if the PAEDP-PAWP gradient is greater than 4 mm Hg,[202] further assessment for possible alveolar compression is warranted. An increase in the PAEDP-PAWP gradient reflects pulmonary vascular compression.[93] If alveolar pressure increases (PEEP) or an extracellular fluid deficit (diuresis, hemorrhage, hypovolemia) occurs, a large portion of the lungs may convert to zone 1 or 2. Therefore, in the clinical setting with a diminished zone 3, it is important to attempt to maximize zone 3 placement by positioning the tip of the catheter below the LA.[336]

PAEDP-PAWP Gradient. Assessment of the PAEDP–PAWP gradient provides information about pulmonary vascular tone, incorrect catheter position, and venous

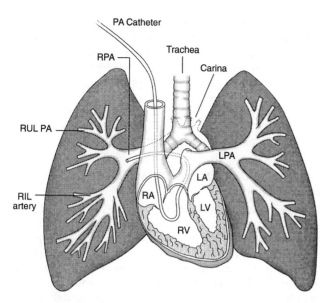

FIGURE 19-21 Schema of the cardiopulmonary structures demonstrating the relationship between the left atrium, pulmonary artery (PA), and pulmonary vasculature, with a correctly positioned PA catheter. RUL PA, right upper lobe PA; RIL, right interlobar PA; RPA, right PA; LPA, left PA; RA, right atrium; LA, left atrium; RV, right ventricle; LV, left ventricle.

obstruction. Normally, there is a 1- to 4-mm Hg pressure gradient between the PAEDP and the PAWP, which is consistent with the forward flow of blood from the PA to the LA.

An increase in this gradient of greater than 5 mm Hg may indicate increased PVR associated with such conditions as pulmonary hypertension, cor pulmonale, pulmonary embolus, hypoxia, Eisenmenger's syndrome,[143] or inadequate time for diastolic equalization of pressures (tachycardia).[36,126,129,336] In these clinical situations, the PAEDP is not an accurate indicator of LA pressure, and the PAWP should be used.

A PAWP that is greater than the PAEDP indicates some form of obstruction between the PA catheter and the LA, such as mitral stenosis, LA myxoma, mitral valve regurgitation (see Fig. 19-14), or nonzone 3 catheter placement.[201,502] In these clinical situations, the PAWP is of limited use as an indicator of LA pressures.

Evaluation of the PAEDP-PAWP gradient is useful in differentiating cardiac and pulmonary pathology:

1. PAEDP = 30 mm Hg; PAWP = 22 mm Hg; PAEDP – PAWP = 8 mm Hg. (Increased LV preload and PVR, e.g., LV failure with pulmonary edema.)
2. PAEDP = 35 mm Hg; PAWP = 13 mm Hg; PAEDP – PAWP = 19 mm Hg. (Increased PVR without an increase in LV volume, e.g., acute pulmonary embolus, addition of PEEP, hypoxia.)
3. PAEDP = 23 mm Hg; PAWP = 20 mm Hg; PAEDP – PAWP = 3 mm Hg. (LV overload without pulmonary involvement. In this situation, the PAEDP is an accurate indirect indicator of LV preload.)

SPONTANEOUS VERSUS MECHANICAL VENTILATION

During spontaneous ventilation, alveolar pressure decreases during inspiration and increases during expiration. During *positive-pressure ventilation,* intrathoracic pressure increases during inspiration and decreases during expiration (the opposite of spontaneous ventilation).[1,53] The changes in intrathoracic pressure are transmitted to the cardiovascular structures in the thorax and are reflected by changes in PA pressure measurements that correspond with inspiration and expiration. During *spontaneous ventilation,* PA pressures decrease during inspiration and increase during expiration; during mechanical ventilation, PA pressures increase during inspiration and decrease during expiration (see Display 19-1). At end-expiration, when no air flow occurs, pleural pressure equals atmospheric pressure regardless of the mode of ventilation and does not affect intracardiac pressures.[25]

Numerous strategies have been suggested to correct for respiratory variation.[336,501] Although measurement of end-expiratory pressure is considered the most accurate method, Wild and Woods[501] identified a marked difference in the pressure measured depending on the technique used, which highlights the need for consistency in the method used when reading PA pressures. Use of airway pressure measurement, a new technique to identify end-expiratory waveforms, has been recommended as a method for increasing the accuracy of pressure measurements,[2] although limited use of this method in practice has not been shown to improve interpretation.[247]

In patients receiving positive-pressure ventilation without PEEP, there are no clinically significant changes in PA pressures on versus off ventilation. Removal from mechanical ventilation for PA pressure measurement usually is not warranted.[95,181,413]

Four studies related to removal from mechanical ventilation with PEEP found that (1) in patients with LV dysfunction, removal was associated with an increased PA pressure and hypoxemia, indicating rebound hypervolemia[276]; (2) in the presence of hypovolemia (>1,000-mL blood volume deficit), PA pressures were lower off mechanical ventilation; and (3) with PEEP greater than 10 cm H_2O, removal was associated with varying responses.[95,159,276] Removal from mechanical ventilation is not recommended because it does not increase the accuracy of PA pressure readings, may further compromise the patient's functional status, and fails to reflect the patient's clinical condition.[292]

At PEEP less than 10 cm H_2O, PAWP is a good indicator of LA pressure.[225,279] Several methods have been suggested to improve accuracy of PAWP as an indicator of LA pressure when high levels of PEEP (>10 cm H_2O) are applied:

1. Place the catheter tip in a position dependent to the LA (zone 3), and verify position with anterior and lateral chest radiographs.[370,409] Pressures from a catheter in zone 1 or 2 tend to be artificially high.
2. Measure extramural pressure with an esophageal balloon. The accuracy of the esophageal balloon may be affected by position and lung volume; therefore, its use in the clinical setting is limited.[164,288,316,336]

3. Analyze pulmonary capillary wedge blood. Although blood gas values that reflect correct pulmonary capillary wedge blood confirm wedging of the PA catheter, they do not ensure that the measured wedge pressure is truly reflective of LA pressure.[213,311]

4. Subtract an estimate of pleural pressure from the measured PAWP. A *rough* estimate of PAWP can be made by subtracting one-half of the applied PEEP.[64,289]

For an example of number 4 above, convert centimeters of water into millimeters of mercury (1.36 cm H_2O = 1 mm Hg). For example, in a patient receiving 20 cm H_2O PEEP with a measured PAWP of 18 mm Hg:

Measured PAWP = 18.0
– ½ applied PEEP = 7.4
───────────────────────
Corrected PAWP = 10.6 mm Hg

This correction reflects the *maximum* pressure change that would result from an increase in PEEP. In patients with decreased lung compliance (e.g., ARDS) a smaller amount (e.g., one-third of the applied PEEP) may be transmitted to the heart. Thus, this correction is the largest pressure change that should be observed. If a larger change occurs, zone 3 placement is questionable and the catheter may need to be repositioned.[336,466] For example, if the applied PEEP was increased by 5 cm H_2O (3.7 mm Hg), and the accompanying increase in PAWP was greater than 1.8 mm Hg (3.7 mm Hg divided by 2 = 1.8 mm Hg), suspect nonzone 3 placement. In this case, the PAWP no longer accurately reflects left heart pressure and the catheter needs to repositioned.

Another option is to position the patient such that the catheter tip is below the LA.[200,201,329,370,409,463] For example, if the catheter tip is in the right PA, positioning the patient in a right lateral position places the catheter tip below the LA. As previously discussed, the use of an angle-specific reference is essential to ensuring the accuracy of the pressure measurements.

RECORDING PULMONARY ARTERY PRESSURES

In patients with respiratory variation, the use of digital readings is unreliable because of the unselective nature of electrical averaging.[57,227,267,280,403,426] In addition, the "stop cursor" method (freezing the monitor screen) is less reliable than the graphic method.[280] The analysis of graphic recordings of the PA pressure waveforms remains the recommended method. Display 19-1 reviews guidelines for recording PA pressure measurements.

Complications/Troubleshooting

Numerous potential complications are associated with PA pressure measurement. A high index of suspicion and attention to detail reduce the risk of complications. Table 19-3 outlines potential complications and actions to take to avoid or resolve them. Table 19-4 summarizes actions for troubleshooting the PA catheter.

TABLE 19-3	**Complications Associated With Pulmonary Artery Monitoring[144]**
Complication	**Nursing Intervention**

Cardiac dysrhythmias
   Endocardial irritation
	Identify patients at high risk: shock, pH < 7.2, PaO_2 < 60 mm Hg, K^+ < 3.5 mEq/L, Ca^{2+} < 8 mg/dL (corrected), Mg^{2+} < 1 mg/dL, myocardial ischemia or infarction, CI < 2.5 L/min/m², prolonged insertion time.[87, 440]
	Prophylactic lidocaine not recommended unless the patient is at high risk.[216, 439, 481]
	Bundle-branch block or complete heart block
	   Right bundle-branch block is usually transient and does not require therapy.[314, 438]
	   Preexisting left bundle-branch block; have method for ventricular pacing immediately available.[382, 438]
	Continuously monitor electrocardiogram during insertion and removal of the catheter.[88]

Pulmonary artery perforation/rupture
   Distal migration of catheter
   Eccentric balloon inflation
   Perforation of wall with catheter tip
   Excessive pressure from balloon
   on vessel wall[15]
	Identify high-risk patients: pulmonary hypertension, age greater than 60 years, use of anticoagulants.[16, 241]
	Withdraw catheter 2 to 4 cm before the initiation of cardiopulmonary bypass.[232, 468]
	Maintain high degree of suspicion whenever a patient presents with hemoptysis.[15]
	Monitor PA waveform continuously during balloon inflation.
	Inflate the balloon gradually to volume (1.25–1.5 mL), at which time the pressure tracing should change from the typical PA waveform to PA wedge pressure.[241, 449] The PA wedge should occur after loss of resistance in the syringe.[296] If "overwedge" pattern occurs (see Fig. 19-20) occurs, STOP IMMEDIATELY.
	Continually monitor PA tracing to detect distal migration.
	Keep wedge time to a minimum (10–15 s).[451]
	Do not inflate the balloon with fluids.
	Follow patient with serial chest radiographic films; if the catheter tip is more than 5 cm from the mediastinum, the catheter should be repositioned.[241]

(continued)

| **TABLE 19-3** | **Complications Associated With Pulmonary Artery Monitoring[145] (Continued)** |

Complication	Nursing Intervention

Pulmonary infarction
  Catheter migration into wedge position
  Balloon left inflated
  Thrombus formation around catheter
	Monitor PA waveform continuously.
	Obtain serial chest radiographs to ensure correct catheter placement (<5 cm from mediastinum.[241]
	Use heparinized flushing solution to maintain catheter patency.

Infection
  Lack of aseptic technique
  Migration of nonsterile portion of catheter
  Prolonged insertion time
  Concomitant infection
  Age (<1 y and > 60 y)
	Use aseptic technique when manipulating stopcock or catheter, even if the sheath is in place.[238,300,301]
	Use single-dose heparin when preparing the flush solution.[238]
	Use normal saline instead of dextrose for the flush solution.[238]
	Monitor insertion site for signs of infection, especially after 72 to 96 h.[88, 213, 355]
	Ensure the catheter is secured to avoid migration.
	Send catheter tip for culture if infection is suspected.

Catheter kinking or knotting
  Excessive insertion of catheter (>15 cm from RA)
  Dilated heart
  Smaller-bore catheter
  Concomitant use of other intracardiac catheters (e.g., pacemaker)
	Monitor catheter length during insertion. The RA should be reached within the following distances: right antecubital fossa (30–40 cm); left antecubital fossa (40–50 cm); internal jugular or subclavian veins (10–15 cm); femoral vein (35–45 cm). The catheter should reach the PA after it is advanced no more than 15 cm from the RA.[450]
	If other lines (pacemaker, indwelling catheters) are in use, insert and remove the PA catheter with the use of fluoroscopy.

Air embolization[40]
  Balloon rupture
  Excessive inflation volume
  Prolonged catheter placement (>48 hours)[450]
  During placement of introducer or insertion of the catheter during insertion
  Catheter removal[481]
    Decreased central venous pressure (hypovolemia, tachycardia)
    Negative intrathoracic pressure (tachypnea, upright position, PA catheter removal during deep inspiration)[40, 310]
    Incompetent valve on introducer[74]
    Right-to-left intracardiac shunt (not required for arterial gas embolism)
	Position the patient in a 20-degree head-down position during insertion.
	Have patient perform Valsalva maneuver, hold breath at critical moments, or administer a positive-pressure ventilation (bag-valve-mask or ventilator).[481]
	Do not exceed recommended balloon inflation volume.
	Use CO_2 for patients with intracardiac shunt.
	Clamp and label the inflation if the balloon is ruptured.
	PA catheter removal
	  Place patient in supine or Trendelenburg position during PA catheter removal.
	  Increase intrathoracic pressure during removal of the catheter (Valsalva maneuver, breath-hold at the end of a deep inspiration, withdraw catheter during positive-pressure ventilation, apply positive-pressure ventilation with a bag-valve device).
	  Apply pressure to insertion site after removal. Apply petroleum jelly gauze to exit site once hemostasis is established (leave in place for a minimum of 24 h).[143, 481]
	  Use obturator after PA catheter removal.

PA, pulmonary artery; RA, right atrium.

Right Ventricular Volumetric Measures

Traditionally, PA pressure monitoring focuses on left heart function. However, research has demonstrated the importance of right heart function, as it affects biventricular function,[207,208] and determines outcomes in patients with trauma, coronary artery disease, septic shock, and pulmonary disease.[32,47,97,114,115,215,362,366,380,407,420,487] In these conditions, an increase in pulmonary pressure results in an increased load on the right heart, which may lead to RV ischemia, dysfunction, or failure.[31,51,127]

The RV ejection catheter is a modified PA catheter (Fig. 19-22) with a rapid-response thermistor that allows for beat-to-beat measurement of changes in PA temperature as observed on a CO thermodilution curve.[98,230,480] The technique for obtaining the RV volumetric measurements is similar to that used to obtain CO measurements with a standard PA catheter (e.g., injection of a cooled or room-temperature [RT] solution into the RA). As demonstrated in Figure 19-23, the computer attached to the catheter system simultaneously records the CO curve and an ECG signal, which allows for the measurement of the RV ejection

(text continues on page 452)

TABLE 19-4	Troubleshooting the Pulmonary Artery Catheter and Measurement Problems		
Clinical Problem	**Implications**	**Possible Causes**	**Interventions**
Overdamped pressure tracing	Falsely low systolic readings Falsely increased diastolic readings	Air bubbles in the pressure tubing or transducer More than three stopcocks between catheter and transducer Loose connections Collection of blood in tubing or in and around transducer Catheter kinked internally or at insertion site Catheter wedged against vessel wall Excessive tubing length (>4 feet) Clot or fibrin deposition on catheter tip	Flush all air from system (including microbubbles). Remove excess stopcocks. Tighten all connections. Flush tubing of all blood (if unable to clear, change transducer–tubing set-up). Maintain pressure in infusion bag at 300 mm Hg. Aspirate blood from catheter if clot suspected (*do not* flush). If PA catheter kinked—notify MD to reposition. If fibrin occluding catheter—catheter may need to be replaced. Use noncompliant/wide-bore tubing.
Underdamped pressure tracing	Overestimation of systolic pressure Underestimation of diastolic pressure	Air bubbles in tubing, stopcocks, or transducer Excessive tubing length (>4 feet) Excess number of stopcocks	Remove all air bubbles from system. Limit tubing to 4 feet (maximum). Remove unnecessary stopcocks. If all attempts to resolve unsuccessful, consider the addition of an in-line damping device.
Catheter whip (fling) or artifact	Overestimation of systolic pressure Underestimation of diastolic pressure Difficult interpretation of waveform	Location of distal tip of PA catheter near pulmonic valve Hyperdynamic heart Looping of PA catheter in RV External disruption of PA catheter system	Assess dynamic response characteristics (troubleshoot system). Notify MD to reposition PA catheter. If fling fails to resolve, use mean pressure.
Absence of PA wedge tracing	Potential for air embolism or blood leaking from balloon port	Balloon rupture Improper positioning of PA catheter	If balloon is inflated without return of air into syringe on passive deflation, assess for signs of air embolism (if present, place in Trendelenburg in left lateral decubitus position—treat symptoms—notify MD). If stable—label balloon port "DO NOT WEDGE." Notify MD of need to replace catheter. If balloon is inflated to 1.5 mL, without change in waveform from PA to PA wedge pattern, notify MD (or, if appropriate, RN) of need to reposition catheter. Once catheter is repositioned, assess amount of air required for wedge (ideal volume 1.25–1.5 mL).
Migration of the PA catheter into the RV	Presence of RV dysrhythmias Decreased diastolic pressure (equal to RAP)	Accidental or spontaneous withdrawal of catheter into the RV	Inflate the balloon fully to engulf the tip of the catheter and reduce ectopy. Notify MD or, if approved for RN, reposition catheter into PA. If compromised by dysrhythmias, ensure balloon is deflated and withdraw catheter into RA (15–20 cm marking on PA catheter and RAP waveform observed from distal port).

(continued)

TABLE 19-4	Troubleshooting the Pulmonary Artery Catheter and Measurement Problems *(Continued)*		
Clinical Problem	**Implications**	**Possible Causes**	**Interventions**
Overwedging	Overwedging (eccentric balloon inflation or inflation in a small vessel) is a potential risk for PA perforation and rupture	Catheter migration Balloon position in small pulmonary vessel	Slowly inflate balloon while constantly observing the waveform. If overwedge pattern observed, immediately stop inflation and allow balloon to deflate passively. Notify MD or, if approved for RN, reposition catheter.
Spontaneous wedge	Potential for loss of blood supply to branch of pulmonary vessel and risk of PA infarction	Catheter migration (Patient movement, warming up of catheter after placement)	Turn patient to side opposite catheter placement. Have patient strengthen arm or turn head to dislodge catheter. Have patient gently cough. Notify MD or, if approved for RN, reposition catheter.

PA, pulmonary artery; RAP, right atrial pressure; RV, right ventricle.
    Modified from Gardner PE: Pulmonary artery pressure monitoring. AACN Clinical Issues in Critical Care Nursing 4: 98–119, 1993.

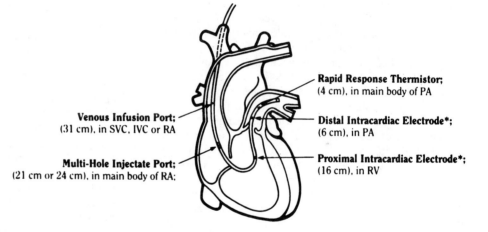

FIGURE 19-22 Swan-Ganz ejection fraction/volumetric catheter characteristics and positioning. (Courtesy of Baxter Healthcare, Edwards Critical-Care Division, Santa Ana, CA.) *Intracardiac electrodes are used for ventricular sensing only and **are not** to be used for pacing.

Venous Infusion Port; (31 cm), in SVC, IVC or RA

Multi-Hole Injectate Port; (21 cm or 24 cm), in main body of RA;

Rapid Response Thermistor; (4 cm), in main body of PA

Distal Intracardiac Electrode*; (6 cm), in PA

Proximal Intracardiac Electrode*; (16 cm), in RV

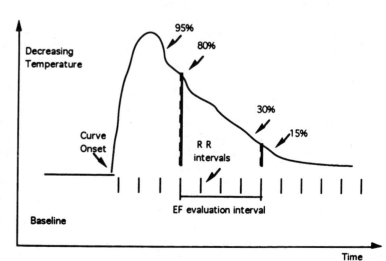

FIGURE 19-23 Determination of ejection fraction (EF). Two reference points on the downslope of the thermodilution curve, one point between 15% and 30% and one between 80% and 95%, correspond to R waves. A curve is fit through these points. Using an exponential method, the slope of the curve is then divided by the number of R-R intervals providing the residual fraction. The value provides the percent of injectate not ejected; therefore, this value is subtracted from one to determine the percentage ejected or EF (1–residual fraction=EF). (Courtesy of Baxter Healthcare, Edwards Critical-Care Division, Santa Ana, CA.)

TABLE 19-5	Right Heart Function Variables
Variable	**Normal**
Stroke volume	60–100 mL/beat
Stroke volume index	33–46 mL/beat/m²
Right ventricular ejection fraction	40%–60% (0.4–0.6)
Right ventricular end-systolic volume index	30–60 mL/m²
Right ventricular end-diastolic volume index	60–100 mL/m²

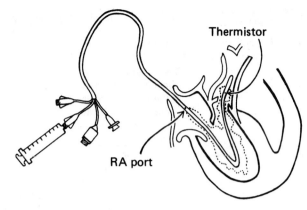

FIGURE 19-24 Injection of iced or room-temperature injectate into the right atrium.

fraction (RVEF), CO, and SV.[230] Using this information, the RV end-diastolic volume (RVEDV = SV/RVEF) and RV end-systolic volume (RVESV = RVEDV – SV) can be calculated[207,215,480] (Table 19-5).

The clinically most useful information obtained from the RVEF catheter is the RVEDV. The RVESV, which is the residual amount of blood left in the ventricle after contraction, is also useful because it provides information regarding the effect of vasodilator and inotropic agents on the ability of the heart to contract effectively and move blood forward into the systemic circulation. The volumetric measurements may overcome the problem caused by the curvilinear pressure—volume relationship, which limits the use of pressure as an indicator of volume change.[466] Direct measurement of heart volumes may provide better insight into the patient's volume status and response to therapy. For example, in a patient who is hypotensive, assessment would include evaluation of the factors that affect CO (SV and HR). Further assessment would include evaluation of the factors that affect SV: preload (RVEDV instead of PAWP), afterload (RVESV, SVR, PVR), and contractility. PAWP remains an important index of the patient's risk for the development of pulmonary edema and should not be ignored.

The RVEDV index has been found to be more highly correlated (*r* = 0.61) to the cardiac index (CI) compared with the PAWP (*r* = 0.35),[99] and has been demonstrated to be a better predictor of a patient's need for and response to volume therapy.[19,321] For example, in only one-half of the patients in a study conducted by Diebel and colleagues[99] did the PAWP predict which patients would respond appropriately to a volume challenge. Conversely, an RVEDV index (RVEDVI) of less than 140 mL/m2 was a markedly better predictor of the need for and response to a volume challenge. The patients with an RVEDVI of less than 140 mL/m² had what Diebel and colleagues[99] termed a "preload recruitable" increase in CI, whereas patients with an EDVI greater than 140 mL/m² did not. Although the validity of this REDVI has been demonstrated in other studies,[63,65,381] it has been recently challenged.[482] The varying results may reflect different techniques or patient populations; however, further research is needed in this area

before practice recommendations can be made for specific patient populations.[361]

TECHNICAL FACTORS

Technical factors that prevent the accurate measurement of RVEF include the inability to sense the R wave, rapid HR (>150 beats/min) or irregularity (atrial fibrillation, frequent ectopy), and faulty injection technique.[215,321]

CARDIAC OUTPUT MEASUREMENT

Measurement of CO by the thermodilution principle (TDCO) was introduced by Fegler[131] in 1954. The TDCO method is based on the injection of a known volume of cold or RT sterile saline or 5% dextrose in water (D₅W) through the proximal port of the PA catheter into the RA (Fig. 19-24). The blood is temporarily cooled by the injectate, and the change in temperature is sensed by the thermistor on the distal end of the PA catheter.[510] A CO computer connected to the PA catheter calculates the area under this curve using the Stewart-Hamilton equation.[121,195,228,368,444,510] Most CO computers display the CO time—temperature curve, and plot the CO over time, which allows for analysis of trends (Fig. 19-25).

Factors Influencing Thermodilution Cardiac Output Measurement

CATHETER POSITION

Although PA measurements vary according to the location of the catheter in the lungs, the distal tip of the catheter may be positioned in the right, left, or main PA when obtaining TDCO.[278] The proximal port (injection port) should be positioned in the RA, which can be determined by observing for an RA waveform from the proximal port. The PA waveform should be monitored continuously on the oscilloscope to ensure proper PA waveform patterns and to detect wedging. A wedged or damped PA waveform may indicate improper catheter position and result in erroneous CO values.

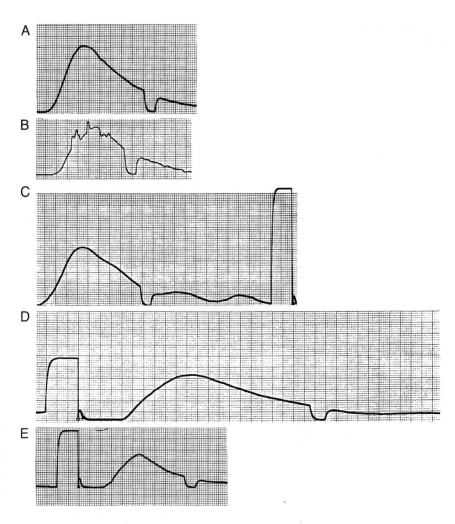

FIGURE 19-25 Cardiac output (CO) curves. Thermodilution time–temperature curves. **(A)** Normal curve configuration. **(B)** Abnormal curve due to faulty injection technique or to a wedged catheter. **(C)** Marked baseline oscillations. **(D)** Prolonged baseline drift. **(E)** Low amplitude of CO curve.

INJECTION PORT

The injectate solution can be injected through the proximal port, the venous infusion port, or right ventricular port, or through any centrally placed catheter that exits into a central vein or the RA.[162,262,291,294,298,360,510] However, injections through the side-port have been found to be less accurate than those from the infusion port,[378] and it has been recommended that the PA catheter be replaced if the proximal injection port is clotted.[156] The exit of the proximal lumen must be located beyond the introducer sheath to avoid retrograde flow from an intravenous line connected to the introducer side port, which may produce falsely high CO values.[142]

CALIBRATION CONSTANT

The CO computer must be presented with an adequate signal (temperature difference)-to-noise (cyclic variations in blood temperature) ratio to sense a temperature change over a period of time. The necessary difference in temperature between injectate solution and blood should be 10° C to obtain accurate TDCO curves.[125] In addition, the accuracy of the TDCO calculation requires the input of information contained in what is known as the calibration or

computation constant.[285,390,391] The calibration constant (a factor that corrects for the gain of heat from the tubing and thermistor) is provided by the manufacturer and is specific for the volume and temperature of injectate solution and the type of PA catheter used. The patient's body temperature and calibration constant are incorporated in the calculation of CO.[510] The calibration coefficient also contains a constant for D_5W; thus, the use of saline as the injectate may introduce a 2% decrease in CO.[266,390,391,510,513]

INJECTION TECHNIQUE

The speed of injection and handling of the injectate syringe can influence the accuracy of thermodilution CO. An injection rate of 4 seconds for 5 or 10 mL of injectate yield accurate results.[26,128,137,141,448] Some investigators recommend the use of an automatic injector to provide consistency as well as to avoid rewarming of injectate by manual handling of the syringe barrel.[101] Although consistency in injection times and flow rates and more reproducible curves were noted with the automatic injector, the CO measurements obtained were not significantly ($P > 0.05$) different from CO measurements obtained using manual injection.[101,325]

DISPLAY 19-4

Protocol for Intermittent Thermodilution Cardiac Output Measurements[144]

1. Set up
   a. Explain procedure to patient.
   b. Set up monitor in accordance with manufacturer's recommendations.
   c. Enter the computation constant (based on temperature and volume of injectate, catheter model, and injectate delivery system).
   d. Remove all vasoactive drips from the proximal port to avoid inadvertent bolus of these medications.
   e. Verify correct position of the PA catheter.
      (1) Proximal port with right atrial waveform.
      (2) Distal port with characteristic PA waveform (not damped or wedged).
   f. Position patient: supine with 20-degree backrest elevation; 20-degree sidelying with 0-degree backrest elevation.
2. Performance of measurement
   a. Determine volume and temperature of injectate and verify temperature
      (1) Iced injectate (0° C–5° C)
         (a) 5 mL ≅ 10 mL
         (b) Low and high CO[377, 483]
         (c) Hyperthermia, 10 mL
         (d) Hyperdynamic patients
         (e) Hypothermia, 10 mL
         (f) 10 mL of iced injectate is considered the standard[434]
      (2) Room temperature (19° C–25° C)
         (a) 10 mL
         (b) CO within normal limits
         (c) Normothermia (5 mL if patient fluid restricted and CO from 5 mL ≅ 10 mL)[157, 354]
         (d) Hyperdynamic patients
         (e) Hypothermia
         (f) It is not necessary to prime the catheter with cold injectate before CO measurements[385]
   b. Activate CO computer in accordance with manufacturer recommendations

c. Inject solution
   (1) Begin injection during same phase of the respiratory cycle (end-expiration or evenly spaced throughout the respiratory cycle)
   (2) Inject smoothly
   (3) Complete injection within 4 seconds
d. Inspect CO curve for the following:
   (1) Smooth, rapid upstroke to peak and gradual downslope to baseline (normal curve; see Fig. 19-25*A*)[26, 266, 278, 285, 391]
   (2) Discard the following waveforms
      (a) Abnormal inflection contour of the wave due to catheter wedging or faulty injection technique (see Fig. 19-25*B*)
      (b) Oscillation of the baseline (±15% of PA temperature) due to hemodynamic and respiratory effects (see Fig. 19-25*C*)[428]
      (c) Prolonged baseline drift due to recirculation of thermal indicator (low-output states; see Fig. 19-25*D*).
      (d) Low-amplitude curve due to small temperature difference (10° C) between injectate solution and blood or thermistor lying against a vessel wall (see Fig. 19-25*E*)[125]
e. Repeat CO procedure
   (1) Allow approximately 60 seconds between injections (computer will indicate when "READY")
   (2) Obtain three measurements that are within 10% of the median value[278, 488] (may require three to five injections); identify median value and include all measurements that are within 10%. Example: median value = 5 L/min; include all values within 4.5 to 5.5 range. Omit all other values and average to obtain CO measurements.

CO, cardiac output; PA, pulmonary artery.

VOLUME AND TEMPERATURE OF INJECTATE

Numerous studies have compared the effects of various volumes and temperature of injectate on TDCO measurements. Regardless of the volume or temperature selected, variations in syringe volume or accidental warming of the injectate by contact with the syringe or delay after withdrawal of the solution from the injectate reservoir lead to inaccurate TDCO values.[285,324,376,511] A summary of the recommendations for volume and temperature is provided in Display 19-4.

Iced Injectate. The rationale for using iced injectate 0° C to 5° C prefilled syringe; 6° C to 12° (CO-Set) is to improve the signal-to-noise ratio (variation in PA blood temperature due to causes other than the injectate).[141] In conditions with high- and low-flow states, the iced injectate

is associated with decreased variability and improved accuracy compared with RT injectate.[377,483] The TDCO measurements obtained with 5 versus 10 mL iced injectate are similar.[92] Further, 10 mL RT injectate is comparable with 5 mL iced injectate; thus, when iced injectate is used, a smaller volume can be used, which is important in patients at risk for volume overload. However, the use of iced injectate is not risk free because bradycardia has been associated with the injection of iced solution into the heart. This bradycardia has not been observed with RT injectate.[198]

Room-Temperature Injectate. The TDCO measurements obtained using RT injectate are highly correlated with measurements using the Fick method.[85] In most critically ill patients, TDCO measurements can be obtained with RT injectate, minimizing the time necessary to achieve the specified temperature of the injectate.[156]

Iced Versus Room-Temperature Injectate. Injection of 10 mL RT and iced injectate were highly correlated ($r = 0.90$) with other CO methods (Fick, dye dilution, and electromagnetic flowmeter).[356] In addition, a very high correlation ($r=0.90$) was also found when TDCO using 10 mL iced and RT injectates were compared in a wide variety of critically ill patients.[17,92,124,214,239,243,254,281,286,324,356,410,411,452,476] Thus, 10 mL iced and RT injectate are interchangeable.

In patients with normal CO, 5 mL iced injectate is comparable with 10 mL RT injectate.[243] However, the results of studies comparing 5 and 10 mL RT injectate versus 10 mL iced solution are variable, with some studies finding increased variability from the RT measures[37,124,476,511] and others with comparable results.[254] The variability associated with RT injections appears to be increased at low COs,[411] resulting in as much as a 25% to 50% overestimation of CO.[511] In addition, there is a decrease in correlation and increased variability in RT CO measures versus iced TDCO measures when a CO–Set (closed system) was used.[17] Finally, the increased variability means that a larger number of measurements must be obtained with RT injectate to provide a satisfactory CO measurement.[37]

There has been some concern that in hypothermia the use of RT injectate decreases the signal (temperature difference) and may yield an erroneous CO value. Despite the decrease in the signal, CO measurements obtained using 10 mL iced and RT injectates were comparable.[411]

RESPIRATORY EFFECTS ON CARDIAC OUTPUT

Pulmonary Artery Temperature Fluctuation. Normally, there is a transient fluctuation in the PA temperature throughout the respiratory cycle ($\pm 0.01°$ C to $0.05°$ C), which is considered physiologic noise and affects the accuracy of TDCO measures.[285,497,498,511] In addition, conditions such as coughing, sudden body movements, alterations in respiratory patterns, and metabolic changes can increase this loss of heat from the respiratory tract and cause wide fluctuations of PA temperature.[222,223] However, temperature variations of 10% to 15% of the patient's baseline temperature have been noted in spontaneously breathing patients and have little effect on the CO value.[498]

Fluctuation in Cardiac Output Due to Respiration. In addition to the effect of the natural fluctuation in PA temperature over the respiratory cycle, the CO varies throughout the respiratory cycle as a result of changes in intrathoracic pressure and thus preload.[222,453] For example, the CO may vary as much as 30% between peak inspiration and peak expiration,[222] and at any given time the CO varies by approximately 6%.[297,396] The effects of a change in intrathoracic pressure are further increased during mechanical ventilation, particularly with PEEP.[109] The respiratory variation in CO can be minimized and the reproducibility of the CO measures can be increased by injecting the indicator during the same phase of the respiratory cycle.[199] As a general rule, the thermodilution injections are timed to begin at the end-expiratory phase of the respiratory cycle.[7,244,251,453,478] The practice of timing injection during the expiratory phase may

result in an overestimation 1.0 to 1.5 times the true CO,[221] but this method is useful for following trends in the CO. If, however, validity (the true change in CO over the respiratory cycle) is desired, then the average of three or four measurement spread evenly (vs. randomly) throughout the respiratory cycle is recommended.[78,220–224,278,432]

EFFECT OF CONCOMITANT INFUSIONS

Several studies have demonstrated an increase in variability in the measured CO with concomitant infusions (central and peripheral infusions).[177,302,492] Many critically ill patients require vasoactive medications for hemodynamic stability and would suffer compromise if these medications were turned off during the measurement procedure. If however, the discontinuation of the infusion would not affect the patient's stability, consideration should be given to turning the infusions off for a short period of time before (30 seconds) and during TDCO measurements,[145,156,211,278,510] or avoid performance of TDCO during rapid volume infusion.[177]

PATIENT POSITION

Thermodilution CO measurements, along with other hemodynamic measurements, are routinely performed with the patient in the flat, supine position. However, reproducible CO measurements have been obtained in patients with 20-degree elevation of backrest position,[103,182,246] while at 45 degrees there are increased differences (–0.06 to –1.09 L/min).[111] The findings from Driscoll and colleagues'[111] study are important because PA pressure measurements are often taken with a backrest elevation of 45 degrees. Thus, the patient may need to be repositioned before initiation of CO and PA pressure measurements. Given the potential variability among patient responses to position, the CO obtained with backrest elevation should be compared with a measurement in the flat, supine position to determine if differences exist, or the position in which CO is measured should be noted in the patient's record.[111,156,157,432]

Patients in lateral recumbent positions yield more variable CO measurements, with measurements taken in the 20- and 45-degree lateral positions significantly different ($P < 0.05$) from those obtained in the supine position with 20-degree backrest elevation.[104,495] The 250- to 500-mL position-related change in CO may be explained by the 1- to 2-mm Hg increase in PAWP that occurs in the lateral position, indicating a position-induced change in volume.[41,348,373] Until further study, it is recommended that CO be measured in the supine position and in the side-lying position, and that the two CO values be compared.

CLOSED INJECTATE SYSTEM

Concerns regarding the contamination of prefilled syringes and injectate warming due to handling led to the creation of closed injectate delivery systems. The obvious advantages are that these systems preclude preparation of individual syringes,[266] eliminate inefficiencies, and reduce multiple entries into a sterile system.[146,326] Several closed injectate delivery systems have been designed. In general, these systems, which are directly connected to the PA catheter and CO computer, incorporate a flow-through temperature probe that measures injectate temperature near the site of injection.

The accuracy of the CO-Set closed system has been examined in several studies, which showed moderate to high correlations between TDCO measures obtained with the iced and RT injectates in modified closed systems versus iced prefilled syringes ($r = 0.64$ to 0.98).[17,145,239,281] Given the relative similarity and the decreased risk of infection between closed system and prefilled syringes, the use of the closed system is recommended.[145,156]

PATHOPHYSIOLOGIC FACTORS

Adequate mixing of the thermal indicator and blood must occur before sensing by the distal thermistor of the PA catheter. Pathophysiologic conditions, such as tricuspid insufficiency and ventricular septal defect, inhibit adequate mixing of indicator and blood and may interfere with accurate TDCO measurements.[273,436] Tricuspid regurgitation results in a small but systematic underestimation of baseline CO values. If this underestimation of CO is taken into account, the presence of tricuspid regurgitation does not necessarily negate the use of TDCO.[194]

Clinically Important Changes in Cardiac Output

In general, a change in CO of greater than 10% to 15% is considered to be physiologically important.[285,443] The 10% value is based on studies that demonstrate that normal physiologic variability is approximately 6.4% in patients with stable (±5% of the mean value) covariables (HR, respiratory rate, MAP, PA mean) and 9.9% in "covariable unstable" patients (covariable change greater than ±5% of the mean).[400] In assessing changes in CO, it is important to evaluate technical (Table 19-6), physiologic, and pathophysiologic (Table 19-7) factors related to the CO.

If the change in CO is determined to be clinically important, steps to determine the cause of the change include[122,467]:

1. Is it a preload problem (volume loss, orthostasis, vasodilator agents)? Assess RAP, PAEDP, PAWP, and volumetric measurements if available.
2. Is it an afterload problem? Assess for changes in blood pressure, pulmonary or systemic vascular resistance, temperature, valvular dysfunction, mistiming of intra-aortic balloon pump (IABP).
3. Is it a contractility problem? Assess SV and stroke work indices, changes in CO without changes in preload or afterload, changes in the characteristics of peripheral pulses, an afterload-induced increase or decrease in force of contraction, change in inotropic, vasoconstrictor, or vasodilator agent.

The direct and derived indices used in a comprehensive hemodynamic assessment are outlined in Table 19-8.

VENTRICULAR FUNCTION CURVES

The interaction between preload, afterload, and contractility and the effects of various disease processes (heart failure, hemorrhage) and therapeutic actions (vasodilator or inotropic drug therapy) can be visualized in a family of ventricular function curves[399] (Fig. 19-26). The family of curves varies for each patient, but is useful in predicting and evaluating the effects of various therapeutic interventions. The curves are constructed by plotting the PAWP (or some measure of end-diastolic volume) on the horizontal axis and the CO, CI, or SV on the vertical axis. The curves demonstrate three primary effects. First, a change in preload is represented by a move up or down a single curve (Frank-Starling principle). For example, an increase in preload related to volume infusion results in movement from point A to point B. However, the curve does not usually demonstrate a descending limb. Second, a change in contractility is represented by an upward or downward shift of the curve. For example, the administration of an inotropic agent (e.g., dobutamine) results in an upward shift of the entire curve, whereas depression of cardiac function (e.g.,

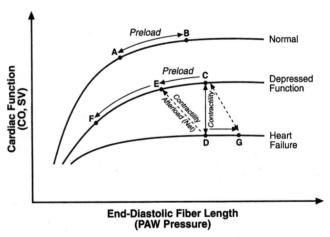

FIGURE 19-26 Family of ventricular function curves. Idealized ventricular function curves representing normal, depressed, and severely depressed function. Point A to Point B and Point B to Point A reflect an increase and decrease, respectively, in preload. Point D to E reflects the net effect of a decrease in afterload on a failing heart. This upward and lateral shift is the result of two actions. Point D to C reflects an increase in force of contraction and Point C to E a decrease in preload due to increased systolic ejection. This shift appears similar to an increase in contractility. A downward shift in the entire curve reflects a decrease in contractility, that is, for any given preload and afterload, the CO is decreased. In a failing heart, an additional effect of decreased contractility is an increase in preload due to decreased systolic ejection; thus, the net effect of a decrease in contractility is to shift the curve down and to the left (Point C to G).

TABLE 19-6	Troubleshooting Guidelines for Cardiac Output Measurement	
Potential Problems Resulting in Erroneous Measurements	**Potential Problems and Contributing Factors**	**Corrective Solutions and Interventions**
Computer and Cable Related		
Wide discrepancy in CO values obtained (>10% median value)	Cables and computer connections not secure; CO computer not plugged into electrical outlet; malfunctioning CO computer	Check and secure all cable and computer connections; plug electrical cord of CO computer into electrical outlet; perform self-test on CO computer; replace CO computer.
No reading on display panel	Cables and computer connections not secure; malfunctioning main cable (broken); malfunctioning CO computer	Check and secure all cable and computer connections; perform self-test on main cable and CO computer; replace main cable or CO computer.
Injectate temperature does not register	Faulty injectate temperature probe; fault in thermistor circuitry	Perform self-test on computer; replace injectate temperature probe.
PA Catheter Related		
PA catheter remains in wedge position or requires less than 0.8 mL of air for balloon inflation	Thermistor of PA catheter against small vessel wall; PA catheter migrated into small pulmonary vessel	Do not perform CO measurement or irrigate PA catheter until catheter is correctly positioned; notify MD to reposition catheter to allow optimal balloon inflation volumes between 1.25 and 1.5 mL; confirm placement of PA catheter on anteroposterior or lateral chest radiograph (catheter tip below level of left atrium).
Clotted proximal lumen	Improper maintenance of the proximal lumen	Maintain patency of the proximal lumen with continuous heparinized intravenous solution; if clotted, alternative methods of injection can be used to obtain CO measurement (venous infusion port or introducer side port if it is exists in the right atrium or lower portion of the vena cava)—correction of computation constant will be needed to account for the added dead space of the catheter; replace the catheter.
Difficulty injecting solution through proximal lumen	Lumen against wall; PA catheter kinked at entrance site or in heart; fibrin growth on catheter	Notify MD to reposition catheter; confirm placement of PA catheter on chest radiograph; tape and secure PA catheter at entrance to introducer to minimize kinking; replace the catheter.
Variations in core temperature	Faulty thermistor; fibrin growth on thermistor; thermistor against vessel wall	Verify core temperature; monitor PA temperature change during CO injection with curve analysis; notify MD of need to reposition catheter; replace catheter.
PA catheter misposition	Proximal port exits in right ventricle because PA catheter advanced too far in PA; distal port exists in right ventricle because of coiling or withdrawal of the catheter	Confirm PA catheter placement on chest radiograph; verify inflation volume of balloon (1.25–1.5 mL); verify presence of correct PA waveforms before and after CO measurement (proximal port with RAP tracing and distal point with undamped PA waveform).
Physiologic and Patient Related		
Variation in serial CO measurement (>10% of median value)	Presence of cardiac dysrhythmias (atrial fibrillation, premature ventricular contractions); catheter whip or artifact due to turbulent flow conditions within heart; patient movement during CO measurement procedure; labile hemodynamics; respiratory effects (mechanical ventilation)	Observe electrocardiogram while doing serial CO measurements; do not inject during or between frequent dysrhythmias; use alternate methods to determine CO; reposition PA catheter; confirm catheter placement on chest radiograph; use 10 mL iced injectate to maximize signal-to-noise ratio; limit patient movement during CO measurement; inject solution at the same point in the respiratory cycle.
Valvular disorders (tricuspid insufficiency) or right-to-left shunts (ventricular septal defect)	Regurgitation or retrograde indicator flow causing recirculation of injectate, resulting in low CO values	Use alternative method to determine CO.

(continued)

TABLE 19-6	Troubleshooting Guidelines for Cardiac Output Measurement *(Continued)*	
Potential Problems Resulting in Erroneous Measurements	**Potential Problems and Contributing Factors**	**Corrective Solutions and Interventions**

Technique Related

CO values too high (high CO does not correspond to patient's clinical presentation)	Incorrect amount of injectate drawn up in syringe (usually less than specified amount); injectate temperature less than specified range; incorrect computation constant (set too high); uneven injection technique	Ensure *exact* amount of injectate volume in syringe (5 or 10 mL) before CO measurement; check temperature of injectate: 　0° C–5° C—10-mL prefilled syringes; 　6° C–12° C—10-mL iced injectate (closed injectate system); Discard CO value if injectate temperature not within specified range (computer will alarm). Correct for error in computation constant: Wrong CO × right constant/wrong constant = right CO. Reset computation constant (based on type of PA catheter, type of injectate system, and volume and temperature of injectate). Perform smooth, even injections within 4 seconds. Verify injection technique with curve analysis (See **Fig. 19–25**).
CO values too low (low CO does not correspond with patient's clinical presentation)	Incorrect amount of injectate drawn up in syringe (usually more than specified amount); solution inadvertently injected before pressing start button on CO computer; injectate temperature exceeds specified range; incorrect computation constant (set too low); prolonged injection delivery (>4 seconds); using NS for injectate solution (NS gives 2% lower reading than D_5W); concomitant infusion at high flow rates (>150 mL/h) proximal lumen or venous infusion port	Ensure *exact* amount of injectate volume in syringe (5 or 10 mL) before CO measurement; check temperature of injectate: 　0° C–5° C—10-mL prefilled syringes; 　6° C–12° C—10-mL iced injectate (closed injectate system); 　8° C–16° C—5-mL iced injectate (closed injectate system). Discard CO value if injectate temperature not within specified range (computer will usually alarm). Add crushed ice and water to closed injectate iced system or change reservoir bag of room temperature closed injectate system; keep reservoir bag away from lights. Correct computation constant. Perform smooth injections within 4 seconds. Verify injection technique with curve analysis. Consider switching to D_5W (depending on patient condition and MD preference). If possible, turn off concomitant infusions during CO measurements.

CO, cardiac output; D_5W, 5% dextrose and water; NS, normal saline; PA, pulmonary artery.
Adapted from Woods SL, Osguthorpe S: Cardiac output determination. AACN Clinical Issues in Critical Care Nursing 4: 81–97, 1993.

heart failure) is represented by a downward shift. Third, a change in afterload results in a shift in the curve that appears similar to that caused by contractility, although the mechanism is different. For example, in a patient with depressed cardiac function, a decrease in afterload has two results. First, a decrease in afterload results in an increase in the velocity of contraction (increased SV; point D to point C). In addition, as a result of the increased SV, the end-diastolic volume decreases (point C to point E). The net effect of the increased force of contraction and decreased end-diastolic volume is reflected by a shift of the curve up and to the left (point D to point E). The effect of afterload on SV depends on filling pressures. Afterload reduction in a patient with increased filling volumes (increased PAWP) and decreased cardiac function results in a shift in the curve up and to the left (point D to point B). However, afterload reduction in a patient with decreased filling pressures results in either no change or a decrease in SV because, as noted, a decrease in afterload is also associated with a decrease in preload. In this case, the patient would move down the ascending limb of the curve, as defined by the Frank-Starling mechanism.

TABLE 19-7 **Hemodynamic Characteristics of Various Pathologic Conditions**

Pathophysiology	Hemodynamic Indices					Additional Findings
	RAP	PAP	PAWP	SV	CO	
Pericardial tamponade	↑	↑	↑	↓	↓	Equalization (within 5 mm Hg) of RAP = PAEDP = PAWP; RAP waveform: prominent x descent with attenuated or absent y descent (d/t decreased ventricular filling); pulsus paradoxus (↓ SBP > 10 mm Hg and ↓ pulse pressure during inspiration; diastolic blood pressure unchanged); pulsus alternans (Fig. 19–18); absent S₃ heart sound; cardiac pressures may be normal if the patient is hypovolemic[5]
Pericardial constriction	↑	↑	↑	↓	N/↓	RAP waveform: steep x and y descent resulting in an "M"- or "W"-shaped waveform; RAP ≈ PAEDP ≈ PAWP (if no tricuspid or mitral regurgitation); decreased respiratory variation in RAP; Kussmaul's sign (inspiratory increase in RAP in severe constriction[437]; pulsus paradoxus (approximately 33% of cases). CO maintained by tachycardia
Massive pulmonary embolism	↑	↑	↑/N/↓	↓	↓	Increased RA v wave with steep y descent due to tricuspid regurgitation, increased alveolar-arterial oxygen gradient (normal value does not rule out pulmonary embolism), tachypnea, dyspnea, increased pulmonic component of S₂, pleuritic chest pain
Mitral regurgitation			↑			If amplitude of V wave 10 mm Hg or more than a wave amplitude, read PAWP at nadir (base) of the x descent (Fig. 19–16C); PAWP > PAEDP (due to regurgitant v wave)
Left ventricular failure	N/↑	↑	↑	↓	↓	Pulmonary congestion or edema, S₃ or S₄, increased a wave height (due to decreased ventricular compliance); increased v wave height due to mitral regurgitation, pulsus alternans
Right ventricular infarction	↑	↓/↑	↓/↑	N/↓	N/↓	RAP > PAWP or RAP 1 to 5 mm Hg > PAWP, or RAP > 10 mm Hg, RA tracing with prominent x and y descent (M configuration), increased jugular venous pressure, systemic venous congestion, right ventricular gallop, split S₂, positive hepatojugular reflux, increased RA a wave, positive Kussmaul's sign (increased RAP with inspiration), right ventricular S₃ or S₄
Acute ventricular septal defect	↑	↑	↑	↓	↓	Acute hypotension and pulmonary congestion, systolic thrill, holosystolic murmur, acute right heart failure with increased jugular venous pressure, late PAWP v wave, oxygen step up of >10% right atrium and PA
Hypovolemia	↓	↓	↓	↓	↓/N	Increased SVR (compensatory), decreased S$\bar{v}O_2$
Septic shock (hyperdynamic)	↓	↓	↑/N/↓	N/↑	N/↑	Systemic hypotension, SBP < 90 mm Hg, metabolic acidosis with compensatory hyperventilation (respiratory alkalosis), decreased SVR, increased S$\bar{v}O_2$
Septic shock (hypodynamic)	↑↓	↑↓	↑↓	↓	↓	Systemic hypotension, SBP < 90 mm Hg, systemic vasoconstriction (increased SVR), decreased S$\bar{v}O_2$

N = normal; ↓, decreased; ↑, increased; CO, cardiac output; PA, pulmonary artery; PAEDP, pulmonary artery end diastolic pressure; PAP, pulmonary artery pressure; PAWP, pulmonary artery wedge pressure; RA, right atrial; RAP, right atrial pressure; SBP, systolic blood pressure; SV, stroke volume; SVR, systemic vascular resistance.

CONTINUOUS CARDIAC OUTPUT

Continuous CO (CCO) is performed using a PA catheter with a heating filament located in the RA or RV (14 to 25 cm from the catheter tip; see Fig. 19-11) that produces pseudorandom heat pulses in an on/off pattern.[107,515] The heat pulses (0.02° C to 0.07° C) are detected by a thermistor on the distal end of the catheter[165,514,515] (Fig. 19-27). The heat pulses replace the cold bolus injection that is normally used for TDCO measurements. The

TABLE 19-8	Hemodynamic Indices	
Indices/Equations	**Normal Values**	**Interpretation**
Preload		
Right atrial pressure (RAP) or central venous pressure (CVP)	2–6 mm Hg	Right ventricular filling pressure.
Pulmonary artery end-diastolic pressure (PAEDP)	8–12 mm Hg	Indirect indicator of left ventricular filling pressure and capillary filling pressure (P_{cap}).
Pulmonary artery wedge pressure (PAWP)	6–12 mm Hg	Indirect indicator of left ventricular filling pressure and capillary filling pressure (P_{cap}).
Afterload		
Systolic blood pressure (SBP)	120 mm Hg	Clinical indicator of pressure that must be overcome during ejection phase of cardiac cycle.
Systemic vascular resistance (SVR) $$\frac{MAP-RAP}{CO} \times 80$$	800–1,200 dynes/sec/cm^{-5}	Measure of systemic vascular tone (one factor that affects afterload; increased SVR manifested by increased MAP).
Systemic vascular resistance index (SVRI)	1,900–2,400 dynes/sec/ cm^{-5}/m^2	SVR indexed to BSA.
Force of contraction		
Stroke volume (SV) $$SV = \frac{CO \times 1,000}{HR}$$	60–180 mL/beat	Amount of blood ejected during each ventricular contraction.
Stroke volume index (SVI) $$SVI = \frac{CI \times 1,000}{HR}$$	33–47 mL/beat/m^2	SV indexed to BSA.
Right ventricular stroke work index (RVSWI) RVSWI = SVI (MAP–CVP)¥0.0136	5–10 gm-m/m2/beat	Work performed by right ventricle to eject blood into the pulmonary vasculature. Stroke work determines the energy expenditure (oxygen consumption) of the heart.
Left ventricular stroke work index (LVSWI) LVSWI = SVI (MAP–PAWP) ×0.0136	45–65 gm-m/m^2/beat	Work performed by the left ventricle to eject the SV into the aorta. The factor 0.0136 converts pressure and volume to units of work. At high filling pressures, this equation may underestimate the amount of work performed.

BSA, body surface area; CI, cardiac index; CO, cardiac output; CVP, central venous pressure; MAP, mean arterial pressure; RAP, right atrial pressure.

CCO computer creates a curve similar to that observed with TDCO measurements. This curve is then used to compute the CO. The CCO measurements are comparable with those obtained by TDCO over a wide range of COs.[10,33,49,94,100,163,192,219,265,271,272,302–304,396,433,461,518]

The CCO measurements can be obtained with blood temperatures between 31° C and 41° C and appear to be more accurate at lower flow rates (2 to 3 L/min),[302,304] less affected by external warming,[433] and more reproducible than TDCO.[264] Caution should be used when interpreting findings comparing CCO with TDCO, because TDCO is simply another method for measuring CO. Comparisons with dye-dilution or the Fick method are still considered the standards for comparison.[156] However, there have been reports that at higher flow rates, there is an increased difference between

CCO and TDCO and dye-dilution measurements; thus, the CCO measurements must be interpreted with caution.[49,218]

The displayed CO is updated every 30 seconds and represents the average CO over the previous 3 to 6 minutes.[515] A limitation of the CCO system is the delay between a change in CO and display of the change.[117,192,259,260,423] For example, the average time to report 75% of a 1 L change in CO was 10.5 minutes, and 90% of the change was reported in 11.8 minutes.[192] Thus, the CCO does not reflect acute changes in CO, and this delay should be considered when monitoring a patient who is unstable or who is undergoing rapid titration of vasoactive medications or modification of supportive therapy (e.g., IABP, ventricular assist device).[423] It has been suggested that more frequent measurements may result in increased "noise" and thus error in the dis-

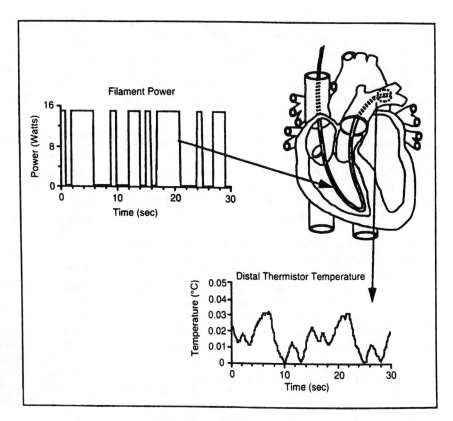

FIGURE 19-27 Cardiac output by continuous thermodilution technique. The continuous cardiac output catheter introduces heat in an on–off pattern to help differentiate temperature changes in the heart due to the heat signal from natural variations in the pulmonary artery (From Gillman P: Continuous measurement of cardiac output: A milestone in hemodynamic monitoring. Focus on Critical Care 19: 155–158, 1992.)

played CO.[148] However, studies demonstrate that the bias (–0.04 to 0.18 L/min) and precision (0.61 L/min) of STAT mode versus TDCO are very small and support the use of the STAT mode.[259]

During the creation of the temperature pulses, the temperature of the catheter increases by 4° C to 7° C. with a maximum temperature of 44° C, which does not damage blood cells or the myocardium.[107,193,269,270,515—517] In addition, the catheters are designed to shut off if filament temperature rises above 44° C (e.g., when CO drops below 1 L/min).[517] To avoid any further potential myocardial injury, the catheter should be free floating in the RV as determined by a chest radiograph.[186]

The CCO system has several limitations. The infusion of a cold solution may result in overestimation of CCO measurements,[192] although CCO measurements are minimally affected by fluctuations in PA temperatures.[302] In addition, fluid boluses result in underestimation of CO in low flow states (CO < 4 L/min), in contrast to TDCO measurements, where the CO is overestimated.[302] The presence of intracardiac shunt (tricuspid regurgitation) also decreases the accuracy of CCO measures, as does incorrect catheter placement (thermal filament in the vena cava or in contact with the heart).[156,302]

The use of CCO offers benefits compared with TDCO in that theoretically it is not subject to the potential technical errors associated with TDCO (e.g., respiratory variation in PA temperature, inaccurate volume, inaccurate calibration coefficient, error in injection technique, avoidance of

additional fluid volume administration).[156,318,445] However, there are no studies indicating that use of CCO improves patient outcomes, and this fact along with the increased cost of CCO must be weighed against less nursing time and potentially earlier detection of changes in determining which patients require this level of monitoring.[30,322]

BIOIMPEDANCE CARDIAC OUTPUT MEASUREMENTS

Thoracic electrical bioimpedance (TEB) is a noninvasive method for measuring CO. The system in general consists of eight specialized electrodes, with two pairs placed laterally on the neck and two pairs at the lateral aspect of the lower thorax (at the level of the xiphosternal junction).[24,470] Additional ECG electrodes are placed in the normal manner.

A small electrical voltage (2 to 4 mA), which is not felt and is safe to the patient, is passed longitudinally through the thorax between electrodes. The voltage is divided by a constant (current) to determine impedance (the resistance to flow of alternating current across a conductor): impedance (Z) = voltage (V)/current (I).[285,347]

The change in impedance is due to the change in blood flow during the cardiac cycle (SV), and respiratory and motion artifact.[285,347] The respiratory and motion artifact can be eliminated; thus, the change in impedance can be used to calculate the SV. Additional information required includes the patient's height, weight, and sex.

Earlier use of TEB technology demonstrated wide disparity with TDCO measurements.[105,108,357,398,424,505,519] However, CO measurements using newer TEB technology are similar to those obtained with TDCO, with improved precision (decreased variability),[419,459,485] although TEB CO measurements are less accurate during the intraoperative and immediate postoperative periods in cardiac surgery patients.[105,460] However, TEB CO measurements cannot be performed in patients with abnormal chest morphology (kyphoscoliosis) or intraoperatively during electrocautery, and TEB CO has decreased accuracy in patients with pleural effusion, low blood flow (<2 L/min), obesity, mechanical ventilation (particularly with PEEP in conjunction with high CO), pulmonary edema, an open thorax, and arrhythmias.[6,55,105,398,417,419,435,505,506]

Thus, the newer versions of TEB CO can be used after the first 12 postoperative hours, but use during surgery and the immediate postoperative periods is not recommended. In addition to the advantages of noninvasive monitoring, TEB CO measurements may be useful in patients who do not require PA pressure monitoring, in following trends or changes in CO, and when beat-to-beat or serial CO measurements are required (e.g., evaluating the effect of various pacing modes).[60,70,347]

Cost and potential improved patient outcomes should be considered in determining the utility of TEB CO.[59,421] The initial outlay for purchase of a TEB device is relatively high ($21,000—1991 cost), but minimal additional costs are required compared with the ongoing costs of the use of various types of PA catheters for TDCO or CCO.[60,70,359] Clancy and associates[70] estimated in 1991 that a single application of TEB CO cost $923.00, whereas the total cost for a single application of TDCO was $1,528.00, and the 1-week cost exceeds $5,000.00.[70,359]

OTHER METHODS FOR CARDIAC OUTPUT MEASUREMENT

Other methods for measurement of CO include echocardiographic Doppler and transtracheal Doppler. Although echocardiographic Doppler measurements of CO are accurate,[68,268,424,505] this technique is not appropriate for ongoing CO measurements, and depends on the expertise of the operator.[192] Transtracheal Doppler is less accurate and is also not appropriate for ongoing CO monitoring.[204,422]

OXYGEN SUPPLY AND DEMAND

Circulatory shock is characterized by tissue hypoperfusion and an imbalance between O_2 supply and demand.[8] However, normalization of the routinely monitored cardiovascular indicators (e.g., urine output, MAP, HR) is poorly related to outcome.[29,355,416—418] The imbalance between supply and demand may result in a conversion from aerobic to anaerobic metabolism, and cellular function is impaired.[75] The impairment of cellular function may ultimately result in organ failure.[355]

To evaluate tissue oxygenation, local and global indices of oxygen transport are measured. Local indices include gastric tonometry and subcutaneous tissue oxygenation. Global indices of oxygenation include lactate, mixed venous oxygen saturation ($S\bar{v}O_2$), and systemic oxygen consumption and oxygen delivery.

Local Indicators

Monitoring of local indices of oxygenation (gut mucosa, subcutaneous tissue) is based on the assumption that these areas serve as early markers of systemic hypoperfusion because hypoperfusion results in the movement of blood away from these areas to more vital areas (i.e., heart, brain).[89,90,187,191,295,299,364]

GASTRIC TONOMETRY

Gastric tonometry is the measurement of intramucosal (pHi) (not intraluminal) using a modified nasogastric tube.[133,455] There is some evidence that there is a relationship between the maintenance of normal pHi and clinical outcomes and survival.[28,71,106,132,188—190,287,299,308,317,386] Use of gastric pHi to guide therapy has been shown to improve outcome in patients whose initial pHi was greater than 7.35.[189,190] Patients with initial gastric pHi of less than 7.35 may require more invasive monitoring (e.g., PA catheter, $S\bar{v}O_2$ monitoring).[375] However, local ischemia does not necessarily indicate a more global problem. In addition, there are still some technical aspects related to this monitoring that require further clarification before recommendations for general use can be made.[178,184,455]

TISSUE OXYGENATION MONITORING

The monitoring of oxygen tension in the tissue is based on the close relationship between oxygen tension in tissues and perfusion. Clinically, hypovolemia is manifested by a decrease in subcutaneous tissue oxygen pressure ($P_{sq}O_2$) and ultimately in a decrease in $S\bar{v}O_2$.[112,176,364,496] In addition, subcutaneous tissue is one of the last areas in the body to regain normal perfusion after restoration of circulation,[176] and therefore may be useful in determining if resuscitation has been adequate. However, this method remains experimental. Current research includes the use of tissue oxygenation monitoring in evaluating postoperative resuscitation in postcardiac surgery patients and on the effects of nursing interventions and activity on wound healing in patients after hip replacement surgery.

Global Indicators of Oxygen Supply and Demand

LACTATE

Serum lactate, which is a byproduct of anaerobic metabolism, is used as an indicator of the adequacy of systemic oxygenation. An increase in lactate and the time the lactate level is increased (>2 mmol/L) is related to oxygen debt (oxygen demand greater than delivery), critical levels of

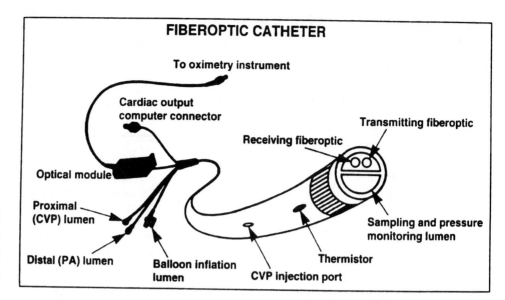

FIGURE 19-28 Diagram of a fiberoptic pulmonary artery catheter and associated interconnections. CVP, central venous pressure. (Courtesy of Abbott Critical Care Systems, Mountain View, CA.)

oxygen delivery, and increased organ failure and mortality.[12,62,374,385,394,465]

Because the liver has a large capacity to oxidize lactate, a normal serum lactate level (<2 mmol/L) does not mean that tissue hypoperfusion and anaerobic metabolism are not occurring. As long as hepatic function is relatively normal, and the CO can increase in response to increased oxygen demands, there will be limited accumulation of lactate, even with a PaO_2 less than 30 mm Hg or with severe anemia.[307] In addition, localized hypoperfusion may be insufficient to increase systemic levels.[345] Conversely, increased lactate production occurs with increased glycolysis (e.g., hypermetabolic state, catecholamine administration, diabetes mellitus, trauma, burns) and hepatic dysfunction.[179] Therefore, lactate is a late, and often insensitive, indicator of hypoperfusion.

As noted, a normal lactate level does not necessarily mean a lack of hypoperfusion. However, an increased lactate level may be considered indicative of hypoperfusion, if the increase is concurrent with signs and symptoms of hypoperfusion (cool, clammy skin, hypotension) and normal hepatic function, and without other conditions that can increase lactate. Sequential monitoring of lactate is useful in assessing the efficacy of resuscitation attempts. A decrease in lactate of 5% to 10% per hour is usually indicative of adequate response to treatment, whereas no change or an increase in lactate level is an ominous sign.[307,350,454,479]

MIXED VENOUS OXYGEN SATURATION

Although CO provides important information about the capacity of the cardiopulmonary system to deliver oxygen to the tissues, it does not necessarily depict the adequacy of oxygen supply at the tissue level. The $S\bar{v}O_2$ is a global measure of the balance between total body oxygen delivery and consumption.[59]

Technical Aspects of $S\bar{v}O_2$ Monitoring. The $S\bar{v}O_2$ is obtained from a blood sample drawn from the distal port of the PA catheter, or from continuous fiberoptic technology in the PA catheter (see Fig. 19-11). The rationale for drawing the sample from the distal port and not the superior vena cava or RA is that the $S\bar{v}O_2$ reflects mixed venous oxygen saturation from the entire body.[327] Samples obtained from the RA give higher venous oxygen determinations.[263,331] To avoid contaminating the specimen, a minimum of 6 mL of blood should be slowly aspirated (30 seconds) from the distal port. A 2-mL sample should then be drawn over a 10-second period. It is also important to ensure that the catheter tip is not wedged or a contaminated specimen may be drawn.[331]

Components of the $S\bar{v}O_2$ monitoring system include the fiberoptic PA catheter, the optical module, and the microprocessor. The fiberoptic catheter is a quadruple-lumen PA catheter with the addition of two fiberoptic channels running the length of the catheter[226] (Fig. 19-28). The optical module contains diodes that emit light pulses at two or three wavelengths through one of the fiberoptic channels in the tip of the catheter.[35,67,160] The second fiberoptic channel returns reflected light to a photodetector in the optical module. The amount of light reflected depends on the amount of saturated hemoglobin (Hgb) because oxygenated and deoxygenated Hgb reflect differently. The light is relayed electronically to the microprocessor, which interprets the light signal and determines the ratio between oxygenated and deoxygenated blood. Based on this ratio, the $S\bar{v}O_2$ is determined.[434]

Preparation of the Equipment. The fiberoptic PA catheter is inserted in the same manner as any PA catheter. The catheter and the optical module must be standardized to an optical reference before the catheter is inserted. A disposable

TABLE 19-9	**Indications for SṼO₂ Monitoring**

High-risk cardiovascular surgery

Advanced heart failure

Acute myocardial infarction

Acute hypoxemic respiratory failure (positive end-expiratory
  pressure)

Severe burns

Multiple organ dysfunction syndrome

Neurosurgery

High-risk obstetrics patients

Monitoring of inotrope therapy in heart failure

For additional information, see
refs.[18,27,56,58,59,81,83,118,206,226,248,249,309,320,332,334,387,430,446,475,493,521]

optical standard is usually included in the packaging of the catheter. If the catheter is already in place, an *in vivo* calibration can be performed according to the manufacturer's instructions. Calibration of the SṼO₂ module is recommended every 24 hours with mixed venous blood gas samples obtained from the distal port of the PA catheter. Recalibration is performed when the calibration datum is lost, when the SṼO₂ measured by the computer differs by greater than 10% from the laboratory interpreted value, or the reported value exceeds the normal range.

INDICATIONS

The indications for SṼO₂ monitoring are summarized in Table 19-9. In addition, continuous SṼO₂ monitoring has been shown to be cost effective and to reduce nursing time compared with intermittent monitoring, thus offsetting the cost of the catheter.[58] However, changes in SṼO₂ are only moderately related to changes in CO in intensive care unit patients (cardiac, respiratory, surgical), postcardiac surgery patients, and patients with advanced heart failure.[155,431,474] Thus, additional monitoring of CO and PA pressures may be required in these cases. In addition, although the Pulmonary Artery Catheter Consensus Conference[351] did not specifically address the utility of SṼO₂ monitoring, the Conference did specify that there is limited research to support use of the catheter as part of a treatment plan aimed at achieving supranormal levels of oxygenation.[250,293]

CLINICAL APPLICATION

The SṼO₂, which is the saturation of the blood returning to the heart, reflects the overall balance between oxygen supply and utilization by the body, and is affected by the factors that affect oxygen delivery (CO, Hgb, SaO₂) and tissue metabolism. The SṼO₂ normally ranges from 60% to 80%, with an average of 75%.[226] An SṼO₂ of 75% is associated with a PvO₂ of 40 mm Hg.

In response to increased oxygen demand, the body either increases CO to deliver more oxygen or increases the extraction of oxygen from the blood. When the SaO₂ is maintained at a high level (near 100%), there is a strong

relationship between the SṼO₂ and the oxygen extraction ratio (OER).[58,323] An increase in oxygen extraction decreases Hgb saturation, which is reflected by a decrease in SṼO₂. As long as oxygen delivery is adequate in meeting tissue oxygen demands, the SṼO₂ remains within 60% to 80%. Decreases in SṼO₂ occur as a result of an increase in oxygen demand (e.g., fever, shivering, pain, seizures, sepsis) or decreased oxygen delivery (e.g., cardiac failure, hemorrhage, hypoxia, hypovolemia, dysrhythmias). Conversely, increased SṼO₂ is the result of decreased oxygen demand (e.g., hypothermia, sedation, neuromuscular blockade) or is an indicator of maldistribution or impaired cellular use of oxygen in sepsis.[61,493] Technical causes of a high SṼO₂ include a wedged PA catheter or deposits of fibrin on the tip of the catheter, and rapid withdrawal of blood from the catheter resulting in a contaminated specimen.[81]

SYSTEMIC OXYGEN CONSUMPTION AND DELIVERY

As noted, the SṼO₂ is affected by factors that affect oxygen delivery (CO, Hgb, and SaO₂) and consumption. The assumption is made that if the Hgb and SaO₂ are not changing, the change in SṼO₂ reflects a change in CO and thus provides an indirect and continuous measurement of CO. However, the clinician must have knowledge of all of the factors that affect SṼO₂. Determination of oxygen delivery (ḊO₂) and oxygen consumption (V̇O₂) provides further insight into the factors that may be responsible for an imbalance between oxygen delivery and consumption.

Oxygen delivery depends on the amount of oxygen in the blood (termed *oxygen-carrying capacity* [CaO₂]) and how much blood is delivered to the tissues (CO). Factors that affect the CaO₂ are Hgb and SaO₂ (Table 19-10). The 1.34 in the CaO₂ equation is the oxygen-carrying capacity of 1 g of fully saturated Hgb.[275] The CaO₂ multiplied times the CO reflects the amount of oxygen delivered to the tissue (ḊO₂). The 10 in the ḊO₂ equation is used to convert the CaO₂, which is reported in mL/100 mL of blood, into mL O₂/L of blood.[209] Thus, a decrease in Hgb, SaO₂, or CO can affect the amount of oxygen delivered to the tissue.

The other half of the delivery/consumption equation is oxygen consumption (V̇O₂) or the oxygen consumption index (V̇O₂I). The normal V̇O₂ is approximately 250 mL/min, with an indexed value of approximately 115 to 165 mL/min/m².[18,275,493] The V̇O₂ cannot be directly measured at the bedside, and therefore derived values (see Table 19-10)[19] are often used.

RESPONSE TO ALTERATIONS IN OXYGEN DELIVERY

In response to an increase in oxygen demand or a decrease in Hgb or SaO₂, the normal compensatory response is to increase CO, such that V̇O₂ is not affected.[333] As the result of this compensation a change in ḊO₂ does not normally result in a decrease in V̇O₂. However, below a critical level (4 to 8 mL O₂/kg/min), as the ḊO₂ decreases, the V̇O₂ decreases (supply dependent).[248,412]

TABLE 19-10	Oxygen Transport Equations	
Variables	**Equation/Example**	**Normal**
Arterial oxygen content (CaO_2)	$(Hgb \times 1.34 \times SaO_2) + (0.003 \times PaO_2)$ $(15 \times 1.34 \times 0.99) + (0.003 \times 100)$	20 mL/dL
Venous oxygen (CvO_2)	$(Hgb \times 1.34 \times S\bar{v}O_2) + (0.003 \times PvO_2)$ $(15 \times 1.34 \times 0.75) + (0.003 \times 40)$	15 mL/dL
Oxygen delivery ($\dot{D}O_2$)	$CO \times CaO_2 \times 10$ $5.0 \times (15 \times 1.34 \times 0.99) \times 10$	1,000 mL/min
Oxygen delivery index ($\dot{D}O_2I$)	$CI \times CaO_2 \times 10$ $3.5.0 \times (15 \times 1.34 \times 0.99) \times 10$	600 mL/min/m²
Oxygen consumption ($\dot{V}O_2$)	$CO \times 1.34 \times Hgb\,(SaO_2 - S\bar{v}O_2)$ $5.0 \times 1.34 \times 15\,(1.0 - 0.75)$	250 mL/min
Oxygen consumption index ($\dot{V}O_2I$)	$CI \times 1.34 \times Hgb\,(SaO_2 - S\bar{v}O_2)$ $3.5 \times 1.34 \times 15\,(1.0 - 0.75)$	120–130 mL/min/m²

CI, cardiac index; CO, cardiac output. Hgb, hemoglobin.

Of the three factors that affect delivery (CO, Hgb, SaO_2), changes in CO and Hgb have the greatest effect, with the changes in Hgb better tolerated than changes in CO.[375,486] This is important in developing a plan of care to optimize oxygen delivery.

Oxygen Extraction Ratio

The normal OER is 25%, which reflects a 4:1 ratio between supply and consumption.[275,493] The 25% OER indicates that 25% of the oxygen is removed from the Hgb, and the Hgb returning to the heart is 75% saturated ($S\bar{v}O_2$). An OER greater than 30% requires further assessment because this value indicates that the oxygen demands of the body are being met by increased oxygen extraction and not by increased delivery.

Clinical Application of $S\bar{v}O_2$ and Oxygen Transport Data

An area where further study is needed is on the effect of oxygen-sensitive nursing and interdisciplinary interventions. For example, as demonstrated in Table 19-11, many commonly performed nursing interventions such as bed bath or positioning may increase oxygen consumption[9,13,14,414,462,489,503] and precipitate the development of an oxygen debt (oxygen demand greater than supply), particularly if the interventions are performed in combination.[493] Modification of the plan of care may be particularly important in patients with increased baseline $\dot{V}O_2$ (sepsis, trauma, pain) who also have limited capacity to increase $\dot{D}O_2$ (heart failure). An interdisciplinary plan of care aimed at balancing oxygen supply and demand may include actions to decrease

TABLE 19-11	Percentage Increase in Resting $S\bar{v}O_2$ Associated with Conditions and Activities			
Conditions	**%**	**Activities**	**%**	
Fever (each 1° C)	10	Dressing change	10	
Fractures (each)	10	Electrocardiogram	16	
Agitation	18	Physical examination	20	
Chest trauma	25	Visitors	22	
Work of breathing	40	Bath	23	
Severe infection	60	Chest radiograph	25	
Shivering	50–100	Endotracheal suctioning	27	
Sepsis	50–100	Nasal intubation	25–40	
Head injury, sedated	89	Turn to side	31	
Head injury, not sedated	138	Chest physiotherapy	35	
Burns	100	Weight on sling scale	36	

From White KM: Using continuous $S\bar{v}O_2$ to assess oxygen supply/demand balance in the critically ill patient. AACN Clinical Issues in Critical Care Nursing 4: 134–147, 1993. With permission.

$\dot{V}O_2$ (antipyretics, pain medications, sedation), and limitation or reorganization of nursing activities (avoiding clustering of activities, e.g., bed bath, linen change, range of motion, weight, repositioning) in high-risk patients.[91,197,284,469] In addition, steps to improve $\dot{D}O_2$ may include increasing CO (volume, inotropes, afterload reduction, HR and arrhythmia control), increasing oxygenation (supplemental oxygen, mechanical ventilation), and increased Hgb.[203,430,457]

There is some evidence that augmenting $\dot{D}O_2$ to "supranormal" levels ($\dot{D}O_2I = 600$ mL/min/m², $\dot{V}O_2I > 160$ mL/min/m²) may improve outcomes in high-risk patients.[11,38,120,190,415,464,521] These recommendations are based in part on findings related to continued regional hypoperfusion after the indices of systemic oxygenation have been normalized.[116] A problem with this definition is that the hypothetical patient with an Hgb = 15 mg/dL, CI = 3 L/min/m², and an SaO_2 = 95% has an $\dot{D}O_2$ of 580 mL/min/m²; thus, the goal of 600 mL/min/m² is normal, not supranormal, and an optimal level for $\dot{D}O_2$ remains to specified.[119,442] In addition, other studies found no evidence of improved outcomes.[34,134,154,521,522] Furthermore, driving up the $\dot{D}O_2$ is not risk free because there have been reports of increased mortality in the subgroup of patients who received catecholamines to increase their $\dot{D}O_2$.[205]

However, other reviews suggest that "supranormal $\dot{D}O_2$ therapy may be effective when used to prevent hypoxia, but does not reduce mortality in patients who are already hypoxic.[392,520] Finally, the Pulmonary Artery Catheter Consensus Conference[351] made the following recommendations: (1) PA catheter-guided hemodynamic interventions to augment $\dot{D}O_2$ to supranormal values in patients with systemic inflammatory response syndrome–related organ dysfunction from sepsis, trauma, or postoperative complications cannot be recommended; and (2) there is inadequate research to support preoperative augmentation of the $\dot{D}O_2$ in high-risk surgical patients. Therefore, further research is needed on the use of supranormal goals before recommendations for practice can be made.

REFERENCES

1. Ahrens T: Effects of mechanical ventilation on hemodynamic waveforms. Crit Care Nurs Clinics of North Am 3: 629–639, 1991
2. Ahrens T: Pulmonary critical care: Airway pressure measurement as an aid to identify end-expiration in hemodynamic. Critical Care Nurse 12(4): 44–48, 1992
3. Ahrens T, Penick J, Tucker M: Frequency requirements for zeroing transducers in hemodynamic monitoring. Am J Crit Care 4: 466–471, 1995
4. Aitken L: Comparison of pulmonary artery pressure measurements in the supine and 60 degrees lateral positions. Aus Crit Care 8(4): 21, 24–29, 1995
5. Antman E, Cargill V, Grossman W: Low-pressure cardiac tamponade. Ann Intern Med 91: 403–406, 1979
6. Appel P, Kram J, MacLabee J et al: Comparison of measurements of cardiac output by bioimpedance and thermodilution in severely ill surgical patients. Crit Care Med 14: 933, 1986
7. Armengol J, Man G, Balsys A et al: Effect of the respiratory cycle on cardiac output measurement: Reproducibility of data by timing the thermodilution injection in dogs. Crit Care Med 9: 852–854, 1982
8. Astiz M, Rackow E, Kaufman B et al: Relationship of oxygen delivery and mixed venous oxygenation to lactic acidosis in patients with sepsis and acute myocardial infarction. Crit Care Med 16: 655–658, 1988
9. Atkins P, Hapshe E, Riegel B: Effects of bedbath on mixed venous oxygen saturation and heart rate in coronary artery bypass graft patients. Am J Crit Care 3: 107–115, 1994
10. Auger S, Hoyt D, Johnson F et al: Continuous cardiac output/mixed venous O_2 monitoring system: A comparative evaluation in critically ill patients (Abstract). Crit Care Med 22: A190, 1994
11. Baigorri F, Russel J: Oxygen delivery in critical illness. Crit Care Clin 12: 971–994, 1996
12. Bakker J, Gris P, Coffernils M et al: Serum blood lactate levels can predict the development of multiple organ failure following septic shock. Am J Surg 171: 221–226, 1996
13. Banasik J. The effect of position on peripheral oxygenation in postoperative CABG patients. Heart Lung 19: 302, 1990
14. Banasik J, Bruya A, Steadman R et al: Effect of position on arterial oxygenation in post-operative coronary revascularization patients. Heart Lung 16: 652–657, 1987
15. Barash N, Nardi D, Hammond G et al: Catheter-induced pulmonary artery perforation: Mechanisms, management, and modifications. J Thorac Cardiovasc Surg 82: 5–12, 1981
16. Barash P, Nardi D, Hammond G et al: Catheter-induced pulmonary artery perforation: Mechanisms, management, and modifications. J Thorac Cardiovasc Surg 82: 5–12, 1981
17. Barcelona M, Patague L, Bunoy M et al: Cardiac output determination by the thermodilution method: Comparison of ice-temperature injectate versus room-temperature injectate contained in prefilled syringes or a closed injectate delivery system. Heart Lung 14: 232–235, 1985
18. Barone J, Snyder A: Treatment strategies in shock: Use of oxygen transport measurements. Heart Lung 20: 81–85, 1991
19. Barron M, Petterson E: Volumetric assessment of cardiac function postcardiopulmonary bypass using a rapid response thermistor Swan-Ganz catheter (Abstract). In Society of Cardiovascular Anesthesiologists Annual Scientific Symposium, New Orleans, 1991
20. Bartz B, Maroun C, Underhill S: Differences in midanteroposterior level and midaxillary level of patients with a range of chest configurations. Heart Lung 17: 309, 1988
21. Batson G, Chandrasekhar K, Payas Y et al: Measurement of pulmonary wedge pressure by the flow directed Swan-Ganz catheter. Cardiovasc Res 6: 748–752, 1972
22. Benumof J, Saidman L, Arkin D et al: Where do pulmonary arterial catheters go: Intrathoracic distribution. Anesthesiology 46: 336–338, 1977
23. Berglund E: Balance of left and right ventricular output: Relation between right and left atrial pressures. Am J Physiol 178: 381, 1954
24. Bernstein D: A new stroke volume equation for the thoracic electrical bioimpedance: Theory and rationale. Crit Care Med 14: 904–909, 1986
25. Berryhill R, Benumof J, Rauscher L: Pulmonary vascular pressure reading at the end of exhalation. Anesthesiology 49: 365–368, 1978
26. Bilfinger T, Lin C, Anagnostopoulos C: In vitro determination of accuracy of cardiac output measurements by thermal dilution. J Surg Res 33: 409–414, 1982
27. Bishop M, Shoemaker W, Appel P et al: Prospective, randomized trail of survivor values of cardiac index, oxygen

delivery, and oxygen consumption as resuscitation endpoints in severe trauma. J Trauma 38: 780–787, 1995

28. Bjork M, Hedberg B: Early detection of major complications after abdominal aortic surgery: Predictive value of sigmoid colon and gastric intramucosal pH monitoring. Br J Surg 81: 25–30, 1994

29. Bland R, Shoemaker W, Abraham E et al: Probability of survival as a prognostic and severity of illness score in critically ill surgical patients. Crit Care Med 13: 9, 1985

30. Boldt J, Heesen M, Muller M et al: Continuous monitoring of critical patients with a newly developed pulmonary arterial catheter. [A cost analysis]. Anaesthesist 44: 423–428, 1995

31. Boldt J, Kling D, Hempelmann G: Right ventricular function after cardiac surgery. Intensive Care Med 14(Suppl 2): 496–498, 1988

32. Boldt J, Kling D, Moosdorf R et al: Influence of acute volume loading on right ventricular function after cardiopulmonary bypass. Crit Care Med 17: 518–522, 1989

33. Boldt Y, Menges T, Wollburck M et al: Is continuous cardiac output measurement using thermodilution reliable in the critically ill patient? Crit Care Med 22: 1913–1918, 1994

34. Bone R, Slotman G, Maunder R et al: The Prostaglandin E$_1$ Study Group: Randomized double-blind, multicenter study of prostaglandin E$_1$ in patients with adult respiratory distress syndrome. Chest 96: 114–119, 1987

35. Bongard F, Lee T, Leighton T et al: Simultaneous in vivo comparison of two– versus three-wavelength mixed venous (SvO$_2$) oximetry catheters. Clin Monitor 11: 329–334, 1995

36. Bouchard R, Gault J, Ross J: Evaluation of pulmonary arterial end-diastolic pressure as an estimate of left ventricular end-diastolic pressure in patients with normal and abnormal left ventricular performance. Circulation 44: 1072–1079, 1971

37. Bourdillon P, Fineberg N. Comparison of iced and room temperature injectate for thermodilution cardiac output. Cathet Cardiovasc Diagn 17: 116–120, 1989

38. Boyd O, Grounds M, Bennett E: A randomized clinical trial of the effect of deliberate perioperative increase of oxygen delivery on mortality in high–risk surgical patients. JAMA 270: 2699–2707, 1993

39. Braunwald E, Brockenbrough E, Frahm C et al: Left atrial and left ventricular pressures in subjects without cardiovascular disease: Observations in eighteen patients studied by transseptal left heart catheterization. Circulation 24: 267–269, 1961

40. Bretz T: Air emboli: A potentially lethal complication of central venous lines. Focus on Critical Care 17: 374–383, 1989

41. Bridges E: Effect of 30-Degree Lateral Recumbent Position on Pulmonary Artery and Pulmonary Artery Wedge Pressures in Critically Ill Adults. Unpublished thesis, University of Washington, Seattle, Washington, 1998

42. Bridges E, Bond E, Ahrens T et al: Ask the experts. Critical Care Nurse 17(6): 96–97, 101–102, 1997

43. Bridges E, Middleton R: Direct arterial vs oscillometric monitoring of blood pressure: Stop comparing and pick one (a decision making algorithm). Crit Care Nurs 17(3): 58–72, 1997

44. Bridges E, Woods S: Cardiovascular chronobiology: Implications for critical care nursing. Crit Care Nurs 18(4): 49–64, 1998

45. Bridges EJ, Woods SL: Pulmonary artery pressure measurement: State of the art. Heart Lung 22: 99–111, 1993

46. Briones T, Dickenson S, Bieberitz R: Effect of positioning on SvO$_2$ and hemodynamic measurements. Heart Lung 20: 297, 1991

47. Brunet F, Dhainut J, Devaux J et al: Right ventricular performance in patients with acute respiratory failure. Intensive Care Med 14(Suppl 2): 474–477, 1988

48. Bryant A, Kennedy G: The effects of lateral body position on pulmonary artery and pulmonary capillary wedge pressure measurements. Circulation 66: II-97, 1982

49. Burchell S, Yu M, Takaguchi S et al: Evaluation of a continuous cardiac output and mixed venous oxygen saturation catheter in critically ill surgical patients. Crit Care Med 25: 388–391, 1997

50. Burrage R: The Effect of Body Position Upon Pulmonary Artery and Pulmonary Capillary Wedge Pressure in Critically Ill Patients. Unpublished thesis, University of Utah, Salt Lake City, UT, 1979

51. Calvin J, Quinn B: Right ventricular pressure overload during acute lung injury: Cardiac mechanics and the pathophysiology of right ventricular systolic dysfunction. J Crit Care 4: 251–265, 1989

52. Campbell B: Arterial waveforms: Monitoring changes in configuration. Heart Lung 26: 204–214, 1997

53. Campbell M, Greenberg C: Reading pulmonary artery wedge pressure at end-expiration. Focus on Critical Care 15: 60–63, 1988

54. Cason CL, Lambert CW, Holland CL et al: Effects of backrest elevation and position on pulmonary artery pressures. Cardiovasc Nurs 26(1): 1–6, 1990

55. Castor G, Molter G, Helms J et al: Determination of cardiac output during positive end-expiratory pressure: Noninvasive electrical bioimpedance compared with standard thermodilution. Crit Care Med 18: 544–546, 1990

56. American Society of Anesthesiologists Task Force on Pulmonary Artery Catheterization: Practice guidelines for pulmonary artery catheterization. Anesthesiology 78: 380–394, 1993

57. Cengiz M, Crapo R, Gardner R: The effect of ventilation on the accuracy of pulmonary artery and wedge pressure measurements. Crit Care Med 11: 502–507, 1983

58. Cernaianu A, DelRossi A, Boatman G et al: Continuous venous oximetry for hemodynamic and oxygen transport stability post cardiac surgery. J Cardiovasc Surg 33: 14–20, 1992

59. Cernaianu A, Nelson L: The significance of mixed venous oxygen saturation and technical aspects of continuous measurement. In Edwards J, Shoemaker W, Vincent J (eds): Oxygen Transport: Principles and Practice, pp 99–124. Philadelphia, WB Saunders, 1993

60. Chalfin D: The pulmonary artery catheter: Economic aspects. New Horizons 5: 292–296, 1997

61. Chan K, Abraham E: Septic shock. In Edwards J, Shoemaker W, Vincent J-L (eds): Oxygen Transport: Principles and Practice, pp 274–293. Philadelphia, WB Saunders, 1993

62. Chan K, Abraham E: Septic shock. In Edwards J, Shoemaker W, Vincent J-L (eds): Oxygen Transport: Principles and Practice, pp 274–293. Philadelphia, WB Saunders, 1993

63. Chang M, Cheatham M, Safcsak K et al: Differences in hemodynamic and oxygen transport variables produced by blood and crystalloid during volume resuscitation (Abstract). Crit Care Med 22: A107, 1994

64. Chapin J, Downs J, Douglas M et al: Lung expansion, airway pressure transmission, and positive end-expiratory pressure. Arch Surg 114: 1193–1197, 1979

65. Cheatham M, Safcsak K, Nelson L: Right ventricular end diastolic volume is superior to cardiac filling pressures in determining preload status. Surgical Forum 95: 79, 1994

66. Chulay M, Miller T: The effect of backrest elevation on pulmonary artery and pulmonary capillary wedge pressures in patients after cardiac surgery. Heart Lung 13: 138–140, 1984

67. Chulay M, Palmer J, Neblett J et al: Clinical comparison of two- and three-wavelength systems for continuous measure-

ment of venous oxygen saturation. Am J Crit Care 1: 69–75, 1992

68. Chunzeng L, Nicolosi G, Burelli C et al: Limitations in the assessment of changes in cardiac output by Doppler echocardiography under various hemodynamic conditions. Am J Cardiol 70: 1370–1374, 1992

69. Civetta J, Gabel J, Lever M: Disparate ventricular function in surgical patients. Surgical Forum 22: 136, 1971

70. Clancy T, Norman K, Reynolds B et al: Cardiac output measurement in critical care patients: Thoracic electrical bioimpedance versus thermodilution. J Trauma 31: 1116–1121, 1991

71. Clark C, Gutierrez G: Gastric intramucosal pH: A noninvasive method for the indirect measurement of tissue oxygenation. Am J Crit Care 1: 53–60, 1992

72. Clark C, Harman E: Hemodynamic monitoring: Arterial catheters. In Taylor R, Civetta J, Kirby R (eds): Techniques and Procedures in Critical Care, pp 218–231. Philadelphia, JB Lippincott, 1990

73. Clochesy J, Hinshaw A, Otto C: Effects of change in position on pulmonary artery and pulmonary capillary wedge pressures in mechanically ventilated patients. NITA 7: 223–225, 1984

74. Conahan T, Barberii J, Calkins J: Valve competence in pulmonary artery catheter introducer. Anesthesiology 58: 189, 1983

75. Connett R, Honig C, Gaveski T et al: Defining hypoxia: A systems review of VO_2, glycolysis, energetics, and intracellular PO_2. J Appl Physiol 68: 833–842, 1990

76. Connors AJ. Right heart catheterization: Is it effective? New Horizons 5: 195–200, 1997

77. Connors AJ, Speroff T, Dawson N et al: The effectiveness of right heart catheterization in the initial care of critically ill patients. JAMA 276: 889–897, 1996

78. Conway J, Lund-Johansen P: Thermodilution method for measuring cardiac output. Eur Heart J 11(Suppl 1): 17–20, 1990

79. Cope D, Allison R, Dumond M et al: Changes in pulmonary pressures following cardiac surgery. J Cardiothora Anes 2: 182–187, 1988

80. Cope D, Grimbert F, Downey J et al: Pulmonary capillary pressure: A review. Crit Care Med 20: 1043–1056, 1992

81. Copel L, Stolarik A: Continuous SvO_2 monitoring: A research review. Dimen of Crit Care Nurs 10: 202–209, 1991

82. Courtois M, Fattal P, Kovacs S et al: Anatomically and physiologically based reference level for measurement of intracardiac pressures. Circulation 92: 1994–2000, 1995

83. Creamer J, Edwards J, Nightingale P: Hemodynamic and oxygen transport variables in cardiogenic shock secondary to acute myocardial infarction, and response to treatment. Am J Cardiol 65: 1297–1300, 1990

84. Cross C, Cain H, Deaton W et al: Vertical relationship of the pulmonary artery catheter tip and transducer reference point in the estimation of left atrial pressure. Am Rev of Respir Dis 117(Suppl): 105, 1978

85. Daily E, Mersch J: Thermodilution cardiac outputs using room and ice temperature injectate: Comparison with the Fick method. Heart Lung 16: 294–300, 1987

86. Dalen J, Bone R: Is it time to pull the pulmonary artery catheter? (Editorial). JAMA 276: 916–918, 1996

87. Damen J: Ventricular arrhythmias during insertion and removal of pulmonary artery catheters. Chest 88: 190–193, 1985

88. Damen J, Bolton D: A prospective analysis of 1,400 pulmonary artery catheterizations in patients undergoing cardiac surgery. Acta Anaesthesiol Scand 30: 386–392, 1986

89. Dantzker D: The gastrointestinal tract: The canary of the body? (Editorial). JAMA 270: 1247–1248, 1993

90. Dantzker D, Gutierrez G: The assessment of tissue oxygenation. Respiratory Care 30: 456–462, 1985

91. Davidson L, Brown S: Continuous SvO_2 monitoring: A tool for analyzing hemodynamic status. Heart Lung 15: 287–292, 1986

92. Davidson L, Killpack A, Woods S et al: Effect of volume and temperature of injectate on thermodilution cardiac output measurements using an open system of injection. Prog Cardiovasc Nurs 2: 86–91, 1987

93. Davidson W, Fee E: Influence of aging on pulmonary hemodynamics in a population free of coronary artery disease. Am J Cardiol 65: 1454–1458, 1990

94. Davis R, Sakuma E: Comparison of semi-continuous thermodilution to intermittent bolus thermodilution cardiac output determinations (Abstract). Anesthesiology 77: A477, 1992

95. Davison R, Parker M, Harrison R: The validity of determination of pulmonary wedge pressure during mechanical ventilation. Chest 73: 352–355, 1978

96. Groot K, Damato M: Monitoring intra-arterial pressure. Critical Care Nurse 6(1): 74–78, 1986

97. Dhainaut J, Lanore J, de Gournay J et al: Right ventricular dysfunction in patients with septic shock. Intensive Care Med 14(Suppl 2): 488–491, 1988

98. Dhainaut J-F, Brunet F, Monsallier J et al: Bedside evaluation of right ventricular performance using a rapid computerized thermodilution method. Crit Care Med 15: 148–152, 1987

99. Diebel L, Wilson R, Tagett M et al: End-diastolic volume: A better indicator of preload in the critically ill. Arch Surg 127: 817–822, 1992

100. Ditmyer C, Shively M, Burns D et al: Comparison of continuous with intermittent bolus thermodilution cardiac output measurement. Am J Crit Care 4: 460–465, 1995

101. Dizon C, Gezari W, Barash P et al: Hand held thermodilution cardiac output injection. Crit Care Med 4: 210–212, 1977

102. Dobbin K, Wallace S, Ahlberg J et al: Pulmonary artery pressure measurement in patients with elevated pressures: Effect of backrest elevation and method of measurement. Am J Crit Care 1: 61–69, 1992

103. Doering L: The effect of positioning on hemodynamics and gas exchange in the critically ill: A review. Am J Crit Care 2: 208–216, 1993

104. Doering L, Dracup K: Comparisons of cardiac output in supine and lateral positions. Nurs Res 37: 114–118, 1988

105. Doering L, Lum E, Dracup K et al: Predictors of between-method differences in cardiac output measurement using thoracic electrical bioimpedance and thermodilution. Crit Care Med 23: 1667–1673, 1995

106. Doglio G, Pusajo J, Egurrola M et al: Gastric intramucosal pH as a prognostic index of mortality in critically ill patients. Crit Care Med 19: 1037–1040, 1991

107. Dollar M, Yelderman M, Quinn M et al: Evaluation of continuous thermodilution cardiac output catheter. ASAIO J 38: M351–M356, 1992

108. Donovan K, Dobb G, Woods W et al: Comparison of transthoracic electrical impedance and thermodilution methods for measuring cardiac output. Crit Care Med 14: 1038–1044, 1986

109. Dorinsky P, Whitcomb M: The effect of PEEP on cardiac output. Chest 84: 210–216, 1983

110. Downes T, Hackshaw B, Kahl F et al: Frequency of large v waves in the pulmonary artery wedge pressure in ventricular septal defect of acquired (during acute myocardial infarction) or congenital origin. Am J Cardiol 60: 415–417, 1987

111. Driscoll A, Shanahan A, Crommy L et al: The effect of patient positioning on the reproducibility of cardiac output measurements. Heart Lung 24: 38–44, 1995

112. Drucker W, Pearce F, Glass-Heidenreich L et al: Subcutaneous tissue oxygen pressure: A reliable index of peripheral perfusion in humans after injury. J Trauma 40: S116–S122, 1996

113. Duke P: Effects of Two Sidelying Positions on the Measurement of Pulmonary Artery Pressures in Critically Ill Adults. Unpublished thesis, University of Washington, Seattle, Washington, 1994

114. Eddy A, Rice C: The right ventricle: An emerging concern in the multiply injured patient. J Crit Care 4: 58–66, 1989

115. Eddy A, Rice C, Anardi D: Right ventricular dysfunction in multiple trauma victims. Am J Surg 155: 712–715, 1988

116. Eduard A, Degremont A, Duranteau J et al: Heterogeneous regional vascular responses to stimulated transient hypovolemia in man. Intensive Care Med 20: 414–420, 1994

117. Edwards J: Continuous thermodilution cardiac output: A significant step forward in hemodynamic monitoring. Crit Care Med 25: 381–382, 1997

118. Edwards J: Oxygen transport in cardiogenic and septic shock. Crit Care Med 19: 658–663, 1991

119. Edwards J: Therapy: Mechanical ventilation, future trends. In Edwards J, Shoemaker W, Vincent J-L (eds): Oxygen Transport: Principles and Practice, pp 139–152. Philadelphia, WB Saunders, 1993

120. Edwards J, Brown C, Nightingale P et al: Use of survivors' cardiorespiratory values as therapeutic goals in septic shock. Crit Care Med 17: 1098–1103, 1989

121. Ehlers K, Mylrea K, Waterson C et al: Cardiac output measurements: A review of current research techniques and research. Ann Biomed Eng 14: 219–239, 1986

122. Eillis M: Low cardiac output following cardiac surgery: critical thinking steps. Dimen of Crit Care Nurs 16: 48–55, 1997

123. Eisenberg P, Jaffe A, Schuster D: Clinical evaluation compared to pulmonary artery catheterization in the hemodynamic assessment of critically ill patients. Crit Care Med 12: 549–553, 1984

124. Elkayam U, Berkley R, Azen S et al: Cardiac output by thermodilution technique: Effect of injectate volume and temperature on accuracy and reproducibility in the critically ill patient. Chest 84: 418–422, 1983

125. Ellis R, Gold J, Rees J et al: Computerized monitoring of cardiac output by thermal dilution. JAMA 220: 507–511, 1972

126. Enger E: Pulmonary artery wedge pressure: When its valid, when its not. Crit Care Nurs Clin of North Am 1: 603–618, 1989

127. Enger E, O'Toole M: Noncardiogenic mechanisms of right heart dysfunction. J Cardiovasc Nurs 6: 54–69, 1991

128. Enghoff E, Sjorgen S: Thermal dilution for measurement of cardiac output in pulmonary artery in man in relation to choice of indicator volume and injectate time. Ups J Med Sci 78: 33–37, 1973

129. Enson Y, Wood J, Mantara N et al: The influence of heart rate on pulmonary artery–left ventricular pressure relationships at end-diastole. Circulation 56: 533–539, 1977

130. Falicov R, Resnekov L: Relationship of the pulmonary artery end-diastolic pressure to left ventricular end-diastolic and mean filling pressures in patients with and without left ventricular dysfunction. Circulation 42: 65–73, 1970

131. Fegler G: Measurement of cardiac output in anesthetized animals by a thermodilution method. Q J Exp Physiol 39: 153–164, 1954

132. Fiddian-Green R, Amelin P, Herrmann J et al: Prediction of the development of sigmoid ischemia on the day of aortic operations. Arch Surg 121: 654–660, 1986

133. Fiddian-Green R, Pittenger G, Whitehouse W: Back-diffusion of CO and its influence on the intramucosal pH in gastric mucosa. J Surg Res 33: 39–48, 1982

134. Fleming A, Bishop M, Shoemaker W et al: Prospective trial of supranormal values as goals for resuscitation in severe trauma. Arch Surg 127: 115–1181, 1992

135. Forrester J, Diamond G, McHugh T et al: Filling pressures in the right and left sides of the heart in acute myocardial infarction: A reappraisal of central-venous pressure monitoring. N Engl J Med 285: 190–192, 1971

136. Forrester J, Diamond G, Swan H: Correlative classification of clinical and hemodynamic function after acute myocardial infarction. Am J Cardiol 39: 137–145, 1977

137. Forrester J, Ganz W, Diamond G et al: Thermodilution cardiac output determination with a single flow-directed catheter. Am Heart J 83: 306–311, 1972

138. Fournier P, Mensche-Dechene J et al: Effects of sitting upon pulmonary blood pressure, flow, and volume in man. J Appl Physiol 46: 36–40, 1979

139. Friedman PJ, Peters RM, Botkin BM et al: Estimation of the lung volume of lung below the left atrium using computed tomography. Crit Care Med 14: 182–187, 1986

140. Gallagher D, O'Rourke M: What is the arterial pressure? In O'Rourke M, Safar M, Dzau V (eds): Arterial Vasodilation: Mechanisms and Therapy, pp 134–148. Philadelphia, Lea & Febiger, 1993

141. Ganz W, Swan H: Measurement of blood flow by thermodilution. Am J Cardiol 29: 241, 1972

142. Gardner P: Cardiac output: Theory, technique, and troubleshooting. Crit Care Nurs Clin of North Am 1: 577–587, 1989

143. Gardner P: Pulmonary artery pressure monitoring. AACN Clin Issues Crit Care Nurs 4: 98–119, 1993

144. Gardner P, Bridges E: Hemodynamic monitoring. In Woods S, Sivarajan Froelicher E, Halpenny C et al (eds): Cardiac Nursing, 3rd ed, pp 424–458. Philadelphia, JB Lippincott, 1995

145. Gardner P, Monat L, Woods S: Accuracy of the closed injectate delivery system in measuring thermodilution cardiac output. Heart Lung 16: 552–560, 1987

146. Gardner P, Monat L, Woods S: Letter to the editor. Heart Lung 15: 108–109, 1987

147. Gardner R: Accuracy and reliability of disposable pressure transducer coupled with modern pressure monitoring. Crit Care Med 24: 879–882, 1996

148. Gardner R: Continuous cardiac output: How accurate and how timely? (Editorial). Crit Care Med 26: 1302–1303, 1998

149. Gardner R: Direct blood pressure measurement: Dynamic response requirements. Anesthesiology 54: 227–236, 1981

150. Gardner R: Hemodynamic monitoring: From catheter to display. Acute Care 12: 3–33, 1986

151. Gardner R: Invasive pressure monitoring. In Civetta J, Taylor R, Kirby R (eds): Critical Care, pp 839–845. Philadelphia, Lippincott–Raven, 1997

152. Gardner R, Hollingsworth K: Optimizing the electrocardiogram and pressure monitoring. Crit Care Med 14: 651–658, 1986

153. Gardner R, Hujcs M: Fundamentals of physiologic monitoring. AACN Clin Issues in Crit Care Nursing 4: 11–24, 1993

154. Gattinoni L, Brazzi I, Pelosi P et al: A trial of goal-oriented hemodynamic therapy in critically ill patients. N Engl J Med 333: 1025–1032, 1995

155. Gawlinski A: Can measurement of mixed venous oxygen saturation replace measurement of cardiac output in patients with advanced heart failure? Am J Crit Care 5: 374–382, 1998

156. Gawlinski A: Cardiac Output Monitoring. Aliso Viejo, CA, American Association of Critical-Care Nurses, 1998

157. Gawlinski A: Facts and fallacies of patient positioning and hemodynamic measurement. J Cardiovasc Nurs 12: 1–15, 1997

158. Geddes L: The significance of a reference in the direct measurement of blood pressure. Med Instrum 20: 331–332, 1986

159. Gershan J: Effect of positive end-expiratory pressure on pulmonary capillary wedge pressure. Heart Lung 12: 143–148, 1983

160. Gettinger A, DeTraglia M, Glass D: In vivo comparison of two mixed venous saturation catheters. Anesthesiology 66: 373–373, 1987

161. Gibbs N, Gardner R: Dynamics of invasive pressure monitoring systems: Clinical and laboratory evaluation. Heart Lung 17: 43–51, 1988

162. Gibney R, Ryan H: Thermodilution cardiac output measurements. Crit Care Med 12: 614–615, 1984

163. Gilbert H, Vender J, Myers P: Evaluation of continuous cardiac output in patients undergoing coronary artery bypass surgery (Abstract). Anesthesiology 77: A42, 1992

164. Gillespie D: Comparison of intraesophageal balloon pressure measurements with a nasogastric-esophageal balloon system in volunteers. Am Re Respir Dis 126: 583–585, 1982

165. Gillman P: Continuous measurement of cardiac output: A milestone in hemodynamic monitoring. Critical Care Nurse 19: 155–158, 1992

166. Ginosar Y, Sprung C: The Swan-Ganz catheter: Twenty-five years of monitoring. Crit Care Clin 12: 771–776, 1996

167. Glenn S: The Effect of Position Upon Pulmonary Artery and Pulmonary Capillary Wedge Pressure in Cardiac Patients. Unpublished thesis, University of Washington, Seattle, Washington, 1975

168. Glenny R, Lamm W, Albert R et al: Gravity is a minor determinant of pulmonary blood flow distribution. J Appl Physiol 71: 620–629, 1991

169. Glenny R, McKinney S, Robertson H: Spatial pattern of pulmonary blood flow distribution is stable over days. J Appl Physiol 82: 902–907, 1997

170. Glenny R, Polissar N, McKinney S et al: Temporal heterogeneity of regional pulmonary perfusion is spatially clustered. J Appl Physiol 79: 986–1001, 1995

171. Glenny R, Roberston H: A computer simulation of pulmonary perfusion in three dimensions. J Appl Physiol 79: 357–369, 1995

172. Glenny R, Robertson H: Fractal modeling of pulmonary blood flow heterogeneity. J Appl Physiol 70: 1024–1030, 1991

173. Glenny R, Robertson H: Fractal properties of pulmonary blood flow: Characterization of spatial heterogeneity. J Appl Physiol 69: 532–545, 1990

174. Gore S, Middleton R, Bridges E: Analysis of an algorithm to guide decision making regarding direct and oscillometric blood pressure measurement (Abstract). Am J Respir Crit Care Med 151: A331, 1995

175. Gorny D: Arterial blood pressure measurement technique. AACN Clinical Issues in Critical Care Nursing 4: 66–80, 1993

176. Gottrup F, Firmin R, Rabkin J et al: Directly measured tissue oxygen tension and arterial oxygen tension assess tissue perfusion. Crit Care Med 15: 1030, 1988

177. Griffin K, DelGiudice R, Schechter C et al: Thermodilution cardiac output measurement during simultaneous volume infusion through the venous infusion port of the pulmonary artery catheter. J Cardiothorac Vasc Anesth 11: 437–439, 1997

178. Groenveld A, Kolkman J: Splanchnic tonometry: A review of physiology, methodology, and clinical applications. J Crit Care 9: 198–210, 1994

179. Groenveld J, Jesterm, ADM, Nauta J et al: Relation of arterial blood lactate to oxygen delivery and hemodynamic variables in human shock states. Circ Shock 22: 35–53, 1987

180. Groom L, Frisch S, Elliott M: Reproducibility and accuracy of pulmonary artery pressure measurement in supine and lateral positions. Heart Lung 19: 147–151, 1990

181. Grose B, Woods S: Effects of mechanical ventilation and backrest position upon pulmonary artery and pulmonary capillary wedge pressure measurements. Am Rev Respir Dis 123: 120, 1981

182. Grose B, Woods S, Laurent D: Effect of backrest position on cardiac output measurement by the thermodilution method in acutely ill patients. Heart Lung 10: 661–665, 1981

183. Grossman W: Pressure measurement. In Baim DS, Grossman W (eds): Cardiac Catheterization, Angiography, and Intervention, 5th ed, pp 125–141. Baltimore, Williams & Wilkins, 1996

184. Guanyuan J, Jie Y, Yueling S et al: Diurnal variation of cardiac output in healthy young people. Prog Clin Biol Res 341B: 613–617, 1990

185. Guenther N, Kay J, Cheng EY et al: Comparing pulmonary artery catheter measurements in the supine, prone and lateral positions. Crit Care Med 15: 383, 1987

186. Guilbeau J, Applegate A: Thermodilution: An advanced technique for measuring continuous cardiac output. Dimensions of Critical Care Nursing 15: 25–30, 1996

187. Gutierez G, Brown S: Gastric tonometry: A monitor of regional dysoxia. New Horizons 4: 413–419, 1996

188. Gutierrez G, Bismar H, Dantzker D et al: Comparison of gastric intramucosal pH with measures of oxygen transport and consumption in critically ill patients. Crit Care Med 20: 451–457, 1992

189. Gutierrez G, Brown S: Gastric tonometry: A new monitoring modality in the intensive care unit. J Intens Care Med 10: 34–44, 1995

190. Gutierrez G, Palizas F, Doglio G et al: Gastric intramucosal pH as a therapeutic index of tissue oxygenation in critically ill patients. Lancet 339: 195–199, 1992

191. Guzman J, Lacoma F, Kruse J: Relationship between systemic oxygen supply dependency and gastric intramucosal PCO_2 during progressive hemorrhage. J Trauma 44: 696–700, 1998

192. Haller M, Zollner C, Briegel J et al: Evaluation of a new continuous thermodilution cardiac output monitor in critically ill patients: A prospective criterion study. Crit Care Med 23: 860–866, 1995

193. Ham T, Shen S, Fleming E et al: Studies in destruction of red blood cells. Blood 3: 373–403, 1948

194. Hamilton M, Stevenson L, Woo M et al: Effect of tricuspid regurgitation on the reliability of thermodilution cardiac output technique in congestive heart failure. Am J Cardiol 64: 945–948, 1989

195. Hamilton W, Moore J, Kinsman J: Further analysis of the injection method and changes in hemodynamics under physiological and pathological conditions. Am J Physiol 99: 534, 1932

196. Hand H: Direct or indirect blood pressure measurement for open heart surgery patients: An algorithm. Critical Care Nurse 12(6): 52–61, 1992

197. Harper J: Third level hemodynamics: Guiding clinical decisions. Dimensions of Critical Care Nursing 11: 130–135, 1992

198. Harris A, Miller C, Beattie C et al: The slowing of sinus rhythm during thermodilution cardiac output determination and the effect of altering injectate temperature. Anesthesiology 63: 540–541, 1985

199. Harris J, Tyler M: The effect of the respiratory cycle on the reliability of thermodilution cardiac output measurements. Heart Lung 19: 306, 1990

200. Hasan F, Malanga A, Braman S et al: Lateral position improves wedge-left atrial pressure during positive-pressure ventilation. Crit Care Med 12: 960–964, 1984

201. Hasan F, Weiss W, Braman S et al: Influence of lung injury on pulmonary wedge-left atrial pressure correlation during positive end–expiratory pressure ventilation. Am Respir Dis 131: 246–250, 1985

202. Haskell R, French W: Accuracy of left atrial and pulmonary artery wedge pressure in pure mitral regurgitation in predicting left ventricular end-diastolic filling pressure. Am J Cardiol 61: 136–141, 1988

203. Haupt M: Therapy: Effects of fluid resuscitation. In Edwards J, Shoemaker W, Vincent J-L (eds): Oxygen Transport: Principles and Practice, pp 175–192. Philadelphia, WB Saunders, 1993

204. Hausen B, Schafers H-J, Rohde R et al: Clinical evaluation of transtracheal Doppler for continuous cardiac output estimation. Anesth Analg 74: 800–804, 1992

205. Hayes M, Timmins A, Yau E et al: Elevation of systemic oxygen delivery in the treatment of critically ill patients. N Engl J Med 330: 1717–1722, 1994

206. Hayes M, Yaym E, Timmins A et al: Response of critically ill patients to treatment aimed at achieving supranormal oxygen delivery and consumption. Chest 103: 886–895, 1993

207. Headley J, Diethorn M: Right ventricular volumetric monitoring. AACN Clin Issues in Crit Care Nursing 4: 120–133, 1993

208. Headley J, Von Reuden K: The right ventricle: Significant anatomy, physiology, and interventricular considerations. J Cardiovasc Nurs 6: 1–11, 1991

209. Henneman E, Gawlinski A: Evaluating cardiopulmonary instability with continuous monitoring of mixed venous oxygen saturation. Crit Care Nurs Clinics of North Am 6: 855–862, 1994

210. Henneman E, Henneman P: Intricacies of blood pressure measurement: Reexamining the rituals. Heart Lung 18: 263–273, 1989

211. Hoel B: Some aspects of the clinical use of thermodilution in measuring cardiac output. Scand J Clin Lab Invest 38: 383–388, 1978

212. Hoppe B: Central venous catheter-related infections: Pathogenesis, predictors, and prevention. Heart Lung 24: 333–340, 1995

213. Hotchkiss R, Datsamouris A, Lappas D et al: Interpretation of pulmonary artery wedge pressure and pullback blood gas determinations during positive end-expiratory pressure ventilation and after exclusion of the bronchial circulation in the dog. Am Rev of Resp Dis 133: 1019–1023, 1986

214. Hruby I, Woods S: Effect of injectate temperature on measurements of thermodilution of cardiac output in cardiac surgery patients (Abstract). Circulation 68: 223, 1983

215. Hurford W, Zapol W: The right ventricle and critical illness: A review of anatomy, physiology, and clinical evaluation of its function. Intensive Care Med 14(Suppl 2): 448–457, 1988

216. Iberti R, Benjamin E, Gruppi L et al: Ventricular arrhythmias during pulmonary artery catheterization in the intensive care unit. Am J Med 48: 451–454, 1985

217. Imperial-Perez F, McRae M: Arterial Pressure Monitoring, pp 1–35. Aliso Viejo, CA, American Association of Critical-Care Nurses, 1998

218. Jacquet L, Hanique G, Glorieux D et al: Analysis of the accuracy of continuous thermodilution cardiac output measurement: Comparison with intermittent thermodilution and Fick cardiac output measurement. Intensive Care Med 22: 1125–1129, 1996

219. Jakobsen C, Melsen NC, Andresen E: Continuous cardiac output measurements in perioperative period. Acta Anaesthesiol Scand 39: 485–488, 1995

220. Jansen J: The thermodilution method for the clinical assessment of cardiac output. Intensive Care Med 21: 691–697, 1995

221. Jansen J, Bogaard J, Vesprille A: Extrapolation of thermodilution curves obtained during a phase in artificial ventilation. J Appl Physiol 63: 1551–1557, 1987

222. Jansen J, Schreuder J, Bogaard J et al: Thermodilution technique for measurement of cardiac output during artificial ventilation. J Appl Physiol 51: 584–591, 1981

223. Jansen J, Vesprille A: Improvement of cardiac output estimation by the thermodilution method during mechanical ventilation. Intens Care Med 12(2): 71–79, 1986

224. Jansen J, Schreuder J, Settels J et al: An adequate strategy for the thermodilution technique in patients during mechanical ventilation. Intensive Care Med 16: 422–425, 1990

225. Jardin R, Farcot J, Boisante L et al: Influence of positive end-expiratory pressure on left ventricular performance. N Engl J Med 304: 387–392, 1981

226. Jesurum J: SvO$_2$ Monitoring. Aliso Viejo, CA, American Association of Critical-Care Nurses, 1998

227. Johnson M, Schumann L: Comparison of three methods of measurement of pulmonary artery catheter readings in critically ill patients. Am J Crit Care 4: 301–307, 1995

228. Kadota L: Theory and application of thermodilution cardiac output measurement: A review. Heart Lung 14: 605–616, 1985

229. Kane P, Askanazi J, Neville J et al: Artifacts in the measurement of pulmonary artery wedge pressure. Crit Care Med 6: 36–38, 1978

230. Kay H, Afshari M, Barash P et al: Measurement of ejection fraction by thermal dilution techniques. J Surg Res 34: 337–346, 1983

231. Kaye W, Dubin H: Vascular cannulation. In Taylor R, Kirby R (eds): Techniques and Procedures in Critical Care, pp 183–217. Philadelphia, JB Lippincott, 1990

232. Kearney T, Shabot M: Pulmonary artery rupture associated with Swan-Ganz catheter. Chest 108: 1349–1352, 1995

233. Keating D, Boylard K, Eichler E et al: The effect of sidelying positions on pulmonary artery pressures. Heart Lung 15: 605–610, 1986

234. Keckeisen M: Pulmonary Artery Pressure Monitoring. Aliso Viejo, CA, American Association of Critical-Care Nurses, 1998

235. Keckeisen M, Monsein S: Techniques for measuring arterial pressure in the postoperative cardiac surgery patient. Crit Care Nurs Clin North Am 3: 699–708, 1991

236. Kee L, Simonson J, Stotts N et al: Echocardiographic determination of left atrial level in relation to patient position. Heart Lung 16: 334, 1987

237. Kee L, Simonson J, Stotts N et al: Echocardiographic determinations of valid zero reference levels in supine and lateral positions. Am J Crit Care 2: 72–80, 1993

238. Keeler C, McLane C, Covey M et al: A review of infection control practices related to intravascular pressure monitoring devices (1975–1985). Heart Lung 16: 201–206, 1987

239. Keen J: The effect of injectate temperature on thermodilution cardiac output measurement in hyperdynamic cirrhotics (Abstract). Heart Lung 15: 312, 1986

240. Kelly R, Gibbs H, O'Rourke M et al: Nitroglycerin has more favourable effects on left ventricular afterload than apparent from measurement of pressure in a peripheral artery. Eur Heart J 11: 138–144, 1990

241. Kelly T, Morris G, Crawford E et al: Perforation of the pulmonary artery with Swan-Ganz catheters. Ann Surg 193: 689–692, 1981

242. Kennedy G, Bryant A, Crawford M: The effects of lateral body positioning on measurement of pulmonary artery and pulmonary artery wedge pressure. Heart Lung 13: 155–158, 1984

243. Killpack A, Davidson L, Woods S et al: Effect of injectate volume and temperature on measurement of thermodilution cardiac output in acutely ill patients (Abstract). Circulation 64: IV-165, 1981

244. Kint P, VanDomburg R, Miy H: Reproducibility of thermodilution cardiac output measurements (Abstract). Circulation Part II 63(4): IV-165, 1981

245. Kirchoff K, Rebenson-Piano M, Patel M: Mean arterial pressure readings: Variations with positions and transducer level. Nurs Res 33: 343–345, 1984

246. Kleven M: Effect of backrest position on thermodilution cardiac output in critically ill patients receiving mechanical ventilation with PEEP. Heart Lung 13: 303–304, 1984

247. Komadina K, Schenk D, LaVeau P et al: Interobserver variability in the interpretation of pulmonary artery catheter pressure tracings. Chest 100: 1647–1654, 1991

248. Komatsu T, Shibutani K, Okamoto K et al: Critical level of oxygen delivery after cardiopulmonary bypass. Crit Care Med 15: 194–197, 1987

249. Kraft P, Steltzer H, Hiesmayr M et al: Mixed venous oxygen saturation in critically ill septic shock patients: The role of defined events. Chest 103: 900–906, 1993

250. Kremzar B, Spec-Marn A, Kompan L et al: Normal values of SvO$_2$ as therapeutic goal in patients with multiple injuries. Intensive Care Med 23: 65–70, 1997

251. Lachenmyer J, Stotts N: Effect of respiratory cycle on reproducibility of thermodilution cardiac output measurements in mechanically ventilated patients (Abstract). Circulation 72: 24, 1985

252. Lange R, Moore D, Cigarroa R: Use of pulmonary capillary wedge pressure to assess severity of mitral stenosis: Is true left atrial pressure needed in this condition. J Am Coll Cardiol 13: 825–829, 1989

253. Larrivee C, Joseph D: Strategies for teaching decision making: discrepancies in cuff versus invasive blood pressure. Dimensions of Critical Care Nursing 11: 278–285, 1992

254. Larson C, Woods S: Effect of injectate volume and temperature on thermodilution cardiac output measurement in critically ill patients (Abstract). Circulation 66: II-98, 1982

255. Larson L, Kyff J: The cost-effectiveness of Oximetrix pulmonary artery catheters in the postoperative care of coronary artery bypass graft surgery patients. Anesth Analg 3: 276–279, 1989

256. Latham R, Slife D: Effects of arterial disease on wave travel and reflection. In O'Rourke M, Safar M, Dzau V (eds): Arterial Vasodilation: Mechanisms and Therapy, pp 41–49. Philadelphia, Lea & Febiger, 1993

257. Laulive J: Pulmonary artery pressure and position changes in the critically ill adult. Dimensions of Critical Care Nursing 1: 28–34, 1982

258. Laxson C, Titler M: Drawing coagulation studies from arterial lines: An integrative literature review. Am J Crit Care 3: 16–22, 1994

259. Lazor M, Pierce E, Stanley G et al: Evaluation of the accuracy and response time of STAT-Mode continuous cardiac output. J Cardiothorac Vasc Anesth 11: 432–436, 1997

260. Lazor M, Stanley G, Cass B et al: Response time of STAT continuous cardiac output to an acute hemodynamic change. Anesth Analg 82: SCA71, 1996

261. Leatherman J, Marini J: Pulmonary artery catheter: Pressure monitoring. In Sprung C (ed): The Pulmonary Artery Catheter: Methodology and Clinical Applications, 2nd ed, pp 119–156. Closter, NJ, Critical Care Research Associates, 1993

262. Lee D, Stevens G: Comparison of thermodilution cardiac output measurement by injection of the proximal lumen versus side port of the Swan-Ganz catheter. Heart Lung 14: 125–127, 1985

263. Lee J, Wright F, Barber R et al: Central venous oxygen saturation in shock: A study in man. Anesthesiology 36: 472–478, 1972

264. LeTulzo Y, Belghith M, Seguin P et al: Reproducibility of thermodilution cardiac output determination in critically ill patients: Comparison between bolus and continuous method. J Clin Monit 12: 379–385, 1996

265. LeTulzo Y, Belghith M, Seguin P et al: Reproducibility of thermodilution cardiac output determination in critically ill patients: Comparison between bolus and continuous method. J Clin Monit 12: 379–385, 1996

266. Levett J, Repogle R: Thermodilution cardiac output: A critical analysis and review of the literature. J Surg Res 27: 392–404, 1979

267. Levine-Silverman S, Johnson J: Pulmonary artery pressure measurements. West J Nurs Res 12: 483–496, 1990

268. Lewis J, Kuo L, Nelson J et al: Pulsed Doppler echocardiographic determination of stroke volume and cardiac output: Clinical validation of two new methods using the apical window. Circulation 70: 425–431, 1984

269. Lichtenthal P, Gordon D: Testing the safety of the Baxter Continuous Cardiac Output monitoring system. J Clin Monit 12: 241–249, 1996

270. Lichtenthal P, Marchand B, Gordon D et al: A safety comparison between a new continuous cardiac output (CCO) monitoring system and a standard pulmonary artery catheter in sheep (Abstract). Anesthesiology 77: A473, 1992

271. Lichtenthal P, Wade L: Accuracy of the Vigilance/Intellicath Continuous cardiac output system during and after cardiac surgery (Abstract). Anesthesiology 79: A474, 1993

272. Lichtenthal P, Wade L: Clinical evaluation of a continuous cardiac output system in post-op cardiac surgical patients (Abstract). Anesthesiology 77: 3, 1992

273. Lipkin D, Poole-Wilson P: Measurement of cardiac output during exercise by the thermodilution and direct Fick techniques in patients with chronic congestive heart failure. Am J Cardiol 56: 321–324, 1985

274. Lipp-Ziff E, Kawanishi D: A technique for improving the accuracy of the pulmonary artery diastolic pressure as an estimate of left ventricular end-diastolic pressure. Heart Lung 20: 107–115, 1991

275. Little R, Edwards J: Applied physiology. In Edwards J, Shoemaker W, Vincent J-L (eds): Oxygen Transport: Principles and Practice, pp 21–40. Philadelphia, WB Saunders, 1993

276. Lookinland S: Comparison of pulmonary vascular pressure based on blood volume and ventilator status. Nurs Res 38: 68–72, 1989

277. Loubser P: Comparison of intra-arterial and automated oscillometric blood pressure measurement methods in postoperative hypertensive patients. Med Instrum 20: 255–259, 1986

278. Loveys B, Woods S: Current recommendations for thermodilution cardiac output measurements. Prog Cardiovasc Nurs 1: 24–32, 1986

279. Lozman J, Powers S, Older T et al: Correlation of pulmonary wedge and left atrial pressures. Arch Surg 109: 270–277, 1974

280. Lundstedt J: Comparison of methods measuring pulmonary artery pressure. Am J Crit Care 6: 324–332, 1997

281. Lyons K, Dalbow M: Room temperature injectate and iced injectate for cardiac output: A comparative study. Crit Care Nurs 6: 48–50, 1983

282. Malanga A, Hasan F, Bramon S et al: The lateral position: An aid in hemodynamic monitoring. Am Rev Respir Dis 127: 88, 1983

283. Mann S, Jones R, Millar-Craig M et al: The safety of ambulatory intra-arterial pressure monitoring: Clinical audit of 1000 studies. Int J Cardiol 5: 585–597, 1984

284. Manthous C, Hall J, Olson D et al: Effect of cooling on oxygen consumption in febrile critically ill patients. Am J Respir Crit Care Med 151: 10–14, 1995

285. Mantin R, Ramsay J: Cardiac output technologies. Int Anesthesiol Clin 34: 79–107, 1996

286. Marcum J, Liberatore K, Willard G: A comparison of varying injectate volumes in determining thermodilution cardiac output in critically ill postsurgical patients (Abstract). Am J Crit Care 2: 262, 1995

287. Marik P: Gastric intramucosal pH: A better predictor of multiorgan dysfunction syndrome and death than oxygen-derived variables in patients with sepsis. Chest 104: 225–229, 1993

288. Marini J: Obtaining meaningful data from the Swan-Ganz catheter. Respir Care 30: 572–585, 1985

289. Marini J, O'Quin R, Culver B et al: Estimation of transmural cardiac pressure during ventilation with PEEP. J Appl Physiol 53: 384–391, 1982

290. Marino P: The ICU Book, 2nd ed. Baltimore, Williams & Wilkins, 1998

291. Martin C, Saux P, Auffray J et al: Thermodilution cardiac output measurement by injection in PA vs CVP catheter. Crit Care Med 11: 460–461, 1983

292. Matthay R, Wiedemann H, Matthay M: Cardiovascular function in the intensive care unit: Invasive and noninvasive monitoring. Respiratory Care 30: 432–455, 1985

293. Matuschak G: Supranormal oxygen delivery in critical illness. New Horizons 5: 233–238, 1997

294. Mault J, Bartlett R, Dechet R et al: Central venous catheters versus proximal injection site for thermodilution cardiac outputs. Crit Care Med 11: 224, 1983

295. Maynard N, Bihari D, Beale R et al: Assessment of splanchnic oxygenation by gastric tonometry in patients with acute circulatory failure. JAMA 270: 1203–1210, 1993

296. McDonald D, Zaidan J: Pressure-volume relationships of the pulmonary artery catheter balloon. Anesthesiology 59: 240–243, 1983

297. McMillan R, Morris D: Effect of respiratory cycle on measurement of cardiac output by thermodilution. Surg Gynecol Obstet 167: 420–422, 1988

298. Medley R, DeLapp T, Fisher D: Comparability of thermodilution cardiac output method: Proximal injectate versus proximal infusion lumens. Heart Lung 21: 12–17, 1992

299. Meier-Helmann A, Hannemann L, Schaffartzik W et al: The relevance of measuring O_2 supply and O_2 consumption for assessment of regional tissue oxygenation. In Vaupel P (ed): Oxygen Transport to Tissue XV, pp 741–746. New York, Plenum, 1994

300. Mermel L, Maki D: Epidemic bloodstream infection from hemodynamic pressure monitoring: Signs of the times. Infect Control Hosp Epidemiol 10(2): 47–53, 1989

301. Mermel L, Maki D: Infectious complications of Swan-Ganz pulmonary artery catheters. Am J Respir Crit Care Med 149: 1020–1036, 1994

302. Mihaljevic T, von Segesser L, Tonz M et al: Continuous versus bolus thermodilution cardiac output measurements: A comparative study. Crit Care Med 23: 944–949, 1995

303. Mihaljevic T, von-Segesser L, Tonz M et al: Continuous thermodilution measurement of cardiac output: In-vitro and in-vivo evaluation. Thorac Cardiovasc Surg 42: 32–35, 1994

304. Mihm F, Gettinger A, Hanson CI et al: A multicenter evaluation of a new continuous cardiac output pulmonary artery catheter system. Crit Care Med 26: 1346–1350, 1998

305. Miller T, Chulay M: Effect of change in body position on pulmonary artery pressures in critically ill patients. In American Association of Critical-Care Nurses International Intensive Care Nursing Conference, London, England, 1982

306. Mimoz O, Rauss A, Rekik N et al: Pulmonary artery catheterization: A prospective analysis of outcome changes associated with catheter-prompted changes in therapy. Crit Care Med 22: 573, 1994

307. Mizock B, Falk J: Lactic acidosis in critical illness. Crit Care Med 20: 80–93, 1992

308. Mohsenifar Z, Hay A, Hay J et al: Gastric intramucosal pH as a predictor of success or failure in weaning patients from mechanical ventilation. Ann Intern Med 119: 794–798, 1994

309. Moore F, Haenel B: Advances in oxygen monitoring in trauma patients. Med Instrum 22: 135–142, 1988

310. Moorthy S, Tinsinai K, Speiser B et al: Cerebral air embolism during removal of a pulmonary artery catheter. Crit Care Med 19: 981–983, 1991

311. Morris A, Chapman R: Wedge pressure confirmation by aspiration of pulmonary capillary blood. Crit Care Med 13: 756–759, 1985

312. Morris A, Chapman R, Gardner R: The frequency of technical problems encountered in the measurement of pulmonary artery wedge pressure. Crit Care Med 12: 164–170, 1984

313. Morris A, Chapman R, Gardner R: Frequency of wedge pressure errors in the ICU. Crit Care Med 13: 705–708, 1985

314. Morris A, Mulvhill D, Lee W: Risk of developing complete heart block during bedside pulmonary artery catheterization in patients in patients with left bundle branch block. Ann Intern Med 98: 2005–2010, 1987

315. Moser D, Woo M: Normal fluctuation in pulmonary artery pressure and cardiac output in patients with severe left ventricular dysfunction. Am J Crit Care 5: 236, 1996

316. Moser K, Spragg R: Use of the balloon-tipped pulmonary artery catheter in pulmonary disease. Ann Intern Med 98: 53–58, 1983

317. Mythen M, Webb A: Intra-operative gut mucosal hypoperfusion is associated with increased postoperative complications and cost. Intensive Care Med 20: 99–104, 1994

318. Nadeau S, Noble W: Limitations of cardiac output by thermodilution. Can Anaesth Soc J 33: 780–784, 1986

319. Nave C, Nave B: Physics for the Health Sciences, 3rd ed, p 421. Philadelphia, WB Saunders, 1980

320. Nelson L: Continuous venous oximetry in surgical patients. Ann Surg 203: 329–333, 1986

321. Nelson L: The new pulmonary artery catheters. Crit Care Clin 12: 795–818, 1996

322. Nelson L: The new pulmonary artery catheters: Continuous venous oximetry, right ventricular ejection fraction, and continuous cardiac output. New Horizons 5: 251–258, 1997

323. Nelson L: Venous oximetry. In Snyder J, Pinsky M (eds): Oxygen Transport in the Critically Ill Patient, pp 235–248. Chicago, Year Book, 1987

324. Nelson L, Anderson H: Patient selection for iced versus room temperature injectate for thermodilution cardiac output determinations. Crit Care Med 13: 182–184, 1985

325. Nelson L, Houtchens B: Automatic versus manual injections for thermodilution cardiac output determinations. Crit Care Med 10: 190–192, 1982

326. Nelson L, Martinez O, Anderson H: Incidence of microbial colonization in open versus closed delivery systems for thermodilution cardiac output. Crit Care Med 14: 291–293, 1986

327. Nelson L, Rutherford E: Monitoring mixed venous oxygen. Respir Care 2: 154–164, 1992

328. Nemens EJ, Woods SL: Normal fluctuations in pulmonary artery and pulmonary capillary wedge pressure in acutely ill patients. Heart Lung 11: 393–398, 1982

329. Neville J, Askanzi J, Mon R et al: Determinants of pulmonary artery wedge pressure. Surgical Forum 2b: 206–208, 1975

330. Nichols W, Avolio A, Kelly R et al: Effects of age and hypertension on wave travel and reflections. In O'Rourke M, Safar M, Dzau V (eds): Arterial Vasodilation: Mechanisms and Therapy, pp 23–40. Philadelphia, Lea & Febiger, 1993

331. Nightingale P: Measurements, technical problems, and inaccuracies. In Edwards J, Shoemaker W, Vincent J-L (eds): Oxygen Transport: Principles and Practice, pp 41–69. Philadelphia, WB Saunders, 1993

332. Noll M, Byers J: Usefulness of SvO_2, SpO_2, vital signs and derived dual oximetry parameters as indicators of arterial blood gas variables during weaning of cardiac surgery patients from mechanical ventilation. Heart Lung 24: 220–227, 1995

333. Noll M, Fountain R, Duncan C et al: Fluctuation in mixed venous oxygen saturation in critically ill medical patients: A pilot study. Am J Crit Care 1: 102–106, 1992

334. Nuez S, Maisel A: Comparison between mixed venous oxygen saturation and thermodilution cardiac output in monitoring patients with severe heart failure treated with milrinone and dobutamine. Am Heart J 5: 383–388, 1998

335. American Association of Critical-Care Nurses: Evaluation of the effects of heparinized and nonheparinized flush solutions on the patency of arterial pressure monitoring lines: The AACN Thunder Project. Am J Crit Care 2: 3–15, 1993

336. O'Quin R, Marini J: Pulmonary artery occlusion pressure: Clinical physiology, measurement, and interpretation. Am Rev Respir Dis 128: 319–326, 1983

337. O'Rourke M: Arterial Function in Health and Disease: Analysis of Arterial Waves, pp 5–128. New York, Churchill Livingston, 1982

338. O'Rourke M: Arterial mechanics and wave reflection with antihypertensive therapy. J Hypertens 10(Suppl 5): S43–S49, 1992

339. O'Rourke M: Towards optimization of wave reflection: Therapeutic goal for tomorrow? Clin Exp Pharmacol Physiol 23(Suppl 1): S11–S15, 1996

340. O'Rourke M: Wave travel and reflection in the arterial system. In O'Rourke M, Safar M, Dzau V (eds): Arterial Vasodilation: Mechanisms and Therapy, pp 10–22. Philadelphia, Lea & Febiger, 1993

341. O'Rourke M: What is blood pressure? Am J Hypertens 3: 803–810, 1990

342. O'Rourke M, Avolio A, Kelly R et al: Difference between central and upper limb pressure wave forms in man. In O'Rourke M, Safar M, Dzau V (eds): Arterial Vasodilation: Mechanisms and Therapy, pp 117–133 Philadelphia, Lea & Febiger, 1993

343. O'Rourke M, Kelly R: Wave reflection in the systemic circulation and its implications in ventricular function. J Hypertens 11: 327–337, 1993

344. O'Rourke R: The measurement of systemic blood pressure: Normal and abnormal pulsations of the arteries and veins. In Hurst J, Schlant R (eds): The Heart, Arteries, and Veins, 7th ed, pp 117–133. New York, McGraw-Hill, 1990

345. Ortiz L, Gutierrez G: The adult respiratory distress syndrome. In Edwards J, Shoemaker W, Vincent J-L (eds): Oxygen Transport: Principles and Practice, pp 294–321. Philadelphia, WB Saunders, 1993

346. Osika C: Measurement of pulmonary artery pressure: Supine versus side-lying head elevated positions. Heart Lung 18: 298, 1989

347. Ovsyshcher I, Furman S: Impedance cardiography for cardiac output estimation in pacemaker patients: Review of the literature. Pacing Clin Electrophysiol 16: 1412–1422, 1993

348. Palacios I, Powers E, Powell W: Effect of end-diastolic volume on the canine left ventricular ejection fraction. Am Heart J 109: 1059–1069, 1985

349. Paolella L, Dortman G, Cronan J et al: Topographic location of the left atrium by computed tomography: Reducing pulmonary artery catheter calibration errors. Crit Care Med 16: 1154–1156, 1988

350. Parker M, Shelhamer J, Natanson C et al: Serial cardiovascular variables in survivors and nonsurvivors of human septic shock: Heart rate as an early predictor of prognosis. Crit Care Med 15: 923–929, 1987

351. Pulmonary Artery Catheter Consensus Conference: Pulmonary artery catheter consensus statement. New Horizons 5: 175–179, 1997

352. Pauca A, Wallenhaupt S, Kon N et al: Does radial artery pressure accurately reflect aortic pressure. Chest 102: 1193–1198, 1992

353. Pearl R, Rostenthal M, Nielson L et al: Effect of injectate volume and temperature on thermodilution cardiac output determination. Anesthesiology 64: 798–801, 1986

354. Pearson M: Guideline for prevention of intravascular device-related infections. Infect Control Hosp Epidemiol 17: 438–473, 1996

355. Peerless J, Alexander J, Pinchak A et al: Oxygen delivery is an important predictor of outcome in patients with ruptured abdominal aortic aneurysms. Ann Surg 227: 726–734, 1998

356. Pelletier C, Dufort G, Fortier P: Cardiac output measurement by thermodilution. Can J Surg 22: 347–350, 1979

357. Perrino A, Lippman A, Ariyan C et al: Intraoperative cardiac output monitoring: Comparison of impedance cardiography and thermodilution. J Cardiothorac Vasc Anesth 8: 24–29, 1994

358. Peruzzi W, Parker M, Lichtenthal P et al: A clinical evaluation of a blood conservation device in medical intensive care unit patients. Crit Care Med 21: 501–506, 1993

359. Pesce R: The Swan-Ganz catheter: It goes through your pulmonary artery and you pay through the nose. Respir Care 34: 784, 1989

360. Pesola G, Rostata H, Carlon G: Room-temperature thermodilution cardiac output: Central venous vs right ventricular port. Am J Crit Care 1: 76–80, 1992

361. Pierson D: Monitoring preload in the ICU: End-diastolic volume or wedge? (Comment). Critical Care Alert 6(3): 17–18, 1998

362. Polak J, Holman B, Wynne J et al: Right ventricular ejection fraction: An indicator of increased mortality in patients with congestive heart failure associated with coronary artery disease. J Am Coll Cardiol 2: 217–224, 1983

363. Potger K, Elliott D: Reproducibility of central venous pressures in supine and lateral positions: A pilot evaluation of the phlebostatic axis in critically ill patients. Heart Lung 23: 285–299, 1994

364. Powell C, Schultz S, Burris D et al: Subcutaneous oxygen tension: A useful adjunct in assessment of perfusion status. Crit Care Med 23: 867, 1995

365. Prakash R, Parmley W, Dikshit K et al: Hemodynamic effects of postural changes in patients with acute myocardial infarction. Chest 64: 7–9, 1973

366. Prewitt R, Ghigon M: Treatment of right ventricular dysfunction in acute respiratory failure. Crit Care Med 11: 346–352, 1983
367. Puri V, Carlson R, Bander J et al: Complications of vascular catheterization in the critically ill: A prospective study. Crit Care Med 8: 495–499, 1980
368. Raffin T: The technique of thermodilution cardiac output measurements. J Crit Illn 2: 73, 1987
369. Rahimtoola S, Loeb H, Ehsani A: Relationship of pulmonary artery to left ventricular diastolic pressures in acute myocardial infarction. Circulation 46: 283–290, 1972
370. Rajacich N, Burchard K, Hasan F et al: Central venous pressure and pulmonary capillary wedge pressure as estimates of left atrial pressure: Effects of positive end-expiratory pressure and catheter tip malposition. Crit Care Med 17: 7–11, 1989
371. Ramsey MI: Blood pressure monitoring: Automated oscillometric devices. J Clin Monit 7: 56–67, 1991
372. Raper R, Sibbald W: Misled by the wedge? The Swan-Ganz catheter and left ventricular preload. Chest 89: 427–434, 1986
373. Raphael L, Mantel J, Moraski R et al: Quantitative assessment of ventricular performance in unstable ischemic heart disease by dextran function curves. Circulation 55: 858–863, 1977
374. Rashkin M, Bosken C, Baughman R: Oxygen delivery in critically ill patients. Chest 87: 580–584, 1985
375. Reed RI: Oxygen consumption and delivery. Curr Opin Anesthesiol 6: 329–334, 1993
376. Reininger E, Troy B: Error in thermodilution cardiac output measurement caused by variation in syringe volume. Cathet Cardiovasc Diagn 2: 415, 1976
377. Renner L, Morton M, Sakuma G: Indicator amount, temperature, and intrinsic cardiac output affect thermodilution cardiac output accuracy and reproducibility. Crit Care Med 21: 586–597, 1993
378. Renner L, Myer L: Injectate port selection affects accuracy and reproducibility of cardiac output measurements with multiport thermodilution pulmonary artery catheters. Am J Crit Care 3: 55–61, 1994
379. Retailliau M, McGregor-Leding M, Woods S: The effect of the backrest position on the measurement of left atrial pressure after cardiac surgery. Heart Lung 14: 477–483, 1985
380. Reuse C, Frank N, Contempre B et al: Right ventricular function in septic shock. Intensive Care Med 14(Suppl 2): 486–487, 1988
381. Reuse C, Vincent J, Pinsky M: Measurement of right ventricular volumes during fluid challenge. Chest 98: 1450–1454, 1990
382. Rosenwasser R, Jallo J, Getch C et al: Complications of Swan-Ganz catheterization for hemodynamic monitoring in patients with subarachnoid hemorrhage. Neurosurgery 37: 872–875, 1995
383. Ross C, Jones R. Comparisons of pulmonary artery pressure measurements in supine and 30 degree lateral positions. Can J Cardiovasc Nurs 6(3–4): 4–8, 1995
384. Roth M: Effects of priming the proximal lumen of a thermodilution catheter with iced injectate on measurement of cardiac output by thermodilution in critically ill adults. Unpublished master's thesis, University of Washington, Seattle, Washington, 1983
385. Roumen R, Redi H, Schlag G et al: Scoring systems and blood lactate concentration in relation to the development of adult respiratory distress syndrome and multiple organ failure in severely traumatized patients. J Trauma 35: 349–355, 1993
386. Roumen R, Vreudge J, Goris J: Gastric tonometry in multiple trauma patients. J Trauma 36: 313–316, 199
387. Routsi C, Vincent J, Bakker J et al: Relation between oxygen consumption and oxygen delivery in patients after cardiac surgery. Anesth Analg 77: 1104–1110, 1993
388. Rowell L: Human Cardiovascular Control, p 500. New York, Oxford University Press, 1993
389. Rowell L: Brengelmann G, Blackmon J et al: Disparities between aortic and peripheral pulse pressures induced by upright exercise and vasomotor changes in man. Circulation 37: 954–964, 1968
390. Runciman W, Itsley A, Roberts J: An evaluation of thermodilution cardiac output measurement using the Swan-Ganz catheter. Anesthesiol Intensive Care 9: 208–220, 1981
391. Runciman W, Itsley A, Roberts J: Thermodilution cardiac output: A systematic error. Anesthesiol Intensive Care 9: 135–139, 1981
392. Russell J: Adding fuel to the fire: The supranormal oxygen delivery trials controversy. Crit Care Med 26: 981–983, 1998
393. Russo P: Comparison of Central Venous Pressures Through the Three Ports of the Triple Lumen Catheter. Unpublished thesis, University of Texas Health Science Center at Houston, Houston, Texas, 1991
394. Rutherford E, Morris J, Reeds G et al: Base deficit stratifies mortality and determines therapy. J Trauma 33: 417–423, 1992
395. Rutten AJ, Nancarrow C, Ilsley AH et al: An assessment of six different pulmonary artery catheters. Crit Care Med 15 : 250–255, 1987
396. Ryan M, Far Y, Lee T et al: Comparison of continuous vs. manual bolus cardiac output following hemodynamic alterations in a porcine model (Abstract). Anesthesiology 79: A469, 1993
397. Saadjian A, Cassot F, Torresani J: Relationship of pulmonary diastolic and pulmonary wedge pressures to left ventricular diastolic pressures: Role of acute myocardial infarction localization. Cardiology 67: 148–163, 1981
398. Sageman W, Amundson D: Thoracic electrical bioimpedance measurement of cardiac output in postaortocoronary bypass patients. Crit Care Med 21: 1139–1142, 1993
399. Sarnoff SJ: Myocardial contractility as described by ventricular function curves: Observations on Starling's Law of the Heart. Physiol Rev 35: 107–122, 1955
400. Sasse S, Chen P, Berry R et al: Variability of cardiac output over time in medical intensive care unit patients. Crit Care Med 22: 225–232, 1994
401. Scheinman M, Evans G, Weiss A et al: Relationship between pulmonary artery end-diastolic pressure and left ventricular filling pressure in patients in shock. Circulation 47: 317–324, 1973
402. Scher A, Feigl E: The heart: Introduction and physical principles. In Patton H, Fuchs A, Hille B et al (eds): Textbook of Physiology, Vol 2, 21st ed, pp 771–781. Philadelphia, WB Saunders, 1989
403. Schmitt E, Brantigan C: Common artifacts of pulmonary artery and pulmonary artery wedge pressures: Recognition and interpretation. J Clin Monit 2: 44–52, 1986
404. Schriner D: Using hemodynamic waveforms to assess cardiopulmonary pathologies. Crit Care Clin North Am 3: 563–575, 1989
405. Scott S, Guiliano K, Pysznik E et al: Influence of port site on central venous pressure measurements from triple-lumen catheters in critically ill adults. Am J Crit Care 7 : 60–63, 1998
406. Seneff M: Arterial line placement and care. In Rippe J, Fink M, Cerra F (eds): Procedures and Techniques in Intensive Care Medicine, pp 36–47. Boston, Little, Brown, 1995

407. Shah P, Maddahi J, Staniloff H et al: Variable spectrum and prognostic implications of left and right ventricular ejection fraction in patients with and without clinical heart failure after acute myocardial infarction. Am J Cardiol 58: 387–393, 1986

408. Sharkey S: Beyond the wedge: Clinical physiology and the Swan-Ganz catheter. Am J Med 83: 111–122, 1987

409. Shasby D, Dauber I, Pfister S et al: Swan-Ganz catheter location and left atrial pressure determine the accuracy of wedge pressure when positive end-expiratory pressure is used. Chest 80: 666–670, 1981

410. Shellock F, Riedinger M: Reproducibility and accuracy of using room temperature versus ice temperature injectate for thermodilution cardiac output determination. Heart Lung 12: 175–176, 1983

411. Shellock F, Riedinger M, Bateman T et al: Thermodilution cardiac output determination in hypothermic post cardiac surgery patients: Room versus ice temperature injection. Crit Care Med 11: 668–670, 1983

412. Shibutani K, Komatsu T, Kubal K et al: Critical level of oxygen delivery in anesthetized man. Crit Care Med 11: 640–643, 1983

413. Shinn J, Woods S, Huseby J: Effect of intermittent positive pressure ventilation upon pulmonary artery and pulmonary capillary wedge pressures in acutely ill patients. Heart Lung 8: 322–327, 1972

414. Shively M: Effect of position change on mixed venous oxygen saturation in coronary artery bypass surgery patients. Heart Lung 17: 51–59, 1988

415. Shoemaker W, Appel H, Kram H: Tissue oxygen debt as a determinant of lethal and nonlethal postoperative organ failure. Crit Care Med 16: 1117–1120, 1988

416. Shoemaker W, Appel P, Kram H: Role of oxygen debt in the development of organ failure sepsis and death in high risk surgical patients. Chest 102: 208–215, 1992

417. Shoemaker W, Appel P, Kram H et al: Multicomponent noninvasive physiologic monitoring of circulatory function. Crit Care Med 16: 482, 1988

418. Shoemaker W, Appel P, Kram H et al: Sequence of physiologic patterns in surgical septic shock. Crit Care Med 21: 1876, 1992

419. Shoemaker W, Wo C, Bishop M et al: Multicenter trial of a new thoracic electrical bioimpedance device for cardiac output estimation. Crit Care Med 22: 1907–1912, 1994

420. Sibbald W, Driedger A, Myers M et al: Biventricular function in the adult respiratory distress syndrome: Hemodynamic and radionuclide assessment with special emphasis on right ventricular function. Chest 84: 126–134, 1983

421. Sibbald W, Eberhard J, Inman K et al: New technologies, critical care, and economic realities. Crit Care Med 21: 1777–1780, 1993

422. Siegel L, Fitzgerald D, Engstrom R: Simultaneous intraoperative measurement of cardiac output by thermodilution and transtracheal Doppler. Anesthesiology 74: 664–669, 1991

423. Siegel L, Hennessey M, Pearl R: Delayed time response of the continuous cardiac output pulmonary artery catheter. Anesthesia Analgesia 83: 1173–1177, 1996

424. Siegel L, Shafer S, Martinez G et al: Simultaneous measurements of cardiac output by thermodilution, esophageal Doppler, and electrical impedance in anesthetized patients. J Cardiothorac Anesth 2: 590–595, 1988

425. Silver M, Jubran H, Stein S et al: Evaluation of a new blood-conserving arterial line system for patients in intensive care units. Crit Care Med 21: 507, 1993

426. Silverman H, Eppler J, Pitman A et al: Measurements of pulmonary capillary wedge pressure from graphic and digital recorders. Chest 86: 335, 1984

427. Simkus G, Fitchett D: Radial arterial pressure may be a poor guide to the beneficial effects of nitroprusside on left ventricular systolic pressure in congestive heart failure. Am J Cardiol 66: 323–326, 1990

428. Singh R, Ranieri A, Vest H et al: Simultaneous determinations of cardiac output by thermodilution, fiberoptic and dye-dilution methods. Am J Cardiol 25: 579–587, 1970

429. Sladen A: Complications of invasive hemodynamic monitoring in the intensive care unit. Curr Probl Surg 25: 74–145, 1988

430. Snell R, Calvin J: Cardiogenic shock: Pathophysiology, management, and treatment. In Edwards J, Shoemaker W, Vincent J-L (eds): Oxygen Transport: Principles and Practice, pp 246–273. Philadelphia, WB Saunders, 1993

431. Sommers M, Stevenson J, Hamlin R: Mixed venous oxygen saturation and oxygen partial pressure as predictors of cardiac index after coronary artery bypass grafting. Heart Lung 22: 112–120, 1993

432. Sommers M, Woods S, Courtade M: Issues in methods and measurement of thermodilution cardiac output. Nurs Res 42: 228–233, 1993

433. Spackman T, Abenstein J: Continuous cardiac output may be more accurate than bolus thermodilution output during the use of an upper-body warming blanket (Abstract). Anesthesiology 79: A473, 1993

434. Sperinde J, Senelly K: The Oximetrix Opticath oximetry system: Theory and development. In Fahey P (ed): Continuous Measurement of Blood Oxygen Saturation in High-Risk Patient, pp 81–89. Mountain View, CA, Abbott Critical Care Systems, 1987

435. Spinale F, Hendrick D, Crawford F et al: Relationship between bioimpedance thermodilution and ventriculographic measurements in experimental congestive heart failure. Cardiovasc Res 24: 423–429, 1990

436. Spinale F, Mukherjee R, Tanaka R et al: The effects of valvular regurgitation on thermodilution ejection fraction measurements. Chest 101: 723–731, 1992

437. Spodick D: Kussmaul's sign. N Engl J Med 293: 1047–1048, 1975

438. Sprung C, Esler B, Schein R: Risk of right bundle branch and complete heart block during pulmonary artery catheterization. Crit Care Med 17: 1–3, 1989

439. Sprung C, Marcia E, Garcia A et al: Prophylactic use of lidocaine to prevent advanced ventricular arrhythmias during pulmonary artery catheterization. Am J Med 75: 906–910, 1983

440. Sprung C, Pozen R, Rozanski J et al: Advanced ventricular arrhythmias during bedside pulmonary artery catheterization. Am J Med 72: 203–208, 1982

441. Steingrub J, Celoria G, Vickers-Lahti M et al: Therapeutic impact of pulmonary artery catheterization in a medical/surgical ICU. Chest 99: 1451, 1991

442. Steltzer H, Hiesmayr M, Mayer N et al: The relationship between oxygen delivery and uptake in critically ill: Is there a critical or optimal therapeutic value? Anaesthesia 49: 229–236, 1994

443. Stetz C, Miller R, Kelly G et al: Reliability of the thermodilution method in the determination of cardiac output in clinical practice. Am Rev Respir Dis 126: 1001–2D1004, 1982

444. Stewart G: Research on the circulation time and on the influences which affect it: IV. The output of the heart. J Physiol (Lond) 22: 159, 1897

445. Stites S, Barnes J, Overman J et al: Impact of injection technique on variability in thermodilution cardiac output (Abstract). Crit Care Med 26 (1 Suppl): A67, 1998

446. Sunimoto T, Takayama Y, Iwasaka T et al: Mixed venous oxygen saturation as a guide to tissue oxygenation and prognosis in patients with acute myocardial infarction. Am Heart J 122: 27–33, 1991

447. Swan H: Monitoring the Seriously Ill Patient with Heart Disease (Including Use of Swan-Ganz Catheter), Vol 2, 7th ed, pp 2072–2077. New York, McGraw-Hill, 1990

448. Swan H: The role of hemodynamic monitoring in the management of the critically ill. Crit Care Med 3: 83–89, 1975

449. Swan H, Ganz W: Use of balloon flotation catheters in critically ill patients. Surg Clin North Am 55: 501–520, 1975

450. Swan H, Ganz W, Forrester W et al: Catheterization of the heart in man with use of a flow-directed balloon-tipped catheter. N Engl J Med 283: 447–451, 1970

451. Swan H, Ganz W: Complications of flow-directed balloon–tipped catheters (Editorial). Ann Intern Med 91: 494, 1979

452. Swinney R, Davenport M, Wagers P et al: Iced versus room temperature injectate for thermodilution cardiac output (Abstract). Crit Care Med 8: 265, 1980

453. Tajiri J, Katsuya H, Okamoto K et al: The effects of respiratory cycle by mechanical ventilation on cardiac output measured using the thermodilution method. Jpn Circ J 48: 328–330, 1984

454. Takala J, Uusaro A, Parvianen I et al: Lactate metabolism and regional lactate exchange after cardiac surgery. New Horizons 4: 483–492, 1996

455. Taylor D, Gutierrez G: Tonometry: A review of clinical studies. Crit Care Clin 12: 1007–1018, 1996

456. Teboul J, Besbes M, Axler D et al: A bedside index for determination of zone III condition of pulmonary artery (PA) catheters tips during mechanical ventilation (Abstract). Am Rev Respir Dis 137: A137, 1988

457. Teboul J-L: Therapy: The effects of vasoactive drugs. In Edwards J, Shoemaker W, Vincent J-L (eds): Oxygen Transport: Principles and Practice, pp 193–208. Philadelphia, WB Saunders, 1993

458. Templin K, Shively M, Riley J: Accuracy of drawing coagulation studies from heparinized arterial lines. Am J Crit Care 2: 88–95, 1993

459. Thangathurai D, Charbonnet C, Roessler P et al: Continuous intraoperative noninvasive cardiac output monitoring using a new thoracic bioimpedance device. J Cardiothorac Vasc Anesth 11: 440–444, 1997

460. Thomas A, Ryan J, Doran B et al: Bioimpedance versus thermodilution cardiac output measurement: The Biomed NCCOM3 after coronary artery bypass surgery. Intensive Care Med 17: 383–386, 1991

461. Thrush D, Downs J, Smith R: Continuous thermodilution cardiac output: Agreement with Fick and bolus thermodilution methods. J Cardiothorac Vasc Anesth 9: 399–404, 1995

462. Tidwell SL, Ryan WJ, Osguthorpe SG et al: Effects of position changes on mixed venous oxygen saturation in patients after coronary revascularization. Heart Lung 19: 574–578, 1990

463. Tooker J, Huseby J, Butler J: The effect of Swan-Ganz catheter height on the wedge pressure-left atrial pressure relationship in edema during positive-pressure ventilation. Am Rev Respir Dis 117: 721–725, 1978

464. Tuchschmidt J, Fried J, Astiz M et al: Elevation of cardiac output and oxygen delivery improves outcome in septic shock. Chest 102: 216–220, 1992

465. Tuchschmidt J, Fried J, Swinney R et al: Early hemodynamic correlates of survival in patients with septic shock. Crit Care Med 17: 719–723, 1989

466. Tuman K, Carroll G, Ivankovich A: Pitfalls in interpretation of pulmonary artery catheter data. J Cardiothorac Anesth 3: 625–641, 1989

467. Urban N: Integrating the hemodynamic profile with clinical assessment. AACN Clin Issues Crit Care Nurs 4: 161–179, 1993

468. Urschel J, Myerowitz P: Catheter-induced pulmonary artery rupture in the setting of cardiopulmonary bypass. Ann Thorac Surg 56: 585–589, 1993

469. van der Linen P, Vincent J-L: The effect of sedative drugs. In Edwards J, Shoemaker W, Vincent J-L (eds): Oxygen Transport: Principles and Practice, pp 209–225. Philadelphia, WB Saunders, 1993

470. van der Meer B, Woltjer H, Sousman A et al: Impedance cardiography: Importance of the equation of the electrode configuration. Intensive Care Med 22: 1120–1124, 1996

471. VanEtta D, Gibbons E, Woods S: Estimation of left atrial location in supine and 30° lateral position. Am J Crit Care 2: 264, 1993

472. VanEtta DJ: Location of the Left Atrium in Thirty-Degree Right- and Thirty-Degree Left Lateral Recumbency in Adults. Unpublished thesis, University of Washington, Seattle, Washington, 1992

473. Varon A: Arterial, central venous, and pulmonary artery catheters. In Civetta J, Taylor R, Kirby R (eds): Critical Care, pp 847–865. Philadelphia, Lippincott–Raven, 1997

474. Vaughn S, Puri V: Cardiac output changes and continuous mixed venous oxygen saturation measurement in critically ill. Crit Care Med 16: 495–498, 1988

475. Vedrinne C, Bastien O, De Varax R et al: Predictive factors for usefulness of fiberoptic pulmonary artery catheter for continuous oxygen saturation in mixed venous blood monitoring in cardiac surgery. Anesth Analg 85: 2–10, 1997

476. Vennix C, Nelson D, Pierpont G: Thermodilution cardiac output in critically ill patients: Comparison of room-temperature and iced injectate. Heart Lung 13: 574–578, 1984

477. Venus B, Mathru M, Smith R et al: Direct versus indirect blood pressure measurements in critically ill patients. Heart Lung 14: 228–231, 1985

478. Versprille A: Reliability of cardiac output estimation by thermodilution (Correspondence). Intensive Care Med 15: 144, 1989

479. Vincent J, Dufaye P, Berre J et al: Serum lactate determination during circulatory shock. Crit Care Med 11: 449–451, 1983

480. Vincent J-L, Thirion M, Brimioulle S et al: Thermodilution measurement of right ventricular ejection fraction with a modified pulmonary artery catheter. Intensive Care Med 12: 33–38, 1986

481. Wadas T: Pulmonary artery catheter removal. Crit Care Nurs 14: 62–72, 1994

482. Wagner J, Leatherman J: Monitoring preload in the ICU: End-diastolic volume or wedge? Chest 113: 1048–1054, 1998

483. Wallace D, Winslow E: Effects of iced and room-temperature injectate on cardiac output measurements in critically ill patients with low and high cardiac outputs. Heart Lung 22: 55–63, 1993

484. Walther S, Domino K, Glenny R et al: Pulmonary blood flow distribution has a hilar-to-peripheral gradient in awake, prone sheep. J Appl Physiol 82: 678–685, 1997

485. Wang X, Sun H, Adamson D et al: Hemodynamic monitoring by impedance cardiography with an improved signal processing technique. Proceedings IEEE Engineering in Medicine and Biology 15: 699–700, 1993

486. Ward M, Magder S, Hussain S: Oxygen delivery: Independent effect of blood flow on diaphragm fatigue. American Review of Respiratory Disease 145: 1058–1063, 1992

487. Weber J, Janicki J, Shroff S et al: The right ventricle: Physiologic and pathophysiologic considerations. Crit Care Med 11: 323–328, 1983

488. Weil M: Measurement of cardiac output. Crit Care Med 5: 117–119, 1977

489. Weissman C, Kemper M, Damask M et al: Effect of routine intensive care interactions on metabolic rate. Chest 86: 815–818, 1984

490. West J, Dollery C, Naimark A: Distribution of blood flow in isolated lung; relation to vascular and alveolar pressures. J Appl Physiol 19: 713–724, 1964

491. Westerhof N, O'Rourke M: Haemodynamic basis for the development of left ventricular failure in systolic hypertension and for its logical therapy. J Hypertens 13: 943–952, 1995

492. Wetzel R, Larson W: Major errors in the thermodilution cardiac output measurements during rapid volume infusion. Anesthesiology 62: 684–687, 1985

493. White K: Using continuous SVO$_2$ to assess oxygen supply/demand balance in the critically ill patient. AACN Clin Issues Crit Care Nurs 4: 134–147, 1993

494. Whitman G: Comparison of pulmonary artery catheter measurements in 20° right and left lateral recumbent positions. In American Association of Critical-Care Nurses International Intensive Care Nursing Conference, 1982, London, 1982

495. Whitman G, Verga T: Comparison of cardiac output measurements in 20-degree supine and 20-degree right and left lateral recumbent positions. Heart Lung 11: 256–257, 1982

496. Whitney J: The measurement of oxygen tension in tissue. Nurs Res 39: 203–205, 1990

497. Wiedemann H, Matthay M, Matthay R: Cardiovascular pulmonary monitoring in the intensive care unit (Part 2). Chest 85: 656–668, 1984

498. Wiedemann H, Matthay M, Matthay R: Cardiovascular-pulmonary monitoring in the intensive care unit (Part 1). Chest 85: 537–549, 1984

499. Wild L: Effect of lateral recumbent positions on measurement of pulmonary artery and pulmonary artery wedge pressures in critically ill adults. Heart Lung 13: 305, 1983

500. Wild L: Effect of Lateral Recumbent Positions on Measurements of Pulmonary Artery and Pulmonary Artery Wedge Pressures in Critically Ill Adults. Unpublished thesis, University of Washington, Seattle, Washington, 1983

501. Wild L, Woods S: Comparison of three methods for interpreting pulmonary artery wedge pressure waveforms with respiratory variation. Heart Lung 14: 308–309, 1985

502. Wilson R, Beckman B, Tyburski J et al: Pulmonary artery diastolic and wedge pressure relationship in critically ill and injured patients. Arch Surg 123: 933–936, 1988

503. Winslow EH, Clark AP, White KM et al: Effect of a lateral turn on mixed venous oxygen saturation and heart rate in critically ill adults. Heart Lung 19: 557–561, 1990

504. Winsor T, Burch G: Phlebostatic level: Reference level for venous pressure measurement in man. Proc Soc Exp Biol Med 58: 165–169, 1945

505. Wong D, Tremper K, Stemmer E et al: Noninvasive cardiac output: Simultaneous comparison of two different methods with thermodilution. Anesthesiology 72: 784–792, 1990

506. Woo M, Stevenson L, Vredevoe D: Comparison of thermodilution and transthoracic electrical bioimpedance cardiac outputs. Heart Lung 20: 357–362, 1991

507. Woods S: Monitoring pulmonary artery pressures. Am J Nurs 76: 1765–1771, 1976

508. Woods S, Grose B, Laurent-Bopp D: Effect of backrest position on pulmonary artery pressures in critically ill patients. Cardiovas Nurs 18 (4): 19–24, 1982

509. Woods S, Mansfield L: Effect of body position upon pulmonary artery pulmonary capillary wedge pressures in noncritically ill patients. Heart Lung 5: 83–90, 1976

510. Woods S, Osguthorpe S: Cardiac output determinations. AACN Clin Issues Crit Care Nursing 4: 81–97, 1993

511. Woog R, McWilliam D: A comparison of methods of cardiac output measurement. Anesth Intensive Care 11: 141–146, 1983

512. Yaginuma T, O'Rourke M: Modification of wave travel and reflection by vasodilator therapy. In O'Rourke M, Safar M, Dzau V (eds): Arterial Vasodilation, pp 50–61. Philadelphia, Lea & Febiger, 1993

513. Yang S, Bentivoglio L, Maranhao V et al (eds): From Cardiac Catheterization Data to Hemodynamic Parameters, 3rd ed. Philadelphia, FA Davis, 1988

514. Yelderman M: Continuous cardiac output by thermodilution. Int Anesthesiol Clin 31: 127–140, 1993

515. Yelderman M: Continuous measurement of cardiac output with the use of stochastic identification techniques. Journal of Clinical Monitoring 6: 322–332, 1990

516. Yelderman M, Quinn M, McKown R: Continuous thermodilution cardiac output measurement in sheep. J Thorac Cardiovasc Surg 104: 315–320, 1992

517. Yelderman M, Quinn M, McKown R: Thermal safety of a filamented pulmonary artery catheter. Journal of Clinical Monitoring 8: 147–149, 1992

518. Yelderman M, Ramsay M, Quinn M et al: Continuous thermodilution cardiac output measurement in intensive care unit patient. J Cardiothorac Vasc Anesth 6: 270–274, 1992

519. Young J, McQuillan P: Comparison of thoracic electrical bioimpedance and thermodilution for the measurement of cardiac index in patients with severe sepsis. Br J Anaesth 70: 58–62, 1993

520. Yu M, Burchell S, Hasaniya N et al: Relationship of mortality to increasing oxygen delivery in patients > 50 years of age: A prospective randomized trial. Crit Care Med 21 1011–1019, 1998

521. Yu M, Levy M, Smith P et al: Effect of maximizing oxygen delivery on morbidity and mortality rates in critically ill patients: A prospective randomized controlled study. Crit Care Med 21: 830–838, 1993

522. Ziegler D, Wright J, Choban P et al: A prospective randomized trial of preoperative "optimization" of cardiac function in patients undergoing elective peripheral vascular surgery. Surgery 122: 584–592, 1997

Treatment of
Heart Disease

20

Myocardial Ischemia and Infarction

SUSANNA CUNNINGHAM
SHERRI DEL BENE
ANNE FALSONE VAUGHAN

PATHOGENESIS OF ATHEROSCLEROSIS

This chapter is divided into four parts: pathogenesis of atherosclerosis; pathophysiology of myocardial ischemia and infarction; diagnosis and management of myocardial ischemia; and diagnosis and management of myocardial infarction. The reader is referred to other chapters for specifics of anatomy, physiology, assessment, treatment, and complications.

The literature contains several terms describing diseases of the arterial wall; there is confusion concerning two terms in particular: arteriosclerosis and atherosclerosis. Some definitions are given later, but the reader needs to determine how each author is using a term because these words are used inconsistently.

Arteriosclerosis means "hardening of the arteries" and is a general term describing three diseases:

1. Atherosclerosis, in which there is a proliferation of smooth muscle cells and accumulation of lipids in the intima of the large and middle-sized muscular arteries
2. Medical calcific sclerosis, or Mönckeberg's sclerosis, in which there is an accumulation of calcium in the media of medium-sized arteries
3. Arteriolar sclerosis, in which there is thickening of the walls and narrowing of the lumen of the small arteries and arterioles, and which is often associated with hypertension

Ischemic heart disease is the most frequent cause of death in the United States and Western Europe, and is projected to be the major cause of death worldwide by 2020. It is an arterial disease, with atherosclerotic plaques most commonly occurring in the aorta and the coronary, cerebral, femoral, and other large or middle-sized arteries. Although infarctions can occur in any organ, myocardial and cerebral infarction (cerebrovascular accident) are two of the major consequences of the disease. Other sequelae of atherosclerotic disease include angina pectoris, heart failure, sudden cardiac arrest, renal failure, and peripheral vascular disease. The occurrence of signs and symptoms related to atherosclerosis is a consequence of two interrelated processes: atherogenesis and thrombogenesis.

The incidence of atherosclerosis increases with age. The major modifiable risk factors are high blood pressure, dyslipidemia, cigarette smoking, and a sedentary lifestyle. Other risk factors include family history/genetics, diabetes mellitus, obesity, hyperhomocysteinemia, infections, and sex. Before the pathogenesis of atherosclerosis is discussed, the morphology of the normal artery and the atherosclerotic lesion are reviewed and the constituents of atherosclerotic plaque are described.

The progress of molecular biology is transforming our understanding of the atherosclerotic process at an astonishing rate. Scientists are exploring the relationships between hundreds of signaling molecules, receptors, coagulation factors, fibrinolytic factors, adhesion molecules, inflammatory and immune cytokines, cell types, and genes. The following discussion summarizes some of this progress and sets the stage for further exploration of the literature by the reader. Research indicates that there are subtle differences between vascular beds in an individual, so the development of atherosclerosis may be somewhat different in different parts of the vasculature.

MORPHOLOGY OF THE NORMAL ARTERIAL WALL

The walls of musculoelastic arteries contain three layers: the intima, the media, and the adventitia (See Figure 2–2). The *intima* is defined as the part of the arterial wall between the lumen and the internal elastic lamina. The three layers of the intima are a layer of endothelial cells; a layer of proteoglycans that contains occasional macrophages and smooth muscle cells; and a musculoelastic layer of smooth muscle cells, elastic fibers, and collagen. Waltner-Romen and colleagues have reported finding T cells, dendritic cells, and mast cells in the intima of children younger than 10 years of age; they are probably also present in adults. The internal elastic lamina, a continuous layer of elastic fibers that marks the boundary between the intima and media, is absent in some vessels, especially in areas where an artery divides (bifurcations). The thickness and exact composition of the intima varies throughout the vasculature. Some thickening of the intima is considered a normal adaptation to mechanical stress and is called either *eccentric* or *diffuse* intimal thickening depending on its distribution in the vessel. Oxygen and nutrients diffuse into the intima from the vessel lumen.

The *media* is mainly smooth muscle cells and extracellular matrix consisting of collagen, elastin, and proteoglycans. The smooth muscle cells have two phenotypes: the contractile phenotype and the synthetic phenotype. The contractile smooth muscle cells contain mainly myofibrils and are involved in regulating vessel diameter, whereas the synthetic smooth muscle cells synthesize the molecules of the extracellular matrix. In the elastic arteries, the media contains multiple layers of elastin known as elastic lamellae.

The *adventitia* is separated from the media by a discontinuous boundary of elastic fibers, the external elastic lamina. The adventitia contains fibroblasts, bundles of collagen fibrils, and elastic fibers along with a few smooth muscle cells. It is well supplied with nerves, lymphatic vessels, and its own blood vessels, the vasa vasorum. In larger arteries, the vasa vasorum extend into the media.

CELLULAR, STRUCTURAL, AND MOLECULAR COMPONENTS OF ATHEROSCLEROTIC PLAQUES

The principal cell types involved in atherosclerosis are endothelial cells, smooth muscle cells, monocyte–macrophages, T cells, and platelets. Extracellular matrix also accumulates within the atherosclerotic plaque. The vasa vasorum supply blood to the walls of larger arteries and have been shown to infiltrate advanced atherosclerotic lesions. A variety of growth factors, cytokines, chemokines, and other molecules (lipids and nitric oxide) have been implicated in plaque development.

Endothelial Cells

The dynamic nature of endothelial cells is increasingly appreciated, and some scientists even consider the endothelium to be the body's largest organ. The endothelium regulates the two-way movement of cells and macromolecules between the blood and tissues; the balance between coagulation and fibrinolysis of the blood; vasomotion or the balance between constriction and dilation; and growth or apoptosis of vascular wall components. Endothelial cells also act as transducers of the mechanical forces within the vasculature. To accomplish these roles, an endothelial cell is continuously up- and downregulating the expression of sur-

face receptors as well as the tightness of the links between adjacent cells. Endothelial cells also secrete components of the extracellular matrix below them, and they release molecules such as von Willebrand factor into the plasma.

Data have been accumulating that indicate the endothelium is dysfunctional in atherosclerosis. For example, rather than promoting the balance between coagulation and fibrinolysis, the endothelium in atherosclerotic areas becomes prothrombotic. Under normal circumstances, tissue factor (the molecule that initiates coagulation in conjunction with activated factor VII) is not expressed on the luminal surface on endothelial cells. However, the endothelium above areas of atherosclerosis does express tissue factor. In addition, the dysfunctional endothelium expresses surface adhesion receptors for monocytes but not neutrophils. During the first 24 hours after tissue injury in normal epithelium, the epithelial cells express receptors that bind neutrophils, and then, over subsequent days, receptors for monocytes are expressed. For reasons that are not yet understood, the dysfunctional endothelium attracts only monocytes. Although the adhesion receptors that attract these monocytes have not yet been positively identified, two candidates are vascular cell adhesion molecule-1 and fibronectin in association with the adhesion molecule β_1-integrin.

One common factor in endothelial dysfunction is minimally modified or oxidized low-density lipoprotein (LDL). As shown in Figure 20–1, entry of LDL into the arterial intima and its subsequent oxidation triggers the endothelial cell to express leukocyte adhesion molecules and release macrophage chemoattractant protein-1 (MCP-1). Research on rabbits indicates that these events occur within weeks after initiation of a high-cholesterol diet. Complement and immunoglobulins were also found in the plaque. Although the cellular results are difficult to confirm in humans, it is known that dietary and drug treatment of dyslipidemia result in improved endothelial function.

Vascular Smooth Muscle Cells

In the normal, mature artery, the primary role of vascular smooth muscle is to regulate vessel diameter by adjusting its state of contraction. If injury occurs, the vascular smooth muscle cell is capable of reversibly switching its phenotype from a contractile type to a synthetic type. The synthetic phenotype of the smooth muscle cell, which has fewer myofibrils and more rough endoplasmic reticulum, can produce constituents of the extracellular matrix such as collagens, elastic fiber proteins, and proteoglycans, as well as growth factors. The contractile and synthetic phenotypes are the opposite extremes of a range of phenotypes that smooth muscle cells can express. As shown in Figure 20–2, numerous environmental stimuli influence which specific phenotype a vascular smooth muscle cell may express in any given situation. In the embryo, vascular smooth muscle cells originate from both the mesoderm and the neuroectoderm, which raises the likelihood that all vascular smooth muscle does not have identical properties.

As atherosclerosis develops, there are two major changes associated with the vascular smooth muscle cells. First, smooth muscle cells migrate from the media through the internal elastic lamina into the subintima. Second, the

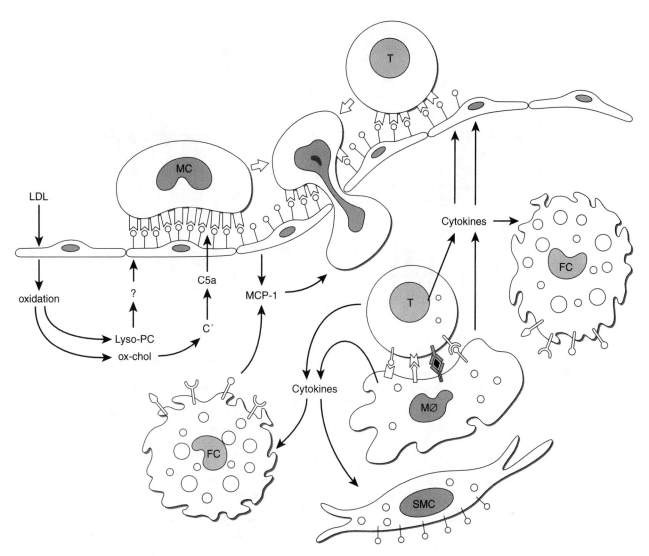

FIGURE 20-1 Postulated recruitment and activation of immunocompetent cells in the early atherosclerotic lesion. Endothelial cells are stimulated to express vascular cell adhesion molecules-1 (VCAM-1), possibly by lysophosphatidylcholine *(Lyso-PC)* or other components of low-density lipoprotein (LDL) oxidized in the intima. Monocytes *(MC)* or T lymphocytes *(T)* adhere to endothelial cells expressing VCAM-1 and other leukocyte adhesion molecules. They are stimulated chemotactically to enter the intima by C5a produced during complement activation *(C')*, which may also be secondary to LDL oxidation *(ox-chol*, oxidized cholesterol). The cytokine, macrophage chemoattractant protein-1 *(MCP-1)*, is another potent chemotactic agent that is produced locally in the atherosclerotic plaque. Antigen-specific T cells are activated by monocyte-derived macrophages *(MØ)* in the lesion. Both cell types produce cytokines that act on endothelial cells *(EC)*, smooth muscle cells *(SMC)*, macrophages, and foam cells *(FC)* to regulate adhesion molecule expression, chemotaxis, procoagulant activity, proliferation, contractility, and cholesterol uptake. In addition, *EC* and *SMC* release cytokines that act on both inflammatory and vascular cells. For the sake of simplicity, vascular-derived cytokines are not indicated in the figure. (From Hansson GK, Libby P: The role of the lymphocyte. In Fuster V, Ross R,Topol EJ [eds]: Atherosclerosis and Coronary Artery Disease, p 564, Philadelphia, Lippincott–Raven, 1996.)

cells switch from a contractile to a synthetic phenotype. It has been shown that these synthetic smooth muscle cells can secrete platelet-derived growth factor (PDGF) and fibroblast growth factor, as well as extracellular matrix. Secretion of both the extracellular matrix and the growth factors then contributes to further growth of the atherosclerotic plaque.

Monocytes—Macrophages

A macrophage is a monocyte that has left the lumen of the blood vessel by first attaching to adhesion molecules (selectins and integrins) on the luminal surface of endothelial cells and then by migrating between the endothelial cells to reach the site of an inflammatory response (extravasation).

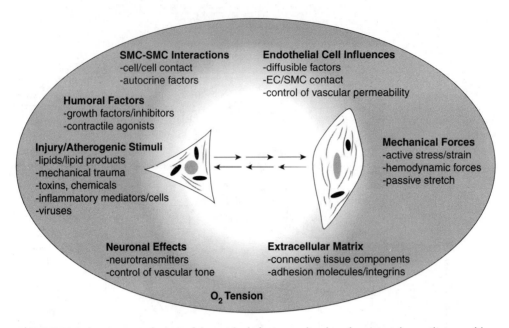

FIGURE 20-2 A summary of some of the extrinsic factors or local environmental cues that are either known or believed to be important in controlling the differentiation/maturation state of the vascular smooth muscle cell *(SMC)*. This figure emphasizes the point that differentiation/maturation of vascular smooth muscle cells depends on the complex interaction of a multitude of local environmental cues, not a single factor, and that a change in any one of these may lead to alterations in the differentiated state of the SMC (i.e., "phenotypic modulation"). Importantly, there appear to be a broad range of different phenotypes that can be exhibited by the SMC, depending on the nature of those environmental changes. This includes a spectrum of phenotypes ranging from the highly synthetic proliferative SMC **(left)** to the highly contractile, fully differentiated/mature SMC **(right)**. The multiple arrows connecting the two cell types are meant to illustrate the multiplicity of phenotypes that are available between these two extremes and the fact that changes appear to be reversible. It cannot be assumed that changes that occur during development are necessarily recapitulated during phenotypic modulation in response to injury, atherogenic stimuli, and the like, and for this reason, two separate pathways are shown between the two representative cell types rather than simply a single reversible pathway. (From Owens GK: Role of alterations in the differentiated state of vascular smooth muscle cells in atherogenesis. In Fuster V, Ross R, Topol EJ [eds]: Atherosclerosis and Coronary Artery Disease, p 409, Philadelphia, Lippincott-Raven, 1996.)

Both monocytes and endothelial cells require stimulation to express the adhesion molecules needed for extravasation. Once a monocyte has left the bloodstream, it alters its phenotype to become a macrophage. Macrophages are normal residents of the vascular media, but their numbers are markedly increased in areas of atherosclerosis. Macrophages are key players in the body's immune and inflammatory defenses against injury and infection. In defense situations, macrophages act as phagocytes, present antigen to lymphocytes, secrete a variety of cytokines, and coordinate wound healing after injury. Once an injury is repaired, macrophages leave the area or undergo apoptosis. Atherosclerotic plaques can be conceptualized as wounds that do not heal.

Macrophages are present in all stages of atherogenesis, from the fatty streak to the complicated lesion. Fatty streaks are mainly composed of lipid-filled macrophages or smooth muscle cells. Macrophages with a variety of phenotypes are found in plaque, which means that their activities are variable. In complicated lesions, activated macrophages are predominantly found in the "shoulder" regions of the plaque, those areas where the crescent-shaped atherosclerotic

lesions join the relatively unaffected portion of the vessel diameter (Fig. 20–3). Plaque rupture occurs most frequently at these shoulder regions, as discussed in the section on Stable and Vulnerable Plaque.

There is a circular relationship between oxidized LDL and macrophages in atherosclerotic plaque. Oxidized LDL in the vessel intima acts as a chemoattractant that brings macrophages to the area (see Fig. 20–1). Once inside the intima, the macrophages ingest the oxidized lipid using their scavenger receptors. This intake of lipid initiates the cell's transformation from a macrophage into a foam cell, a key component of atherosclerotic lesions. Macrophages in their capacity as phagocytes release oxidizing agents that increase the conversion of LDL to oxidized LDL. LDL movement into the intima is increased in people with hypercholesterolemia. Macrophages along with the endothelial cells and smooth muscle cells produce the chemokine MCP-1, a powerful factor that increases monocyte extravasation into the atherosclerotic lesion.

Macrophages produce enzymes called matrix metalloproteinases (MMPs) that digest extracellular matrix con-

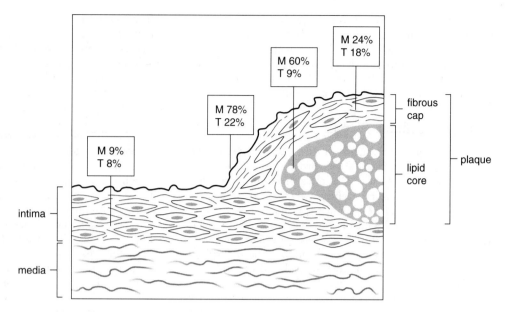

FIGURE 20-3 Monocyte-derived macrophages *(M)* and T lymphocytes *(T)* in an advanced atherosclerotic plaque. Values are expressed as percentages of total cells in different regions of the plaque and are based on immunohistochemical analyses of endarterectomy specimens (Reprinted from Hansson et al: T lymphocytes inhibit the vascular response to injury. *Proc Natl Acad Sci* U S A 88: 10530-10534, 1991, with permission of the American Heart Association.)

stituents such as collagen, proteoglycans, and elastin. One MMP, stromelysin-3, has been found in advanced plaques but not normal arteries or fatty streaks. When macrophages are participating in infection control and wound healing, the MMPs help in the removal of damaged tissue and facilitate the growth of new blood vessels and tissue. In normal tissue repair, the actions of these enzymes are limited to the injury site by substances called tissue inhibitors of metalloproteinases (TIMPs). In the atherosclerotic plaque, however, the MMP enzymes are thought to be harmful because they weaken the fibrotic cap of the atherosclerotic plaque, thus increasing the likelihood of plaque rupture. Studies have shown that exposing cultured macrophages to oxidized LDL causes increased production of MMPs but not TIMPs, thus predisposing the extracellular matrix to breakdown. It has also been shown that foam cells increase their surface expression of tissue factor, the molecule that activates the coagulation cascade.

Lymphocytes

Both helper (CD4+) and cytotoxic (CD8+) T lymphocytes are found in atherosclerotic plaques. The location and density of T cells in the wall of an atherosclerotic artery are shown in Figure 20–3 The antigens in the atherosclerotic plaque that activate both helper and cytotoxic T cells have not been identified. However, it is known that macrophages, endothelial cells, and smooth muscle cells in the plaque all express major histocompatibility class II proteins, which are also needed for helper T-cell activation. Under normal conditions, neither endothelial cells nor smooth muscle cells are capable of activating T cells. Although B cells are not commonly found in the atherosclerotic plaque, antibodies to oxidized LDL are found there. It is hypothesized that helper T cells migrate through the lymphatics from the atherosclerotic plaque to regional lymph nodes, where the B cells are activated and stimulated to produce antibodies. The precise role of lymphocytes in the development of atherosclerotic plaque is still not clear, but it is hoped that further understanding will be a step toward developing new therapeutic interventions.

Platelets

Platelets participate in both the atherosclerotic and thrombotic phases of atherosclerotic cardiovascular disease. Platelets are activated by some of the major cardiovascular risk factors, specifically hypercholesteremia and smoking. In arterial areas such as bifurcations and curved parts of vessels, the local decrease in shear stress may allow these activated platelets to adhere to the surface of the endothelium. Platelets also adhere to any areas of endothelial injury (see section on Theories of Atherosclerosis Pathogenesis, later). In tissue culture, platelets attach to endothelial cells and then stimulate them to release MCP-1 and express intracellular adhesion molecule-1 on their luminal surface. As a result of these activities, monocytes are attracted to the area and migrate into the vessel intima. Electron micrographs have shown that when monocytes migrate into the intima, they may be coated with activated platelets.

When platelets bind to the endothelium or enter the intima, the growth factors released when the platelets degranulate include PDGF, epidermal growth factor, transforming growth factor-α, a platelet-derived endothelial cell growth factor, transforming growth factor-β, and serotonin. These growth factors act as mitogens to stimulate the migration and proliferation of smooth muscle cells in the atherosclerotic plaque. Platelets also produce oxidizing agents that participate in converting LDL into an oxidized form that binds with the scavenger receptor on macrophages. Entry of oxidized LDL into the macrophages is one of the factors involved in the conversion of macrophages into foam cells. Conversely, it also has been shown that oxidized LDL activates platelets.

Platelets have a central role in the thrombotic phase of cardiovascular disease. This role has been confirmed by the success of both aspirin and blockers of the platelet glycoprotein IIb/IIIa receptor in preventing cardiovascular morbidity and mortality in patients with known atherosclerotic disease and after revascularization procedures.

The Extracellular Matrix

The four major components of the vascular extracellular matrix are collagen, elastic fibers, proteoglycans, and glycoproteins. In each of these categories there are several subtypes of macromolecules; each subtype may be expressed in a variety of forms. The components of the vascular extracellular matrix are important for two major reasons: they provide much of the strength, elasticity, flexibility, and compressibility of the blood vessels; and they have a role in regulating the adhesion, migration, proliferation, and activity of the cells in the vascular wall. The amounts and types of extracellular matrix macromolecules vary in different layers and regions of normal arteries. It is also clear that alterations in the expression of these macromolecules occur in atherosclerosis and in other vascular diseases such as Marfan's syndrome.

Of the 19 different types of collagen found in the human body, 6 (types I, II, IV, V, VI, and VIII) are found in the vascular extracellular matrix, with types I and III accounting for 89% to 90% of the total. Vascular smooth muscle cells make the collagens of the intima and media. In atherosclerosis there is an increase in the production of type I collagen, which binds both normal and oxidized LDL. With plaque rupture, exposure of the blood to the collagen is one of the factors that activates platelets and initiates thrombosis.

Vascular smooth muscle cells produce elastic fibers mainly during fetal development and in early childhood, with very little produced in adulthood. The largest amounts of elastic fibers are found in large arteries such as the aorta, where they have an important role in transforming the pulsatile blood flow produced by the pumping action of the heart into the smoother blood flow supplied to the body tissues. With atherosclerosis, elastic fiber is both lost and fragmented, probably because of the action of the MMPs such as stromelysin and gelatinase B. It has also been observed that the elastic fibers in atherosclerotic plaque bind lipid and calcium. These changes in the elastic fibers all contribute to the increased stiffness of atherosclerotic arteries.

Proteoglycans are long polymers of disaccharides (sugars) attached to a core of glycoprotein, except for hyaluronan (formerly known as hyaluronic acid), which does not have a core glycoprotein. These proteoglycans provide turgor and viscoelasticity to the vessel walls. Proteoglycans have been reclassified, so names that the reader may recognize, such as chondroitin sulfate, heparan sulfate, keratan, sulfate, and dermatan sulfate, have been replaced with names such as versican, decorin, biglycan, lumican, and perlecan. The proteoglycan macromolecules are synthesized by vascular smooth muscle cells and endothelial cells under normal circumstances, but can also be produced by cells from the blood (mast cells, lymphocytes, and monocytes) that have moved into the arterial wall. It has been found that, as monocytes differentiate into macrophages with the atherosclerotic plaque, they increase their production of proteoglycans. As atherosclerosis develops, the amount and distribution of proteoglycans change. Lipoproteins that bind to proteoglycans also are more likely to be oxidized and be engulfed by macrophages.

The five major glycoproteins of the vascular wall are osteopontin, tenascin, laminin, fibronectin, and thrombospondin. The glycoproteins provide a framework to which the vascular cells attach and on which the cells can move. In addition, the glycoproteins play a role in regulating the integrity of the extracellular matrix itself and can influence the phenotypes expressed by vascular smooth muscle. Although it is not clear what role most of the glycoproteins have in atherosclerosis, it is known that osteopontin is present only in atherosclerotic vessels, where it is produced by both vascular smooth muscle and by endothelial cells. Osteopontin is a chemotactic agent that attracts smooth muscle cells; it may also have a role in the calcification of advanced atherosclerotic lesions.

Vasa Vasorum

In 1981, Heistad hypothesized that because atherosclerosis thickens the intima, it would not be possible for the media to obtain its oxygen supply from the lumen by diffusion, and therefore the density of the vasa vasorum may be increased. Studying normal and atherosclerotic cynomolgus monkeys, Heistad and colleagues found blood flow in the vasa vasorum was increased three to eight times greater than normal in atherosclerotic aortas. These researchers later demonstrated that if atherosclerotic monkeys were fed a low-fat diet there was regression of the atherosclerosis and a loss of the vasa vasorum. The density of the vasa vasorum is also increased in atherosclerotic coronary arteries. Areas of atherosclerotic plaque have been shown to become vascularized, with most of the new vessels coming from the vasa vasorum in the adventitia. Other work has found dendritic cells (cells derived from macrophages that present antigen to T cells) associated with the adventitial vasa vasorum. In larger arteries, the vasa vasorum may contribute to the hemorrhage and thrombosis associated with unstable or vulnerable plaques.

Growth Factors and Cytokines

Cells communicate by releasing and binding a variety of molecules. Several classes of these molecules—cytokines, interleukins, growth factors, and others—play important roles in the development and progression of atherosclerotic plaque. The activity of these molecules depends both on their local concentration and on the number of receptors for that molecule expressed on the surface of the cell being influenced. To simplify the multiple factors involved in both normal arteries and atherosclerotic plaques, it helps to consider the various categories of agents. These categories are chemokines, growth factors (mitogens), vasoactive substances, cytokines, procoagulant and anticoagulant factors, and enzymes (MMPs). Because these molecules are often pleiotropic (have more than one function), it is possible that any given molecule may be included in several categories.

Some of the chemokines known to play a role in attracting monocytes and T cells to areas where fatty streaks and plaques develop are oxidized LDL, MCP-1, osteopontin, pulmonary and activation-regulated chemokine, and EBI1-ligand chemokine. Chemokines are secreted by activated endothelial cells, smooth muscle cells, and macrophages. PDGF acts as a chemokine to attract vascular smooth muscle cells to migrate from the media to the intima of vessels. Elevated serum levels of PDGF have been found in patients with hypercholesterolemia, and lipoprotein(a) can induce endothelial cells to secrete MCP-1.

Growth factors are molecules that can either stimulate or inhibit cell proliferation. Another term for factors that stimulate cell growth is *mitogen*. Both the growth-regulatory molecules and their receptors are tightly but independently regulated. Some of the molecules that are potentially important in cell proliferation include PDGF, MCP-1, basic fibroblast growth factor, insulin-like growth factor-1, macrophage colony-stimulating factor, granulocyte–macrophage colony-stimulating factor, interleukin-1 (IL-1), tumor necrosis factor-α (TNF-α), and TNF-β. These growth factors that induce the proliferation of smooth muscle cells, macrophages, and T cells usually are not expressed in the normal artery; however, they are upregulated in atherosclerosis.

Many of the major risk factors for atherosclerotic cardiovascular disease influence the release of vasoactive molecules by the endothelium. Nitric oxide is a major vasoactive agent produced by the endothelium, although many of the molecules discussed in this section also have vasoactive properties. In addition, many circulating vasoactive agents such as catecholamines, endothelin, vasopressin, prostaglandins, prostacyclins, kinins, and serotonin influence the contractility of vascular smooth muscle.

With the explosion of knowledge about the inflammatory and immune responses and the recognition that atherosclerosis is an inflammatory disease, it has been recognized that many cytokines are involved. Some of these include IL-1, IL-2, IL-4, IL-8, interferon-η, TNF-α, and transforming growth factor-β.

The blood and vascular endothelium are continuously adjusting the balance of procoagulant and anticoagulant factors to keep the blood flowing and yet prevent hemorrhage. The expression of both tissue factor and tissue factor pathway inhibitor are increased in atherosclerotic plaques. It has been hypothesized that the increased expression of tissue factor in the plaque increases the probability of thrombosis after plaque rupture or endothelial erosion.

As discussed in the section on Monocytes–Macrophages, the production of MMPs is increased in the shoulder regions of complicated lesions. Inhibitors of the MMPs are also produced with the plaque, and the balance between the enzymes and their inhibitors may have a major role in determining whether plaque is stable or vulnerable.

MORPHOLOGY OF THE ATHEROSCLEROTIC LESION

Classification of the morphology of atherosclerotic lesions is evolving with visualization techniques and molecular biology. As the field has developed, several concepts have become clear. First, there is variability in lesion morphology both between individuals as well as within each individual. Second, different types of plaques are more common in different vessels. Third, the probability that a plaque will cause signs and symptoms may be more closely associated with the internal structure of the lesion than with the degree of stenosis. Last, as plaque accumulates in an artery, the vessel remodels so that there is no major change in the vessel lumen until the lesion occupies more than 40% of the luminal area.

Atherosclerotic lesions are not evenly distributed throughout the arteries. Extensive pathologic research has shown that lesions are more common at arterial bifurcations, at places where smaller arteries branch off a main vessel, and in areas where vessels curve. All of these are places where blood flow is nonlaminar and turbulent, leading to a reduction in the shear stress to which the endothelium is exposed. It has been demonstrated that shear stress is one factor that contributes to tight adhesion between endothelial cells. In addition, turbulence and decreased shear stress favor the attachment of blood cells such as monocytes and platelets to the endothelium. Therefore, if shear stress is decreased, vascular permeability is increased and the migration into the intima of cells known to contribute to the formation of atherosclerotic plaque may be enhanced. Examination of femoral arteries has revealed that atherosclerotic lesions are distributed in a helical or spiral fashion down the vessel, possibly as a result of hemodynamic patterns.

The classification of atherosclerotic plaque morphology presented in this section is a synthesis of several published schemes. Early schemes for grading atherosclerotic vessels were developed by the World Health Organization and groups of researchers in the United States. In the mid-1990s, the American Heart Association's Committee on Vascular Lesions published three reports defining lesions. A summary diagram of the Committee on Vascular Lesions' classification is shown in Figure 20–4. Modifications to the Committee's classification have subsequently been proposed. Because the information presented here is an integrated summary of these prior reports, the reader is encouraged to consult them for additional information.

Fatty Streaks

The fatty streak is a yellowish, smooth lesion protruding slightly into the arterial lumen. It does not obstruct blood flow and is not associated with any clinical symptoms. The lesion is characterized histologically by aggregations of lipid-containing macrophages or smooth muscle cells in the arterial intima. The lipid is mostly cholesterol and cholesterol esters. T cells have also been found in the streaks. Fatty streaks are classified as type I and type II lesions in the American Heart Association's classification.

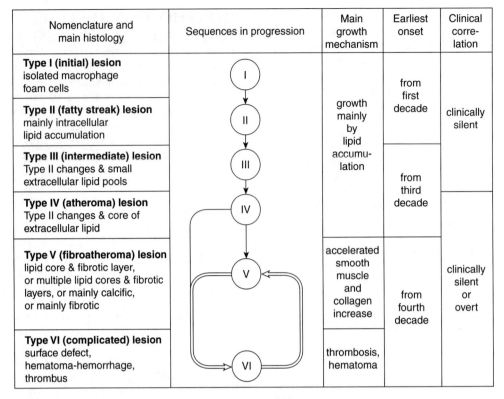

Nomenclature and main histology	Sequences in progression	Main growth mechanism	Earliest onset	Clinical correlation
Type I (initial) lesion isolated macrophage foam cells	I	growth mainly by lipid accumulation	from first decade	clinically silent
Type II (fatty streak) lesion mainly intracellular lipid accumulation	II			
Type III (intermediate) lesion Type II changes & small extracellular lipid pools	III		from third decade	
Type IV (atheroma) lesion Type II changes & core of extracellular lipid	IV			
Type V (fibroatheroma) lesion lipid core & fibrotic layer, or multiple lipid cores & fibrotic layers, or mainly calcific, or mainly fibrotic	V	accelerated smooth muscle and collagen increase	from fourth decade	clinically silent or overt
Type VI (complicated) lesion surface defect, hematoma-hemorrhage, thrombus	VI	thrombosis, hematoma		

FIGURE 20-4 Flow diagram in center column indicates pathways in evolution and progression of human atherosclerotic lesions. Roman numerals indicate histologic characteristics of types of lesions defined in left column. The direction of arrows indicates sequence in which characteristic morphologies may change. From type I to type IV, changes in lesion morphology occur primarily because of increasing accumulation of lipid. The loops between types V and VI illustrate how lesions increase in thickness when thrombotic deposits form on their surfaces. Thrombotic deposits may form repeatedly over varied periods in the same location and may be the principal mechanism for gradual occlusion of medium-sized arteries. (From Stary HC, Chandler AB, Dinsmore RE et al: A definition of advanced types of atherosclerotic lesions and a histological classification of atherosclerosis: A report from the Committee on Vascular Lesions of the Council on Arteriosclerosis, American Heart Association. Arterioscler Thromb Vasc Biol 15: 1520, 1995.)

Fatty streaks have been observed in people of all ages, from premature infants to the elderly. In a study of fetal aortas from spontaneous abortions or infants who died within 12 hours of birth, the size of the fetal lesions was correlated with the presence of hypercholesterolemia in the mothers. The prevalence of fatty streaks in children between 1 month and 1 year of age was found to be approximately 45%, and after 1 year it was 100%. In the Pathobiologic Determinants of Atherosclerosis in Youth (PDAY) Study, 100% of the aortas and between 57% and 83% of the right coronary arteries of 2,876 people between 15 and 34 years of age who had died in accidents were found to have fatty streaks.

Whether fatty streaks are irreversible and whether they are the precursors of more advanced plaques are controversial points. Data from monkeys and humans have provided evidence that some degree of regression is possible. It is generally, but not universally, believed that fatty streaks develop into more advanced lesions.

Fatty Plaque

Based on their analyses of the right coronary arteries and aortas from over 2,000 people, the PDAY investigators have defined a new category of atherosclerotic lesion, the fatty plaque. These investigators believe that this type of plaque is intermediate between the fatty streak and fibrous plaque. The variability in the cellular composition of the fatty plaque led the PDAY investigators to define four types of fatty plaque. In the type 1 fatty plaque, most of the lipid is contained within smooth muscle cells, and macrophages are relatively rare. The type 2 fatty plaque is made up of extracellular lipid, numerous smooth muscle cells, many of which do not contain lipid, and a few macrophages. In the type 3 fatty plaque, there are many cells, the lipid is intracellular, and at least 20% of the cells are macrophage foam cells. The relatively rare type 4 fatty plaques are similar to type 3 lesions, except lymphocytes are present in the lesion.

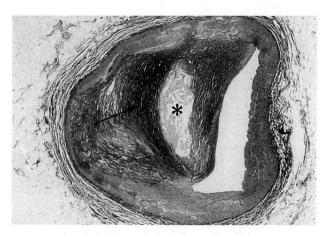

FIGURE 20-5 Histologic cross-section of coronary artery illustrating the two main components of mature atherosclerotic plaques: soft, lipid-rich atheromatous "gruel" (asterick) and hard, collagen-rich sclerotic tissue (arrow). The sclerotic component usually is, like here, by far the most voluminous plaque component, but the atheromatous component is most dangerous because it may destabilize a plaque, making it vulnerable to rupture. This plaque is probably relatively stable because the soft "gruel" is separated from the vascular lumen by a thick cap of fibrous tissue. Trichrome, staining collagen blue. (From Falk E, Shah PK, Fuster V. Pathogenesis of Plaque Disruption. In Fuster V, Ross R, Topol EJ (eds): Atherosclerosis and Coronary Artery Disease, p 491–507. Philadelphia, Lippincott-Raven, 1996.)

Fibrous Plaque

The category of fibrous plaque includes types IV (atheroma) and V (fibroatheroma) described by the Committee on Vascular Lesions. The type IV lesion has an extracellular lipid core in addition to the smooth muscle cells, macrophages, foam cells, and extracellular matrix found in fatty plaques (Fig. 20–5). The lipid is predominantly cholesterol ester, with some in the form of cholesterol crystals. Although some of the pool of lipid may originate from lipid-filled smooth muscle cells or foam cells that have died, some is thought to have been directly deposited in the extracellular space. When there are dead smooth muscle or foam cells in the lipid core, it is labeled as necrotic core. This core is described as having the consistency of toothpaste when examined at autopsy.

A type V lesion or fibroatheroma is similar to the type IV lesion except that more fibrous connective tissue has formed between the lipid core of the plaque and the endothelium. This fibrous connective tissue consists of collagen plus the smooth muscle cells that secrete the collagen. Some of these lesions have multiple lipid cores with layers of connective tissue between the layers. In addition, some type V lesions are calcified, whereas others are not. In both types of fibrous plaque, vasa vasorum are seen extending into the lesion up to the margins of the lipid cores.

Various components of the plasma have been found in the fibrous plaque, including fibrin, fibrinogen, albumin, white blood cells, and lipoproteins. All the serum lipids have been found in fibrous plaques except the large chylomicrons.

Complicated Lesions

Complicated lesions are also known as advanced lesions or type VI lesions. These lesions are structurally similar to fibrous plaques or type IV and V lesions, but also include endothelial erosions, hemorrhage within the plaque, and luminal thrombosis. Some classifications also include heavily calcified lesions in this category.

Stable and Vulnerable Plaques

Subsequent to the development of the classification schemes described previously, it was recognized that some plaques are more prone to rupture than others. This recognition has led to exploration of the concept that some plaques are considered stable and unlikely to rupture, whereas others are thought to be at high risk of rupturing. Vulnerable plaques are those with a thin layer of fibrous cap over the lipid core (Fig. 20–6). These plaques tend to have increased concentrations of macrophages and T cells in what are called their "shoulder" regions, where the atherosclerotic part of the artery is adjacent to the relatively normal part of the vessel wall. Vulnerable plaques tend to rupture at these shoulder regions. As discussed in the previous section, activated macrophages produce enzymes known as MMPs that break down connective tissue. In contrast, stable plaques have thick fibrous caps over the lipid core. Thus, the key factors in categorizing a plaque as stable or vulnerable are the nature of the fibrous cap and whether there is a high degree of inflammatory activity at the shoulder regions of the cap. Display 20–1 lists features of rupture-prone plaques.

Vascular Remodeling

In 1987, Glagov demonstrated that as plaque accumulates in an artery, the vessel remodels its wall so that the size of the vessels stays relatively constant until the plaque fills approximately 40% of the potential luminal area (Fig. 20–7). This finding led to an examination of the value of angiography in atherosclerosis. New technologies such as intravascular ultrasound and positron emission tomography are being studied to determine their usefulness as diagnostic tools. In a study of 36 people, endothelial dysfunction was associated with vascular remodeling.

THEORIES OF ATHEROSCLEROSIS PATHOGENESIS

Over the past 100 years, many theories have been advanced in an attempt to explain the evolution of atherosclerosis.

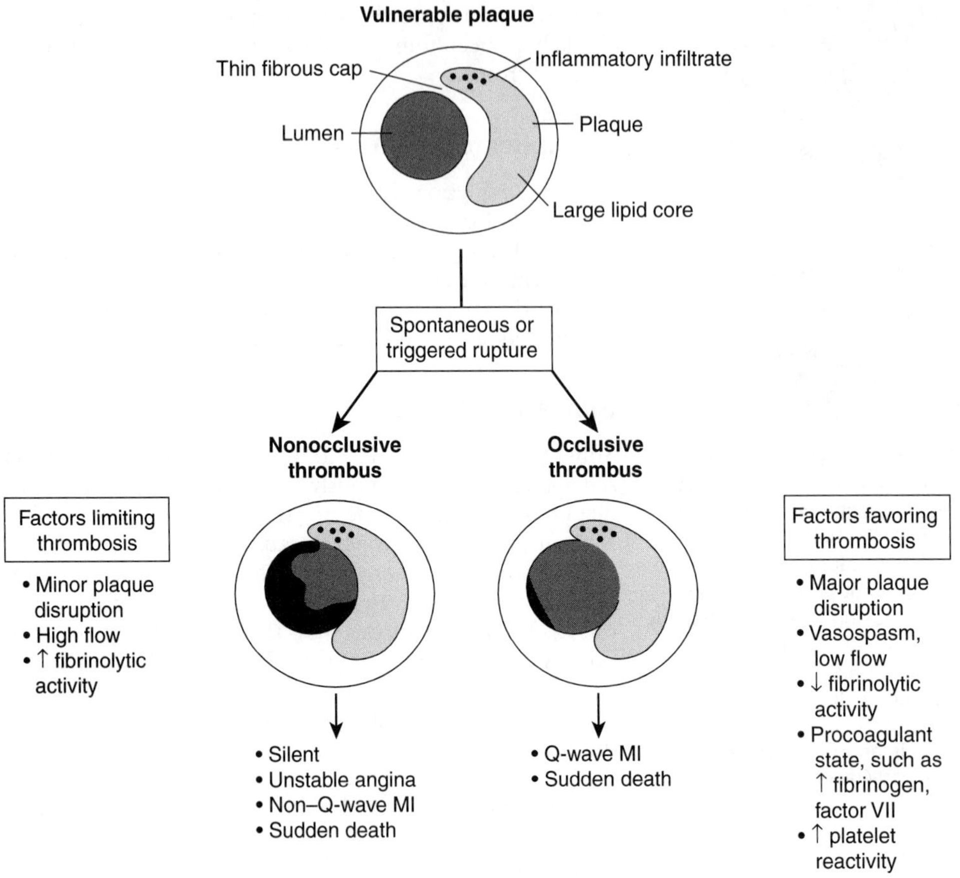

Vulnerable plaque

Thin fibrous cap — Inflammatory infiltrate

Lumen — Plaque

Large lipid core

Spontaneous or
triggered rupture

**Nonocclusive
thrombus**

**Occlusive
thrombus**

Factors limiting
thrombosis

• Minor plaque
  disruption
• High flow
• ↑ fibrinolytic
  activity

Factors favoring
thrombosis

• Major plaque
  disruption
• Vasospasm,
  low flow
• ↓ fibrinolytic
  activity
• Procoagulant
  state, such as
  ↑ fibrinogen,
  factor VII
• ↑ platelet
  reactivity

• Silent
• Unstable angina
• Non–Q-wave MI
• Sudden death

• Q-wave MI
• Sudden death

FIGURE 20-6 Vulnerable plaque. (From Kullo IJ, Edwards WD, Schwartz RS: Vulnerable plaque: Pathobiology and clinical implications. Ann Intern Med 129: 1051, 1998.)

Until recently, the most studied were the response-to-injury, monoclonal, and hemodynamic hypotheses. Advances have led to a consolidation of theories into the inflammatory response hypothesis.

The Inflammatory Response Hypothesis

Evidence has accumulated connecting the development of atherosclerotic plaque with the inflammatory response. It is hypothesized that through a variety of means, cardiovascular risk factors injure the endothelium, leading to endothelial dysfunction. The dysfunctional endothelium then undergoes changes that activate the inflammatory response. If the injury to the endothelium persists, the ongoing

---

DISPLAY 20-1

Features of Rupture-Prone Plaques

Structural
    Large lipid-rich core
    Thin fibrous cap
    Reduced collagen content
Cellular
    Local chronic inflammation
    Increased macrophage density and activity
    T-lymphocyte accumulation near sites of rupture
    Increased neovascularization
    Reduced density of smooth muscle cells
    Increased number and activity of mast cells
    Expression of markers of inflammatory activation
Molecular
    Matrix metalloproteinase secretion
    Increased tissue factor expression

From Kullo IJ, Edwards WD, Schwartz RS: Vulnerable plaque: pathobiology and clinical implications. Ann Intern Med 129: 1050–1060, 1998, table 1.

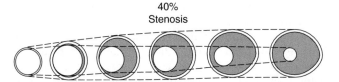

40%
Stenosis

FIGURE 20-7 Diagrammatic representation of a possible sequence of changes in atherosclerotic arteries leading eventually to lumen narrowing. The artery enlarges initially (left to right in diagram) in association with plaque accumulation to maintain an adequate, if not normal, lumen area. Early stages of lesion development may be associated with overcompensation. At more than 40% stenosis, however, the plaque area continues to increase to involve the entire circumference of the vessel, and the artery no longer enlarges at a rate to prevent significant narrowing of the lumen. (From Glagov S, Weisenberg E, Zarins CK et al: Compensatory enlargement of human atherosclerotic coronary arteries. N Engl J Med 316: 1374, 1987.)

inflammation contributes to the formation of atherosclerotic plaque. It is hoped that research into the inflammatory response hypothesis of atherosclerosis will lead to new treatments and preventive strategies.

There is a growing body of evidence demonstrating that the traditional cardiovascular risk factors, including age, dyslipidemia, smoking, hypertension, and a sedentary lifestyle, contribute to endothelial dysfunction. Some of the emerging risk factors such as hyperhomocysteinemia and infection have also been shown to damage the endothelium.

The changes in the dysfunctional epithelium that contribute to the development of the atherosclerotic plaque are increased permeability; increased expression of adhesion molecules that bind monoctyes, T cells, and platelets; and secretion of growth factors such as PDGF that lead to vascular remodeling. As the endothelium becomes more permeable, serum lipids predominantly move into the vascular intima. (Figure 20-1) Either during transcytosis across the endothelial cell or after entering the intima, the LDL becomes oxidized. Once oxidized, the LDL becomes a chemoattractant for monocytes and is also easier for the already present macrophages to ingest through their scavenger receptors. As the macrophages take up oxidized LDL, they become the foam cells that form the fatty streak. Interactions between the macrophage/foam cells and the T cells lead to activation of both types of cell. As these cells become activated, the inflammatory response is established.

Progression from the fatty streak to complicated lesions is associated with continuation of the inflammatory response plus plaque rupture accompanied by hemorrhage from the disrupted vasa vasorum or formation of a mural thrombus. It is hypothesized that multiple rupture events contribute to growth of the lesion until the resulting thrombus is large enough to occlude the vessels and cause symptoms.

It is hoped that recognition of atherosclerosis as an inflammatory disease will lead to research into new methods of prevention and treatment. As the inflammatory hypothesis has developed, related research has shown that links exist between infectious diseases and atherosclerosis. Saikku, Grayston, and others have demonstrated a relationship between *Chlamydia pneumoniae* infection and coronary heart disease (CHD). Subsequently, other infections as well as markers of infections have been found to be associated with the incidence of atherosclerotic disease.

REFERENCES

1. Anderson TJ, Meredith IT, Yeung AC et al: The effect of cholesterol-lowering and antioxidant therapy on endothelium-dependent coronary vasomotion. N Engl J Med 332: 488–493, 1995
2. Aviram M: LDL-platelet interaction under oxidative stress induces macrophage foam cell formation. Thromb Haemost 74: 560–564, 1995
3. Aviram M, Brook JG: Platelet activation by plasma lipoproteins. Prog Cardiovasc Dis 30: 61–72, 1987
4. Bataineh A, Raij L: Angiotensin II, nitric oxide, and end-organ damage in hypertension, Kidney Int Suppl 68: S14–19, 1998
5. Bath PM, Martin JF: Serum platelet-derived growth factor and endothelin concentrations in human hypercholesterolaemia. J Intern Med 230: 313–317, 1991
6. Benzuly KH, Padgett RC, Kaul S et al: Functional improvement precedes structural regression of atherosclerosis [published erratum appears in Circulation 1994 Sept 90(3):1585]. Circ 89: 1810–1818, 1994
7. Blankenhorn DH, Azen SP, Kramsch DM et al: Coronary angiographic changes with lovastatin therapy: The Monitored Atherosclerosis Regression Study (MARS). Ann Intern Med 119: 969–976, 1993
8. Blankenhorn DH, Nessim SA, Johnson RL et al: Beneficial effects of combined colestipol-niacin therapy on coronary atherosclerosis and coronary venous bypass grafts. JAMA 257: 3233–3240, 1987
9. Blann AD, Kirkpatrick U, Devine C et al: The influence of acute smoking on leucocytes, platelets and the endothelium. Atherosclerosis 141: 133–139, 1998
10. Bobryshev YV, Lord RS: Mapping of vascular dendritic cells in atherosclerotic arteries suggests their environment in local immune-inflammatory reactions. Cardiovasc Res 37: 799–810, 1998
11. Boot RG, van Achterberg TA, van Aken BE et al: Strong induction of members of the chitinase family of proteins in atherosclerosis: Chitotriosidase and human cartilage gp-39 expressed in lesion macrophages. Arterioscler Thromb Vasc Biol 19: 687–694, 1999
12. Burke AP, Farb A, Malcom GT et al: Coronary risk factors and plaque morphology in men with coronary disease who died suddenly. N Eng J Med 336: 1276–1282, 1997
13. Caplice NM, Mueske CS, Kleppe LS et al: Presence of tissue factor pathway inhibitor in human atherosclerotic plaques is associated with reduced tissue factor activity. Circ 98: 1051–1057, 1998
14. Cashuin-Hemphill L, Mack WJ, Pogoda JM et al: Beneficial effects of colestipolniacin on coronary atherosclerosis: A 4-year follow-up. JAMA 264: 3013–3017, 1990
15. Celermajer DS, Adams MR, Clarkson P et al: Passive smoking and impaired endothelium-dependent arterial dilatation in healthy young adults. N Engl J Med 334: 150–154, 1996
16. Danesh J, Collins R, Peto R: Chronic infections and coronary heart disease: Is there a link? Lancet 350: 430–436, 1997
17. Davies MJ, Woolf N, Rowles PM et al: Morphology of the endothelium over athersclerotic plaques in human coronary arteries. Br Heart J 60: 459–464, 1988
18. DiCorleto PE, Gimbrone Jr MA: Vascular endothelium. In Fuster V, Ross R, Topol EJ (eds): Atherosclerosis and Coronary Artery Disease, pp. 387–399. Philadelphia, Lippincott-Raven, 1996
19. Eggen DA, Strong JP, Newman WP et al: Regression of experimental atherosclerosis lesions in rhesus monkeys consuming a high saturated fat diet. Arteriosclerosis 7: 125–134, 1987
20. Faggiotto A, Ross R: Studies of hypercholesterolemia in the nonhuman primate: Fatty streak conversion to fibrous plaque. Arteriosclerosis 4: 341–356, 1984
21. Farstad M: The role of blood platelets in coronary atherosclerosis and thrombosis. Scand J Clin Lab Invest 58: 1–10, 1998
22. Ferri C, Bellini C, Desideri G et al: Clustering of endothelial markers of vascular damage in human salt-sensitive hypertension: Influence of dietary sodium load and depletion. Hypertension 32: 862–868, 1998
23. Fishman MC: Assembly of blood vessels in the embryo. In Fuster V, Ross R, Topol EJ (eds): Athersclerosis and Coronary Artery Disease, pp. 379–383. Philadelphia, Lippincott-Raven, 1996
24. Frostegard J, Nilsson J, Haegerstrand A et al: Oxidized low density lipoprotein induces differentiation and adhesion of human monocytes and the monocytic cell line U937. Proc Natl Acad Sci USA 87: 904–908, 1090

25. Fusegawa Y, Goto S, Handa S et al: Platelet spontaneous aggregation in platelet-rich plasma is increased in habitual smokers. Thromb Res 93: 271–278, 1999

26. Fuster V: Connor Memorial Lecture. Mechanisms leading to myocardial infarction: Insights from studies of vascular biology. Circ 90: 2126–2146 [published erratum appears in Circulation 1995 Jan 1: 91(1) 256, 1994

27. Fuster V: Human lesion studies. Ann NY Acad Sci 811: 207–224; discussion 224–225, 1997

28. Fuster V, Badimon L, Badimon JJ et al: The pathogenesis of coronary artery disease and the acute coronary syndromes (2). N Engl J Med 326: 310–318, 1992

29. Fuster V, Badimon L, Badimon JJ et al: The pathogenesis of coronary artery disease and the acute coronary syndromes (1). N Engl J Med 326: 242–250, 1992

30. Giachelli CM, Liaw L, Murry CE et al: Osteopontin expression in cardiovascular diseases. Ann NY Acad Sci 760: 109–126, 1995

31. Gibbons GH, Dzau VJ: The emerging concept of vascular remodeling. N Engl J Med 330: 1431–1438, 1994

32. Glagov S, Weisenberg E, Zarins CK et al: Compensatory enlargement of human atherosclerotic coronary arteries. N Engl J Med 316: 1371–1375, 1987

33. Glagov S, Zarins C, Giddens DP et al: Hemodynamics and atherosclerosis. Insights and perspectives gained from studies of human arteries. Arch Pathol Lab Med 112: 1018–1031, 1988

34. Gonzales RS, Wick TM: Hemodynamic modulation of monocytic cell adherence to vascular endothelium. Ann Biomed Eng 24: 382–393, 1996

35. Gould KL: New concepts and paradigms in cardiovascular medicine: The noninvasive management of coronary artery disease. Am J Med 104: 2S–17S, 1998

36. Grayston JT: Chlamydia pneumoniae and athersclerosis. Rev Med Interne 17: 45S–47S, 1996

37. Gronholdt ML: Ultrasound and lipoprotiens as predictors of lipid-rich, rupture-prone plaques in the carotid artery. Arterioscler Thromb Vasc Biol 19: 2–13, 1999

38. Gurfinkel E, Bozovich G, Daroca A et al: Randomised trial of roxithromycin in non-Q-wave coronary syndromes: ROXIS pilot study. Lancet 350: 404–407, 1997

39. Guyton JR, Klemp KF: Development of the atherosclerotic lesions from human aorta. Arterioscler Thromb 14: 1305–1314, 1994

40. Haller H, Schaper D, Ziegler W et al: Low-density lipoprotein induces vascular adhesion molecule expression on human endothelial cells. Hypertension 25 [part 1]: 511–516, 1995

41. Hambrecht R, Fiehn E, Weigl C et al: Regular physical exercise corrects endothelial dysfunction and improves exercise capacity in patients with chronic heart failure. Circ 98: 2709–2715, 1998

42. Hansson GK, Holm J, Jonasson L: Detection of activated T lymphocytes in the human athersclotic plaque. AM J Pathol 135: 169–175, 1989

43. Hansson GK, Libby P: The role of the lymphocyte. In Fuster V, Ross R, Topol EJ (eds): Atherosclerosis and Coronary Artery Disease, pp. 557–568. Philadelphia, Lippincott-Raven, 1996

44. Haskell WL, Alderman EL, Fair JM et al: Effects of intensive multiple risk factor reduction on coronary athesclerosis and clinical cardiac events in men and women with coronary artery disease: The Stanford Coronary Risk Intervention Project (SCRIP). Circ 89: 975–990, 1994

45. Heistad DD, Armstrong ML, Marcus ML: Hyperemia of the aortic wall in atgherosclerotic monkeys. Circ Res 48: 669–675, 1981

46. Henney AM, Wakeley PR, Davies MJ et al: Localization of stromelysin gene expression in atherosclerotic plaques by in situ hybridization. Proc Natl Acad Sci USA 88: 8154–8158, 1991

47. Higashi Y, Oshima T, Ozono R et al: Aging and severity of hypertension attenuate endothelium-dependent renal vascular relaxation in humans. Hypertension 30: 252–258, 1997

48. Holman RH, McGill Jr HC, Strong JP et al: The natural history of atherosclerosis: the early aortic lesions as seen in New Orleans in the middle of the 20th century. Am J Pathol 34: 209–235, 1959

49. Kane JP, Malloy MJ, Ports TA et al: Regression of coronary atherosclerosis during treatment of familial hypercholesterolemia with combined drug regimens. JAMA 264: 3007–3012, 1990

50. Kocher O, Gabbiani F, Gabbiani G et al: Phenotypic features of smooth muscle cells during the evolution of experimental cartoid artery intimal thickening. Biochemical and morphologic studies. Lab Invest 65: 459–470, 1991

51. Krettek A, Fager G, Lindmark H et al: Effect of phenotype on the transcription of the genes for platelet-derived growth factor (PDGF) isoforms in human smooth muscle cells, monocyte-derived macrophages, and endothelial cells in vitro. Arterioscler Thromb Vasc Biol 17: 2897–2903, 1997

52. Kullo IJ, Edwards WD, Schwartz RS: Vulnerable plaque: pathobiology in human coronary atherosclerosis: Its origin and pathophysical significance. Hum Pathol 26: 450–456, 1995

53. Kumamoto M, Nakashima Y, Sueishi K: Intimal neovascularization in human coronary atherosclerosis: Its origin and pathophysical significance. Hum Pathol 26: 450–456, 1995

54. Kuo CC, Gown AM, Benditt EP et al: Detection of Chlamydia pneumoniae in aortic lesions of atherosclerosis: Its origin and pathophysical significance. Hum Pathol 26: 450–456, 1995

55. Kwon HM, Sangiorgi G, Ritman EL et al: Enhanced coronary vasa vasorum neovascularization in experimental hypercholesterolemia. J Clin Invest 101: 1551–1556, 1998

56. Lerman A, Cannan CR, Higano SH et al: Coronary vascular remodeling in association with endothelial dysfunction. AM J Cardiol 81: 1105–1109, 1998

57. Li H, Cybulsky MI, Gimbrone Jr MA et al: An atherogenic diet rapidly induces VCAM-1, a cytokine-regulatable mononuclear leukocyte adhesion molecule, in rabbit aortic endothelium. Arterioscler Thromb 13: 197–204, 1993

58. Libby P, Geng YJ, Aikawa M et al: Macrophages and atherosclerotic plaque stability. Curr Opin Lipidol 7: 330–335, 1996

59. Libby P, Hansson GK: Involvement of the immune system in human atherogenesis: Current knowledge and unanswered questions. Lab Invest 64: 5–15, 1991

60. Libby P, Schoenbeck U, Mach F et al: Current concepts in cardiovascular pathology: The role of LDL cholesterol in plaque rupture and stabilization. Am J Med 104: 14S–18S, 1998

61. Loscalzo J: Nitric oxide and vascular disease. N Engl J Med 333: 251–253, 1995

62. Magnusson MK, Mosher DF: Fibronectin: Structure, assembly, and cardiovascular implications. Arterioscler Thromb Vasc Biol 18: 1363–1370, 1998

63. Mannucci PM: von Willebrand factor: A marker of endothelial damage? Arterioscler Thromb Vasc Biol 18: 1359–1362, 1998

64. Manson JE, Stampfer MJ, Colditz GA et al: A prospective study of aspirin use and primary prevention of cardiovascular disease in women. JAMA 266: 521–527, 1991

65. Moreau M, Brocheriou I, Petit L et al: Interleukin-8 mediates downregulation of tissue inhibitor of metalloproteinase-1 expression in cholesterol-loaded human macrophages: Relevance to stability of atherosclerotic plaque. Circ 99: 420–426, 1999

66. Murray CJ, Lopez AD: Alternative projections of mortality and disability by cause 1990–2020: Global Burden of Disease Study. Lancet 349: 1498–1504, 1997

67. Napoli C, D'Armiento FP, Mancini FP et al: Fatty streak formation occurs in human fetal aortas and is greatly enhanced by maternal hypercholesterolemia. Intimal accumulation of low density lipoprotein and its oxidation precede monocyte recruitment into early atherosclerotic lesions. J Clin Invest 100: 2680–2690, 1997

68. Narahara N, Enden T, Wiiger M et al: Polar expression of tissue factor in human umbilical vein endothelial cells. Arterioscler Thromb 14: 1815–1820, 1994

69. Nelken NA, Coughlin SR, Gordon D et al: Monocyte chemoattractant protein-1 in human atheromatous plaques. J Clin Invest 88: 1121–1127, 1991

70. Okano M, Yoshida Y: Junction complexes of endothelial cells in atherosclerosis-prone and atherosclerosis-resistant regions on flow dividers of brachiocephalic bifurcations in the rabbit aorta. Biorheology 31: 155–161, 1994

71. Ornish D, Brown SE, Scherwitz LW et al: Can lifestyle changes reverse coronary heart disease? Lancet 336: 129–133, 1990

72. Owens GK: Role of alterations in the differentiated state of vascular smooth muscle cells in atherogenesis. In Fuster V, Ross R, Topol EJ (eds): Atherosclerosis and Coronary Artery Disease, pp. 409–420. Philadelphia, Lippincott-Raven, 1996

73. Panza JA: Endothelial dysfunction in essential hypertension. Clin Cardiol 20: II-26–33, 1997

74. Pasterkamp G, Schoneveld AH, van der Wal AC et al: Inflammation of the atherosclerotic cap and shoulder of the plaque is a common and locally observed feature in unruptured plaques of femoral and coronary arteries. Arterioscler Thromb Vasc Biol 19: 54–58, 1999

75. Petit L, Lesnik P, Dachet C et al: Tissue factor pathway inhibitor is expressed by human monocyte-derived macrophages: relationship to tissue factor induction by cholesterol and oxidized LDL. Arterioscler Thromb Vasc Biol 19: 309–315, 1999

76. Poon M, Zhang X, Dunsky KG et al: Apolipoprotein(a) induces monocyte chemotactic activity in human vascular endothelial cells. Circ 96: 2514–2519, 1997

77. Porreca E, Di Febbo C, Reale M et al: Monocyte chemotactic protein 1 (MCP-1) is a mitogen for cultured rat vascular smooth muscle cells. J Vasc Res 34: 58–65, 1997

78. Reape TJ, Rayner K, Manning CD et al: Expression and cellular localization of the CC chemokines PARC and ELC in human atherosclerotic plaques. Am J Pathol 154: 365–374, 1999

79. Ridker PM, Cushman M, Stampfer MJ et al: Inflammation, aspirin, and the risk of cardiovascular disease in apparently healthy men. N Engl J Med 336: 973–979, 1997

80. Ridker PM, Cushman M, Stampfer MJ et al: Plasma concentration of C-reactive protein and risk of developing peripheral vascular disease. Circ 97: 425–428, 1998

81. Ross R: The pathogenesis of atherosclerosis. In Braunwald E (ed): Heart Disease: A Textbook of Cardiovascular Medicine, pp. 1105–1125. Philadelphia, W. B. Saunders, 1997

82. Ross R: Atherosclerosis—an inflammatory disease. N Engl J Med 340: 115–126, 1999

83. Ross R, Glomset JA: Atherosclerosis and the arterial smooth muscle cell: Proliferation of smooth muscle is a key event in the genesis of the lesions of atherosclerosis. Science 180: 1332–1339, 1973

84. Ross R, Masuda J, Raines EW: Cellular interactions, growth factors, and smooth muscle proliferation in atherogenesis. Ann N Y Acad Sci 598: 102–112, 1990

85. Saikku P, Leinonen M, Mattila K et al: Serological evidence of an association of a novel Chlamydia, TWAR, with chronic coronary heart disease and acute myocardial infarction. Lancet 2: 983–986, 1988

86. Salonen JT, Yla-Herttuala S, Yamamoto R et al: Autoantibody against oxidised LDL and progression of carotid atherosclerosis. Lancet 339: 883–887, 1992

87. Schmitz G, Herr AS, Rothe G: T-lymphocytes and monocytes in atherogenesis. Herz 23: 168–177, 1998

88. Schoenbeck U, Mach F, Sukhova GK et al: Expression of stromelysin-3 in atherosclerotic lesions: regulation via CD40-CD40 ligand signaling in vitro and in vivo. J Exp Med 189: 843–853, 1999

89. Schwartz CJ, Ardie NG, Carter RF et al: Gross aortic sudanophilia and hemosiderin deposition. A study on infants, children, and young adults. Arch Pathol 83: 325–332, 1967

90. Shih PT, Elices MJ, Fang ZT et al: Minimally modified low-density lipoprotein induces monocyte adhesion to endothelial connecting segment-1 by activating beta-1 integrin. J Clin Invest 103: 613–625, 1999

91. Stary HC: Evolution and progression of atherosclerotic lesions in coronary arteries of children and young adults. Arteriosclerosis 9: I19–32, 1989

92. Stary HC: The histological classification of atherosclerotic lesions in human coronary arteries. In Fuster V, Ross R, Topol EJ (eds): Atherosclerosis and Coronary Artery Disease, pp. 463–474. Philadelphia, Lippincott-Raven, 1996

93. Stary HC, Blankenhorn DH, Chandler AB et al: A definition of the intima of human arteries and of its atherosclerosis-prone regions. A report from the Committee on Vascular Lesions of the Council on Arteriosclerosis, American Heart Associaton. Circ 85: 391–405, 1992

94. Stary HC, Chandler AB, Dinsmore RE et al: A definition of advanced types of atherosclerotic lesions and a histological classification of atherosclerosis. A report from the Committee on Vascular Lesions of the Council on Arteriosclerosis, American Heart Association. Arterioscler Thromb Vasc Biol 15: 1512–1531, 1995

95. Stary HC, Chandler AB, Glagov S et al: A definition of initial, fatty streak, and intermediate lesions of atherosclerosis. A report from the Committee on Vascular Lesions of the Council on Arteriosclerosis, American Heart Association. Circ 89: 2462–2478, 1994

96. Stemme S, Faber B, Holm J et al: T lymphocytes from human atherosclerotic plaques recognize oxidized low density lipoprotein. Proc Natl Acad Sci USA 92: 3893–3897, 1995

97. Strong JP, Bhattacharyya AK, Eggen DA et al: Long-term induction and regression of diet-induced atherosclerotic lesions in rhesus monkeys. II. Morphometric evaluation of lesions by light microscopy in coronary and carotid arteries. Arterioscler Thromb 14: 2007–2016, 1994

98. Strong JP, Malcom GT, McMahan CA et al: Prevalence and extent of atherosclerosis in adolescents and young adults: Implications for prevention from the Pathobiological Determinants of Atherosclerosis in Youth Study. JAMA 281: 727–735, 1999

99. Taddei S, Virdis A, Mattei P et al: Defective l-arginine-nitric oxide pathway in offspring of essential hypertensive patients. Circ 94: 1298–1303, 1996

100. Terkeltaub R, Boisvert WA, Curtiss LK: Chemokines and atherosclerosis. Curr Opin Lipidol 9: 397–405, 1998

101. The Dutch TIA Trial Study Group: A comparison of two doses of aspirin (30 mg vs. 283 mg a day) in patients after a transient ischemic attack or minor ischemic stroke. N Engl J Med 325: 1261–1266, 1991

102. Thom DH, Wang SP, Grayston JT et al: Chlamydia pneumoniae strain TWAR antibody and angiographically demonstrated coronary artery disease. Arterioscler Thromb 11: 547–551, 1991

103. Topol EJ, Califf RM, Weisman JF et al: Randomised trial of coronary intervention with antibody against platelet

IIIb/IIIa integrin for reduction of clinical restenosis: Results at six months. Lancet 343(8902): 881–886, 1994

104. Toschi V, Gallo R, Lettino M et al: Tissue factor modulates the thrombogenicity of human atherosclerotic plaques. Circ 95: 594–599, 1997

105. Traub O, Berk BC: Laminar shear stress: Mechanisms by which endothelial cells transduce an atheroprotective force. Arterioscler Thromb Vasc Biol 18: 677–685, 1998

106. Treasure CB, Klein JL, Weintraub WS et al: Beneficial effects of cholesterol-lowering therapy on the coronary endothelium in patients with coronary artery disease. N Engl J Med 332: 481–487, 1995

107. Tsao PS, Niebauer J, Buitrago R et al: Interaction of diabetes and hypertension on determinants of endothelial adhesiveness. Arterioscler Thromb Vasc Biol 18: 947–953, 1998

108. Uemura K, Sternby N, Vanecek R et al: Grading atherosclerosis in aorta and coronary arteries obtained at autopsy. Bulletin World Health Organization 31: 297–320, 1964

109. Vogel RA, Corretti MC, Gellman J: Cholesterol, cholesterol lowering, and endothelial function. Prog Cardiovasc Dis 41: 117–136, 1998

110. Waltner-Romen M, Falkensammer G, Rabl W et al: A previously unrecognized site of local accumulation of mononu-

clear cells. The vascular-associated lymphoid tissue. J Histochem Cytochem 46: 1347–1350, 1998

111. Wensing PJ, Meiss L, Mali WP et al: Early atherosclerotic lesions spiraling through the femoral artery. Arterioscler Thromb Vasc Biol 18: 1554–1558, 1998

112. Wight TN: The vascular extracellular matrix. In Fuster V, Ross R, Topol EJ (eds): Atherosclerosis and Coronary Artery Disease, pp. 421–440. Philadelphia, Lippincott-Raven, 1996

113. Wissler RW, Hiltscher L, Oinuma T et al: The lesions of atherosclerosis in the young: From Fatty streaks to intermediate lesions. In Fuster V, Ross R, Topol EJ (eds): Atherosclerosis and Coronary Artery Disease, pp. 475–489. Philadelphia, Lippincott-Raven, 1996

114. Wissler RW, Vesselinovitch D: Can atherosclerotic plaques regress? Anatomic and biochemical evidence from nonhuman animal models. Am J Cardiol 65: 33F–40F, 1990

115. Yoshida Y, Okano M, Wang S et al: Hemodynamic–force-induced difference of interendothelial junctional complexes. Ann N Y Acad Sci 748: 104–120, 1995

116. Zeiher AM, Schachinger V, Minners J: Long-term cigarette smoking impairs endothelium-dependent coronary arterial vasodilator function. Circ 92: 1094–1100, 1995

SUSANNA CUNNINGHAM*

PATHOPHYSIOLOGY OF MYOCARDIAL ISCHEMIA AND INFARCTION

The pathophysiologic events that occur with CHD range from reversible injury of the muscle cells to the irreversible destruction of all cellular components in a tissue area. Ischemia results from an imbalance between the flow of blood to the myocardium (supply) and the metabolic needs of the myocardium (demand) (Fig. 20–8). *Supply ischemia* results from functional or structural abnormalities in the coronary arteries, reducing blood flow in the region perfused by the vessels. *Demand ischemia* results from increased heart rate, contractility, or heart size, such as with exercise, sympathetic stimulation, and hypertrophic cardiomyopathy. Myocardial ischemia is, by definition, reversible and presents clinically as angina pectoris. Severe and prolonged myocardial ischemia results in irreversible injury or infarction of tissue.[9,21,26]

As discussed in the previous section, both atherosclerotic plaque and thrombosis can contribute to reductions in coronary vessel lumina and thus in myocardial perfusion. When endothelial rupture or erosion results in platelet aggregation at a site, a thrombus develops and vasoconstrictors are released, which can cause further platelet aggregation and vasospasm. Thus, atherosclerosis leads to thrombosis, which leads to spasm and further tissue hypoxia, setting up a vicious cycle of damage.[30]

Coronary heart disease follows a nonlinear course; plaque rupture and occlusion are highly unpredictable, and acute ischemic events commonly result from disruption of only mild to moderate lesions.[51] Factors that influence the amount of ischemia include the size of the vessel, the adequacy of collateral flow, the status of the intrinsic fibrinolytic system, alterations in vascular tone, and myocardial oxygen demand.[31,32,33]

The pathologic evolution of a myocardial infarction (MI) involves infiltration by neutrophils and then macrophages, necrotic tissue removal, and scar formation. The repair process ends when damaged muscle is replaced by fibrous scar tissue. Although the heart is healed, the noncontractile scar creates functional abnormalities.

The development and resolution of an area of MI can be divided into four pathologic phases: ischemic insult, coagulation necrosis, healing, and scarring.[26] The morphologic characteristics of the phases are shown in Figure 20–9. The ischemic insult phase lasts 4 hours from the time blood flow ceases. Within this period, some of the tissue in the infarct area may be saved from necrosis if reperfusion occurs. Dur-

ing the ischemic phase, the earliest histologic changes of irreversible injury, wavy myofibers, become apparent. The wavy myocytes (muscle cells) are seen because the dying infarcted cells are pulled into thinner sections by neighboring functional myocytes.[8]

In the ischemic phase, as the myocardium ceases beating, the cells become functionally and electrically silent.[33] This change begins in the subendocardium within 20 minutes after occlusion and progresses to major subendocardial necrosis within 60 minutes.[80] The "wavefront" of this necrotic zone progresses from the subendocardium to the epicardium in 1 to 6 hours.

The phase of coagulation necrosis last from 4 to 48 hours after infarction. Reperfusion during this period does not result in the salvage of any myocytes. At 6 hours after occlusion, the staining characteristics of the myocyte nucleus begin changing, and by 24 hours the myocyte nuclei have disappeared.[26]

Healing of the infarcted area begins approximately 48 hours after the occlusive event and lasts until the seventh day. During this time, the center of the infarcted area appears yellow because of loss of myoglobin from the dying myocytes, whereas the periphery or margins are red because of the local inflammation. This inflammation causes local blood vessels to dilate and leads to accumulation of macrophages, T cells, and plasma cells. In cases of transmural MI, damage to the epicardium may allow lymphocytes and fibrin to enter the pericardial space as well. Fibrous pericarditis may then result and may become apparent during this phase.[56] Fibroblasts appear after 4 days and synthesize collagen matrix. Small capillaries bud from surviving vessels and grow into the damaged zone.[26,53,55]

The healing phase is when the infarcted area is most likely to rupture because of myocyte necrosis and breakdown of the connective tissue caused by the enzymes released by the macrophages (mononuclear cells) that are coordinating the healing process. It is also the time when aneurysms may form as the necrotic tissue is stretched and thinned by the remaining viable myocardium.

The scarring phase begins at approximately 1 week after the infarction. Because the duration of this phase depends on infarct size, it may last from 2 weeks to months. In the healing phase, the necrotic myocytes are replaced with connective tissue scar. Over many years after the infarct, the scar tissue is slowly but continuously remodeled, and it may eventually disappear. Grossly visible signs of scarring are present from the second through the fourth weeks. The bulk of the necrotic cells is removed, and the density of capillaries increases.[56] The endocardium overlying the MI may gradually increase in thickness.[22]

*This section was revised by Susanna Cunningham. The work of Sharon Jensen for the 3rd edition is acknowledged.

495

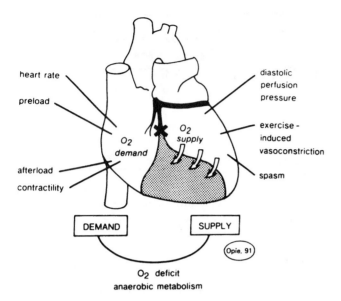

FIGURE 20-8 Myocardial oxygen balance. When the oxygen demand is increased, as in exercise, in the face of coronary artery disease, angina may be precipitated. When the supply is decreased abruptly, as in angina caused by coronary artery spasm or when a thrombus occludes the artery, angina at rest may be precipitated. (From Opie LH: The Heart: Physiology and Metabolism, p 18. New York, Raven Press, 1991.)

The final product of the repair process is a tough, white, fibrous scar. The time it takes for the MI to form a mature scar varies. Estimates based on autopsy data and healing from experimental MIs range from 2 to 3 months. Very large infarcts may have some necrotic muscle bundles in the central zone for longer periods. Between 3 and 6 months, the scar contracts.[26,53,56]

Progressive increase in the function of normal muscle and stabilization of the infarcted zone usually occur as scar formation evolves. End-diastolic dimensions decrease in the central zone. Dyskinesia (outward movement) of this area may evolve into akinesia (absent movement).[81] Stiffening of this zone may improve left ventricular (LV) performance because the loss in compliance may prevent systolic bulging, energy loss, and sequestration of blood.[6] A gradual increase in the dimensions of normal tissue takes place, possibly due to compensatory lengthening or hypertrophy of muscle.[81]

CAUSES AND CLASSIFICATIONS OF ISCHEMIA AND INFARCTION

Most ischemia and infarction are the consequence of atherosclerotic cardiovascular disease, as described in the previous section. Ischemia can also be caused by cardiomyopathy, sudden cardiac arrest, and embolism. The classification schemes for ischemia and infarction are described in the sections on Diagnosis and Management of Myocardial Ischemia and Diagnosis and Management of Myocardial Infarction. The only cause of ischemia, infarction, and myopathy that is not discussed in these other sections is related to the use of cocaine.

Cocaine

Cocaine use has been associated with myocardial ischemia, MI, arrhythmias, sudden death, cardiomyopathy, and accelerated atherosclerosis.[6] It increases heart rate and blood pressure, reduces coronary caliber and blood flow, and increases coronary vascular resistance. Thus, cocaine increases oxygen demand at the same time it reduces supply.[50]

Cocaine increases the release of stored catecholamines from both peripheral and central stores, and it also blocks the reuptake of these catecholamines. The excess catecholamine accumulation results in stimulation not only of the central nervous system, but of the heart muscle and vascular smooth muscle.[7] Increased levels of norepinephrine result in stimulation of β–adrenergic receptors, causing vasoconstriction.

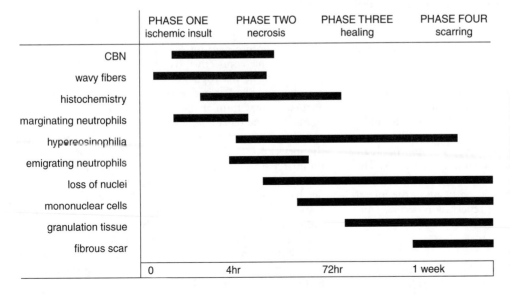

FIGURE 20-9 Major morphologic features of each phase of myocardial infarction that may be helpful in dating an infarct. The best site to observe these findings is at the periphery of the infarct zone. CBN, contraction band necrosis. (From Fallon JT: Pathophysiology of myocardial infarction and reperfusion. In Fuster V, Ross R, Topol EJ [eds]: Atherosclerosis and Coronary Artery Disease, p 795. Philadelphia, Lippincott-Raven, 1996.)

β-Adrenergic receptors are stimulated by epinephrine, resulting in increased heart rate, a positive inotropic effect, and increased cardiac automaticity.

Cocaine has a local anesthetic effect, blocking the fast sodium channel and resulting in a depression of depolarization and a slowing of conduction velocity. The PR, QRS, and QT intervals are prolonged, and the refractory periods of atrial and ventricular muscle are prolonged.[42] In addition, cocaine may increase platelet aggregation[93] and deregulate the renin–angiotensin system,[97] contributing to cardiotoxicity.

Patients with cocaine-related cardiovascular symptoms such as MI commonly inhale, inject, or smoke the drug. The time of symptom onset from cocaine use ranges from minutes to several hours. Chronic cocaine use causes ischemia that may continue for up to 6 weeks after use.[85] Approximately one third of the patients with fatal MI have normal coronary arteries. The Cocaine-Associated Myocardial Infarction Study Group found that underlying atherosclerotic disease is more likely in cocaine abusers with MI who are older, have other cardiovascular risk factors, and who have bradyarrhythmias (Hollander, 1997). Most patients with MI do not demonstrate typical plaque fissuring; alternatively, marked thickening of the walls of the intramural coronary arteries is more common.[55] This fibroproliferative pathophysiology of MI in the setting of cocaine use may, therefore, be different from that observed in noncocaine users.[50]

ALTERATIONS IN CORONARY BLOOD FLOW

Flow in Stenotic Vessels

Normal coronary vessels match blood flow with metabolic requirements of the myocardium. A vessel whose cross-sectional area is reduced by 75% (75% stenosis) severely restricts flow to distal beds.[9,40] Coronary stenoses may either be eccentric, occupying part of the vessel wall circumference, or concentric, occupying the whole circumference. Vessels distal to a coronary artery with concentric stenosis may adapt by maximally dilating, even when the person is at resting levels of oxygen consumption. In this case, further vasodilatation may not occur when metabolic demands increase (as in stable angina), or when the driving pressure falls (as in systemic arterial hypotension). Thus, during periods of increased demand, the myocardium distal to the stenotic artery becomes ischemic. An eccentric lesion has a vessel with part of its circumference capable of tonal variations; it may respond to vasodilating agents and may increase flow to distal beds when myocardial oxygen consumption ($M\dot{V}O_2$) rises. However, eccentric vessels are also capable of spasm, a condition detrimental to acutely ischemic tissue.[9,39]

Collateral Vessels

The outcome of redistribution patterns of flow in the heart during ischemia and after MI depends on collateralization as well as on cardiac metabolic demands. Collateral vessels serve as alternative interconnecting channels and may be recruited when a parent vessel is unable to meet flow requirements.[41] Collateral vessels are either preformed but dormant vessels that expand and grow when the need arises, or they may grow in response to angiogenic cytokines released during periods of ischemia.[3,95] Enlargement of collateral vessels is often demonstrated by coronary arteriography in patients with CHD, ventricular hypertrophy, and cor pulmonale.[13] Regression of collateral vessels has been demonstrated with successful intracoronary streptokinase therapy and with percutaneous transluminal coronary angioplasty (PTCA).[98] To stimulate the growth of collaterals in men with myocardial ischemia who were not candidates for other interventions, researchers are experimenting with gene therapy using the gene for vascular endothelial growth factor.[54]

The interest in collateral vessels stems from the role they may play in limiting or preventing necrosis in the at-risk myocardium threatened by inadequate blood flow from a parent vessel. Autopsy studies have demonstrated totally occluded coronary vessels without infarction, suggesting that collateral vessels protect the myocardium.[4] Further, infarct size is smaller than the area supplied by an occluded vessel, presumably because the tissue at risk is partly reperfused by collateral flow.[13,58] Higher ejection fractions, better regional wall motion, and fewer MIs have also been observed in patients with well developed collaterals.[86]

Competitive Redistribution of Coronary Blood Flow

Competitive redistribution is another mechanism by which flow can be altered in the ischemic myocardium. As metabolism accelerates, increased blood flow through normal vessels may alter flow through collaterals. Autoregulation in normal coronaries lowers the resistance in the large vessels from which distal collaterals are fed. Lower resistance, in turn, reduces the driving pressure of blood through the collaterals so that flow through them decreases. In effect, normal vessels may "steal" flow from collaterals during times of increased $M\dot{V}O_2$, such as with exercise or sympathetic stimulation.

ENDOTHELIAL AND BLOOD CELL INTERACTIONS

With the inflammation that occurs from damaged endothelium, leukocytes migrate to the injured area, adhere to the endothelial cells, migrate through the cell junctions, and accumulate in the injured area. Within seconds of their activation, neutrophils increase their oxygen consumption nearly 100-fold.[60] Stimulated leukocytes release leukotrienes, oxygen-free radicals, and proteolytic enzymes. These substances cause endothelial damage and contraction of smooth muscle, and induce an increase in vascular permeability. They may therefore reduce local blood flow and lead to further ischemia, which may slow tissue repair.[35] Accumulated neutrophils may relate to the loss of coronary vasodilator reserve, arrhythmias, and myocardial stunning. However, neutrophils also mediate plasmin-independent fibrinolysis and scavenge dead tissue. Thus, they provide a defense against thrombosis and participate in remodeling.[23]

On contact with the endothelium, platelets are rapidly activated and produce procoagulants, potent vasoconstrictors, leukocyte stimulants, and a variety of growth factors. Activated platelets cause relaxation of intact endothelium; however, in damaged endothelium, platelets constrict smooth muscle.[45] This action is mediated through the release of thromboxane A_2 and serotonin. PDGF is a potent vasoconstrictor produced by platelets, and is also important to the maintenance of the endothelial barrier.[82]

Myocardial ischemia and necrosis also activate an inflammatory response. Inflammatory mediators such as IL-1, IL-6, IL-10, TNF-α, E-selectin, intercellular adhesion molecule-1, and C-reactive protein are released from macrophages and injured vascular endothelium.[36] These mediators cause low-grade fever, leukocytosis, and increased erythrocyte sedimentation rate (from the synthesis of proteins).[23] Anti-inflammatory interventions are being explored as possible treatments for myocardial ischemia and infarction.[67]

LOCAL PHYSIOLOGIC ALTERATIONS IN ISCHEMIA

Metabolism in Ischemic Myocardium

The metabolic consequences of ischemia include inadequate myocardial oxygenation and supply of nutrients, depletion of tissue myoglobin, and local accumulation of metabolic waste products (Fig. 20–10). The heart depends on an adequate supply of oxygen and on dietary substrates to form adenosine triphosphate (ATP). Breakdown of ATP into adenosine diphosphate and inorganic phosphate liberates the energy used for a number of metabolic and reparative processes. Within seconds after onset of ischemia, the myocardium converts to anaerobic metabolism, ceases contracting, and manifests electrophysiologic changes.[26]

ANAEROBIC METABOLISM

Ischemia results in a shift from aerobic to anaerobic metabolism. Immediately after the onset of ischemia, ATP levels are maintained by accelerated use of ATP and creatinine phosphate stores. Within seconds, these resources are expended, and glycolysis of glycogen increases. Glycogen depletion occurs minutes later, but anaerobic glycolysis of free fatty acids continues slowly for an additional 40 to 60 minutes.[47] With anaerobic glycolysis, pyruvate is not metabolized to acetyl coenzyme A, and pyruvate levels rise. This rise in pyruvate stimulates the reaction to form lactate, catalyzed by lactate dehydrogenase. Although energy production through anaerobic glycolysis is only 5% of that from oxidative metabolism, it is critical to the survival of ischemic tissue.[67,71,73]

CONSEQUENCES OF ANAEROBIC GLYCOLYSIS

An important sequel to deficient energy supplies is the inhibition of intracellular ion pumps. The sodium–potassium (Na^+-K^+) pump uses ATP to maintain high K^+ and low Na^+ intracellular concentrations. Defective pumping leads to

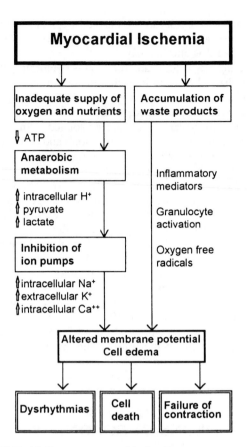

FIGURE 20-10 Consequences of ischemia

equilibration of ions, intracellular Na^+ accumulation, and efflux of K^+ from the cell. Intracellular calcium (Ca^{2+}) also accumulates in the cell in ischemia because of activation of the Na^+-Ca^{2+} pump, Ca^{2+} leakage from the sarcoplasmic reticulum, and alterations in Ca^{2+} channels and Ca^{2+}-ATPase pumps on the cell membranes. Consequences of this altered ionic ratio include membrane depolarization and conduction abnormalities, inhibition of contractile processes, cell edema, and membrane leak.[69]

Failure of Contraction

The size of an MI is the most important determinant of power failure, except for instances of particular sites of damage (e.g., papillary muscle rupture) that lead to acute heart failure. Methods used to quantify size are discussed in Chapter 16. The most frequent and hemodynamically significant MIs involve the left ventricle. Necrosis of 40% of the left ventricle is usually associated with fatal cardiogenic shock.[1] A transmural MI is more likely to produce changes in stroke volume (SV) and LV end-diastolic volume than is an MI confined to the subendocardium. Moreover, loss of functional muscle from previous MIs has additive effects on impairment from subsequent MIs.

Right ventricular (RV) infarction may contribute to biventricular or isolated ventricular failure. In isolated RV MI, the SV of the right ventricle decreases, diastolic filling of the left ventricle is limited, and forward cardiac output subsequently falls; hypotension and sympathetic compensatory mechanisms ensue. In addition to decreased systolic function and ventricular contraction, diastolic relaxation is inhibited, resulting in a stiff ventricle; this causes increased diastolic pressure and jugular venous pressure.[72]

CELLULAR CHANGES

Although anaerobic glycolysis is vital, it does create environmental consequences for the ischemic myocardial cell. Accelerated production of lactate and accumulation of inorganic phosphate from hydrolysis of ATP leads to an excess of hydrogen ions (H^+), and acidosis results.[66] Contractile changes occur because of the buildup of protons and inorganic phosphate that desensitize the contractile elements to Ca^{2+}. Abnormal relaxation develops secondary to prolonged tension of the cross-bridges that become permanently attached and form rigor bridges. This abnormal relaxation is due to decreased uptake of Ca^{2+} by the sarcoplasmic reticulum or insufficient supply of ATP to reconstitute the binding state of the contractile elements.[66,69]

CONTRACTILE FAILURE: THE FLACCID HEART

The functional changes that occur with an MI originate in the contractile elements and vary on a continuum from mild to severe alterations in hemodynamics. Contractility diminishes within seconds after a coronary occlusion and occurs *before* ST segment elevation.[77,81,90] A mixture of normal and necrotic fibers in the marginal zone produces a hypokinetic area.[81] This alteration creates asynergy of contractile proteins, and wasted contractile effort results.

Abnormal contraction of these elements, with holosystolic expansion in the central zone, creates asynchronous movement. Aortic flow decreases and further ischemia can result.[12] The most marked contractile changes take place in the subendocardium, because its perfusion is most compromised by compression during systole.[26] Impeded shortening of muscle fibers reduces the development of contractile tension. In addition, passive lengthening of necrotic fibers replaces shortening during systole.[96] Increased diastolic length and systolic shortening in normal muscle may compensate for the contractile defects in injured muscle.[81]

Hibernating myocardium refers to ischemic myocardium in which the cells remain viable but contraction is chronically (as opposed to acutely) depressed. This depressed contraction reduces $M\dot{V}O_2$ and may serve to protect the vulnerable myocytes. Myocardial hibernation occurs during ischemia, and recovery may be delayed as long as the ischemia persists.[16]

ABNORMAL RELAXATION: THE STIFF HEART

Abnormal relaxation can be caused by either an impairment in the relaxation process or stiffening of the ventricles.[81] The decline in relaxation velocity parallels contractile dysfunction. However, the reversal of relaxation impairment is more prolonged than recovery of contractility after reperfusion takes place. Wall stiffness describes the passive stress character, or compliance, of the ventricle and is a determinant of diastolic pressure.[22] Thinning of the wall, scar tissue formation, tissue edema, and muscle fiber disarray increase stiffness.[81]

Changes in contractility and compliance can alter the ventricular function curve (see Chapter 19). A contractility change may signal a need for alteration in medical therapy. A change in compliance due to wall stiffness, however, is often transient and is part of the process of scar tissue formation.[22] Compliance changes can also follow alterations in ventricular size and geometry. The differentiation of these mechanisms partly accounts for the increased use of hemodynamic monitoring in the patient with acute MI (AMI).

CHANGE IN LEFT AND RIGHT VENTRICULAR PARAMETERS

In general, the changes in LV parameters that result from ischemia and infarction parallel the alterations in contractility and compliance. The rate of pressure development correlates with shortening velocity; both are depressed after MI. The amplitude of systolic pressure may decrease (because of decreased contractility), increase (because of catecholamine release), or remain the same. As a consequence of depressed contractility and ejection speed, the fraction of blood expelled with each ventricular contraction diminishes, SV decreases, and an increase in end-diastolic volume and fiber length results. Indirect indicators of LV function may also change. Left atrial, pulmonary artery wedge pressure (PAWP), and pulmonary artery end-diastolic pressures may increase as contractility and compliance decrease.[6,77]

Isolated RV infarction can present with increased central venous and RV end-diastolic pressures and with normal pulmonary artery systolic and wedge pressures.[12,14,15] More commonly, RV dysfunction is a companion of LV MI in the inferoposterior location.[72]

SYSTEMIC HEMODYNAMIC CHANGES

The diversity of systemic hemodynamic patterns after an MI may be due largely to variations in systemic vascular resistance (SVR). Transient hypertension with elevated SVR and normal cardiac output has been noted and may be due to catecholamine excess. The resultant increase in afterload may depress SV while increasing $M\dot{V}O_2$. The hypotension with normal cardiac output and normal or decreased SVR that is sometimes observed may represent active vasodilatation of peripheral arterioles or decreased sympathetic tone.

Most often, changes in LV contractility and compliance precipitate the onset of sympathetic compensation. Increases in heart rate help to maintain cardiac output. Elevations in SVR help sustain arterial blood pressure. If contractility is severely depressed, compensatory mechanisms fail. As peripheral resistance and afterload increase, $M\dot{V}O_2$ rises, more ischemia ensues because of inadequate perfusion, and contractility is further depressed. This process is cyclical and leads to pump failure and cardiogenic shock (see Chapters 22 and 24).

Electrophysiologic Alterations

CHANGES IN THE SINGLE CELL

Alterations in the cardiac resting potential and action potential are a consequence of ischemia (Fig. 20–11). These

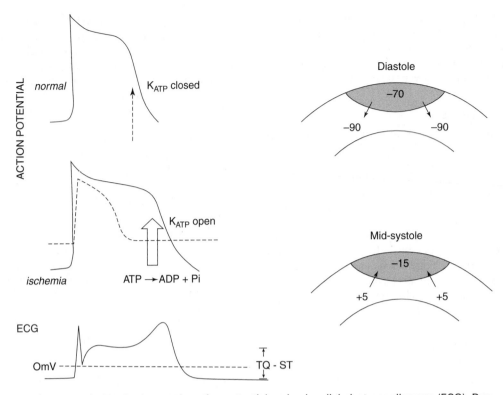

FIGURE 20-11 Ischemic changes in action potential and epicardial electrocardiogram (ECG). During the normal action potential **(top left)**, the adenosine triphosphate–sensitive potassium channel is closed. During ischemia, the resting membrane potential is less negative, with a slow rate of depolarization and early return to a higher resting level. Thus, there is shortening of the action potential duration and plateau. During diastole **(top right)**, ischemic depolarization causes a less negative value in the ischemic zone (stipples). Current therefore flows from the ischemic to the nonischemic zone, causing depression of the TQ segment. During mid-systole, however, the changes in the action potential duration mean that the ischemic zone is more negative than the nonischemic zone (compare dashed and solid lines in middle left panel). Therefore, during systole, current flows from the ischemic to the nonischemic tissue, which is reflected as ST segment elevation. Thus, as shown in the bottom left panel, there are two components for the apparent ST segment elevation of the epicardial ECG, namely true TQ depression (which is dominant) and true ST elevation. (From Opie LH: The Heart: Physiology from Cell to Circulation, 3rd ed, p 531. Philadelphia, Lippincott-Raven, 1998.)

changes are due to abnormal permeability of cell membranes and diminished ATP supplies, leading to defects in the Na⁺-K⁺ and Ca²⁺ pumps. The ischemic cell has a decreased resting membrane potential,[17] decreased conduction velocity,[90] slowed phase 0 depolarization, reduced action potential duration and amplitude, and increased phase 4 depolarization (see Chapter 1). The composite of electrical alterations in these cells is manifested by morphologic changes in the surface electrocardiogram (ECG), conduction abnormalities, and arrhythmias.

ELECTROCARDIOGRAPHIC CHANGES

In the necrotic zone, cells are equally permeable to Na⁺ and K⁺, and ionic equilibration occurs. Because the necrotic zone is electrically silent, it produces ECG changes correlating with the ischemic location. Thus, the changes in the ischemic cardiac cell correlate to specific alterations in the ECG (see Fig. 20–11). Reduction of the resting membrane potential may be associated with TQ depression. ST segment elevation relates to reduced amplitude and duration of

the action potential and delayed depolarization. T-wave inversion results from prolonged repolarization in ischemic cells relative to repolarization in normal tissue.[29,69]

MECHANISMS OF ARRHYTHMIAS

In general, conducting tissue is resistant to ischemia because of its relatively low oxygen consumption and high supply of glycogen. Purkinje cells have longer survival than the surrounding muscle because of their proximity to oxygenated ventricular cavity blood. These variations in ischemia and survival times set the stage for arrhythmias. Variations in depolarization, duration of action potential, and refractoriness contribute to random dispersal of electrical impulses in areas where ischemic and normal cells are intermixed, thus producing arrhythmias.[18,77]

Reentry and increased automaticity are the primary mechanisms responsible for electrical disturbances (Chapter 14). The influence of these mechanisms may be related to the site as well as the extent of injury in the ischemic myocardium.[18,77] The resulting arrhythmias can be significant because they may alter hemodynamics. In addition, they may extend an MI by increasing the energy imbalance in the heart. Tachycardias may also increase the amount of potassium lost to the extracellular space.

Reentry. Reentry is the most common cause of ectopy and is noted in the earliest period after MI because of the instability of collateral flow to the ischemic cells. The normal heart acts as a syncytium, in which electrically coupled cells pass impulses without decrement. The ischemic heart, however, has adjacent zones of cells that are unequal in refractoriness and excitability.[18,70] The abnormal conduction in these adjacent zones is the mechanism responsible for reentry (Chapter 14).

Recurrence of arrhythmias, caused by reentry days to weeks after the acute event, may be due to the permanent functional damage of Purkinje cells.[18,77]

Automaticity. Automaticity is a property of pacemaker cells and is due to a spontaneous loss of diastolic potential[37] (see Chapters 1 and 14).

Increased or decreased automaticity may account for arrhythmias in the period 12 to 24 hours after AMI,[18] and also in the later recovery period.[100] The slope of phase 4 depolarization determines heart rate, bringing the cell close to threshold in a cyclic manner. This slope increases in the ischemic pacemaker cell, possibly because of the influence of cyclic adenosine monophosphate (cAMP) and catecholamines, bringing the cell close to threshold sooner than normal. Spontaneous depolarization can also be initiated in nonpacemaker tissue (e.g., Purkinje cells) when the resting potential decreases, bringing the cell closer to threshold at rest. These sources of automaticity may generate *tachyarrhythmias.*[70,77]

Alternatively, a decreased slope of phase 4 depolarization sometimes may follow pronounced vagal activity after MI, causing decreased automaticity. Bradycardia and escape rhythms may subsequently occur. Early and delayed afterdepolarizations in ischemic cells may contribute to the development of automatic dysrhythmias.[64]

MECHANISMS FOR THE STRESS RESPONSE

Sympathetic Nervous System

Pain, anxiety, anger, and reflex activation of the sympathetic nervous system result in enhanced sympathetic nerve input directly to the heart, in addition to increased systemic catecholamine release.[85] Local acidosis, accumulation of metabolites, and increased wall stretch also contribute to the sympathetic response in ischemia. With progressive ischemia, the myocardium becomes increasingly overwhelmed with extracellular catecholamines. In addition, there is enhanced responsiveness of the myocardium to the catecholamines. The combination of increased catecholamines and increased sensitivity to them contribute to the propagation of the wavefront of irreversible cell death.[80]

The net effect of plasma catecholamine activity on the ischemic myocardium is related to the degree of α-, and particularly β-adrenergic overload. The positive inotropic actions of norepinephrine and epinephrine increase $M\dot{V}O_2$. α-Adrenergic stimulation elevates SVR and systolic blood pressure. Afterload increases, and cardiac work is further extended. Epinephrine stimulates β-adrenergic activity, increasing heart rate and contractility. The rate of Ca^{2+} uptake and release from the sarcoplasmic reticulum is increased, resulting in increased force (and $M\dot{V}O_2$).[68,70]

Even in humans with augmented collateral flow, a stress-induced increase in myocardial metabolism produces ischemic changes in the ECG.[98] Ischemia has also been documented as a result of mental stress, possibly due to elevating afterload and contractility. Transient vasoconstriction in stenosed arteries has also been observed. These effects are similar in magnitude to the effects observed with exercise.[83] Measurement of circulating catecholamines demonstrates peaks in norepinephrine and epinephrine within the first few hours after MI[49] and after transfer from cardiac to intermediate care units.[87,89]

Arrhythmias may be generated because of catecholamine excess. Sympathetic stimulation can lead to tachycardia and increased automaticity of nonpacemaker cells.[29] This mechanism is due to an increased inward Ca^{2+} current, which elevates the action potential plateau; enhanced K^+ current, which shortens the action potential; and increased cAMP production. The increase in cAMP enhances diastolic depolarization in the sinus node, thereby increasing heart rate, and causes hyperpolarization in the Purkinje fibers, thereby increasing automaticity.[91] The refractory period may not be uniformly shortened throughout the ischemic myocardium, resulting in initiation of reentrant arrhythmias.[18,77]

Catecholamines also induce lipolysis and enhance platelet clumping. Products of lipolysis and free fatty acid metabolism may have potentially harmful effects on the cell membranes.[63] The stress response elevates epinephrine, serotonin, and adenosine diphosphate levels, which enhance platelet clumping.[57] Significant increases in circulating platelet microthrombi have been documented in patients during the acute period of MI.[61] Thus, disrupted flow due to an occlusion and increased catecholamine activity may induce platelet aggregation and contribute to extension of the infarction.

Parasympathetic Nervous System

Increased parasympathetic activity after MI may be a protective mechanism. By decreasing heart rate and contractility, it lowers $M\dot{V}O_2$ and may protect against arrhythmias.[27] Enhanced parasympathetic stimulation may be beneficial in opposing sympathetic stimulation and preventing excessive elevations in heart rate that may jeopardize myocardial tissue in advancing ischemia.[25] Heart rate variability (normal variation in R-R interval) is considered a clinical measure of parasympathetic control. Decreased heart rate variability places patients with a history of MI[48] and sudden cardiac arrest[14] at risk for subsequent sudden cardiac arrest.

A subgroup of patients after AMI have increased vagal activity; this is most frequent after inferoposterior MI. These patients have bradycardia, atrioventricular (AV) block, and an inappropriately low SVR with normal or low cardiac output.[10]

The LV stretch receptors may be activated in the ischemic zone, leading to increased vagal afferent activity and causing symptoms of excess parasympathetic activity.[27]

MECHANISMS FOR PAIN

Ischemia activates chemoreceptors and mechanoreceptors in the myocardium. A kinin activation sequence is initiated in response to tissue injury; the bradykinin produced may activate chemoreceptors.[94] In addition, serotonin may sensitize pain receptors to bradykinin.[96] Stretch of the myocardium due to ischemic injury, edema formation, and altered local contractility may stimulate mechanoreceptors.[19] Mechanoreceptors may also be stimulated directly from alterations in the coronary vessels.[2]

Once the pain receptor is stimulated, impulses are carried by the visceral afferent fibers accompanying the sympathetic nerves. They enter the spinal cord through the eighth cervical to the first four thoracic dorsal root ganglia. The dermatomes (peripheral axonal fields supplied by single dorsal roots) innervating the heart are also shared by other cutaneous and somatic structures. When the brain receives a pain impulse from those dermatomes, the input may be registered as coming from any of those structures. Because neck or arm pain is more commonly experienced than is cardiac visceral pain, the cardiac afferent input may be interpreted as jaw, neck, or arm discomfort. This explains the mechanism of referred pain frequently observed with angina associated with MI. In addition, the brain uses past experience to integrate information; this central processing of pain may either excite or inhibit nociception.[5]

Silent Myocardial Ischemia

Approximately 70% of ischemic episodes in patients with CHD are silent,[88] making silent ischemia a more common occurrence than angina. In addition, up to 30% of symptomatic MIs are silent.[96] Ischemia is more likely to be silent when it occurs in the setting of decreased coronary blood flow as opposed to increased demand, such as in exercise.[59] In patients who have both painful and silent ischemia, the painful episodes are more likely to involve more severe and longer periods of ischemia.[78] Silent ischemia has outcomes similar to those of painful ischemia, however.[5]

Silent ischemia is particularly common among patients with diabetes, possibly because of a neuropathy that inhibits pain perception.[43] Ischemia may be silent when it involves the afferent pain fiber, effectively denervating the area.[46] Some patients with silent ischemia have an increased pain threshold and tolerance and reduced pain sensitivity, contributing to a "defective pain warning system."[24] Perception of ischemic pain may, therefore, be diminished at the point of origin, in the transmission of pain, or in the central processing of pain.[5]

CIRCADIAN RHYTHMICITY

The frequency of ischemic episodes increases between 7 to 8 AM, reaches a plateau at 1 PM, and gradually decreases thereafter, with possibly a second peak at approximately 6 PM.[74,79] Heart rate,[62] blood pressure, and contractility

(measured indirectly as plasma epinephrine level) [92] peak between 7 AM and noon, contributing to increased $M\dot{V}O_2$. Plasma norepinephrine levels[121] and renin activity[38] are also increased in the early morning, contributing to vasoconstriction. The increased plasma cortisol levels that occur in the early morning have a synergistic effect on the action of catecholamines.[99]

Platelet aggregation is greater in the early morning,[92] and the intrinsic fibrinolytic activity of blood is lowest in the morning. These factors contribute to the circadian pattern of increased ischemia in the early morning, which may be amplified by the assumption of upright posture.

CONSEQUENCES OF REPERFUSION

Local Consequences of Reperfusion

Reperfusion or restoration of flow to previously ischemic myocardium after a period of occlusion has been the subject of inquiry since the advent of techniques to reduce infarct size. Reperfusion also occurs each time coronary spasm is relieved or angina secondary to increased $M\dot{V}O_2$ (in the setting of fixed stenotic coronary lesions) subsides. Reperfusion can influence viability only for those myocardial cells not irreversibly injured; therefore, the potential benefits of reperfusion are time dependent (see Fig. 20–10). Histochemical studies suggest early reperfusion leads to smaller infarcts and structural recovery of ischemic myocytes, whereas late reperfusion (3 hours of coronary artery occlusion) accelerates myocyte degeneration.[84] Therefore, reperfusion of injured cells has both beneficial and harmful effects.[51]

Reperfusion Injury

The act of reperfusion may independently contribute to ischemia by creating postischemic cardiac dysfunction, irreversible injury, and reperfusion arrhythmias.[36] However, it is difficult to differentiate reperfusion injury due to oxygen-free radicals (OFRs) from the acceleration of the necrotic process due to ischemia.[51] Transient worsening of the ECG, acceleration of Q-wave development, and an early CK rise reflect damage from ischemia; these signs do not indicate injury from reperfusion.[69]

Reperfusion of the ischemic myocardium results in an explosive production of OFRs, peaking in the first minute of reperfusion, and continuing for hours after reperfusion.[35] The radicals are produced by endothelial cells, granulocytes, mitochondria, and catecholamines. OFRs are highly toxic to endothelia, mitochondria, and collagen, and cause severe tissue injury. Early effects of OFRs may be mediated by changes in the lipid environment of the membrane proteins or by direct oxidation of amino acids and proteins. This causes loss of enzyme activity and altered function of ion channels, transporters, and receptors. Late effects may be caused by disruption of the sarcolemma in myocytes.[37]

In reperfusion injury, damage occurs not only to the myocytes, but also to the microvasculature. This damage causes the "no-reflow phenomenon," which refers to blood flow not returning to its preischemic level.[66] The no-reflow phenomenon occurs in areas of myocardium where endothelial cells undergo irreversible injury. The microvascular damage probably prevents flow to jeopardized myocytes and contributes to necrosis. With the damaged endothelium, production of the vasodilator, nitric oxide, may be inhibited, production of endothelin may be stimulated, and neutrophils and platelets may be activated, contributing to the no-reflow phenomenon.[75]

Reperfusion arrhythmias may be due to either overload of calcium or formation of OFRs. Because ischemia is also responsible for calcium overload and arrhythmias are an insensitive marker for reperfusion in the setting of MI, it is difficult to separate the arrhythmias due to reperfusion from those due to ischemia.[51] Of interest, however, is the role that reperfusion arrhythmias play in sudden cardiac arrest in patients with variant angina, stable angina, unstable angina, and silent ischemia, and after restoration of blood flow to the heart after cardiopulmonary bypass.[64]

Stunned myocardium is viable myocardial tissue that has been salvaged by coronary reperfusion but exhibits prolonged postischemic contraction dysfunction.[16,66] Stunned myocardium returns to normal function within hours to weeks. The myofilaments exhibit depressed sensitivity and reduced force in response to calcium, possibly because of the effect of OFRs on the myofilaments.

RESTENOSIS AND REOCCLUSION

Restenosis of a vessel is due to the buildup of atherosclerotic plaque, whereas reocclusion of a vessel is usually due to thrombus formation. In the acute situation, occlusion or reocclusion of the vessel with thrombus is most likely to occur. Angioplasty may lead to intimal tears that extend even deeper than those naturally occurring; these sites are at risk for formation of hematomas that extend into, and may obstruct, the vessel lumen.[20] With thrombolysis, the residual thrombus creates increased shear forces, which facilitate the activation and deposition of platelets on the lesion. In addition, thrombi that undergo lysis expose a highly thrombogenic surface to the blood, activating platelets and the coagulation system once again, and potentially leading to thrombotic reocclusion.[34] This same mechanism accounts for late reocclusion of the vessel.

With restenosis, the endothelial damage causes thrombus formation, followed by an accelerated fibroproliferative response.[28] Platelets adhered to the vessel wall produce PDGFs, which stimulate smooth muscle cell migration within 48 hours of injury. The inflammatory cells that respond to the injury secrete and release membrane growth factors up to 1 to 2 weeks after the injury. Smooth muscle and endothelial cells proliferate and produce other growth factors that stimulate production of an extracellular matrix. This matrix accumulates in the subintima over the next 3 to 6 months, and may contribute to late restenosis. Gradually, the matrix evolves to consist primarily of collagen, producing the raised scar at the site of injury.[11]

IMPLICATIONS FOR NURSING

Ischemia is a condition that is influenced by alterations of either the *supply* of oxygen and nutrients to the myocardium, or *demand* of the myocardium for oxygen and nutrients. The extent of symptoms resulting from supply or demand depends on the specific pathophysiologic process in the individual patient. Supply of oxygen and nutrients may be altered by *functional* or *mechanical* conditions, or a combination of both. The extent of functional versus mechanical alteration also depends on the patient's specific pathophysiologic process.

The consequences of ischemia include contractile failure, dysrhythmias, sympathetic nervous system stimulation, and pain. When the normal physiologic response to injury becomes pathophysiologic and contributes to dysfunction, nursing interventions are indicated. Nurses can plan to prevent ischemia from occurring, identify early symptoms of ischemia, intervene to salvage myocardium at risk, and evaluate the effectiveness of the interventions for future modification. Thus, knowledge of ischemic pathophysiology contributes to nursing care at every step of the process. This knowledge therefore can improve the nursing care delivered to the individual patient and promote positive outcomes and responses to cardiac ischemia.

REFERENCES

1. Alonso DR, Scheidt S, Post M, Killip T: Pathophysiology of cardiogenic shock: Quantification of myocardial necrosis, clinical, pathologic and electrocardiographic correlations. Circulation 48: 588–596, 1973
2. Baker DG, Coleridge HM, Coleridge JC et al: Search for a cardiac nociceptor: Stimulation of bradykinin of sympathetic nerve endings in the heart of the cat. J Physiol (Lond) 306: 519–536, 1980
3. Banai S, Jaklitsch MT, Shou M et al: Angiogenic-induced enhancement of collateral blood flow to ischemic myocardium by vascular endothelial growth factor in dogs. Circulation 89: 2183–2189, 1994
4. Baroldi G: Coronary thrombosis: Facts and beliefs. Am Heart J 91: 683–688, 1976
5. Barsky AJ, Hochstrasser B, Coles NA et al: Silent myocardial ischemia. Is the person or the event silent? JAMA 264: 1132–1135, 1990
6. Bertrand ME, Rousseau MF, LaBlanche JM: Cineangiographic assessment of left ventricular function in the acute phase of transmural myocardial infarction. Am J Cardiol 43: 472–480, 1979
7. Billman GE: Mechanisms responsible for the cardiotoxic effects of cocaine. FASEB J 4: 2469–2475, 1990
8. Bouchardy B, Majno G: Histopathology of early myocardial infarcts: A new approach. Am J Pathol 74: 301–330, 1974
9. Brown BG, Bolson EL, Dodge HT: Dynamic mechanisms in human coronary stenosis. Circulation 70: 917–922, 1984
10. Bulkley BH: Site and sequelae of myocardial infarction. N Engl J Med 305: 337–338, 1981
11. Cercek B, Sharifi B, Barath P et al: Growth factors in pathogenesis of coronary arterial restenosis. Am J Cardiol 68: 24C–33C, 1991
12. Cintron GB, Hernandez E, Linares E et al: Bedside recognition, incidence and clinical course of right ventricular infarction. Am J Cardiol 47: 224–227, 1981
13. Cohen MV: The functional value of coronary collaterals in myocardial ischemia and therapeutic approach to enhance collateral flow. Am Heart J 95: 396–404, 1978
14. Cohn JN, Guiha NH, Broder MI: Right ventricular infarction: Clinical and hemodynamic features. Am J Cardiol 32: 209–214, 1974
15. Cohn JN: Right ventricular infarction revisited. Am J Cardiol 43: 666–668, 1979

16. Conti CR: The stunned and hibernating myocardium: A brief review. Clin Cardiol 14: 708–712, 1991

17. Corr PB, Sobel BE: The importance of metabolites in the genesis of ventricular dysrhythmias induced by ischemia: I. Electrophysiological considerations. Modern Concepts of Cardiovascular Disease 48(8): 34–47, 1979

18. Corr PB, Sobel BE: The importance of metabolites in the genesis of ventricular dysrhythmias induced by ischemia: II. Biochemical factors. Modern Concepts of Cardiovascular Disease 48(9): 48–52, 1979

19. Davies GJ, Bencivelli W, Fragasso G et al: Sequence and magnitude of ventricular volume changes in painful and painless myocardial ischemia. Circulation 78: 310–319, 1988

20. Davies MJ: A macro and micro view of coronary vascular insult in ischemic heart disease. Circulation, 82(Suppl 3): II38–II46, 1990

21. DeWood MA, Spores J, Notske R et al: Prevalence of total coronary occlusion during the early hours of transmural myocardial infarction. N Engl J Med 303: 897–902, 1980

22. Diamond G, Forrester JS: Effect of coronary artery disease and acute myocardial infarction on left ventricular compliance in man. Circulation 45: 11–19, 1972

23. Dinerman JL, Mehta JL: Endothelial, platelet, and leukocyte interactions in ischemic heart disease: Insights into potential mechanisms and their clinical relevance. J Am Coll Cardiol 16: 207–222, 1990

24. Droste C, Greenlee MW, Roskamm H: A defective angina pectoris pain warning system: Experimental findings of ischemic and electrical pain test. Pain 26: 199–209, 1986

25. Eckberg DL, Drabinsky M, Braunwald E: Defective cardiac parasympathetic control in patients with heart disease. N Engl J Med 285: 877–884, 1971

26. Fallon JT: Pathology of myocardial infarction and reperfusion. In Fuster V, Ross R, Topol EJ (eds): Atherosclerosis and Coronary Artery Disease, pp 791–796. Philadelphia, Lippincott-Raven, 1996

27. Feola M, Arbel ER, Glick G et al: Attenuation of cardiac sympathetic drive in experimental myocardial ischemia in dogs. Am Heart J 93: 82–88, 1977

28. Forrester J: Intimal disruption and coronary thrombosis: Its role in the pathogenesis of human coronary disease. Am J Cardiol 68: 69B–77B, 1991

29. Fozzard HA, Makielski JC: The electrophysiology of acute myocardial ischemia. Annu Rev Med 36: 275–284, 1985

30. Fuster V: Conner Memorial Lecture. Mechanisms leading to myocardial infarction: Insights from studies of vascular biology. Circulation 90: 2126–2146 [published erratum appears in Circulation 91: 256 1995, 1994

31. Fuster V: Human lesion studies. Ann N Y Acad Sci 811: 207–224; 1997

32. Fuster V, Badimon L, Badimon JJ et al: The pathogenesis of coronary artery disease and the acute coronary syndromes: Part 2. N Engl J Med 326: 310–318, 1992

33. Fuster V, Badimon L, Badimon JJ et al: The pathogenesis of coronary artery disease and the acute coronary syndromes: Part 1. N Engl J Med 326: 242–250, 1992

34. Fuster V, Stein B, Ambrose JA et al: Atherosclerotic plaque rupture and thrombosis: Evolving concepts. Circulation 82: II47–II59, 1990

35. Garcia-Dorado D, Oliveras J: Myocardial oedema: A preventable cause of reperfusion injury? Cardiovasc Res 27: 1555–1563, 1993

36. Glasako GI: Cocaine, a risk factor for myocardial infarction. Journal of Cardiovascular Risk 4: 185–190, 1997

37. Goldhaber JI, Weiss JN: Oxygen free radicals and cardiac reperfusion abnormalities. Hypertension 20: 118–127, 1992

38. Gordon RD, Wolfe LK, Island DP et al: A diurnal rhythm in plasma renin activity in man. J Clin Invest 45: 1587–1592, 1966

39. Gorlin R: Role of coronary vasospasm in the pathogenesis of myocardial ischemia and angina pectoris. Am Heart J 103: 598–603, 1982

40. Gotlieb AI, Langille BL: The Role of Rheology in Atherosclerotic Coronary Artery Disease. In Fuster V, Ross R, Topol EJ (eds): Atherosclerosis and Coronary Artery Disease, pp 595–606. Philadelphia, Lippincott-Raven, 1996

41. Gregg DE: The natural history of coronary collateral development. Circ Res 35: 335–344, 1974

42. Hale SL, Lehmann MH, Kloner RA: Electrocardiographic abnormalities after acute administration of cocaine in the rat. Am J Cardiol 63: 1529–1530, 1989

43. Hikita II, Kurita A, Takase B et al: Usefulness of plasma beta-endorphin level, pain threshold and autonomic function in assessing silent myocardial ischemia in patients with and without diabetes mellitus. Am J Cardiol 72: 140–143, 1993

44. Hollander JE, Shih RD, Hoffman RS et al: Predictors of coronary artery disease in patients with cocaine-associated myocardial infarction: Cocaine-Associated Myocardial Infarction (CAMI) Study Group. Am J Med 102: 158–163, 1997

45. Houston DS, Shepherd JT, Vanhoutte PM: Aggregating human platelets cause direct contraction and endothelium-dependent relaxation of isolated canine coronary arteries: Role of serotonin, thromboxane A_2 and and adenine nucleotides. J Clin Invest 78: 539–544, 1986

46. Inoue H, Skale BT, Zipes DP: Effects of ischemia on cardiac afferent sympathetic and vagal reflexes in dog. Am J Physiol 255: H26–H35, 1988

47. Jennings RB, Murry CE, Steenbergen C Jr et al: Development of cell injury in sustained acute ischemia. Circulation 82(Suppl 3): II2–II12, 1990

48. Kleiger RE, Miller JP, Bigger JT Jr, et al, and The Multicenter Post-Infarction Research Group: Decreased heart rate variability and its association with increased mortality after acute myocardial infarction. Am J Cardiol 59: 256–262, 1987

49. Klein RF, Troyer WG, Thompson HK: Catecholamine excretion in myocardial infarction. Arch Intern Med 122: 476–482, 1968

50. Kloner RA, Hale S, Alker K et al: The effects of acute and chronic cocaine use on the heart. Circulation 85: 407–419, 1992

51. Kloner RA: Does reperfusion injury exist in humans? J Am Coll Cardiol 21: 537–545, 1993

52. Kullo IJ, Edwards WD, Schwartz RS: Vulnerable plaque: Pathobiology and clinical implications. Ann Intern Med 129: 1050–1060, 1998

53. Lodge-Patch I: The ageing of cardiac infarcts, and its influence on cardiac rupture. Br Heart J 13: 37–42, 1951

54. Losordo DW, Vale PR, Symes JF et al: Gene therapy for myocardial angiogenesis: Initial clinical results with direct myocardial injection of phVEGF165 as sole therapy for myocardial ischemia. Circulation 98: 2800–2804, 1998

55. Majid PA, Patel B, Kim HS et al: An angiographic and histologic study of cocaine-induced chest pain. Am J Cardiol 65: 812–814, 1990

56. Mallory GK, White PD, Salcedo-Salgar J: The speed and healing of myocardial infarction. Am Heart J 18: 647–658, 1939

57. Marcus AJ: Platelet Activation. In Fuster V, Ross R, Topol EJ (eds): Artherosclerosis and Coronary Artery Disease, pp 607–637. Philadelphia, Lippincott-Raven, 1996

58. Marvoka Y, Tomoike H, Kawachi Y et al: Relations between collateral flow and tissue salvage in the risk area after acute coronary occlusion in dogs: A topographical analysis. Br J Exp Pathol 67: 33–42, 1986

59. Maseri A, Parodi O, Severi S et al: Transient transmural reduction of myocardial blood flow demonstrated by thallium-201 scintigraphy, as a cause of variant angina. Circulation 54: 280–288, 1976

60. Mehta JL, Nichols WW, Mehta P: Neutrophils as potential participants in acute myocardial ischemia: Relevance to reperfusion. J Am Coll Cardiol 11: 1309–1316, 1988

61. Mehta M, Mehta J: Platelet function studies in coronary artery disease: Evidence for enhanced platelet microthrombus formation activity in acute myocardial infarction. Am J Cardiol 43: 757–760, 1979

62. Milar-Craig MW, Bishop CN, Raftery EB: Circadian variation of blood pressure. Lancet 1: 795–797, 1978

63. Mueller HS, Ayres SM: Metabolic responses of the heart in acute myocardial infarction in man. Am J Cardiol 42: 363–371, 1978

64. Myerburg RJ, Kessler KM, Castellanos A: Pathophysiology of sudden cardiac death. Pacing Clin Electrophysiol 14: 935–943, 1991

65. Nademanee K, Gorelick DA, Josephson MA et al: Myocardial ischemia during cocaine withdrawal. Ann Intern Med 111: 876–880, 1989

66. Naka Y, Stern DM, Pinsky DJ: The pathophysiology and biochemistry of myocardial ischemia, necrosis, and reperfusion. In Fuster V, Ross R, Topol EJ (eds): Atherosclerosis and Coronary Artery Disease, pp 807–817. Philadelphia, Lippincott-Raven, 1996

67. Ohnishi M, Yamada K, Morooka S et al: Inhibition of P-selectin attenuates neutrophil-mediated myocardial dysfunction in isolated rat heart. Eur J Pharmacol 5: 271–279, 1999

68. Oliver MF: The metabolic response to a heart attack. Heart Lung 4: 57–60, 1975

69. Opie, LH: The Heart: Physiology from Cell to Circulation, pp 515–541. New York, Raven Press, 1991

70. Opie LH, Nathan D, Lubbe WF: Biochemical aspects of arrhythmogenesis and ventricular fibrillation. Am J Cardiol 432: 131–148, 1979

71. Opie LH, Owen P, Lubbe W: Estimated glycolytic flux in infarcting heart. Recent Advances in Studies of Cardiac Structure and Metabolism 7: 249–255, 1976

72. O'Rourke RA, Dell'Italia LJ: Right Ventricular Myocardial Infarction. In Fuster V, Ross R, Topol EJ (eds): Artherosclerosis and Coronary Artery Disease, pp 1079–1096. Philadelphia Lippincott-Raven, 1996

73. Page E, Polimeni PI: Ultrastructural changes in the ischemic zone bordering experimental infarcts in rat left ventricles. Am J Pathol 87: 81–92, 1977

74. Pelter MM, Adams MG, Wung SF et al: Peak time of occurrence of myocardial ischemia in the coronary care unit. Am J Crit Care 7: 411–417, 1998

75. Pinsky DJ, Oz MC, Koga S et al: Cardiac preservation is enhanced in a heterotopic rat transplant model by supplementing the nitric oxide pathway. J Clin Invest 93: 2291–2297, 1994

76. Pudil R, Pidrman V, Krejsek J et al: Cytokines and adhesion molecules in the course of acute myocardial infarction. Clin Chim Acta 280: 127–134, 1999

77. Puri PS: Correlation between biochemical and contractile changes after myocardial ischemia and revascularization. Recent Advances in Studies on Cardiac Structure and Metabolism 7: 161–169, 1976

78. Quyyumi AA, Mockus L, Wright C et al: Morphology of ambulatory ST segment changes in patients with varying severity of coronary artery disease: Investigation of the frequency of nocturnal ischaemia and coronary spasm. Br Heart J 53: 186–193, 1985

79. Quyyumi AA: Current concepts of pathophysiology, circadian patterns, and vasoreactive factors associated with myocardial ischemia detected by ambulatory electrocardiography. Cardiol Clin 10: 403–415, 1992

80. Reimer KA, Jennings RB: The "wavefront phenomenon" of myocardial ischemic cell death: II. Transmural progression of necrosis within the framework of ischemic bed size (myocardium at risk) and collateral flow. Lab Invest 40 : 633–644, 1979

81. Ross J, Franklin D: Analysis of regional myocardial function, dimensions, and wall thickness in the characterization of myocardial ischemia and infarction. Circulation 53(Suppl I): 188–192, 1976

82. Ross R: Platelet derived growth factor. Lancet 1: 1179–1182, 1989

83. Rozanski A, Bairey CN, Krantz DS et al: Mental stress and the induction of silent myocardial ischemia in patients with coronary artery disease. N Engl J Med 318: 1005–1012, 1988

84. Schaper J, Schaper W: Reperfusion of ischemic myocardium: Ultrastructural and histochemical aspects. J Am Coll Cardiol 1: 1037–1046, 1983

85. Schöming A: Catecholamines in myocardial ischemia: Systemic and cardiac release. Circulation 82: II13–II22, 1990

86. Schwarz F, Flameng W, Ensslen R et al: Effect of coronary collaterals on left ventricular function at rest and during stress. Am Heart J 95: 570–577, 1978

87. Shannon VJ: The transfer process: An area for concern for the CCU nurse. Heart Lung 2: 364–367, 1973

88. Shea MJ, Deanfield JE, Wilson R et al: Transient ischemia in angina pectoris: Frequent silent events with every day activities. J Am Coll Cardiol 56: 34E–38E, 1985

89. Siggers DC, Salter C, Fluck DC: Serial plasma adrenaline and noradrenaline levels in myocardial infarction using a new double isotope technique. Br Heart J 33: 878–883, 1971

90. Smith HJ, Kent KM, Epstein SE: Relationship between regional contractile function and S-T segment elevation after experimental coronary artery occlusion in the dog. Cardiovasc Res 12: 444–448, 1978

91. Thandroyen FT, Muntz KH, Buja LM et al: Alterations in β-adrenergic receptors, adenylate cyclase, and cyclic AMP concentrations during acute myocardial ischemia and reperfusion. Circulation 83: II30–II37, 1990

92. Tofler GH, Brezinski D, Schafer AI et al: Concurrent morning increase in platelet aggregability and the risk of myocardial infarction and sudden cardiac death. N Engl J Med 316: 1514–1518, 1987

93. Togna G, Tempesta E, Togna AR et al: Platelet responsiveness and biosynthesis of thromboxane and prostacyclin in response to in vitro cocaine treatment. Haemostasis 15: 100–107, 1985

94. Torstila I: The plasma kinin system in acute myocardial infarction. Acta Medica Scandinavica Supplementum 620: 1–62, 1978

95. Unger EF, Banai S, Shou M et al: Basic fibroblast growth enhances myocardial collateral flow in a canine model. Am J Physiol 266: H1588–H1595, 1994

96. Uretsky BF, Farquhar OS, Berezin AF et al: Symptomatic myocardial infarction without chest pain: Prevalence and clinical course. Am J Cardiol 40: 498–503, 1977

97. Van de Kar LD, Levy AD, Rittenhouse PA et al: Cocaine-induced suppression of renin secretion is mediated in the brain: Investigation of cardiovascular and local anesthetic mechanisms. Brain Res Bull 28: 837–842, 1992

98. Wahr DW, Ports TA, Botvinick EH et al: The effects of coronary angioplasty and reperfusion on distribution of myocardial flow. Circulation 72: 334–343, 1985

99. Weitzman ED, Fukshinma D, Nogeire C et al: Twenty-four patterns of the episodic secretion of cortisol in normal subjects. J Clin Endocrinol Metab 33: 14–22, 1971

100. Wit AL, Bigger JT: Possible electrophysiological mechanisms for lethal arrhythmias accompanying myocardial ischemia and infarction. Circulation 51(Suppl III): III96–III115, 1975

DIAGNOSIS AND MANAGEMENT OF MYOCARDIAL ISCHEMIA

Myocardial oxygen demand is increased by exercise, emotional stress, smoking tobacco, eating heavy meals, and exposure to cold weather or extreme humidity.[22] As long as coronary vasodilation increases blood supply, this extra demand can be met. Coronary atherosclerosis or vasospasm, however, may prevent adequate coronary vasodilation, which may result in myocardial ischemia. Ischemia is reversible, but if myocardial blood flow is not increased or myocardial oxygen demands are not reduced, ischemia can progress to cell death (MI).

Angina pectoris, literally "strangling of the chest," is a symptom of myocardial ischemia. Myocardial ischemia can occur without angina, however, and is referred to as *silent ischemia*.

EPIDEMIOLOGY

Although mortality from CHD continues to decrease, MI is still the leading cause of death in the United States.[6] Eighty percent of all coronary deaths occur in patients 65 years of age and older.[17] Unstable angina accounts for approximately 50% of all admissions to coronary care units in the United States,[1] and approximately 60% of the people admitted to the hospital with unstable angina are older than 65 years of age. Each year, approximately 1 to 1.5 million Americans have an MI,[5,9] and the mortality rate is approximately 33%. Fifty percent of victims wait 2 hours after the onset of pain before deciding to seek medical help, and approximately 300,000 people per year die from MI before reaching the hospital. The mortality rate for patients who reach the hospital is 10% to 15%.[7]

CLASSIFICATION OF ANGINA

There are a variety of categorization systems for angina. For example, the Canadian system[22] is based on functional capacity and applies to all types of angina (Display 20–2). Other systems have been developed specifically for unstable angina (Table 20–1).

Stable (Classic) Angina

Stable angina is characterized by transient episodes of substernal chest pain or discomfort (which may be accompanied by arm or jaw pain) related to activities that increase myocardial oxygen demand (Fig. 20–12). Its patterns are usually predictable. Rest or sublingual nitroglycerin usually relieves the discomfort within a few minutes.

Anginal equivalents are characterized by a sensation of dyspnea, excessive fatigue or weakness, or isolated arm or jaw pain as the major manifestation of cardiac ischemia. The elderly are likely to experience the anginal equivalents already described, or palpitations, excessive sweating, dizziness, or syncope as manifestations of angina.[17]

Variant Angina (Prinzmetal's Angina)

Variant angina, a less common form of angina, is characterized by episodes of chest pain that occur at rest. This discomfort tends to be prolonged, severe, and not readily relieved by nitroglycerin. Variant angina is caused by spasm of the coronary arteries and can be accompanied by transient elevation of the ST segment. The *transient* ST segment elevation recorded during an episode of variant angina should not be confused with the ST segment elevation recorded in the acute phase of MI.

Unstable Angina

Unstable angina is a syndrome classified as intermediate in severity between stable angina and MI.[3] The main features are recent onset of angina, prolonged angina at rest, or a change in the pattern of angina.[21,22] One classification system describing the severity of unstable angina is given in Table 20–1. It is believed that unstable angina usually results from rupture of an atherosclerotic plaque, which partially thromboses a coronary artery.[8] In addition, certain signs and symptoms suggestive of unstable angina may be used to determine the likelihood of having significant coronary disease (Table 20–2) and the risk of sudden death (Table 20–3).

DIAGNOSIS

Myocardial ischemia can be diagnosed by patient history, ECG, stress testing, cardiac imaging, echocardiography, and coronary angiography. Patients with chest pain may be stratified into low- or high-risk groups for myocardial ischemia on the basis of history and laboratory findings.

History

DURATION AND QUALITY

Angina is a subjective symptom that usually lasts 2 to 5 minutes if the precipitating factor is relieved. It can occasionally last 5 to 15 minutes, and rarely 15 to 30 minutes. Patients

DISPLAY 20-2

Canadian Cardiovascular Society Classification for Angina Pectoris

Class I	*Ordinary physical activity* (such as walking or climbing stairs) *does not cause angina.* Angina may occur with strenuous, rapid, or prolonged exertion (work or recreation).
Class II	There is *slight limitation of ordinary activity.* Angina may occur with walking or climbing stairs rapidly; walking uphill; walking or stair climbing after meals or in the cold, in the wind, or under emotional stress; walking more than two blocks on the level and climbing one flight of stairs at a normal pace under normal conditions.
Class III	There is *marked limitation of ordinary physical activity.* Angina may occur after walking one or two blocks on the level or climbing one flight of stairs in normal conditions at a normal pace.
Class IV	There is *inability to carry on any physical activity without discomfort; angina* may be present *at rest.*

From Canadian Cardiovascular Society Classification for Angina Pectoris. Courtesy of the Canadian Cardiovascular Society. Shub C, Click RL, & McGoon MD: Myocardial ischemia clinical syndromes, p. 1164. Mayo Clinic Practice of Cardiology (3rd Ed.) Mosby, St. Louis, 1996.

sign). Asymptomatic, or silent, ischemia may also occur. Angina also may be associated with many other conditions (Display 20–3). Differentiation of CHD pain from other causes of chest discomfort can be difficult.

ANATOMIC LOCATION

Discomfort is usually described in the retrosternal region, although it may occur anywhere in the chest. It usually radiates down the left arm, but occasionally may radiate down both. The pain may radiate to the jaw or mouth, or the neck. The patient may complain of an aching shoulder, wrist, elbow, or forearm, which may be significant when it is not related to effort involving that shoulder or arm. Sometimes, patients experience discomfort only in the area of radiated pain (e.g., arm or jaw) without discomfort in the chest (see Fig. 20–12). A circumscribed painful area smaller than the size of a fingertip usually does not indicate myocardial ischemia.

PRECIPITATING FACTORS

Stable angina occurs during physical exertion, usually at a defined exercise level, and is relieved by rest or nitroglycerin. Occasionally, a patient may experience a *second-wind phenomenon*, characterized by discomfort that develops during exertion but disappears while the activity is continued. Early-morning activity after a night's sleep sometimes precipitates angina that the same level of activity later in the day does not.

Angina may result from eating a heavy meal because of increased gastrointestinal oxygen demand. Smoking tobacco may result in angina by increasing myocardial work from the release of endogenous catecholamines, or by causing coronary artery spasm.

Emotional tension is a frequent precursor of angina. Catecholamine release increases heart rate and systemic blood pressure, thereby increasing the work of the heart.

do not always describe chest "pain." Common descriptions of anginal discomfort include sensations of chest heaviness, tightness, squeezing, pressing, aching, burning, or even indigestion. A patient may clench his or her fist over his or her sternum when describing the discomfort (Levine's

TABLE 20-1	Classification of Unstable Angina		
	Clinical Circumstances		
Severity	**A. Develops in Presence of Extracardiac Condition That Intensifies Myocardial Ischemia (Secondary UA)**	**B. Develops in Absence of Extracardiac Condition (Primary UA)**	**C. Develops Within 2 wk After AMI (Postinfarction UA)**
I. New onset of severe angina or accelerated angina; no rest pain	IA	IB	IC
II. Angina at rest within past month but not within preceding 48 h (Angina at rest, subacute)	IIA	IIB	IIC
III. Angina at rest within 48 h (Angina at rest, acute)	IIIA	IIIB	IIIC

UA, unstable angina; AMI, acute myocardial infarction.

Patients with UA may also be divided into three groups depending on whether UA occurs (1) in the absence of treatment for chronic stable angina, (2) during treatment for chronic stable angina, or (3) despite maximal anti-ischemic drug therapy. These three groups may be designated by subscripts 1, 2, or 3, respectively.

Patients with UA may be further divided into those with and without transient ST-T–wave changes during pain.

From Braunwald E: Unstable Angina: A classification. Circulation 80(2): 411, August 1989.

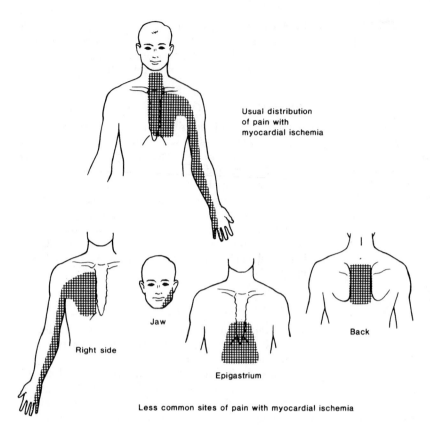

Usual distribution
of pain with
myocardial ischemia

Jaw

Right side

Epigastrium

Back

Less common sites of pain with myocardial ischemia

FIGURE 20-12 Pain patterns with myocardial ischemia. The usual distribution is referral to all or part of the sternal region, the left side of the chest, the neck, and down the ulnar side of the left forearm and hand. With severe ischemic pain, the right chest and right arm are often involved as well, although isolated involvement of these areas is rare. Other sites sometimes involved, either alone or together with pain in other sites, are the jaw, epigastrium, and back. (From Horwitz LD, Groves BM: Signs and Symptoms in Cardiology, p 9. Philadelphia, JB Lippincott, 1985)

Chest discomfort from emotional stress tends to persist longer than that produced by physical stress, probably because emotions are not as easily controlled or abated as activity.[12,22]

ALLEVIATING FACTORS

Stable angina is often relieved by rest. Nitroglycerin also often relieves angina, and relief by nitroglycerin may help in diag-

nosing the cause of chest pain. However, these features alone are not sufficient for diagnosis because chest pain caused by esophageal spasm may also be relieved by nitroglycerin.

Physical Assessment

A generalized physical assessment may also provide helpful diagnostic information. The presence of xanthomas, for example, especially in a young client, may indicate hypercho-

TABLE 20-2	**Likelihood of Significant Coronary Artery Disease in Patients With Symptoms Suggesting Unstable Angina**	
High Likelihood	**Intermediate Likelihood**	**Low Likelihood**
Any of the following features	Absence of high likelihood features and any of the following	Absence of high or intermediate likelihood features but may have
Known history of coronary artery disease	Definite angina: mean <60 or women <70 years of age	Chest pain, probably not angina
Definite angina: men ≥ 60 or women ≥ 70 years of age	Probable angina: men >60 or women >70 years of age	One risk factor but not diabetes
Hemodynamic changes or ECG changes with pain	Probably not angina in diabetics or in nondiabetics with two or more other risk factors*	T wave flat or inverted <1 mm in leads with dominant R waves
Variant angina	Extracardiac vascular disease	Normal ECG
ST increase or decrease ≥1 mm	ST depression 0.05 to 1 mm	
Marked symmetric T-wave inversion in multiple precordial leads	T-wave inversion ≥1 mm in leads with dominant R waves	

ECG, electrocardiogram.
*Coronary artery disease risk factors include diabetes, smoking, hypertension, and elevated cholesterol.
From Braunwald E, Jones RH, Mark DB et al: Diagnosing and managing unstable angina. Circulation 90(1): 617, July 1994.

TABLE 20-3	Short-Term Risk of Death or Nonfatal Myocardial Infarction in Patients With Symptoms Suggesting Unstable Angina	
High Risk	**Intermediate Risk**	**Low Risk**
At least one of the following features must be present	No high-risk features but must have any of the following	No high- or intermediate-risk features but may have any of the following
Prolonged ongoing (>20 min) rest pain	Rest angina now resolved but not low likelihood of CAD	Increased angina frequency, severity, or duration
Pulmonary edema	Rest angina (>20 min or relieved with rest or nitroglycerin)	Angina provoked at a lower threshold
Angina with new or worsening mitral regurgitation murmurs	Angina with dynamic T-wave changes	New-onset angina within 2 wk to 2 mo
Rest angina with dynamic ST changes ≥1 mm	Nocturnal angina	Normal or unchanged electrocardiogram
Angina with S$_3$ or rales	New-onset CCSC III or IV angina in past 2 wk but not low likelihood of CAD	
Angina with hypotension	Q waves or ST depression ≥1 mm in multiple leads	
	Age >65 y	

CAD, coronary artery disease; CCSC, Canadian Cardiovascular Society Classification.

From Hurst JW: Artherosclerotic coronary heart disease: Historical benchmarks, methods of study and clinical features, differential diagnosis and clinical spectrum. In Hurst JW, Schlant RC, Rackley CE (eds): The Heart, 7th ed, p 938. New York, McGraw-Hill, 1990.

lesterolemia. Systemic hypertension is known to accelerate the development of atherosclerosis. Carotid or femoral bruits may indicate diffuse arteriosclerosis and increase the possibility of obstructive coronary artery disease being present.

During an anginal event, the patient may exhibit pallor, cold, clammy skin, an increased heart rate, and pulsus alternans. Systemic blood pressure may be elevated at the onset of the event.

A paradoxically split S$_2$ or an S$_3$ may be auscultated, suggesting LV failure. An S$_4$ may be noted, indicating decreased LV compliance. The murmur of mitral regurgitation secondary to ischemia of the papillary muscle may be present.[12] The presence of any of these findings may lead the examiner to the diagnosis of CHD.

Diagnostic Tests

ELECTROCARDIOGRAM

The ECG remains a standard diagnostic test for patients with angina. Possible abnormal findings include pathologic Q waves, (indicative of prior MI), ST-T abnormalities, (indicative of ischemia), and conduction abnormalities, such as AV block or bundle-branch blocks.[22] These findings are not specific for CHD, however. For example, ST-T abnormalities can also be seen in mitral valve prolapse, another common cause of chest pain.[22] A resting ECG in a patient with CHD may be normal.

An ECG that shows ST-T abnormalities during an episode of chest pain can be extremely helpful in diagnosing angina due either to CHD or coronary spasm. ST segment depression of at least 1 mm is evidence of ischemia. T-wave flattening or inversion is a more nonspecific diagnostic finding (see Chapter 13). Ambulatory ECG monitoring (Holter monitoring) can also be used to aid in diagnosing ischemia or CHD, and may be particularly helpful in

patients who have pain only at rest or are suspected of having silent ischemia.[21]

STRESS TEST

The purpose of the stress test is to increase cardiac workload under direct observation and controlled conditions. The exercise treadmill test is recommended for patients with a normal ECG who are not taking digoxin.[4] The patient is assessed by continuous ECG monitoring during a period of progressively graded exercise. The variables assessed include ST segment and T-wave changes, heart rate and blood pressure response, and the presence or absence of arrhythmias and anginal symptoms[22] (see Chapter 17).

For patients unable to exercise (e.g., because of obesity, chronic obstructive pulmonary disease [COPD], or degenerative joint disease), pharmacologic stress testing can be carried out with intravenous (IV) infusions of dipyridamole, adenosine, or dobutamine. Each of these medications increases the work of the heart, thereby increasing myocardial oxygen demand, while the patient remains stationary.

CARDIAC IMAGING

Cardiac imaging techniques are described in Chapter 16.

Chest radiographs are usually the initial imaging tests obtained in patients with suspected CHD. Radiography is of limited value in the diagnosis of CHD, but is of great value in excluding other potential causes of chest pain (e.g., pneumonia, pneumothorax, congestive heart failure [CHF]; see Chapter 12).

Radionuclides such as thallium-201 or technetium-99m sestamibi can be used in association with exercise or pharmacologic stress testing to detect myocardial perfusion defects. The radionuclide is injected intravenously during maximal stress. Its distribution in the myocardium is proportional to

Conditions Associated With Chest Discomfort

"Emotional" and psychiatric causes of chest discomfort
  Anxiety states (neurocirculatory asthenia)
  Depression
  Cardiac psychosis
  Self-gain
Noncoronary cardiovascular causes of chest discomfort
  Premature beats
  Acute pericarditis
  Postmyocardial infarction syndrome
  Myocarditis and cardiomyopathy
  Valve disease
  Right ventricular hypertension
  Dissecting aneurysm of the aorta
  Superficial thrombophlebitis of the precordial veins
  Pulmonary embolism
  Vasoregulatory asthenia
  Paroxysmal hepatic engorgement
Gastrointestinal causes of chest discomfort
  Reflux esophagitis and hiatal hernia
  Diffuse esophageal spasm
  Cholecystitis and cholelithiasis
  Acute pancreatitis
  The "café coronary"
  Distention of the splenic flexure of the colon
Pulmonary causes of chest discomfort
  Pulmonary hypertension pain
  Pulmonary embolism
  Postmyocardial infarction syndrome
  Mediastinal emphysema (Hamman's disease)
  Spontaneous pneumothorax
Neuromuscular–skeletal causes of chest discomfort
  Thoracic outlet syndrome
  Tietze's syndrome
  Herpes zoster
  Chest wall pain and tenderness

From Hurst JW: Atherosclerotic coronary heart disease: Historical benchmarks, methods of study and clinical features, differential diagnosis, and clinical spectrum. In Hurst JW, Schlant RC, Rackley CE (eds): The Heart, 7th ed, p 983. New York, McGraw-Hill, 1990.

myocardial blood flow. Thallium or sestamibi *single-photon emission computed tomography* provides a multiplanar evaluation of myocardial perfusion and may reveal areas of stress-induced ischemia. When this information is combined with the hemodynamic and ECG data, it offers a more complete evaluation of the patient[11,18,25,26] (see Chapter 16).

Positron emission tomography (PET) may also be used to differentiate ischemic from infarcted myocardium. Cardiac PET uses radiolabeled glucose, which may provide more specific information about myocardial viability than thallium or sestamibi. PET has the significant disadvantages of very high cost and very limited availability.[1,24,26,28]

Echocardiography can be used to detect transient or permanent segmental ventricular wall motion abnormalities or reduced ejection fractions associated with CHD. It may also detect areas of myocardial thinning from old MI, ventricular aneurysms, or valvular heart disease that may contribute to angina. Echocardiography in conjunction with pharma-

cologic stress can be used to detect stress-induced wall motion abnormalities indicative of significant ischemia.

Magnetic resonance imaging coronary angiography is a promising emerging noninvasive technology that may eventually replace conventional coronary angiography. At the time of this writing, it is still in the experimental stage.[23]

CARDIAC CATHETERIZATION AND CORONARY ANGIOGRAPHY

Cardiac catheterization is the most reliable as well as the most invasive diagnostic procedure to evaluate chest pain. Coronary angiography is indicated to confirm or exclude the diagnosis of CHD when noninvasive tests have been equivocal, when disabling angina has been unresponsive to medical therapy, in unstable angina, postinfarction angina, recurrent angina at rest, or ischemia accompanied by an S_3 gallop or definite ECG changes[4] (see Chapter 18).

The extent and severity of CHD, along with LV function, greatly influence a patient's survival. Whether patients are then managed medically or surgically depends on angiographic findings and many other factors that are discussed in the next section. In many centers, angiography offers the significant advantage of endovascular intervention (angioplasty, stenting), which may help to avoid surgery in selected cases (see Chapter 21).

MEDICAL MANAGEMENT

Treatment goals for all patients with angina include relieving anginal symptoms and decreasing the risk of MI. Treatment is based on increasing myocardial oxygen supply or decreasing myocardial oxygen demand.

The comparative effects of surgical and medical therapies on survival in patients with stable angina have been examined in three large, randomized, prospective studies: the Veterans Administration Randomized Study, the European Coronary Surgery Study, and the Coronary Artery Surgery Study.

Data from the Veterans Administration Randomized Study showed significantly improved survival rates at 6-year follow-up for patients with three-vessel disease undergoing coronary artery bypass graft (CABG) surgery compared with patients managed with medical therapy. Surgical patients with three-vessel disease and LV dysfunction also had improved survival rates at 7-year follow-up. At 11 years, however, there was no difference in survival rates between medically and surgically treated patients.[24,29]

The data from the European Coronary Surgery Study showed that for all surgically treated patients, 5-year survival rates were significantly increased compared with the medically treated group. In addition, surgical patients had a significant advantage in symptom relief after 2 years compared with medical patients. At 8 years, survival remained statistically improved for surgical patients compared with medical patients.[30]

The Coronary Artery Surgery Study examined a subset of patients with chronic, stable angina and mild symptoms. This study revealed that 5-year survival rates were only slightly improved for surgical patients compared with medical patients. For patients with three-vessel disease and diminished LV function, survival rates were statistically greater for surgical patients.[14,31]

Recommendations for Chronic Stable (Classic) Angina

The goals of therapy in managing chronic, stable angina are to prolong survival, reduce disease progression, and alleviate symptoms. Lifestyle adjustment is necessary in most patients with angina. This adjustment may include an individually prescribed exercise program, a decrease in dietary intake of cholesterol and saturated fats, smoking cessation, control of hypertension, weight reduction, and stress management.[8] Other medical conditions that may exacerbate angina (e.g., anemia or COPD) may also require treatment.

MEDICAL THERAPY

Medical treatment is the initial treatment for most patients with chronic, stable angina. Treatment may include the nonpharmacologic interventions mentioned previously, and the use of one or more medications, including nitrates, beta blockers, or calcium antagonists (presented later in this chapter). If medical therapy is unsuccessful, myocardial revascularization may be necessary.

MYOCARDIAL REVASCULARIZATION

Revascularization procedures include both PTCA and CABG. The primary goal of PTCA (see Chapter 21) is to increase blood flow to ischemic areas by dilating coronary artery stenoses. The long-term efficacy of balloon angioplasty in patients with chronic ischemic heart disease is well documented.[10,13,27] However, the long-term efficacy in patients with multivessel disease remains controversial and is the subject of several ongoing research studies.[8] Potential complications include acute vessel occlusion and groin hematomas.

Intracoronary stenting during PTCA can be used to dilate lesions resistant to balloon angioplasty. It involves insertion of a wire mesh stent that holds open the stenotic segment. Potential complications include acute thrombosis or progressive restenosis of the stented segment.

Coronary artery bypass grafting (see Chapter 23) is the most widely accepted treatment for patients with severe anginal symptoms unrelieved by medical therapy, although its role remains controversial in stable angina. It is primarily indicated for patients with left main coronary artery disease, three-vessel disease with LV dysfunction, worsening angina, or disabling symptoms.[8,29,30] The more severe the heart disease, the greater the survival advantage of CABG over PTCA.[19] Potential complications of CABG include bleeding, failure of the bypass graft, and graft stenosis.

INVESTIGATIONAL PROCEDURES

Investigational procedures include laser angioplasty and transmyocardial revascularization. Laser angioplasty is under investigation as adjunctive therapy to PTCA and CABG. It involves the use of a laser to vaporize coronary obstruction during CABG or PTCA.[8] Transmyocardial revascularization is being researched as a treatment for medically refractory angina that is not amenable to the current established treatment methods. Transmyocardial revascularization uses a high-powered carbon dioxide laser to create transmural channels that directly perfuse the ischemic myocardium.[2]

Recommendations for Unstable Angina

Patients with unstable angina require hospitalization with cardiac monitoring, immediate bed rest, and correction of reversible precipitating factors (e.g., hypertension, anemia). The patient should receive nitroglycerin sublingually until it can be administered intravenously. Anticoagulant and antiplatelet therapy must also be initiated.[2,8] Thrombolytic therapy (e.g., urokinase, tissue plasminogen activator) has shown no significant clinical advantage over standard anticoagulation and antiplatelet therapy (i.e., aspirin and heparin).[8] If symptoms are controlled, these patients are treated as if they have chronic, stable angina. If symptoms persist, the use of β-adrenergic blockers and possibly calcium antagonists may be considered. If symptoms are still not relieved, intra-aortic balloon counterpulsation can be considered, followed by coronary angiography.

Cardiac catheterization may also be considered after symptoms are controlled because there is a high prevalence of left main and three-vessel coronary artery disease in patients with unstable angina. If either is demonstrated by cardiac catheterization, PTCA or CABG is indicated.

Recommendations for Variant Angina

Patients with variant (Prinzmetal's) angina usually require hospitalization and intense medical therapy. Both nitrates and calcium channel blocking agents are effective in controlling symptoms,[16] although calcium channel blockers are often more successful. If symptoms are not controlled adequately with these medications, β-adrenergic blocking agents may be beneficial. The response to beta blockers is variable because blockade of the β_2 receptors may allow unopposed α-receptor-mediated coronary vasoconstriction.[22] Surgery and PTCA usually are not indicated in patients with isolated coronary artery spasm unless it occurs in conjunction with marked coronary atherosclerosis.[22]

PROGNOSIS

The most important determinants of outcome are the extent of coronary artery obstruction and the severity of LV dysfunction. The presence of hypertension, resting ECG abnormalities, marked ST segment changes during an anginal episode, cardiomegaly, and three-vessel or left main coronary artery disease are indicators of adverse prognosis in the patient with angina.

NURSING MANAGEMENT

Nursing care in the acute situation should be aimed toward minimizing or eliminating myocardial ischemia and preventing progression to infarction. The nurse also aids in reducing the patient's anxiety related to the anginal episode.

In the chronic situation, nurses must assist the patient and family to identify lifestyle changes to reduce or eliminate angina. Sudden bursts of activity should be avoided, especially after prolonged rest periods, because they may precipitate an anginal episode. Patients should be coached in ways to control emotional reactions to stressful situations by way of biofeedback or relaxation therapy. Paradoxically, sexual activity may be encouraged, perhaps with prophylactic use of sublingual nitroglycerin.[15,20]

Patients should be instructed in the importance of adhering to the prescribed medication regimen to minimize pain and myocardial damage. The proper use of sublingual nitroglycerin should be stressed. The patient should be taught to recognize symptoms of worsening ischemia, and instructed to seek prompt medical assistance if indicated.

REFERENCES

1. Albert NM: High risk unstable angina: Keeping pace with current research findings. AACN Clinical Issues 6(1): 110–120, 1995
2. Ballard JC, Wood LL, Lansing AM: Transmyocardial revascularization: Criteria for selecting patients, treatment, and nursing care. Critical Care Nurse 17(1): 42–49, 59, 1997
3. Braunwald E: Unstable angina: A classification. Circulation 80: 410–414, 1989
4. Braunwald E, Jones RH, Mark DB et al: Diagnosing and managing unstable angina. Circulation 90: 613–622, 1994
5. Burke JA: Emergency: Cardiogenic shock. Hospital Medicine 37–43, 1994
6. Casey K, Bedker DL, Roussel-McElmeel PL: Myocardial infarction: Review of clinical trials and treatment strategies. Critical Care Nurse 18(2): 39–52, 1998
7. Cercek B, Shah PK: Complicated acute myocardial infarction: Heart failure, shock, mechanical complications. Cardiol Clin 9: 569–593, 1991
8. Fleury J: Long term management of the patient with stable angina. Nurs Clin North Am 27: 205–230, 1992
9. Folta A, Potempa K: Reduced cardiac output and exercise capacity in patients after MI. J Cardiovasc Nurs 6(4): 71–77, 1992
10. Hamm CW, Riemers J, Ischinger T et al: A randomized study of coronary angioplasty compared with bypass surgery in patients with symptomatic multivessel coronary disease: German Angioplasty Bypass Surgery Investigation. N Engl J Med 331: 1037–1043, 1994
11. Hayes JT, Mahmarian JJ, Cochran AJ et al: Dobutamine thallium-201 tomography for evaluating patients with suspected coronary artery disease unable to undergo exercise or vasodilator pharmacologic stress testing. J Am Coll Cardiol 21: 1583–1590, 1993
12. Hurst JW: Atherosclerotic coronary heart disease: Historical benchmarks, methods of study and clinical features, differential diagnosis, and clinical spectrum. In Hurst JW, Schlant RC, Rackley CE (eds): The Heart, 7th ed, pp 961–1001. New York, McGraw-Hill, 1990
13. Jeurgens CP, Whitbourn RJ, Yeung AC et al: Primary angioplasty for acute myocardial infarction. Vasc Med 2: 327–334, 1997
14. Killip T, Passamani E, Davis K et al: Coronary Artery Surgery Study (CASS): A randomized trial of coronary bypass surgery. Eight year follow-up and survival of patients with reduced ejection fraction. Circulation 72: V102–V109, 1985
15. Malan SS: Psychosocial adjustment following MI: Current views and nursing implications. J Cardiovasc Nurs 6(4): 57–70, 1992
16. McGoon MD, Shub C: Myocardial ischemia clinical syndromes, c. antianginal agents. In Giuliani ER, Gersh BJ, McGoon MD et al: Mayo Clinic Practice of Cardiology, 3rd ed, pp 1191–1215. St. Louis, Mosby, 1996
17. Olson HG, Aronow WS: Medical management of stable angina and unstable angina in the elderly with coronary artery disease. Clin Geriatr Med 12: 121–140, 1996
18. Pennell DJ, Underwood SR, Swanton RH et al: Dobutamine thallium myocardial perfusion tomography. J Am Coll Cardiol 18: 1471–1479, 1991
19. Petticrew M, Turner-Boutle M, Sheldon T: The management of stable angina. Health Service Journal 107(5577): 37–38, 1997
20. Riegel B, Thomason T, Carlson B: Nursing care of patients with acute myocardial infarction: Results of a national survey. Critical Care Nurse 17(5): 23–33, 1997
21. Schroeder JS: Unstable angina and non-Q wave myocardial infarction. In Alpert JS (ed): Cardiology for the Primary Care Physician, pp 143–148. St. Louis, Mosby, 1996
22. Shub C, Click RL, McGoon MD: Myocardial ischemia clinical syndromes, b. angina pectoris and coronary heart disease. In Giuliani ER, Gersh BJ, McGoon MD et al: Mayo Clinic Practice of Cardiology, 3rd ed, pp 1160–1190. St. Louis, Mosby, 1996
23. Steinberg EP: Magnetic resonance coronary angiography: Assessing an emerging technology. N Engl J Med 328: 879–880, 1993
24. Takaro T, Hultgren H, Detre K et al: The Veterans Administration Cooperative Study of stable angina: Current status. Circulation 65(Suppl II): 60–67, 1982
25. Verani MS: Thallium-201 single photon emission computed tomography (SPECT) in the assessment of coronary artery disease. Am J Cardiol 70: 4E–9E, 1992
26. Wackers FJT: Comparison of thallium-201 and technetium-99m methoxyisobutyl isonitril. Am J Cardiol 70: 30E–34E, 1992
27. Weaver WD, Simes RJ, Betriu A: Comparison of primary coronary angioplasty and intravenous thrombolytic therapy for acute myocardial infarction: A quantitative review. JAMA 278: 2093–2098, 1997
28. Zellner JL, Elliott BM, Robinson JG et al: Preoperative evaluation of cardiac risk using dobutamine thallium imaging in vascular surgery. Ann Vasc Surg 4: 238–243, 1990
29. Veterans Administration Coronary Bypass Surgery Cooperative Study Group: Eleven year survival in the Veterans Administration randomized trial of coronary bypass surgery for stable angina: Veterans Administration Coronary Bypass Surgery Cooperative Study Group. N Engl J Med 311: 1333–1339, 1984
30. European Coronary Surgery Study Group: Long term results of a prospective randomized study of coronary artery bypass surgery in stable angina pectoris. Lancet 2: 1173–1180, 1982
31. Myocardial infarction and mortality in the Coronary Artery Surgery Study (CASS) randomized trial. N Engl J Med 310: 750–758, 1984

SHERRI DEL BENE
ANNE VAUGHAN

DIAGNOSIS AND MANAGEMENT OF MYOCARDIAL INFARCTION

Acute MI occurs as a result of prolonged myocardial ischemia that leads to irreversible injury and necrosis. The pain associated with an MI usually lasts longer than 30 minutes and, although occasionally mild and even absent, is typically the most severe pain a person has ever experienced. The diagnosis of AMI is based on patient history, the presence of ST segment elevation, or Q waves on the 12-lead ECG and serial markers of myocardial necrosis.[45] In 1995, 1 of every 4.8 deaths in the United States was caused by CHD.[4] The mortality rate from an MI is highest within the first few hours after the onset of symptoms. Early diagnosis of an MI permits early treatment with reperfusion therapies such as thrombolysis and primary angioplasty, which can preserve myocardial function. People who are suspected of having an AMI should be admitted to a cardiac intensive care unit (CICU), where complications can be identified and acted on quickly. The focus of care for a patient with an AMI has changed from bed rest to early intervention. Attention is given to treatment that can possibly alter the course of necrosis and subsequent healing. The options are drug therapy, interventional procedures, and surgery. The appropriate therapy needs to be tailored for each specific patient. All patients with clinically suspected MI should be treated for AMI until proven otherwise.

CLASSIFICATION OF MYOCARDIAL INFARCTIONS

Classification of MI is based on location of the infarction and the layers of the heart involved. Because the three major branches of the coronary arteries almost always supply the regions of the left ventricle, which have the greatest oxygen need, most MIs involve the left ventricle. Coronary occlusions that also jeopardize perfusion of other cardiac structures (i.e., right ventricle, AV node) can cause more extensive damage. LV infarctions are usually classified as anterior, inferior, posterior, or lateral based on the location of the tissue damage. MI can occur in the subendocardium or epicardium or can be transmural, involving all three layers of the heart. Ischemia and infarction result in decreased contractility and asynchronous contraction. Heart failure may result from large areas of myocardium with decreased or absent contraction.

Left Ventricular Myocardial Infarction

The portion of the left ventricle damaged by MI is largely determined by the anatomic distribution of the occluded coronary artery. In multivessel coronary disease, the extent of damage may exceed the distribution of a single major artery.

ANTERIOR MYOCARDIAL INFARCTION

Anterior MIs occur with occlusion of the left anterior descending coronary artery (LAD), a major supplier of blood to the anterior wall of the left ventricle. Complications of an anterior MI may include severe LV dysfunction, resulting in CHF and cardiogenic shock. Because the LAD supplies the anterior two thirds of the intraventricular septum, its occlusion can produce variable degrees of fascicular or AV block. Sinus tachycardia is a common finding and may be related to a neurohormonal sympathetic response to reduced cardiac output or blood pressure.

INFERIOR/POSTERIOR MYOCARDIAL INFARCTION

Inferior or posterior MIs result from occlusion of the right coronary artery (RCA), which supplies these regions in 80% to 90% of patients. In the remaining 10% to 20% of patients, these MIs result from occlusion of the left circumflex artery. The extent of LV damage ranges from apical diaphragmatic through posterobasal involvement. Sinus node block and atrial arrhythmias may develop. Varying degrees of heart block, especially second-degree AV block, type I (Wenckebach), are common and are usually transient. Parasympathetic overactivity may also occur, manifested by sinus bradycardia and hypotension. Other symptoms of parasympathetic activity, such as hiccuping, nausea, vomiting, or an urge to defecate, are seen frequently in the patient with an inferior or posterior MI.

LATERAL MYOCARDIAL INFARCTION

Lateral MIs result from occlusion of coronary branches supplying the lateral wall of the left ventricle. Typically, this is the left circumflex branch of the main left coronary artery, although diagonal branches of the LAD and terminal branches of the RCA may supply the lateral wall. Because the left circumflex artery supplies the AV junction, His bundle, and anterior and posterior papillary muscles in 10% of the population, its occlusion may be associated with conduction abnormalities or with mitral valve insufficiency due to papillary muscle dysfunction.

Right Ventricular Myocardial Infarction

Myocardial infarction traditionally has been considered an affliction of the left ventricle. RV dysfunction secondary to RV infarction, however, is now known to be an entity with important clinical correlates and potentially deleterious consequences. RV infarction chiefly occurs in association with inferior LV infarction. Associated damage usually includes transmural infarction of the adjacent inferior intraventricular septum. The primary cause of RV infarction is occlusion of the RCA proximal to the three acute marginal branches of the RCA supply to the RV free wall.[53] The extent of RV damage is usually transmural, primarily involving the posterior RV wall, although there may be extension into the anterolateral free wall. MI of the RV anterior free wall is uncommon because of the dual blood supply from the moderator band artery of the LAD and the conus branch of the RCA to this area.

Autopsy studies have documented a 5% to 41% incidence of RV infarction in patients who died from AMI and a 24% incidence in patients who died from posterior MI.[36,53] One clinical study reported a 40% incidence of predominant RV dysfunction in acute inferior MI based on radionuclide studies. This high incidence may reflect detection of ischemic dysfunction in addition to infarction-related dysfunction and also includes patients with RV infarction who survive.[75] In addition, one pathologic study reported a much higher incidence (78.6%) of RV infarction in the setting of inferior MI in patients with preexistent RV hypertrophy secondary to chronic lung disease.[57]

Right ventricular infarction usually occurs in conjunction with an inferior LV infarction; therefore, some degree of LV impairment may be present. The hemodynamic alterations in RV infarction, however, primarily reflect impaired contractility of the right ventricle. With predominant RV dysfunction, the right and left heart filling pressures, or right atrial pressure and PAWP, tend to be elevated to the same degree. The right ventricle has difficulty generating pressure and SV, reflected as a decrease in pulmonary artery pulse pressure, with subsequent difficulty adequately filling the left ventricle. The cardiac output decreases, possibly to critical levels. As a compensatory mechanism, the right ventricle dilates, but if dysfunction is severe, the chamber may behave only as a passive conduit that depends on a high filling pressure to sustain SV. Other additional mechanisms for the low-cardiac-output state have been suggested. A state of increased RV volume in association with posterior septal infarction may contribute to bulging of the intraventricular septum into the left ventricle during diastole, thus distorting LV size and decreasing its end-diastolic volume. This phenomenon may be promoted by a restraining effect of the pericardium. Acute dilation of the right ventricle increases intrapericardial pressure, which consequently diminishes LV distending pressure. Diastolic expansion of the left ventricle is sacrificed because of limited pericardial space.[75]

Q-Wave and Non–Q-Wave Infarction

Damage to the heart occurs in a continuum that progresses from the subendocardium to the epicardium (Fig. 20–13). The subendocardium is particularly vulnerable to changes in LV dynamics. As the damage approaches the full thickness of the myocardium, Q waves appear on the 12-lead ECG. Non–Q-wave MIs occur with damage to the subendocardium and may be associated with nondiagnostic ECG changes such as ST segment depression and T-wave abnormalities. Forty percent of patients who have an MI present with ST segment depression, T-wave abnormalities, or other, nonspecific ECG changes.[74] Q-wave MIs are associated with higher in-hospital mortality rates and may result in signs and symptoms of heart failure, mural thrombi, and pericarditis. However, patients with non–Q-wave MIs frequently experience recurrent ischemia, MI, and death in the weeks and months after discharge.[46] Indeed, the cumulative mortality rate after non–Q-wave MI is comparable with that of Q-wave MI after 2 years.[73] Non–Q-wave MIs are more common in elderly patients and those with prior MIs.

DIAGNOSIS

The diagnosis of MI is based on the history, serial ECGs, and serum enzyme changes indicative of cardiac muscle necrosis.[47] A definite AMI is diagnosed by the presence of unequivocal ECG changes or unequivocal enzyme changes, or both. The patient may present with a typical history of severe, prolonged chest pain or an atypical history of mild or no chest pain. A possible MI is diagnosed on the basis of equivocal ECG changes that persist longer than 24 hours, with or without equivocal enzyme changes.[3]

History

Chest discomfort is present in 75% to 80% of patients with AMI. The pain may resemble classic angina pectoris but occurs at rest or with less than usual activity.[8] Typically, the pain is severe and prolonged and may be described as crushing, constricting, or oppressive. The pain may radiate down the ulnar aspect of the left arm and be associated with tingling in the wrist, hand, and finger. The pain may also radiate into the neck, jaw, and interscapular region. Pain may occur in the epigastric region and may simulate gastrointestinal disorders. Chest discomfort may be associated with indigestion, nausea and vomiting, diaphoresis, palpitations, or dyspnea. In 15% to 25% of patients, chest discomfort is absent. These patients may present with "anginal equivalent" symptoms such as dyspnea, palpitations, or arrhythmias. Older patients, patients with diabetes mellitus, and women are more likely to present in an atypical manner.[32,45,65] Older patients more often experience complaints of stroke, confusion, and syncope with AMI (Gibler, 1998).[45]

Physical Assessment

Unless marked cardiac dysfunction is present, physical assessment of the patient with AMI is often unremarkable. However, it is important to establish baseline data. The patient may appear pale, anxious, and in distress. Cold per-

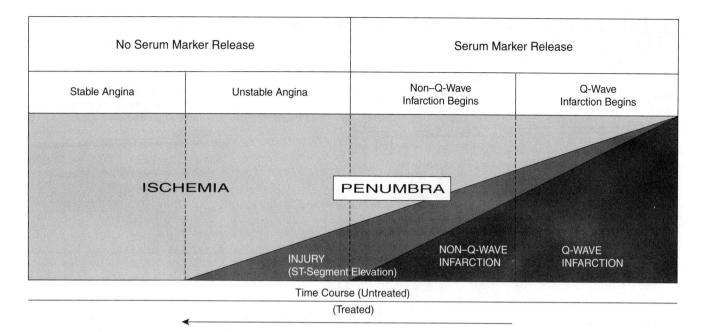

No Serum Marker Release		Serum Marker Release	
Stable Angina	Unstable Angina	Non–Q-Wave Infarction Begins	Q-Wave Infarction Begins

ISCHEMIA PENUMBRA

INJURY (ST-Segment Elevation) NON–Q-WAVE INFARCTION Q-WAVE INFARCTION

Time Course (Untreated)

(Treated)

FIGURE 20-13 Schematic drawing showing the overlapping relationships of the acute coronary syndromes. The areas of ischemia and injury represent compromised but salvageable tissue in zones of reduced blood flow. In this zone, called the *penumbra*, the blood supply is inadequate to maintain normal myocardial functions. The penumbra is viable up to several hours from the primary onset of artial occlusion. The myocardium in the penumbra dies (infarcts) if not salvaged by reperfusion strategies such as thrombolytic agents or angioplasty. (From Cummins RO, Ornato JP, Abramson NS et al: Advanced Cardiac Life Support, p 9–3. Dallas, American Heart Association, 1997.)

spiration may be present on the skin. The patient may present with crackles in the lung bases and an S₃ gallop, indicating LV failure. The patient may also exhibit a productive cough with pink, frothy, or blood-tinged sputum. An S₄ heart sound may also be present and indicates decreased LV compliance. A systolic murmur may indicate mitral valve regurgitation secondary to papillary muscle dysfunction. With the development of worsening LV dysfunction and subsequent cardiogenic shock, hypotension, oliguria, pallor, and confusion may become evident (Display 20–4).

In RV infarction, the abnormalities noted on physical examination depend on the degree of RV dysfunction. RV failure produces signs of systemic venous congestion and poor systemic perfusion (Table 20–4). Elevated RV filling pressure is clinically manifested as jugular venous distention. An inspiratory rise in jugular venous pressure (Kussmaul's sign) and pulsus paradoxus may be present. In RV infarction, Kussmaul's sign reflects the inability of the right ventricle to manage augmented venous return that normally accompanies inspiration. Hepatomegaly and peripheral edema may develop from persistently elevated systemic venous pressure. The lung fields are usually clear, a finding in sharp contrast to the pulmonary congestion usually noted with LV dysfunction.

DISPLAY 20-4

Common Physical Presentation of the Patient With Acute Myocardial Infarction

General	Alert, anxious, restless, often fatigued
Skin	Cool, clammy, diaphoretic
Heart/cardiovascular	S₃ or S₄ gallop may or may not be present; dysrhythmias or murmurs
	Jugular venous distention may be seen in the presence of pump failure
Lungs	Dyspnea, tachypnea, rales (crackles) suggest pulmonary congestion and heart failure
Gastrointestinal	Nausea and vomiting may be associated with chest pain
Circulatory	Peripheral pulses may be pounding or thready, regular or irregular

From Gardiner-Caldwell SynerMed: Nursing Management in Thrombolytic Therapy: A Slide/Lecture Guide. San Francisco, Genentech, Inc., 1989.

TABLE 20-4	Major Differences in the Low-Cardiac-Output Syndromes of Predominant Right Ventricular Versus Left Ventricular Infarction	
	Right Ventricle	**Left Ventricle**
Physical examination	Clear lungs Systemic venous congestion Jugular venous distention S_3 or S_4 may be present Tricuspid regurgitation	Crackles, pulmonary edema No systemic venous congestion Normal jugular veins S_3 or S_4 Mitral regurgitation may be present
Hemodynamic profile	CI < 2.2 L/min/m² PAWP < 18 mm Hg	CI < 2.2 L/min/m² PAWP > 18 mm Hg
Initial treatment	↑ Preload: Aggressive volume expansion	↓ Preload: Limited volume administration Diuretic therapy

CI, cardiac index; PAWP, pulmonary artery wedge pressure; ↑, increased; ↓, decreased.

Diagnostic Tests

ELECTROCARDIOGRAPHIC CHANGES WITH MYOCARDIAL INFARCTION

The 12-lead ECG is central to the diagnosis of MI because patients with ST segment elevation or new bundle-branch block should receive immediate reperfusion therapy.[74] Unequivocal ECG changes include the development of abnormal, persistent Q waves; presence of a QS complex in two or more leads; or an evolving injury current pattern lasting longer than 1 day. The presence of Q waves indicates infarcted tissue that extends at least halfway through the myocardial wall. Q waves may appear within hours of MI. The presence of Q waves, however, does not indicate when the MI occurred. Myocardial injury that occurs when ischemia is prolonged more than a few minutes is reflected by ST segment elevation.

Equivocal ECG changes are not diagnostic but are suggestive of MI and consist of ST segment elevation and T-wave inversion in the leads facing the damaged zone, an abnormal Q wave, or conduction disturbances. The diagnosis of AMI becomes difficult or impossible when there are preexisting ECG abnormalities such as left bundle-branch block, an old MI in the same area, ventricular hypertrophy, and Wolff-Parkinson-White syndrome. Other disorders, such as cardiomyopathies, pulmonary embolism, pericarditis, and subarachnoid hemorrhage, may mimic the ST segment and T-wave abnormalities of an MI.

The standard 12-lead ECG does not provide specific diagnostic clues to acute RV infarction. Frequently, the ECG demonstrates the evolution of a concomitant acute inferior or posterior LV infarction. Although RV necrosis may produce ST segment elevation in leads V_1 through V_4, these changes also occur in both anteroseptal and anterior injury and infarction, and therefore may be misleading.[23,40,43,58] The right precordial ECG may be helpful in the detection of RV infarction. An ECG pattern sometimes seen in inferior MI with posterior LV and RV involvement is illustrated in Figure 20–14. ST segment elevation may be of short duration, possibly disappearing in less than 10 hours from onset of chest pain; however it may persist for longer than 24 hours.[14,55] Therefore, early recording of right precordial ECG is essential. Arrhythmias typically associated with inferior infarction may also be evident, and include bradycardia and first-, second-, or third-degree AV block.

SERUM MARKERS ASSOCIATED WITH MYOCARDIAL INFARCTION

Certain serum markers rise in the patient after an MI. Each marker has a typical period of appearance and return to normal (see Chapter 11). CK and CK-MB, enzymes released with tissue necrosis, rise 4 to 6 hours after MI, whereas lactate dehydrogenase peaks later, at 36 hours after MI. The measurement of CK and CK-MB levels is the gold standard for serum markers of MI. Newer markers are also used in conjunction with measurement of CK and CK-MB enzymes. Myoglobin, a heme protein, found in all striated tissue and released from myocytes after injury, rises within 1 to 2 hours after MI, and thus is useful in the early diagnosis of MI. Myoglobin, however, is not specific to cardiac tissue and may be elevated for reasons other than MI.[67]

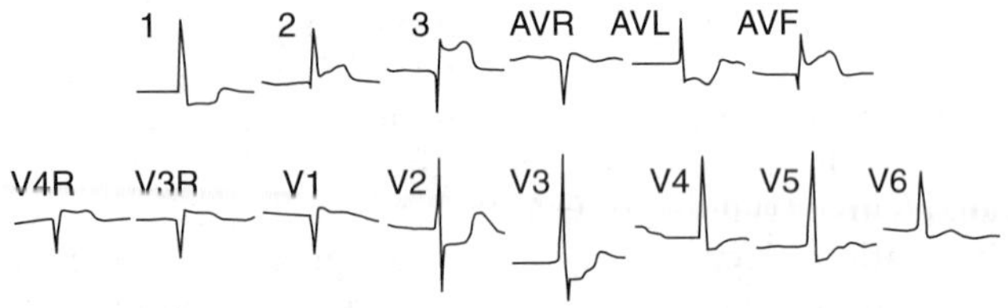

FIGURE 20-14 Electrocardiogram demonstrating an evolving inferior myocardial infarction with ST segment elevation and QS pattern in leads V_3R and V_4R suggestive of right ventricular involvement. (From Morgera T, Alberti E, Silvestri F et al; Right precordial ST and QRS changes in the diagnosis of right ventricular infarction. Am Heart J 108:13, 1984.)

Troponin T or troponin I is also used in the diagnosis of an AMI because both are specific to cardiac necrosis and rise 6 to 8 hours after the onset of ischemia. The half-life of the troponins is long and they are not used for diagnosis for reinfarction in the period after an MI. In one study, the most powerful predictors of high (three-fold) mortality rate during the first 30 days after an MI were an elevated troponin T level (0.1 mg/mL) and ST segment elevation.[68]

HEMODYNAMIC MONITORING

Hemodynamic monitoring of pulmonary artery pressures is not indicated in patients with uncomplicated MI. However, for patients with complicated MI, knowledge of pulmonary artery pressure and PAWP is important for prescribing treatment. Indications for placement of a pulmonary artery catheter include (1) severe or progressive CHF or pulmonary edema; (2) cardiogenic shock or progressive hypotension; and (3) suspected mechanical complications of AMI, such as ventricular septal defect, papillary muscle rupture, or pericardial tamponade.[58] The central venous pressure, PAWP, and cardiac output guide treatment decisions by helping distinguish the patient with inadequate intravascular volume or RV infarct and low filling pressures who requires fluid, from the patient with high filling pressures who requires diuresis, inotropes, or afterload reduction (see Chapter 19).

The hemodynamic profile characteristic of RV dysfunction includes (1) elevated right atrial pressure; (2) normal to modestly elevated RV and pulmonary arterial pressures; (3) increased RV end-diastolic pressure; (4) low, normal, or minimally elevated PAWP depending on the degree of LV dysfunction; (5) narrow RV pulse pressure; and (6) low cardiac index (2.2 L/min/m²). Occurrence of these characteristic findings and criteria is variable and is primarily determined by the degree of RV dysfunction present. The degree of LV impairment also influences the clinical findings.

ECHOCARDIOGRAPHY

Echocardiography is useful in the diagnosis and evaluation of AMI. Regional wall motion abnormalities are associated with MI in 90% to 100% of patients with a transmural MI.[56] Echocardiography allows for identification of regions of abnormal wall motion and is useful in ruling out other causes for hemodynamic compromise, such as a pericardial effusion and mitral insufficiency. When RV infarct is suspected, echocardiography may be used to compare RV and LV dimensions and determine wall motion abnormalities.[30] In some cases, two-dimensional echocardiography has been found to be significantly more sensitive in detecting MI than the initial ECG.[56] Echocardiography may facilitate the diagnosis of MI in cases in which the ECG in nondiagnostic. The echocardiogram may further provide information about the location and extent of the MI and thereby affect treatment. Absence of regional wall motion abnormalities on echocardiography may also provide data needed to rule out the diagnosis of MI (see Chapter 16).[77]

CARDIAC IMAGING

Radionuclide studies may be performed to identify areas of myocardium at risk as well as tissue necrosis. Technetium-99m sestamibi is a radioisotope that is taken up by myocardial tissue in proportion to blood flow in the region and may be used to identify areas of tissue viability.[62] Like echocardiography, the technetium-99m sestamibi study may be useful as an aid to rule out the diagnosis of AMI when the ECG is normal or nondiagnostic. Imaging can be delayed several hours after the injection of the radioisotope, but the scan still reflects myocardial perfusion at the time of injection.[10] Sestamibi scans performed before and after reperfusion therapy may also be used to evaluate the effectiveness of reperfusion strategies on regional blood flow to the myocardium.

COMPLICATIONS OF ACUTE MYOCARDIAL INFARCTION

Patients with AMI are prone to a variety of complications. Some of these (e.g., sudden death) may occur before the patient reaches the hospital. Additional complications may occur simply as a result of the hospitalization itself (nosocomial infection) or may be more likely in elderly patients, particularly those requiring intensive care (delirium, pressure ulcers).[61] This section discusses only those complications occurring during the initial hospitalization.

Arrhythmias

Arrhythmias may occur early in the course of the event because of electrophysiologic alterations in ischemic myocardium, pharmacotherapy, electrolyte disturbances, or endogenous epinephrine release. Arrhythmias that occur later may be secondary to other complications (e.g., CHF or ventricular aneurysm).

TACHYARRHYTHMIAS

Ventricular Tachyarrhythmias. Greater than 90% of patients with AMI experience premature ventricular contractions,[22] which in themselves do not require therapy but may herald the onset of more dangerous arrhythmias. Approximately 7% of patients with AMI experience ventricular fibrillation, and a similar number experience recurrent ventricular tachycardia. Lidocaine and other antiarrhythmics are used to suppress these potentially fatal arrhythmias (see Chapters 14 and 25).

Atrial Tachyarrhythmias. Less than 10% of patients with AMI experience sustained supraventricular tachycardia, atrial fibrillation, or atrial flutter.[22] These arrhythmias may exacerbate myocardial ischemia by increasing the heart rate. Their presence often indicates a worse prognosis because they occur most often in patients with significant heart failure. Heart failure should be suspected in any patient with AMI in whom a sustained atrial tachyarrhythmia develops.[22] These arrhythmias may also occur in patients with atrial infarctions and RCA occlusions, but do not necessarily herald a worse prognosis in these cases.

BRADYARRHYTHMIAS

Bradyarrhythmias are in general more common with inferior wall MI, with sinus bradycardia, sinus arrest, second- and third-degree AV block occurring more commonly in RV infarction. Complete heart block occurs in up to 20% of patients with acute RV infarcts.[22] These bradyarrhythmias are usually treated with atropine, although they may also require transvenous pacing.

Anterior wall MI is much more likely to cause infranodal conduction disturbances. These patients experience wide-complex idioventricular rhythms, which carry a much worse prognosis because they are associated with large infarcts. They are typically treated acutely with transvenous pacing.

Left Ventricular Failure

Left ventricular failure ranges from mild decreases in LV ejection fraction to cardiogenic shock, which may occur in 5% to 20% of patients with AMI.[19] The degree of hemodynamic compromise parallels the degree of LV dysfunction, as do the clinical manifestations.

LEFT VENTRICULAR DYSFUNCTION

Ischemic myocardial segments have diminished (or absent) contractility, and depending on the size of the segment and the degree of decreased contractility, LV ejection fraction is compromised. Diminished contractility places an increased burden on the remaining functioning myocardium, some of which may also be supplied by stenotic coronary vessels. The left ventricle may dilate in an effort to preserve SV despite a decrease in ejection fraction, which in turn increases oxygen demand and LV end-diastolic pressure.[21] Increases in LV end-diastolic pressure lead to varying degrees of pulmonary interstitial edema.

Myocardial ischemia not only impairs LV contraction and therefore peripheral perfusion (systolic dysfunction), but the ischemic segment may initially become stiff and noncompliant (diastolic dysfunction),[50] which also increases the LV end-diastolic pressure.

HEMODYNAMIC ALTERATIONS

Some investigators have grouped patients with AMI into clinical subsets based on the predominance of peripheral hypoperfusion or pulmonary venous hypertension[21,22] those with no significant manifestation of either (subset 1), those with primarily pulmonary manifestations (subset 2), those with primarily peripheral hypoperfusion (subset 3), and those with manifestation of both (subset 4). These subsets may be separately recognized by physical examination and monitored by specific hemodynamic parameters, and each requires different treatment.

Subset 1: Up to 50% of patients with AMI may have no clinical evidence of LV dysfunction. They require no additional hemodynamic monitoring.

Subset 2: Patients with primarily pulmonary manifestations can be further divided according to the severity of pulmonary symptoms. Those with mild venous congestion can be managed with supplemental oxygen, diuretics, morphine, and careful use of vasodilators, without invasive monitoring. Those with more severe manifestations may require ventilatory support, and invasive hemodynamic monitoring (which usually reveals a PAWP 25 mm Hg) to guide vasodilator and other pharmacotherapy.

Subset 3: Signs and symptoms of peripheral hypoperfusion (hypotension, peripheral vasoconstriction, impaired mental status, and decreased urine output) without pulmonary symptoms usually occur in the setting of RV infarction or hypovolemic shock.[22] These patients require invasive monitoring to guide the use of rehydration and inotropics or vasodilators.

Subset 4: Patients with signs of hypoperfusion and pulmonary venous congestion require use of invasive monitoring to guide the use of inotropics, diuretics, and possibly vasodilators.

Cardiogenic shock is a clinical syndrome characterized by hypoperfusion and hypotension in conjunction with pulmonary edema (see Chapter 24). Clinical evaluation of these patients reveals signs and symptoms of decreased peripheral perfusion, including hypotension, impaired mental status, decreased urine output, and peripheral vasoconstriction. Cardiac index is markedly diminished (2.2 L/min), PAWP is elevated (18 mm Hg), and SVR may be elevated or remain within the normal range. Cardiogenic shock results from severe LV dysfunction, usually caused by large infarcts with transmural necrosis (35% to 40% of LV mass), and is highly correlated with three-vessel disease.[22] Cardiogenic shock may occur at the onset or within a few hours of AMI, or later as a consequence of mechanical complications. Mortality rates in patients with early cardiogenic shock may be as high as 80% to 100% without aggressive revascularization. Therapy includes cautious use of sympathomimetics, vasodilators, and intra-aortic balloon pumps. Aggressive revascularization, with either PTCA or surgery, may decrease the mortality rate to 25% to 50%.[21]

Infarct Expansion/Left Ventricular Remodeling

Through mechanisms that are not completely understood, the infarcted segment of myocardium may increase its surface area, thereby increasing LV volume.[50] LV volume may also increase in an attempt to preserve SV despite a falling ejection fraction.[21] Increased LV volume increases the oxygen requirement of the remaining viable tissue and requires gradual lengthening of the remaining muscle, placing it at a mechanical disadvantage. The use of inotropic agents and afterload reduction may help optimize myocardial performance, but this can become a progressive cycle, leading to a dilated, poorly contractile LV.

Left Ventricular Aneurysms

In addition to global ventricular dilation, more localized dilation or aneurysm formation can occur. The two types of aneurysms are termed *true* and *false*.

TRUE ANEURYSMS

True LV aneurysms are broad-necked, localized dilations of the left ventricle. The LV wall segment, although likely a noncontractile fibrous scar, remains intact. They tend to involve the apex, may calcify over time, and may accumulate thrombus, although clinically recognized embolization is uncommon (2% to 5%).[21] They are not prone to rupture, but cause morbidity and mortality because of recurrent ventricular arrhythmias, thought to be incited at the junction of the aneurysm with adjacent, normal myocardium.

FALSE ANEURYSMS

False aneurysms (pseudoaneurysms) result from myocardial ruptures that are contained by the pericardium. The wall of these narrow-necked aneurysms is composed of pericardium and adhesions,[50] and they are usually lined by thrombus. These aneurysms have a tendency to rupture, with a uniformly fatal outcome. Surgical resection is always recommended.

Mechanical Complications

MITRAL REGURGITATION

Mitral regurgitation may occur early in the course of AMI secondary to ischemia and dysfunction (or necrosis and rupture) of one of the papillary muscles that support the chordae tendineae of the mitral valve (see Chapter 27). It most commonly affects the posteromedial papillary muscle and is seen most often with inferior wall MI.[50] It may occur with subendocardial (non–Q-wave) MI.[71] Mitral regurgitation tends to occur between 2 and 7 days after MI, but may occur within the first 24 hours (20%).[21] With ischemia and dysfunction, the resultant pulmonary congestion may be intermittent or persistent, and the diagnosis can be confirmed by echocardiography.[71] These patients require relatively prompt revascularization. Papillary muscle rupture is usually a catastrophic event, with sudden-onset pulmonary edema. The mortality rate without prompt surgical correction is 50% in 24 hours and 94% within 8 weeks.[21]

VENTRICULAR SEPTAL RUPTURE

Septal rupture may occur with anterior MI, producing apical septal rupture, or with inferior wall MI, with rupture occurring at the base of the septum.[71] It is seen with transmural infarction, and occurs in 1% to 3% of AMIs.[50] It tends to occur between 3 and 7 days after infarction. Ventricular septal rupture produces a loud, holosystolic murmur and causes systemic hypoperfusion due to left-to-right shunting. Prompt diagnosis and surgical intervention is

required because the mortality rate is 24% in 24 hours and 46% in 1 week.[21]

VENTRICULAR FREE WALL RUPTURE

Free wall rupture complicates anterior and inferior MIs with equal frequency, occurring typically from 2 to 8 days postinfarction, although up to 30% may develop in the first 24 hours.[21] It may account for up to 10% of AMI-associated mortality.[71] Clinically, it manifests as sudden death with pulseless electrical activity (PEA), and attempts at resuscitation usually are futile. Occasionally, patients present with a syndrome of subacute rupture, with pericardial pain, ECG evidence of pericarditis, and echocardiographic evidence of localized pericardial effusion or even pseudoaneurysm.[71] Such a scenario is unfortunately rare, and accurately identifying patients at high risk for rupture is extremely difficult.

Right Ventricular Myocardial Infarction

Right ventricular MI may occur to some degree in 30% to 40% of patients with inferior wall MI,[21] but hemodynamically significant RV infarction occurs in less than 10% of patients with inferior wall MI.[71] RV failure results in underfilling of the left atrium and ventricle, reducing pump efficiency and SV. Resultant peripheral hypoperfusion may be exacerbated by concomitant bradyarrhythmia.[2] It is recognized clinically as a triad of hypotension, jugular venous distention, and clear lungs in a patient with inferior wall MI.[71] ST segment elevation may be seen in lead V_4R, and RV dysfunction can be confirmed by echocardiography. Because these patients require fluid resuscitation, invasive hemodynamic monitoring is necessary. PAWP is usually low, and fluid resuscitation is continued until PAWP reaches 18 to 20 mm Hg.[71] Diuretics and afterload-reducing agents must be avoided. Aggressive reperfusion should be considered for patients who fail to improve with standard therapies.

Pericarditis

Pericarditis most commonly occurs several weeks after MI (Dressler's syndrome). However, in some patients it may occur acutely, usually within 3 days of the event, sometimes as early as the first day. In these cases, it is often localized to the pericardium adjacent to the infarcted segment and results from transmural infarction extending to the epicardial surface, inciting a localized inflammatory response. The diagnosis is made clinically by history, physical examination, and ECG. The pain is typically sharp, severe, and substernal, radiating to the neck, shoulders, and back. The pain is exacerbated with inspiration and with reclining. A pericardial friction rub may be present on auscultation. The classic ECG changes (ST segment elevation in multiple chest leads) are not usually present with localized pericarditis. The incidence of acute pericarditis has decreased by almost 50% with the use of thrombolytic therapy.[50]

MEDICAL MANAGEMENT

Treatment of MI is based on rapidly increasing myocardial blood and oxygen supply, reducing myocardial oxygen demand, and limiting infarct size (Display 20–5). Treatment goals include (1) restoring coronary blood flow and minimizing infarct size, (2) maintaining adequate oxygenation, (3) administering appropriate fluid therapy, (4) improving ventricular performance to maximize oxygen supply-and-demand ratio, (5) giving appropriate drug therapy, (6) detecting and managing complications early, and (7) assessing risk after infarction. A calm, quiet atmosphere should be maintained and explanations should be given to the patient with the goal of reducing anxiety. Figure 20–15 illustrates the American Heart Association's recommended algorithm for management of acute ischemic chest pain.[27]

DISPLAY 20-5

Selected Therapies to Reduce Ischemia and Infarction

DECREASE MYOCARDIAL O₂ CONSUMPTION

Rest with backrest elevation 20–30 degrees
Selected diet (small, frequent, easily digested meals)
Nitroglycerin and long-acting nitrates
Narcotic analgesics
Beta-blocking agents
Calcium channel blocking agents
Vasodilators
Sedatives and tranquilizers
Stool softeners and laxatives
Diuretics
Antihypertensive agents
Stress management
Exercise program
Risk factor modification

INCREASE CORONARY BLOOD AND O₂ SUPPLY

Oxygen
Nitroglycerin
Calcium channel blocking agents
Revascularization
　Thrombolysis
　Percutaneous transluminal coronary angioplasty
　Coronary artery bypass surgery
Vasoactive drugs that improve systemic hemodynamics
Anticoagulants and antiplatelet agents
Antilipid agents (long term)
Exercise program
Risk factor modification

From Woods SL, Underhill SL: Coronary heart disease: Myocardial ischemia and infarction. In Patrick M., Woods SL, Craven RF et al (eds): Medical Surgical Nursing: Pathophysiological Concepts, p 522. Philadelphia, JB Lippincott, 1986.

Included in this section are overviews of interventional cardiology techniques; prehospital, emergency department, and CICU care; other therapies to reduce infarct size; and pharmacologic management.

Interventional Cardiology Techniques

THROMBOLYTIC THERAPY

Thrombolytic therapy is recommended for patients without contraindications to restore coronary blood flow, improve coronary oxygen supply-and-demand ratio, and minimize infarct size. Optimal candidates for thrombolytic therapy include patients with ST segment elevation or bundle-branch block. Absolute and relative contraindications to thrombolytic therapy, recommendations for administration, and a listing of thrombolytic agents may be found in Chapter 21. Nurses should be alert to physiologic signs of reperfusion, including relief of chest pain; resolution of ST segment changes, cardiac arrhythmias, or conduction abnormalities; and early rise of CK and CK-MB.

PRIMARY CORONARY ANGIOPLASTY

Angioplasty has been associated with lower early mortality rates and better long-term outcome compared with thrombolysis.[77A] However, these results have been obtained only when the delay is minimal. Therefore, primary PTCA is a class I recommendation as an alternative to thrombolytic therapy only if performed in a timely manner by surgeons skilled in the procedure and supported by experienced personnel in high-volume centers.[74] Primary PTCA is a class IIa recommendation in patients who are candidates for reperfusion but who are at risk for bleeding and for patients in cardiogenic shock, and a class IIb recommendation for patients who do not qualify for thrombolysis for reasons other than bleeding. Primary PTCA is recommended only if (1) balloon dilation can take place within 60 to 90 minutes of the diagnosis of AMI, and (2) the center in which it is performed achieves a documented success rate with TIMI (Thrombolysis in Myocardial Infarction)[74A] grade II or III flow in more than 90% of patients without resultant CABG, stroke, or death.

Prehospital Care

Prehospital treatment includes reducing mortality from MI, reducing infarct size, and preserving LV function. One goal of the Emergency Medical System is to minimize the delay between the patient's onset of symptoms and initiation of reperfusion strategies, such as thrombolysis or primary angioplasty. Over half of patients who die from MI, die from ventricular fibrillation before they reach the hospital.[69] Early initial intervention can be achieved by a prehospital community system of cardiac life support. Basic to an effective community-wide emergency cardiac care system is an informed public, an efficient communication center, trained medical and paramedical teams, and appropriate vehicles with appropriate equipment. The emergency cardiac care system provides for early access to the Emergency Medical

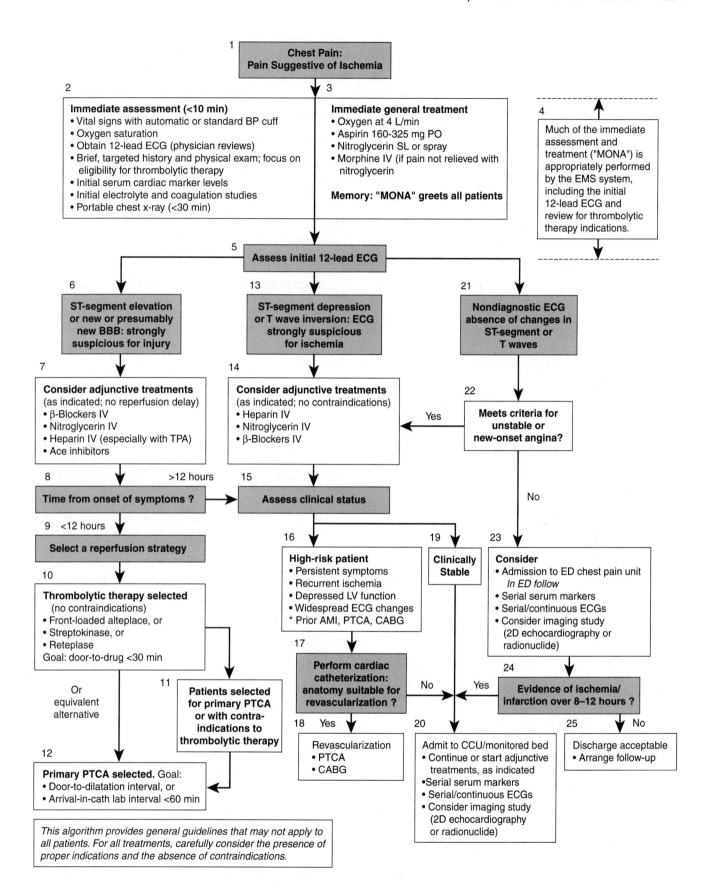

FIGURE 20-15 Ischemic chest pain algorithm. (From Cummins RO, Ornato JP, Abramson NS et al: Advanced Cardiac Life Support, p 9-12. Dallas, American Heart Association, 1997.)

System, early basic life support, early defibrillation, and early advanced cardiac life support.

Although an effective emergency cardiac care system is an important factor in reducing the delay between the patient's onset of symptoms and treatment, the patient and family play an important role. Of all patients with MI, one fourth to one half delay longer than 6 hours from onset of symptoms before seeking treatment.[33] Dracup found that the mean time from onset of symptoms until arrival in the emergency department averaged 110 minutes. Patients who are most likely to delay seeking treatment include the elderly, people with lower incomes, people with diabetes, those who experienced symptoms at home, those who did not appraise symptoms as serious or heart related, and those who had intermittent symptoms. Interventions, such as teaching the patient and family about symptoms of MI and initial steps to take with onset of symptoms, should be targeted at groups who delay. The National Heart, Lung and Blood Institute recommends that all patients be counseled to call 911 at the onset of symptoms of MI.[5]

Emergency Department Care

Treatment in the emergency department focuses on a rapid, targeted history and physical assessment, initial treatment, and triage of the patient with an AMI. Patients with complicated MIs and symptoms of CHF and life-threatening arrhythmias should be admitted directly to the CICU. A 12-lead ECG should be performed and interpreted within 10 minutes of arrival in the emergency department on all patients with suspected MI.[8] If the ECG shows either ST segment elevation of 1 mm or more in two contiguous leads, or left bundle-branch block, screening for contraindications to thrombolytic therapy should be initiated. If the patient is eligible for thrombolytic therapy, it should be started within 30 minutes of arrival in the hospital.[44] All patients should receive cardiac monitoring. Patients with ST segment depression or T-wave inversion should be treated as though they are experiencing an MI.

Initial therapy should be started in the emergency department. Treatment priorities include pain relief with morphine and nitroglycerin, oxygen therapy, and the administration of 160 to 325 mg of aspirin. Beta-blocker therapy may also be initiated. At least one IV line should be started. Two IV lines should be started if the patient is a candidate for thrombolytic therapy.

The development of the "chest pain" emergency department represents an attempt to balance the risk of unnecessary and costly admissions of patients to the CICU who eventually are ruled out for an MI with the risk of sending the patient experiencing an MI home. Of the patients admitted to the CICU for suspected MI, 70% eventually are ruled out for an MI.[11] On the other hand, 2.9% to 10% of patients who present with chest pain with AMI are sent home.[45] The chest pain unit focuses on rapid diagnosis of the patient experiencing chest discomfort with nondiagnostic ECG changes. Rapid diagnosis is accomplished by assessment of serial markers of myocardial necrosis such as CK-MB and myoglobin. With more rapid testing of CK-MB available, the diagnosis of an AMI can

be determined within 4 to 5 hours after onset of symptoms.[45] Other tests used in the early diagnosis of an AMI include two-dimensional echocardiography and radionuclide scanning.

Coronary Intensive Care Unit (CICU) Care

Since its inception in the early 1960s, the focus of the CICU has evolved from the monitoring and rapid treatment of arrhythmias to aggressive intervention and alteration of the underlying disease process.[38] The CICU is equipped with cardiac monitoring equipment and has the capability to provide intensive observation and highly technical interventions for patients. It is staffed by registered nurses with specialized knowledge about the care of the critically ill cardiac patient and with skills in the use of complex technologies. Since the advent of the CICU, mortality rates of cardiac patients have decreased dramatically, initially because of the early detection and treatment of arrhythmias. Later, advanced hemodynamic monitoring became possible with the development of the flow-directed pulmonary artery catheter. The use of cardiac medications, such as thrombolytics and beta blockers, further decreased mortality rates.[9,16]

The CICU is usually a confined area with limited access from other parts of the hospital. Increasingly, families are present with the patients. Liberalized visiting policies can be helpful for many patients; family visits have not been found to have a greater negative impact on heart rate, blood pressure, or the occurrence of ventricular ectopy than other social situations. Length of stay in the CICU is based on the patient's condition. After their stay in the CICU, patients may be transferred to a telemetry unit, where they may gradually increase their physical activity with close monitoring of heart rate, blood pressure, and symptoms. Patients at low risk for complications may be discharged within 72 hours of admission.[15]

Standard admission orders for patients with suspected MI should facilitate early decision making and administration of, or monitoring the response to, thrombolytic agents. Other important considerations include vital sign observations; ECG monitoring; oxygen; monitoring of intake and output and weight; IV fluids; diet; medications for anticoagulation, pain, anxiety, or nausea or vomiting; bowel management; sleep; activity using a cardiac rehabilitation approach; and appropriate laboratory tests including the 12-lead ECG, chest radiography, serum markers of MI, electrolytes, glucose, creatinine, blood urea nitrogen, coagulation studies, arterial blood gases, and urinalysis. Each patient should be asked if there are written advance directives and about personal preferences for life support in an emergency situation.

For the initial admission assessment, priorities include vital signs, oxygen saturation, initiating or confirming IV access, initiating cardiac monitoring, and obtaining a 12-lead ECG in the patient with chest pain. If the patient is a direct admit to CICU, completing a brief targeted history and physical examination, deciding on patient eligibility for thrombolytic therapy,[74] and obtaining a chest radiograph, serum electrolytes, serum markers of MI, and coagulation studies are priorities.

The brief history should be targeted to (1) identify and define the patient's complaint of chest pain, and (2) review personal and family health history to identify risk factors for cardiovascular disease, including previous cardiac problems, allergies, smoking history, and current medications. Because chest pain is the most common symptom of AMI, a "PQRST" format for eliciting pain information ensures a complete pain history.[42A] Questions should be directed to determine pain characteristic in terms of *P* (placement and provocation), *Q* (quality), *R* (radiation), *S* (severity), and *T* (time) of unrelenting pain onset. Concurrent physical examination allow early evaluation and decision making related to thrombolysis.

Cardiac monitoring should be initiated immediately because of the high incidence of ventricular fibrillation and other arrhythmias in the initial hours after MI (Pantridge, 1975 #100). The patient without complications should be monitored for 3 days after presentation in the emergency department.[8] Cardiac monitoring should be continued for a longer period for patients with complications such as arrhythmias, conduction defects, pump failure, silent ischemia, and shock. Five lead wires are typically used to monitor the patient. An electrode is placed on the right arm, the left arm, the right leg, the left leg, and the chest. Accurate lead placement is illustrated in Figure 20–16. When five leads are used, only one precordial lead can be selected. This lead may be either V_1 or V_6. V_1 is the preferred choice of precordial leads because it allows for detection of right bundle-branch block and the distinction between ventricular tachycardia and supraventricular tachycardia.[35] Many cardiac monitors can display two leads simultaneously. In this case, a precordial lead and a limb lead, such as lead II, may be monitored.

In select leads, ST segment abnormalities may be seen depending on the area of ischemia and injury. The lead chosen for monitoring in the patient with an MI should reflect the area of ischemia and location of the coronary artery occlusion.[34] The 12-lead ECG, taken during the initial period after an MI, provides the best information about which leads to monitor. For example, the most sensitive leads in detecting ischemia caused by a occlusion of the RCA are leads II, III, and aVF.[78]

Modified chest lead 1 (MCL_1) is the preferred choice of leads if the cardiac monitor or telemetry unit has only three lead wires. MCL_6 or M_3 may also be used. The following are directions for converting a standard lead system (leads I, II, III) into a modified lead system (leads MCL_1, MCL_6, M_3) using three electrodes.

- When the monitor lead selector switch is turned to lead I and you want to obtain MCL_1, MCL_6, or M_3, place:
  LA (positive) electrode on the V_1 or V_6 position, or the left upper abdomen, respectively
  RA (negative) electrode on the left posterior shoulder
  RL (ground) electrode on the right posterior shoulder
- When the monitor lead selector switch is turned to lead II and you want to obtain MCL_1, MCL_6, or M_3, place:
  LL (positive) electrode on the V_1 or V_6 position, or the left upper abdomen, respectively
  RA (negative) electrode on the left posterior shoulder
  RL (ground) electrode on the right posterior shoulder

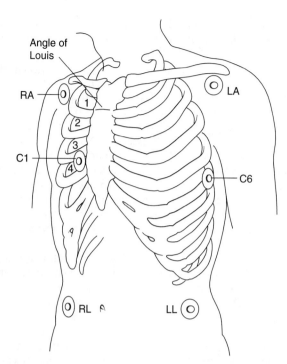

FIGURE 20-16 Proper electrode placement for obtaining V_1, as well as the six limb leads. Electrodes designated for the limbs are placed close to where each limb joins the torso, and the chest electrode is placed in the fourth intercostal space at the right sternal border (C_1). Because patients vary with respect to body shape, it is difficult to palpate the first intercostal space with any accuracy. Thus, the fourth intercostal space is located by first palpating the little bony prominence, called the angle of Louis, where the body of the sternum joins the manubrium. This rise in the sternum identifies the second rib, and the space below it is the second intercostal space. To obtain V_6, the chest electrode is moved to the mid-axillary line at the level of the fifth intercostal space (C_6). (From Drew BJ: Bedside electrocardiogram monitoring. *AACN Clinical Issues* 4(1): 26, 1993.)

- When the monitor lead selector switch is turned to lead III and you want to obtain MCL_1, MCL_6, or M_3, place:
  LL (positive) electrode on the V_1 or V_6 position, or the left upper abdomen, respectively
  LA (negative) electrode on the left posterior shoulder
  RL (ground) electrode on the right posterior shoulder

The electrode sites on the skin should be clean, dry, and relatively flat. Hair should be shaved and the skin mildly abraded (use gauze or abrading pad on electrode packaging). The pregelled electrodes are then applied to the chest. The audio switch in the patient's room may be turned off depending on the patient's status, and the alarm system turned on. Electrodes should be changed often enough to prevent skin breakdown and provide artifact-free tracings. By placing electrodes on the posterior shoulder, skin breakdown over the subclavicular area, which is often used for percutaneous catheter insertion, is avoided. The patient and family should be given a brief explanation of the purpose of cardiac monitoring and the patient and family's questions answered.

Newer monitors provide capability for ST segment monitoring at the bedside. ST segment deviation is the number of millimeters the ST segment is displaced from the isoelectric line. ST segment displacement of a minimum of 1 mm from the patient's baseline or isoelectric line for at least 1 minute is indicative of ischemia.[78] ST segment elevation is associated with MI more frequently than ST segment depression. ST segment monitoring may assist in detecting silent ischemia and recurrent ischemia after an MI, as well as the effectiveness of reperfusion therapy. ST segment monitoring may also provide the means to assess the effect of nursing care and self-care activities on the incidence of ischemia.[12]

Intravenous access is required for drug administration and blood draws if the patients has received thrombolytic therapy. As one or more stable IV lines are established, blood for laboratory tests should be obtained through the IV catheter to prevent additional venipuncture sites that may bleed after thrombolytic therapy. One IV catheter may be capped to provide access for direct blood sampling, and 1 mL of saline can be injected every 8 hours and after injection of medication to maintain patency. If thrombolytic or vasoactive agents are infusing, an additional IV catheter is needed for administration of pain medications and emergency cardiac drugs. For the patient who is admitted to the CICU with an IV line in place, the line's patency, the conditions under which the line was inserted, and the appropriateness of the placement site should be assessed. The insertion site should be inspected daily for signs of inflammation.

Oxygen therapy is beneficial for patients with MI who are hypoxemic. Hypoxia is common in patients with AMI and is usually the result of ventilation-perfusion abnormalities.[37] Some evidence suggests that oxygen therapy may reduce ischemia and limit infarct size.[63] If the patient's oxygen saturation is less than 90%, supplemental oxygen therapy should be given.[74] Four to 6 L/min of 100% oxygen by nasal prongs or mask may be administered for 2 to 3 days.[5] Pulse oximetry can be used to monitor oxygen saturation, particularly in patients receiving thrombolytic therapy.

Efforts have been made to standardize care and reduce practice variations in the care of patients who sustain a MI. The development and implementation of clinical pathways, care maps, and practice guidelines represent an attempt to provide high-quality care and to reduce the costs associated with unnecessary tests and treatments. Clinical pathways and care maps reflect optimal management strategies as defined by a consensus of experts in a particular health care organization and outline goals for the patient as well as ideal sequencing and timing of interventions to meet goals with maximal efficiency.[70] The purpose of critical pathways is to (1) reduce practice variation; (2) minimize delay in treatment; (3) decrease resource use; and (4) improve or maintain the quality of care.[51]

Clinical practice guidelines have also been developed by panels of experts in cardiology, cardiovascular nursing, and related fields. These clinical practice guidelines also represent an attempt to provide a framework for the standardization of care for patients with AMI, based on clinical evidence of effective diagnosis and treatment and expert opinion. Thus, these guidelines are "evidence based" and define optimal care with the goal of reducing the frequency of unnecessary tests and treatment. The American Heart Association and the American College of Cardiology initially developed practice guidelines for the management of patients with AMI in 1990. These practice guidelines were revised in 1996. The guidelines are intended as a guide for management rather than a strict prescription, and are to be altered based on clinical judgment, individual patient needs, and new findings.[74]

Limitation of Infarct Size

Strategies to limit infarct size and decrease morbidity and mortality after AMI include early reperfusion, reducing myocardial oxygen demands, and the manipulation of sources of energy production in the myocardium.[8] Early reperfusion with thrombolytics, primary PTCA, or CABG results in restored blood flow to the myocardium and improved hemodynamics. Restored blood flow prevents the extension of the existing infarction and reinfarction. Therapies that reduce myocardial oxygen demands include beta blockers, pain relief and sedation, and providing the patient with a restful, quiet environment. Hypertension and tachycardias increase myocardial oxygen demand and place the patient at risk. Associated clinical conditions that increase myocardial oxygen demand, such as fever and infection, should be treated.

Other therapies may improve the supply of oxygen to the myocardium. Supplemental oxygen has been shown to decrease acute ischemia injury and development of myocardial necrosis in an experimental model.[63] Supplemental oxygen is recommended for all patients with AMI for the first 2 to 3 hours and in patients with arterial oxygen saturation levels of less than 90%.[74] Anemia should be treated promptly. The administration of IV nitroglycerin during AMI has been found to limit infarct size and improve LV function.[49]

Cardiac rehabilitation is the process of actively assisting the cardiac patient to achieve and maintain optimal health. Components of a cardiac rehabilitation program are the education of the patient and family and prescription for activity and exercise. Before discharge, patients should receive detailed instructions regarding follow-up medical care, including activity and exercise, medications and risk factor modification, and when to seek help (see chapters in Part V of this book).

PAIN MANAGEMENT

Because pain increases myocardial oxygen demands, pain management is a priority for the patient with AMI. Pain management strategies focus on increasing oxygen supply to the heart and reducing oxygen demand. Interventions include nitrates, narcotic analgesics, oxygen therapy, and beta blockers in conjunction with reperfusion therapies such as thrombolysis and primary PTCA.[8] Sublingual nitroglycerin may be tried first if the patient's systolic blood pressure is at least 90 mm Hg and the heart rate is between 50 and 100 beats/min.[74]

Nitrates result in dilation the coronary arteries to enhance collateral flow to the ischemic myocardium; dilation of the venous bed, which decreases ventricular preload; and reduction of coronary spasm. An IV nitroglycerin drip may be initiated because long-acting nitrates should be avoided in the management of early MI. Nitroglycerin, however, should not be used as a substitute for narcotic analgesics.[74]

Morphine sulfate relieves pain and anxiety and reduces the patient's restlessness. Morphine also reduces the activity of the sympathetic nervous system with a resultant decrease in myocardial oxygen consumption by a decrease in heart rate and blood pressure. It also dilates the venous and arterial bed, reduces ventricular preload, and may relieve symptoms of pulmonary edema.[1] Morphine sulfate may be given in doses of 2 to 4 mg IV every 5 minutes until the pain is relieved or problematic side effects such as respiratory depression or hypotension occur. Some patients require as much as 25 to 30 mg IV to relieve pain and anxiety. Morphine-related hypotension is mainly seen in the setting of orthostatic volume depletion, and may be prevented by maintaining the patient in a supine position as tolerated.[8] In patients with morphine sensitivity, IV meperidine may be used.

PHYSICAL ACTIVITY

The plan for physical activity after AMI should be individualized based on the patient's condition. Specific activities should be stopped for increasing shortness of breath, the patient's perception of fatigue, or an increase in heart rate of greater than 20 to 30 beats/min.[8] The patient may eat unassisted with back and arms supported. Feeding and other low-level activities such as toileting and positioning are safe for most patients after AMI because they require low energy expenditure.[72]

In general, patients with uncomplicated MI should not be confined to bed for more than 12 hours if they are hemodynamically stable. After 12 hours, the patient who is hemodynamically stable may transfer from bed to chair and remain in the chair for 1 to 2 hours per day. On days 3 and 4, the patient may bathe and dress himself or herself, sitting on the side of the bed, transfer from bed to chair as desired, and ambulate in the room. Prescriptions for activity and exercise after MI are components of a cardiac rehabilitation program (see Chapter 34).

"Coronary precautions," introduced in the 1960s, have been widely practiced despite a lack of literature to support their use.[72] Examples of coronary precautions include the limitation of hot and iced fluids, avoidance of rectal temperatures, limitation of caffeinated beverages, and avoidance of the Valsalva maneuver. The only coronary precaution supported by literature is avoidance of the Valsalva maneuver. In the Valsalva maneuver, air is trapped in the lungs by a closed glottis and intrathoracic pressure increased by expiratory mechanisms, causing sudden and intense changes in systolic blood pressure and heart rate. Increased intrathoracic pressure results in a decreased venous return to the heart (decreased preload), decreased SV, decreased cardiac output, and an increase in heart rate and peripheral vasoconstriction. When the trapped air is released, the intrathoracic pressure is decreased and preload is increased, resulting in an increased workload for the heart.

Assisted use of both bedside commode and a bedpan results in minimal energy cost and cardiovascular stress to most patients.[80] The position a person assumes when using a commode is more natural and allows for appropriate and optimal use of the muscles of defecation (abdominal and rectal), which may reduce the resultant straining usually associated with the Valsalva maneuver. Therefore, the use of the commode is recommended for patients without specific contraindications to postural change. Stool softeners should also be given to avoiding straining while defecating.

DIET

The patient's diet should consist of foods high in fiber, potassium, and magnesium (except in the presence of renal failure) and low in sodium, and should include plenty of fresh fruits and vegetables. No more than 30% of total calories should come from fat. Small meals should be provided on a frequent basis.[8]

The literature does not support limiting beverages containing caffeine. Blood pressure changes related to caffeine consumption are not significant until at least 400 mg of caffeine is consumed. Moderate consumption of caffeine does not increase the likelihood of ventricular arrhythmias or coronary events.[60] People who routinely drink caffeinated beverages develop a tolerance, and withdrawal from caffeine can cause headaches and an increase in heart rate.[74] Thus, routine coffee drinkers may safely drink four to five cups of coffee per day in the CICU or on the telemetry unit.[60]

TREATMENT OF HEMODYNAMIC DISTURBANCES

After AMI, patients may be classified into one of four hemodynamic subsets: (1) normal perfusion (cardiac output) and no pulmonary congestion (normal PAWP); (2) normal perfusion and pulmonary artery congestion (high PAWP); (3) low perfusion (low cardiac output) without pulmonary congestion; and (4) low perfusion (low cardiac output) and pulmonary congestion (high PAWP).[41,42] Therapy is tailored to the patient's hemodynamic profile and the patient may move between hemodynamic subsets as a result of therapy. In all cases, therapies are designed to maintain ventricular performance, support hemodynamics, and protect the ischemic myocardium.

Right heart catheterization at the bedside with a pulmonary artery catheter may provide valuable diagnostic information in select patients with hemodynamic disturbances. Indications for insertion of a pulmonary artery catheter in the patient after AMI include (1) hypotension not corrected by volume administration; (2) hypotension in the presence of CHF; (3) hemodynamic compromise requiring vasoactive drugs or balloon counterpulsation; and (4) mechanical lesions such as cardiac tamponade, severe mitral valve regurgitation, RV infarction, or ruptured ventricular septum.[8,66] Use of the pulmonary artery catheter may also be helpful in distinguishing between cardiac and noncardiac etiologies of pulmonary edema.

TREATMENT OF RIGHT VENTRICULAR INFARCTION

The presence of RV infarction associated with inferior MI has been associated with an in-hospital mortality rate seven to eight times that of patients with inferior MI alone.[82] RV infarction is also an independent predictor of mortality in elderly patients with their first inferior MI.[18] Early diagnosis is key to effective treatment, and a right-sided ECG should be obtained on all patients presenting with signs and symptoms of an inferior MI. Right ventricular involvement has been associated with inferior MI in up to 50% of cases.[54]

The treatment of RV MI differs from that of LV MI and includes (1) early reperfusion with thrombolytics or primary PTCA, (2) volume administration to maintain RV preload, (3) the administration of inotropic medications such as dobutamine, (4) the reduction of RV afterload, and (5) the insertion of a pacemaker in cases of AV block. The administration of fluids increases cardiac output by increasing RV preload. In some cases, however, volume administration may increase RV dilation and decrease cardiac output.[31] Drugs such as nitroglycerin and diuretics, which decrease preload, are usually avoided.[74]

If the cardiac output has not improved after 1 to 2 L of fluid, inotropic drugs such as dobutamine or dopamine should be administered.[74] Dobutamine may markedly improve RV and LV systolic performance through improved contractility of hypokinetic wall segments.[31]

The reduction of RV afterload in the setting of LV dysfunction, by reducing LV afterload, may also improve cardiac output. Judicious use of vasodilators such as sodium nitroprusside has been recommended to increase the pressure gradient from the right to the left side of the heart, thereby promoting passive flow through the pulmonary vascular system and increasing LV filling.[25] Sodium nitroprusside dilates both the pulmonary and the systemic vascular bed and decreases LV and RV afterload.[81] In the setting of LV dysfunction, the use of an intra-aortic balloon pump may improve cardiac output by decreasing LV afterload and improving LV performance, thereby decreasing RV afterload and improving forward flow.[74]

Patients with RV infarction are predisposed to sinus bradycardia and high-grade AV block.[74] An external pacemaker may be used in emergency situations. However, AV pacing is considered optimal. Preservation of synchronous atrial contraction (atrial kick) is considered especially important in RV infarction for three reasons: (1) to maintain adequate RV preload by maximizing presystolic stretch of damaged RV myocardial fibers, (2) to propel blood forward into the pulmonary circuit in the absence of effective RV contraction, and (3) to avoid further pericardial restriction by preventing simultaneous atrial and ventricular diastole. For example, if filling of the atria and ventricles coincides, ventricular end-diastolic volume is further reduced because of the limited pericardial space available for chamber distention.[54] Up to one third of patients with RV infarction may experience atrial fibrillation because of atrial infarction or right atrial chamber enlargement.[54] These patients should be cardioverted as soon as possible to preserve atrial function and optimize cardiac output.

PHARMACOLOGIC MANAGEMENT

A summary of action, indications, contraindications, and nursing implications for aspirin, heparin, nitrates, beta blockers, calcium channel blockers, angiotensin-converting enzyme (ACE) inhibitors, and warfarin sodium (Coumadin; Du Pont Pharma, Wilmington, DE) follows. The reader is referred to Chapter 21 for thrombolytic agents, Chapter 14 for antiarrhythmics, Chapter 23 for drugs used in the perioperative period, and Chapter 25 for drugs used in management of cardiac arrest.

Aspirin

ACTION/INDICATIONS

Platelet activity is increased in the setting of AMI. Platelets are initially involved in thrombus at the site of the ruptured atherosclerotic plaque.[6] Aspirin inhibits cyclooxygenase-dependent platelet aggregation and inhibits platelet activity.[52] Moreover, aspirin appears to damage platelets permanently, and restoration of normal hemostatic function occurs only after the damaged platelets have been replaced by normal ones (2 to 7 days).

The International Study of Infarct Survival (ISIS) trial found that the administration of 162 mg of enteric-coated aspirin alone resulted in a 23% reduction in the odds of death compared with placebo in the setting of AMI.[52] The risk of reinfarction, cardiac arrest, and stroke were also significantly reduced in the group receiving aspirin alone. In addition, this study demonstrated decreased mortality rates when aspirin was used in conjunction with streptokinase. The dosage required to achieve total platelet inhibition is only 40 mg/d. However, the administration of 162 mg initially in the setting of MI results in more rapid onset of action. Patients with suspected MI or unstable angina should be given aspirin immediately and should continue to receive it for several years.[26]

CONTRAINDICATIONS/ADVERSE REACTIONS

Aspirin is contraindicated for patients with a known sensitivity to the drug, history of gastrointestinal bleeding, and intrinsic coagulation defects.

NURSING IMPLICATIONS

Aspirin may also be taken with meals or milk to avoid gastric irritation. Monitoring for bleeding tendencies and a periodic check of hemoglobin and hematocrit for anemia are recommended.

Heparin

ACTION/INDICATIONS

Heparin is an antithrombin that prevents coagulation by interfering with the formation of thrombin from prothrombin, preventing thrombin from supporting or allowing the conversion of fibrinogen to fibrin. Although it has no effect on existing clots, heparin does interfere with platelet function and is the anticoagulant of choice to treat MI as well as ischemic heart disease, pulmonary emboli, and deep vein thrombosis.[20] The accumulation of thrombin at sites of endothelial injury promotes platelet aggregation, vasoconstriction, and the conversion of fibrinogen to fibrin. Heparin alone, or administered in conjunction with aspirin, has been shown to reduce the frequency of MI when given to patients in the acute phase of unstable angina.[2,79A] The goal of heparin therapy is to prevent the extension of thrombus. The therapeutic activated partial thromboplastin time (aPTT) threshold (1.5 to 2.5 times the control value) should be reached within 24 hours of initiating therapy.

CONTRAINDICATIONS/ADVERSE REACTIONS

Heparin may be contraindicated in patients with heparin allergy, acute cerebrovascular accident, or a history of life-threatening gastrointestinal bleeding, or who are thrombocytopenic or coagulopathic on another basis. Heparin can induce thrombocytopenia, and patients should be monitored closely for signs and symptoms.

NURSING IMPLICATIONS

A baseline aPTT should be obtained before therapy is begun, 6 hours after therapy is initiated, any time a dose change occurs, and every 6 hours until the therapeutic level is obtained on two consecutive aPTTs. The aPTT may then be drawn every 24 hours for 3 days. Therapy should be discontinued after 3 to 5 days or if bleeding occurs. A patient receiving heparin therapy should be frequently assessed for hemorrhage and thrombocytopenia. A baseline platelet count and hemoglobin and hematocrit should be obtained and monitored daily. Hemodynamic monitoring may aid in the early detection of occult hemorrhage. Heparin should not be abruptly discontinued because MI can develop quickly, especially in the absence of aspirin.[17]

Nitrates

ACTION/INDICATIONS

In the setting of AMI, nitrates are effective in treating ischemic chest pain and hypertension and reducing pulmonary congestion. Nitrates decrease preload by peripheral vasodilation. A reduction in preload results because of the decreased venous return, reduced filling pressures, and reduced intracardiac volumes of the right and left sides of the heart. At higher doses, arterial vasodilation results in a decreased afterload. In the coronary circulation, nitrates increase coronary vasodilation, reverse coronary vasoconstriction, and cause dilation of the collateral vessels. Nitroglycerin may also inhibit platelet activation and aggregation.[1] Despite their effectiveness in the treatment of ischemic chest pain, at least two large studies have failed to find a reduction in mortality rates associated with the use of nitrates after AMI. In ISIS-4, patients who presented within 24 hours of onset of symptoms were randomized to oral controlled-release isosorbide mononitrate or placebo. A nonsignificant 3% reduction in mortality rate was found at 35 days.[52] In GISSI 3, patients were randomized to IV nitroglycerin for 24 hours, followed by transdermal nitroglycerin or usual care. The mortality rate in the nitrate group was reduced by 6%,

which was not significant. However, patients experienced lower rates of postinfarction angina ($P = 0.033$) and reduced rates of cardiogenic shock ($P = 0.009$).[48] Nitroglycerin is recommended for the first 24 to 48 hours in patients with AMI and CHF, persistent ischemia, or hypertension, and beyond 48 hours in patients with recurrent angina or persistent pulmonary congestion.[74] Nitroglycerin should be used with caution in patients with RV MI because of the reduction in preload.

CONTRAINDICATIONS/ADVERSE REACTIONS

The contraindications for nitrates include hypotension, hypovolemia, increased intracranial pressure, constrictive pericarditis, pericardial tamponade, and known hypersensitivity or known idiosyncratic response to organic nitrates. Tolerance, requiring increased dosage of medication, may develop as soon as 12 hours after the start of the infusion. Tolerance may be minimized by providing a period without nitrates or by using the smallest therapeutic dose and alternating nitrates with other vasodilators. To minimize tolerance, a nitroglycerin patch should be worn only for 12 to 14 hours, followed by a patch-free interval of 10 to 12 hours.[1]

NURSING IMPLICATIONS

The use of nitroglycerin in patients with AMI may result in hypotension, causing a reduction in coronary perfusion pressure and a consequent increase in myocardial ischemia. These effects may be potentiated by saline depletion secondary to diuretic agents. The nurse should monitor the patient's heart rate and blood pressure, keeping in mind the onset of action and the occurrence of the peak effect for the particular mode of therapy being used.

β-Adrenergic Blocking Agents

ACTION/INDICATIONS

The cardiovascular system's response to catecholamines is mediated by specific cell membrane receptors. The action of a specific beta blocker is determined by the type and site of receptor with which it interacts. Stimulation of β_1 receptors, which are located primarily in the myocardium, increases cardiac contractility, sinus discharge rate, and AV node conduction velocity, and decreases AV node refractoriness. Stimulation of β_2 receptors, the predominant β-adrenergic receptor in vascular and bronchial tissue, mediates arteriolar dilation and bronchial smooth muscle relaxation. Beta blockers are used in the management of angina and after MI because of their ability to inhibit the chronotropic and inotropic responses to catecholamines.[64] Their use has been shown to improve postinfarction survival rates.[7,24]

Blocking sympathetic stimulation of β-adrenergic receptors decreases myocardial contractility, slows the heart rate, and decreases systolic blood pressure, decreasing myocardial oxygen demand.[2,20,24,39] A slower heart rate also provides a longer diastole, thereby increasing coronary artery blood flow and myocardial oxygen supply. Beta blockers are classified by cardioselectivity, duration of action, membrane-stabilizing activities, and lipophilic properties.[39,79A] β_1-Selective beta blockers, such as atenolol, esmolol, and metoprolol, are considered "cardioselective" and are recommended for use in patients who have a history of obstructive pulmonary disease or mild CHF because they are less likely to cause bronchospasm. Certain beta blockers (i.e., propranolol and metoprolol) have the secondary properties of inhibiting platelet aggregation and desensitizing activated platelets.[2] Beta blockers are classified as class II antiarrhythmics according to the Vaughn Williams' classification (see Chapter 14). Propranolol, nadolol, timolol, pindolol, atenolol, nietoprolol, esmolol, and labetalol are a few examples of beta blocking agents.

CONTRAINDICATIONS/ADVERSE REACTIONS

The use of beta blockers is contraindicated in patients with moderate to severe CHF, pulmonary edema, LV dysfunction, obstructive pulmonary disease, cardiogenic shock, and severe peripheral vascular disease.[7,17,79A] In patients with impaired LV function, CHF may occur or intensify, although it may be controlled with the use of digitalis or diuretics.[39] The use of beta blockers is contraindicated in variant angina because coronary artery spasm is likely to worsen. Caution should be used when administering beta blockers to patients with first-degree AV block, a bifascicular block, or sick sinus syndrome.[24] Chronic administration of beta blockers has been associated with unfavorable effects on plasma lipid and lipoprotein levels, including a decrease in high-density lipoprotein cholesterol.[39] Some adverse reactions associated with beta-blocker therapy include bradycardia, heart block, bronchospasm, fatigue, dyspepsia, diarrhea or constipation, mental disturbances such as mood changes, and nightmares.[68A]

NURSING IMPLICATIONS

When beta blockade is initiated, a patient should have continuous ECG monitoring. The target heart rate is 50 to 60 beats/min, although the medication should not be initiated if the heart rate is less than 60 beats/min. Beta blockers should be avoided if the PR interval is more than 0.24 second, or if second- or third-degree AV block is present.[17] Because a major effect of beta blockade is a decrease in systolic blood pressure, patients must be monitored for hypotension, and therapy should not be initiated if systolic blood pressure is less than 90 mm Hg. Beta blockers should not be administered to patients with known or suspected coronary artery vasospasm because they allow unopposed α-adrenergic stimulation and may intensify the frequency and severity of coronary artery spasm.[2] Nurses must be aware that sudden withdrawal of beta blockers may result in exaggerated cardiac β-adrenergic responsiveness, producing an exacerbation of angina and precipitating arrhythmias or AMI. The mechanism for the rebound effect after abrupt withdrawal is unknown, although it is suspected to be related to increased myocardial sensitivity to catecholamines on

the removal of beta blockade.[39,68A] Elderly patients may have occult sinus or AV node disease unmasked by the use of beta blockers, and therefore must be monitored carefully on initiation of therapy and followed closely for signs of conduction delay.[68A] Patients of Chinese descent tend to have an increased sensitivity to beta blockers and therefore may have good results achieved with lower-than-expected doses. Beta blockers are generally avoided in people with insulin-dependent diabetes mellitus because symptoms of hypoglycemia may be masked. Their use in non-insulin-dependent diabetes mellitus is considered more appropriate because hypoglycemia is less of a threat.

Calcium Antagonists

ACTION/INDICATIONS

Calcium antagonists, or calcium channel blockers, are often considered for patients with contraindications to beta blockers. They are potent vasodilators that block the calcium inflow in smooth muscle cells, dilating coronary arteries and thereby increasing myocardial oxygen supply.[39] The relaxation of coronary arteries may be especially beneficial in patients with Prinzmetal's angina. Calcium antagonists also decrease heart rate and AV node conduction rate, increasing diastolic filling time and thereby increasing myocardial oxygen supply. They effectively decrease myocardial oxygen demand by decreasing SVR and myocardial contractility. Calcium channel agents are also thought to interfere with thrombus formation by reducing platelet aggregation. Calcium channel blockers are usually considered a better choice than beta blockers for people with asthma or COPD. Diltiazem and verapamil should be avoided in patients with bradycardia or heart block because of their negative chronotropic effects, but remain good choices for patients with tachycardia (Cody, 1993). Nifedipine, amlodipine, nicardipine, verapamil, and diltiazem are a few examples of calcium channel blocking agents.

CONTRAINDICATIONS/ADVERSE REACTIONS

Calcium channel agents should be avoided in patients with evidence of significant LV dysfunction (LV ejection fraction 40%), and pulmonary edema.[17] Adverse reactions include dizziness, headache, flushing, peripheral edema, bradycardia, nausea, or constipation.

NURSING IMPLICATIONS

As with beta blockers, when therapy with calcium channel blockers is initiated, patients should receive continuous ECG monitoring and be closely monitored for hypotension and conduction disturbances. Unlike beta blockers, calcium channel agents can be used safely in patients with COPD, and their vasodilating effects may be critical in patients with Prinzmetal's angina.

Angiotensin-Converting Enzyme Inhibitors

ACTION/INDICATIONS

Angiotensin-converting enzyme inhibitors are a class of drug that blocks the conversion of angiotensin I, which is a weak vasoconstrictor, to angiotensin II, a potent vasoconstrictor. Their use in AMI has been shown to reduce postinfarction mortality rates if therapy is begun within 24 hours of hospital admission.[20,76A] Their vasodilating effects help to reduce afterload, thereby reducing the work of the heart. Long-term use (6 to 12 months) of ACE inhibitors may improve the endothelium in abnormal segments of coronary arteries. They have also been shown to prevent or retard development of LV dysfunction.[76A] Examples of ACE inhibitors include captopril, enalapril, and lisinopril.

CONTRAINDICATIONS/ADVERSE REACTIONS

Angiotensin-converting enzyme inhibitors should be used very cautiously in patients who are hemodynamically unstable, particularly in the presence of hypovolemia, because the vasodilation caused with ACE inhibitor therapy can produce a marked hypotension. If diuretic dosages are decreased during the first 48 to 72 hours of initiating ACE inhibitor therapy, hypotension can often be avoided.[76A] Cautious use of ACE inhibitors is recommended for patients with renal insufficiency. Therapy is contraindicated in patients with renal artery stenosis because very rapid and significant elevations of creatinine levels may occur. In general, therapy can be initiated safely if serum creatinine is less than 2.5 mg/dL.

NURSING IMPLICATIONS

Before initiation of therapy, a baseline serum creatinine level should be drawn and baseline blood pressure obtained. It is of utmost importance that patients receiving ACE inhibitor therapy be monitored closely for hypotension, especially on initiation of therapy. Serum creatinine levels should also be monitored closely, and a significant elevation in serum creatinine should receive prompt attention.

Warfarin Sodium

ACTION/INDICATIONS

Warfarin sodium (Coumadin) is an oral anticoagulant that competes with vitamin K, which is essential for the liver to manufacture clotting factors II, VII, IX, and X. Warfarin is bound to albumin in the blood, with very little of the drug remaining "free." It is this free warfarin, however, that provides the drug's therapeutic effect. When initiating warfarin therapy, it is important to know that a lag time of 48 to 72 hours occurs between the initiation of therapy and the achievement of therapeutic levels. This lag time signifies the gradual disappearance of the clotting factors. Warfarin is prescribed for patients who require long-term anti-coagulation, as in atrial fibrillation, or patients who have had a CK of more than 1,000 U/L with AMI. In the latter population, warfarin is usually prescribed for 3 to 6 months after MI.

CONTRAINDICATIONS/ADVERSE REACTIONS

Patients with a history of alcohol abuse, those requiring aspirin therapy, and those with malignant hypertension or active tuberculosis should not receive warfarin because of their increased risk of bleeding.

NURSING IMPLICATIONS

The effectiveness of warfarin is measured by the prothrombin time (PT). Before therapy is initiated, a baseline PT should be obtained and levels should be checked daily. Once a patient's response to therapy has been established, PT can be checked less frequently, and is typically checked once a month when a maintenance dose has been established. Patients must be educated about safety precautions while taking warfarin, such as using electric shavers instead of razors, wearing gloves while gardening, using a soft-bristle toothbrush, and avoiding contact sports. Urine and stool color should be checked daily, and epistaxis, bleeding gums, and bruising should be immediately reported. It is suggested that a PT be checked 1 week after any new medication is begun while taking warfarin because many drugs may interact unfavorably with it. Warfarin should be stored in a cool, dry place because it loses its potency when exposed to high heat.

NURSING MANAGEMENT

Nursing management of the patient with CHD or MI may involve caring for the patient in varying stages of the disease process: during the acute chest discomfort before or during CICU admission, as the diagnosis or angina pectoris or MI is confirmed, at hospital discharge, during convalescence, or on an ongoing basis with the goal of preventing episodes of angina or another MI. Refer to Nursing Care Plan 20–1 for management of the patient with AMI. The focus of this section is on the nursing management of angina pectoris or the acute phase of MI. This section includes examples of nursing diagnoses for problems associated with angina and MI.

Chest Discomfort

DIAGNOSIS

Chest discomfort, related to an imbalance between myocardial oxygen supply and demand, manifested by patient complaints of chest discomfort, with or without radiation to arms, neck, back, or jaw, by nonverbal expressions of discomfort (facial grimacing, Levine sign), and by increases in heart rate, blood pressure, and respiratory rate and by cool, clammy skin.

NURSING CARE PLAN 20–1 ◆ The Patient With Acute Myocardial Infarction

Nursing Diagnosis:	Inadequate myocardial tissue perfusion relative to myocardial oxygen demand, related to coronary artery narrowing from atherosclerosis, spasm, and thrombosis, manifested by chest discomfort, arrhythmias and conduction disturbances, and heart failure
Nursing Goal:	To detect early the manifestations of inadequate myocardial tissue perfusion
Outcome Criteria:	1. Chest discomfort is detected at its onset. Effects of chest discomfort on cardiovascular hemodynamics reported within 15 minutes of the onset of pain.
	2. Marked changes in heart rate, rhythm, and conduction, and the effects of these changes on hemodynamics are detected at their onset and reported to the physician.
	3. The following signs and symptoms of left ventricular (LV) failure are detected and reported to the physician at their onset:

- Complaints of shortness of breath, dyspnea on exertion, orthopnea, and paroxysmal nocturnal dyspnea
- Heart rate greater than 100 beats/min, irregular rhythm, and blood pressure outside acceptable limits for this patient
- S_3 and S_4 gallops
- New systolic murmur
- Respiratory rate greater than 20/min with physical activity and greater than 16 min with rest
- Cheyne-Stokes breathing pattern
- Crackles and wheezes
- Buccal cyanosis
- Dyspnea at rest or with minimal exertion

4. The signs and symptoms of right ventricular (RV) failure are detected and reported to the physician at their onset:
- Jugular venous distention greater than 10 cm
- Dependent edema
- Weight gain

NURSING INTERVENTIONS	RATIONALE
1. On admission, assess, document, and report to the physician the following:	1. These data assist in determining the cause and effect of the chest discomfort and provide a baseline so that post-therapy symptoms can be compared.
a. The patient's description of chest discomfort, including: location, radiation, duration of pain, and factors that affect it	a. There are many conditions associated with chest discomfort. Characteristic clinical findings of ischemic pain are described in the clinical manifestations section of this chapter.
b. The effect of chest discomfort on cardiovascular hemodynamic perfusion to the heart (heart rate, rhythm and conduction, blood pressure), to the brain (mentation), to the kidneys (urine output, creatinine–blood urea nitrogen ratio), and to the skin (color, temperature, moisture)	b. Myocardial infarction decreases myocardial contractility and ventricular compliance and may produce arrhythmias by promoting reentry and increased automacity. Cardiac output is reduced, resulting in reduced blood pressure and decreased organ perfusion. The heart rate may increase as a compensatory mechanism to maintain cardiac output. An electrocardiogram in patients with pain may be useful in the diagnosis of myocardial ischemia (classic or variant angina), injury, and infarction.

(continued)

NURSING CARE PLAN 20–1 ◆ The Patient With Acute Myocardial Infarction (*Continued*)

NURSING INTERVENTIONS	RATIONALE
2. Using a cardiac monitor, assess continuously and document the heart rate, rhythm, and conduction every 4 hours and before administration of medications that have a cardiovascular effect. Determine the effect of the arrhythmia or conduction disturbance on the patient's blood pressure and perfusion to the heart, brain, and kidneys and report marked changes to the physician. Obtain a 12-lead ECG with any marked change in heart rate, rhythm, or conduction.	2. Early detection of arrhythmias and conduction disturbances allows initiation of therapy and may prevent a lethal arrhythmia. Arrhythmias and conduction disturbances can result in reduced cardiac output, hypotension, and reduced perfusion to vital organs. Rhythms that do not result in a pulse have no cardiac output (cardiac arrest). A 12-lead ECG assists in the diagnosis of arrhythmias and conduction disturbances and of further myocardial damage.
3. On admission, every 4 hours, and with onset of chest discomfort, or any other new symptom, assess, document, and report to the physician the following signs and symptoms of left heart failure: complaints of shortness of breath; changes in heart rate and rhythm; abnormal heart sounds (particularly S_3 and S_4 gallops and the systolic murmur of LV papillary muscle dysfunction); abnormal blood pressure; abnormal respiratory rate and rhythm; abnormal breath sounds; central cyanosis; and specific activities that result in dyspnea. Initially, every 4 hours, and with chest discomfort, assess, document, and report to the physician the following signs and symptoms of right heart failure: jugular venous distention and dependent edema. In addition, weigh the patient on admission and daily.	3. These data are useful in diagnosing LV and RV failure. (Refer to Chapter 22 for the rationale for the signs and symptoms of heart failure.)

Nursing Goal 2: To reduce, eliminate, or prevent the manisfestations of inadequate myocardial tissue perfusion

Outcome Criteria:
1. Patient reports relief of chest discomfort within 15 to 30 minutes. Patient appears comfortable:
   a. Restful
   b. Respiratory rate returns to prediscomfort rate
   c. Skin is warm and dry
2. Ideally, normal sinus rhythm without arrhythmia is maintained or restored, or the patient's baseline heart rate, rhythm, and conduction are maintained or restored.
3. Patient reports absence of shortness of breath, dyspnea on exertion, orthopnea, and paroxysmal nocturnal dyspnea. Heart rate is less than 100 beats/min. Rhythm regular. Blood pressure within normal limits for this patient. Absence of S_3 and S_4 gallops and systolic murmur. Respiratory rate is less than 20/per min with physical activity and greater than 16/per min with rest. Regular rhythm. No adventitious breath sounds or a reduction in crackles and wheezes. No cyanosis. No dyspnea with rest or with mild exertion. No jugular venous distention.

NURSING INTERVENTIONS	RATIONALE
1. Administer oxygen as ordered.	1. Most patients with acute myocardial infarction have hypoxemia. Oxygen increases the oxygen supply to the myocardium.
2. Administer narcotic analgesic as ordered for chest discomfort and evaluate continuously the patient's response.	2. Narcotics are central nervous system depressants that are useful in alleviating chest discomfort, decreasing anxiety, and increasing sense of well-being. In addition, morphine sulfate is a venodilator, thereby decreasing preload, which reduces myocardial oxygen consumption.

(continued)

NURSING CARE PLAN 20–1 ◆ The Patient With Acute Myocardial Infarction (*Continued*)

NURSING INTERVENTIONS	RATIONALE
3. Administer nitroglycerin as ordered for chest discomfort.	3. Nitroglycerin is primarily a venodilator, reducing preload and therefore reducing myocardial oxygen consumption. In addition, it dilates arterioles and relieves spasm, thus increasing blood flow to the myocardium.
4. Administer antiarrhythmic and other medications as ordered or according to hospital policy and evaluate continuously the patient's response to therapy.	4. Antiarrhythmic medications decrease automaticity and conductivity of myocardium.

5. After appropriate treatment of arrhythmia, assess, document, and report to the physician causes of the arrhythmias or conduction disturbances.
  a. Perform a cardiac assessment.
  b. Obtain a chest radiograph.
	5. a., b. Data obtained from the history of physical and laboratory studies can assist in the diagnosis of disease processes (LV failure or pulmonary embolism) that can cause arrhythmias by the mechanisms of hypoxemia or myocardial stretch. Placement of catheters within the heart can be seen on chest radiograph.

c. Obtain blood specimens for electrolytes (especially potassium and calcium), hemoglobin, appropriate drug levels, and for blood gases.	c. Electrolyte imbalance (especially potassium or calcium) can cause arrhythmias and conduction disturbances. Reduced hemoglobin decreases the oxygen-carrying capacity of the blood. Hypoxia, acidosis and alkalosis, and concurrent drug toxicity or subtherapeutic drug levels can cause arrhythmias and conduction disturbances.

6. Teach patient:
  a. To adhere to the prescribed diet (e.g., low sodium, low cholesterol and saturated fats, low calories)
  b. To adhere to activity prescription.
	6. Low sodium diet may reduce extracellular volume, thus reducing preload and afterload and thus myocardial oxygen consumption. Decreased cholesterol and saturated fat intake results in reduced serum cholesterol levels. In the obese patient, weight reduction may decrease cardiac work and improve tidal volume. The activity prescription is determined individually to maintain the heart rate and blood pressure within normal limits.

7. Plan nursing care to reduce myocardial oxygen need: assist patient to the bedside commode; elevate backrest to comfort; provide a full liquid diet as tolerated; support arms during upper extremity activity; use stool softener to prevent straining at stool; teach patient to exhale with physical movement to avoid a Valsalva maneuver and to practice the relaxation response; individualize visitor privileges based on patient response (e.g., appears restful, no increase in chest discomfort, arrhythmias, or pulse rate).	7. Physical rest reduces the myocardial oxygen consumption. See text for rationale for specific interventions. Fear and anxiety precipitate the stress response, which results in increased levels of endogenous catecholamines. With increased epinephrine, the pain threshold is decreased; more pain further increases myocardial oxygen consumption.
8. Promote the patient's physical comfort by providing individualized basic nursing care.	8. Physical comfort promotes the patient's sense of well-being and reduces anxiety.

GOALS

1. To detect early chest discomfort and associated ECG and hemodynamic changes
2. To reduce or eliminate chest discomfort
3. To prevent the occurrence of chest discomfort

INTERVENTIONS

Interventions are prescribed to meet each goal and are directed toward assessment and improvement of the balance between myocardial supply and demand. The balance between myocardial supply and demand can be improved by interventions that

decrease myocardial oxygen consumption or increase coronary blood flow. Examples of nursing interventions for the hospitalized patient with angina or AMI follow.

For Goal 1. Instruct the patient to report chest discomfort immediately (based on a scale of 1 to 10, with 10 being as bad as it could be) at onset of discomfort; and (1) assess and document the patient's description of chest discomfort, including location, radiation, duration, and the factors that affect it; (2) assess blood pressure, heart rate and rhythm, and respiratory rate and rhythm; (3) assess the skin for temperature and moistness; (4) obtain a 12-lead ECG during chest discomfort; and (4) report the findings of these assessments to the physician. In patients with angina pectoris, if MI is suspected, immediately draw baseline CK and CK isoenzymes, and for recurrent chest discomfort in patients with MI, repeat CK and CK isoenzymes, as ordered.

For Goal 2. Immediately reduce patient's physical activity to the level of activity before occurrence of chest discomfort; administer oxygen, morphine sulfate, nitroglycerin, or other medications as ordered, and continuously evaluate the patient's response to therapy; provide a restful environment; and promote the patient's physical comfort by elevating head of bed to 20 to 30 degrees or higher and by individualizing basic nursing care.

For Goal 3. (1) Provide care in a calm, competent manner; (2) provide a restful, quiet environment; (3) provide small portions of easily digested food; (4) assist the patient with activities of daily living; (5) teach the patient to exhale with physical movement and, as necessary, offer stool softeners and laxatives to prevent straining with bowel movements; (6) teach the patient to recognize precipitating factors and alter behavior accordingly; and (7) teach the patient to practice relaxation techniques.

OUTCOME CRITERIA

Specific outcome criteria are written for each goal statement.

For Goal 1. Chest discomfort, changes in the 12-lead ECG, and hemodynamic responses are detected at onset.

For Goal 2. Within 5 minutes of intervention: patient states that chest discomfort is relieved or reduced; patient appears comfortable; heart and respiratory rates and blood pressure are returning or have returned to baseline level before the onset of chest discomfort; ST segments and T waves revert to pattern seen before onset of chest discomfort; and skin is warm and dry.

For Goal 3. Patient denies chest discomfort; patient appears comfortable; heart and respiratory rates and blood pressure are within patient's normal range; and skin is warm and dry.

Decreased Myocardial Tissue Perfusion

DIAGNOSIS

Decreased myocardial tissue perfusion related to an imbalance between myocardial oxygen supply and demand and manifested by chest discomfort, arrhythmias, conduction disturbances, or heart failure. Refer to previous diagnosis of chest discomfort for goals, interventions, and outcome criteria for chest discomfort.

GOALS

Goals for this diagnosis include:

1. To detect early manifestations (specify) and etiologies of decreased myocardial tissue perfusion
2. To reduce or eliminate manifestations (specify) of decreased myocardial tissue perfusion

3. To prevent, when possible, manifestations (specify) of decreased myocardial tissue perfusion and extension of MI or progression to infarction in patients with angina

INTERVENTIONS

Interventions are designed to detect manifestations of the imbalance between myocardial oxygen supply and demand and to improve this imbalance. Interventions to meet each goal include the following.

For Goal 1. The patient's heart rate and rhythm should be monitored during the acute phase of MI. Assess and document cardiac rhythm every 1 to 4 hours depending on the patient's condition, before and after each dose of antiarrhythmic or vasoactive drug (or any drug with cardiovascular effects), and when the patient's status indicates. Assess blood pressure and obtain 12-lead ECG with changes in cardiac rhythm or if the patient complains of palpitations.

If the patient experiences arrhythmias, perform a cardiovascular physical examination; obtain venous blood for electrolytes, hemoglobin, and, if appropriate, drug levels; obtain arterial blood for blood gas analysis; and obtain a chest radiograph as ordered by the physician.

Initially, every 4 to 8 hours, and during chest discomfort, assess, document, and report to the physician the following: new S_3 or S_4 gallops or a new murmur of mitral regurgitation; new or increasing crackles; and reduced activity tolerance.

For Goal 2. Immediately reduce patient's physical activity to the level before occurrence of manifestations of decreased myocardial tissue perfusion; administer oxygen and antiarrhythmic and other medications (positive inotropic, afterload-reducing, and preload-reducing agents) as ordered, and continuously evaluate the patient's response to therapy; provide a restful environment; and promote the patient's physical comfort by elevating head of bed to 20 to 30 degrees or higher and providing individualized basic nursing care.

For Goal 3. Provide small portions of easily digested, low-sodium, low-saturated-fat foods; provide a restful environment; as needed, assist the patient in a supportive, calm, competent manner with activities of daily living; teach patient to exhale with physical movement; as necessary, offer stool softeners and laxatives to prevent straining with bowel movements; and teach patient to practice relaxation techniques.

OUTCOME CRITERIA

Specific outcome criteria are written for each goal statement.

For Goal 1. Arrhythmias and conduction disturbances and signs and symptoms of heart failure are detected at onset.

For Goal 2. Immediately after intervention, the patient's cardiac rate and rhythm return to patient's normal range; patient states that palpitations are relieved or reduced; patient appears comfortable; blood pressure is returning or has returned to baseline level; S_3 or S_4 gallops or the murmur of mitral regurgitation disappear or do not increase in intensity; crackles are eliminated or reduced; activity tolerance is maintained or improved.

For Goal 3. Patient denies chest discomfort; patient appears comfortable; heart and respiratory rates and blood pressure are within patient's normal range; skin is warm and dry; no S_3 or S_4 gallops; no murmur of mitral regurgitation; no crackles; and activity tolerance is maintained.

Decreased Systemic Tissue Perfusion

DIAGNOSIS

Decreased systemic tissue perfusion related to a decrease in cardiac output from arrhythmias and conduction disturbances and from heart failure, manifested by abnormal pulse rate and rhythm; abnormal respiratory rate and rhythm; deterioration of other hemodynamic parameters; decreased mentation; decreased urine output; individually defined undue or excess fatigue; and moist, cool, cyanotic skin.

GOALS

1. To detect early manifestations and etiologies of decreased systemic tissue perfusion
2. To reduce or eliminate manifestations of decreased systemic tissue perfusion
3. To prevent, when possible, manifestations of decreased systemic tissue perfusion

INTERVENTIONS

Interventions are designed to detect the manifestations of the imbalance between systemic oxygen supply and demand and to improve this imbalance by restoring the balance between myocardial oxygen supply and demand. Interventions to meet each goal include the following.

For Goal 1. On admission, every 4 hours, and during chest discomfort, assess, document, and report to the physician the following: abnormal heart rate and rhythm; hypotension; narrowing pulse pressure; abnormal respiratory rate and rhythm; decreased mentation; decreased urine output; increasing fatigue; and moist, cool, cyanotic skin.

For Goal 2. Immediately reduce patient's physical activity to the level before occurrence of manifestations of decreased systemic tissue perfusion; administer oxygen and antiarrhythmic and other medications (positive inotropic, afterload-reducing, and preload-reducing agents) as ordered, and continuously evaluate the patient's response to therapy; provide a restful environment; and promote the patient's physical comfort by elevating head of bed to 20 to 30 degrees or higher, or by providing a cardiac chair (depending on blood pressure response), and by giving individualized basic nursing care.

For Goal 3. Provide small portions of easily digested, low-sodium, low-saturated-fat foods; provide a restful environment; as needed, assist the patient in a supportive, calm, competent manner with activities of daily living; teach patient to exhale with physical movement; as necessary, offer stool softeners and laxatives to prevent straining with bowel movements; teach patient to recognize precipitating factors of decreased systemic tissue perfusion and to alter behavior accordingly; and teach patient to practice relaxation techniques.

OUTCOME CRITERIA

Specific outcome criteria are written for each goal statement.

For Goal 1. Signs and symptoms of decreased systemic tissue perfusion are detected early.

For Goal 2. Immediately after intervention, ideally normal sinus rhythm without arrhythmia or conduction disturbance returns; blood pressure and pulse pressure are returning or have returned to baseline level; respiratory rate and rhythm are returning or have returned to patient's baseline; patient remains fully alert and oriented, without personality change; urine output remains greater than 250 mL/8 h; patient's complaints of fatigue are reduced; patient is able to carry out activities of daily living within prescribed activity limits; and extremities remain warm, dry, and of normal color.

For Goal 3. Normal sinus rhythm without arrhythmia or conduction disturbance is maintained; blood pressure and pulse pressure are maintained at patient's baseline level; respiratory rate and rhythm are maintained at patient's baseline; patient remains fully alert and oriented, without personality change; urine output remains greater than 250 mL/8 h; patient does not complain of worsening fatigue; patient is able to carry out activities of daily living within prescribed activity limits; and extremities remain warm, dry, and of normal color.

Fear or Anxiety

DIAGNOSIS

Fear or anxiety related to diagnosis, treatment, and prognosis of angina or AMI, manifested by abnormal rate and rhythm of pulse and respiration, elevated blood pressure, subjective complaints of fear and anxiety from patient and family, restlessness, and sleeplessness.

GOALS

1. To detect early manifestations of fear and anxiety
2. To reduce or eliminate fear and anxiety
3. To prevent, when possible, fear and anxiety

INTERVENTIONS

Interventions are directed at reducing fear and anxiety in the patient and family. Patients with angina or AMI are understandably frightened and concerned. They frequently associate the occurrence of chest pain or heart attack with impending death. Most people have had relatives or friends who died suddenly from heart problems. The acute onset of symptoms, the decision to seek medical help, transportation to the hospital, the admission procedure, and the rapid, frequently invasive therapeutics are extremely stressful. During this time, the patient is required to make rapid, important decisions regarding care. In addition, many patients need to make major lifestyle changes to manage manifestations of CHD. Fear and anxiety perpetuate the ischemic process by increasing sympathetic nervous system responses, resulting in elevated serum catecholamines, which increase myocardial oxygen consumption. The increased myocardial oxygen consumption can precipitate an attack of angina and jeopardizes ischemic myocardium in patients with AMI, increasing pain and further increasing anxiety. Anxiety causes patients to focus their attention on their hearts, resulting in escalation of the severity of the symptoms in patients with angina. The nursing role includes interventions aimed at reducing anxiety in the patient and family. Interventions to meet each goal include the following.

For Goal 1. Assess and document the patient's and family's level of fear and anxiety and effectiveness of coping mechanisms.

For Goals 2 and 3. (1) Treat promptly chest discomfort or any other manifestations of angina or AMI; (2) provide a restful environment; (3) provide individualized basic nursing care in a supportive, calm, and competent manner; (4) show genuine interest and concern; (5) provide a conducive atmosphere for communication; facilitate communication (listen, reflect, guide); (6) answer questions and discuss with the patient diagnostic procedures and interventions and describe sensations that the patient may experience during procedures; (7) teach stress reduction techniques; and (8) assess the need for spiritual counseling and refer as appropriate.

OUTCOME CRITERIA

Specific outcome criteria are written for each goal statement.

For Goal 1. Abnormal rate and rhythm of pulse and respiration, elevated blood pressure, and subjective complaints of fear and anxiety, restlessness, and sleeplessness are detected early.

For Goal 2. Rate and rhythm of pulse and respiration and blood pressure are normal or are approaching normal, and subjective complaints of fear, anxiety, restlessness, and sleeplessness are reduced or absent.

For Goal 3. Rate and rhythm of pulse and respiration and blood pressure remain normal, and subjective complaints of fear, anxiety, restlessness, and sleeplessness are absent.

Knowledge Deficit

DIAGNOSIS

Knowledge deficit about AMI and CHD, medical or surgical management plan, risk factor modification, or return to usual activities of daily living; related to fear and anxiety, lack of exposure, lack of recall, nonuse of information, misinterpretation, cognitive limitations, disinterest, lack of familiarity with available resources, or denial of angina or AMI; manifested by the patient being unable to describe the disease process, unable to explain the rationale behind the diagnosis, treatment, and prognosis of AMI and CHD, unaware of activity limitations and prescribed medications, unaware of cardiac risk factors in general, or unaware of specific risk factors and how to modify them.

GOALS

General goals are early detection, reduction or elimination, and prevention of the specific knowledge deficit and maintenance of heart-healthy behaviors in the patient and family. Specific goals should be based on each identified knowledge deficit.

INTERVENTIONS

Development of a teaching plan enables the nurse to provide standardized content to each patient. When angina occurs during hospitalization, teach the patient to rest and relax, take nitroglycerin as prescribed, and notify the nurse. In preparation for discharge, teach the patient to rest and relax when angina occurs; take nitroglycerin and other antianginal medications, as prescribed; immediately seek medical attention if no relief of chest discomfort has occurred within 30 minutes; and call the physician if there is a change in the pattern of angina.

- ◆ Diagnostic procedures and interventions may be a source of anxiety and fear. Provide concrete information about procedures and describe sensory experiences that they may have, such as "the dye (during cardiac catheterization) will make you feel hot and flushed for approximately 15 seconds" or "the room (cardiac catheterization laboratory) will be dimly lit and cool."
- ◆ Teach the patient and family the content necessary for them to modify their lifestyles. Provide information about modification of risk factors such as elevated cholesterol levels, smoking, hypertension, and sedentary lifestyle. Advise the patient to adhere to the prescribed therapeutic plan (diet, medication, and activity level). Teach stress reduction techniques, and encourage active participation in cardiac rehabilitation programs.
- ◆ To prevent myocardial ischemia from progressing to infarction or reinfarction, teach the patient to be aware of physiologic (e.g., activity during cold weather, after a heavy meal, or with sexual intercourse) and psychological (e.g., anger or grief) precipitating factors; teach the patient to reduce precipitating factors by taking prophylactic nitroglycerin, reducing specific physical activities and psychological stresses that often result in chest discomfort, and countering emotional stress by regular physical exercise.

OUTCOME CRITERIA

Outcome criteria for the patient with a knowledge deficit may include the patient and family being able to describe the disease process; being able to explain the rationale behind the diagnosis, treatment, and prognosis of AMI and CHD; being aware of activity limitations and prescribed medications; and being aware of general and specific cardiac risk factors and how to modify them.

Nursing Management Plan for Patients With Right Ventricular Infarction: Analysis of Medical and Nursing Assessment Data and Formulation of Nursing Diagnoses

The management of a patient with an RV infarction is illustrated in Nursing Care Plan 20–2. An important initial

NURSING CARE PLAN 20–2 ◆ The Patient with Right Ventricular Infarction

Nursing Diagnosis: Decreased cardiac output, related to dilated and noncompliant right ventricle, manifested by decreased blood pressure, decreased pulmonary artery wedge pressure (PAWP), decreased urine output, cool moist skin, cyanosis, mental confusion

Nursing Goal 1: To detect early the signs of right ventricular (RV) dysfunction secondary to RV infarction

Outcome Criteria: During hospitalization, the following signs are detected, documented, and immediately reported to the physician:

1. Physical assessment features: jugular venous distention, RV S_3 or S_4 gallop, systolic murmur of tricuspid regurgitation, hepatomegaly, peripheral edema, hypotension, urine output less than 0.5 mL/kg/h or 4 mL/k/8 h, cool, moist skin, cyanosis, mentation change

2. Right precordial electrocardiographic (ECG) features:
   ST elevation of ≥0.5–1 mm in lead V_4R
   ST elevation of ≥1 mm in leads V_4R–V_6R or V_6R only
   QS pattern in lead V_4R or V_3R–V_4R
   ST elevation in lead V_4R that is greater than the ST elevation in V_1–V_3
   ST depression in lead V_2 that is 50% or less than the magnitude of ST elevation in aVF

3. Hemodynamic profile characteristics:
   RA pressure >10 mm Hg and RA: PAWP ratio ≥0.8
   RA waveform: prominent *y* descent that is at least as great as the *x* descent
   RV waveform: diastolic dip–plateau pattern ("square-root sign")
   Cardiac index <2.2 L/min/m²

NURSING INTERVENTIONS	RATIONALE

1. On admission, every 4 hours, and with chest pain, assess, document, and report to the physician the following:
  a. Jugular venous distention
  b. RV S_3 or S_4 gallop
  c. Systolic murmur of tricuspid regurgitation
  d. Hepatomegaly
  e. Peripheral edema
  f. Clear lungs
  g. Hypotension
  h. Urine output less than 0.5 mL/kg/h or 4 mL/k/8 h
  i. Cool, moist, cyanotic extremities
  j. Mentation change
	1. These clinical features may develop secondary to a dilated and noncompliant right ventricle that is unable to contract adequately, resulting in elevated systemic venous pressure, inadequate left ventricular (LV) preload, and reduced stroke volume and cardiac output.

2. On admission, every 8 hours the first 24 hours, and every 24 hours for at least 3 days obtain standard 12-lead ECG and right precordial ECG.	2. ST segment elevation suggestive of RV infarction may disappear in less than 10 hours from onset of chest pain, necessitating frequent serial recordings to allow documentation.
3. Continually monitor the V_4R lead in addition to conventional leads, and record a rhythm strip every 4 hours and during chest discomfort.	3. ST segment and QRS morphologic changes thought to be indicative of RV infarction frequently involve lead V_4R. Continual monitoring of this lead may provide early ECG clues to the occurrence of RV infarction and subsequently expedite appropriate treatment.

4. Assess serial (as stated in number 2) right precordial ECG for the following changes:
  a. ST elevation of ≥0.5–1 mm in lead V_4R
  b. ST elevation of ≥1 mm in V_4R–V_6R or V_6R only
  c. QS pattern in lead V_4R or V_3–V_4R
  d. ST elevation in V_4R greater than the ST elevation in V_1–V_3
  e. ST depression in V_2 that is 50% or less than the magnitude of ST elevation in aVF
	4. Clinical studies suggest that these ECG features may suggest an evolving RV infarction.

(continued)

NURSING CARE PLAN 20-2 ◆ **The Patient with Right Ventricular Infarction (***Continued***)**

NURSING INTERVENTIONS	RATIONALE
5. Record and document pressures and obtain pressure tracings as the pulmonary artery catheter is inserted into the RA, RV, pulmonary artery, and wedge position.	5. These measurements and tracings serve as a baseline for comparison of later data. Also, the hemodynamic diagnosis of RV infarction may be missed with exclusion of this step, precluding prompt treatment.
6. Measure RA pressure, PAWP, and cardiac index, and derive pulmonary and systemic vascular resistance every hour.	6. Early frequent recordings of hemodynamic parameters may aid in the recognition of low cardiac output secondary to RV infarction.
7. Observe, document, and report the following hemodynamic patterns:	7. Investigative reports suggest that these hemodynamic criteria may be indicative of RV infarction.
a. RA pressure >10 mm Hg and RA:PAWP ratio of ≥0.8	
b. RA waveform: prominent *y* descent that is at least as great as the *x* descent	
c. RV waveform: diastolic dip-plateau pattern ("square-root sign")	
d. Cardiac index <2.2 L/min/m²	

Nursing Goal 2:	To eliminate the signs of RV dysfunction secondary to RV infarction
Outcome Criteria:	During hospitalization, the following signs are observed and documented: Systolic blood pressure >90 mm Hg PAWP of 15–20 mm Hg Urine output = at least 0.5 mL/kg/h or 4 mL/kg/8h Cardiac index >2.2 L/min/m² Skin pink, warm, dry Mentation unchanged

NURSING INTERVENTIONS	RATIONALE
1. Infuse intravenous fluid bolus per physician protocol to attain a PAWP of 15–20 mm Hg.	1. Initial rapid volume expansion increases RV end-diastolic volume, which may optimize contractility of a diastolic noncompliant RV.
2. Administer positive inotropic agents such as dobutamine or dopamine per physician protocol. Monitor heart rate and rhythm for development of tachycardia or tachyarrhythmias.	2. Dobutamine (2–20 µg/kg/min) and dopamine (2–10 vg/kg/min) directly stimulate β-adrenergic myocardial receptors, resulting in increased contractility and cardiac output. Although dobutamine is less arrhythmogenic than dopamine, both agents may precipitate tachycardia and tachyarrhythmias, resulting in decreased diastolic filling and reduced cardiac output.
3. Administer peripheral vasodilators such as nitroprusside or hydralazine per physician protocol. Monitor pulmonary and systemic vascular resistance at least every hour.	3. These agents decrease RV and LV afterload, thereby enhancing RV and LV stroke volume. Hydralazine may be preferable because it selectively vasodilates arterioles and should not decrease preload.[139] Pulmonary and systemic vascular resistance parameters are necessary to optimize preload and afterload.
4. When pacing therapy is indicated, institute atrial or atrioventricular sequential method per physician protocol.	4. Preservation of atrioventricular synchronous contraction maximizes contractility and cardiac output.

5. Avoid administration of drugs and performance of maneuvers that decrease preload:
  a. Diuretics
  b. Venodilators (nitroglycerin, morphine)
  c. Sitting up in bed
  d. Valsalva maneuver
	5. Filling of the left ventricle is dependent on distention of the right ventricle.[31] These actions decrease preload, thereby reducing stretch of the RV myocardial fibers and further compromising the ability of the noncompliant chamber to propel blood forward. Reduced cardiac output results.

nursing consideration is to suspect RV infarction in any person admitted to an intensive care unit with an acute inferior or posterior LV infarction. A right-sided ECG should be obtained for any patient with evidence of an inferior MI. Initial clues to the development of RV dysfunction may be subtle. In addition, the low-cardiac-output syndrome may be thought secondary to primary LV dysfunction. The major differences between the low-cardiac-output states of predominant RV and LV infarction are listed in Table 20–4. Critical care nurses can facilitate the diagnosis and appropriate management of patients with RV infarction through awareness of the usual clinical features and ECG changes associated with an RV infarction and the systematic and continual assessment of these features as well as the evaluation of the patient's response to therapy.

Patients with RV infarction experience alterations in functional health status similar to those with LV infarction. In the setting of RV infarction, however, decreased cardiac output is a potential nursing problem that requires a different approach in terms of detection, assessment, and treatment.

Right ventricular infarction represents a unique clinical syndrome that may exhibit a spectrum of hemodynamic alterations depending on the extent of RV dysfunction. Early detection of RV dysfunction secondary to RV infarction is crucial to the institution of appropriate therapy and subsequent resolution of an existing low-cardiac-output state.

REFERENCES

1. Abrams J (1995). The role of nitrates in coronary heart disease. Archives of Internal Medicine, *155*(4): 357
2. Albert, NM. High risk unstable angina: Keeping pace with current research findings. AACN Clinical Issues. 1995 Feb;6(1): 110–120
3. Alpert J, Rippe J: Manual of Cardiovascular Diagnosis and Therapy. Boston: Little, Brown & Company, 1980
4. American Heart Association (1997). Heart and stroke fact statistics. Dallas: American Heart Association
5. American Heart Association (1992). American Heart Association guidelines for cardiopulmonary resuscitation and emerging cardiac care III, Adult advanced cardiac life support. JAMA, 268, 2199–2242
6. Anderson HV, Willerson JT (1993). Current Concepts: Thrombolysis in Acute Myocardial Infarction. New England Journal of Medicine, *329*(10), 703–709
7. Andresen D, Ehlers H, Wiedemann M, Bruggemann T. Beta Blockers: Evidence versus wishful thinking. American Journal of Cardiology 1999, March 11, 83(5B): 64D–66D
8. Antman EM, Braunwald E: Myocardial Infarction. In E. Braunwald (Ed.), Heart Disease: a Textbook of Cardiovascular Medicine (5 ed., Vol. 2, pp. 1184–1274). Philadelphia: Saunders, 1997
9. Armstrong PW (1996). Evolution of the CCU from rhythm, Function and protection to reperfusion and beyond: A personal journey and perspective. Canadian Journal of Cardiology, 12(10), 909–913
10. Arrighi JA, Dilsizian V: Identification of Viable, Nonfunctioning Myocardium. In D. L. Brown (Ed.), Cardiac Intensive Care (pp. 307–327). Philadelphia: W. B. Saunders, 1998
11. Bahr R (1998). The concept and the development of chest pain emergency departments as a strategy in the war against heart attack. Critical Care Nursing Clinics of North America, 10(1), 41–51
12. Bell NN (1992). Clinical Significance of ST-Segment Monitoring. Critical Care Nursing Clinics of North America, *4*(2), 313–323
13. Berger C, Murabito J, Evans J, Anderson K, Levy D (1992). Prognosis after first myocardial infarction: comparison of Q-wave myocardial infarction in the Framingham Heart Study. JAMA, *268*, 1545–1551
14. Braat S, Brugada P, DeZwaan C, et al (1983). Value of electrocardiogram in diagnosing right ventricular involvement in patients with an acute inferior wall myocardial infarction. British Heart Journal, 49, 368
15. Braunwald E (1998). Evolution of the management of acute myocardial infarction: a 20th century sage. The lancet, 352(9142), 1771–1774
16. Braunwald E, Antman E (1997). Evidence-Based Coronary Care. Annals of Internal Medicine, 126(7), 551–553
17. Braunwald E, Jones RH, Mark DB, et al. Diagnosing and managing unstable angina. Circulation 1994 Jul 90(1):613–623
18. Bueno H, Lopez-Palop R, Bermejo J, Lopez-Sendon JL, Delcan J (1997). In-Hospital Outcome of Elderly Patients With Acute Inferior Myocardial Infarction and Right Ventricular Involvement. Circulation, 96(2), 436–441
19. Burke James A. Emergency: Cardiogenic shock. Hospital Medicine. June, 1994, 37–43
20. Casey M, Bedker DL, Roussel-McElmeel PL. Myocardial infarction: Review of clinical trials and treatment strategies. Critical Care Nurse 1998 April 18(2) 39–52
21. Cercek B, Shah PK. Complicated acute myocardial infarction: Heart failure, shock, mechanical complications. Cardiology Clinics 1991 Nov; 9(4):569–593
22. Chatterjie K. Complications of acute myocardial infarction. Current Problems in Cardiology. 1993 Jan; 18(1):1–79
23. Chou T, Van Der Bel-Kahn J, Allen J, et al (1981). Electrocardiographic diagnosis of right ventricular infarction. American Journal of Medicine, 70(1175)
24. Cody RJ, Conti R Jr, Samet P. Managing angina and concomitant disease. Patient Care 1993, July. 45–72
25. Cohn J, Guiha N, Broda M, et al (1974). Right ventricular infarction: Clinical and hemodynamic features. American Journal of Cardiology, 33, 209–214
26. Collins R, Peto R, Baigent C, Sleight P (1997). Drug Therapy: Aspirin, Heparin, and Fibrinolytic Therapy in Suspected Myocardial Infarction. New England Journal of Medicine, 336(12), 847–860
27. Cummins RO, Ornato JP, Abramson NS, et al (1997). Advanced Cardiac Life Support. Dallas, American Heart Association
28. Cushinotto, NM. Pharmacology update: Clinical considerations of Heparinization. Journal of the American Academy of Nurse Practitioners 1997 June 9(6) 273–276
29. Daily E (1991). Clinical Management of patients receiving thrombolytic therapy. Heart and Lung, *20*, 52–565
30. D'Arcy B, Nanda N (1982). Two-dimensional echocardiographic features of right ventricular infarction. Circulation, 65, 167
31. Dell'Italia L, Starling M, Blumhardt R (1985). Comparative Effects of volume loading, dobutamine and nitroprusside in patients with predominant right ventricular infarction. Circulation, 72, 1327
32. Douglas PS, Ginsburg GS (1996). Current Concepts: The evaluation of chest pain in women. New England Journal of Medicine, 334(20), 1311–1315
33. Dracup K, Moser DK (1997). Beyond sociodemographics: Factors influencing the decision to seek treatment for symptoms of acute myocardial infarction. Heart and Lung, *26*, 253–262

34. Drew BJ (1991). Bedside electrocardiographic monitoring: state of the art for the 1990s. Heart and Lung, 20, 610–623

35. Drew BJ (1993). Bedside Electrocardiogram Monitoring. AACN Clinical Issues, 4(1), 25–33

36. Efhardt J, Young J (1974). Clinical and pathological observations in different types of acute myocardial infarction. Acta Medica Scandinavia, Supplement 560, 1

37. Fillmore S, Shapiro M, Killip T (1970). Arterial Oxygen Tension in acute myocardial infarction: Serial analysis of clinical state and blood gas changes. American Heart Journal, 79, 620

38. Fleischmann KE, Lee TH: The evolution of the coronary care unit: past, present and future. In D. L. Brown (Ed.), Intensive Cardiac Care (pp. 3–5). Philadelphia: W. B. Saunders, 1998

39. Fleury J. Long term management of the patient with stable angina. Nursing Clinics of North America. 1992 Mar; 27(1):205–230

40. Forman M, Goodin J, Phelan B, et al (1984). Electrocardiographic changes associated with isolated right ventricular infarction. Journal of the American College of Cardiology, 4(640)

41. Forrester J, Diamond G, Chatterjie K (1976a). Medical Therapy of acute myocardial infarction by application of hemodynamic subsets (first of two parts). New England Journal of Medicine, 295, 1356

42. Forrester J, Diamond G, Chatterjie K (1976b). Medical Therapy of acute myocardial infarction by application of hemodynamic subsets (second of two parts). New England Journal of Medicine, 295, 1404

42A. Gardiner-Caldwell. Synermed: Nursing Management in Thrombolytic Therapy: A Slide/Lecture Guide. San Francisco, Genentech, Inc. 1989

43. Geft I, Shah P, Rodriguez L, et al (1984). ST elevation in leads V1 to V5 may be caused by right coronary artery occlusion and acute right ventricular infarction. American Journal of Cardiology, 53, 991

44. Gershlick AH, More RS (1998). Recent Advances: Treatment of myocardial infarction. British Medical Journal, 316, 280–284

45. Gibler WB (1998). Diagnosis of Acute Coronary Syndromes in the emergency department: Evolution of chest pain centers. In E. J. Topol (Ed.), Acute Coronary Syndromes. New York Basel Hong Kong: Marcel Dekker, Inc

46. Gibson R (1989). Non-Q wave myocardial infarction: pathophysiology, prognosis, and therapeutic strategy. Annual Review of Medicine, 40(395–410)

47. Gillum R, Fortmann S, Prineas R, Kottke T (1984). International diagnostic criteria for acute myocardial infarction and acute stroke. American Heart Journal, 108(1), 150–158

48. G1551-3 (1994). Gissi-3: effects of lisinopril and transdermal glyceryl trinitrate singly and together on 6-week mortality and ventricular function after acute myocardial infarction. Lancet, 343 1115–1122

49. Hennekens CH, Albert CM, Godfried SL, Gaziano JM, Burning JE (1996). Adjunctive Drug Therapy of Acute Myocardial Infarction Evidence from Clinical Trials. New England Journal of Medicine, 335(22), 1660–1667

50. Hochman JS, Gerch BJ. Acute Myocardial Infarction. Ch 18, Textbook of Cardiovascular medicine. 1998, Lippincott-Raven, Philadelphia pp437–480

51. Ireson CL (1997). Critical Pathways: Effectiveness in Achieving Patient Outcomes, JONA, 27(6)

52. 1515-4 (1995). ISIS-4; a randomised factorial trail assessing early oral captopril, oral mononitrate, and intravenous magnesium sulphate in 58,050 patients with suspected acute myocardial infarction. Lancet, 345, 669–686

53. Isner J, Roberts W (1978). Right ventricular infarction complicating left ventricular infarction secondary to coronary heart disease. American Journal of Cardiology, 42, 885

54. Kinch JWM, Ryan TJ (1994). Right Ventricular Infarction. New England Journal of Medicine, 330(17), 1211–1217

55. Klein H, Tordjman T, Ninio R, et al (1983). The early recognition of right ventricular infarction: Diagnostic accuracy of the electrocardiographic V4R lead. Circulation, 67 558

56. Kontos MC, Arrowood JA, Paulsen WHJ, Nixon J (1998). Early Echocardiography Can Predict Cardiac Events in Emergency Department Patients with chest pain. Annals of Emergency Medicine, 31(5), 550–557

57. Kopelman H, Forman M, Wilson B, et al (1985). Right ventricular myocardial infarction in patients with chronic lung disease: possible role of right ventricular hypertrophy. Journal of the American College of Cardiology, 5, 1302

58. Lopez-Sendon J, Coma-Canella I, Gamallo C, et al (1985). Electrocardiographic findings in acute right ventricular infarction: Sensitivity and specificity of electrocardiographic alterations in right precordial leads V4R, V3R, V1, V2, and V3. Journal of the American College of Cardiology, 6 1273

59. Love J, Haffajee C, JM, G, et al (1984). Reversibility of hypotension and shock by atrial or atrioventricular pacing in patients with right ventricular infarction. American Heart Journal, 108, 5

60. Lynn LAM, Kissinger JF (1992). Coronary Precautions: Should caffeine by restricted in patients after myocardial infarction? Heart and Lung, 21, 365–370

61. Malone ML, Rosen LB, Goodwin JS. Complications of acute myocardial infarction in patients >90 years of age. American Journal of Cardiology. 1998 Mar; 81;638–41

62. Marcassa C, Galli M, Temporelli PL, Campini R, Orrego PS, Zoccarato O, Giordano A, Giannuzii P (1995). Technetium-99m Sestamibi Tomographic Evaluation of Residual Ischemia After Anterior Myocardial Infarction. Journal of the American College of Cardiology, 25, 590–596

63. Maroko P, Radvany P, Braunwald E, Hale S (1975). Reduction of Infarct Size by Oxygen Inhalation following Acute Coronary Occlusion. Circulation, 52, 360–368

64. McGoon MD, Shub C. Myocardial ischemia clinical syndromes. Mayo Clinic Practice of Cardiology Mosby, St. Louis 1996 3rd Ed.; Ch 29C.: 1160–90

65. Mosca L, Manson JE, Sutherland SE, Langer, Manolio T, Barret-Connor E (1997). Cardiovascular Disease in Women: A Statement for Healthcare Professionals From the American Heart Association. Circulation, 96(7), 2468–2482

66. Mueller HS, Chatterjee K, Davis K, Fifer MA, Franklin C, Greenberg MA, Labovitz A, Shah PK, Tuman K, Weil MH, Weintraub W (1998). Present Use of Bedside Right Heart Catheterization in Patients With Cardiac Disease. JACC, 32(3), 840–864

67. Newby LK, Ohman EM, Christenson RH (1998). The role of troponin and other markers for myocardial necrosis in risk stratification. In E. J. Topol (Ed.), Acute Coronary Syndromes. New York: Marcel Dekker, Inc

68. Ohman D, Amstron P, Christenson R, et al (1996). Cardiac troponin t-levels for risk stratification in acute myocardial ischemia. New England Journal of Medicine, 335, 1333–1341

68A. Olson HG, Aronow WS. Medical management of stable angina and unstable angina in the elderly with coronary artery disease. Clinics in Geriatric Medicine 1996 Feb; 12(1): 121–140

69. Pantridge J, Geddes J (1967). A mobile intensive-care unit in the management of myocardial infarction. Lancet, 2, 271–273

70. Pearson SD, Goulart-Fisher D, Lee TH (1995). Critical Pathways as a Strategy for Improving Care: Problems and Potential. Annals of Internal Medicine, 123, 941–948

71. Reeder GS. Identification and Treatment of Complications of Myocardial Infarction. Mayo Clinic Proceedings 1995; 70:880-4

72. Riegel B, Thomason T, Carlson B, Gocka I (1996). Are Nurses Still Practicing Coronary Precautions? A National Survey of Nursing Care of Acute Myocardial Infarction Patients. American Journal of Critical Care, 5(2), 91–98

73. Rogers WJ (1995). Contemporary Management of Acute Myocardial Infarction. American Journal of Medicine, 99(2), 195–206

74. Ryan TJ, Anderson JL, Antman EM, et al (1996). ACC/AHA Guidelines for the Management of Patients With Acute Myocardial Infarction: A Report of the American Cardiology/American Heart Association Task Force on Practice Guidelines (Committee on Management of Acute Myocardial Infarction. JACC, 28(5), 1328–1428

74A. Schweiger MJ, McMahon RP, Terrin ML, Raocco NA, Porway MN, Wiseman AH, Knalterud GL, Braunwald E (1994). Comparison of patients with < 60% to > or = 60% diameter narrowing of the myocardial infarct-related artery after thrombolysis. The TIMI Investigators. American Journal of Cardiology, 74, 105–110

75. Shah P, J, M, Berman D, et al (1985). Scintigraphically detected predominant right ventricular dysfunction in acute myocardial infarction: Clinical and hemodynamic correlates and implications for therapy and prognosis. Journal of the American College of Cardiology, 6, 1264

76. Simpson T (1990). Cardiovascular responses to family visits in coronary care unit patients. Heart and Lung, 19, 344–351

76A. Smith SC. ACE inhibitor therapy: Benefits and underuse. American Family Physician 1999, Jan 1, 59(1) 35–38

77. Sobel JL, Dittrich HC, Keen WD: Echocardiography in the Cardiac Intensive Care Unit. In D. L. Brown (Ed.), Cardiac Intensive Care. Philadelphia: W. B. Saunders Company, 1998

77A. Stone GW, Grines CL (1997). Primary Coronary Angioplasty Versus Thrombolysis. New England Journal of Medicine 337, 1168–1170

78. Tisdale LA, Drew BJ (1993). ST Segment Monitoring for Myocardial Ischemia. AACN Clinical Issues, 4(1), 34–43

79. Wellens HJJ (1993). Right ventricular infarction. New England Journal of Medicine, 328(14), 1036–1038

79A. Willerson JT. Recognition and Treatment of Unstable Angina, Cardiac Intensive Care Saunders, Philadelphia, 337–346, 1998

80. Winslow E, Lane L, Gaffney A (1984). Oxygen Uptake and cardiovascular response in patients and normal adults during in-bed toileting. Journal of Cardiac Rehabilitation, 4, 346–354

81. Yager M (1996). Right ventricular infarction in the emergency department: A review of pathophysiology, assessment, diagnosis, treatment and nursing care. Journal of Emergency Nursing, 22(4), 288–292

82. Zebender M, Kasper W, Kauder E. Schonthaler M, Geibel A, Olschewski M, Just M (1993). Right ventricular infarction as an independent predictor of prognosis after acute inferior myocardial infarction. New England Journal of Medicine, 328, 481–488

21

Interventional Cardiology Techniques

MICHAELENE HARGROVE DEELSTRA

Since the early 1970s, the goal of acute care for patients with myocardial ischemia due to coronary heart disease (CHD) has shifted from reducing risks associated with acute myocardial infarction (MI) to improving myocardial blood flow by reperfusion or revascularization of the myocardium. Restoration of perfusion to ischemic or at-risk myocardium may be achieved through thrombolysis, angioplasty, atherectomy, placement of an intracoronary stent, antiplatelet therapy, or a combination of these interventions.

THROMBOLYTIC THERAPY

In 1980, Dewood and colleagues[22] reported a high prevalence of coronary artery thrombosis in acute MI, establishing the pathophysiologic basis for thrombolytic therapy of patients with acute MI. Subsequently, research has attempted to determine the most efficacious means of early clot lysis, including studies of exogenously administered thrombolytic agents.

Thrombolytic Agents

Thrombolytic agents can be divided into two major categories: *fibrin selective,* characterized by activation of fibrin-bound plasminogen and a high velocity of clot lysis, and *nonselective,* characterized by systemic plasminogenolysis and fibrinogenolysis, somewhat slower clot lysis, and a more prolonged systemic lytic state.[72] Fibrin-selective agents include tissue-type plasminogen activator (t-PA), recombinant tissue plasminogen activator (alteplase [generic] activase; rt-PA), recombinant plasminogen activator (reteplase; r-PA), and single-chain urokinase plasminogen activator (scu-PA or prourokinase). Nonselective agents include streptokinase (SK), anisoylated plasminogen streptokinase activator complex (APSAC), and urokinase (UK). The most commonly used thrombolytics for intravenous administration in the setting of acute MI are discussed in the following sections.

STREPTOKINASE

Streptokinase is a nonenzymatic protein product of β-hemolytic streptococci. Exogenously administered SK combines with circulating plasminogen, forming complexes that catalyze plasmin formation (see Chapter 20). The resultant excessive circulating plasmin then creates a systemic lytic state, with dissolution of all recent thrombi, depletion of circulating fibrinogen, plasminogen, factor V and VIII, and accumulation of fibrin(ogen) degradation products.

Streptokinase is given in a dose of 1.5 million units infused over 30 to 60 minutes. Reported 90-minute angiographic patency of the infarct-related artery after this dose of SK ranges from 42% to 58%.[16,48] Because of its foreign protein origins, SK may trigger an antigenic response. Some type of allergic reaction was reported to occur in 3.6% of patients receiving SK in a large, multicenter study.[47] Pruritus, fever, nausea, flushing, urticaria, headache, and malaise are common symptoms, with bronchospasm and angioedema rarely reported.

People with anti-SK antibodies may not attain full therapeutic benefit from the SK, and therefore patients with known recent streptococcal infection or those who received SK within the last 5 days to 6 months should not be treated with an SK-based drug. Variable degrees of hypotension may also occur with administration of SK, presumably owing to plasmin-mediated activation of kinins and the complement system,[72] although hypotension may also be related to hemodynamic changes associated with acute myocardial ischemia. The Third International Study of Infarct Survival (ISIS-3) investigators reported hypotension in 11.8% of patients receiving SK, with 6.7% requiring pharmacologic intervention for hypotension.[42]

ANISOYLATED PLASMINOGEN STREPTOKINASE ACTIVATOR COMPLEX

Anisoylated plasminogen streptokinase activator complex is a chemically altered form of SK, created by the addition of an acyl group to an SK and lys-plasminogen activator complex. In the circulation, the activator complex converts circulating and fibrin-bound plasminogen into plasmin. APSAC has a relatively long half-life and results in pronounced fibrinogenolysis.

Anisoylated plasminogen streptokinase activator complex is administered as a bolus of 30 U over 2 to 5 minutes. The reported 90-minute angiographic patency from APSAC ranges from 72% to 90%.[9,48] Because APSAC is a form of SK, it possesses the same antigenic properties of SK. Allergic symptoms occurred in 5.1% of patients receiving APSAC in the ISIS-3 study.[42] Hypotension may occur in about 12% of patients[47] and is more pronounced if the drug is administered rapidly.

TISSUE-TYPE PLASMINOGEN ACTIVATOR

Endogenous t-PA is a serine protease produced by vascular endothelial cells. t-PA exhibits marked affinity for fibrin, primarily activating fibrin-bound plasminogen. Exogenously administered t-PA for clinical use is produced by recombinant DNA techniques. Alteplase (rt-PA) standard-dose accelerated regimen includes a 15-mg bolus, 50 mg or 0.75 mg/kg body weight over 30 minutes, and 35 mg or 0.50 mg/kg body weight over 60 minutes[43] for a total maximum dose 100 mg. Weight adjustment for patients who weigh less than 65 kg is recommended.[37] The half-life is 5 minutes. The reported 90-minute angiographic patency from 100 mg of rt-PA ranges from 61% to 89%.[65,75]

Reteplase (r-PA) is a modified recombinant form of rt-PA with a longer half-life (15 minutes) that can be given as two 10-megaunit (MU) bolus doses 30 minutes apart. The randomized comparison of coronary thrombolysis achieved with double-bolus Reteplase™ and front-loaded accelerated alteplase in patients with acute myocardial infarction. (RAPID II) trial showed higher patency rates with reteplase over alteplase (100 mg/90 minutes) at 60- and 90-minute intervals of reperfusion. However, follow-up angiography indicated similar overall patency rates in the alteplase and reteplase groups and did not show differences in mortality and patient outcome.[8] Dosing strategies may continue to evolve.

The unique activity and short half-lives of rt-PA and r-PA result in an increased likelihood of arterial reocclusion. Systemic anticoagulation with continuous intravenous heparin to maintain the activated partial thromboplastin time (aPTT) within a therapeutic range is recommended to sustain arterial patency after rt-PA and r-PA.[39] Allergic symptoms and hypotensive events have also been reported with t-PA.[42]

Patient Selection

The accepted indication for intravenous thrombolysis is chest pain suggestive of myocardial ischemia associated with acute ST segment elevation on 12-lead electrocardiogram (ECG) or a presumed new left bundle-branch block. The duration of symptoms or "window of opportunity" has been an issue of controversy. In the 1986 Gruppo Italiano per lo Studio della Streptochinasi nell'Infarcto Miocardico study,[33] patients who received SK 6 hours or more after the onset of symptoms had no improvement in mor-

---

DISPLAY 21-1

Recommendations for Administration of Thrombolytic Therapy in Acute Myocardial Infarction

Patients without contraindications to thrombolytic therapy:

CLASS I

1. Patients younger than 75 years of age presenting with ST elevation greater than 0.1 mV in two or more contiguous leads; time to therapy 12 hours or less.
2. Patients with bundle-branch block (obscuring ST segment analysis) and a history suggesting acute MI.

CLASS IIa

1. Patients older than 75 years of age presenting with ST elevation greater than 0.1 mV in two or more contiguous leads; time to therapy 12 hours or less.

CLASS IIb

1. Patients presenting with ST elevation greater than 0.1 mV in two or more contiguous leads; time to therapy greater than 12 to 24 hours.
2. Patients with blood pressure on presentation greater than 180 mm Hg systolic or greater than 110 mm Hg diastolic associated with high-risk MI.

CLASS III

1. Patient presenting with ST elevation; time to therapy greater than 24 hours and ischemic pain resolved.
2. Patients with ST segment depression only.

MI, myocardial infarction.
Adapted from Ryan T, Anderson J, Antman E, et al: ACC/AHA Task Force Report on Practice Guidelines: Management of acute myocardial infarction. J Am Coll Cardiol 28: 1328–428, 1996.

---

tality compared with patients who received placebo. In contrast, patients who received SK within 6 hours of symptom onset demonstrated reduced mortality compared with patients who received placebo, with the greatest mortality difference noted in patients treated within 1 hour of symptom onset. These findings were consistent with a general belief that there is a limited time before the myocardium supplied by the occluded artery suffers irreversible ischemic damage and that thrombolytic reperfusion is of no benefit after that time. Consequently, many thrombolytic trials and institutional protocols excluded patients who presented 4 to 6 hours or more after symptom onset. The ISIS-2 studies, however, which admitted patients up to 24 hours after symptom onset, demonstrated treatment benefit in patients presenting 6 to 24 hours after symptoms began.[41] Recommendations for patient selection are summarized in Display 21-1.

The original investigations of thrombolytic agents in acute MI excluded patients deemed at risk for bleeding,

DISPLAY 21-2

Contraindications and Cautions for Thrombolytic Use in Myocardial Infarction

CONTRAINDICATIONS

- Previous hemorrhagic stroke at any time; other strokes or cerebrovascular events within 1 year
- Known intracranial neoplasm
- Active internal bleeding (does not include menses)
- Suspected aortic dissection

CAUTIONS/RELATIVE CONTRAINDICATIONS

- Severe, uncontrolled hypertension on presentation (blood pressure >180/110 mm Hg)
- History of prior cerebrovascular accident or known intracerebral lesion not covered in contradictions
- Current use of anticoagulants in therapeutic doses (international normalized ratio >2–3); known bleeding diathesis
- Recent trauma (within 2–4 weeks), including head trauma or traumatic or prolonged (>10 minutes) cardiopulmonary resuscitation or major surgery (<3 weeks)
- Noncompressible vascular punctures
- Recent (within 2–4 weeks) internal bleeding
- For streptokinase/antistreplase: prior exposure (especially within 5 days to 2 years) or prior allergic reaction
- Pregnancy
- Active peptic ulcer
- History of chronic severe hypertension

Adapted from Ryan T, Anderson J, Antman E, et al: ACC/AHA Task Force Report on Practice Guidelines: Management of acute myocardial infarction. J Am Coll Cardiol 28: 1328–428, 1996.

including patients with previous cerebrovascular accident, patients with severe hypertension, patients who received cardiopulmonary resuscitation, and patients older than 75 years of age. Strict application of these contraindications excludes approximately 30% of patients from consideration for thrombolytic therapy despite proven mortality reduction.[72] Therefore, many of the contraindications have been challenged, particularly the upper age limit and hypertension. In general, the risk of uncontrollable bleeding is weighed against the potential benefit of thrombolytic therapy to the patient with acute MI. The established absolute and relative contraindications to the drugs are outlined in Display 21-2.

Patient Outcome

A number of mortality studies have evaluated the efficacy of thrombolysis for acute MI. Topol[72] performed a meta-analysis of trials comparing SK, t-PA, or APSAC to placebo and noted that the reported mortality risk reductions in the various studies overlap at 27%. In ISIS-3, patients were randomized to receive SK, double-chain t-PA, or APSAC with and without subcutaneous heparin to determine if one

thrombolytic agent offered a clear benefit in mortality reduction.[41] The mortality rates in the groups were 10.6%, 10.3%, and 10.5%, respectively. These differences were not statistically significant. The ISIS-3 trial has been criticized for not using continuous, monitored intravenous heparin therapy after thrombolysis, which may have introduced bias in favor of the nonselective agents SK and APSAC. The Global Utilization of SK and rt-PA in Occluded Coronary Arteries (GUSTO) trial randomized 41,021 patients to one of four treatment arms: accelerated-dose rt-PA plus intravenous heparin, SK plus intravenous heparin, SK plus subcutaneous heparin, or a combination of rt-PA, SK, and intravenous heparin.[33] The 30-day mortality rate of the accelerated rt-PA group was 6.3%, compared with 7.2% for the SK plus subcutaneous heparin group ($P = 0.009$), 7.4% for the SK plus intravenous heparin group ($P = 0.003$), and 7% for the rt-PA plus SK plus intravenous heparin group ($P = 0.04$). This was a significant reduction in mortality with the accelerated-dose rt-PA, suggesting rapid and complete reperfusion improves overall outcome and survival.

Bleeding is the most serious complication from thrombolytic therapy and relates to the dissolution of protective vascular thrombi as well as the delayed blood coagulation from circulating fibrin(ogen) degradation products and heparin. Most commonly, bleeding occurs at vascular access sites. In one study of 20,768 patients receiving SK or t-PA with or without subcutaneous heparin, major bleeds (bleeding requiring transfusion of 2 U or more) occurred in approximately 0.8% of patients. Hemorrhagic stroke occurred in approximately 0.4%.[40] Hemorrhagic stroke was more common in patients receiving t-PA than in patients receiving either SK or APSAC in the ISIS-3 trial (0.66% vs. 0.24% vs. 0.55% in ISIS-3).[42] In the GUSTO trial, clinically important bleeding (bleeding requiring transfusion, intracerebral bleeding, or bleeding causing hemodynamic compromise) occurred in 5.4% to 6.8% of patients. Hemorrhagic stroke was significantly more common in the accelerated t-PA plus heparin group compared with both SK groups (0.72% accelerated t-PA plus heparin, 0.49% SK plus subcutaneous heparin, 0.54% SK plus intravenous heparin; $P = 0.03$). The combined t-PA, SK, and intravenous heparin group had the highest overall rate of hemorrhagic stroke at 0.94%.[33]

Because most patients presenting with acute MI have a coronary stenosis with underlying thrombosis and ongoing stimulus to form clot, reocclusion is a risk and occurs in approximately 12% to 29% of patients, depending on the timing of follow-up angiography.[1,53] Reinfarction due to reocclusion was reported to occur in 2.9% to 3.6% of patients in the ISIS-3 trial.[42]

The Thrombolysis and Angioplasty in Myocardial Infarction study demonstrated no benefit in immediate angioplasty after successful thrombolysis compared with a more conservative approach of delayed elective angioplasty.[73] However, rescue angioplasty for failed thrombolysis may prove a beneficial strategy. Unfortunately, no reliable noninvasive means of early determination of thrombolytic success has been established. The clinical events of relief of chest pain and resolution of ST segment elevations and arrhythmia were noted to occur with reperfusion, but lack adequate predictive value.[12] Early peaking of the plasma level of the myocardial band of creatine kinase (CK-MB) is associated with reperfusion.[56]

Selection of a thrombolytic agent is based on its adverse effects as well as its efficacy. The t-PA type of thrombolytic has a more rapid rate of reperfusion but a higher frequency of hemorrhagic stroke compared with SK. The 10-fold cost of t-PA over SK must be considered. The dose regimens may also factor into selection choice because simplicity of dosing would be a consideration for administration by emergency medical personnel.

Prethrombolysis and Post-thrombolysis Management

The prevailing goal when treating a patient with acute MI is to attempt rapid reperfusion by the best means available. To this end, most institutions have developed protocols, checklists, or standing orders to facilitate patient selection and reduce delays in thrombolytic treatment.[19] At minimum, institutions must (1) establish patient selection criteria; (2) delineate the medical staff responsible for the decision to administer a thrombolytic agent; (3) determine which agent or agents will be available in the institution; (4) determine where thrombolytic drugs will be stored; (5) delineate responsibility for mixing, delivering, and administering the drug; and (6) establish the parameters of monitoring and intervention during and after thrombolytic administration. General aspects of care common to most patients receiving thrombolytic therapy for acute MI are discussed further.

Before thrombolysis, a brief, focused history and physical examination are necessary to establish the presence of any absolute or relative contraindications to thrombolytic therapy (see Display 21-2) and to determine the characteristics and duration of symptoms. A 12-lead ECG is obtained. ECG criteria indicative of acute myocardial injury include greater than 0.1 mV of ST segment elevation in two or more contiguous leads, new or presumed new left bundle-branch block, or ST segment depression with a prominent R wave in precordial leads V_2 and V_3 if thought to be indicative of posterior infarction.[6] Sublingual nitroglycerin may be administered to rule out myocardial ischemia primarily due to spasm. Baseline laboratory tests are obtained, including complete blood count, chemistry profile, aPTT, cardiac enzymes, and type and crossmatch (patient specific). The treatment is explained to the patient, and thrombolytics are administered as prescribed. Chewable aspirin (acetylsalicylic acid [ASA]), 160 or 325 mg, is given with the thrombolytic drug and continued on a daily basis. Continuous intravenous heparin is initiated during or after infusion of the thrombolytic agent and adjusted to maintain a therapeutic aPTT. Additional therapies such as intravenous nitroglycerin, lidocaine, atropine, morphine sulfate, and β-adrenergic blocking agents may be given as described in Chapter 20. Continuous ECG monitoring in a lead appropriate for identification of ongoing cardiac ischemia and arrhythmia detection aids in monitoring response to thrombolysis as well as identification of reocclusion.

INTERVENTIONAL DEVICES

The expansion of interventional cardiology devices has provided multiple treatment options for patients with CHD, including percutaneous transluminal coronary angioplasty (PTCA), atherectomy, intracoronary stents, and laser angioplasty. Percutaneous interventions have increased in frequency because of advanced technology, minimal invasiveness, increased success rates, and decreased complications. Intracoronary stenting has become the most frequently used procedure because of the superior final results and clinical evidence of reductions in abrupt closure and long-term restenosis.

Percutaneous Transluminal Coronary Angioplasty

The technique of PTCA was initially applied to human coronary arteries in late 1977 by Andreas Gruentzig.

PATHOPHYSIOLOGY

The desired therapeutic effect of balloon angioplasty is the enlargement of the internal luminal diameter of the treated coronary vessel. Balloon pressure to an area of atherosclerotic stenosis results in plaque rupture, disruption of endothelium, and stretching of unaffected vessel segments, thus enlarging the lumen.

PATIENT SELECTION

The decision to perform PTCA in a patient with atherosclerotic coronary disease is based on an assessment of the potential benefit compared with the associated risks. PTCA risks are determined by technical and clinical factors. Technical risks based on lesion characteristics as assessed by angiography are delineated in Display 21-3. Improvements in angioplasty technologies continue to alter risk statistics related to lesion morphology and location. Clinical risks include age older than 65 years, female sex, unstable angina, congestive heart failure, and chronic renal failure. Angiographic risk factors include three-vessel disease, left main coronary artery disease or left main equivalent (severe stenosis of the left anterior descending and circumflex arteries proximal to any major branches), ejection fraction less than 30%, high percentage of myocardium at risk, proximal right coronary stenosis, and collaterals originating from dilated vessel.[5]

PROCEDURE

Percutaneous transluminal coronary angioplasty may be performed at the time of the initial diagnostic cardiac catheterization, electively at some time after catheterization, or urgently in the setting of acute MI. In all circumstances, an initial complete cardiac catheterization is performed as described in Chapter 18.

Percutaneous transluminal coronary angioplasty is performed by the cardiologist in the cardiac catheterization laboratory. A sheath is inserted into the femoral, brachial, or radial artery and a guide catheter is passed through the sheath into the coronary artery. A balloon system (guide wire and angioplasty balloon) is passed through the guide catheter and positioned across the lesion. Multiple balloon inflations of variable pressure and duration are used to achieve at least 20% improvement in the diameter and residual narrowing of less than 50% of the arterial segment (Fig. 21-1). Balloon inflation results in occlusion of the coronary artery and ischemia of the subtended myocardium. Some patients may require temporary transvenous pacing, intra-aortic balloon counterpulsation, or femorofemoral cardiopulmonary bypass circulatory support during PTCA.

PATIENT OUTCOME

The immediate success rate for PTCA performed by an experienced interventional cardiologist with proper patient selection is greater than 90%.[46] Major acute complications associated with PTCA include abrupt closure, MI, emergency coronary artery bypass graft (CABG) surgery, and death. The patient is also at risk for all complications associated with cardiac catheterization.

Trauma to the vessel during PTCA may trigger abrupt closure due to thrombus formation, obstruction from intimal or medial flaps, or elastic recoil of the media, with most incidents occurring in the catheterization laboratory. Sequelae to abrupt closure included MI, emergency CABG, and death.[29]

Restenosis is a clinical and angiographic syndrome resulting from a combination of elastic recoil and neointimal hyperplasia. Restenosis is a response to arterial injury incurred during revascularization. The physiologic process of repairing intracoronary injury involves multiple steps. The healing process appears to be initiated by platelet deposition along the subendothelial surface, which releases other agonists—adenosine diphosphate, serotonin, thromboxane A_2, and platelet-derived growth factor—that stimulate further platelet aggregation. Smooth muscle cell migration and proliferation occur at the injury site, causing neointimal hyperplasia. Some coronary artery injuries from PTCA heal with minimal neointima, whereas others heal with prolific neointima, resulting in restenosis.

The Multi-Hospital Eastern Atlantic Restenosis Trial investigators observed an overall restenosis rate of 39.6%, noting that restenosis rate varied markedly depending on lesion location, lesion length, percentage of stenosis existing before and after angioplasty, and arterial diameter.[37] The reported incidence of restenosis varies depending on the definition used, the method of measurement, and the timing and completeness of angiographic follow-up.[24]

PREPROCEDURE AND POSTPROCEDURE MANAGEMENT

Percutaneous transluminal coronary angioplasty is primarily performed electively as an alternative to medical or surgical management of symptomatic CHD, but may also be done urgently in the setting of acute MI or unstable angina. Before the procedure, the patient must give informed consent to PTCA. Consent for CABG is usually obtained provisionally at the same time. Elective PTCA patients receive antiplatelet therapy, commonly ASA, the day before and the day of the procedure. Patients treated urgently receive ASA before the procedure. Other preprocedure medical therapy depends on individual patient needs.

During PTCA, nitroglycerin is frequently administered into the coronary artery to dilate the artery and prevent reactive spasm after balloon inflation. If acute thrombus is also present, a glycoprotein (GP) IIb/IIIa inhibitor (see section on Antiplatelet Therapy) or intracoronary thrombolytic agent may be given. Anticoagulation with intravenous heparin is maintained throughout the PTCA procedure to prevent thrombus formation on angioplasty catheters and wires, and at areas of vascular damage due to balloon inflations.

After the procedure, the patient is monitored for manifestations of myocardial ischemia such as chest pain, ECG changes, arrhythmias, or hemodynamic instability. A 12-lead ECG is usually obtained to establish a baseline for

CORONARY ANGIOPLASTY

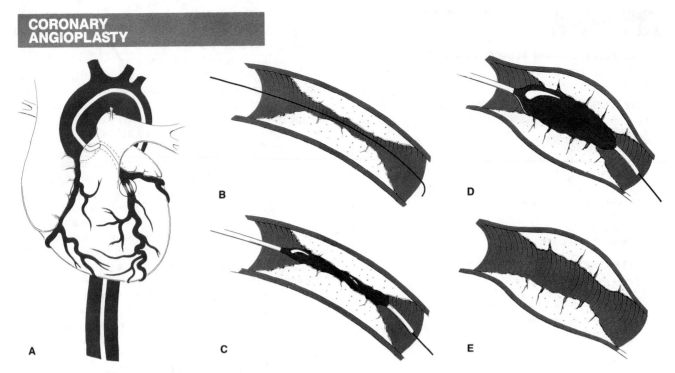

FIGURE 21-1 Mechanism of intracoronary balloon angioplasty. **(A)** A balloon catheter is introduced into the coronary artery through a guide catheter in the aorta. **(B)** A guide wire is advanced across the area of narrowing. **(C)** The balloon catheter is advanced over the wire across the lesion. **(D)** The balloon is inflated. **(E)** Coronary artery after dilation. (Courtesy of Boston Scientific Corporation, Maple Grove, MN.)

further comparison. Patients experiencing prolonged angina during PTCA are evaluated for acute MI with serial cardiac enzyme determinations and ECGs. Patients may be relatively volume depleted after PTCA because of NPO status, radiographic contrast-induced diuresis, and the effects of vasodilating drugs. Hydration is maintained through intravenous fluids until oral intake is sufficient to meet the patient's requirements.

Heparin anticoagulation is routinely discontinued after PTCA for sheath removal. GP IIb/IIIa inhibitors are continued per protocol. Heparin is restarted in patients considered to be at high risk for acute thrombus formation. ASA is continued in the acute postprocedure period and indefinitely. Nitrates and calcium channel blocking agents may be continued for 24 to 48 hours after PTCA to prevent arterial spasm. These agents may be empirically continued after discharge, although long-term benefits have not been demonstrated.

The site of vascular access is monitored for complications such as bleeding or hematoma formation. Distal limb perfusion is also monitored through frequent evaluation of pulses, skin and nail bed color, and sensation. Vascular sheaths are removed as soon as possible after the discontinuation of heparin therapy. Sheath management and removal are guided by institutional protocols.

LIMITATIONS

Despite the advances in PTCA technique and technology, with increased immediate success rates of 90% to 95%, there are still limitations to treatment. The following major limitations have prompted the development of alternative interventional devices to treat coronary lesions:

1. Abrupt closure, occurring in up to 7.3% of patients[21]
2. Restenosis, defined as a loss of more than 50% of the initial improvement in the cross-sectional diameter of the coronary lumen occurring over a period of 3 to 6 months
3. Anatomically unsuitable angioplasty lesions or lesions that carry a high risk of dissection or restenosis, such as eccentric lesions, tandem lesions, ostial lesions, and lesions at bifurcations or on a bend, which are difficult to approach with angioplasty catheters[5] (see Display 21-3)
4. Chronic total occlusions that are difficult to cross reliably with a wire and have reported restenosis rates of greater than 45%[74]
5. Unsatisfactory results in patients with prior CABG surgery or saphenous vein graft (SVG) lesions, with restenosis rates of 45% to 58%, depending on location[52]

Coronary Atherectomy

The atherectomy catheters reduce the severity of coronary stenoses by removing the atheromatous plaque rather than compressing or fracturing the plaque or stretching the arterial wall. In theory, this approach permits a more controlled vascular injury and minimizes the degree of

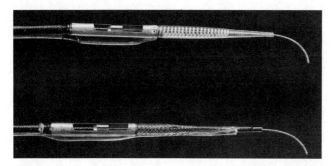

FIGURE 21-2 Directional coronary atherectomy catheters: Simpson Coronary AtheroCaths. (Courtesy of Guidant/ Advanced Cardiovascular Systems, Santa Clara, CA.)

arterial mural stretch. Removal of plaque creates a smoother surface by debulking the vessel and removes atherosclerotic plaque that is frequently resistant to balloon dilatation.

DIRECTIONAL CORONARY ATHERECTOMY

The directional coronary atherectomy (DCA) catheter, or Simpson AtheroCath (Guidant/Advanced Cardiovascular Systems, Santa Clara, CA), consists of a catheter-mounted, cylindric metallic housing unit (i.e., collection chamber, window, and cup-shaped cutter) and a small balloon attached to the housing (Fig. 21-2). A hand-held motor-drive unit is attached to the proximal end of the catheter, and the cutter in the housing is rotated at 2,000 rpm through the driving cable.[39] When this catheter is placed at the stenotic lesion, a balloon is inflated at low pressure against one wall of the vessel to stabilize the housing chamber and the window against the opposite vessel wall of atherosclerotic plaque. Plaque that protrudes into the housing unit through the window is then excised with the rotating cutter, which is advanced manually. The device is then rotated and plaque is excised from around the vessel lumen. The material removed from coronary lesions during DCA procedures has been used histologically to study the obstructive and stenotic tissue matrix and enhance research on restenosis.

In September 1990, the U.S. Food and Drug Administration (FDA) approved the use of DCA for treatment of patients with discrete subtotal stenoses in native vessels or SVGs. DCA is indicated for lesions with calcification or thrombus, and those at the ostium of the vessel. To assess the benefit of DCA relative to PTCA, a randomized trial was undertaken involving 35 sites from the United States, Germany, The Netherlands, and Belgium. The Coronary Angioplasty Versus Excisional Atherectomy Trial (CAVEAT) failed to show restenosis benefit over PTCA.[15] The optimal DCA technique evaluated in the Balloon Versus Optimal Atherectomy Trial (BOAT) showed higher success rates, and removal of coronary artery plaque with DCA led to a larger postprocedure luminal diameter. The larger lumen postprocedure lowered restenosis rates to 32% for DCA. However, with more aggressive plaque removal, there was increased evidence of MI and a moderate increase in CK-MB with DCA.[7]

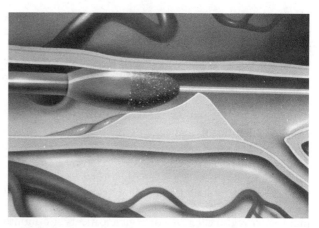

FIGURE 21-3 Rotational ablation catheter. The diamond-coated tip preferentially ablates inelastic plaque. (Courtesy fo SCIMED/ Boston Scientific Corporation, Maple Grove, MN.)

ROTATIONAL ABLATION

The rotational atherectomy device (Rotablator) was developed by David Auth (SCIMED/Boston Scientific, Maple Grove, MN) and approved for clinical use in 1993. The Rotablator is a flexible catheter-deliverable system that can be used transluminally. The Rotablator system uses a high-speed, rotating, elliptical bur coated with diamond chips 20 to 30 μm in diameter that form an abrasive surface (Fig. 21-3). When the bur is spun at a high speed (140,000 to 180,000 rpm, depending on bur size), it preferentially removes atheroma because of its selective differential cutting of inelastic plaque rather than elastic normal tissue. The process involves a stepwise incremental increase in bur size to provide a "sanding effect" (Fig. 21-4). Gradual advancement and withdrawal of the bur in 2- to 5-second intervals for up to 20 to 30 seconds in the lesion allows for heat dissipation, improved distal perfusion, and washout of particulate debris. The postablation vessel diameter is equal to the largest bur size used. Adjunctive PTCA is frequently used to maximize final coronary artery luminal diameter or stent placement.

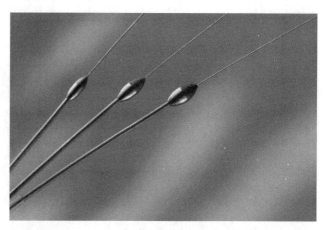

FIGURE 21-4 Rotational ablation catheters in different sizes. (Courtesy of SCIMED/Boston Scientific Corporation, Maple Grove, MN.)

The debris emitted from the Rotablator ablation process is released into the coronary bloodstream as pulverized microparticles. Results of *in vitro* analysis of the debris produced during ablation indicated that 90% of particles were smaller than 8 to 12 μm, a size suitable to traverse the capillary bed without causing significant vascular occlusions.[90] Vascular tracking of arterially injected, technetium 99m-labeled atherectomized microparticles into the femoral arteries of dogs indicated passage through the peripheral microcirculation and subsequent uptake by the reticuloendothelial system of the lungs, spleen, and liver.[3]

Diabetic patients, lesion length greater than 10 mm, and eccentricity of lesion morphology increased the risk of a major complication. The restenosis rate reported from the multicenter registry for 78% of eligible patients at 6-month follow-up was 39%.[10]

Rotational atherectomy has been shown to be particularly effective in the treatment of calcified coronary lesions by ablating the fibrocalcific plaque, which is difficult to dilate with an angioplasty balloon.[38,71] To maximize luminal diameter, stent implantation is used adjunctively after ablation. Rotational ablation has also been used for in-stent restenosis.

TRANSLUMINAL EXTRACTION ATHERECTOMY

The transluminal extraction catheter (TEC) was developed by Interventional Technologies, Inc. (San Diego, CA) and approved for clinical use in 1993. The device consists of a motorized, rotating, hollow catheter equipped with a distal cone-shaped head. The cutting head is mounted on a flexible torque tube, which incorporates a vacuum system that allows retrieval of the excised material. As the cone is rotated at 750 rpm, continuous suction is applied at the proximal end of the catheter, thereby removing the atheromatous debris, which is flushed with saline through the central lumen of the drive shaft and collected in a vacuum bottle[80,67,78] (Fig. 21-5).

The TEC catheter produces a lumen size as large as its nominal size. Adjunctive PTCA and stent placement are used frequently to increase luminal diameter. Lesions previously identified as high risk for PTCA that responded favorably to the TEC device included native coronaries and SVGs with intraluminal thrombus.[54,66] A randomized trial, TEC or PTCA in Thrombus (TOPIT), indicated a decreased risk of postprocedure CK-MB elevation with TEC procedures of

native coronaries in acute coronary syndromes.[45] Degenerated SVG lesions with angiographically apparent thrombus had a lower incidence of distal embolization with TEC than with PTCA. The overall restenosis rate is approximately 45% for patients undergoing TEC.[66]

COMPLICATIONS ASSOCIATED WITH ATHERECTOMY

Vascular spasm at the site or distal to the treated site is a potential cause of acute ischemia during or after treatment with rotablator. It may occur at the treated site, in the proximal vessel secondary to guide catheter-related injury, or in the distal vessels. It can be attributed to high-speed rotation of the rotablator device and vibrations transmitted to the guide wire. Vascular spasm is usually transient and relieved with intracoronary nitroglycerin or a low-pressure balloon. When using a rotational atherectomy device, waiting between ablations frequently allows full reversal of spasm and debris clearance. Vessel spasm after the procedure potentially causes a recurrence of chest discomfort. If it is spasm, it usually is relieved rapidly by an increase in nitroglycerin or calcium channel blocker. Intravenous fluids are frequently required to maintain an adequate blood pressure during an episode of vascular spasm. Patients are occasionally maintained on a nitroglycerin drip for 12 to 24 hours for its vasodilatory effects. Calcium channel blockers may be continued after the procedure to prevent vasospasmodic activity.[20]

Myocardial necrosis represented by an elevation in CK-MB occurs in approximately 6% to 26% of patients after percutaneous intervention. The most common causes for elevated enzymes after procedures include minor branch occlusion, evidence of thrombus, intimal dissection, coronary spasm, and distal embolization. Distal embolization is more common in patients with an acute ischemic syndrome and those undergoing percutaneous interventions in SVGs.[4] Patients with CK-MB elevations of threefold or more after percutaneous intervention should be treated as per MI protocol.[11] Elevated enzymes are associated with a higher risk of death, subsequent MI, and a need for repeat revascularization procedures. An ECG should be obtained before and after the preprocedure, and routine measurement of CK and CK-MB are recommended. Administration of GP IIb/IIIa inhibitors during interventional procedures reduces myocardial necrosis by preventing platelet aggregation or thrombosis formation.[26,27]

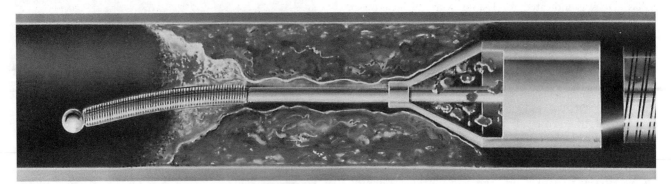

FIGURE 21-5 Distal end of the Transluminal Extraction Catheter (TEC) coaxially placed over the TEC guide wire. (Courtesy of InterVentional Technologies, Inc., San Diego, CA.)

An infrequent but devastating complication of atherectomy devices is vessel perforation. Perforation may occur because of deep cuts by the atherectomy catheter into the normal segment of the vessel wall, extending into the adventitia. Perforation has also been seen with rotational atherectomy in lesions that are eccentric, tortuous, and longer than 10 mm. Angiographic evidence of perforation is rare, occurring in 0.5% of cases.[36] Management of coronary perforation includes reversal of anticoagulation, preferably by discontinuation of heparin. If this is not adequate, protamine may be given. Balloon inflation should be performed as soon as perforation is recognized to occlude the leak, prevent further extravasation, and attempt to self-seal the defect. Patients who have limited pericardial blood can be managed conservatively. Cardiac tamponade may occur if there is significant leakage into the pericardial space, requiring pericardiocentesis. Active bleeding from the artery requires emergent CABG surgery.

Groin complications and the potential for bleeding are increased because of the increased size of the vascular sheaths (8 to 10 Fr) needed to accommodate the atherectomy devices. Groin care is discussed in the section on Patient Care Issues.

Coronary Laser Angioplasty

The concept of applying laser energy to remove, in a percutaneous manner, atherosclerotic coronary obstructions first emerged in the early 1980s. The Advanced Interventional Systems excimer laser angioplasty technology received FDA premarket approval for selected application in coronary arteries in January 1992. In theory, laser treatment removes or debulks the fibrous inner cap of the atherosclerotic lesion, resulting in softer, more pliable lesions that yield to the forces of balloon expansion.[49]

Laser energy is delivered over a small fraction of the lasing cycle, with heat dissipating between pulses. The excimer laser energy is absorbed by atherosclerotic plaque, creates precise ablation without thermal injury, and can ablate calcified plaque.

Laser angioplasty has been used for treatment of total occlusions and in-stent restenosis. The most important complication with laser ablation involves minor or major coronary dissection of treated lesions. Limitations to laser use include the expense of the units and a high rate of restenosis (>40%).[47,49]

Coronary Stents

The concept of stenting an injured vessel was first demonstrated by Dotter in 1969.[7] In 1986, percutaneous implantation of metallic stents in coronary vessels was first reported in humans by Sigwart and coworkers[64] with the Wallstent. The development of intravascular stents was initiated to provide structural support to an artery opposing elastic recoil, to prevent vasoconstriction, and to prevent or treat dissections of the arterial wall. The success of a vascular stent depends on minimal thrombosis and rapid endothelialization.[60] The initial stent trials were hindered by a high rate of subacute stent thrombosis, embolization of stents, and difficulty in placement.

The first stent approved by the FDA for clinical use was the Gianturco-Roubin Flex-Stent in June 1993 for acute and threatened closure of coronary arteries, reducing the incidence of emergent CABG surgery associated with PTCA.[57] The Gianturco-Roubin coronary stent (Cook, Inc., Bloomington, IN) is balloon expandable and consists of surgical stainless steel that is 0.006″ thick and wrapped cylindrically, with bends that make an inverted "U" configuration every 360 degrees (Fig. 21-6).

The Palmaz-Schatz coronary stent was approved in 1994. The original stent design, developed by Palmaz, consists of a single, rigid, slotted, stainless steel tube. This design was modified by Schatz for use in coronary arteries (Palmaz-Schatz Stent, Cordis/Johnson & Johnson, Warren, NJ) and consists of two 7-mm tubes connected by a central bridging 1-mm strut (Fig. 21-7). The stent fits over an angioplasty balloon for deployment. When the balloon is inflated, the struts of the stent take on a diamond configuration, with a high open space-to-metal ratio. The articulation point of the stent imparts longitudinal flexibility, which enhances passage.[58,63]

STENT CLINICAL TRIALS

Two landmark trials that empowered the stent revolution were randomized trials comparing the Palmaz-Schatz Stent with PTCA. The Stent Restenosis Trial (STRESS) found that patients with an intracoronary stent in a *de novo* lesion had a higher procedural success rate and a less frequent need for revascularization. The angiographic restenosis rate was 31.6% for stents and 42.1% for PTCA, with similar rates of clinical events after 6 months.[31] In the Belgium Netherlands Stent Trial (Benestent), over a 7-month follow-up, clinical and angiographic outcomes were better in patients who received a stent rather than PTCA, with restenosis rates of 22% for stents and 32% for PTCA.[72] However, this benefit was achieved at the cost of a significantly higher risk of vascular bleeding complications and a longer hospital stay.[31,72] An aggressive regimen of adjunctive pharmacologic agents was used during these trials and during the initial experience of stenting, including ASA, dipyridamole, coumarin drugs, heparin, and dextran.[14] Two major advances that influenced the evolution of stenting and procedural and postprocedural treatment are intravascular ultrasound (IVUS) and antiplatelet therapy.

Intravascular Ultrasound. Intravascular ultrasound imaging provides a detailed cross-sectional image of the vessel

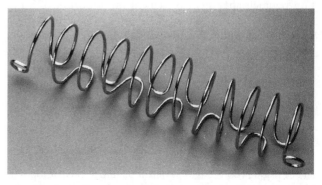

FIGURE 21-6 The Gianturco-Roubin Flex-Stent. (Courtesy of Cook, Inc., Bloomington, IN.)

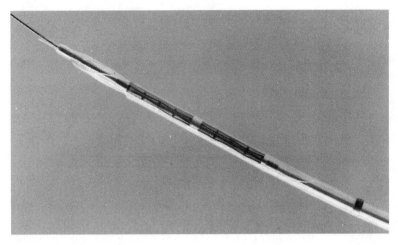

FIGURE 21-7 The Palmaz-Schatz stent. (Courtesy of Cordis Endovascular Systems, Warren, NJ.)

wall. This method of direct visualization of the arterial wall lesion at the site of a planned intervention has improved clinical and angiographic outcomes. A miniaturized ultrasound transducer is placed on the distal end of a flexible catheter and advanced down the coronary artery. IVUS can be used during cardiac catheterization to evaluate plaque and tissue characteristics and during interventional procedures to verify adequate results and stent deployment. Colombo and associates[17] recognized with the use of IVUS that stent deployment techniques were inadequate and that the stents frequently were not completely expanded in the vessel, contributing to subacute closure. As a result of these findings, the use of high-pressure balloon dilatation after stent deployment to ensure full stent expansion was instituted. This had a significant effect on stenting practices and decreased thrombotic complications (Fig. 21-8).

Antiplatelet Therapy. As stenting techniques improved with the use of IVUS, the need for aggressive anticoagulation to prevent abrupt closure was reduced. The Intracoronary Stenting and Antithrombotic Regimen trial compared the outcomes of two different antithrombotic regimens after placement of coronary stents. The combined antiplatelet therapy with ticopidine plus ASA was superior to therapy with heparin, warfarin, and ASA in reducing cardiac events and hemorrhagic and vascular complications after stenting. This change in therapy decreased length of stay and cost of hospitalization.[59] Antiplatelet therapy is continued for 4 weeks after stenting. The current medication regimen after stent placement includes ASA 325 mg daily or bid and ticopidine 250 mg bid for 1 month. Side effects of ticopidine include allergy, rash, gastrointestinal upset, and neutropenia. A complete blood count with differential should be done at 10 days after starting Ticopidine to rule out neutropenia. Patients who are allergic to or intolerant of ticopidine are prescribed clopidogrel 75 mg daily for 1 month in addition to ASA.

GLYCOPROTEIN IIB/IIIA RECEPTOR INHIBITORS. The GP IIb/IIIa receptor inhibitors are a new class of drugs used in interventional cardiology. Platelet aggregation at the site of plaque rupture is a dominant feature in the pathophysiology of unstable angina, MI, and associated treatment with PTCA and interventional procedures. The final common pathway to platelet aggregation and coronary thrombus involves the activation of the platelet GP IIb/IIIa receptor. After platelet activation, GP IIb/IIIa becomes a receptor for fibrinogen and von Willebrand factor. There are three GP IIb/IIIa receptor inhibitors available for intravenous use to block platelet aggregation: abciximab, tirofiban, and eptifibatide.

Abciximab (Reopro), the first agent approved for use by the FDA, is an antigen-binding fragment of the chimeric human-murine monoclonal antibody 7E3. Intravenous administration of abciximab as a 0.25 mg/kg bolus followed by a 10 μg/kg/min infusion for 12 hours produces sustained GP IIb/IIIa receptor blockade (>80%) and inhibition of platelets for the duration of the infusion. Low levels of GP IIb/IIIa receptor blockade are present for more than 10 days after cessation of the infusion. Complications associated with administration include bleeding, thrombocytopenia, intracranial hemorrhage, and allergic reactions. Platelet infusion may be needed in excess bleeding or for urgent surgery.[1]

The first trial to demonstrate conclusively that GP IIb/IIIa receptor blockade can prevent ischemic events in high-risk patients undergoing percutaneous intervention was the Evaluation of 7E3 for the Prevention of Ischemic Complications (EPIC) trial.[26] Abciximab bolus plus a 12-hour infusion was found to reduce the risk of death, MI, or need for urgent repeat revascularization, and this benefit was maintained for 3 years of follow-up. All patients received ASA and intravenous, non–weight-based heparin. This therapeutic benefit was achieved at the cost of a significant increase in major bleeding complications (10.6% for abciximab vs. 3.3% for placebo).

The second trial, platelet glycoprotein IIb/IIIa receptor blockade and low-dose heparin during percutaneous coronary revascularization. (EPILOG) confirmed the clinical benefits of abciximab in all patients undergoing percutaneous interventions. This study introduced procedural changes at the time of intervention, including the use of low-dose, weight-adjusted heparin regimens and abciximab infusion doses, elimination of postprocedural heparin infusions, early femoral sheath removal, and careful patient and access site management. The changes in therapy reduced the rate of major bleeding complications to 1.1%.[27] The first randomized, placebo-controlled trial of abciximab before and during coronary intervention in refractory unstable angina (CAPTURE) found that treatment during the 24 hours before PTCA reduces preprocedural and periprocedural events.[13] This trial expanded the use of GP IIb/IIIa receptor inhibitors.

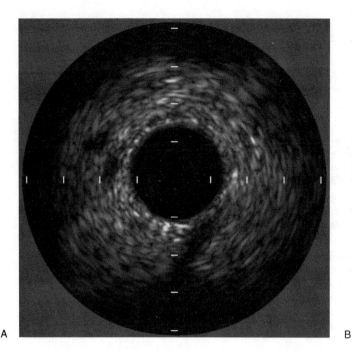

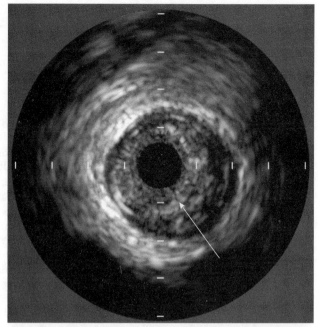

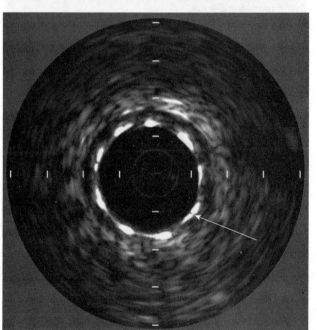

FIGURE 21-8 Intravascular ultrasound: **(A)** Normal coronary artery, **(B)** Concentric atherosclerotic plaque inside coronary artery, **(C)** Cornary artery after stent placement. *Arrow* indicates stent struts. (Courtesy of ENDOSONICS Corporation, Rancho Cordova, CA.)

Tirofiban (Aggrastat) is a nonpeptide mimetic antagonist of the GP IIb/IIIa receptor. The Patients Limited by Unstable Signs and Symptoms (PRISM-PLUS) trial indicated that tirofiban in combination with heparin and ASA was associated with a lower incidence of ischemic events in patients with acute coronary syndromes.[56]

Eptifibatide (Integrilin) is a cyclic heptapeptide inhibitor of the GP IIb/IIIa receptor. The Platelet IIb/IIIa in Unstable Angina: Receptor Suppression Using Integrilin Therapy (PURSUIT) trial evaluated the effects of eptifibatide bolus plus infusion in unstable angina/non–Q-wave MI.[34] Compared with placebo, eptifibatide reduced the incidence of death and MI early during treatment (30 days).

The nonpeptide and peptide synthetic compounds have the advantage of a short half-life, rapid onset of action, and return of normal platelet function in 2 to 4 hours. This provides reversal of platelet function in the event of emergency surgery or significant bleeding. The disadvantage is a shorter inhibition of platelet aggregation.

STENT TECHNOLOGY

Stent technology has improved, leading to better stent designs and the availability of multiple products. The optimal stent should be easily and safely deliverable to various locations in coronary arteries. It should be flexible, low

TABLE 21-1	Balloon-Expandable Stents					
				Stent-Specific Issues		
Stent	**Design**	**Metal**	**Manufacturer**	Radiopaque	Deliverability	Radial Strength
Gianturco-Roubin	Coil	Stainless steel	Cook, Inc.	+	+++	+
Gianturco-Roubin II	Coil	Stainless steel	Cook, Inc.	+	+++	+
Palmaz-Schatz (PS153)	Slotted tube	Stainless steel	Cordis/Johnson & Johnson†	+	++	+++
Crown	Slotted tube	Stainless steel	Cordis/Johnson & Johnson	++	+	++++
Micro-Stent II	Coil	Stainless steel	Arterial Vascular Engineering‡	++	+++	++
GFX-Micro II	Multicellular	Stainless steel	Arterial Vascular Engineering	+++	++++	++
NIR	Multicellular	Stainless steel	SCIMED/Boston Scientific§	++	++++	+++
Multilink	Multicellular	Stainless steel	Guidant/Advanced Cardiovascular Systems‖	++	+++	+++
Wiktor	Coil	Tantalum	Medtronic¶/Minn, MN	++++	++	+
Self-Expanding Stents						
Magic Wallstent	Slotted tube	Cobalt alloy/ platinum	SCIMED/Boston Scientific	++	++	+++
Radius	Slotted tube	Nitinol	SCIMED/Boston Scientific	+++	+++	++

+Bloomington, IN
†Warren, NJ
‡Santa Rosa, CA
§Maple Grove, MN
‖Santa Clara, CA

profile, radiopaque, smooth contoured, of sufficient radial strength, and tissue and blood compatible. Materials used for stents include stainless steel, tantalum, and nitinol, each of which has its own properties (Table 21-1). Stent categories and commonly used stents are discussed in the following sections; this is only a sampling of the stents currently available (Figs. 21-9 and 21-10).

Balloon-Expandable Stents. Balloon-expandable coil stents are more flexible by design. Open spaces in the coils allow for accessibility to treat a side branch adjacent to the target lesion. Coil development has improved since the Gianturco-Roubin Flex-Stent. The second-generation Gianturco-Roubin II has a backbone structure to prevent stent deformity. The disadvantages of the coil stent are less radial strength, smaller postdeployment luminal diameter, and plaque herniation between coils, which has been implicated in stent restenosis.

Balloon-expandable tubular or multicellular stents provide more radial strength and cover the lesion with more metal. The Palmaz-Schatz stent (PS153) was designed with an articulation joint to provide flexibility. This articulation joint was a site of plaque herniation and a common site of restenosis. The next generation of stents has improved design features with improved technology.

Self-Expanding Stents. Self-expanding stents are able to expand without balloon dilatation. The stents are covered by a retaining sheath that, when removed, allows the stent to expand. The protective membrane covering the stent allows passage through tortuous segments of preformed catheters and the coronary vasculature.[70] Once at the site of the coronary stenosis, the retaining sheath is gradually removed, allowing the stent to expand fully, and its residual elastic force dilates the artery. Dilatation continues until an equilibrium is reached between the circumferential elastic resistance of the vessel and the dilating force of the stent. To achieve optimal coronary dilatation, balloon expansion of the device is commonly performed.[62] The Radius Stent is a self-expanding system approved by the FDA in 1998. This stent system deploys without high pressure and trauma. It is made of nitinol alloy, which conforms to the vessel curvature (Fig. 21-11).

COMPLICATIONS ASSOCIATED WITH STENTS

Thrombotic occlusion of stents is a major and potentially life-threatening complication that can occur with all stents regardless of design or composition. Stenting activates expression of the GP IIb/IIIa receptor on the platelet sur-

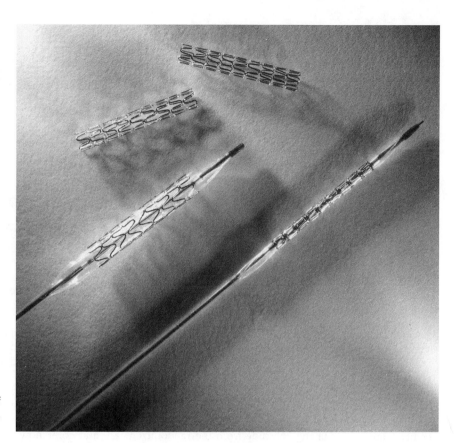

FIGURE 21-9 The GFX stent. (Courtesy of Arterial Vascular Engineering, Santa Rosa, CA.)

face and predisposes to subacute thrombosis. This mechanism can lead to death or MI and occurs in 1% to 3% of patients 7 to 10 days after stent implantation. Improved stent deployment, IVUS, and antiplatelet medications have decreased the incidence. The Evaluation of IIb/IIIa Platelet Inhibitor for Stenting (EPISTENT) trial found reduced incidence of death, MI, or urgent intervention when abciximab is used with stenting.[28]

In-stent restenosis is another problem associated with the use of stents.[25] Treatment options include PTCA, rotational ablation, and laser angioplasty.[69]

PATIENT CARE ISSUES

Vascular Sheaths. Sheath removal, mobilization, and ambulation protocols vary according to the device protocol and different management strategies as mandated by hospital policy. In general, the sheaths are removed 4 to 6 hours after the procedure, when the activated clotting time falls to less than 150 to 180 seconds. Pressure is applied for at least 20 minutes or longer, as warranted, with strict attention to distal circulation. Pressure devices (C-Clamp or Fem-Stop), dressings, and sand bags are frequently applied to groin sites after removal to decrease the incidence of femoral artery complications.

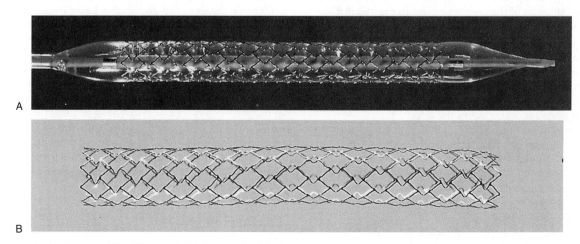

A

B

FIGURE 21-10 The NIR stent. **(A)** Stent expanded on delivery balloon; **(B)** Stent fully expanded. (Courtesy of SCIMED/Boston Scientific Corporation, Maple Grove, MN.)

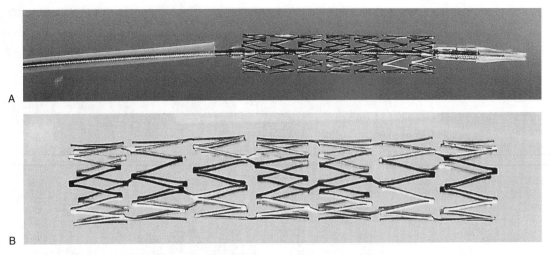

FIGURE 21-11 The Radius stent. **(A)** Stent expanded with delivery sheath pulled back; **(B)** Stent fully expanded. (Courtesy of SCIMED/Boston Scientific Corporation, Maple Grove, MN.)

Vascular closure devices available for femoral artery puncture sites include the Angioseal, Vasoceal, and the Purclose.

Groin Complications. The incidence of vascular complications has increased with the use of larger arterial sheaths, anticoagulation, and antiplatelet or thrombolytic agents. Recognition and treatment are essential to prevent peripheral vascular injuries. A nursing substudy from the randomized placebo-controlled trial of the effect of eptifibatide on complications of percutaneous coronary intervention (IMPACT-II) trial called Standards of Angioplasty Nursing Techniques to Diminish Bleeding around the Groin (SANDBAG) investigated nursing interventions to minimize vascular bleeding with PTCA. Findings associated with an increased incidence of bleeding included a nurse-to-patient ratio of 1 : 6 and a nurse removing the vascular sheath using manual pressure. Other interventions that made no difference in access site bleeding included patient activity, restraint of the affected leg, type of groin dressing used after sheath removal, and frequency of groin assessment.[44]

Hematoma formation is frequent and self-limiting. Large hematomas dissecting into the retroperitoneum are life threatening. Puncture site of the artery proximal to the inguinal ligament, which involves the external iliac artery is frequently the cause. There is less supporting tissue in this area, and therefore it is more difficult to compress the puncture site. Retroperitoneal bleeding is characterized by lumbar or groin pain and a significant drop in hematocrit. Diagnosis is confirmed by a computed tomography scan. Treatment involves transfusion and occasionally surgical repair of the artery.

Arterial thrombosis at the puncture site may lead to occlusion of the artery or distal thrombosis into the extremity. Preexisting peripheral vascular disease increases the risk of a thromboembolic event. Surveillance of distal circulation and sensory checks should be continued after sheath removal. Signs of loss of pulse, color changes, decreased sensation, decreased temperature, or decreased motor function are potential indicators of thrombosis.

A pseudoaneurysm is an extraluminal cavity in communication with an adjacent artery, usually the femoral artery.

Inadvertent puncture of the superficial femoral or profunda femoris artery increases the incidence of arterial complications. Contributing factors include inadequate compression of the puncture site, heparin use, intramural arterial calcifications, and hypertension. On physical examination, the patient may have a pulsatile mass, systolic bruit, normal distal arterial pulses, and pain in the groin. Doppler ultrasound and color flow imaging are used to confirm the diagnosis and delineate the location and size of the pseudoaneurysm. Although most small pseudoaneurysms (<3.5 cm) spontaneously close in 4 to 8 weeks without sequelae, they may enlarge or hemorrhage, especially in patients with prolonged anticoagulation. Treatment includes surgical closure or ultrasound-guided compression.[2]

Arteriovenous fistula is a communication between an artery and vein. The mechanism of injury involves a puncture through both the femoral artery and vein, which results in a false communication. On physical examination, the patient may have a pulsatile mass in the groin and a continuous systolic-diastolic bruit; temperature of the extremity may be decreased owing to high flow through the fistula and ischemia of the extremity; a thrill may be present at the site; and congestive heart failure may result if the fistula is persistent. Diagnosis is confirmed by Doppler ultrasound and color flow imaging. Surgical treatment is necessary for closure and repair of the peripheral vasculature.

Septic endarteritis has been implicated in chronic intimal damage and stasis due to flow turbulence in the region of pseudoaneurysm or arteriovenous fistula, multiple procedures through same access, or sheaths left in place for 24 to 72 hours. Intravenous antibiotics are started before the procedure and continued until sheath removal, or for 24 hours in high-risk patients.[31] Discharge teaching and planning are essential to prevent vascular complications.

Future Research

Interventional cardiology has expanded to provide the cardiologist with an array of options for treating CHD.

Devices play a complementary or synergistic role in allowing revascularization in the catheterization laboratory and treating atherosclerotic disease. Research has indicated higher costs associated with newer interventional devices compared with PTCA[68] and with GP IIb/IIIa inhibitors.[1] Restenosis is the most important problem that continues to complicate treatment with interventional devices. Endovascular radiation therapy to prevent intimal hyperplasia and restenosis after coronary interventions is promising therapy. Radiation can be delivered by catheter-based systems or the placement of radioactive stents. Both β and γ isotopes are of value, although β radiation is safer and easier to use. Multiple clinical trials are underway studying the effects of radiation after PTCA and PTCA with stenting.[76] The future will probably see a combined approach of mechanical and pharmacologic interventions, with possible radiation therapy to maintain coronary artery patency, prolong long-term effects, and ultimately improve quality of life.

NURSING MANAGEMENT

Nursing management focuses on identification and preparation of eligible patients before treatment and on prevention, detection, and treatment of potential complications after interventional cardiology measures.

Analysis of Medical and Nursing Assessment Data and Formulation of Nursing Diagnoses

Common complications and major areas of assessment from which nursing diagnoses are derived were previously discussed. Possible nursing diagnoses include the following:

Anxiety related to unfamiliar environment, unfamiliar treatment modality, and uncertainty of outcome manifested by restlessness; increased pulse rate, respiratory rate, and blood pressure; inability to focus attention; and statements of anxiousness

Chest pain related to myocardial ischemia manifested by complaints of chest pain; restlessness; facial grimacing; hand clutched to chest; increased pulse rate, respiratory rate, and blood pressure; and moaning

High risk for fluid volume deficit related to contrast-induced diuresis, restricted oral intake before elective procedures, or vasodilator therapies

High risk for fluid volume deficit: hemorrhage related to delayed coagulation or lysis of protective clots; hemorrhage other than that occurring at the site of vascular sheaths is primarily a risk for patients receiving thrombolytic drugs that may lyse protective clots and antiplatelet medications

High risk for altered cerebral tissue perfusion related to intracranial hemorrhage (thrombolytic therapy recipients and GP IIb/IIIa only)

High risk for decreased cardiac output related to arrhythmias

High risk for altered myocardial tissue perfusion related to reocclusion of a coronary artery after discontinu-

ation of thrombolytic therapy or abrupt closure after PTCA, atherectomy, intracoronary stenting, or laser angioplasty

ANXIETY AND CHEST PAIN

At the time of admission, primary nursing diagnoses are anxiety related to unfamiliar environment, unfamiliar treatment modality, and uncertainty of outcome; and chest pain related to myocardial ischemia if the patient is in the acute phase of MI or unstable angina.

Goals. The goals of nursing intervention are to provide the patient and family with sufficient information to allow decision making and to reduce anxiety.

Interventions. Concise, precise explanations of all procedures and a calm, organized delivery of care aid in alleviation of anxiety. History and physical assessment of the patient under consideration for thrombolytic therapy focus on inclusion and exclusion criteria to expedite selection of appropriate treatment. Baseline ECG and laboratory data are obtained. Conventional measures to relieve ischemic chest pain are implemented (see Chapter 20). Many indices of anxiety are also cues to pain, and skilled assessment is necessary to distinguish pain from anxiety. Anxiety also increases myocardial oxygen demand and may contribute to ischemic pain. For patients admitted for elective intervention, an assessment of the level of understanding is necessary to guide patient teaching. The focus of teaching is to enhance patient and family knowledge of the procedure and postprocedure care. Risks, potential complications, and alternative therapies are part of informed consent and should be addressed by the cardiologist.

Outcome Criteria. Outcome criteria to measure alleviation of anxiety include reduction in magnitude and numbers of verbal and nonverbal indices of anxiousness. The patient and family report that questions are satisfactorily answered, and informed decision making occurs.

HIGH RISK FOR FLUID VOLUME DEFICIT RELATED TO CONTRAST-INDUCED DIURESIS, RESTRICTED ORAL INTAKE BEFORE ELECTIVE PROCEDURES, OR VASODILATORS

Goals. Nursing goals are prevention, early detection, and treatment of fluid volume deficit.

Interventions. Ongoing patient assessment is necessary to prevent and detect fluid volume deficit. Infuse hydrating intravenous fluids as ordered and provide plenty of fluid to drink unless contraindicated. Monitor patient response to oral and intravenous fluid by evaluating patient complaints of thirst, intake and output, body weight, blood pressure, heart rate and rhythm, and pulmonary artery pressures if applicable. If parameters indicate inadequate intravascular volume, notify the physician and obtain a prescription for appropriate volume replacement.

Outcome Criterion. The outcome criterion for prevention of fluid volume deficit is the absence of subjective and objective indicators of volume deficit. Early detection of volume deficit is achieved when signs of volume deficit are recognized and reported within 60 minutes. Effectiveness of dependent nursing functions to treat volume deficit is determined by continued monitoring and reporting of indices of volume status.

HIGH RISK FOR FLUID VOLUME DEFICIT: HEMORRHAGE RELATED TO DELAYED CLOT FORMATION OR LYSIS OF PROTECTIVE CLOTS

Aggressive anticoagulation and vessel trauma from the large-diameter intravascular sheaths for mechanical interventions place the patient at risk for periaccess bleeding. Also, hemorrhage is the most frequent complication of thrombolytic therapy and manifests differently depending on the site, extent, and organ system involved.

Goals and Interventions

PUNCTURE SITES. Patients receiving thrombolytic agents are likely to experience dissolution of all protective hemostatic clots. Prevention of unnecessary bleeding from arterial and venous puncture sites after thrombolytic therapy involves establishment of a saline-flushed intravenous line for all blood draws, keeping vascular punctures to a minimum, using small-gauge cannulae and needles for intravenous lines, and leaving femoral arterial sheaths and disused intravenous cannulae in place until systemic lysis has ceased. Oozing from puncture sites is detected by monitoring all sites every 15 to 30 minutes. Pressure is maintained over oozing puncture sites for a minimum of 5 to 10 minutes or until bleeding ceases.

More commonly, severe bleeding at puncture sites occurs from vascular trauma due to diagnostic angiography or mechanical interventions (e.g., PTCA, atherectomy). This type of periaccess bleeding is a risk for all patients receiving some type of interventional cardiac therapy because aggressive postprocedure anticoagulation and antiplatelet therapies result in delayed clot formation. Periaccess bleeding ranges from oozing at the site of puncture to hematoma formation or retroperitoneal bleeding if the femoral approach is used.

Prevention of periaccess bleeding may involve leaving arterial and venous sheaths in place until heparin anticoagulation can be interrupted or discontinued. Systematic monitoring and assessment of access sites and serial laboratory evaluation of patient hemoglobin and hematocrit levels aid in detection of overt or occult periaccess bleeding. Care is also guided by institutional protocols and standing orders specific to each type of intervention.

GASTROINTESTINAL BLEEDING. Prevention of gastrointestinal bleeding is achieved by careful patient selection and minimization of procedural or pharmacologic trauma to the gastrointestinal tract. All nasogastric drainage and feces are tested to detect occult bleeding. Treatment depends on the severity of bleeding but may require discontinuance of thrombolytic and anticoagulant therapy and transfusion of blood products.

OTHER CAUSES OF HEMORRHAGE. Hemorrhage into soft tissue may be prevented minimizing handling and transfer of the patient. Intramuscular and subcutaneous injections are contraindicated. Constant monitoring for ecchymosis, petechiae, or oozing from mucous membranes aids in early detection of soft tissue bleeding. Treatment depends on severity of bleeding and results of laboratory tests of coagulation.

Outcome Criterion. The outcome criterion for prevention of hemorrhage is absence of all subjective and objective signs of puncture site, gastrointestinal, or soft tissue hemorrhage. Early detection of hemorrhage is achieved by recognition of subjective or objective indices of severe bleeding within 15 minutes of onset. Criteria for evaluation of treatment specify effectiveness of dependent and independent nursing functions in controlling hemorrhage and maintaining hemodynamic stability.

ALTERED CEREBRAL TISSUE PERFUSION RELATED TO INTRACRANIAL HEMORRHAGE

Although rare, cerebral bleeding is a potentially devastating complication of thrombolytic therapy. Severity of injury ranges from transient neurologic dysfunction to permanent impairment or death.

Goals. Nursing interventions are directed at prevention, early detection, and treatment of cerebral hemorrhage.

Interventions. Careful patient selection and frequent assessment of central nervous system function are necessary for prevention and detection of cerebral bleeding. If signs and symptoms of neurologic impairment manifest, thrombolytic and anticoagulant therapies are discontinued.

Outcome Criterion. The outcome criterion for measurement of prevention of cerebral hemorrhage is the absence of subjective and objective indices of altered central nervous system function. Changes in neurologic assessment are noted and reported within 30 minutes of onset, and treatment is initiated to control bleeding so that central nervous system function does not deteriorate.

HIGH RISK FOR DECREASED CARDIAC OUTPUT RELATED TO ARRHYTHMIAS

Cardiac ischemia, reperfusion, injection of contrast, and fluctuating fluid and electrolyte status place patients receiving interventional cardiac therapies at risk for cardiac arrhythmias. The severity of the drop in cardiac output determines the patient's response to arrhythmias. Some arrhythmias are well tolerated and require only identification, assessment of hemodynamic response, and documentation.

Goals. Goals of nursing intervention are early detection, identification, and treatment of arrhythmias, and assessment and treatment of hemodynamic response to arrhythmias.

Interventions. Continuous cardiac monitoring is necessary to detect arrhythmias after interventional cardiac therapy. Appropriate assessment includes identification and documentation of the arrhythmia and the associated hemodynamic response. The most common reperfusion arrhythmia is a well-tolerated accelerated idioventricular rhythm requiring no additional intervention. Also common are ventricular tachycardia responsive to lidocaine infusion and cardioversion; ventricular fibrillation requiring countershock therapy; and bradyarrhythmia and atrioventricular blocks responsive to atropine. Specific therapies are determined by the type of arrhythmia and severity of alteration in cardiac output.

Outcome Criteria. Outcome criteria for the patient with decreased cardiac output due to arrhythmias include the detection at onset of arrhythmias and accompanying hemodynamic response and immediate institution of appropriate interventions to stop the arrhythmia or stabilize hemodynamic parameters.

HIGH RISK FOR ALTERED MYOCARDIAL TISSUE PERFUSION RELATED TO REOCCLUSION OF A CORONARY ARTERY

Reocclusion continues to be an early complication after successful reperfusion or revascularization by cardiac interventional techniques.

Goals. Nursing goals are prevention, detection, and treatment of inadequate myocardial tissue perfusion.

Interventions. Prevention of myocardial ischemia requires maintenance of thrombolytic and anticoagulant infusions as prescribed and monitoring of ordered coagulation tests. Reocclusion of the stenotic coronary artery is signaled by fresh onset of chest pain and return of ST segment elevation on the ECG. Lead selection for continuous ECG monitoring should be based on knowledge of the involved vessels to allow early detection of ST segment changes that may occur in the absence of chest pain. Treatment is the same as described for the patient with myocardial ischemia in Chapter 20.

Outcome Criteria. Outcome criteria for prevention of altered myocardial tissue perfusion are coagulation tests remain within therapeutic range, and the patient remains free of chest pain and ECG manifestations of acute injury. Early detection necessitates that chest pain and ECG and hemodynamic changes are noted and reported within 15 minutes of onset.

Summary of Nursing Diagnoses

The preceding is a partial list of nursing diagnoses and management principles. Institutional protocols concerning thrombolytic therapy and other interventional cardiac techniques vary; therefore, nurses must familiarize themselves with the protocols of their institution. In addition, new techniques are under investigation. There is insufficient information about these investigational therapies to address nursing management specific to them.

REFERENCES

1. Adgey AA: An overview of the results of clinical trials with glycoprotein IIb/IIIa inhibitors. Am Heart J 135: S43, 1998
2. Agrawal SK, Pinheiro L, Roubin GS et al: Nonsurgical closure of femoral pseudoaneurysms complicating cardiac catheterization and percutaneous transluminal coronary angioplasty. J Am Coll Cardiol 20: 610, 1992
3. Ahn SS, Auth D, Marcus DR: Removal of focal atheromatous lesions by angioscopically guided high-speed rotary atherectomy: Preliminary experimental observations. J Vasc Surg 7: 292, 1988
4. Altman DB, Popma JJ, Hong MK et al: CPK-MB elevation after angioplasty of saphenous vein grafts. J Am Coll Cardiol 21: 232A, 1993
5. American College of Cardiology/American Heart Association Task Force on Assessment of Diagnostic and Therapeutic Cardiovascular Procedures (Subcommittee on Percutaneous Transluminal Coronary Angioplasty): Guidelines for percutaneous coronary angioplasty. J Am Coll Cardiol 22: 2033, 1993
6. Anderson HV, Willerson JT: Thrombolysis in acute myocardial infarction. N Engl J Med 329: 703, 1993
7. Baim DS, Cutlip D, Ho KK et al: Acute results of directional coronary atherectomy in the Balloon Versus Optimal Atherectomy Trial (BOAT) pilot phase. Coron Artery Dis 7: 290, 1996
8. Bode C, Smalling RW, Berg G et al: Randomized comparison of coronary thrombolysis achieved with double-bolus retaplase (recombinant plasminogen activator) and front-loaded, accelerated alteplase (recombinant tissue plasminogen activator) in patients with acute myocardial infarction. Circulation 94: 891, 1996
9. Brochier ML, Quillet L, Kulbertus H et al: Intravenous APSAC versus intravenous streptokinase in evolving myocardial infarction. Drugs 33(Suppl 3): 140, 1987
10. Buchbinder M, Leon M, Warth DC et al: Multicenter registry of percutaneous coronary rotational ablation using the Rotablator. J Am Coll Cardiol 19: 333A, 1992
11. Califf RM, Abdelmeguid AE, Kuntz RE et al: Myonecrosis after revascularization procedures. J Am Coll Cardiol 31: 241, 1998
12. Califf RM, O'Neill, Stack RS et al: Failure of simple clinical measurements to predict perfusion status after intravenous thrombolysis. Ann Intern Med 108: 658, 1988
13. The CAPTURE Investigators: Randomized placebo-controlled trial of abciximab before and during coronary intervention in refractory unstable angina. Lancet 349: 1429, 1997
14. Carrozza JP, Kuntz RE, Levine MJ et al: Angiographic and clinical outcome of intracoronary stenting: Immediate and long-term results from a large single-center experience. J Am Coll Cardiol 20: 328, 1992
15. CAVEAT Investigators: The coronary angioplasty versus excisional atherectomy trial (CAVEAT) preliminary results. Circulation 86(Suppl 1): I-341, 1992
16. Chesebro JH, Knatterud G, Roberts R et al: Thrombolysis in Myocardial Infarction (TIMI) Trial, phase I: A comparison between intravenous tissue plasminogen activator and intravenous streptokinase. Circulation 76: 142, 1987
17. Colombo A, Hall P, Nakamura S et al: Intracoronary stenting without anticoagulation accomplished with intravascular ultrasound guidance. Circulation 91: 1676, 1995
18. Cowley MJ, DiSciascio G: Directional coronary atherectomy for saphenous vein disease. Cathet Cardiovasc Diagn (Suppl 1): 10, 1993
19. Daily EK: Clinical management of patients receiving thrombolytic therapy. Heart Lung 20: 552, 1991

20. Deelstra MH: Coronary rotational ablation: An overview with related nursing interventions. Am J Crit Care 2: 16, 1993

21. Detre KM, Holmes DR, Holubkov R et al: Incidence and consequences of periprocedural occlusion. Circulation 82: 739, 1990

22. DeWood MA, Spores J, Notske R: Prevalence of total coronary occlusion during the early hours of transmural myocardial infarction. N Engl J Med 303: 897, 1980

23. Dotter CT: Transluminally placed coilspring endarterial tube grafts: Long-term patency in canine popliteal artery. Invest Radiol 4: 329, 1969

24. Ellis SG, Muller DWM: Arterial injury and the enigma of coronary restenosis. J Am Coll Cardiol 19: 275, 1992

25. Ellis SG, Savage M, Fischman D et al: Restenosis after placement of Palmaz-Schatz stents in native coronary arteries. Circulation 86: 1836, 1992

26. The EPIC Investigators: Use of a monoclonal antibody directed against the platelet glycoprotein IIb/IIIa receptor in high-risk coronary angioplasty. N Engl J Med 330: 956, 1994

27. The EPILOG Investigators: Platelet glycoprotein IIb/IIIa receptor blockade and low-dose heparin during percutaneous coronary revascularization. N Engl J Med 336: 1689, 1997

28. The EPISTENT Investigators: Randomised placebo-controlled and balloon-angioplasty-controlled trial to assess safety of coronary stenting with use of platelet glycoprotein-IIb/IIIa blockade. Lancet 352: 87, 1998

29. de Feyter PJ, van den Brand M, Jaarman GJ et al: Acute coronary artery occlusion during and after percutaneous transluminal coronary angioplasty. Circulation 83: 927, 1991

30. Fischman DL, Leon MB, Baim DS et al: A randomised comparison of coronary-stent placement and balloon angioplasty in the treatment of coronary artery disease. N Engl J Med 331: 496, 1994

31. Frazee BW, Flajhert JP: Septic endarteritis of the femoral artery following angioplasty. Rev Infect Dis 13: 620, 1991

32. Gruppo Italiano per lo Studio Della Streptochinasi nell' Infarcto Miocardico: Effectiveness of intravenous thrombolytic treatment in acute myocardial infarction. Lancet 1: 397, 1986

33. Gusto Investigators: An international trial comparing four thrombolytic strategies for acute myocardial infarction. N Engl J Med 329: 673, 1993

34. Harrington R: Design and methodology of the PURSUIT trial: Evaluating eptifibatide for acute ischemic coronary syndromes. Am J Cardiol 80(Suppl 4A): 34B, 1997

35. Hinohara T, Robertson GC, Selmon MR et al: Directional coronary atherectomy complications and management. Cathet Cardiovasc Diagn (Suppl 1): 61, 1993

36. Hinohara T, Selmon MR, Robertson GC et al: Directional atherectomy: New approaches for treatment of obstructive coronary and peripheral vascular disease. Circulation 81(Suppl 4): 79, 1990

37. Hirshfeld JW, Schwartz S, Jugo R et al: Restenosis after coronary angioplasty: A multivariate statistical model to relate lesion and procedure variables to restenosis. J Am Coll Cardiol 18: 647, 1991

38. Hong MK, Mintz GS, Popma JJ et al: Safety and efficacy of elective stent implantation following rotational atherectomy in large calcified coronary arteries. Cathet Cardiovasc Diagn (Suppl 3): 50, 1996

39. Hsia J, Hamilton WP, Kleiman N et al: A comparison between heparin and low-dose aspirin as adjunctive therapy with tissue plasminogen activator for acute myocardial infarction. N Engl J Med 323: 1433, 1990

40. International Study Group: In-hospital mortality and clinical course of 20,891 patients with suspected acute myocardial infarction randomized between alteplase and streptokinase with or without heparin. Lancet 336: 71, 1990

41. ISIS-2 (Second International Study of Infarct Survival) Collaborative Study Group: Randomized trial of intravenous streptokinase, oral aspirin, both or neither among 17,187 cases of suspected acute myocardial infarction. Lancet 2: 349, 1988

42. ISIS-3 (Third International Study of Infarct Survival) Collaborative Group: A randomized comparison of streptokinase vs tissue plasminogen activator vs anistreplase and of aspirin plus heparin vs aspirin alone among 41,299 cases of suspected acute myocardial infarction. Lancet 339: 753, 1992

43. de Jaegere PP, Serruys PW, Bertrand M et al: Wiktor stent implantation in patients with restenosis following balloon angioplasty of a native coronary artery. Am J Cardiol 69: 598, 1992

44. Juran N, Deluca S, Rouse C et al: Nursing interventions post PTCA: Do they make a difference? Abstract 25th National Teaching Institute and Critical Care Exposition, Los Angeles, CA, 1998

45. Kaplan BM, Gregory M, Schreiber TL et al: Transluminal extraction atherectomy versus balloon angioplasty in acute ischemic syndromes: An interim analysis of the Topit trial. Circulation 94(Suppl 8): 1-3171, 1996

46. Kulick DL, Kawanishi DT: Percutaneous transluminal coronary angioplasty. In Kulick DL, Rahimtoola SH (eds): Techniques and Applications in Interventional Cardiology, p 43. St. Louis, Mosby-Year Book, 1991

47. Litvak F, Marglis J, Cummins R et al: Excimer laser coronary (ECLA) registry: Report of the first 2080 patients. J Am Coll Cardiol 19: 276A, 1992

48. Lopez-Sendon J, Seabra-Gomes R, Martin Santos F et al: Intravenous anisoylated plasminogen streptokinase activator complex (APSAC) versus intravenous streptokinase (SK) in myocardial infarction (AMI): A randomized multicentre trial. Eur Heart J 9(Suppl A): 10, 1988

49. Margolis JR, Mehta S: Excimer Xaser coronary angioplasty. J Am Coll Cardiol 69:3F, 1992

50. Mehta S, Kramer B, Margolis JR: Transluminal extraction. Coron Artery Dis 3: 887, 1992

51. Meijer A, Verheugt FWA, Werter CJPJ et al: Aspirin versus Coumadin in the prevention of reocclusion and recurrent ischemia after successful thrombolysis: A prospective placebo-controlled angiographic study. Circulation 87: 1524, 1993

52. Misumi K, Matthews RV, Sun GW et al: Reduced distal embolization with transluminal extraction atherectomy compared to balloon angioplasty for saphenous vein graft disease. Cathet Cardiovasc Diagn 39: 246, 1996

53. Ohman EM, Califf RM, Topol EJ et al: Consequences of reocclusion after successful reperfusion therapy in acute myocardial infarction. Circulation 82: 781, 1990

54. O'Neill W, Kramer B, Sketch M et al: Mechanical extraction atherectomy: Report of the U. S. transluminal extraction catheter investigation. Circulation 86: 779A, 1992

55. The PRISM-PLUS Investigators: Inhibition of the platelet glycoprotein IIb/IIIa receptor with tirofiban in unstable angina and non-Q wave myocardial infarction. N Engl J Med 338: 1488, 1998

56. Puleo PR, Perryman MB: Noninvasive detection of reperfusion in acute myocardial infarction based on plasma activity of creatine kinase MB subforms. J Am Coll Cardiol 17: 1047, 1991

57. Roubin GS, Cannon AD, Agrawal SK et al: Intracoronary stenting for acute and threatened closure complicating percutaneous transluminal coronary angioplasty. Circulation 85: 916, 1992

58. Schatz RA, Baim DS, Leon M et al: Clinical experience with the Palmaz-Schatz coronary stent: Initial results of a multicenter study. Circulation 83: 148, 1991

59. Schomig A, Neumnn FJ, Kastrati A et al: A randomized comparison of antiplatelet and anticoagulant therapy after the placement of coronary-artery stents. N Engl J Med 34: 1084, 1996

60. Scott S, King S: Coronary stents. Coron Artery Dis 3: 901, 1992

61. Serruys PW, De Jaegere P, Kiemeneij F et al: A comparison of balloon-expandable-stent implantation with balloon angioplasty in patients with coronary artery disease. N Engl J Med 331: 489, 1994

62. Serruys PW, Strauss BH, Beatt KJ et al: Angiographic follow-up after placement of self-expanding coronary artery stent. N Engl J Med 324: 13, 1991

63. Shaknovik A, Lieberman SM, Moses JW: Clinical and angiographic outcomes of native coronary stenting with single Palmaz-Schatz stents: Update of US multicenter experience. J Am Coll Cardiol 21(Suppl A): 29A, 1993

64. Sigwart U, Puel J, Mirkovitch V et al: Intravascular stents to prevent occlusion and restenosis after transluminal angioplasty. N Engl J Med 316: 13, 1987

65. Simoons ML, Arnold AER, Betriu A et al: Thrombolysis with rt-PA in acute myocardial infarction: No beneficial effects of immediate PTCA. Lancet 1: 197, 1988

66. Sketch MH, O'Neill WW, Galichia JP et al: Restenosis following coronary transluminal extraction-endarterectomy: The final analysis of a multicenter registry. J Am Coll Cardiol 19: 277A, 1992

67. Sketch M, Phillips J, Myoung-Mook L et al: Coronary transluminal extraction/endarterectomy. Inv Cardiol 3: 13, 1991

68. Steekiste AR, Baim DS, Sipperly ME et al: The NACI Registry: An instrument for the evaluation of new approaches to coronary intervention. Cathet Cardiovasc Diagn 23: 270, 1991

69. Stone GW: Rotational atherectomy for treatment of in-stent restenosis: Role of intracoronary ultrasound guidance. Cathet Cardiovasc Diagn (Suppl 3): 73, 1996

70. Strauss BH, Serruys BW, Bertrand ME et al: Quantitative angiographic follow-up of coronary Wallstent in native vessels and bypass grafts. Am J Cardiol 69: 475, 1992

71. Terstein PS, Warth DC, Haq N et al: High speed rotational coronary atherectomy for patients with diffuse coronary artery disease. J Am Coll Cardiol 18: 1694, 1991

72. Topol EJ: Thrombolytic intervention. In Topol EJ (ed): Textbook of Interventional Cardiology, p 76. Philadelphia, WB Saunders, 1990

73. Topol EJ, Califf RM, George BS et al: A randomized trial of immediate versus delayed elective angioplasty after intravenous tissue plasminogen activator in acute myocardial infarction. N Engl J Med 317: 581, 1987

74. Topol EJ, Leya F, Pinkerton CA et al: A comparison of directional atherectomy with comparison of coronary angioplasty in patients with coronary artery disease. N Engl J Med 329: 221, 1993

75. Verstraete M, Brower RW, Collen D et al: Double-blind randomised trial of intravenous tissue-type plasminogen activator versus placebo in acute myocardial infarction. Lancet 2: 965, 1985

76. Williams D: Radiation vascular therapy: A novel approach to preventing restenosis. Am J Cardiol 81(Suppl 7A): 18E, 1998

77. Zacca NM, Raizner AE, Noon GP et al: Short term follow-up of patients treated with a recently developed rotational atherectomy device and in-vivo assessment of the particles generated. J Am Coll Cardiol II (2):109A, 1998

Heart Failure

DEBRA LAURENT-BOPP

Heart failure (HF) is the pathophysiologic state in which an abnormality of cardiac function is responsible for the failure of the heart to pump blood at a rate adequate to meet the requirements of the tissue, either at rest or exercise. Although this syndrome has been extensively researched and intensively treated, it remains a leading cause of death. There is an increasing incidence of HF in the aging population, with a prevalence of approximately 10% by the age of 75 years. The quality of life, exercise capacity, and perhaps the life expectancy of patients with HF may be altered by the introduction of appropriate medical and nursing therapy at the appropriate time in the course of the patient's heart disease. This chapter reviews major physiologic and pathophysiologic concepts of HF as a basis for understanding its underlying causes as well as its clinical and physical findings. Emphasis also is placed on the various diagnostic tests, the vast array of pharmacologic agents, and other medical and nursing interventions. With this knowledge, the nurse is able to implement a plan of care, which may involve restriction of activity and diet, medications, and coping strategies for patients and families to adapt effectively to an acute or chronic illness.

DEFINITION AND CLASSIFICATIONS

Heart failure is a complex clinical syndrome manifested by shortness of breath, fatigue, and abnormal heart function. HF is not a diagnosis, and its etiology should be sought carefully. Any disorder that places the heart under a chronically increased volume or pressure load or that produces primary damage or an increased metabolic demand on the myocardium may result in HF[18,19,44,46] (Table 22-1).

Heart failure has been subdivided into different classifications to describe the pathology of HF, and each system of classification reveals a theory about the cause of HF.[6,61] Classifications include backward and forward failure, acute and chronic HF, left-sided and right-sided failure, low-

output and high-output syndrome, shock, and systolic and diastolic dysfunction.

Backward and Forward Failure

In 1832, James Hope first described *backward failure* as the failure that results as the ventricle fails to pump its volume, causing blood accumulation and subsequent rise in ventricular, atrial, and venous pressures.[6,27] A primary etiology of backward failure is mechanical cardiac obstruction.

The term *forward failure*, proposed by MacKenzie in 1913, is applied to a situation in which the primary pathologic process is decreased cardiac output, which ultimately leads to a decrease in vital organ perfusion.[6,61] Both backward and forward failure are seen in most patients with chronic HF.

Acute and Chronic Failure

The clinical manifestations of acute and chronic failure depend on how rapidly the syndrome of HF develops. *Acute HF* may be the initial manifestation of heart disease or may indicate exacerbation of a chronic cardiac condition. The marked decrease in left ventricular (LV) function may be due to acute myocardial infarction (MI) or acute valvular dysfunction. The events occur so rapidly that the sympathetic nervous system compensation is ineffective, resulting in the rapid development of pulmonary edema and circulatory collapse (cardiogenic shock). *Chronic HF* develops over time and is usually the end result of an increasing inability of physiologic mechanisms to compensate. It can be caused by valvular disease, high blood pressure, or chronic obstructive pulmonary disease.[6,27,36,44]

Left-Sided and Right-Sided Failure

The right and left sides of the heart are independent circuits and can fail independently. It is, however, unusual for left-sided failure not to progress to biventricular failure.

Left-sided HF exists when LV stroke volume is reduced and blood accumulates in the left ventricle, left

TABLE 22-1	Conditions That Cause Heart Failure			
Abnormal Volume Load	**Abnormal Pressure Load**	**Myocardial Dysfunction**	**Filling Disorders**	**Increased Metabolic Demand**
Aortic incompetence	Aortic stenosis	Cardiomyopathy	Mitral stenosis	Anemias
Mitral incompetence	Hypertrophic cardiomyopathy	Myocarditis	Tricuspid stenosis	Thyrotoxicosis
Tricuspid incompetence	Coarctation of the aorta	Coronary heart disease	Cardiac tamponade	Fever
Overtransfusion	Hypertension	Ischemia	Restrictive pericarditis	Beriberi
Left-to-right shunts	Primary	Infarction		Paget's disease
Secondary hypervolemia	Secondary	Arrhythmias		Arteriovenous fistulas
		Toxic disorders		

From Michaelson CR (ed): Congestive Heart Failure, p 45. St Louis, CV Mosby, 1983.

atrium, and pulmonary circulation, which causes elevated pulmonary venous pressure and reduced cardiac output. LV failure is by far the most frequent of the two instances in which only one side of the heart is affected. It can be caused by arterial high blood pressure, myocardial ischemia or MI, aortic valve incompetence or stenosis, or mitral valve incompetence or stenosis. People with chronic volume overload, high-output states, cardiomyopathies, or arrhythmias demonstrate signs of LV failure before those of right HF.[44,61]

Inability of the right heart to empty its blood volume results in blood backing up into the systemic circulation. LV failure is the most common cause of right ventricular (RV) failure. Sustained pulmonary hypertension also causes RV failure. Pulmonary hypertension occurs in patients with congenital anomalies (tetralogy of Fallot or ventricular septal defect), severe pulmonary infections, massive pulmonary embolization, or mitral or aortic stenosis.[44,61]

Low and High Cardiac Output Syndrome

In response to high blood pressure and hypovolemia, low cardiac output syndrome appears. The word *syndrome* implies that the failure represents a reaction rather than a primary pathologic process. Low cardiac output syndrome is evidenced by impaired peripheral circulation and peripheral vasoconstriction.

Any condition that causes the heart to work harder to supply blood may be categorized as high cardiac output syndrome. High cardiac output states require an increased oxygen supply to the peripheral tissues, which can occur only with an increased cardiac output. Reduced systemic vascular resistance (SVR) is characteristic of this condition and augments peripheral circulation and venous return, which in turn increases stroke volume and cardiac output. High cardiac output states may be caused by increased metabolic requirements, as seen in hyperthyroidism, fever, and pregnancy, or may be triggered by hyperkinetic conditions such as arteriovenous fistulas, anemia, and beriberi.[6,27,44]

Shock

Shock describes a syndrome in which tissue perfusion is inadequate to meet the needs of cells, thus representing the extreme end of the forward failure continuum. Any factor that lowers cardiac output predisposes a person to shock (see Chapter 24).

Systolic and Diastolic Dysfunction

Systolic dysfunction is determined by an impaired pump function with reduced ejection fraction and an enlarged end-diastolic chamber volume.[23] The main etiologies are coronary heart disease, dilated cardiomyopathy, and hypertension.[53] *Diastolic dysfunction* implies normal systolic function in the presence of clinical HF and is characterized by an increased resistance to filling with increased filling pressures.[27] LV failure is caused by diastolic dysfunction in up to 40% of cases, mainly due to long-standing hypertension. Coronary heart disease is secondary; hypertrophic and restrictive cardiomyopathies and aortic valve diseases are less frequent. Increased age also appears to be a factor.[23,71]

During the last 20 years, the role of diastolic dysfunction has been increasingly recognized. The different pathophysiologic processes behind systolic and diastolic dysfunction affect prognosis and treatment and are addressed in the following sections.

PATHOPHYSIOLOGY

Before the pathogenesis of systolic and diastolic HF is presented, it is necessary to understand the determinants of ventricular performance. Cardiac output depends on the relation between heart rate and stroke volume; it is the product of these two variables. The *stroke volume* is the amount of blood ejected by a ventricle during each systolic contraction. Several factors influence cardiac output and stroke volume: heart rate, preload, afterload, and contractility.

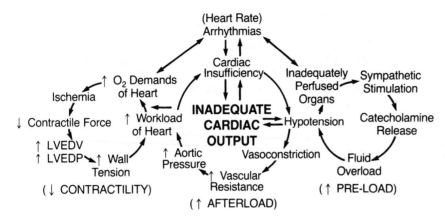

FIGURE 22-1 Cycle of heart failure. The determinants of ventricular performance, heart rate, contractility, afterload, and preload are altered in heart failure. In an attempt to compensate for an inadequate cardiac output, these determinants set up a number of positive-feedback mechanisms that contribute to an increased oxygen demand on the heart, eventually causing further reduction in cardiac output. LVEDP, left ventricular end-diastolic pressure; LVEDV, left ventricular end-diastolic volume.

Compensatory Mechanisms

When the heart is presented with an increased workload, a number of physiologic alterations are evoked in an attempt to maintain normal cardiac pumping function. These compensatory mechanisms include[6,27]:

1. Sympathetic nervous system response to baroreceptors or chemoreceptors
2. Renal compensation: retention of sodium and water and peripheral vasoconstriction
3. Ventricular dilatation to accommodate increased volume (Frank-Starling response)
4. Myocardial hypertrophy
5. Increased tissue oxygen extraction
6. Neurohormonal response

The syndrome of HF, as recognized clinically, represents the combination of a number of positive-feedback mechanisms involving the heart, the peripheral circulation, and a number of vital organ systems. During the course of HF, the mechanisms of compensation promoting cardiac and peripheral circulatory adjustments may lead to a number of positive-feedback mechanisms. Because all of these contribute to an increase in myocardial oxygen consumption, they may eventually have deleterious effects on pump function[6,8,44,61] (Fig. 22-1).

SYMPATHETIC NERVOUS SYSTEM RESPONSE

In HF, stimulation of the sympathetic nervous system represents the most immediately responsive mechanism of compensation. Stimulation of the β-adrenergic receptors in the heart causes an elevation in heart rate and contractility to raise stroke volume and cardiac output. Sympathetic effects on the peripheral vascular system increase vascular tone to raise SVR and mean systemic filling pressure, thereby augmenting venous return, preload, and afterload. The next stage of compensation occurs as a result of partial recovery of the heart and renal conservation of fluid.[6,27]

RENAL COMPENSATION

Renal compensation is triggered initially by a drop in kidney perfusion, which decreases glomerular filtration and activates the renin–angiotensin–aldosterone mechanisms, resulting in an increased SVR and increased sodium and water absorption. The renal compensatory mechanisms augment blood volume and increase systemic filling pressure and venous return. This renal compensation results in enhanced preload, afterload, and contractility.[6,15,61,68]

Ventricular Preload. The elevated preload seen in HF is caused by a number of factors. Impaired emptying of the left ventricles leaves a larger end-diastolic volume and pressure than in the normally functioning left ventricle. Sodium retention caused by abnormalities of renal perfusion leads to expansion of plasma volume. Decreased venous compliance reduces the capacitance of the venous system and may contribute to the rise in venous pressure. A high LV preload contributes to the pulmonary venous congestion and probably plays an important role in precipitating the breathlessness that limits exercise tolerance.[6,63]

Sodium Retention. Hormonal and hemodynamic factors appear to contribute to sodium retention. Hormonal factors, including the sympathetic nervous system and the renin–angiotensin–aldosterone system, probably contribute in part to the functional abnormality of the kidney.[6,15,27,44] Decreased renal perfusion appears to play a critical role in the abnormalities of sodium excretion.

Peripheral Edema. Peripheral edema develops owing to an elevated venous pressure, either at rest or during exercise. A number of additional factors also may contribute to the development of edema. Increased hydrostatic pressure and decreased plasma oncotic pressure contribute to the transudation of fluid out of the capillary bed. Abnormalities of lymphatic drainage related to an elevated central venous pressure and resultant inhibition of thoracic duct drainage also may contribute to the development of dependent edema.

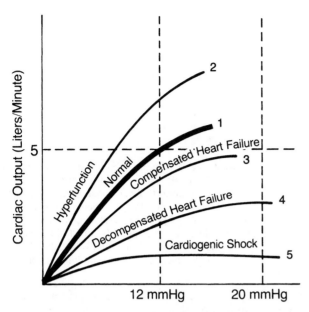

FIGURE 22-2 Left ventricular function curves. *Curve 1:* Normal function curve, with a normal cardiac output at optimal filling pressures. *Curve 2:* Cardiac hyperfunction, with an increased cardiac output at optimal filling pressures. *Curve 3:* Compensated heart failure, with normal cardiac outputs at higher filling pressures. *Curve 4:* Decompensated heart failure, with a decrease in cardiac output and elevated filling pressures. *Curve 5:* Cardiogenic shock, with extremely depressed cardiac output and marked increase in filling pressures. (Adapted from Michaelson CR: Congestive Heart Failure, p 61. St. Louis, CV Mosby, 1983.)

VENTRICULAR DILATATION

As diastolic filling increases, ventricular dilatation occurs. Renal compensatory mechanisms cause sympathetic stimulation, thus increasing the end-diastolic volume or preload. The Frank-Starling response is immediately activated as a consequence of increased diastolic volume. According to the Frank-Starling law of the heart, stretching of the myocardial fibers during diastole increases the force of contraction during systole. The increased preload augmenting contractility is the major mechanism by which the ventricles maintain an equal output as their stroke volumes vary.[6,27,61] It may be useful to consider normal and impaired myocardial function within the framework of the Frank-Starling mechanism, as illustrated by analysis of LV function curves (Fig. 22-2). Cardiac output or cardiac index is used as a measure of ventricular work; LV end-diastolic pressure or pulmonary artery wedge pressure (PAWP) is used as a reflection of preload.[6] The normal relation between ventricular end-diastolic volume and ventricular work is shown in Figure 22-2 by *curve 1.* Optimal contractility occurs at a diastolic volume of 12 to 18 mm Hg.[6,61] If the heart is stressed initially, as occurs in acute MI, the initial drop in cardiac output stimulates the sympathetic nervous system. An increase in sympathetic tone elevates both heart rate and

contractility, illustrated in Figure 22-2 by *curve 2.* As the cardiac workload increases and myocardial dysfunction persists, HF progresses, which is reflected by further elevation of end-diastolic volume (preload) and ventricular dilatation. This increased preload, in turn, may further contribute to depressed ventricular contractility and the development of congestive symptoms (see Fig. 22-2, *curve 3*).

Aortic Impedance. The normal left ventricle is able to adjust to large changes in aortic impedance with small changes in output, in part by calling on the Frank-Starling response and, perhaps, by augmenting the contractile force as an intrinsic property of the normal myocardium. In contrast, the damaged left ventricle loses this compensatory ability and becomes sensitive to even small changes in impedance.[27] Because increased activity of the sympathetic nervous system or the renin–angiotensin–aldosterone system results in vasoconstriction of the small arteries and arterioles, an increased impedance of LV filling is imposed, decreasing the stroke volume and cardiac output.[15,68] Because HF is characterized by heightened activity of these neurohormonal vasoconstrictor systems, a positive-feedback loop can be generated in which impaired pump performance increases impedance to LV ejection, further impairing the pump performance.

MYOCARDIAL HYPERTROPHY

Myocardial hypertrophy with or without chamber dilatation is a compensatory mechanism in which the heart increases its muscle mass and alters its geometric configuration. In response to pressure overload, concentric hypertrophy produces an increase in the thickness of the ventricular wall without dilatation of the ventricular chamber. Concentric hypertrophy may be caused, for example, by high blood pressure or aortic stenosis. Eccentric hypertrophy produces a proportional increase in ventricular wall thickness and dilatation of the ventricular chamber in response to diastolic volume overload. Conditions that cause eccentric hypertrophy include arteriovenous fistulas and mitral or tricuspid incompetence.[6,27,61]

Ventricular Remodeling. The pressure- and volume-overloaded ventricle responds to these abnormal loads by myocardial hypertrophy. With time, hypertrophy may lead to further impairment of pump performance because of either diastolic compliance changes (a result of a thickened ventricular wall) or impaired systolic pump performance (caused by impaired muscle function and the growth of collagen).[6,27] Because failure induces hypertrophy, and hypertrophy may thus induce failure, another positive-feedback mechanism may be identified.

Hypertrophy alters cardiac function by its depressant effect on ventricular compliance and rate and force of ventricular contraction.[5,61–63] As HF progresses, the compensatory mechanism of sympathetic stimulation, renal conservation of fluid, in addition to myocardial hypertrophy, causes a further shift to the right of the ventricular function curve, reflecting a more pronounced increase in ventricular filling pressure with no further increase in cardiac performance

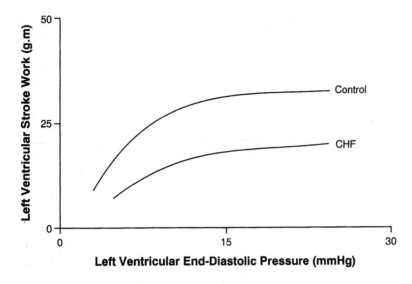

FIGURE 22-3 The Frank-Starling mechanism is altered in heart failure. The failing ventricle is unable to respond to an increase in preload with a normal increase in left ventricular stroke work. (From Francis GS: Pathosphysiology of the heart failure clinical syndrome. In Topol EJ [ed]: Textbook of Cardiovascular Medicine, pp 2179–2203. Philadelphia, Lippincott-Raven, 1998, with permission.)

(see Fig. 22-2, *curve 4*). When cardiac performance fails to satisfy the requirements of the peripheral tissues even at rest, and the pulmonary artery (PA) pressure is elevated to levels that result in pulmonary edema, cardiogenic shock develops (see Fig. 22-2, *curve 5*).

INCREASED TISSUE OXYGEN EXTRACTION

In HF, blood flow to the peripheral tissues usually is diminished, secondary to a drop in cardiac output and perfusion pressure. Tissues compensate for this slow circulation time by increasing tissue oxygen extraction.

Myocardial Ischemia. Normally, the subendocardium is perfused during diastole with a fairly low effective perfusion pressure. If ventricular diastolic pressure rises to abnormal levels, it is transmitted into the subendocardium and compresses the subendocardial vessels, reducing subendocardial perfusion. This abnormality may be a particularly important mechanism of ischemia in patients with proximal coronary artery stenosis. Even in the presence of normal coronary arteries, however, subendocardial ischemia can be induced by experimental elevation of the LV diastolic pressure.[61] Because myocardial ischemia can induce a rise in cardiac filling pressure by virtue of a decrease in compliance of the ventricle, and because an elevated ventricular filling pressure can induce ischemia by virtue of subendocardial underperfusion, it is clear that a potential positive-feedback cycle may be generated by the coexistence of both ischemia and poor ventricular function.

NEUROHORMONAL RESPONSE

Heart failure frequently is accompanied by a depletion of cardiac norepinephrine stores and a reduction of the inotropic response to impulses in the cardiac adrenergic nerves. Ventricular performance cannot be elevated to normal levels by the adrenergic nervous system, and the normal improvement of contractility that takes place during exercise is attenuated or even prevented.[6,10] Although the plasma renin activity often is elevated to high levels in HF, in some patients, plasma renin activity is normal or even depressed. Therefore, it is likely that in at least some patients with HF, activation of the renin–angiotensin–

aldosterone system represents another compensatory mechanism.[15,68] Studies demonstrate that plasma arginine vasopressin levels also are increased in patients with HF.[32] Because vasopressin is a potent vasoconstrictor as well as an antidiuretic hormone, the participation of this system in the neurohormonal response to HF may represent further the body's effort to constrict the peripheral vessels in an effort to support blood pressure. Activation of all these systems may be inappropriate on the basis of previous comments regarding aortic impedance.

Atrial natriuretic peptide (ANP), or atrial natriuretic factor, has emerged as an important hormone participating in the regulation of cardiovascular volume homeostasis. An increase in atrial distending pressure, however produced, leads to the release of ANP. ANP is a counter-regulatory hormone that opposes many of the effects of the adrenergic, renin–angiotensin–aldosterone, and arginine vasopressor systems. Therefore, ANP may protect the central circulation from volume overload and reduces tachycardia by modulating baroreceptor function. Plasma ANP is clearly increased in acute HF. Recent evidence shows, however, that chronic congestive HF may be a state of relative ANP deficiency or depletion, which would not counteract the volume overload or tachycardia.[6,57,61]

Systolic Dysfunction

A reduction in systolic performance begins after a loss of muscle cells, decrease in contractility, or structural changes of the myocardium with an increase in interstitial fibrosis or LV remodeling. The fundamental problem is impaired LV contractility with a subsequent fall in cardiac output. This fall in cardiac output is counteracted by numerous compensatory mechanisms, as previously described.

Decreased LV contractility, increased cardiac volume and pressure, decreased responsiveness to increased preload (Fig. 22-3), and increased sensitivity to increased afterload (Fig. 22-4) eventually produce a situation in which the heart cannot meet the metabolic demands of the tissue.[27] The result is a patient with systemic hypoperfusion, severe vasoconstriction, congested lungs, and poor pump performance.[31]

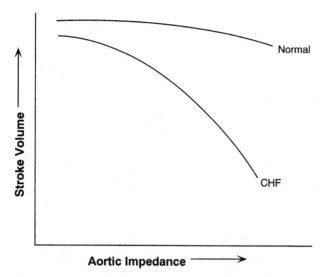

FIGURE 22-4 A hallmark of heart failure is the exquisite sensitivity of the left ventricle to an afterload stress. As impedance to ejection is raised, there is an impressive reduction in left ventricular performance. (From Francis GS: Pathophysiology of the heart failure clinical syndrome. In Topol EJ [ed]: Textbook of Cardiovascular Medicine, pp 2179–2203. Philadelphia, Lippincott-Raven, 1998, with permission.)

Diastolic Dysfunction

Isolated diastolic dysfunction is characterized by a preserved ejection fraction (normal or even enhanced contractile function. The ventricles are capable of responding to an increase in preload, and there is no undue sensitivity of systolic performance to increased afterload.[27] The fundamental problem is that diastolic dysfunction impairs ventricular filling by diminished relaxation (during early diastole) or reducing compliance (during early to late diastole) of the ventricle, or both.[7,71] This leads to an abnormal diastolic pressure–volume relationship, shifting the pressure–volume curve to the left and producing a higher pressure for a given diastolic volume (Fig. 22-5). This elevated pressure is transmitted backward to the atria and the pulmonary and systemic circuits. These effects limit cardiac output and cause dyspnea during exercise and fatigue.[7,27,31]

The pathophysiologic processes behind diastolic dysfunction are more diverse than those of systolic dysfunction. The functional abnormalities are slowed or incomplete relaxation (as in hypertrophic cardiomyopathy), impaired myocardial relaxation (as in ischemia and hypertrophy), myocardial scar (as in ischemia or endomyocardial fibrosis), and pericardial restriction (as in constrictive pericardial disease).[7,23,31,71]

CLINICAL MANIFESTATIONS

Most patients with HF have reduced LV systolic function and variable degrees of diastolic dysfunction. The predominant symptom is breathlessness or dyspnea. Orthopnea and paroxysmal nocturnal dyspnea occur in the more advanced stages of HF. *Systolic dysfunction* is characterized by occurrence of HF in the presence of marked cardiomegaly, whereas *dias-*

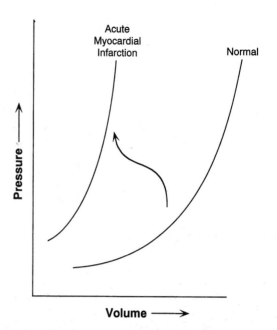

FIGURE 22-5 The fundamental consequence of diastolic heart failure is a shift in the pressure–volume relationship of the left ventricle, so that for any given volume, there is a much higher left ventricular end-diastolic pressure. (From Francis GS: Pathophysiology of the heart failure clinical syndrome. In Topol EJ (ed): Textbook of Cardiovascular Medicine, pp 2179–2203. Philadelphia, Lippincott-Raven, 1998, with permission.)

tolic dysfunction is associated with pulmonary congestion and a normal or only slightly enlarged ventricle.[27,36]

The signs and symptoms that characterize HF can be considered in the context of the four components of the syndrome: failure of the left ventricle as a pump, failure of the right ventricle as a pump, pulmonary venous congestion, and systemic venous congestion. Symptoms are often described as those due to left- or right-sided HF, and although the symptoms of both types overlap, they are addressed separately in the following for discussion[4,8,27,29,63] (Fig. 22-6).

Related to Left-Sided Heart Failure

Left-sided HF, associated with elevated pulmonary venous pressure and decreased cardiac output, appears clinically as breathlessness, weakness, fatigue, dizziness, confusion, pulmonary congestion, hypotension, and death.

Weakness or fatigue is precipitated by decreased perfusion to the muscles. Patients describe a feeling of heaviness in their arms and legs.

Decreased cerebral perfusion due to low cardiac output leads to changes in mental status, such as restlessness, insomnia, nightmares, or memory loss. Anxiety, agitation, paranoia, and fear of impending doom may develop as the syndrome progresses.

During the course of HF, pulmonary congestion progresses through three stages: stage 1, early pulmonary congestion; stage 2, interstitial edema; and stage 3, alveolar edema.[5,63] During the early phase, little measurable increase in interstitial lung fluid is noted. There are few clinical manifestations during this phase.

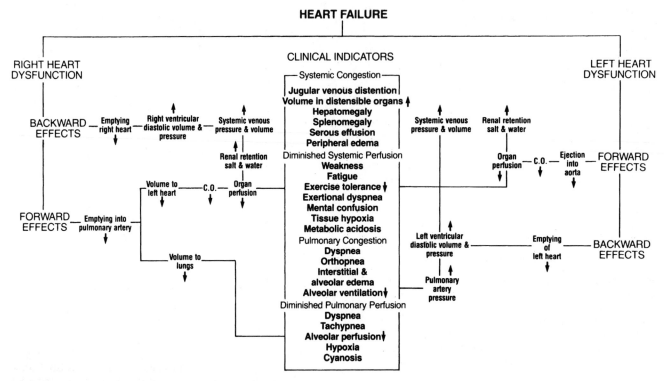

FIGURE 22-6 Heart failure flow chart, with complex interaction of forward and backward effects of right and left ventricular failure. The clinical indicators arise from systemic and pulmonary congestion and from diminished systemic and pulmonary perfusion. (From Michaelson CR: Congestive Heart Failure, p 52. St Louis, CV Mosby, 1983.)

Interstitial edema occurs when the PAWP exceeds 18 mm Hg, leading to a net filtration of fluid into the interstitial space. Clinical manifestations of interstitial edema are varied.[5,44,63] Engorged pulmonary vessels, elevated PA pressure, and reduced lung compliance cause increased exertional dyspnea. If the left ventricle is severely impaired, orthopnea or a nonproductive cough may be present. Paroxysmal nocturnal dyspnea may also occur because of postural redistribution of blood flow that increases venous return and pulmonary vascular pressure when the patient is in a recumbent position. Congestion of the bronchial mucosa that increases airway resistance and the work of breathing may also contribute to paroxysmal nocturnal dyspnea. Pulmonary crackles are first noted over the lung bases, and as the PAWP ranges between 18 and 25 mm Hg, they progress toward the apices.[5,44,63]

Stage 3 occurs when the PAWP rises to 25 to 28 mm Hg, causing rapid movement of fluid out of the intravascular and interstitial spaces into the alveoli. As the edema progresses, the alveoli no longer remain open owing to the large fluid accumulation. At this point, the alveolar–capillary membrane is disrupted, fluid invades the large airways, and the patient expectorates frothy, pink-tinged sputum. Acute pulmonary edema is a catastrophic indicator of HF.

Related to Right-Sided Heart Failure

Right-sided HF, associated with increased systemic venous pressure, gives rise to the clinical signs of jugular venous distention, hepatomegaly, dependent peripheral edema, and ascites.[5,58,62]

Dependent ascending peripheral edema is a manifestation in which edema begins in the lower legs and ascends to the thighs, genitalia, and abdominal wall. Patients may notice their shoes fitting tightly or marks left on the feet from their shoes or socks. Weight gain is what most patients recognize, and consistent morning daily weights help to detect any sudden weight gain. An adult may retain 10 to 15 lb (4 to 7 L) of fluid before pitting edema occurs.

Congestive hepatomegaly, characterized by a large, tender, pulsating liver, and ascites also occur. Liver engorgement is caused by venous engorgement, whereas ascites results from transudation of fluid from the capillaries into the abdominal cavity. Gastrointestinal complaints of nausea and anorexia may be a direct consequence of the increased intra-abdominal pressure.

Another finding related to fluid retention is diuresis at rest. When at rest, the body's metabolic requirements are decreased, and cardiac function improves. This decreases systemic venous pressure, allowing edema fluid to be mobilized and excreted. Table 22-2 lists the various subjective and objective indicators for LV and RV failure.

TABLE 22-2 Clinical Indicators and Physical Findings of Left and Right Ventricular Failure

Left Ventricular Failure	Right Ventricular Failure
Subjective Findings	
Breathlessness	Weight gain
Cough	Transient ankle swelling
Fatigue and weakness	Abdominal distention
Memory loss and confusion	Gastric distress
Diaphoresis	Anorexia, nausea
Palpitations	
Anorexia	
Insomnia	
Objective Findings	
Tachycardia	Neck vein pulsations and distention
Decreased S_1	Increased jugular venous pressure (increased central venous pressure), direct and indirect measurement
S_3 and S_4 gallops	
Crackles (rales)	
Pleural effusion	
Diaphoresis	Edema
Pulsus alternans	Hepatomegaly
Increased pulmonary artery wedge pressure	Positive hepatojugular reflux
	Ascites
Decreased cardiac index	
Increased systemic vascular resistance	

MEDICAL MANAGEMENT

The American College of Cardiology and the American Heart Association (ACC/AHA) have been involved in the joint development of practice guidelines for the evaluation and management of HF.[36]

Diagnostic Evaluation

All patients presenting with HF should undergo a diagnostic evaluation to (1) determine the type of cardiac dysfunction, (2) uncover correctable etiologic factors, (3) determine prognosis, and (4) guide treatment. Recognition of signs and symptoms resulting from an inadequate cardiac output and from systemic and pulmonary congestion is accomplished through a careful history, physical examination, routine laboratory analyses, and diagnostic studies.[27,36] Transthoracic Doppler two-dimensional echocardiography is of particular benefit for specifically assessing ventricular mass, chamber size, and systolic and diastolic dysfunction.[36,62,63]

PHYSICAL ASSESSMENT

A major goal in assessing the patient with HF is to determine the type and severity of the underlying disease causing HF and the extent of the HF syndrome. Physical examination of the patient with HF focuses on the cardiovascular and pulmonary systems and relevant aspects of gastrointestinal and skin assessment.[10,27,29]

Cardiovascular Assessment. Determination of the rate, rhythm, and character of the pulse is important in patients with HF. The pulse rate is usually elevated in response to a low cardiac output. Pulsus alternans (alternating pulse) is characterized by an altering strong and weak pulse with a normal rate and interval. Pulsus alternans is associated with altered functioning of the left ventricle causing variance in LV preload.

Increased heart size is common in patients with HF. This cardiac enlargement is detected by precordial palpation, with the apical impulse displaced laterally to the left and downward.

In patients with HF, there is a third heart sound (S_3) that is associated with a reduced ejection fraction and impaired diastolic function as determined by the peak filling rate.[54] A fourth heart sound (S_4) may occur, although it is not in itself a sign of failure but rather a reflection of decreased ventricular compliance associated with ischemic heart disease, high blood pressure, or hypertrophy. When the heart rate is rapid, these two diastolic sounds may merge into a single loud or summation gallop. Patients with HF frequently have a murmur of mitral regurgitation, which radiates to the axilla.[27]

Jugular venous pulses are a means of estimating venous pressure. The a and v waves both rise as the mean right atrial pressure rises. The hepatojugular reflux is also assessed. When the abdomen of a patient with RV failure is compressed, there is an increase in the forward flow of blood to the right atrium, causing the right atrial pressure to rise.

Pulmonary Examination. Persistently elevated PA pressures result in the transudation of fluid from the capillaries into the interstitial spaces and, eventually, into the alveolar spaces. The accumulated fluid results in pulmonary crackles. Initially, the crackles are heard at the most dependent portions of the lungs, but later, as pulmonary congestion increases, crackles become diffuse and are heard over the entire chest.

Integumentary Assessment. Patients with HF often present with dependent symmetric edema. It is most often detected in the feet, ankles, or sacral area. Color and temperature of the skin are also assessed, with major findings being pallor, decreased temperature, cyanosis, and diaphoresis.

Gastrointestinal Assessment. Characteristically, HF results in hepatomegaly. The liver span is increased and the liver is usually palpable well below the right costal margin. An enlarged spleen may also be palpated in advanced HF.

LABORATORY AND DIAGNOSTIC TESTS

A number of routine laboratory tests useful in the evaluation of HF are suggested in Table 22-3.[36,39] A chest radiograph

TABLE 22-3	Recommended Tests for Patients with Signs or Symptoms of Heart Failure[39]	
Test Recommendation	**Finding**	**Suspected Diagnosis**
Electrocardiogram	Acute ST–T wave changes	Myocardial ischemia
	Atrial fibrillation, other tachyarrhythmia	Thyroid disease or heart failure due to rapid ventricular rate
	Bradyarrhythmias	Heart failure due to low heart rate
	Previous myocardial infarction (e.g., Q waves)	Heart failure due to reduced left ventricular performance
	Low voltage	Pericardial effusion
	Left ventricular hypertrophy	Diastolic dysfunction
Complete blood count	Anemia	Heart failure due to or aggravated by decreased oxygen-carrying capacity
Urinalysis	Proteinuria	Nephrotic syndrome
	Red blood cells or cellular casts	Glomerulonephritis
Serum creatinine	Elevated	Volume overload due to renal failure
Serum albumin	Decreased	Increased extravascular volume due to hypoalbuminemia
T_4 and TSH (obtain only if atrial fibrillation, evidence of thyroid disease, or patient age >65 y)	Abnormal T_4 or TSH	Heart failure due to or aggravated by hypothyroidism/hyperthyroidism

T_4, thyroxine; TSH, thyroid-stimulating hormone.

should also be included to assess the size of the heart and the pulmonic vascular markings. The electrocardiogram (ECG) is not helpful in assessing the presence or degree of HF, but it demonstrates patterns of ventricular hypertrophy, arrhythmias, and any degree of myocardial ischemia, injury, or infarction.[31,62,63]

Laboratory tests include blood chemistries, complete blood count, and urinalysis. Electrolyte imbalances in HF reflect complications of failure as well as the use of diuretics and other drug therapy. Disturbances in sodium, potassium, and magnesium are particularly significant. In patients with severe HF, an increase in total-body water dilutes body fluid and is reflected by a decrease in the serum sodium. Diuretics may also contribute to this low serum sodium if fluid intake is not restricted. Hypokalemia, or low serum potassium level, and low serum magnesium may complicate HF as the result of the use of diuretics such as thiazides and furosemides because these diuretics may lead to excessive excretion of potassium and magnesium.[29,51] Hyperkalemia, or elevated potassium level, may occur secondary to depressed effective renal blood flow and low glomerular filtration rate.[29,63]

Any impairment of kidney function may be reflected by elevated blood urea nitrogen (BUN), creatinine, and uric acid. Elevated levels of bilirubin, serum glutamic oxaloacetic transaminase, and lactate dehydrogenase result from hepatic congestion. Urinalysis may reveal proteinuria, red blood cells, and high specific gravity.[29] Thyroid-stimulating hormone in patients with atrial fibrillation and unexplained HF may also be helpful.[36,39]

The arterial blood gases usually show a drop in PaO_2 (hypoxemia) and a low $PaCO_2$. In the clinical situation of

HF, the alveoli become filled with fluid, causing a decrease in PaO_2, whereas the compensatory attempt to increase the PO_2 by hyperventilating causes a decrease in the PCO_2, resulting in a mild respiratory alkalosis. Later changes due to decreased peripheral perfusion result in a build-up of lactic acid, causing metabolic acidosis.[63]

The cornerstone of evaluation is the transthoracic Doppler two-dimensional echocardiography. The echocardiogram is useful in diagnosing cardiac valvular changes, pericardial effusion, chamber enlargement, and ventricular hypertrophy. Radionuclide studies are a more precise and reliable measurement of ejection fraction (technetium pyrophosphate imaging or thallium scintigraphy) and have also become important in providing clues to the presence and etiology of HF[36,39] (Table 22-4). Both these studies are valuable in assessing systolic function and diastolic dysfunction.[31,36,58,63] Systolic dysfunction is defined as an ejection fraction of less than 35% to 40%. Diastolic dysfunction appears with concentric LV hypertrophy, left atrial enlargement, an ejection fraction of 45% to 55%, a reduced rate of LV filling, and a prolonged time to peak filling.[7,31]

If systolic function is normal, additional steps must be taken to diagnose diastolic dysfunction. Exclusion of other significant causes of dyspnea is important, and appropriate studies may include pulmonary function testing, noninvasive testing, and cardiac catheterization/coronary arteriography.

Noninvasive stress testing is used to detect ischemia in patients without angina, but with high probability of coronary artery disease (CAD) who would be candidates for revascularization. Cardiac catheterization/coronary arteriography is used in patients with angina or large areas of ischemic or hibernating myocardium. This is also the best

TABLE 22-4	Echocardiography and Radionuclide Ventriculography Compared in Evaluation of Left Ventricular Performance[39]	
Test	**Advantages**	**Disadvantages**
Echocardiogram	Permits concomitant assessment of valvular disease, left ventricular hypertrophy, and left atrial size Less expensive than radionuclide ventriculography in most areas Able to detect pericardial effusion and ventricular thrombus More generally available	Difficult to perform in patients with lung disease Usually only semiquantitative estimate of ejection fraction provided Technically inadequate in up to 18% of patients under optimal circumstances
Radionuclide ventriculogram	More precise and reliable measurement of ejection fraction Better assessment of right ventricular function	Required venipuncture and radiation exposure Limited assessment of valvular heart disease and left ventricular hypertrophy

quantitative evaluation of diastolic dysfunction and shows an increase in PAWP or LV end-diastolic pressure during exercise or volume loading.[36,39]

HEMODYNAMIC MONITORING

In seriously ill patients, direct determination of intra-arterial pressure with an arterial line is necessary because systemic arterial pressure determines the perfusion pressure of various organ systems and is predominantly the product of the cardiac output and SVR. In HF, a drop in cardiac output is compensated for by an increased SVR in an attempt to maintain the arterial blood pressure in normal range.[6,27,63]

Right-sided heart catheterization with a PA quadruple-lumen thermodilution catheter can aid in the diagnosis and assessment of the severity of HF.[24,25] The hemodynamic variables measured by this catheter are cardiac output by thermodilution, right atrial pressure, and PA systolic, diastolic, and wedge pressures. The cardiac output is decreased in HF, whereas the right atrial pressure or central venous pressure is either normal in LV failure or elevated in right HF. The PAWP indirectly measures the LV end-diastolic pressure, which is a measure of end-diastolic volume or preload and is elevated in HF.[24,73]

Derived parameters that may be obtained by the use of the PA catheter include cardiac index (CI) and SVR. Body surface area (BSA), measured in square meters, is correlated with the volume of cardiac output (CO) to establish the CI:

$$CI = \frac{CO}{BSA}$$

Systemic vascular resistance (SVR), measured in dynes/second/cm^{-5}, reflects the pressure difference of the systemic arteries to the veins.[36]

$$SVR = \frac{MAP - RAP}{CO} \times 80$$

where MAP is mean arterial pressure and RAP is right atrial pressure.

Besides offering diagnostic information, hemodynamic variables show a strong prognostic value for short-term survival. Forrester and colleagues[22] classified patients with acute MI into four subsets with different mortality rates (Table 22-5). They showed that clinical signs of hypoperfusion occur with a cardiac index of less than 2.2 L/min/m². Also, clinical signs of pulmonary congestion occur with a PAWP greater than 18 mm Hg. Subset II describes the patient in pulmonary edema with an elevated PAWP but

TABLE 22-5	Forrester Subsets: Relation of Hemodynamics to the Clinical State				
Subset	**Pulmonary Congestion**	**Peripheral Hypoperfusion**	**Cardiac Index**	**PAWP**	**% Mortality**
I	−	−	Normal	Normal	3
II	+	−	Normal	↑	9
III	−	+	↓	Normal	23
IV	+	+	↓	↑	51

−, without; +, with; ↑, increased; ↓, decreased; PAWP, pulmonary artery wedge pressure.
From Forrester JS, Diamond G, Chatterjee K et al: Medical therapy of acute myocardial infarction by application of hemodynamic subsets. N Engl J Med 295: 1362–1386, 1404–1413, 1976. Copyright © 1974 Massachussetts Medical Society. All rights reserved.

without peripheral hypoperfusion. Subset IV describes the patient with pulmonary edema with hypoperfusion (i.e., cardiogenic shock).[22,23]

Assessment of tissue metabolism, which is determined by mixed venous oxygen saturation, conventionally required sending a PA blood sample to the laboratory for interpretation. Some PA catheters are designed with a fiberoptic photometric lumen, allowing for continuous monitoring of mixed venous oxygen saturation.

CLASSIFICATION

After the history and physical examination are completed, the patient may be categorized according to the New York Heart Association's (NYHA) Cardiac Status and Prognosis Classification.[45] The four subdivisions are:

Cardiac Status	Prognosis
1. Uncompromised	1. Good
2. Slightly compromised	2. Good with therapy
3. Moderately compromised	3. Fair with therapy
4. Severely compromised	

The NYHA's Functional and Therapeutic Classification is still being used in the clinical setting.[20,45]

Treatment

Three major approaches have been developed for treating patients with HF.[9,36,58,62,63] The first is removal of the underlying cause, which may include surgical correction of structural abnormalities and medical treatment of such conditions as infective endocarditis and hypertension. The second approach is the removal of the precipitating cause, such as infections, arrhythmias, and pulmonary emboli. The third is the treatment and control of HF. Therapy for HF is directed at reducing the workload of the heart and manipulating the various factors that determine cardiac performance, such as contractility, heart rate, preload, and afterload.[29,53,62,63,74] Treatment of HF is based on the manner in which patients clinically present, which may encompass the extremes from acute HF with shock to asymptomatic LV dysfunction.

ACUTE HEART FAILURE IN ADULTS

Acute HF can be grouped clinically into acute cardiogenic pulmonary edema, cardiogenic shock, and acute decompensation of chronic left HF.[36] A detailed section on specific management is found in Chapter 24.

CHRONIC AND STABILIZED ACUTE HEART FAILURE IN ADULTS

Systolic Dysfunction. Coronary heart disease, hypertension, and dilated cardiomyopathy are the most commonly identified causes of LV systolic dysfunction. The combination of ischemia and LV dysfunction carries a poor prognosis, and it is this group that may benefit from revascularization.[35] Figure 22-7 presents the Agency for Health Care Policy and Research (AHCPR) guideline regarding evaluation and treatment of CAD in patients with HF.[39]

An additional, innovative treatment option for selected patients with advanced HF has been proposed. Partial left ventriculectomy (or volume reduction surgery) in patients with dilated hearts due to cardiomyopathy has improved clinical outcomes.[65] Cardiac transplantation plays a role in end-stage patients without contraindications to this operation.[74]

Pharmacologic approaches are presented in Figure 22-8, which reviews the AHCPR algorithm for drug management.[39,74] For mild dyspnea on exertion but no fluid overload, it is recommended to begin with a titrated dose of angiotensin-converting enzyme (ACE) inhibitor.[18,30,41,59,64]

Hydralazine and isosorbide dinitrate are used in patients who cannot take ACE inhibitors. Patients with mild dyspnea on exertion and volume overload should be initiated on both an ACE inhibitor and a diuretic.[17–19,41,64] Digoxin should be added for those patients not adequately responsive to ACE inhibitors and diuretic agents. Digoxin also should be considered in those patients with atrial fibrillation and rapid ventricular response.[1,76] In patients who do not respond to triple therapy, acceleration of diuretic therapy is recommended. Long-acting nitrates, with consideration of other therapies, such as peripheral alpha blocker (Prazosin; Pfizer Laboratories, New York, NY) or an angiotensin II receptor blocker (Losartan), may be appropriate.[47,74] Any patient with angina should use nitrates and aspirin. Table 22-6 list medications commonly used in HF.[39]

Routine anticoagulation with warfarin is not recommended but is appropriate for patients with atrial fibrillation, a previous history of systemic pulmonary embolism, or mobile ventricular thrombi.[36,39]

Beta blocker therapy for HF shows promise as a result of growing evidence that this group of drugs can reverse or slow the progressive LV dilatation that characterizes HF.[14,30,37,40] Carvedilol, a nonselective β-adrenergic blocker with peripheral vasodilating properties, may be added to the regimens of patients who are stabilized on a regimen of ACE inhibitors, diuretics, and digoxin and who are NYHA functional class 1 and 3.[4] Research studies are ongoing and will continue to change the official status of the use of this category of drugs.

Calcium channel blockers are not of proven benefit for patients with systolic dysfunction and may be harmful. Such risks may not extend to the use of longer-acting calcium channel blockers (e.g., amlodipine), which are undergoing further evaluation.[36,38] Low-dose dobutamine or milrinone on an outpatient basis may benefit patients with refractory HF.[3]

Diastolic Dysfunction. The treatment of HF due to diastolic dysfunction has both similarities and dissimilarities to the treatment of HF due to systolic dysfunction.[36,71] The first step is the treatment of the underlying cause. Ischemia is relieved through standard medical management and revascularization for CAD.[36,39] Control of systemic hypertension is important, with ACE inhibitors assisting in normalizing blood pressure and reducing LV mass in patients with hypertension-induced LV hypertrophy. When appropriate anticoagulation and antiarrhythmic agents are recommended for both systolic and diastolic dysfunction. Both calcium chan-

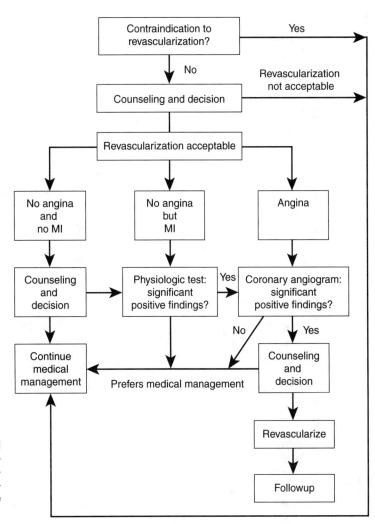

FIGURE 22-7 The Agency for Health Care Policy and Research (AHCPR) algorithm for evaluation and treatment of coronary artery disease patients with heart failure. The algorithm emphasizes the importance of determining if ischemic myocardium is present, so it can be addressed with revascularization.[39]

nel blockers and β-adrenergic blockers are useful in maintaining normal heart rates. The difference in pharmacologic therapy is that the goal of drug therapy in diastolic dysfunction is to reduce symptoms by lowering the elevated filling pressures without significantly reducing cardiac output.[7,36,71,74] Careful titration of low doses of diuretic drugs and nitrates can be used initially in symptomatic patients. Calcium channel blockers have important lusitropic effects that enhance ventricular relaxation, with verapamil usually the drug of choice.[7,23,31] β-adrenergic blockers also improve LV relaxation by decreasing myocardial oxygen consumption and ischemia.[14,40] Agents with positive inotropic actions are not indicated if systolic function is normal.[7,36,71]

SPECIFIC STRATEGIES

Angiotensin-Converting Enzyme Inhibitors.
The use of ACE inhibitors, such as captopril or enalapril, may be the most effective treatment of advanced congestive HF because ACE inhibitors block the formation of angiotensin II (reducing afterload), inhibit the release of aldosterone (inhibiting sodium retention), and produce venodilation (reducing preload).[47,56] The administration of captopril or enalapril also reduces the frequency and complexity of ventricular arrhythmias and is associated with an increase in total-body and cir-

culating levels of potassium and a decrease in circulating catecholamines.[11,12,60,69] These agents are the only drugs used in the treatment of chronic HF that have been shown both to improve symptoms and prolong life.[18,19,34,41,64] The unique characteristics of the ACE inhibitors support the use of captopril or enalapril as first-line drugs in all patients with HF, regardless of the severity of symptoms.[36,39,50,62,64,74]

Diuretics.
Diuretics and dietary salt restriction exert their primary benefit by decreasing extracellular water and intravascular blood volume.[9,48,72] The elimination of dependent edema helps reduce tissue pressure, opposing venous pooling and therefore improving the capacitance of the venous system. Similarly, the decrease in intravascular volume also reduces ventricular preload directly and thereby helps to diminish the filling pressures in both the pulmonary and systemic circulations.[9] Mechanical removal of fluid usually is not required in acute HF, but it may be required in chronic failure. If fluid collects in serous cavities, thoracentesis, paracentesis, or dialysis may be necessary. Phlebotomy is a technique rarely used.

Positive Inotropics.
Myocardial contractility can be enhanced by the use of inotropic agents that, in the presence of HF, increase cardiac output and decrease ventricular filling pressure.[28,40] The agents used for a positive inotropic

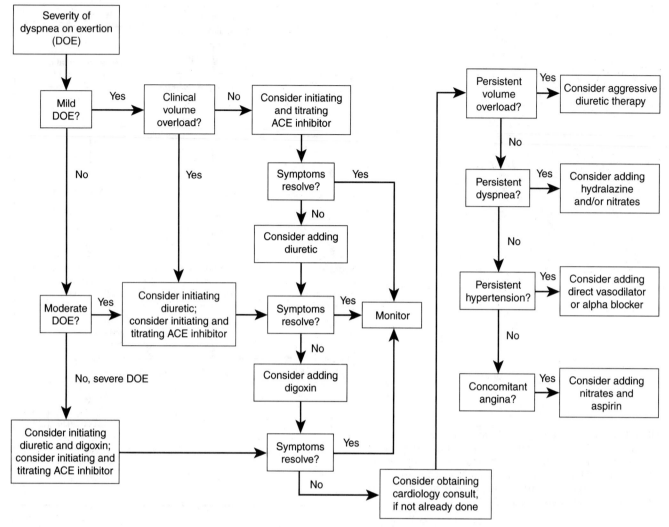

FIGURE 22-8 The AHCPR algorithm for pharmacologic management of heart failure patients focuses largely on symptomatic out-of-hospital patients with suspected heart failure. In these patients, initiating diuretic and ACE inhibitor therapy is initially recommended, with addition of digoxin and other vasodilating agents.

effect are (1) digitalis glycosides; (2) sympathomimetic agents, such as dopamine or dobutamine; and (3) phosphodiesterase inhibitors, such as amrinone or milrinone.[4]

Digitalis is given to improve contractility and increase cardiac output, which results in reduction of pulmonary vascular congestion and central venous pressure.[1,9,28,42,43,76] Sympathomimetic agents, such as dobutamine, produce systemic vasodilatation as well as having a powerful inotropic effect, which increases cardiac output and significantly decreases ventricular filling pressure. In contrast, dopamine, which tends to liberate norepinephrine and thereby increase systemic impedance, increases cardiac output in some patients with HF but provides little change or an increase in ventricular filling pressure. Sympathomimetic agents are most effective in cases in which the β-adrenergic receptors are fully responsive.[43] In severe chronic failure, when a β-adrenergic receptor response is lost, phosphodiesterase inhibitors may have a role. These agents, such as amrinone

and milrinone, with mixed inotropic–vasodilator effects ("inodilators"), inhibit the breakdown of cyclic adenosine monophosphate in cardiac and peripheral vascular smooth muscle, resulting in augmented myocardial contractility and peripheral arterial and venous vasodilatation.[3,22,43]

**Vasodilator Therapy.** The venous and arterial beds are often inappropriately constricted. Venoconstriction tends to displace blood in the thorax, causing pulmonary congestion, whereas arteriolar constriction increases the impedance to LV emptying. Arteriolar dilatation results in a reduction of afterload and may augment cardiac output, whereas venodilatation tends to produce a reduction in preload, lower ventricular filling pressure, and reduce symptoms of pulmonary congestion. Vasodilators may be separated into three categories: venous dilators (preload reducers), arterial dilators (afterload reducers), and mixed venous and arterial dilators (preload and afterload reducers).[8,9,13]

TABLE 22-6	Medications Commonly Used for Heart Failure[39]			
Drug	**Initial Dose (mg)**	**Target Dosage (mg)**	**Recommended Maximal Dosage (mg)**	**Major Adverse Reactions**
Thiazide diuretics				Postural hypotension, hypokalemia, hyperglycemia, hyperuricemia, rash. Rare severe reaction includes pancreatitis, bone marrow suppression, and anaphylaxis.
Hydrochlorothiazide	25 qd	As needed	50 qd	
Chlorthalidone	25 qd	As needed	50 qd	
Loop diuretics				
Furosemide	10–40 qd	As needed	240 bid	Same as thiazide diuretics.
Bumetanide	0.5–1.0 qd	As needed	10 qd	
Ethacrynic acid	50 qd	As needed	200 bid	
Thiazide-related diuretic				
Metolazone	2.5*	As needed	10 qd	Same as thiazide diuretics.
Potassium-sparing diuretics				
Spironolactone	25 qd	As needed	100 bid	Hyperkalemia, especially if administered with ACE inhibitor; rash; gynecomastia (spironolactone only).
Triamterene	50 qd	As needed	100 bid	
Amiloride	5 qd	As needed	40 qd	
ACE inhibitors				
Enalapril	2.5 bid	10 bid	20 bid	Hypotension, hyperkalemia, renal insufficiency, cough, skin rash, angioedema, neutropenia.
Captopril	6.25–12.5 tid	50 tid	100 tid	
Lisinopril	5 qd	20 qd	40 qd	
Quinapril	5 bid	20 bid	20 bid	
Digoxin	0.125 qd	As needed	As needed	Cardiotoxicity, confusion, nausea, anorexia, visual disturbances.
Hydralazine	10–25 tid	75 tid	100 tid	Headache, nausea, dizziness, tachycardia, lupus-like syndrome.
Isosorbide dinitrate	10 tid	40 tid	80 tid	Headache, hypotension, flushing.

ACE, angiotensin-converting enzyme.
  *Given as a single test dose initially.

VENOUS DILATORS. Nitroglycerin and the closely related isosorbide dinitrate are primarily reducers of preload because they dilate the systemic veins and reduce venous return, ultimately to reduce LV filling pressure.[2,52,66]

ARTERIAL DILATORS. As a direct arteriolar vasodilator with direct inotropic effects, hydralazine can improve LV function by reducing afterload and myocardial oxygen consumption, augment stroke volume, and improve cardiac output.[18,47,74]

MIXED VENOUS AND ARTERIAL DILATORS. Other vasodilators that provide combined preload and afterload reduction include ACE inhibitors, such as captopril or enalapril, prazosin, and nitroprusside.[47] Prazosin, an α-adrenergic blocking agent established for hypertension, has been tried in refractory HF. Acting as an "oral nitroprusside," prazosin dilates peripheral arterial and venous systems. Prazosin, however, produces neither symptomatic nor prognostic benefits in HF.[20,41,50]

Intravenous nitroprusside remains the drug of choice for severe, low-output, left-sided HF because it acts rapidly and has a balanced effect, dilating both veins and arterioles.[26] It is particularly useful in severe refractory HF caused by aortic or mitral valve incompetence.[47]

The combined effect of preload and afterload reduction can also be achieved by the administration of both hydralazine and isosorbide dinitrate. Giving this combination to patients with mild to moderate HF maintained on a regimen of diuretics and digoxin produced moderate but clinically significant improvement in survival. This benefit was particularly prominent in younger patients with a low ejection fraction, those with a history of hypertension, and those without a history of alcohol abuse.[16,17,41]

Table 22-7 compares the effects of selected agents that unload the heart and are used in HF.

Angiotensin II Receptor Blocker. An alternative to an ACE inhibitor may be a specific angiotensin II receptor blocker.[14,37] Hemodynamic effects are similar to those of ACE inhibitors with respect to reducing preload and afterload and increasing cardiac output. Losartan is usually started at an initial dose of 25 mg qd and titrated between 50 to 100 mg qd. Several large-scale studies are ongoing that may answer many questions concerning this group of agents.[21,47,74]

β-Adrenergic Blockers. Excessive neurohormonal activity in HF can be blunted by β-adrenergic blocker.[14,37] As a result of increased myocardial interstitial norepinephrine concentration, poor LV dysfunction is associated with several changes in the β-adrenergic receptor complex. These include β_1 receptor downregulation and uncoupling of the

TABLE 22-7   **Comparative Effects of Agents for Unloading the Heart and for Heart Failure**

Agent	Preload (Peripheral Veins)	Afterload (Peripheral Arteries)	Direct Inotropic Effect	Heart Rate	Proposed Indication
Nitrates	+++	+	0	↑ or 0	Backward LV failure; pulmonary edema
Hydralazine (Apresoline)	0	+++	+	↑ or 0 (↑↑ if no failure)	Chronic forward failure (except valvular stenosis)
Nifedipine (Procardia)	+	+++	0	↑ or 0	Acute LV failure with pulmonary edema
Nitroprusside (Nipride)	+++	+++	0	0	Heart failure of acute myocardial infarction or regurgitant valves
Captopril (Capoten)	+	+	0	↑	LV failure
Prazosin (Minipress)	+	+	0	↓ or 0	Forward and backward failure (except valvular stenosis)

+, dilatation; ↑, increase; ↓, decrease; LV, left ventricular.

Adapted from Opie LH: Drugs for the heart: Vasodilating drugs. Lancet (8175): 968, 1980, and Opie LH (ed): Drugs for the Heart, pp 135–137. Orlando, Grune & Stratton, 1984.

β_2 receptor.[27] In patients with HF, the outcome of these changes is a reduction in myocyte contractility with an associated diminished ability to respond to dynamic stress, resulting in chronic fatigue. Carvedilol, a nonselective β-adrenergic blocker with α_1-adrenergic receptor blockade, reduces mortality, slows progression of disease, and improves quality of life in patients with HF when added to standard therapy. Indicated for NYHA functional class 2 to 3 patients with systolic dysfunction, this medication is titrated for patients who are receiving standard therapy and are clinically stable. The starting dose is 3.125 mg bid for 2 weeks. It may be doubled every 2 weeks to a maximum of 50 mg bid in patients weighing more than 85 kg, or 25 mg bid in those weighing less than 85 kg.[4,74]

Calcium Channel Blockers. The net benefits of calcium channel blocker use lay in their ability to decrease afterload and their anti-ischemic effects.[38,55] Calcium channel blockers are a diverse group of agents with complex actions. They do not seem to have a place in systolic dysfunction and may be harmful, although risks may not accompany the use of the longer-acting agent, amlodipine, which is undergoing further evaluation.[36,39,74] Calcium channel blockers may be of benefit in diastolic dysfunction because of improvement of diastolic relaxation, control of blood pressure, and prevention of myocardial ischemia, and they may reverse LV hypertrophy.[7,36,38,71]

Antiarrhythmics. Heart failure is the most arrhythmogenic disorder in cardiovascular disease.[51] Management of arrhythmias in this group of patients is difficult and remains far from satisfactory. Nearly all patients with HF experience frequent and complex ventricular tachyarrhythmias, and the imminent risk of sudden death appears to be present for all patients with HF.[36,49,74] Experimental and clinical evidence indicates that circulatory neurohormones and electrolyte deficits (potassium and magnesium) interact to provoke malignant ventricular ectopic rhythms. Intravenous magnesium administration has been shown to decrease the frequency of ventricular arrhythmias, but the use of oral magnesium needs more investigation.[33] In addition to oral magnesium supplements, use of amiodarone and beta blockers in the prevention of sudden cardiac death is being explored, although use of beta blockers in HF remains controversial.[37,75] Class 1 antiarrhythmics appear unpromising or even harmful.[70,75] If the use of antiarrhythmic agents is considered, the ventricular contractile depressant effects of many antiarrhythmics must be considered and may best be guided with an antiarrhythmic drug selected by invasive electrophysiologic testing. Nonpharmacologic therapy for symptomatic ventricular tachyarrhythmias may include implantation of an automatic implantable cardioverter-defibrillator, radiofrequency ablation therapy of ectopic foci, or arrhythmia surgery.[67]

Patients with HF and atrial fibrillation should have their ventricular rate controlled. Multiple drugs may be necessary, such as digoxin, diltiazem, or a β-adrenergic blocker. Positive inotropics should be avoided in diastolic dysfunction if possible.[36,71] New-onset atrial fibrillation should be converted to normal sinus rhythm.

Amiodarone or catheter ablation or modification of the atrioventricular node with use of a pacemaker may be necessary.

Prognosis

The prognosis of systolic dysfunction is poor, with a 5-year survival rate of approximately 40% in most studies, compared with 70% with isolated diastolic dysfunction. Diastolic dysfunction often precedes systolic dysfunction. However, when systolic dysfunction ensues, the HF is usually in the advanced state and has a poor outcome.[23]

NURSING MANAGEMENT

Whether the setting is a clinic, hospital, nursing home, or patient's home, the nurse cares for patients in some phase of HF. The nurse may be the first person to assess the presence of HF. The best means of controlling HF is through early detection and treatment of predisposing factors. Early detection of high blood pressure, arteriosclerosis and atherosclerosis, valvular disorders, and congenital anomalies may ensure early treatment of the patient and prevention of complications.

A major goal of assessing the patient in HF is to determine the type and severity of the underlying disease and the extent of the syndrome. Identification of the early onset of HF may allow therapeutic means to be instituted on an ambulatory basis. When the client is admitted to the hospital, the problems associated with HF may have become more advanced and may require supervised administration of medications as well as other measures to reduce edema and improve myocardial performance.

The overall plan of care for patients with HF is to reduce cardiac workload, improve cardiac output, prevent complications, and educate the patient regarding follow-up care. Display 22-1 presents topics for patient, family, and caregiver education from the AHCPR guidelines.[39]

Analysis of Medical and Nursing Assessment Data and Formulation of Nursing Diagnoses

Based on the assessment data, including medical and nursing histories, physical examination, hemodynamic monitoring, and diagnostic tests, the most common nursing diagnoses for the patient with HF are (1) decreased cardiac output; (2) altered respiratory function, including ineffective breathing patterns, ineffective airway clearance, and impaired gas exchange; (3) fluid volume excess; and (4) altered nutrition: less than body requirements.

DECREASED CARDIAC OUTPUT

Diagnosis. This diagnosis can be stated as: decreased cardiac output, related to an inability of the heart to pump effectively associated with myocardial damage or hypertrophy, manifested by decrease in blood pressure; increase in heart rate; cool, clammy skin; decreased urine output; and decreased level of consciousness.

Goals. Possible goals for this diagnosis include:

1. To detect specific early manifestations of decreased cardiac output
2. To reduce or eliminate specific manifestations of decreased cardiac output
3. To prevent symptoms of decreased cardiac output

Interventions. Interventions are designed to detect the manifestations of the imbalance between myocardial oxygen supply and demand and to improve cardiac output. Interventions to meet this goal include the following.

FOR GOAL 1. Assess the blood pressure, apical-radial heart rate, cardiac rhythm, lung sounds, heart sounds, level of consciousness, urine output, and condition of the skin every 4 hours or more frequently as indicated by the patient's condition. Monitor ECG readings, continuously assessing heart rate and rhythm, and document ECG

DISPLAY 22-1

Suggested Topics for Patient, Family, and Caregiver Education and Counseling[39]

GENERAL COUNSELING

Explanation of heart failure and the reason for symptoms
Cause or probable cause of heart failure
Expected symptoms
Symptoms of worsening heart failure
What to do if symptoms worsen
Self-monitoring with daily weights
Explanation of treatment/care plan
Clarification of patient's responsibilities
Importance of cessation of tobacco use
Role of family members or other caregivers in the treatment/care plan
Availability and value of qualified local support group
Importance of obtaining vaccinations against influenza and pneumococcal disease

PROGNOSIS

Life expectancy
Advance directives
Advice for family members in the event of sudden death

ACTIVITY RECOMMENDATIONS

Recreation, leisure, and work activity
Exercise
Sex, sexual difficulties, and coping strategies

DIETARY RECOMMENDATIONS

Sodium restriction
Avoidance of excessive fluid intake
Fluid restriction (if required)
Alcohol restriction

MEDICATIONS

Effects of medications on quality of life and survival
Dosing
Likely side effects and what to do if they occur
Coping mechanisms for complicated medical regimens
Availability of lower-cost medications or financial assistance

IMPORTANCE OF COMPLIANCE WITH THE TREATMENT/CARE PLAN

---

rhythm strips every 4 hours and with conduction disturbances or arrhythmias. Obtain a chest radiograph. For patients with hemodynamic monitoring with a PA catheter, assess the preload and afterload parameters by obtaining right atrial or PA diastolic or wedge pressures, and the derived parameters of SVR. Obtain cardiac output readings in relation to other physical findings and in relation to titration of vasoactive medications. Assess, document, and report to the physician the following: drop of 20 mm Hg in systolic pressure, a systolic pressure below 80 mm Hg, or a mean arterial pressure less than 60 mm Hg; presence of new S_3 or S_4 gallops; new or increasing crackles; urine output less than 30 mL/h; decreased cardiac output (<4 L/min) or cardiac index (<2.2 L/min/m²); increased PAWP (>18 mm Hg); and significant change in mental status.

FOR GOAL 2. Perform actions to reduce cardiac workload. Place the patient in a semi- to high Fowler's position; administer oxygen and other medications, including positive inotropic agents (to improve contractility), venodilators (to reduce preload), arterial dilators (to decrease afterload), balanced vasodilators (to decrease preload and afterload), and ACE inhibitors (to decrease SVR and venous tone) as ordered and evaluate the patient's response to therapy; and provide a restful environment.

FOR GOAL 3. Instruct the patient to avoid activities that create a Valsalva response; provide frequent, small meals low in sodium; discourage smoking and intake of caffeine-containing foods and beverages; and gradually increase activities of daily living.

Outcome Criteria. Outcome criteria are written for each goal statement.

FOR GOAL 1. Signs and symptoms of HF are detected at onset.

FOR GOAL 2. Immediately after intervention, the client has improved cardiac output as evidenced by blood pressure within normal range for patient; apical pulse audible, regular, and between 60 and 100 beats/min; resolution of S_3 or S_4 gallops, which disappear or do not increase in intensity; crackles absent or reduced; urine output at least 30 mL/h; decrease in peripheral edema; mental status improving; and hemodynamic parameters returning to a normal range.

FOR GOAL 3. Patient appears comfortable; heart rate, respiratory rates, blood pressure, and hemodynamic parameters are within patient's normal range; no S_3 or S_4 gallops; skin is warm and dry and without edema; no crackles; and activity tolerance is maintained.

ALTERED RESPIRATORY FUNCTION

Diagnosis. This diagnosis includes the following diagnostic labels: ineffective breathing pattern, ineffective airway clearance, and impaired gas exchange. This diagnosis can be stated three ways:

1. Ineffective breathing pattern related to loss of alveolar elasticity owing to vascular engorgement, restricted lung expansion from pleural effusion, and respiratory depressant effect of hypoxia or hypercapnia, as manifested by tachypnea, orthopnea, or hyperventilation
2. Ineffective airway clearance related to fluid accumulation associated with pulmonary edema, as manifested by ineffective cough, dyspnea, cyanosis, pallor, and abnormal breath sounds
3. Impaired gas exchange related to ineffective breathing patterns and airway clearance and decreased systemic tissue perfusion associated with decreased cardiac output, as manifested by decreased oxygen content, increased PCO_2, cyanosis, lethargy, and fatigue

Goals. Goals for this diagnosis include:

1. To detect specific early manifestations and etiologies of altered respiratory function
2. To reduce or eliminate specific manifestations of altered respiratory function
3. To prevent when possible specific manifestations of altered respiratory function

Interventions. Interventions are designed to detect the manifestations of alterations in respiratory function and maintain adequate ventilatory exchange. Interventions to meet each goal include the following.

FOR GOAL 1. On admission, every 4 hours, and during respiratory distress, assess, document, and report to the physician the following: abnormal arterial blood gases; diminished or absent breath sounds; adventitious breath sounds (crackles, wheezes, rhonchi); dyspnea or orthopnea; confusion or somnolence; and persistent cough productive of frothy or blood-tinged sputum.

FOR GOAL 2. Immediately implement measures to improve respiratory status. Place the patient in a semi- to high Fowler's position; administer oxygen; instruct patient to deep breathe every hour; and perform actions to improve cardiac status. (Refer to first diagnosis in this section.) Monitor for therapeutic and nontherapeutic effects of the following if administered: medications to improve cardiac output (refer to first diagnosis in this section); diuretics (decrease pulmonary fluid accumulation); morphine sulfate (decreases pulmonary vascular congestion); and aminophylline (dilates bronchioles, promotes diuresis).

FOR GOAL 3. To facilitate removal of pulmonary secretions: instruct and assist patient to cough every 1 to 2 hours; humidify inspired air as ordered; assist with administration of mucolytic agents by nebulizer; assist with or perform postural drainage; and perform tracheal suctioning if needed. Instruct the patient to avoid intake of gas-forming foods and large meals to prevent gastric distention and a further increase in pressure on the diaphragm.

Outcome Criteria. Specific outcome criteria are written for each goal statement.

FOR GOAL 1. Specific signs and symptoms of alteration in respiratory function are detected within 4 hours of onset of respiratory distress.

FOR GOAL 2. After interventions, the patient experiences adequate respiratory function as evidenced by normal rate, rhythm, and depth of respirations; decreased dyspnea; usual or improved breath sounds; and improving blood gases.

FOR GOAL 3. Patient denies dyspnea, orthopnea, shortness of breath; patient appears comfortable; respiratory rate, rhythm, and depth are within normal range; no adventitious breath sounds are heard; skin color is normal, and skin is warm and dry; and blood gases are within normal range.

FLUID VOLUME EXCESS

Diagnosis. This diagnosis can be stated as: fluid volume excess related to high levels of aldosterone and antidiuretic hormone associated with decreased renal blood flow, manifested by edema, weight gain, increased venous filling pressures, and intake greater than output.

Goals. Goals for this diagnosis include:

1. To detect early specific manifestations and etiologies of fluid volume excess
2. To reduce or eliminate specific manifestations of fluid volume excess
3. To prevent when possible specific manifestations of fluid volume excess

Interventions. Interventions are designed to detect the manifestations of fluid volume overload and to stabilize the fluid volume. Interventions to meet each goal include the following.

FOR GOAL 1. On admission and every 4 hours, assess, document, and report to the physician the following: history of significant weight gain (>0.5 kg/d); developing or worsening S_3; intake greater than output; low serum osmolality; distended neck veins; dyspnea, orthopnea; rales and diminished or absent breath sounds; and peripheral edema.

FOR GOAL 2. Implement measures to reduce fluid volume excess, including: maintain fluid restriction as ordered; and restrict sodium intake as ordered (usually 2 to 3 g/d). Monitor for therapeutic and nontherapeutic effects of diuretics (to increase excretion of water) and positive inotropic agents and arterial dilators (to improve renal blood flow).

FOR GOAL 3. Teach dietary restrictions of sodium and fluid intake, provide a diet high in protein; instruct patient to record weight daily; and assist the patient with activities of daily living.

Outcome Criteria. Outcome criteria are written for each goal statement.

FOR GOAL 1. Signs and symptoms of fluid overload are detected on onset.

FOR GOAL 2. After intervention, the patient shows resolution of fluid imbalance as evidenced by decline in weight toward patient's normal; resolution of S_3; less labored respirations; improved breath sounds; further balancing of intake and output; resolution of peripheral edema and neck vein distention; and serum osmolality returning to normal range.

FOR GOAL 3. Patient maintains normal weight; no S_3; no crackles; balanced intake and output; no peripheral edema; and normal serum osmolality.

ALTERED NUTRITION: LESS THAN BODY REQUIREMENTS

Diagnosis. The diagnosis can be stated as: altered nutrition: less than body requirements related to decreased oral intake, loss of nutrients with vomiting, and impaired absorption and transport of nutrients, manifested by anorexia, nausea, weakness, fatigue, and decreased serum albumin.

Goals. Goals for this diagnosis include:

1. To detect early the signs and symptoms of malnutrition
2. To reduce or eliminate malnutrition
3. To prevent malnutrition, when possible

Interventions. Interventions are designed to detect the manifestations of malnutrition and to improve the nutritional status of the patient.

FOR GOAL 1. On admission, assess the patient for signs and symptoms of malnutrition, including dry weight below normal for patient's age, height, and build; decreased BUN and serum albumin; and weakness and fatigue.

FOR GOAL 2. Implement measures to improve oral intake; implement measures to relieve nausea and vomiting; provide oral care before meals; serve small portions of nutritious foods and fluids within dietary restrictions of sodium management; place client in high Fowler's position for meals; and allow adequate time for meals.

FOR GOAL 3. Instruct patient to use herbs, spices, and salt substitutes rather than salt; encourage rest periods before meals; and obtain a dietary consult if necessary to assist patient in selecting foods and fluids.

Outcome Criteria. Specific outcome criteria are written for each goal statement.

FOR GOAL 1. Specific signs and symptoms of malnutrition are detected within 24 hours of admission.

FOR GOAL 2. After intervention, the patient progresses toward an adequate nutritional state as evidenced by dry weight within normal range for patient's age, height, and build (dry weight is achieved after fluid volume excess has been resolved); BUN and serum albumin are normal; and strength and activity tolerance are improved.

FOR GOAL 3. The patient maintains an adequate nutritional status and verbalizes an understanding of the rationale for and constituents of a diet low in sodium, saturated fat, and cholesterol but adequate in protein.

REFERENCES

1. Antman EM, Smith TW: Pharmacokinetics of digitalis glycosides. In Smith TW (ed): Digitalis Glycosides. Orlando, Grune & Stratton, 1985
2. Armstrong PW, Armstrong JA, Marks GS: Pharmacokinetic-hemodynamic studies of intravenous nitroglycerin in congestive heart failure. Circulation 62: 160–166, 1980
3. Benotti JR, Grossman W, Braunwald E: Hemodynamic assessment of amrinone: A new inotropic agent. N Engl J Med 299: 1373–1378, 1978
4. Bleske BE, Gilbert EM, Munger MA: Carvedilol: Therapeutic application and practice guidelines. Pharmacotherapy 18: 729–737, 1998

5. Braunwald E: Clinical aspects of heart failure. In Braunwald E (ed): Heart Disease: A Textbook of Cardiovascular Medicine, pp 444–463. Philadelphia, WB Saunders, 1992

6. Braunwald E: Pathophysiology of heart failure. In Braunwald E (ed): Heart Disease: A Textbook of Cardiovascular Medicine, pp 393–418. Philadelphia, WB Saunders, 1992

7. Cash LA: Heart failure from diastolic dysfunction. Dimensions of Critical Care Nursing 15(4): 170–177, 1996

8. Chatterjee K: Vasodilator therapy for heart failure. In Cohn JN (ed): Drug Treatment of Heart Failure, pp 151–173. New York, Yorke Medical Books, 1983

9. Chesebro J: Cardiac failure: Medical management. In Giuliani ER, Fuster V, Gersch BJ, et al (eds): Cardiology: Fundamentals and Practice, pp 814–846. St. Louis, Mosby-Year Book, 1991

10. Chesebro J, Burnett JC: Cardiac failure: Characteristics and clinical manifestations. In Giuliani ER, Fuster V, Gersch BJ, et al (eds): Cardiology: Fundamentals and Practice, pp 793–813. St. Louis, Mosby-Year Book, 1991

11. Cleland JGF, Dargie HJ, Ball SG et al: Effects of enalapril in heart failure: A double blind study of effects on exercise performance, renal function, hormones, and metabolic state. Br Heart J 54: 305–312, 1985

12. Cleland JGF, Dargie HJ, Hadsman GP et al: Captopril in heart failure: A double blind controlled trial. Br Heart J 52: 530–535, 1980

13. Cody RJ, Laragh JH: The role of the renin-angiotensin-aldosterone system in the pathophysiology of chronic heart failure. In Cohn JN (ed): Drug Treatment of Heart Failure, pp 35–51. New York, Yorke Medical Books, 1983

14. Cohn JN: Beta-blockers in heart failure. Eur Heart J 19(Suppl F): F52–F55, 1998

15. Cohn JN: Future directions in vasodilator therapy for heart failure. Am Heart J 123: 969–974, 1991

16. Cohn JN, Archibald DG, Francis GS et al: Veterans Administration Cooperative Study on vasodilator therapy of heart failure: Influence of prerandomization variables on the reduction of mortality by treatment with hydralazine and isosorbide dinitrate. Circulation 75(5) (Part II): 49–54, 1987

17. Cohn JN, Archibald DG, Ziesche S et al: Effects of vasodilator therapy on mortality in chronic congestive heart failure: Results of a Veterans Administration Cooperative Study. N Engl J Med 314: 1547–1552, 1986

18. Cohn JN, Johnson G, Ziesche S et al: A comparison of enalapril with hydralazine-isosorbide dinitrate in the treatment of chronic congestive heart failure. N Engl J Med 325: 303–310, 1991

19. CONSENSUS Trial Study Group: Effects of enalapril on mortality of chronic congestive heart failure: Results of a Cooperative North Scandinavian Enalapril Survival Study. N Engl J Med 316: 1429, 1987

20. Colucci WS: Alpha adrenergic receptor blockade with prazosin. Ann Intern Med 97: 67–77, 1982

21. Crozier I, Ikram H, Anwan N et al: Losartan in heart failure: Hemodynamic effects and tolerability. Losartan Hemodynamic Study Group. Circulation 91:291–297, 1995

22. DiBianco R, Shabetai R, Kostuk W et al: A comparison of oral milrinone, digoxin and their combination in the treatment of patients with chronic heart failure. N Engl J Med 320: 677–683, 1989

23. Federman M, Hess OM: Differentiation between systolic and diastolic dysfunction. Eur Heart J 15(Suppl D): D2–D6, 1994

24. Forrester JS, Diamond G, Chatterjee K et al: Medical therapy of acute myocardial infarction by application of hemodynamic subsets. N Engl J Med 295: 1362–1386, 1404–1413, 1976

25. Forrester J, Walter D: Hospital treatment of congestive heart failure: Management of hemodynamic profile. Am J Med 65: 173–179, 1978

26. Franciosa JA, Dunkman WB, Wilen W et al: Optimal left ventricular filling pressure during nitroprusside infusion for congestive heart failure. Am J Med 74: 457–464, 1983

27. Francis GS: Pathophysiology of the heart failure clinical syndrome. In Topol EJ (ed): Textbook of Cardiovascular Medicine, pp 2179–2203. Philadelphia, Lippincott-Raven, 1998

28. Francis GS: The role of inotropic agents in the management of heart failure. In Cohn JN (ed): Drug Treatment of Heart Failure, pp 73–89. New York, Yorke Medical Books, 1983

29. Gazes PC: Cardiac failure in adults. In Gazes PC (ed): Clinical Cardiology, 3rd ed, pp 469–522. Chicago, Year Book, 1990

30. Gheorghiade M, Benatar D, Konstam MA et al: Pharmacotherapy for systolic dysfunction: A review of randomized clinical trials. Am J Cardiol 80(Suppl 8B): 14H–27H, 1997

31. Goldsmith SR, Dick C: Differentiating systolic from diastolic heart failure: Pathophysiologic and therapeutic considerations. Am J Med 95:645–654, 1993

32. Goldsmith SR, Francis GS, Cowley AW et al: Increased plasma arginine vasopressin in patients with congestive heart failure. J Am Coll Cardiol 1: 1385–1390, 1983

33. Gottlieb SS, Fisher ML, Pressel MD et al: Effects of intravenous magnesium sulfate on arrhythmias in patients with congestive heart failure. Am Heart J 125: 1645–1650, 1993

34. Gorkin L, Norvell NK, Rosen RC et al: Assessment of quality of life as observed from the baseline data of the Studies of Left Ventricular Dysfunction (SOLVD) trial quality-of-life substudy. Am J Cardiol 71: 1069–1073, 1993

35. Guidelines and indications for coronary artery bypass graft surgery: A report of the American College of Cardiology/American Heart Association Task Force on Assessment of Diagnostic and Therapeutic Cardiovascular Procedures. J Am Coll Cardiol 17: 543–89, 1991

36. Guidelines for the evaluation and management of heart failure: A report of the American College of Cardiology/American Heart Association Task Force on Practice Guidelines (Committee on Evaluation and Management of Heart Failure). J Am Coll Cardiol 26: 1376–1398, 1995

37. Ikram H, Fitzpatrick D, Crozier IG: Therapeutic controversies with use of beta-adrenoreceptor blockade in heart failure. Am J Cardiol 71: 54C–60C, 1993

38. Iliceto S: Left ventricular dysfunction: Which role for calcium antagonist? Eur Heart J 18(Suppl A): A87–A91, 1997

39. Konstam M, Dracup K, Baker D et al: Heart failure: Management of patients with left-ventricular systolic dysfunction. Quick Reference Guide for Clinicians No. 11. AHCPR publication no. 94-0613. Rockville, MD, Agency for Health Care Policy and Research, Public Health Service, U.S. Department of Health and Human Services, June 1994

40. Lechat P, Packer M, Chalon S et al: Clinical effects of β-adrenergic blockade in chronic heart failure: A meta-analysis of double blind, placebo-controlled, randomized trials. Circulation 98: 1184–1191, 1998

41. Loeb HS, Johnson G, Henrick A et al: Effect of enalapril, hydralazine plus isosorbide dinitrate, and prazosin on hospitalization in patients with chronic congestive heart failure: The V-HeFT VA Cooperative Studies Group. Circulation 87 (Suppl 6): VI78–V187, 1993

42. Marcus FI: The use of digitalis for the treatment of congestive heart failure: A tale of its decline and resurrection. Cardiovasc Drug Ther 3: 473–476, 1989

43. Marcus FI, Opie LH, Sonnenblick EH: Digitalis and other inotropes. In Opie LH (ed): Drugs for the Heart, pp 129–154. Philadelphia, WB Saunders, 1991

44. Michaelson CR: Pathophysiology of heart failure: A conceptual framework for understanding clinical indicators and therapeutic modalities. In Michaelson CR (ed): Congestive Heart Failure, pp 44–83. St Louis, CV Mosby, 1983

45. New York Heart Association Criteria Committee: Major changes made by Criteria Committee of the New York Heart Association. Circulation 49: 390, 1974

46. Opie LH: The Heart, pp 301–313. London, Grune & Stratton, 1984

47. Opie LH, Chatterjee K, Poole-Wilson PA: Angiotensin converting enzyme inhibitors and conventional vasodilators. In Opie LH (ed): Drugs for the Heart, pp 100–128. Philadelphia, WB Saunders, 1991

48. Opie LH, Kaplan NM: Diuretics. In Opie LH (ed): Drugs for the Heart, pp 74–99. Philadelphia, WB Saunders, 1991

49. Packer M: Sudden unexpected death in patients with congestive heart failure: A second frontier. Circulation 72: 681–685, 1985

50. Packer M: Therapeutic options in the management of chronic heart failure: Is there a drug of first choice? Circulation 79: 198–204, 1989

51. Packer M, Gottlieb SS, Kessler PD: Hormone–electrolyte interactions in the pathogenesis of lethal cardiac arrhythmias in patients with congestive heart failure. Am J Med 80(Suppl 4A): 23–29, 1986

52. Packer M, Lee WH, Kessler PD et al: Prevention and reversal of nitrate tolerance in patients with congestive heart failure. N Engl J Med 317: 799–804, 1987

53. Parmley WW: Pathophysiology of congestive heart failure. Clin Cardiol 15 (Suppl I): I-5–I-12, 1992

54. Patel R: Implications of an audible third heart sound in evaluating cardiac function. West J Med 158: 606–609, 1993

55. Polese A, Fiorentini C, Olivari MT et al: Clinical use of a calcium antagonist (nifedipine) in acute dyspnea edema. Am J Med 66: 825–830, 1979

56. Pouler H. Angiotensin-converting enzyme inhibitors in the treatment of clinical heart failure. Basic Res Cardiol 88(Suppl 1): 203–209, 1993

57. Raine AEG, Phil D, Hu DC et al: Atrial natriuretic peptide and atrial pressure in patients with congestive heart failure. N Engl J Med 315: 533–537, 1986

58. Rapaport E: Congestive heart failure: Diagnosis and principles of treatment. In Cohn JN (ed): Drug Treatment of Heart Failure, pp 73–89. New York, Yorke Medical Books, 1983

59. Riegger GA: Ace inhibitors in early stages of heart failure. Circulation 87(Suppl 10): IV117–IV119, 1993

60. Riegger GA: Lessons from recent randomized controlled trials for the management of congestive heart failure. Am J Cardiol 71(Suppl 17): 38E–40E, 1993

61. Schlant RC, Sonneblick EH: Pathophysiology of heart failure. In Hurst JW (ed): The Heart, 7th ed, pp 387–418. New York, McGraw-Hill, 1990

62. Smith TW, Braunwald E, Kelly RA: The management of heart failure. In Braunwald E (ed): Heart Disease: A Textbook of Cardiovascular Medicine, pp 465–559. Philadelphia, WB Saunders, 1992

63. Spann JF, Hurst JW: The recognition and management of heart failure. In Hurst JW (ed): The Heart, 7th ed, pp 418–441. New York, McGraw-Hill, 1990

64. SOLVD Investigators: Effect of enalapril on survival in patients with reduced left ventricular ejection fraction and congestive heart failure. N Engl J Med 325(5): 293–302, 1991

65. Starling RC, Young JB, Scalia GM, et al: Preliminary observations with ventricular remodeling surgery for refractory congestive heart failure. J Am Coll Cardiol 29: 2A–64A, 1997

66. Thandi U, Opie LH: Nitrates. In Opie LH (ed): Drugs for the Heart, pp 26–41. Philadelphia, WB Saunders, 1991

67. Vargo R, Dimengo JM: Surgical alternatives for patients with heart failure. AACN Clinical Issues in Critical Care Nursing 4: 244–260, 1993

68. Weber KT, Villarreal D: Role of aldosterone in congestive heart failure. Postgrad Med 93: 203–218, 1993

69. Webster MWI, Fitzpatrick A, Nicholls MG et al: Effect of enalapril on ventricular arrhythmia's in congestive heart failure. Am J Cardiol 57: 577–579, 1985

70. Weintraub NL, Chaitman BR: Newer concepts in the medical management of patients with congestive heart failure. Clin Cardiol 16: 380–390, 1993

71. Wigle ED: Diastolic dysfunction: Pathophysiology and treatment options. In Dhalla NS, Beamish RE, Takeda N et al (eds): The Failing Heart, pp 79–94. Philadelphia, Lippincott-Raven, 1995

72. Wilcox CS: Diuretics. In Brenner BM, Rector FC (eds): The Kidney, 4th ed, pp 2123–2147. Philadelphia, WB Saunders, 1991

73. Woods SL: Monitoring pulmonary artery pressure. Am J Nurs 76): 1766–1771, 1976

74. Young JB: Chronic heart failure management. In Topol EJ (ed): Textbook of Cardiovascular Medicine, pp 2273–2307. Philadelphia, Lippincott-Raven, 1998

75. Yusef S: Clinical experience in protecting the failing heart. Clin Cardiol 16(5 Suppl 2): II25–II29, 1993

76. Yusef S: Digoxin in heart failure: Results of the recent digoxin investigation group trial I the context of other treatments for heart failure. Eur Heart J 18:1685–1688, 1997

Cardiac Surgery

DENISE LEDOUX[*]
HELEN LUIKART[†]

Surgical intervention continues to be a mainstay of treatment for heart disease even though catheter-based interventional cardiology techniques have continued to expand and medical management has improved. This chapter focuses on surgical interventions for acquired heart disease, including coronary artery bypass grafting (CABG), minimally invasive cardiac surgery, transmyocardial revascularization, cardiomyoplasty, aortic surgery, and cardiac transplantation. Surgical intervention for valvular heart disease is briefly discussed in this chapter and is more extensively covered in Chapter 27.

EVOLVING TRENDS IN CARDIAC SURGERY

Cardiac surgical operative techniques continue to evolve. Myocardial protection approaches involve both antegrade and retrograde delivery of cardioplegia solution as well as refined reperfusion strategies.[49] Arterial bypass conduits such as the internal mammary artery (IMA) are the preferred graft because of excellent long-term patency. Additional arterial conduits have expanded to include gastroepiploic artery (GEA) and radial artery grafts. Spawned by laparoscopic approaches in other surgical subspecialties, minimally invasive cardiac surgery (with and without cardiopulmonary bypass [CPB]) has rapidly developed and promises to be the one of the greatest advances in cardiac surgery. Shorter intubation times and "rapid recovery" programs have led to shorter intensive care unit stays with overall reduced length of stay and decreased cost associated with cardiac surgery.

As cardiac surgery techniques evolve, the population changes as well. Interventional cardiology approaches such as coronary angioplasty, atherectomy, and stenting have delayed or replaced surgical revascularization in patients with coronary lesions amenable to catheter-based interventions. Many investigators have found an increase in the age

of surgical candidates, more women, less severe angina but greater incidence of recent myocardial infarction (MI), more left ventricular dysfunction, a higher rate of surgical candidates with three-vessel disease, and more comorbidity such as diabetes, arrhythmias, and heart failure.[51] The mean age of CABG surgical candidates has increased from 50 years in 1967 to 66 years today, and nearly 30% of patients are older than 70 years of age.[49]

PREOPERATIVE ASSESSMENT AND PREPARATION

Before referral for cardiac surgery, patients complete their cardiac work-up, which includes cardiac catheterization to define coronary artery anatomy and target vessels for revascularization; stress testing to verify areas of ischemia; nuclear scans to identify areas of myocardial viability and ventricular function; and echocardiography to delineate valvular lesions, ventricular function, and focal wall motion abnormalities. Usually, most of the preoperative medical evaluation is completed before the patient enters the hospital. Before cardiac surgery, the patient should have a complete physical examination with special attention given to the cardiovascular examination. A new history and physical examination, chest radiograph, electrocardiogram (ECG), complete blood count, serum electrolytes, coagulation screen, and typing and crossmatching of blood are done. These data provide information about other disease conditions and cardiac problems. Patients are admitted to the hospital early on the morning of their surgery. Patients with symptomatic carotid bruits should undergo carotid duplex to assess for carotid stenosis. Patients with chronic lung disease should undergo pulmonary function testing and arterial blood gas testing because they may have difficulty weaning from the ventilator. Patients undergoing valve surgery should complete a dental evaluation and work before valve repair or replacement to reduce the chance of dental disease being a source of bacteremia and possible prosthetic valve endocarditis.

Patients are maintained on antianginal, antihypertensive, and heart failure medications until surgery. Antiplatelet medications are usually discontinued before surgery: aspirin

---

[*]Author of the section on cardiac surgery.
[†]Author of the section on cardiac transplantation.

SURGICAL TECHNIQUES

Minimally Invasive Techniques

In standard cardiac surgery, the heart is arrested and circulation is maintained by placing the patient on CPB (Fig. 23-1). Although this procedure has been used successfully for over three decades, it has drawbacks such as physiologic derangements associated with CPB and long hospital stays. Minimally invasive cardiac surgery has evolved out of laparoscopic techniques originally used in general and gynecologic surgery. The term *minimally invasive* covers a variety of techniques rather than referring only to one surgical procedure. Minimally invasive techniques include CABG surgery done by standard sternotomy but without the use of CPB (off-pump or beating heart bypass), CABG surgery done off-pump through a small left anterior thoracotomy (minimally invasive direct coronary artery bypass [MIDCAB]), valve surgery done on-pump but through "ministernotomy," and port-access techniques that allow CABG and valve replacement to be done on-pump through a small incision with videoscopic assistance and femorofemoral bypass (Fig. 23-2). Techniques are rapidly evolving that are geared toward multivessel revascularization through port access on a beating heart. Rather than just one approach for all patients, cardiac surgeons have a variety of surgical techniques available depending on the patient's anatomy, medical history, and comorbid conditions. Further discussion of these surgical methodologies is found in the coronary bypass and valve surgery sections of this chapter.

Cardiopulmonary Bypass

Cardiopulmonary bypass has been the standard method used during cardiac surgical procedures for diverting blood from the heart and lungs to provide a stationary, bloodless surgical field and to promote preservation of optimal organ function. Blood is removed from the right atrium or vena cava by one or two cannulae, routed through the CPB machine, and returned to the patient by a cannula in the ascending aorta or the femoral artery. The CPB machine has several components, including venous and arterial cannulae; a bubble or membrane oxygenator that allows oxygenation of blood, removal of carbon dioxide, and delivery of anesthetic gases; a heat exchanger that allows the blood to be heated or cooled; a pump, which keeps the blood moving at a constant speed; filters, which remove particulate or air emboli and plasma protein or platelet aggregates; a left ventricular vent to prevent distention of the left ventricle during aortic cross-clamp; cardiotomy suction to aspirate blood from the operative field; and sensors, which detect air bubbles, low levels of oxygen saturation, and low levels of blood in collection chambers.[20,26,33] Heparin is used for anticoagulation during CPB to prevent clotting in the CPB circuit. Before initiation of CPB, a heparin dose of 3 mg/kg is given through a central line. Activated clotting time is monitored a minimum of every 30 minutes during CPB. If the activated clotting time is less than 480 seconds, additional heparin is given. Once CPB is completed,

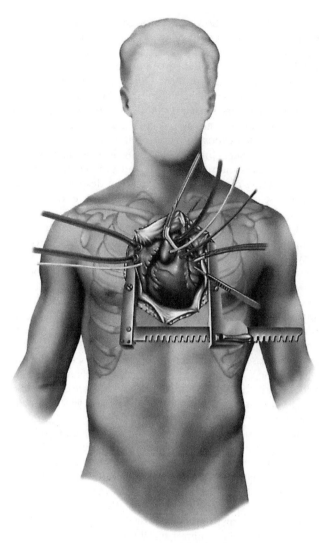

FIGURE 23-1 Approach for conventional cardiac surgery using median sternotomy and cannulae placed for cardiopulmonary bypass (Courtesy of Heartport, Inc.)

and nonsteroidal anti-inflammatory agents should be stopped 7 to 10 days before surgery; dipyridamole usually is stopped 2 to 3 days before surgery. If a patient is receiving sodium warfarin, it should be discontinued 3 to 5 days before surgery.[20]

The preoperative nursing assessment should be thorough and well documented because it provides baseline data for postoperative comparison. The history should include a social assessment of family roles and support systems and a description of the patient's usual functional level and typical activities. Elderly patients or those with limited social and emotional support may need additional assistance from social service for effective discharge and rehabilitation planning. The patient with acute coronary heart disease (CHD) may be hospitalized for only hours or days before surgery. An MI may have occurred, or the patient may be experiencing unstable angina. In either case, if CABG surgery is being considered, a cardiac catheterization is performed to determine if surgery is indicated.

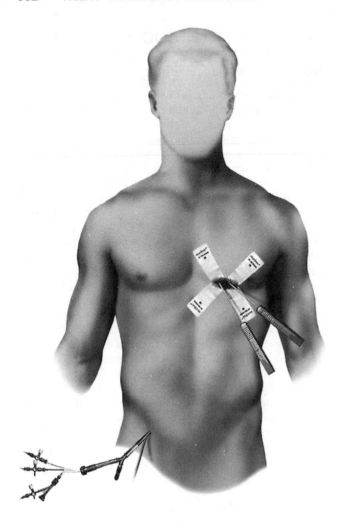

FIGURE 23-2 Port access approach for cardiac surgery using femerofemoral bypass and endoaortic technology. Coronary artery bypass or valve surgery is accomplished through small chest wall incisions with videoscopic assistance. (Courtesy of Heartport, Inc.)

heparin is reversed using protamine sulfate.[5] Care is taken to administer protamine slowly and watch for a possible protamine reaction, which may vary from mild hypotension to full-blown anaphylaxis. Patients at greater risk for protamine reaction include those with insulin-dependent diabetes and those with a fish allergy.

While the patient is connected to the CPB machine, the surgeon, anesthetist, and CPB perfusionist control many physiologic variables. A hemodilution technique is used to decrease the patient's hematocrit, thereby decreasing blood viscosity and the tendency of blood to hemolyze[41] or form microemboli.[76] The patient's hematocrit is decreased to 18% to 20% by the infusion of crystalloid solution, such as Ringer's lactate.[20,33,42,76] Patient hypothermia, induced by cooling the patient's blood and body surfaces, causes a 50% to 80% decrease in cellular oxygen consumption.[20] During the common hypothermia protocol, moderate hypothermia, the patient's core temperature is decreased to 28° C to

30° C.[20,33,76] Blood flow rates through the CPB machine are usually controlled to maintain a mean arterial pressure of approximately 70 mm Hg, a cardiac index of approximately 2.1 L/min/m², and an adequate urine output.[42]

Blood passing through the CPB machine is affected by contact with nonendothelial surfaces, by acceleration and deceleration stresses that result from movement through the blood pumps, and by incorporation of abnormal substances.[42] When exposed to the foreign surfaces of the CPB machine, platelets clump together. A decrease in the number of platelets and the aggregate and adhesive functions of the remaining platelets occurs.[76] Platelet destruction causes the release of vasoactive substances.[42] Exposure to a foreign surface causes the breakdown (denaturing) of a variety of plasma proteins, including γ-globulins, carrier proteins, and complement glycoproteins.[42] Denaturing of these proteins may cause the following to occur: release of fat microemboli (due to release of lipoprotein and fat when protein breakdown occurs),[42] a defect in cellular immunity (due to destruction of γ-globulins),[42] microcoagulation and consumption of clotting factors (due to activation of the coagulation cascade),[43] a whole-body immune response (due to activation of the complement glycoprotein system),[42] and increased vascular permeability (due to increased production of bradykinin).[42] The acceleration and deceleration stresses produced by the CPB machine destroy or decrease the functional capacity of leukocytes and erythrocytes.[42] Finally, when blood passes through the CPB machine, air bubbles, fibrin, or tissue debris may become incorporated into it.[42]

Cardiopulmonary bypass produces a systemic inflammatory response that releases biologically active substances that impair coagulation and the immune response.[26] Other responses to CPB include an increase in venous tone; a large release of catecholamines; changes in body fluid and electrolyte status; myocardial cellular dysfunction, injury, or necrosis; and mild pulmonary dysfunction.[42] Plasma epinephrine levels increase when CPB begins and return to normal after CPB ends. Patients who are hypertensive after surgery have epinephrine levels that remain elevated after surgery and have abnormal increases in norepinephrine levels.[42] In response to the vascular permeability changes that occur with CPB and to the decrease in plasma oncotic pressure that occurs with hemodilution, large amounts of fluid move from intravascular to interstitial spaces. A decrease in intracellular and extracellular potassium accompanies these fluid volume changes.[4] The imbalance between ventricular subendocardial oxygen supply and demand that occurs during CPB may result in myocardial edema, dysfunction, or necrosis.[42] Mild pulmonary dysfunction occurs commonly after CPB because of an increase in extravascular lung water, leukocyte aggregation and deposition in the pulmonary microcirculation,[42] and deactivation of pulmonary surfactant (resulting from the decrease in pulmonary ventilation that occurs during CPB).[65] The most apparent sequela of CPB for most patients, the edema caused by movement of fluid into the interstitial spaces, may resolve spontaneously within 2 to 3 days.[76] Other minor symptoms, such as leukocytosis, fever, and mild renal dysfunction, are common. Severe sequelae, including noncardiac pulmonary edema (a pulmonary edema that results from capillary permeability changes), severe bleeding tendencies, and neurologic dysfunction, occur rarely.[42] The longer the CPB time, the more severe the physiologic derangements.

Systemic warming is started approximately 30 minutes before the anticipated time of discontinuing CPB. If the left atrium, left ventricle, or aorta has been entered, air must be evacuated before aortic cross-clamp removal to prevent air embolism. The heart is warmed and resumes spontaneous rhythm or is paced with epicardial wires. Ventricular fibrillation may occur and is converted with internal defibrillation. Under the direction of the surgeon and anesthesiologist, CPB weaning begins by ventilation of the lungs. CPB is gradually weaned by decreasing the amount of blood diverted through the CPB circuit. When the heart is functioning normally with adequate blood pressure and adequate cardiac index, CPB is discontinued, heparin is reversed, and cannulae are removed. If the heart cannot support an adequate cardiac index and mean arterial pressure after weaning from CPB, the patient may have to be placed back on CPB to rest the heart, and other measures for heart failure may need to be instituted, such as inotropic treatment or intra-aortic balloon pump. In patients who continue to have severe hemodynamic compromise, ventricular assist devices may be used.

Myocardial Protection

Myocardial protection can be defined as the specific intraoperative strategies designed to protect the myocardium from tissue damage resulting from the ischemic state that occurs with extracorporeal circulation.[25] Advances in myocardial protection in cardiac surgery have been instrumental in achieving successful outcomes.[22] Cardioplegia is infused to arrest the heart and provide a bloodless, motionless operative field as well as protect the heart during cardiac surgery. Cardioplegic solution is infused into the aorta or coronary sinus or into the coronary arteries themselves to cause cardiac arrest. Debate continues over the best type of cardioplegia, what is the best temperature (hypothermic vs. normothermic), whether cardioplegia should be infused antegrade or retrograde, and timing of infusion (intermittent or continuous). Most cardiac surgery programs use a combination of the myocardial protection techniques discussed here.

Cardioplegia solutions are made of crystalloid, oxygenated crystalloid, or crystalloid–blood mixtures. Standard crystalloid solutions can deplete adenosine triphosphate stores because they carry insufficient oxygen and substrates to replenish myocardial stores.[66] Blood cardioplegia (one part cardioplegia to four parts blood) provides oxygen-carrying capability and maintains oncotic pressure, resulting in less myocardial edema. Blood proteins furnish buffering and contain oxygen free radical scavengers that can decrease oxygen-mediated injury with reperfusion.[66] Although cardioplegic solutions vary widely, typical components include potassium, magnesium, or procaine to provide immediate diastolic arrest; oxygen, glucose, glutamate, or aspartate as energy substrate; bicarbonate or phosphate to buffer acidosis; and calcium, steroids, or procaine to stabilize membranes. The solution should be hyperosmolar to prevent edema. Cardioplegia is infused continuously or intermittently. Generally, cardioplegia delivered by antegrade method is infused intermittently, and cardioplegia delivered retrograde is infused continuously.[22]

Cardioplegia can be normothermic or hypothermic. Hypothermic techniques were originally used as a means to reduce metabolic demands during arrest. A cooled, nonbeating heart uses less oxygen than a warm, beating, or fibrillating heart. Cold cardioplegic solutions are commonly cooled to 15° C to 20° C to reduced oxygen demand. Deep hypothermia can increase edema because of activation of the sodium–potassium pump, alter function of platelets and leukocytes, produce arrhythmias, prolong bleeding times, alter membrane stability, and impair calcium influx, thus affecting systolic function.[66] Normothermic cardioplegia has been used at both the induction of cardioplegic arrest and at the termination of arrest. Warm, oxygenated, hyperkalemic blood cardioplegia maintains arrest while supplying oxygenated blood to myocardial cells. "Hot shots" are warm cardioplegic infusions given at the end of the surgical procedure, before removal of the aortic cross-clamp. Warm cardioplegia has been associated with an increased incidence of total neurologic and perioperative cerebral vascular accidents.[54] Because hypothermia reduces cerebral oxygen demand, cerebral protection is improved and transient injury from emboli and ischemia is better tolerated and less likely to result in permanent damage.[22]

Cardioplegia solution can be delivered antegrade into the ascending aorta proximal to the aortic cross-clamp,[66] after which it flows through the coronary circulation and returns to the heart through the coronary sinus. Although antegrade cardioplegia has been the standard in cardiac surgery for many years, its delivery may be inadequate. Antegrade cardioplegia infusion through coronary arteries that are severely stenosed or occluded is uneven. Hearts with left ventricular hypertrophy may receive incomplete delivery to the subendocardium. In patients with aortic insufficiency, the left ventricle may become distended because of the retrograde flow of cardioplegia across the valve. Although cardioplegia can be delivered through saphenous vein grafts, it cannot be delivered through IMA grafts. Insufficient delivery of cardioplegia results in poor myocardial protection, which results in postoperative myocardial damage and dysfunction. Because of inadequate delivery using antegrade techniques, retrograde delivery systems were developed. Retrograde cardioplegia is infused under low pressure through catheters inserted directly into the coronary sinus. Cardioplegia flows retrograde through the coronary veins to capillaries to the coronary arterial bed, and exits at the coronary ostia, where effluent is removed by vent and suction. Retrograde and combined retrograde–antegrade techniques allow for optimal delivery and myocardial protection.

Deep Hypothermic Circulatory Arrest

Circulatory arrest (interruption of circulation through the ascending aorta for an extended period of time) may be necessary in procedures involving the ascending aorta and aortic arch. Profound hypothermia is used to protect the brain and other vital organs. The patient's body temperature is lowered to 18° C and CPB is stopped. Operative procedures are carried out expediently because of the interruption of circulation to vital organs. In general, deep hyperthermic arrest can be used up to 60 minutes.[36] After repair, the patient is placed back on CPB and is gradually rewarmed.

CARDIAC SURGERY PROCEDURES FOR CORONARY ARTERY REVASCULARIZATION

Coronary Artery Bypass Surgery

INDICATIONS FOR SURGICAL REVASCULARIZATION

Coronary artery bypass graft surgery is done primarily to alleviate anginal symptoms as well as improve survival. Indications for CABG surgery evolved from large, randomized, prospective clinical trials designed to compare the efficacy of medical and surgical management of CHD. In the 1970s, studies such as the Coronary Artery Surgery Study, the Veterans Administration Cooperative Trial, and the European Coronary Artery Surgery Study Group helped define which patients would benefit from surgical rather than medical therapy.[19,24,40] Recommendations for CABG vary depending on which coronary arteries are stenosed, whether the patient has lesions that could be treated with catheter-based interventions such as percutaneous transluminal coronary angioplasty (PTCA) or stenting, the number of coronary arteries involved, ventricular function, response to medical therapy, and the relative risk of impending MI without intervention. Indications for CABG surgery include left main coronary artery stenosis of 50% or greater, patients with proximal three-vessel disease (>50% stenosis of three main coronary arteries), and patients with multivessel disease and decreased left ventricular function, unstable angina, and chronic stable angina that is lifestyle limiting and unresponsive to medical therapy or interventional techniques.

RELATIVE CONTRAINDICATIONS

Conditions that greatly increase the mortality risk during surgery and anatomic limitations are relative contraindications to CABG surgery. Lack of adequate conduit, coronary arteries distal to the stenosis smaller than 1 to 1.5 mm, and severe aortic sclerosis are all anatomic abnormalities that may limit the success of the revascularization for technical reasons. Severe left ventricular failure and coexisting pulmonary, renal, carotid, and peripheral vascular disease may significantly increase the risk of surgery by predisposing to complications during the perioperative period.[23]

BYPASS CONDUITS

Coronary artery revascularization is accomplished most commonly with the IMA in combination with saphenous vein grafts. Because of the excellent patency associated with IMA grafts, other arterial conduits are now accepted for bypass surgery. Use of the right GEA as a pedicle graft to

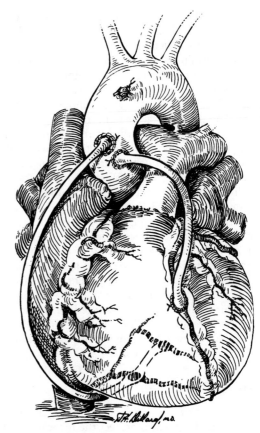

FIGURE 23-3 Completed saphenous vein bypass grafts. Vein graft to the left anterior descending coronary artery is a simple graft. Vein graft to the right coronary artery is a sequential graft, supplying two branches of the right coronary artery. Note suture at aortic cannulation site. (From Dillard DH, Miller DW: Atlas of Cardiac Surgery. New York, Macmillan, 1983.)

the right coronary or as a free graft to the left coronary system requires a more extensive surgery because the abdomen must be entered. Radial artery grafts were initially used in the early 1970s but were abandoned because of their tendency to spasm and their poor short-term patency. With the advent of calcium channel blockers, radial artery grafts have enjoyed renewed interest, although their long-term patency has yet to be shown. Greater saphenous vein from the legs is the most commonly used venous conduit (Fig. 23-3). Because of patient anatomy, history of vein stripping, or previous revascularizations, alternative conduits may be necessary. Veins harvested from the arms, such as the cephalic or basilic, make poor bypass conduits because of their caliber and high incidence of aneurysm formation. Lesser saphenous vein located on the posterior aspect of the lower leg may be used, but may be small caliber and difficult to harvest. Synthetic bypass grafts have also been used but are not in common use owing to poor patency rates.[15] Cryopreserved vein grafts harvested from cadavers also appears to have high early and midterm occlusion rates.[14]

Although the choice of conduit has no effect on early patency of bypass grafts, IMA grafts have demonstrated longer patency rates (up to 96% at 10 years) than saphenous vein grafts (81% at 10 years).[50] The IMA graft has demonstrated a 27% reduction in 15-year mortality rates compared with saphenous vein grafts.[17] Because of long-term patency, the left IMA is most commonly used to bypass the left anterior descending (LAD) artery. The right IMA may also be used to bypass the LAD artery as well as the posterior descending or right coronary artery.[69] When multiple grafts are required, single or bilateral IMA grafts in combination with other arterial conduit and saphenous vein grafts can be used to accomplish complete revascularization. Many authors recommended complete arterial revascularization in young patients in hopes of avoiding redo revascularizations later in life.

Saphenous Vein Bypass Grafts. While the sternal incision is made and the patient is readied for CPB, the saphenous vein is prepared. Traditionally, saphenous vein is harvested using standard incisions. With the advent of minimally invasive surgery, saphenous vein can be harvested using endoscopic techniques and small incisions. A long segment of vein is carefully exposed, the branches are ligated and divided, and the vein is removed. The vein is flushed with a cold heparinized solution and checked for leaks. One side of the untwisted vein is marked with a surgical pencil, and the vein is filled with and stored in a cold solution. CPB is instituted, a clamp is placed across the distal aorta, and cold cardioplegia is injected into the aortic root. Portions of saphenous vein are sutured to coronary arteries beyond the arterial stenoses. Distal anastomoses to the LAD artery are usually made first, followed by distal anastomoses to the coronary arteries located on the back of the heart. After all distal anastomoses are completed, the aortic cross-clamp is removed and patient warming is begun. Small openings in the ascending aorta are made with a punch, and the proximal end of the saphenous vein is anastomosed to the aorta. After the proximal anastomoses are completed, CPB is discontinued and the chest is closed.[41] Alternatively, proximal graft anastomoses may be completed before distal ones.[20]

Internal Mammary Artery Bypass Grafts. Harvesting the IMA is technically more difficult than harvesting the saphenous vein graft. After the sternum is cut open, the IMA is dissected away from the chest wall. A 2-cm–wide pedicle strip is removed from the chest wall muscle, fat, and pleura that surround the IMA. The pedicle strip, with the IMA lying in the center, is exposed from the IMA origin at the subclavian artery down to the level of the fourth to sixth intercostal space. The branches of the IMA are exposed, divided, and ligated. The IMA and pedicle are cut and clamped, and the end of the IMA is dissected free of the pedicle. A small cut is made in the artery (usually the LAD), and the IMA graft is sutured in place[20,41] (Fig. 23-4). The IMA can be used as a free graft rather than a pedicle graft if it is not long enough to reach the target. Bilateral IMA grafting has been associated with an increased incidence of sternal wound infection.[60]

Radial Artery Bypass Grafts. The radial artery graft is used for bypass conduit only after collateral circulation of the ulnar artery has been assessed by vascular ultrasound or

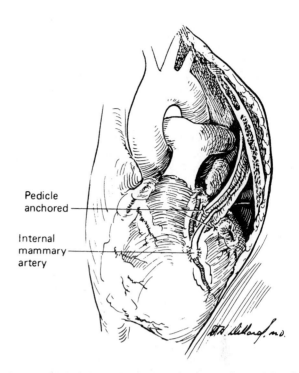

Pedicle anchored

Internal mammary artery

FIGURE 23-4 Left internal mammary bypass graft supplying the left anterior descending coronary artery. (From Dillard DH, Miller DW: Atlas of Cardiac Surgery. New York, Macmillan, 1983.)

Allen's test. Although both radial arteries can be used, the radial artery from the patient's nondominant hand is the usual choice and can be harvested before the chest is opened. Because the radial artery is very thick walled and prone to spasm, after harvesting, papaverine is used to flush and dilate the artery before grafting. During and after surgery, calcium channel blockers are used to prevent spasm. The radial graft is a desirable conduit because of its length and ability to reach most distal targets. Patency rates are less than for IMA grafts but have been reported to be as high as 90% at 9 to 14 months.[56] Further outcome studies are needed to establish long-term patency. Postoperative nursing care includes evaluation of ulnar pulse and distal circulation.

Gastroepiploic Graft. The right GEA is a branch of the gastroduodenal artery that supplies blood to the greater curvature of the stomach. The GEA can be used as an *in situ* graft on the posterior surfaces of the heart or as a free graft to other vessels. Harvesting of the GEA graft requires laparotomy in addition to the sternotomy or thoracotomy incisions required for CABG. Longer operative times and abdominal surgery increase the complexity of the surgery. Because of its excellent flow and resistance to atherosclerosis, it is hoped that the GEA will have long-term patency similar to that of IMA grafts.[64] The inferior epigastric artery may also be used as bypass conduit. Because of its length (only 10 to 12 cm), it can be used only as a free graft.[60]

OPERATIVE RESULTS

Coronary bypass surgery is done to improve quality of life by relieving anginal symptoms, or to prolong life.[79]

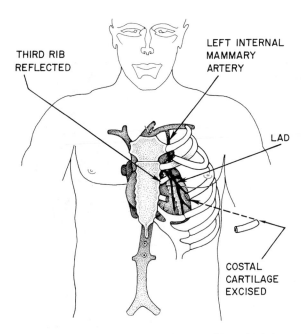

THIRD RIB
REFLECTED

LEFT INTERNAL
MAMMARY
ARTERY

LAD

COSTAL
CARTILAGE
EXCISED

FIGURE 23-5 Minimally invasive direct grafting of left internal mammary bypass graft to left anterior descending coronary artery (LAD). (From Hannan RL, Kron IL: Minimally invasive coronary artery bypass grafting. In Kaiser LR, Kron IL, Spray TL [eds]: Mastery of Cardiothoracic Surgery. Philadelphia, Lippincott–Raven, 1998.)

Although angina pectoris is relieved in more than 90% of patients who undergo CABG surgery, Canadian Cardiovascular Society class III angina reoccurs in 5% to 10% of patients at 3 years and gradually increases because of graft stenosis or progression of native disease.[12] Although the operative mortality rates in the 1980s were approximately 1%, operative mortality rates for CABG surgery approached 3% in the early 1990s, with rates of 1% to 1.5% for uncomplicated patients with stable angina.[12] Clinical variables most predictive for mortality are age, female sex, increased heart size, and congestive heart failure.[41] The overall rate is thought to have increased because of the changing population referred for cardiac surgery. With the advent of interventional cardiology and improved medical management, patients now referred for CABG surgery are older, sicker, and have more complex disease.

Minimally Invasive Coronary Artery Bypass Surgery

Minimally invasive direct coronary artery bypass is CABG surgery done through a left anterior small thoracotomy (LAST), a short parasternal incision, or small incisions using port access and video-assisted technology (Fig. 23-5). Because the small incisions limit the surgical approach, MIDCAB is usually confined to proximal disease of the LAD or right coronary artery with IMAs as conduits to these sites. Radial artery, GEA, and saphenous vein grafts have also been used if the IMA graft could not be used or

if more distal targets required grafting. Surgery is performed on the beating heart. To allow suturing of the graft anastomosis to the beating heart, pharmacologic measures such as adenosine and beta-blockers are used to slow or temporarily stop the heart, in conjunction with mechanical stabilizers that immobilize the portion of the coronary artery where the graft anastomosis is sutured. Blood flow through the target vessel is temporarily interrupted with padded snares or luminal occluders.[75] Transesophageal echocardiography is used to assess for wall motion abnormalities that would signal ischemia. CPB is on standby during each MIDCAB procedure if emergent conversion to standard sternotomy and CPB is required. The advantages of MIDCAB surgery are coronary revascularization without the physiologic derangements of CPB and avoidance of the traditional sternotomy incision. As a result, patients have less pain, need fewer blood transfusions, and have reduced overall length of hospital stay. With shortened length of stay, MIDCAB procedures have become a competitive alternative to PTCA or stenting of proximal coronary artery lesions.

Coronary artery bypass surgery done by median sternotomy but without the use of CPB is known as off-pump CABG. Like MIDCAB, grafts are done on the beating heart. Avoidance of CPB and aortic cross-clamping may be desirable in patients with poor ventricular function or severe atherosclerosis of the aorta who may not tolerate aortic cross-clamping. Median sternotomy allows for better exposure than in MIDCAB techniques. In a study by Tasdemir and colleagues[71] that reviewed 2,052 CABG cases done off-pump, 74.2% did not require transfusion, the overall mortality rate was 1.9%, and the perioperative MI rate was 2.9%.

Despite comparable mortality results, a study by Gundry and colleagues[32] suggested that off-pump CABG was twice as likely to require repeat catheterization (30% vs. 16%) and had a much higher rate of repeat intervention (20% vs. 7%).

OPERATIVE RESULTS FOR MIDCAB

Midterm results in patients undergoing MIDCAB through LAST and using the left IMA have been encouraging. In a series by Calafiore and associates[9] (n = 460), 71.2% of patients were extubated by the second postoperative hour, the mean intensive care unit stay was 4.2 ± 4.5 hours, and the mean postoperative hospital length of stay was 66 ± 29 hours. In the study, 5.7% of patients required conversion from the LAST approach to standard sternotomy, the 30 day mortality rate was 1.1%, and the late mortality rate was 1.4%. At 29 months after surgery, the survival rate was 97.1% ± 0.7% (95% confidence interval, 90.5% to 100%), and the event-free survival rate was 89.4% ± 1.2% (95% confidence interval, 78.2% to 100%).[9] Because MIDCAB surgical approaches have been available only for a short time, no long-term results of graft patency and mortality are available. Because operative techniques that involve minimally invasive incisions, port access, and operation on a beating heart have a learning curve, results associated with new operative technology are expected to improve over time.

Transmyocardial Laser Revascularization

Transmyocardial laser revascularization (TMLR) is a technique under investigation in patients with refractory angina. In TMLR, carbon dioxide, holmium-YAG (yttrium-aluminum garnet), or excimer lasers[27] are used to produce multiple channels from the endocardial surface of the ventricular wall in an effort directly to improve blood flow to areas of myocardium that cannot be revascularized using traditional techniques. It has also been postulated that myocardial blood flow is enhanced by angiogenesis that occurs with TMLR, although this is still unproven. Left anterolateral thoracotomy is most often used to provide exposure, although TMLR can also be done by standard median sternotomy if it is done at the same time as standard CABG to other vessels. TMLR is done on a beating heart. The laser is synchronized with the patient's ECG to provide the laser pulse with the R wave so that firing occurs during end-diastole, thus minimizing the risk of ventricular dysrhythmias.[52] Transesophageal echocardiography is used to detect steam or bubbles that verify channel creation. Epicardial surface seals off with gentle pressure, leaving an endocardial channel in which blood flows.

Patients selected for TMLR have severe CHD with Canadian Cardiovascular Society functional class III or IV[52]; viable myocardium with reversible ischemia as evidenced by radionuclide myocardial scan; left ventricular ejection fraction of 20% or more; diffuse coronary disease; or target vessels too small for catheter-based intervention or CABG. Studies continue to evaluate its efficacy and its role in revascularization strategies.[17] Research strategies are aimed at defining which laser works best and which patients benefit the most in terms of anginal relief, and developing transvenous approaches of TMLR. Nursing care and recovery after TMLR are similar to those in patients who have had MIDCAB.

OPERATIVE RESULTS AND FUTURE TRENDS

Clinical studies involving TMLR have demonstrated a decrease in angina by more than two Canadian Cardiovascular Society classes, improved clinical status, mild to moderate improvement in regional cardiac perfusion, and exercise tolerance for more than 2 years.[27] The 1-year mortality rate of patients undergoing TMLR is the same as or less than that of control patients undergoing maximal medical management (12% to 15%).[27] Although TMLR clinical trials have established it as a low-risk therapy for patients with end-stage ischemic CHD, it has been more effective in improving quality of life for these patients than in improving survival.[27] Clinical trials are being carried out by cardiologists using transluminal catheter-based technology through a percutaneous approach, creating laser channels from within the ventricular cavity. The ability to deliver TMLR by a less invasive means will broaden its applications and increase its availability to patients with depressed cardiac function who would not be eligible for the current thoracotomy approach.

CARDIAC SURGERY PROCEDURES FOR ACQUIRED STRUCTURAL HEART DISEASE

Acquired Valvular Heart Disease

VALVULAR REPAIR

Surgical repair of a stenotic or incompetent mitral valve is performed frequently. The reparative surgeries, mitral commissurotomy (in which the fused valve cusps are split open) and annuloplasty (in which the large orifice of an incompetent valve is made smaller) are discussed in Chapter 27. Care of the patient after surgical repair of valves is similar to that of the patient after CABG surgery.

VALVULAR REPLACEMENT

If a dysfunctional mitral or aortic valve is not suitable for repair, valve replacement is undertaken. Valvular heart surgery can be accomplished through a standard median sternotomy incision, through a small parasternal incision, or through port access using small incisions and endoscopic techniques. Because valve surgery requires an arrested, open heart, CPB must be used and can be done by the standard method or by femorofemoral cannulation. Surgical techniques for mitral valve replacement (MVR) and aortic valve replacement (AVR), types of prosthetic heart valves, and indications for valvular replacement are discussed in Chapter 27.

Mitral Valve Replacement. The routine medical care after MVR surgery is similar to that after CABG surgery. Early after MVR surgery, a patient is more likely to have important cardiovascular or pulmonary dysfunction than a patient who has undergone CABG surgery. Late after surgery, problems related to the prosthetic device may occur. Prognosis and outcome after MVR are related to severity of the left ventricular and right ventricular dysfunction before surgery.

Most patients have an improvement in symptoms, cardiac hemodynamics, and left and right heart function after MVR surgery.[6,42] Symptoms may gradually develop years after valve replacement because of progression of rheumatic cardiomyopathy, progression of disease in the native valves, or prosthetic valve dysfunction.[42] Hospital mortality rates after MVR range from 2% to 7%.[42]

Aortic Valve Replacement. The routine medical care after AVR surgery is similar to that after CABG surgery. Early after AVR surgery, a patient is more likely to have arrhythmia, decreased cardiac output, or neurologic dysfunction than a patient who has undergone CABG surgery. Late after surgery, arrhythmia, heart failure, or problems related to the prosthetic device may occur. Prognosis and outcome after AVR are related to severity of left ventricular dysfunction before surgery.

Most patients have an improvement in cardiac hemodynamics,[61] left ventricular function, symptoms, and exercise tolerance after AVR surgery. The presence of preoperative left ventricular dysfunction, ventricular arrhythmias,[30] or untreated CHD adversely affect long-term survival. Eighty-five percent of patients are alive 5 years after an AVR.[42]

Surgical Techniques for the Failing Heart

Dynamic cardiomyoplasty is an alternative to heart transplantation for patients with end-stage heart failure. Skeletal muscle from the latissimus dorsi is wrapped around the weakened heart muscle and paced in synchrony with the heart to strengthen ventricular contraction.[73] Surgery is accomplished through a left thoracotomy incision, and CPB is not required. The latissimus dorsi muscle is placed into the thoracic cavity through a space where the second rib has been resected. Intramuscular pacing electrodes are inserted in the proximal portion of the muscle. The patient is then repositioned and a sternal incision is made to complete the muscle wrap around the heart. A cardiomyostimulator (a pacemaker especially designed for cardiomyoplasty) is implanted beneath the rectus muscle and activated 2 weeks after surgery, allowing the muscle to rest and develop collateral circulation before pacing is started. Stimulation is gradually introduced by a stimulated pulse synchronized to every other cardiac cycle. Over the next 7 to 8 weeks, amplitude and number of pulses are increased to every cycle.[29] Clinical improvements appear to plateau at 6 to 12 months.[29] The operative mortality rate with cardiomyoplasty has been reported at approximately 10%, with more than 80% of patients experiencing functional improvement greater than that of the control group, which was treated medically.[13]

Although cardiomyoplasty is not a replacement for cardiac transplantation, it may have a role in patients who would not be candidates for transplantation.

The reduction ventriculoplasty was pioneered by Battitista as a surgical option for patients with cardiomyopathy who cannot undergo cardiac transplantation. To decrease wall tension and ventricular size in the dilated left ventricular, an oval-shaped portion of myocardium is removed from apex to base (Fig. 23-6). Although Battitista reports encouraging results in his own series, this procedure has only recently been introduced in the United States and is awaiting validation.[23]

Acquired Ventricular Septal Defect Repair

Rupture of the intraventricular septum after MI is a rare complication that occurs in only 0.5% to 2% of patients with acute MI.[55] The infarct that accompanies ventricular septal defect (VSD) is usually extensive and transmural. Thinning and dilatation of the infarcted portion of septum, which evolves to rupture 1 to 7 days after MI, causes biventricular failure as the left ventricle shunts blood into the right ventricle, causing right-sided heart failure and pulmonary edema. Clinical signs of acquired VSD include rapid-onset biventricular failure or cardiogenic shock, pansystolic murmur, and a sequential increase in venous oxygen saturation from the right atrium to the pulmonary artery. Bedside cardiac output measures done with the pulmonary artery catheter by thermodilution are falsely elevated owing to the left-to-right ventricular shunt. The anatomy and size of the septal rupture is diagnosed by echocardiography and

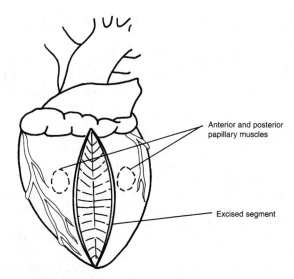

FIGURE 23-6 Reduction ventriculoplasty procedure pioneered by Battitista. To reduce left ventricular size and wall tension in the dilated, failing heart, an oval of myocardium is resected. (From Elefteriades JA, Zaret BL: Coronary bypass: The bad ventricle. In Kaiser LR, Kron IL, Spray TL [eds]: Mastery of Cardiothoracic Surgery, pp 409–419. Philadelphia, Lippincott–Raven, 1998.)

cardiac catheterization. Approximately 60% of septal ruptures occur with anterior wall MI and 40% with posterior or inferior wall MI.[38]

Stabilization of the patient with septal rupture is aimed at afterload reduction. Using pharmacologic vasodilators and intra-aortic balloon pumping, forward flow is improved and the left-to-right shunt fraction is reduced. If the patient can be hemodynamically stabilized, surgery is postponed for 2 to 3 weeks because the edges for the defect will be tougher and the repair will be more secure.[41] If the patient is hemodynamically unstable, emergent surgical repair of the VSD is advised because the mortality rate with medical therapy only exceeds 80%.[37] The VSD is repaired by patching the defect with a Dacron-covered patch, which is then lined, if possible, with pericardium to make it leakproof. In patients with significant coronary artery stenosis, CABG surgery may also be added to the operative procedure.[44]

Even with surgical repair, the hospital mortality rate after VSD repair is approximately 35%. The most important risk factors associated with early death are poor preoperative hemodynamic state and acute right ventricular dysfunction.

Repair of Ascending Aortic Aneurysm or Dissection

Aortic aneurysm is used to describe localized dilatation of the aorta. Causes of ascending aortic aneurysm include hypertension, Marfan's syndrome, and cystic medial necrosis. The likelihood of aortic aneurysm rupture is related to size. The more the aorta is stretched, the greater the tension and wall stress forces. If the ascending aorta is aneurysmal, the cusps of the aorta may be distorted, resulting in aortic insufficiency and acute or chronic heart failure.

Aortic dissection occurs secondary to disruption of the intimal layer of the aorta and is a true medical emergency. Blood enters the intimal tear and dissects a false lumen in the abnormal medial layer, with blood flowing retrograde and antegrade, separating layers of the intimal and adventitial layers. The dissection is propagated by hypertension and elevated force of contraction. In the Stanford classification, type A describes dissection of the ascending aorta and transverse arch, whereas type B is used to describe dissections of the descending thoracic aorta. Aortic dissection has a grave prognosis and requires prompt surgical intervention.

Ascending aortic dissection and aneurysm are treated with surgical resection of the involved portion of aorta and replacement with prosthetic tubular graft. In ascending aortic aneurysm or type A dissection, if the aortic valve is regurgitant, it is replaced. In the case of aneurysm alone, it may be possible to spare the aortic valve by resuspending it within the prosthetic graft of the ascending aorta (David procedure). If surgery involves the aortic arch, deep hypothermic circulatory arrest is used (see section on Surgical Techniques).

Routine Postoperative Care

Immediate postoperative care is similar for patients undergoing any cardiac surgical procedure, including CABG, MIDCAB, valve repair or replacement, and cardiac transplantation. After cardiac surgery, the patient is admitted to an intensive care unit for close monitoring for 12 to 24 hours after surgery. On arrival in the intensive care unit, the critical care nurse performs a number of rapid assessments to ensure patient stability (Table 23-1). Routine care includes continuous ECG monitoring, measurement of blood pressure by arterial line, pulse oximetry, and body temperature measurement. Intermittent measures include pulmonary artery pressure to estimate preload and cardiac output measurement as well as calculation of derived hemodynamic parameters, such as afterload, cardiac index, and contractility indices. Specialty pulmonary artery catheters, such as the continuous cardiac output pulmonary artery catheter, may be used to evaluate minute-to-minute changes in cardiac output. Oximetry pulmonary artery catheters may be used continuously to monitor mixed venous oxygen concentration, and values can be used to calculate oxygen consumption and delivery parameters during periods of critical illness.

Sinus bradycardia or junctional rhythm, with heart rates of less than 70 beats/min, usually is treated with an atrial or atrioventricular pacemaker set at a rate of 90 or 100 beats/min.[42] Heart block may occur after valve repair or replacement owing to edema and trauma at the suture lines close to the conduction system. Mild systolic hypertension is common after CABG surgery; hypertension occurs in 48%[62] to 55%[28] of patients during the first 4 to

6 hours after surgery. Postoperative hypertension is associated with elevated systemic vascular resistance and elevated levels of plasma renin and plasma catecholamines.[62] High blood pressure increases the aortic wall tension, which increases myocardial oxygen demand, making myocardial ischemia more likely to occur, and places increased stresses on aortic suture lines, making bleeding more likely to occur.[44] Hypotension occurs often during the first 12 hours after surgery as the patient warms and as systemic vascular resistance decreases to normal levels. If mean arterial blood pressure remains above 70 mm Hg and preload and cardiac output remain normal, no treatment or treatment with low-dose dopamine (2 mg/kg/min) may be ordered.[42] Hypovolemia (right or left atrial or pulmonary artery wedge pressure of less than 8 to 10 mm Hg) may be present owing to the fluid volume alterations that occur with CPB or to diuretic administration at the end of CPB. Hypovolemia may be treated with crystalloid or colloid volume expanders, such as 5% albumin or hetastarch. If the patient's hemoglobin is less than 8 g/dL, packed red blood cells or whole blood may be administered. Blood may be recovered through the chest tubes for autotransfusion during the first 4 to 12 hours after surgery. If patients are normovolemic, they are usually placed on a salt and free-water restriction. Potassium replacement is often necessary. Patients are usually maintained on a respirator for the first 1 or 2 hours after surgery, until the effects of anesthesia are reversed. Patients are on prophylactic antibiotics, usually a second-generation cephalosporin, to prevent wound infection. Antibiotic prophylaxis beyond 48 hours is not associated with decreased infections.[45]

Because of improved anesthesia and surgical techniques and a shift from acute care resulting from changes in reimbursement, cardiac surgery has evolved to include same-day admission and shortened length of stay. Stable, uncomplicated patients are earmarked to "fast track" by extubating early and minimizing their intensive care unit and hospital stay. Patient care is directed by an established care map or "roadmap." In the operating room, patients receive lower doses of opioids with the aim of extubation within 1 or 2 hours after arrival in the intensive care unit. The patient is kept sedated with short-acting agents such as propofol or midazolam intravenous infusions. When the patient is hemodynamically stable, awake and responsive without neurologic complications, and normothermic, pain is controlled, and mediastinal bleeding is minimal, the patient is extubated.[70] As a result, cardiac surgery patients may stay in the intensive care unit as little as 8 to 12 hours, thus freeing up critical care beds and reducing costs to the patient. Patients who are "fast tracked" in rapid recovery programs are discharged 3 to 5 days after surgery. Cardiac surgery patients may be managed by nurse practitioners or physician assistants in collaboration with the physician. Atrial arrhythmias and pulmonary complications are the most common variances that keep patients in hospital longer than planned by the care map. Elderly patients are also difficult to discharge within 5 days after surgery because of comorbid conditions and social issues related to discharge.[74]

TABLE 23-1	Postoperative Admission Procedure for Patients Undergoing Cardiac Surgical Procedures

Nursing Actions	Rationale
Immediately on arrival, assess skin color and observe for presence of bilateral chest excursion.	The endotracheal tube may become displaced during transport.
Assess the arterial pressure and cardiac rhythm on the transport monitor.	Because of alterations in the patient's physiologic status or displacement of the tubes, lines, or infusions, hemodynamic instability, arrhythmias, or both may develop during transport.
Assess the patient's level of consciousness. Inform the patient that the surgery is over and he or she is in the ICU.	The patient may be awake and able to hear on arrival. Reassurance reduces anxiety.
Obtain a report from the surgeon, anesthesiologist, or both.	Preoperative or intraoperative events may affect the patient's postoperative course.
Auscultate both lung fields as soon as the endotracheal tube is attached to the ventilator (usually the anesthesiologist or respiratory therapist adjusts ventilator settings).	The endotrachial tube may have entered the right main-stem bronchus during transport or during attachment to the ventilator.
Attach the patient cable to the bedside ECG monitor. Set the upper and lower rate alarm limits. Evaluate the cardiac rhythm.	Arrhythmias are common in the early postoperative period.
Auscultate heart sounds for quality, extra sounds, murmurs, or rubs.	Baseline heart sounds are essential for future comparison.
Attach the intravascular lines to the bedside monitor. Zero and calibrate the systems. Observe the waveform tracings. Set alarm limits. Document the following parameters: systolic blood pressure, diastolic blood pressure, mean arterial blood pressure, central venous pressure, right atrial pressure, pulmonary artery pressure, pulmonary artery wedge pressure, and left atrial pressure (if available).	Hemodynamic instability is common in the early postoperative period. Accuracy of hemodynamic pressures is essential for accurate assessment and treatment of postoperative complications.
Connect chest tubes to suction. Note the location, number, and type of tubes. Note and record the amount and type of drainage from each.	One or two mediastinal chest tubes are inserted during surgery to facilitate intrathoracic drainage (if the internal mammary artery was used for bypass grafting, a pleural tube also is present).
Assess all intravascular lines for patency, flow rates, and drugs being infused. Use rate control devices for all vasoactive and antiarrhythmic drugs.	Intravascular lines may have become displaced or flow rates of fluids or drugs may have been altered during transport.
Empty the urinary drainage bag. Note amount, color, and consistency of urine.	Accurate hourly urinary outputs are essential to evaluate fluid status and renal perfusion.
Obtain the patient's temperature using the pulmonary artery catheter or rectally.	Postoperative patients are frequently hypothermic on arrival in the ICU.
Obtain thermodilution cardiac output measurement (when available) and calculate derived hemodynamic parameters: cardiac index and systemic vascular resistance.	Baseline cardiac output, cardiac index, and systemic vascular resistance measurements are important to determine the patient's hemodynamic stability and response to therapy.
Perform and document an admission assessment, including the following systems: neurologic, respiratory, cardiovascular, gastrointestinal, and renal.	Baseline assessment information is vital to determine the patient's hemodynamic stability and response to therapy.
Obtain blood laboratory studies, chest radiograph, and 12-lead ECG.	Baseline laboratory studies are essential to assess fluid and electrolyte and respiratory status. The ECG is helpful in determining perioperative ischemic events, whereas the chest radiograph is used to determine correct placement of lines and tubes as well as to assess the lungs.
Allow family and close friends to visit as soon as the patient is admitted and stabilized.	Early visitation may reduce both patient and family anxiety.

ECG, electrocardiogram; ICU, intensive care unit.

Early Complications After Cardiac Surgery

CARDIOVASCULAR

Cardiovascular dysfunction or low cardiac output syndrome can occur after cardiac surgery. Low cardiac output syndrome may be related to decreased preload, increased afterload, arrhythmias, cardiac tamponade, or myocardial depression with or without myocardial necrosis.[42] Excessive bleeding can occur secondary to coagulopathy, uncontrolled hypertension, or inadequate hemostasis. Perioperative MI and pericarditis can occur as a result of cardiac surgery.

Postoperative Bleeding. Pleural and mediastinal tubes are attached to water-seal and 20-cm suction to drain mediastinal shed blood. Although blood may clot in these chest tubes, they should not be stripped because stripping may cause excessive suction, which may increase bleeding or cause damage to grafts.[21] Excessive postoperative bleeding (mediastinal drainage of >500 mL for the first hour after surgery or drainage, totaling >200 mL/h thereafter) usually is mechanical in nature and due to bleeding from suture lines, but it may be due to the presence of pericardial adhesions from an earlier surgery or to a coagulopathy. Postoperative bleeding is usually venous rather than arterial. Coagulopathies may occur in patients with prolonged CPB times or excessive intraoperative bleeding. Coagulation panels should be obtained immediately in patients with excessive bleeding. Ideally, platelet counts should be kept higher than 100,000, and prothrombin time and partial prothrombin time should be less than 1.2 times the control value.[18] The thromboelastogram is used as a measure of whole blood clotting and is abnormal if there are qualitative or quantitative coagulation disorders of any kind. Bleeding in the face of a normal thromboelastogram suggests surgical bleeding rather than coagulopathy.[70] Coagulopathies due to depletion of factors should be treated with administration of depleted factors, such as fresh-frozen plasma, platelets, and cryoprecipitate. Autotransfusion may be used to replete red blood cells, but filtered blood lacks adequate clotting factors.

Pharmacologic means of controlling postoperative hemorrhage include a variety of nonhematogenous therapies. Aprotinin, a serine protease inhibitor, inhibits plasmin. Aprotinin also preserves platelet function during bypass and, like the antifibrinolytics, has been shown to reduce postoperative bleeding[70] and decrease the need for blood transfusion. Aprotinin is used in high-risk operations in which bleeding is anticipated (such as reoperations or when prolonged CPB is expected), and may be used in the Jehovah's Witness patient to reduce blood loss. Aminocaproic acid (Amicar; Lederle Laboratories, Pearl River, NY) is an antifibrinolytic medication that inhibits conversion of plasminogen to plasmin. Aminocaproic acid is loaded intravenously in a 5-g dose over 5 minutes and is then followed by a 1 g/h infusion for up to 6 hours.[18] Desmopressin (DDAVP) may be infused intravenously in patients with severe platelet dysfunction after prolonged CPB. DDAVP shortens bleeding time and improves platelet function by increasing circulating levels of von Willebrand factor. DDAVP also increases factor VIII:C levels, which shortens the partial prothrombin time. Protamine also may be given intravenously in patients who had inadequate reversal of heparin or in those with heparin rebound. Protamine must be given as a slow intravenous infusion to prevent hypotension. Patients with insulin-dependent diabetes or fish allergy are more likely to have allergic reactions to protamine. If postoperative bleeding continues and coagulation tests are normal, bleeding may be mechanical or may result from suture line or venous bleeding. By increasing the patient's positive end-expiratory pressure on the ventilator, diffuse mediastinal bleeding may be controlled.[2] Adequate control of hypertension with sodium nitroprusside may also help control bleeding. If coagulopathies were corrected and bleeding continues, mediastinal reexploration is advised to decrease the risk of cardiac tamponade. Reoperation for bleeding is necessary after 1% to 2% of cardiac surgeries.[42]

Cardiac Tamponade. Cardiac tamponade is suspected as a cause of low cardiac output if right and left heart pressures increase and equalize; cardiac output index decreases; rapidly accumulating mediastinal drainage suddenly decreases or stops; mediastinal drainage that has been of normal volume abruptly increases; radiography shows widening of the cardiac silhouette or neck vein distention; a pulsus paradoxus is noted by arterial line or auscultation; or narrow pulse pressure is present. Although tachycardia is a sign of classic tamponade, the cardiac surgical patient may be unable to generate a compensatory tachycardia because of heart block or previously administered beta blockers or calcium channel blockers. Because the cardiac silhouette is frequently widened on chest radiography, bedside echocardiography can better define tamponade. When cardiac tamponade occurs, the patient often becomes unresponsive to inotropic medications, and unless urgent surgical exploration is done, death ensues.[42] The incidence of pericardial tamponade is reported to be less than 1%[77] during the first several days after cardiac surgery.

Myocardial Depression. Myocardial depression (impaired myocardial contractility) may be reversible or irreversible after cardiac surgery. Acute, reversible depression of ventricular function also is known as *stunned myocardium*. Metabolic or respiratory acidosis or hypoxemia may cause a reversible depression of myocardial contractility.[53] If a patient is not acidotic or hypoxemic and has evidence of decreased cardiac contractility, myocardial cell dysfunction or necrosis is suspected. A temporary form of myocardial dysfunction can affect myocardial contractility in the first 6 to 18 hours after surgery; this decreased contractility is not associated with clinical evidence of myocardial necrosis and usually improves without treatment.[42] Myocardial depression occurs secondary to myocardial necrosis in 15% of patients after CABG surgery (as evidenced by an increase in cardiac isoenzyme levels without ECG evidence of a transmural MI);[42] myocardial depression occurs secondary to MI in 0.1% to 4% of patients after CABG surgery.[16,63] Treatment of low cardiac output secondary to myocardial dysfunction first involves treatment of hypoxemia, acidosis, heart rate and rhythm abnormalities, decreased preload, and increased afterload. If a patient continues to have a low cardiac output after these maneuvers, inotropes or intra-aortic balloon pump therapy is instituted. Dobutamine, dopamine, epinephrine, norepinephrine, and milrinone intravenous infusions are frequently used for inotropic support of myocardial depression after cardiac surgery. A variety of vasodilating agents such as sodium nitroprusside, nitroglycerin, and angiotensin-converting enzyme inhibitors may be used to reduce afterload in low cardiac output syndrome. Intra-aortic balloon pump therapy is the treatment of choice for patients with severe cardiac dysfunction and evidence of myocardial ischemia or ventricular arrhythmias.[42]

Perioperative Myocardial Infarction.

Despite improved methods of myocardial protection, perioperative MI continues to be a serious complication. At the consensus meeting of the National Institutes of Health, it was determined that the rate of perioperative MI may be expected to be as high as 5% for patients with stable angina and 10% for those with unstable angina.[3] Risk factors for perioperative MI include elevated left ventricular end-diastolic pressure, cardiomegaly, long operative time (longer CPB time, multiple grafts), multiple stenotic vessels, and lack of collaterals.[3] Mechanisms of MI include graft spasm, embolization of air or debris into coronary artery or graft, and inadequate myocardial protection.[3]

Diagnosis of perioperative MI is made from a variety of diagnostic tests. New Q-wave development on ECG is relied on more than any other test for the diagnosis of perioperative MI.[3] Creatine kinase (CK) is routinely elevated immediately after cardiac surgery and usually drops after 12 to 16 hours. CK peaks associated with perioperative MI occur 16 to 24 hours after surgery.[3] CK-MB levels that indicate possible MI are established by individual institutions based on average CK elevations on uncomplicated, consec-utively operated cohorts with no ECG abnormalities.[3] New wall motion abnormalities noted on echocardiography are another way to verify perioperative MI. Postoperative pericarditis may mimic myocardial ischemia with chest pain and widespread ST segment elevation. ECG changes associated with pericarditis are J-point changes, concave rather than convex, and do not result in pathologic Q waves.

Arrhythmias.

Arrhythmias are common after cardiac surgery and are a prevalent cause of increased length of stay after cardiac surgery. Although there is no single cause of atrial fibrillation, etiologies include increased circulating catecholamines, electrolyte or metabolic imbalances, atrial volume and pressure overload, myocardial ischemia or MI, and alterations in autonomic nervous system tone.[1] Atrial arrhythmias are the most common after cardiac surgery, occurring in approximately 20% to 40% of patients.[39] Atrial tachyarrhythmias may occur any time during the first 2 to 3 weeks after cardiac surgery. The peak incidence occurs at postoperative days 3 through 5.[31] The onset of tachyarrhythmias is often preceded by frequent premature atrial contractions. Postoperative arrhythmia diagnosis and treatment is facilitated by the presence of atrial epicardial pacemaker wires. Atrial activity is more pronounced when recorded in atrial ECGs than when recorded in a normal surface ECG (Fig. 23-7). When atrial activity is accentuated, differentiation between supraventricular and ventricular arrhythmias, and atrial fibrillation and flutter is made easier. If the ventricular response to atrial fibrillation exceeds 110 beats/min, the patient's rate should be controlled. Medications commonly used to control the ventricular response in atrial fibrillation and flutter include diltiazem (either intravenous drip or orally), digoxin, and beta blockers (orally or by intravenous drip, such as esmolol). Medications used to convert atrial fibrillation include procainamide, amiodarone, and sotalol.

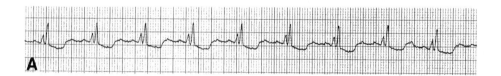

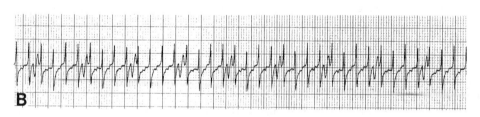

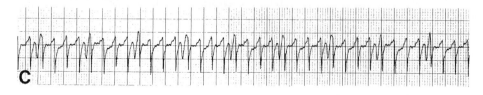

FIGURE 23-7 Atrial electrocardiography (ECG) is done by attaching limb leads and V_1 in standard fashion and then attaching V_2 and V_3 directly to the atrial pacing wires with alligator clips. Simultaneous surface lead and unipolar atrial lead ECG recordings are obtained. **(A)** Lead V_1 is the surface or reference lead. There is no atrial enhancement. **(B, C)** Leads V_2 and V_3 are unipolar atrial leads that accentuate the atrial activity and demonstrate an atrial rate of approximately 300 beats/min that was not apparent on the surface lead or standard 12-lead ECG.

If pharmacologic modalities fail to convert the patient to a sinus rhythm, electrical therapies may be used. Atrial flutter may be converted using rapid atrial pacing. To perform rapid atrial pacing, both atrial epicardial wires are connected to the rapid atrial pacemaker. The pacemaker output is set between 10 and 20, and the pacemaker rate is set approximately 20% faster than the existing atrial rate (atrial rate can be determined on the atrial ECG). Rapid atrial pacing continues for 30 seconds or until the atrial ECG complex changes from a negative to a positive deflection in lead II. Rapid atrial pacing is then abruptly discontinued, which allows the atria to resume a normal sinus rhythm (Fig. 23-8). Patients with chronic atrial fibrillation may be refractory to either pharmacologic or electrical conversion. If the atrial fibrillation is new in onset (<1 year), the patient may be successfully cardioverted by synchronized cardioversion. If the patient has been in atrial fibrillation or flutter longer than 48 hours or the atrial fibrillation remains paroxysmal, it is desirable to anticoagulate for 3 to 4 weeks to prevent thromboembolism,[31] and then have the patient return for elective cardioversion.

Ventricular arrhythmias requiring medical treatment are described in 8.9% to 24% of patients after CABG surgery.[63] Causes of ventricular arrhythmias include hypoxia, metabolic or electrolyte abnormalities, myocardial ischemia, hypertension, fear, pain, or increased catecholamine levels.[53] If ventricular ectopy occurs, causes should be diagnosed and eliminated. Premature ventricular beats, if more frequent than 6 beats/min, may be treated with lidocaine or procainamide. Ventricular tachycardia is usually treated initially with lidocaine. If the patient is compromised hemodynamically by ventricular tachycardia or if ventricular fibrillation occurs, countershock is used.[42]

PULMONARY

Pulmonary complications after cardiac surgery are a substantial cause of morbidity. Routinely, patients are intubated and ventilated for 2 to 4 hours after cardiac surgery. Pulmonary function is monitored with continuous pulse oximetry as well as intermittent arterial blood gases and chest radiographs. Mild pulmonary dysfunction is common after cardiac surgery. Pathophysiologic changes that occur after CPB include increased capillary permeability, increased pulmonary vascular resistance, and intrapulmonary aggregation of leukocytes and platelets. Severe pulmonary dysfunction is uncommon and may be related to preexisting lung disease. A noncardiac pulmonary edema may occur immediately after CPB or during the first several days after surgery. After CPB, protein-rich fluid is able to migrate through the abnormally permeable pulmonary capillaries into the alveoli. Fulminating pulmonary edema may result; the edema fluid may clear within 1 to 2 hours or may require treatment with continued intubation and aggressive pulmonary toilet for several days. Alternatively, noncardiac pulmonary edema may be manifested by a normal chest radiograph and hypoxemia that begins shortly after surgery. Two or 3 days after surgery, the patient begins to cough up thick, proteinaceous fluid, and hypoxia improves.[42] Chest radiographs should be done as part of the fever work-up to rule out atelectasis and pneumonia. Bronchial breath sounds may reflect atelectasis, which occurs in up to 70% of patients.[58] Atelectasis may occur secondary to hypoventilation related to sternal incision discomfort. Pain from chest tubes and sternotomy incision interferes with normal respiration and pulmonary toilet, making adequate pain control a high priority. Diminished breath sounds and lung fields at the bases that are dull to percussion indicate significant pleural effusions. Pneumothorax may occur any time during the postoperative period or at the time of pleural chest tube removal. Phrenic nerve damage may result in diaphragmatic paralysis or dysfunction.

Pulmonary emboli are uncommon after cardiac surgery. Factors associated with a higher incidence of pulmonary emboli include atrial fibrillation, heart failure, obesity, hypercoaguable states, and immobilization. Diagnostic work-up for pulmonary emboli includes arterial blood gas, ventilation perfusion scan, or pulmonary angiogram. Treatment with continuous intravenous heparin is begun once the diagnosis of pulmonary emboli is established, and warfarin is started for long-term anticoagulation. In patients in whom anticoagulation is contraindicated, an inferior vena caval filter may be placed. Surgical pulmonary embolectomy may be used in patients with large pulmonary emboli and associated clinical presentation of right-sided heart failure.

RENAL

Patients who undergo cardiac surgery experience reduced glomerular filtration and renal blood flow as a result of CPB and anesthesia.[1] Renal blood flow and glomerular filtration are reduced by 25% to 75% during bypass because of renal artery vasoconstriction, hyperthermia, and loss of pulsatile perfusion during CPB.[58] Radiocontrast used during coronary

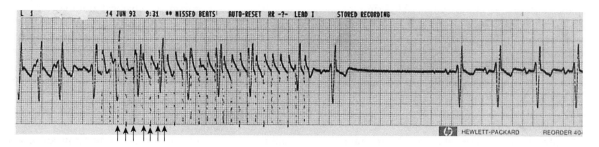

FIGURE 23-8 Recording of a burst of rapid atrial pacing used to overdrive and convert this atrial flutter to sinus rhythm. Arrows denote atrial pacing spikes.

angiography before cardiac surgery can further reduce renal function. Although minor renal impairment occurs in as much as 30% of cases,[58] renal dysfunction that progresses to acute renal failure occurs at a rate of 0.1% to 0.7%.[42,62] Patients older than 60 years of age are reported to have a higher incidence of renal failure than younger adult patients (6% vs. 0.7%; $P = 0.03$).[62] Low cardiac output during the perioperative period can lead to the development of renal dysfunction 12 to 18 hours after surgery.[42,46] Acute renal dysfunction is manifested by oliguria that occurs despite adequate preload and cardiac output.[42] If the renal dysfunction is detected early, treatment with diuretics and renal-dose dopamine may improve renal blood flow, increase the glomerular filtration rate, and increase urinary output.[48] If renal dysfunction progresses to oliguric renal failure, serum potassium levels may rise rapidly and maintenance of normovolemia may be difficult without hemofiltration or dialysis. Nephrotoxic medications such as aminoglycoside antibiotics, radiographic contrast, and nonsteroidal anti-inflammatory drugs must be avoided in postoperative renal failure, and many other medications, such as antibiotics and digoxin, must be adjusted for decreased renal clearance. Even with adequate supportive therapy, including dialysis and nutritional support, patients with oliguric renal failure after cardiac surgery have mortality rates of 70% to 100%.[46]

GASTROINTESTINAL

Perioperative dysfunction of all organs of the gastrointestinal tract has been reported after cardiac surgery.[11] Abdominal distention occurs occasionally during the first several days after surgery. If ileus and abdominal distention do not resolve with fasting and suppository or enema treatments, the etiology of the distention should be explored further. Anesthetics and potent analgesics can cause self-limited ileus and nausea.[11] Gastroduodenal bleeding can result from erosive gastritis or esophagitis, or frank ulceration, especially in patients with a previous history of peptic ulcer disease. Patients after cardiac surgery usually are placed on prophylactic gastrointestinal agents such as antacids, sucralfate, or histamine blockers such as famotidine or ranitidine. Cholecystitis presents with right upper quadrant pain and can be evaluated with abdominal ultrasound. After cardiac surgery or critical illness, cholecystitis commonly occurs in its acalculous (no stones) form. Mild elevations of hepatic transaminases also occur commonly after CPB. Severe hepatic dysfunction or "shock liver syndrome" with massive increases in liver enzymes most often occurs as a result of global hypoperfusion and end-organ damage. Acute hemorrhagic pancreatitis is uncommon after CABG surgery, but it has high rates of mortality and morbidity. Pancreatitis is noted more frequently in patients who require inotropic support and have evidence of poor perioperative tissue perfusion. Pancreatitis is usually managed with adequate fluid and nutritional support and careful use of analgesics.[67] Mesenteric ischemia may result secondary to hypoperfusion or embolization and is a grave complication.[68] If the patient continues to remain acidotic and the diagnostic work-up fails to identify another cause, abdominal exploration is done in the hope of finding a correctable source such as necrotic bowel. Both bowel infarction and ulceration are

treated surgically, and both diseases have high associated mortality rates.[42]

Diarrhea may occur with enteral feedings and medications such as quinidine or procainamide, or may be the result of *Clostridium difficile* infection. Patients with diarrhea should have stool samples sent to test for *C. difficile* toxin and are treated with oral administration of metronidazole or vancomycin.

NEUROPSYCHOLOGICAL

Neurologic complications are among the most devastating after cardiac surgery because they may have long-lasting effects on the patient and family and may require lengthy hospitalization and rehabilitation.[59] Neuropsychological dysfunction after cardiac surgery can be either central or peripheral. Symptoms of central nervous system deficits due to cerebral ischemia, infarction, or emboli are detected in 0.8% to 2.8% of patients after CABG surgery.[16,63] The highest risk of postoperative central nervous system dysfunction is associated with long CPB times, perioperative hypotension,[47] preoperative neurologic disease, or carotid artery disease. In the elderly, neurologic complications increase disproportionately to cardiac risk with advancing age.[72] Signs of focal or generalized neurologic damage usually are apparent soon after surgery.

Postcardiotomy delirium occurs 2 to 5 days after cardiac surgery and is manifested as mild confusion, somnolence, agitation, or hallucinations. Haloperidol is often used for sedation. Serious postcardiotomy delirium may include a mixture of abnormal patient sensations and behaviors; hallucinations and delusional or psychotic behavior may occur.[42,56] The etiology of postcardiotomy delirium is complex; a combination of preoperative patient characteristics, CPB cerebral injury, and perioperative environmental factors has been implicated.[56] Roberts and colleagues[63] documented a 7.8% incidence of severe postcardiotomy delirium (delirium lasting longer than 24 hours) in adult patients younger than 60 years of age; the incidence in patients older than 60 years of age was 44%. Symptoms of postcardiotomy delirium usually disappear within 1 to 2 days to 2 weeks after a patient is transferred out of the intensive care unit.[53]

Two types of peripheral neurologic deficits, brachial plexus injury and ulnar nerve injury, are described after cardiac surgery. Brachial plexus injury, with symptoms ranging from mild clumsiness to marked weakness of the hand associated with a mild numbness to a severe burning pain, was found in 5% of patients studied after cardiac surgery.[34] This neurologic dysfunction involves the C8 and T1 vertebral levels and results from mechanical trauma due to sternal retraction, but may also be due to penetration by a posterior fractured segment of the first rib during cannulation of the internal jugular.[58] Ulnar nerve injury, a result of nerve compression, is frequently described by patients after cardiac surgery. Ulnar nerve injury may be prevented by proper patient positioning during surgery; a position in which the arms are bent at the elbow and abducted less than 90 degrees, and the hands are elevated and supported by pillows close to the head was found to produce no ulnar nerve deficits.[78] The symptoms of ulnar nerve injury—numbness and tingling in the fourth and fifth digits of the affected hand—usually disappear within 3 months without treatment.[57]

Late Postoperative Complications

After the fourth postoperative day, most cardiac surgery patients have short, uncomplicated hospital stays and are discharged to home. However, postpericardiotomy syndrome, cardiac tamponade, or incisional wound infection may occur during the last postoperative period.

Postpericardiotomy syndrome may occur several weeks to several months after cardiac surgery.[42] The postpericardiotomy syndrome occurs when traumatized tissue in the pericardial cavity triggers an autoimmune response. The resulting inflammation of the pleura and pericardium causes aching pericardial pain and severe pleuritic pain. Pleural and pericardial effusions may accompany the inflammation. Treatment is with ibuprofen, indomethacin, or a brief course of prednisone. Large or symptomatic pleural effusions should be drained by thoracentesis (Fig. 23-9).

Cardiac tamponade, when seen 1 to 3 weeks after surgery, is associated with the administration of anticoagulant[7,42] or antiplatelet[8] medications to patients with a pericardial effusion. Borkon and colleagues[7] found a 1.3% incidence of late cardiac tamponade (occurring an average of 13 days after surgery) in a large group of patients receiving warfarin. The diagnosis of cardiac tamponade was made from the combination of nonspecific symptoms, including fever, lethargy, oliguria, dysphagia, epigastric or sternal pain, and a widening cardiac silhouette on chest radiography. If diagnosis is made promptly, surgery or pericardiocentesis is usually effective; if diagnosis is delayed, cardiac tamponade is associated with a high mortality rate.[7]

Wound infection after CABG surgery occurs despite perioperative antibiotics and aseptic technique. Sternal wound infections and mediastinitis occur in 0.4% to 5% of patients after sternotomy, associated with risk factors such as prolonged intubation, bilateral IMA grafting, pneumonia, diabetes, emergency surgery, postoperative bleeding, and surgical reexploration.[58] Sternal wound infections typically present 4 to 14 days after surgery with fever, leukocytosis, and inflammatory wound with purulent drainage. Sternal wounds are often associated with a sternal click and sternal instability. Staphylococci are the most common causative organisms. Superficial chest wounds are treated with antibiotics and local drainage. Deep sternal wounds and mediastinitis are treated with surgical débridement and closure or plastic surgical closure with muscle flap. Infections at the venectomy donor sites may also occur and are usually treatable with oral antibiotics.

CARDIAC TRANSPLANTATION

Cardiac transplantation is an accepted therapy for end-stage heart disease. Impressive improvements in survival, refinement of immunosuppressive therapy, and improvements in

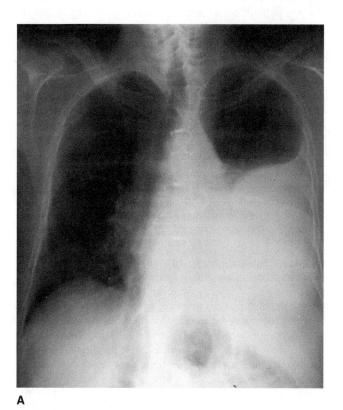 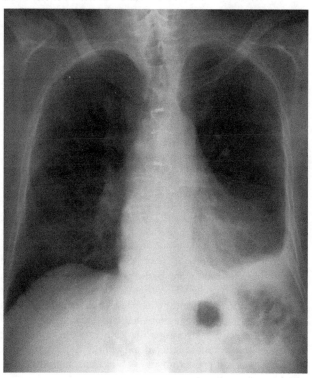

A   **B**

FIGURE 23-9 Left pleural effusion after coronary bypass surgery. **(A)** Chest radiograph shows large pleural effusion obscuring the left heart border. **(B)** Chest radiograph film shows decrease in effusion after 1,500 ml of serosanguineous fluid was aspirated by thoracentesis.

monitoring techniques have prompted many new centers to initiate cardiac transplantation programs. Worldwide, 40,700 heart transplantations have been performed, 3,048 in 1996.[21] The 1-year actuarial survival rate for patients after heart transplantation is 79%, the 5-year survival rate is 63%, and the 10-year survival rate is 43%. These figures represent patients who underwent transplantation from 1987 through 1997.[21] This section outlines expectations, therapeutic treatment regimes, and a plan of nursing care.

Progress in Cardiac Transplantation

One-year survival rates after cardiac transplantation have improved from 22% in 1968 to over 80% in 1997.[21] In 1974, major changes in survival were attributed to the introduction of the endomyocardial biopsy technique for monitoring rejection, to the treatment of rejection, and to the introduction of polyclonal antibodies. Survival results took another upward leap after the introduction of cyclosporine therapy in 1980. We are now benefiting from better prevention, diagnosis, and management of rejection and the complications of immunosuppressive therapy.

Cyclosporine is one of the most effective immunosuppressant drugs available and is capable of specific immunosuppressant activity to control rejection without totally suppressing the body's ability to fight infection.[6,17,19] It contributed to an approximate 20% increase in 1-year patient survival in the early 1980s. This is due in large part to its superior ability selectively to inhibit T-cell proliferation and reduce the incidence of rejection.

Improved survival has led to alterations in patient selection criteria with respect to age. Other selection criteria have changed little since the earlier years of cardiac transplantation. Before the introduction of cyclosporine therapy, an upper age limit of 50 years and a lower age limit of adult-sized adolescence was followed. Earlier data indicated that patients older than 50 years of age did not tolerate immunosuppression and had poorer survival.[24] Because cyclosporine does not totally suppress the entire immune system, older patients now are being considered for transplantation. The general trend is to define the upper age limit as 60 to 65 years. The current age range is from newborn to 75.3 years, with a mean age of 45 years.[21] Before 1980, children younger than 10 years of age were not considered to be transplantation candidates. This criterion is being reevaluated. Before 1980, each year, fewer than five children (18 years of age or younger) underwent heart transplantation. In 1996, 78 transplantations were performed in children from newborn to 1 year of age, and 170 transplantations were performed in children between 1 and 18 years of age.[21] There remains some concern about the effect of chronic immunosuppressive therapy on growth (steroids), an apparent higher incidence of lymphoma and leukemia in recipients younger than 20 years of age, and the availability of donors for the young child.[44]

Distant organ procurement enables transplantation centers to increase the number of transplantations performed. A surgical team can be dispatched from the transplantation center and can travel up to 500 miles to retrieve the needed heart. An ischemic time of up to 4 hours is considered acceptable. This allows for an approximate travel time of 2.5 hours, with the remaining time required to implant the heart into the patient. Greater public awareness and media attention focused on the need for donors have also contributed to an increase in the available donor pool and transplantation activity. Legislation in some states requires that a family of a potentially eligible donor be asked if that person wished organ donation. However, the limiting factor in solid organ transplantation continues to be organ donation. The success of heart transplantation has created an ever-increasing gap between the number of transplantation candidates and usable heart donors. In 1996, there were 3,700 patients waiting for a heart donor and 2,343 transplantations in the United States.[1] Transplant centers and organ procurement organizations work together to promote organ donation by public and health care professional education.[7]

With a greater number of centers involved in transplantation and listing potential recipients in organ registries, the average wait for a donor heart has increased dramatically. As a result, the patients often become sicker while waiting. In 1996, the United Network for Organ Sharing Transplantation Registry reported that 9% of patients were status I (patient hospitalized and on inotropic or mechanical support) at the time of transplantation, 57% of patients were listed as status II (all other active candidates), and 34% are inactive candidates. Because of the increasingly sophisticated management of the patient with heart failure, the use of beta blockers to produce hemodynamic and symptomatic improvement, and the pressure for transplant physicians to manage patients on an outpatient basis, status II patients are waiting longer for available donors.[34]

Evaluation of Recipients

Patients who are acceptable candidates for cardiac transplantation must have end-stage cardiac disease not amenable to further medical or surgical therapy.[22,25,35,48] The prognosis for these patients must be limited to 6 to 12 months to live without transplantation. The most frequent medical diagnoses of these patients are cardiomyopathy of various origins (idiopathic, viral, or valvular) and ischemic heart disease.[26,45] Candidate criteria have been established for use in the evaluation process to identify patients most likely to benefit from the operation. Table 23-2 outlines contraindications to cardiac transplantation.

Pediatric patients who may benefit from cardiac transplantation include those with cardiomyopathy and those with structural heart disease without severe pulmonary vascular disease.[36] These patients might have been treated surgically initially, but progressive, severe ventricular dysfunction or progressive pulmonary vascular disease limits further therapeutic options. A child with severe pulmonary vascular disease is not a cardiac transplantation candidate owing to the likelihood of irreversible right ventricular failure after transplantation. Neonatal transplantation has been performed on a small scale.[3,44] It is difficult to ascertain the availability of donors for this age group. It appears that the largest population of donors for neonates may be the sudden infant death group.[36] Once a child reaches late adolescence,

TABLE 23-2	Contraindications to Cardiac Transplantation
Condition	**Rationale**
Age greater than 65 years	Older patients do not tolerate immunosuppression well, and poor survival is likely.
Severe pulmonary vascular hypertension	Normal transplanted right ventricle fails when faced with acute, severe increase in workload.
Irreversible renal and hepatic failure	Organs are damaged further by immunosuppressive therapy; poor survival is likely.
Malignancy, severe peripheral or cerebrovascular disease	These conditions limit long-term survival.
Active peptic ulcer disease and insulin-dependent diabetes	Conditions are exacerbated by steroid therapy. Diabetic patients are prone to poor wound healing and may be more prone to infection.
Active infection	Infection is exacerbated by immunosuppression; poor risk for survival.
Potential sites of infection (recent pulmonary infarction, embolus, open wounds)	High risk of infection.
History of substance abuse that resulted in previous noncompliance with a medical regime or interfered with work performance or family relationships. Careful individual evaluation indicated.	A history of poor compliance and disruption of work and family relationships may indicate the patient is at high risk for future noncompliance. This may not be a contraindication if patient has successfully recovered from previous substance abuse problem.

it becomes feasible to use adult donor hearts, and organ procurement is no more difficult than it is with adults.

As previously indicated, the potential transplant recipient must not have fixed, irreversible pulmonary hypertension. This is defined as a pulmonary vascular resistance greater than 6 to 8 Wood units. The presence of severe pulmonary hypertension would result in certain right ventricular failure in a newly transplanted heart. The transplanted heart is developed normally and not accustomed to pumping against such elevated pressures. Irreversible hepatic and renal failure also may preclude transplantation. Some dysfunction may exist, but this should be due to the patient's low cardiac output and is expected to reverse with replacement with a healthy heart. Cyclosporine and azathioprine have untoward side effects on renal and hepatic function, respectively. Irreversible failure in either organ limits the possibility of survival.

Other systemic conditions that contraindicate transplantation include malignancy, severe peripheral or cerebrovascular disease, and active peptic ulcer disease. Insulin-

dependent diabetes does not appear to effect outcome and does not contraindicate transplantation unless associated with severe end-organ disease.[13] Patients with mild diabetes may be candidates. Some centers also view cured (no evidence of disease for more than 5 years), nonmetastatic malignancies as a relative contraindication.[10,11] All these conditions may limit long-term survival, and the required steroid therapy would exacerbate active peptic ulcer disease and insulin-dependent diabetes. Any active infection would progress rapidly after immunosuppression; patients with active infection are excluded for that reason. Any patient with a condition that places him or her at high risk for infection is also excluded. Because the lungs are the most frequent site of infections, patients who had a recent pulmonary infarction or embolus are excluded until these conditions resolve.

Donor Characteristics

It is widely recognized that pronouncement of death can be based on neurologic criteria.[51] People who have sustained complete and irreversible destruction of the brain and have met the criteria for brain death may become heart donors. The most common causes of brain death among heart donors are blunt head trauma, gunshot wounds, intracerebral hemorrhage, and cerebral anoxia. Donors are typically men younger than 30 years of age. Donor age ranges from newborn to 70 years of age, with the average being 26.7 years. Seventy percent of donors are male.[21] Male heart donors may be considered up to the age of 35 years.[14] Female heart donors are accepted up to 40 years of age.[14] Older donors are considered based on need and a negative cardiac history.

Nurses play an important role in managing the care of heart donors. Once brain death has occurred, hemodynamic instability potentially can develop in donors owing to several factors. Hypotension in a donor may be caused by multiple contributing clinical conditions. Preexisting fluid deficits may be present in donors who were treated with diuretics to decrease cerebral edema and may precipitate hypotension. In addition, with the death of the brainstem and loss of the vasomotor center, vascular tone is lost, resulting in vascular dilatation and subsequent hypotension. It is crucial to restore intravascular volume to avoid serious hypotension. With loss of pituitary function, antidiuretic hormone secretion ceases. This change contributes to the development of diabetes insipidus and subsequent decreased intravascular volume. After correcting intravascular volume deficits with fluid administration, vasomotor tone may be supported with a vasopressor agent. Dopamine hydrochloride is used most often owing to its property of renovascular dilatation and its beneficial effects on renal perfusion. Diabetes insipidus is treated with aqueous vasopressin (Pitressin; Parke-Davis, Morris Plains, NJ), which increases reabsorption of water by the renal tubules.

Surgical Procedure

Once accepted into a transplantation program, the recipient must wait for the donor heart. This requires a residence close to the hospital. Recipients often carry telepagers or beepers and are "on call" for a donor heart. When a donor is available, the recipient is admitted rapidly to the hospital and prepared for surgery. Because little time is available for preoperative teaching and preparation for the recovery process, the major portion of that is done during the initial candidacy evaluation and during the process of informed consent.

Donor and recipient are matched by ABO blood group, weight, and body size. Lymphocyte crossmatch is necessary for those recipients whose lymphocytes react to crossmatch testing (performed when recipients are accepted as transplantation candidates) against standard pools of lymphocytes from multiple serum donors.[14]

The original surgical technique for orthotopic heart transplantation described by Shumway and colleagues[43] in 1960 has remained the standard procedure. After a median sternotomy and the initiation of CPB, the recipient's heart is removed, leaving the posterior walls of the atria intact (Fig. 23-10). The inflows of the two venae cavae and the pulmonary veins are left in place and unaltered. Both the aorta and pulmonary artery are transected. Then the atrial walls of the donor heart are anastomosed to the recipient atria, with care taken to avoid injury to the donor heart's sinus node. After atrial anastomosis, the donor pulmonary artery and aorta are anastomosed to the recipient vessels. On completion of the procedure, temporary epicardial atrial and frequently ventricular pacing wires are placed. Before closing the chest, mediastinal drainage tubes are secured as with any cardiac surgical procedure.

An alternative technique is referred to as total orthotopic heart transplantation or the bicaval and pulmonary venous anastomosis. The basic features of the bicaval method are complete excision of the recipient atria and donor heart implantation with bicaval end-to-end anastomosis. Proponents of this technique cite the potential for more synchronous atrial contraction, reduction of pacemaker implantation, and atrioventricular valve regurgitation.[49]

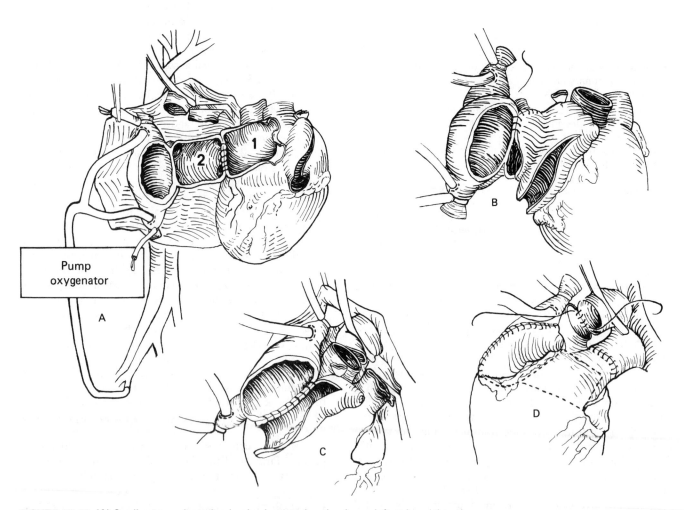

FIGURE 23-10 (A) Cardiac transplantation begins by suturing the donor left atrium (*1*) to the posterior wall of the recipient left atrium (*2*). **(B)** The intra-atrial septa are anastomosed, followed by **(C)** anastomosis of the right atrial wall. **(D)** The final step is the anastomosis of the donor and recipient great vessels. (Adapted from Cooley DA, Norman JL: Techniques in Cardiac Surgery, p 220. Houston, Texas Medical Press, 1975.)

Medical Management

In the immediate postoperative period, postoperative care is similar to that of any cardiac surgical patient. Transplant recipients are intubated and mechanically ventilated for 12 to 24 hours and require hemodynamic stabilization. Differences in care revolve around the patient's likely debilitated preoperative status, potential manifestations of ischemia in the donor heart, potential cardiac rejection, and immunosuppression.

IMPACT OF PREOPERATIVE STATUS

Cardiac transplant recipients were in chronic low cardiac output states before transplantation surgery. They likely had poor nutritional status and were relatively immobile. Many were hospitalized with an acute exacerbation of heart failure and, in some cases, cardiogenic shock. Maintenance of adequate nutrition during the preoperative phase is difficult owing to the anorexia, nausea, and impaired digestion and absorption associated with serious cardiac failure.

After transplantation, interventions to improve nutritional status are important because the patient is immunosuppressed. Postoperative basal metabolic requirements are increased at the same time corticosteroid therapy is accelerating protein catabolism. Maintaining adequate nutrition is important to minimize postoperative complications and to facilitate recovery and rehabilitation.[12] Diet becomes an important factor in minimizing some of the side effects of corticosteroid therapy.[42] Diet can be supplemented with hyperalimentation and intravenous lipid preparations in sicker patients.

Preoperative cardiac failure potentially contributes to postoperative renal and hepatic dysfunction as a result of the chronic low cardiac output state. Renal dysfunction is evidenced by elevated serum creatinine levels. Because cyclosporine may induce nephrotoxicity, careful attention must be given to monitoring renal status. An elevated preoperative serum creatinine may be an indication to reduce cyclosporine dosage or even delay by a few days postoperative administration of the drug. Weekly urine creatinine clearance tests are ordered to follow postoperative renal function.

Preoperative hepatomegaly from chronic heart failure may precipitate postoperative bleeding due to clotting deficiencies associated with compromised hepatic function. Vitamin K deficiency also may contribute to the problem. It is fairly routine to administer fresh-frozen plasma and vitamin K before transplantation to minimize the expected coagulopathy. The risk of bleeding is increased slightly in patients who have had previous cardiac surgery. Previous surgery usually requires more dissection through adhesions that formed during the previous healing process. Coagulation status and blood loss are monitored carefully during the postoperative period. Treatment of coagulopathy is usually addressed with the administration of fresh-frozen plasma and platelets. Autotransfusion is the preferred approach to blood replacement. If additional replacement is required, consideration is given to the recipient's cytomegalovirus (CMV) titer. If the titer is negative, the patient should receive only blood that also has a negative CMV titer to avoid the possibility of introducing an opportunistic infection.

CARDIAC FUNCTION

Although the donor heart is protected from ischemia with cold saline immersion and cardioplegia, it may still incur some ischemia that is evident during the immediate postoperative period. The transplanted heart benefits from pharmacologic ß-receptor stimulation in the early postoperative period. Isoproterenol is used routinely for up to 4 days to augment contractility, atrioventricular conduction, and heart rate. The denervated heart cannot respond to the autonomic nervous system and depends on circulating catecholamines. Underlying bradycardia and junctional rhythms are not uncommon during this time. Sinus node dysfunction can occur as a result of injury during procurement, surgery, or distortion of the atria with transplantation, or it may be acquired as the result of cardiac rejection.[4] Temporary atrial pacing may be used during the immediate postoperative period. Once the heart has recovered from the trauma of surgery, a normal intrinsic heart rate of approximately 100 beats/min becomes evident. Sinus node dysfunction is common, and 6% to 10% of patients may require permanent pacemaker implantation.[9]

Blood pressure control with sodium nitroprusside therapy is usually required for the first 24 to 48 hours after surgery. In patients with high preoperative pulmonary artery pressures, prostaglandin E_1 therapy may be used to dilate the pulmonary vascular bed and reduce afterload in the donor right ventricle. Pulmonary artery pressures decrease over the next few days, while the right ventricle adjusts to its new workload. Dopamine hydrochloride is administered at doses of 3 µg/kg/min or less to enhance renal vascular blood flow. This drug is usually discontinued after the first 24 to 48 hours. Table 23-3 outlines hemodynamic support in the immediate postoperative period.

TABLE 23-3	Hemodynamic Support in the Immediate Postoperative Period
Heart rate and rhythm	Isoproterenol titrated to maintain heart rate >100 beats/min Range 0.5 to 1 µg/min Atrial pacing to maintain sinus rhythm
Contractility	Isoproterenol as above maintained for 4 postoperative days
Renal perfusion	Dopamine hydrochloride 3 µg/kg/min May be increased for inotropic effect
Blood pressure control	Sodium nitroprusside titrated to maintain mean arterial pressure between 65 and 85 mm Hg. Maximum dose 5 µg/kg/min
Volume therapy	Normal saline, plasma expanders, or blood products to maintain central venous pressure 8–12 mm Hg
Pulmonary vasodilation	Prostaglandin E_1 used for elevated pulmonary vascular resistance or long donor ischemic times associated with right ventricular dysfunction

MONITORING REJECTION

Rejection of the heart is triggered by the presence of antigens on the surface of the cells of the transplanted heart. There are three forms of rejection: hyperacute, acute, and chronic.

Hyperacute rejection occurs when the recipient has preformed cytotoxic antibodies to the donor antigens.[39] Hyperacute rejection may result from ABO blood group incompatibility. This origin of rejection is prevented by matching the donor and recipient ABO blood group. The potential recipient is screened for the presence of preformed cytotoxic antibodies by mixing the recipient's serum with a known pool of different antigens. Results of the antibody screening are reported as percentage of reactive antibody (%PRA). If the recipient has cytotoxic antibodies present, more specific testing for compatibility with a specific donor heart can be done by mixing recipient serum with that donor's lymphocytes. This testing identifies if the potential recipient has cytotoxic antibodies that will react to that specific donor heart. Hyperacute rejection results in immediate, irreversible heart failure and can be treated only by retransplantation.

Acute rejection is the most frequently occurring form of rejection and is a major cause of death within the first year after transplantation.[55,90] Preoperative immunosuppressive therapy is begun in anticipation of acute cardiac rejection. Routine monitoring for acute rejection is centered around endomyocardial biopsy. With cyclosporine therapy, there are few clinically evident signs and symptoms of acute rejection. The objective is to detect acute rejection in its early stages at a time when the process can be reversed, thus preventing serious, permanent damage to the new heart. Therefore, biopsy remains the gold standard for monitoring and early detection of acute rejection. Because acute rejection is expected to occur during the first 3 months after surgery, biopsy is performed within the first 14 days after transplantation, and then up to once a week during this crucial time interval. Any time that rejection is present, biopsies are done frequently to monitor the progress of antirejection treatment. By 1 month, the biopsy schedule is tapered to every other week, then once per month after the third month. Patients are then monitored indefinitely by biopsy every 4 months to annually, depending on the transplant center.

The biopsy procedure may be done in the operating room, echocardiography laboratory, or catheterization laboratory for hospitalized patients and usually in the cardiac catheterization laboratory for outpatients. It can be performed in 15 minutes and requires only local anesthesia. Figure 23-11 illustrates the technique of endocardial specimen retrieval from the right ventricle. Mild rejection may resolve spontaneously and is often not treated. It is characterized by endocardial and interstitial infiltrate, International Society of Heart and Lung Transplantation (ISHLT) grade 1A, 1B, and 2. Moderate rejection is characterized by the presence of myocyte necrosis and perivascular, endocardial, and interstitial infiltration of immunoblasts (ISHLT grade 3A, 3B).[39] Severe rejection results in myocyte and vascular necrosis with hemorrhage and a mixed infiltrate of immunoblasts and neutrophils (ISHLT grade 4).[39] Resolv-

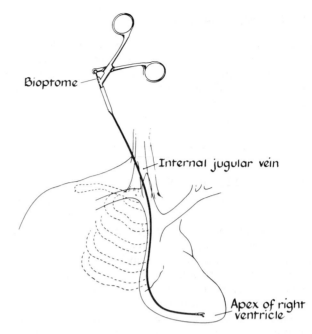

FIGURE 23-11 To perform a biopsy, a bioptome is introduced by way of the internal jugular vein and advanced to the right ventricular apex, where several pieces of tissue are retrieved for analysis.

ing rejection is evidenced by active fibrosis, which represents reparative changes. Table 23-4 outlines the heart biopsy grading system adopted by the ISHLT in 1990.[5] Treatment of rejection depends on the grade of rejection, length of time from transplantation, clinical findings, symptoms, and the presence or absence of hemodynamic compromise.

Accelerated graft coronary artery disease or graft atherosclerosis, often referred to as *chronic rejection,* may be present in up to 50% of patients 5 years after transplantation.[16] This type of rejection is thought to be caused by immune-mediated injury to the coronary arteries and results in diffuse obliterative vascular lesions.[39] Severe myocardial fibrosis occurs as a result and can cause serious myocardial dysfunction. Occlusive lesions also may precipitate MI. Exercise stress testing and annual cardiac catheterization are used to monitor for the development or progression of this

TABLE 23-4	International Society of Heart and Lung Transplantation Standard Grading of Cardiac Rejection[5]

Grade	Nomenclature
0	No rejection
1	A, Focal, mild
	B, Diffuse, mild
2	One aggressive infiltrate, focal moderate
3	A, Multifocal aggressive, moderate
	B, Diffuse inflammatory process
4	Diffuse, aggressive, with necrosis, severe acute rejection

condition. These are necessary owing to the denervated state of the heart. The patient does not experience the early warning signs of angina if arterial occlusions are causing ischemia. Chronic rejection is treated with retransplantation. The diffuse nature of the condition precludes the use of CABG or angioplasty as treatment options.

MONITORING FOR INFECTION

Infection is an ever-present threat to the immunosuppressed cardiac transplant recipient and is almost inevitable at some point during the postoperative course. It is a major cause of morbidity and mortality.[7,24,20,22] Patients on multiple immunosuppressants at high doses are at greater risk. Bacterial infections are the most common form of infection. Fungal, viral, and protozoan infections are the most difficult to treat. Prophylactic regimes have been shown to be effective in transplant recipients to prevent or attenuate opportunistic infections. Trimethtoprim-sulfamethoxazole is used against *Pneumocystis carinii*,[50] and intravenous gancyclovir is used after surgery for 4 to 6 weeks against CMV activation or reactivation; in addition, hyperimmune globulin may be used in CMV-seronegative recipients of a seropositve donor.[33]

Handwashing and universal precautions are used as the mainstays of protection in the hospitalized patient. A retrospective review of 51 patients transplanted using isolation and 55 patients cared for without isolation revealed that the change had no impact on morbidity or mortality associated with infection.[15]

Infection is monitored for closely. Because the lungs are the primary site of infection, daily chest radiographs are done immediately after surgery, as well as chest auscultation every 4 hours. Good pulmonary assessment is extremely important. Incentive spirometry, early mobility, and coughing and deep breathing are used to minimize atelectasis and possible infection. A temperature rise over 37° C, changes on the chest radiograph, or development of a cough are indications for obtaining sputum cultures. A temperature rise over 38° C is an indication for blood cultures. Otherwise, routine laboratory screening for infection is done on a weekly basis, except white blood cell counts, which are done daily.

MONITORING FOR IMMUNOSUPPRESSIVE DRUG SIDE EFFECTS

Specific adverse effects and clinical manifestations of common immunosuppressive drugs are outlined in Table 23-5. Several side effects have implications for patient teaching and coaching and warrant further discussion. Nurses play a key role in providing patients with knowledge of drug side effects and methods of self-monitoring. It is important that patients are able to detect problems that can be injurious to their health and know when to seek medical attention. A knowledgeable patient also can take steps to minimize some of these problems. Some of the drug side effects may be particularly emotionally troublesome for patients. Nurses can do much to prepare them for this and assist them with strategies for coping with these side effects.

Cyclosporine. Cyclosporine (Sandimmune, Neoral) is a natural metabolite found in a fungus. It is a lymphokine synthesis inhibitor that profoundly inhibits cell-mediated immunity. It also impairs interleukin secretion by macrophages. Cyclosporine selectively interferes in the immune system, specifically targeting T cells; this specificity allows the body to retain some ability to protect itself from infection.[23,47] The drug must be used cautiously and monitored closely. Cyclosporine is nephrotoxic, leading to a decrease in glomerular filtration rate, renal plasma, and blood flow.[18,29,31,32,35] Cyclosporine-induced arterial hypertension has been reported to be as high as 100% and is a difficult problem to control in the long-term survivor.[35,48] It is important to maintain a consistent administration time for cyclosporine. Equally important is timely acquisition of blood specimens for cyclosporine levels after the last dose of the drug. Cyclosporine has numerous drug interactions with common medications. Cyclosporine is metabolized by the cytochrome P-450 system, so drugs that affect the P-450 system alter the metabolism of cyclosporine.[52] It is extremely important for nurses to know most of these interactions to avoid adverse side effects, in addition to understanding the pharmacology of cyclosporine. Patients are taught to take this drug after meals to decrease the possibility of gastrointestinal intolerance and to promote absorption.

Hypertension is a serious side effect that often is difficult to control. Patients need to monitor their hypertension and should be taught how to take an accurate blood pressure. They are also sent home with an understanding of what symptoms, such as headaches, may indicate their hypertension has become uncontrolled.

Cyclosporine therapy does result in changed bodily appearance, particularly diffuse increased hair growth. Changed bodily appearance was reported in 34% of 44 patients on cyclosporine and corticosteroid protocols.[27,28] Excessive hair growth was reported in 45% of the patients. Nurses can coach patients to prepare for this side effect and provide ideas for managing this problem. Cyclosporine can also cause neurotoxicity, and patients may exhibit tremors and complain of headache.

Tacrolimus. Tacrolimus (Prograf), formally referred to as FK506, is a potent immunosuppressive macrolide antibiotic. Tacrolimus acts by inhibition of the earliest steps of T-cell activation in a manner similar to that of cyclosporine. It was initially used in liver and kidney transplantation with successful results, and it is now used as a frequent alternative to cyclosporine. It is used as an effective agent for rescue therapy in refractory cardiac rejection and as a primary immunosuppressant in some centers.[37]

Tacrolimus has demonstrated that it is well tolerated in general. It is nephrotoxic, as is cyclosporine, and has a slightly higher diabetogenic effect.[2] Tacrolimus does not cause hirsutism, gingival hyperplasia, or facial dysmorphism as cyclosporine does. Its primary side effects are headache, nausea, and tremors. It is important to monitor patient blood levels, kidney function, and blood glucose. Tacrolimus is also similar to cyclosporine in that it is metabolized through the P-450 system; therefore, similar drug interactions are present.[52]

TABLE 23-5 | Major Adverse Side Effects of Immunosuppressive Agents and Clinical Manifestations

Drug	Adverse Effects	Clinical Manifestations
Cyclosporine	Nephrotoxicity	Elevated BUN and creatinine Decreased urine output Weight gain, edema
	Hypertension	Elevated blood pressure
	Hepatotoxicity	Elevated bilirubin Elevated alkaline phosphatase, AST, and ALT levels Jaundice
	Hypertrichosis	Excessive hair growth all over body
	Tremors, seizures	Fine motor tremors, especially hands Associated paresthesias Seizure activity
	Increased risk of malignancy when associated with high doses of multiple agents	Dependent on type and location of malignancy
	Gingival hyperplasia	Growth of gums over teeth Bleeding of gums
Corticosteroids	Aseptic necrosis of bone, osteoporosis	Pain in weight-bearing joints Pathologic fractures
	Hyperglycemia, steroid-induced diabetes mellitus	Elevated serum glucose Polydipsia, polyuria
	Salt and water retention	Weight gain or fluctuations associated with edema
	Hypertension	Elevated blood pressure
	Skin alterations	
	Acne	Rash or pimples on face and trunk
	Sun sensitivity	Susceptibility to sunburn Skin malignancies
	Hirsutism	Excessive hair growth on face, trunk, and extremities
	Growth retardation in children	Failure to reach normal height for age
	Gastritis/gastrointestinal ulcerations	Abdominal pain, dysphagia Hematemesis, guaiac-positive stools
	Cataracts	Visual acuity problems
Azathioprine	Bone marrow depression	Leukopenia, thrombocytopenia, anemia
	Hepatotoxicity	Elevated bilirubin Elevated alkaline phosphatase, AST, and ALT levels Jaundice
	Increased risk of malignancy when associated with high doses of multiple agents	Dependent on type and location of malignancy
	Sun sensitivity of skin	Susceptibility to sunburn Skin malignancies
Orthoclone OKT3	Pyrexia, malaise	Fever, chills, influenza-like symptoms Headache, diarrhea
	Respiratory distress associated with initial doses and fluid overload	Chest tightness, dyspnea, wheezing
	Increased risk of malignancy when associated with high doses of multiple agents	Dependent on type and location of malignancy
Antithymocyte preparations	Anaphylactic reactions	Hypotension, dyspnea, wheezing, fever, chills
	Serum sickness associated with antibody formation to foreign protein	Fever, joint pain Elevation of BUN and creatinine
	Bone marrow depression associated with prolonged use in conjunction with azathioprine	Leukopenia Thrombocytopenia Anemia
	Local inflammatory reactions associated with intramuscular administration	Pain, redness, extreme muscle soreness, swelling
	Increased risk of malignancy when associated with high doses of multiple agents	Dependent on type and location of malignancy
Tacrolimus	Nephrotoxicity associated with high doses	Elevated BUN and creatinine Decreased urine output
	Hyperkalemia	Elevated potassium levels
	Insomnia	Sleep disturbances
	Malaise	Headaches, nausea, and vomiting associated with IV administration

ALT, alanine aminotransferase; AST, aspartate aminotransferase; BUN, blood urea nitrogen.
From Luikart H, Shinn J, Willis B: Transplantation. In Thelan L, Davie J, Urden L et al (eds): Critical Care Nursing: Diagnosis and Management, 2nd ed, pp 834–836. St Louis, CV Mosby. 1994.

Corticosteroids. The anti-inflammatory actions of corticosteroids provide important protection of the transplanted heart against damage from rejection. Steroids impair the sensitivity of T cells to the foreign antigen, decrease proliferation of sensitized T cells, and decrease macrophage mobility. Long-term corticosteroid therapy may be associated with several side effects that require monitoring. Glucose intolerance may develop during hospitalization and persist long enough to require insulin therapy. Insulin coverage is initiated for serum glucose levels in excess of 200 to 250 mg/dL. This necessitates patient instruction on diet management and self-administration of insulin. Weight gain is problematic for many patients. Diet instruction and initiation of exercise programs may help minimize this problem. Regular exercise is also thought to be important in minimizing the calcium loss from bone associated with long-term corticosteroid therapy. Stress ulceration is a concern in patients on higher doses of corticosteroid therapy for long periods. Nurses need to be aware of the possibility and be alert to signs or symptoms that may indicate a problem. It is also necessary to teach the importance of good skin care. Fragile skin that heals poorly may become a problem with the long-term patient. Patients should be taught to monitor the condition of their skin and be alert for lesions that do not heal well or that become infected.

Fragile skin and bruising were reported to occur often or always in up to 60% of patients on corticosteroid and azathioprine protocols.[27,28] Changed facial and bodily appearance were reported by 43%. Poor vision, a problem associated with corticosteroid therapy, was "quite a bit" or "extremely" upsetting to 30% of patients.[27,28]

Azathioprine. Azathioprine (Imuran) is used as a maintenance drug to prevent activation and proliferation of T cells in response to the foreign antigen or the transplanted heart. It is an antimetabolite that interferes with purine synthesis. Purine synthesis is necessary for antibody production and for synthesis of nucleic acids in rapidly proliferating cells, such as the cells of the immune system.[8] Prevention of this cell proliferation can also impair other rapidly proliferating cells in the body and cause conditions such as leukopenia, thrombocytopenia, and anemia. It is important to monitor the patient's white blood cell count closely and titrate the dose of the drug accordingly.

Mycophenolate Mofetil. Mycophenolate mofetil (Cellcept) is a new immunosuppressive agent that inhibits the *de novo* pathway of purine synthesis in activated lymphocytes. Mycophenolate mofetil works at a late stage in T-cell activation, in contrast to cyclosporine and tacrolimus, which inhibit the earliest events.[2] Mycophenolate mofetil has been shown to have activity against B cells and therefore may have a role in preventing graft atherosclerosis.[52]

Multicenter trials have shown that mycophenolate mofetil is an effective immunosuppressant, safe and well tolerated in kidney and heart transplant recipients. It is less myelosuppressive than azathioprine, thereby avoiding the neutropenia and anemia, and less hepatotoxic as well. Its major side effects are gastrointestinal disturbances. Nausea, vomiting, and diarrhea are the most frequently reported complaints. These symptoms are usually self-limiting and dose dependent.[24]

Orthoclone OKT3. Orthoclone OKT3 is a monoclonal antibody that is targeted to remove T cells from circulation through the formation of antigen–antibody complexes.[8] It can be used initially after transplantation to eliminate the T-cell response in the first 14 postoperative days, or can be used to treat a later rejection episode. Patients can acquire sensitivity to the drug and form antibodies against the foreign protein. For that reason, usually only one 7-day course of the drug is given. Adverse effects are caused by the massive lysis of T cells, resulting in general malaise, fever, and chills.

Antithymocyte Preparations. Like orthoclone OKT3, antithymocyte preparations are antibodies produced by animals in response to foreign human T cells. They are polyclonal preparations pooled from multiple animals, however, with much variation in potency, and are not specific for the T cell most important in the rejection process. These preparations are used only to treat severe rejection after standard antirejection therapy has failed. The course of therapy is typically 5 days. As with orthoclone OKT3, adverse effects are associated with the massive lysis of T cells, causing fever and chills.[8] Although rare, patients can have anaphylactic reactions to the foreign animal protein.

Other Complications

Sexual dysfunction is a prevalent problem in cardiac transplantation recipients. Impotence is not uncommon, and much of it can be attributed to the requirement for antihypertensive therapy. In a survey of 31 patients on conventional immunosuppression without cyclosporine, impotence was reported by 28% and decreased interest in sex by 27% of patients.[27] Impotence and decreased interest in sex were reported to be "quite a bit" or "extremely" upsetting by 41% and 30%, respectively.[27] This is a strong indication that preparation for this potential problem should begin during hospitalization. Patients would benefit from knowing that these occurrences are not uncommon. They need to feel comfortable voicing concerns and reporting future problems so that appropriate counseling or other assistance can be provided.

Conditioning and Exercise Training

Physical rehabilitation is a necessary part of the posttransplantation patient recovery program. Physical therapy is needed to ameliorate the deconditioning of the pretransplantation, heart failure state and to decrease the sequelae of the immunosuppressants and surgical procedure.[40] Low-level exercise is begun with extremity and shoulder flexion, extension, and abduction exercises. The intensity and duration are progressed to the patient's tolerance.[41] These low-level exercises serve as warm-up for more intensive exercises once the patient can complete the low-level program without undue fatigue or balance loss.

Bicycle ergometry is usually introduced within 3 days. Intensity and duration are gradually progressed according to patient response. By discharge, most patients are able to cycle for 20 minutes without resistance and for 5 minutes with resistance. With cardiac denervation, heart rate response to exercise is abnormal.

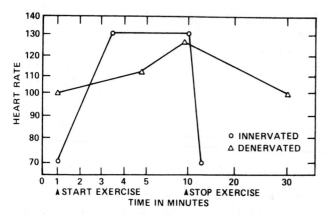

FIGURE 23-12 Sample differences in response to exercise between an innervated and denervated heart. (From McKelvey SA: Effects of denervation in the cardiac transplant recipient. In Douglas MK, Shinn JA [eds]: Advances in Cardiovascular Nursing, p 201. Rockville, MD, Aspen Systems, 1985.)

TABLE 23-6	Cardiac Transplant Recipients' Dyspnea Index for Exercise Training
Level 0	No shortness of breath Can count to 15 without taking a breath
Level 1	Mild shortness of breath Counts to 15 and requires one breath in the sequence: continue at this intensity
Level 2	Moderate shortness of breath Counts to 15 and requires two breaths in the same sequence; this is the desired level of intensity
Level 3	Definite shortness of breath Must take three breaths in the sequence of counting to 15; reduce the intensity of exercise
Level 4	Severe shortness of breath Unable to count or speak; cease activity

Adapted with permission from Sadowsky HS, Rohrkemper KF, Quon S: Rehabilitation of Cardiac and Cardiopulmonary Recipients, Appendix 1. Stanford, CA, Stanford University Hospital, 1986.

The ability to perform any exercise beyond mild in intensity depends on circulating catecholamines to increase heart rate, contractility, and cardiac output. The normal, immediate increase in heart rate induced by exercise is absent in the denervated heart, and several minutes are required before heart rate can increase.[30] Warm-up exercise is necessary before vigorous activity, and its duration should be approximately 5 minutes. Deceleration of heart rate after exercise is prolonged. The patient's heart rate may not return to resting levels for up to 20 minutes after cessation of the activity. Prolonged cool-down periods are also necessary. Figure 23-12 illustrates a typical response to exercise.

Patients need to understand how their response to exercise is different after transplantation. Self-monitoring techniques are taught before discharge, and continued regular exercise is encouraged. Patients are taught to use dyspnea as a guide for activity intensity rather than heart rate. The dyspnea index is presented in Table 23-6. Patients are coached not to exceed a dyspnea index greater than level 2. The rating of perceived exertion is a widely used self-monitoring tool for transplant recipient. The Borg scale is a rating of perceived exertion that is scaled from 6 (very, very easy) to 12 to 14 (somewhat hard), to 15 to 20 (very, very hard) Patients are instructed to continue their exertion until they perceive their exercise has become somewhat hard.[40] Patients are also counseled to decrease their duration of exercise if they experience excessive fatigue during or after exercise.

Corticosteroid therapy, cyclosporine, and tacrolimus are detrimental to bone density and structure. Potential corticosteroid-induced osteoporosis puts the patient in greater jeopardy of bone fractures. Several types of medications are available to treat transplantation osteoporosis such as bisphosphonates, calcitonin, estrogen, and vitamin D. Bisphosphonates, such as alendronate, inhibit bone resorption and can prevent bone loss. Calcitonin is another antiresorptive drug. Estrogen therapy effectively prevents bone loss related to estrogen deficiency.[38]

Regular exercise programs help patients to control weight and to minimize calcium loss from bone. Approximately 86% of transplant recipients are considered to have class I New York Heart Association functional status.[21] They are capable of performing most recreational activities and are advised against contact sports or other sports with high risk of injury, such as alpine skiing, unless the recipient was previously accomplished in the sport. Physician approval is recommended if patients wish to pursue vigorous running or jogging. The additional benefit of improved collateral circulation is important if chronic rejection develops at a later time.

Preparation for Discharge

Patient preparation for discharge begins in the intensive care unit and continues until discharge. It is important that patients fully understand their condition and the implications of cardiac denervation. They need to adapt to a new medical regime and must understand its importance in maintaining their state of health. Patients are discharged with multiple medications and must understand their purpose, actions, and side effects. By discharge, it is important that they assume total responsibility for self-care. Bedside flow sheets can be used by the nursing staff to indicate the progress of the patient's learning. Patients are taught how to detect signs of infection and to monitor their temperature. Cardiac risk factors should be evaluated with the patient so that strategies can be outlined to decrease risk. In addition to the primary nurse, dietitians, social workers, physical therapists, and the nurse transplantation coordinators can all contribute to patient instruction. It is important for a nurse to have good teaching skills, a sensitivity to the patient's psychological needs, and an ability to communicate. These skills can greatly enhance the patient's success in learning.

Nursing Management Plan

Nursing care of the transplant recipient is, for the most part, interdependent with medical management. The exception to this is the provision of patient teaching. Nonetheless, several nursing diagnoses can be identified for the patient after cardiac transplantation. This management plan focuses on diagnoses, goals, and interventions unique to the transplant recipient. Because this patient has undergone cardiac surgery, many diagnoses used for the cardiac surgical patient can be used with the transplant recipient. Nursing Care Plan 23-1 is an outline of a nursing management plan for an uncomplicated cardiac transplantation recipient.

Sample nursing diagnoses are presented. Not all possibilities have been discussed. Other diagnoses that the nurse may assess for include:

Potential fluid volume excess related to sodium and water retention from corticosteroid therapy

Potential altered nutrition: more than body requirement related to appetite increase from corticosteroid therapy

Potential fear or anxiety related to the possibility of rejection and death from complications

Altered family processes related to disruption of family life from prolonged hospitalization

Potential for noncompliance related to the complexity of the prescribed medical regime

---

NURSING CARE PLAN 23-1 ◆ The Patient With Uncomplicated Cardiac Transplantation

Nursing Diagnosis 1: Decreased cardiac output in the immediate postoperative period related to cardiac denervation and ischemia during transplantation, manifested by bradycardia and hypotension.

Nursing Goal 1: To detect early manifestations of decreased cardiac output

Outcome Criteria:
1. Patient will maintain a mean arterial blood pressure (MAP) between 70 and 90 mm Hg.
2. Patient will maintain a sinus rhythm with a heart rate (HR) of 100 to 110 beats/min.
3. Changes in above conditions will be detected within 20 minutes of occurrence.
4. Patient's skin will be warm, dry, and normal in color.
5. Nail beds will return to normal color after blanching from pressure over the capillary bed.
6. All peripheral pulses will be palpable. Urine output will be >30 mL/h.
7. Changes in 4, 5, and 6 above will be detected within an hour of occurrence.

NURSING INTERVENTIONS	RATIONALE
1. Assess and document MAP, HR, and rhythm continuously.	1. Required to detect changes.
2. Report any HR < 100, loss of sinus rhythm, or MAP < 70 mm Hg to physician.	2. An HR < 100 may be considered bradycardic for the immediate postoperative transplantation period and may indicate the need for more isoproterenol support. Myocardial edema and manipulation of the heart during surgery increase the risk of bradycardia.[4,35] Junctional rhythms occur at lesser degrees of bradycardia in the transplant recipient and loss of sinus rhythm may indicate the need for atrial pacing.[27] Loss of blood pressure may be a result of bradycardia or loss of sinus rhythm.
3. Evaluate volume status; a central venous pressure (CVP) < 8 mm Hg may indicate need for fluid. If MAP < 60 mm Hg with an adequate CVP, hypotension may be a result of decreased contractility. Notify physician if these findings occur.	3. Hypotension also may be an indication of hypovolemia or a depressed inotropic state related to ischemia incurred during surgery and organ donation. Further evaluation is required.
4. Assess and document skin temperature, color, moisture, capillary filling, quality of peripheral pulses, and urine output hourly as needed. Report abnormal findings to physician.	4. Low cardiac output will be manifested by decreased peripheral perfusion and decreased renal vascular blood flow, resulting in decreased glomerular filtration and subsequent urine output.

(continued)

NURSING CARE PLAN 23-1 ◆ **The Patient With Uncomplicated Cardiac Transplantation** *(Continued)*

| **Nursing Goal 2:** | To reduce or eliminate manifestations of decreased cardiac output specifically bradycardia or hypotension |

Outcome Criteria:	1. Within 15 minutes of intervention, HR returns to >100 beats/min.
	2. Within 15 minutes of intervention, MAP returns to >70 mm Hg.
	3. Within 30 minutes of intervention, good peripheral pulses are present, skin is warm, dry, and of normal color.

NURSING INTERVENTIONS	**RATIONALE**
1. Evaluate isoproterenol infusion and titrate within ordered parameters to a level that raises HR to 100 beats/min minimum.	1. Isoproterenol has positive chronotropic effects that increase heart rate.
2. Notify physician if intervention is not successful and connect pacing wires to a temporary pacemaker. Obtain an order for pacing support and appropriate settings.	2. Temporary pacing may be indicated to maintain an HR in the prescribed parameters.
3. Notify physician if a junctional rhythm develops and results in bradycardia or hypotension.	3. Sinus node function may be impaired due to myocardial edema in the area of the sinus node. Atrial pacing may be indicated.
4. Verify that CVP is between 8 and 12 mm Hg and administer ordered replacement fluid if CVP is below ordered minimum (usually < 8 mm Hg).	4. Hypotension may be the result of hypovolemia: a denervated heart depends on a large stroke volume to stretch myocardial fibers (Sarling mechanism) and produce a strong contraction.
5. Notify physician if hypotension does not respond to volume therapy or is present with an adequate CVP.	5. Hypotension may be the result of decreased contractility, and further inotropic support is needed.

| **Nursing Diagnosis 2:** | Potential for infection related to immunosuppression manifested by a temperature > 37.5° C, a rising white blood cell count, or a change in pulmonary secretions. |

| **Nursing Goal 1:** | To prevent conditions and situations that predispose the patient to increased risk of infection |

Outcome Criteria:	1. Patient will maintain a temperature < 37° C.
	2. Patient will maintain a white blood cell count between 5,000 and 10,000.
	3. Patient will have normal breath sounds without cough and a clear chest radiograph.

NURSING INTERVENTIONS	**RATIONALE**
1. Maintain protective protocols and monitor protective technique of all visitors and staff entering the patient's room.	1. Poor technique may put the patient at risk for infection by organisms carried in the room from the outside environment.
2. Restrict plants, flowers, and unpeeled fruit from the room.	2. Plants, flowers, and unpeeled fruit, such as oranges, may harbor fungus and put the patient at risk for fungal infection.
3. Teach each patient technique for wearing mask when leaving the room. Explain rationale. (May not be required in all institutions.)	3. It is important for the patient to begin to assume responsibility for health maintenance. The hospital environment is contaminated with multiple organisms and potentially resistant strains that may jeopardize the patient not knowledgeable in precautionary techniques.
4. Monitor visitors and personnel for signs of infection and decline entry into room.	4. Some visitors and personnel may be unaware of the potential threat of a seemingly benign infection. Viral infections such as herpes simplex or colds, or infected cuts and other skin lesions, are of particular concern.
5. Change all wound, CVP insertion site, and pacemaker wire exit site dressings daily. Use absolute sterile technique.	5. Conscientious attention to potential ports of entry reduces the potential for wound , systemic, or pacemaker wire–borne infection.

(continued)

NURSING CARE PLAN 23-1 ◆ The Patient With Uncomplicated Cardiac Transplantation *(Continued)*

NURSING INTERVENTIONS	RATIONALE
6. Change all intravenous solutions, tubings, stopcocks, and any heparin-locked lines daily. (Individual program guidelines may vary from 24 to 48 hours.)	6. Intravenous lines that are frequently accessed for specimens and medications increase risk of introducing organisms into the bloodstream.
7. Monitor patient technique of self-administration of antibiotic and antifungal mouthwashes. Ensure that mouthwashes are swished throughout the mouth, are allowed to linger, and are taken after meals. Teach patient not to perform toothbrushing or eat immediately after the administration of mouthwashes.	7. The patient is at risk for opportunistic oral infection, and care must be taken to ensure that medications are used appropriately. Mouthwashes should be allowed to linger and not be followed by eating, drinking, or other rinsing, which reduce mouthwash effectiveness.
8. Restrict patient to room during rejection or if daily white blood cell count returns below target suppression level (less than 5,000). Notify physician if white blood cell count falls below 5,000.	8. Patient is at greatest risk for infection during augmented immunosuppression and any time the white blood cell count falls below target suppression level. A fall in this count indicates a need for adjustment of azathioprine dosage.
9. Provide aggressive pulmonary care, including inspirometers, deep breathing, coughing, and early mobility to prevent atelectasis.	9. Atelectasis is a risk after surgery, and its development increases the risk of pulmonary infection.

Nursing Goal 2: To detect early manifestations of infection to ensure prompt medical attention and Intervention

Outcome Criteria:
1. Patient will have negative cultures 7 days after course of antimicrobial therapy.
2. Patient will have a white blood cell count between 5,000 and 10,000 after antimicrobial therapy.
3. Patient's temperature will return to less than 37° C after antimicrobial therapy.

NURSING INTERVENTIONS	RATIONALE
1. Obtain weekly urine, sputum, and viral cultures as ordered. Ensure that daily white blood cell counts and chest radiographs are obtained.	1. Absolute vigilance in monitoring for infection and identifying organisms is crucial to successful, early treatment of infection.
2. Auscultate breath sounds every 4 hours. Document and immediately report changes in secretions or aeration.	2-4. Nurses are often the first to identify changes in pulmonary status. The lungs are a likely site of infection, and prompt medical evaluation is important. Cultures are necessary to identify appropriate antimicrobial therapy.
3. Monitor for and report any productive or nonproductive cough.	
4. Obtain sputum cultures if quantity, composition, color, or odor changes dramatically.	
5. Observe all wound, intravenous, and pacemaker wire sites daily for signs of suspect drainage, redness, swelling, or heat, and report any of these findings to the physician.	5-6. Wound and insertion site infections can be well established by the time overt signs are present in the immunosuppressed patient. Prompt treatment and insertion site changes are indicated.
6. Obtain cultures of any suspicious drainage.	
7. Obtain temperature every 4 hours. Immediately document and report any temperature greater than 37° C.	7-8. Corticosteroid therapy reduces normal basal and maximal body temperature. A temperature rise greater than 37° C may indicate the presence of systemic infection. It is important to obtain cultures when the temperature elevation occurs to identify possible organisms and appropriate antimicrobial therapy.
8. Obtain aerobic and anaerobic blood cultures if temperature is greater than 37° C.	

(continued)

NURSING CARE PLAN 23-1 ◆ **The Patient With Uncomplicated Cardiac Transplantation** *(Continued)*

Nursing Diagnosis 3:	Activity intolerance related to preoperative deconditioned state manifested by easy fatigue, decreased muscle strength, and inability to ambulate outside of room without assistance.
Nursing Goal:	To increase activity intolerance and muscle strength to level compatible with requirements for activities of daily living and recreational exercise
Outcome Criteria:	1. Patient will be able to ambulate independently in room by fourth postoperative day and out of room by sixth postoperative day. 2. Patient will be able to cycle on stationary bicycle for 20 minutes at dyspnea level 2 by discharge (see Table 23-6). 3. Patient will self-monitor exercise tolerance by discharge.

NURSING INTERVENTIONS	**RATIONALE**
1. Obtain physical therapy consult and evaluation 2 days after transplantation.	1. Reconditioning exercises can begin as soon as the patient is alert, extubated, and hemodynamically stable. Further inactivity may contribute to existing deconditioned state.
2. Begin supine in-bed exercises on first postoperative day after extubation (one session per day).	2. Patients are mobile enough to perform ankle pumps and flexion and abduction of hips and shoulders.
3. Progress patient activity to include shoulder circles, trunk rotation, and knee flexion and extension when stable in a sitting position (one session per day).	3–6. Slow progression of conditioning can coincide with increasing patient strength and endurance. Progression cam be guided by patient tolerance and is only decreased during rejection episodes. Once rejection resolves, activity progression resumes.
4. When patient is able to stand with sufficient balance, include toe raises, trunk lateral flexion, backward and forward bends, and arm circles in the exercise program (one session per day).	
5. When able to complete previous activities without undue fatigue or balance loss, initiate light weight resistance exercises, and stationary cycling (two sessions per day).	

6. Monitor and document blood pressure, dyspnea, and heart rate response to exercise. Monitor and document symptom occurrence with exercise. Stop exercise:[41]
   a. Systolic blood pressure increases greater than 40 mm Hg or decreases more than 15 mm Hg from baseline.
   b. HR increases greater than 30 beats/min over baseline.
   c. Dyspnea index is greater than level 2.
   d. Patient has vertigo, excessive fatigue, or ST segment increase or decrease greater than 1 mm. Report any findings to physician, and reevaluate exercise progression with physical therapist.	

7. Revert to I low-level activity if moderate or severe rejection occurs, and consult physician for guidelines.	7. It is important to limit the amount of stress on the rejecting heart. Exercise capacity is decreased during this time.
8. Teach patient the dyspnea index and how to obtain a pulse. Assess and document patient learning.	8. Patient must acquire self-monitoring skills for continuation of safe exercise after discharge.

(continued)

Nursing Diagnosis 4:	Potential disturbance in self-concept related to changes in facial appearance secondary to immunosuppressive drug therapy, manifested by subjective complaints.
Nursing Goal:	To assist patient with identifying strategies to enhance appearance and self-esteem
Outcome Criteria:	1. Patient will identify methods to minimize hirsutism and increased body hair. 2. Patient will identify methods to deemphasize cushingoid facial features. 3. Patient will remain socially involved. 4. Patient will take initiative to seek resources for enhancing appearance if desired.

NURSING INTERVENTIONS

1. Introduce patient to a transplantation support group or to other patients who have had a cardiac transplantation.
2. Allow male patients time to shave more frequently if bothered by increased facial hair growth. Allow female patients extra time for grooming.
3. Offer female patients possible solutions to increased body hair growth and hirsutism if perceived as disturbing. Shaving, bleaching, and cream hair removers may be suggested. Caution patient not to apply to inflamed, broken, or chapped skin.
4. In response to expressed concerns, arrange for patients to meet with other patients or hairstyle and makeup experts to provide possible suggestions for enhancing facial features. Seek patient's agreement before initiating.
5. Allow patients to initiate any changes; merely offer ideas and resources that have been helpful to others. Avoid introducing personal values and feelings about patient's change in appearance.

RATIONALE

1. Transplant recipients achieve a better understanding of positive adaptive measures used by other patients who have experienced transplantation.
2–3. Cyclosporine stimulates hair follicles, causing a diffuse increase in hair growth (hypertrichosis). Corticosteroid steroid therapy contributes to the development of hirsutism. Male patients may not view this as problematic, but female patients may find this side effect to be troublesome.[27,28]

4. Hairstyle and makeup application changes can deemphasize cushingoid facial features and enhance self-confidence and self-esteem. Men may choose to grow a beard to mask cushingoid features.
5. Patients are likely to have different values about their appearance, and changes may not be problematic to all. A nurse's eagerness to intervene may hinder a patient's adaptation to this alteration in appearance.

Nursing Diagnosis 5:	Potential knowledge deficit about medications related to lack of familiarity, manifested by inability to self-administer medications correctly.
Nursing Goal:	To provide patient with knowledge and skills that will allow patient to self-administer medications correctly by discharge
Outcome Criteria:	1. Patient will identify each medication by name, proper dose, dosage schedule, and potential side effects by discharge. 2. Patients will self-administer medications at correct time on a consistent basis by discharge.

NURSING INTERVENTIONS

1. Set realistic goals for self-administration. Consider patient's previous experience with self-medication, present state of recovery, ability to concentrate and read printed material. Include patient in planning realistic time frames.

2. Tape sample medications to a poster accompanied by the medication's name. Once the patient learns this, add side effects of the medication. Progressive information can be added as patient accomplishes learning of previous material.
3. Provide patient with a variety of materials to assist with learning, such as flashcards, posters, and written material.

RATIONALE

1. It is unrealistic to expect patients to learn multiple medications in a short time. They also may not be feeling well and may not be able to concentrate on instruction while still experiencing discomforts from surgery. Rushing learning may only increase anxiety about their capabilities.
2–3. A poster allows the patient visual and written information about medications. Its format allows for independent review at the patient's directed pace. Learning is more successful when a variety of materials are used.

(continued)

NURSING CARE PLAN 23-1 ♦ The Patient With Uncomplicated Cardiac Transplantation *(Continued)*

NURSING INTERVENTIONS	RATIONALE
4. Allow patient to assume gradually total responsibility for self-administration of medication. Acknowledge accomplishments.	4. Positive reinforcement will help the patient feel more fully functional and capable before assuming total responsibility.
5. Monitor patient's progress in ability to self-administer medications and document.	5. Documentation assists other staff in following the teaching plan and focusing on areas in which knowledge deficit still exists.

NOTE: There are many other areas of potential knowledge deficit. These include:

Prevention of infection
Signs and symptoms of infection
Monitoring activity progression at home
Diet
Treatment of rejection
Seeking medical attention for illness or unusual symptoms
Follow-up care
Management of health care insurance and other financial issues
Return to work

REFERENCES FOR CARDIAC SURGERY

1. Antman EM: Medical management of the patient undergoing cardiac surgery. In Braunwald E (ed): Heart Disease, 4th ed, pp 1670–1693. Philadelphia, WB Saunders, 1992
2. Banasik JL, Tyler ML: The effect of prophylactic positive end expiratory pressure on mediastinal bleeding after coronary revascularization surgery. Heart Lung 15(1): 43–48, 1986
3. Bateman TM, Gray RJ: Perioperative myocardial infarction. In Gray RJ, Matlof JM (eds): Medical Management of the Cardiac Surgical Patient, pp 12–26. Baltimore, Williams & Wilkins, 1990
4. Beattie HW, Evans G, Garnett ES et al: Sustained hypovolemia and extracellular fluid volume expansion following cardiopulmonary bypass. Surgery 71(6): 891–897, 1972
5. Blanche C, Matloff JM, MacKay DA: Technical aspects of cardiopulmonary bypass. In Gray RJ, Matloff JM (eds): Medical Management of the Cardiac Surgical Patient, pp 55–68. Baltimore, Williams & Wilkins, 1990
6. Boncheck LI: The basis for selecting a valve prosthesis. In McCauley KM, Brest AN, McGoon DC (eds): McGoon's Cardiac Surgery: An Interdisciplinary Approach to Patient Care, pp 103–116. Philadelphia, FA Davis, 1985
7. Borkon AM, Schaff HV, Gardner TJ et al: Diagnosis and management of postoperative pericardial effusions and late cardiac tamponade following open-heart surgery. Ann Thorac Surg 31(6): 512–519, 1981
8. Breyer RH, Rosou JA, Engelman RM et al: Late postoperative tamponade following coronary artery bypass grafting in patients on antiplatelet therapy. Ann Thorac Surg 39(1): 27–29, 1985
9. Calafiore AM, Giammarco GD, Teodori G et al: Midterm results after minimally invasive coronary surgery (LAST operation). J Thorac Cardiovasc Surg 115: 763–771, 1998
10. Cameron A, Davis KB, Green G et al: Coronary bypass surgery with internal thoracic artery grafts: Effects on survival over a 15-year period. N Engl J Med 334: 216–219, 1996
11. Casale AS, Ullrich S: Complications in other organ systems. In Baugartner WA, Owen SG, Cameron DE et al (eds): The Johns Hopkins Manual of Cardiac Surgical Care, pp 271–286. St. Louis, Mosby, 1994
12. Chatterjee K: Recognition and management of patients with stable angina pectoris. In Goldman L, Braunwald E (eds): Primary Cardiology, pp 234–256. Philadelphia, WB Saunders, 1998
13. Chiu RC: Cardiomyoplasty. In Edmunds LH (ed): Cardiac Surgery in the Adult, pp 1491–1504. New York, McGraw-Hill, 1997
14. Cho PW, Finney RCS, Gardner TJ: Ischemic heart disease and its complications. In Baugartner WA, Owen SG, Cameron DE et al (eds): The Johns Hopkins Manual of Cardiac Surgical Care, pp 335–364. St. Louis, Mosby, 1994
15. Coleman B, Coughlan Lavieri M, Gross S: Patients undergoing cardiac surgery. In Clochesy JM, Breu C, Cardin S et al (eds): Critical Care Nursing, pp 385–436. Philadelphia, WB Saunders, 1993
16. Cosgrove DM, Loop FD, Lytle BW et al: Does mammary artery grafting increase surgical risk? Circulation 72: II-170, 1985
17. Cuffe Carlson P: Patient care and expectations for recovery after transmyocardial laser revascularization. AACN Clinical Issues 8: 33–40, 1997
18. Czer LSC: Mediastinal bleeding, blood conversation techniques, and transfusion practices. In Gray RJ, Matloff JM (eds): Medical Management of the Cardiac Surgical Patient, pp 55–68. Baltimore, Williams & Wilkins, 1990
19. Detre KM, Takaro T, Hultgren H et al: Long-term mortality and morbidity results of the Veterans Administration randomized trial of coronary artery bypass surgery. Circulation 72: V-84, 1985
20. Dillard DH, Miller DW: Atlas of Cardiac Surgery. New York, Macmillan, 1983
21. Duncan C, Erickson R: Pressures associated with chest tube stripping. Heart Lung 11(2): 166–171, 1982
22. Earp JK, Mallia G: Myocardial protection for cardiac surgery: The nursing perspective. AACN Clinical Issues 8: 20–32, 1997

23. Elefteriades JA, Zaret B L: Coronary bypass: The bad ventricle. In Kaiser LR, Kron IL, Spray TL (eds): Mastery of Cardiothoracic Surgery, pp 409–419. Philadelphia, Lippincott–Raven, 1998

24. European Coronary Surgery Study Group: Long-term results of prospective randomized study of coronary artery bypass surgery in stable angina pectoris. Lancet 2: 1172–1180, 1982

25. Finkelmeier BA: Myocardial preservation. In Finkelmeier BA (ed): Cardiothoracic Surgical Nursing, pp 121–125. Philadelphia, JB Lippincott, 1995

26. Finkelmeier BA: Cardiopulmonary bypass. In Finkelmeier BA (ed): Cardiothoracic Surgical Nursing, pp 113–120. Philadelphia, JB Lippincott, 1995

27. Frazier OH, Kadipasaoglu KA, Cooley DA: Transmyocardial laser revascularization: Does it have a role in treatment of ischemic heart disease? Tex Heart Inst J 25: 24–29, 1998

28. Fremes SE, Weisel RD, Mickle DAG et al: A comparison of nitroglycerin and nitroprusside: I. Treatment of postoperative hypertension. Ann Thoracic Surg 39(1): 53–60, 1985

29. Futterman LG, Lemberg L: Cardiomyoplasty: A potential alternative to cardiac transplantation. Am J Crit Care 5: 80–86, 1996

30. Gradman AH, Harbison MA, Berger HJ et al: Ventricular arrhythmias late after aortic valve replacement and their relation to left ventricular performance. Am J Cardiol 48(5): 824–831, 1981

31. Gray RJ, Mandel WJ: Management of common postoperative arrhythmias. In Gray RJ, Matlof JM (eds): Medical Management of the Cardiac Surgical Patient, pp 12–26. Baltimore, Williams & Wilkins, 1990

32. Gundry SR, Romano MA, Shattuck OH et al: Seven-year follow-up of coronary artery bypasses performed with and without cardiopulmonary bypass. J Thorac Cardiovasc Surg 115: 1273–1278, 1998

33. Guyton RA, Williams WH, Hatcher CR: Techniques of cardiopulmonary bypass. In Hurst JW, Logue RB, Rackley CE et al (eds): The Heart, Arteries and Veins, 6th ed, pp 2025–2029. New York, McGraw-Hill, 1986

34. Hanson MR, Breuer AC, Furlan AJ et al: Mechanism and frequency of brachial plexus injury in open-heart surgery: A prospective analysis. Ann Thorac Surg 36(6): 675–679, 1983

35. Hayes EC, L'Ecuyer KM: A standard of care for radial artery grafting. Am J Crit Care 7: 429–435, 1998

36. Heitmiller ES, Thompson S, Michael K et al: Multidisciplinary care in conducting the operation. In Baugartner WA, Owen SG, Cameron DE et al (eds): The Johns Hopkins Manual of Cardiac Surgical Care, pp 335–364. St. Louis, Mosby, 1994

37. Hurst JW, King SB, Friesinger GC et al: Atherosclerotic coronary heart disease: Recognition, prognosis, and treatment. In Hurst JW, Logue RB, Rackley CE et al (eds): The Heart, Arteries and Veins, 6th ed, pp 882–1008. New York, McGraw-Hill, 1986

38. Jones EL, Hatcher CR: Techniques for surgical treatment of atherosclerotic coronary artery disease and its complications. In Hurst JW, Logue RB, Rackley CE et al (eds): The Heart, Arteries and Veins, 6th ed, pp 2036–2051. New York, McGraw-Hill, 1986

39. Kern LS: Management of postoperative atrial fibrillation. J Cardiovasc Nurs 12(3), 57–77, 1998

40. Killip T, Passamani E, Davis K: Coronary artery surgery study (CASS): A randomized trial of coronary artery bypass surgery. Eight years follow-up and survival in patients with reduced ejection fraction. Circulation 72: V-102, 1984

41. Kirklin JW, Barratt-Boyes BG: Cardiac Surgery, 2nd ed, pp 285–382, 403–413. New York, Churchill Livingstone, 1993

42. Kirklin JW, Barratt-Boyes BG: Cardiac Surgery, pp 29–44, 139–147, 207–278, 323–420. New York, John Wiley & Sons, 1986

43. Kirklin JW, Westaby S, Blackstone EH et al: Complement and the damaging effects of cardiopulmonary bypass. J Thorac Cardiovasc Surg 86(6): 845–857, 1983

44. Krantz DS, Arbian JM, Davia JE et al: Type A behavior and coronary artery bypass surgery: Intraoperative behavior and perioperative complications. Psychosom Med 44(3): 273–284, 1982

45. Kreter B, Woods M: Antibiotic prophylaxis for cardiothoracic operations. J Thorac Cardiovasc Surg 104(3): 590–599, 1992

46. Kron IL, Joob AW, Van Meter C: Acute renal failure in the cardiovascular surgical patient. Ann Thorac Surg 39(6): 590–598, 1985

47. Lee WH, Brady MP, Rowe JM et al: Effects of extracorporeal circulation upon behavior, personality, and brain function: Part II. Hemodynamic, metabolic, and psychometric correlations. Ann Surg 173(6): 1013–1023, 1971

48. Lindner A, Cutler RE, Goodman WG et al: Synergism of dopamine plus furosemide in preventing acute renal failure in the dog. Kidney Int 16(2): 158–166, 1979

49. Loop FD: Coronary artery bypass surgery. In Topol EJ (ed): Textbook of Cardiovascular Medicine, pp 2011–2030. Philadelphia, Lippincott–Raven, 1998

50. Loop FD, Lytle BW, Cosgrove DM et al: Influence of the internal-mammary-artery graft on 10-year survival and other cardiac events. N Engl J Med 314(1): 1–6, 1986

51. Loop FD, Muehrcke DD: Surgical treatment of atherosclerotic coronary heart disease. In Alexander RW, Schlant RC, Fuster V (eds): Hurst's The Heart, Arteries, and Veins, 9th ed, pp 1473–1487. New York, McGraw-Hill, 1998

52. Lynn-McHale DJ, Hambach C, Carter T et al: Transmyocardial laser revascularization. J Cardiovasc Nurs 12(3), 17–28, 1998

53. Markmann PJ, Wallace P: Nursing care in the intensive care unit. In McCauley KM, Brest AN, McGoon DC (eds): McGoon's Cardiac Surgery: An Interprofessional Approach to Patient Care, pp 319–354. Philadelphia, FA Davis, 1985

54. Martin T, Craver J, Gott J et al: Prospective randomized trial of retrograde warm blood cardioplegia: Myocardial benefit and neurological threat. Ann Thorac Surg 57: 298–304, 1994

55. Matlof JM: Current indications for coronary pass and/or valvular surgery. In Gray RJ, Matlof JM (eds): Medical Management of the Cardiac Surgical Patient, pp 12–26. Baltimore, Williams & Wilkins, 1990

56. Meyendorf R: Visual disturbances after open-heart surgery. In Becker R, Katz J, Polonius MJ et al (eds): Proceedings of the Second International Symposium of Psychopathological and Neurological Dysfunctions Following Open-Heart Surgery, Milwaukee WI, 1980, pp 16–31. Berlin, Springer-Verlag, 1982

57. Morin JE, Long R, Elleker MG: Upper extremity neuropathies following median sternotomy. Ann Thorac Surg 34(2): 181–185, 1982

58. Morris DC, Clements SD, Hug CC Jr: Management of the patient after cardiac surgery. In Alexander RW, Sclant RC, Fuster V (eds): Hurst's The Heart, Arteries, and Veins, 9th ed, pp 1489–1500. New York, McGraw-Hill, 1998

59. Mravinac, CM: Neurologic dysfunctions following cardiac surgery. Critical Care Nursing Clinics of North America 3: 691–697, 1991

60. Pym J, Luffman B, Parry M: Total arterial revascularization of the heart: Intentional or inevitable. AACN Clinical Issues 8: 9–19, 1997

61. Rahimtoola SH: Outcome of aortic valve surgery. Circulation 60: 1191–1195, 1979

62. Roberts AJ, Niarchos AP, Subramanian VA et al: Systemic hypertension associated with coronary artery bypass surgery: Predisposing factors, hemodynamic characteristics, humoral profile, and treatment. J Thorac Cardiovasc Surg 74(6): 846–859, 1977

63. Roberts AJ, Woodhall DD, Conti CR et al: Mortality, morbidity, and cost-accounting related to coronary artery bypass graft surgery in the elderly. Ann Thorac Surg 39(5): 426–432, 1985

64. Rosborough D: Surgical myocardial revascularization in the 1990's. AACN Clinical Issues 4: 219–226, 1993

65. Schlenker JD, Hubay CA: The pathogenesis of post-operative atelectasis. Arch Surg 107(6): 846–850, 1973

66. Seifert PC: Advances in myocardial protection. J Cardiovasc Nurs 12(3): 29–38, 1998

67. Severance SR: Pancreatitis. In Zschoche DA (ed): Mosby's Comprehensive Review of Critical Care, pp 559–567. St Louis, CV Mosby, 1986

68. Shapiro SJ, Gordon LA: General surgery complications following cardiac surgery. In Gray RJ, Matloff JM (eds): Medical Management of the Cardiac Surgical Patient, pp 271–279. Baltimore, Williams & Wilkins, 1990

69. Shinn J: Management of a patient undergoing myocardial revascularization: Coronary artery bypass graft surgery. Nurs Clin North Am 27: 243–256, 1992

70. Staples JR, Ramsay JG: Advances in anesthesia for cardiac surgery: An overview for the 1990's. AACN Clinical Issues 8: 41–49, 1997

71. Tasdemir Q, Vurnal KM, Karagoz H et al: Coronary artery bypass grafting on the beating heart without use of extracorporeal circulation: Review of 2052 cases. J Thorac Cardiovasc Surg 116: 68–73, 1998

72. Tuman KJ, McCarthy RJ, Najafi H et al: Differential effects of advanced age on neurologic and cardiac risks of coronary artery operations. J Thorac Cardiovasc Surg 104(6): 1510–1517, 1992

73. Vargo R, Dimengo J: Surgical alternatives for patients with heart failure. AACN Clinical Issues 4: 244–259, 1993

74. Verrier ED, Wright IH, Cochran RP et al: Changes in cardiovascular surgical approaches to achieve early extubation. J Cardiothorac Vasc Anesth 9(Suppl 1): 10–15, 1995

75. Vitello-Cicciu J, Fitzgerald C, Whalen D: On the horizon: Minimally invasive cardiac surgery. J Cardiovasc Nurs 12(3): 1–16, 1998

76. Weiland AP, Walker WE: Physiological principles and clinical sequelae of cardiopulmonary bypass. Heart Lung 15(1): 34–39, 1986

77. Weitzman LB, Tinker WP, Kronzon I et al: The incidence and natural history of pericardial effusion after cardiac surgery: An echocardiographic study. Circulation 69(3): 506–511, 1984

78. Wey JM, Guinn GA: Ulnar nerve injury with open-heart surgery. Ann Thorac Surg 39(4): 359–360, 1985

79. Yusuf S, Zucker D, Peduzzi P et al: Effect of coronary bypass graft surgery on survival: Overview of 10-year results from randomized trials by the Coronary Artery Bypass Graft Surgery Trialists Collaboration. Lancet 344: 563–570, 1994

REFERENCES FOR CARDIAC TRANSPLANTATION

1. 1997 Annual Report. The U.S. Scientific Registry of Transplant Recipients and the Organ Procurement and Transplantation Network. SR AR 1988–1996. United Network for Organ Sharing (UNOS); Health Resources and Services Administration/Department of Health and Human Services, Office of Special Programs, Division of Tranplantation, Rockville, MD; UNOS, Richmond, VA.

2. Armitage JM, Kormos RL, Morita S et al. Clinical trial of FK506 Immunosuppressive in adult Cardiac transplantation. Ann Thorac Surg 54: 205–211, 1992

3. Backer CL, Zales VR, Harrison HL et al: Intermediate term results of infant orthotopic cardiac transplantation from two centers. J Thorac Cardiovasc Surg 101: 826–832, 1991

4. Bexton RS, Nathan AW, Hellestrand KJ et al: Sinoatrial function after cardiac transplantation. J Am Coll Cardiol 13: 712–723, 1984

5. Billingham ME, Cary NRB, Hammond ME et al: A working formulation for the standardization of nomenclature in the diagnosis of heart and lung rejection: Heart rejection study group. J Heart Transplant 9: 587–591, 1990

6. Bolman RM, Elick B, Oilvari MT et al: Improved immunosuppression for heart transplantation. Heart Transplantation 4: 315–318, 1985

7. Brown M: Thoracic transplantation: Procurement and organization. In Shumway NE, Shumway SJ (eds): Thoracic Transplantation, pp 79–83. Cambridge, MA, Blackwell Science, 1995

8. Crandell B: Immunosuppression. In Sigardson-Poor KM, Haggerty LM (eds): Nursing Care of the Transplant Recipient, pp 53–85. Philadelphia, WB Saunders, 1990

9. DiBiase A, Tse TM, Schnittger I et al: Frequency and mechanism of bradycardia in cardiac transplant recipients and need for pacemakers. Am J Cardiol 67: 1385–1389, 1991

10. Dillon TA, Sullivan M, Schatzlein MH et al: Cardiac transplantation in patients with preexisting malignancies. Transplantation 52: 82–85, 1991

11. Edwards BS, Hunt SA, Fowler MB et al: Cardiac transplantation in patients with preexisting neoplastic diseases. Am J Cardiol 65: 501–504, 1990

12. Frazier DH, VanBuren CT, Poindexter SM et al: Nutritional management of the heart transplant recipient. Heart Transplantation 4: 450–452, 1985

13. Frazier OH: patient selection for heart transplantation. In Frazier OH, Macris MP Radovancevic B (eds): Support and Replacement of the Failing Heart, pp 59–68. Philadelphia, JB Lippincott, 1996

14. Funk M: Heart transplantation: Postoperative care during the acute period. Critical Care Nurse 6(2): 27–45, 1986

15. Gamberg P, Miller J, Lough M: Impact of protective isolation on the incidence of infection after heart transplantation. Heart Transplantation 6: 147–149, 1987

16. Gao S, Hunt SA, Schroeder JS: Accelerated graft coronary artery disease. In Shumway NE, Shumway SJ (eds): Thoracic Transplantation, pp 273–289. Cambridge, MA, Blackwell Science, 1995

17. Goldman MH, Barnhart G, Mohanakumar T et al: Cyclosporine in cardiac transplantation. Surg Clin North Am 65: 637–659, 1985

18. Griffith BP, Hardesty RL, Bahnson HT: Powerful but limited immunosuppression for cardiac transplantation with cyclosporin and low-dose steroid. J Thorac Cardiovasc Surg 87: 35–42, 1984

19. Harwood CH, Cook CV: Cyclosporin in transplantation. Heart Lung 14: 529–540, 1985

20. Hunt SA: Complications of heart transplantation. Heart Transplantation 3: 70–74, 1983

21. Hosenpud JD, Bennet LE, Berkley MK et al: The Registry of the International Society for Heart and Lung Transplantation: Fifteenth Official Report—1998. J Heart Lung Transplant 17: 656–668, 1998

22. Jamieson SW, Oyer P, Baldwin J et al: Heart transplantation for end-stage ischemic heart disease: The Stanford experience. Heart Transplantation 3: 224–227, 1984

23. Kahan BD, Van Buren CT: The new Immunosuppressants. In Frazier OH, Macris MP, Raclovancevic B (eds): Support and Replacement of the Failing Heart, pp 309–326. Philadelphia, JB Lippincott, 1996

24. Kirklin JK, Bourge RC, Naftel DC: Treatment of recurrent heart rejection with mycophenolate mofetil (RS-61443): Initial clinical experience. J Heart Lung Transplant 13: 444–450, 1994

25. Levett JM, Karp RB: Heart transplantation. Surg Clin North Am 65: 613–635, 1985

26. Losse B: Indications and selection criteria for cardiac transplantation. Thorac Cardiovasc Surg 38: 276–279, 1990

27. Lough ME, Lindsey AM, Shinn JA et al: Impact of symptom frequency and symptom distress on self-reported quality of life in heart transplant recipients. Heart Lung 16: 193–200, 1987

28. Lough ME, Lindsey AM, Shinn JA et al: Life satisfaction following heart transplantation. Heart Transplantation 4: 446–449, 1985

29. McGregor CG, Jamieson JW, Oyer PE et al: Heart transplantation at Stanford University. Heart Transplantation 4: 31–32, 1984

30. McKelvey SA: Effects of denervation in the cardiac transplant recipient. In Douglas MK, Shinn JA (eds): Advances in Cardiovascular Nursing, pp 197–209. Rockville, MD, Aspen Systems, 1985

31. Moran M, Tomlanovich S, Myers BD: Cyclosporin-induced nephropathy in human recipients of cardiac allografts. Transplant Proc 17(Suppl 1): 185–190, 1985

32. Myers BD, Ross J, Newton L et al: Cyclosporin associated chronic nephrotoxicity. N Engl J Med 311: 699–705, 1984

33. Olsen SL, Eastburn TE, Renlund DG et al: Trimethoprim sulfamethoxazole prevents *Pneumocystis carinii* pneumonia in cardiac transplant recipients. J Heart Transplan 9: 49–57, 1990

34. Packa M, Bristow MR, Cohn JN et al: The effect of carvedilol on morbidity and mortality in patients with chronic heart failure. N Engl J Med 334: 1349–1355, 1996

35. Painvin GA, Frazier OH, Chandler LB et al: Cardiac transplantation: Indications, procurement, operation and management. Heart Lung 14: 484–489, 1985

36. Penkoske PA, Freedom RM, Rowe RD et al: The future of heart and heart-lung transplantation in children. Heart Transplantation 3: 233–238, 1984

37. Przepiorka D: Tacrolimus: Preclinical and clinical experience. In Przepioka D, Sollinger H (eds): Recent Developments in Transplantation Medicine: New Immunosuppressive Drugs, pp 29–50. Glenview, IL, Physicians and Scientist Publishing, 1992

38. Rodino, MA, Shane E: Osteoporosis after organ transplantation. Am J Med 104(5): 459–469, 1998

39. Rose AG: Endomyocardial biopsy diagnosis of cardiac rejection. Heart Failure 2(2): 64–72, 1986

40. Sadowsky HS: Cardiac Transplantation: A review. Phys Ther 76: 498–515, 1996

41 Sadowsky HS, Fries K: Introduction to the Treatment of Cardiac and Cardiopulmonary Transplant Patients. Stanford, CA, Stanford University Hospital, Department of Physical and Occupational Therapy, 1986

42. Shinn JA: New issues in cardiac transplantation. In Douglas MK, Shinn JA (eds): Advances in Cardiovascular Nursing, pp 185–195. Rockville, MD, Aspen Systems, 1985

43. Shumway NE, Lower RR, Stofer C: Transplantation of the heart. Adv Surg 2: 265–284, 1966

44. Starnes VA, Bernstein D, Oyer PE et al: Heart transplantation in children. J Heart Transplant 8: 20–26, 1989

45. Stevenson LW, Laks H, Terasaki PI et al: Cardiac transplant selection, immunosuppression and survival. West J Med 149: 572–582, 1988

46. Strong AG, Sneed NV: Clinical evaluation of a critical path for coronary artery bypass patients. Prog Cardiovasc Nurs 6(1): 29–37, 1991

47. Thelan LA, Urden LD, Lough ME et al (eds): Critical Care Nursing: Diagnosis and Management, 3rd ed, pp 1179–1184. St. Louis: Mosby, 1998

48. Thompson ME, Shapiro ME, Johnsen AM et al: New onset of hypertension following cardiac transplantation. Transplant Proc 25(Suppl 1): 2573–2577, 1983

49. Trento A, Takkenberg JM, Czer LSC et al: Clinical experience with one hundred consecutive patients undergoing orthotopic heart transplantation with bicaval and pulmonary venous anastomosis. J Thorac Cardiovasc Surg 112: 1496–1503, 1996

50. Valantine HA: Prevention and treatment of cytomegalovirus disease in thoracic organ transplant patients: Evidence for a beneficial effect of hyperimmune globulin. Transplant Proc 27: 49–57, 1995

51. Veith FJ, Fein JM, Tendler MD et al: Brain death: I. A status report of medical and ethical considerations. JAMA 238: 1651–1655, 1978

52. Wagoner LW: Management of the cardiac transplant recipient: Roles of the transplant cardiologist and primary care physician. Am J Med Sci 324: 173–184, 1997.

24

Shock

DEBRA LAURENT-BOPP
JULIE A. SHINN

DATABASE FOR NURSING MANAGEMENT

Shock is a complex clinical syndrome characterized by impaired cellular metabolism due to decreased tissue perfusion. This inadequacy of tissue perfusion results in cellular hypoxia, the accumulation of cellular metabolic wastes, cellular destruction, and, ultimately, organ and system failure. The syndrome begins as an adaptive response to some insult or injury and progresses to multiple organ system failure.[6,8,38,44,59] The pathophysiologic mechanisms of shock include decreased circulating blood volume, decreased cardiac contractility, and increased venous capacitance. One of these mechanisms predominates in each type of shock; however, the mechanisms are interactive, with more than one occurring in each of the shock syndromes.

Classification

This chapter discusses three basic types of shock: hypovolemic, cardiogenic, and vasogenic. Hypovolemic shock exists when there is a decrease in the circulating blood volume. Losses of blood volume may be external (e.g., hemorrhage) or internal (e.g., sequestration of fluid in the abdomen secondary to intestinal obstruction). Cardiogenic shock is characterized by a decreased strength of contraction of myocardial fibers, leading to a decreased cardiac output. The decrease in myocardial contractile strength may be due to ischemia, infarction, trauma, myocarditis, or cardiomyopathy. Distributive or vasogenic shock is characterized by vasodilation in response to neurologic or hormonal stimuli. Profound vasodilation results in an inequality between the circulating blood volume and the capacity of the vascular bed. Septic shock is the most often encountered form of distributive shock and is the representative form discussed in this chapter. Two other forms of distributive shock are anaphylactic and neurogenic.[38,51,59]

A variety of labels can be found in the literature to describe the various types of shock. Display 24-1 classifies the types of shock according to the primary physiologic deficit.

Pathophysiology

Although the clinical syndrome of shock has various etiologies and basic pathophysiologic defects, all three types are characterized by tissue hypoperfusion, which, if untreated or inadequately treated, results in generalized cellular and systemic dysfunction. In response to tissue hypoperfusion, compensatory mechanisms are activated and are directed at the restoration and maintenance of adequate blood volume and pressure and at the adequate perfusion of the heart and brain. If the basic physiologic defect is not corrected, compensatory mechanisms become counterproductive, resulting in the vicious cycle of irreversible shock.[18,38,51]

Clinical shock is a dynamic continuum. The prominence of its features and compensatory mechanisms varies with time and with treatment. Although other features (e.g., low blood pressure or decreased cardiac output) are present, the basic problem is acute, generalized tissue hypoperfusion.

HYPOVOLEMIC SHOCK

Hypovolemic shock exists when the volume of blood is inadequate to fill the intravascular space. A significant reduction in the venous return to the right heart results in a decreased cardiac output, a reduced mean arterial blood pressure (MAP), and renal hypoperfusion. A 10% reduction in blood volume initiates compensatory mechanisms, and a rapid reduction of 20% of blood volume produces the clinical signs and symptoms of hypovolemic shock.[18,51,64]

CARDIOGENIC SHOCK

Cardiogenic shock results from the impaired ability of the heart to pump blood.[38,51] As the endpoint on the clinical continuum of left ventricular (LV) failure, cardiogenic shock includes shock due to ineffective cardiac contractility and myocardial failure. This can happen with a myocardial infarction (MI) when there is inadequate contractility of the heart muscle (pump failure), or when the heart rate and rhythm are disrupted and the efficiency of myocardial contractions is impaired (power failure). MI usually involves the left ventricle, but a small percentage of patients have damage to the right ventricle. Right ventricular infarctions can lead to cardiogenic shock because the damaged right ventricle does not propel sufficient blood to the left ventricle, resulting in a decreased cardiac output and inadequate systemic circulation.[51] Cardiogenic shock may also occur after cardiac surgery, in association with episodes of cardiac tamponade, or as a result of severe heart failure (HF) due to coronary heart disease, myocardial disease (e.g., the cardiomyopathies), or valvular dysfunction. Acute HF can be grouped clinically into acute cardiogenic pulmonary edema, cardiogenic shock, and acute decompensation of chronic HF.[21]

DISTRIBUTIVE SHOCK

Massive peripheral vasodilation causes shock because the blood volume, although within normal limits, is insufficient to fill the enlarged vascular capacity. This leads to a decreased venous return and a diminished cardiac output.[38] Several types of distributive shock exist, including septic, anaphylactic, and neurogenic shock.

Septic Shock. In septic shock, cellular derangements precede and contribute to cardiovascular abnormalities.[5] Any type of microorganism can produce septic shock, including gram-negative bacteria, gram-positive bacteria, viruses, fungi, and rickettsiae; however, gram-negative bacteria are the most common cause, producing more than two-thirds of the reported cases.[51] The gram-negative bacteria include *Escherichia coli*, *Klebsiella*, *Enterobacter*, and *Serratia* species, *Pseudomonas aeruginosa*, and *Bacteroides* and *Proteus* species. A complex hormonal and chemical release of substances is produced through the body's immune system in response to the adverse effects of endotoxins. The invading microorganisms elaborate vasoactive toxins (histamine and kinins), which results in selective but profound vasodilation. In addition, the pathogens create a focus of inflammation, which creates a high-flow, low-resistance state.[51,58]

There is a persistent decreased ability to extract oxygen from inspired air and from the blood, which results in tissue hypoxia. These abnormalities in oxygen diffusion result from destruction of pulmonary alveolar type I and II cells, a reduction in 2,3-diphosphoglycerate, and a shift of the oxyhemoglobin dissociation curve to the left.[18,38] In late stages (see section on Irreversible Stage), septic shock is remarkably similar to cardiogenic and hypovolemic shock, with hypotension, vasoconstriction, decreased cardiac output, hypoxia, and acidosis.[15,58,59]

Anaphylactic Shock. Anaphylactic shock is the result of a severe allergic, antigen–antibody reaction. Examples of substances that can act as antigens include drugs, contrast media, transfused blood and blood products, and insect venoms.[51,59] This reaction results in the release of histamine, serotonin, and bradykinin, causing direct vasodilation and increased capillary permeability. Slow-reacting substances of anaphylaxis are also released, causing bronchoconstriction.[38,44,51]

Neurogenic Shock. In neurogenic shock, there is a reduction of vasomotor tone, which occurs at the level of the vasomotor centers in the brainstem and causes decreased vasoconstriction, resulting in generalized systemic vasodilation. This form of shock can develop with spinal anesthesia, spinal cord injury, or altered function of the vasomotor center in response to low blood sugar or drugs, including sedatives, barbiturates, and narcotics.[38,51]

Compensatory Mechanisms

The following equations illustrate the physiologic relation of the hemodynamic variables. Here, CO = cardiac output, SV = stroke volume, HR = heart rate, MAP = mean arterial pressure, and SVR = systemic vascular resistance:

$$CO = SV \times HR$$
$$MAP = CO \times SVR$$

In the pathophysiologic state of shock, the decrease in MAP is brought about by an alteration in one of the variables. In hypovolemic and cardiogenic shock, the reduction in MAP results from a decrease in stroke volume, whereas in distributive shock, the reduction in MAP results from a decrease in systemic vascular resistance:

1. Hypovolemic:

$$CO = {\downarrow}SV \times HR; {\downarrow}MAP = {\downarrow}CO \times SVR$$

2. Cardiogenic:

$${\downarrow}CO = {\downarrow}SV \times HR; {\downarrow}MAP = {\downarrow}CO \times SVR$$

3. Vasogenic:

$$CO = SV \times HR; {\downarrow}MAP = CO \times {\downarrow}SVR$$

Compensatory mechanisms consist of reflex reactions to an initial fall in blood pressure. They are activated immediately and increase in intensity in an attempt to restore adequate tissue perfusion. The compensatory mechanisms are directed at the restoration and maintenance of adequate blood volume, cardiac output, and vascular tone. The initial compensatory mechanisms vary with the primary pathophysiologic derangement, but the intermediate and final stages are similar. The initial compensatory mechanisms in hypovolemic and cardiogenic shock are increased heart rate and increased systemic vascular resistance. In vasogenic shock, the initial compensatory mechanism is increased heart rate and cardiac output.[38,51,59]

INITIAL STAGE

The initial stage of hypovolemic shock is characterized by selective venoconstriction of the renal, cutaneous, muscular, and splanchnic beds, with preservation of circulation to the heart and brain.[38,53]

In cardiogenic shock, the decreased coronary blood flow results in profound local compensatory events. There is an increase in myocardial oxygen extraction and dilation of the coronary arteries. The myocardial cells shift to anaerobic metabolism and use glycolysis in the production of adenosine triphosphate (ATP).[38,53] These events occur immediately in response to myocardial ischemia. If inadequate, myocardial contractility decreases, leading to a fall in cardiac output and systemic hypoperfusion.

The initial stage of septic shock is characterized by a hyperdynamic cardiovascular and metabolic state. This hyperdynamism results from the interrelation between the inflammatory responses and those caused by the endotoxins. Various vasoactive substances (e.g., vasodilators, histamine, and kinins) are released early in septic shock.[38,53,59] It is in the late stages of sepsis that a hypodynamic state characterized by reduced cardiac output, vasoconstriction, and additional blood shunting occurs and initiates compensatory mechanisms similar to those in cardiogenic and hypovolemic shock (Fig. 24-1).

A reduction in arterial blood pressure secondary to decreased blood volume, decreased cardiac output, or increased venous capacitance initiates the body's compensatory mechanisms to maintain adequate tissue perfusion. These mechanisms serve to increase cardiac output and arterial blood pressure through increasing heart rate, enhancing myocardial contractility, providing selective vasoconstriction, conserving sodium and water, and shifting fluid from the interstitial to the intravascular space.[53,59,60]

Specialized nerve endings (mechanoreceptors) in the carotid sinus, aortic arch, heart, and lungs sense the decrease in blood pressure and transmit their impulses to the vasomotor center. The vasomotor center stimulates the sympathetic nervous system, inhibits the parasympathetic, and initiates the secretion of catecholamines from the adrenal gland. Sympathetic nervous system stimulation unopposed by parasympathetic effects results in increased heart rate, increased myocardial contractility, and selective

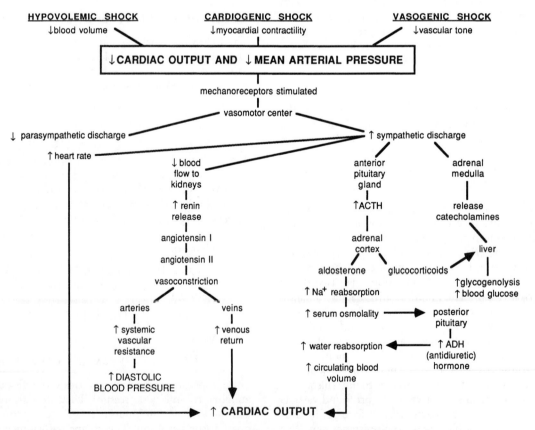

FIGURE 24-1 In the initial stage of shock, all three types of shock lead to a decrease in mean arterial pressure. Compensatory mechanisms attempt to reduce the effects of this decreased mean arterial pressure and, if successful, lead to an increase in cardiac output and mean arterial pressure.

vasoconstriction. Reflexes of the sympathetic nervous system are active within 30 seconds of an acute decrease in circulating blood volume and are able to compensate for a 20% loss in blood volume by increasing cardiac output by 20% to 25%.[18,58]

In response to ischemia and sympathetic stimulation, hormones are released from the adrenal medulla, adrenal cortex, anterior and posterior pituitary gland, and kidney, which further compensate for decreased circulating blood volume. The adrenal medulla releases epinephrine and norepinephrine, which enhance vasoconstriction, myocardial contractility, and heart rate. Epinephrine and norepinephrine also stimulate glycogenolysis, thus increasing serum glucose. The adrenal cortex releases glucocorticoids, which also increase serum glucose. Decreased renal blood flow results in the release of renin, which initiates a series of reactions in the liver and elsewhere, resulting in the production of angiotensin. Angiotensin promotes the release of aldosterone by the adrenal cortex and, in situations of hypovolemia, promotes profound vasoconstriction. Aldosterone enhances renal sodium reabsorption accompanied by increased water reabsorption. Antidiuretic hormone is released from the posterior pituitary and further enhances renal water reabsorption. Thirst is stimulated and also causes increased fluid intake.[18,53,60] As a result of decreased capillary pressure, Starling capillary balance is shifted, and fluid is transferred from the interstitial space to the capillary.

INTERMEDIATE STAGE

If shock is not recognized and reversed in the initial compensatory stage, it progresses. Compensatory mechanisms are no longer able to maintain homeostasis and may become counterproductive. For example, continued profound vasoconstriction in the presence of decreased MAP promotes inadequate tissue perfusion and cellular hypoxia[6,8,53] (Fig. 24-2).

Decreased delivery of oxygen and nutrients causes cells to shift to anaerobic metabolic pathways.[5,18] Increasing amounts of lactic acid are produced and accumulate in the cells owing to decreased perfusion.[36] Because anaerobic metabolism is less efficient in meeting the energy requirements of the cells, ATP is depleted. Reduction in the available ATP results in failure of the membrane transport mechanisms, intracellular edema, and rupture of the cell membrane. Progressive tissue ischemia results in increased anaerobic metabolism and the further production of metabolic acidosis.

Impairment of cellular function disrupts all body organs and organ systems. Splanchnic ischemia results in the release of endotoxin from the intestine. The reticuloendothelial (tissue macrophage) system (RES) is suppressed by splenic and hepatic ischemia. The continued renal response to ischemia leads to further vasoconstriction, stimulating the release of aldosterone from the adrenal gland and promoting the reabsorption of sodium in the kidney.

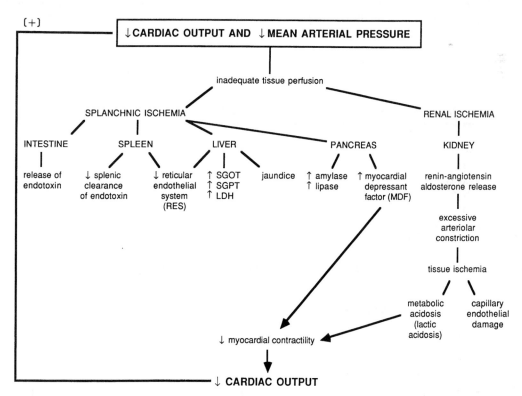

FIGURE 24-2 In the intermediate stage of shock, compensatory mechanisms fail, resulting in decreased tissue perfusion and organ function. Decreased myocardial contractility leading to a decrease in cardiac output sets up a positive feedback mechanism (+) to decrease further cardiac output and mean arterial pressure. SGOT, serum glutamic oxaloacetic transaminase; SGPT, serum glutamic pyruvic transaminase; LDH, lactate dehydrogenase.

This response is no longer useful because the increased volume cannot be pumped by the failing heart and results in ventilatory failure. The increased volume begins to pool in tissues secondary to profound venoconstriction and increased capillary permeability.[53,59]

Myocardial ischemia results in the deterioration of cardiac function. In addition to the direct detrimental effects of myocardial ischemia, there is some evidence that a peptide secreted by the pancreas, the myocardial depressant factor (MDF), may further depress myocardial function.[58] MDF has been identified in the serum of patients in the early stages of septic shock.[42] Its presence in other forms of shock remains controversial.

IRREVERSIBLE STAGE

In this stage, the compensatory mechanisms are nonfunctioning or no longer effective, and hypotension has reached the critical level of adversely affecting the heart and brain (Fig. 24-3). Myocardial hypoperfusion, resulting from hypotension and tachycardia, produces acidosis, which leads to further depression of myocardial function. Decreased cerebral blood flow leads to depressed neuronal function and activity and loss of the central neuronal compensatory mechanisms.[6,8,53]

The progressive general hypoxia and reduction in cardiac output further deprive body cells of oxygen and nutrients needed for cell growth and result in microcirculatory insufficiency. The microcirculation responds by vasodilation to secure the necessary nutrients and oxygen for the deprived cells. Microcirculatory vasodilation in association with systemic vasoconstriction results in the sequestration of blood in the capillary beds, further limiting the volume of blood returning to the systemic circulation. This loss of circulating blood volume and impaired capillary flow result in reduced venous return, further reducing cardiac output and arterial pressure. This situation creates a positive feedback mechanism in which the low-flow state produces a further reduction in flow.[18]

CLINICAL MANIFESTATIONS

Patients in the initial stages of shock exhibit a variety of behavioral and physiologic symptoms, depending on the cause of shock. Changes noted on physical examination during the initial stages are primarily due to sympathetic stimulation. Regardless of the classification of shock, the principal physiologic defect remains the same: reduced cellular perfusion. Continued tissue hypoxia and acidosis affect specific vital organs in specific ways.

Brain. Decreased cerebral blood flow and coagulopathy can lead to a cerebral infarction or cerebral thrombus formation. Alterations in cellular metabolism throughout the body, metabolic acidosis, and the accumulation of toxins further depress cerebral function. Lethargy, stupor, and coma develop as shock progresses. Finally, in the irreversible stage of shock, the vasomotor center in the brain is disrupted, causing failure of the circulatory mechanisms.[53,59]

Myocardium. Because it cannot greatly increase oxygen extraction as other organs and tissues can, the myocardium is

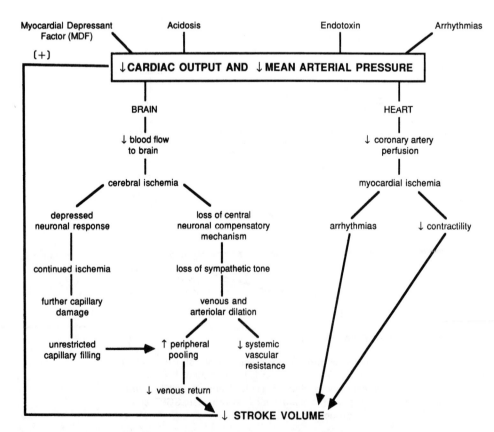

FIGURE 24-3 In the irreversible stage of shock, a prolonged decrease in cardiac output and mean arterial pressure leads to cellular necrosis and multiple organ failure.

more vulnerable to the effects of decreased blood flow. A drop in aortic pressure decreases coronary perfusion pressure. Myocardial cells convert to anaerobic metabolism due to the underperfused hypoxic myocardium, and lactate production increases. The normal functioning of the sodium–potassium pump is disrupted. Because of ischemia and necrosis of the pancreas, MDF is released and has a direct negative inotropic effect on the myocardium, contributing to further ischemia. MDF is thought to interfere with calcium in coupling electrical excitation with contraction of the heart.[42,58]

Kidney. Adequate renal perfusion produces a minimum of 400 mL urine/24 hours, or 20 mL/h. Impaired renal perfusion in shock results in hourly urine outputs of less than 20 mL/h.[53,59,64] The excretion of high volumes of low-solute urine may also represent renal hypoperfusion. Prolonged hypoperfusion may lead to acute tubular necrosis and acute renal failure.

Gastrointestinal Tract. Compensatory vasoconstriction in shock may result in mucosal ischemia, an ileus, and full-thickness gangrene of the bowel. If the bowel wall becomes disrupted, the normal bacterial flora of the intestines enter the abdomen and can then enter the circulation. Gastrointestinal bleeding may also occur.[8,53]

Liver. Factors that cause damage to the liver include decreased blood flow, splanchnic vasoconstriction, pooling of blood in the microcirculation, right HF, and bacterial invasion. The subsequent changes include a loss of RES function, increasing the risk of infection; a decreased lactic acid conversion, contributing to metabolic acidosis; altered protein, fat, and carbohydrate metabolism; and altered bilirubin function.

Jaundice, increased serum bilirubin levels, and increased serum enzymes are early indicators of liver damage associated with shock. Serum globulin is increased, and serum albumin is decreased.[53]

Lungs. The lung is fairly resistant to short-term ischemia. Thus, it is unlikely that low blood flow is the sole cause of pulmonary insufficiency associated with shock. Other contributory factors have been implicated, including thromboemboli or fat emboli in the pulmonary tree, the toxic effect of fibrin degradation products resulting from intravascular coagulation, serum complement depletion with sequestration of granulocytes in the lung, and sepsis.[6,8,53] These factors lead to increased pulmonary capillary permeability. As the ensuing alveolar edema impairs surfactant production, massive atelectasis develops. Clinically, this is called shock lung, adult respiratory distress syndrome (ARDS), or primary pulmonary edema and is characterized by severe hypoxemia, dyspnea, a marked reduction in lung compliance, and the presence of extensive lung infiltrates.

In cardiogenic shock, failure of the left ventricle leads to acute cardiogenic pulmonary edema. Because of the increase in LV end-diastolic pressure, there is an increase in left atrial pressure and dilation. Pressure is increased within the pulmonary capillary bed, forcing plasma or whole blood into the pulmonary interstitial compartment and, finally, into the pulmonary alveoli.

Coagulation. Disseminated intravascular coagulation is a disorder characterized by simultaneous thrombosis and hemorrhage, which occurs in the stage of irreversible shock. Procoagulants initiate uncontrolled microcirculatory clotting. The rapid thrombin formation causes three major problems: fibrin deposits in the microcirculation, consumption of clotting factors, and provocation of the fibrinolytic system. The prothrombin time and the partial thromboplastin time are prolonged, the platelet count and fibrinogen levels are decreased, and the fibrin degradation products are increased. Diffuse bleeding, which may ultimately lead to massive bleeding, may occur from the mucosal surfaces in the trachea, gastrointestinal tract, or urinary tract.

Immune System. Patients sustaining shock or trauma are at heightened risk of serious infection. The RES function is depressed in shock. The ability of the RES to clear damaged red cells, fibrin degradation products, and bacteria is impaired and contributes to the increased susceptibility to infection.[6,8,44,53]

Physical Assessment

Ongoing assessment of the patient at risk for or in shock, with early detection of subtle changes in the patient's condition, is essential. Subjective and objective data must be correlated with adjunctive clinical measurements such as the measurement of cardiac output and oxygen consumption. The clinical assessment of the patient provides the basis for medical and nursing intervention.[4]

INTEGUMENTARY

Skin appearance and temperature provide a clinical measure of peripheral circulation. Progressive peripheral vasoconstriction results in a change from the initial normal skin appearance to cool, moist, pale skin with mottling. In cardiogenic shock, cool, moist skin with barely perceptible peripheral pulses is commonly observed. Patients with vasogenic shock initially appear flushed, followed by pallor and mottling as shock progresses. Capillary refill and peripheral pulses are other indicators of the relative adequacy of cardiac output. Normal capillary refill is almost instantaneous; in cardiogenic and hypovolemic shock, capillary refill is often prolonged. Dry mucous membranes and thirst may be seen in association with an elevated serum sodium.[8,50,59]

CIRCULATORY

Blood pressure is one of the defining characteristics of shock. A MAP of 65 to 75 mm Hg is required to maintain myocardial and renal perfusion.[18,58] Shock is defined clinically as the pathophysiologic state that results from a MAP of less than 65 mm Hg over time. Narrowing of the pulse pressure indicates arteriolar vasoconstriction and a decreasing cardiac output.

Pulse rate usually increases in response to sympathetic stimulation to compensate for decreased stroke volume and to maintain cardiac output. In vasogenic shock, the pulse may be full and bounding; in hypovolemic and cardiogenic shock, the pulse is weak and thready.

Jugular veins are flat in hypovolemic and vasogenic shock. Distended neck veins may be seen with cardiogenic shock associated with right ventricular failure.

NEUROREGULATORY

Level of consciousness is an indicator of the adequacy of cerebral blood flow. With cerebral ischemia, the patient initially exhibits hypervigilance, restlessness, agitation, and mild confusion. Persistent cerebral hypoxia results in progressive unresponsiveness to verbal stimuli with eventual coma.[50,59]

RENAL

Urine output is an indicator of the adequacy of renal perfusion and may decrease early in hypovolemic and cardiogenic shock. Distributive shock may initially cause polyuria. Oliguria is defined by a urine output of less than 20 mL/h. Urine osmolarity and specific gravity increase, and urine sodium decreases with decreased urine output. Nonoliguric renal insufficiency is characterized by the output of large volumes of urine with low specific gravity. An elevated serum creatinine is an early, nonspecific indicator of impaired renal perfusion.[8,50]

PULMONARY

Respiratory rate and depth are initially increased in all forms of shock, and patients may experience dyspnea or air hunger. This increased ventilation represents the body's attempt to eliminate lactic acid resulting from decreased tissue perfusion. Increased respiratory depth also enhances blood return to the right heart. Arterial blood gases initially reveal respiratory alkalosis. As shock progresses, this is followed by a combined metabolic and respiratory acidosis.

Medical Management Plan

DIAGNOSIS

The diagnosis of shock is made by the history, physical examination, and collection of data from adjunctive diagnostic tests. The primary measurements that document the relative adequacy of blood flow include continuous monitoring of arterial blood pressure and central venous pressure (CVP), monitoring of the electrocardiogram (ECG), and repeated measurements of pulmonary artery wedge pressure (PAWP) and of cardiac output by thermal dilution technique.[6,8,50,59]

Continuous measurement of urine output and urine studies is the best indicator of adequate organ perfusion because the kidney is sensitive to decreased blood flow. Serial measurements of arterial blood gases reflect the overall metabolic state of the patient, the adequacy of ventilation, and the adequacy of the circulation in providing for oxygen and metabolic needs. Measurement of mixed venous oxygen content ($S\bar{v}O_2$) by direct blood sampling or by continuous invasive monitoring reflects peripheral oxygen extraction and use. Serial arterial lactate levels can also be measured because the presence of lactic acidosis helps identify critical hypoperfusion as marked by anaerobic metabolism.[3,36,49] Elevation of other substances in the blood that reflect the function of specific organs, such as blood urea nitrogen, creatinine, biliru-

bin, aspartate aminotransferase, and lactate dehydrogenase, may be useful in the diagnosis of shock.[8,50]

Hypovolemic Shock. Hypovolemic shock is a diagnosis based on the history and clinical assessment. Patients admitted after injury or surgery and those experiencing dehydration, gastrointestinal hemorrhage or obstruction, burns, liver disease, or peritonitis are all at risk for development of hypovolemic shock. In the initial stages of hypovolemia, interstitial fluids tend to move into the capillaries. The hematocrit value reflects the relation between red cells and intravascular fluid and drops 6 to 8 hours after hemorrhage. Hematocrit initially is stable in hemorrhage because both red cells and plasma are lost. It is elevated in situations in which intravascular fluid is sequestered in the abdomen or selectively lost from the body, as in burns. If the fluid volume is monitored invasively, a worsening fluid volume deficit is indicated by a sustained decrease in CVP or PAWP.

Cardiogenic Shock. Cardiogenic shock is diagnosed by the presence of systemic and pulmonary hemodynamic alterations and neurohormonal mechanisms that reflect ventricular failure and result in an inadequate cardiac output and the retention of sodium and water. Primary indicators of cardiogenic shock include a systolic blood pressure less than 85 mm Hg or a MAP less than 65 mm Hg; cardiac index less than 2.2 L/min/m²; and an elevated PAWP greater than 18 mm Hg[16,60] (Forrester subset IV; Fig. 24-4). Noninvasive

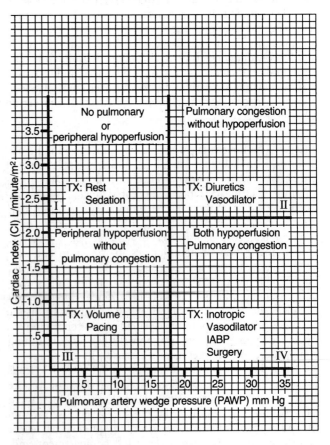

FIGURE 24-4 Forrester subsets: Clinical states and therapy. IABP, intra-aortic balloon pumping.

assessments of a rapid, thready pulse, arrhythmias, oliguria, and decreased mentation are important clinical indices of an inadequate cardiac output.

Radiographically, the heart may be enlarged, and there may be evidence of pulmonary congestion. The arterial blood gases frequently show a decreased PaO_2, which provides an important indicator of intrapulmonary shunting.

Septic Shock. Septic shock has no universal pattern of signs and symptoms. Its many variations make it difficult to diagnose. The diagnosis is confirmed by microbiologic data, usually from two sets of blood cultures and cultures of sputum and urine.[15,44,50]

PROGNOSIS

The stages of shock depict a series of pathophysiologic changes that occur if medical and nursing interventions are delayed or inappropriate. The stages do not progress at the same speed in all patients. The length of time tissues are hypoxic is a major factor in determining the occurrence of complications. The early and intermediate stages of shock are reversible with aggressive management. The irreversible stage, due to cellular necrosis and multiple organ failure, is not. The chance of recovery in the irreversible stage without permanent injury is low.

In cardiogenic shock, patients with a cardiac index less than 1.81 L/min/m^2 have a 70% mortality rate.[16] Patients with an $S\overline{v}O_2$ less than 55% also have a high mortality rate.[36] Patients in septic shock are at greater risk for development of disseminated intravascular coagulation and ARDS than are patients with cardiogenic or hypovolemic shock. The survival rate with ARDS varies from 50% to 70% and depends on early recognition and management.

TREATMENT

The main goal of treatment of the metabolic defects produced by shock is the restoration of adequate tissue perfusion. Treatment should be aimed at (1) restoring the blood volume, (2) strengthening the heart, and (3) restoring the normal luminal size of blood vessels. Depending on the cause of shock, treatment must revolve around the manipulation of one or more of these three mechanisms.[6,8,15,26,38,52,64]

Hypovolemic Shock. Hypovolemic shock requires restoration of fluids and the circulating plasma volume. The amount of fluids and the speed at which they are infused is dictated by the severity of the loss and clinical status of each patient. Parental fluids used in shock include blood and blood products, colloids (e.g., dextran, hespan, albumin, or plasma protein fraction [Plasmanate]), and crystalloids (e.g., normal saline or lactated Ringer's solution).[19,29,52]

After severe hypotension from massive hemorrhage, volume replacement should be given rapidly enough to maintain the systolic pressure greater than 100 mm Hg and the MAP greater than 80 mm Hg. To maximally augment stroke volume, the CVP should be raised to 15 cm H_2O or the PAWP to 16 to 20 mm Hg.

The type of fluid to be given is determined by the type lost, although opinions vary as to the amount and type.[20,22,29,52] Crystalloid solutions such as lactated Ringer's are the most appropriate replacement solutions in hypovolemia due to vomiting, intestinal obstruction, or other sequestration of fluids. Much work has focused on the efficacy of hypertonic saline solutions (3%, 5%, and 7.5%) for fluid resuscitation in various forms of circulatory shock.[20,26,68] Volume replacement with hypertonic solutions was reduced, but careful monitoring was essential to avoid complications. Until more studies are conclusive regarding the safety and efficacy of hypertonic saline solutions, they should not be considered for widespread clinical use.[26]

Crystalloid solutions can be given initially while blood is being crossmatched for the patient who has hemorrhaged, and resuscitation with Ringer's alone may be adequate if blood loss is 20% or less.[29] When acute hemorrhage reaches 20% to 50% blood loss, nonprotein plasma expanders (e.g., dextran) are indicated. Major losses of whole blood (>50%) should be replaced with whole blood and fresh or frozen plasma to maintain a hematocrit of at least 24% and a hemoglobin of 8 g/dL.[29,41,52] Packed cells should be used if the CVP is high or if myocardial failure limits the amount and speed of fluid resuscitation. If the blood loss exceeds 80%, for every 5 units of blood, 1 to 2 units of fresh frozen plasma and 1 to 2 units of platelets should be given to prevent hemodilution of clotting factors and bleeding.[26,29,37,41,52]

Cardiogenic Shock. Cardiogenic shock requires the institution of therapeutic measures to protect the ischemic myocardium. The three major goals of treatment are (1) to increase the oxygen supply to the myocardium, (2) to maximize the cardiac output, and (3) to decrease the workload of the left ventricle.[10,16]

1. *Increase the oxygen supply to the myocardium.* Increased inspired oxygen concentrations, including the institution of mechanical ventilation with positive end-expiratory pressure, may be required to maintain arterial blood gases within normal limits. Narcotic analgesics are used to control the patient's pain and aid in reducing myocardial oxygen demands. Reperfusion of the coronary arteries can be undertaken by invasive and noninvasive approaches, including percutaneous transluminal coronary angioplasty, atherectomy or stent placement, coronary artery bypass grafting, and thrombolytic therapy.

2. *Maximize the cardiac output.* Because the cardiac output is already compromised, arrhythmias, which occur as a result of ischemia, acid–base alterations, or MI, can cause a further decline in cardiac output. Antiarrhythmic agents, pacing, or cardioversion may be used to maintain a stable heart rhythm. Volume loading is undertaken with caution and in the presence of adequate hemodynamic monitoring. Optimal preload (LV end-diastolic pressure) ranges between 14 and 18 mm Hg.[16] However, fluid loading must be abandoned when the increase in filling pressure occurs without increase in cardiac output. A diuretic such as furosemide is given when symptoms of pulmonary edema occur. Pharmacologic agents are also used in an attempt to increase the cardiac output. Sympathomimetic amines such as dopamine, epinephrine, and norepinephrine may

improve contractility and cardiac output; however, the peripheral vasoconstriction and increase in myocardial oxygen requirements associated with these agents may outweigh the benefit and prove deleterious. Other agents used for positive inotropic effect include dobutamine and the phosphodiesterase inhibitors, such as amrinone or milrinone.[52]

3. *Decrease the LV workload.* The efficacy of vasodilators has been shown in the treatment of cardiogenic shock. The major physiologic effect of vasodilators is a reduction in LV end-diastolic pressure and systemic vascular resistance, with a subsequent increase in stroke volume and improved LV function.[10,38] Intravenous nitroprusside remains the drug of choice in cardiogenic shock because it acts rapidly and has a balanced effect, dilating both veins and arterioles, thereby reducing both preload and afterload.[14] Other vasodilators that provide a reduction in preload, afterload, or a combined effect include nitroglycerin, hydralazine, captopril, and enalapril. Mechanical support of circulation may be used in the reduction of LV workload in cardiogenic shock. The intra-aortic balloon pump (IABP) is used to reduce afterload at the time of systolic contraction and to increase myocardial perfusion during diastole. Other mechanical assist devices may be used. An in-depth discussion of circulatory assist devices follows this treatment section.

DISPLAY 24-2

Initial Management of Acute Cardiogenic Pulmonary Edema

Sublingual nitroglycerin
    0.4 mg every 5 min
Intravenous nitroglycerin
    Start at 0.2 to 0.4 µg/kg/min
Intravenous furosemide
    20 to 40 mg intravenously
    Follow volume status closely
Nitroprusside if further afterload reduction required
Supplemental oxygen/mechanical ventilation as guided by arterial blood gas analysis
Consider intravenous morphine (2 to 6 mg) if no pulmonary contraindication
Electrocardiogram
    Exclude myocardial infarction
Echocardiography
    Evaluate ventricular function, valvular status
Proceed with urgent coronary angiography if reperfusion therapy indicated

From Hass GJ, Young JB: Acute heart failure management. In Topol EJ (ed): Textbook of Cardiovascular Medicine, p 2247–2271. Philadelphia, Lippincott-Raven, 1998.

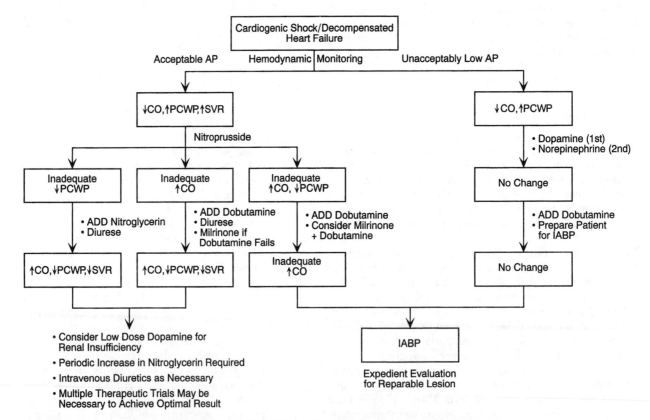

FIGURE 24-5 Algorithm for hemodynamically directed pharmacologic support of cardiogenic shock and decompensated heart failure. AP, arterial pressure; CO, cardiac output; PCWP, pulmonary capillary wedge pressure; SVR, systemic vascular resistance; IABP, intra-aortic balloon pump. (From Haas GJ, Young JB: Acute heart failure management. In Topol EJ [ed]: Textbook of Cardiovascular Medicine, p 2262. Philadelphia, Lippincott–Raven, 1998.)

DISPLAY 24-3

Hemodynamically Directed Protocol for Decompensated Heart Failure Therapy

I. General hemodynamic goals
  RAP ≤ 7 mm Hg
  PAWP ≤ 15 mm Hg
  SVR 1,000 to 1,200 dyne/sec/cm^5
  CI > 2.5 L/min/m^2
  "Optimum" systolic or mean BP is the lowest
    pressure that adequately supports renal function and
    central nervous system activity without significant
    orthostatic symptoms (systolic BP usually > 80 to
    90 mm Hg)
II. Patient-specific hemodynamic goals
  "Optimum filling pressure" (PAWP): lowest PAWP
    that can be maintained without preload-related
    decline in systolic BP or CI. A higher PAWP
    (18 to 20 mm Hg) is usually required in acute
    myocardial injury
  "Optimum afterload" (SVR): lowest SVR that leads to
    reasonable cardiac index while maintaining adequate
    systolic BP (usually > 80 mm Hg) and renal perfusion
    (urine output > 0.5 mL/kg/h)

III. Specific intravenous pharmacologic therapy
  Nitroprusside: begin when combined preload and
    afterload reduction is most important hemodynamic goal
    Start at 0.1 to 0.2 µg/kg/min
    Titrate upward by 0.2 µg/kg/min at 3- to 5-min intervals
    Target hemodynamics (Section I)
    Hemodynamic effects resolve rapidly when
      infusion stopped
  Nitroglycerin: begin when preload reduction is primarily desired
    Start at 0.2 to 0.3 µg/kg/min
    Titrate at 3- to 5-min intervals
    Be aware of tolerance
    Target hemodynamics (Section I)
    Effects resolve rapidly when infusion stopped
  Dobutamine: begin when both inotropic and vasodilating
    effects desired but inotropic effects most important
    Start at 2.5 µg/kg/min
    Attempt to keep dose < 15 µg/kg/min; avoid
      significant tachycardia
    Consider adding low-dose dopamine or milrinone to
      assist with augmenting renal perfusion or achieving
      hemodynamic endpoints
    Hemodynamic effects resolve over minutes to hours
      when infusion stopped, but benefits occasionally
      persist longer
  Milrinone: begin when both vasodilating and inotropic
    effects desired
    Dose range is 0.375 to 0.75 µg/kg/min (usual is
      0.5 µg/kg/min)
    Target hemodynamics (Section I)
    Excessive hypotension with loading dose; would
      avoid loading in acute heart failure
    Prolonged hemodynamic effects after drug is stopped

BP, blood pressure; CI, cardiac index; PAWP, pulmonary artery wedge pressure; RAP, right atrial pressure; SVR,
  systemic vascular resistance. From Hass GJ, Young JB: Acute heart failure management. In Topol EJ (ed):
  Textbook of Cardiovascular Medicine, p 2247–2271. Philadelphia, Lippincott-Raven, 1998.

ACUTE PULMONARY EDEMA. The Forrester subsets (see Fig. 24-4) can be used as guidelines for the patient in cardiogenic pulmonary edema.[16,17] In subset II, the goal of therapy is to reduce the PAWP below a level that causes pulmonary congestion but above a level that causes a deleterious reduction in cardiac output by the Starling mechanism. There are several options, because diuretics, peripheral vasodilators, and inotropic agents all reduce PAWP. The management strategy for the patient in acute cardiogenic pulmonary edema is outlined in Display 24-2.

CARDIOGENIC SHOCK AND DECOMPENSATED HEART FAILURE. In the high-risk Forrester subset IV (see Fig. 24-4), simultaneous improvement of both cardiac index and PAWP is the goal of therapy. Afterload reduction by peripheral vasodilators appears particularly well suited to this goal. Inotropic agents are also used to increase systemic and coronary artery perfusion pressure. IABP counterpulsation may also be indicated.[16,17] Figure 24-5 provides a general approach to the selection of specific intravenous pharmacologic agents based on hemodynamic profile.[23]

The initial therapeutic decision is influenced by the systemic arterial pressure. Display 24-3 reviews the hemodynamically directed protocol for decompensated HF.[21,23]

Septic Shock. Treatment of septic shock has two primary therapeutic goals: (1) to eradicate the causative organism and (2) to support vital life functions compromised by circulatory failure.[15,38,52] Interventions directed at identifying, localizing, and controlling the microorganisms include surgery, removal of the source of the contaminating organisms, and antimicrobial drugs.

Fluid replacement is the most common therapy used to support vital functions in septic shock. As with hypovolemic shock, there is disagreement about which fluid to use. Advantages of one fluid type over another have not been conclusively demonstrated.[25] Two types of fluids are used: crystalloids (e.g., lactated Ringer's, normal saline) and colloids (e.g., Plasmanate, hespan, or dextran).[20,24,26] Weil and Shubin[66] advocate a "7/3 rule" for fluid replacement. They give fluid challenges of 5 to 20 mL/min for 10 min. If the

PAWP reading is elevated more than 7 mm Hg above the beginning level, the infusion is stopped. If the PAWP or pulmonary artery diastolic pressure rises only 3 mm Hg above the starting point, or decreases, another fluid challenge is given.[66]

Inotropic agents are sometimes indicated to maximize cardiac output. The most commonly recommended inotropic agent in septic shock is dopamine. Dobutamine is not an optimal drug for this clinical setting owing to its peripheral vasodilator effects. Epinephrine has been shown to be effective in dopamine-resistant septic shock.[38]

Clinical research studies report conflicting results from the use of steroids in septic shock. Steroids at high doses appear to block inhibition of gluconeogenesis by endotoxin and thus prevent intracellular hypoglycemia.[15,38,60] Other actions of steroids include reduction of lactic acid concentration and stabilization of the endothelial wall of the pulmonary microcirculation. Future therapies will focus on the immune system, with interferon and the prostaglandins as agents involved in the immune response.[38,52,59]

One of the greatest challenges in septic shock is maintaining adequate tissue oxygenation. A recent study addressed the optimization of oxygen delivery ($\dot{D}O_2$) to "supranormal" levels, with the $\dot{D}O_2$ indexed goal of 600 mL/min/m².[69] This study suggested that the standard of care of treating these critically ill patients to a normal indexed $\dot{D}O_2$ of 450 to 550 mL/min/m² should be reconsidered.

CIRCULATORY ASSIST DEVICES

Circulatory assist devices have been clinically used, in various forms, since the mid-1960s. IABP counterpulsation is now commonly used in a variety of hospital centers for both medical and surgical patients. Temporary extracorporeal circulatory support devices, once restricted to a few large centers, are now used with increasing frequency in most larger hospitals as an adjunct to cardiovascular surgery programs. Such devices are used to support circulation temporarily when the injured myocardium cannot generate adequate cardiac output. In centers with heart transplantation programs, these devices are being used temporarily to support patients with end-stage HF until a donor heart becomes available. One such device has been used successfully to support patients for over 2 years. We are on the horizon of the clinical application of chronic, long-term support of circulation with totally implantable devices for situations in which myocardial recovery is not expected to occur. It is estimated that 17,000 to 35,000 patients younger than 70 years of age could benefit from the increased life span with an acceptable quality of life provided by implantable, long-term circulatory support devices.[65]

With early recognition, the rapid deterioration of patients with acute LV failure can be arrested with circulatory assist devices. The type of device used depends on the degree of myocardial injury and the degree to which LV function is compromised. The purpose of therapy is to stabilize the patient until (1) the left ventricle recovers from acute injury, (2) mechanical problems causing acute failure (e.g., ruptured ventricular septum) can be surgically corrected, or (3) possible heart transplantation can be performed. As implied, the goal of any circulatory assist device is to arrest deterioration and to stabilize or improve hemodynamics and secondary organ function. The major principles governing all devices are that they (1) decrease LV workload, (2) partially or totally support the systemic circulation, and (3) enhance oxygen supply to the injured myocardium. The extent to which each principle is achieved depends on the type of device used. The IABP offers only partial support, whereas an implantable LV assist device (LVAD) can assume the total workload of the left ventricle.

Most cardiovascular critical care nurses encounter patients requiring IABP support, which is the emphasis of this chapter. For completeness, examples of various other types of circulatory assist devices and a nursing care plan are included. Because LV support is used most commonly, examples are limited to this scenario.

Intra-aortic Balloon Pump Counterpulsation. The IABP was introduced clinically in the late 1960s as a therapy for cardiogenic shock after MI.[28] Since then, its application has expanded to include patients with acute LV failure after cardiac surgery and potential heart transplant recipients whose end-stage condition begins to deteriorate. Another large group of patients who benefit from IABP therapy are those with unstable angina that is refractory to pharmacologic therapy.[67] In most of these patients, IABP therapy eliminates rest pain accompanied by ischemic ECG changes and allows for surgical revascularization under less emergent conditions. IABP therapy also may be used to stabilize patients with papillary muscle rupture or ventricular septal rupture after MI, allowing for safer anesthesia induction before the surgical repair of these injuries. Major indications are summarized in Display 24-4.

DESCRIPTION. The intra-aortic balloon is constructed of biocompatible polyurethane and mounted on a catheter constructed of the same material. Perforation at the catheter–balloon connection allows pressurized gas to move in and out of the balloon, causing inflation and deflation to occur. Helium is preferred as the inflating gas. Properly positioned, the balloon catheter rests just distal to the left subclavian artery and proximal to the renal arteries. Figure 24-6 illustrates proper anatomic position of the IABP catheter. The catheter is inserted by way of a direct femoral or iliac

---

DISPLAY 24-4

Major Indications for Intra-aortic Balloon Pump Therapy

Postcardiotomy support
Severe unstable angina
Cardiogenic shock after myocardial infarction
Postinfarction ventricular septal defect or mitral regurgitation resulting in shock
Emergency support after injury during percutaneous transluminal coronary angioplasty or cardiac catheterization
Hemodynamic deterioration in patients awaiting heart transplantation

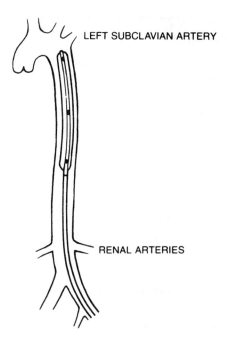

LEFT SUBCLAVIAN ARTERY

RENAL ARTERIES

FIGURE 24-6 Proper placement of the balloon catheter is just distal to the left subclavian artery and proximal to the renal arteries. (From Shinn JA: Intra-aortic balloon pump counterpulsation. In Hudak CM, Gallo BM, Lohr TS [eds]: Critical Care Nursing: A Holistic Approach, 4th ed, p 190. Philadelphia, JB Lippincott, 1986.)

arteriotomy or by percutaneous insertion using a Seldinger technique. It can also be inserted through a femoral artery sheath or introducer. A direct arteriotomy approach is used infrequently today; it was once the only method available owing to previous catheter designs. It may still be the choice for a patient with serious peripheral vascular disease when direct visualization is desired, or in pediatric patients. The approach requires an incision in the groin for access to the femoral or iliac artery. A major disadvantage of this technique is its increased invasiveness, the required surgical procedure for removal, and the time required for insertion. The percutaneous technique allows for more rapid insertion and is less invasive. Catheters used for this technique are designed especially for this approach and can be passed through a large-bore sheath that has been placed in the artery. The balloon is wrapped tightly around its own guide wire so that it slides easily through the sheath. Once in proper position, the balloon is unwrapped in the aorta, allowing inflation and deflation to commence. This catheter is secured in place by suturing it to the skin. Figure 24-7 illustrates the percutaneous insertion technique.

PHYSIOLOGIC PRINCIPLES. Goals of IABP therapy are to increase coronary artery perfusion pressure and thus coronary artery blood flow and to decrease LV workload. These goals are achieved by displacement of volume in the aorta during systole and diastole with alternating inflation and deflation of the balloon. A typical adult-sized balloon contains 40 mL of gas or volume. For smaller patients, a 34-mL balloon is available. The size of the catheter ranges from 7 to 9 French.

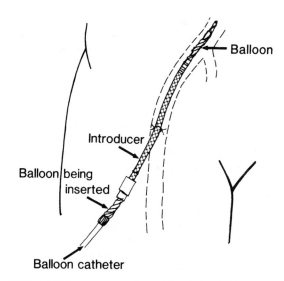

Balloon

Introducer

Balloon being inserted

Balloon catheter

FIGURE 24-7 Percutaneous insertion of the balloon catheter through an introducer or sheath. Note the right wrap of the balloon. (From Bull SO: Principles and techniques of intra-aortic balloon counterpulsation. In Woods SL [ed]: Cardiovascular Critical Care Nursing, p 171. New York, Churchill Livingstone, 1983.)

When the balloon is rapidly inflated at the onset of diastole, 40 mL of volume is suddenly added to the aorta. This acute increase in volume creates a pressure rise in the aorta and generates retrograde flow toward the aortic valve. The increase in aortic pressure early in diastole effectively increases pressure at the aortic root, where the coronary ostia are located. As a result, the perfusion pressure of the coronary arteries is increased. Figure 24-8 illustrates this effect. The objective is to increase coronary artery perfusion

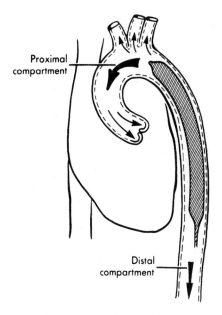

Proximal compartment

Distal compartment

FIGURE 24-8 Balloon inflation during diastole displaces volume retrograde toward the aortic root. The result is increased coronary artery perfusion pressure. Enhanced distal flow may also occur. (From Quaal SJ: Comprehensive Intra-Aortic Balloon Pumping, p 82. St. Louis, CV Mosby, 1984.)

and subsequently oxygen delivery to the ischemic ventricle. The desired outcome is decreased ischemia. The period of time early in diastole in which diastolic pressure is enhanced is referred to as *diastolic augmentation*. Diastolic augmentation also contributes to enhanced flow to other organs. Diastolic pressure gradually tapers off, as it normally does when diastolic run-off occurs.

Rapid evacuation of the 40 mL of gas out of the balloon during deflation displaces 40 mL of volume out of the aorta. This sudden drop in aortic volume rapidly decreases pressure. Deflation is timed to occur at the end of diastole, just before the patient's next systole. Effective deflation, which decreases end-diastolic pressure, decreases the impedance or resistance to systolic ejection. Impedance to ejection is what determines the amount of wall tension (afterload) that the ventricle must generate to force the aortic valve open and to sustain ejection during systole. The greater the impedance, the greater the LV workload. In shock states, high systemic vascular resistance contributes to greater impedance, resulting in a greater workload for the failing left ventricle. With properly timed deflation, which lowers end-diastolic pressure and impedance to ejection, the LV workload requirement is reduced. In this situation, it is not necessary for the ventricle to generate higher degrees of wall tension or to maintain high pressures to sustain ejection. Figure 24-9 illustrates this effect. Systolic pressure is actually decreased when deflation of the balloon is timed properly. As a result of decreased afterload, contractility improves and there is more effective forward flow during systole. Improved forward flow contributes to decreased end-systolic volume in the ventricle. Improved emptying leads to decreased subsequent preload. A decrease in excessive preload also contributes to decreasing LV workload. Improved forward flow results in increased cardiac output with a resultant increase in blood pressure. Tachycardia that resulted from decreased

stroke volume in the shock state is not necessary for compensation as forward flow (stroke volume) improves. As a result, rapid heart rate should diminish, decreasing oxygen demand. Better systemic perfusion helps to reverse the acidosis often seen in shock states and improves secondary organ dysfunction related to the previous hypoperfused state. Displays 24-5 and 24-6 summarize the physiologic effects of IABP therapy.

CONTRAINDICATIONS. Inflation of the balloon during diastole dictates that the aortic valve be competent. If aortic regurgitation is present, inflation serves to generate

---

DISPLAY 24-5

Physiologic Effects and Expected Clinical Outcomes of Balloon Inflation

PHYSIOLOGIC EFFECTS
Increased early diastolic pressure
  Diastolic augmentation
Increased aortic root pressure
Enhanced coronary artery perfusion pressure
Improved oxygen delivery
Decreased ischemia

CLINICAL OUTCOME
Early diastolic pressure ≥ systolic pressure
Decreased angina
Decreased signs of ischemia on the electrocardiogram
Decreased ventricular ectopy of ischemic origin

DISPLAY 24-6

Physiologic Effects and Expected Clinical Outcomes of Balloon Deflation

PHYSIOLOGIC EFFECTS
End-diastolic drop in aortic pressure
Decreased afterload requirement
Lower systolic pressure requirement
Improved contractility
Increased forward flow during systole
Improved secondary organ perfusion
Increased efficiency of left ventricular work (decreased oxygen demand)

CLINICAL OUTCOMES
Improved forward flow
  Decreased preload
  Decreased pulmonary artery wedge pressure
  Decreased rales
Increased cardiac output
Increased mean blood pressure
Improved urine output
Improved peripheral pulses and warm skin temperature
Clearer sensorium
Decreased heart rate

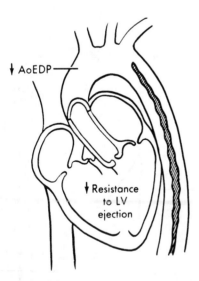

FIGURE 24-9 Impedence or resistance to left ventricular (LV) ejection is decreased by abrupt balloon deflation before systole. Properly timed deflation decreases aortic end-diastolic pressure (A$_0$EDP), which decreases the workload of the left ventricle. (From Quaal SJ: Comprehensive Intra-Aortic Balloon Pumping, p 83. St. Louis, CV Mosby, 1984.)

more aortic regurgitation because of the increased pressure and retrograde flow against the aortic valve. This effect actually increases the workload of the ventricle. Thus, IABP therapy is of no benefit to this patient and actually may contribute to further deterioration of the patient's condition.

The presence of an aortic aneurysm also contraindicates IABP therapy. First, the tip of the catheter may advance into the aneurysm during insertion, resulting in perforation of the weakened wall or dislodgement of thrombus. A second concern is the effect of inflation and deflation adjacent to the thrombotic debris that accumulates in the aneurysm. There is a great potential for thrombus material to break free, resulting in emboli and possibly precipitating a catastrophic event.

Severe peripheral vascular occlusive disease is considered a contraindication to IABP therapy. More accurately, a femoral or iliac artery insertion site is the actual contraindication. Catheter insertion may be difficult or impossible in this situation. There is a potential for dislodgement of plaque from the vessel wall, which can embolize and totally disrupt distal flow. Dissection of the vessel is also possible in this situation. Another possibility is disruption of flow caused by the presence of the catheter in an already compromised vessel. Such a situation jeopardizes the distal extremity by depriving it of oxygen. This potential problem can be avoided by selecting an alternate method of insertion. In the cardiac surgery patient, the catheter may be inserted directly into the thoracic aorta. The obvious disadvantage of this approach is the requirement for reopening the sternotomy incision to remove the catheter. Another, less conventional approach is antegrade aortic insertion of the balloon catheter by way of the right subclavian artery.[33] This approach requires a subperiosteal clavicular resection to access the artery, but is less invasive than a sternotomy incision. Newer catheters of smaller diameter minimize the risk of occluding distal blood flow. When distal flow to the extremity is threatened by iliac or femoral insertion and other options are not ideal, femoro-femoral crossover Dacron grafts have been used to shunt arterial flow from one femoral artery to the femoral artery compromised by the presence of the catheter.[2] In this way, blood flow to the affected extremity can be maintained.

A final contraindication is balloon catheter insertion in any patient who has a terminal condition in which no medical or surgical therapy exists that might alter the outcome. It would serve no purpose to introduce more aggressive therapy to support such a patient. The only time this may be considered is when the patient meets the criteria for heart transplantation.

PROPER TIMING TO ACHIEVE EXPECTED CLINICAL OUTCOMES. Proper timing of IABP therapy is crucial to achieving the beneficial hemodynamics previously outlined. Proper timing requires coordination of inflation and deflation of the balloon with the patient's cardiac cycle. The R wave from the ECG, pacemaker spikes on the ECG, or the arterial systolic pressure are used to identify individual cardiac cycles. All these act as signals to the IABP console to discriminate systole from diastole. The R wave signals the onset of electrical depolarization, which precedes mechanical systole. A ventricular pacemaker spike essentially represents the same event. Arterial systolic pressure signals the

onset of mechanical systole. Any of these can be used as a reference point to determine when deflation of the balloon should optimally occur. An arterial waveform is necessary to determine the onset of mechanical diastole and systole and to verify timing. Diastole has begun when the dicrotic notch appears on the arterial waveform. Balloon inflation is timed to occur at this point in the cardiac cycle. The deflation point can be optimally adjusted by observing the end-diastolic drop in pressure created by balloon deflation. The goal is to create the greatest pressure drop possible. Ideally, the difference between end-diastolic pressure without the balloon effect and end-diastolic pressure created by balloon deflation is at least 10 mm Hg. Evidence that afterload reduction has occurred is seen in the following systolic pressure. With afterload reduction, the next systolic pressure after balloon deflation is lower than the systolic pressure with no balloon effect. This is evidence that LV workload has been decreased.

To evaluate balloon timing properly, the assist ratio is set at 1 : 2, meaning the balloon is assisting every other cardiac cycle. In this way, the observer can compare the effect of balloon inflation and deflation with unassisted beats. Most patients tolerate this well for a brief period. Five criteria can be used to determine the effectiveness of IABP timing, as illustrated on the arterial pressure tracing (Fig. 24-10).

The first step is to ensure that inflation occurs at the dicrotic notch, the beginning of diastole. Inflation should actually be timed to obliterate the notch. The interval between the onset of systolic upstroke and the point of balloon inflation should not be shorter than the interval between the systolic upstroke and dicrotic notch on the

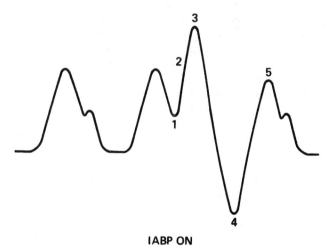

IABP ON

FIGURE 24-10 Criteria for effective intra-aortic balloon pump (IABP) timing: (*1*) inflation occurs at the dicrotic notch; (*2*) the slope of rise of balloon inflation is straight and runs parallel with the preceding systolic upstroke; (*3*) augmented diastolic pressure is at least equal to the preceding systolic pressure; (*4*) end-diastolic pressure at balloon deflation is lower than the preceding unassisted end-diastolic pressure; (*5*) the next systolic pressure is assisted systole and is lower than the preceding systole, which was not affected by balloon deflation. (From Shinn JA: Intra-aortic balloon pump counterpulsation. In Hudak CM, Gallo BM, Lohr TS [eds]: Critical Care Nursing: A Holistic Approach, 5th ed, p 213. Philadelphia, JB Lippincott, 1990.)

unassisted beat. Inflation that occurs too early is detrimental to the patient because the abrupt increase in diastolic pressure may force the aortic valve closed prematurely. Complete ejection may be impaired. Late inflation, past the dicrotic notch, does not harm the patient, but the duration of assistance is unnecessarily shortened so that maximal benefit from augmented pressure is not achieved.

Next, the upstroke of balloon inflation should be sharp and parallel with the preceding systolic upstroke. This creates a V-shaped appearance on the ECG, with the nadir of the V being the point of inflation. The sharp upslope ensures that maximal early augmentation is occurring. A slope that is not straight may indicate that the balloon is inflating late, perhaps off of some other artifact during early diastole. In this case, the loss of the V configuration also is evident.

The third criterion is that the augmented diastolic pressure peak be at least equal to the preceding systolic pressure peak. A decrease in this pressure peak may indicate gas loss from the balloon. This loss can occur by natural diffusion. A balloon normally requires refilling every 2 to 4 hours because of natural diffusion of gas through the membrane. Most consoles automatically purge and refill the balloon and catheter every 2 hours. An abrupt loss of the pressure peak may indicate the development of a leak in the balloon or the catheter. Occasionally, augmentation greater than the systolic pressure is not achievable owing to the size of the balloon relative to the size of the aorta. To fit properly, the balloon should occlude 80% of the aorta when inflated. If a smaller balloon was used because of insertion difficulties, or if the aorta is dilated, diastolic augmentation may be less than the patient's systole. In this instance, balloon inflation does not generate as much volume displacement or rise in aortic pressure during diastole.

The fourth point to evaluate is balloon deflation at the end of diastole. Proper deflation results in a drop in pressure at the end of diastole. This drop in pressure creates an end-diastolic pressure much lower than diastolic pressure without the balloon effect. Timing is adjusted so that the lowest pressure possible is achieved. It is important to make sure that the systolic upstroke that follows is straight and that a sharp, V-shaped configuration is present. The V shape indicates that systole began immediately after deflation. Any plateau indicates that deflation occurred too early. In this case, early deflation does not relieve the ventricle of impedance, and afterload reduction does not occur. Late deflation results in higher impedance because the balloon remains inflated at the onset of systolic ejection. An end-diastolic pressure that is the same or greater than the end-diastolic pressure without balloon assistance is evidence of late deflation. The following systolic pressure is the same as the unassisted systole because no afterload reduction has occurred. It can also be lower than the unassisted systole because of the inability of the failing ventricle to work against the higher impedance to ejection.

Finally, the observer should note what effect balloon deflation has on the next systolic pressure, for reasons just described. The goal is to ensure that the lower systolic pressure that follows balloon deflation is caused by afterload reduction and not by improper timing, which resulted in late deflation. Proper balloon fit has an impact on the abil-

ity to achieve afterload reduction. If the balloon size is small, volume displacement may have less of an effect on lowering end-diastolic pressure. Figure 24-11 illustrates the four possible errors that can occur with timing.

COMPLICATIONS. Intra-aortic balloon pump therapy carries a relatively low risk of morbidity given the clinical condition of the patient. Most complications are vascular. The incidence has been reported to be 10% to 45%.[1,19,27,57] Vascular injuries that may occur during insertion include plaque dislodgement, dissection, laceration, and compromised circulation to the distal extremity. If a cutdown was used during insertion, peripheral nerve injury is another complication that may be incurred during the insertion procedure. Compromised circulation can occur any time during IABP therapy as a result of the presence of the indwelling catheter, compartment syndrome, or embolus from thrombus formation along the catheter or on the balloon.[11,47,61] These complications occur with greater frequency in patients with peripheral vascular occlusive disease, in women with small vessels, and in patients with insulin-dependent diabetes.[19] Nursing functions involved in monitoring or preventing compromised circulation include careful assessment of peripheral perfusion; preventing the patient from flexing the hip of the affected extremity, which may compromise blood flow; and maintaining coagulation times within prescribed parameters by careful titration of anticoagulants. The nurse should be aware that multiple or prolonged attempts at insertion increase the risk of vascular injury and thrombus formation.

Infection is reported to occur in approximately 0.2% of patients.[57] Insertion site infections may dictate the removal of the IABP catheter. Careful efforts must be made to maintain the sterility of insertion site dressings. Other problems

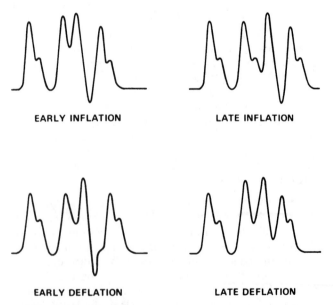

EARLY INFLATION   **LATE INFLATION**

EARLY DEFLATION   **LATE DEFLATION**

FIGURE 24-11 Possible errors in balloon timing. (From Shinn JA: Intra-aortic balloon pump counterpulsation. In Hudak CM, Gallo BM, Lohr TS [eds]: Critical Care Nursing: A Holistic Approach, 4th ed, p 198. Philadelphia, JB Lippincott, 1986.)

that may be encountered include thrombocytopenia; compromised circulation to the left subclavian, renal, or mesenteric arteries owing to balloon malposition; and bleeding from the insertion site or other line insertion sites. Mechanical problems related to the balloon include improper timing or a leak or perforation in the balloon, necessitating its removal. A leak in the balloon becomes evident as augmentation becomes less effective. Eventually, blood backs up in the catheter and can be detected. When a leak has occurred, the balloon must be removed immediately to avoid the possibility of gas embolus.

NURSING MANAGEMENT PLAN. Good cardiovascular assessment of the patient provides indicators that IABP therapy is effectively assisting LV function. Assessment includes vital signs, cardiac output, heart rhythm, heart regularity, heart ischemia, urine output, color, peripheral perfusion, and mentation. All these parameters should reflect an improvement in the patient's condition. The patient on IABP therapy is relatively immobile owing to the need to avoid hip flexion and to multiple invasive monitoring and infusion lines. Often, the patient requires endotracheal intubation and ventilator support. Care must be taken to prevent or minimize extensive atelectasis. These patients also are at greater risk for respiratory tract infection. Careful suctioning technique and prevention of aspiration reduce this risk. Prolonged hypotension from the shock state may jeopardize renal function. Monitoring urine output and quality closely may contribute to early recognition and treatment of renal dysfunction, thus avoiding acute renal failure. Psychosocial support of both the patient and family is important. The patient requires interventions that minimize stress, disorientation, and sleep deprivation. Families benefit from honest communication and help with the interpretation of the patient's condition. Nursing Care Plan 24-1 outlines a plan of care for the patient on IABP therapy. Because this patient is experiencing acute LV failure or cardiogenic shock, many nursing diagnoses used for those conditions apply. The plan of care that is outlined focuses on issues unique to IABP therapy.

Left Ventricular Assist Devices.

In patients who have catastrophic myocardial injury or deteriorating end-stage HF, IABP therapy may provide inadequate support. IABP therapy depends on ventricular function to maintain systemic blood pressure. The IABP is not capable of contributing to cardiac output directly. With profound ventricular failure, mean blood pressure is less than 60 mm Hg, systolic blood pressure is less than 90 mm Hg, and the cardiac index typically is less than 1.8 L/min/m².[7,30,45] IABP therapy increases cardiac output only marginally (500 to 800 mL/min), and the expectation of long-term support in this scenario is unrealistic.[13] Therefore, more aggressive therapy with an LVAD, which can provide a physiologic cardiac output, is warranted.

PATIENT INDICATIONS. The most frequent indications for use of an LVAD are to support a patient awaiting a donor for heart transplantation or for patients who cannot be weaned from cardiopulmonary bypass after conventional treatment, including IABP therapy. Approximately 1% to 4%

of cardiac surgery patients cannot be weaned from cardiopulmonary bypass after major myocardial injury.[31,34,43] Between 30% and 50% of those patients may survive with LVAD support.[45,55] Some centers use LVADs to support the patient in cardiogenic shock after MI. The LVAD is used to decrease LV work and to maintain systemic blood pressure while the left ventricle recovers from injury. If allowed to rest for 48 to 96 hours, there is potential for myocardial function to return.[7] Indications of initial ventricular recovery should appear within 24 hours.[31] The decision to insert an LVAD must be made quickly but carefully. The longer the patient remains on cardiopulmonary bypass, the more likely the patient is to have profound coagulopathy, which may become difficult or impossible to amend. Situations that may contraindicate LVAD placement include preexisting disease states, severe debilitation making recovery unlikely, massive myocardial injury in which recovery is not possible, multisystem organ failure, and prolonged cardiac arrest associated with neurologic damage.[31] Unless cardiac transplantation is an option, a major factor in the decision-making process is to select patients in whom recovery is possible, thus avoiding a situation in which the patient becomes totally LVAD dependent without potential for weaning.

MECHANISM OF SUPPORT. Left ventricular assist devices are designed temporarily to replace the pumping function of the left ventricle by being placed in the circuit of normal blood flow. Blood is diverted from the left atrium or left ventricle and shunted to the LVAD by the pressure gradient between those chambers and the LVAD. Blood is returned to the aorta with continuous flow from the LVAD or in a pulsatile fashion with pump ejection occurring during the patient's diastole or asynchronous to the patient's cardiac cycle. Available pumps are divided into two categories: continuous-flow pumps and pulsatile pumps.

Continuous-flow pumps are continuously filled by left atrial blood flow, and blood is returned to the aorta at a continuous rate. There is no ability to mimic systole or diastole, but constant flow rates and mean blood pressure are maintained. Left atrial blood flow is captured by a cannula placed in the chamber. As a result, LV preload is markedly diminished, and LV workload is reduced. Continuous-flow pumps are capable of flow rates of up to 6 L/min.[34,45]

Pulsatile pumps are filled during atrial contraction or ventricular systole, depending on whether the LVAD inflow cannula is placed in the left atrium or left ventricle. In the latter case, the LV acts as an "atrium" to fill the LVAD, and filling of the LVAD occurs during the patient's native systole. Because the LVAD is empty before LV contraction, impedance to LV ejection is reduced dramatically, and minimal work is required to fill the pump. LV pressures as low as 10 mm Hg may be all that is required to fill the LVAD. The aortic valve remains closed, and no blood is ejected from the ventricle into the aorta during systole. Once the LVAD is filled, ejection from the LVAD pump into the aorta occurs. This coincides with the patient's native diastole. The LVAD is in counterpulsation with the patient's heart. It is in its filling phase during LV contraction and is ejecting during LV relaxation. Blood pressure during true diastole in these patients actually is higher than blood

(text continued on page 633)

NURSING CARE PLAN 24-1 ◆ The Patient with an Intra-aortic Balloon Pump

Nursing Diagnosis 1: Potential decreased tissue perfusion in the lower extremities related to possible catheter obstruction, emboli, or thrombosis, manifested by signs and symptoms of decreased perfusion in legs.

Nursing Goal 1: To minimize risk of decreased tissue perfusion in lower extremities

Outcome Criteria:
1. Appropriate level of anticoagulation will be maintained as prescribed.
2. Dorsalis pedis and posterior tibial pulses will be palpable and of equivalent strength of baseline assessment.
3. Patient's skin will be warm, dry, and of normal color.
4. Patient will be knowledgeable about proper hip position.

NURSING INTERVENTIONS	RATIONALE
1. Record quality of peripheral pulses before insertion of the intra-aortic balloon pump (IABP) catheter.	1. Required to establish a baseline so changes will be detectable.
2. Evaluate quality of peripheral pulses, skin color, capillary refill, and temperature at least hourly.	2. Required to detect changes.
3. Maintain anticoagulation level at prescribed range by accurate monitoring of heparin or dextran infusion.	3. Thrombus could form along catheter or on balloon if anticoagulation falls below therapeutic range. Any thrombus may potentially break loose with balloon movement, causing emboli.
4. Assist patient with ankle flexion and extension every 1 to 2 hours.	4. Exercise of calf muscles will minimize venous stasis and potential for deep venous thrombosis.
5. Maintain cannulated extremity in a straight position, avoiding hip flexion. Use a brace or soft restraint as needed.	5–7. Hip flexion will decrease flow in the cannulated artery, potentially compromising distal circulation.
6. Keep head of bed at a 15-degree backrest position or lower.	
7. If patient is alert, instruct patient in importance of avoiding hip flexion.	
8. Maintain continuous alternating inflation and deflation of the balloon.	8. Continuous motion minimizes the possibility of thrombus formation on the balloon. Thrombus can occur rapidly on a motionless balloon, with subsequent risk of vascular occlusion or embolization.

Nursing Goal 2: To detect early manifestations of decreased tissue perfusion in lower extremities

Outcome Criteria:
1. Patient will maintain palpable dorsalis pedis and posterior tibial pulses equivalent to baseline.
2. Patient's skin will be warm, dry, and of normal color.
3. These changes will be detected within 1 hour of occurrence.

NURSING INTERVENTIONS	RATIONALE
1. Monitor quality of peripheral pulses, capillary refill, skin temperature, and color hourly.	1. Required to detect changes.
2. Notify physician if pulses diminish or become absent in the cannulated extremity.	2. Circulatory compromise may progress slowly as thrombus grows larger or rapidly as a result of an embolus.
3. If patient complains of leg pain, promptly evaluate peripheral perfusion. Notify physician of any changes.	3. Leg pain may be occurring as a result of ischemia. Ischemia is an indication for removal of the IABP catheter.
4. Monitor for swollen limb that is tense on palpation, patient complaints of continuous pressure, and pain induced with passive stretching of the affected muscle.	4. These signs and symptoms may indicate the presence of compartment syndrome.

(continued)

NURSING CARE PLAN 24-1 ◆ The Patient with an Intra-aortic Balloon Pump *(Continued)*

Nursing Diagnosis 2:	Decreased cardiac output related to suboptimal IABP therapy, manifested by lowered mean arterial blood pressure with requirement for high-dose inotropic support.
Nursing Goal 1:	To prevent decreases in cardiac output as a result of suboptimal IABP therapy
Outcome Criteria:	1. Mean arterial blood pressure will be 60 to 70 mm Hg or better.

2. IABP timing will be correct with:
   Inflation occurring at the dicrotic notch
   Optimal diastolic augmentation
   Deflation at end-diastole with a drop in pressure of at least 8 to 10 mm Hg below unassisted end-diastole
3. Balloon will be refilled before large gas losses secondary to diffusion.
4. Patient will have decreasing requirements for inotropic support over the course of IABP assistance.

NURSING INTERVENTIONS	RATIONALE
1. Verify correct timing of IABP hourly. Make corrections as needed.	1. Timing may be altered if the heart rate changes or systolic function improves.
2. Document settings for inflation, deflation, and systolic, end-diastolic, and mean arterial pressures with IABP assistance.	2. Documentation will illustrate trends, improvement, and necessary interventions to achieve optimal assistance.
3. Document level of diastolic augmentation. Evaluate for a decrease in augmentation.	3–4. A decrease in diastolic augmentation indicates a need to refill the balloon. A major loss of diastolic augmentation in a short time may indicate a tear or leak in the balloon. (Check catheter for evidence of blood backing up from aorta.)
4. Maintain proper volume of balloon to ensure optimal diastolic augmentation.	
5. Refill balloon every 2 to 4 hours according to unit protocol. Use automatic filling mode if available.	5. An optimally filled balloon is necessary for optimal diastolic augmentation.

Nursing Goal 2:	To reduce or eliminate situations that will interfere with maintenance of proper IABP timing assist ratio (i.e., assistance of every beat).
Outcome Criteria:	1. Patient will have a regular heart rhythm.

2. There will be no interference of trigger signal to IABP console.
3. Timing will be corrected with changes in heart rate.
4. Balloon will be free of kinking.

NURSING INTERVENTIONS	RATIONALE
1. Reevaluate timing anytime there is a greater than a 10- to 20-beat change in heart rate or onset of new dysrhythmias.	1. A 10- to 20-beat or greater change in heart rate alters the systole-to-diastole ratio in each cardiac cycle. Previous inflation and deflation settings may be inappropriate for a change in this ratio (i.e., the time spent in diastole is longer at slower heart rates and shorter at rapid heart rates).
2. Maintain adequate electrocardiogram (ECG) trigger signals to IABP console. Change any ECG electrodes that become loose, placing new ones on clean, dry skin.	2. Loss of trigger signals impairs IABP ability to assist the heart with each cardiac cycle.
3. Notify physician of any dysrhythmias. Secure cardiac pacing parameters if dysrhythmia is irregular and is impairing IABP tracking. Administer antiarrhythmic agents as ordered.	3. Irregular dysrhythmias may impair IABP ability to assist each cardiac cycle. Pacing can stabilize this situation so that systole-to-diastole ratio is the same for each cardiac cycle. The pacemaker spike may be used as the trigger for IABP timing.

(continued)

NURSING CARE PLAN 24-1 ◆ The Patient with an Intra-aortic Balloon Pump *(Continued)*

NURSING INTERVENTIONS	RATIONALE
4. Maintain patient in proper body position (head of bed 15 degrees and no hip flexion). Use leg brace and soft restraint as necessary. Log roll patient when turning. 5. Instruct radiologists and other personnel not to sit patient upright.	4–5. Sitting the patient upright or elevating head of bed may cause hip flexion and subsequent catheter kinking. Kinking impairs the flow of gas in and out of balloon. An upright position also may cause the catheter to advance up the aorta with potential migration into an aortic arch vessel.

Nursing Diagnosis 3: Sensory/perceptual alterations: sensory overload related to intensive care unit environment and the need for frequent monitoring, manifested by disorientation, anxiety, restlessness, and sleeplessness.

Nursing Goal 1: To reduce or eliminate excessive sensory stimuli that might impair sleep–wake cycles

Outcome Criteria:
1. There will be no excessive or unnecessary noise in patient's environment.
2. Patient will have progressive blocks of undisturbed time for sleep.

NURSING INTERVENTIONS	RATIONALE
1. Maintain monitor "bleep" volume at lowest audible level. 2. Minimize amount of extraneous noise from other equipment in patient's room. 3. Minimize unnecessary noise caused by staff conversations in patient's room. 4. Turn down lights in patient's room during the night. 5. Organize nursing care so patient has uninterrupted time for sleep during the night, amount to be determined by patient's condition.	1–3. Unnecessary noise disturbs patient's sleep and creates higher levels of stress during wakefulness. 4. Darkening the room during the night helps patient distinguish day from night and provides a better environment for sleep at night. 5. Organized care can provide patients with up to 2-hour periods when it is unnecessary directly to touch the patient. As the patient's condition improves, longer blocks of time are feasible.

Nursing Goal 2: To assist patient with maintaining orientation and some degree of control of self

Outcome Criteria:
1. Patient will be oriented to date, time, and place.
2. Patient will be able appropriately to interpret his or her environment.

NURSING INTERVENTIONS	RATIONALE
1. Talk with patient while administering care. Explain noises, activity, and procedures to be done. 2. Involve patient in decision making about care if possible (e.g., which direction to turn next). When patient is able, teach patient to do ankle flexion exercises and deep breathing exercises, which can be done independently by patient. 3. Frequently inform patient of the time and date and orient to surroundings. 4. Place familiar objects such as pictures within patient view; involve family in the process.	1. Explanations assist the patient to interpret the environment appropriately and minimize stress and anxiety associated with a fear of the unknown. 2. Involvement in decisions helps the patient maintain some degree of control. 3. Frequently reorienting the patient helps prevent disorientation. 4. Familiar objects may help maintain orientation.

(continued)

NURSING CARE PLAN 24-1 ◆ The Patient with an Intra-aortic Balloon Pump *(Continued)*

Nursing Diagnosis 4:	Ineffective family coping related to inadequate support, knowledge deficit, fear of patient dying, and fear of the intensive care unit environment, manifested by requests for help or inappropriate behavior.
Nursing Goal:	To assist family with development of ability to cope
Outcome Criteria:	1. The family members will acknowledge their fears and concerns. 2. The family will verbalize a decrease in their level of fear and will appear calmer. 3. The family will demonstrate an ability to cope effectively.

NURSING INTERVENTIONS	**RATIONALE**
1. Encourage family members to express feelings, and convey understanding of their concerns and emotional stress.	1. Expression of concerns promotes effective coping.
2. Provide the family with honest information about the patient's condition to reduce fears. Keep the family informed of changes.	2–3. Fear is reduced by clarifying misunderstandings. Information decreases fear of the unknown.
3. Set aside time during visiting hours to spend with the family, and encourage family members to ask questions. Offer explanations about the intensive care unit environment.	
4. Encourage realistic hope based on the patient's progress. Point out progress to the family.	4. Hope helps the family with coping.
5. Allow family to participate in care as appropriate.	5. Participation decreases feelings of helplessness in aiding the recovery of the patient.
6. Determine how the family has coped with previous stressful situations.	6. It is important to identify previous effective coping mechanisms and to promote the use of these mechanisms.

pressure during true systole. Pumps can also run in a fill-to-empty mode, with ejection occuring any time the pump is fully filled. The LVAD is capable of assuming total responsibility for maintaining physiologic cardiac output.

TYPES OF CONTINUOUS-FLOW DEVICES. One type of device provides continuous flow by means of a roller pump. This pump is filled from a left atrial cannula, and flow is returned to the ascending aorta after passing through the roller pump (Fig. 24-12). Long cannulas are required that create high resistance to blood flow. This high resistance necessitates the use of high pressure to maintain flow. Tubing occlusion that causes a pressure back-up is one of the disadvantages of this system. Heparinization is required to prevent thrombus formation along the long cannulas.[32,34] Roller pumps also traumatize blood cells, causing hemolysis. This device is best applied for short-term situations. After long periods, hemolysis and coagulopathies become problematic. An example of this support would be the maintenance of partial cardiopulmonary bypass after a cardiac surgical procedure.

The centrifugal-kinetic energy pump is an example of a frequently used continuous-flow LVAD (Fig. 24-13). The Bio-Medicus pump is an example of this type of device. With this system, blood is taken from the left atrium and returned to the aorta. The major advantage of such a device is the ability to function at low pressure while delivering high volume or flow. As blood enters the pump, it is whirled by centrifugal force, creating a vortex or tornado effect.[32] The higher the

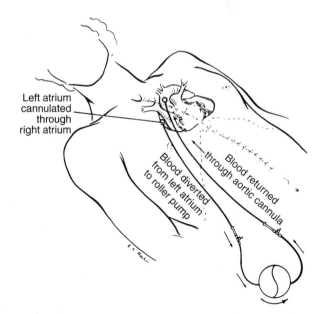

Left atrium cannulated through right atrium

Blood diverted from left atrium to roller pump

Blood returned through aortic cannula

FIGURE 24-12 Continuous flow to the aorta is provided by a roller pump. Cannulas are tunneled through the abdominal wall to the external roller pump. (From Litwak RS, Koffsky RM, Lukban SB et al: Implanted heart assist devices after intracardiac surgery. N Engl J Med 291: 1342, 1974. Copyright © 1974 Massachusetts Medical Society. All rights reserved.)

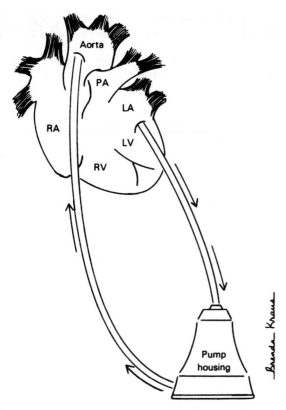

FIGURE 24-13 Continuous-flow centrifugal-kinetic energy pump. PA, pulmonary artery; LA, left atrium; LV, left ventricle; RA, right atrium; RV, right ventricle. (From Marchetta S, Stennis E: Ventricular assist devices: Applications for critical care. J Cardiovasc Nurs 2[2]: 45, 1988.)

speed of the pump (revolutions per minute), the greater the centrifugal force and the greater the output of the pump. Thus, flow rates are controlled by the number of revolutions per minute that the pump spins. An advantage of this design is that any air accumulates at the top of the vortex while blood accumulates at the bottom, thus avoiding the possibility of air microembolus. Chipping from the inner surfaces of the tubing or other wear and tear on the tubing does not occur with this pump design. Trauma to blood cells is markedly decreased, compared to cardiopulmonary bypass. Heparinization is not required for up to 48 hours, as long as flow rates are kept at greater than 1 L/min.[31] This pump also minimizes the buildup of excessive outflow pressure that can result in tubing disconnections. These devices can support patients for longer times than roller pump designs, primarily owing to the decreased trauma to blood cells.

A new device undergoing clinical trials also works in series with the native heart, like IABP therapy. This device, called the Hemopump (Johnson & Johnson), is capable of generating up to 3.5 L/min of continual, nonpulsatile blood flow, which more effectively rests the left ventricle.[56] This device is classified as an axial flow pump. The pump is mounted in a cannula that is inserted through the femoral artery and passed up the aorta. The tip of the cannula crosses the aortic valve and is positioned in the LV chamber (Fig. 24-14). Axial flow is achieved by rotating blades contained within the pump housing, which rotate at speeds of up to 25,000 rpm.[56] This action draws blood from the left ventricle and propels it into the systemic circulation. Nonrotating blades placed more distally in the cannula maintain unidirectional flow. An external motor magnet is connected to a drive shaft, which is housed in the inner lumen of the cannula. This drive shaft connects to the pump and provides it with a means to turn the pump's rotating blades. A newer version of the Hemopump is being developed by Thermo Cardiosystems Inc., (Woburn, MA) that is totally implantable.

Advantages of this system are that it does not have to be synchronized with a cardiac cycle, so its function does not depend on secure ECG electrode placement or nursing time for timing adjustments. Its insertion and removal are also relatively minor procedures (except the implanted design), which make it more available to medical patients. Its major

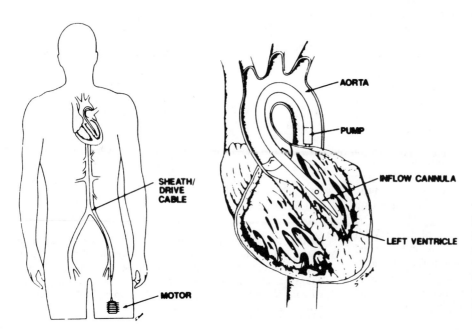

FIGURE 24-14 Placement of the Hemopump cannula in the left ventricle, with exit out the femoral artery. The driving motor is located externally. (From Rutan PM, Roundtree WD, Myers KK et al: Initial experience with the hemopump. Critical Care Nursing Clinics of North America 1: 527–534, 1989.)

disadvantage, which may exclude smaller patients, is the size of the cannula. The patient's femoral anatomy must be able to accommodate a large cannula. Because of the size, there is also risk of compromised distal blood flow. All placements require arteriotomy under direct vision using a cutdown technique.

TYPES OF PULSATILE PUMPS. Pulsatile LVAD pumps are either pneumatic (air driven) or electric. Either can be used as temporary support, but the electrically driven pump has the potential to be totally implantable.

The Thoratec pump (Thoratec Laboratories, Inc., Pleasanton, CA) is an example of a pneumatic system. Pulsatile flow is created by air compression of a polyurethane sac that contains up to 65 mL of blood. Positive air pressure compresses the sac, causing ejection from the LVAD to the aorta. Negative pressure is applied after ejection, causing the blood sac to fill. Backward flow is prevented by placement of inflow and outflow disk valves in the pump. The blood sac is filled by means of a cannula placed in either the left atrium or left ventricle. It can be controlled by three modes: (1) a fixed rate that is asynchronous with the patient's heart and delivers variable stroke volumes, (2) triggering of the pump by the R wave of the ECG (not practical for long-term support), or (3) triggering of pump ejection by reaching full fill (also called *fill-to-empty mode*).[30,39] A major advantage is pulsatile flow, which allows for longer term support. Pulsatile flow provides better kidney perfusion, decreases peripheral vascular resistance, and increases systemic circulation.[32] A major disadvantage is the risk of infection associated with a pump that is placed externally. Conduits from the atrium and to the aorta are tunneled through the chest and connected to the external pump (Fig. 24-15). Epithelial cells ingrow into the Dacron-covered conduits. Tissue ingrowth acts as a seal from the surface of the body.

Another pulsatile pump is the Novacor pump (Baxter Healthcare Corporation, Oakland, CA). This electrically driven pump is designed to be totally implanted in a preperitoneal pocket just anterior to the posterior rectus sheath. Chronic support is possible because electrical energy can be stored in battery cells that are small enough to implant, although the electric power unit currently used is an exchangeable five hour battery. Filling of the pump occurs from a cannula that is placed in the LV apex. The cannula is tunneled through to the abdomen, where the pump is implanted. Blood is returned to the ascending aorta through another cannula. The device also uses inflow and outflow valves. Ejection is triggered by either a fixed rate, changes in the velocity of filling, or in a fill-to-empty mode. When the blood sac is filled, or the trigger is recognized, two electrically powered pusher plates compress the blood sac, which is located between the two plates. Ejection occurs when the sac is compressed.[61] The major advantage of this system is the ability to implant the device, eliminating much of the risk of infection. Another major advantage is the potential for storing and implanting the energy source. Figure 24-16 illustrates the

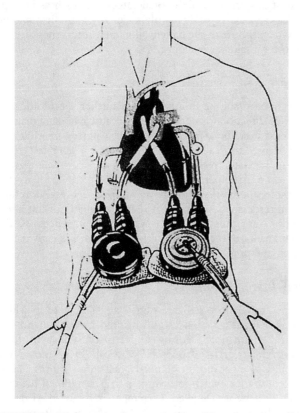

FIGURE 24-15 Cannula placement of two Thoratec pumps during support of both right and left ventricles. Arrows indicate direction of blood flow. (From Ruzevich SA, Swartz MI, Pennington DG: Nursing care of the patient with a pneumatic ventricular assist device. Heart Lung 17: 399–405, 1988.)

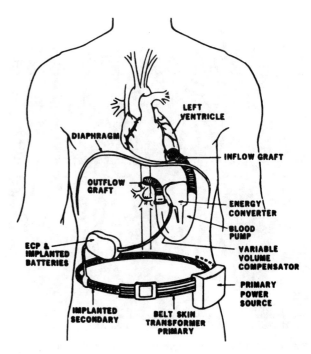

FIGURE 24-16 Illustration of the Novacor left ventricular assist device shows the design of the totally implanted system. Power is transmitted from the belt, through the skin, to the implanted controller (ECP) and storage batteries. (From Ream AK, Portner PM: Cardiac assist devices and the artificial heart. In Ream AK, Fogdall RP [eds]: Acute Cardiovascular Management, Anesthesia, and Intensive Care, p 864. Philadelphia, JB Lippincott, 1982.)

appearance of the device in its totally implantable form. In the device's current configuration, patients must wear the controller on a belt and carry a power source with them. The controller and battery packs can also be carried in a shoulder bag or in specially designed vests that have pockets for the controller and two battery packs. One battery serves as a reserve supply when the patient switches from AC power to battery operation, and vice versa. The other primary battery pack can supply power for up to 5 hours, allowing the patient freedom from a tethered set-up. Figure 24-17 shows the first patient in the United States who is ambulatory with the wearable system.

Another pump that can also be totally implanted is the Heartmate implantable pneumatic system (Thermo Cardiosystems, Inc., Woburn, MA). With this design, an external source of pressurized air is used to pressurize the chamber housing the blood sac. With pressure, the blood sac is compressed by a single pusher plate, causing ejection to occur. A second Heartmate pump is electrically driven, with a controller and battery pack system similar to those of the Novacor pump. Ejection occurs as a result of compression of the blood sac by a single, motor-driven pusher plate.[25]

Both the Novacor and Heartmate systems can support patients for extended periods with a relatively low risk of thromboembolism or mechanical problems. All are used to support patients awaiting heart transplantation. The portability of the systems allows patients to be ambulatory and care for themselves. As a result, these patients are now routinely discharged from the hospital while they wait for suitable donor hearts.[40,46]

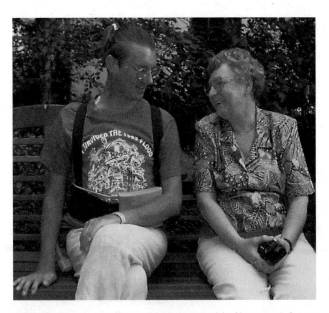

FIGURE 24-17 A patient with the wearable Novacor left ventricular assist system. The patient carries a 5-hour battery pack on a specially designed belt, allowing him to be totally untethered to a heavy operating console, as with many other types of devices. This patient is shown at approximately 3 weeks after implantation and is waiting for a donor heart.

NURSING MANAGEMENT PLAN FOR THE PATIENT IN SHOCK

When caring for the acutely ill patient in shock, the goals of nursing and medicine merge to preserve life through the maintenance of oxygenation and circulation. In addition, the nurse considers the human responses to shock and the extent to which normal daily activities must be supplemented by nursing care.[9] This is done through a careful functional assessment of the individual patient. Cues are collected within functional categories, and patterns are recognized, which provide the basis for nursing diagnosis and intervention. Altered tissue perfusion, self-care deficit, and altered family processes are among the nursing diagnoses encountered in association with shock.[9,35]

Decreased Cardiac Output

Decreased cardiac output is a clinical problem requiring the specialized intervention of nursing and medicine for resolution. Both disciplines possess the knowledge necessary to recognize the signs and symptoms and to diagnose the problem. The accepted therapy (e.g., fluid replacement, inotropes, vasopressors, IABP) legally falls within the definition of medical practice. The physician must define the parameters of therapy. The nurse uses knowledge and judgment in administering the prescribed therapy.[12] In addition, the nurse considers the impact that a reduction in cardiac output has on other functional categories, such as perceptual awareness or activity tolerance. After confirming the specific response of the patient, the nurse intervenes directly to foster a salutary response.[9,35]

Decreased Tissue Perfusion

Decreased tissue perfusion requires further specification to provide direction for nursing care. Because a nursing diagnosis must describe a problem for which nurses are educated and licensed to treat, use of the customary "related to" clause is inappropriate. Instead, the nurse must specify the impact of decreased tissue perfusion on the health of the patient—for example, altered tissue perfusion: decreased, cerebral, resulting in restlessness, agitation. The independent nursing interventions are then directed toward patient protection, the maintenance of the current level of function, and early recognition and prevention of further deterioration.

Self-Care Deficit

Carpenito[9] defines self-care deficit as "The state in which the individual experiences an impaired motor function or cognitive function, causing a decreased ability to feed, bathe, dress, or toilet oneself." Critical illness implies the inability to meet one's care needs. Self-care requires energy and endurance, which may surpass the strengths of the critically ill patient. Detailed assessment is required to determine the scope and extent of the deficit and to provide appropriate supportive or supplemental intervention. Nursing activities designed to meet these needs include turning, positioning,[63] bathing, massaging, and communicating. Knowing when to help and when to refrain from helping are equally important. There is an interrelatedness among the self-care deficits—feeding, bathing, toileting—and interventions instituted in one category may affect other categories.

Altered Family Processes Related to an Ill Family Member

This nursing diagnosis refers to the state in which a normally supportive family experiences a stressor that challenges its previously effective functioning ability.[9] It is frequently seen in caring for people who are critically ill, with the stressors being the critical illness and the intensive care environment.[54] Defining characteristics include a family system that cannot, or does not (1) meet the physical, emotional, or spiritual needs of its members; (2) accept or express a full range of feelings; (3) seek or accept help appropriately; (4) communicate openly with its members; or (5) adapt constructively to crisis. Nursing interventions must be individualized but may include actions such as conducting family orientation to the hospital, providing a private place for family to wait, providing information regarding changes in the patient's condition or treatment, acknowledging family strengths, and facilitating the expression of feelings.

REFERENCES

1. Alderman JD, Giabliani G, McCabe C et al: Incidence and management of limb ischemia with percutaneous wire-guided intra-aortic balloon catheters. Am J Crit Care 9: 524–529, 1989
2. Alpert J, Parsonnet V, Goldenkranz RJ et al: Limb ischemia during intraaortic balloon pumping: Indications for femoro-femoral cross over graft. J Thorac Cardiovasc Surg 79: 729–737, 1980
3. Astiz ME, Rackow: Assessing perfusion failure during circulatory shock. Crit Care Clin 9: 299–309, 1993
4. Bates B: A Guide to Physical Examination, 5th ed. Philadelphia, JB Lippincott, 1991
5. Baue AE: Metabolic abnormalities of shock. Surg Clin North Am 56(5): 1059–1071, 1976
6. Bordicks KJ: Patterns of Shock, 2nd ed. New York, Macmillan, 1980
7. Brannon PHB, Towner SB: Ventricular failure: New therapy using the mechanical assist device. Crit Care Nurse 6(2): 70–84, 1986
8. Bruya MA: Shock. In Patrick ML, Woods SL, Craven RF et al. (eds): Medical-Surgical Nursing: Pathophysiological Concepts, pp 282–293. Philadelphia, JB Lippincott, 1986
9. Carpenito LJ: Nursing Diagnosis: Application to Clinical Practice. Philadelphia, JB Lippincott, 1992
10. Chatterjee K, Parmly WW, Swan W et al: Hemodynamic and metabolic responses of vasodilator therapy in acute myocardial infarction. Circulation 48(6): 1183–1193, 1973
11. Conry K: Compartment syndrome: A complication of IABP. Dimensions in Critical Care Nursing 4: 274–284, 1985
12. Coombs M: Hemodynamic profiles and the critical care nurse. Intensive Crit Care Nurs 9(1): 11–26, 1993
13. Copeland JG, Emery RW, Leivinson MM et al: The role of mechanical support and transplantation in treatment of patients with end-stage cardiomyopathy. Circulation 72(Suppl II): 7–12, 1985
14. Durrer J: Effect of sodium nitroprusside on mortality in acute myocardial infarction. N Engl J Med 306(19): 1121–1128, 1982
15. Eskridge RA: Septic shock. Crit Care Quart 4: 55–68, 1982
16. Forrest JS, Diamond G, Chatterjee K et al: Medical therapy of acute myocardial infarction by application of hemodynamic subsets. N Engl J Med 295: 1362–1386, 1404–1413, 1976
17. Forrester J, Walter D: Hospital treatment of congestive heart failure: Management of hemodynamic profile. Am J Med 65: 173–179, 1978
18. Ganong WF: Review of Medical Physiology. Los Altos, CA, Lange, 1989
19. Goran SF: Vascular complications of the patient undergoing intra-aortic balloon pumping. Crit Care Nurs Clin North Am 1: 459–467, 1989
20. Griffel MI, Kaufman BS: Pharmacology of colloids and crystalloids. Crit Care Clin 8: 235–248, 1992
21. Guidelines for the Evaluation and Management of Heart Failure. Report of the American College of Cardiology/American Heart Association Task Force on Practice Guidelines (Committee on Evaluation and Management of Heart Failure). J Am Coll Cardiol 26: 1376–1398, 1996
22. Haljamae H: Volume substitution in shock. Acta Anaesthesiol Scand Suppl 98: 25–28, 1993
23. Haas GJ, Young JB: Acute heart failure management. In Topol EJ (ed): Textbook of Cardiovascular Medicine, pp 2247–2271. Philadelphia, Lippincott–Raven, 1998
24. Haupt MI, Kaufman BS, Carlson RW: Fluid resuscitation in patients with increased vascular permeability. Crit Care Clin 8: 341–352, 1992
25. Hunt SA, Frazier OH, Myers TJ. Mechanical circulatory support and cardiac transplantation. Circulation 97: 2079–2090, 1998.
26. Imm A, Carlson RW: Fluid resuscitation in circulatory shock. Crit Care Clin 9(2): 313–333, 1993
27. Iverson L, Herfindahl G, Eicher R et al: Vascular complications of intra-aortic balloon counterpulsation. Am J Surg 154: 99–123, 1987
28. Kantrowitz A: Clinical experience with cardiac assistance by means of intra aortic place-shift balloon pumping. Transactions of the American Society for Artificial Internal Organs 14: 344–348, 1968
29. Kuhn MM: Colloids versus crystalloids. Critical Care Nurse 11(5): 37–52, 1993
30. Ley SJ: The Thoratec ventricular assist device: Nursing guidelines. Clin Issues Crit Care Nurs 2: 529–544, 1991
31. Magovern GJ, Park SB, Maher TD: Use of a centrifugal pump without anticoagulants for postoperative left ventricular assist. World J Surg 9(1): 25–36, 1985
32. Marchetta S, Stennis E: Ventricular assist devices: Applications for critical care. Cardiovascular Nursing 2(2): 39–51, 1988
33. Mayer JH: Subclavian artery approach for insertion of intra-aortic balloon. J Thorac Cardiovasc Surg 76: 61–63, 1978
34. Miller CA, Pae WE, Pierce WS: Combined registry for the clinical use of mechanical ventricular assist devices: Postcardiotomy cardiogenic shock. Transactions of the American Society for Artificial Internal Organs 36: 43–46, 1990
35. Mitchell PH: Diagnostic reasoning in the critical care setting. In Carnevali DL, Mitchell PH, Woods NF et al (eds): Diagnostic Reasoning in Nursing, pp 159–174. Philadelphia, JB Lippincott, 1984

36. Mizock BA, Falk JL: Lactic acidosis in critical illness. Crit Care Med 20: 80–91,1992

37. Moss GS, Lowe RJ, Jilek J et al: Colloid or crystalloid in the resuscitation of hemorrhagic shock: A controlled clinical trial. Surgery 89(4): 434–438, 1981

38. Mouchawar A, Rosenthal M: A pathophysiologic approach to the patient in shock. Int Anesthesiol Clin 31: 1–17, 1993

39. Mulford E: Nursing perspectives for the patient receiving post-operative ventricular assistance in the critical care unit. Heart Lung 16: 246–255, 1987

40. Myers TJ, Catanese KA, Vargo RL et al: Extended cardiac support with a portable left ventricular assist system in the home. ASAIO J 42: M576–M579, 1996.

41. Nacht A: The use of blood products in shock. Crit Care Clin 8: 255–291, 1992

42. Parrillo JE, Burch C, Shelhamer JH et al: A circulating myocardial depressant substance in humans with septic shock. J Clin Invest 76(4): 1539–1553, 1985

43. Pennock JL, Pierce WS, Wisman CB et al: Survival and complications following ventricular assist pumping for cardiogenic shock. Ann Surg 198: 469–478, 1983

44. Perry AG, Potter PA (eds): Shock: Comprehensive Nursing Management. St. Louis, CV Mosby, 1983

45. Pierce WS, Parr GVS, Myers JL et al: Ventricular assist pumping in patients with cardiogenic shock after cardiac operations. N Engl J Med 305: 1606–1610, 1981

46. Pristas JM, Winowich S, Nastala CJ et al: Protocol for releasing Novacor left ventricular assist system patients out-of-hospital. ASAIO J 41: M539–M543, 1995.

47. Quaal SJ: Comprehensive Intra-aortic Balloon Pumping. St. Louis, CV Mosby, 1984

48. Quaal SJ: Treatment of the failing heart. In Kern LS (ed): Cardiac Critical Care Nursing, pp 397–452. Rockville, MD, Aspen, 1988

49. Rady MY: The role of central venous oximetry, lactic acid concentration and shock index in the evaluation of clinical shock: A review. Resuscitation 24: 55–60, 1992

50. Rice V: Shock, a clinical syndrome: An update. Part four: Nursing care of the shock patient. Critical Care Nurse 11(7): 28–39, 1991

51. Rice V: Shock, a clinical syndrome: An update. Part one: An overview of shock. Critical Care Nurse 11(4): 20–27, 1991

52. Rice V: Shock, a clinical syndrome: An update. Part three: Therapeutic management. Critical Care Nurse 11(6): 34–39, 1991

53. Rice V: Shock, a clinical syndrome: An update. Part two: The stages of shock. Critical Care Nurse 11(5): 75–85, 1991

54. Rodgers CD: Needs of relatives of cardiac surgery patients during the critical care phase. FOCUS 10(5): 50–55, 1983

55. Rose DM, Culliford A, Cunningham J et al: Late functional and hemodynamic status of surviving patients following insertion of a left heart assist device. J Thorac Cardiovasc Surg 86: 639–645, 1983

56. Rountree DW: The Hemopump temporary cardiac assist system. Clinical Issues in Critical Care Nursing 2: 562–574, 1991

57. Sanfelippo RM, Baker NH, Ewy HG et al: Experience with intra aortic balloon counterpulsation. Ann Thorac Surg 41: 36–42, 1986

58. Schlant RC, Sonnenblick EH: Normal physiology of the cardiovascular system. In Hurst JW (ed): The Heart, Vol 1, 7th ed., p 35–71. New York, McGraw-Hill, 1991

59. Schuster DP, Lefrak SS: Shock. In Civetta JM, Taylor RW, Kirby RR (eds): Critical Care, 2nd ed, pp 407–422. Philadelphia, JB Lippincott, 1992

60. Shatney CH: Pathophysiology and treatment of circulatory shock. In Zschoche DA (ed): Comprehensive Review of Critical Care, 3rd ed., pp 177–217. St. Louis, CV Mosby, 1986

61. Shinn JA, Oyer PE: Novacor ventricular assist system. In Quaal S (ed): Cardiac Mechanical Assist Beyond Balloon Pumping, pp 99–115. St. Louis, CV Mosby, 1993

62. Shinn JA: Intra-aortic balloon pump counterpulsation. In Hudak CM, Gallo BM, Lohr TS (eds): Critical Care Nursing: A Holistic Approach, 4th ed, pp 189–201. Philadelphia, JB Lippincott, 1986

63. Taylor J, Weil MH: Failure of the Trendelenburg position to improve circulation during clinical shock. Surg Gynecol Obstet 124(5): 1005–1010, 1967

64. Thal AP, Brown EB, Hermreck AS et al: Shock: A Physiologic Basis for Treatment. Chicago, Year Book, 1971

65. Van Citters RL, Bauer CB, Christopherson LK et al: Artificial heart and assist devices: Directions, needs, costs, societal and ethical issues. Artif Organs 9: 375–415, 1985

66. Weil MH, Shubin H: The "VIP" approach to the bedside management of shock. JAMA 207(2): 337–340, 1969

67. Weintraub RM, Thurer RL: The intra-aortic balloon pump: A ten-year experience. Heart Transplantation 3: 8–15, 1983

68. Younes RN, Aun F, Accioly CQ et al: Hypertonic solution in the treatment of hypovolemic shock: A prospective, randomized study in patients admitted to the emergency room. Surgery 111: 380–385, 1992

69. Yu Mihae, Levy MM, Smith P et al: Effect of maximizing oxygen delivery on morbidity and mortality rates in critically ill patients: A prospective randomized, controlled study. Crit Care Med 21: 834–838, 1993

Sudden Cardiac Death and Cardiac Arrest

CAROLYN CHANDLER MAIN
DONNA GERITY

Sudden cardiac death (SCD) is a major clinical and public health problem in the United States, accounting for approximately 300,000 deaths annually.[87,101] Despite the reduction of total cardiac mortality, the proportion of SCD remains unchanged. Depending on the availability of emergency medical services, 40% or more of SCD victims die before reaching the hospital.[4,12,73,77,83,109] Only 25% to 30% of out-of-hospital sudden cardiac arrest victims survive to discharge.[18] Survivors of sudden cardiac arrest have a high risk for future events. Myocardial revascularization, implantable cardiac defibrillators, ablation procedures, and amiodarone therapy have improved the long-term care of these patients.[96] However, there are still no highly reliable physiologic predictors available to foretell the first event of ventricular fibrillation (VF).

DEFINITION OF SUDDEN DEATH

Sudden cardiac death is defined as an unexpected death due to cardiac causes that occurs within 1 hour of symptom onset. The person may or may not have known of preexisting heart disease. Cardiac arrest, usually due to cardiac arrhythmias, is the term used to describe the sudden collapse, loss of consciousness, and loss of effective circulation that precedes biologic death.[62,87]

Ventricular Fibrillation

Ventricular fibrillation is the rhythm most commonly found in adult cardiac arrest.[8,17,54,56,88] Associations between acute and chronic premature ventricular contractions (PVCs) and the occurrence of sustained ventricular tachycardia (VT) and VF have been documented. An increased risk for development of VT and VF has been identified when complex forms of ventricular ectopy were recorded during ambulatory monitoring.[9,23,51,72,102] These observations led to a view that VF is an "electrophysiologic accident"[90] caused by the presence of ventricular ectopy.

The theory that PVCs accidentally cause VF and sudden cardiac arrest expanded as additional clinical and experimental observations were recorded. It was recognized that a transitional event was required to cause nonlethal PVCs to initiate VF. In 1989, Myerburg and colleagues[90] described a biologic model of SCD (Fig. 25-1). In this model, the concept that PVCs cause VT and VF remains important and is integrated into a scheme of structure and function. For a PVC to initiate VT or VF, cardiac structural abnormalities (usually chronic conditions) must be present to interact with transient functional factors. These transient functional changes alter the stable structural abnormality and convert it to an unstable pathophysiologic state. Examples of structural abnormality include myocardial infarction (MI), cardiomyopathies, left ventricular (LV) hypertrophy, and abnormal electrical structures such as bypass tracts. Examples of functional abnormalities include hemodynamic changes, electrolyte imbalances, hypoxemia, acidosis, and proarrhythmic drug effects.[2,35,90] Although it reported an absence of simple causal relationships between PVCs and VT/VF, the Cardiac Arrhythmia Suppression Trial (CAST) supports this theory. In the experimental group, cardiac antiarrhythmic drugs successfully suppressed PVCs. However, compared with the placebo group, the experimental group still had a much higher incidence of SCD.[35,40]

PATHOLOGY AND PATHOPHYSIOLOGY OF SUDDEN CARDIAC ARREST

Structural Abnormalities

Coronary heart disease (CHD) is the major structural abnormality found in most sudden cardiac arrest victims.[6,75,102,123] In an early study of cardiac arrest survivors, 78% of patients with CHD reported previous histories of old MI, angina, congestive heart failure, or hypertension before the arrest. For the remaining 22% of survivors, the

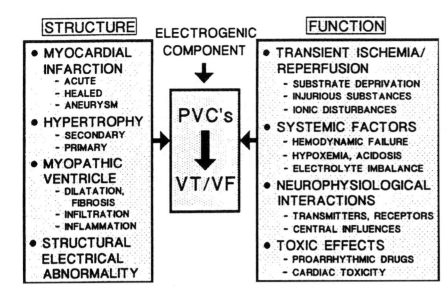

FIGURE 25-1 Short- or long-term structural abnormalities and functional modulations interact to influence the propensity for premature ventricular contractions (PVCs) to initiate a ventricular tachycardia or fibrillation (VT or VF). The four major categories of structural abnormalities may be influenced by one or more functional events, as outlined. (From Myerburg RJ, Kessler KM, Bassett AL et al: A biological approach to sudden cardiac death: Structure, function, and cause. Am J Cardiol 63: 1513, 1989.)

sudden cardiac arrest was their first manifestation of CHD.[21] In another study, 81% of 220 sudden cardiac arrest victims had CHD as a major causative factor.[75] Prior healed MI has been reported in as many as 75% of hearts examined at autopsy after SCD. However, the 20% to 30% frequency of pathologic evidence of acute MI after SCD is relatively low.[52,79,93,102] Other causes of sudden death are listed in Display 25-1.

Up to 75% of SCD victims have been reported as having advanced, chronic, atherosclerotic coronary artery lesions. Severe CHD is defined as one or more coronary vessels with 75% or greater stenosis. In a sample of (87) people who died suddenly, 59% had an old complete occlusion in one or more coronary vessels; 8% had single-vessel stenosis of over 90%; 18% had double-vessel stenosis of over 90%; and 13% had triple-vessel stenosis of over 90%. Only 8% did not have significant CHD.[102] Several studies have demonstrated no correlation between the anatomic pattern or distribution of the coronary artery lesion and the risk for SCD.[75,120]

There is some evidence that acute, thrombotic coronary lesions may be related to the occurrence of sudden cardiac arrest.[34] Acute coronary lesions are defined as plaque fissuring, platelet aggregation, acute thrombi, or any combination of these. In one study, acute coronary lesions were found in 95 of 100 autopsies of SCD victims. Thus, coronary spasm at or distal to the site of an acute thrombosis may be the factor associated with the creation of myocardial electrical disturbances and the development of VT.[34] Sudden cardiac arrest has been described as an event that may follow acute myocardial ischemia resulting from an episode of coronary artery plaque instability and thrombosis.[33] Sudden cardiac arrest also may be part of a spectrum of unstable angina and acute MI. Therefore, if the plaque were restabilized and antegrade blood flow through the coronary artery was maintained or rapidly restored, evidence for a transmural MI would not necessarily be present.[33]

Left ventricular hypertrophy has been established as an independent risk factor for SCD, regardless of the presence of CHD.[63] Increased ventricular ectopy has also been associated with electrocardiographic patterns of LV hypertro-

phy as well as increased myocardial mass documented by echocardiography.[82] Heart weights are higher among SCD victims than among those who did not die suddenly.[52] The underlying causes for myocardial hypertrophy include hypertensive or valvular heart disease, obstructive and

---

DISPLAY 25-1

Causes of Sudden Death

CARDIAC CAUSES

Atherosclerotic coronary heart disease
    Myocardial Infarction
    Coronary artery spasm
Aortic stenosis
Cardiomyopathies
    Idiopathic hypertrophic subaortic stenosis
Acute myocarditis
Aortic or ventricular aneurysm with dissection or rupture
Congenital heart disease
Prolapsed mitral valve syndrome
Iatrogenic causes: Digitalis, quinidine, and other drug causes
Conduction defects: Wolff-Parkinson-White syndrome, prolonged QT syndrome, complete atrioventricular block

NONCARDIAC CAUSES

Pulmonary hypertension (primary, particularly during pregnancy)
Pulmonary embolism
Cerebral or subarachnoid hemorrhage
Sudden infant death syndrome (should at least in part be included in cardiac causes)
Choking
Jervell and Lange-Nielson syndrome (syndrome of prolonged QT interval, congenital deafness, syncope, and ventricular fibrillation after emotional or physical stresses)
Romano-Ward syndrome (similar to Jervell and Lange-Nielson syndrome, without congenital deafness)
Electrolyte abnormalities (i.e., hypokalemia)
Acid–base abnormalities (i.e., alkalosis)

nonobstructive hypertrophic cardiomyopathy, and right ventricular hypertrophy secondary to pulmonary hypertension or congenital heart disease. All of these conditions are associated with increased risk of SCD, but it has been suggested that people with severely hypertrophic ventricles are especially susceptible to SCD.[2]

Abnormal Ventricular Function

Because of the relationship of premature ventricular beats to abnormal ventricular function, it is not clear if abnormal LV function is an independent predictor of SCD. Patients with an ejection fraction no greater than 0.40 had a higher prevalence of complex ventricular arrhythmias and a higher postinfarction mortality rate than those patients with ejection fractions greater than 0.40. The mean ejection fraction in patients without complex ventricular arrhythmias was greater than 0.40. An analysis of the relationships among LV dysfunction, ventricular arrhythmias, and subsequent mortality in 766 patients post-MI revealed that an LV ejection fraction below 0.30 and the presence of ventricular arrhythmias were independently related to an increased mortality risk post-MI.[9]

Severe LV wall motion abnormalities were reported in patients who had been resuscitated from VF, especially in those patients who had sudden cardiac arrest recurrences at a later time.[124] There appears to be a relationship between LV dysfunction and SCD.[12] In a study involving exercise testing of 1,852 men with CHD, 115 (6.2%) died suddenly.[12] Cardiomegaly, exercise duration of less than 3 minutes (or failure to attain level II on the Bruce protocol), and exertional hypotension or failure to increase systolic pressure above 130 mm Hg were studied and positively related to the risk of SCD.

Mechanisms Involved in the Initiation of Cardiac Arrest

Each of the four functional factors illustrated in Figure 25-1—(1) transient ischemia and reperfusion; (2) systemic, metabolic, and hemodynamic factors; (3) neurochemical and neurophysiologic interactions; and (4) toxic effects—may interact with any of the structural abnormalities to lead to regional membrane instability and cause VF or VT.[87,91] CHD causes steady-state reductions in regional myocardial blood flow. Whereas myocardial cells are free of electrical instability most of the time, they are more susceptible to the changes that may occur than if the structural lesions were not present. The mechanism by which these functional modifications might cause ventricular arrhythmias in a heart with underlying structural abnormalities is illustrated in Figure 25-2.

Exercise-induced arrhythmias and subsequent cardiac arrest may be the result of an increase in myocardial oxygen demand in a part of the heart that is served by a vessel that can deliver only a fixed blood supply.[20,80] Coronary artery spasm may subject the heart to the deleterious effects of both ischemia and reperfusion.[107] Platelet aggregation and thrombosis may play a key role in the initiation of VF. When endothelial damage occurs in the presence of chronic atherosclerotic lesions, plaque fissuring and platelet activation and aggregation are followed by thrombosis.[34] Platelet activation also produces a series of biochemical reactions and may enhance myocardial susceptibility to VF by causing vasomotor modulation.[60] Ischemia causes a large number of regional and global changes that may destabilize myocardial membrane integrity and make the myocardium more likely to fibrillate in the face of an electrical triggering event.[62]

Neurophysiologic interactions, including central nervous system influences, circulating catecholamines, and disturbed adrenergic function, have been studied in relation to myocardial structural changes associated with VF induction. Autonomic nervous system function can be reflected in heart rate variability[69,81] and baroreceptor reflex changes.[72] Decreased heart rate variability has been identified as a possible marker for increased sudden cardiac arrest risk.[69] For survivors of acute MI (n = 808), the relative risk of mortality was 5.3 times greater in patients with heart rate variability less than 50 milliseconds compared with greater than 100 milliseconds.[74] Thus, decreased heart rate variability may be associated with either increased sympathetic tone or decreased vagal tone, or

FIGURE 25-2 Cascade for the genesis of ventricular arrhythmia in the anatomic substrate. The existing abnormal myocardium is converted from a stable electrophysiologic status to an unstable one because of its functional modulation (*e.g.*, ischemia or reperfusion). This unstable status causes changes in the membrane channels, receptors, and pumps that lead to electrophysiologic dysfunction. The latter may be manifested as automatic activity or reentrant circuits that form the electrophysiologic basis for ventricular arrhythmias. (From Myerburg RJ, Kessler KM, Castellanos A: Pathophysiology of sudden cardiac death. Pacing Clin Electrophysiol 14: 935–943, 1991. With permission.)

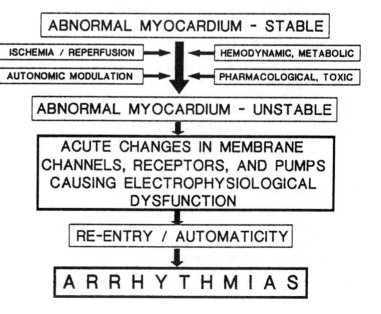

both and might predispose the heart to VF. Likewise, depressed baroreceptor reflexes after MI were also associated with an increased risk of subsequent cardiac arrest.[74]

Mechanisms of Ventricular Fibrillation

The mechanisms of VF have not been established. Automaticity or reentrant mechanisms, or both, could be involved. It is well established that nonuniform cardiac recovery properties reduce the threshold for VF. A variety of states, including ischemia and sympathetic stimulation, increase the degree of inequality of refractory periods in ventricular muscle. Although the mechanism of VF is not known, it is likely that the degree of inequality of recovery times is related to the duration of the vulnerable period and to the occurrence of excitation propagating in a nonuniform manner. Therefore, reentry may occur at varying cardiac locations.

Ventricular arrhythmias that occur within minutes of coronary occlusion are due to the multiple effects on the electrical properties of cardiac fibers of hypoxia, pH changes, anaerobic metabolites, adenosine, potassium, calcium, and catecholamines. An abnormal "slow response" action potential of myocardial cells induced by calcium, potassium, and catecholamines may be one of the causes of VF in cardiac arrest.[126] An increased interstitial potassium concentration may exist because of the leakage of potassium out of the injured myocardial cell. The increased interstitial potassium concentration causes the resting membrane potential to become less negative, inactivating the sodium channels. Thus, no "normal" action potential can be generated. In the presence of a less negative membrane potential caused by high extracellular potassium concentration and increased concentration of catecholamines, the voltage threshold of the calcium channel (approximately –40 mV) is activated. Hence, the slow inward Ca^{2+} current produces the slow response action potential. In addition to being propagated slowly, the slow response action potential also promotes unidirectional block. These characteristics allow reentry to occur in very short conduction path lengths. The slow response action potential is blocked by verapamil and magnesium, which are specific calcium channel blockers.

Automaticity describes the behavior of cardiac cells that can spontaneously depolarize during diastole and generate action potentials. Normal automaticity can be enhanced in the His-Purkinje system by an increased catecholamine concentration or in tissues adjacent to an ischemic zone.[126]

Environmental stress of diverse types can affect the heart, lower the threshold of vulnerability to VF, and, in animals with coronary occlusion, provoke VF. Undue anxiety and bereavement appear to increase vulnerability to SCD in humans.[76]

Risk Factors for Recurrent Cardiac Arrest

There is a high incidence of recurrent cardiac arrest, particularly in the first 1 to 2 years after resuscitation. Patients resuscitated from VF without associated acute MI had a 47% mortality rate within 2 years after resuscitation. To the contrary, those who had been resuscitated from VF secondary to acute MI had a mortality rate of only 14% after 2 years. Although a lower mortality rate in sequential years

has been reported by others, a high incidence of recurrence within the first 2 years still was seen.[17]

There are six major univariate predictors of recurrence of the SCD syndrome in patients with CHD:[19] (1) abnormal LV function as evidenced by a history of remote MI before VF, a history of congestive heart failure before VF, and segmental LV dysfunction and reduced ejection fraction; (2) extensive coronary artery obstruction; (3) VF not precipitated by acute infarction; (4) complex or high frequency of ventricular ectopic activity; (5) age; and (6) exercise-evoked hypotension or angina.

MANAGEMENT OF SUDDEN CARDIAC ARREST

Ventricular fibrillation is the initial rhythm most often identified by rescuers in cardiac arrest. The outcome of cardiac arrest is determined by how promptly treatment is initiated (advanced cardiac life support [ACLS]). To improve outcome from sudden cardiac arrests, the following must occur as rapidly as possible: (1) early recognition of warning signs, (2) early activation of the emergency medical system, (3) early basic cardiopulmonary resuscitation (CPR), (4) early defibrillation, and (5) early ACLS. These events have been described as "links in a chain of survival" because they are all connected and indispensable to the overall success of emergency cardiac care.[29,46,115]

Although this section summarizes ACLS recommendations for the adult patient, it is not a complete reference. For each cardiac nurse, ACLS provider certification by the American Heart Association is strongly recommended. In addition, the most current version of *Emergency Cardiac Care*,[43] *Basic Life Support for Healthcare Providers*,[6] and *The Textbook of Advanced Cardiac Life Support*[115] should be used as definitive references.

Adult Advanced Cardiac Life Support

Advanced cardiac life support[43,45] includes basic life support, the use of airway and circulation adjuncts, cardiac monitoring, and defibrillation and other arrhythmia control techniques. ACLS also includes establishment of intravenous access, drug therapy, and postresuscitation care. This section focuses on defibrillation and ACLS management of cardiac arrest due to VF and VT. Postresuscitation management of sudden cardiac arrest survivors is also included. For discussions of basic and complex arrhythmia and conduction disturbances, electrophysiologic studies, acute MI and thrombolytic therapy, hemodynamic monitoring, pacemakers, and implantable defibrillators, respectively, refer to Chapters 14, 15, 20, 21, 19, and 26.

ELECTRICAL THERAPY OF MALIGNANT ARRHYTHMIAS

Defibrillation and cardioversion are attempts completely to depolarize the myocardium and allow the sinus node to resume its function as the pacemaker for the heart. The two types of electrical therapy use defibrillators; defibrillation is, by definition, the therapy for VF, and cardioversion is the electrical therapy for all other malignant arrhythmias. Transcutaneous and transvenous pacing are additional types of electrical therapy used in ACLS for patients with hemodynamically compromised bradycardias (see Chapter 26).

EARLY DEFIBRILLATION

Ventricular tachycardia and VF cause 80% to 90% of nontraumatic adult cardiac arrests.[8,56] Defibrillation is the definitive therapy for cardiac arrest due to VF. Rapid, early defibrillation is a key step and the most important intervention likely to save lives.[16,25,29,30,41,113,114,115,121,123] That most cardiac arrests occur outside of the hospital is a major obstacle to rapid, early defibrillation.[1] The widespread use of automated external defibrillators (AEDs) helps to make early defibrillation a reality by expanding the number of rescuers available to treat SCD. Only minimal training is required. The American Heart Association has now integrated the use of AEDs into the *Textbook of Basic Life Support for Healthcare Providers,* acknowledging the importance of early defibrillation and the increased availability of AEDs[6,70] (Fig. 25-3).

Defibrillators. Defibrillators are the power source used to deliver the electrical therapy. Direct-current defibrillators contain a transformer, an alternating-current-to-direct-current converter, a capacitor to store direct current, a charge switch, and discharge switches to complete the circuit from the capacitor to the electrodes. Portable defibrillators derive their power from a battery, which must be kept charged. Electrical output of defibrillators is quantified in terms of joules (J), or watt-seconds, of energy.[115]

Most available commercial defibrillators use a half-sinusoid waveform when delivering external defibrillation. Alternative waveforms for transthoracic defibrillation such as biphasic waveforms have also been approved for use. Studies show that biphasic waveforms achieve shock success rates at substantially lower energies (in the range of 150 J).[64] Lower energy requirements reduce the size and weight of the defibrillator, which in turn increases public access to AEDs because they are easier to handle, less expensive, and more convenient to keep available.[125]

Rapid defibrillation can be performed with manual, automatic, or semiautomatic external defibrillators. Manual defibrillators must be operated by well-trained personnel, often ACLS responders, who are able to interpret cardiac rhythms on a rhythm strip or monitor. Automatic advisory or semiautomatic external defibrillators have been developed for use by first responders. AEDs are accurate and easy to use and, unlike standard defibrillators, have detection systems that analyze the rhythm and advise the operator to shock when VF/VT characteristics are determined. Thus, successful defibrillation can be achieved without requiring the operator to have rhythm recognition skills. AEDs are attached to the patient with the use of adhesive sternal apex pads that are connected to a cable, allowing for "hands-free defibrillation."[6,115] AEDs were shown to help emergency personnel deliver the first shock on an average of 1 minute sooner than personnel using conventional defibrillators.[113]

DEFIBRILLATION

Transthoracic Resistance. The ability to defibrillate requires the passage of sufficient electric current through the heart. Current flow is determined by transthoracic impedance, or resistance to current flow, and the selected energy (joules). If transthoracic resistance is high, a low-energy shock may fail to produce enough current to defibrillate. The factors that determine transthoracic resistance include energy selected, electrode size and composition, electrode–skin interface, number of and time interval between previous electrical discharges, electrode pressure, ventilation phase, and interelectrode distance.

Resistance between the electrode and the chest wall must be minimized. Bare electrodes produce high resistance to electrical flow.[22,48,49] Electrode gel, some commercial electrode pads, and gauze pads moistened with normal saline decrease electrical impedance. Self-adhesive monitor or defibrillator pads are also available and very effective. They can be used in any of the aforementioned locations.[68]

Repeat defibrillator shocks decrease transthoracic resistance.[31,53] Transthoracic resistance is lowered by approximately 8% after the second shock. In hand-held paddles, the amount of paddle pressure applied to the chest influences the transthoracic resistance by ensuring good electrode–skin contact.[65] Current recommendations are to apply 25 pounds of pressure per paddle.[115] Minimum transthoracic resistance occurs in the end-expiratory phase of the respiratory cycle. A short interelectrode distance reduces transthoracic resistance as well. The optimal paddle size for both hand-held and self-adhesive electrodes is 8 to 12 cm in diameter.[65,68,112]

Energy Requirements. Selection of the appropriate energy is one of the factors that determines success of defibrillation. A shock with insufficient energy and current fails to defibrillate. Myocardial damage may occur if energy and current are too high.[32,67]

Once VF or pulseless VT has been identified (Fig. 25-4), immediate defibrillation must be carried out. Three shocks at 200 J, 200 to 300 J, and up to 360 J are delivered, one after the other. The defibrillator paddles should be left on the chest between shocks. The rescuers should *not* perform CPR between shocks. While the defibrillator is recharging, the rhythm should be rechecked. It is not necessary to perform pulse checks between shocks if a properly connected monitor shows persistent VF and VT. Rescuers who perform defibrillation must announce that they are about to deliver a shock. They must then check that all personnel are clear of the patient and stretcher before defibrillating.

If the first or second shocks are successful, but the patient subsequently refibrillates, the energy should be kept at the last successful level rather than increased to 360 J.[115] Because the most important determinant of survival in VF is *rapid* defibrillation, the shocks should be given as soon as the defibrillator arrives.[41,114]

Electrode Position. Electrode placement is critical in ensuring that a critical mass of myocardium is depolarized. Any of three electrode positions may be used. *Standard* or *anterolateral* electrode placement involves one electrode being placed to the right of the upper sternum just below the right clavicle. The other electrode is placed just to the left of the left nipple, with the center of the electrode in the mid-axillary line (Fig. 25-5). *Anterior-posterior* electrode placement involves one paddle positioned anteriorly over the precordium, just to the left of the lower sternal border.

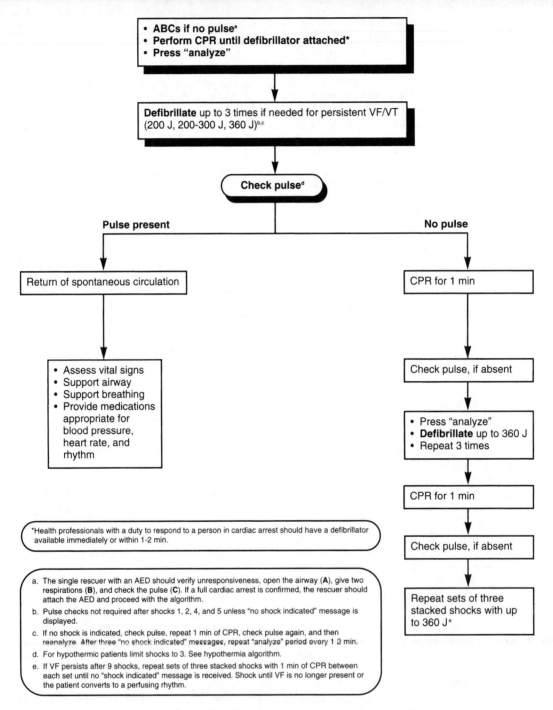

Automated External Defibrillation (AED) Treatment Algorithm
Emergency cardiac care pending arrival of ACLS personnel

- **ABCs if no pulse**[a]
- **Perform CPR until defibrillator attached***
- **Press "analyze"**

Defibrillate up to 3 times if needed for persistent VF/VT (200 J, 200-300 J, 360 J)[b,c]

Check pulse[d]

Pulse present

Return of spontaneous circulation

- Assess vital signs
- Support airway
- Support breathing
- Provide medications appropriate for blood pressure, heart rate, and rhythm

No pulse

CPR for 1 min

Check pulse, if absent

- Press "analyze"
- **Defibrillate** up to 360 J
- Repeat 3 times

CPR for 1 min

Check pulse, if absent

Repeat sets of three stacked shocks with up to 360 J[e]

*Health professionals with a duty to respond to a person in cardiac arrest should have a defibrillator available immediately or within 1-2 min.

a. The single rescuer with an AED should verify unresponsiveness, open the airway (**A**), give two respirations (**B**), and check the pulse (**C**). If a full cardiac arrest is confirmed, the rescuer should attach the AED and proceed with the algorithm.

b. Pulse checks not required after shocks 1, 2, 4, and 5 unless "no shock indicated" message is displayed.

c. If no shock is indicated, check pulse, repeat 1 min of CPR, check pulse again, and then reanalyze. After three "no shock indicated" messages, repeat "analyze" period every 1-2 min.

d. For hypothermic patients limit shocks to 3. See hypothermia algorithm.

e. If VF persists after 9 shocks, repeat sets of three stacked shocks with 1 min of CPR between each set until no "shock indicated" message is received. Shock until VF is no longer present or the patient converts to a perfusing rhythm.

FIGURE 25-3 Algorithm for automatic external defibrillation (AED): recommendations for ventricular tachycardia/fibrillation (UT/VF) before arrival of advanced cardiac life support personnel. (From Advanced Cardiac Life Support. American Heart Association: 1–13. Dallas, AHA 1997. Copyright 1997 AHA.)

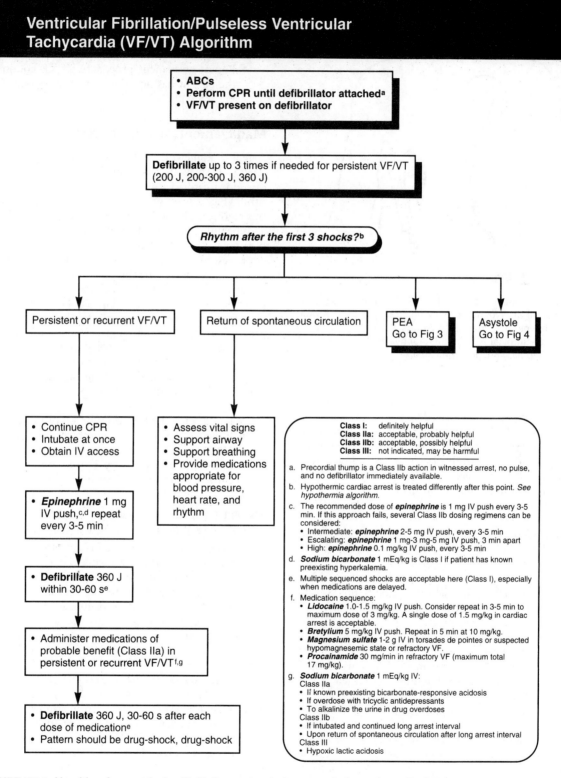

FIGURE 25-4 Algorithm for ventricular fibrillation and pulseless ventricular tachycardia (*VF* and *VT*). (From American Heart Association: Advanced Cardiac Life Support, pp. 1–17. Dallas, AHA, 1997. Copyright 1997, AHA.)

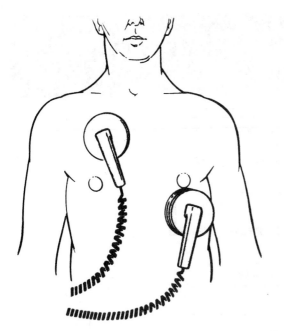

FIGURE 25-5 Standard positioning of defibrillator paddles. (From Underhill SL, Woods SL: Nursing strategies for common cardiac problems. In Patrick ML, Woods SL, Craven RF et al (eds): Medical–Surgical Nursing: Pathophysiological Concepts, p 498. Philadelphia, JB Lippincott, 1986.)

The other electrode is positioned posteriorly behind the heart.[115] A third alternative for paddle placement is to place the posterior paddle in the right infrascapular location and the anterior paddle over the left apex.[66] In patients with permanent pacemakers, electrode placement should be at least 5 inches from the pacemaker pulse generator.[115] Refer to Chapter 26 for information on paddle placement for patients with implantable cardioverter-defibrillators (ICDs).

Procedure. Identify the rhythm as VF. If the rhythm appears to be asystole, check the rhythm in another lead to confirm that the rhythm is not fine VF.

◆ Apply conductive material to electrodes, unless using conductive pads. Position electrodes on the chest.
◆ Turn on the defibrillator.
◆ Set energy level to 200 J.
◆ Charge capacitors. Charging may take several seconds. Many defibrillators emit a sound or light signal, or both, to indicate that the unit has charged.
◆ Ensure proper electrode placement on chest.
◆ Apply pressure of 25 pounds per paddle. Do not lean forward because of the danger of the paddles slipping.
◆ Scan the area to ensure that no personnel are in contact directly or indirectly with the patient. Indicate that you are about to shock the patient by yelling "all clear."
◆ Reassess rhythm.
◆ Deliver countershock by depressing both buttons simultaneously on the paddles.
◆ Reassess rhythm. Do not remove the paddles from the chest. If VF persists, shock a second time at 200 to 300 J. Scan for personnel in contact with the

patient, indicate you are about to reshock, and reshock immediately.
◆ Repeat assessment procedure. If necessary, increase the energy to 360 J. Scan for personnel in contact with the patient, indicate you are about to reshock, and reshock immediately.
◆ Repeat assessment procedure. If VF continues or if the patient has no pulse, start (or resume) CPR (see Fig. 25-4).

Management of Cardiac Arrest

A general framework for the use of ACLS algorithms is outlined in Display 25-2. The initial approach to management of sudden cardiac arrest is outlined in the Universal Algorithm (Fig. 25-6). ACLS providers must always start with this algorithm by activating the emergency medical system and beginning basic life support. The basics of airway, breathing, and circulation remain important during the entire resuscitation continuum. Once the patient is attached to a monitor, determine the rhythm and potential cause for the arrest. If VF or pulseless VT is present, go to the VF and pulseless VT algorithm (see Fig. 25-4). If electrical activity is present without a pulse, go to the pulseless electrical activity (PEA) algorithm (Fig. 25-7). If the monitor displays asystole, go to the asystole algorithm (Fig. 25-8).

Cardiac arrest should be managed by an ACLS team composed of a team leader and one or more team members. Priorities for resuscitation are:[115]

◆ Rapid, early defibrillation for VF or pulseless VT
◆ Effective CPR with endotracheal intubation and 100% oxygen delivery
◆ Epinephrine given every 3 to 5 minutes to maintain coronary and cerebral perfusion

VENTRICULAR FIBRILLATION AND PULSELESS VENTRICULAR TACHYCARDIA

Rapid countershock is the determinant of survival in VF and pulseless VT. If the arrest was witnessed and a defibrillator is not immediately available, a precordial thump may be effective in terminating VT and, rarely, VF.[13,84,98] A precordial thump must never be allowed to delay defibrillation when a defibrillator is available. Because a precordial thump may convert VT to VF, asystole, or electromechanical dissociation, it should not be used in a patient who has VT with a pulse unless a defibrillator and external pacemaker are present.[13,84,127]

If three shocks fail to convert the patient, the VF and pulseless VT algorithm (see Fig. 25-4) directs rescuers to give epinephrine. Epinephrine remains an extremely important drug for patients in cardiac arrest. It is given for its β-adrenergic property of peripheral vasoconstriction, which increases aortic diastolic pressure, coronary perfusion pressure, and coronary blood flow.[97,115] Defibrillation at 360 J should be performed within 30 to 60 seconds after administration of all drugs in ACLS. If VF and VT are still present after CPR, intubation, ventilation, four shocks, and epinephrine administration, then rescuers are dealing with refractory VF. An antifibrillatory drug such as lidocaine, bretylium, or procainamide should be administered in bolus

---

DISPLAY 25-2

The Algorithm Approach to Emergency Cardiac Care

The American Heart Association guidelines use algorithms as an educational tool. They are an illustrative method to summarize information. Providers of emergency care should view algorithms as a summary and a memory aid. They provide ways to treat a broad range of patients. Algorithms by nature oversimplify. The effective teacher and care provider uses them wisely, not blindly. Some patients may require care not specified in the algorithms. When clinically appropriate, flexibility is accepted and encouraged. Many interventions and actions are listed as "considerations" to help providers think. These lists should not be considered endorsements or requirements or "standard of care" in a legal sense. Algorithms do not replace clinical understanding. Although the algorithms provide a good "cookbook," the patient always requires a "thinking cook."
    The following clinical recommendations apply to all treatment algorithms:

- First, treat the patient, not the monitor.
- Algorithms for cardiac arrest presume that the condition under discussion continually persists, that the patient remains in cardiac arrest, and that cardiopulmonary resuscitation is always performed.
- Apply different interventions whenever appropriate indications exist.
- The flow diagrams present mostly class I (acceptable, definitely effective) interventions. The footnotes present class IIa (acceptable, probably effective), class IIb (acceptable, possibly effective), and class III (not indicated, may be harmful) interventions.
- Adequate airway, ventilation, oxygenation, chest compressions, and defibrillation are more important than administration of medications and take precedence over initiating an intravenous line or injecting pharmacologic agents.
- Several medications (epinephrine, lidocaine, and atropine) can be administered by the endotracheal tube, but the dosage should be 2 to 2.5 times the intravenous dose.
- With a few exceptions, intravenous medications should always be administered rapidly, by a bolus method.
- After each intravenous medication, give a 20- to 30-mL bolus of intravenous fluid and immediately elevate the extremity. This technique enhances delivery of drugs to the central circulation, which may take 1 to 2 minutes.
- Last, treat the patient, not the monitor.

From American Heart Association: Advanced Cardiac Life Support, pp 1–11. Dallas, AHA, 1997. Copyright 1997, AHA.

---

form. Only after a return of spontaneous circulation should a constant infusion be started.

ASYSTOLE

The prognosis for patients in asystole is extremely poor.[3,35] Asystole usually is the result of end-stage heart disease or prolonged cardiac arrest. CPR, intubation, epinephrine, and atropine are the treatment options in cardiac arrest with asystole (see Fig. 25-8). Shocking asystole has been discouraged. Electric shocks can cause parasympathetic discharge and may, in fact, prevent a return of spontaneous cardiac electrical activity.[119] There have been no studies that have documented an improvement in survival by shocking asystole.[111,116]

Transcutaneous pacing must be performed early. It is rarely effective in the out-of-hospital setting.[27,28] Transcutaneous pacing is most likely to benefit those patients in whom a bradysystolic arrest or asystole develops from vagal discharge after defibrillation.[10]

PULSELESS ELECTRICAL ACTIVITY

Pulseless electrical activity includes electromechanical dissociation, pseudo-electromechanical dissociation, idioventricular rhythms, ventricular escape rhythms, postdefibrillation idioventricular rhythms, and bradysystolic rhythms[45,115] (see Fig. 25-7). Prognosis of patients with electromechanical dissociation is very poor unless the underlying cause can be identified and treated appropriately.[3] Therefore, the highest priority is to find the correctable cause while maintaining the patient's airway, breathing, and circulation. Common correctable causes of electromechanical dissociation include hypovolemia, cardiac tamponade, tension pneumothorax, hypoxemia, and acidosis. Massive damage from MI, prolonged ischemia during resuscitation, and pulmonary embolism are less correctable causes. Patients in profound shock of any etiology initially may present with PEA. Hypovolemia is assessed by history and lack of neck vein distention; it is treated by volume replacement. Tension pneumothorax is assessed by history and neck vein distention; it is treated by needle aspiration, chest tube insertion, or both. Cardiac tamponade is assessed by history and neck vein distention; it is treated by pericardiocentesis or thoracotomy. Hypoxemia is assessed by history and arterial blood gases; it is treated by improving oxygenation and ventilation. Acidosis is assessed by history and arterial blood gases; it is treated by improving CPR technique and hyperventilating the patient. If bradycardia is present, atropine may be administered in an attempt to increase heart rate.[45,115]

Management of Impending Cardiac Arrest

VENTRICULAR AND SUPRAVENTRICULAR TACHYCARDIA

The tachycardia treatment algorithm (Fig. 25-9) directs rescuers to focus on the causes of a tachyarrhythmia and the hemodynamic stability of the patient. Electrical cardioversion is the therapy of choice for poorly tolerated,

(text continued on page 649)

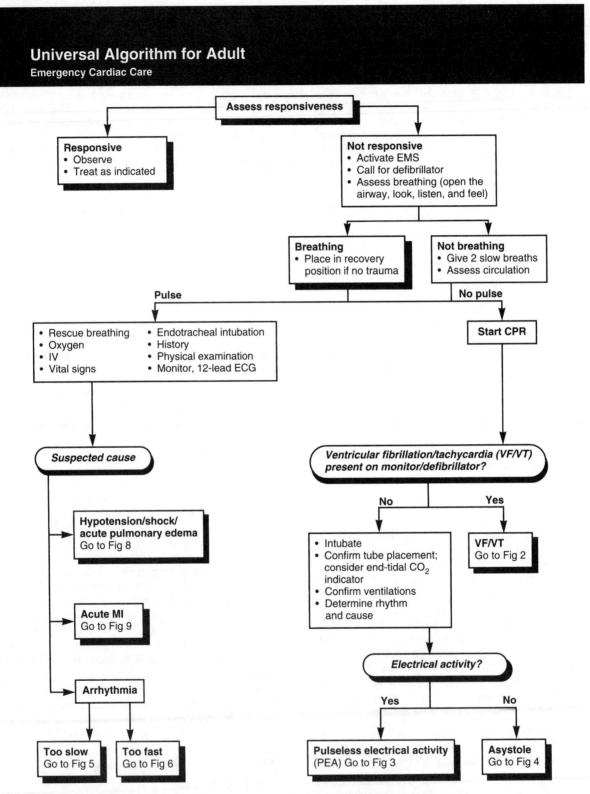

FIGURE 25-6 Universal algorithm for adult emergency cardiac care (ECC). (From American Heart Association: Advanced Cardiac Life Support, pp. 1–12. Dallas, AHA, 1997. Copyright 1997, AHA.)

Pulseless Electrical Activity (PEA) Algorithm
(Electromechanical Dissociation [EMD])

Includes
- Electromechanical dissociation (EMD)
- Pseudo-EMD
- Idioventricular rhythms
- Ventricular escape rhythms
- Bradyasystolic rhythms
- Postdefibrillation idioventricular rhythms

- Continue CPR
- Intubate at once
- Obtain IV access

- Assess blood flow using Doppler ultrasound, end-tidal CO_2, echocardiography, or arterial line

---

Consider possible causes
(Parentheses = possible therapies and treatments)

- Hypovolemia (volume infusion)
- Hypoxia (ventilation)
- Cardiac tamponade (pericardiocentesis)
- Tension pneumothorax (needle decompression)
- Hypothermia (see hypothermia algorithm)
- Massive pulmonary embolism (surgery, *thrombolytics*)

- Drug overdoses such as tricyclics, digitalis, β-blockers, calcium channel blockers
- Hyperkalemia[a]
- Acidosis[b]
- Massive acute myocardial infarction (go to Fig 9)

- *Epinephrine* 1 mg IV push,[a,c] repeat every 3-5 min

- If absolute bradycardia (<60 BPM) or relative bradycardia, give *atropine* 1 mg IV
- Repeat every 3-5 min to a total of 0.03-0.04 mg/kg[d]

Class I: definitely helpful
Class IIa: acceptable, probably helpful
Class IIb: acceptable, possibly helpful
Class III: not indicated, may be harmful

a. *Sodium bicarbonate* 1 mEq/kg is Class I if patient has known preexisting hyperkalemia.
b. *Sodium bicarbonate* 1 mEq/kg:
   Class IIa
   - If known preexisting bicarbonate-responsive acidosis
   - If overdose with tricyclic antidepressants
   - To alkalinize the urine in drug overdoses
   Class IIb
   - If intubated and continued long arrest interval
   - Upon return of spontaneous circulation after long arrest interval
   Class III
   - Hypoxic lactic acidosis
c. The recommended dose of *epinephrine* is 1 mg IV push every 3-5 min. If this approach fails, several Class IIb dosing regimen can be considered:
   - Intermediate: *epinephrine* 2-5 mg IV push, every 3-5 min
   - Escalating: *epinephrine* 1 mg-3 mg-5 mg IV push, 3 min apart
   - High: *epinephrine* 0.1 mg/kg IV push, every 3-5 min
d. The shorter *atropine* dosing interval (3 min) is possibly helpful in cardiac arrest (Class IIb).

FIGURE 25-7 Algorithm for pulseless electrical activity (PEA). (*electromechanical dissociation EMD*) (From American Heart Association: Advanced Cardiac Life Support, pp. 1–22. Dallas, AHA, 1997. Copyright 1997, AHA.)

---

malignant ventricular and supraventricular tachyarrhythmias with a heart rate greater than 150 beats/min. When the heart rate is less than 150 beats/min, a trial of medications may be indicated. With R-wave synchronous cardioversion, the defibrillator is programmed to fire on the R wave, thus avoiding the vulnerable period of cardiac repolarization, which is the downslope of the T wave. If the electrical shock were delivered on the downslope of the T wave, the patient's rhythm probably would deteriorate into VF.

When pulseless, the patient is treated as if in VF; thus, R-wave asynchronous cardioversion is not used. (Refer to

(text continued on page 652)

Asystole Treatment Algorithm

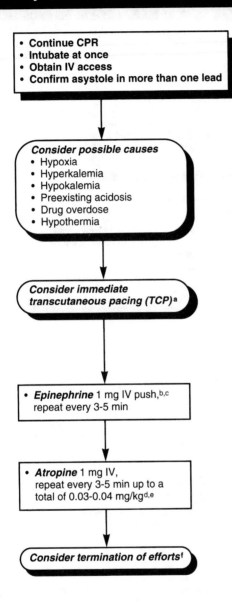

- **Continue CPR**
- **Intubate at once**
- **Obtain IV access**
- **Confirm asystole in more than one lead**

⬇

Consider possible causes
- Hypoxia
- Hyperkalemia
- Hypokalemia
- Preexisting acidosis
- Drug overdose
- Hypothermia

⬇

Consider immediate transcutaneous pacing (TCP)[a]

⬇

- **Epinephrine** 1 mg IV push,[b,c] repeat every 3-5 min

⬇

- **Atropine** 1 mg IV, repeat every 3-5 min up to a total of 0.03-0.04 mg/kg[d,e]

⬇

Consider termination of efforts[f]

Class I: definitely helpful
Class IIa: acceptable, probably helpful
Class IIb: acceptable, possibly helpful
Class III: not indicated, may be harmful

a. TCP is a Class IIb intervention. Lack of success may be due to delays in pacing. To be effective TCP must be performed early, simultaneously with drugs. Evidence does not support routine use of TCP for asystole.

b. The recommended dose of **epinephrine** is 1 mg IV push every 3-5 min. If this approach fails, several Class IIb dosing regimens can be considered:
   - Intermediate: **epinephrine** 2-5 mg IV push, every 3-5 min
   - Escalating: **epinephrine** 1 mg-3 mg-5 mg IV push, 3 min apart
   - High: **epinephrine** 0.1 mg/kg IV push, every 3-5 min

c. **Sodium bicarbonate** 1 mEq/kg is Class I if patient has known preexisting hyperkalemia.

d. The shorter **atropine** dosing interval (3 min) is Class IIb in asystolic arrest.

e. **Sodium bicarbonate** 1 mEq/kg:
   Class IIa
   - If known preexisting bicarbonate-responsive acidosis
   - If overdose with tricyclic antidepressants
   - To alkalinize the urine in drug overdoses
   Class IIb
   - If intubated and continued long arrest interval
   - Upon return of spontaneous circulation after long arrest interval
   Class III
   - Hypoxic lactic acidosis

f. If patient remains in asystole or other agonal rhythm after successful intubation and initial medications and no reversible causes are identified, consider termination of resuscitative efforts by a physician. Consider interval since arrest.

FIGURE 25-8 Asystole treatment algorithm. (From American Heart Association: Advanced Cardiac Life Support, pp. 1–24. Dallas, AHA, 1997. Copyright 1997, AHA.)

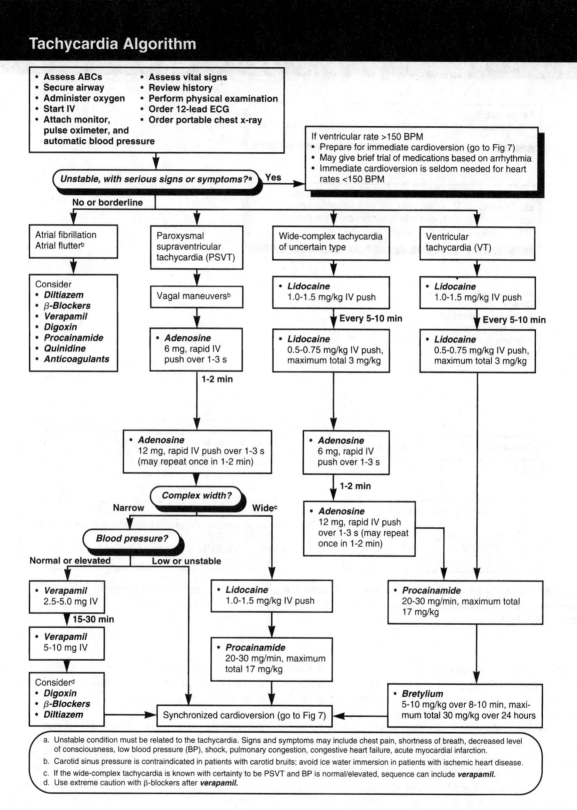

FIGURE 25-9 Tachycardia algorithm. (From American Heart Association: Advanced Cardiac Life Support, pp. 1–33. Dallas, AHA, 1997. Copyright 1997, AHA.)

Electrical Cardioversion Algorithm
(Patient is not in cardiac arrest)

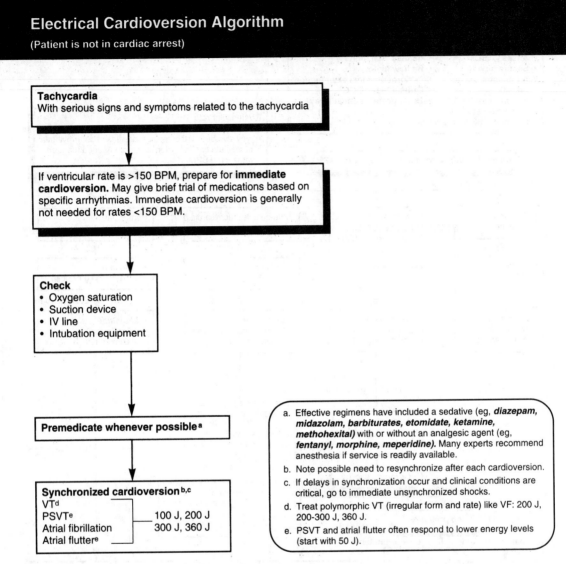

Tachycardia
With serious signs and symptoms related to the tachycardia

↓

If ventricular rate is >150 BPM, prepare for **immediate cardioversion.** May give brief trial of medications based on specific arrhythmias. Immediate cardioversion is generally not needed for rates <150 BPM.

↓

Check
• Oxygen saturation
• Suction device
• IV line
• Intubation equipment

↓

Premedicate whenever possible[a]

↓

Synchronized cardioversion[b,c]
VT[d]
PSVT[e]   100 J, 200 J
Atrial fibrillation   300 J, 360 J
Atrial flutter[e]

---

a. Effective regimens have included a sedative (eg, *diazepam, midazolam, barbiturates, etomidate, ketamine, methohexital)* with or without an analgesic agent (eg, *fentanyl, morphine, meperidine).* Many experts recommend anesthesia if service is readily available.

b. Note possible need to resynchronize after each cardioversion.

c. If delays in synchronization occur and clinical conditions are critical, go to immediate unsynchronized shocks.

d. Treat polymorphic VT (irregular form and rate) like VF: 200 J, 200-300 J, 360 J.

e. PSVT and atrial flutter often respond to lower energy levels (start with 50 J).

FIGURE 25-10 Electrical cardioversion algorithm (with the patient not in cardiac arrest). (From American Heart Association: Advanced Cardiac Life Support, pp. 1–34. Dallas, AHA, 1997. Copyright 1997, AHA.)

Figure 25-4 and the procedure for defibrillation.) If the patient is severely unstable (e.g., in acute pulmonary edema, having chest pain, or unconscious or hypotensive), unsynchronized cardioversion is recommended. Not only can there be considerable time delays with synchronized cardioversion, but in patients with extremely rapid VT, asynchronous cardioversion actually may be safer[45,47,115] because at rapid rates, the synchronizer may not be able to distinguish the T wave from the QRS complex. In this instance, an asynchronous shock may have less likelihood of falling on the T wave than a synchronous shock.[45,115]

Urgent R-wave synchronous cardioversion is indicated in the management of patients with hemodynamically unstable ventricular or supraventricular tachycardias. Elective R-wave synchronous cardioversion is indicated in patients with hemodynamically stable ventricular or supraventricular tachyarrhythmias unresponsive to vagal maneuvers and drug therapy.[115]

Energy Requirements. Figure 25-10 summarizes the electrical cardioversion algorithm. Energy requirements are variable depending on the rhythm and the number of cardioversion attempts. Rhythms that tend to be organized (i.e., VT, atrial flutter) usually require less energy than unorganized rhythms (i.e., VF, atrial fibrillation).

The energy requirements for cardioverting VT depend on the rate and morphology of the arrhythmia. The operator should start at 100 J for an organized, monomorphic VT with or without a pulse. Polymorphic VT requires an initial shock energy of 200 J. The electrical cardioversion algorithm recommends a 100-, 200-, 300-, and 360-J sequence for synchronized cardioversion.

Procedure for Urgent Synchronized Cardioversion.
Because the patient is conscious, anesthesia or analgesia is necessary. Except for the following points, the procedure for urgent synchronized cardioversion is the same as for defibrillation:

◆ Turn on the synchronizer.
◆ Select the appropriate energy level.
◆ Look for the synchronizer indicator on the screen, usually a spike or dot highlighted on the R wave. If you are unable to get a highlighted indicator, consider switching leads. Some older defibrillator or cardioverter units require an upright R wave for synchronization.
◆ Reassess rhythm.
◆ Expect a slight delay (milliseconds) from the time the buttons are pushed to the delivered shock.
◆ If the defibrillator does not fire, reassess rhythm. If the patient has reverted to VF, there is no R wave with which to synchronize. Therefore, the unit will not fire. Immediately turn the synchronizer off, adjust the energy level, and proceed to defibrillate the patient.
◆ If VF develops in the patient after the synchronous shock, immediately turn the synchronizer off, adjust the energy level, and proceed to defibrillate the patient.

SYMPTOMATIC BRADYCARDIA

The bradycardia algorithm (Fig. 25-11) outlines the approach to management of symptomatic bradyarrhythmias. Symptoms resulting from bradycardia (heart rate < 60 beats/min) include chest pain, dyspnea, lightheadedness, hypotension, or ventricular ectopy. An external pacemaker is always appropriate for use in symptomatic bradycardias and should be used immediately for patients who do not respond to atropine. Atropine must be used with caution in patients with acute MI who have third-degree heart block and ventricular escape beats or Mobitz type II heart block. Dopamine and epinephrine should be added as the patient's condition worsens. Isoproterenol increases myocardial oxygen consumption and peripheral vasodilatation. It should be used only with extreme caution.[45,115]

SURVIVORS OF CARDIAC ARREST

Prognosis

Prognosis of survivors is affected by how promptly definitive therapy is initiated, the rhythm or conduction disturbance initially recognized after cardiac arrest, and whether the patient also has sustained an acute MI. For patients whose initially recognized rhythm is asystole or PEA, prognosis is dismal.[3,35] Survival rates for patients found in asystole or PEA are only 1% to 6%, compared with 25% for

those patients found in VT/VF.[35] Despite early CPR and advanced life support, which have substantially improved initial resuscitation success rates up to 50%, only approximately half of these patients are discharged home. Most of these patients succumb either to cardiogenic shock, congestive heart failure, respiratory complications, or sepsis.[35,53,62]

Survivors of SCD are at high risk for future events. An epidemiologic study reported recurrence rates of 30% to 50% during a 2-year follow-up.[91] However, in recent years, SCD survivors have received benefits from revascularization procedures, ICDs, antiarrhythmic drugs, radiofrequency ablation of VT, or any combined therapies.[11,37,96] Ongoing research is also focused on identifying patients with CHD who are at high risk for future SCD.[11,14,37]

Medical Management of Survivors of Cardiac Arrest

IMMEDIATE POSTRESUSCITATION GOALS

◆ Provide cardiac and respiratory support to provide optimal tissue perfusion, especially to the brain.
◆ Transfer the patient to the nearest appropriately equipped emergency department and then to a critical care unit.
◆ Identify the causes of the arrest.
◆ Institute medical therapy to prevent arrhythmia recurrence, such as antiarrhythmic drug therapy and correction of underlying abnormalities that may have precipitated the cardiac arrest.
◆ Treat complications of resuscitation.

CEREBRAL RESUSCITATION

The primary goal of cardiopulmonary-cerebral resuscitation is to retain healthy brain function. In normothermic cardiac arrests, complete recovery of the heart and brain takes place within the same approximate time frame, between 10 and 20 minutes. Improvement in cerebral recovery after cardiac arrest results when cardiac arrest and CPR times are short, spontaneous normotension is restored, brain-oriented standard support of extracerebral organs is used, controlled brief hypertension is followed by normotension, and moderate normovolemic hemodilution is used. Brain-oriented standard support of extracerebral organs requires rescuers to:[105]

Control mean arterial pressure and normalize blood volume.
Maintain controlled ventilation for at least 2 hours after arrest. Immobilize the patient with less than fully paralyzing doses of muscle relaxants during controlled ventilation.
Control or prevent restlessness, straining, seizures.
Maintain arterial PCO_2 during controlled ventilation and spontaneous breathing at 25 to 35 mm Hg and 20 to 40 mm Hg, respectively.
Maintain arterial pH at 7.3 to 7.6.
Maintain arterial PO_2 over 100 mm Hg with an inspired oxygen concentration of 0.9 to 1.0 during first hour after arrest, and with an inspired oxygen concentration of 0.5 after 1 hour to 6 hours.

(text continued on page 655)

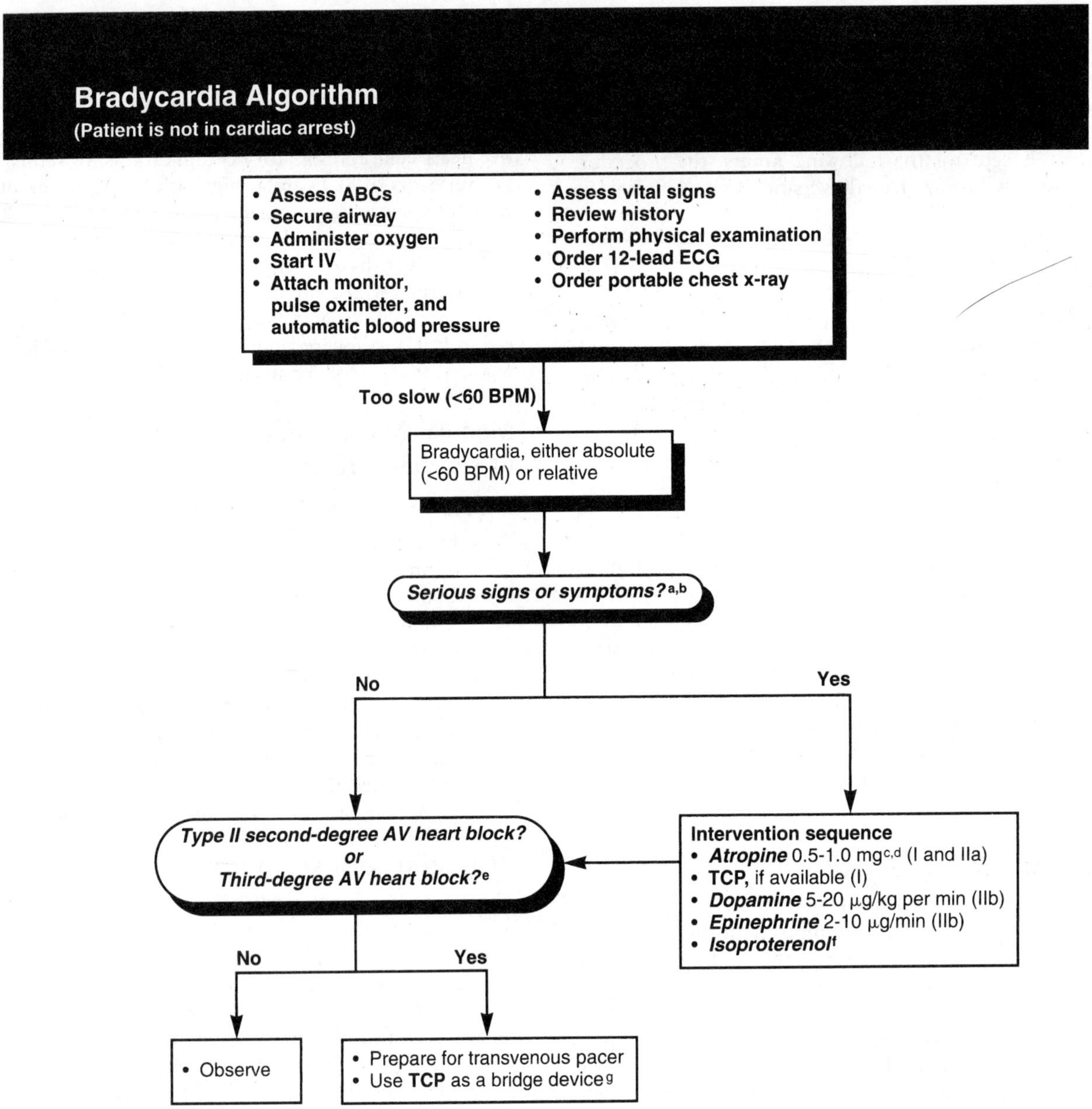

Bradycardia Algorithm
(Patient is not in cardiac arrest)

- **Assess ABCs**
- **Secure airway**
- **Administer oxygen**
- **Start IV**
- **Attach monitor, pulse oximeter, and automatic blood pressure**

- **Assess vital signs**
- **Review history**
- **Perform physical examination**
- **Order 12-lead ECG**
- **Order portable chest x-ray**

↓

Too slow (<60 BPM)

Bradycardia, either absolute (<60 BPM) or relative

↓

Serious signs or symptoms?[a,b]

No / **Yes**

No →

Type II second-degree AV heart block?
or
Third-degree AV heart block?[e]

→ ← **Yes**

Intervention sequence
- *Atropine* 0.5-1.0 mg[c,d] (I and IIa)
- **TCP,** if available (I)
- *Dopamine* 5-20 μg/kg per min (IIb)
- *Epinephrine* 2-10 μg/min (IIb)
- *Isoproterenol*[f]

No / **Yes**

- Observe

- Prepare for transvenous pacer
- Use **TCP** as a bridge device[g]

---

a. Serious signs or symptoms must be related to the slow rate. Clinical manifestations include
   - Symptoms (chest pain, shortness of breath, decreased level of consciousness)
   - Signs (low BP, shock, pulmonary congestion, CHF, acute MI)

b. Do not delay TCP while awaiting IV access or for *atropine* to take effect if patient is symptomatic.

c. Denervated transplanted hearts will not respond to *atropine.* Go at once to pacing, *catecholamine* infusion, or both.

d. *Atropine* should be given in repeat doses every 3-5 min up to total of 0.03-0.04 mg/kg. Use the shorter dosing interval (3 min) in severe clinical conditions. It has been suggested that *atropine* should be used with caution in atrioventricular (AV) block at the His-Purkinje level (type II AV block and new third-degree block with wide QRS complexes) (Class IIb).

e. Never treat third-degree heart block plus ventricular escape beats with *lidocaine.*

f. *Isoproterenol* should be used, if at all, with extreme caution. At low doses it is Class IIb (possibly helpful); at higher doses it is Class III (harmful).

g. Verify patient tolerance and mechanical capture. Use analgesia and sedation as needed.

FIGURE 25-11 Bradycardia algorithm (with the patient not in cardiac arrest). (From American Heart Association: Advanced Cardiac Life Support, pp. 1–29. Dallas, AHA, 1997. Copyright 1997, AHA.)

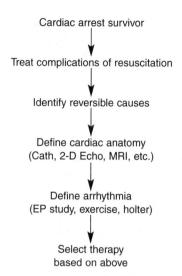

FIGURE 25-12 Management of the cardiac arrest survivor. (From Dimarco JP: Work–up and management of sudden cardiac death survivors. Cardiol Clin 11: 11–19, 1993.)

Administer corticosteroid (optional).
Control blood variables:
Hematocrit 30% to 35%, with normal electrolytes
Serum osmolality 280 to 330 mOsm/L
Glucose 100 to 300 mg/dL
Maintain normothermia.
Give intravenous fluids, avoiding dextrose-in-water
  solutions.

ONGOING MEDICAL CARE

Medical management of survivors of cardiac arrest depends on the patient's central nervous system function and known preexisting factors. Management includes diagnostic evaluation and therapy directed toward ischemia, LV dysfunction, structural abnormalities, arrhythmias, and other concurrent medical conditions. The evaluation process for the SCD survivor is summarized in Figure 25-12. In the evaluation of the SCD patient, the electrophysiology study, the degree and type of underlying structural heart disease, and

the status of the LV function are used to determine further management and therapies (Fig. 25-13).

Diagnostic Evaluation. If central nervous system functioning is limited, extensive evaluation usually is not done. If the patient sustained cardiac arrest as a result of acute MI, evaluation and treatment are no different from those in any other patient with acute MI.[92] If the arrest is attributable to proarrhythmic drug effects or electrolyte disturbances, extensive evaluation usually is not indicated. Aggressive evaluation is warranted for most patients whose cardiac arrest was precipitated by coronary atherosclerosis not associated with acute transmural MI, or with other heart disease that can be managed medically or surgically. Diagnostic tests include cardiac catheterization, radionuclide stress testing, echocardiography, electrophysiologic studies, and possibly magnetic resonance imaging if arrhythmogenic right ventricular dysplasia is suspected.[85,35]

Reduction of Ischemia. Depending on the anatomy and physiology of the disease process, either medical or surgical therapy is used. Medical therapy includes β-adrenergic blocking agents, calcium channel blocking agents, and angiotensin-converting enzyme (ACE) inhibitors, alone or in combination. One important study, the Beta-blocker Heart Attack Trial (BHAT), a randomized, double-blind, placebo-controlled study, tested whether the use of beta blockers in patients with a history of at least one MI could reduce subsequent mortality.[14,37] The study was stopped 9 months early because of significant improvement in total mortality in the beta-blocker treatment group. SCD was significantly less frequent in the beta-blocker group (3.3% vs. 4.6%). Patients with a history of congestive heart failure who were treated with beta blockers experienced a more dramatic reduction in SCD (10.4% vs. 4.4%). ACE inhibitor use also may reduce SCD, as evidenced by the Trandolapril Cardiac Evaluation Trial (TRACE).[37,71]

Myocardial revascularization has been shown to reduce the incidence of SCD in patients with heart disease, both in primary and secondary prevention of SCD.[14] Surgery is indicated for those patients with conventional criteria (i.e., uncontrolled angina or left main or multiple-vessel CHD)

FIGURE 25-13 Illustrative algorithm showing treatment strategy for cardiac arrest survivors. Patients with reversible causes of cardiac arrest should receive specific therapy to prevent recurrence. The results of the electrophysiology study divide the remainder of patients into two categories. VT, ventricular tachycardia; VF, ventricular fibrillation; LVEF, left ventricular ejection fraction; CAR, coronary artery revascularization; ICD, implantable cardioverter defibrillator; MI, myocardial infarction; LV Func, left ventricular function. (From Knilans TK, Prystowsky EN: Antiarrhythmic drug therapy in the management of cardiac arrest survivors. Circulation 85 [Suppl I]: 118–124, 1992.)

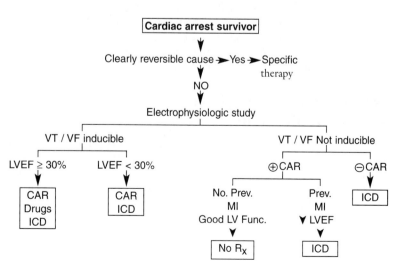

or with specific criteria for antiarrhythmic surgery (i.e., discrete ventricular aneurysms or inducible, potentially lethal, arrhythmias not controlled by medication).[89]

Antiarrhythmic Therapy. Premature ventricular contractions in the absence of structural heart disease are benign, but are a risk factor in patients after MI.[9] However, unlike beta blockers and ACE inhibitors, certain antiarrhythmics, particularly class I drugs, have been associated with increased mortality rates despite suppressing ventricular ectopy.[14] Increased mortality was seen in the CAST study with the use of encainide and flecainide in the patient post-acute MI. CAST II showed increased mortality rates in this same group with the use of moricizine.[14,37,40] In contrast, several trials have shown a beneficial effect on mortality with the use of amiodarone, a class III drug, in patients post-MI. Properties of amiodarone that may help reduce mortality after MI are coronary vasodilation and heart rate reduction, which serve to reduce ischemia.[14,37]

Implantable Cardioverter-Defibrillators. Electrophysiologic studies are used to determine inducibility or noninducibility of the potentially lethal arrhythmia. Patients whose arrhythmias continue to be inducible in spite of antiarrhythmic therapy have a higher mortality rate (43%) than those patients whose arrhythmias are no longer inducible (9%).[89] The ICD has emerged as the preferred mode of therapy for most patients who have life-threatening ventricular tachyarrhythmias.[96] Factors that favor ICD therapy include the reported success in preventing SCD, dramatic technological improvements, reduced mortality and morbidity associated with ICD implantation, and the low efficacy of many available antiarrhythmics.[11,14,37] The Multicenter Automatic Defibrillator Implantable Trial (MADIT) compared prophylactic therapy with an ICD to conventional medical therapy in patients with prior history of MI who were at high risk for ventricular arrhythmias. The patients were randomly assigned to receive an ICD or conventional medical therapy. The trial was stopped early because of a highly significant reduction in mortality in the ICD group.[86] Several other ongoing trials are addressing the potential benefits of prophylactic implantation of ICD devices in other high-risk patient populations. Treatment of life-threatening ventricular arrhythmias will most likely remain the domain of the ICD in the future. Antiarrhythmic drugs and catheter ablation will continue to complement the ICD, decreasing the frequency of ICD discharges and, it is hoped, improving quality of life.[11]

Nursing Management of Sudden Cardiac Death Survivors

Survivors of cardiac arrest and their families have physiologic, psychological, and educational needs that differ from those of the patient with acute myocardial ischemia and infarction. However, if the underlying etiology includes ischemia, management of the patient with ischemia and infarction should be included in nursing care.

PHYSIOLOGIC NURSING MANAGEMENT

After cardiac arrest, patients are admitted to the cardiac care unit. At this time, the same priorities of care exist for these patients as for patients with acute MI. Once acute ischemia and infarction have been ruled out, activity restrictions related to reduction of infarct size may be discontinued. Because of the danger of recurrent VF, the patient continues to be monitored electrocardiographically. An intravenous line is left in place for immediate venous access. Time of hospital discharge is related to the etiology of the cardiac arrest, the type of diagnostic studies required, and the eventual therapies selected by the patient and family. If the patient will be receiving an ICD, the implications of having an ICD must be discussed thoroughly. As much education and support as possible should be provided about the ICD (see Chapter 26).

EMOTIONAL SUPPORT

Emotional support given to patients and their families affects their quality of life. Fear of recurrent cardiac arrest is experienced by patients and their families. Fear is exacerbated further at the time of transfer out of the cardiac care unit to a step-down unit, and further still at the time of discharge from the hospital. Patients who experience cardiac arrest with no known (and, therefore, treatable) etiology may require more emotional support than do patients who can receive treatment to correct or modify the causative factor. Anxiety, insomnia, restlessness, irritability,[38] fear of being alone,[58] and fear of death during sexual intercourse[100] continue to persist. Anxiety, fear, memory difficulties, loss of sexual interest, trouble concentrating, and perceived lifestyle changes have also been reported.[39,50] Denial, isolation, projection, and hallucinatory or delusional behavior have been identified as coping mechanisms used by survivors.[38]

Should VF recur in the hospital, it is important to realize that some patients retain auditory function during cardiac arrest. Therefore, refrain from negative, ominous, or derogatory remarks during the arrest.[95] If the family members are present at the time of arrest, direct someone to take them to a private waiting room, stay with them, and, if requested, help them to contact a member of the clergy. After a successful resuscitation, allow family members to see the patient as soon as possible.[117] Listen to the patient's recollections of the arrest[95] and to any accounts of near-death phenomena in an objective, nonjudgmental way.[95]

PATIENT AND FAMILY EDUCATION

Next to competent resuscitative and emotional care, education of the patient and family may do the most to relieve fear of, and prevent death from, recurrent cardiac arrest. Assess readiness to learn. Teach at an appropriate level, taking into account any learning disabilities from central nervous system dysfunction that may have resulted from the arrest. Content that should be presented and understood before discharge includes normal cardiac anatomy and physiology; pathophysiology related to CHD in general and to the arrest in particular; ICD teaching for those patients who receive an ICD, including implications, follow-up care, and what to do if they receive an ICD shock; CHD risk factor modification; medications; activity prescription; importance and dates of return appointments; how to activate the emergency medical system; cough CPR; and CPR. Specific recommendations about teaching CPR to families have been made: teach only one-rescuer CPR; teach CPR in short segments, with reinforcement of each segment before progression to the next; and emphasize the need to teach neighbors and coworkers.[36,115]

All of this information is overwhelming and almost impossible to remember without teaching aids such as booklets, charts, and pictures. Family members may also feel particularly overwhelmed by the thought of recurring episodes. Support groups provide invaluable services to patients and their families. They allow the patient and family members to ask questions and discuss issues related to devices and heart disease, as well as providing the chance for them to meet and talk to others with similar circumstances.

REFERENCES

1. American College of Emergency Physicians EMS Committee: Prehospital defibrillation by basic level emergency medical technicians. Ann Emerg Med 13: 974, 1984
2. Anderson KP: Sudden death, hypertension, and hypertrophy. J Cardiovasc Pharmacol 6: S498–S503, 1984
3. Atkins JM: Emergency medical service systems in acute cardiac care: State of the art. Circulation 74(6 part 2): IV-4–IV-8, 1986
4. Bainton CR, Peterson DR: Deaths from coronary heart disease in persons fifty years of age and younger. N Engl J Med 268: 569–575, 1963
5. Baroldi G, Falzi G, Mariani F: Sudden coronary death: A postmortem study in 208 selected cases compared to 97 "control" subjects. Am Heart J 98: 20–31, 1979
6. Basic Life Support for Healthcare Providers. Dallas, American Heart Association, 1997
7. Baum R, Alvarez H, Cobb L: Survival after resuscitation from out-of-hospital ventricular fibrillation. Circulation 50: 1213–1235, 1974
8. Bayes de Luna A, Coumel P, Leclercq JF: Ambulatory sudden cardiac death: Mechanisms of production of fatal arrhythmia on the basis of data from 157 cases. Am Heart J 117: 151–159, 1989
9. Bigger JT, Fleiss JL, Kleiger R et al: The relationships among ventricular arrhythmias, left ventricular dysfunction, and mortality in the 2 years after myocardial infarction. Circulation 69: 250–258, 1984
10. Bocka JJ: External transcutaneous pacemakers. Ann Emerg Med 18: 1280–1286, 1989
11. Bocker D, Block M, Hindricks G et al: Antiarrhythmic therapy: Future trends and forecast for the 21st century. Am J Cardiol 80: 99G–104G, 1997
12. Bruce R, DeRouen T, Peterson D et al: Non-invasive predictors of sudden cardiac death in men with coronary artery disease. Am J Cardiol 39: 833–840, 1977
13. Caldwell G, Millar G, Quinn E et al: Simple mechanical methods for cardioversion: Defense of the precordial thump and cough version. BMJ 291: 627–630, 1985
14. Chang D, Goldstein S: Sudden cardiac death in ischemic heart disease. Compr Ther 23: 95–103, 1997
15. Cobb LA, Baum RS, Alvarez H et al: Resuscitation from out-of-hospital ventricular fibrillation: 4-year follow-up. Circulation 52(Suppl III): 223, 1975
16. Cobb LA, Eliastam M, Kerber RE et al: Report of the American Heart Association Task Force on the future of cardiopulmonary resuscitation: Special report. Circulation 85: 2346–2355, 1992
17. Cobb L, Hallstrom AP, Weaver WD, Copass MK, Haynes RE (eds): Clinical predictors and characteristics of the sudden cardiac death syndrome. In Proceedings USA-USSR First Joint Symposium on Sudden Death. DHEW Publication No. (NIH): pp 99–117 1977
18. Cobb LA, Hallstrom AP: Community-based cardiopulmonary resuscitation: What have we learned? Ann NY Acad Sci 382: 330–341, 1982
19. Cobb LA, Hallstrom AP, Weaver WD et al: Considerations in the long-term management of survivors of cardiac arrest. Ann NY Acad Sci 432: 247–257, 1984
20. Cobb LA, Weaver WD: Exercise: A risk for sudden death in patients with coronary heart disease. J Am Coll Cardiol 7: 215–219, 1986
21. Cobb LA, Werner JA: Predictors and prevention of sudden cardiac death. In Hurst JW (ed): The Heart, pp 538–546. New York, McGraw-Hill, 1982
22. Connell PN, Ewy GA, Dahl CF et al: Transthoracic impedance to defibrillation discharge: Effect of electrode size and electrode chest wall interface. J Electrocardiol 6: 313, 1973
23. The Coronary Drug Project Research Group: Prognostic importance of premature beats following myocardial infarction: Experience in the Coronary Drug Project. JAMA 223: 1116–1124, 1973
24. Criley JM, Blaufuss AJ, Kissel GL: Cough induced cardiac compression. JAMA 263: 1246, 1976
25. Cummins RO: From concept to standard of care? Review of the clinical experience with automated external defibrillators. Ann Emerg Med 18: 1269–1275, 1989
26. Cummins RO, Eisenberg MS, Litwin PE et al: Automatic external defibrillators used by emergency medical technicians: A controlled clinical trial. JAMA 257: 1605–1610, 1987
27. Cummins R, Graves J, Horan S. et al: Prehospital transcutaneous pacing of significant bradycardias by paramedics: Clinical and system effectiveness. Prehospital Disaster Medicine 4: 70, 1989
28. Cummins R, Graves J, Horan S et al: Prehospital use of transcutaneous pacing for asystolic cardiac arrest (Abstract). Ann Emerg Med 19: 239, 1990
29. Cummins RO, Ornato JP, Thies WH et al: Improving survival from sudden cardiac arrest: The "Chain of Survival" concept. A statement for health professionals from the Advanced Cardiac Life Support Subcommittee and the Emergency Cardiac Care Committee, American Heart Association. Circulation 83: 1832–1847, 1991
30. Cummins RO, Thies WH: Encouraging early defibrillation: The American Heart Association and automated external defibrillators. Ann Emerg Med 19: 1245–248, 1990
31. Dahl CF, Ewy GA, Ewy MD et al: Transthoracic impedance to direct current discharge: Effect of repeated countershocks. Medical Medical Instrumentation 10: 151, 1976
32. Dahl CF, Ewy GA, Warner ED et al: Myocardial necrosis from direct current countershock. Circulation 50: 956–961, 1974
33. Davies MJ: Anatomic features in victims of sudden coronary death. Circulation 85(Suppl I): I-19–I-24, 1992

34. Davies MJ, Thomas A: Thrombosis and acute coronary lesions in sudden cardiac ischemic death. N Engl J Med 310: 1137–1140, 1984

35. Deshpande S, Vora A, Axtell K et al: Sudden cardiac death. In Brown D (ed): Cardiac Intensive Care, pp 391–404. Philadelphia, WB Saunders, 1998

36. Dracup K, Breu C: Teaching and retention of cardiopulmonary resuscitation skills for families of high-risk patients with cardiac disease. Focus on Critical Care 14(1): 67–72, 1987

37. Domanski MJ, Zipes DP, Schron MS: Treatment of sudden cardiac death: Current understandings from randomized trials and future research directions. Circulation 95: 2694–2699, 1997

38. Druss RG, Kornfeld DS: The survivors of cardiac arrest. JAMA 201: 291, 1967

39. Dunnington CS, Johnson NJ, Finkelmeier BA et al: Patients with heart rhythm disturbances: Variables associated with increased psychologic distress. Heart Lung 17: 381–89, 1988

40. Echt DS, Liebson PR, Mitchell LB et al: Mortality and morbidity in patients receiving encainide, flecainide, or placebo: The Cardiac Arrhythmia Suppression Trial. N Engl J Med 324: 781–788, 1991

41. Eisenberg MS, Copass MK, Hallstrom AP et al: Treatment of out-of-hospital cardiac arrests with rapid defibrillation by emergency medical technicians. N Engl J Med 302: 1379–1383, 1980

42. Emberson JW, Nuir AR: Changes in the ultrastructure of rat myocardium induced by hypokalemia. Quarterly Journal of Experimental Physiology 54: 36–40, 1969

43. Emergency Cardiac Care Committee and Subcommittees, American Heart Association: Guidelines for cardiopulmonary resuscitation and emergency cardiac care. JAMA 268: 2172–2298, 1992

44. Emergency Cardiac Care Committee and Subcommittees, American Heart Association: Guidelines for cardiopulmonary resuscitation and emergency cardiac care: II. Adult basic life support. JAMA 268: 2184–2198, 1992

45. Emergency Cardiac Care Committee and Subcommittees, American Heart Association: Guidelines for cardiopulmonary resuscitation and emergency cardiac care: III. Adult advanced cardiac life support. JAMA 268: 2199–2241, 1992

46. Emergency Cardiac Care Committee and Subcommittees, American Heart Association: Guidelines for cardiopulmonary resuscitation and emergency cardiac care: IX. Ensuring effectiveness of communitywide emergency cardiac care. JAMA 268: 2289–2295, 1992

47. Ewy G: Electrical therapy of cardiovascular emergencies. Circulation 74(Suppl IV): IV-111, 1986

48. Ewy GA, Taren DT: Impedance of transthoracic direct current discharge: A model for testing interface material. Medical Instrumentation 12: 47, 1978

49. Ewy GA, Taren DT: Comparison of paddle electrode pastes used for defibrillation. Heart Lung 6: 847, 1977

50. Finkelmeier BA, Kenwood NJ, Summers C: Psychologic ramifications of survival from sudden cardiac death. Critical Care Quarterly 7: 71–79, 1984

51. Follansbee WP, Michelson EL, Morganroth J: Nonsustained ventricular tachycardia in ambulatory patients: Characteristics and association with sudden cardiac death. Ann Intern Med 92: 741–747, 1980

52. Freidman M, Manwaring J, Rosenmann R et al: Instantaneous and sudden deaths: Clinical and pathological differentiation in coronary artery disease. JAMA 255: 1319–1328, 1973

53. Geddes LA, Tacker WA, Cabler DP et al: The decrease in transthoracic impedance during successive ventricular defibrillation trials. Medical Instrumentation 9: 179, 1975

54. Gradman AH, Bell PA, DeBusk RF: Sudden death during ambulatory monitoring. Circulation 55: 210–211, 1977

55. Grayboys TB, Lown B, Podrid PJ et al: Long-term survival of patients with malignant ventricular arrhythmia treated with antiarrhythmic drugs. Am J Cardiol 50: 437–443, 1982

56. Greene HL: Sudden arrhythmic cardiac death: Mechanisms, resuscitation, and classification. Am J Cardiol 65: 4B–12B, 1990

57. Groh WJ, Foreman LD, Zipes DP: Advances in the treatment of arrhythmias: Implantable cardioverter-defibrillators. Am Fam Physician 57: 297–307, 1998

58. Hackett TP, Cassem NH: Psychological reactions to life-threatening illness-acute myocardial infarction. In Abram HS (ed): Psychological Aspects of Stress, pp 29–43. Springfield, IL, Charles C Thomas, 1970

59. Halperin HR, Tsitlik JE, Guerci AD et al: Determinants of blood flow to vital organs during cardiopulmonary resuscitation in dogs. Circulation 73: 539–550, 1986

60. Hammon JW, Oates JA: Interaction of platelets with the vessel wall in the pathophysiology of sudden cardiac death. Circulation 73: 224–226, 1986

61. Instructors Manual for Basic Life Support. Dallas, American Heart Association, 1985

62. Jimenez RA, Myerburg RJ: Sudden cardiac death: Magnitude of the problem, substrate/trigger interaction, and populations at high risk. Cardiol Clin 11: 1–9, 1993

63. Kannel WB, Thomas HE: Sudden coronary death: The Framingham Study. Ann NY Acad Sci 38: 3–21, 1982.

64. Kerber RE, Becker LB, Bourland JD et al: Automatic external defibrillators for public access defibrillation: Recommendations for specifying and reporting arrhythmia analysis algorithm performance, incorporating new waveforms, and enhancing safety. AHA Scientific Statement. Circulation 95: 1677–1681, 1997

65. Kerber RE, Grayzel J, Hoyt R et al: Transthoracic resistance in human defibrillation: Influence of body weight, chest size, serial shocks, paddle size, and paddle contact pressure. Circulation 63: 676, 1981

66. Kerber RE, Jensen SR, Grayzel J et al: Elective cardioversion: Influence of paddle-electrode location and size on success rates and energy requirements. N Engl J Med 305: 658–662, 1981

67. Kerber RE, Kouba C, Martins JB et al: Energy, current, and success in defibrillation and cardioversion: Clinical studies using an automated impedance-based method of energy adjustment. Circulation 77: 1038–1046, 1988

68. Kerber RE, Martins JB, Kelly KJ et al: Self-adhesive preapplied electrode pads for defibrillation and cardioversion. J Am Coll Cardiol 3: 815–820, 1984

69. Kleiger RE, Miller JP, Bigger JT et al: Decreased heart rate variability and its association with increased mortality after acute myocardial infarction. Am J Cardiol 59: 256–262, 1987

70. Kloeck W, Cummins RO, Chamberlain D et al: Early defibrillation: An advisory statement from the advanced life support working group of the international liaison committee on resuscitation. Circulation 95: 2183–2184, 1997

71. Kober L, Torp-Pederson C, Carlsen JE et al, for the Trandolapril Cardiac Evaluation (TRACE) Study Group: A clinical trial for the ACE inhibitor trandolapril in patients with left ventricular dysfunction after myocardial infarction. N Engl J Med. 333: 1670–1676, 1995

72. Kotler MN, Tabatznik B, Mower MM et al: Prognostic significance of ventricular ectopic beats with respect to sudden

death in the late postinfarction period. Circulation 47: 959–966, 1973

73. Kuller LH: Sudden death definition and epidemiologic considerations. Prog Cardiovasc Dis 23: 1–12, 1980

74. LaRovere MT, Specchia G, Mortara A et al: Baroreflex sensitivity, clinical correlates, and cardiovascular mortality among patients with a first myocardial infarction: A prospective study. Circulation 78: 816–824, 1988

75. Liberthson RR, Nagel EL, Hirschman JC et al: Pathophysiologic observations in prehospital ventricular fibrillation and sudden cardiac death. Circulation 49: 790–798, 1974

76. Lown B, Verrier RL, Rabinowitz SH: Neural psychologic mechanisms and the problem of sudden cardiac death. Am J Cardiol 39: 890–902, 1977

77. Lown R, Wolf M: Approaches to sudden death from coronary heart disease. Circulation 44: 130, 1971

78. Maier GW, Tyson GS, Olsen CO et al: The physiology of external cardiac massage: High-impulse cardiopulmonary resuscitation. Circulation 70: 86–101, 1984

79. Malliani A, Recordati G, Schwartz PJ: Nervous activity of afferent cardiac sympathetic fibers with atrial and ventricular endings. J Physiol 229: 457–469, 1973

80. Maron BJ, Epstein SE, Roberts WC: Causes of sudden death in competitive athletes. J Am Coll Cardiol 7: 204–214, 1986

81. Martin GJ, Magid NM, Myers G et al: Heart rate variability and sudden death secondary to coronary artery disease during ambulatory electrocardiographic monitoring. Am J Cardiol 60: 86–89, 1987

82. Lenachen JM, Henderson E, Morris KI et al: Ventricular arrhythmias in patients with hypertensive left ventricular hypertrophy. N Engl J Med 317: 787, 1987

83. McNally RH, Pemberton J: Duration of last attack in 998 fatal cases of coronary artery disease and its relation to possible cardiac resuscitation. BMJ 3: 129–142, 1968

84. Miller J, Tresch D, Horowitz et al: The precordial thump. Ann Emerg Med 13: 791–794, 1984

85. Moore JE, Eisenberg MS, Andresen E et al: Home placement of automatic external defibrillators among survivors of ventricular fibrillation. Ann Emerg Med 15: 811–812, 1986

86. Moss A, Hall J, Cannom D et al, for the Multicenter Automatic Defibrillator Implantation Trial: Improved survival with an implanted defibrillator in patients with coronary disease at high risk for ventricular arrhythmia. N Engl J Med 335: 1933–1940, 1996.

87. Myerburg RJ, Castellanos A: Cardiac arrest and sudden cardiac death. In Braunwald E (ed): Heart Disease: A Textbook of Cardiovascular Medicine, 5th ed, pp 742–779. Philadelphia, WB Saunders, 1997

88. Myerburg RJ, Conde CA, Sung RJ et al: Clinical, electrophysiologic, and hemodynamic profile of patients resuscitated from prehospital cardiac arrest. Am J Med 68: 568–576, 1980

89. Myerberg RJ, Kessler KM: Management of patients who survive cardiac arrest. Modern Concepts in Cardiovascular Disease 55(12): 61–66, 1986

90. Myerburg RJ, Kessler KM, Bassett AL et al: A biological approach to sudden cardiac death: Structure, function and cause. Am J Cardiol 63: 1512–1516, 1989

91. Myerburg RJ, Kessler KM, Castellanos A: Sudden cardiac death: Structure, function, and time-dependence of risk. Circulation 85(Suppl I): I-2–I-10, 1992

92. Myerberg RJ, Kessler KM, Zaman L et al: Survivors of prehospital cardiac arrest. JAMA 247: 1485–1490, 1982

93. Newman WP, Strong JP, Johnson WD et al: Community pathology of atherosclerosis and coronary heart disease in New Orleans: Morphologic findings in young black and white men. Lab Invest 44: 496–501, 1981

94. Niemann JT, Rosborough JP, Hausknecht M et al: Cough CPR: Documentation of systemic perfusion in man and in an experimental model: A "window" to the mechanism of blood flow in external CPR. Crit Care Med 8: 141–146, 1980

95. Oakes A: The Lazarus syndrome: Caring for patients who have returned from the dead. RN 41: 54, 1978

96. O'Callaghan P, Ruskin J: Current status of implantable cardioverter-defibrillators. Curr Probl Cardiol 22: 645–707, 1997

97. Otto CW: Cardiovascular pharmacology: II. The use of catecholamines, pressor agents, digitalis, and corticosteroids in CPR in emergency cardiac care. Circulation 74(6 part 2): IV-80–IV-85, 1986

98. Pennington JE, Taylor J, Lown B: Chest thump for reverting ventricular tachycardia. N Engl J Med 283: 1192–1195, 1970

99. Perper JA, Kuller LH, Cooper M: Arteriosclerosis of coronary arteries in sudden, unexpected deaths. Circulation 52(Suppl III): 27–33, 1975

100. Puksta NS: All about sex . . . after a coronary. Am J Nurs 77: 602, 1977

101. Patient Oriented Research–Fundamental and Applied, Sudden Cardiac Death. Report of the Working Group on Arteriosclerosis of the National Heart, Lung, and Blood Institute, Vol 2, pp 114–122. DHEW, NIH Publication No. 82-2035. Bethesda, MD, 1981

102. Reichenbach D, Moss N, Meyer E: Pathology of the heart in sudden cardiac death. Am J Cardiol 39: 865–872, 1977

103. Ruberman W, Weinblatt E, Goldberg JD et al: Ventricular premature beats and mortality after myocardial infarction. Circulation 64: 297–305, 1981

104. Rudikoff MT, Maughan WL, Effron M et al: Mechanisms of blood flow during cardiopulmonary resuscitation. Circulation 61: 345, 1980

105. Safar P: Cerebral resuscitation after cardiac arrest: A review. Circulation 74(6 part 2): IV-138–IV-153, 1986

106. Schaffer WA, Cobb LA: Recurrent ventricular fibrillation and modes of death in survivors of out-of-hospital ventricular fibrillation. N Engl J Med 293: 259–262, 1975

107. Schamroth L: Mechanism of lethal arrhythmias in sudden death: Possible role of vasospasm and release. Practical Cardiology 7: 105–115, 1981

108. Schulze RA, Strauss HW, Pitt B: Sudden death in the year following myocardial infarction: Relation to ventricular premature contractions in the late hospital phase and left ventricular ejection fraction. Am J Med 62: 192–199, 1977

109. Sellick BA: Cricoid pressure to control regurgitation of stomach contents during induction of anesthesia. Lancet 2: 404–406, 1961

110. Spiekerman RE, Brandenberg JT, Achor RWP et al: The spectrum of coronary heart disease in a community of 30,000: A clinic pathologic study. Circulation 25: 57–65, 1962

111. Stults KR, Brown DD: Converting asystole. Emergency Medi Ser 9: 38–39, 1984

112. Stults KR, Brown DD, Cooley F et al: Self-adhesive monitor/defibrillation pads improve prehospital defibrillation success. Ann Emerg Med 16: 872–877, 1987

113. Stults KR, Brown DD, Kerber RE: Efficacy of an automated external defibrillator in the management of out-of-hospital cardiac arrest: Validation of the diagnostic algorithm and initial clinical experience in a rural environment. Circulation 73: 701–709, 1986

114. Stults KR, Brown DD, Schug VL et al: Prehospital defibrillation performed by emergency medical technicians in rural communities. N Engl J Med 310: 219–223, 1984

115. Textbook of Advanced Cardiac Life Support. Dallas, American Heart Association, 1997

116. Thompson BM, Brooks RC, Pionkowski RS et al: Immediate countershock treatment of asystole. Ann Emerg Med 13: 827–829, 1984

117. Tuggle DJ: Meeting the emotional needs of survivors of sudden cardiac arrest. Cardiovascular Nurse 18(5): 25–30, 1982

118. Underhill SL, Woods SL, Froelicher ES et al: Cardiovascular Medications for Cardiac Nursing. Philadelphia, JB Lippincott, 1990

119. Vassalle M: On the mechanisms underlying cardiac standstill: Factors determining success or failure of escape pacemakers in the heart. J Am Coll Cardiol 5: 35B–42B, 1985

120. Warnes CA, Roberts WC: Sudden coronary death: Relation of amount and distribution of coronary narrowing at necropsy to previous symptoms of myocardial ischemia, left ventricular scarring and heart weight. Am J Cardiol: 54: 65, 1984

121. Weaver WD, Copass MK, Bufi D et al: Improved neurologic recovery and survival after early defibrillation. Circulation 69: 943–948, 1984

122. Weaver WD, Hill DL, Bolles J et al: Training families of victims at risk for cardiac arrest in the use of an automatic external defibrillator (Abstract). Circulation 72: 111–119, 1985

123. Weaver WD, Hill D, Fahrenbruch CE et al: Use of the automatic external defibrillator in the management of out-of-hospital cardiac arrest. N Engl J Med 319: 661–666, 1988

124. Weaver WD, Lorch GS, Alvarez HA et al: Angiographic findings and prognostic indicators in patients resuscitated from sudden cardiac death. Circulation 54: 895–900, 1976

125. Weisfeldt ML, Kerver RE, McGoldrick RP et al: American Heart Association Report on Public Access Defibrillation Conference, December 8–10 1994. Circulation 92: 2740–2747, 1995

126. Wit A, Bigger JT: Possible electrophysiological mechanisms for lethal arrhythmias accompanying myocardial ischemia and infarction. Circulation 52(Suppl III): 96–115, 1975

127. Yakaitis RW, Redding JS: Precordial thumping during cardiac resuscitation. Crit Care Med 1: 22–26, 1973

26

Pacemakers and Implantable Defibrillators*

CAROL JACOBSON
DONNA GERITY

PACEMAKERS

Arrhythmia device therapy has become common and very complex, requiring health care workers to have more knowledge and greater responsibilities than ever before. Early pacemakers were single-chamber devices designed to pace only in the ventricle, and the only programmable parameters were pacing rate and output. With the introduction of dual-chamber pacemakers with the capability of pacing the atria and the ventricles, the number of programmable parameters increased dramatically. Rate-responsive pacemakers came next and are capable of increasing the pacing rate in response to the body's need for increased cardiac output. Antitachycardia devices were developed to terminate both supraventricular and ventricular tachyarrhythmias using pacing techniques, cardioversion, or defibrillation. There have been tremendous advances in technology of devices for both bradycardia and antitachycardia therapy in recent years, with even more complex devices coming in the future. Given the number of companies in the arrhythmia device market and the increasing complexity of the devices themselves, it has become very difficult for nurses to stay abreast of device features and function. The goal of this chapter is to present generic concepts of pacemaker and implantable defibrillator function to provide a basic knowledge background on which cardiac nurses can build to enhance their understanding of antiarrhythmia devices.

Indications for Pacing

The purpose of a cardiac pacemaker is to provide an artificial electrical stimulus to the heart muscle when the heart rate fails to provide a cardiac output adequate to meet physiologic demands, or to stimulate the heart in an effort to

*The section on pacemakers was written by Carol Jacobson. The section on implantable defibrillators was written by Donna Gerity.

terminate tachyarrhythmias. Pacemakers were originally designed to treat disorders of impulse initiation and conduction resulting in symptomatic bradycardia. *Symptomatic bradycardia* is a term used to define a bradycardia that is directly responsible for symptoms such as syncope, near syncope, transient dizziness or light-headedness, and confusion resulting from cerebral hypoperfusion due to slow heart rate.[4,10,14] Other symptoms such as fatigue, exercise intolerance, congestive heart failure (CHF), dyspnea, and hypotension can also result from bradycardia.

In addition to treating symptomatic bradycardia, current pacemaker therapy can have beneficial effects on hemodynamics and clinical status by providing rate response for patients with *chronotropic incompetence,* meaning that the sinus node is not capable of increasing its rate appropriately in response to the body's need for increased cardiac output.[6,7,9,12,13,16] Dual-chamber pacemaker therapy is also useful in preserving stroke volume in patients with left ventricular dysfunction by ensuring atrioventricular (AV) synchrony and providing optimal AV intervals to enhance ventricular filling.[1,4,16,17] An additional benefit of atrial or dual-chamber pacing is preservation of atrial electrical stability, which reduces the incidence of atrial fibrillation.[17]

The American College of Cardiology and American Heart Association task force on pacemaker implantation has published guidelines for implantation of permanent pacemakers and antiarrhythmia devices.[10] Display 26-1 lists the class I indications for permanent pacing according to the guidelines. Refer to the guidelines for class II indications.

Temporary pacing is indicated to treat symptomatic bradycardia after acute myocardial infarction (MI) or associated with hyperkalemia, drug toxicity, bradycardia-dependent ventricular tachycardia (VT); before permanent pacemaker implantation in symptomatic patients; and sometimes in myocarditis.[3,11,14] Temporary pacing in acute MI is still controversial. Inferior MI results in intranodal block

---

DISPLAY 26-1

Class I Indications for Permanent Pacing in Adults

ACQUIRED AV BLOCK

1. Third-degree AV block at any anatomic level associated with any one of the following conditions:
   a. Bradycardia with symptoms presumed to be due to AV block.
   b. Arrhythmias and other medical conditions that require drugs that result in symptomatic bradycardia.
   c. Documented periods of asystole >3.0 seconds or any escape rate <40 bpm in awake, symptom-free patients.
   d. After catheter ablation of the AV junction.
   e. Postoperative AV block that is not expected to resolve.
   f. Neuromuscular diseases with AV block.
2. Second-degree AV block regardless of type or site of block, with associated symptomatic bradycardia.

PACING FOR CHRONIC BIFASCICULAR AND TRIFASCICULAR BLOCK

1. Intermittent third-degree AV block
2. Type II second-degree AV block

PACING FOR AV BLOCK ASSOCIATED WITH ACUTE MYOCARDIAL INFARCTION

1. Persistent second-degree AV block in the His-Purkinje system with bilateral bundle-branch block or third-degree AV block within or below the His-Purkinje system after acute myocardial infarction.
2. Transient advanced (second- or third-degree) infranodal AV block and associated bundle-branch block.
3. Persistent and symptomatic second- or third-degree AV block.

PACING IN SINUS NODE DYSFUNCTION

1. Sinus node dysfunction with documented symptomatic bradycardia, including frequent sinus pauses that produce symptoms. In some patients, bradycardia is iatrogenic and occurs as a consequence of essential long-term drug therapy of a type and dose for which there are no acceptable alternatives.
2. Symptomatic chronotropic incompetence.

PACEMAKERS THAT AUTOMATICALLY DETECT AND PACE TO TERMINATE TACHYCARDIA

1. Symptomatic recurrent supraventricular tachycardia that is reproducibly terminated by pacing after drugs and catheter ablation fail to control the arrhythmia or produce intolerable side effects.
2. Symptomatic recurrent sustained VT as part of an automatic defibrillator system.

PACING TO PREVENT TACHYCARDIA

1. Sustained, pause-dependent VT, with or without prolonged QT, in which the efficacy of pacing is thoroughly documented.

PACING IN HYPERSENSITIVE CAROTID SINUS SYNDROME AND NEURALLY MEDIATED SYNCOPE

1. Recurrent syncope caused by carotid sinus stimulation; minimal carotid sinus pressure induces ventricular asystole of >3 seconds' duration in the absence of any medication that depresses the sinus node or AV conduction.

PACING FOR HYPERTROPHIC CARDIOMYOPATHY OR DILATED CARDIOMYOPATHY

1. Class I indications for sinus node dysfunction or AV block as previously described.

AV, atrioventricular; VT, ventricular tachycardia.
From Gregoratos G, Cheitlin MD, Conill A et al: ACC/AHA guidelines for implantation of cardiac pacemakers and antiarrhythmic devices: Executive summary. Circulation 971: 1325–1335, 1998.

---

that is usually benign and temporary, and requires pacing only if it results in symptomatic bradycardia or bradycardia-dependent VT. When AV block occurs in anterior MI, it is usually infranodal, involves a large amount of myocardium, and is often symptomatic. Second- or third-degree AV block associated with anterior MI and bundle-branch block usually requires temporary pacing, but the mortality rate is high because of left ventricular dysfunction secondary to the large infarction rather than to the conduction disturbance. Prophylactic temporary pacing is often done in the presence of new right bundle-branch block with either anterior or posterior hemiblock, in left bundle-branch block with first-degree AV block, and in alternating right and left bundle-branch block.[3]

Temporary pacing is also used after cardiac surgery to treat or prevent symptomatic bradycardia and is sometimes used prophylactically in high-risk patients during cardiac catheterization or after cardioversion.[3,11,14] Overdrive atrial pacing is sometimes used in an attempt to terminate atrial flutter or fibrillation after cardiac surgery when atrial epicardial wires are in place.[8,11]

Types of Pacemakers

Refer to Displays 26-2 and 26-3 for definitions of single- and dual-chamber pacemaker terminology. The terms defined there are used throughout the pacemaker section of this chapter and are not defined in the text unless necessary.

(Text continues on page xx)

DISPLAY 26-2

Single-Chamber Pacing Terminology

Asynchronous (Fixed-Rate) Pacing The pacemaker releases a pacing stimulus at the programmed rate regardless of the heart's intrinsic activity. No sensing occurs, so the pacemaker fires in competition with the heart's natural rhythm. Examples of asynchronous modes are AOO, VOO, DOO.

Automatic Interval The period between two consecutive paced events without an intervening sensed event. Also known as the **basic interval** or **pacing interval.**

Base Rate The rate at which the pacemaker paces when no intrinsic cardiac activity is present. Also called the **minimum rate** or **lower rate.**

Bipolar Having two poles. (1) A pacing lead with two electrical poles. The negative pole is the distal tip of the lead and the positive pole is a metal ring located a few millimeters proximal to the distal tip. The stimulating pulse is delivered through the distal tip electrode. (2) A pacing system with both electrical poles in or on the heart.

Capture Ability of the pacing stimulus to depolarize the chamber being paced. Capture is recognized on the electrocardiogram whenever the pacing spike is followed immediately by the appropriate waveform: an atrial spike followed by a P wave or a ventricular spike followed by a wide QRS.

Demand Pacing The pacemaker paces only when the heart's intrinsic rate is below the pacemaker's programmed rate (only when necessary, or on demand). This mode means that the pacemaker senses intrinsic cardiac activity and inhibits its output when intrinsic activity is present.

Electrode The exposed metal tip of a pacing lead that contacts myocardium and directly transmits the pacing stimulus to cardiac tissue.

Electromagnetic Interference Electrical signals from the environment (i.e., radiofrequency waves) that can be sensed by the pacemaker and interfere with pacer function. Abbreviated **EMI.**

Escape Interval The period between a sensed cardiac event and the next pacemaker output. The escape interval is usually equal to the basic pacing rate, but it can be programmed longer in some pacemakers (hysteresis).

Fusion Beat A cardiac depolarization (either atrial or ventricular) that results from two foci both contributing to depolarization of the chamber. In pacing, a fusion beat results when an intrinsic depolarization and a pacing stimulus occur simultaneously and both contribute to depolarization (usually seen in the ventricle).

Hysteresis A programmable feature in some pacemakers that allows the escape interval to be programmed longer than the basic pacing interval (the pacing interval after a sensed beat is longer than the basic pacing interval). This allows more time for the heart's intrinsic activity to occur.

Inhibited Response A type of response to sensing that inhibits pacemaker output when an intrinsic beat is sensed. This results in demand pacing, or pacing only when the heart's intrinsic activity is slower than the basic pacing rate.

Lead The insulated wire and its electrode that transmits the pacing stimulus from the pulse generator to the heart and relays sensed intrinsic activity back to the pulse generator. A single-chamber pacemaker uses one lead and a dual-chamber pacemaker usually uses two leads, one in the atrium and one in the ventricle.

Magnet Mode The pacemaker's response when a magnet is placed over the pulse generator. A magnet inactivates the sensing circuitry and causes a pacemaker to function asynchronously at a predetermined rate and in a preset manner. The magnet mode differs among manufacturers in pacing rate and number of impulses delivered with the magnet in place. A change in magnet-induced pacing rate is often an indicator of battery depletion and warrants pulse generator replacement.

Myopotential An electrical signal generated by muscle movement. Myopotentials are sometimes sensed by the pacemaker and cause inhibition of pacemaker output.

Output The electrical stimulus delivered by the pulse generator, usually defined in terms of pulse amplitude (volts) and pulse width (milliseconds).

Oversensing Detection of inappropriate electrical signals by the pacemaker's sensing circuit, resulting in inappropriate inhibition of pacer output. Sources of oversensing can include electromagnetic interference, myopotentials, T waves, or crosstalk between atrial and ventricular channels in dual-chamber pacemakers.

Pacemaker Syndrome Adverse clinical signs and symptoms due to inadequate timing of atrial and ventricular contraction. The syndrome can be due to loss of atrioventricular (AV) synchrony in VVI pacing, inappropriate AV interval in dual-chamber pacing, or inappropriate rate modulation. Symptoms include fatigue, confusion, unpleasant pulsations in neck or chest, limited exercise capacity, congestive heart failure, hypotension, and syncope or near syncope.

Pacing Interval The time between two consecutive paced events without an intervening sensed event. Measured in milliseconds. AA interval = atrial pacing interval, VV interval = ventricular pacing interval.

Pacing Spike The small vertical "blip" recorded on the electrocardiogram with every pacemaker output pulse. The presence of a pacing spike indicates that a stimulus was released by the pacemaker.

Pseudofusion Beat An electrocardiographic phenomenon resulting from delivery of a pacemaker spike into an intrinsic event. In the ventricle, it appears as a pacing spike in an intrinsic QRS complex, but because the ventricle is already depolarized, the spike is ineffective but may distort the QRS complex on the electrocardiogram.

(continued)

DISPLAY 26-2 *(CONTINUED)*

Single-Chamber Pacing Terminology

Pulse Generator The device that contains the power source (battery) and the electronic circuits that control pacemaker function. The term *pacemaker* is commonly used for the pulse generator.

Rate Modulation The ability of a pacemaker to increase the pacing rate in response to physical activity or metabolic demand. The pacemaker uses some type of physiologic sensor to determine the need for increased pacing rate. The most commonly used sensors are motion sensors and minute ventilation sensors. Also called **rate adaptation** or **rate response.**

Refractory Period (1) In the heart, the period of time that the myocardium is incapable of responding to a stimulus. (2) In the pacemaker, an interval or timing cycle following a sensed or paced event during which the pacemaker does not respond to incoming signals. A single-chamber pacemaker has one refractory period, and a dual-chamber pacemaker has an atrial refractory and a ventricular refractory period.

Sensing The ability of the pacemaker to recognize and respond to intrinsic cardiac depolarization.

Sensing Threshold The smallest intrinsic atrial or ventricular signal (measured in millivolts) that can be consistently sensed by the pacemaker.

Stimulation Threshold The minimum amount of voltage necessary to capture the heart consistently. Also called **capture threshold** or **pacing threshold.**

Undersensing Failure of a pacemaker to sense intrinsic cardiac depolarizations. This can result in competition between the pacemaker and the intrinsic rhythm.

Unipolar Having one pole. (1) A unipolar lead has only one pole, located at the distal tip. (2) A pacing system with one pole in or on the heart and the second pole located remote from the heart to complete the circuit. Permanent unipolar systems use the back of the pulse generator as the second pole. Temporary epicardial pacing systems use a ground wire in subcutaneous tissue as the second pole.

DISPLAY 26-3

Dual-Chamber Pacemaker Terminology

Adaptive Atrioventricular (AV) Delay (or Rate-Adaptive AV Delay) See AV Interval.

Alert Period The portion of the pulse generator's timing cycle during which it can sense and respond to intrinsic cardiac activity. The alert period follows the refractory period.

Atrial Escape Interval Period from a sensed or paced ventricular event to the next paced atrial event. Also called the **V-A interval.**

Atrial Refractory Period Period of time during which the atrial channel is unable to respond to sensed signals. In dual-chamber pacemakers, the total atrial refractory period is divided into two parts: the atrioventricular interval and the postventricular atrial refractory period (PVARP).

Atrial Tracking A state of pacing in which sensed atrial activity triggers a ventricular pacing output at the end of the programmed atrioventricular delay. Also known simply as **tracking.**

Atrioventricular (AV) Interval (or AV Delay) The "electronic PR interval," or the length of time between a sensed or paced atrial event and the delivery of the ventricular pacing output. The AV interval is programmable and is measured in milliseconds (e.g., an AV interval of 120 ms = a PR interval of 0.12 second). Many pacemakers have an **adaptive AV delay,** meaning that the AV delay can be programmed to shorten when the intrinsic atrial rate increases, thus mimicking the heart's own physiologic increase in AV conduction as the heart rate increases. Many devices also have a **differential AV delay,** meaning that the AV interval can be programmed to be longer on an atrial paced beat than on an atrial sensed beat (e.g., 200 ms when the atrium is paced and 150 ms when P waves are sensed).

Blanking Period A very short ventricular refractory period that occurs simultaneously with every atrial pacing output to prevent the ventricle from sensing the atrial stimulus. It is intended to prevent inhibition of ventricular output due to crosstalk (see definition). Many pacemakers allow the blanking period to be programmed longer to prevent crosstalk.

Crosstalk The sensing of a signal in one chamber by the sensing circuit in the other chamber, usually used in reference to the sensing of the atrial output pulse by the ventricular channel. Crosstalk due to sensing of atrial signals by the ventricular channel causes inhibition of ventricular pacing output because the ventricular channel interprets the atrial output as a ventricular event.

Differential Atrioventricular (AV) Delay See AV Interval.

Endless-Loop Tachycardia See Pacemaker-Mediated Tachycardia.

Maximum Tracking Rate (MTR) The programmable upper rate limit of a dual-chamber pacemaker that determines the fastest rate at which 1 : 1 tracking of atrial sensed events occurs. The MTR prevents the ventricular channel from pacing faster than the upper rate limit when the intrinsic atrial rate exceeds the programmed MTR. When the intrinsic atrial rate is faster than the upper rate limit, the pacemaker reverts to its "upper-rate response" (see later) to prevent the ventricular rate from exceeding the MTR. Also called the **ventricular tracking limit** or **upper rate limit.**

(continued)

DISPLAY 26-3 *(CONTINUED)*

Dual-Chamber Pacemaker Terminology

Pacemaker-Mediated Tachycardia A tachycardia induced by competition between the pacemaker and the intrinsic rhythm and sustained by the continued participation of the pacemaker. Most commonly used to describe the endless-loop tachycardia that results when there is retrograde conduction from the ventricles to the atria, sensing of the retrograde P wave by the atrial channel, and pacing in the ventricle in response to the sensed P wave. This results in a reentry tachycardia in which the pacemaker serves as the antegrade limb of the circuit and the intrinsic conduction system serves as the retrograde limb. Also known as **endless-loop tachycardia** or **pacemaker reentry tachycardia.**

Pseudofusion Beat An electrocardiographic phenomenon in which an atrial pacing spike is superimposed on a native QRS complex. The atrial pacing spike cannot contribute to ventricular depolarization, but the presence of the spike can distort the native QRS complex on the electrocardiogram.

PVARP (Postventricular Atrial Refractory Period) Part of the total atrial refractory period that begins with a sensed or paced ventricular event. PVARP is a programmable parameter and is intended to prevent the atrial channel from sensing far-field ventricular signals, such as T waves or local myocardial potentials. PVARP can also be programmed to prevent the atrial channel from sensing retrograde P waves, thus preventing pacemaker-mediated tachycardia.

Rate Response Ability of the pacemaker to increase its pacing rate in response to physical activity or increased metabolic demand. Rate-responsive pacemakers have some type of sensor that detects physical activity or a physiologic parameter that indicates the need for increased heart rate. The sensors most commonly used are vibration or motion sensors and minute ventilation sensors. Other sensors being evaluated include blood temperature, blood oxygen content, QT interval, and stroke volume. Also known as **rate modulation** or **rate adaptation.**

Rate Smoothing A programmable function that prevents excessive cycle-to-cycle changes in pacing rate. Atrial tracking and rate response can occur, but no sudden acceleration or deceleration in pacing rate can occur.

Safety Pacing The delivery of a ventricular output at a short atrioventricular (AV) interval whenever a signal is sensed early in the AV delay. The purpose of safety pacing is to prevent crosstalk inhibition of ventricular output. Also called **nonphysiologic AV delay** or **ventricular safety standby.**

Total Atrial Refractory Period (TARP) Timing cycle that determines the total length of time that the atrial channel is unresponsive to signals (in effect, "has its eyes closed"). TARP is composed of two separately programmable timing cycles during which the atrial channel is refractory: the atrioventricular interval and the postventricular atrial refractory period.

Ventricular Refractory Period The amount of time after a ventricular sensed or paced event during which the ventricular channel cannot respond to signals (in effect, "has its eyes closed"). The purpose is to prevent the ventricular channel from seeing large repolarization signals (T waves) or other local myocardial signals.

PERMANENT PACEMAKERS

Permanent pacemakers are usually implanted under local anesthesia either in the operating room or the cardiac catheterization laboratory. The pulse generator is placed in a subcutaneous pocket in the pectoral area and the pacing lead is inserted either through the cephalic vein or the subclavian vein into the right ventricular apex (Fig. 26-1). If a dual-chamber pacemaker is implanted, a second lead is placed in the right atrial appendage. Permanent pulse generators are powered by lithium batteries with a life span of approximately 10 years depending on many factors, including how the pacemaker is programmed and the percentage of time that it paces.[7,9]

TEMPORARY PACEMAKERS

Temporary pacing can be accomplished with transvenous, epicardial, or transcutaneous methods. Temporary pacing can be done in both emergency and elective situations, and is usually done in a monitored unit such as critical care or telemetry unit. Transcutaneous pacing can also be done by paramedics or other trained personnel in emergency response vehicles or in the field.

Transvenous Pacing. Transvenous pacing is usually done by percutaneous puncture of the internal jugular, subclavian, antecubital, or femoral vein and threading a pacing wire into the apex of the right ventricle for ventricular pacing, the right atrium for atrial pacing, or both chambers for dual-chamber

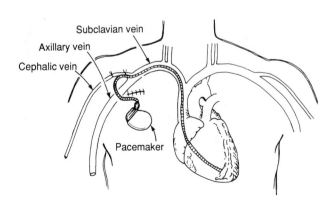

FIGURE 26-1 Transvenous installation of a permanent pacemaker. For dual-chamber pacing, a separate pacing wire would be in the antrum.

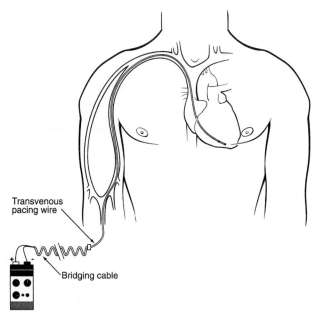

FIGURE 26-2 Temporary transvenous pacing wire in right ventricle inserted through antecubital vein.

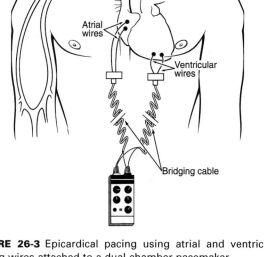

FIGURE 26-3 Epicardical pacing using atrial and ventricular pacing wires attached to a dual-chamber pacemaker.

pacing (Fig. 26-2). The transvenous pacing wire is attached to an external pulse generator that is kept either on the patient or at the bedside. The procedure can be done under fluoroscopy in a cardiac catheterization laboratory or without fluoroscopy at the bedside. Transvenous pacing is usually necessary only for a few days until the rhythm returns to normal or a permanent pacemaker is inserted. Instructions for initiating transvenous pacing are covered later in this chapter.

Epicardial Pacing. Epicardial pacing is done through electrodes placed on the atria or ventricles during cardiac surgery. The pacing electrode end of the wire is looped through or loosely sutured to the epicardial surface of the atria or ventricles and the other end is pulled through the chest wall, sutured to the skin, and attached to an external pulse

generator. A ground wire is often placed subcutaneously in the chest wall and pulled through with the other wires. The number and placement of wires varies with the surgeon; there may be one or two atrial wires, one or two ventricular wires, and one, two, or no ground wires (Fig. 26-3). Instructions for initiating epicardial pacing are covered later in this chapter.

Transcutaneous Pacing. Transcutaneous pacing is a noninvasive method of pacing used as a temporary measure in emergency situations for treatment of asystole, severe bradycardia, or overdrive pacing for tachyarrhythmias until a transvenous pacing wire can be inserted. Large-surface adhesive electrodes are attached to the anterior and posterior chest wall and connected to an external pacing unit (Fig. 26-4). The pacing current passes through skin and

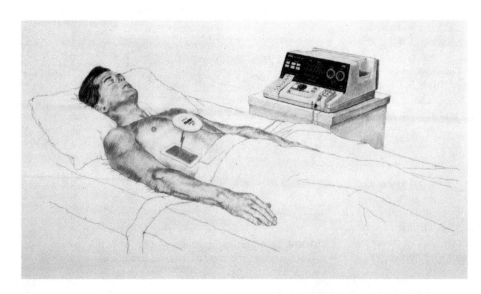

FIGURE 26-4 Transcutaneous pacing. Electrodes are placed on anterior and posterior chest wall and attached to the external pacing unit.

TABLE 26-1	**Five Letter Pacemaker Code**			
First Letter: **Chamber Paced**	**Second Letter:** **Chamber Sensed**	**Third Letter:** **Response to Sensing**	**Fourth Letter:** **Programmability,** **Rate Modulation**	**Fifth Letter:** **Antitachycardia** **Pacing Functions**
O = None	O = None	O = None	O = None	O = None
A = Atrium	A = Atrium	I = Inhibited	P = Simple programmable	P = Pacing (antitachycardia)
V = Ventricle	V = Ventricle	T = Triggered	M = Multiprogrammable	S = Shock
D = Dual (A and V)	D = Dual (A and V)	D = Dual (I and T)	C = Communicating	D = Dual (P and S)
			R = Rate modulation	

chest wall structures to reach the heart; therefore, large energies are required to achieve capture and sedation is usually needed to minimize the discomfort felt during pacing.

SINGLE-CHAMBER PACING

Single-chamber pacing means that only the atria or the ventricles, but not both, are paced. This requires only one pacing wire inserted into the desired chamber. Single-chamber ventricular pacing is the most frequently used temporary transvenous type of pacing and is also often used for permanent pacing. Single-chamber atrial or ventricular pacing can be done using epicardial pacing wires.

DUAL-CHAMBER PACING

Dual-chamber pacing means that both the atria and the ventricles can be paced. Dual-chamber pacing is a frequently used method of permanent pacing and can also be used with epicardial pacing wires. Temporary transvenous dual-chamber pacing can be done, but it is difficult to place temporary atrial wires and it is not as reliable as ventricular pacing.

RATE-ADAPTIVE PACING

Rate-adaptive pacing is used when the heart is unable to increase its rate appropriately when the body's need for cardiac output increases (chronotropic incompetence).[6,7,9,13] The pacing system contains a physiologic sensor that tells the pacemaker to pace faster in response to the sensed parameter. The most frequently used sensors at this time are motion sensors and minute ventilation sensors. Motion sensors are activated by body movement, such as occurs with exercise, and signal the pacemaker to pace faster. Minute ventilation sensors measure transthoracic impedance and increase the pacing rate when the respiratory rate is increased in response to exercise. Other technologies being investigated include sensors for metabolic parameters like blood temperature and venous oxygen saturation, and sensors of cardiac indices like QT interval, ventricular depolarization gradient, pre-ejection interval, stroke volume, and rate of myocardial wall tension development.[6,9,13] It is likely that future pacemakers will combine two or more sensors to get the most physiologic response to the body's needs for increased cardiac output.

ATRIAL OVERDRIVE PACING

Atrial pacing at rapid rates of 200 to 500 impulses/min is used in an attempt to terminate atrial tachyarrhythmias such as atrial tachycardia, atrial flutter, and atrial fibrillation. This type of pacing is most frequently done using a temporary pulse generator and pacing through epicardial wires in cardiac surgery patients. It can also be done with a transvenous atrial wire, but this is less effective. A special atrial asynchronous pacemaker is available for this purpose, and the newer dual-chamber temporary pulse generators also have overdrive pacing capability.

ANTITACHYCARDIA PACING

Antitachycardia pacing involves the delivery of one to several paced impulses to the atria or the ventricles in an attempt to terminate tachycardias.[8,9] This type of pacing is most often done in the ventricle to terminate VT, and most antitachycardia pacing is incorporated into implantable defibrillator devices, which are covered later in this chapter.

Classification of Pacemakers

Pacemakers are classified with a generic five-letter code that is universally used to describe the expected function of the device according to the site of the pacing electrodes and the mode of pacing. The first letter describes the chamber that is paced: A = atrium, V = ventricle, D = dual (both atrium and ventricle), O = none. The second letter describes the chamber where intrinsic electrical activity is sensed: A = atrium, V = ventricle, D = dual (both atrium and ventricle), O = none. The third letter describes the pacemaker's response to sensing of intrinsic electrical activity: I = inhibited, T = triggered, D = dual (inhibits or triggers), O = none. The fourth and fifth letters describe additional functions but are not usually used, except for the letter R in the fourth position, which indicates that the pacemaker is a rate-adaptive device. Table 26-1 illustrates the pacemaker code in detail.

The most commonly used pacing modes are VVI and DDD. The VVI mode means that the electrode is in the ventricle and paces the ventricle (first V), senses ventricular activity (second V), and inhibits its output when it senses intrinsic ventricular depolarization (I in third position). VVI is the most commonly used mode of pacing with temporary transvenous wires because it is the quickest and easiest method of pacing in an emergency, and it is difficult to get a temporary atrial wire to stay in place. VVI is also often used with epicardial wires after cardiac surgery, especially if third-degree AV block is present, and is the mode that has to be used for permanent pacing in patients with chronic

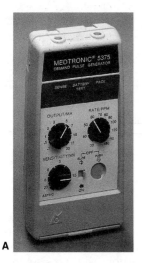
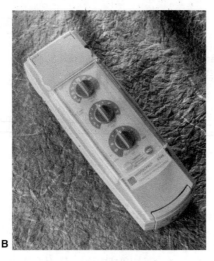
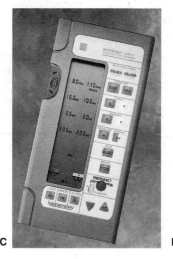
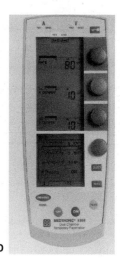

FIGURE 26-5 Examples of temporary pulse generators. **(A, B)** Single-chamber pulse generators. **(C, D)** Dual-chamber pulse generators.

atrial fibrillation. The DDD mode means that both atrial and ventricular electrodes are present and both chambers are paced (first D), both chambers are sensed (second D), and the device either inhibits or triggers an output in response to sensed intrinsic activity (D in third position means dual response to sensing). DDD is the most frequently used permanent pacing mode, unless the patient has chronic atrial fibrillation or flutter.

Other pacing modes that are sometimes used are AOO, AAI, DVI, DDI, and VDD.

Basics of Pacemaker Operation

Electrical current flows in a closed-loop circuit between two pieces of metal (poles). For current to flow, there must be conductive material (i.e., a wire, muscle, or conductive solution) between the two poles. In the heart, the pacing wire, cardiac muscle, and body tissues serve as conducting material for the flow of electrical current in the pacing system. The pacing circuit consists of the pacemaker (the power source), the conducting wire (pacing lead), and the myocardium. The electrical stimulus travels from the pulse generator through the pacing lead to the myocardium, through the myocardium, and back to the pulse generator, thus completing the circuit.

COMPONENTS OF A PACING SYSTEM

The three basic components of a cardiac pacing system are the pulse generator, the pacing lead, and the myocardium. The *pulse generator* contains the power source (battery) and all of the electronic circuitry that controls pacemaker function. Most pacemakers are powered by a lithium battery. The pulse generator of a permanent pacemaker is small and thin and is implanted in the pectoral area or sometimes in the abdominal area (see Fig. 26-1). Once a permanent pulse generator is implanted, the only way to alter its pacing parameters is with a programmer that communicates with the pacemaker through a wand placed over the pulse generator. A temporary pulse generator is a box that is kept at the

bedside of the patient and is usually powered by a regular 9-volt battery. It has controls on the front that allow the operator to set certain pacing parameters easily (Fig. 26-5).

The *pacing lead* is an insulated wire used to transmit the electrical current from the pulse generator to the myocardium. A unipolar lead contains a single wire and a bipolar lead contains two wires that are insulated from each other. In a unipolar lead, the electrode is an exposed metal tip at the end of the wire that contacts the myocardium and serves as the negative pole of the pacing circuit. In a bipolar lead, the end of the wire is a metal tip that contacts myocardium and serves as the negative pole, and the positive pole is an exposed metal ring located a few millimeters proximal to the distal tip. Permanent pacing leads can be unipolar or bipolar, but bipolar is more commonly used. Permanent leads have some type of fixation device on the end of the lead that helps keep the tip in contact with myocardium. Passive-fixation leads usually have tines on the end that get caught in the trabeculae of the right ventricle and keep the lead in position. Active-fixation leads have a screw on the end that is screwed into the ventricular muscle to hold the lead in place (Fig. 26-6). Occasionally, epicardial leads with a screw-type fixation are used in permanent pacing, especially in children and with implantable defibrillators. Temporary transvenous pacing leads are insulated wires (usually bipolar) with a no-fixation device, making them more prone to dislodgment. Temporary epicardial pacing leads are unipolar wires with one end looped through the myocardium and the wires then pulled through the chest wall for easy access.

A *bridging cable* is usually used to connect a temporary pacemaker pulse generator to the pacemaker lead, similar to an extension cord. This enhances patient comfort by allowing the pulse generator to be kept at the bedside rather than being strapped to the patient.

BIPOLAR PACEMAKER OPERATION

In any pacing system, there are two metal poles that make up the pacing circuit. The term *bipolar* means that both of

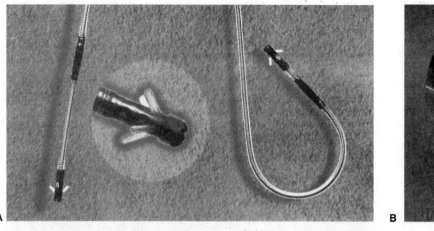

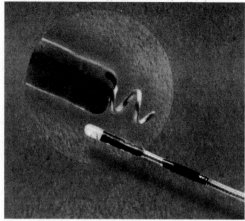

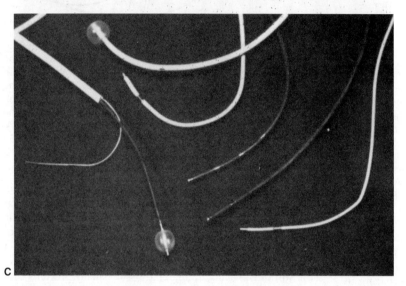

FIGURE 26-6 Pacing leads. **(A)** Passive fixation leads with silicone or polyurethane tines that help hold the lead in place. **(B)** Active fixation lead with screw tip to secure lead to myocardium. **(C)** Temporary transvenous pacing leads. Atrial leads are J-shaped. Some leads have a balloon tip for flotation. (A and B are from Sultzer Intermedics, Angleton, TX, Concepts of Cardiac Pacing, p. 7, 1998. C is from Furman S, Hayes DL, Holmes DR: A Practice of Cardiac Pacing, Armonk, NY, Futura Publishing Co, p. 138, 1986.)

these poles are in or on the heart. In a bipolar system, the pulse generator initiates the electrical impulse and delivers it out the negative terminal of the pacemaker to the pacing lead. The impulse travels down the lead to the distal electrode (negative pole) that is in contact with myocardium. As the impulse reaches the tip, it travels through the myocardium and returns to the positive pole of the system, completing the circuit. In a bipolar system, the positive pole is the proximal ring located a few millimeters proximal to the distal tip. As illustrated in Figure 26-7, the circuit over which the electrical impulse travels in a bipolar system is small because the two poles are located close together. This results in a small pacing spike on the electrocardiogram (ECG) as the pacing stimulus travels between the two poles. If the stimulus is strong enough to depolarize the myocardium, the pacing spike is immediately followed by a P wave if the wire is in the atrium, or a wide QRS complex if the wire is in the ventricle.

UNIPOLAR PACEMAKER OPERATION

A unipolar system has only one of the two poles in or on the heart. In a permanent unipolar pacing system, the back of the pulse generator serves as the second pole. In a temporary epicardial pacing system, a ground wire placed in the subcutaneous tissue in the mediastinum serves as the second pole. Unipolar pacemakers work the same way as bipolar systems, but the circuit over which the impulse travels is much larger because of the distance between the two poles (Fig. 26-8). This results in a large pacing spike on the ECG as the impulse travels between the two poles.

ASYNCHRONOUS (FIXED-RATE) PACING MODE

A pacemaker programmed to an asynchronous mode paces at the programmed rate regardless of intrinsic cardiac activity. This can result in competition between the pacemaker

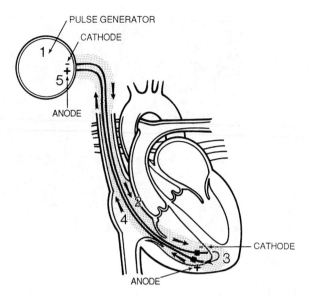

FIGURE 26-7 Bipolar pacing system. (1) The pulse generator delivers an electrical stimulus at a predetermined rate. (2) The stimulus travels down the negative electrode wire. (For learning purposes, the positive and negative wires are exposed; normally, they are insulated from each other and encased in a single catheter.) (3) The electrical stimulus is delivered to the myocardium. (The catheter is positioned at the apex of the right ventricle.) (4) Current spreads through cardiac muscle and then to the positive electrode wire. (5) Current returns to the pulse generator, completing the circuit. (From Purcell JA, Burrows SG: A pacemaker primer. Am J Nurs 85: 553–568, 1985.)

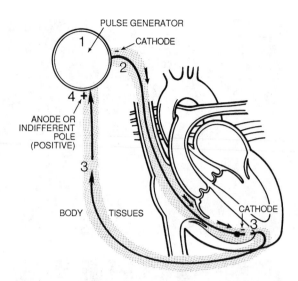

FIGURE 26-8 Unipolar pacing system. (1) The pulse generator delivers an electrical impulse. (2) The stimulus travels from the negative terminal to the electrode at the tip of the catheter. (3) Current exits through the electrode tip, stimulates the myocardium, and completes the circuit by traveling through body tissues to the positive terminal. (4) A metal plate on the pulse generator serves as the positive terminal (From Purcell JA, Burrows SG: A pacemaker primer. Am J Nurs 85: 553–568, 1985.)

and the heart's own electrical activity. Asynchronous pacing in the ventricle is unsafe because of the potential for pacing stimuli to fall in the vulnerable period of repolarization and cause ventricular fibrillation (VF). Asynchronous pacing in the atria is less dangerous but can cause atrial fibrillation.

DEMAND MODE

The term *demand* means that the pacemaker paces only when the heart fails to depolarize on its own, that is, the pacemaker fires only "on demand." In the demand mode, the pacemaker's sensing circuit is capable of sensing intrinsic cardiac activity and inhibiting pacer output when intrinsic activity is present. Sensing takes place between the two poles of the pacemaker. A bipolar system senses over a small area because the poles are close together, and this can result in "undersensing" of intrinsic signals. A unipolar system senses over a large area because the poles are far apart, and this can result in "oversensing." A unipolar system is more likely to sense myopotentials caused by muscle movement and inappropriately inhibit pacemaker output, potentially resulting in periods of asystole. The demand mode should always be used for ventricular pacing to avoid the possibility of VF.

CAPTURE

Capture means that a pacing stimulus results in depolarization of the chamber being paced. Capture is determined

by the strength of the stimulus, which is measured in milliamperes (mA), the amount of time the stimulus is applied to the heart (pulse width), and by contact of the pacing electrode with the myocardium. Capture cannot occur unless the distal tip of the pacing lead is in contact with healthy myocardium that is capable of responding to the stimulus. Pacing in infarcted tissue usually prevents capture. Similarly, if the catheter is floating in the cavity of the ventricle and not in direct contact with myocardium, capture will not occur.

In permanent pacing systems, stimulus strength is programmed at implant and can be changed as necessary by using a pacemaker programmer. In temporary pacing, the output dial on the face of the pulse generator controls stimulus strength, and can be set and changed easily by the operator. Temporary pulse generators usually are capable of delivering a stimulus of from 0.1 to 20 mA.

SENSING

The sensing circuit controls how sensitive the pacemaker is to intrinsic cardiac depolarizations. Intrinsic activity is measured in millivolts (mV), and the higher the number, the larger the intrinsic signal. For example, a 10-mV QRS complex is larger than a 2-mV QRS. When pacemaker sensitivity needs to be increased to make the pacemaker "see" smaller signals, the sensitivity number must be decreased. For example, a sensitivity of 2 mV is more sensitive than one of 5 mV.

A fence analogy may help explain sensitivity. Think of sensitivity as a fence standing between the pacemaker and what it wants to see—the ventricle, for example. If there is

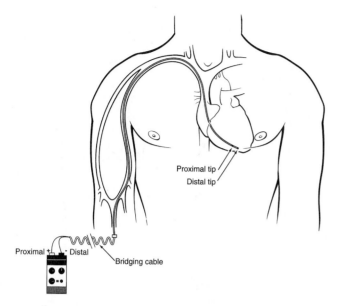

Proximal tip

Distal tip

Proximal + – Distal

Bridging cable

FIGURE 26-9 Initiating temporary transvenous pacing. The distal tail of the pacing wire is connected to the negative terminal of the pacemaker, and the proximal tail of the pacing wire is connected to the positive terminal of the pacemaker.

a 10-foot-high fence (or a 10-mV sensitivity) between the two, the pacemaker may not see what the ventricle is doing. To make the pacemaker able to see, the fence needs to be lowered. Lowering the fence to 2 feet would probably enable the pacemaker to see the ventricle. Changing the sensitivity from 10 to 2 mV is like lowering the fence—the pacemaker becomes more sensitive and is able to "see" intrinsic activity more easily. Thus, to increase the sensitivity of a pacemaker, the millivolt number (fence) must be decreased.

Initiating Temporary Pacing

TRANSVENOUS VENTRICULAR PACING

A transvenous pacing wire is inserted through a peripheral vein, either antecubital or femoral, or through the internal jugular or subclavian vein, and threaded into the apex of the right ventricle. The wire is sutured in place at its insertion site and a dressing is applied. Temporary transvenous pacing wires are bipolar and have two tails, one marked "positive" or "proximal" and the other marked "negative" or "distal," that are connected to the pulse generator. To initiate ventricular pacing using a transvenous wire (Fig. 26-9):

1. Connect the negative terminal of the pulse generator to the distal end of the pacing wire.
2. Connect the positive terminal of the pulse generator to the proximal end of the pacing wire.
3. Set the rate at 70 to 80 beats/min or as ordered by physician.
4. Set the output at 5 mA and adjust according to stimulation threshold.

5. Set the sensitivity at 2 mV and adjust according to sensitivity threshold.

See the section on Nursing Considerations for the procedure for performing stimulation and sensitivity threshold tests.

EPICARDIAL PACING

The number and location of epicardial wires placed in surgery determines connections for epicardial pacing. There may be one or two atrial or ventricular wires with a ground or no ground wire. If only one wire is on a chamber, unipolar pacing is done. If there are two wires on a chamber, bipolar pacing can be done.

To initiate unipolar atrial or ventricular pacing (Fig. 26-10*A*):

1. Connect the negative terminal of the pulse generator to the wire on the chamber to be paced (atrial wire for atrial pacing, ventricular wire for ventricular pacing).
2. Connect the positive terminal of the pulse generator to the ground wire.
3. Set the rate at 70 to 80 beats/min or as ordered by physician.
4. Set the output at 10 mA for atrial pacing and 5 mA for ventricular pacing, then determine stimulation threshold and set two to three times higher.
5. Set the sensitivity at the lowest possible number for atrial pacing and at 2 mV for ventricular pacing.

To initiate bipolar atrial or ventricular pacing (see Fig. 26-10*B*):

1. Connect the negative terminal of the pulse generator to one of the wires on the chamber to be paced (atrial wire for atrial pacing, ventricular wire for ventricular pacing)
2. Connect the positive terminal of the pulse generator to the other wire on the chamber to be paced.
3. Set the rate at 70 to 80 beats/min or as ordered.
4. Set the output at 10 mA for atrial pacing and 5 mA for ventricular pacing, then determine stimulation threshold and set two to three times higher.
5. Set the sensitivity at the lowest possible number for atrial pacing and at 2 mV for ventricular pacing.

DUAL-CHAMBER TEMPORARY PACING

Dual-chamber pacing can be done through epicardial pacing wires or with transvenous atrial and ventricular wires. Transvenous dual-chamber pacing is not often done because of difficulties in placing temporary atrial wires and the unreliable stability of atrial wires. Epicardial dual-chamber pacing is often done after cardiac surgery, but should be done only when there are two ventricular wires in place. Two ventricular wires allow for bipolar ventricular pacing and sensing, thus reducing the possibility that the ventricular wire will sense atrial output and inappropriately inhibit ventricular pacing (crosstalk).

Dual-chamber pacing modes available depend on the type of pulse generator used for pacing. Older dual-

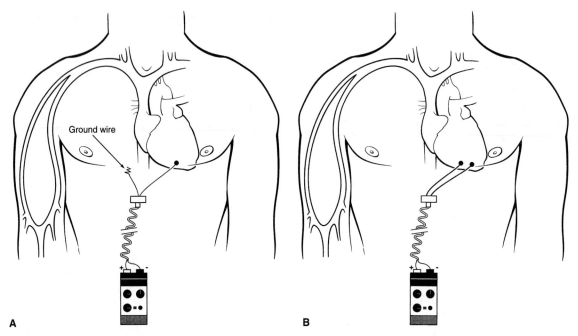

FIGURE 26-10 Initiating epicardial pacing. **(A)** Unipolar epicardial pacing. The ventricular wire (or atrial wire for atrial pacing) is connected to the negative terminal of the pacemaker and the ground wire is connected to the positive terminal. **(B)** Biopolar epicardial pacing. One ventricular wire is connected to the positive terminal and one to the negative terminal of the pacemaker. (For atrial pacing, either atrial wire is connected to the positive terminal and the other atrial wire to the negative terminal of the pacemaker.)

chamber temporary pulse generators (like that shown in Fig. 26-5*B*) allow only DVI pacing. The newer dual-chamber units allow for DDD, DVI, and VDD pacing in addition to the single-chamber options AAI, AOO, and VVI.

To initiate dual-chamber pacing with epicardial wires:

1. Connect atrial wires:
   a. If two atrial wires are present, connect one to the positive atrial terminal and the other to the negative atrial terminal on the pulse generator.
   b. If only one atrial wire is present, connect it to the negative atrial terminal on the pulse generator.
2. Connect ventricular wires.
3. Connect one wire to the negative ventricular terminal and the other to the positive ventricular terminal on the pulse generator.
4. Select dual-chamber pacing mode desired (if option is provided): DDD, DVI, VDD. The DDD mode is almost always used.
5. Set AV delay at 150 milliseconds or as ordered.
6. Set atrial output at 10 mA and ventricular output at 5 mA, then determine stimulation thresholds for both chambers and set output two to three times higher than threshold.
7. Set atrial or ventricular sensitivity as necessary, depending on pacing mode selected. (Atrial sensing occurs only in DDD or VDD dual-chamber modes.)

a. Set atrial sensitivity as 0.5 mV.
b. Set ventricular sensitivity at 2 mV.

Nursing Considerations

Nursing care of patients with pacemakers requires an understanding of how pacemakers work and what to expect the pacemaker to do depending on how it is programmed. Nurses must be able to evaluate appropriate pacemaker function by looking at the ECG or rhythm strips. Evaluating pacemaker function is covered in the next section of this chapter.

PERMANENT PACEMAKERS

Implantation of a permanent pacemaker is often done on an outpatient basis, but many patients are kept overnight for observation. The procedure is done under local anesthesia in the cardiac catheterization laboratory or the operating room, and may take only 1 or 2 hours to complete. In addition to routine postoperative care given to any surgical patient, permanent pacemaker insertion usually requires that the patient immobilize the operative arm in a sling for the first 24 hours to prevent lead dislodgment. The nurse must be aware of the potential complications of pacemaker insertion, including the potential for cardiac perforation leading to tamponade, and monitor for those complications. Patient teaching includes information about pacemaker function, how to count the pulse, and importance of follow-up visits to the physician. Because patients are discharged so soon after the procedure, they should be told to take their temperature and monitor the insertion site for signs of infection.

Occasionally the nurse is asked to place a pacemaker magnet over the permanent pulse generator. Use of a magnet usually requires a physician's order or is covered by a written protocol detailing conditions under which a magnet can be used without a direct order.

A magnet inactivates the sensing circuit of a permanent pacemaker and causes it to revert to the fixed-rate mode of pacing. This may be done to verify a pacemaker's ability to pace when it is being inhibited by a patient's own natural rhythm. With a magnet in place, the pacemaker paces at the automatic rate in competition with the patient's rhythm, thus verifying the pacemaker's ability to deliver pacing stimuli. When a paced impulse happens to fall at a time when the ventricle is able to respond, capture should occur, verifying the pacemaker's ability to capture. A magnet may also be used to evaluate battery status if a pacemaker is nearing its end of service. Often the primary indicator of battery depletion is a change in the magnet-induced pacing rate. Another indication for magnet use is to terminate a pacemaker-mediated tachycardia (PMT) in a dual-chamber pacemaker (see section on Dual-Chamber Pacing). When using the magnet, the nurse should have the patient on a cardiac monitor and must be aware of the potential danger of a pacing spike falling in the vulnerable period and causing ventricular arrhythmias.

TEMPORARY PACEMAKERS

In the care of patients with temporary pacemakers, the following additional considerations become important.

Insertion Site Care. A temporary pacing catheter is usually inserted through a venous sheath that is sutured to the skin and treated as any central venous catheter. Maintaining a clean insertion site is important to prevent infection, and hospital policies governing the care of central venous catheters and dressings should be followed.

Care of Epicardial Wires. Epicardial wires exit through the chest and unless they are being used for pacing, they are usually coiled and placed in a gauze dressing until needed. The exit site should be cleaned with a liquid iodine preparation daily and covered with a dressing. Wires are easily dislodged, so care must be taken when handling them not to pull them out. Because the exposed metal end of the wires is a direct route for electrical current from the environment to conduct directly to the heart, care must be taken to insulate the wires to prevent cardiac arrhythmias, especially VF (see the section on Electrical Safety, next, for more information).

Electrical Safety. A temporary pacing wire provides a direct pathway for stray electrical current to reach the heart without the protective resistance of the skin. Even a very small electrical current can initiate atrial fibrillation or VF if it is conducted directly to the heart by pacing wires.

Some considerations for electrical safety when caring for patients with temporary pacing wires include:

1. Wear gloves when handling pacing wires.
2. Make sure that all connections between the pulse generator and bridging cable and between bridging cable and pacing wires are tight and inserted completely into their receptacles so no metal is exposed.
3. If using a bridging cable with an alligator clip connector, wrap a glove around the connections in such a way that they are separated and insulated from each other and from the environment.
4. Cover exposed metal ends of pacing wires that are not in use with some type of insulating material.
   a. Wrap a glove around the ends of transvenous wires and tape loosely.
   b. Place the ends of epicardial wires in a glove (or cut a finger from a glove and place them inside) or place the metal end of each individual wire in a needle cover, small syringe, or some other insulating material.
5. Keep dressings over pacing wire insertion sites dry. Wet dressings conduct electricity more easily.
6. Make sure all electrical equipment in the room is grounded and in good working order.
7. Be aware of your own body's static electricity, especially if your unit is carpeted.
   a. Never let the pacing system be the first thing you touch when entering a patient's room
   b. Be especially careful when using slider boards to transfer patients into and out of bed because they generate static electricity.

Stimulation Threshold Test. The stimulation threshold is the minimum pacemaker output necessary to capture the heart consistently. The contact of the pacing lead with the myocardium causes local tissue edema and inflammation that impedes the delivery of current to the myocardium. Peak thresholds occur approximately 3 to 4 weeks after permanent lead placement, and chronic stable thresholds are usually reached at approximately 3 months.[6,9] Stimulation threshold testing with a temporary pacing system should be done every shift to ensure an adequate safety margin for capture. The procedure for performing a stimulation threshold test is as follows:

1. Verify that the patient is in a paced rhythm. Pacing rate may need to be temporarily increased to override an intrinsic rhythm.
2. Watch the cardiac monitor continuously while gradually decreasing output.
3. Note when loss of capture occurs (pacing spike not followed by appropriate waveform; P wave for atrial pacing, QRS for ventricular pacing).
4. Gradually turn output up until 1 : 1 capture resumes—this is the stimulation threshold.
5. Set the output two to three times higher than threshold to ensure adequate safety margin. For example, if consistent capture is regained at 2 mA, set the output at 4 to 6 mA.

Sensitivity Threshold Testing. The sensitivity threshold is the minimum voltage of intrinsic cardiac activity that can be sensed by the pacemaker. The pacemaker becomes more sensitive (can sense smaller signals) as the number on the sensitivity control gets smaller (see section on Sensing, earlier, for further explanation).

Sensitivity testing can be done only if the patient has a hemodynamically stable underlying rhythm. If the patient is completely pacemaker dependent or has a very slow underlying rate, do not perform sensitivity threshold testing. The procedure for performing a sensitivity threshold test is as follows:

1. Verify that the patient has an intrinsic rhythm (is not being paced). This may require temporarily decreasing the pacing rate to allow the underlying rhythm to emerge.
2. Slowly decrease the pacemaker's sensitivity (by *increasing* the number on the sensitivity control) while watching the sense indicator light on the pulse generator or watching the cardiac monitor.
   a. The sense indicator light flashes with each sensed P wave (for atrial pacing) or QRS (for ventricular pacing).
   b. Pacing remains inhibited and there are no pacing spikes seen on the monitor as long as sensing continues.
3. Note when the sense indicator fails to flash with each P wave or QRS and when pacing spikes begin to appear in competition with the intrinsic rhythm. This is the sensitivity threshold.
4. Set the sensitivity at one-half the identified threshold to ensure an adequate safety margin. For example, it the threshold is 5 mV, set the sensitivity at 2.5 mV.

Evaluating Pacemaker Function

This section is directed primarily at temporary pacemakers because nurses can interact more directly with them than with permanent pacemakers. The same concepts apply to permanent pacemakers, but corrective measures require the use of a pacemaker programmer or an actual surgical procedure to reposition pacing leads or replace the pulse generator.

Evaluation of pacemaker function requires knowledge of the mode of pacing expected (e.g., VVI, AAI, DDD); the minimum rate of the pacemaker, or pacing interval; and any other programmed parameters in the pacemaker. The basic functions of a pacemaker include stimulus release, capture, and sensing, and should be evaluated for both temporary and permanent pacemakers. *Stimulus release* refers to pacemaker output, or the ability of the pacemaker to generate and release a pacing impulse. *Capture* is the ability of the pacing stimulus to cause depolarization of the chamber being paced. *Sensing* is the ability of the pacemaker to recognize and respond to intrinsic electrical activity in the heart. Pacemaker operation is evaluated by assessing these three functions. Single-chamber pacemaker evaluation is much less complicated than dual-chamber evaluation. Because ventricular pacing is the most common type of single-chamber pacing, evaluation of VVI pacemakers is discussed here. The concepts presented for ventricular pacemaker evaluation can also be applied to atrial pacemaker evaluation.

A VVI pacemaker is expected to pace the ventricle at the set rate unless spontaneous ventricular activity occurs to inhibit pacing. The minimum rate of the pacemaker, or pacing interval, is measured from one pacing stimulus to the next consecutive pacing stimulus with no intervening sensed beats between the two. In a normally functioning VVI pacemaker, pacing spikes occur at the preset pacing interval and each spike results in a ventricular depolarization (capture). If spontaneous ventricular activity occurs (either a normally conducted QRS or a premature ventricular contraction [PVC]), that activity is sensed, the next pacing stimulus is inhibited, and the pacing interval timing cycle is reset. If no intrinsic ventricular activity occurs, a pacing stimulus is released at the end of the timing cycle. Figure 26-11 shows normal VVI pacemaker function.

The pacemaker has a *refractory period*, which is a period of time after either pacing or sensing in the ventricle during which the pacemaker is unable to respond to intrinsic activity. During the refractory period, the pacemaker in effect has its "eyes closed" and is not able to sense spontaneous activity. If an intrinsic QRS should occur during the pacemaker's refractory period, it is not sensed because the pacemaker is "blind" at that time.

STIMULUS RELEASE

Stimulus release is verified on the ECG by the presence of a pacing spike. A pacing spike indicates that the pacemaker battery has enough power to initiate a stimulus and that the stimulus was delivered into the body. When evaluating a temporary pacing system, the presence of a pacing spike indicates that the connections between the pulse generator and the bridging cable and between the bridging cable and the pacing wires are intact. If any part of the system becomes disconnected, the stimulus cannot reach the body and a pacing spike is not seen. The presence of a pacing spike alone does not indicate where the stimulus was delivered, only that it entered the body somewhere.

Absence of pacing stimuli when they should be present can indicate a faulty pulse generator or battery, or a break or disconnection in the lead system. Pacing stimuli can also be absent when pacing is inhibited by the sensing of extraneous electrical signals, such as electromagnetic interference (EMI) or myopotentials. Figure 26-12 illustrates total loss of stimulus release in a patient whose permanent pacemaker battery was dead.

CAPTURE

Capture is indicated by a wide QRS complex immediately after the pacemaker spike and represents the ability of the pacing stimulus to depolarize the ventricle. Loss of capture is recognized by the presence of pacing spikes that are not followed by paced ventricular complexes (Fig. 26-13). Causes of loss of capture include:

1. Inadequate stimulus strength, which can be corrected by increasing the electrical output of the pacemaker (turning up the milliamperage).
2. Pacing wire out of position and not in contact with myocardium, which can sometimes be corrected by

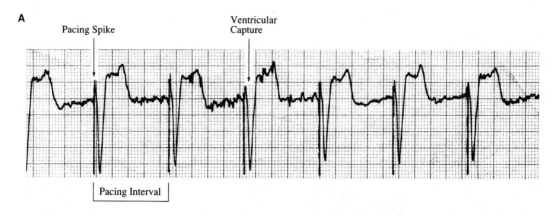

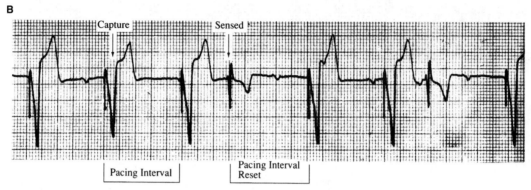

FIGURE 26-11 Normal VVI pacemaker function. **(A)** Capture is good, but sensing cannot be evaluated because no intrinsic QRS complexes are present. **(B)** Capture and sensing both normal. The two intrinsic QRS complexes are sensed, inhibit ventricular pacing output, and reset the pacing interval. (From Chulay M, Guzzetta C, Dossey B: AACN Handbook of Critical Care Nursing, Stamford, CT, Appleton Lange, p. 448, 1997.)

repositioning the patient. Repositioning the pacing wire is usually not a nursing function and must be performed by a physician or someone trained in intracardiac catheter manipulation.

3. Pacing lead positioned in infarcted tissue, which can be corrected by repositioning the wire to a place where myocardium is healthy and capable of responding to the stimulus.

4. Electrolyte imbalances or drugs that alter the ability of the heart to respond to the pacing stimulus.

5. Delivery of a pacing stimulus during the ventricle's refractory period when the heart is physiologically unable to respond to the stimulus. This problem occurs with loss of sensing (undersensing) and can be prevented by correcting the sensing problem (Fig. 26-15A).

Loss of capture in a totally pacemaker-dependent patient is an emergency because without an effective underlying rhythm, the patient may be asystolic or severely symptomatic because of slow, ineffective rate. If the underlying rhythm is ineffective or absent, cardiopulmonary resuscitation must be performed until the capture problem is corrected or until emergency transcutaneous pacing can be instituted. If loss of capture is intermittent, it may not result in symptoms but should be corrected as soon as possible.

SENSING

Sensing of intrinsic ventricular electrical activity inhibits the next pacing stimulus and resets the pacing interval. Sensing cannot occur unless the pacemaker is given the opportunity to sense. It must be in the demand mode and there must be

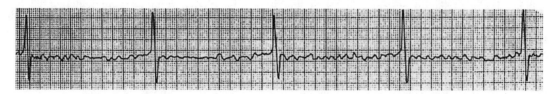

FIGURE 26-12 Absence of stimulus release in a patient with a permanent pacemaker. Underlying rhythm is atrial fibrillation with complete atrioventricular block and a very slow ventricular rate. The battery in the pacemaker generator was at end of service. (From Chulay M, Guzzetta C, Dossey B: AACN Handbook of Critical Care Nursing, Stamford, CT, Appleton Lange, p. 448, 1997.)

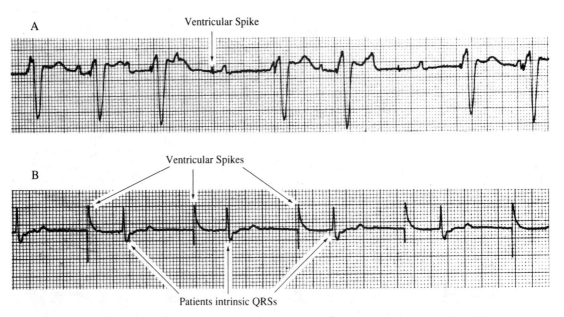

FIGURE 26-13 **(A)** VVI pacemaker with intermittent loss of capture. **(B)** VVI pacemaker with total loss of capture. (From Chulay M, Guzzetta C, Dossey B: AACN Handbook of Critical Care Nursing, Stamford, CT, Appleton Lange, p. 449, 1997.)

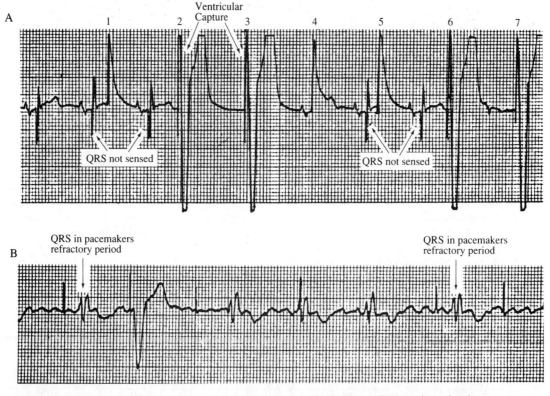

FIGURE 26-14 **(A)** Intermittent loss of sensing in a VVI pacemaker. Delivery of the pacing stimulus during the heart's refractory period makes it appear that capture is lost as well. Because the heart is physiologically unable to respond to the pacing stimulus when it falls in the refractory period, this is not a problem. Pacing spikes 1, 2, 5, and 6 should not have occurred; their presence is due to loss of sensing. Pacing spike 4 occurred coincident with the normal QRS complex, resulting in a "pseudofusion" beat, and does not represent loss of sensing. **(B)** Loss of capture in a VVI pacemaker. Only one pacing spike captures the ventricle. Two QRS complexes occur during the pacemaker's refractory period and thus are not sensed. This does not represent loss of sensing because the pacemaker has its "eye closed" during the time intrinsic ventricular activity occurred. (From Chulay M, Guzzetta C, Dossey B: AACN Handbook of Critical Care Nursing, Stamford, CT, Appleton Lange, p. 450, 1997.)

intrinsic ventricular activity for the pacemaker to have an opportunity to sense. In Figure 26-11*A*, sensing cannot be evaluated because there is no intrinsic ventricular activity, and therefore the pacemaker is not given an opportunity to sense. In Figure 26-11*B*, the occurrence of two spontaneous QRS complexes provides the opportunity to sense. In this example, sensing occurred normally, as indicated by the absence of the next expected pacing stimulus and resetting of the pacing interval from the intrinsic QRS complex.

Undersensing. *Undersensing* means that the pacemaker fails to sense intrinsic activity that is present. This can be due to:

1. Asynchronous (fixed-rate) pacing mode in which the sensing circuit is off. This problem can be corrected by turning the sensitivity control to the demand mode.
2. Pacing catheter out of position or lying in infarcted tissue, which can be corrected by repositioning the wire. Wire repositioning must be done by a physician; however, turning the patient to the side sometimes temporarily works when the pacing wire loses contact with the ventricle.
3. Intrinsic QRS voltage may be too low to be sensed by the pacemaker. Increasing the pacemaker's sensitivity (by decreasing the number on the sensitivity control) allows it to see smaller intrinsic signals and may solve the problem.
4. Break in connections, battery failure, or faulty pulse generator. Check and tighten all connections along the pacing system, and replace the battery if it is low. A chest radiograph may detect wire fracture. Change the pulse generator if problems cannot be corrected any other way.
5. Intrinsic ventricular activity falling in the pacemaker's refractory period. If a spontaneous QRS complex occurs during the time the pacemaker has its "eyes" closed, the pacemaker cannot see it. This may occur when the pacemaker fails to capture, which can allow an intrinsic QRS to occur during the pacemaker's refractory period. This problem is due to loss of capture and does not reflect a sensing malfunction (see Fig. 26-15*B*).

Oversensing. *Oversensing* means that the pacemaker is so sensitive that it inappropriately senses internal or external signals as QRS complexes and inhibits its output. Common sources of external signals that can interfere with pacemaker function include electromagnetic or radiofrequency signals or electronic equipment in use near the pacemaker. Internal sources of interference can include large P waves, large T-wave voltage, local myopotentials in the heart, or skeletal muscle potentials. Figure 26-15*B* illustrates oversensing in a temporary pacemaker. Because a VVI pacemaker is programmed to inhibit its output when it senses, oversensing can be a dangerous situation in a pacemaker-dependent patient, resulting in a dangerously slow rate or ventricular asystole. Oversensing is usually due to the sensitivity being set too high, which can be corrected by reducing the pacemaker's sensitivity by increasing the number on the sensitivity control. For example, if sensitivity is set at 0.5 mV,

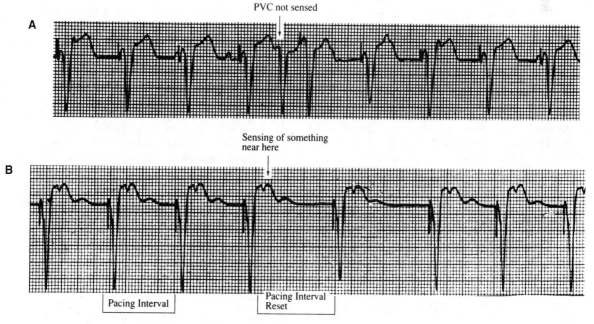

FIGURE 26-15 (A) Undersensing in a VVI pacemaker. The premature ventricular contraction (PVC) is not sensed and pacing occurs at the programmed pacing interval, resulting is a spike on the T wave of the PVC. **(B)** Oversensing in a VVI pacemaker. The pacing rate slows for two intervals, presumably because the device sensed something near the T wave that reset the pacing interval from the point where sensing occurred. (From Chulay M, Guzzetta C, Dossey B: AACN Handbook of Critical Care Nursing, Stamford, CT, Appleton Lange, p. 451, 1997.)

TABLE 26-2   Dual-Chamber Pacing Modes

Mode	Chambers Paced	Chambers Sensed	Response to Sensing
DVI	Atrium and ventricle	Ventricle	Ventricular sensing inhibits atrial and ventricular pacing
VDD	Ventricle	Atrium and ventricle	Atrial sensing—triggers ventricular pacing Ventricular sensing—inhibits ventricular pacing
DDI	Atrium and ventricle	Atrium and ventricle	Atrial sensing inhibits atrial pacing Ventricular sensing inhibits ventricular pacing
DDD	Atrium and ventricle	Atrium and ventricle	Atrial sensing—inhibits atrial pacing, triggers ventricular pacing Ventricular sensing—inhibits atrial and ventricular pacing

changing it to 2 mV decreases the sensitivity of the pacemaker. For ventricular pacing, a sensitivity of 2 mV is usually safe and can always be changed if needed to correct sensing problems.

Dual-Chamber Pacemaker Operation

Dual-chamber pacemakers have become very complicated, with multiple programmable parameters and varying functions, depending on the manufacturer. Because it is impossible to present a detailed explanation of all aspects of dual-chamber pacing in a single chapter, this section concentrates on basic dual-chamber pacing concepts that apply to all manufacturers' products. More detailed information is best obtained by attending a formal pacing program sponsored by a pacemaker manufacturer or from a pacemaker technical manual. Dual-chamber pacemakers can function in a variety of modes, depending on how they are programmed (Table 26-2). Because the DDD mode is most commonly used, basic DDD function is described here. Display 26-3 defines terms commonly used in dual-chamber pacing.

DUAL-CHAMBER TIMING CYCLES

According to the pacemaker code, DDD means that both chambers (atria and ventricles) are paced, both chambers are sensed, and the mode of response to sensed events is either inhibited or triggered, depending on which chamber is sensed. When atrial activity is sensed, atrial pacing is inhibited and ventricular pacing is triggered at the end of the programmed AV delay. When ventricular activity is sensed, all pacemaker output is inhibited. The following timing cycles determine how a dual-chamber pacemaker functions, and Figure 26-16 illustrates many of these timing cycles:

1. Pacing interval (or lower rate limit)—the base rate of the pacemaker, measured between two consecutive atrial pacing stimuli with no intervening sensed events. The pacing interval is a programmable parameter and determines the minimum rate at which the pacemaker paces in the absence of intrinsic cardiac activity.
2. AV delay (or AV interval)—the amount of time between atrial and ventricular pacing, or the "electronic PR interval." This is measured from the atrial pacing spike to the ventricular pacing spike and is a programmable parameter. The AV delay timer is initiated by a paced or sensed atrial event, and if no intrinsic conduction occurs to the ventricle within that time, a ventricular pacing spike occurs at the end of the programmed AV delay.
3. Atrial escape interval (or ventriculoatrial [VA]) interval—the interval from a sensed or paced ventricular event to the next atrial pacing output. The VA interval represents the amount of time the pacemaker waits after it paces in the ventricle or senses ventricular activity before pacing the atrium. The atrial escape interval is not a programmed parameter, but is derived by subtracting the AV delay from the pacing interval. Its length can be estimated by measuring from a ventricular spike to the next atrial pacing spike.
4. Total atrial refractory period—the period of time after a sensed wave or a paced atrial event during which the atrial channel does not respond to sensed events. The total atrial refractory period consists of the AV delay and the postventricular atrial refractory period (PVARP).
5. PVARP—the period of time after an intrinsic QRS or a paced ventricular beat during which the atrial channel is refractory and does not respond to sensed atrial activity. PVARP is a programmable parameter but is not evident on a rhythm strip.
6. Blanking period—the very short ventricular refractory period that occurs with every atrial pacemaker output. The ventricular channel "blinks its eyes" so it will not sense the atrial output and inappropriately inhibit ventricular pacing. The blanking period is a programmable parameter but is not evident on a rhythm strip.
7. Ventricular refractory period—the period of time after a ventricular pacing output or a sensed QRS during which the ventricular channel ignores intrinsic ventricular activity. Ventricular refractory period is a programmable parameter but is not evident on a rhythm strip.
8. Maximum tracking interval (or upper rate limit)—the maximum rate at which the ventricular channel tracks atrial activity. The upper rate limit prevents rapid ventricular pacing in response to very rapid atrial activity, such as atrial tachycardia or atrial flutter. The maximum tracking interval is a programmable parameter and usually is set according to how active a patient is expected to be and how fast a ventricular rate is likely to be tolerated.

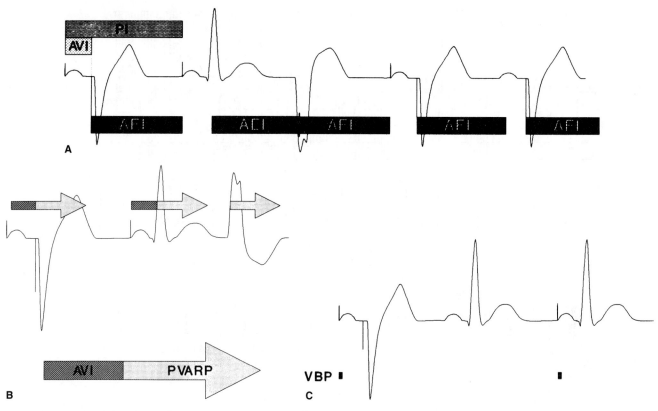

FIGURE 26-16 Dual-chamber pacemaker timing cycles. **(A)** The pacing interval (PI) represents the minimum pacing rate and is measured from one atrial pacing spike to the next consecutive atrial pacing spike. The atrioventricular interval (AVI) is measured from the atrial pacing spike to the ventricular pacing spike. The atrial escape interval (AEI) is the interval from a sensed or paced ventricular event to the next atrial pacing output and determines when the next atrial output is due. **(B)** The arrows represent the total atrial refractory period, which is composed of the AVI, begins with an atrial output or sensed P wave, and the post ventricular atrial refractory period (PVARP) begins with a paced or sensed ventricular event. **(C)** The ventricular blanking period (VBP) is a brief ventricular refractory period that occurs with every atrial pacer output to prevent sensing of atrial output by the ventricular channel (crosstalk). The ventricular refractory period (VRP) begins with a paced or sensed ventricular event. (From Pacemaker Technology, p. 71, 54, 66, with permission from St. Jude Medical Cardiac Rhythm Management Division, Sylmar, CA.)

THE FOUR STATES OF DUAL-CHAMBER PACING

When programmed to the DDD mode, dual-chamber pacemakers are capable of functioning in four main ways, depending on intrinsic cardiac activity and conduction capability. Each of the four states of pacing is described in the following sections.

Atrioventricular Sequential Pacing State (Atrial and Ventricular Pacing). Atrial and ventricular pacing (AV sequential pacing state) occurs at the minimum rate (Fig. 26-17*A*). Atrial pacing occurs at the lower rate limit, followed by ventricular pacing at the end of the programmed AV delay. This type of pacing would occur if the underlying cardiac rhythm were sinus bradycardia with AV block or asystole.

Atrial Pacing State (Atrial Pacing with Ventricular Sensing). Atrial pacing occurs at the minimum rate, but normal conduction to the ventricle occurs before the AV delay times out, resulting in intrinsic QRS complexes after the paced atrial beats (see Fig. 26-17*B*). This type of pacing would occur if the underlying rhythm were sinus bradycardia with normal conduction through the AV node.

Atrial Tracking State (Atrial Sensing with Ventricular Pacing). Intrinsic P waves are followed by paced ventricular beats (see Fig. 26-17*C*). Intrinsic atrial activity is sensed by the pacemaker and starts the AV delay. No intrinsic ventricular activity occurs before the AV delay times out, so a ventricular output is released at the end of the programmed AV delay. This type of pacing would occur if the underlying rhythm were sinus rhythm with complete AV block.

Inhibited State (Atrial and Ventricular Sensing). No pacing occurs in either chamber because intrinsic atrial and ventricular activity is present at a rate faster than the minimum pacing rate (see Fig. 26-17*D*). This occurs when the underlying rhythm is normal sinus rhythm.

The pacemaker is capable of switching from one state of pacing to another on a beat-to-beat basis depending on

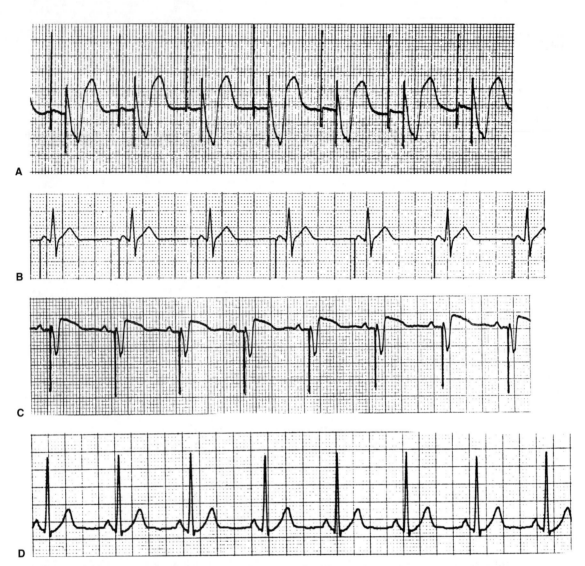

FIGURE 26-17 The four states of dual-chamber pacing. **(A)** Atrioventricular (AV) sequential pacing state with atrial and ventricular pacing at the minimum pacing rate. **(B)** Atrial pacing state with atrial pacing at the minimum rate and normal conduction to the ventricles, which inhibits ventricular output and terminates the AV delay. **(C)** Atrial tracking state. The pacemaker senses the patient's intrinsic P waves and paces the ventricle at the end of the AV delay. **(D)** Inhibited state with all pacing inhibited by normal sinus rhythm.

intrinsic activity. Figure 26-18 illustrates a DDD pacemaker operating in all four pacing states within a short period of time.

Evaluating Dual-Chamber Pacemaker Function

Because a dual-chamber pacemaker has both atrial and ventricular pacing and sensing functions, evaluation includes assessing atrial capture, atrial sensing, ventricular capture, and ventricular sensing. To evaluate pacemaker function, it is necessary to know the programmed mode (e.g., DDD, DVI), the minimum rate, the upper rate limit, the programmed AV delay, and refractory periods for both channels.[5,12] In reality, the only time all of this information is available is immediately after an implant, when the final programmed parameters are in the current patient chart, or in the physician's office

records. Therefore, in the real world of bedside nursing, we have to rely on a basic understanding of the issues involved in pacemaker evaluation, often without having all of the necessary information at hand. Some of the needed information can be determined by measuring intervals on a rhythm strip. For example, the AV delay can be measured from atrial spike to ventricular spike if there are any AV sequentially paced beats present. The minimum rate can be determined by measuring the interval between two consecutive atrial pacing spikes, if present. The following sections briefly discuss the issues of assessing atrial and ventricular capture and sensing in a dual-chamber pacing system.

ATRIAL CAPTURE

Atrial capture can be verified by seeing a P wave in response to every atrial pacing spike, although this is not always easy to see. The atrial response to pacing is often so small that it

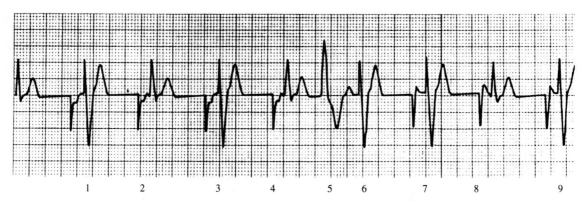

FIGURE 26-18 DDD pacemaker operating in all four states of pacing (stimulated strip). Beat 1 = atrioventricular (AV) sequential pacing; beat 2 = atrial pace, ventricular sense; beat 3 = AV sequential pacing; beat 4 = atrial pace, ventricular sense; beat 5 = premature ventricular contraction; beat 6 = atrial sense, ventricular pace; beat 7 = AV sequential pacing; beat 8 = atrial pace, ventricular sense; beat 9 = AV sequential pacing. Atrial capture is proven by beats 2, 4, and 8 (atrial spike followed by normal QRS within the programmed AV delay). Atrial sensing is proven by beat 6 (normal P followed by paced V at end of AV delay). Ventricular capture is verified by beats 1, 3, 6, 7, and 9 (wide paced QRS following ventricular pacing spike). Ventricular sensing is proven by beats 2, 4, and 8 (atrial spike followed by normal QRS, which inhibited ventricular pacing spike).

cannot be seen in many monitoring leads, so we cannot rely on the presence of a P wave after atrial pacing spikes as evidence of atrial capture. In the absence of a clear P wave, atrial capture can be assumed only when an atrial pacing spike is followed by a normally conducted QRS complex within the programmed AV delay. If the atrial spike captures the atrium and there is intact AV conduction, the presence of the normal QRS indicates that the atrium must have been captured for conduction to have occurred into the ventricles before the ventricular pacing stimulus was delivered. Because a DDD pacemaker paces the ventricle at a preset AV delay after atrial pacing, the presence of a ventricular paced beat after an atrial paced beat does not verify capture because the ventricle paces at the end of the AV delay regardless of whether atrial capture occurs. Therefore, atrial capture can be assumed only when there is an obvious P wave after every atrial pacing spike or when an atrial pacing spike is followed by a normal QRS within the programmed AV delay (see Figs. 26-17*B* and 26-18).

ATRIAL SENSING

Atrial sensing is verified by the presence of an intrinsic P wave that is followed by a paced ventricular beat at the end of the programmed AV delay. If a P wave is sensed, it starts the AV delay and ventricular pacing is triggered at the end of the AV delay, unless AV conduction is intact and results in a normal QRS. The presence of a normal P wave followed by a normal QRS proves only that AV conduction is intact, not that the P wave was sensed by the pacemaker. Therefore, atrial sensing is verified by an intrinsic P wave followed by a paced QRS (see Figs. 26-17*C* and 26-18).

VENTRICULAR CAPTURE

Ventricular capture is recognized by a wide QRS immediately after a ventricular pacing spike. Ventricular capture is much easier to recognize than atrial capture and is

the same as with single-chamber ventricular pacing (see Figs. 26-17*A* and *D* and 26-18).

VENTRICULAR SENSING

Ventricular sensing can be assessed only if there is intrinsic ventricular activity present for the pacemaker to sense. Ventricular sensing is verified by an atrial pacing spike followed by a normal QRS that inhibits the ventricular pacing spike, which is the same event that proves atrial capture (see Figs. 26-17*B* and 26-18). If a QRS is sensed before the next atrial pacing spike is due, both the atrial and ventricular pacing stimuli are inhibited and the VA interval (atrial escape interval) is reset.

Other Functions of Dual-Chamber Pacemakers

UPPER-RATE BEHAVIOR

To avoid rapid ventricular pacing in response to atrial arrhythmias, dual-chamber pacemakers have an *upper rate limit* or *maximal tracking rate* that limits the rate at which ventricular pacing occurs in response to sensed atrial activity. This upper rate limit applies only to paced tachycardias, not to intrinsic tachycardias. That is, tachycardias that are due to ventricular pacing in response to rapid atrial rhythms should not exceed the upper rate limit of the pacemaker. However, spontaneous VT or supraventricular tachycardia that conducts to the ventricle through the normal AV node or across an accessory pathway may result in ventricular rates that exceed the upper rate limit of the pacemaker. When an atrial rate being tracked by the ventricular channel of the pacemaker exceeds the upper rate limit, the pacemaker is programmed to limit the ventricular rate. Upper rate responses can be used alone or in combination and include Wenckebach response, block response, fall-back, or rate smoothing.

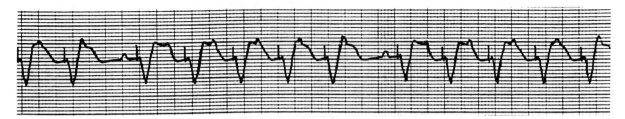

FIGURE 26-19 Wenckebach upper-rate response. Sinus tachycardia at a rate of 115 beats/min is present and the upper rate limit programmed in the pacemaker is 110 beats/min. The pacemaker tracks the intrinsic P waves and ventricular pacing occurs at the upper rate limit of 110, with occasional pauses. Note that the atrioventricular delay prolongs on consecutive beats until a P wave falls in the postventricular atrial refractory period, causing a pause in the ventricular paced rhythm. (From Pacemaker Technology, p. 71, 54, 66, with permission from St. Jude Medical Cardiac Rhythm Management Division, Sylmar, CA.)

Wenckebach response is the most commonly used upper rate response. As the atrial rate increases above the upper rate limit, P waves fall progressively closer to the preceding ventricular paced beat and the AV interval gets progressively longer. Eventually, a P wave falls in PVARP, where it cannot be sensed. The unsensed P wave does not start an AV delay, and therefore there is no ventricular paced beat after that P wave, and the resulting pause causes the ventricular paced rate to remain at or below the upper rate limit. The ECG shows a gradual lengthening of the AV interval and pauses whenever a P wave falls in PVARP (Fig. 26-19). This pattern presents as group beating just like AV Wenckebach, but the R-R intervals are constant instead of getting shorter. The atrial rate, the upper rate limit, and the PVARP determine the degree of block (e.g., 3 : 2, 5 : 4).

In *block response*, 1 : 1 tracking occurs at a constant AV delay until the atrial rate reaches a critical rate at which a P wave falls in PVARP and sudden block develops. As the atrial rate increases, P waves fall closer to the preceding ventricular paced beat, and eventually a P wave lands in PVARP where it cannot be sensed. The unsensed P wave does not start an AV delay; therefore, there is no ventricular paced beat after that P wave and the resulting pause keeps the ventricular paced rate below the upper rate limit. The ECG shows constant AV intervals with sudden block, often in a 2 : 1 ratio (Fig. 26-20). This type of response causes an abrupt rate change rather than a more gradual rate change, as occurs with the Wenckebach response.

Fall-back response is believed to be a more physiologic, but also more complex type of response. When atrial tachycardia is first recognized by the atrial channel, ventricular pacing synchronizes with atrial activity for a programmable amount of time, after which the atrial and ventricular channels dissociate. From then on, the ventricular pulse interval (distance between two paced beats) lengthens. The pacing rate eventually slows down to the programmed fall-back rate, a process taking as long as several minutes. While the ventricular rate slows gradually, the atrial rate is still monitored. When the atrial rate falls below the upper rate limit, the pacemaker returns to its original mode of pacing. This type of rate response provides a more comfortable hemodynamic transition from a rapid to a lower rate of ventricular pacing. AV synchrony, however, is not maintained by the fall-back response (Fig. 26-21).

Rate smoothing is not truly an upper-rate response but rather a programmed parameter used to prevent the ventricular pacing rate from changing by more than a predetermined percentage from one cardiac cycle to the next. This response prevents the pacemaker from tracking rapid atrial rates at the onset or if the rapid atrial rate stops abruptly. With this type of response, when the atrial rate exceeds the upper rate limit, a Wenckebach response is observed. When the tachycardia stops abruptly, pacing resumes at a rate faster than the lower rate limit to prevent an abrupt decrease in ventricular rate (Fig. 26-22).

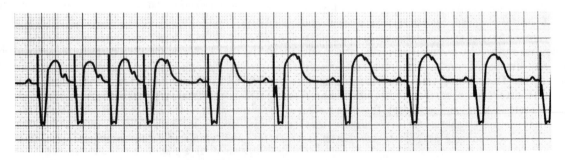

FIGURE 26-20 Atrioventricular block upper-rate response (stimulated strip). Sinus tachycardia is present at a rate of approximately 120 beats/min and the upper rate limit is 120 beats/min. Atrial tracking occurs at the beginning of the strip. As the sinus rate increases slightly, 2 : 1 block develops as every other P wave falls in the postventricular atrial refractory period. (From Sultzer Intermedics, Angleton, TX, Concepts of Cardiac Pacing, p. 144, 1998.)

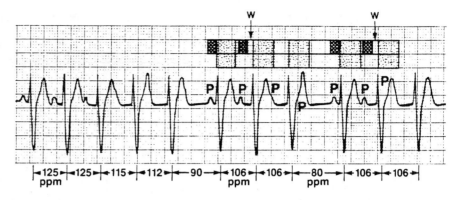

FIGURE 26-21 Fall-back response from an atrial tachycardia of 125 pulses/min to the nominal programmed fall-back rate of 100 pulses/min seen in the strip as falling between 80 to 106 pulses/min. P, P waves; heavy stippling, atrioventricular delay; light stippling, postventricular refractory periods; no stippling, alert periods; W, ventricular channel wall, cannot pace in the ventricle faster than the nominal fall-back rate. (From Isicoff C: Understanding upper rate responses of DDD pacers. Heart Lung 14: 327–334, 1985.)

PACEMAKER-MEDIATED TACHYCARDIA

Pacemaker-mediated tachycardia (PMT, also called *endless-loop tachycardia*) is rapid ventricular pacing, usually at the upper rate limit, that can occur in patients with dual-chamber pacemakers when retrograde conduction is present in the normal conduction system or in an accessory pathway. Retrograde conduction means that impulses can conduct backward from ventricle to atrium. Pacemaker units that detect intrinsic atrial activity and stimulate the ventricle after an appropriate AV delay (VDD and DDD modes) can participate in the maintenance of a PMT. The tachycardia circuit consists of the patient's normal AV conduction system (or an accessory pathway) that is capable of retrograde conduction, and the pacemaker's atrial sensing and ventricular output circuits (Fig. 26-23A). Retrograde conduction results in a sensed atrial depolarization, which in turn triggers the ventricular output channel. If this sequence is repeated, a tachycardia is maintained indefinitely until the retrograde pathway fatigues or the tachycardia is terminated by inactivating the atrial sensing circuit (see Fig. 26-23B). Placing a magnet over the pulse generator inactivates the atrial sensing circuit and terminates PMT.

Conditions necessary for initiation of PMT include loss of AV synchrony, intact retrograde conduction, and VA conduction times longer than PVARP.[2,6,9] Any condition that results in the atrium being repolarized and ready to respond to retrograde conduction can initiate PMT. Common initiators include loss of atrial capture, PVCs with retrograde conduction, premature atrial contractions, myopotential or EMI tracking, magnet application and removal, and reprogramming from asynchronous to synchronous mode.[2,6] Most newer dual-chamber pacemakers incorporate PMT prevention algorithms, such as extending PVARP after a PVC or temporarily inactivating the atrial sensing circuit after a PVC, in an attempt to prevent the initiation of PMT. Many devices also have PMT termination algorithms that attempt to break the tachycardia if it occurs.

CROSSTALK

Crosstalk refers to the sensing of activity in one channel by the other channel's sensing circuit. The most common and potentially dangerous type of crosstalk is sensing of the atrial output pulse by the ventricular channel, resulting in inhibition of ventricular output. If the ventricular channel senses the atrial pacing stimulus, it thinks it sees a ventricular event and thus inhibits its next output. This could result in total ventricular asystole in a patient who has no underlying ventricular rhythm (Fig. 26-24). Other manifestations of crosstalk include atrial pacing at a rate faster than the programmed rate and a longer distance from the atrial pacing spike to the conducted QRS than is programmed for the AV delay[15] (see Fig. 26-24).

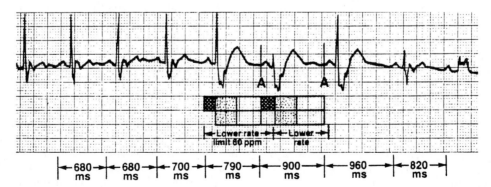

FIGURE 26-22 Electrocardiogram strip and timing cycle of rate smoothing as the intrinsic rate decreases. Atrial pacing is seen before the programmed lower rate limit of 60 pulses/min because the pacer does not allow P-P or R-R intervals to change by more than 12.5% (program smoothing constant) from one beat to the next. ms, milliseconds; A, atrial output pulse; heavy stippling, atrioventricular delay; light stippling, postventricular refractory periods; no stippling, alert periods. (From Isicoff C: Understanding upper rate responses of DDD pacers. Heart Lung 14: 327–334, 1985.)

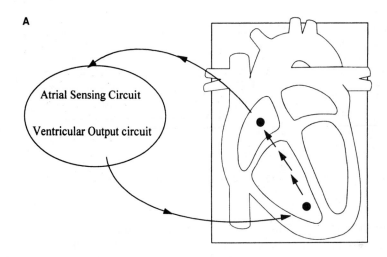

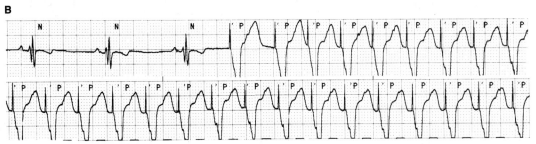

FIGURE 26-23 (A) Diagram illustrating the mechanism of pacemaker-mediated tachycardia (PMT). Retrograde ventriculoatrial conduction is represented by the dashed line. The retrograde P wave is sensed by the atrial channel of the pacemaker and a ventricular output is delivered at the end of the programmed atrioventricular delay. The reentry circuit consists of the intrinsic conduction system as the retrograde limb and the pacemaker as the antegrade limb. **(B)** Rhythm strip of PMT. Sinus rhythm is present, and then a ventricular paced beat occurs, probably in response to an extraneous signal (e.g., myopotential or electromagnetic interference from something in the environment). Retrograde conduction occurs to the atria (seen as a P wave after the first ventricular paced beat), which then initiates PMT. On the rhythm strip, N is the rhythm strip recorder's annotation of a "normal" beat, and P is the annotation of a "paced" beat (however, the Ps happen to coincide with the retrograde P waves seen on the rhythm strip).

Blanking Period. The ventricular blanking period is one method of trying to eliminate crosstalk. The blanking period is a very short refractory period that occurs on the ventricular channel during delivery of the atrial output pulse (see Figs. 26-16C and 26-24A). The blanking period "blinds" the ventricular channel for a short time so it cannot see the atrial pacing output. This should prevent crosstalk, but if the blanking period is too short, it may still be possible for the ventricular channel to sense the end of the atrial output pulse. In most pacemakers, the blanking period is programmable and can be made longer if necessary to prevent crosstalk.

Safety Pacing (Nonphysiologic Atrioventricular Delay). Safety pacing is a mechanism used by some pacemakers to prevent the inhibition of ventricular output when crosstalk occurs. Safety pacing results in the delivery of a ventricular pacing spike at a short AV delay (e.g., 100 milliseconds) whenever the ventricular channel senses any signal immediately after the blanking period. Safety pacing prevents inhibition of ventricular pacing and the short AV delay prevents delivery of the ventricular pacing spike on a T wave (Fig. 26-25).

Potential Complications of Pacing

Early complications of temporary or permanent pacemaker insertion include pneumothorax, lead perforation, and ventricular arrhythmias. Complications occurring later can include infection at the insertion site, endocarditis, hematoma formation, thrombosis, skin erosion over a permanent pulse generator, pacemaker failure, lead dislodgment, Twiddler's syndrome, and symptoms from pacemaker syndrome.[2,9]

Pneumothorax can occur when the subclavian vein is used for lead insertion because the apex of the lung is located very near the subclavian vein, and lung injury is a possibility when accessing the vein. Pneumothorax may become manifest immediately or as long as 48 hours after implantation.[9] Clinical signs of pneumothorax can include respiratory distress, absence of lung sounds on the affected side, chest pain, hypotension, elevated neck veins, and hypoxia.

Lead perforation may be asymptomatic or it can lead to cardiac tamponade if there is rapid accumulation of blood in the pericardium secondary to perforation of the right ventricular wall. If the pacing lead perforates the septum and

FIGURE 26-24 Crosstalk. **(A)** Lower diagram illustrates the normal programmed A-A interval (minimum pacing rate), atrioventricular (AV) delay (measure from A spike to V spike), atrial escape interval (AEI), ventricular refractory period (VRP), and ventricular blanking period (small square in front of the VRP arrows). The upper diagram shows possible manifestations of crosstalk due to ventricular sensing of atrial output: (1) shortening of the A-A interval, seen as atrial pacing at a rate faster than programmed, (2) prolongation of the A-R interval (time from atrial pace to intrinsic R wave) seen in the first two beats, and (3) inhibition of ventricular output, seen in the middle of the strip. **(B)** Crosstalk inhibition of ventricular pacing. Atrial pacing spikes are present followed by paced P waves. No ventricular output is delivered at the end of the AV delay because the ventricular channel senses the atrial output, interprets it as a ventricular event, and inhibits ventricular output. The wide QRS complexes represent an underlying ventricular escape rhythm. (A is from Pacemaker Technology, p. 75, with permission from St. Jude Medical Cardiac Rhythm Management Division, Sylmar, CA. B is from Sultzer Intermedics, Angleton, TX, Concepts of Cardiac Pacing, p. 131, 1998.)

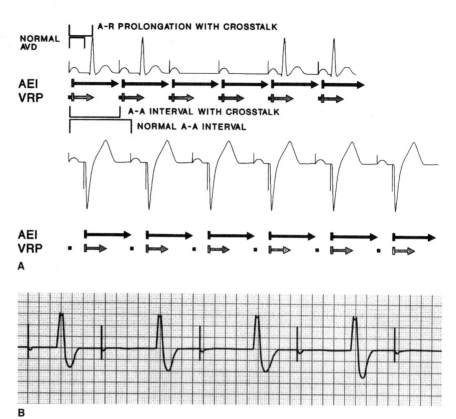

FIGURE 26-25 (A) Safety pacing due to crosstalk. The programmed atrioventricular (AV) interval is 150 milliseconds (ms). The pacemaker is in the AV sequential pacing state with an AV delay of approximately 100 ms due to crosstalk. **(B)** Safety pacing due to sensing early in the AV delay. The first two beats are AV sequential paced beats with an AV delay of approximately 150 ms. The ventricular channel blanking period occurs with the delivery of each atrial pacing spike and prevents the ventricular channel from sensing atrial output. The third beat is a premature ventricular contraction (PVC) that occurs immediately after the atrial pacing spike. When the ventricular channel "opened its eyes" after the blanking period, it saw the PVC very early in the AV delay, and rather than inhibit its output, it paced the safety pacing AV delay of approximately 100 ms. Safety pacing prevents inappropriate inhibition of ventricular pacing but delivers the ventricular output early enough to avoid the T wave of the PVC. (From Furman S, Hayes DL, Holmes DR: A Practice of Cardiac Pacing, Armonk, NY, Futura Publishing Co., p. 313, 1989.)

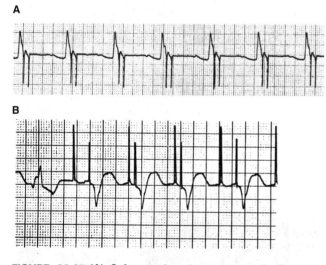

enters the left ventricle, the ECG may show a right bundle-branch block pattern rather than the usual left bundle-branch block pattern that results from pacing the right ventricular apex. Intercostal muscle or diaphragmatic stimulation by a perforated lead can cause hiccups or muscle twitching in the chest wall. The presence of a friction rub after implantation can indicate pericarditis or pericardial effusion due to lead perforation.

Ventricular arrhythmias, either PVCs or runs of VT, can result from irritation of the ventricle by the pacing lead. PVCs that are due to pacing wire irritation have the same morphology as paced beats because they originate from the same spot (see Figure 26-14*A*). Wire-induced arrhythmias most often occur within 24 to 48 hours of lead placement and usually resolve spontaneously.[9]

Twiddler's syndrome is manipulation of a permanent pulse generator within its pocket by the patient. This can lead to rotation of the pacemaker and twisting of the leads, which can result in lead fracture or dislodgment.

Pacemaker syndrome refers to a constellation of symptoms resulting from inadequate timing of atrial and ventricular contraction. Symptoms include fatigue, jugular venous distention and pulsations in the neck, weakness, dizziness or near-syncope, hypotension, CHF, and pounding in the chest. Symptoms may occur during periods of VVI pacing because of loss of AV synchrony or when retrograde conduction to the atria occurs, causing the atria to contract against closed AV valves. Contraction of the atria at a time when the AV valves are closed due to ventricular systole can activate stretch receptors in the atrial wall and pulmonary veins, resulting in a reflex vasodilation that causes hypotension and dizziness.

The loss of AV synchrony causes loss of atrial contribution to ventricular filling and may be another cause of symptoms.

IMPLANTABLE CARDIOVERTER-DEFIBRILLATORS

Sudden cardiac death (SCD) continues to claim approximately 300,000 lives each year, with most deaths related to VF or VT.[31,33] The implantable cardioverter-defibrillator (ICD) terminates VF/VT automatically, preventing sudden death. Clinical trials have shown that the ICD is better than antiarrhythmic therapy in preventing sudden death from ventricular arrhythmias.[29,41]

Development

The implantable defibrillator was the brainstorm of Dr. Michel Mirowki. In the late 1960s, Mirowki conceived the idea of an automatic implantable defibrillator after a close friend died from repeated episodes of ventricular arrhythmias. The first experimental model was tested successfully in 1969 in a dog. After many years, and much refining, the ICD was first implanted in humans in 1980.[26] The device was experimental until 1985, when it gained full U.S. Food and Drug Administration approval. The first-generation devices were large (weighing 250 g and occupying a volume of 145 mL), requiring implantation in a subcutaneous abdominal pocket. The earliest ICD systems required a thoracotomy because patch electrodes were sutured to the pericardium over the apex of the heart, and either epicardial screw-in leads or an endocardial lead was placed for rate sensing and pacing (Fig. 26-26). The leads were then tunneled to the pulse generator in the abdominal pocket.[28,32,43] The need for thoracotomy increased morbidity and mortality associated with ICD implantation and limited use in high-risk patients.

The first ICD was a nonprogrammable, committed, shock-only device intended to treat VF, but was quickly modified to a second-generation device that had cardioversion capabilities.[30,32,43] The current generations of defibrillators have evolved into a smaller, sophisticated device (Fig. 26-27). ICDs can deliver either high-energy or low-energy shocks, demand and rate-responsive pacing, antitachycardic pacing, and noninvasive electrical stimulation for electrophysiology studies (EPS), have extensive programmability allowing for tiered therapy, and have the ability to record and store electrograms of tachycardic episodes. Lead technology and the use of biphasic waveforms have made transvenous, nonthoracotomy systems the standard, eliminating the need for open heart surgery.[30]

Indications for Use

Initial indications for an ICD during clinical trials in 1980 were quite stringent. To meet criteria for receiving an ICD, the patient had to have survived at least two episodes of cardiac arrest not associated with an acute MI. Documentation of VF had to occur on at least one occasion, and the patient had to have been treated with antiarrhythmics on one

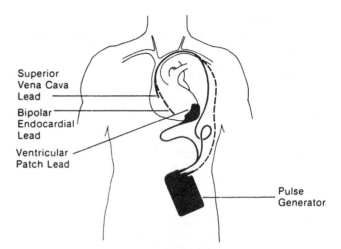

FIGURE 26-26 Diagram of automatic implantable cardioverter-defibrillator with placement in abdominal region. (From Physician's Manual for the Automatic Implantable Cardioverter Defibrillator, p 1. St. Paul, MN, Cardiac Pacemakers, Inc., 1986.)

episode.[32] Since 1980, guidelines have been updated several times by expert panels of the American College of Cardiology/American Heart Association Task Force and the North American Society of Pacing and Electrophysiology. The most current guidelines were published in 1998. The most recent guidelines are no longer based on the assumption that first-line therapy for VF or symptomatic sustained VT should be guided by drug therapy. Current recommendations are evidenced based whenever possible and are given rankings of level A, B, and C.[16] Level A indicates that data were derived from multiple, randomized clinical trials involving a large number of subjects. Level B indicates data were derived from a limited number of trials involving comparatively small numbers of patients or from well-designed, nonrandomized studies or observational data registries. Level C indicates that the consensus opinion of experts was the primary source of the recommendation[16] (Display 26-4).

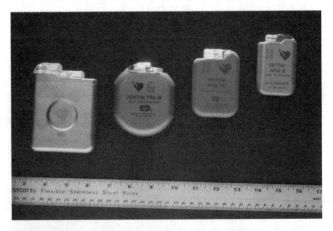

FIGURE 26-27 Assortment of implantable cardioverter-defibrillators, showing the evolution to smaller and more efficient devices.

DISPLAY 26-4

1998 Indications for Implantable Cardioverter-Defibrillator Therapy–American College of Cardiology/American Heart Association (ACC/AHA) Practice Guidelines

CLASS I INDICATIONS

Indications per level of evidence–A, B, or C

A: Data were derived from multiple *randomized* clinical trials involving a large number of subjects.

B: Data were derived from a limited number of trials involving comparatively small numbers of patients from well-designed data analysis of *nonrandomized* studies or *observational* data registries.

C: Consensus of expert opinion was the primary source or recommendation.

1. Cardiac arrest due to VF or VT–not due to a transient or reversible cause. *(Level A)*
2. Spontaneous sustained VT. *(Level B)*
3. Syncope of undetermined origin with sustained VT or induced with EP study when drug therapy is ineffective, not tolerated, or not preferred. *(Level B)*
4. Nonsustained VT with coronary disease, prior MI, LV dysfunction, and inducible VF or sustained VT at EP study that is not suppressible by class I antiarrhythmic drug. *(Level B)*

CLASS II INDICATIONS

1. Cardiac arrest presumed to be due to VF when EP testing is precluded by other medical conditions. *(Level C)*
2. Symptomatic sustained ventricular arrhythmia while awaiting heart transplantation. *(Level C)*
3. Familial or inherited conditions with a high risk for life-threatening arrhythmias such as long QT syndrome or hypertrophic cardiomyopathy. *(Level B)*
4. Nonsustained VT with CAD, prior MI, and LV dysfunction, with EP-induced VT or VF. *(Level B)*
5. Recurrent syncope of undetermined etiology in the presence of ventricular dysfunction and inducible EP study, when other causes of syncope have been excluded.

CLASS III INDICATIONS†

1. Syncope of undetermined cause in patient without EP-induced arrhythmias. *(Level C)*
2. Incessant VT or VT. *(Level C)*
3. VF or VT resulting from arrhythmias that are amenable to ablation (e.g., Wolff-Parkinson-White syndrome, right ventricular outflow tachycardia, fascicular VT). *(Level C)*
4. Ventricular arrhythmias due to reversible causes. *(Level C)*
5. Significant psychiatric illnesses that may be aggravated by ICD implantation, or systematic follow-up. *(Level C)*
6. Terminal illness with life expectancy < 6 months. *(Level C)*
7. Patients with CAD and LV dysfunction with prolonged QRS duration in the absence of spontaneous or inducible VT who are undergoing coronary artery bypass surgery. *(Level B)*
8. New York Heart Association class IV drug-refractory congestive heart failure in patients who are not candidates for heart transplantation. *(Level C)*

CAD, coronary artery disease; EP, electrophysiology; ICD, implantable cardioverter-defibrillator; LV, left ventricle; MI, myocardial infarction; VF, ventricular fibrillation; VT, ventricular tachycardia.
*Change–this is the first time guidelines for ICDs have included a primary prevention indication.
†Class III indications are patients in whom ICD therapy is not appropriate.
Adapted from Guidelines for Implantation of Cardiac Pacemakers and Antiarrhythmia Devices–ACC/AHA Practice Guidelines, 1998.

The rapid evolution of ICD technology, with the results of studies documenting efficacy of the ICD over drugs in both secondary and primary prevention of SCD, has led to the expansion of indications for the ICD.[21,32] Patients who receive an ICD usually fall into one of four categories: cardiac arrest survivors; those with spontaneous sustained VT; those with syncope of unknown origin with inducible VT/VF per electrophysiologic testing; and patients at high risk for future, life-threatening arrhythmic events.

SUDDEN CARDIAC DEATH SURVIVORS

Ventricular arrhythmias are the cause of most sudden cardiac arrests.[4,8,14,15] Survivors of cardiac arrest, in the absence of acute MI, are at risk for a future event. Cobb and associates[7] report a 36% 1-year mortality rate in untreated patients who were successfully resuscitated, hospitalized, and discharged home. The Antiarrhythmics Versus Implantable Defibrillator (AVID) study confirmed that the ICD is superior to antiarrhythmic drugs in decreasing overall and cardiac mortality rates in patients with known life-threatening ventricular arrhythmias. In this study, 1,016 patients at risk for cardiac arrest because of a history of VF or sustained VT and low ejection fraction were randomized to receive either an ICD or antiarrhythmic drug therapy, primarily empiric amiodarone therapy. The study was stopped early because of a statistically significant benefit of the ICD compared with drug therapy. Based on the results of AVID, the ICD is superior to antiarrhythmic drugs and is considered the preferred treatment in patients with documented symptomatic VT or VF.[12,17,41]

Work-up of the sudden cardiac arrest survivor includes an assessment of left ventricular function, coronary angiography, echocardiography, and EPS (see Chapter 25, Sudden Cardiac Arrest). If test results do not uncover any treatable cause of cardiac arrest, such as preexcitation, ICD implantation is advised. The ICD is the best available therapy for preventing sudden death.

SUSTAINED VENTRICULAR TACHYCARDIA

The ICD is also used in the patient who has spontaneous or EPS-induced sustained monomorphic VT. In this group of patients, other treatment options may be available, such as (1) antiarrhythmic drug therapy guided by EPS or Holter monitoring, (2) surgical aneurysmectomy when a ventricular aneurysm is the substrate for VT; and (3) radiofrequency catheter ablation of the VT foci.[11,32] A combination of ICD therapy with drugs and ablation is also used.[16]

In patients with poor left ventricular function and rapid VT, who are syncopal or near syncopal, the ICD is often used as first-line therapy. The antitachycardic pacing mode (ATP) delivers an effective therapy in terminating monomorphic VT. ATP is particularly effective with slower VT, and when delivered is usually imperceptible to the patient. Low-energy cardioversion or high-energy cardioversion-defibrillation is also programmed into the ICD. The ATP feature leads to fewer shocks, is more comfortable for the patient, and enhances the patient's acceptance of the device.[19,32,43]

SYNCOPE OF UNKNOWN ORIGIN

Syncope in the setting of structural heart disease and inducible VT per electrophysiologic testing carries a high risk of SCD. A sudden death rate of 48% at 3 years in patients with syncope of unknown origin and inducible sustained VT, compared with only 9% in patients with a negative EP study, was reported by Bass and colleagues.[3] Syncope with induced VT/VF is considered a class I indication for an ICD with the 1998 revised guidelines. Evidence supporting the use of the ICD in this group of patients was reported in a study of 50 patients who received an ICD for syncope of unknown origin and inducible ventricular arrhythmias. Most (n = 36) of the patients had a sustained monomorphic VT induced, 9 patients had a VF induced, and 5 patients had a nonsustained VT induced. During a 2-year follow–up period, 18 of the 50 patients (36%) experienced appropriate ICD discharges.[24]

HIGH-RISK PATIENTS

The most notable change in the revised guidelines for ICDs is that prophylactic ICD implantation is now justified in patients who are considered at high risk but have never had a spontaneous episode of sustained VT or VF. The goal in this group of patients is to prevent sudden death.

The first randomized study to report primary prevention of SCD with direct comparison between the ICD and antiarrhythmic drugs was the Multicenter Automatic Defibrillator Implantation Trial (MADIT).[29] MADIT was designed as a prophylactic trial to determine if patients with coronary heart disease, left ventricular dysfunction, and asymptotic nonsustained VT would have a better survival rate than those patients who were treated with conventional medical therapy. Eligible patients had inducible, sustained, nonsuppressible VT during electrophysiologic testing. During a 5-year time span, 196 patients were enrolled, 95 to the ICD group and 101 patients to the conventional group. The study was stopped early on advice of the Data and Safety Monitoring Board because the patients randomized to the ICD arm were found to have a 54% reduction in all-cause mortality compared with the patients receiving conventional therapy.[29,30,32]

The MADIT study showed that prophylactic use of ICDs saves lives in patients with heart disease. Those selected patients with coronary heart disease, severe left ventricular dysfunction, and nonsustained VT certainly may benefit from ICD therapy before sustaining a sudden cardiac arrest. Other groups of patients may also benefit from prophylactic ICD therapy. Those patients with idiopathic dilated cardiomyopathy, hypertrophic cardiomyopathy, long QT syndrome, and arrhythmogenic right ventricular dysplasia have been shown to have better survival rates when treated with an ICD.[16]

Functional Characteristics

The ICD system consists of a pulse generator and defibrillation lead electrodes for arrhythmia detection and therapy delivery. New ICD systems are implanted transvenously, like pacemakers, and no longer require cardiac surgery. However, devices that use defibrillation patches on the ventricle are still in use, and if these leads are still functional at the time of generator change for depleted battery, the original leads are retained and used.[17,22] The newest ICD systems consist of a unipolar system that uses the pectorally implanted pulse generator as part of the electrical circuit, further simplifying implantation (Fig. 26-28). In addition to internal defibrillation, today's ICD provides synchronized cardioversion, ATP, VVI, and DDDR pacing, telemetry, episode history logs, and electrograms. An example of device diagnostics is shown in Figure 26-29.

The pulse generator is essentially a self-powered computer in a hermetically sealed titanium can. The operational circuitry consists of a battery, sense amplifier, control circuits (microprocessors, logic, and memory), high-voltage charging circuits, defibrillation energy-storing capacitor, and a high-voltage output switch circuit. A header made of epoxy is the interface between the generator and the leads.[22,32,43]

The lead system connects the generator to the heart. Lead technology has markedly improved over the 1990s. Most new ICDs require only one lead that is placed into the right ventricle in the same manner as a pacemaker lead. The lead has sensing and pacing capabilities similar to pacing leads, but also has a large electrical surface area for delivering high-energy shocks. If a dual-chamber ICD is placed, a second lead is placed in the atrium.[32,34] The defibrillation pathway that was used with the initial pectoral implants consisted of a right ventricle–to–superior vena cava coil. If defibrillation thresholds (DFTs) were not acceptable with this configuration, a patch electrode was placed. More

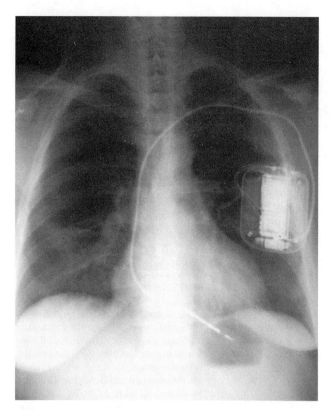

FIGURE 26-28 Radiograph of transvenous lead placed in the right ventricle and a pectorally placed active can. (Medtronic Transvene lead with Medtronic Jewel Active Can Pectoral ICD system. Photo reproduced with permission from Gust H. Bardy, MD.)

```
Therapy History          Data Since Counters Cleared on: 28-MAY-98
Nonsustained Episode(s) Have Occurred Since Last Cleared

Episode Counters

                                 Since Last      Device
                                  Cleared        Totals
                                 28-MAY-98
Treated
  VF Therapy                         0              3
  VT Therapy                         0              9
  VT-1 Therapy                       0              0
  Commanded Therapy                  0              0
Nontreated
  No Therapy Programmed              0              0
  Nonsustained Episodes             1             13
Total Episodes                      1             25

Device Parameter Summary      Tachy Mode =      Monitor+Therapy

VF    1.0 sec                         29J/ 33J/ 33J X 3
─ 200 bpm
VT    2.5 sec                 ATP1x OFF  1.1J/ 33J/ 33J X 3
                             ATP2x OFF
─ 145 bpm
BRADY           VVI   40 bpm   4.0  volts and  0.50 ms
POST-SHOCK      VVI   40 bpm   7.5  volts and  1.00 ms

Change Tachy Mode with Magnet                     OFF
Beep During Capacitor Charge                      OFF
Beep on Sensed Events and Paced Events            OFF
Beep when ERI is Reached                          ON
Electrogram Storage                               ON
```

```
Episodes:        1 to 24
Dates:    28-JAN-97 to 17-SEP-98

** Gaps in episode numbers
   indicate episodes that did
   not meet initial duration.

Epsd #    Date      R-Rs EGMs Saved  Comments

  24    11-APR-98   x    x           Spontaneous, 1 Att, Shk
  22    27-MAR-98   x    x           Spontaneous, 2 Att, Shk
  19    14-JAN-98   x    x           Spontaneous, 1 Att
  18    17-NOV-97   x    x           Spontaneous, 1 Att, Shk
  17    16-AUG-97   x    x           Spontaneous, 3 Att, Shk
  16    12-AUG-97   x    x           Spontaneous, 1 Att, Shk
  14    26-JUL-97   x    x           Spontaneous, 1 Att
  13    26-JUL-97   x    x           Spontaneous, 1 Att, Shk
  11    10-JUN-97   x    x           Spontaneous, 1 Att
  10    10-JUN-97   x    x           Spontaneous, 1 Att
   9    10-JUN-97   x    x           Spontaneous, 1 Att, Shk
   8    10-JUN-97   x                Spontaneous, 1 Att
   6    10-JUN-97   x                Spontaneous, 1 Att, Shk
   4    10-MAY-97   x                Spontaneous, 1 Att, Shk
   3    28-JAN-97   x                Induced, 1 Att, Shk
   2    28-JAN-97   x                Induced, 1 Att, Shk
   1    28-JAN-97   x                Spontaneous, 1 Att, Shk

End of Report
```

FIGURE 26-29 Printout of episode counters and device parameter summary from CPI Ventak Mini–model 1746. Episode logs provide valuable information about the patient's arrhythmias and are used to help assess the efficacy of medical treatment.

recently, a unipolar defibrillation system has been introduced. The titanium case of the pulse generator acts as a large–surface-area defibrillation electrode, like a patch, simplifying implantation.[2,38]

Early ICDs delivered shocks with a monophasic waveform, which was a single pulse at a given polarity and duration. Today's ICDs deliver shocks with a biphasic waveform. A biphasic shock has a negative and positive pulse, which has lowered DFTs significantly. Lower thresholds result in higher rates of successful defibrillation, a higher margin of safety, and prolonged battery life.[2]

SENSING AND DETECTION

Recognizing ventricular arrhythmias is essential for the ICD; it is the *sensing* that measures the intracardiac electrogram signal from the lead electrodes. The sensing electrodes transmit each ventricular depolarization (R-wave) signal to the sense amplifier of the ICD. The main challenge for the sensing system is twofold. It must detect the very low amplitudes of VF, while avoiding oversensing of T waves during repolarization and P waves during atrial depolarization. Other incoming signals that can be sensed include low-frequency noise, skeletal myopotentials, and EMI. Newer ICD systems have either an automatic gain control or an autoadjusting threshold feature that helps with proper sensing.[17,32]

The ICD primarily *detects* arrhythmias by looking at the cycle length, which is the time between R waves produced by ventricular depolarization. The cycle length represents the heart rate. The ICD can also be programmed to look at signal morphology, which helps in arrhythmia detection.[32,43] For VF, ICD devices use rate criteria as the sole detection method. The use of rate criteria results in maximal sensitivity. The ICD charges the capacitor once the programmed amount of intervals is met (e.g., 8 to 12 intervals of a rate of 180 beats/min). The ICD then delivers the shock after reconfirming the rate. If rate criteria are not met, the shock is aborted. The reconfirmation prevents unnecessary shocks for nonsustained events.

A VT zone can also be programmed into the ICD. Once again, rate is the primary detection method, but other detection enhancements can be programmed to increase specificity of VT detection, thus decreasing

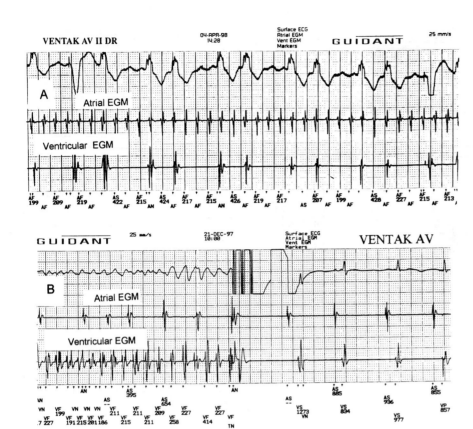

FIGURE 26-30 (A) Tracing of atrial fibrillation (AF). The atrial electrogram (EGM) shows the rapid atrial response of AF and the much slower ventricular response. **(B)** A tracing of induced ventricular fibrillation (VF), with the ventricular rate much faster than the atrial rate. Marker annotations for Guidant/CPI AV and AV II DR: AF, atrial fibrillation sense; AS, atrial sense; AN, atrial noise; VF, ventricular fibrillation; VN, ventricular noise; VP, ventricular pace.

inappropriate shocks for supraventricular tachycardia and atrial fibrillation.[25] These optional detection features include a sudden-onset criterion, an R-R interval stability criterion, an electrogram width criterion, and sustained-rate duration. The new dual-chambered pacemaker-defibrillator also looks at atrial rate data (Fig. 26-30) and has a V rate greater than A rate override feature to help deliver appropriate therapy.[27,34]

Onset criterion is a feature used to distinguish sinus tachycardia from VT. When the patient is exercising and the ventricular rate increases gradually and subsequently goes into the VT zone, the ICD does not classify the tachycardia as VT. The ICD compares each cycle length interval and determines if the rate has increased faster than would be expected for a sinus increase.[25,32]

The rate stability criterion is used to help differentiate atrial fibrillation from VT. Atrial fibrillation has a large cycle length variability, whereas VT cycle length varies minimally. When a fast ventricular response from atrial fibrillation meets the VT criteria and rate stability is programmed on, the ICD does not classify the fast rate as VT because it varies more than VT would.[25,32]

The electrogram width criterion measures the intracardiac electrogram and inhibits the ICD from detecting sinus tachycardia as VT. The ICD compares the width of the R wave with a programmed value. If the R wave is narrow, the ICD classifies the tachycardia as sinus. If the R wave is wide, the ICD treats the tachycardia as VT.[25]

Modes of Operation

Implantable cardioverter-defibrillators can be programmed to detect one to three zones, one zone for VF and two different zones for VT. Therapies are programmed according to the detection zone. ICDs offer different types of tachyarrhythmia therapy depending on the manufacturer, including burst pacing, adaptive burst pacing or ramp pacing, incremental/decremental bursts, low-energy cardioversion, and defibrillation. Different zones allow the ICD to be programmed in a tiered- or staged-therapy approach, allowing for maximum safety in the VF zone and less aggressive and less painful therapies in the VT zones. In addition to VT/VF therapy, the ICD has pacemaking abilities. Depending on the ICD system implanted, VVI pacing or DDDR pacing with mode switching is available[39] (Table 26-3).

All ICDs have a magnet mode, a feature that is activated when a magnet is placed over the pulse generator. The magnet is usually located in the upper right hand corner or over either end of the unit, depending on the manufacturer. Magnet modes allow for therapy to be suppressed in emergency situations when the patient is receiving inappropriate shocks. Audible tones are emitted by some generators when a magnet is placed over the unit. Some of the newer devices offer the option of programming the device temporarily to inhibit therapy, or turn off therapies with magnet application. ICDs also provide noninvasive EPS capabilities that help confirm the inducibility of the patient's clinical arrhythmia and evaluate the effectiveness of various therapies.

TABLE 26-3 Current Implantable Cardioverter-Defibrillators

Manufacturer	Device Name (Model No.)	Volume	Energy	Description	Longevity*	Magnet Response
Guidant/CPI (St. Paul, MN)	Ventak AV III DR (1831/1836)	58 cc	31 J stored	ICD with DDDR pacing and Atrial View, three VT/VF zones, five different detection enhancements, details V>A, ATR trigger, noninvasive A & V EPS capabilities, up to 16 min EGM, therapy episode, P/S histograms, biphasic waveform and programmable polarity	5.0–6.1 y	Beeps when magnet applied, can program to inhibit therapy temporarily with magnet or turn off with magnet, no effect on brady pacing
Guidant/CPI	Mini III / Mini III+ (1782/1783/1786)	48 cc/53 cc	33 J stored	ICD with VVI pacing, three VT/VF zones, three detection enhancements, up to 16 min stored electrograms, noninvasive EPS capabilities, biphasic waveform and programmable polarity	5.0–8.0 y	Beeps when magnet applied, can program to inhibit therapy temporarily with magnet or turn off with magnet, no effect on brady pacing
Intermedic	Res-Q Micron *Advantage* (101-10)	68 cc	32 J delivered	ICD with VVI pacing, three VT/VF zones, true atrial discrimination, atrial EGMs present, five different detection criteria, history on all episodes, 5 min of EGM available, noninvasive EPS capabilities, biphasic waveform and programmable polarity	5.0–8.6 y	Audible tone when magnet applied, allows evaluation of battery status/pacing threshold, temporarily inhibits detections and therapies
Medtronic (Minneapolis, Mn)	Micro Jewel II (7223Cx)	54 cc	30 J delivered	ICD with VVI pacing, three VT/VF zones, three detection enhancements, up to 15 min stored EGM, event trends reports, 12,000 R-Rs, 150 episodes, noninvasive EPS capabilities, biphasic waveform and programmable polarity	4.9–9.0 y	No beeps/tones with magnet, temporarily inhibits detections and therapies, no effect on brady pacing
Medtronic	Gem SR/Gem DR (7227/7271)	49 cc/62 cc	35 J delivered	ICD with VVIR (7227) pacing and DDDR (7271) pacing and mode switching, three VT/VF zones, five different detection enhancements, noninvasive EPS capabilities, multiple diagnostic schemes, up to 22 min EGM, biphasic waveform and programmable polarity	5.5–11.0 y	No beeps/tones with magnet unless programmed with Patient Alert, audible tone will then be present with magnet application, temporarily inhibits detections, no effect on brady pacing
Ventritex	Contour II (V185)	57 cc	38 J delivered	ICD with VVI pacing, three VT/VF zones, 16 min EGM available–fully annotated, 59 episodes, no R-R, noninvasive EPS capabilities, biphasic waveform	3.5–6.5 y	No beeps/tones with magnet, temporarily inhibits detections and therapies, no effect on brady pacing

*Dependent on shocks and percentage pacing.

A, atrium; ATR, atrial tachycardia response (mode switching); DDDR, dual-chamber rate-responsive pacing; EMG, electromyogram; EPS, electrophysiology study; ICD, implantable cardioverter-defibrillator; P/S, paced/sensed; V, ventricle; VF, ventricular fibrillation; VT, ventricular tachycardia; VVI, ventricular demand pacing; VVIR, ventricular rate-responsive pacing.

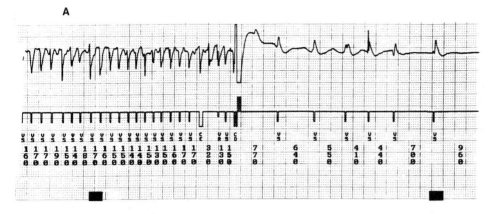

SUMMARY

Type:	VF
Average Cycle(ms):	160
Last Therapy:	VF Rx 1, Successful
Duration:	11 sec

DETECTION SETTINGS

Detection Intervals(ms):	VF=310	VT=400
NID Initial:	VF=18	VT=16
NID Redetect:	VF=12	VT=12
Stability:	ON	
Onset:	OFF	

FIGURE 26-31 (A) An episode of ventricular fibrillation (VF) detected and successfully converted with 33-J shock. **(B)** A summary of the episode. The device (Medtronic 7221) was set with VF and ventricular tachycardia zones. The arrhythmia was rapid and was detected in the VF zone.

All newer devices have memory and electrogram storage capability. The ICD continuously stores parameter setting, device status, and significant information about the patient's arrhythmia. When the ICD programmer retrieves the data, it summarizes the data for display and printout. For each episode, up to maximum storage capacity, the ICD stores the ventricular electrogram for the single-chamber devices and stores atrial and ventricular electrograms for the dual-chamber devices. The ability to review stored electrograms from an episode has been especially helpful in differentiating between appropriate and inappropriate shocks.[17,25,34]

VENTRICULAR FIBRILLATION THERAPY

Implantable cardioverter-defibrillators use defibrillation as the sole therapy option for arrhythmias in the VF zone (Fig. 26-31). Programming of the shock energy is based on DFT testing. The DFT is the minimum effective energy required to defibrillate the heart. To ensure that the ICD is effective, ICD shocks must be programmed above the DFT. Historically, a safety margin of 10 joules (J) has been used, and therefore, the first therapy is usually set between 20 and 34 J in the VF zone.[38] The ICD reconfirms that the patient is still in VF before delivering the first shock. If the patient has returned to sinus rhythm during the charging time, the first VF therapy is aborted. The ICD attempts to deliver a synchronized shock to the R wave, but if it cannot, therapy is delivered anyway.[25]

VENTRICULAR TACHYCARDIA THERAPY

In contrast to treating arrhythmias in the VF zone, there are many more options when the ICD is programmed in the VT zone. Each VT episode can be treated with multiple therapies and is often treated in a stepwise fashion. The first therapy is often ATP, followed by low-energy cardioversion, and finally by defibrillation if necessary to terminate the episode.[32]

Most sustained monomorphic VTs are due to reentry and can be terminated by a timed pacing sequence. Pacing at a faster rate than the VT increases the probability of VT termination. ATP offers the patient the ability to terminate a tachycardia without a shock. The downside of ATP is the risk of acceleration to an unstable faster rhythm and is the reason high-energy shocks are also programmed into the VT zone. When VT is induced, ATP successfully terminates the VT 65% to 90% of the time and accelerates VT 3% to 21% of the time.[32,37]

Antitachycardic pacing mode therapies can be set in the electrophysiology laboratory after VT has been induced and a specific ATP therapy has been proven successful in terminating the tachycardia. Another approach is programming the ICD empirically, modifying it if needed, after the patient has a spontaneous VT event.[32] A variety of pacing modes can be used to terminate the tachycardia. Each manufacturer has a slightly different approach to programming ATP. A common form of ATP is burst pacing, where a group of paced beats is delivered at equal or fixed-cycle intervals that exceed the rate of the tachycardia. The number of beats in each burst and the number of burst sequences are programmed, and vary from device to device. Adaptive bursts, also called *ramp pacing*, is another frequently used ATP method. A ramp sequence consists of a set of pulses delivered at decreasing intervals to treat a detected episode of VT. Incremental/decremental bursts is another form of burst pacing in which the bursts alternate between incremental and decremental cycle lengths.[19,32]

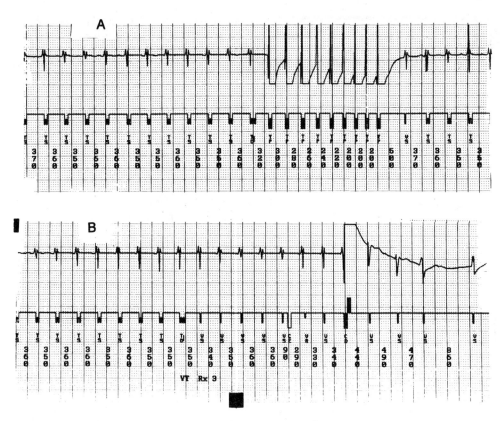

FIGURE 26-32 Electrogram tracing shows unsuccessful ramp pacing series **(A)**, followed by successful low-energy cardioversion terminating the ventricular tachycardia **(B)**.

Low-energy cardioversion is available on all devices and can be set as low as 0.1 J. The very–low-energy therapies are often determined by electrophysiology testing.

Shocks that are under 2 J are much more comfortable for the patient and usually are perceived as small shocks.[10] Low-energy shocks often are delivered after ATP therapy has failed (Fig. 26-32), but may also be programmed as the initial therapy to terminate the tachycardia. Another advantage of cardioversion is that it can be delivered more rapidly than repeated ATP sequences. If low-energy cardioversion is unsuccessful, a high-energy shock is delivered.[19,32,39]

BRADYCARDIA PACING

Bradycardia pacing (VVI) is a standard feature available on all ICDs. Dual-chamber pacing has become available as well, reducing the need for separate pacemaker implantation in pacemaker-dependent patients.[26,34] Pacing rate, hysteresis, sensitivity, pulse width, pulse amplitude, and blanking after pace are all programmable. In the dual-chamber device, atrial tachycardia rate and mode-switch capabilities can also be programmed. Pacing thresholds during VT and after defibrillation are usually higher than needed for bradycardia pacing, and they can be independently programmed in some of the devices.

Device Implantation

Most ICD implants consist of the unipolar system, which is implanted in the left pectoral region and is referred to as the *active can* or *hot-can*. The lead is inserted in either the subclavian vein or the cephalic vein and advanced to the right ventricular apex, using techniques similar to those for permanent pacemaker implantation. Defibrillation testing is completed once the lead is secured and is done with either an external device or with the device itself. VF is induced to test whether the programmed energy level converts the VF to sinus rhythm. If the first shock fails, a second shock at maximum output is delivered. If the second shock fails, a 360-J external shock is delivered. The ICD is implanted only if sensing during sinus rhythm and VF is acceptable, if pacing thresholds and impedances are within normal limits, and if an adequate safety margin is demonstrated by DFT testing.[38] With the current unipolar pectoral ICDs and biphasic waveform, it is very rare for implant criteria not to be met.[2,38] The ICD may be implanted in the electrophysiology laboratory, catherization laboratory, or operating room. Anesthesia can be local or general, and the device can be placed subcutaneously or submuscularly.[32,39]

Most patients with an ICD placed transvenously in the pectoral position are discharged on the day after surgery. A postimplantation noninvasive study is often performed before discharge.[30]

Complications

Postoperative complications have been reduced with the advent of the transvenous pectoral technique for ICD implantation. Complications postimplantation resemble those observed with permanent pacemaker implantation.[32,39] Potential complications of ICD implantation are listed in Display 26-5.

Potential Complications of Implantable Cardioverter-Defibrillator

ADVERSE EVENTS ASSOCIATED WITH SURGERY
Acceleration of arrhythmia
Air embolism
Bleeding
Hemothorax
Perforation of the myocardium
Pneumothorax
Puncture of subclavian artery
Thromboemboli
Venous occlusion

ADVERSE EVENTS AFTER SYSTEM IN PLACE
Chronic nerve damage
Diaphragmatic stimulation
Erosion of pulse generator
Formation of pocket hematoma
Fluid accumulation/seroma
Infection of the pocket/system
Keloid formation
Lead dislodgment
Lead fractures and insulation breaks
Venous thrombosis

One of the most serious complications is infection of the ICD system. Explantation of the entire ICD system is mandatory, and a long course of antibiotics is necessary.

Surgical revision of the ICD system may be necessary after lead dislodgment in the early recovery period (24 to 72 hours) or lead fracture, which is seen in long-term follow-up. Lead-related problems have been reported to occur in 5.8% to 7.8% of patients with transvenous ICD implants.[23]

Electromagnetic interference can result in inappropriate discharge or inhibition of the ICD. These problems can be temporary or permanent.[25,32,34,35] The delivery of inappropriate therapy can actually produce tachyarrhythmias. Sources of interference include, but are not limited to, electrocautery, diathermy, hydraulic shock-wave lithotripsy, current-carrying conductors, arc welders, electrical smelting furnaces, radiofrequency transmitters such as radar, high-voltage systems, theft prevention equipment, and high-powered electromagnetic fields. Magnetic resonance imaging is contraindicated because it may cause permanent damage to the ICD. Inadvertent contact between the generator and magnets should be avoided because changes in the magnetic field may inactivate the pulse generator or cause erratic functioning.[25,28,32] Tachyarrhythmia detection must be programmed *OFF* before subjecting the patient to procedures that induce strong EMI.[25,32] If detections are turned OFF, the patient should be monitored. Once the procedure is completed, the ICD should be reprogrammed to the active mode.

Antiarrhythmic medications can result in complications by changing the appearance or rate of the arrhythmia or by altering the DFT. The arrhythmia rate also may be slowed below the cut-off rate so that the ICD fails to identify VT. The DFT could be changed by drugs, resulting in ineffective shocks. Amiodarone, for example, increases the threshold. Repeat EPS testing is often performed after the addition of antiarrhythmic drugs.[21,28,32,39]

Standard Precautions

EXTERNAL DEFIBRILLATION

Implantable cardioverter-defibrillators are designed to withstand external defibrillation. However, possible circuit damage or loss of output may occur if the external paddle is placed within 15 cm of the device. Direct defibrillation within 3 cm could cause permanent damage to the ICD or the implanted leads. Effectiveness of transthoracic defibrillation may also be affected by the implanted ICD system. Therefore, standard defibrillator protocols may need to be altered depending on the type of lead system used. If the patient has an older system with patches, paddle electrode placement should be perpendicular to an imaginary line drawn between the patches. The silicone rubber insulation on the back of the defibrillating patches effectively blocks current from passing through them.[32] After any external defibrillation, the ICD should be interrogated and checked to ensure proper function.

PACEMAKER INTERACTION

If a patient has an older-model ICD in place and requires a temporary or permanent pacemaker in conjunction with the ICD, special care is required. For those patients who may still have an older system in place, unipolar pacemakers are contraindicated because the larger pacing pulse associated with unipolar lead systems may be mistaken by the ICD for the patient's intrinsic rhythm.[42,43] Three unique complications have been observed in patients with both a permanent pacemaker and an ICD[32]: failure of the ICD to cardiovert VT; double counting of pacing spikes and QRS complexes, exceeding the rate cut-off and resulting in discharge; and misinterpretation of ST segment elevation as a sinusoid pattern, resulting in discharge.

To avoid potential complications with older-generation ICDs, single-chamber pacemakers with bipolar leads and lower voltages have been used. The newer generation of ICDs has eliminated the problem of potential interaction between an ICD and a pacemaker by adding the VVI pacing mode. The newest ICD models have DDD capabilities, eliminating the need for a second device when symptomatic bradycardia is present.[27]

Preoperative and Postoperative Nursing Care

Consideration of the emotional response of the patient and family to the ICD is an important part of nursing care.

Before surgery, an assessment of the patient's (and family's) knowledge level, support systems, and usual coping mechanisms should be made. Patients may have a high anxiety level owing to categorization as a high-risk patient,

EPS, impending surgery, and the ICD unit. Anxiety may be reduced through provision of competent care, education, and permission to express feelings.[21]

Patient education is very important. The patient should understand why the ICD is recommended and how it functions. ICD system models and patient education videotapes are available from the ICD manufacturers and are useful tools in providing visual and general information.[18] The patient and family members should also understand that the ICD does not prevent arrhythmias from occurring, but is there to correct the arrhythmia. The surgical procedure, where the ICD is placed, and the need to restrict overhead arm movements after surgery should be reviewed with the patient.

Because of the many life-threatening issues the patient may face, preoperative counseling by a psychiatrist or clinical psychologist may be beneficial.[9,42] The patient may be fearful of future SCD events, be anxious, have feelings of powerlessness, and have a component of depression.[21]

Postoperative care of the patient with an ICD is similar to the care of the patient after permanent pacemaker implantation. The patient should be informed that mild or moderate pain will be felt at the incision site. The patient's pain level and the incision site should be assessed and pain medications administered as needed. The patient should be instructed to minimize arm movements for the first 24 hours after implantation.

Discharge instructions are an important aspect of postoperative nursing care. With transvenous ICD implants, hospital stays are much shorter, which limits the time available to teach patients. Written discharge instructions should be supplied to the patient and should include instructions about pain management, site assessment and care, what to do in the event of receiving a shock, when to notify the physician, the importance of carrying proper identification that allows medical personnel quickly to check the ICD with the correct programmer, avoiding magnetic fields, and cardiopulmonary resuscitation, as well as information regarding support groups[10,18,21,28] (Table 26-4).

Instructions regarding ICD discharges should be thoroughly reviewed and understood because at least one spontaneous discharge occurs in approximately 50% of patients during the first year after receiving an ICD.[5] With ICD discharges, the patient may have symptoms of dizziness or loss of consciousness. Patients revive immediately, reporting feelings of well-being.[26] Patient perceptions of the discharge vary from none to very painful. Descriptions are usually of a strong blow to the chest, occurring rapidly and without sequelae. Patients with VF or a rapid VT are usually unconscious by the time the generator discharges.[42] Routine emergency protocols should be administered as needed. People who touch the patient as the unit discharges do not get hurt; at most, they feel a slight buzz or tingling.[10,21]

Psychosocial Issues

AUTOMOBILE DRIVING

Patients with an ICD who are SCD survivors may be restricted from driving for at least 6 months. The main concern is the risk of an arrhythmic event or the delivery of a shock while driving. The length of the driving restriction depends on where the patient resides and state/country regulations. Driving restrictions can cause feelings of isolation, anger, and loss of autonomy because driving is an important part of maintaining independence.[6,21] It is important for the patient to realize that it is the symptoms associated with ventricular arrhythmias, and not ICDs, that make driving potentially dangerous. After 6 months, if the patient has not had an ICD discharge, he or she may resume noncommercial driving. Patients who have had their ICD placed for prophylactic reasons and have not had a documented spontaneous episode of ventricular tachyarrhythmia should not be prohibited from driving.[32]

QUALITY OF LIFE

Implantable cardioverter-defibrillators therapy may be the primary treatment for life-threatening ventricular arrhythmias, but its impact on quality of life should be considered. Factors that affect quality of life include frequent or inappropriate shocks, device malfunction, or product recall.[32,40]

Sometimes, patients may think that they have received a shock, but when the ICD is interrogated, there is no record that a discharge has occurred. This phenomenon is known as a *phantom shock*. Phantom shocks are fairly common, often occurring as the patient is drifting off to sleep.[17,21] It is important to spend time reassuring the patient and family and reviewing the interrogated follow-up printouts with them.

An ICD discharge can be frightening for both the patient and spouse, particularly if the shock occurs with sexual activity. The patient may need to have the tachycardia detection rate increased if sexual activity increases the heart rate enough to meet the detection criteria. Education and support regarding shocks should be provided to the patient. Professional counseling should be recommended for the patient and spouse with emotional concerns. Many implanting centers have ICD support groups that can be very helpful to the ICD recipient and family. The support group provides a forum for the patients to discuss their concerns and fears with one another and provides the nurse with an excellent opportunity for patient education.[21,32]

Follow-up Care

Regular ICD follow-up is necessary to assess the patient's clinical status, ICD battery status, and device function and to review stored data that provide diagnostic information for treated episodes of tachyarrhythmias. Patients are followed every 3 to 6 months at an outpatient clinic. Capacitor reformation ("cap-reform") is necessary to prevent prolonged charge times. Older devices required manual cap-reform, but all new devices have an automatic cap-reform feature that is programmed for 3 to 6 months, depending on the manufacturer's recommendation.

The ICD lead system is evaluated by testing lead impedance, completing pacing thresholds, and determining appropriate R-wave sensing. R-wave sensing is checked by evaluating the marker channel and real-time electrograms. Potential for lead problems can be identified if inappropriate sensing is noted. Chest radiographs showing the ICD system should be taken annually.[32]

TABLE 26-4	Patient Discharge Instruction for Implantable Cardioverter-Defibrillator (ICD)			
Topic	**Instruction/Information**	**Patient Understands**	**Patient Initials**	**Nurse Initials**
Site care	• Keep site dry for 72 hours. • Change dressing daily. • Report drainage, redness, swelling, and symptoms of infection to your doctor.	Yes/No		
Activity restriction	• Avoid lifting arm on ICD side overhead, and no lifting with that arm until approved by your doctor. • Avoid pushing, pulling, or twisting. • Discuss resuming sexual activity with your doctor. Most patients resume sexual activity when their incisions are healed.	Yes/No		
Driving	• Avoid driving until given approval from your doctor.	Yes/No		
ICD discharges Your ICD will deliver therapy for a rate of _____	• If you get a shock, call your doctor immediately. • If you get a shock and do not feel well, call 911. • If you get two or more shocks, call 911.	Yes/No		
ICD identification Medical information	• Always carry your ICD identification card with you. Use the temporary card for now; your ICD company will mail you a permanent one. • It is advisable to wear a Medic Alert ID bracelet or necklace. • Keep a current list of the medications you take.	Yes/No		
Magnetic fields	• Avoid large magnets and strong electromagnetic fields–see patient booklet. • You **cannot** have a magnetic resonance imaging (MRI) scan. • Always tell medical personnel that you have an ICD. Your ICD will need to be turned off for some procedures.	Yes/No		
CPR	• In the event of future emergencies, family members should learn CPR.	Yes/No		
Support group	• Offers you a chance to meet others who have an ICD. • See the flyer in your packet for meeting times and location.	Yes/No		
Emergency numbers	• Doctor: _____ • Family member:			

CPR, cardiopulmonary resuscitation.

Battery status is monitored at each follow-up visit. If the device is close to its elective replacement indicator (ERI), more frequent visits may be required. Almost all patients should be considered for pulse generator replacement when the device ERI is reached.[32]

Episode data are reviewed and compared with the patient's clinical symptoms. Stored electrograms provide trending information on the frequency and severity, if any, of spontaneous ventricular arrhythmias.

TROUBLESHOOTING

Differentiating appropriate from inappropriate device function when a patient receives an ICD discharge or experiences symptoms such as syncope or palpitations can be challenging. Evaluation of a single ICD shock is usually performed in the outpatient clinic. Multiple, successive shocks constitute a medical emergency and require an in-hospital evaluation.[17]

The initial approach is to *identify* the problem, placing the problem in one of five categories: 1) appropriate therapy, 2) suspected inappropriate therapy, 3) failure to deliver therapy, 4) ineffective therapy, and 5) device deactivation. The second step is to *analyze* the problem by completing a full interrogation of the device to determine if the therapy was appropriate or inappropriate. The third step is to use a *systematic approach* to determine the cause for device deactivation or failure.[39] Approximately 20% of patients with ICDs that use heart rate only as the detection criterion receive an inappropriate shock, most commonly from atrial fibrillation or sinus tachycardia.[32,39] The newer devices that provide detection enhancement criteria can reduce this problem considerably. When stored electrograms are available, the appropriateness of ICD therapy can be checked immediately. The ICD also tracks nonsustained episodes, allowing the health care provider to know the frequency and severity of arrhythmias. If the patient is receiving multiple ICD discharges and not having clinical symptoms,

A

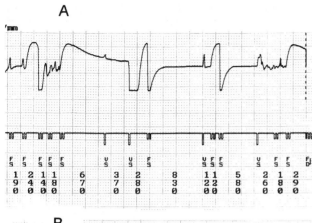

B

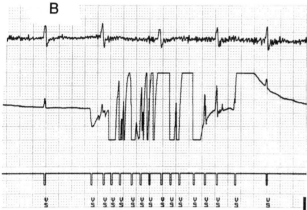

FIGURE 26-33 Electrogram tracings showing artifact due to fractured lead. **(A)** Intracardiac signals from stored electrograms showing artifact signals and irregular cycle length. **(B)** Real-time recording while patient moved arm with detections suspended to reproduce artifact. Marker annotations for Medtronic Jewel CD 7202: FS, fibrillation sense; VS, ventricular sense; FD, fibrillation detection–charge initiated.

dislodged lead, fractured lead, or double counting of QRS and T waves should be suspected. The patient should be instructed to call emergency medical services or go to the hospital in case of multiple shocks. When electrograms are available, interrogation of ICD can confirm fractured lead artifact (Fig. 26-33). In an emergency situation, the ICD can be deactivated by placing a large ICD/pacemaker magnet over the ICD. The magnet suspends tachycardia detection and inhibits therapy on all ICD devices. Some devices may be permanently placed in the inactive mode with a magnet, and therefore all ICDs should be interrogated whenever a magnet has been placed over the device. Magnets do not inhibit the bradycardia therapy that is programmed into the ICD. A chest radiograph may be able to provide information on lead fracture or insulation breaks and can diagnose a dislodged lead.[10,17,32]

Failure to deliver therapy is caused by failure to detect the arrhythmia. This could be due to a sensitivity problem, a change in VT rate, deactivation of the device, or system failure. Inadvertent deactivation of the ICD is rare, but potentially devastating.[39] The device could be inadvertently deactivated during a programming session. Therefore, a final interrogation with a printout should always be per-

formed. Some ICDs (Guidant-CPI; St. Paul, MN) can be deactivated after a magnet has been placed over the ICD for approximately 30 seconds. Rarely, exposure to a strong magnetic field results in deactivation. Battery depletion and circuit failure could be other causes for the ICD failing to deliver therapy.

Frequent and thorough follow-up care can help detect potential problems early, preventing devastating results.[10,39]

REFERENCES FOR PACEMAKERS

1. Auricchio A, Sommariva A, Salo RW et al: Improvement of cardiac function in patients with severe congestive heart failure and coronary artery disease by dual chamber pacing with shortened AV delay. Pacing Clin Electrophysiol 16: 2034–2043, 1993
2. Barold SS: Complications of pacemaker implantation and troubleshooting. In Singer I (ed): Interventional Electrophysiology, pp 935–1054. Baltimore, Williams & Wilkins, 1997
3. Barold SS, Zipes DP: Cardiac pacemakers and antiarrhythmic devices. In Braunwald E (ed): Heart Disease, 5th ed., pp 705–741. Philadelphia, WB Saunders, 1997
4. Brinker JA: Indications for permanent cardiac pacing. In Singer I (ed): Interventional Electrophysiology, pp 879–912. Baltimore, Williams & Wilkins, 1997
5. Catania SL: Cordis Guide to Interpretation of DDD Pacer ECGs. Miami, FL, Cordis Corporation, 1984
6. Concepts of Permanent Cardiac Pacing. Educational manual provided by Educational Services, Angleton, TX, Sulzer Intermedics, 1998
7. Finkelmeier NE: Pacemaker technology: an overview. AACN Clinical Issues in Critical Care Nursing 2: 99–106, 1991
8. Fisher JD, Kim SG, Mercando AD: Electrical devices for treatment of arrhythmias. Am J Cardiol 61: 45A–57A, 1988
9. Furman S, Hayes DL, Holmes DR: A Practice of Cardiac Pacing, 2nd ed. Mount Kisco, NY, Futura, 1989
10. Gregoratos G, Cheitlin MD, Conill A et al: ACC/AHA Guidelines for implantation of cardiac pacemakers and antiarrhythmia devices: executive summary. Circulation 97(13): 1325–1335, 1998
11. Hickey CS: Temporary cardiac pacing. AACN Clinical Issues in Critical Care Nursing 2: 107–117, 1991
12. McErlean ES: Dual-chamber pacing. AACN Clinical Issues in Critical Care Nursing 2: 126–131, 1991
13. Morton PG: Rate-responsive cardiac pacemakers. AACN Clinical Issues in Critical Care Nursing 2: 140–149, 1991
14. Moses HW, Schneider JA, Miller BD et al: Practical Guide to Cardiac Pacing, 3rd ed. Boston, Little, Brown, 1991
15. Pacemaker Technology for Nurses and Allied Health Professionals. Siemens Pacesetter Education Department, Sylmar, CA
16. Ridgely P, Edery T, Dinicola D et al: The Hemodynamics of Pacing: Choosing a Pacing Mode. Technical Concept Paper. Minneapolis, MN, Medtronic, Inc., 1991
17. Ridgely P: Pacing Indications: Elements of Optimal Physiologic Therapy. Technical Concept Paper. Minneapolis, MN, Medtronic, Inc., 1991

REFERENCES FOR IMPLANTABLE DEFIBRILLATORS

1. Akhtar M, Jazayeri MR, Sra JS et al: Implantable cardioverter-defibrillator therapy for prevention of sudden cardiac death. Cardiol Clin 11: 97–108, 1993
2. Bardy GH, Johnson G, Poole JE et al: A simplified, single-lead unipolar transvenous cardioversion-defibrillation system. Circulation 88: 543–547, 1993

3. Bass EB, Elson JJ, Fogoros RN et al: Long-term prognosis of patients undergoing electrophysiologic studies for syncope of unknown origin. Am J Cardiol 62: 1186–1191, 1988

4. Bayes de Luna A, Coumel P, Leclercq JF: Ambulatory sudden cardiac death: Mechanisms of production of fatal arrhythmia on the basis of data from 157 cases. Am Heart 117: 151–159, 1989

5. Bocker D, Block M, Isbruch F et al: Do patients with an implantable defibrillator live longer? J Am Coll Cardiol 21: 1638–1644, 1993

6. Cambre S, Silverman ME: Is it safe to drive with an automatic implantable cardioverter defibrillator or a history of recurrent symptomatic ventricular arrhythmias? Heart Disease and Stroke 2: 179–181, 1993

7. Cobb LA, Baum RS, Alvarez H et al: Resuscitation from out-of-hospital ventricular fibrillation: 4-Year follow-up. Circulation 52(Suppl III): 223, 1975

8. Cobb L, Hallstrom AP: Clinical predictors and characteristics of the sudden cardiac death syndrome. In Proceedings USA-USSR First Joint Symposium on Sudden Death. DHEW Publication No. (NIH) 78-1470. Washington, DC, 1977

9. Cooper D, Luceri RM, Thurer RJ et al: The impact of the automatic implantable defibrillator on quality of life. Circulation 72: 24, 1985

10. Davidson T, Van Riper S, Harper P et al: Implantable cardioverter defibrillators: A guide for clinicians. Heart Lung 23: 205–215, 1994

11. Deshpande S, Vora A, Axtell K et al: Sudden cardiac death. In Brown D (ed): Cardiac Intensive Care, pp 391–404. Philadelphia, WB Saunders, 1998

12. Domanski MJ, Zipes DP, Schron MS: Treatment of sudden cardiac death: Current understandings from randomized trials and future research directions. Circulation 95: 2694–2699, 1997

13. Goodman LR, Troup PJ, Thorsen MK et al: Automatic implantable cardioverter-defibrillator: Radiographic appearance. Radiology 155: 571–573, 1985

14. Gradman AH, Bell PA, DeBusk RF: Sudden death during ambulatory monitoring. Circulation 55: 210–211, 1977

15. Greene HL: Sudden arrhythmic cardiac death: Mechanisms, resuscitation, and classification. Am J Cardiol 65: 4B–12B, 1990

16. Gregoratos G, Cheitlin MD, Conill A et al: ACC/AHA Guidelines for Implantation of Cardiac Pacemakers and Antiarrhythmia Devices: Executive Summary: A report of the American College of Cardiology/American Heart Association Task Force on Practice Guidelines (Committee on Pacemaker Implantation). J Am Coll Cardiol 31: 1175–1206, 1998

17. Groh WJ, Foreman LD, Zipes DP: Advances in the treatment of arrhythmias: Implantable cardioverter-defibrillators. Am Fam Physician 57: 297–307, 1998

18. Harper P, VanRiper S: Implantable cardioverter defibrillator: A patient education model for the illiterate patient. Critical Care Nurse 13(2): 55–59, 1993

19. Jung W, Luderitz B: Antitachycardia pacemakers: Patient selection, appropriate programming, and testing. In Singer I (ed): Interventional Electrophysiology, pp 825–859. Baltimore, Williams & Wilkins, 1997

20. Kelly PA, Cannom DS, Garan H: Predictors of automatic implantable cardioverter defibrillator discharge for life-threatening arrhythmias. Am J Cardiol 62: 83–87, 1988

21. Knight L, Livingston NA, Gawlinski A et al: Caring for patients with third-generation implantable cardioverter defibrillators: From decision to implant to patient's return home. Critical Care Nurse 17(5): 51–65, 1997

22. Kuck KH, Cappato R, Siebels J: ICD therapy. In Camm JA (ed): Approaches to Tachyarrhythmias, pp 1–69. New York, Futura, 1996

23. Lawton JS, Wood MA, Gilligan DM et al: Implantable trans-venous cardioverter defibrillator leads: The dark side (Guest Editorial). Pacing Clin Electrophysiol 19: 1273–1278, 1996

24. Link MS, Costeas XF, Griffith JL et al: High incidence of appropriate implantable cardioverter-defibrillator therapy in patients with syncope of unknown etiology and inducible ventricular arrhythmias. J Am Coll Cardiol 29: 370–375, 1997

25. Medtronic System Reference Guide: A guide to the operation and programming of the 7223 Micro Jewel II Arrhythmia Management Device. Minneapolis, MN, Medtronic, Inc., 1996

26. Mirowski M: The automatic implantable cardioverter-defibrillator: An overview. J Am Coll Cardiol 6: 461–466, 1985

27. Mortensen PT, Pedersen KA: An overview of the Ventak AV AICD European Clinical Review. Guidant/AICD Advances pp 2–5, 1997

28. Moser SA, Crawford D, Thomas A: Updated guidelines for patients with automatic implantable cardioverter defibrillators. Critical Care Nurse 13(2): 62–73, 1993

29. Moss A, Hall J, Cannom D et al, for the Multicenter Automatic Defibrillator Implantation Trial: Improved survival with an implanted defibrillator in patients with coronary disease at high risk for ventricular arrhythmia. N Engl J Med 335: 1933–1940, 1996

30. Moss AJ, Zareba W: Implantable defibrillators for prevention of sudden cardiac death. Updates 1(1): 1–12, 1998

31. Myerburg RJ, Castellanos A: Cardiac arrest and sudden cardiac death. In Braunwald E (ed): Heart Disease: A Textbook of Cardiovascular Medicine, 5th ed, pp 742–779. Philadelphia, WB Saunders, 1997

32. O'Callaghan P, Ruskin J: Current status of implantable cardioverter-defibrillators. Curr Probl Cardiol 22: 645–707, 1997

33. Patient Oriented Research–Fundamental and Applied, Sudden Cardiac Death. Report of the Working Group on Arteriosclerosis of the National Heart, Lung, and Blood Institute, Vol 2, pp 114–122. DHEW, NIH Publication No. 82-2035. Washington, DC, National Institute of Health, 1981

34. Physician's System Manual for the Ventak Mini. St. Paul, MN, Guidant Corp. (CPI), 1998

35. Physician's Manual for the Ventak AV II–1820/1825. St. Paul, MN, Guidant Corp. (CPI), 1998

36. Physician's Manual for the Contour-ICD System. Sunnyvale, CA, Ventritex, 1997

37. Rosenqvist M: Pacing techniques to terminate ventricular tachycardia. Pacing Clin Electrophysiol 18: 592–598, 1995

38. Singer I: Defibrillation threshold testing and intraoperative ICD evaluation. In Singer I (ed): Interventional Electrophysiology, pp 741–762. Baltimore, Williams & Wilkins, 1997

39. Singer I: Complications of cardioverter defibrillator surgery, postoperative care, and patient follow-up. In Singer I (ed): Interventional Electrophysiology, pp 765–792. Baltimore, Williams & Wilkins, 1997

40. Sneed NV, Finch NJ, Leman RB: The impact of device recall on patients and family members of patients with automatic implantable cardioverter defibrillators. Heart Lung 23: 317–322, 1994

41. The Antiarrhythmics vs. Implantable Defibrillators (AVID) Investigators: A comparison of antiarrhythmic drug therapy with implantable defibrillators in patients resuscitated from near fatal ventricular arrhythmias. N Engl J Med 337: 1576–1583, 1997

42. Winkle RA, Stinson EB, Echt DS et al: Practical aspects of automatic implantable cardioverter-defibrillator implantation. Am Heart J 108: 1335–1346, 1984

43. Wolfe DA, Kosinski D, Grubb BP: Update on implantable cardioverter-defibrillators: New, safer devices have led to changes in indications. Postgrad Med 103: 115–130, 1998

Acquired Valvular Heart Disease

DENISE LeDOUX

DATABASE FOR NURSING MANAGEMENT

Definition, Classification, and Epidemiology

Valvular heart disease continues to be a common source of cardiac dysfunction and mortality. Competent cardiac valves maintain a unidirectional flow of blood through the heart as well as to the pulmonary and systemic circulations. Diseased cardiac valves that restrict the forward flow of blood because they are unable to open fully are referred to as *stenotic*. Stenotic valves elevate afterload and cause hypertrophy of the atria or ventricles pumping against the increased pressure. Cardiac valves that close incompetently and permit the backward flow of blood are refereed to as *regurgitant, incompetent,* or *insufficient.* Regurgitant valves cause an elevated volume load and dilation of the cardiac chambers receiving the blood reflux. Valvular dysfunction may be primarily stenotic or regurgitant, or it be a "mixed" lesion, a valve that neither opens nor closes adequately.

Valvular heart disease is usually described by the duration of the dysfunction (acute vs. chronic), the valves involved, and the nature of the valvular dysfunction (stenosis, insufficiency, or a combination of stenosis and insufficiency). The degree of cardiac dysfunction is defined by the New York Heart Association's (NYHA) Functional and Therapeutic Classification. Acquired valvular heart disease most commonly affects, and is most symptomatic with, the aortic and mitral valves. This chapter focuses on the mitral and aortic valves, with a brief discussion of tricuspid valve disease. Because the etiology of pulmonic disease is primarily congenital, it is not presented.

Etiologies of Acquired Valvular Heart Disease

RHEUMATIC HEART DISEASE

Rheumatic fever is the most commonly acquired cause of valvular heart disease in childhood.[31] Rheumatic fever is an acute inflammatory disease that damages the collagen fibrils and the ground substance of connective tissue (especially in the heart).[49] Tissues involved in rheumatic fever include the lining and valves of the heart, the skin, and connective tissue (Fig. 27-1). Rheumatic fever is a complication of group A streptococcal upper respiratory tract infections, occurring in approximately 3% of those with streptococcal pharyngitis 2 to 3 weeks after acute rheumatic fever. Group A streptococcal throat infection is responsible for both initial and recurrent attacks of rheumatic fever. Lymphatic channels from the tonsils are thought to transmit group A streptococci to the heart. Acute rheumatic fever probably results from a hyperimmune reaction to a bacterial allergy or an autoimmune reaction.[49]

Although acute rheumatic fever is still common in other countries, it has declined in frequency in the United States since mid-century, even though there is a persistently high frequency of streptococcal pharyngitis.[7] Reasons for the decline in rheumatic fever include the use of antibiotics to treat and prevent streptococcal infections, as well as improved social conditions such as decreased crowding, better housing and sanitation, and access to health care. Rheumatic fever persists in underdeveloped countries in which socioeconomic conditions enable the spread of streptococcal bacteria as well as limit access to adequate health care.

Acute rheumatic fever involves diffuse exudative and proliferative inflammatory reactions in the heart, joints, and skin. Major diagnostic criteria include carditis, polyarthritis, chorea, subcutaneous nodules, and erythema marginatum (pink, circinate skin rash). Those manifestations with minor diagnostic importance are fever, migratory arthralgias, acute-phase reactants in the blood (C-reactive protein) leukocytosis, and an elevated erythrocyte sedimentation rate, prolonged PR interval on the electrocardiogram (ECG), heart block, and a history of acute rheumatic fever or rheumatic heart disease.[49]

Carditis is the most important clinical manifestation of acute rheumatic fever, causing inflammation of the endocardium, myocardium, and pericardium. Myocarditis is characterized by interstitial inflammation that may affect cardiac conduction. Pericardial inflammation may result in

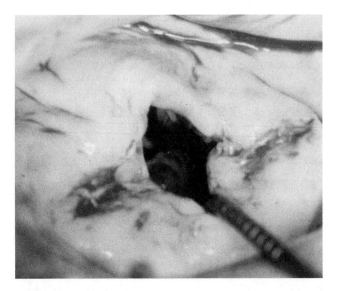

FIGURE 27-1 Rheumatic mitral valve with leaflet thickening and commissural fusion. (From Alpert JS, Sabick J, Cosgrove DM: Mitral valve disease. In Topol EJ, Califf RM, Isner JM et al [eds]: Textbook of Cardiovascular Medicine, p 511. Philadelphia, Lippincott–Raven, 1998.)

a fibrinous exudate as well as small to moderate amounts of serous fluid in the pericardial sac.[2] Endocarditis causes extensive inflammatory changes, resulting in scarring of the heart valves and acute heart failure. Warty lesions of eosinophilic material build up at the bases and edges of the valves. As the lesions progress, granulation tissue and subsequent vascularization develop, and fibrosis occurs. The annulus, cusps, and chordae tendineae are scarred and, as a result, they thicken and shorten. Acute heart failure develops because of interstitial myocarditis. Fibrinoid degeneration develops, followed by the appearance of Aschoff nodules, the characteristic pathologic lesion of acute rheumatic fever. As Aschoff nodules heal, fibrous scars remain. In severe cases, death from acute heart failure may result. Carditis frequently does not cause any symptoms and is detected only when the patient seeks help because of arthritis or chorea. Diagnostic criteria of rheumatic carditis are new organic heart murmur, cardiomegaly, heart failure, or pericarditis.[49]

Auscultatory signs of aortic and mitral insufficiency are frequently apparent. In over 90% of patients with carditis, the mitral valve is affected. When the mitral valve is affected, there may be a high-pitched, blowing, pansystolic murmur. A Carey-Coombs murmur, a low pitched, mid-diastolic murmur of short duration, may be noted at the apex. The Carey-Coombs murmur may be attributed to swelling and stiffening of mitral valve leaflets, increased flow across the valve, and alteration in left ventricular compliance. The regurgitation of the aortic valve results in diastolic murmurs, whereas involvement of the tricuspid valve is rarely appreciated during the acute phase.[2]

Rheumatic fever can be prevented by aggressive treatment of the initial episode of streptococcal pharyngitis: penicillin G, 500 mg as the first dose and then 250 mg four times daily for a duration of 10 days. If a patient is penicillin allergic, clarithromycin 500 mg twice daily for 7 to 14 days or clindamycin 150 mg every 8 hours can be substituted.[31]

INFECTIVE ENDOCARDITIS

Infective endocarditis is an infection of the endocardial surface of the heart, including the valves. Infective endocarditis is a serious illness and carries a mortality rate as high as 20% to 30% in the general population, and 40% to 70% in the elderly.[50] Rheumatic heart disease, as well as other cardiac lesions such as calcific aortic stenosis, hypertrophic cardiomyopathy, and congenital heart disease, as well as the presence of prosthetic heart valves, predispose to endocarditis. Intravenous drug abusers are also at high risk for endocarditis due to bacteremias caused by direct injection from contaminated needles and local infections at injection sites.[20] In patients with community-acquired, native valve endocarditis, *Staphylococcus aureus* is the predominant cause of acute disease.[29,32] Pathogens that are most commonly responsible for subacute endocarditis include streptococci, enterococci, coagulase-negative staphylococci, and the HACEK group of organisms (*Hemophilus* species, *Actinobacillus actinomycetemcomitans*, *Cardiobacterium hominis*, *Eikenella* species, and *Kingella kingae*). The *S. aureus* infecting intravenous drug users is frequently methicillin resistant.[29]

Clinical presentations of endocarditis range from fever and malaise to symptoms related to systemic emboli (Table 27-1).

The pathologic process of endocarditis requires that several conditions exist to permit infection to grow in the heart as well as to promote an environment that supports growth on the endocardial surface. For endocarditis to occur, there must be (1) endocardial surface injury, (2) thrombus formation at the site of injury, (3) bacteria in the circulation, and (4) bacterial adherence to the injured endocardial surface.[11] Acute endocarditis can also occur in normal heart valves from infection somewhere else in the body, resulting in extensive damage and valvular dysfunction that may cause severe cardiac failure and death within days to weeks.[50]

TABLE 27-1	**Clinical Manifestations of Infective Endocarditis**
Symptoms	**Physical Examination Findings**
Fever	Fever
Chills and sweats	Changing or new heart murmur
Malaise	Evidence of systemic emboli
Weight loss	Splenomegaly
Anorexia	Janeway lesions (small hemorrhages on palms or soles of feet)
Stroke symptoms	
Myalgias	
Arthralgias	Splinter hemorrhages (hemorrhagic streaks at fingernail tips)
Confusion	Osler's nodules (small, tender nodules on finger or toe pads)
Congestive heart failure	

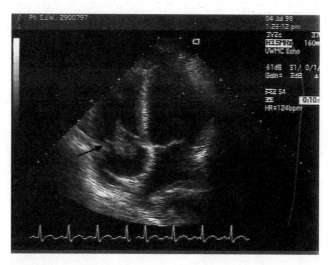

FIGURE 27-2 Two-dimensional echocardiogram view of vegetation on tricuspid valve in 27-year-old woman with endocarditis (*arrow*).

Blood cultures are an essential diagnostic tool in infective endocarditis. Three separate sets of blood cultures drawn from different venipuncture sites, obtained over 24 hours, usually identify the organism. Patients with infective endocarditis that remain culture negative may have fastidious organisms or may have received intravenous antibiotics before blood samples were drawn. In acute endocarditis, antibiotic therapy should be started after blood cultures have been obtained. The clinical approach in acute endocarditis includes appropriate antibiotics and monitoring for complications (Display 27-1). The usual course is 6 full weeks of intravenous antibiotics. Patients who do not respond well to standard antibiotic therapy may be referred for surgical valve replacement (Display 27-2).

Echocardiography is frequently used to verify the presence of vegetations on the valves (Fig. 27-2). Transthoracic echocardiography is less sensitive than transesophageal echocardiography in identifying vegetations (45% to 75% vs. 90% to 94%).[29] Transesophageal echocardiography is also useful to identify paravalvular leaks and annular abscesses seen in prosthetic valve endocarditis.

Prevention of endocarditis in high-risk populations, such as those with rheumatic heart disease or structural valve disease, is essential. Patients at risk (Display 27-3) who are undergoing procedures that may cause a transit bacteremia, such as dental or genitourinary procedures, should be treated prophylactically using recommended guidelines. (For complete guidelines, refer to *Prevention of Bacterial Endocarditis: Recommendations by the American Heart Association*.[17]) The treatment for infective endocarditis is prolonged high-dose antibiotic therapy and valve replacement for those who have evidence of severe valve dysfunction.[11]

MISCELLANEOUS ETIOLOGIES OF VALVULAR DISEASE

In addition to rheumatic fever and endocarditis, there are other etiologies of acquired valvular heart disease. Degenerative changes of the tissue, such as myxomatous degeneration, calcification, and those associated with Marfan's syndrome, can cause valvular dysfunction. Trauma or infection may affect the supportive or subvalvular apparatus. Dilation of the ventricles due to chronically elevated preloading may dilate an atrioventricular valve opening to the point the leaflets no longer approximate and the valve becomes incompetent. Coronary heart disease (CHD) and myocardial infarction (MI) can affect the papillary muscles of both the right and left ventricles, causing either dysfunction due to ischemia or frank flail of atrioventricular valve leaflets due to papillary muscle rupture. Systemic diseases such as lupus erythematosus and scleroderma may also cause valvular dysfunction.

Diagnostic Testing for Valvular Heart Disease

The diagnosis of valvular heart disease is based on patient history, physical assessment, and diagnostic testing. Some tests, such as the ECG and the chest radiograph, may be relatively insensitive in diagnosing valvular heart disease even though they are part of standard screening tests in patients with heart dysfunction. Diagnostic tests that are more specific and quantitative for valvular dysfunction include echocardiography (M-mode, two-dimensional, Doppler ultrasonography, or transesophageal), right and left heart catheterization, nuclear imaging, and exercise testing.[6] Diagnostic findings for specific valvular lesions are noted in the sections discussing each abnormality.

Mitral Stenosis

ETIOLOGY

The predominant cause of mitral stenosis is rheumatic fever. Rheumatic fever causes thickening and decreased mobility of the mitral valve leaflets associated with fusion of the commissures. Uncommon, nonrheumatic causes of mitral stenosis include malignant carcinoid syndrome, severe mitral annular or leaflet calcification, congenital absence of one of the papillary muscles, resulting in a parachute deformity of the mitral valve, neoplasm, endocardial vegetations, and degenerative calcification of an implanted tissue prosthetic heart valve.[22]

PATHOLOGY

The rheumatic process causes the mitral valve to become fibrinous, resulting in leaflet thickening, commissural or chordal fusion, and calcification. As a result, the mitral valve apparatus becomes funnel shaped with a narrowed orifice. Fusion of the mitral valve commisures results in narrowing of the principal orifice, whereas interchordal fusion obliterates the secondary orifices.

PATHOPHYSIOLOGY

The normal mitral valve area is 4 to 6 cm². Once the cross-sectional area of the mitral valve is reduced to 2 cm² or less, a pressure gradient between the left atrium and left ventricle occurs. Left atrial emptying is impeded by the reduced orifice. Increased left atrial pressure and dilation occurs along with left atrial hypertrophy in an attempt to maintain normal diastolic flow into the left ventricle. Increased left atrial pressure is transmitted to the pulmonary circuit, resulting in pulmonary hypertension and pulmonary congestion. As the left atrium distends and pressure rises, atrial conduction fibers are stretched, stimulating onset of atrial fibrillation.[11] Patients have left-sided congestive heart failure

(CHF) without left ventricular dysfunction. Mitral stenosis has a sparing effect on the left ventricle. Symptoms of mitral stenosis are usually related to obstruction of the mitral valve rather than ventricular dysfunction. As pulmonary pressure increases, right-sided heart failure may occur.

CLINICAL MANIFESTATIONS

Women have mitral stenosis four times more frequently than men.[5] Women may first become symptomatic with mitral stenosis during pregnancy when they decompensate hemodynamically.[9] Most patients remain asymptomatic for several years and may not have symptoms until the fourth or fifth decades of life.[9]

Mild dyspnea on exertion occurs as the most common symptom of mild mitral stenosis (valve area of 1.6 to 2.0 cm²). As mitral stenosis becomes more severe (valve area of 1 to 1.5 cm²), dyspnea, fatigue, paroxysmal nocturnal dyspnea, and atrial fibrillation may occur. When mitral stenosis becomes severe (valve area of 1 cm² or less), symptoms include fatigue and dyspnea with mild exertion or rest. Patients often have a cough or hoarseness and may have hemoptysis.[31] With advanced mitral stenosis, pulmonary hypertension and symptoms of right-sided heart failure occur (i.e., edema, hepatomegaly, ascites, elevated jugular venous pressure). Increased left atrial pressure, atrial fibrillation, and stagnation of left atrial blood flow can result in formation of mural thrombi, with resultant embolic events, including cerebral vascular accidents.

PHYSICAL ASSESSMENT

In severe mitral stenosis, on auscultation, there are four typical findings including: (1) an accentuated S_1; (2) an opening diastolic snap; (3) a mid-diastolic rumble noted best at the apex (in sinus rhythm, followed by presystolic accentuation); and (4) an increased pulmonic S_2 intensity associated with pulmonary hypertension (Table 27-2). It usually takes 2 or more years after the rheumatic episode for development of the typical murmur of mitral stenosis.[31]

Patients with mitral stenosis may exhibit malar blush (pinkish discoloration of the cheeks). Patients with severe mitral stenosis may have weak pulses secondary to reduced cardiac output. The apical pulse is tapping in quality and is nondisplaced. A lower left parasternal lift or heave due to right ventricular hypertrophy may be present. Cardiac rhythm is often irregular, indicating atrial fibrillation.

DIAGNOSTIC TESTS

Echocardiography is used in the evaluation of mitral stenosis to (1) quantify the valve area and gradient; (2) quantify the degree of mitral insufficiency; (3) define the degree of left atrial enlargement; (4) assess mitral annular calcification; (5) assess pulmonary artery pressures and degree of pulmonary hypertension; and (6) evaluate right- and left-sided ventricular function.

Cardiac catheterization is used less in diagnosis of mitral stenosis as echocardiography techniques improve. Cardiac catheterization does allow for accurate assessment of valve area and can also identify associated mitral regurgitation.

TABLE 27-2 | Diastolic Murmurs in Acquired Valvular Heart Disease

Origin of Murmur	Auscultatory Location and Radiation	Configuration	Quality and Frequency	Maneuvers That Alter Intensity
Aortic insufficiency	Third and fourth left intercostal spaces	Decrescendo S_1 $S_2 S_1$	Blowing High pitched	Increases with isometric exercise and squatting Decreases with amyl nitrate and Valsalva maneuver
Mitral stenosis	Apex	Decrescendo Opening snap OS S_1 S_2 S_1	Rumbling Low pitched	Increases with expiration, squatting, amyl nitrate, and isometric exercise Decreases with Valsalva maneuver
Pulmonic insufficiency	Second left intercostal space	Crescendo-decrescendo S_1 $S_2 S_1$	Blowing High pitched	Increases with inspiration and amyl nitrate Decreases with Valsalva maneuver
Tricuspid stenosis	Parasternal at left fourth and fifth intercostal spaces	Decrescendo S_1 $S_2 S_1$	Rumbling Low pitched	Increases with inspiration, squatting, and amyl nitrate Decreases with Valsalva maneuver

For patients with known or suspected CHD, coronary angiography can delineate coronary anatomy. Right heart catheterization can evaluate right heart and pulmonary artery pressures.

Electrocardiography is nonspecific and does not indicate the severity of mitral stenosis. If the patient remains in sinus rhythm and left atrial enlargement has occurred, characteristic P mitrale (broad, bifid P waves in leads II and V_1) may be identified. Right axis deviation and right ventricular hypertrophy may be noted in severe mitral stenosis. Atrial fibrillation is common in patients with long-standing mitral stenosis and is usually coarse in appearance.

Chest radiography correlates with the degree of mitral stenosis. As mitral stenosis becomes more severe, the chest radiograph demonstrates straightening of the left heart border due to left atrial enlargement, elevation of the left mainstem bronchus caused by distention of the left atrium, and distribution of blood flow from the lower to upper lobes. Although heart size remains normal, central pulmonary arteries become prominent. Kerley B lines and interstitial edema are often present.

MEDICAL MANAGEMENT

Patients who have asymptomatic mitral stenosis require only antibiotic prophylaxis. Patients with mild pulmonary congestion can be managed with diuretics alone. Beta blockers can be used to reduce heart rate and improve diastolic filling time. When patients have atrial fibrillation, digoxin, beta blockers, or calcium channel blockers can be used for ventricular response rate control. Patients with atrial fibrillation require anticoagulation to prevent thrombus formation in the atrium. Once the patient has symptoms of NYHA functional class III or IV despite adequate medical management, mechanical correction of mitral stenosis by balloon valvuloplasty or surgery should be done.

INTERVENTIONAL AND SURGICAL MANAGEMENT

Percutaneous Mitral Catheter Balloon Valvuloplasty. Percutaneous mitral catheter balloon valvuloplasty is an alternative, less invasive procedure than surgical treatment for mitral stenosis. Balloon valvuloplasty is performed in the cardiac catheterization laboratory by a cardiologist experienced with invasive techniques. A small balloon valvuloplasty catheter is introduced percutaneously at the femoral vein and passed into the right atrium. The catheter is then directed transseptally and positioned across the mitral valve. Inflation of either one large balloon (23 to 25 mm) or two smaller balloons (12 to 18 mm) stretches the valve leaflets (Fig. 27-3). Separation of the commissures and fracture of nodule calcium are the apparent mechanisms that improve valve movement and function.[4] The best results from this technique to date have been in patients with rheumatic mitral stenosis with commissural fusion. After the procedure, the patient may be maintained on chronic aspirin therapy or may not require any antithrombotic medicines. Prophylactic measures to prevent endocarditis remain necessary.[16,38,44] Results have been promising, with the average gradient reduction being approximately 18 to 6 mm Hg and, on the average, an increase in calculated valve area of 50% to 100%. The overall mortality rate from the procedure ranges from 0% to 4%. Complications include embolic events, regurgitation, and cardiac perforation. As many as 35% of patients are left with a persistent, residual atrial septal defect that is rarely large enough to precipitate right-sided heart failure.[4]

Surgical Treatment. Surgical replacement of the mitral valve is required when there is severe mitral regurgitation coexisting with mitral stenosis. Although some valves with mitral stenosis may be repaired by open commissurotomy

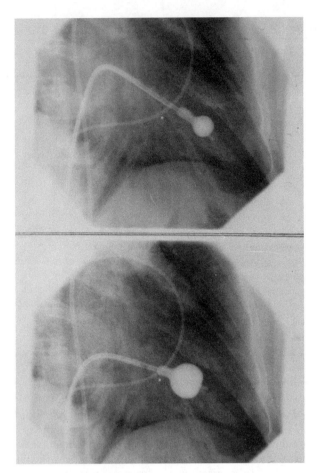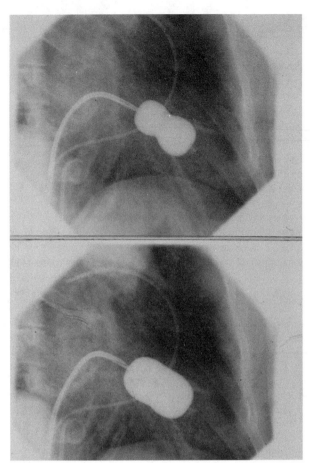

FIGURE 27-3 Mitral valvuloplasty: Inoue's technique. (*A*) Inflation of distal portion of balloon, which is then pulled back and anchored at the mitral valve. (*B*) Inflation of proximal and middle portions of balloon. At full inflation, the narrowed "waist" of the balloon has disappeared. (From Vahanian AS: Valvuloplasty. In Topol EJ, Califf RM, Isner JM et al [eds]: Textbook of Cardiovascular Medicine, p 2157. Philadelphia, Lippincott–Raven, 1998.)

and reconstruction, heavily calcified rheumatic mitral valves often are beyond the point of repair. The usual prosthetic valve of choice in mitral stenosis is a mechanical prosthesis because patients already require life-long anticoagulation because of atrial fibrillation. For young women who wish to become pregnant, a bioprosthesis may be recommended.

Tricuspid Valve Disease

Tricuspid stenosis is primarily due to rheumatic heart disease and has a pathologic process similar to that of mitral stenosis. The murmur of tricuspid stenosis is similar to the murmur of mitral stenosis, but it increases with inspiration.[11] Common symptoms of tricuspid stenosis include fatigue, minimal orthopnea, paroxysmal nocturnal dyspnea, hepatomegaly, and anasarca. Patients may have peripheral cyanosis, neck vein distention with prominent A waves, and a right ventricular lift.[4] The murmur of tricuspid stenosis is a diastolic decrescendo murmur along the left sternal border (Table 27-3).

Tricuspid regurgitation is primarily "functional" rather than structural and occurs secondary to dilation of the right ventricle and the annulus of the tricuspid valve. Functional tricuspid regurgitation frequently accompanies mitral stenosis and pulmonary hypertension because of the increased

pressure and volume load on the right ventricle. Symptoms include signs of ride-sided heart failure, large V waves in their right atrial or central venous pressure trace, and pulsatile neck veins. Other causes of tricuspid regurgitation include trauma, infective endocarditis, right atrial tumor, and tricuspid valve prolapse. The murmur of tricuspid regurgitation is a holosystolic murmur heard along the left sternal border (see Table 27-3).

Patients with mild tricuspid regurgitation normally do not require treatment. Severely stenotic tricuspid valves may undergo balloon valvuloplasty or may be surgically reconstructed or repaired rather than replaced. Surgical repair of the tricuspid valve most frequently occurs as an additional procedure for the patient with rheumatic heart disease undergoing a repair or replacement of the aortic or mitral valve, or both.

Prosthetic Valves

Prosthetic cardiac valves have been used since the mid-1960s to treat acquired valvular heart disease. Because no "perfect" prosthetic valve exists, the patient with valvular heart disease is managed medically as long as it is safely feasible. Timing of valve replacement depends on the patient's functional status, ventricular dysfunction, and the natural course of the lesion.

TABLE 27-3	Systolic Murmurs Related to Acquired Valvular Heart Disease			
Origin of Murmur	**Auscultatory Location and Radiation**	**Configuration**	**Quality and Frequency**	**Maneuvers That Alter Intensity**
Aortic stenosis	Right second intercostal space. Radiates to carotid arteries and apex	Crescendo-decrescendo "Diamond shaped" S_1 ◆ S_2	Harsh High pitched	Increases with squatting, amyl nitrate Decreases with standing, Valsalva maneuver, and isometric exercise
Mitral regurgitation	Apex. Radiates to axilla and back	Holosystolic S_1 ▬ S_2	Harsh or blowing High pitched	Increases with expiration, squatting, and isometric exercise Decreases with Valsalva maneuver, standing, and amyl nitrate
Mitral valve prolapse	Apex. Radiates to axilla and back	Mid- to late systolic, with systolic click S_1 click S_2	Harsh High pitched	Increases with Valsalva maneuver, amyl nitrate, and inspiration Decreases with squatting, standing, and isometric exercise
Tricuspid regurgitation	Fourth and fifth left intercostal spaces. Radiates to right parasternal border	Holosystolic S_1 ▬ S_2	Harsh High pitched	Increases with amyl nitrate and inspiration Decreases with Valsalva maneuver and standing
Pulmonic stenosis	Second left intercostal space. Radiates to back	Crescendo-decrescendo "Diamond shaped" S_1 ◆ S_2	Harsh High Pitched	Increases with amyl nitrate, squatting, and inspiration Decreases with Valsalva maneuver and standing

Before a decision is made to use a particular valve, factors in valve design, specifically durability, thrombogenic potential, and hemodynamic properties, are weighed against annulus size and certain clinical conditions such as the desirability of long-term anticoagulation. Table 27-4 summarizes the characteristics considered in selection of prosthetic valves. Because of their proven durability, mechanical valves are most often chosen for patients younger than 65 to 70 years of age, unless contraindicated (e.g., previous bleeding problems, desire to become pregnant, or poor compliance with medication and follow-up). Prosthetic heart valves differ in design, echocardiography image, and radiologic appearance (Fig. 27-4).

MECHANICAL VALVES

Mechanical (nonbiologic) valves have excellent durability but are usually thrombogenic. Bileaflet and tilting-disk valves are the mechanical valves in common use today. Caged-ball valves are used less frequently in the United States, but may be used in other areas of the world. In patients with aneurysm or dissection of the ascending aorta, composite grafts of conduit and mechanical valves may be used.

Bileaflet valves, such as St. Jude, ATS (Advancing the Standard), Edwards Tekna, and the CarboMedic are low-profile valves that have centrally mounted leaflets attached to the seating ring with butterfly hinges. These hinges allow the leaflets to open to 85 degrees, making these valves the least obstructive of the mechanical valves. Made of pyrolytic carbon, these valves produce nearly central flow with little turbulence.[21] The two leaflets swing open in systole, resulting in three separate flow areas.[26] With adequate anticoagulation, thromboembolic risk is low with bileaflet valves.

The *tilting-disk valve* is a low-profile valve consisting of a disk that sits in a seating ring; the flat or convexoconcave disk tilts in response to pressure changes. The

TABLE 27-4	Selection of Type of Prosthetic Valve Based on Patient Characteristics	
Biologic Valve		**Mechanical Valve**
History of bleeding		Age <65 y
Inability to take warfarin		Already on anticoagulation
Desire to become pregnant		History of embolic cerebral vascular accident
History of thrombosis with mechanical valve		History of atrial fibrillation
Age >65 y		

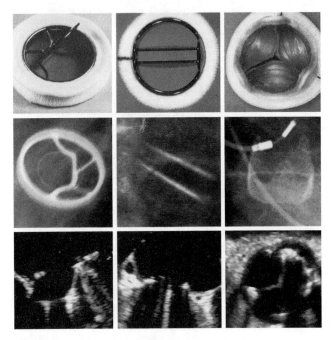

FIGURE 27-4 Photographic (*top row*), radiographic (*middle row*), and echocardiographic (*bottom row*) appearance of prosthetic valves. From left to right: Bjork-Shiley single tilting disk, St. Jude's Medical bileaflet mechanical valve, and Carpentier-Edwards xenograft (radiographs courtesy of Dr. Carolyn van Dyke). (Adapted from Garcia ML: Prosthetic valve disease. In Topol EJ, Califf RM, Isner JM et al [eds]: Textbook of Cardiovascular Medicine, p 580. Philadelphia, Lippincott–Raven, 1998.)

Medtronic Hall valve is a tilting-disk valve commonly used today. Tilting-disk valves open to an angle of 60 to 75 degrees in relation to the seating ring. When open, tilting-disk valves produce a minor and major orifice for blood to pass through. Tilting disks have more central flow, but usually more turbulence, than caged-ball valves. Tilting disks close with an audible click. The technology for production of tilting-disk valves has evolved so that a single piece of metal is used to avoid welded struts. In the past, welded struts fractured and caused fatal results, as did the older Bjork-Shiley convexoconcave valve (no longer manufactured or implanted).[21]

Caged-ball valves have been used since the 1960s and have an excellent durability record. Changes in pressure cause the ball to move forward and back within its caged structure. Flow is directed laterally through the valve rather than centrally. Because of its high profile, the caged-ball valve prosthesis can become obstructive, especially when used in patients with small aortic roots or small left ventricles. The Starr-Edwards and Sutter (formerly Smeloff-Cutter) are two of the most common caged-ball valves used. Caged-ball prostheses have been largely abandoned in favor of lower profile bileaflet valves.

TISSUE VALVES

Tissue (biologic) valves are characterized by having low rates of thrombotic episodes associated with their use. Porcine or bovine tissue is strengthened and made nonviable by treat-

ment with glutaraldehyde. Homografts are tissue valves from cadavers. They are preserved cryogenically, but are difficult to procure, and their longevity has not been well proven. The main advantages of tissue valves are the associated low rates of thromboembolism and the subsequent decrease in patient morbidity when anticoagulant therapy is not required. Non-thrombogenicity is particularly important for those patients in whom long-term anticoagulation should be avoided, such as children, young adult women, patients older than 70 years of age, or people with a history of bleeding.

The Hancock porcine valve and the Carpentier-Edwards porcine valve are xenografts using preserved porcine aortic valves mounted on a stent. More recently, stentless bioprosthetic xenograft valves have been developed to improve the durability and enhance the hemodynamic performance of porcine aortic valves. Because of the structural similarity to aortic allografts, stentless bioprostheses adapt to the aortic root and reproduce the anatomy of the native aortic valve.[34] In the United States, the Toronto stentless porcine valve has demonstrated excellent freedom from valve-related events.[34] Use of stentless aortic bioprostheses has resulted in enhanced survival and hemodynamic superiority.[18] It is expected that reducing mechanical stress on valve leaflets, and the associated degeneration of the bioprosthesis, may be slowed. Thus, stentless xenografts may prove more durable than commonly used stented valves.[34] The Carpentier-Edwards pericardial bioprosthesis is made of leaflets fashioned from bovine pericardium fixed without pressure in glutaraldehyde.

Homografts or *allografts* from human cadavers are virtually free of any associated thrombosis. They are especially useful in patients with small aortic roots or in patients with active endocarditis. Earlier homografts were preserved with glutaraldehyde and demonstrated early failure. Homografts are now stored "fresh" after harvesting in an antibiotic solution and are then cryopreserved, increasing their longevity to at least 10 years. Valve failure is uncommon and usually the result of progressive valve incompetence.[19] Even though the homografts are human tissue, there does not appear to be any problem with antigenicity.[51] Aortic allografts have demonstrated excellent freedom from thromboembolism, endocarditis, and progressive valve incompetence.[19] Because of lack of availability, use of homografts has been limited.

In the *Ross procedure* (also known as pulmonary autograft), the aortic valve is replaced with a pulmonary autograft, and the native pulmonary valve is replaced with a pulmonic allograft. Although this procedure was originally developed for pediatric application, it has been expanded to adult surgery as well. In patients undergoing the Ross procedure, the native pulmonary valve is excised and then implanted in the aortic position (autograft); a pulmonary homograft (allograft) is implanted into the pulmonic position (Fig. 27-5). The pulmonary autograft has been shown to be resistant to degeneration and calcification.[39] Potential clinical and hemodynamic advantages of the pulmonary autograft over the aortic homograft include potential for growth when used in the pediatric population, increased cellular viability, enhanced durability, and possibly internal innervation of the cusps.[45] Although the Ross procedure is gaining acceptance, especially in young adults who wish to avoid anticoagulation, there is concern that it offers no better result than the aortic

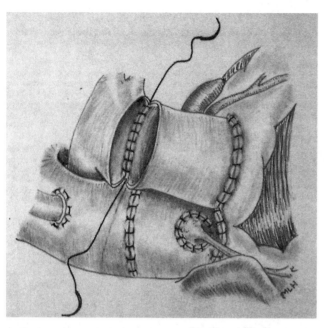

FIGURE 27-5 Illustration of Ross procedure. Suture line of pulmonary homograft is shown. (From Elkins RC: Valve repair and valve replacement in children, including the Ross procedure. In Kaiser LR, Kron IL, Spray TL [eds]: Mastery of Cardiothoracic Surgery, p 947. Philadelphia, Lippincott–Raven, 1998.)

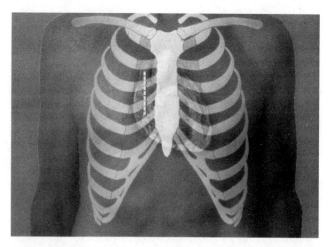

FIGURE 27-6 Example of one approach to minimally invasive mitral valve surgery. An 8- to 10-cm incision is made from the lower border of the second costal cartilage to the upper border of the fifth costal cartilage. (From Alpert JS, Sabick J, Cosgrove DM: Mitral valve disease. In Topol EJ, Califf RM, Isner JM et al [eds]: Textbook of Cardiovascular Medicine, p 526. Philadelphia, Lippincott–Raven, 1998.)

homograft, which is a simpler procedure, with less morbidity. Pulmonary autografts require significantly longer operating time but do not seem to affect early and midterm outcomes compared with aortic homografts.[45]

MINIMALLY INVASIVE VALVE SURGERY

Minimally invasive valve surgery is now used for both aortic valve replacement and mitral valve repair and replacement. Minimally invasive surgical approaches are possible because a wide assortment of technological advances, such as endoscopic and surgical equipment, have been developed. Although patients undergoing minimally invasive valve surgery still require cardiopulmonary bypass, classic median sternotomy may be avoided, thus reducing pain, improving cosmetic results, and expediting recovery. These patients have a lower requirement for erythrocytes, express greater satisfaction, and have lower hospital charges (approximately 20% less than in patients with standard mitral valve and aortic valve approaches).[13] As minimally invasive valve surgery continues to evolve, it will likely become a mainstay in the treatment of valvular heart surgery.

Aortic valve replacement can be done through an upper "T" ministernotomy without intraoperative difficulties. Postoperative pain is reduced and recovery is expedited, with patients discharged to home as early as postoperative day 3.[27] Two minimally invasive techniques for mitral valve surgery have been used: a right parasternal approach (Fig. 27-6) developed at the Cleveland Clinic, and a minithoracotomy.[12] Compared with patients with median sternotomy, patients undergoing mitral valve replacement through the right parasternal approach had a shortened length of stay

and reduced direct hospital costs.[15] The minithoracotomy approach with video assistance can be used safely in patients undergoing mitral valve repair or replacement; compared with standard techniques, the minithoracotomy resulted in less morbidity, earlier discharge, and lower cost.[12]

COMPLICATIONS OF PROSTHETIC VALVES

Thromboembolism remains the most common complication of patients with prosthetic valves. Anticoagulant therapy with warfarin is begun on all patients 48 hours after surgery and continued for 6 to 12 weeks. All patients with mechanical valves require life-long anticoagulation because of the risk of thrombosis and embolization. The highest thromboembolic risk for both mechanical and biologic valves occurs in the first few days to months after implantation, before the valve is fully endothelialized. Even with anticoagulation, the risk of thromboembolism is 1% to 2% per year for patients with mechanical valves.[35] Optimal anticoagulation recommended for patients with mechanical valves is a target international normalized ratio of 3.0 to 4.0.[8] Of mechanical valves, the caged-ball valves have the highest rate of thromboembolism and the St. Jude's valves have the lowest.[25] Tissue valves other than homografts also usually require anticoagulation for 6 to 12 weeks after surgery, after which patients may be converted to aspirin. The overall risk of thromboembolism with biologic valves is 0.6% to 0.7% per year.[35] Homografts or the Ross procedure require no anticoagulation.

Prosthetic valvular thrombosis is a serious complication and can result in severe hemodynamic compromise. In patients with prosthetic valves who are not anticoagulated into a therapeutic range, thrombosis of the prosthetic valve can occur. Valve thrombosis can occur with either mechanical or bioprosthetic heart valves, but occurs most often in prosthetic valves in the mitral position.[25] Thrombus or pannus formation on the valve may occlude the orifice or entrap the pivoting mechanisms, causing acute stenosis or regurgitation. Symptoms of valve thrombosis include embolic events and CHF. Valve thrombosis can be diagnosed with transesophageal echocardiography.[35] Emergent valve replacement usually is indicated for large thrombi, but if the patient is not a surgical candidate, thrombolytic agents may be used.[25]

The rate of *bacterial endocarditis* is approximately 3% the first year after valve replacement and 0.5% each year thereafter.[35] Although symptoms of prosthetic valve endocarditis are similar to those of native valve endocarditis, the infection may be difficult to control with antibiotics alone because of prosthetic material involved.

Early prosthetic valve endocarditis (within the first 60 days) carries a high mortality rate of 20% to 70%.[25] The most common organism in early prosthetic valve endocarditis is *Staphylococcus epidermidis*. Eighty percent of these staphylococci are methicillin resistant, suggesting that these infections may be nosocomial in nature.[25] Fever, heart failure, new murmur, and embolic events are common manifestations. *Late prosthetic valve endocarditis* (≥60 days after surgery) occurs most commonly in patients with bioprosthetic valves in the aortic position.[25] Urinary infection, dental procedures, and urologic procedures are the most common sources identified.[25]

Compared with mitral valve endocarditis, medical treatment of prosthetic valve endocarditis requires a longer course of antibiotic therapy and is less successful.[25] For patients who do not respond to antibiotic therapy or who have local invasion of the annulus, embolic events, fungal infection, heart failure, or prosthetic valve dysfunction, repeat valvular replacement is indicated.[35]

Prosthesis malfunction is uncommon for the first 10 years after mechanical valve implantation. The best known problems with mechanical failures were those affecting the Bjork-Shiley convexoconcave tilting-disk valves first manufactured in 1978, with the peak incidence of valve failure in the 1981 to 1982 models. Subsequent modifications improved the valve area but also increased stress forces. As a result, by 1994, 564 strut fractures were reported in these Bjork-Shiley valves; two-thirds of those strut fractures were fatal.[25] Although these valves have been withdrawn from the market, approximately 40,000 had been implanted worldwide. Because acute valve strut fracture can be fatal, patients with these valves should be evaluated for partial strut fracture using high-resolution cineradiography and should be considered for valve replacement.[25]

Valve degeneration is the primary complication of patients with tissue prostheses. Degeneration of biologic prostheses can occur as lipid or calcium deposits cause valve cusps to stiffen and stenose. The incidence of structural failure requiring replacement is approximately 30% at 10 years after valve replacement.[25] Failure of tissue valves often occurs slowly over months to years and presents as progressive heart failure. Prosthetic valve degeneration and failure are most easily diagnosed with echocardiography.

Paravalvular leaks between the prosthetic ring and the annulus occur because of tearing of the suture line, sponta-neously or after infection. Presence of a new murmur and signs of heart failure alert the clinician to paravalvular leaks. The patient's clinical course should be followed; when the leak becomes significant, surgical repair or replacement is indicated. Hemolysis may also accompany paravalvular leaks.

Hemolytic anemia is a consequence of shortened red cell survival time in all patients with prosthetic valves. Movement of the valve ball or disk causes varying degrees of destruction of the red blood cells. Hemolysis may also occur with paravalvular leak. Commonly, hemolysis is mild and the patient can compensate by increasing red blood cell production. Rarely, hemolytic anemia occurs. Chronic intravascular hemolysis results in loss of iron in the urine; iron deficiency anemia may result after several years.

Mitral Insufficiency

ETIOLOGY

Mitral insufficiency (also termed *regurgitation*) may be either chronic or acute (Table 27-5). Acute mitral regurgitation is caused by MI, mitral valve prolapse, and endocarditis.[32] Chronic mitral regurgitation may be the result of a number of abnormalities, including rheumatic heart disease, ischemic damage to the subvalvular apparatus, infective endocarditis, myxomatous degeneration, hypertrophic cardiomyopathy, or marked left ventricular dilation.[11,23]

PATHOLOGY

Primary mitral regurgitation occurs when the mitral valve annulus, leaflets, chordae, or papillary muscles are affected by ischemia, collagen disease, infection, calcification, trauma, or degenerative changes, causing incompetent

TABLE 27-5	Etiologies of Acquired Mitral Regurgiation
Chronic Mitral Regurgitation	**Acute Mitral Regurgitation**
Rheumatic heart disease	Myocardial infarction causing:
Ischemia to subvalvular apparatus	Papillary muscle rupture or dysfunction
Infective endocarditis	Rupture of chordae
Myxomatous degeneration	Infective endocarditis
Hypertrophic cardiomyopathy	Trauma
Left ventricular dilation	Myxomatous degeneration with chordal rupture
Systemic lupus erythematosus	
Marfan's syndrome	
Calcification of annulus	
Ankylosing spondylitis	
Scleroderma	
Ehlers-Danlos syndrome	
Prosthetic paravalvular leak	
Deterioration of prosthetic mitral valve	

coaptation of the mitral leaflets. Secondary mitral regurgitation occurs with ventricular dilation when ventricular geometry is changed, causing malalignment of the papillary muscles. Although it is sometimes difficult to distinguish between primary and secondary regurgitation, primary regurgitation is often more severe than insufficiency secondary to annular dilation.[4]

PATHOPHYSIOLOGY

Mitral regurgitation occurs as the result of inadequate closure of the mitral valve, allowing regurgitant flow back into the left atrium during each left ventricular systole. Its severity depends on the volume of regurgitant flow. Regurgitant flow into the left atrium reduces forward flow, stroke volume, and cardiac output.[31] Regurgitant flow also increases left atrial pressure, causing left atrial dilation and pulmonary congestion. During diastole, the regurgitant volume returns to the left ventricle and increases its volume load.

In chronic mitral regurgitation, persistent volume overload results in progressive ventricular dilation and mild hypertrophy. Although ventricular dilation and hypertrophy are initially compensatory, over time, chronic volume overload may result in decreased systolic function of the left ventricle and lead to heart failure.[31] In acute mitral regurgitation, neither the left atrium nor ventricle have had sufficient time to adjust to the increased volume load. Left atrial pressure rises quickly, resulting in pulmonary congestion and edema.

CLINICAL MANIFESTATIONS

Patients in acute versus chronic mitral regurgitation vary in both clinical presentation and physical examination findings. In acute mitral regurgitation, symptoms progress rapidly. Symptoms are typically those of left ventricular failure. The patient is usually tachycardic to compensate for the reduced forward stroke volume. Patients are dyspneic secondary to pulmonary congestion and edema; they are often orthopneic and have paroxysmal nocturnal dyspnea and poor exercise tolerance. Patients may also have signs of biventricular failure because right-sided failure may occur secondary to pulmonary hypertension. Patients in acute mitral regurgitation often present acutely to the emergency room with complaints of inability to breathe. New-onset atrial fibrillation can occur. Patients with ischemic mitral insufficiency or papillary muscle rupture may also complain of chest pain.

During the compensatory phase of chronic mitral regurgitation, patients may be relatively asymptomatic for years. Initial signs of mitral regurgitation include exertional dyspnea, orthopnea, paroxysmal nocturnal dyspnea, cough, palpitations, new atrial fibrillation, and lower extremity edema. Symptoms may occur so gradually that patients may present subacutely to the clinic with complaints as vague as fatigue and inability to sleep.

PHYSICAL ASSESSMENT

On examination, the most easily noted characteristic of either chronic or acute mitral regurgitation is the holosystolic murmur, which is heard best at the apex and radiates to the axilla (see Table 27-3). The murmur of mitral regurgitation may vary somewhat depending on the underlying etiology. Patients may have an S_3 gallop in moderate to severe regurgitation due to high diastolic flow into the ventricle. An S_4 gallop is uncommon in chronic mitral regurgitation; however, in acute mitral regurgitation, an S_4 gallop is common because the left atrium and ventricle are noncompliant. The patient with rheumatic heart disease may also have a diastolic murmur related to coexisting mitral stenosis.

Because of left ventricular dilation, patients with chronic mitral regurgitation have an easily palpated, left laterally displaced point of maximal impulse. Patients with a markedly enlarged left atrium may have a left parasternal lift because of anterior displacement of the apex. Patients with acute or decompensated chronic mitral regurgitation may be anxious and diaphoretic because of left ventricular failure. Blood pressure may be normal to low and pulse pressure may be narrowed secondary to decreased stroke volume. Jugular venous pressure can be normal or elevated in the patient with right-sided heart failure. Breath sounds can range from basilar crackles to dullness secondary to pleural effusion. In addition, hepatosplenomegaly, hepatojugular reflux, peripheral edema, and ascites may be present in the patient with right-sided heart failure.

DIAGNOSTIC TESTS

Transthoracic echocardiography can identify the structural cause of the mitral regurgitation as well as gauge left atrial size, left ventricular dimensions and performance, pulmonary artery pressures, and right heart function. Color flow Doppler allows for assessment of severity of regurgitation. *Transesophageal echocardiography* is better than transthoracic echocardiography for defining mitral valve anatomy and discriminating prosthetic valves and paravalvular leaks.

Cardiac catheterization is used to identify coexisting coronary artery disease and to grade the severity of mitral regurgitation. Left ventriculography can assess left ventricular function and distinguish any wall motion abnormalities. Right heart catheterization quantifies pulmonary artery pressures and allows for evaluation of the large V waves in the pulmonary artery wedge tracing (see Chapter 18).

Electrocardiography in chronic mitral regurgitation may demonstrate left ventricular hypertrophy and left atrial enlargement or P mitrale (characterized by M-shaped P waves). Atrial fibrillation may occur with both acute and chronic mitral regurgitation. Patients with ischemic papillary muscle dysfunction may demonstrate ischemic changes, and patients with papillary muscle rupture can show acute inferior, posterior, or anterior MI.

Chest radiography in chronic mitral regurgitation shows left ventricular hypertrophy and left atrial enlargement. Calcification of the mitral valve annulus and apparatus may also be seen. In acute or decompensated chronic mitral regurgitation, pulmonary vascular redistribution and pulmonary edema can be observed. If the heart is normal sized, the degree of mitral regurgitation is so mild or so acute that eccentric left ventricular hypertrophy has not had time to develop.

MEDICAL MANAGEMENT

Medical therapy for mitral regurgitation is geared toward afterload reduction to promote forward flow and minimize regurgitation back into the left atrium and pulmonary vasculature. In patients with acute or decompensated chronic mitral regurgitation, intravenous vasodilators such as nitroprusside can reduce filling pressures and ventricular cavity size, and promote forward flow with afterload reduction. Intravenous diuretics are used to reduce volume overload. In acutely ill patients refractory to medications, intra-aortic balloon counterpulsation can be used further to reduce afterload, while maintaining coronary perfusion with diastolic augmentation.

In patients with chronic mitral regurgitation or those in acute heart failure who are being weaned from intravenous inotropes and vasodilators, other afterload-reducing agents, such as angiotensin-converting enzyme (ACE) inhibitors, nitrates, or hydralazine may be used. Chronic and acute volume overload can be treated by diuretics. Some practitioners continue to advocate the use of digoxin, especially for patients in atrial fibrillation. In the patient with chronic but compensated mitral valve regurgitation, mitral surgery can be safely deferred or avoided. The patient should be carefully monitored, however, and referred for mitral valve repair or replacement before significant left ventricular dysfunction or pulmonary hypertension occur.

SURGICAL MANAGEMENT

Surgical Intervention. Two surgical approaches are used to treat mitral regurgitation. Mitral valve repair uses reconstructive techniques as well as a rigid prosthetic ring to repair the mitral valve apparatus, thus sparing the valve and avoiding the consequences of valve replacement (Fig. 27-7). Mitral valve replacement involves implantation of a prosthetic valve with attempted preservation of at least part of the mitral valve apparatus, which contributes to left ventricular function (Fig. 27-8).

In patients with chronic mitral regurgitation, mitral replacement should occur before the patient has had irreversible left ventricular dysfunction. Mitral valve replacement or repair can preserve left ventricular function and ejection fraction. Patients with NYHA class II symptoms should be considered for surgery. Factors contributing to increased operative risk include reduced left ventricular ejection fraction, increased left ventricular end-systolic volume, older age, concomitant coronary artery disease, previous cardiac surgery, and pulmonary hypertension.[4,22]

Mitral Valve Repair. In selected patients, mitral valve repair may be undertaken for patients with mitral insufficiency as an alternative to replacement. Surgical techniques involve reconstructing the leaflets and annulus in such a way as to narrow the orifice. These procedures consist of direct suture of the valve cusps, repair of the elongated or ruptured chordae tendineae (chordoplasty), or repair of the valve annulus (annuloplasty). With an annuloplasty, the incompetent valve is remodeled using a ring prosthesis attached to the leaflets and the annulus.

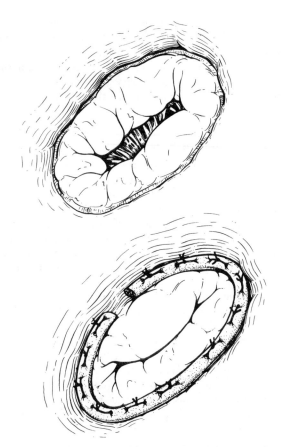

FIGURE 27-7 (*Top*) Regurgitant mitral valve (note large primary orifice). (*Bottom*) Completed mitral valve annuloplasty with ring sutured in place.

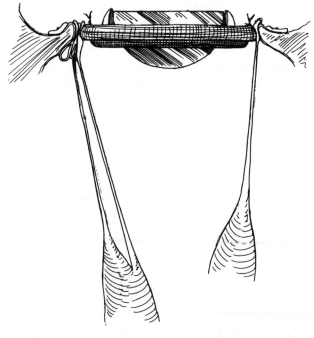

FIGURE 27-8 Valve replacement with chordal preservation. (From Chitwood WR: Mitral valve repair: Ischemic. In Kaiser LR, Kron IL, Spray TL [eds]: Mastery of Cardiothoracic Surgery, p 321. Philadelphia, Lippincott–Raven, 1998.)

Mitral Valve Replacement. In patients with acute mitral regurgitation secondary to MI, coronary angiography should be done to define coronary anatomy for concomitant coronary bypass surgery at the time of mitral valve repair or replacement. In patients with acute mitral regurgitation secondary to MI, the mortality rate can be as high as 50% secondary to acute left ventricular failure.[22]

Mitral Valve Prolapse

ETIOLOGY

Mitral valve prolapse refers to a number of conditions in which one or both of the mitral valve leaflets becomes superior to the plane of the annulus during systole.[5] The posterior leaflet is most often affected. Mitral valve prolapse is also known as Barlow's syndrome or click-murmur syndrome. It is the most common cause of significant isolated mitral regurgitation[30] and has been reported to be one of the most common heart disorders, with estimates commonly ranging from 5% to 10% of the U.S. population.[31] Although mitral valve prolapse occurs most commonly in women, with a peak incidence in the fourth decade of life, severe mitral regurgitation associated with mitral valve prolapse is more common in men.[22] The most common cause of mitral valve prolapse is myxomatous degeneration. Marfan's syndrome, Ehlers-Danlos syndrome, rheumatic heart disease, and ischemic papillary muscle dysfunction also cause mitral valve prolapse. In addition, mitral valve prolapse has a hereditary component transmitted as an autosomal dominant trait.[4]

PATHOLOGY

Patients with mitral valve prolapse have redundant myxomatous tissue with excess deposits of proteoglycans in the middle or spongiosa layer of the valve.

Histologically, collagen fragmentation and disorganization as well as elastic fiber are present. Acid mucopolysaccharide material accumulates in the valve leaflets. The mitral valve leaflets, annulus, and chordae tendineae may also demonstrate disrupted collagen structure and extensive myxomatous change. Myxomatous changes may also occur in the tricuspid, aortic, and pulmonic valves.[1]

PATHOPHYSIOLOGY

Enlargement of the valve leaflets related to myxomatous degeneration causes systolic prolapse of one or both leaflets into the left atrium. Patients with mitral valve prolapse may have mitral regurgitation ranging in severity from none to severe. Persistent billowing of the valve causes stress to the underlying chordae and papillary muscles. Progressive mitral valvular degeneration can result in increasingly severe mitral regurgitation. If chordal rupture occurs, severe mitral regurgitation develops.

Supraventricular tachycardias (i.e., premature atrial contractions and paroxysmal supraventricular tachycardias) and ventricular arrhythmias may occur in patients with mitral valve prolapse. Although some patients with mitral valve prolapse have had sudden cardiac death, it is unclear what

role mitral valve prolapse has in the etiology. Some investigators believe that patients with mitral valve prolapse, history of syncope, complex ventricular arrhythmias, significant mitral regurgitation, and prolonged QT interval are at increased risk for sudden death.[33] Patients with mitral valve prolapse may also have autonomic nervous system dysfunction; specifically, midbrain control of adrenergic and vagal responses may be abnormal. Heightened sympathetic nervous system tone may lead to a decease in left ventricular preload, resulting in mitral valve prolapse.[1]

CLINICAL MANIFESTATIONS

Most patients with mitral valve prolapse are asymptomatic. Patients may complain of sharp, localized chest pain that is usually brief in duration. Although the etiology of this chest pain is unclear if the patient does not have CHD, some authorities have suggested that the chest pain is cardiac in origin and is related to abnormal traction and tension on the papillary muscles.[37] Patients may have equivocal complaints of anxiety, fatigue, palpitations, and orthostatic hypotension. As mitral regurgitation progresses, patients may note increasing dyspnea, fatigue, decreased exercise tolerance, orthopnea, and paroxysmal nocturnal dyspnea. Ruptured chordae with leaflet flail and acute mitral regurgitation result in symptoms of severe left ventricular failure.

PHYSICAL ASSESSMENT

The classic auscultatory finding of mitral valve prolapse is mid-systolic click with mid- to late systolic murmur (see Table 27-3). The click of mitral valve prolapse occurs when the elongated mitral valve apparatus reaches the end of its tether in mid-systole.[9] The murmur occurs secondary to regurgitant flow when the mitral valve leaflets fail to approximate. Patients with mitral valve prolapse may have either the murmur or click, or both. Findings may also vary over time. When the degree of mitral regurgitation is mild to moderate or less, heart rate and blood pressure may be normal. Additional physical findings may include thin body habitus, pectus excavatum, straight-back syndrome, and scoliosis.

DIAGNOSTIC TESTS

Echocardiography plays a key role in the diagnosis of mitral valve prolapse. Abnormal systolic motion of one or both of the mitral valve leaflets superior to the annular plane can be seen (Fig. 27-9). Doppler echocardiography gives additional evidence of valve regurgitation.

Cardiac catheterization can be used to rule out CHD as the origin of chest pain. Left ventriculography can demonstrate abnormal motion of the mitral valve and help determine the degree of regurgitation.

Electrocardiography is nondiagnostic. The ECG may be normal or have nonspecific ST-T–wave changes in the inferior leads (II, III, and aVF) and occasionally in the anterolateral leads (V_4 through V_6). The ST-T–wave changes may become more notable with exercise. Some have suggested that these changes occur secondary to ischemia from increased tension on the papillary muscles.[41] Premature atrial and ventricular complexes may also be identified

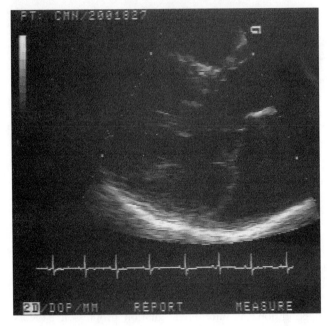

A

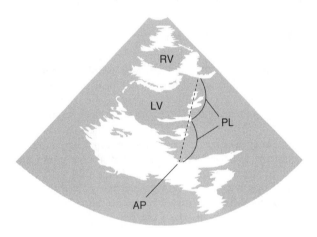

B

FIGURE 27-9 (*A*) Long-axis echocardiographic view of mitral valve with bileaflet prolapse above the annular plane into the left atrium. (*B*) Illustration corresponding to echocardiogram. RV, right ventricle; LV, left ventricle; AP, annular plane; PL, prolapsing leaflet.

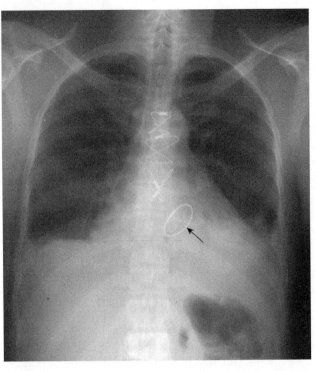

FIGURE 27-10 Chest radiograph of 51-year-old man with history of mitral valve prolapse and repair (note annuloplasty ring marked with *arrow*). Patient's valve repair has failed and his mitral regurgitation is now severe. Patient is now in severe heart failure with notable bilateral pleural effusions and cardiomegaly.

Exercise testing may be used to help rule out the etiology of the chest pain.

Chest radiography is often normal and is usually nondiagnostic for mitral valve prolapse. Patients with acute mitral regurgitation secondary to chordal rupture have pulmonary congestion but not cardiomegaly. Patients with chronic severe mitral regurgitation have an enlarged cardiac silhouette secondary to left atrial and left ventricular enlargement in addition to pulmonary congestion (Fig. 27-10).

MEDICAL AND SURGICAL MANAGEMENT

Medical Treatment. Asymptomatic patients with mitral valve prolapse require no therapy other than antibiotic prophylaxis. Opinions remain divided on whether patients with isolated click without murmur require antibiotic prophylaxis. Patients with the murmur of mitral regurgitation or echocardiographic evidence of mitral regurgitation are recommended to have antibiotic prophylaxis. Beta blockers or calcium channel blockers may be used to help alleviate palpitations or chest pain syndrome.

Surgical Treatment. Patients with mitral valve prolapse and severe mitral regurgitation or flail leaflet(s) should be evaluated for surgery. They can often undergo repair rather than replacement. For discussion of surgical options, refer to the section on surgical intervention for mitral regurgitation.

Prognosis. Mitral valve prolapse is usually a benign condition. Most patients remain asymptomatic for their entire lives. However, in a small subset of patients, sudden cardiac death may occur secondary to arrhythmias. Patients with palpitations, syncope, or dizziness should be further evaluated and considered for treatment of arrhythmias.[47]

Aortic Stenosis

ETIOLOGY

Aortic stenosis is characterized by obstruction of the left ventricular outflow tract. Most commonly, left ventricular outflow obstruction is valvular, but it may be either supravalvular or subvalvular. The age at which aortic stenosis becomes symptomatic is determined by the underlying cause. Aortic stenosis occurring from age 1 to 30 years usually represents congenital aortic stenosis. Aortic stenosis presenting at the ages of 40 to 60 years is primarily rheumatic in origin or secondary to calcific aortic stenosis in a congenitally bicusp aortic valve. Past the age of 60 to 70 years, calcific degenerative stenosis is the most prevalent etiology. Of the causes of aortic stenosis, senile/degenerative calcific aortic stenosis is most common.

PATHOLOGY

In senile/degenerative calcific aortic stenosis, cumulative wear and tear leads to calcification on an otherwise normal aortic valve. Calcific deposits prevent the cusps from opening normally in systole, resulting in stenosis. Both hypercholesterolemia and diabetes are risk factors for development of senile/degenerative calcific aortic stenosis.[4] In patients with congenitally bicuspid aortic valves, abnormal flow through the valve leads to calcium deposition and restriction of cusp opening. In rheumatic aortic stenosis, inflammation and fibrosis of the valve result in fusion of the commisures as well as calcified masses in the aortic cusp.[11]

PATHOPHYSIOLOGY

Aortic stenosis typically progresses over a period of years. As the valve cusps become less mobile, the valve orifice decreases in size, resulting in an increasingly higher left ventricular systolic pressure necessary to eject blood across the stenosed valve. This increased left ventricular afterload results first in compensatory concentric left ventricular hypertrophy. Although initially adaptive in aortic stenosis, left ventricular hypertrophy leads to decreased ventricular compliance and diastolic dysfunction. As aortic stenosis becomes severe, left ventricular systolic function may also decline, resulting in CHF. Late in the course, any coexisting mitral regurgitation increases because of an increased pressure gradient, which drives blood from the left ventricle into the left atrium.[4]

Angina may result even in the absence of CHD because of an imbalance in myocardial oxygen supply and demand. Myocardial oxygen demand is increased secondary to increased left ventricular wall stress and muscle mass. Myocardial oxygen delivery is reduced as a result of decreased coronary perfusion pressure.

Syncope or near syncope can result secondary to reduced cerebral perfusion pressure, inappropriate left ventricular baroreceptor response, or arrhythmia. Orthostatic blood pressure changes may occur during exertion when arterial pressure drops due to systemic vasodilation in the setting of a fixed cardiac output. Increased left ventricular pressure may result in inappropriate baroreceptor response. Rapid atrial arrhythmias or ventricular arrhythmias may also cause "graying out" spells or frank syncopal episodes.[4]

CLINICAL MANIFESTATIONS

Patients with mild to moderate aortic stenosis are usually asymptomatic. As severe aortic stenosis develops, the most common initial complaint is dyspnea on exertion, followed by angina and near syncope or syncope. CHF also may occur as a result of ventricular dysfunction or increasing mitral regurgitation. Less commonly, sudden death, probably due to ventricular fibrillation, may be the presenting clinical feature. Aortic stenosis is rated in severity by valve area, with valve areas of greater than 1.5 cm², 1.1 to 1.5 cm², and less than or equal to 0.8 to 1.0 cm² described as mild, moderate, and severe stenosis, respectively.[43]

PHYSICAL ASSESSMENT

Aortic stenosis is most readily detected by auscultation of its classic mid-systolic (systolic ejection) murmur (see Table 27-3). As aortic stenosis progresses, the murmur peaks progressively later in systole and decreases in intensity as cardiac output falls. The murmur may decrease or disappear over the sternum and reappear at the apex, causing the incorrect impression of mitral regurgitation (Gallivardin's phenomenon).[9] An S_4 gallop is usually present. The point of maximal intensity is sustained but may not be displaced.

Blood pressure is normal to hypertensive until late in the disease progress. Jugular venous pressure is normal in most patients except those with severe aortic stenosis associated with heart failure. Reduction in stroke volume and cardiac output may cause diminished carotid upstrokes and late systolic peak (tardus) in severe or critical aortic stenosis.

DIAGNOSTIC TESTS

Echocardiography is the principal modality used to diagnose and quantify aortic stenosis. Two-dimensional echocardiography defines valve leaflet thickening and cusp movement restriction as well as gauging left ventricular hypertrophy and evaluating ventricular function.[9] Aortic valve pressure gradient can be measured, aortic valve area calculated, and pulmonary artery pressures estimated.

Cardiac catheterization is done in patients with aortic stenosis primarily to rule out concomitant CHD. Left ventriculography can quantify the left ventricular ejection fraction. The transvalvular gradient can be established by direct pressure measurement. Right heart catheterization can better quantify pulmonary artery pressures and cardiac output.

Electrocardiography often shows a pattern of left ventricular hypertrophy, although its absence does not exclude the presence of critical aortic stenosis. In addition to QRS amplitude changes typically associated with left ventricular hypertrophy, the patient with aortic stenosis may demonstrate ST-T–wave changes typical of left ventricular strain.[4]

Exercise testing in patients with mild to moderate aortic stenosis with equivocal symptoms may be cautiously accomplished in the hands of a cardiologist and can provide relevant information regarding exercise tolerance. In patients with known severe aortic stenosis and classic symptoms such as syncope, dyspnea, and chest pain, exercise testing is unnecessary and carries increased risk of ventricular tachyarrhythmias and ventricular fibrillation.[10,28]

Gated blood pool radionuclide scans provide information regarding ventricular function similar to echocardiography and left ventriculography. Gated pool scans may be useful in patients in whom left ventriculography cannot be done (i.e., patients with elevated creatinine), or in those in whom the left ventricle cannot be clearly imaged with echocardiography.

Chest radiography may be negative even in advanced disease. Heart size may be normal or only minimally enlarged. The left ventricular border and apex may be rounded, demonstrating a boot-shaped silhouette. Identifiable calcification of the aortic valve and aorta may be present. As disease progresses, left atrial enlargement, pulmonary hypertension, and CHF may become evident. Poststenotic dilation of the proximal ascending aorta may be noted along the right heart border in the posteroanterior chest radiograph (Fig. 27-11).

MEDICAL MANAGEMENT

Aside from antibiotic prophylaxis to prevent endocarditis, there is no effective medical management of aortic stenosis.[9] Because the course of aortic stenosis varies in its progression, patients should be carefully followed by their health care providers with serial physical examinations and periodic echocardiography. Patients with mild aortic stenosis undergo echocardiography every 2 years. Patients with asymptomatic severe aortic stenosis are followed with serial echocardiograms every 6 to 12 months. Patients are instructed regarding symptoms of aortic stenosis, including dyspnea,

decreased exercise tolerance, shortness of breath, chest pain, near syncope and syncope.[4] Beta blockers, diuretics, nitrates, and ACE inhibitors must be used with caution because they may precipitate syncope or even cardiovascular collapse in the patient with severe aortic stenosis.[9]

INTERVENTIONAL AND SURGICAL MANAGEMENT

Percutaneous Aortic Catheter Balloon Valvuloplasty.
Percutaneous aortic catheter balloon valvuloplasty is accomplished by passing a guide wire across the stenotic aortic valve into the apex of the left ventricle. A balloon-tipped catheter is advanced retrograde across the stenotic valve. The balloon is inflated, fracturing calcified nodules and separating the fused commissures. The aortic valve ring is also stretched to increase the size of the aortic valve orifice. Although results vary, aortic balloon valvuloplasty has been shown, on average, to increase aortic valve area from 0.5 to 0.8 cm^2 and decrease the gradient from 60 to 30 mm Hg. In addition, left ventricular ejection fraction tends to rise in those patients with depressed left ventricular function.[4]

Restenosis is a major problem in balloon aortic valvuloplasty in adults, occurring in approximately half of the patients within 6 months. Approximately one-third of patients have recurrence of symptoms within 6 months. Because of the high restenosis rate, aortic balloon valvuloplasty in adults is reserved for those candidates unsuitable for surgery (i.e., the elderly with heart failure or pregnant

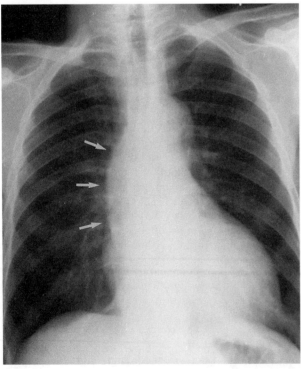

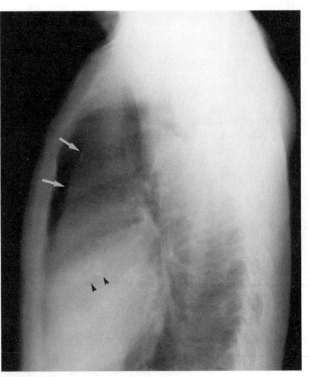

A   **B**

FIGURE 27-11 (*A*) Posteroanterior chest radiograph showing rounded border of left ventricle (*arrows*). (*B*) Lateral chest radiograph showing calcified aortic valve (*arrowheads*) and filling of the retrosternal airspace with dilated ascending aorta (*arrows*). (From Boxt LM: Plain film examination of the chest. In Topol EJ, Califf RM Isner JM et al [eds]: Textbook of Cardiovascular Medicine, p 511. Philadelphia, Lippincott–Raven, 1998.)

women). Aortic balloon valvuloplasty may be used as a bridge or palliative procedure in these populations, and surgical replacement may be considered for a later time.[4]

Aortic Valve Replacement. Aortic valve replacement is the only effective treatment for advanced aortic stenosis.[11] The natural history of aortic stenosis is used as a guide to determine the timing of aortic valve replacement surgery. Patients with asymptomatic aortic stenosis have nearly the same survival rate as the age-matched general population. Once the patient experiences symptoms of angina, syncope, or heart failure, there is an abrupt decline in survival rate. In patients presenting with CHF, only 50% survive 2 years. For patients who present with syncope, the 3-year survival rate is only 50% without aortic valve replacement. The average life expectancy of patients with apnea is only 5 years without aortic valve replacement.[40] Aortic valve replacement is recommended in all patients with severe, symptomatic aortic stenosis. Although the average perioperative mortality rate in most centers ranges from 2% to 8%,[4] perioperative mortality rates range from less than 5% in young, healthy patients to as high as 30% in the frail elderly.[36] Factors that increase the mortality risk at the time of aortic valve replacement include class III or IV heart failure, emergency surgery, aortic insufficiency, and cardiomegaly.[48] Even in patients with severe left ventricular dysfunction, improvement of symptoms and left ventricular ejection fraction occurs in most.[14] Selection of aortic valve prostheses was discussed earlier in this chapter.

Aortic Insufficiency

ETIOLOGY

Aortic regurgitation may be due either to intrinsic abnormalities of the aortic valve leaflets or disease of the aortic root. In rheumatic fever and endocarditis, the aortic leaflets are directly affected. In congenitally bicuspid valves, the larger cusp may become redundant, resulting in diastolic prolapse and progressive aortic regurgitation. The aortic valve may also become incompetent due to aortic root dilation. As the aortic root dilates, the aortic annulus becomes so large that the valve cusps no longer approximate, resulting in regurgitation.

Aortic root dilation is seen in patients with Marfan's syndrome, rheumatic arthritis, ankylosing spondylitis, annuloaortic ectasia (associated with hypertension and aging), aortic dissection, syphilitic aortitis, and collagen vascular disease.

PATHOLOGY

Rheumatic fever leads to fibrinous infiltrates on the valve cusps, causing them to contract and become malaligned and incompetent. Patients with rheumatic disease may have a "mixed lesion" that includes both aortic regurgitation and aortic stenosis. In acute or subacute infective endocarditis of the aortic valve, tissue destruction of the leaflets causes cusp perforation or prolapse. Vegetations adherent to the aortic valve may also interfere with valve closure, causing incompetence. In patients with aortic root dilation or ascending aortic dissection, the aortic annulus becomes

greatly enlarged, the aortic leaflets separate, and aortic incompetence follows.

PATHOPHYSIOLOGY

Volume overload occurs secondary to regurgitant volume reentering the left ventricle from the aorta through the incompetent aortic valve. Retrograde flow occurs during diastole when left ventricular pressure is low and aortic pressure is high. The left ventricle is forced to pump the normal volume received from the left atrium as well as the regurgitant volume from the aorta. The severity of aortic regurgitation is determined by the size of the regurgitant orifice, the pressure gradient across the aortic valve during diastole, and the duration of diastole.[19]

Similar to mitral regurgitation, the hemodynamic presentation and the heart's ability to compensate differ depending on whether the aortic insufficiency is acute or chronic. In chronic aortic regurgitation, the left ventricle is subjected to both a pressure and volume overload. As a result, the left ventricle develops mild concentric hypertrophy to accommodate the pressure load and eccentric hypertrophy to compensate for the increased volume load. Patients with chronic aortic regurgitation may remain asymptomatic for years, until progressive left ventricular dilation and dysfunction result in CHF. In patients with acute aortic regurgitation, the left ventricle has not had time to compensate with either concentric or eccentric hypertrophy and cannot accommodate the large volume caused by acute aortic regurgitation. As a result, left ventricular and left atrial pressures rise sharply, causing acute CHF and pulmonary edema. Patients with acute aortic regurgitation usually require surgical intervention.

CLINICAL MANIFESTATIONS

Patients with chronic aortic regurgitation are often asymptomatic for many years. Common symptoms of aortic regurgitation include fatigue and exertional dyspnea. Patients may complain of palpitations, dizziness, and the sensation of a forceful heartbeat, especially when lying on their left side. Angina may also be noted, but it occurs less frequently in aortic regurgitation than in aortic stenosis. As heart failure ensures, patients experience orthopnea, paroxysmal nocturnal dyspnea, and cough related to left-sided heart failure. With acute aortic regurgitation, symptoms of left-sided heart failure develop rapidly.

PHYSICAL ASSESSMENT

The typical murmur of aortic regurgitation is a high-pitched, early diastolic decrescendo murmur with a blowing quality (see Table 27-2). Patients may also have a physiologic murmur of mitral stenosis due to the regurgitant aortic jet, which partially prevents mitral valve closure (Austin Flint murmur). As the severity of aortic regurgitation increases, the murmur becomes louder and longer. In chronic aortic regurgitation, the point of maximal impulse is displaced laterally. Systolic hypertension and decreased diastolic pressure create a widened pulse pressure. Patients with chronic aortic regurgitation may have a host of other physical findings that may not be present in acute aortic regurgitation (Table 27-6).

TABLE 27-6	Specific Physical Examination Findings in Aortic Regurgitation
Sign	**Physical Description**
Quincke's sign	Pulsatile flushing/blanching of nail bed with application of gentle pressure
de Musset's sign	Bobbing of head with each pulse
Corrigan's pulse (waterhammer)	Sharp systolic upstroke and diastolic collapse of pulse
Müller's sign	Bobbing of uvula with each pulse
Traube's sign	"Pistol shot" sound auscultated over the femoral arteries
Duroziez's sign	Biphasic femoral bruit auscultated with mild pressure
Hill's sign	Blood pressure higher in arms than legs

DIAGNOSTIC TESTS

Echocardiography is helpful in identifying the cause of aortic regurgitation. Echocardiography can indicate left ventricular volume overload by the increased internal diameter of the ventricular chamber during both systole and diastole. Doppler echocardiography is the best noninvasive means to detect aortic regurgitation. Transesophageal echocardiography is especially useful in imaging both the ascending and descending aorta in patients with suspected aortic dissection.

Cardiac catheterization should be performed to visualize and quantify the extent of regurgitation before surgery. However, physical findings and noninvasive tests are sufficient to establish the diagnosis of aortic insufficiency. In patients with known or suspected CHD, coronary angiography should be done. In patients with aortic root dilation, aortic root angiography may be done concurrently with coronary angiography.

Radionuclide imaging can be used to estimate ejection fraction and determine myocardial perfusion defects in patients with concomitant CHD.

Exercise testing may be used to establish exercise tolerance and to evaluate asymptomatic patients.

Electrocardiography may be normal in patients with acute aortic regurgitation or in patients with mild to moderate chronic regurgitation. Patients with moderate to severe chronic regurgitation may have left axis deviation and a pattern of left ventricular strain (Q waves in I, aVL, and V_3 to V_6, with small R wave in V_1). Intraventricular conduction defects may occur with left ventricular dysfunction or annular abscess.

Chest radiography may show only CHF in the patient with acute aortic regurgitation because compensatory left ventricular dilation has not yet occurred. In chronic aortic regurgitation, the chest radiograph demonstrates marked cardiomegaly with inferior and leftward displacement of the apex.[4] Dilation of the ascending aorta and a widened mediastinum may be noted in patients with aortic dissection. In patients with a dilated aortic root or dissection, computed tomography or magnetic resonance imaging may be necessary to delineate better the ascending aorta, transverse arch, and proximal descending aorta.

MEDICAL MANAGEMENT

Patients who have asymptomatic aortic regurgitation should receive appropriate antibiotic prophylaxis as well as afterload reduction with vasodilators. In patients with asymptomatic, chronic, severe aortic regurgitation and normal left ventricular function, nifedipine reduced left ventricular size and mass, and further improved left ventricular function,[46] thus reducing and delaying the need for aortic valve replacement. Nifedipine is superior to hydralazine, which does not decrease left ventricular mass or reduce left ventricular dimension.[31] Diltiazem and verapamil are contraindicated in aortic regurgitation because they have a more potent negative inotropic effect and may produce bradycardia, which may worsen heart failure. It is probably reasonable to substitute other dihydropyridine calcium channel blockers if nifedipine is poorly tolerated.[9] ACE inhibitors may be used to reduce afterload, although they are not as well studied in this population of patients. Patients with moderate to severe aortic regurgitation should not participate in severe exercise or competitive sports. Patients with chronic severe aortic regurgitation should be followed with physical examination and echocardiography every 6 to 12 months.[42]

Sodium nitroprusside reduces both preload and afterload and can be used to stabilize patients with acute aortic regurgitation before surgery. Intra-aortic balloon counterpulsation cannot be used because inflation of the balloon during diastole would increase the regurgitant volume into the left ventricle, which acutely worsens left ventricular dilation and heart failure.

SURGICAL MANAGEMENT

Acute aortic regurgitation requires urgent aortic valve replacement. Without adequate time for compensatory mechanisms to develop, aortic regurgitation triggers rapid onset of CHF, tachycardia, and diminished cardiac output. It is desirable to treat patients with acute aortic regurgitation secondary to infective endocarditis with a minimum of 48 hours of appropriate intravenous antibiotics before implanting a prosthetic valve. In patients with active endocarditis who are hemodynamically unstable, use of cadaveric human aortic homografts may minimize the risk of prosthetic valve endocarditis. Patients who have aortic regurgitation due to ascending aortic dissection or dilation require replacement of the ascending aorta as well.

In chronic aortic regurgitation, the aortic valve must be replaced before irreversible left ventricular dysfunction. In asymptomatic patients, it is usually recommended that the aortic valve be replaced when left ventricular function begins to deteriorate. Surgery is recommended when the echocardiographic left ventricular ejection fraction is 55% or less, the end-diastolic diameter approaches 75 mm, or the end-systolic diameter reaches 50 mm. When symptoms of heart failure develop, aortic valve surgery should be performed regardless of echocardiography findings, because new-onset heart failure indicates the heart has met the limits of compensation.[9]

REFERENCES

1. Alpert JS, Sabick J, Cosgrove DM: Mitral valve disease. In Topol EJ, Califf RM, Isner JM et al (eds): Textbook of Cardiovascular Medicine, pp 503–532. Philadelphia, Lippincott–Raven, 1998

2. Abraham MT, Cherin G: Rheumatic fever. In Chatterjee K, Cheitlin MD, Karliner J et al (eds): Cardiology: An Illustrated Text/Reference, pp 10.98–10.106. Philadelphia, JB Lippincott, 1991

3. Anderson ET, Hancock EW: Long-term follow-up of aortic valve replacement with the mesh aortic homograft. J Thorac Cardiovasc Surg 72: 150–156, 1976

4. Braunwald E: Valvular heart disease. In Braunwald E (ed): Heart Disease: A Textbook of Cardiovascular Medicine, 4th ed, pp 1007–1077. Philadelphia, WB Saunders, 1992

5. Braunwald E: Valvular heart disease. In Fauci AS, Braunwald E, Isselbacher KJ (eds): Harrison's Principles of Internal Medicine. 14th ed, pp 1311–1324. New York, McGraw-Hill, 1998

6. Buccino D, Tu AS, Come PC: Diagnostic imaging and catheterization techniques. In Lilly LS (ed): Pathophysiology of Heart Disease, pp 130–146. Philadelphia, Lea & Febiger, 1993

7. Burge DJ, DeHoratius RJ: Acute rheumatic fever. In Brest AN (ed): Valvular Heart Disease: Comprehensive Evaluation and Treatment, 2nd ed, pp 3–7. Philadelphia, FA Davis, 1993

8. Cannegieter SC, Rosendaal FR, Wintzen AR et al: Optimal oral anticoagulation therapy in patients with mechanical heart valves. N Engl J Med 333: 11–17, 1995

9. Carabello BA: Recognition and management of patients with valvular heart disease. In Goldman L, Braunwald E (eds): Primary Cardiology, pp 370–389. Philadelphia, WB Saunders, 1998

10. Carabello BA: The timing of valve surgery. In Smith TW, Antman EM, Bittl JA et al (eds): Cardiovascular Therapeutics: A Companion to Braunwald's Heart Disease, pp 628–642. Philadelphia, WB Saunders, 1996

11. Chan E, Duh E, Stidham B et al: Valvular heart disease. In Lilly LS (ed): Pathophysiology of Heart Disease, pp 130–146. Philadelphia, Lea & Febiger, 1993

12. Chitwood WR, Wixon CL, Elbeery JR: Video-assited minimally invasive mitral valve surgery. J Thorac Cardiovasc Surg 114: 773–781, 1997

13. Cohn LH, Adams DH, Couper GS et al: Minimally invasive cardiac valve surgery improves patient satisfaction while reducing costs of cardiac valve replacement and repair. Ann Surg 226: 421–426, 1997

14. Connolly HM, Oh JK, Orszulak TA et al: Aortic valve replacement for aortic stenosis with severe left ventricular dysfunction: Prognostic Indicators. Circulation 95: 2395–2399, 1997

15. Cosgrove DM, Sabik JF, Navia JL: Minimally invasive valve operations. Ann Thorac Surg 65: 1538–1539, 1998

16. Cullen L, Laxson C: Ballooning open a stenotic valve. Am J Nurs (7): 987–992, 1988

17. Dajani AS, Taubert KA, Wilson W et al: Prevention of bacterial endocarditis: Recommendations by the American Heart Association. Circulation 96: 358–366, 1997

18. David TE, Puschmann R, Ivanov J, et al: Aortic valve replacement with the stentless and stented porcine valves: A case-match study. J Thorac Cardiovasc Surg 116: 236–240, 1998

19. Doty JR, Salazar JD, Liddicoat JR et al: Aortic valve replacement with cryopreserved aortic allograft: Ten year experience. J Thorac Cardiovasc Surg 115: 371–379, 1998

20. Durack DT, MB, Phil D: Endocarditis. In Hurst JW, Logue RB, Rackey CE et al (eds): The Heart, 6th ed, pp 1130–1157. New York, McGraw-Hill, 1986

21. Edmunds LH, Addonizio VP, Tepe NA: Valvular heart disease: Prosthetic valve replacement. In Chatterjee K, Cheitlin MD, Karliner J et al (eds): Cardiology: An Illustrated Text/Reference, pp 940–941. Philadelphia, JB Lippincott, 1991

22. Fann JI, Ingels NB, Miller DC: Pathophysiology of mitral valve disease and operative indications. In Edmunds LH (ed): Cardiac Surgery in the Adult, pp 959–990. New York, McGraw-Hill, 1997

23. Finkelmeier BA: Surgical treatment of valvular heart disease. In Finkelmeier BA: Cardiothoracic Surgical Nursing, pp 149–163. Philadelphia, JB Lippincott, 1995

24. Friedman WF: Congenital heart disease in infancy and childhood. In Braunwald E (ed): Heart Disease: A Textbook of Cardiovascular Medicine, 2nd ed, pp 941–1023. Philadelphia, WB Saunders, 1984

25. Garcia MJ: Prosthetic valve disease. In Topol EJ, Califf RM, Isner JM et al (eds): Textbook of Cardiovascular Medicine, pp 579–605. Philadelphia, Lippincott–Raven, 1998.

26. Grunkemeier GL, Starr A, Rahimtoola SH: Replacement heart valves. In O'Rourke RA (ed): Hurst's The Heart: Update I, pp 98–123. New York, McGraw-Hill, 1994

27. Izzat MB, Yim AP, El-Zufari et al: Upper T mini-sternotomy for aortic valve operations. Chest 114: 291–294, 1998

28. Kaplan EL: Prevention of bacterial endocarditis (Abstract). Circulation 56(1): 139a–143a, 1977

29. Karchmer AW: Approach to the patient with infective endocarditis. In Goldman L, Braunwald E (eds): Primary Cardiology, pp 201–218. Philadelphia, WB Saunders, 1998

30. Karon BL: Valvular regurgitation. In Murphy JG (ed): Mayo Clinic Cardiology Review, pp 533–554. Armonk, NY, Futura, 1997

31. Khan MG: Valvular heart disease and rheumatic fever. In Khan MG (ed): Heart Disease Diagnosis and Therapy: A Practical Approach, pp 415–460. Baltimore, Williams & Wilkins, 1996

32. Khan MG: Infective endocarditis. In Khan MG (ed): Heart Disease Diagnosis and Therapy: A Practical Approach, pp 461–476. Baltimore, Williams & Wilkins, 1996

33. Kligfield P, Devereux RB: Arrhythmia in mitral valve prolapse. In Podrid PR, Kowey PR (eds): Cardiac Arrhythmia: Mechanisms, Diagnosis, and Management, pp 1253–1260. Baltimore, Williams & Wilkins, 1995

34. Luciani GB, Bertolini P, Vecchi B et al: Midterm results after aortic valve replacement with freehand stentless xenografts: A comparison of three prostheses. J Thorac Cardiovasc Surg 115: 1287–1296, 1998

35. McAnulty JH, Rahimtoola SH. Antithrombotic therapy and valvular heart disease. In Alexander RW, Sclant RC, Fuster V (eds): Hurst's The Heart, 9th ed, pp 1759–1787. New York, McGraw-Hill, 1998

36. Nishimura RA: Valvular stenosis. In Murphy JG (ed): Mayo Clinic Cardiology Review, pp 521–532. Armonk, NY, Futura, 1997

37. O'Rourke RA. Mitral valve prolapse syndrome. In Alexander RW, Sclant RC, Fuster V (eds): Hurst's The Heart, 9th ed, pp 1821–1831. New York, McGraw-Hill, 1998

38. Palacios I, Block PVC, Brandi S et al: Percutaneous balloon valvotomy for patients with severe mitral stenosis. Circulation 75: 778–784, 1987

39. Ross DN, Jackson M, Davies J: Pulmonary autograft aortic valve replacement. Circulation 75: 895–901, 1987

40. Ross J Jr, Braunwald E: Aortic stenosis. Circulation (Suppl V): 38: 61–67, 1968

41. Pape LA, Price JM, Alpert JS et al: Relation of left atrial size to pulmonary capillary wedge pressure in severe mitral regurgitation. Cardiology 78: 297–303, 1991

42. Rahimtoola SH: Aortic valve disease. In Alexander RW, Sclant RC, Fuster V (eds): Hurst's The Heart, 9th ed, pp 1759–1787. New York, McGraw-Hill, 1998

43. Rahimtoola SH: Perspective on valvular heart disease: Update II. In Knobel S (ed): Era in Cardiovascular Medicine, pp 45–70. New York, Elsevier, 1991

44. Rahimtoola SH: Catheter balloon valvuloplasty of aortic and mitral stenosis in adults. Circulation 75: 895–901, 1987

45. Santini F, Dyke C, Edwards S et al: Pulmonary autograft versus homograft replacement of the aortic valve: A prospective randomized trial. J Thorac Cardiovasc Surg 113: 894–899, 1997

46. Scognamiglio R, Rahimtoola SH, Fasoli G et al: Nifedipine in asymptomatic patients with severe aortic regurgitation and normal left ventricular function. N Engl J Med 331: 689–694, 1994

47. Shah PM: Mitral valve prolapse. In Chatterjee K, Cheitlin MD, Karliner J et al (eds): Cardiology: An Illustrated Text/Reference, pp 9.30–9.39. Philadelphia, JB Lippincott, 1991

48. Shine L, Howland-Gradman J: Aortic stenosis in the elderly: Valvuloplasty vs surgery. Am J Nurs (Suppl to May): 7–11 1996

49. Stollerman GH: Rheumatic Fever and other rheumatic diseases of the heart. In Braunwald E (ed): Heart Disease: A Textbook of Cardiovascular Medicine, 4th ed, pp 1721–1738. Philadelphia, WB Saunders, 1992

50. Trausch PA: Infective endocarditis: Nursing care and prevention. Prog Cardiovasc Nurs 3: 45–51, 1988

51. Whittlesay D, Geha AS: Selection and complications of cardiac valvular prosthesis. In Baue AE, Geha AS, Hammond GL et al (eds): Glenn's Thoracic and Cardiovascular Surgery, 5th ed, pp 1719–1728. Norwalk, CT, Appleton & Lange, 1991

Pericardial, Myocardial, and Endocardial Disease

MARGARET M. MCNEILL

Diseases of the pericardium, myocardium, and endo-cardium have a major impact on cardiac function, and therefore quality of life. For this reason, and because of wide-ranging economic ramifications, it is imperative that nurses have a comprehensive understanding of these condi-tions and provide care that optimizes outcomes for patients and families.

PERICARDIAL DISEASE

The pericardium is composed of two layers, the *serosa* and the *fibrosa*, which contain nerves, blood vessels, and lym-phatics.[117] The fibrous outer layer, also called the parietal pericardium, is discretely attached to the sternum, great ves-sels, and diaphragm.[97,117] It is lined by a serosal layer of cuboidal cells one cell layer thick. The monocellular serosa directly covers the heart surfaces and is also known as the *visceral pericardium* or the *epicardium*. The phrenic nerves supply most of the parietal pericardium. The pericardial space between the layers normally contains 15 to 35 mL of serous pericardial fluid, an ultrafiltrate of the blood plasma.[117]

The pericardium serves several functions, yet cardiac activity is normal if it is missing because of congenital absence or surgical removal. The pericardium is a relatively inelastic covering and it exerts a powerful restraining effect on the size of the heart in situations of acute volume over-load.[97,118] The pericardium maintains the heart in a compar-atively stable position and functionally optimum shape in the mediastinum. It acts as a barrier to inflammation from adjacent structures and contains defensive immunologic constituents. The pericardial fluid reduces friction on the pericardium.

Almost every known pathologic process, medical and sur-gical, can contribute to pericardial disease, either primarily involving the pericardium or with an indirect pericardial impact.[108] For unknown reasons, there is a predominance of men with pericardial disease.[112] The many types and descrip-tions of pericardial diseases are given in Table 28-1, and the major primary congenital abnormalities are listed in Display 28-1.[108]

Pericarditis

The clinically most significant pericardial condition is peri-carditis, an inflammation of the pericardium.

ETIOLOGY

The major causes of pericarditis are given in Display 28-2.[5,39,97,108] Direct or indirect trauma to the chest, as well as injuries caused by pacing wires and migrating or misplaced central catheters, can lead to pericarditis. Viral pathogens and dis-eases include but are not limited to coxsackievirus, infec-tious mononucleosis, influenza, chickenpox, and acquired immunodeficiency syndrome (AIDS). In AIDS, oppor-tunistic infections, such as tuberculosis, or neoplasms are the most likely etiologies of pericardial disease. Some of the bacteria causing pericarditis include *Staphylococcus, Pneumo-coccus,* and *Streptococcus* species, and *Mycobacterium tuber-culosis.* Aspergillosis and histoplasmosis are among the fun-gal infections that can cause pericarditis.

Abnormalities of the myocardium, pleura, lungs, diaphragm, esophagus, and mediastinal lymph nodes all may directly involve the pericardium because of its proxim-ity or by transmission through lymphatic or blood circula-tion. Transmural myocardial infarction (MI) frequently involves the pericardium, but this is not detected in more than half of the cases.[108] Metastatic cancers, including bronchogenic carcinoma, breast cancer, lymphoma, leukemia, and melanoma, can all cause pericarditis, as can some of the treatments for these conditions. Pericarditis has been linked to end-stage renal disease related to both uremia and dialysis. Uremic pericarditis is usually found in patients with newly diagnosed chronic renal failure who have never been dialyzed. Dialysis-associated pericarditis could be related to infection, heparin, and elevations of

TABLE 28-1	Acquired Pericardial Disease
Condition	**Description**
Pericarditis	Inflammation of the pericardium
Myopericarditis	Inflammation of both the myocardium and the pericardium
Pericardial fat necrosis	Rare condition sometimes causing chest pain
Pericardial effusion	Excess pericardial fluid produced by the pericardium
Polyserositis	Multiple serous membrane inflammation
Hemopericardium	Frank bleeding into the pericardium
Chylopericardium	Results from extravasation of chyle (milklike contents of the lacteals and lymphatic vessels, carried by the lymphatic vessels to the thoracic duct and to the left subclavian vein) due to a neoplasm or abnormal communication between pericardium and the thoracic duct
Cholesterol pericarditis	High concentration of cholesterol in the pericardial fluid
Lymphopericardium	Rare lesion related to lymphangiectasis, a dilation of the lymphatic vessels
Pneumopericardium	Air or gas in the pericardium caused by trauma or communication between the esophagus, stomach, or lungs and the pericardium
Pneumohydropericardium	Air and fluid accumulation in the pericardium

blood urea nitrogen (BUN), creatinine, and uric acid.[5] Most chronic inflammatory disorders of the vasculitis–connective tissue disease group, which share the common feature of inflammation tending to damage blood vessel walls, can cause pericarditis, pericardial effusion, pericardial adhesions, and constriction.[115] The vasculitis seen in this group of diseases probably is primarily due to deposition of immune complexes resulting in inflammatory cell infiltration in blood vessels and the pericardium. Systemic lupus erythematosus (SLE), rheumatoid arthritis, and progressive systemic sclerosis are just a few of the syndromes related to pericarditis.[115] SLE causes many anatomic and pathophysiologic pericardial abnormalities, including acute, clinically dry pericarditis and exudative (serous, serosanguineous, or hemorrhagic) pericardial effusions. SLE should be suspected in all women with acute pericarditis until disproved, because this may be its first manifestation.[115] Drug-induced SLE, caused by medications such as procainamide, isoniazid, hydralazine, methyldopa, or penicillin, also produces pericarditis.

Acute Clinically Noneffusive Pericarditis. Noneffusive or "dry" pericarditis refers to pericardial inflammation without significant symptom-causing effusion. This is the most commonly recognized pericarditis. Frequently, the patient's history indicates that a viral infection preceded the pericarditis, or sometimes the pericarditis itself is the first presenting symptom of a systemic disease, as in SLE or malignancy. Viral infection is often presumed rather than definitively diagnosed, so many cases are classified as idiopathic.[97]

DISPLAY 28-1

Major Primary Congenital Abnormalities of the Pericardium

Pericardial (celomic) cysts
Pericardial absence
    Complete
    Partial
Teratomas
Lymphangiomas
Diverticulum

DISPLAY 28-2

Major Causes of Pericarditis

Idiopathic
Trauma
    Direct
    Indirect
Infections
    Viral
    Bacterial
    Parasitic
    Fungal
Radiation
Immunologic conditions
Connective tissue diseases
    Systemic lupus erythematosus
    Vasculitis
Metabolic disorders
    Uremia
Myocardial infarction
Dissecting aneurysm
Drugs/anticoagulants

ASSESSMENT FINDINGS. The onset of symptoms can be acute, as is commonly seen in viral pericarditis, or insidious, as in uremic pericarditis. Acute viral pericarditis is nearly always preceded by a recent respiratory, gastrointestinal, or "flulike" illness.[109] This prodromal illness may be characterized by fever and myalgia.

The characteristic symptom of pericarditis is chest pain, although sometimes pain is absent. Initially, the pain of acute pericarditis tends to be sharp, precordial, and pleuritic, exacerbated by inspiration and lying down. The patient often sits up and leans forward to achieve relief. The pain can radiate in a manner similar to angina, confusing the diagnosis. Trapezius ridge pain is almost pathognomonic for pericardial irritation, and in some patients this is the only area of pain.[109] It is transmitted through the phrenic nerves, and usually is seen on the left side. Shoulder pain should be distinguished from trapezius ridge pain by having the patient physically point to the specific site of pain. Frequently the chest pain caused by pericarditis induces shallow tachypnea as patients attempt to splint their chest movement.[109] Fever, usually below 39° C, is also very common in acute pericarditis.

The hallmark sign of acute pericarditis is the pericardial friction rub, a superficial, scratchy, or creaky, mostly high-pitched sound, most commonly heard between the middle to lower left sternal edge and the cardiac apex.[97] The sounds can be very distant and faint, or loud and even palpable, especially in uremic pericarditis.[110] Pericardial rubs are thought to be due to friction between pericardial surfaces. The sound can be heard throughout the cardiac cycle, can come and go, and can change in quality and intensity. Auscultation for a pericardial friction rub is accomplished with the diaphragm of the stethoscope at the left middle to lower sternal border during both inspiration and expiration, while the patient changes positions. Sometimes the rub can be heard best while the patient is in the sitting position. Rubs in acute pericarditis may disappear or persist regardless of the presence of a large effusion or tamponade. Pericardial rubs are most often triphasic, then biphasic, and monophasic approximately 10% of the time. The classic pericardial friction rub is triphasic, with components during atrial systole, ventricular systole, and ventricular diastole.[55,110]

The pericardium itself does not produce electrical activity. The electrocardiographic (ECG) changes seen in pericarditis are a result of superficial inflammation of the myocardium underneath the pericardium. The ECG of a patient with pericarditis may be normal, atypically abnormal with nonspecific changes, or have a four-stage sequence that is diagnostic.

In stage I, there are ST segment deviations, primarily due to inflammation on the ventricular surfaces. PR segment deviations also usually are present. Stage I is virtually pathognomonic of acute pericarditis when it involves all or almost all leads with earliest ST junction elevations that produce an appearance of T waves "jacked-up" on the QRS interval, but that is otherwise normal.[114] The ST segment is always depressed in aVR. In early stage II, the ST segments return to baseline, and PR segments may now be depressed. In late stage II, the T waves flatten and then invert. In stage III, the

ECG is characteristic of diffuse myocardial injury. In stage IV, the ECG evolves back to the prepericarditis state.[98,114]

The changes seen in the ECG of a patient with pericarditis can occur over hours, particularly from stage I to II, or can take place over days or weeks, most often as stage III evolves to stage IV. The ST elevation seen in pericarditis is usually distinguished from that of acute MI by the absence of Q waves, upward ST segments, and the absence of associated T-wave inversion.[97]

Evaluation of laboratory results almost always reveals an elevated erythrocyte sedimentation rate. Leukocytosis is present early but, depending on etiology, may give way to lymphocytosis. Serum cardiac enzymes are frequently normal unless the myocardium is involved, and then they give some indication as to the degree of involvement.

MEDICAL MANAGEMENT. In pericarditis, the goal of treatment is to eliminate the underlying cause and relieve symptoms. Analgesics and bed rest are used to treat pain. Nonsteroidal anti-inflammatory drugs (NSAIDs) are the mainstay of treatment.[97,109] Gastrointestinal mucosa protectants guard against the side effects, but close monitoring is essential. Colchicine may be added to an NSAID or given as monotherapy for both the initial attack and to prevent recurrences.[109] Corticosteroids are used only if other treatments fail, and then only in minimally effective dosages. The use of these agents is controversial. The patient with pericarditis is also closely observed for development of the complications of pericardial effusion or cardiac tamponade.

Constrictive Pericarditis.
The pericardium loses its flexibility and elasticity and becomes scarred and rigid in constrictive pericarditis. As a result, the heart is compressed and its function is disturbed. Advances in diagnostic testing as well as in our understanding of hemodynamics have improved early diagnosis.[113] Traditionally, constriction has been chronic, with sometimes surprising pericardial thickness. Recently, relatively thinner constricting pericardia are increasingly evident, perhaps because of earlier diagnoses and a shift in recognizable etiologies.[113] The etiology of constrictive pericarditis is often undetermined, but it can result from almost all the conditions that also cause acute pericarditis.

PATHOPHYSIOLOGY. The essential pathologic process is healing, resulting in a scar, thick or thin, that restricts cardiac filling, particularly that of the ventricles.[113] A constricting pericardial scar accentuates the ventricular pressure–volume relationship and increases ventricular coupling while restricting filling of the ventricles progressively earlier in diastole, until 70% to 80% of the reduced filling occurs in the first 25% to 30% of diastole.[113] The filling pressures of the two sides of the heart become equilibrated. Elevated arterial pressures reflect elevated ventricular diastolic pressures. Because of constriction, cardiac output (CO) decreases, and tachycardia occurs in an attempt to compensate. The syndrome of increased ventricular diastolic pressure, low CO, and increased systemic vascular resistance mimics cardiac failure.[97] The thickened pericardium effectively isolates the heart from normal respiratory swings in pressure.[55]

ASSESSMENT FINDINGS. A history of antecedent pericarditis or drugs or procedures that induce pericarditis may indicate constrictive pericarditis. Many abnormal findings can be seen on the echocardiogram that indicate constrictive pericarditis, such as premature opening of the pulmonic valve and rapid posterior motion of the left ventricular posterior wall in early diastole, with little or no posterior motion during the rest of diastole. However, these findings are not specific for constrictive pericarditis and can be caused by other conditions, such as severe mitral regurgitation.[17]

Pericardial thickening is best demonstrated by magnetic resonance imaging (MRI) and computed tomography. These tests are more specific than echocardiography in differentiating scarring from fluid or tumor. Constrictive pericardia may be too thin to be seen with any available imaging techniques.[120]

On cardiac catheterization, the major finding is near-equalization of all diastolic chamber pressures and venous pressures. Both left and right ventricular traces have a dip and plateau, the "square root" configuration, more pronounced in the right ventricle, because of the sharp, short, early diastolic decrease toward zero pressure (dip), increasing rapidly to a restrictive plateau as the relaxing ventricles rapidly reach the tight, limiting pericardium.[113] There is equalization of the right atrial and pulmonary wedge pressures.[96] The central venous pressure is elevated and shows no respiratory deviation except in the depth of the y descent. During classic constriction, *Kussmaul's* sign, inspiratory jugular venous distention, replaces the normal inspiratory venous "collapse" that reflects a normal inspiratory decrease of 3 to 7 mm Hg in right atrial pressure.[113] This is a hallmark of constrictive pericarditis.

Severe compression causes signs and symptoms of heart failure: dyspnea, ascites, leg edema, neck vein distention, organomegaly, and decreased coronary, cerebral, and renal perfusion.[87,113] The patient can display tachycardia, atrial fibrillation, and other signs of decreased CO such as cool extremities, peripheral cyanosis, and jaundice due to liver involvement. Blood pressure may be normal, hypotensive, and sometimes hypertensive. Early diastolic thrust corresponds to a rapid ventricular filling pressure and coincides with a loud abnormal S_3 produced in both ventricles, sometimes with a "knocking" quality. S_1 and S_2 can be muted because of hemodynamic compromise.

Laboratory tests often reveal normocytic normochromic anemia, abnormal liver function tests, and hypoalbuminemia.

The ECG is nonspecifically abnormal. The T waves are usually flat or low and sometimes inverted. The QRS interval and T waves may show decreased voltage. Interatrial block is common, indicated by widened, notched P waves.

MEDICAL MANAGEMENT. Medical management does not relieve constriction. Surgical pericardectomy is the definitive treatment. It is more easily accomplished if done early in the course of the disease, when the patient has less systemic disease and before calcification and myocardial abnormalities develop.[55] Preventing the development of constrictive pericarditis is the optimal method to combat this condition, through adequate treatment of pericarditis, and draining of fluid and pus if indicated.

Pericarditis Associated With Myocardial Infarction

EARLY ACUTE POSTMYOCARDIAL INFARCTION PERICARDITIS. In the 2 to 3 days after MI, an early pericardial syndrome may develop and then resolve over a period of approximately 1 week. A pericardial rub may be evident, and there is pericardial-type pain in approximately 50% of cases.[83] The course is usually benign, and treatment consists of aspirin or other NSAIDs. Because of an unknown mechanism, when thrombolytics are given and successfully treat MI, pericarditis rarely develops.[83]

DRESSLER'S SYNDROME. Dressler's syndrome of chest pain, pleurisy, pericarditis with friction rub, severe malaise, and moderate fever and leukocytosis occurs 3 weeks to several months post-MI. The underlying pathologic process is unknown, but many believe an autoimmune reaction occurs secondary to the infarct. Patients with Dressler's syndrome can have recurrent ischemia, significant pericardial effusion, bacterial superinfection, and hemorrhagic complications.[55] The ECG shows a typical pattern of pericarditis and should be helpful in differentiating between pericardial and ischemic pain.

Pericardial Effusion

Pericardial effusion is the excess accumulation of fluid, blood, pus, or a combination of all three, in the pericardium. If the rate of exudation is slow enough to allow the pericardium to stretch, even large amounts of fluid might not compromise cardiac function.

ETIOLOGY

Pericardial effusions are caused by pericardial irritation and inflammation. Congestive heart failure (CHF) contributes to many small- and moderate-sized effusions.[116] There is a high incidence of pericardial effusion in patients infected with the human immunodeficiency virus (HIV), and the presence of effusions is associated with shortened survival and suggests end-stage HIV disease.[47]

ASSESSMENT FINDINGS

"Noncompressing" effusions do not produce changes in CO, nor pulsus paradoxus. If the effusions are caused by a systemic disease, then the symptoms are related to that disease. A pericardial rub may or may not be appreciated. The ECG shows reduced voltage, and these changes are nonspecific and unreliable for diagnosis. Electrical alternans is a marker of massive pericardial effusion.[55] Chest radiographs are at best suggestive and nonspecific. If the effusion is visible on radiography, then there is at least 250 mL of fluid accumulated.[116]

On echocardiography, both normal and excess fluid can be seen. The size of the effusion can be estimated, giving a powerful predictor of prognosis in hospitalized patients. Echocardiography is the mainstay of diagnosis and the tool of choice.[55,116] Computed tomography and MRI can also aid in diagnosis.

MEDICAL MANAGEMENT

In the absence of tamponade or pyopericardium, there are few absolute indications for drainage. Successful treatment of the cause should lead to resolution of the effusion. Persistent illness without etiologic diagnosis indicates need for surgical tissue and fluid sampling. Techniques include sub-xyphoid incision and video-assisted thoracoscopic pericardial resection and drainage, which allows for removal of thrombi, adhesions, and fibrinous material. Fluid can be drained by pericardiocentesis. However, when used for diagnostic purposes, pericardiocentesis often yields poor results.[116] Patients must be monitored after drainage for decompensation secondary to cardiac dilation, which can take place once the effusion that was compressing the heart is removed.

Cardiac Tamponade

Cardiac tamponade is defined as significant compression of the heart by accumulating pericardial content. Cardiac tamponade can be of varying degrees and can be caused by varying amounts of fluid. The speed of accumulation usually affects the severity of symptoms. Any scarring or thickening of the pericardium serves to amplify the effects of excess fluid on the heart.

ETIOLOGY

Any disease affecting the pericardium can cause effusion that can be complicated by cardiac tamponade. The common causes are idiopathic or viral pericarditis, neoplastic invasion of the pericardium, and nephrogenic pericardial disease. Acute tamponade is frequently caused by trauma, which may be iatrogenic, or by aortic rupture or rupture of the heart after MI.[97]

ASSESSMENT FINDINGS

Symptoms are related to the degree of cardiac impairment. It may be difficult to diagnose cardiac tamponade if the patient initially presents in cardiogenic shock or cardiopulmonary failure. Symptoms include tachypnea and dyspnea on exertion, progressing to air hunger at rest. Cough and dysphagia may be early symptoms but often are not recognized as indicating tamponade. Oliguria occurs as the tamponade worsens in severity. Syncope and convulsions can develop.

If the patient has pericarditis, a pericardial friction rub may be detectable. Heart sounds may be muffled because of excess fluid and impaired cardiac function. The venous pressure is elevated in all except the mildest cases of tamponade, or if hypovolemia is present. Jugular venous pressure is elevated. Central venous pressure can be as high as 30 mm Hg.[98]

Hypotension is produced by significant tamponade, leading to symptoms of poor perfusion.

Pulsus paradoxus develops when tamponade becomes moderately severe. Pulsus paradoxus is present when systemic arterial pressure drops 10 mm Hg or more during inspiration. It is easily observed on arterial line tracings and can be detected by using a sphygmomanometer. To measure the blood pressure change using a blood pressure cuff,

inflate the cuff to 15 mm Hg above the highest systolic reading. The cuff is slowly deflated until the first Korotkoff sounds are heard. The sounds are heard only with some heart beats; these are the ones occurring during expiration at that pressure. The other sounds are heard at a lower pressure during inspiration. Slowly deflate the cuff until all of the Korotkoff sounds can be heard. The difference between these two readings gives the size of the pulsus.[111] The pulse pressure also decreases during inspiration, reflecting decreased stroke volume.[98]

The mechanism of pulsus paradoxus is related to competition between the two sides of the compressed heart for the severely restricted space. During inspiration, the expansion of the right heart volume impairs left heart stroke volume.[98] Experimental observations indicate that this is only part of the explanation for pulsus paradoxus in cardiac tamponade.[99] Pulsus paradoxus is multifactorial and still incompletely understood.[119]

In moderate to severe tamponade, right atrial, right ventricular diastolic, and pulmonary artery wedge and diastolic pressures are all equal.[98] Exceptions are commonly seen and are due to underlying cardiac disease.

The ECG usually does not show diagnostic features. Electrical alternans of the P wave, QRS complex, and T wave are highly suggestive of cardiac tamponade, but are uncommon.[98]

MEDICAL MANAGEMENT

Cardiac tamponade is usually an indication for pericardiocentesis, drainage of the fluid accumulated in the pericardium. If tamponade recurs, open drainage may be indicated and is safer, particularly if tissue samples are needed.[97] If cardiac tamponade is caused by bleeding, the bleeding may actually be slowed by tamponade pressure. In this case, open surgical drainage and treatment of the bleeding source is superior to pericardiocentesis.[119] Continuous hemodynamic monitoring of the effects of the procedure is critical.

Nursing Management in Pericardial Disease

The nurse is in a prime position to recognize the symptoms of pericardial disease and the complications that may develop. A careful and skilled assessment is critical and often crucial to the medical diagnosis.

The nurse who is knowledgeable of pericardial disease is able to identify the patients most at risk, such as those with renal failure or MI. The subtle characteristics of pericardial pain, including the location, quality, and the effect of position changes, are aspects of the patient's condition that nurses are best suited to assess. As the member of the health care team who is consistently evaluating the patient, the nurse is most likely to find a pericardial friction rub because the sound is likely to come and go, and change in quality. Evaluation of laboratory results, ECGs, and vital signs are key nursing interventions that have an enormous impact on the outcome of care. If the patient with pericardial disease is uremic, then he or she is prepared for increased dialysis.

Emotional support and education can serve to decrease patient anxiety. Consistent care and a caring demeanor can encourage both the patient and family members to verbalize their fears. Listening to concerns and questions and providing information bolsters coping. Teaching about diagnostic tests can allay fears. The nurse intervenes with many measures that promote patient comfort, including narcotics and NSAIDs, positioning, diversion, and bed rest or limitation of activities.

It is critical that the patient maintain an adequate CO. The nurse evaluates the patient's hemodynamic state and implements any interventions that increase cardiac function, including vasoactive medications, decreasing anxiety and stress, and detection of pulsus paradoxus and jugular venous distension.

Nurses monitor for cardiac arrhythmias and evaluate their effects on the patient. It is imperative that cardiac tamponade be diagnosed early, before a crisis ensues. If a patient is at risk, the nurse has the equipment readily available for an emergency pericardiocentesis. Monitoring the patient's condition during and after the procedure detects any other complications.

If a patient is to have surgery, preoperative teaching and preparation are a key nursing responsibility. Letting the patient and family know what to expect can help them deal with this frightening event. If a patient has a pericardectomy or a pericardial window, close monitoring of hemodynamics after surgery is important. Volume expanders and vasopressors may both be needed to maintain CO. Accurate hemodynamic readings are the nurse's responsibility and guide many treatment decisions. The nurse must provide respiratory care to prevent atelectasis and pneumonia and monitor the surgical incision for infection. The nurse also monitors the effects of any therapy, such as NSAIDs, and is vigilant for side effects such as gastrointestinal upset or bleeding. The physician is notified if the desired effects of medical interventions are not being achieved or if side effects or complications arise.

CARDIOMYOPATHIES

Cardiomyopathy is an irreversible primary disease of the heart muscle. Cardiomyopathy affects the myocardial layer of the heart, but it can also affect the endocardial, subendocardial, and pericardial layers. Cardiomyopathies used to be defined as heart muscle disease of unknown cause, but in recent years much has been learned about some of the etiologies of these diseases.[82] The condition is characterized by chamber dilation, wall thickening (hypertrophy), decreased contractility, and conduction disturbances.[16] The end result is usually severe dysfunction of the heart muscle, resulting in terminal heart failure.[40]

The World Health Organization classified three types of cardiomyopathy according to anatomic and pathophysiologic characteristics: dilated, hypertrophic, and restrictive.[82] Dilated cardiomyopathy (DCM) is the most common type of cardiomyopathy, followed by hypertrophic cardiomyopathy (HCM), and then restrictive cardiomyopathy (RCM), which is quite rare, particularly in the United States.

Dilated Cardiomyopathy

Dilated cardiomyopathy is a primary disease of the ventricular myocardium characterized by decreased systolic function and increased ventricular volumes without a proportionate increase in ventricular wall thickness.[121] Stroke volume is initially maintained despite a reduced ejection fraction because the decrease in systolic function is accompanied by an increase in end-systolic and end-diastolic volumes. Therefore, there is compensation early in the disease. Eventually, the ejection fraction deteriorates, myocardial contractility is further depressed, and severe dysfunction of the heart muscle leads to heart failure.[40,121]

ETIOLOGIES

Myocarditis, inflammation of the myocardium, is thought to be the major cause of DCM. Discussed in greater depth later in this chapter, the causes of myocarditis are many, and thus so are the causes of DCM. The etiologies are listed in Display 28-3.[121] Half of the patients with DCM are diagnosed with idiopathic DCM, isolated heart failure of unknown etiology.[77] This condition affects 5 to 8 of 100,000 people.[52,63] Genetic factors make idiopathic DCM hereditary in approximately 20% of cases.[75] Studies support the hypothesis that alcohol is one of many triggers for the development of DCM in a susceptible person.[72] Cocaine abuse can also lead to DCM, as well as CHF and endocarditis.[81] Many chemotherapeutic agents, such as doxorubicin, daunorubicin, and cyclophosphamide have been linked to DCM.[60]

The pathogenesis of DCM is controversial and is believed to include genetic disposition, viral infection, and autoimmunity. It has been proposed that diminished cardiac function in inflammatory myocarditis and DCM might be mediated by the release of cytokines in the myocardium.[40] Further research in this area may lead to new treatments.

ASSESSMENT FINDINGS

Clinical manifestations of DCM reflect right and left ventricular dysfunction, a combination of inadequate CO and perfusion, and excessive congestion of the pulmonary and systemic venous circulations. Orthopnea, nocturnal cough, and dyspnea may present if DCM progresses slowly. Abdominal distention, right upper quadrant pain, and nau-

---

DISPLAY 28-3

Etiologies of Dilated Cardiomyopathy

Idiopathic
Inflammatory
  Infectious
    Noninfectious
Toxic
Metabolic
Familial
Abnormal coronary vasculature

sea secondary to systemic congestion can be the dominant symptoms if DCM progresses rapidly. Physical signs often depend on how long the patient has had DCM, and this usually relates to the severity of the condition.

Specific findings include a point of maximal intensity away from the normal position, at the fifth intercostal space mid-clavicular line. Auscultation of heart sounds may reveal an S₃, indicating failure, or a murmur, signifying mitral regurgitation or tricuspid regurgitation. Mitral regurgitation is common even if a murmur is not heard. Peripheral edema and jugular venous distention may be apparent. Because stroke volume and CO are decreased, blood pressure may be low and pulse pressure may be decreased. Extremities are cool and clammy, and peripheral pulses are decreased. There may be evidence of systemic emboli secondary to endocardial thrombi that are most likely to lodge in the apex of the left ventricle.

The ECG of a patient with DCM may show nonspecific ST segment and T-wave abnormalities or may indicate bundle-branch blocks and supraventricular and ventricular arrhythmias. Echocardiography reveals dilated chambers with normal or decreased wall thickness. Symptomatic patients frequently have an ejection fraction of less than 30%. Radiography shows cardiomegaly with ventricular enlargement.

Laboratory values reflect the impact of DCM on other organs. Liver functions test results are elevated, as are the BUN and creatinine.

MEDICAL MANAGEMENT

Fifty percent of all deaths in patients with DCM occur suddenly. A 5-year mortality rate of 50% has been reported for DCM of various etiologies with ejection fractions below 50%.[121] Ventricular arrhythmias are possibly the major cause, but clots and hemorrhages secondary to treatment or bradyarrhythmias may also contribute to deaths in DCM.

If the etiology of the DCM can be determined, treatment focuses on eliminating the cause. Otherwise, general principles of medical care include maximizing ventricular function and exercise performance, reducing associated risks, and, late in the disease, consideration for cardiac transplantation.[121] The suppression of premature ventricular contractions may be associated with improvement of left ventricular function in patients with presumed idiopathic DCM.[30] Medications such as digoxin and dobutamine are administered to increase contractility. Vasodilators are given to decrease afterload and therefore left ventricular work, and increase CO. Heparin and warfarin for long-term anticoagulant therapy, are given to prevent clot formation in the dilated left ventricle and if atrial fibrillation is present. Fluid and sodium restriction, along with administration of diuretics, maintain fluid balance. Daily weights assist in monitoring fluid status.

A preliminary study on the intermittent home administration of the inotrope/vasodilator milrinone in patients with end-stage heart failure secondary to DCM showed multiple benefits.[16] Intermittent infusions limited the toxicity and tachyphylaxis seen previously in outpatient use. Another study found that continuous inotropic therapy was best suited to those patients with idiopathic DCM who were not able to be weaned while hospitalized, and helped to manage these patients at decreased hospital stays, until transplantation was available.[103]

Implantation of left ventricular assist devices is becoming more common for patients with end-stage disease awaiting transplantation.[102] In the future, these devices may be considered for patients who are not transplantation candidates.[19]

Cardiac transplantation prolongs the lives of patients with DCM, but not every patient is a candidate for the procedure. Cardiac transplantation is done approximately 2,300 times per year in the United States, but each year 3,700 people are on the waiting list.[78] Many patients die before a heart becomes available.

Dynamic cardiomyoplasty is an experimental alternative to transplantation. The procedure involves the use of an autologous latissimus dorsi muscle graft that is wrapped around the ventricles by pericardial attachment. The muscle graft is then stimulated by specialized synchronous train impulses from a cardiomyostimulator; the resultant muscle graft contractions provide support for ventricular function.[127]

Hypertrophic Cardiomyopathy

Hypertrophic cardiomyopathy (HCM), also known as idiopathic hypertrophic subaortic stenosis, is a disorder of cardiac muscle characterized by diastolic dysfunction and hypertrophy without dilation.[125] It occurs without any systemic precipitating factors. The left ventricle is the predominant site of involvement, but hypertrophy of the right ventricle may occur.[74,91] Different areas of the ventricle can be affected, and some studies have indicated that the extent of hypertrophy correlates with manifestation of symptoms, whereas others show no relationship.[53,91] Histologic characteristics of this condition are myocardial fiber disarray, loose intercellular connective tissue with fibrosis, and abnormal intramural coronary arteries.[67,91,125]

ETIOLOGY

The etiology of HCM is thought to be mutations in genes encoding several cardiac sarcomeric proteins.[73] As many as 60% to 80% of cases are inherited through autosomal dominant transmission, but it is usually undetected until adulthood.

PATHOPHYSIOLOGY

Hypertrophic cardiomyopathy produces both diastolic and systolic abnormalities. The compliance of the left ventricle decreases because of an increased muscle mass and fibrosis.[125] The stiffness impairs ventricular filling during diastole and is often evidenced by high left ventricular end-diastolic pressure. Because of this, atrial contraction is extremely important in patients with significant impairment of diastolic filling. The heart attempts to compensate by increasing the force of left atrial contraction. If the atria dilate under increased pressure load or atrial fibrillation or flutter develops, filling and preload are further reduced and hemodynamic compromise results.[53]

Approximately 25% of patients with HCM also have left ventricular outflow tract obstruction (LVOTO) caused by a markedly hypertrophic, asymmetric septal wall that is out of proportion to the remainder of the chamber.[59] This changes the shape of the left ventricular cavity, causing the papillary muscles to become misaligned. During contraction, the papillary muscle abnormally pulls the anterior mitral leaflet toward the ventricular septum; this is known as systolic anterior motion of the mitral valve. Together, the displaced papillary muscle, mitral valve leaflet, and septal hypertrophy cause a left ventricular outflow gradient.[92] This pressure gradient increases myocardial oxygen demand and left ventricular systolic pressures. The combination of decreased left ventricular chamber size, elevated systolic and end-diastolic pressures, and decreased blood volume leads to further hypertrophy and possible myocardial ischemia.[53]

There are many potential complications of HCM, with sudden death being the most important.[64] It occurs throughout life with an annual incidence (in referral populations) of 4% to 6% in children and 6% in adults.[74] One study found that patients who die suddenly commonly have marked and diffuse left ventricular hypertrophy.[107] However, sudden death has been reported in an active, healthy, and symptom-free 16-year-old boy without left ventricular hypertrophy but with histologic abnormalities.[67] Syncope has been identified as a risk factor for sudden death in the younger age group.[91] Infective endocarditis risk is slightly increased in patients with resting LVOTO, so antibiotic prophylaxis is indicated for these patients undergoing high-risk procedures such as dental surgery.[91] Another complication is atrial fibrillation, which can have a major impact on CO. Ventricular arrhythmias as well as conduction system disease can occur.[74,91]

ASSESSMENT FINDINGS

Hypertrophic cardiomyopathy may present in sudden death with no prior indication of the disease, or it can evolve with increasing symptoms. A systolic murmur heard at the lower left sternal border and apex may be the only physical sign of HCM.[66] The murmur may occur with or without obstruction, and usually is of a higher grade (III to IV/VI) if there is LVOTO.[91] Dyspnea is the most common symptom and appears to be related to the elevated left ventricular end-diastolic pressure. Fatigue, chest pain, dizziness, syncope, palpitations, CHF, and sudden death can present at any age.[65,74] Angina is common and seems to be related to myocardial ischemia due to the combination of LVOTO and diminished myocardial blood flow.[74] A heavy apical pulse and S_4 are also common findings, reflecting atrial systole into a noncompliant and stiff left ventricle.[100] The carotid pulse in patients with HCM is characteristically brisk and bifid.[91]

A thorough family history is imperative because of the strong genetic component of HCM.

The standard diagnostic technique is echocardiography, which has been invaluable in the diagnosis of patients at risk without symptoms. The ECG in HCM is usually abnormal, but it is not diagnostic or prognostic.[66] The most common abnormalities seen are ST segment and T-wave changes.[91] Q waves in the inferior and lateral leads reflect septal hypertrophy, not MI. Tall precordial R waves also reflect hypertrophy.[35,91] Conduction abnormalities can also be seen on the ECG.

MEDICAL MANAGEMENT

The main goals of management of patients with HCM are to decrease the risk of sudden cardiac death and treat symptoms of dyspnea, angina, fatigue, and syncope.[34,53,74] An automatic implantable cardioverter-defibrillator has been used with success after sudden death was the presenting symptom.[123] Thus far, cardiac rhythm disturbances are believed to be the most common cause of sudden cardiac death in HCM.[28] Nonsustained ventricular tachycardia has been frequently found on 24-hour Holter monitoring. Ventricular fibrillation and ventricular tachycardia have also been implicated, especially when patients have a history of syncope, presyncope, or prior cardiac arrest.[28]

Medical management includes the use of beta blockers, calcium channel blockers, and antiarrhythmics.

Beta blockers, such as propranolol hydrochloride, decrease outflow tract obstruction and the heart rate, allowing greater time for filling of the chambers. Oxygen demand is decreased, therefore decreasing angina.[125] The rationale for beta blocker use is inhibition of sympathetic stimulation of the heart, resulting in diminished left ventricular contractility and reduced myocardial oxygen demand at rest and during exercise.[91] Beta blockers can relieve most symptoms of HCM, including angina, dyspnea, presyncope, or syncope. However, beta blockers have not produced sustained effects on HCM in many patients, and frequently deterioration results.[7,91] In a review and analysis of the use of beta blockers in HCM, McKenna[73] concluded that propranolol exerted no significant effect on the incidence of sudden death.

Calcium channel blockers improve the rate of relaxation and decrease heart rate and blood pressure.[125] Calcium channel blockers, such as verapamil, reduce LVOTO.[49] A decrease in systolic function and an improvement in diastolic relaxation and filling results from calcium channel blocker use.[28] However, long-term success has also been a problem with these agents.

Quinidine and procainamide hydrochloride have been used to suppress ventricular arrhythmias.[129] Disopyramide, a type I antiarrhythmic with negative inotropic properties, has been advocated for patients with HCM and LVOTO. Varying results with its use have been reported, but long-term results, as with the other therapies, have shown symptom improvement for some patients.[7] Amiodarone is a potent class III antiarrhythmic agent that shows slow calcium channel, fast sodium channel, and β-adrenergic blocking properties. It has been shown to lessen symptoms caused by LVOTO, to increase exercise tolerance, and to improve left ventricular compliance and diastolic filling in patients with HCM.[7,28] Some studies have shown proarrhythmic effects, whereas others have shown a marked reduction in ventricular tachycardia.[28] One study, however, suggested empiric use of amiodarone may be associated with increased rather than reduced mortality in patients with HCM.[36]

Dual-chamber, sequential atrioventricular (AV) pacing has been used in patients who have not responded to medical therapies.[35,93,128] The exact mechanism by which dual-chamber pacing improves the clinical status of patients with LVOTO is unknown. One possibility is that the beneficial effect is due to modification of the ventricular activation sequence.[51] It also has been reported that systolic anterior motion is smaller secondary to the effect of pacing on septal movement. It is important that AV synchrony be maintained because although the left atrial contribution to CO is only 20% to 30% in the normal heart, it becomes a major factor to the total CO in a patient with LVOTO. Ventricular pacing without synchrony results in either AV dissociation or retrograde ventriculoatrial conduction, causing hemodynamic deterioration.[93] The AV interval must be individualized and of sufficient length to permit left atrial emptying into a ventricle with increased filling pressures.[93] This reduces the intraventricular pressure gradient and improves functional tolerance.[51]

Surgical therapy for HCM has included ventricular septal myotomy–myectomy as well as mitral valve replacement in selected patients.[28] The advantage to incision (myotomy) or excision (myectomy) of hypertrophied septal tissue in the left ventricular outflow tract is that it decreases the amount of obstruction and results in clinical improvement.[25] Surgery is not curative; the goal is to improve quality of life.[125] The surgical experience at the National Institutes of Health demonstrated that 90% of patients had short-term improvement in functional status, and 70% maintained this benefit over the long term.[65]

Treatment options include percutaneous laser myoplasty, an investigational procedure that may benefit patients who are refractory to medical treatment, have persistent symptoms, and are poor surgical risks.[35] Percutaneous septal myocyte injury by alcohol infusion is undergoing intensive clinical investigation at several centers throughout the United States, and it may prove to be a valuable alternative to surgery for patients with a significant obstructive component.[74]

Restrictive Cardiomyopathy

PATHOPHYSIOLOGY AND ETIOLOGY

Restrictive cardiomyopathy is the least common type of cardiomyopathy seen in Western countries. It is more common in Africa than in other parts of the world.[60] RCM is characterized by a primary abnormality of diastolic ventricular function with normal to near-normal systolic function and normal ventricular internal dimensions.[18] Diminished ventricular distensibility, due to thickened, rigid ventricular walls, is manifested functionally by a disproportionate increase in diastolic pressure for a given increased diastolic volume. The result is an abnormally steep slope of the diastolic pressure–volume curve known as the *square root* hemodynamic pattern.[18,55] RCM is frequently mistaken for constrictive pericarditis.[18,45] RCM can be idiopathic and sometimes genetically linked. It is seen in amyloidosis, sarcoidosis, endomyocardial fibrosis, and other infiltrative diseases.[18,60]

ASSESSMENT FINDINGS

Clinical signs and symptoms are those of high systemic and pulmonary venous pressure. Peripheral edema and ascites may be evident. There is a normal left ventricular systolic impulse and a prominent S_3. Auscultation frequently reveals AV valve regurgitation.[18,55] Biatrial enlargement due to rigid ventricular walls is seen, and atrial fibrillation is common.[55]

MEDICAL MANAGEMENT

There is no known treatment for RCM, so therapy is supportive. It includes diuretics, corticosteroids, or anticoagulants, depending on the etiology and manifestations. Fluid restriction, oxygen, and positive inotropes may also be used to treat the symptoms.

Myocarditis

Myocarditis is an inflammation of the myocardium. It is usually diagnosed when it leads to significant cardiac dysfunction. Myocarditis can cause considerable morbidity and mortality and is implicated in the development of DCM.[131] Unsuspected myocarditis is detected in almost 10% of routine autopsies.[126]

ETIOLOGY

Myocarditis can be caused by a variety of agents. Display 28-4 gives a list of the etiologies.[9,10,41,44]

DISPLAY 28-4

Etiologies of Myocarditis

Infections
  Viral
    Coxsackievirus
    Poliomyelitis
    Mumps
    Rubella
    Epstein-Barr
    Human immunodeficiency virus
  Bacterial
    Tuberculosis
    Tetanus
    Staphylococcal
    Pneumococcal
  Fungal
  Parasitic
    Toxoplasmosis
    Cytomegalovirus
  Pharmacologic agents
    Inotropes
  Radiation therapy
  Chemical poisons
  Peripartum condition
  Autoimmune
    Eosinophilia
    Asthma

Viral myocarditis is considered the most common type and is estimated to affect at least 1 in 10,000 of the U. S. population each year, frequently striking children, young adults, and pregnant women.[122]

PATHOPHYSIOLOGY

Myocarditis is usually characterized by necrosis and cell injury associated with inflammation of the heart muscle and lymphocytic inflammation in the absence of an ischemic episode.[15] As the myocardium becomes infected and necrosis occurs, an immune response is initiated and cytokines are produced. The viral infection persists, and an autoimmune response is initiated, causing the body to attack its own cells. These mechanisms and the viral attack of vascular endothelium, causing microvascular spasm and reperfusion injury, are thought to produce the myocardial damage that occurs in myocarditis. Cardiac tissues show multiple focal areas of myocyte loss, sheets of fibrosis, and calcified deposits diffusely distributed across all cardiac muscle layers and chambers.[106]

ASSESSMENT FINDINGS

Myocarditis classically presents with nonspecific symptoms such as fatigue, dyspnea, and palpitations, along with viral illness symptoms, including fever. If the disease has progressed, symptoms of heart failure present, such as tachycardia, pulmonary edema, diaphoresis, neck vein distention, and cardiomegaly. Symptoms of poor perfusion or cardiogenic shock can also be manifested, such as hypotension, cool, clammy extremities, decreased urine output, and decreased level of consciousness.

Cardiac function is evaluated through echocardiography, ECG, nuclear scans, and cardiac catheterization with endomyocardial biopsy. The latter test remains the gold standard for diagnosis of myocarditis, although results remain controversial and it is invasive and costly.[41,50,131] One study indicated that MRI may serve as a powerful, noninvasive diagnostic tool in myocarditis.[41] In myocarditis, the ECG can show low-voltage QRS complexes, ST segment elevation, or heart block. Nonsustained atrial or ventricular arrhythmias are common. An S_4 and systolic ejection murmurs may be heard on auscultation.

MEDICAL MANAGEMENT

Management of myocarditis is focused on support. Heart failure is treated and arrhythmias are controlled.

Inotropic support of cardiac function with amrinone, dopamine, or dobutamine may be used. Nitroprusside and nitroglycerin may be used to reduce afterload. Bed rest is used to promote healing and minimize myocardial oxygen consumption. Intubation, ventilation, and sedation may be necessary to decrease cardiac workload.[56,89,121] Extracorporeal membrane oxygenation has been used in 50 cases of pediatric and neonatal myocarditis, with a 54% survival rate.[90] Mechanical assist devices such as intra-aortic balloon pulsation and left ventricular assist devices have been used to improve CO in myocarditis.[102] Another important aspect of management is prevention of complications. If the ejection fraction is low

and there is blood stasis in the chambers, anticoagulant therapy is necessary to prevent thrombus formation.

The use of immunosuppression in the treatment of myocarditis is controversial. An immunosuppressive therapy trial of myocarditis demonstrated no beneficial effects.[69] However, immunosuppression during the autoimmune phase of myocarditis may be effective.[50]

Nursing Management in Dilated Cardiomyopathy

The nurse can help in identifying the cause of DCM through a careful and detailed nursing history.

The nurse is also in the best position to monitor the patient for worsening of symptoms and for response to medical treatments. Evaluation of heart sounds, lung sounds, vital signs, and peripheral perfusion, as well as interpretation of laboratory results, are key nursing responsibilities. Signs of congestion and decreased CO must be detected and reported early to provide the most effective treatment. The nurse titrates medications to increase left heart function, monitoring the effects and side effects. If a left ventricular assist device is used, the nurse monitors the effects of this therapy as well.[84,102] Reduction of afterload and filling pressures is accomplished with diuretics and vasodilators given and monitored by the nurse. The nurse optimizes the patient's oxygenation through position changes, pulmonary toilet, monitoring and interpretation of arterial blood gases, and oxygen administration or ventilator management. Recognition of symptoms of excess use of cocaine or alcohol or withdrawal from these substances is necessary.[81]

Sudden position changes, strenuous exercise, and Valsalva maneuvers can worsen signs and symptoms.[46] The patient and his or her family must be educated about DCM and its treatments and possible complications. Each test that is done should be explained to the patient. The plan of care needs to be discussed and agreed on. If anticoagulants are used, side effects and their symptoms, as well as dietary interactions need to be explained. Other dietary considerations must be addressed, such as fluid and salt restriction, and the nurse as a leader of the multidisciplinary team can ensure that the patient's multiple needs are met. Emotional needs are particularly significant in DCM because of its wide-ranging impact on the lives of both the patient and family. Physical limitation was a significant predictor of less effective psychosocial adjustment for patients studied with DCM.[8,42] A study on couples dealing with severe cardiomyopathy found they experienced considerable psychosocial distress attributable to illness. DCM affects the entire family, and adequate information about the illness and treatment, along with emotional support, can facilitate adaptation and coping.[8] Individual counseling, support groups, or both can be effective.

When the patient is to have surgery, preoperative education can allay many fears if the patient and family have an opportunity to ask questions and are prepared for the postoperative course.[95] Teaching needs to be individualized, with determination of the best method for the patient and family. The nurse is responsible for postoperative hemodynamic monitoring, pain control, and respiratory care. Infection control is also critical.

Nursing Management in Hypertrophic Cardiomyopathy

Hypertrophic cardiomyopathy is a condition that limits activity and is potentially life threatening. It is associated with substantial restrictions in health-related quality of life.[23] It is often diagnosed after another family member has died a sudden death. While a patient is grieving for a family member, he may also be coping with his or her own new diagnosis. To make the diagnosis, the patient undergoes many tests, such as echocardiography and cardiac catheterization. Emotional support and education are key components of nursing care of patients with HCM.

The other goals of nursing care for patients with HCM are to assess and observe for complications and to promote comfort. After surgery or pacemaker insertion, careful monitoring of hemodynamic status and prompt detection of decreased blood pressure and CO, CHF, arrhythmias, and bleeding are important. Conduction defects are common after surgery. It is crucial that the patient wear a medical alert bracelet in case of emergency and that family members be trained in basic life support techniques.[127]

Nursing Management in Myocarditis

Psychological support is an important aspect of care because the patient and family are faced with a sudden and devastating illness. They may need assistance coping with this stressful crisis. Providing education and accurate information on the condition, medications, test, and treatments is an important intervention. Nutrition is another important aspect of care that the nurse must evaluate, along with the dietitian. As a leader of the health care team, the nurse can alert social workers, chaplains, mental health professionals, and others of the patient's needs and coordinate the multidisciplinary care.

The nurse is responsible for oxygenation and ventilation management, fluid balance and electrolyte monitoring, and prevention of infection. Accurate hemodynamic monitoring is essential. Skin care of the patient on bed rest with decreased CO can be a difficult challenge.[2] The nurse must detect arrhythmias immediately and respond appropriately. AV block and ventricular tachyarrhythmias are among those that can occur.[79] Emergency equipment should be readily available.

ENDOCARDIAL DISEASE

Infectious Endocarditis

Infectious endocarditis (IE) is a disease in which infective organisms invade the endothelial lining of the heart, usually involving one or more valves. This is the major endocardial disease. The endocardium covers the valves and surrounds the chordae tendineae. The infection that forms, usually on the valve of the heart, is called a *vegetation*.

EPIDEMIOLOGY

The incidence of IE is not known accurately because it is not a notifiable disease and the case definitions have varied over time and among authors and different medical centers.[32,96] A recent study in the eastern United States showed the estimated rate was 11.6 cases per 100,000 per year.[6] This rate was influenced by a high number of intravenous drug users and may be somewhat lower in other areas.[32]

Since World War II, advances in the use of antibiotics, the evolution of cardiac surgery, and the advent of improved diagnostic techniques have changed the trends of IE. The patients are older, more often male, and have acute IE more often than subacute IE. Streptococcal cases have decreased, whereas staphylococcal cases have increased. Many more organisms have been found to cause IE, including rare and unusual microbes, and HIV infection has also been implicated.[32] The number of drug users has increased, as has the incidence of HIV infection in this population, and older substance abusers continue to inject drugs.[22] Rheumatic valvular disease has steadily decreased in developing countries, and at the same time, the number of children with congenital heart disease surviving palliative or corrective surgery has increased.[3,32] The congenital heart defects of greatest risk are those in an area of high turbulence, such as septal defects, valvular abnormalities under high pressure, prosthetic valves and conduits, cyanotic defects, and palliative shunts. The rate of prosthetic valve IE is also on the rise.[32,48] HCM with LVOTO also is a risk for IE.[3,58] Despite many improvements in diagnostics and therapy, IE remains a disease with high morbidity and mortality.[96] Display 28-5 lists predisposing factors for IE.[3,32]

TYPES

In the past, IE has been divided into three categories, acute, subacute, and chronic, according to the presentation and condition of the patient. The lines separating these categories are blurred, and the same organisms can produce sudden, severe disease as well as slowly progressing disease in different cases.[96] IE can be better classified by site of

---

DISPLAY 28-5

Predisposing Factors for Infectious Endocarditis

Male sex
Rheumatic heart disease
Degenerative valvular disease
Aortic or mitral valve disease
    Mitral valve prolapse
Prosthetic cardiac valve
Congenital heart disease
    Ventricular septal defect
    Coarctation of the aorta
    Patent ductus arteriosus
Hypertrophic cardiomyopathy with left ventricular outflow tract obstruction
Intravenous drug use
Diabetes mellitus
Pregnancy
Marfan's syndrome
Central venous and pulmonary artery catheters

involvement, such as native valve versus prosthetic valve; by type of pathogen; and definitiveness of the diagnosis, such as possible, probable, or definite.[76]

Native valve endocarditis (NVE) is an infection seen in patients without prosthetic valves but who usually have valvular or heart disease that predisposes them to IE. One study compared NVE in elderly and younger adults, excluding intravenous drug users. Most of the cases were caused by *Streptococcus viridans* and *Staphylococcus aureus* in similar rates in each population. The signs and symptoms were also similar in both groups.[43]

The clinical index for suspicion is much higher for *prosthetic valve endocarditis* (PVE). IE occurs in 1% to 6% of all patients with prosthetic cardiac valves.[14,71] The rates of infection of mechanical and tissue valves are similar.[38] The mortality rate in patients with PVE was found to be 55% in a study published in 1982.[123] A more recent study showed an overall in-hospital mortality rate of 10% to 20%, possibly reflecting a more aggressive approach to treatment of PVE.[61,62]

Nosocomial endocarditis is usually a complication of bacteremia induced by an invasive procedure or a vascular device and accounts for nearly 10% of IE in some areas.[6,29] IE can occur after pacemaker implantation and has a mortality rate as high as 24%.[6] Another study found the hospital mortality rate to be 7.6% and the overall mortality rate to be 26.9% for patients with IE secondary to pacemaker implantation.[1]

Other research concluded that strong evidence supports the theory that pacemaker-related infections are mainly due to local contamination during implantation.[25]

PATHOGENESIS AND PATHOLOGY

Based on results of experimental and clinical studies, it is known that IE results from a complex interaction between damaged vascular endothelium, local hemodynamic abnormalities, circulating bacteria, and local and systemic host defenses.[3] Platelets and fibrin from the circulation accumulate at the site of endothelial damage on the surface of the heart valve.[68] The endothelial damage is thought to be due to an abnormally high-velocity jet stream of blood. The lesions thus formed are called *nonbacterial thrombotic endocarditis* (NBTE) lesions. Intracardiac pressure monitoring catheters can also produce identical lesions.[89] This lesion is usually a prerequisite of IE, although it is thought that highly invasive organisms can directly invade the endocardium.[3] The NBTE lesion is then attacked by bacteria in the bloodstream. Bacteremia often occurs after manipulation of the oropharyngeal, gastrointestinal, and genitourinary tracts. The bacteremia in postoperative and intensive care patients usually occurs secondary to intravenous lines, invasive monitoring devices, wound infections, pneumonia, and urinary tract infections.[76] Bacteremia can occur after urethral catheterization, labor and delivery, and abortion.

The ability to adhere to fibrin correlates with the ability of microbes to cause IE.[32] Dextran-producing strains avidly bind to the fibrin–platelet aggregate on the cardiac valves. Fibronectin is produced by damaged endothelial cells. Fibronectin receptors have been demonstrated on the surface of several organisms that cause IE.[3] Once the bacteria

adhere to the NBTE lesion and multiply, they stimulate inflammatory responses. Cytokines and tumor necrosis factor may be involved in the systemic manifestations of IE.[11]

Almost any type of bacteria can cause IE. Most, 80% to 85% of cases, are caused by streptococci and staphylococci. Fifty percent of NVE is caused by *S. viridans;* 20% is caused by *S. aureus.* In intravenous drug users, *S. aureus* is the cause in 57% of cases.[3,76] In patients with prosthetic valves, 33% of the early cases, which occur within 2 months of valve replacement surgery, are caused by *Staphylococcus epidermidis.* *S. aureus* causes 15% of these cases, and gram-negative bacteria cause 17% of the cases. In late PVE, the same organisms at the same rates as seen in NVE are found.[3]

ASSESSMENT FINDINGS

According to the Duke criteria, persistent bacteremia with organisms typical for endocarditis and an oscillating mass on a valve (vegetation) make a clinically definitive diagnosis of IE. In the course of clinical practice, the diagnosis is suspected more often than it is confirmed. The Duke criteria include several minor criteria that also suggest IE, such as predisposition, fever, vascular phenomena such as septic pulmonary infarcts, and immunologic phenomena such as Osler's nodes.[33] In one study, the diagnosis was not established until 3 to 4 weeks after onset of symptoms and 2 weeks after admission to the hospital.[54]

Transthoracic echocardiography with Doppler flow studies should be performed in everyone suspected of having endocarditis. If the clinical suspicion is high and the transthoracic echocardiogram is negative or inconclusive, a transesophageal echocardiogram should be obtained.[96] Transesophageal echocardiography is of great value in assessment of tricuspid valve endocarditis and tricuspid regurgitation, and is superior to transthoracic echocardiography in left-sided endocarditis as well.[3]

Blood cultures should be drawn from three different sites with 1 hour between each draw or, if time is limited, a total of 1 hour between the first and the last draw.[3,32] Blood cultures isolate the organism. Other laboratory findings seen in IE can include normocytic anemia, elevated white blood cell count, elevated erythrocyte sedimentation rate in almost all cases, proteinuria, hematuria, elevated BUN and creatinine possibly secondary to embolization, and positive rheumatoid factor in approximately 50% of cases.[21]

The virulence of the organism usually determines the acuteness of the presentation. The illness may be characterized by subtle chronic fatigue with low-grade fevers, weight loss, and malaise, or abrupt fulminating and acute pulmonary edema brought on by massive acute aortic regurgitation.[94] The symptoms seen are a reflection of the effects of infective vegetations in the heart and throughout the body.

Symptoms include fever, chills, rigors, weight loss, fatigue, loss of appetite, weakness, myalgias, arthralgias, and back pains. Splenomegaly and metastatic infections may become evident.

The symptoms can be distinguished by the effect the IE has on the heart and the effect emboli from the vegetations have on the lungs or other organs. Intracardiac symptoms most often come from regurgitant aortic or mitral valves, on the most frequently affected left side of the heart. Tachy-

TABLE 28-2	Immunologic Manifestations of Infectious Endocarditis	
Finding	Description	Occurrence
Petechiae	Red, flat, 1 to 2-mm, nontender lesions	50% of patients
Splinter hemorrhages	Linear, black, longitudinal streaks on distal tip of nail bed	20% of patients with subacute IE
Osler's nodes	Red, swollen lesions with white centers 1 to 10 mm in size, most commonly found on the pads of the fingers or toes, palms, soles of feet or thighs	10%–20% of patients with subacute IE
Janeway lesions	Nontender, purple or red lesion 1 to 5 mm in size, found on arms, legs, palms, and soles of feet	Not known
Conjunctival petechiae	Caused by microemboli	Not known
Roth's spots	Small, 3 to 10-mm white spots in the retina close to the optic disc, often encircled by hemorrhages	Not known

IE, infectious endocarditis.

cardia, gallop rhythm, dyspnea, crackles, and hypotension due to decreased CO can result from left-sided IE. Up to 15% of patients do not have a murmur when first seen.[33] Intracardiac complications of IE include valvular destruction with regurgitation and heart failure, ring abscesses with first- or second-degree heart block, and valve perforations.

The complications from systemic emboli that can accompany left-sided IE include hemiplegia and paralysis, mental status changes, visual defects and blindness, MI, intra-abdominal disaster, and renal failure. These symptoms are caused by infarcts of the spinal cord, brain, retina, heart, bowel, spleen, or kidney. When an arterial wall is damaged by septic emboli, mycotic aneurysms can form and are subject to sudden bleeding. Patients can have toxic metabolic encephalopathy, meningitis, brain abscesses, seizures, and headache from sepsis and septic emboli. Myocarditis and pericarditis can also result from IE.

Right-sided IE is not as common as left-sided IE and is usually seen in intravenous drug users. When the tricuspid valve is effected, the symptoms that are produced include peripheral edema, neck vein distention, hepatomegaly, ascites, and atrial arrhythmias. Pulmonary emboli that accompany right-sided IE result in chest pain, cough, hemoptysis, tachycardia, pneumothorax, pleural effusions, and pneumonia.

The circulating immune complexes in IE produce the symptoms of glomerulonephritis, petechiae, Osler's nodes, and arthritis.[3,21,32] Table 28-2 lists the common immunologic manifestations of IE.[32,76,80]

MEDICAL MANAGEMENT

The cornerstone of treatment of IE is early recognition and elimination of the infecting organism. Timely surgical intervention and anticipation and treatment of complications are also key concepts in the care of these patients.[37] Antibiotics are usually bactericidal whenever possible.[33] First-line treat-

ment is usually a combination of penicillin and an aminoglycoside, usually gentamicin. Published experience can guide specific therapeutic regimens.[101,124,130] Antibiotics often are given from 4 to 6 weeks, and longer courses are sometimes necessary. Outpatient intravenous antibiotic therapy has been successful in stable patients with endocarditis in limited trials.[12] Others have experienced problems with safety and efficacy and have called for controlled clinical trials to determine if home- versus hospital-based antimicrobial therapy have similar outcomes.[20]

Surgery is indicated in IE if the patient has heart failure that is not responding to medical management; recurrent infection; infection of prosthetic valves, especially if the valve is malfunctioning; large aortic valve vegetations; or recurrent systemic embolization.[3] Most patients with PVE require valve replacement. Urgent surgery is indicated for severe CHF secondary to significant aortic regurgitation.[3] Valve replacement has become the routine in the management of patients with IE and should be undertaken as soon as signs and symptoms of failure appear.[96] Surgical correction of tricuspid valves through valvuloplasty, which allows for débridement of vegetation, is usually successful, especially if a single leaflet is involved.[85]

PREVENTION

Prevention of IE remains the standard of care. Meticulous dental hygiene may be just as important as antibiotic prophylaxis in the prevention of IE.[96] The American Heart Association and European experts have published guidelines for antimicrobial prophylaxis for IE.[26,86] It is generally agreed that patients with prosthetic valves and a prior episode of IE are at increased risk for IE. Because patients who are at risk for development of IE have been identified, the usual practice is to prescribe prophylactic antibiotics if these patients are to undergo procedures that are likely to produce bacteremia. A recent meta-analysis suggests that systemic antibiotic prophylaxis significantly reduces the incidence of potentially serious infective complications after permanent pacemaker implantation.[24] However, there is varied scientific evidence that antibiotic prophylaxis is effective.[96]

Nursing Management in Infectious Endocarditis

Nurses need to be knowledgeable about IE and its symptoms and complications, the difficulty in making the diagnosis, and its far-reaching effects. A detailed history reveals risk factors, symptoms, prodromal illness, recent antibiotic therapy, and preexisting renal disease. This information aids in the medical diagnosis. A careful physical examination may reveal the signs of IE, such as a murmur secondary to new-onset regurgitation.[13,94]

Once the patient is diagnosed, the plan of care should be discussed with the patient and family. The nurse can be the leader on the health care team to make sure the multiple needs of the patient with IE are addressed and met by all disciplines.[68] A lengthy hospitalization is likely, and patients need assistance with coping with this and the illness.

This illness is life threatening, so information and emotional support are crucial in facilitating coping mechanisms.[124] If it is indicated, a referral for drug addiction treatment should be completed. Drug addiction and alcohol abuse frequently engender strong negative feelings among nurses and physicians. The nurse must make care decisions in an ethical, professional manner, even when caring for patients who use intravenous drugs, do not follow recommendations, or do not take the prescribed medications.[70]

The nurse manages oxygen therapy, ventilator care, and vasoactive medications and monitors fluid balance and ECGs. The nurse often obtains the blood for laboratory tests and blood cultures, and then interprets the results. The nurse is responsible for proper administration of antibiotics and monitoring for therapeutic levels and side effects. The nurse also manages the intravenous lines for the long course of antibiotics. If a pulmonary artery catheter is in place, accurate measurements and interpretations guide medical care. Infection control and early removal of invasive lines, chest tubes, and pacing wires help prevent nosocomial IE.[38,105]

A general systems approach to assessment facilitates detection of complications.[57] Knowing the indications for surgery may prove life saving.[105] Preoperative teaching is necessary to prepare the patient undergoing surgery. During surgery, it is desirable to keep the family informed of the progress. After surgery, as the nurse rewarms the patient, intravenous fluids must be available to give in response to vasodilation.[37] Pulmonary hygiene is crucial, as is monitoring for potential drug withdrawal if the patient is an intravenous drug user. The signs include restlessness, insomnia, diaphoresis, chills, diarrhea, tachycardia, hypertension, pupillary dilation, and tachypnea.[85]

Once the patient is ready for discharge, education is critical because the patient must be knowledgeable about recurrence of symptoms, such as fever and weight loss, antibiotic prophylaxis for certain high-risk procedures, and the need for keeping all health care providers informed that he or she is at increased risk for IE. The nurse should stress the impor-

tance of postdischarge follow-up and inform the patient about the need to obtain medical alert identification. The importance of proper oral hygiene should also be stressed.[27]

REFERENCES

1. Arber N, Pras E, Copperman Y et al: Pacemaker endocarditis: Report of 44 cases and review of the literature. Medicine 73: 299, 1994
2. Baker A: Acquired heart disease in infants and children. Critical Care Clinics of North America 6(1):175, 1994
3. Bansal RC: Infectious endocarditis. Med Clin North Am 79: 1205, 1995
4. Bennett SJ: Pericarditis: Nursing care makes the difference. Advancing Clinical Care Nov/Dec 5(6): 32, 1990
5. Berg J: Assessing pericarditis in the end-stage renal disease patient. Dimensions of Critical Care Nursing 9: 266, 1990
6. Berlin JA, Abrutyn E, Strom BL et al: Incidence of infectious endocarditis in the Delaware Valley 1988–1990. Am J Cardiol 76: 933, 1995
7. Blanchard DG, Ross J: Hypertrophic cardiomyopathy: Prognosis with medical or surgical therapy. Clin Cardiol 14: 11, 1991
8. Bohachick P, Anton BB: Psychosocial adjustment of patients and spouses to severe cardiomyopathy. Res Nurs Health 13: 385, 1990
9. Borczuk AC, van Hoeven KH, Factors M: Review and hypothesis: The eosinophil and peripartum heart disease (myocarditis and coronary artery dissection)—coincidence or pathogenetic significance? Cardiovasc Res 33: 527, 1997
10. Brown CS, Bertolet BD: Peripartum cardiomyopathy: A comprehensive review. Am J Obstet Gynecol 2: 409, 1998
11. Brown M, Griffin GE: Immune responses in endocarditis. Heart 79: 1, 1998
12. Brown RB: Selection and training of patients for outpatient intravenous antibiotics. Rev Infect Dis 13(Suppl 12): 5147, 1991
13. Burden LL, Rodgers JC: Endocarditis: When bacteria invade the heart. RN 51(12):38–46, 1988
14. Calderwood SB, Swinski LA, Waternaux CM et al: Risk factors for the development of prosthetic valve endocarditis. Circulation 72: 31, 1985
15. Carthy CM, Yang D, Anderson DR et al: Myocarditis as systemic disease: New perspectives on pathogenesis. Clin Exp Pharmacol Physiol 24: 997, 1997
16. Cesario D, Clark J, Maisel A: Beneficial effects of intermittent home administration of the inotrope/vasodilator milrinone in patients with end-stage congestive heart failure: A preliminary study. Am Heart J 135: 121, 1998
17. Chandraratna PAN: Echocardiography and Doppler ultrasound in the evaluation of pericardial disease. Circulation 84(Suppl I): I-303, 1991
18. Child JS, Perloff JK: The restrictive cardiomyopathies. Cardiol Clin 6: 266, 1988
19. Chillcott SR, Atkins PJ, Adamson RM: Left ventricular assist is a viable alternative for cardiac transplantation. Critical Care Nursing Quarterly 20(4): 64, 1998
20. Colford JM, Corelli RL, Ganz JW: Home antibiotic therapy for streptococcal endocarditis: A call for a controlled trial. Am J Med 94: 111, 1993
21. Conlon PJ, Jeffries F, Krigman HR et al: Predictors of prognosis and risk of acute renal failure in bacterial endocarditis. Clin Nephrol 49: 96, 1998
22. Contoreggi C, Rexroad V, Lange WR: Current management of infectious complications in the injecting drug user. J Subst Abuse Treat 15: 95, 1998

23. Cox S, O'Donoghue AC, McKenna WJ et al: Health related quality of life and psychological wellbeing in patients with hypertrophic cardiomyopathy. Heart 78: 182, 1997

24. DaCosta A, Kirkorian G, Cucherat M: Antibiotic prophylaxis for permanent pacemaker implantation. Circulation 97: 1796, 1998

25. DaCosta A, Lelievre H, Kirkorian G: Role of preaxillary flora in pacemaker infections. Circulation 97: 1791, 1998

26. Dajani AS, Taubart KA, Watson W et al: Preventing bacterial endocarditis. Recommendations by the American Heart Association. JAMA 277: 1794, 1997

27. DeJong MJ: Infectious endocarditis. Am J Nurs 98(5): 34, 1998

28. DeRose JJ, Banas JS, Winters SL: Current perspectives on sudden cardiac death in hypertrophic cardiomyopathy. Prog Cardiovasc Dis 36: 475, 1994

29. Dodds GA, Sexton DJ, Durack DT: Negative predictive value of the Duke criteria for infectious endocarditis. Am J Cardiol 77: 403, 1996

30. Duffee DF, Shen WK, Smith HC: Suppression of frequent premature ventricular contractions and improvement of left ventricular function in patients with presumed idiopathic dilated cardiomyopathy. Mayo Clin Proc 73: 430, 1998

31. Dugan KJ: Caring for patients with pericarditis. Nursing 3: 50, 1998

32. Durack DT: Infectious endocarditis. In Alexander RW, Schlant RC, Fuster V et al (eds): Hurst's The Heart, pp 2205–2239. New York, McGraw-Hill, 1998

33. Durack DT, Bright DK, Lukes AS: Duke endocarditis service new criteria for diagnosis of infective endocarditis: Utilization of specific echocardiographic findings. Am J Med 96: 200, 1994

34. Elliot PM, McKenna WJ: Management of hypertrophic cardiomyopathy. Br J Hosp Med 55: 419, 1996

35. Enfanto PA, Pickett S, Pieczeu AM et al: Percutaneous laser myoplasty, nursing care implications. Critical Care Nurse 14(3): 94, 1994

36. Fananapazur L, Leon MD, Bannon RO et al: Sudden death during empiric amiodarone therapy in symptomatic hypertrophic cardiomyopathy. Am J Cardiol 67: 161, 1991

37. Finkelmeier BA, Hartz RS, Fisher EB et al: Implications of prosthetic valve implantation: An 8-year follow-up of patients with porcine bioprostheses. Heart Lung 18: 564, 1989

38. Fitzgerald CA: Current perspectives on prosthetic heart valves and valve repair. AACN Clinical Issues 4: 228, 1993

39. Fowler NO: Pericardial disease. Heart Disease and Stroke March/April(2): 85, 1992

40. Francis SE, Holden H, Holt CM et al: Interleukin-1 in myocardium and coronary arteries of patients with dilated cardiomyopathy. J Mol Cell Cardiol 30: 215, 1998

41. Friedrich MG, Strohm O, Shulz-Menger J et al: Contrast media-enhanced magnetic resonance imaging visualizes myocardial changes in the course of viral myocarditis. Circulation 97: 1802, 1998

42. Frost MH, Kelly AW, Mangan DB et al: An analysis of factors influencing psychosocial adjustment to cardiomyopathy. Cardiovasc Nurs 30: 1, 1994

43. Gagliardi JP, Nettles RE, McCarty DE et al: Native valve infectious endocarditis in elderly and younger adult patients: Comparison of clinical features and outcomes with the use of the Duke criteria and the Duke endocarditis database. Clin Infect Dis 26: 1165, 1998

44. Galiuto L, Enriquez-Sarano M, Reeder GS et al: Eosinophilic myocarditis manifesting as myocardial infarction: Early diagnosis and successful treatment. Mayo Clin Proc 72: 603, 1997

45. Handerhan B: Managing patients with cardiomyopathy. Nursing 1: 32C, 1995

46. Handerhan B: Staying alert for endocarditis. Nursing 7: 14, 1991

47. Heidenreich PA, Eisenberg MJ, Keel L et al: Pericardial effusion in AIDS: Incidence and survival. Circulation 92: 3229, 1995

48. Higgins SS: Long-term follow-up of the postoperative patient with congestive heart disease. Nurs Clin North Am 29: 221, 1994

49. Hopf R, Kaltenbach M: Management of hypertrophic cardiomyopathy. Annu Rev Med 41: 75, 1990

50. James KB, Ratliff N, Starling R et al: Inflammatory cardiomyopathy. Rheum Dis Clin North Am 23: 333, 1997

51. Jeanrenaud X, Goy JJ, Kappenberger L: Effects of dual-chamber pacing in hypertrophic obstructive cardiomyopathy. Lancet 339: 1318, 1992

52. Kasper EK, Agema WR, Hutchins GM et al: The causes of dilated cardiomyopathy: A clinicopathologic review of 673 consecutive patients. J Am Coll Cardiol 23: 586, 1994

53. Katz JR, Kraft P, Fox K: Assessing a murmur, saving a life: Current trends in the management of hypertrophic cardiomyopathy. Nurse Pract 21: 62, 1996

54. Kjerulf A, Tvede M, Aldershvile et al: Bacterial endocarditis at a tertiary hospital: How do we improve diagnosis and delay of treatment? Cardiology 89: 79, 1998

55. Klein AL, Scalia GM: Diseases of the pericardium, restrictive cardiomyopathy and diastolic dysfunction. In Topol EJ (ed): Comprehensive Cardiovascular Medicine, pp 639–705. Philadelphia, Lippincott-Raven, 1998

56. Ledford DK: Immunologic aspects of vasculitis and cardiovascular disease, JAMA 278: 1962, 1997

57. Leith B, Furimsky I: A nursing case history: The patient with mycotic aneurysm secondary to endocarditis. AXON 16(3): 63–67, 1995

58. Li W, Somerville J: Infectious endocarditis in the grown-up congenital heart (GUCH) population. Eur Heart J 19: 166, 1998

59. Louie EK, Edwards LC: Hypertrophic cardiomyopathy. Prog Cardiovasc Dis 36: 275, 1994

60. Luquire R, Houston S: Cardiomyopathy: How to buy time. RN 5: 28, 1993

61. Lutwick LI, Vaghjimal A, Connolly MW: Postcardiac surgery infections. Crit Care Clin 14: 249, 1998

62. Lytle BW, Priest BP, Taylor PC et al: Surgical treatment of prosthetic valve endocarditis. J Thorac Cardiovasc Surg 111: 198, 1997

63. Manolio TA, Baughman KL, Rodeheffer R et al: Idiopathic dilated cardiomyopathy, prevalence and etiology: Summary of a National Heart, Lung, and Blood Institute workshop. Am J Cardiol 69: 1458, 1992

64. Maron BJ: Hypertrophic cardiomyopathy in athletes, catching a killer. The Physician and Sports Medicine 21(9): 83, 1993

65. Maron B, Epstein S, Morrow A: Symptomatic status and prognosis of patients after operations for hypertrophic obstructive cardiomyopathy. Eur Heart J 4: 175, 1983

66. Maron BJ, Hecht G, Klues HG et al: Both aborted sudden cardiac death and end-stage phase in hypertrophic cardiomyopathy. Am J Cardiol 72: 363, 1993

67. Maron BJ, Kragel AH, Roberts WC: Sudden death in hypertrophic cardiomyopathy with normal ventricular mass. Br Heart J 63: 308, 1990

68. Marrie TJ: Infectious endocarditis: A serious and changing disease. Critical Care Nurse 7(2): 31, 1987

69. Mason JW, O'Connel JB, Herskowitz A et al: A clinical trial of immunosuppressive therapy for myocarditis. N Engl J Med 333: 269, 1995

70. Maupin CR: The potential for noncaring when dealing with difficult patients: Strategies for moral decision making. J Cardiovasc Nurs 9(3): 11–22, 1995

71. Mayer KH, Schoenbaum SC: Evaluation and management of prosthetic valve endocarditis. Prog Cardiovasc Dis 24: 43, 1982

72. McKenna CJ, Codd MB, McCann HA et al: Alcohol consumption and idiopathic dilated cardiomyopathy: A case control study. Am Heart J 135: 833, 1998

73. McKenna WJ: The natural history of hypertrophic cardiomyopathy. Cardiovascular Clinics 19: 135, 1998

74. McKenna, WJ, Elliot PM: Hypertrophic cardiomyopthy. In Topol EJ (ed): Comprehensive Cardiovascular Medicine, pp 745–768. Philadelphia, Lippincott-Raven, 1998

75. Michels VV, Moll PP, Miller FA et al: The frequency of familial dilated cardiomyopathy in a series of patients with idiopathic dilated cardiomyopathy. N Engl J Med 326: 77, 1992

76. Miner PD: Infective endocarditis: Implications for care of the adult with congenital heart disease. Nurs Clin North Am 29: 269, 1994

77. Olson TM, Michels VV, Thibideau SN: Actin mutations in dilated cardiomyopathy: A heritable form of heart failure. Science 280: 750, 1998

78. Organ Procurement and Transplantation Network/SR 1996 Annual Report. United Network for Organ Sharing (UNOS) Scientific Registry. Richmond, VA, UNOS, April 15, 1997

79. Owens-Jones S, Hopp L: Viral myocarditis. Focus on Critical Care 15: 25, 1988

80. Page JG, Hubble MW: Recognizing infectious endocarditis: Case study of a 28-year-old. J of Emerg Nurs 22: 24, 1996

81. Paul S, York D: Cocaine abuse: An expanding health care problem for the 1990s. Am J Crit Care 1: 109, 1992

82. Perloff JK: Cardiomyopathies: Introduction. Cardiology Clinics 6: 185, 1998

83. Pierce CD: Acute post-MI pericarditis. J Cardiovasc Nurs 6(4): 46, 1992

84. Purcell JA: Advances in treatment of dilated cardiomyopathy. AACN Clinical Issues in Critical Care Nursing 1: 31, 1990

85. Relf MV: Surgical intervention for tricuspid valve endocarditis: Vegetectomy, valve excision, or valve replacement? J Cardiovasc Nurs 7(2): 71, 1993

86. Rey JR, Axon A, Budzynska A et al: Guidelines of the European Society of Gastrointestinal Endoscopy (ESGE): Antibiotic prophylaxis for gastrointestinal endoscopy. Endoscopy 30: 318, 1998

87. Rodgers ML: Pericarditis: A different kind of heart disease. Nursing 2: 53, 1990

88. Rowe GT: Hypertrophic cardiomyopathy in pregnancy: A case study. J Cardiovasc Nurs 8(2): 69–73, 1994

89. Rowley KM, Clubb KS, Smith GJ et al: Right-sided infective endocarditis as a consequence of flow-directed pulmonary artery catheterization: A clinicopathological study of 55 autopsied patients. N Engl J Med 311: 1152, 1984

90. Sandberg M, Singh A, Graves P: Extracorporeal membrane oxygenation as therapy in refractory reversible myocarditis. Critical Care Nurse 15: 53, 1995

91. Sasson Z, Rakowski H, Wigle ED: Hypertrophic cardiomyopathy. Cardiology Clinics 6: 233, 1988

92. Schactman, M, Cote PM, Ramza B: The importance of atrial contribution: A case study of dual-chamber pacing in hypertrophic obstructive cardiomyopathy. Heart Lung 26: 345, 1997

93. Schmidt J, Boilanger M, Abbott S: Peripartum cardiomyopathy. J Obstet Gynecol Neonatal Nurs Nov/Dec 18(6): 465–472 1989

94. Scrima DA: Infective endocarditis: Nursing considerations. Critical Care Nurse 7(2): 47, 1987

95. Sedlacek JA, Huffman M: The challenge of performing three heart transplantations in one day. AORN J 61: 712, 1995

96. Sexton DJ, Bashore TM: Infectious endocarditis. In Topol EJ (ed): Comprehensive Cardiovascular Medicine, pp 607–637. Philadelphia, Lippincott-Raven, 1998

97. Shebatai R: Diseases of the pericardium. In Alexander RW, Schlant RC, Fuster V (eds): Hurst's The Heart, p 2169. New York, McGraw-Hill, 1998

98. Shebatai R: Pericardial disease. In Brown DL (ed): Cardiac Intensive Care, p 469. Philadelphia, WB Saunders, 1998

99. Shebatai R, Fowler NO, Fenton JC et al: Pulsus paradoxus. J Clin Invest 44: 1882, 1965

100. Shenoy MM, Khanna A, Ansari M: Hypertrophic cardiomyopathy: Why is it often overlooked in elderly patients? Postgrad Med 90(5): 187, 1991

101. Simmons NA, Ball AP, Eykyn SJ et al: Amoxycillin prophylaxis for endocarditis prevention. Br Dent J 184(15): 208, 1998

102. Simpson M, Luquire R, Dewitt l et al: TCI left ventricular assist device: Nursing implications. Dimensions of Critical Care Nursing 9: 318, 1990

103. Sindone AP, Keogh AM, MacDonald PS et al: Continuous home ambulatory intravenous inotropic drug therapy in severe heart failure: Safety and cost efficiency. Am Heart J 134: 889, 1997

104. Smith SH: Uremic pericarditis in chronic renal failure: Nursing implications. American Nephrology Nurses Association Journal 20: 432, 1993

105. Snelson C, Cline BA, Luby C: Infective endocarditis: A challenging diagnosis. Dimensions of Critical Care Nursing 12: 4, 1993

106. Sole MJ, Liu P: Viral myocarditis: A paradigm for understanding the pathogenesis and treatment of dilated cardiomyopathy. J Am Coll Cardiol 22: 99A, 1993

107. Spirito P, Maron BJ: Relation between extent of left ventricular hypertrophy and occurrence of sudden death in hypertrophic cardiomyopathy. J Am Coll Cardiol 15: 1521, 1990

108. Spodick DH: Acquired pericardial disease: Pathogenesis and overview. In Spodick DH (ed): The Pericardium: A Comprehensive Textbook, pp 76–93. New York, Marcel Dekker, 1997

109. Spodick DH: Acute, clinically noneffusive ("dry") pericarditis. In Spodick DH (ed): The Pericardium: A Comprehensive Textbook, pp 94–113. New York, Marcel Dekker, 1997

110. Spodick DH: Auscultatory phenomena in pericardial disease. In Spodick DH (ed): The Pericardium: A Comprehensive Textbook, pp 27–39. New York, Marcel Dekker, 1997

111. Spodick DH: Cardiac tamponade: Clinical characteristics, diagnosis, and management. In Spodick DH (ed): The Pericardium: A Comprehensive Textbook, pp 153–179. New York, Marcel Dekker, 1997

112. Spodick DH: Congenital abnormalities of the pericardium. In Spodick DH (ed): The Pericardium: A Comprehensive Textbook, pp 65–75. New York, Marcel Dekker, 1997

113. Spodick DH: Constrictive pericarditis. In Spodick DH (ed): The Pericardium: A Comprehensive Textbook, pp 214–259. New York, Marcel Dekker, 1997

114. Spodick DH: Electricocardiographic abnormalities in pericardial disease. In Spodick DH (ed): The Pericardium: A Comprehensive Textbook, pp 40–64. New York, Marcel Dekker, 1997

115. Spodick DH: Pericardial disease in the vasculitis-connective tissue disease group. In Spodick DH (ed): The Pericardium: A Comprehensive Textbook, pp 314–333. New York, Marcel Dekker, 1997

116. Spodick DH: Pericardial effusion and hydropericardium without tamponade. In Spodick DH (ed): The Pericardium: A Comprehensive Textbook, pp 126–152. New York, Marcel Dekker, 1997

117. Spodick DH: Pericardial macro- and microanatomy: A synopsis. In Spodick DH (ed): The Pericardium: A Comprehensive Textbook, pp 7–14. New York, Marcel Dekker, 1997

118. Spodick DH: Physiology of the normal pericardium: Functions of the normal pericardium. In Spodick DH (ed): The Pericardium: A Comprehensive Textbook, pp 15–26. New York, Marcel Dekker, 1997

119. Spodick DH: Pulsus paradoxus. In Spodick DH (ed): The Pericardium: A Comprehensive Textbook, pp 191–199. New York, Marcel Dekker, 1997

120. Soulen RL: Magnetic resonance imaging of great vessel, myocardial and pericardial disease. Circulation 84(Suppl I): 311-I, 1991

121. Stevenson LW, Perloff JK: The dilated cardiomyopathies: Clinical aspects. Cardiology Clin 6: 187, 1988

122. Suddaby EC: Viral myocarditis in children. Critical Care Nurse 16: 73, 1996

123. Talard P, Levy S, Bonal J et al: Sudden death as a presenting symptom of hypertrophic cardiomyopathy: Treatment with an implantable cardioverter defibrillator. Pacing Clin Electrophysiol 19: 1264, 1996

124. Trausch PA: Infective endocarditis: Nursing care and prevention. Prog Cardiovasc Nurs 3(2): 45–53, 1988

125. Uszenski HJ, Booker SM, Goliash IB et al: Hypertrophic cardiomyopathy: Medical, surgical, and nursing management. J Cardiovasc Nurs 7(2): 13, 1993

126. Vasiljevic JD, Kanjuh V, Seferovic P: The incidence of myocarditis in endomyocardial biopsy of patients with congestive heart failure. Am Heart J 12: 1370, 1990

127. Vollman MW: Dynamic cardiomyoplasty: Perspectives on nursing care and collaborative management. Prog Cardiovasc Nurs 10(2): 15, 1995

128. Wackowski CA, Bierman PQ: Dual chamber pacing in patients with hypertrophic obstructive cardiomyopathy: A case study. Am J Crit Care 4: 165, 1995

129. Wilson WR, Danielson GK, Giuliani ER et al: Prosthetic valve endocarditis. Mayo Clin Proc 57: 255, 1982

130. Wilson WR, Karchmer AW, Dajani AS et al: Adults with infective endocarditis due to streptococci, enterococci, staphylococci, and HACEK microorganisms. JAMA 274: 1706, 1995

131. Zales VR, Wright KL: Endocarditis, pericarditis, myocarditis. Pediatr Ann 26: 116, 1997

Health Promotion and Disease Prevention

Coronary Heart Disease Risk Factors

KATHERINE M. NEWTON
ERIKA SIVARAJAN FROELICHER

Coronary heart disease (CHD) is usually associated with one or more characteristics known as risk factors. A risk factor is "an aspect of personal behavior or lifestyle, an environmental exposure or an inborn or inherited characteristic, which on the basis of epidemiologic evidence is known to be associated with" the occurrence of disease.[80]

Several aspects of the association between a potential risk factor and the disease are evaluated before an association is considered causal. These include the strength or magnitude of the association, the consistency or repeatability of the association, temporality (the cause precedes the disease), dose response (greater dose leads to greater likelihood of disease), the biologic and epidemiologic plausibility of the association, coherence of the potential cause with what is known about the disease, a decrease in the incidence of disease when the potential cause is eliminated, and experimental evidence.[69,122] Although few potential risk factors meet all of these criteria, the goal of epidemiologic investigations is to establish these characteristics.

The results of epidemiologic studies of disease etiology are frequently presented either as disease rates or as a relative risk. Relative risk is the rate of disease in a group exposed to a potential risk factor, divided by the rate of disease in an otherwise similar group that is unexposed to the risk factor.[122] For example, if the rate of fatal myocardial infarction (MI) in a group of smokers was 120/100,000 per year, and the rate in comparable nonsmokers was 60/100,000 per year, the relative risk associated with smoking would be:

Relative risk = rate in exposed / rate in unexposed = $(120/[100,000/\text{yr}])/(60/[100,000/\text{yr}]) = 2.0$

The risk of MI is thus doubled in the smokers, or a 200% increase in risk compared with nonsmokers. A relative risk of 1.30 represents a 30% increase in risk; a relative risk of 3.0 represents a 300% increase, or a tripling of risk.

United States death rates in 1994 to 1995 from all cardiovascular diseases combined, acute MI, cancer, and other causes, for African-American and white women and men are presented in Figure 29-1.[22] Cardiovascular disease continues to be the leading cause of death for African-American and white men and women throughout their life spans. Death rates from MI increase with age in men and women, with rates for women lagging 5 to 10 years behind those for men (Fig. 29-2). The rate of acute MI is higher in African-American women than white women throughout their life span, whereas MI rates in white and African-American men are similar until age 65 years, when the rate in white men exceeds that in African-American men. In the Third National Health and Nutrition Examination Survey (NHANES III), the prevalence of a personal history of MI was higher for men than women among whites and Mexican Americans, but this difference was less pronounced among African Americans (Table 29-1).

Coronary heart disease mortality rates have declined steadily since the late 1960s. From 1968 to 1984, CHD mortality declined at an average rate of 2% to 3% per year in all age groups, in both sexes, and in blacks and whites.[127] From 1979 to 1985, the average annual percentage change in CHD mortality, for people aged 35 to 74 years, was −2.59% for white women, −3.37% for white men, −2.0% for African-American women, and −2.84% for African-American men.[127] From 1987 to 1994, the average annual percentage change in CHD mortality, for people aged 35 to 74 years, was −4.5% for white women, −4.7% for white men, −4.1% for African-American women, and −2.5% for African-American men.[118] There is ongoing speculation as to the cause of this decline in

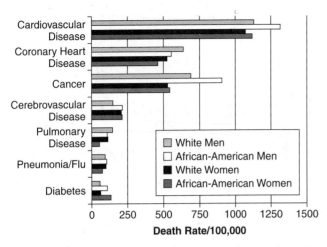

FIGURE 29-1 U.S. death rates per 100,000 population for major causes of death, by gender, and race/ethnicity. (From Centers for Disease Control and Prevention: CDC Wonder. Available: *http://wonder.cdc.gov/WONDER/mort.oo.ex./*.October, 1998.)

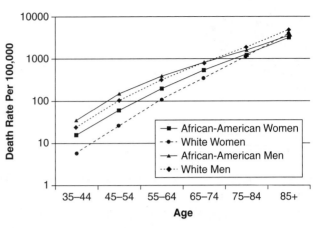

FIGURE 29-2 U.S. coronary heart disease death rate per 100,000 population by age, gender, and race/ethnicity. (From Centers for Disease Control and Prevention: CDC Wonder. Available: *http://wonder.cdc.gov/WONDER/mort.oo.ex./*.October, 1998.)

CHD mortality, although multiple causes are likely. Small, population-wide behavior changes leading to lower serum cholesterol, lower smoking rates, and lower blood pressure may account for as much as 50% of the decrease.[127] Decreases in case fatality rates also have been documented. This indicates that changes in patient management, including more rapid access to emergency care and interventions that reduce infarct size and prevent death due to arrhythmias, may account for some of the decline in CHD mortality.[109]

Cardiovascular disease risk factors have additive effects. The MI risk in a person with three major risk factors is higher than that of a person with two or one[61] (Fig. 29-3). Furthermore, for any given combination of risk factors, at a given age, the risk is lower in women than men (Fig. 29-4).

In this chapter, the major known risk factors for cardiovascular disease are briefly reviewed. Data from NHANES III is used to demonstrate the prevalence of CHD risk factors in U.S. women and men.

DEMOGRAPHIC CHARACTERISTICS

Coronary heart disease mortality rates rise exponentially with age for men and women (see Fig. 29-2). Until the seventh decade of life, African-American men have the highest rates of CHD mortality, followed by white men, African-American women, and white women. The rates in men converge at approximately the seventh decade, and those in women converge in the ninth decade. Further data about CHD rates by race/ethnicity come from analysis of death rates in California from 1985 to 1990[156]. The CHD death rates per 100,000 population were as follows: white women, 143; white men, 302; Hispanic women, 97; Hispanic men, 175; African-American women, 214; African-American men, 316; Chinese women, 73; Chinese men, 155; Japanese women, 67; Japanese men, 146; Asian Indian women, 110; and Asian Indian men 258.[156] Thus, within all

TABLE 29-1	Personal History of Myocardial Infarction Among U.S. Women and Men by Age and Race/Ethnicity					
	White		**African American**		**Mexican American**	
Age Group (y)	Women (%)	Men (%)	Women (%)	Men (%)	Women (%)	Men (%)
20–29	0.0	0.2	0.1	0.9	0.1	0.4
30–39	0.0	0.7	0.1	0.2	0.7	0.8
40–49	0.5	2.7	1.7	2.2	0.5	2.6
50–59	1.9	6.4	5.2	7.3	3.3	6.4
60–69	5.9	13.3	8.3	10.5	4.0	8.8
≥70	11.9	18.8	11.1	11.1	6.6	12.1

From the National Center for Health Statistics: National Health and Nutrition Examination Survey, III. Rockville, MD 1988–1994.

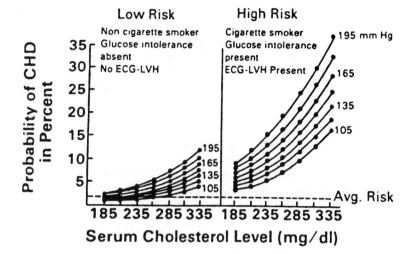

FIGURE 29-3 Risk of coronary heart disease as it relates to cholesterol levels in the absence (*left*) or presence (*right*) of additional risk factors. ECG-LVH, left ventricular hypertrophy. (From Kannell WB et al: Report of Inter-Society Commission for Heart Disease Resource: Optimal resource for primary prevention of atherosclerotic diseases. Circulation 70: 181A, 1984.) By permission of the American Heart Association, Inc.

groups, CHD rates are lower in women than in men, although African-American women have CHD death rates far exceeding those for women in other groups. The reasons behind these differences in rates have not been well studied and are poorly understood.

Lower socioeconomic status[73,94] and low income[104] are associated with increased CHD mortality in men and women, probably due in part to the higher prevalence of CHD risk factors among those of lower socioeconomic status. Perceived financial status is also associated with MI and coronary death in women.[33] Higher systolic blood pressure, higher low-density lipoprotein (LDL) cholesterol, higher fasting glucose levels and 2-hour insulin values, higher body mass index (BMI), and lower high-density lipoprotein (HDL) cholesterol are all associated with lower socioeconomic status.[94] Educational attainment, which often determines socioeconomic status, is inversely related to CHD risk in African-American and white women and white men, but is positively associated with CHD in African-American men.[33,34,66,71,79,104] Women of lower educational attainment are more often smokers, sedentary, angry, pessimistic, depressed, and dissatisfied with their work, and have less social support and self-esteem.[94] Educational incongruity with the spouse is associated with increased risk of sudden cardiac death and MI in women.[146,147] Among men, the 10-year incidence of CHD increases with the wife's education level for those whose wives are employed outside the home, but not for those whose wives are homemakers.[62]

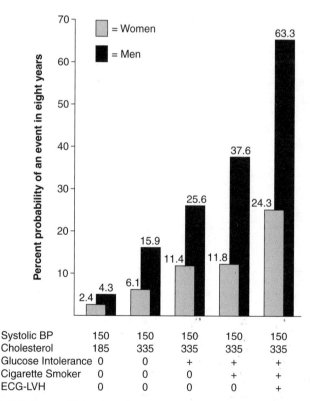

Systolic BP	150	150	150	150	150
Cholesterol	185	335	335	335	335
Glucose Intolerance	0	0	+	+	+
Cigarette Smoker	0	0	0	+	+
ECG-LVH	0	0	0	0	+

FIGURE 29-4 Risk of cardiovascular disease at systolic blood pressure of 150 mm Hg according to intensity of other known risk factors in subjects aged 45 years, Framingham Heart Study. (Adapted from Kannell WB et al: Report of Inter-Society Commission for Heart Disease Resources: Optimal resources for primary prevention of atherosclerotic diseases. Circulation 70: 181A, 1984. By permission of the American Heart Association, Inc.)

FAMILY HISTORY OF CARDIOVASCULAR DISEASE

A family history of CHD puts women and men at increased risk for CHD, probably from a combination of genetic and environmental factors.[19,59,104,116] A history of MI in one first-degree relative doubles, and in two or more first-degree relatives triples MI risk.[116] MI risk is strongest when MI in relatives occurs before age 55 years but is still present when MI occurs after age 55 years.[116] The risk associated with a positive family history is independent of other known CHD risk factors. In the Nurses Health Study, women with a family history of parental MI at or below 60 years of age had 2.8 times the risk of nonfatal MI, 5 times the risk of fatal CHD, and 3.4 times the risk for angina pectoris compared with women without a history of parental MI.[135] For women with a history of parental MI after age 60 years, there was no increase in risk for nonfatal CHD, but risk for fatal CHD was increased 2.6 times, and for angina pectoris it was increased 1.9 times compared with women with no family history of CHD.[135] In contrast, a study of older women found no increase in CHD risk with a family history of heart attack.[7]

Twin studies shed further light on the influence of family history on CHD risk. In a study of male and female Swedish monozygotic and dizygotic twins, among male twins the relative risk of CHD for monozygotic twins was 8.1 and the relative risk for dizygotic twins was 3.8 when one twin died of CHD before age 55 years.[93] Among female twins, the relative risk of CHD for monozygotic twins was 15 and the relative risk for dizygotic twins was 2.6 when one twin died of CHD before age 55 years. In both monozygotic and dizygotic twins, as the age at which one twin died increased, the risk for CHD among the remaining twin decreased.[93]

CIGARETTE SMOKING

In 1995, 47 million adults were current smokers, or 24.7% of the adult U.S population (27.1% of men and 24.1% of women).[38] Smoking prevalence varies markedly by race/ethnicity and age (Fig. 29-5). In 1995, smoking rates by race/ethnicity were as follows: Native Americans/Alaskan Natives, 36.2%; African Americans, 25.8%; non-Hispanic whites, 25.6%; Hispanics, 18.3%; and Asians/Pacific Islanders 16.6%.[38] From 1965 to 1985, the prevalence of smoking in men and women decreased at a rate of 0.5% per year. From 1987 through 1990, smoking prevalence decreased at an even faster rate of 1.1% per year, although smoking prevalence was the same in 1991 as in 1990 for white men.[37] For African Americans and women, the smok-

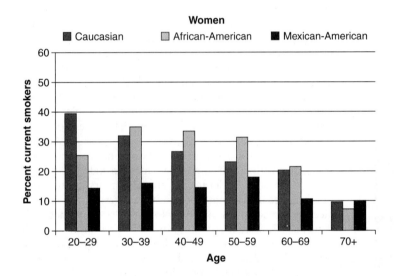

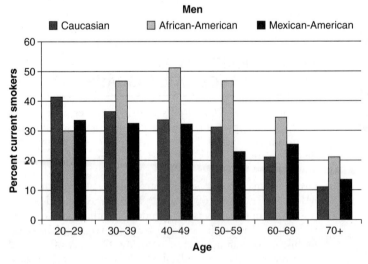

Source: National Center for Health Statistics. National Health and Nutrition Examination Survey, III 1988-1994.

FIGURE 29-5 Prevalence of current smoking among U.S. women and men by age and race/ethnicity.[100]

ing prevalence was actually higher in 1991 than in 1990.[36] The initiation of smoking from 1974 to 1987 among people 20 to 24 years of age decreased among men but remained relatively unchanged among women. By 1987, the proportion of men and women aged 20 to 24 years who initiated smoking was virtually identical.[103] However, the absolute number of smokers aged 25 to 44 years increased by 54%, and the number of smokers aged 65 or older increased by 47%, whereas the number of smokers aged 45 to 64 years remained stable.

Smoking and Coronary Heart Disease

Cigarette smoking is perhaps the most preventable known cause of CHD today, leading to more deaths from CHD than from either lung cancer or chronic obstructive pulmonary disease.[42] CHD risk increases with number of cigarettes smoked, longer duration of smoking, and younger age at initiation of smoking.[55,133]

The CHD risk of male cigarette smokers is two (aged 60 years and older) to three (aged 30 to 59 years) times that of nonsmokers,[30] whereas women who are current smokers have up to four times the risk of first MI of those who have never smoked.[26,82,121] In the Nurses Health Study, cigarette smoking was associated with a fivefold increase in the risk for fatal CHD and nonfatal MI, and tripled the risk of angina.[157] This elevation in risk of MI and CHD death is sustained from youth into advanced age for men and women.[78,133] Smoking low-tar (<17.6 mg), low-nicotine (<1.2 mg), or filter cigarettes does not lower the risk of MI compared with high-tar, high-nicotine, or nonfiltered cigarettes.[61,65]

Smoking cessation confers benefit regardless of sex, age, or presence of CHD. Men and women of all ages with documented CHD who quit smoking have half the risk of mortality compared with those who continue to smoke.[50,82,123] For women who quit smoking, MI risk is indistinguishable from that of nonsmokers within 3 to 5 years of smoking cessation.[77,121,135] There are many successful approaches to smoking cessation, and these interventions are less costly than many other preventive interventions.[27] The simple advice from health care providers to smokers to quit smoking increases smoking cessation rates by 30%.[38] Thus smoking cessation should be encouraged regardless of age, sex, or the presence of established disease.

Environmental Tobacco Smoke

It is estimated that 53,000 deaths annually are attributable to environmental tobacco smoke (ETS), making it the third leading preventable cause of death in the Unites States.[42] Ten times as many of these deaths are due to CHD as lung cancer.[42] Exposure of nonsmokers to ETS from a spouse who smokes increases the risk of CHD death by 30% in men and women. This risk increases with the amount smoked by the spouse.[42] ETS causes arterial endothelial damage, may initiate or accelerate the development of atherosclerosis, and increases platelet aggregation, which may result in coronary thrombosis.[42] Thus, the effects of ETS are similar to those of smoking cigarettes.

HIGH BLOOD PRESSURE

High blood pressure, or hypertension (systolic blood pressure ≥140 mm Hg or diastolic blood pressure ≥90 mm Hg) carries particular importance as a cardiovascular risk factor for several reasons. It is highly prevalent, it is relatively simple to identify, it is a major risk for devastating cardiovascular outcomes, and control of high blood pressure is known to decrease its risk.[63] Prevalence of high blood pressure increases with age among whites, African Americans, and Mexican Americans[22] (Fig. 29-6). The prevalence of high blood pressure is highest among African Americans at all ages, whereas prevalence rates in whites and Mexican Americans are similar among men and women (NHANES III data, 1988 to 1994).

High blood pressure is associated with three- to four-fold increases in the risk of CHD, stroke, and MI,[30,55,82] and it also increases the risk of peripheral vascular disease, renal failure, and congestive heart failure in men and women across the life span.[4,30] The normalization of blood pressure dramatically decreases the risk of stroke, renal failure, cardiac failure, and coronary events.[54,97,111] Even in the elderly, control of high blood pressure confers major benefits against stroke, coronary events, and all cardiovascular events.[98,128] High blood pressure and the nurse's role in its management are discussed in detail in Chapter 32.

SERUM LIPIDS AND LIPOPROTEINS

Elevated serum total cholesterol and LDL cholesterol are associated with an increased risk of CHD in men and women of all ages.[20,89,160] The prevalence of hypercholesterolemia is higher in U.S. women than men, and higher in whites and African Americans than in Mexican Americans[100] (Table 29-2). In the Framingham Heart Study, women and men with serum cholesterol concentrations greater than 295 mg/dL had over three times the risk of MI and definite coronary events than those with cholesterol concentrations less than 204 mg/dL.[20] CHD rates are lower for women than men at any given level of serum cholesterol.[20]

Serum HDL cholesterol has a protective effect against CHD. A 1 mg/dL increment in HDL is associated with a 2% (men) to 3% (women) decrement in total CHD risk, and a 3.7% (men) to 4.7% (women) decrement in CHD mortality.[44] At any given level of LDL, higher levels of HDL confer protection against CHD.[62]

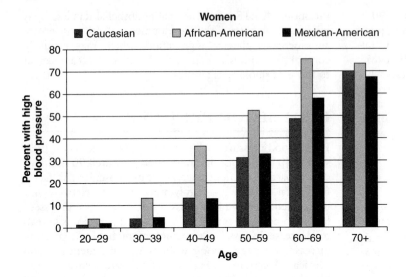

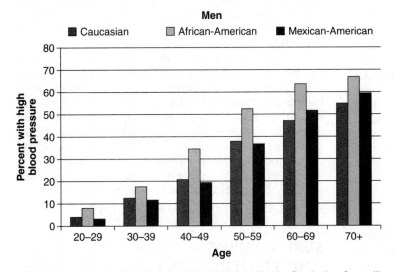

Source: National Center for Health Statistics. National Health and Nutrition Examinations Survey, III 1988-1994. ªDiastolic (≥90 mg/dL), or Systolic (≥ 140 mg/dL), or self-reported use of anti-hypertensive medication.

FIGURE 29-6 Prevalence of high blood pressure among U.S. women and men by age and race/ethnicity.

TABLE 29-2	**Prevalence of Hypercholesterolemia* Among U.S. Women and Men by Age and Race/Ethnicity**

	White		African American		Mexican American	
Age Group (y)	Women (%)	Men (%)	Women (%)	Men (%)	Women (%)	Men (%)
20–29	6.9	4.6	7.3	7.3	7.2	7 7
30–39	7.8	17.8	7.3	9.7	8.8	18.0
40–49	20.3	25.0	16.4	19.2	16.8	20.6
50–59	39.1	26.6	35.1	26.9	27.3	26.9
60–69	44.2	29.4	47.8	28.3	39.7	33.8
≥70	43.4	23.6	39.6	23.6	28.9	18.1

From the National Center for Health Statistics, U.S. Department of Health and Human Services (DHHS). Third National Health and Nutrition Examination Survey, 1988–1994, NHANES III Data File (CD-ROM Series II, NO 1). Public Use Data File, Hyattsville, MD: Centers for Disease Control and Prevention, 1997.

*Based on self-reported use of cholesterol-lowering medication or a total serum cholesterol value of ≥240 mg/dL.

Attention has been focused on subfractions of HDL and LDL, the apolipoproteins (apo AI, apo AII, apo B) and lipoprotein(a) (Lp[a]). In a study of the predictors of premature CHD at coronary arteriography, Kwiterovich and associates[76] found that apo B was more strongly associated with an increase in CHD risk in women (relative risk = 1.7; 95% confidence interval [CI], 1.0 to 2.9) than in men (relative risk = 1.4; 95% CI, 0.8 to 2.6), whereas Apo AI was more strongly associated with a decrease in CHD risk in men (relative risk = 0.5; 95% CI, 0.3 to 1.0) than in women (relative risk = 0.9; 95% CI, 0.6 to 1.4). Increasing levels of Lp(a) are also associated with an increase in CHD risk.[5,15,16,28,141] In the Framingham Heart Study, the relative risk for CHD associated with elevated Lp(a) was 1.6 (95% CI, 1.1 to 2.3) in women[15] and 1.9 (95% CI, 1.2 to 2.9) in men.[16] LDL subclass patterns also influence CHD risk. Compared with light, buoyant LDL, small, dense LDL is associated with a threefold increase in risk of MI.[5]

Reproductive hormones have a major impact on serum lipid levels in women. During menopause, total serum cholesterol concentrations rise by an average of 19%.[151] This change is reversed by postmenopausal estrogen replacement, which increases HDL cholesterol from 9% to 13% and lowers LDL 4% to 10%.[20]

Serum cholesterol levels influence prognosis after MI. The risk for reinfarction is 3.7 (men) to 9.2 (women) times as great when serum cholesterol levels are 275 mg/dL or greater, compared with levels of less than 200 mg/dL.[162] There is evidence that normalization of serum lipids and lipoproteins reduces the CHD mortality rate.[18] Hyperlipoproteinemia and its management are discussed in more detail in Chapter 33.

PHYSICAL ACTIVITY

The roles of physical activity and physical fitness in preventing cardiovascular disease and controlling cardiovascular disease risk factors are well established. The 1996 Surgeon General's Report on Physical Activity and Health recommends that children and adults accumulate at least 30 minutes of moderate-intensity physical activity most days of the week.[150] Applying this definition to NHANES III data (Figs. 29-7, 29-8) shows that only approximately half of

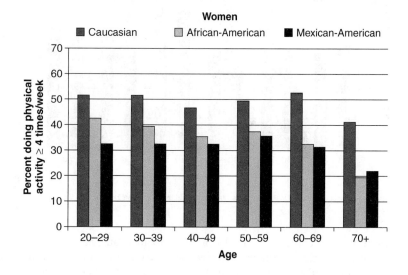

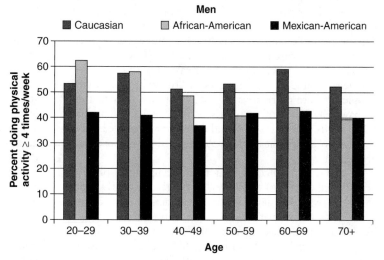

FIGURE 29-7 Prevalence of physical activity at least four times per week among U.S. women and men by age and race/ethnicity.

*Physical activity = walking, jogging or running, bicycling, swimming, aerobics, dancing, calisthenics, garden/yard work, and/or lifting weights.
Source: National center for Health Statistics. National Health and Nutrition Examination Survey, III 1988–1994.

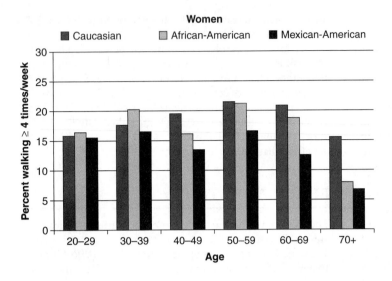

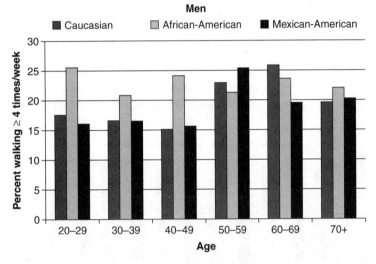

Source: National Center for Health Statistics. National Health and Nutrition Examination Survey, III 1988-994.

FIGURE 29-8 Prevalence of walking at least 1 mile without stopping at least four times per week among U.S. women and men by age and race/ethnicity.

white women and less than 40% of African-American and Mexican-American women are physically active four or more times per week, and less than 25% of women walk at least four times per week. The proportions are only slightly higher for American men. Thus, a large proportion of the American public could be targeted for public health interventions to increase physical activity.

The effects on cardiovascular disease of both on-the-job and leisure-time activity have been studied.[48] In general, people who are more physically active or physically fit tend to have CHD less often than sedentary or less fit people. CHD tends to be less severe and occurs at a later age among those who are physically active compared with those who are sedentary.[48]

When data from cohort studies of occupational physical activity and CHD risk were pooled, the risk for CHD death for those with low-level occupational activity was almost twice that of those with high-level activity, and MI risk was 40% higher in the sedentary group.[13] Analysis of studies of nonoccupational activity showed a 60% increase in risk of CHD death for low compared with high activity and a tripling of the risk of MI.[13] There was a 30% to 40% increase in risk of CHD death and MI for moderate occupational

and nonoccupational activity compared with high activity.[13] In the five studies that included women, the risk for angina pectoris, MI, and sudden death was two to three times higher among women in the lowest compared with the highest activity level.[32]

An important addition to understanding the benefits of fitness has been made by studies that measure physical fitness using standardized exercise tests and then compare fitness with later cardiovascular outcomes.[14,35,131,134] In these studies, a higher level of fitness was associated with a significantly lower rate of cardiovascular disease mortality in men and women,[14,134] all-cause mortality in men and women,[14] and ischemic heart disease (fatal and nonfatal MI plus sudden death) in men.[134]

There are insufficient data to determine whether physical conditioning reduces reinfarction or mortality in people with established CHD.[48] Although pooled analyses from randomized trials of comprehensive cardiac rehabilitation suggest a 19% to 25% reduction in mortality rates associated with rehabilitation, it is difficult to dissociate the benefits of the exercise component of these programs from other lifestyle changes.[105,149] However, the potential benefits of a program of regular exercise after MI include an increase in exercise capacity, decrease in angina, improved control of other cardiovascular disease risk factors, decreased anxiety and depression, and increased self-esteem and sense of well-being.[149]

The Protective Effect of Physical Activity

Regular physical exercise has favorable effects on many CHD risk factors, including hypertension, plasma lipid, insulin and glucose levels, and coagulation and fibrinolysis.[23,48] The level of regular physical activity or fitness is inversely related to risk for development of hypertension, and in people at high risk for hypertension, a program of regular exercise decreases that risk.[23,48] In people with established hypertension, starting a program of low to moderate regular endurance exercise lowers the blood pressure 5% to 10%.[23,48]

High-density lipoprotein is increased, whereas LDL, very–low-density lipoprotein, and triglyceride levels are decreased by regular exercise.[48] This response appears to be related to the intensity, duration, and frequency of exercise. Insulin levels are reduced, and insulin resistance and glucose intolerance are improved by regular exercise. Exercise also promotes favorable effects on coagulation by decreasing platelet aggregatability, lowering plasma fibrinogen concentration, and enhancing tissue plasminogen activator activity.[23,48] Last, even a moderate level of regular exercise is an important adjunct to weight reduction.

DIABETES MELLITUS

The American Diabetes Association diagnostic criteria for diabetes mellitus are a random blood glucose of at least 200 mg/dL or a fasting blood glucose of at least 126 mg/dL.[39] In the NHANES III study, using the criteria of self-reported diabetes or a fasting plasma glucose of at least 126 mg/dL, the prevalence of diabetes in African-American and Hispanic women is two to three times that of white women in the United States (Fig. 29-9). By 60 to 69 years of age, approximately 11% of white women, 13% of white men, 27% of African-American and Hispanic women, 18% of African-American men, and 24% of Hispanic men have diabetes.

Diabetes mellitus is associated with an increase in the incidence of CHD in men and women across the life span.[30]

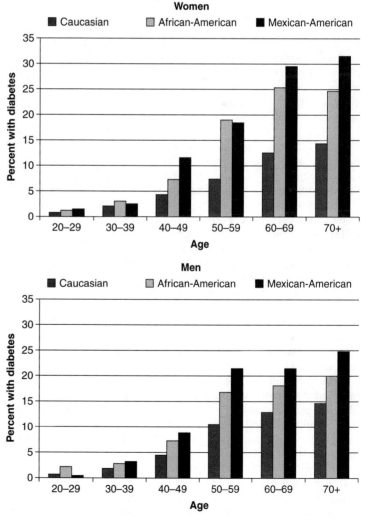

FIGURE 29-9 Prevalence of diabetes among U.S. women and men by age and race/ethnicity.

Source: National Center for Health Statistics. National Health and Nutrition Examination Survey, III 1988-1994. ªBased on self report, fasting glucose levels (≥ 126 mg/dL), and random (non-fasting) glucose levels (≥ 200 mg/dL)

In men, diabetes is associated with a doubling in CHD incidence and, in women with diabetes, CHD incidence is five to seven times that of nondiabetic people.[30,135] Diabetes doubles the rate of MI in men and increases the rate of MI in women four- to sixfold.[30,82,135] CHD and MI rates in diabetic women approach those of men of similar age, essentially eliminating the advantage found in nondiabetic women compared with men. This is true for white,[107] Mexican-American,[99] and Japanese[72] women. Ischemic heart disease mortality is doubled in men with diabetes and tripled in women with diabetes.[8]

Rates of other atherosclerotic manifestations such as atherothrombotic stroke and peripheral vascular disease are also higher in diabetic people.[30] The incidence of peripheral vascular disease is five times higher in men and eight times higher in women with diabetes compared with nondiabetic people. Diabetes is associated with a three- to fivefold increase in the incidence of atherothrombotic stroke in men and women.[30,90]

After MI or the diagnosis of CHD, diabetic patients have a significantly poorer prognosis than nondiabetic patients, and this effect is particularly pronounced for women.[70,161] Diabetic patients with MI are two to four times as likely to die in hospital, more often have congestive heart failure and postinfarction angina pectoris, and more often extend their infarct than nondiabetic patients.[145] Among survivors of an initial MI, the incidence of recurrent MI is increased by 30% in diabetic men and almost tripled in diabetic women, whereas fatal CHD is doubled in men and women.[1] During follow-up after MI, total mortality among diabetic patients is 1.5 times to 3 times that of nondiabetic patients.[145] Whether the degree of control of diabetes after MI affects survival after MI is unknown.

Insulin resistance, the primary pathologic process in type II diabetes, may also be associated with CHD. Among nondiabetic adults in the Atherosclerosis Risk in Communities Study (ARIC), women in the highest quintile of fasting insulin had a threefold increase in CHD risk compared with women in the lowest quintile of fasting insulin; however, fasting insulin was not associated with CHD risk in men.[40] In contrast, a study of Finnish men and women found that CHD prevalence increased with increasing fasting plasma insulin levels in both diabetic and nondiabetic men and women.[117] A prospective study in the England found a 60% increase in risk of fatal and nonfatal MI among men in the 10th decile of serum insulin compared with the 1st to 9th deciles.[110] The differences in these findings in men appear to be related to the degree of insulin elevation; only severe elevations are related to increased risk.

The mechanisms responsible for the acceleration of myocardial dysfunction and atherosclerosis associated with diabetes are the subject of great scrutiny.[64,130] Diabetes, hyperinsulinemia, and insulin resistance are associated with higher relative weight (specifically with a central body fat distribution); higher systolic and diastolic blood pressure; lower levels of HDL; and higher total cholesterol, HDL, and triglyceride levels.[30,61,91,130] These disturbances appear to be linked through a complex set of genetic and environmental factors, and hypotheses about these associations are still being explored.

The Diabetes Control and Complications Trial was the first randomized trial to show that intensive therapy to improve glycemic control reduced the risk of laser treatment of retinopathy, clinical neuropathy, and microalbuminuria in patients with type I diabetes.[31] There was also a trend toward the reduction of macrovascular events. Although clinical trials are underway, there is no evidence that interventions to improve diabetic control in patients with type II diabetes prevent CHD events. However, because other CHD risk factors cluster in people with diabetes, attention should focus on altering those risk factors where change is known to make a difference in CHD risk, including hypertension, hypercholesterolemia, and smoking.

OBESITY, WEIGHT DISTRIBUTION, AND WEIGHT CHANGE

The proportion of U.S. adults characterized as overweight is steadily increasing. Overweight is defined as a BMI greater than 27.2 kg/m^2 for women and greater than 27.8 kg/m^2 for men. This represents the 85th percentile of weight for adults 20 to 29 years of age in the NHANES II study, or 120% of desirable weight for medium-framed adults from the 1983 Metropolitan Life Insurance Tables. In the NHANES I study (1960 to 1962), the age-adjusted prevalence of overweight was 23.6% among white women, 23.0% among white men, 41.6% among African-American women, and 41.6% among African-American men. By the time of the NHANES III study (1988 to 1991), 33.2% of white women, 32% of white men, 48.6% of African-American women, and 31.8% of African-American men were overweight.[74] Overweight increases with age, peaking at midlife. By 50 to 59 years of age, the proportions classified as overweight in the NHANES III study were 47.6% of white women, 41.5% of white men, 66.4% of African-American women, 40.4% of African-American men, 65.1% of Mexican-American women, and 54.8% of Mexican-American men (Fig. 29-10).

A positive association between obesity and CHD is expected. Hypertension, diabetes, and hypercholesterolemia are all more common in overweight people,[153] and weight reduction is an important therapy in the management of all CHD risk factors. Nevertheless, findings about the association between body weight and CHD risk are inconsistent. For example, despite the fact that body weight increased for African-American and white men and women from 1962 through 1980, cardiovascular mortality, stroke, and MI all decreased during this same time.[9]

In the Framingham Heart Study, men younger than 50 years of age who were greater than 30% above ideal weight (determined by Metropolitan Life Insurance tables) had twice the incidence of CHD and acute MI compared with those less than 10% above ideal weight.[52] The findings were similar but of lower magnitude in those older than 50 years of age.[52] In a Dutch study of BMI measured at 18 years of age in men, the 32-year CHD mortality rate was more than doubled in those in the highest BMI category.[51] Others have found no relationship between BMI and CHD mortality among white men, but a 70% increase in CHD mortality in African-American men in the 90th percentile of

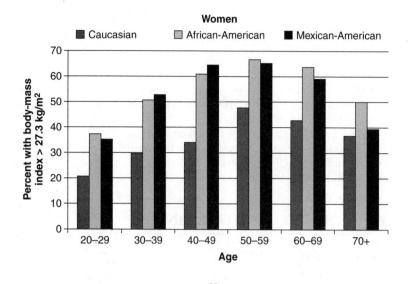

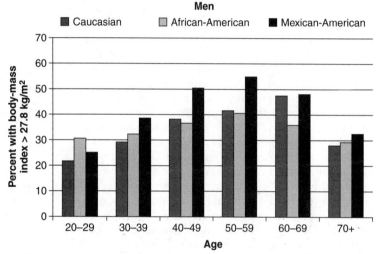

FIGURE 29-10 Prevalence of obesity among U.S. women and men by age and race/ethnicity.

Source: National Center for Health Statistics. National Health and Nutrition Examination Survey, III 1988-1994.

BMI compared with the 50th percentile.[144] Still other investigators have found no association between BMI and CHD death rates in African-American or white men.[67]

In women, relative weight predicts angina pectoris, CHD other than angina, CHD death, stroke, and congestive heart failure.[52] In the Nurses Health Study, women in the highest quartile of BMI (>29 kg/m²) had a relative risk of nonfatal MI and fatal CHD of 1.8, and double the risk of angina pectoris compared with women in the lowest BMI quartile.[91] These relationships hold even among women of normal or near-normal weight, where those with a BMI of 25 to 28.9 kg/m² and 23 to 24.9 kg/m² had a relative risk for CHD of 2.06 and 1.45, respectively, compared with women with a BMI less than 21 kg/m².[158] In the Framingham Heart Study, obese women (Metropolitan Relative Weight ≥130%) aged 50 years or younger had a 2.4-fold increase in CHD risk over 26 years of follow-up compared with lean women (Metropolitan Relative Weight <110%).[52] The relationship between overweight and CHD is weaker, perhaps absent, among African-American women. In African-American women, BMI is unrelated to MI,[58,67,144]

CHD death,[67,144] and all-cause mortality.[58,144] Overweight also has a role in secondary prevention. Among women who have survived a first MI, a 1-unit increase in BMI is associated with a 3% increase in risk of reinfarction.[102]

Overweight continues to play a role in the elderly. Among men and women 65 years of age and older, the total mortality rate is as much as doubled in those above the 70th percentile of BMI compared with those in the 10th to 29th percentile, and the CHD mortality rate is increased by 50% in men and doubled in women.[47]

Weight gain after the young adult years increases the risk of CHD in men and women.[52,91] In the Nurses Health Study, women who gained 20 to 35 kg after 18 years of age had double the risk of nonfatal MI and fatal CHD compared with those who gained less than 3 kg.[91]

The role of the distribution of body weight has attracted increasing attention. The primary hypothesis is that a central body weight distribution, often measured as waist-to-hip ratio, increases CHD risk to a greater degree than a more peripheral body weight distribution. In white men, abdominal girth was not associated with total or CHD mortality, although African-American men in the 90th percentile for abdominal girth had almost double the rate of CHD mortality compared with those in the 50th percentile.[144] These results were reversed in women. There was no association between abdominal circumference and all-cause or CHD mortality in African-American women, but white women in the 85th percentile of abdominal circumference had a 50% increase in all-cause and CHD mortality compared with those in the 15th percentile.[144]

We are unaware of trials of the effects of weight loss on CHD risk. Nevertheless, weight loss is frequently recommended for its beneficial effects on cholesterol, blood pressure, insulin resistance, and glycemic control.

REPRODUCTIVE HORMONES

Reproductive History

Blood pressure and blood lipids change in relation to reproductive events. It is thus reasonable to investigate the potential impact of these events on the risk of CHD in women. Few studies have examined these factors, and their findings are contradictory. Nulliparous women appear to be at lower risk of CHD than parous women, and a woman's risk of CHD may increase with younger age at first birth.[12,81,108] Increasing parity may also increase CHD risk, perhaps because of the large changes in hormones associated with pregnancy.[108] Others, however, have found no differences in risk with parity and number of births.[24]

Earlier age at menopause increases CHD risk regardless of the mechanism of menopause. Among women who undergo bilateral oophorectomy, those younger than 35 years of age have almost eight times the risk for nonfatal MI compared with natural menopause.[136] Premenopausal women of any age who undergo bilateral oophorectomy without estrogen replacement therapy have twice the risk of nonfatal MI and fatal CHD compared with premenopausal women of the same age, whereas those who receive estrogen replacement therapy have no increase in risk.[137] At menopause, serum HDL levels decline and LDL levels increase, compared with premenopausal values,[83,95] and these unfavorable lipid changes may be prevented by hormone replacement therapy (HRT).[95]

Oral Contraceptives

The increased risk for fatal and nonfatal MI in users of oral contraceptives (OC) was first established in the 1960s and early 1970s. In these early studies, OC use was associated with an increased risk of nonfatal and fatal MI in young women. In women aged 30 to 39 years, the risk of fatal and nonfatal MI among OC users was three times that of nonusers. For women aged 40 to 44 years, risk of fatal MI was 5.7 times,[88] and risk of nonfatal MI 4.7 times[87] that of nonusers. Concurrent cigarette smoking acts synergistically with the risk from OCs, with the greatest risk occurring in women who smoke and are older than 35 years of age.[26,57] The risk in past users was similar to that in women who had never used OCs.[87,88,132,138] When duration of past use was examined, use of 5 to 9 years increased the risk of nonfatal

MI by 50%, and 10 or more years of use more than doubled the risk.[132] Smoking did not amplify this effect of past use.

There are at least two mechanisms for the risk of cardiovascular events associated with OCs. First, OCs increase the risk of arterial and venous thromboembolism. The risk of arterial and venous thrombosis increases with the dosage of estrogen, whereas higher dosages of progestogens increase only the risk of arterial thrombosis.[68,96] The second possible mechanism for the association between OCs and CHD risk is the promotion of atherogenesis through unfavorable effects on blood pressure, serum lipids, and glucose tolerance.[120]

Dosages of estrogen and progestin in current OCs are considerably lower than those of the 1970s, and there appears to be little or no risk of MI or CHD death among users of newer OC formulations.[92,129,138,139] The exception is the finding in some,[26,92] but not all[129] studies of continued high risk among women who are heavy cigarette smokers and OC users. A prospective cohort study in England and Scotland found a fivefold increase in risk of MI among current smokers who used OCs.[92] It has been estimated that 9.7% of cases of nonfatal MI among women 35 to 44 years of age in the United States are due to the combination of smoking and OC use.[43] However, a U.S. case-control study of low-dose OCs and MI risk in women aged 18 to 44 years found no increase in risk among smokers.[129] Overall, OCs appear to offer a safe contraceptive alternative in terms of cardiovascular disease risk.

Postmenopausal Hormone Replacement Therapy

There are numerous plausible biologic mechanisms whereby HRT (postmenopausal estrogen with progestins) might reduce the risk of CHD in postmenopausal women. HRT promotes a favorable lipid profile, decreasing LDL and total cholesterol while increasing HDL cholesterol and triglycerides.[21,85,163,164] The effect of HRT on blood pressure varies with the type and dosage of estrogen preparation and whether progestins are also taken. However, it appears that unopposed estrogen replacement therapy does not raise blood pressure and may even decrease blood pressure.[85,163,164] HRT may also attenuate postmenopausal weight gain.[6,56,155,164] Animal and human studies further suggest that estrogen has important beneficial effects on arterial endothelium, including plaque reduction and the favorable modulation of vascular responsiveness in diseased coronary arteries.[2,25,112,119,159]

Despite these favorable intermediate end points, and the consistent findings of observational studies that HRT is associated with a 30% to 50% reduction in CHD events in women with[101] and without[45] preexisting CHD, the results of the first randomized trial of the effects of HRT on CHD risk found no benefit.[53] The Heart and Estrogen/Progestin Replacement Study (HERS) randomized 2,763 women to placebo or 0.625 mg of conjugated equine estrogens plus 2.5 mg of medroxyprogesterone acetate daily. After 4.1 years of follow-up, the relative risk for MI or CHD death was 0.99, or no difference between the placebo and control groups. In their first year in the trial, women assigned to HRT had a 50% increase in MI and CHD death compared with women assigned to placebo. By years 4 and 5, these relationships were reversed and women assigned to HRT had a 33% reduction in CHD risk compared with women on placebo. These results seem to support the concerns of some that the benefit of HRT found in observational studies was due to the association of HRT with other factors that favorably affect CHD risk. For example, women taking HRT are more likely to practice health promotion behaviors such as exercise and dietary changes, more likely to use health screening,[10] and are younger and of lower weight[46] than women not taking HRT. The authors of the HERS trial recommend that, based on their findings, women with CHD not be started on HRT, but that it may be appropriate for women in whom CHD develops while taking HRT to continue its use.[53] Those interested in this important question now await the results of other randomized trials such as the Women's Health Initiative, a large, long-term, randomized trial designed to assess the effects of HRT on coronary disease, breast cancer, and fracture risk.

FOLATE AND HOMOCYSTEINE

Homocysteine is an amino acid that is an intermediate byproduct of the metabolism of the dietary protein methionine. Homocysteine levels are higher in postmenopausal than premenopausal women, lower in women than in men, positively correlated with age, and negatively correlated with serum folate and dietary folate intake.[11,29,126] Methylenetetrahydrofolate (MTHFR) is an enzyme that contributes to the remethylation of homocysteine to methionine. This reaction requires folate as the substrate, and levels of dietary and blood folate are strong determinants of homocysteine levels.[124] Normally present in only small amounts (<10 μmol/mL), homocysteine is highly toxic to the vascular endothelium. People with homocysteinuria, a rare autosomal recessive condition in which homocysteine levels are severely elevated, are at extremely high risk for premature atherosclerosis. A common variation in MTHFR, thermolabile MTHFR, is associated with reduced MTHFR activity and mild elevations in homocysteine.[124]

Even mild elevations in homocysteine appear to increase CHD risk. In a case-control study of MI among women younger than 45 years of age, those in the highest quartile (>15.6 μmol/L) of homocysteine had 2.3 times the risk of MI compared with those in the lowest quartile (<10 μmol/L). This relationship was reversed for serum folate; women in the highest quartile of folate had half the risk of those in the lowest quartile.[124] Among French Canadians with CHD, 44% of women and 18.1% of men had homocysteine levels greater than the 90th percentile of control levels.[29] Mean homocysteine levels of those with and without CHD were 12.0 ± 6.3 μmol/L versus 7.6 ± 4.1 μmol/L for women, and 11.7 ± 5.8 μmol/L versus 9.7 ± 4.9 μmol/L in men.[29]

Homocysteine levels are higher in women and men with angiographically confirmed obstruction of one or more major coronary arteries than in those with normal coronaries.[60,115] In the Framingham Heart Study, high plasma homocysteine concentrations and low concentrations of folate were associated with increased risk of extracranial carotid artery stenosis.[125] In ARIC, the relative risk for carotid artery intimal-medial wall thickening among participants in the highest versus the lowest quintiles of plasma homocysteine was 3.2.[86]

Increasing homocysteine after menopause may partially explain the increase in CHD risk associated with aging. Postmenopausal women have an excessive rise in homocysteine after a methionine load compared with premenopausal women, and folic acid supplementation decreases this rise in homocysteine after methionine loading.[17] In a 2-year, prospective study, HRT was associated with an 11% decrease in homocysteine. The decrease was 17% in women with high homocysteine levels, whereas levels in women with low homocysteine did not change.[152]

ANTIOXIDANTS

Epidemiologic findings that antioxidants decrease CHD risk are supported by evidence that oxidized LDL is present in atherosclerotic lesions.[142] The accumulation of cholesterol in the arterial intima is the hallmark of early atherosclerotic lesions, and oxidation of LDL appears to enhance the accumulation of cholesterol in atherosclerotic lesions.[142] Interest in the effects of antioxidants and CHD risk has centered on vitamins E and C, and β-carotene. Although observational studies suggested that consumption of foods high in β-carotene might reduce CHD risk,[41,148] the results of randomized trials in men[3,49] and men and women[106] show no benefit of β-carotene supplementation on CHD risk. Similarly, evidence that vitamin C reduces CHD risk is weak or lacking.[41,75,114]

There is emerging evidence of cardiovascular benefit associated with vitamin E.[113,140] In the Nurses Health Study, the rate of major CHD was 35% lower among women in the highest quintile of vitamin E consumption compared with women in the lowest quintile.[140] The authors found that most of the variability in vitamin E consumption was due to supplements. In the Iowa Women's Health Study, among women who did not use supplements, women in the highest quintile of Vitamin E intake had a 60% reduction in CHD death compared with women in the lowest quintile, but there was no association between vitamin A or vitamin C intake and CHD risk.[75] There is evidence from both observational studies and randomized trials of a beneficial effect of increased vitamin E intake in men. Among U.S. male health professionals, there was a 36% reduction in CHD risk among those who consumed more than 60 IU vitamin E per day compared with those who consumed less than 7.5 IU/d.[113] There was a similar reduction in risk among men who took at least 100 IU/d in supplements, compared with those who did not. These beneficial effects of vitamin E appear to reduce CHD risk even in the elderly. Users of vitamin E supplements in the Established Populations for Epidemiologic Studies of the Elderly had a 67% reduction in risk for CHD mortality compared with nonusers.[84] Finally, a randomized trial of 50 mg of vitamin

E in male smokers found only a 4% reduction in major coronary events,[154] whereas in a trial of patients with angiographically proven CHD, supplementation with 400 to 800 IU of vitamin E resulted in a 75% reduction in nonfatal MI compared with placebo.[143] These trials imply that only supplementation at high doses may yield CHD protection.

Further randomized trials of the effect of vitamin E on the primary and secondary prevention of CHD in women and men are underway. Recommendations about the use of vitamin E for CHD prevention should await the results of these trials.

CONCLUSIONS

Outstanding progress has been made in our understanding of CHD risk factors and their management. The evidence against cigarette smoking, elevated serum cholesterol, and high blood pressure is strong, and sustained campaigns are underway to prevent and appropriately manage them. The importance of adequate physical activity and weight control is acknowledged, and the American Heart Association now features sedentary lifestyle fourth in its list of risk factors for CHD. Research in progress will contribute to our understanding of the role of reproductive and postmenopausal hormones in the etiology of CHD in women. The focus of future research will be on clarifying the role of these factors, particularly for women and ethnic minorities.

REFERENCES

1. Abbott RD, Donahue RP, Kannell WB et al: The impact of diabetes on survival following myocardial infarction in men vs women: The Framingham Study. JAMA 260: 3456–3460, 1988
2. Al-Khalili F, Eriksson M, Landgren BM et al: Effect of conjugated estrogen on peripheral flow-mediated vasodilation in postmenopausal women. Am J Cardiol 82: 215–218, 1998
3. Alpha Tocopherol, Beta Carotene Cancer Prevention Study Group: The effect of vitamin E and beta carotene on the incidence of lung cancer and other cancers in male smokers. N Engl J Med 330: 1029–1035, 1994
4. Anastos K, Charney P, Charon RA et al: Hypertension in women: What is really known? The Women's Caucus, Working Group on Women's Health of the Society of General Internal Medicine. Ann Intern Med 115: 287–293, 1991
5. Austin MA, Breslow JL, Hennekens CH et al: Low-density lipoprotein subclass patterns and risk of myocardial infarction. JAMA 260: 1917–1921, 1988
6. Barrett-Connor E, Brown W, Turner J et al: Heart disease risk factors and hormone use in postmenopausal women. JAMA 241: 2167–2169, 1979
7. Barrett-Connor E, Khaw KT, Wingard DL: A ten-year prospective study of coronary heart disease mortality among Rancho Bernardo women. In Eaker ED, Packard B, Wenger NK et al (eds): Coronary Heart Disease in Women, pp 117–121. New York, Haymarket Doyma, 1987
8. Barrett-Connor E, Wingard DL: Sex differential in ischemic heart disease mortality in diabetics: A prospective population-based study. Am J Epidemiol 118: 489–496, 1983
9. Barrett-Connor EL: Obesity, atherosclerosis, and coronary artery disease. Ann Intern Med 103: 1010–1019, 1985
10. Barrett-Connor EL: Postmenopausal estrogen and prevention bias. Ann Intern Med 115: 455–456, 1991
11. Bates CJ, Mansoor MA, van der Pols J et al: Plasma total homocysteine in a representative sample of 972 British men and women aged 65 and over. Eur J Clin Nutr 51: 691–697, 1997
12. Beard DM, Fuster V, Annergers JF: Reproductive history in women with coronary heart disease: A case-control study. Am J Epidemiol 120: 108–114, 1984
13. Berlin JA, Colditz GA: A meta-analysis of physical activity in the prevention of coronary heart disease. Am J Epidemiol 132: 612–628, 1990
14. Blair SN, Kohl HW, Paffenbarger RS et al: Physical fitness and all-cause mortality: A prospective study of healthy men and women. JAMA 262: 2395–2401, 1989
15. Bostom AG, Cupples LA, Jenner JL et al: Elevated plasma lipoprotein(a) and coronary heart disease in men aged 55 years and younger: A prospective study. JAMA 276: 544–548, 1996
16. Bostom AG, Gagnon DR, Cupples LA et al: A prospective investigation of elevated lipoprotein(a) detected by electrophoresis and cardiovascular disease in women: The Framingham Heart Study. Circulation 90: 1688–1695, 1994
17. Brattstrom LE, Hultberg BL, Hardebo JE: Folic acid responsive postmenopausal homocysteinemia. Metabolism 34: 1073–1077, 1985
18. Brown G, Albers JJ, Fisher LD et al: Regression of coronary artery disease as a result of intensive lipid-lowering therapy in men with high levels of apolipoprotein B. N Engl J Med 323: 1289–1298, 1990
19. Burke GL, Savage PJ, Sprafka JM et al: Relation of risk factor levels in young adulthood to parental history of disease. The CARDIA study. Circulation 84: 1176–1187, 1991
20. Bush TL, Fried LP, Barrett-Connor E: Cholesterol, lipoproteins and coronary heart disease in women. Clin Chem 34: 660–670, 1988
21. Cauley JA, LaPorte RE, Kuller LH et al: Menopausal estrogen use, high density lipoprotein cholesterol subfractions and liver function. Atherosclerosis 49: 31–39, 1983
22. Centers for Disease Control and Prevention: CDC Wonder. Mortality. Available: http://wonder.CDC.gov/WONDER. October, 1998
23. Chandrashekhar Y, Amand IS: Exercise as a coronary protective factor. Am Heart J 122: 1723–1739, 1991
24. Colditz, GA, Willett WC, Stampfer MJ et al: A prospective study of age at menarche, parity, age at first birth, and coronary heart disease in women. Am J Epidemiol 126: 861–870, 1987
25. Collins P, Rosano GMC, Sarrel PM et al: 17β-estradiol attenuates acetylcholine-induced coronary arterial constriction in women but not men with coronary heart disease. Circulation 92: 24–30, 1995
26. Croft P, Hannaford PC: Risk factors for acute myocardial infarction in women: Evidence from the Royal College of General Practitioners' oral contraception study. BMJ 298: 165–168, 1989
27. Cromwell J, Bartosch WJ, Fiore MC et al: Cost-effectiveness of the clinical practice recommendations in the AHCPR guideline for smoking cessation. JAMA 278: 1759–1766, 1997
28. Dahlen GH, Guyton JR, Attar M et al: Association of levels of lipoprotein Lp(a), plasma lipids, and other lipoproteins with coronary artery disease documented by angiography. Circulation 74: 758–765, 1986
29. Dalery K, Lussier-Cacan S, Selhub J et al: Homocysteine and coronary artery disease in French Canadian subjects: Relation with vitamins B_{12}, B_6, pyridoxal phosphate, and folate. Am J Cardiol 75: 1107–1111, 1995

30. Dawber TR: The Framingham Study: The Epidemiology of Atherosclerotic Disease. Cambridge, MA, Harvard University Press, 1980

31. Diabetes Control and Complications Trial Research Group: The effect of intensive treatment of diabetes on the development and progression of long-term complications in insulin-dependent diabetes mellitus: The Diabetes Control and Complications Trial Research Group. N Engl J Med 329: 977–986, 1993

32. Douglas PS, Clarkson TB, Flowers NC et al: Exercise and atherosclerotic heart disease in women. Med Sci Sports Exerc 23(Suppl): S266–S276, 1992

33. Eaker ED, Pinsky J, Castelli WP: Myocardial infarction and coronary death among women: Psychosocial predictors from a 20-year follow-up of women in the Framingham Study. Am J Epidemiol 135: 854–864, 1992

34. Eaker ED: Psychosocial factors in the epidemiology of coronary heart disease in women. Psychiatr Clin North Am 12: 167–173, 1989

35. Ekelund LG, Haskell WL, Johnson JL et al: Physical fitness as a predictor of cardiovascular mortality in asymptomatic North American men: The Lipid Research Clinics mortality follow-up study. N Engl J Med 319: 1379–1384, 1988

36. Epidemiology Branch, Office on Smoking and Health, National Center for Chronic Disease Prevention and Health Promotion, Division of Health Interview Statistics, National Center for Health Statistics: Cigarette smoking among adults: United States, 1991. MMWR 42: 230–233, 1993

37. Epidemiology Branch, Office on Smoking and Health, National Center for Chronic Disease Prevention and Health Promotion, Centers for Disease Control: Surveillance for selected tobacco-use behaviors: United States, 1900–1994. MMWR 43: SS-3, 1994

38. Epidemiology Branch, Office on Smoking and Health, National Center for Chronic Disease Prevention and Health Promotion, Centers for Disease Control: Cigarette smoking among adults: United States, 1995. MMWR 46: 1217–1220, 1997

39. The Expert Committee on the Diagnosis and Classification of Diabetes Mellitus: Report of the Expert Committee on the Diagnosis and Classification of Diabetes Mellitus. Diabetes Care 20: 1183–1197, 1997

40. Folsom AR, Szklo M, Stevens J et al: A prospective study of coronary heart disease in relation to fasting insulin, glucose, and diabetes. Diabetes Care 20: 935–942, 1997

41. Gaziano JM: Antioxidant vitamins and coronary artery disease risk. Am J Med 97: 3A-18S–3A-28S, 1994

42. Glantz SA, Parmley WW: Passive smoking and heart disease: Epidemiology, physiology and biochemistry. Circulation 83: 1–12, 1991

43. Goldbaum GM, Kendrick JS, Hogelin GC et al: The relative impact of smoking and oral contraceptive use on women in the United States. JAMA 258: 1339–1342, 1987

44. Gordon DJ, Probstfield JL, Garrison RJ et al: High-density lipoprotein cholesterol and cardiovascular disease: Four prospective American studies. Circulation 79: 8–15, 1989

45. Grodstein F, Stampfer M: The epidemiology of coronary heart disease and estrogen replacement in postmenopausal women. Prog Cardiovasc Dis 38: 199–210, 1995

46. Harris RB, Laws A, Reddy VM et al: Are women using postmenopausal estrogens? A community survey. Am J Public Health 80: 1266–1268, 1990

47. Harris T, Cook EF, Garrison R et al: Body mass index and mortality among nonsmoking older persons: The Framingham Heart Study. JAMA 259: 1520–1524, 1988

48. Haskell WL, Leon AS, Caspersen CJ et al: Cardiovascular benefits and assessment of physical activity and physical fitness in adults. Med Sci Sports Exerc 24(Suppl): S201–S220, 1992

49. Hennekens CH, Buring JE, Manson JE et al: Lack of effect of long-term supplementation with beta carotene on the incidence of malignant neoplasms and cardiovascular disease. N Engl J Med 334: 1145–1149, 1996

50. Hermanson B, Omenn GS, Kronmal RA et al: Beneficial six-year outcome of smoking cessation in older men and women with coronary artery disease: Results from the CASS registry. N Engl J Med 319: 1365–1369, 1988

51. Hoffmans MDAF, Kromhout D, De Lezenne Coulander C: Body mass index at the age of 18 and its effects on 32-year-mortality from coronary heart disease and cancer. J Clin Epidemiol 42: 513–520, 1989

52. Hubert HB, Feinleib M, McNamara PM et al: Obesity as an independent risk factor for cardiovascular disease: A 26-year follow-up of participants in the Framingham Heart Study. Circulation 67: 968–977, 1983

53. Hully S, Grady D, Bush T et al: Randomized trial of estrogen and progestin for secondary prevention of coronary heart disease in postmenopausal women. JAMA 1998: 605–618, 1998

54. Hypertension Detection and Follow-up Program Cooperative Group: Persistence of reduction in blood pressure and mortality of participants in the hypertension detection and follow-up program. JAMA 259: 2113–2122, 1988

55. Jensen G, Nyboe J, Appleyard M et al: Risk factors for acute myocardial infarction in Copenhagen: II. Smoking, alcohol intake, physical activity, obesity, oral contraception, diabetes, lipids, and blood pressure. Eur Heart J 12: 298–308, 1991

56. Jensen J, Riis BJ, Strom V et al: Long-term effects of percutaneous estrogens and oral progesterone on serum lipoproteins in postmenopausal women. Am J Obstet Gynecol 156: 66–71, 1987

57. Jick H, Dinan B, Rothman KJ: Oral contraceptives and non-fatal myocardial infarction. JAMA 239: 1403–1406, 1978

58. Johnson JL, Heineman EF, Heiss G et al: Cardiovascular disease risk factors and mortality among black women and white women aged 40–64 years in Evans County, Georgia. Am J Epidemiol 123: 209–220, 1986

59. Jousilahti P, Puska P, Vartiainen E et al: Parental history of premature coronary heart disease: An independent risk factor of myocardial infarction. J Clin Epidemiol 49: 497–503, 1996

60. Kang S, Wong PWK, Cook HY et al: Protein-bound homocysteine, a possible risk factor for coronary artery disease. J Clin Invest 77: 1482–1486, 1986

61. Kannel WB et al: Report of Inter-Society Commission for Heart Disease Resources: Optimal resources for primary prevention of atherosclerotic diseases. Circulation 70: 181A, 1984

62. Kannel WB: New perspectives of cardiovascular risk factors. Am Heart J 114: 213–219, 1987

63. Kannel WB: Status of risk factors and their consideration in antihypertensive therapy. Am J Cardiol 59: 80A–90A, 1987

64. Kaplan NM: The deadly quartet: Upper-body obesity, glucose intolerance, hypertriglyceridemia, and hypertension. Arch Intern Med 149: 1514–1520, 1989

65. Kaufman DW, Helmrich SP, Rosenberg L et al: Nicotine and carbon monoxide content of cigarette smoke and the risk of myocardial infarction in young men. N Engl J Med 308: 409–413, 1983

66. Keil JE, Gazes PC, Loadholt CB et al: Coronary heart disease mortality and its predictors among women in Charleston, South Carolina. In Eaker ED, Packard B, Wenger NK et al (eds): Coronary Heart Disease in Women, pp 90–98. New York, Haymarket Doyma, 1987

67. Keil JE, Sutherland SE, Knapp RG et al: Mortality rates and risk factors for coronary disease in black as compared with white men and women. N Engl J Med 329: 73–78, 1993

68. Kelleher CC: Clinical aspects of the relationship between oral contraceptives and abnormalities of the hemostatic system: Relation to the development of cardiovascular disease. Am J Obstet Gynecol 163: 392–395, 1990

69. Kelsey JL, Thompson WD, Evans AS: Methods in Observational Epidemiology. New York, Oxford University Press, 1986

70. Khaw KT, Barrett-Connor E: Prognostic factors for mortality in a population-based study of men and women with a history of heart disease. J Cardiopulm Rehabil 6: 474–480, 1986

71. Kitagawa WM, Hauser PM: Differential Mortality in the United States: A Study of Socioeconomic Epidemiology. Cambridge, MA, Harvard University Press, 1973

72. Kodama K, Sasakli H, Shimizu Y: Trend of coronary heart disease and its relationship to risk factors in a Japanese population: A 26 year follow-up, Hiroshima/Nagasaki Study. Jpn Circ J 54: 414–421, 1990

73. Kraus JF, Borhani NO, Franci CE: Socioeconomic status, ethnicity, and risk of coronary heart disease. Am J Epidemiol 111: 407–414, 1980

74. Kuczmarski RJ, Flegal KM, Campbell SM et al: Increasing prevalence of overweight among US adults: The National Health and Nutrition Examination Surveys, 1960 to 1991. JAMA 272: 205–211, 1994

75. Kushi LH, Folsom AR, Prineas RJ et al: Dietary antioxidant vitamins and death from coronary heart disease in postmenopausal women. N Engl J Med 334: 1156–1162, 1996

76. Kwiterovich PO, Coresh J, Smith HH et al: Comparison of the plasma levels of apolipoproteins B and A-1, and other risk factors in men and women with premature coronary artery disease. Am J Cardiol 69: 1015–1021, 1992

77. LaCroix AZ, Lang J, Scherr P et al: Smoking and mortality among older men and women in three communities. N Engl J Med 324: 1619–1625, 1991

78. LaCroix AZ, Omenn GS: Older adults and smoking. Clin Geriatr Med 8: 69–87, 1992

79. Lapidus L, Bengtsson C: Socioeconomic factors and physical activity in relation to cardiovascular disease and death: A 12 year follow-up of participants in a population study of women in Gothenburg, Sweden. Br Heart J 55: 295–301, 1986

80. Last JM: A Dictionary of Epidemiology, 2nd ed. New York, Oxford University Press, 1988

81. LaVecchia C, DeCarli A, Franceshi S et al: Menstrual and reproductive factors and the risk of myocardial infarction in women under fifty-five years of age. Am J Obstet Gynecol 157: 1108–1112, 1987

82. LaVecchia C, Franceshi S, Decarli A et al: Risk factors for myocardial infarction in young women. Am J Epidemiol 125: 832–843, 1987

83. Lindquist O, Bengtsson C, Lapidus L: Relationships between the menopause and risk factors for ischaemic heart disease. Acta Obstet Gynecol Scand Suppl 130: 43–47, 1985

84. Losonczy KG, Harris TB, Havlik RJ: Vitamin E and vitamin C supplement use and risk of all-cause and coronary heart disease mortality in older persons: The Established Populations for Epidemiologic Studies of the Elderly. Am J Clin Nutr 64: 190–196, 1996

85. Luotola H, Pyorala T, Loikkanen M: Effects of natural oestrogen/progestogen substitution therapy on carbohydrate and lipid metabolism in post-menopausal women. Maturitas 8: 245–253, 1986

86. Malinow MR, Nieto FJ, Szklo M et al: Carotid artery intimal-medial wall thickening and plasma homocysteine in asymptomatic adults. Circulation 87: 1107–1113, 1993

87. Mann JI, Inman WHW: Oral contraceptives and death from myocardial infarction. BMJ 2: 245–248, 1975

88. Mann JI, Vessey MP, Thorogood M et al: Myocardial infarction in young women with special reference to oral contraceptive practice. BMJ 2: 241–245, 1975

89. Manolio TA, Pearson TA, Wenger NK et al: Cholesterol and heart disease in older persons and women: Review of an NHLBI workshop. Ann Epidemiol 2: 161–176, 1992

90. Manson JE, Colditz GA, Stampfer MJ et al: A prospective study of maturity-onset diabetes mellitus and risk of coronary heart disease and stroke in women. Arch Intern Med 151: 1141–1147, 1991

91. Manson JE, Colditz GA, Stampfer MJ et al: A prospective study of obesity and risk of coronary heart disease in women. N Engl J Med 322: 882–889, 1990

92. Mant J, Painter R, Vessey M: Risk of myocardial infarction, angina and stroke in users of oral contraceptives: An updated analysis of a cohort study. Br J Obstet Gynaecol 105: 890–896, 1998

93. Marenberg ME, Risch N, Berkman LF et al: Genetic susceptibility to death from coronary heart disease in a study of twins. N Engl J Med 330, 1041–1046, 1994

94. Matthews KA, Kelsey SF, Meilhan EN et al: Educational attainment and behavioral and biologic risk factors for coronary heart disease in middle-aged women. Am J Epidemiol 129: 1132–1144, 1989

95. Matthews KA, Meilhan E, Kuller LH et al: Menopause a risk factor for coronary heart disease. N Engl J Med 321: 641–646, 1989

96. Meade TW: Risks and mechanisms of cardiovascular events in users of oral contraceptives. Am J Obstet Gynecol 158: 1646–1652, 1988

97. Medical Research Council Working Party: Medical research council trial of treatment of hypertension in older adults: Principal results. BMJ 304: 405–412, 1992

98. Medical Research Council Working Party: MRC trial of treatment of mild hypertension: Principal results. BMJ 291: 97–104, 1985

99. Mitchell BD, Haffner SM, Huzuda HP, Patterson JK et al: Diabetes and coronary heart disease risk in Mexican-Americans. Ann Epidemiol 2: 101–106, 1992

100. National Center for Health Statistics, U.S. of Health and Human Services (DHHS). Third National Health and Nutrition Examination Survey, 1988–1994, NHANES III Data File (CD-ROM Series II, No 1). Public Use Data File, Hyattsville, MD: Centers for Disease Control and Prevention, 1997.

101. Newton KM, LaCroix AZ, McKnight B et al: Estrogen replacement therapy and prognosis after first myocardial infarction. Am J Epidemiol 145: 269–277, 1997

102. Newton KM, LaCroix AZ: Association of body mass index with reinfarction and survival after first myocardial infarction in women. J Womens Health 5: 133–444, 1996

103. Novotny TE, Fiore MC, Hatziandreu EJ et al: Trends in smoking by age and sex, United States, 1974–1987: The implications for disease impact. Prev Med 19: 552–561, 1990

104. Nyboe J, Jensen G, Appleyard M et al: Risk factors for acute myocardial infarction in Copenhagen: I. Hereditary, educational and socioeconomic factors. Copenhagen City Heart Study. Eur Heart J 10: 910–916, 1989

105. Oldridge NB, Guyatt GH, Fischer ME et al: Cardiac rehabilitation after myocardial infarction, combined experience of randomized clinical trials. JAMA 260: 945–950, 1988

106. Omenn GS, Goodman GE, Thornquist MD et al: Effects of a combination of beta carotene and vitamin A on lung cancer and cardiovascular disease. N Engl J Med 334: 1150–1155, 1996

107. Orchard TJ: The impact of gender and general risk factors on the occurrence of atherosclerotic vascular disease in non-insulin-dependent diabetes mellitus. Ann Med 28: 323–333, 1996

108. Palmer JR, Rosenberg L, Shapiro S: Reproductive factors and risk of myocardial infarction. Am J Epidemiol 136: 408–416, 1992

109. Pell S, Fayerweather WE: Trends in the incidence of myocardial infarction and associated mortality and morbidity in a large employed population, 1957–1983. N Engl J Med 312: 1005–1011, 1985

110. Perry IJ, Wannamethee SG, Whincup PH et al: Serum insulin and incident coronary heart disease in middle-aged British men. Am J Epidemiol 144: 224–234, 1996

111. Ramsay LE, Yeo WW: Hypertension and coronary artery disease: An unsolved problem. J Cardiovasc Pharmacol 18(Suppl): S31–S34, 1991

112. Reis SE, Gloth ST, Blumenthal RS et al: Ethinyl estradiol acutely attenuates abnormal coronary vasomotor responses to acetylcholine in postmenopausal women. Circulation 89: 52–60, 1994

113. Rimm EB, Stampfer M, Ascherio A et al: Vitamin E consumption and the risk of coronary heart disease in men. N Engl J Med 328: 1450–1456, 1993

114. Rimm EB, Stampfer MJ: The role of antioxidants in preventive cardiology. Curr Opin Cardiol 12: 188–194, 1997

115. Robinson K, Mayer EL, Miller DP et al: Hyperhomocysteinemia and low pyridoxal phosphate, common and independent reversible risk factors for coronary artery disease. Circulation 92: 2825–2830, 1995

116. Roncaglioni MC, Santoro L, D'Avanzo B et al: Role of family history in patient with myocardial infarction: An Italian case-control study. GISSI-EFRIM investigators. Circulation 85: 2065–2072, 1992

117. Rönnemaa T, Kaakso M, Pyörälä K et al: High fasting plasma insulin is an indicator of coronary heart disease in non-insulin-dependent diabetic patients and nondiabetic subjects. Arteriosclerosis and Thrombosis 11: 80–90, 1991

118. Rosamond WD, Chambless LE, Folsom AR et al: Trends in the incidence of myocardial infarction and in mortality due to coronary heart disease, 1987 to 1994. N Engl J Med 339: 861–867, 1998

119. Rosano GMC, Sarrell PM, Collins P: Beneficial effect of oestrogen on exercise-induced myocardial ischaemia in women with coronary artery disease. Lancet 342: 133–136, 1993

120. Rosenberg L, Palmer JR, Lesko SM et al: Oral contraceptive use and the risk of myocardial infarction. Am J Epidemiol 131: 1009–1016, 1990

121. Rosenberg L, Palmer JR, Shapiro S: Decline in the risk of myocardial infarction among women who stop smoking. N Engl J Med 322: 213–217, 1990

122. Rothman KJ: Modern Epidemiology. Boston, Little, Brown, 1986

123. Salonen JT: Stopping smoking and long-term mortality after acute myocardial infarction. Br Heart J 43: 463–469, 1980

124. Schwartz SM, Siscovick DS, Malinow MR et al: Myocardial infarction in young women in relation to plasma total homocysteine, folate, and a common variant in the methylenetetrahydrofolate reductase gene. Circulation 96: 412–417, 1997

125. Selhub J, Jacques PF, Bostom AG et al: Association between plasma homocysteine concentrations and extracranial carotid-artery stenosis. N Engl J Med 332: 286–291, 1995

126. Selhub J, Jacques PF, Wilson PWF et al: Vitamin status and intake as primary determinants of homocysteinemia in an elderly population. JAMA 270: 2693–2698, 1993

127. Sempos C, Cooper R, Kovar MG et al: Divergence of the recent trends in coronary mortality for the four major race-sex groups in the United States. Am J Public Health 78: 1422–1427, 1988

128. SHEP Cooperative Research Group: Prevention of stroke by antihypertensive drug treatment in older persons with isolated systolic hypertension: Final results of the systolic hypertension in the elderly program (SHEP). JAMA 265: 3255–3264, 1991

129. Sidney S, Siscovick DS, Petitti DB et al: Myocardial infarction and use of low-dose oral contraceptives: A pooled analysis of 2 US studies. Circulation 98: 1058–1063, 1998

130. Simonson DC, Dzau VJ: Workshop IX: Lipids, insulin, diabetes. Am J Med 90(Suppl 2A): 85S–86S, 1991

131. Slattery ML, Jacobs DR: Physical fitness and cardiovascular disease mortality: The US Railroad Study. Am J Epidemiol 127: 571–580, 1988

132. Slone D, Kaufman DW, Shapiro S et al: Risk of myocardial infarction in relation to current and discontinued oral-contraceptive use. N Engl J Med 305: 420–424, 1981

133. Slone D, Shapiro S, Rosenberg L et al: Relation of cigarette smoking to myocardial infarction in young women. N Engl J Med 298: 1273–1276, 1978

134. Sobolski J, Kornitzer M, Backer GD et al: Protection against ischemic heart disease in the Belgian physical fitness study: Physical fitness rather than physical activity? Am J Epidemiol 125: 601–610, 1987

135. Stampfer MJ, Colditz GA, Willett WC et al: Coronary heart disease risk factors in women: The Nurses' Health Study experience. In Eaker ED, Packard B, Wenger NK et al (eds): Coronary Heart Disease in Women, pp 112–116. New York, Haymarket Doyma, 1987

136. Stampfer MJ, Colditz GA, Willett WC: Menopause and heart disease: A review. Ann N Y Acad Sci 592: 193–203, 1990

137. Stampfer MJ, Colditz GA: Estrogen replacement therapy and coronary heart disease: A quantitative assessment of the epidemiologic evidence. Prev Med 20: 47–63, 1991

138. Stampfer MJ, Willett WC, Colditz GC et al: A prospective study of past use of oral contraceptive agents and risk of cardiovascular diseases. N Engl J Med 319: 1313–1317, 1988

139. Stampfer MJ, Willett WC, Colditz GC et al: Past use of oral contraceptives and cardiovascular disease: A meta-analysis in the context of the Nurses' Health Study. Am J Obstet Gynecol 163: 285–291, 1990

140. Stampfer MU, Hennekens Ch, Manson JE et al: Vitamin E consumption and the risk of coronary disease in women. N Engl J Med 328: 1444–1449, 1993

141. Stein JH, Rosenson RS: Lipoprotein Lp(a) excess and coronary heart disease: Arch Intern Med 157: 1170–1176, 1997

142. Steinbrecher UP: Dietary antioxidants and cardioprotection: Fact or fallacy? Can J Physiol Pharmacol 75: 228–233, 1997

143. Stephens NG, Parsons A, Schofiled PM et al: Randomised controlled trial of vitamin E in patient with coronary disease: Cambridge Heart Antioxidant Study. Lancet 347: 781–786, 1996

144. Stevens J, Keil JE, Rust PF et al: Body mass index and body girths as predictors of mortality in black and white women. Arch Intern Med 152: 1257–1262, 1992

145. Stone PH, Muller JE, Hartwell T et al: The effect of diabetes mellitus on prognosis and serial left ventricular function after acute myocardial infarction: Contribution of both coronary disease and diastolic left ventricular dysfunction to the adverse prognosis. J Am Coll Cardiol 12: 49–57, 1989

146. Szklo M, Tonascia J, Gordis L: Psychosocial factors and the risk of myocardial infarction in white women. Am J Epidemiol 103: 312–320, 1976

147. Talbott E, Kuller LH, Detre K et al: Biologic and psychosocial risk factors for sudden death from coronary disease in white women. Am J Cardiol 39: 858–864, 1977

148. Tavani A, Negri E, Avanzo BD et al: Beta-carotene intake and risk of nonfatal acute myocardial infarction in women. Eur J Epidemiol 13: 631–637, 1997

149. Thompson PD: The benefits and risks of exercise training in patients with chronic coronary artery disease. JAMA 259: 1537–1540, 1988

150. U.S. Department of Health and Human Services: Physical Activity and Health: A Report of the Surgeon General. Atlanta, GA: U.S. Department of Health and Human Services, Centers for Disease Control and Prevention, National Center for Chronic Disease Prevention and Health Promotion, 1996

151. Van Berestejin ECH, Korevaar JC, Hujibregts PCW et al: Perimenopausal increase in serum cholesterol: A 10-year longitudinal study. Am J Epidemiol 137: 383–392, 1993

152. Van Der Mooren MJ, Wouters MG, Blom HJ et al: Hormone replacement therapy may reduce high serum homocysteine in postmenopausal women. Eur J Clin Invest 24: 733–736, 1994

153. Van Itallie TB: Health implication of overweight and obesity in the United States. Ann Intern Med 103: 983–988, 1985

154. Vitamo J, Rapola MJ, Ripatti S et al: Effect of vitamin E and beta carotene on the incidence of primary nonfatal myocardial infarction and fatal coronary heart disease. Arch Intern Med 158: 668–675, 1998

155. Wallace RB, Heiss G, Burrows B et al: Contrasting diet and body mass among users and nonusers of oral contraceptives and exogenous estrogens: The Lipid Research Clinics Program Prevalence Study. Am J Epidemiol 125: 854–859, 1987

156. Wild SH, Laws A, Fortmann SP et al: Mortality for coronary heart disease and stroke for six ethnic groups in California, 1985 to 1990. Ann Epidemiol 5: 432–439, 1995

157. Willett WC, Green A, Stampfer MJ: Relative and absolute excess risks of coronary heart disease among women who smoke cigarettes. N Engl J Med 317: 1303–1309, 1987

158. Willett WC, Manson JE, Stampfer MJ et al: Weight, weight changes, and coronary heart disease in women, risk within the "normal" weight range. JAMA 273: 461–465, 1995

159. Williams JK, Adams MR, Klopfenstein HS: Estrogen modulates responses of atherosclerotic coronary arteries. Circulation 81: 1680–1687, 1990

160. Wilson PWF: High-density lipoprotein, low-density lipoprotein and coronary artery disease. Am J Cardiol 66: 7A–10A, 1990

161. Wong ND, Cupples LA, Ostfeld AM et al: Risk factors for long-term coronary prognosis after initial myocardial infarction: The Framingham Study. Am J Epidemiol 130: 469–480, 1989

162. Wong ND, Wilson PWF, Kannel WB: Serum cholesterol as a prognostic factor after myocardial infarction: The Framingham Study. Ann Intern Med 115: 687–693, 1991

163. Wren BG, Routledge AD: The effect of type and dose of oestrogen on the blood pressure of post-menopausal women. Maturitas 5: 135–142, 1983

164. Writing Group for the PEPI Trial: Effects of estrogen or estrogen/progestin regimens on heart disease risk factors in postmenopausal women. JAMA 273: 199–208, 1995

30

Psychosocial Interventions

JOAN M. FAIR
ERIKA SIVARAJAN FROELICHER

Over the past several decades, much wisdom and knowledge has been gained about coronary heart disease (CHD). Despite enormous research efforts, traditional risk factors and genetics fail fully to explain either the development or the course of the disease. Consistent with biopsychosocial models of health, studies have now demonstrated that psychological and social factors are also related to both the development of and recovery from heart disease. In health schemas that consider the mind and body, emotion and feelings have usually been linked to aspects of the body. Our language is full of expressions that describe this attachment: "feelings of joy that make your heart flutter" or anxiety that causes "butterflies in your stomach." Since early times, emotions have also been specifically attached to the heart. William Harvey (1578–1657), who first described the circulatory system, wrote that "every affliction of the mind that is attended with either pain or pleasure, hope or fear, is the cause of an agitation whose influence extends to the heart" (cited in Jenkins[29]). This chapter explores the evidence relating psychological and social factors to CHD and describes strategies to promote cardiovascular and psychosocial health.

Several factors have been put forth as critical psychosocial concepts influencing health and disease. At a minimum, these can be classified as those relating to stress and coping, and those relating to personality predispositions, including both personality traits and transient psychological states.

STRESS

Physiologic Effects

Historically, *stress* has been defined as a state of physiologic arousal engendered in response to real or imagined threats (stressors).[42] The physiologic responses to stressors have been described as the "fight-or-flight" responses.[57] Neuroendocrine response systems are activated, triggering the release of cortisol and catecholamines (epinephrine [adrenaline] and norepinephrine) that initiate a variety of physiologic responses (Fig. 30-1). Circulating levels of plasma lipids are also increased; platelet and macrophage cells are activated to release chemotactic and cytotoxic substances. Cardiovascular responses include increased heart rate, blood pressure, and muscle and myocardial oxygen demands, and accelerated blood flow. Increased blood flow triggers a cascade of endothelial vascular responses, including release of nitric oxide to promote vasodilation, stimulation of platelets to release chemoattractants and promote thrombosis, and activation of macrophages. Activated macrophages have enhanced phagocytic activity and have been implicated in the development of atherosclerotic foam cells and the destabilization and rupture of the fibrous cap surrounding atherosclerotic plaque. (For more detailed discussions of these physiologic responses, see reviews by Adams[1] and McCarty and Gold.[47])

Stress and Coronary Heart Disease

As with cigarette smoking, the effects of exposure to severe stress cannot be ethically evaluated in experimental human studies. However, several observational studies provide evidence associating stress with the precipitation of coronary events. In experimental animal studies, cynomolgus monkeys were exposed to stress by having their normal social housing patterns disrupted.[31] Monkeys exposed to this stress had significantly more atherosclerosis compared with monkeys without this stress. Further studies elucidated that social status, as determined by dominance, was also a major predictor of atherosclerotic development; dominant males and females had less atherosclerosis than their subordinate counterparts. Some have suggested that these findings support the association of lower socioeconomic status and increased incidence of CHD observed in human population studies. Although it can be argued that lower social class reflects less dominance and control over the environment, other factors, such as lack of access to medical care or engaging in unhealthy lifestyle behaviors, may partially account for these findings. Perhaps the strongest support for the association of socioeconomic status and the development of CHD is found in a study of

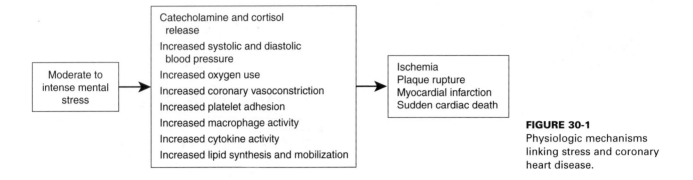

FIGURE 30-1
Physiologic mechanisms linking stress and coronary heart disease.

more than 1,100 Finish men, in which socioeconomic status was related to the degree of carotid artery stenosis after accounting for traditional coronary risk factors.[45]

Acute stress is considered a trigger for ischemia. Evaluation of angina includes determining if the event was triggered by physical exertion, eating, exposure to cold, or emotion. Among coronary patients, the physiologic effects of mental stress have also been studied by correlating cardiac ischemia, measured by ambulatory electrocardiographic monitoring, with daily life experiences. Carefully recorded diaries were used to identify ischemia triggered by physical activity and by specific emotions.[21,25] Both moderate and intense physical and mental activities were associated with ischemic episodes. Estimates suggest that in the hour after high levels of negative emotions, the risk for ischemia doubles.[25] The effects of mental stress have also been evaluated during angiography. Using arithmetic as an acute mental stressor, Yeung and colleagues[66] found that stenosed coronary artery segments responded to mental stress by constricting, whereas normal segments typically responded by dilating. Studies using challenging, timed video games have demonstrated similar results. Comparisons of mental and physical activity stress tests found that mental stress produces higher diastolic blood pressure, similar systolic blood pressure, and lower heart rate responses than physical activity.[53] These studies suggest that ischemia occurring in response to mental stress might be accounted for by inappropriate vasoconstrictor responses.

Observational studies have also examined the incidence of cardiac events and exposure to sudden stresses such as natural disasters. The incidence of fatal and nonfatal myocardial infarction (MI) in Los Angeles County significantly increased on the day of the Northridge earthquake compared with rates before and after the earthquake.[38] In contrast, mortality rates for other types of heart disease, such as cardiomyopathy or cerebrovascular disease, were not increased. Similar increases were observed after major Japanese earthquakes and the 1991 Gulf War missile attacks in Israel. It should be noted that these studies are not able to exclude the effects of increased physical stress brought on by exertion. Interestingly, data from both the Israel missile attacks and from Japanese earthquakes suggest that the incidence of MI and CHD mortality was greater in women than in men. Post-traumatic stress scores were also higher in Japanese women than in men, suggesting that mental stress could be a trigger of these coronary events.[33,63]

Job Strain

Several observational studies have attempted to associate chronic work stress with the precipitation of coronary events. Intriguing data show that MIs occur in circadian patterns. Daily peaks occur in the early morning hours and are associated with morning increases in catecholamines. Weekly patterns suggest approximately a 20% increase in MI incidence on Mondays, with the lowest rates occurring on Saturdays and Sundays.[61] Some relate this increased incidence with return to a stressful workplace environment; others have suggested that lifestyle habits associated with work versus weekend leisure time account for this difference.

Occupational stress has been posited as the explanation for the increase in CHD mortality observed among blue-collar workers. As more women enter the workforce, some have suggested that women will experience increased cardiovascular events. When CHD risk factors were examined in middle-aged women in Rancho Bernardo, California, employed women had significantly lower lipids and glucose levels than unemployed women. In this same study, although the finding was not statistically significant, employed women smoked fewer cigarettes and exercised more than unemployed women.[39] This suggests that factors other than employment status explain observed associations.

Analysis of the Framingham Heart Study data in the early 1970s found that female secretaries and clerks who reported having an unsupportive boss had a higher incidence of CHD events.[26] Low levels of support from coworkers and supervisors have also been associated with elevated blood pressure after accounting for factors such as cigarette smoking.[46] Such findings led theorists to hypothesize that workers who have job strain (high job demands and a low amount of control) would be more likely to acquire CHD.[56] Studies using this assessment of "job strain" have, however, shown both positive and negative associations with CHD mortality,[28,32] leading researchers to suggest that other job factors, including support from coworkers, job security, and juggling family and job demands, likely influence whether employment is experienced as a stress. Similarly, what one person experiences as stress, another may view as a stimulating and exciting experience. This is likely to be particularly true when different cultures and sexes are compared. Nevertheless, it is likely that chronic stress, including stresses experienced in the workplace, promotes biologic responses that can lead to the development of CHD.

SOCIAL SUPPORT

Theoretical concepts of stress suggest that a person's coping resources modulate biologic and cognitive responses to stressors. One coping mechanism, social support, has received considerable attention as a buffering agent against the effects of environmental stresses. Social support is assessed by evaluating the structure and function of social relationships. Structural support reflects social interactions, social ties, and networks. Functional support focuses on the specific function of the support—consider the differences in function of support that provides resources or tangible aid and support that provides emotional comfort and care. Some researchers consider structural support as a quantitative analysis of social networks (i.e., the number or frequency of supports) and functional support as a qualitative analysis (i.e., the value or importance of the support).[3,59] Research that considers only structural and functional support, however, fails to account for individual perceptions and beliefs about the support. As with the concept of stress, what one person considers valuable support may engender feelings of obligation or guilt in another.

Despite a lack of consensus regarding the assessment of social support, some important studies deserve review. Case and colleagues[10] examined social networks by comparing recurrent cardiac events in patients post-MI. In this study, those patients who lived alone had more than a 50% increased risk for a subsequent event. Studies of patients with MI or congestive heart failure, or both, found that patients who report little or no sources of emotional support have more than a twofold increase in risk of a subsequent event.[5,40] Clearly, social isolation has negative health consequences. Although we lack a clear understanding of how social support protects the patient with CHD, it appears such protection exists.

PERSONALITY FACTORS

Personality factors, including personality predispositions and psychological states and traits, have been linked to development and recovery from CHD. Personality predispositions are considered more stable traits, whereas psychological states may be more transient and acute.[54] Anger and hostility are usually considered personality traits, whereas depression and anxiety are usually considered psychological states.

Personality Traits

In the 1980s, much of the research focused on describing a coronary-prone personality or set of psychosocial behaviors that would lead to the development of CHD. Friedman and Rosenman[51] described a set of observable behaviors that encompassed aspects of time urgency, hard-driving and competitive behaviors, and elements of free-floating hostility. This constellation of behaviors became known as type A behavior. Studies undertaken to assess the independent CHD risk associated with this behavior type showed mixed results. For example, the Western Collaborative Group Study showed that type A behavior conferred twice the risk for development of CHD,[52] whereas the Multiple Risk Factor Intervention Trial (MRFIT) failed to establish an association of type A behavior and CHD death.[58] Similarly, cross-sectional angiographic studies examining type A behavior and the presence and severity of CHD have not found a consistent relationship between angiographic extent of disease and type A behavior.[6,27,60] During the late 1980s, further investigations delineated hostility and anger expression as key dimensions of type A behavior. A meta-analysis of available early research studies found that measures of hostility had the greatest effect on subsequent development of CHD and the largest effect size across all studies, and the relationship was at least as strong in women as in men. Thus, these early studies found that personality characteristics, such as the type A behavior pattern, were inconsistently related to the development of CHD, perhaps in part because the personality components were not appropriately defined.

Hostility/Anger and Coronary Heart Disease

Based on the results from these early studies, the construct of hostility has been redefined to include behavioral, affective, and cognitive components. *Expressive hostility* refers to the expression of overt behaviors, such as anger expression, aggressive or rude behaviors, or assaultive behaviors. *Potential for hostility* refers to the tendency to experience anger and resentment in daily life.[60] Hostility is frequently measured by self-rating scales such as the Cook and Medley Hostility Inventory or by a structured interview refined from the type A structured interview.

Several lines of inquiry have been used to investigate the association of hostility and anger with the development of CHD, including laboratory studies and population studies. Laboratory studies have focused on evaluating the physiologic and cardiovascular effects in hostile personality types. People with hostile personalities usually have greater blood pressure, heart rate, and neuroendocrine responses, such as cortisol release, when challenged with a frustrating or harassing situation.[60] It has been hypothesized that the increased "reactivity" over the course of life events promotes the atherosclerotic process.

To elucidate the relationship between hostility and CHD development, researchers have examined this construct among children and adolescents.[23] In young adults, high hostility levels have been related to unhealthy lifestyle habits later in life. For example, the Coronary Artery Risk Development in Young Adults (CARDIA) study found a positive relationship between hostility and lifestyle behaviors such as cigarette smoking, body weight, and alcohol consumption.[55] Similarly, studies in adults also support that the association between CHD mortality and morbidity might be mediated by behavioral risk factors. The Finnish Kuopio Study found that men with high hostility scores followed for 9 years had more than a twofold risk for MI, although accounting for the behavioral risk factors of smoking, alcohol intake, and body mass index substantially reduced the risk.[14] In contrast, prospective studies reported that high levels of anger and hostility were associated with as much as a twofold increase in risk of a coronary event compared with low levels.[35,48] High levels of hostility were also predictive of restenosis after angioplasty.[22] Perhaps the most compelling evidence associating anger and hostility with the development of CHD is from a study of Finnish men who were followed with serial carotid ultrasound. In this study, a twofold increase in carotid artery disease over a 2-year period was observed in men reporting high levels of cynical distrust and anger control.[30]

In summary, studies continue to observe an inconsistent relationship between the development of CHD and type A behavior or specific constructs such as hostility and anger. However, the link between the personality traits of anger and hostility with cardiac reactivity suggests an important physiologic pathway for triggering cardiovascular events.

Psychological States: Depression and Anxiety

In the 1970s, with the advent of coronary care units and continuous electrocardiographic monitoring, a psychological model was proposed that linked emotional responses to the time course of MI.[11] This model suggested that during the initial period of this critical and life-threatening event, patients experience 1 to 2 days of heightened anxiety followed by 3 to 5 days of depression. In reaction to these strong emotions, denial occurred and served as a coping mechanism. During this time, it was implied that the severity of the disease and the hospitalization caused the emotional response.

More recent investigations suggest that these emotions influence both the development and recovery from CHD. Several population studies have demonstrated a relationship between high levels of the negative emotion of anxiety and an increased incidence of heart disease. The Normative Aging Study followed 2,271 men for 32 years and found that men reporting two or more symptoms of anxiety at baseline were three times more likely to have a fatal coronary event than men without symptoms of anxiety.[36] Similar associations have been reported for phobic anxiety symptoms and for high levels of chronic worry.[34,41] In a community study of Danish men and women, a high score for depressive symptoms was associated with an increased risk of acute MI and CHD death during the 27-year follow-up period.[4] Although there is little evidence that depression leads to the development of CHD, it is considerably more prevalent in CHD populations. Depression is found in approximately 6% of the overall population, but its incidence ranges from 16% to 25% in CHD populations.[8,20]

Negative emotions have also been linked to a worse prognosis once heart disease is established. During recovery from an acute MI, high levels of anxiety were associated with increased in-hospital complications, including acute ischemia, arrhythmias, reinfarction, and cardiac death.[49] After controlling for indicators of disease severity, patients with major depression have been reported to be three to four times more likely to die in the first year after infarction compared with those with little or no depression.[19] When the negative emotions of depression, anger, and anxiety were simultaneously evaluated in the same group of patients with MI, both depression and anxiety were significant independent predictors of subsequent cardiac events.[20] In this study, the authors divided events into thrombogenic events (infarction or unstable angina) or arrhythmic events, and found that anxiety and a past history of depression were associated with thrombogenic events, whereas current depression and anger were associated with arrhythmic events.[20] The study authors speculate that mechanisms such as enhanced platelet adhesion leading to plaque instability and thrombosis might account for these results. These biologic pathways have yet to be tested, however. Nevertheless, the aforementioned studies suggested that negative emotions adversely influence recovery.

PSYCHOSOCIAL INTERVENTIONS

During recovery from coronary events, nurses have many opportunities to facilitate and provide psychosocial interventions. During the course of caring for the cardiac patient, it is important to evaluate the patient's sources of social support, as well as the presence of high levels of negative emotional states, including anxiety, depression, and anger. Several brief screening inventories have been developed that can reliably identify patients with psychosocial risks. The most rigorously developed assessment tools are those for depression, such as the Guidelines for Detection and Treatment of Depression developed by the Agency for Health Care and Policy Research.[2] Some research studies have evaluated anxiety by positive responses to simple questions such as, "During the past month have you been bothered by nervousness or your nerves?"[34]; others have used more formal inventories, such as the anxiety subscale of the Brief Symptom Inventory.[49,62] During this evaluation process, it may be appropriate to consult a psychologist or psychiatrist to evaluate fully the degree of psychosocial risk.

Social Support Interventions

Nurses can provide functional support in terms of education and knowledge. Anticipatory guidance regarding the disease and recovery process can alleviate both patient and family stress. However, it is important to assess the patient's needs and desire for knowledge. This is illustrated by research observations of patients with a repressive coping style. Those who were provided high levels of information had a higher frequency of heart alarms and more medical complications.[13] Patients who actively deny they have had a heart attack are not ready to receive high levels of information. Open-ended questions that allow the patient to direct the flow of information should be used. Behavioral strategies that allow the patient and family to rehearse or model experiences are also useful. For example, predischarge treadmill exercise testing observed by the spouse has been shown to enhance the patient's self-esteem and to reduce spousal anxiety.[64] Rather than being overprotective in the recovery period, the spouse can provide positive support. The nurse is also in a position to provide emotional support. Cardiac hospitalizations invoke apprehension and fear in most patients. Allowing the patient an opportunity to express these concerns can be beneficial for both the patient and their family.

Because people with few social ties and little structural support have a significantly poorer prognosis than those with complex social networks, the size and quality of the patient's network should be evaluated. If the patient lives alone, he or she should be asked if they have someone who usually provides support for them (e.g., driving them to a doctor's appointment). Questions such as, "how may times a week do you visit with friends or relatives," or "how many times a week do you attend a community or social event, such as church" can provide key information for evaluating social support. For patients with few social ties, referral to cardiac rehabilitation programs or to Mended Hearts may provide increased community contacts. Patients referred to cardiac rehabilitation benefit from observing other patients' recoveries, and from the continuing contact with health care staff. Many patients in rehabilitation programs develop lasting friendships with their counterparts. Such ties serve as a buffer from the stresses of daily life.

Because it is impossible totally to avoid mental stress in daily life, control of other coronary risk factors is especially important. Mental stress results in elevations in blood pressure and low-density lipoprotein and very-low-density lipoprotein cholesterol levels, highlighting the importance of controlling these risk factors. In response to mental stress, blood pressure surges that can occur at relatively low heart rates can be partially ameliorated by beta blockers. Aspirin may also provide some protection by counteracting the platelet aggregation effects generated in response to stress. These pharmacologic interventions should be considered in all coronary patients.

Intervention Strategies for Anger and Hostility

Only a few studies have tested interventions for type A behaviors, hostility, or anger. Most interventions use group therapy programs with educational and behavioral strategies to assist patients in identifying and modifying their behaviors. For example, a patient might identify routine time-urgent behaviors such as speeding up at a yellow light or passing cars. These patients would be instructed to modify their behavior by purposefully driving in the slow lane. This type of program, although costly and time consuming, has been shown to reduce type A and hostility ratings and recurrent coronary events.[50]

Because hostility and anger have been linked to adverse coronary risk factor profiles, attention should be paid to modifying all coronary risk factors. Some studies have suggested that people with high levels of these negative personality characteristics may be less compliant with risk factor modification and medical regimes. For example, studies have found that when patients use smoking to relieve symptoms experienced during episodes of anger or frustration, quit rates are lower.[44] In contrast, however, a hypertensive drug study found that people with high hostility showed the greatest decline in pressure, independent of the type of blood pressure medication.[43] It is also observed that people with type A behavior may strive for a greater treatment response and, in fact, be more adherent. Evaluating adherence and applying problem-solving strategies is important

in all coronary patients, but may be particularly important in people with high hostility and anger ratings.

Intervention Strategies for Depression and Anxiety

It is possible that adverse lifestyle behaviors may be more prevalent in people experiencing higher levels of anxiety or depression. Depressed noncardiac patients are reported to have higher low-density lipoprotein levels and decreased glucose utilization.[16] Depressed patients with CHD consistently report higher smoking rates compared with nondepressed patients with CHD.[9,44] Other evidence suggests that depressed and anxious patients have more difficulty adopting healthy lifestyle behaviors. For example, in elderly patients post-MI, depression scores predicted the performance of self-care behaviors related to risk reduction.[12] In cardiac rehabilitation patients, anxiety, depression, and coping abilities predicted leisure-time activity and smoking cessation at 1-year follow-up.[24] Other evidence suggests that depressed patients are less likely to adhere to medical or behavioral regimes. Medication compliance is lower in both depressed and hostile patients.[8,43] Compliance with an aspirin regime was measured using electronic medication bottlecap monitoring; it was found that depressed elderly patients adhered 45% of days, whereas nondepressed elderly patients adhered 65% of days.[7] Although some evidence suggests that depression may affect adherence to risk reduction interventions, other studies have suggested that adherence may, in fact, improve these emotional states. In an exercise study, those who adhered to exercise had greater reductions in anxiety and depression scores than nonadherers.[17] The relation between adherence to exercise and improvement in psychological variables was extended in a community study of older adults randomly assigned to high- or low-intensity exercise training or control conditions.[37] Exercise participation, independent of randomized condition or change in physical fitness, was significantly related to lower depressive and anxiety scores. These data support the inclusion of exercise training programs as an intervention strategy for anxious or depressed patients. Many cardiac rehabilitation programs also include relaxation techniques as an integral part of the program that may be particularly useful in the patient with anxiety. These data also suggest that all interventions should include adherence counseling. Although behavioral strategies such as education, emotional support, and risk reduction may improve emotional states, consideration should also be given to use of pharmacologic interventions. Newer classes of drugs such as the serotonin reuptake inhibitors are effective and safe for use in cardiac patients.

All psychosocial interventions should be implemented only after fully considering the needs and beliefs of the individual patient. Data have shown that a psychosocial intervention delivered by nurses during home visits was ineffective in reducing recurrent events, and in fact may be detrimental for women.[18] Although these results are not fully understood, this study, along with other studies, failed to find differences in psychological variables between treatment and control groups.[15,65] Studies that report benefits related to prognosis and recurrent events also included substantial risk factor reduction strategies.[15,65] Thus, a multifactorial program that includes both psychosocial and traditional risk reduction strategies may provide the greatest overall benefit for both men and women with CHD.

In summary, important components of psychosocial interventions relate first to the recognition of the psychological and social needs of each patient. Education, emotional support, and specific behavioral strategies can influence a patient's response to psychosocial factors. Consistent with a nursing perspective, it is important to treat the person as a whole. Management of the coronary patient calls for attention to all cardiovascular risk factors, including psychosocial factors.

REFERENCES

1. Adams DO: Molecular biology of macrophage activation: A pathway whereby psychosocial factors can potentially affect health. Psychosom Med 56: 316–327, 1994
2. Agency for Health Care Policy and Research: Depression in primary care: Detection, diagnosis and treatment. Rockville, MD, U.S. Department of Health and Human Services, 1993
3. Antonucci TC, Johnson EH: Conceptualization and methods in social support theory and research as related to cardiovascular disease. In Shumacker SA, Czajkowski SM (eds): Social Support and Cardiovascular Disease, pp 21–39. New York, Plenum, 1994
4. Barefoot JC, Schroll M: Symptoms of depression, acute myocardial infarction, and total mortality in a community sample. Circulation 93: 1976–1980, 1996
5. Berkman LF, Leo-Summers L, Horwitz RI: Emotional support and survival after myocardial infarction. Ann Intern Med 117: 1003–1009, 1992
6. Booth-Kewley S, Friedman HS: Psychological predictors of heart disease: A quantitative review. Psychol Bull 101: 343–362, 1987
7. Carney RM, Freeland K, Eisen R et al: Depression as a risk factor for cardiac events in established coronary heart disease: A review of possible mechanisms. Ann Behav Med 17: 142–149, 1995
8. Carney RM, Rich MW, Freeland KE et al: Major depressive disorder predicts cardiac events in patients with coronary artery disease. Psychosom Med 50: 627–633, 1988
9. Carney RM, Rich MW, Tevelde A et al: Major depressive disorder in coronary artery disease. Am J Cardiol 60: 1273–1275, 1987
10. Case RB, Moss AJ, Care N et al: Living alone after myocardial infarction: Impact on prognosis. JAMA 267: 515–519, 1992
11. Cassem NH, Hackett TP: Psychological rehabilitation of myocardial infarction patients in the acute phase. Heart Lung 2: 382–388, 1973
12. Conn VS, Taylor SG, Wiman O. Anxiety, depression, quality of life, and self-care among survivors of myocardial infarction. Issues in Mental Health Nursing 12: 321–331, 1991
13. Ell K, Dunkel-Schetter C: Social support and adjustment to myocardial infarction, angioplasty and coronary artery bypass surgery. In Shumacker SA, Czajkowski SM (eds): Social Support and Cardiovascular Disease., pp. 301–322 New York, Plenum, 1994
14. Everson SA, Kauhanen J, Kaplan GA et al: Hostility and increased risk of mortality and acute myocardial infarction: The mediating role of behavioral risk factors. Am J Epidemiol 146: 142–152, 1997
15. Fair JM: Psychosocial Responses to Multifactor Coronary Risk Reduction. Ann Arbor, Michigan, UMI Dissertation Abstracts International, 1996
16. Fielding R: Depression and acute myocardial infarction: A review and reinterpretation. Soc Sci Med 32: 1017–1027, 1991
17. Fontana AF, Kerns R, Rosenberg R et al: Exercise training for cardiac patients: Adherence, fitness and benefits. J Cardiopulm Rehabil 6: 4–15, 1986
18. Frasure-Smith N, Lesperance F, Prince RH: Randomised trial of home-based psychosocial nursing intervention for patients recovering from myocardial infarction. Lancet 350: 473–479, 1998
19. Frasure-Smith N, Lesperance F, Talajic M: The impact of negative emotions on prognosis following myocardial infarction: Is it more than depression? Health Psychol 14: 388–398, 1995
20. Frasure-Smith N, Lesperance F, Talajic M: Major depression before and after myocardial infarction: Its nature and consequences. Psychosom Med 58: 99–110, 1996
21. Gabbay F, Krantz D, Kop W et al: Triggers of myocardial ischemia during daily life in patients with coronary artery disease: Physical and mental activities, anger and smoking. J Am Coll Cardiol 27: 585–592, 1996
22. Goodman M, Quigley J, Moran G et al: Hostility predicts restenosis after percutaneous transluminal coronary angioplasty. Mayo Clin Proc 71: 729–734, 1996
23. Grunbaum JA, Vernon SW, Clasen CM: The association between anger and hostility and risk factors for coronary heart disease in children and adolescents: A review. Ann Behav Med 19: 179–189, 1997
24. Guiry E, Conroy RM, Hickey N et al: Psychological response to an acute coronary event and its effect on subsequent rehabilitation and lifestyle change. Clin Cardiol 10: 256–260, 1987
25. Gullette E, Blumenthal J, Babyak M et al: effects of mental stress on myocardial ischemia during daily life. JAMA 277: 1521–1526, 1997
26. Haynes S, Feinleib M: Women, work, and coronary heart disease: Prospective findings from the Framingham Heart Study. Am J Public Health 70: 133–141, 1980
27. Helmer DC, Ragland DR, Syme SL: Hostility and coronary artery disease. Am J Epidemiol 133: 112–122, 1991
28. Hlatky MA, Lam LC, Lee K et al: Job strain and the prevalence and outcome of coronary artery disease. Circulation 92: 327–333, 1995
29. Jenkins CD: Behavioral risk factors in coronary artery disease. Annu Rev Med 29: 543–563, 1978
30. Julkunen J, Salonen R, Kaplan GA et al: Hostility and the progression of carotid atherosclerosis. Psychosom Med 56: 519–525, 1994
31. Kaplan JR, Adams MR, Clarkson TB et al: Psychosocial factors, sex differences, and atherosclerosis: Lessons learned from animal models. Psychosom Med 58: 598–611, 1996
32. Karasek R, Baker D, Marxer F et al: Job decision latitude, job demands and cardiovascular disease: A prospective study of Swedish men. Am J Public Health 71: 694–705, 1981
33. Kark JD, Goldman S, Epstein L: Iraqi missile attacks on Israel. JAMA 273: 1208–1210, 1995
34. Kawachi I, Colditz GA, Ascherio A et al: Prospective study of phobic anxiety and risk of coronary heart disease in men. Circulation 89: 1992–1997, 1994
35. Kawachi I, Sparrow D, Spiro A et al: A prospective study of anger and coronary heart disease. Circulation 94: 2090–2095, 1996
36. Kawachi I, Sparrow D, Vokona SPS et al: Symptoms of anxiety and risk of coronary heart disease: The Normative Aging Study. Circulation 90: 2225–2229, 1994
37. King A, Taylor CB, Haskell W: The effects of differing intensities and formats of twelve months of exercise training on psychological outcomes. Health Psychol 12: 292–302, 1993

38. Kloner RA, Leor J, Poole WK et al: Population-based analysis of the effect of the Northridge earthquake on cardiac death in Los Angeles County. J Am Coll Cardiol 30: 1174–1180, 1997

39. Kritz-Silverstein D, Wingard D, Barrett-Connor E: Employment status and heart disease risk factors in middle-aged women: The Rancho Bernardo Study. Am J Public Health 82: 215–219, 1992

40. Krumholz HM, Butler J, Miller J et al: Prognostic importance of emotional support for elderly patients hospitalized with heart failure. Circulation 97: 958–964, 1998

41. Kubzansky LD, Kawachi I, Spiro III A et al: Is worrying bad for your heart? Circulation 95: 818–824, 1997

42. Lazarus RS, Folkman S: Stress, Appraisal, and Coping. New York, Springer-Verlag, 1984

43. Lee D, Mendes de Leon CF, Jenkins CD et al: Relation of hostility to medication adherence, symptom complaints and blood pressure reduction in a clinical field trial of antihypertensive medication. J Psychosom Res 36: 181–190, 1992

44. Littman AB: Review of psychosomatic aspects of cardiovascular disease. Psychother Psychosom 60: 148–167, 1993

45. Lynch J, Kaplan G, Salonen R et al: Socioeconomic status and carotid atherosclerosis. Circulation 92: 1786–1792, 1995

46. Matthews K, Cottington E, Talbot E et al: Stressful work conditions and diastolic blood pressure among blue collar factory workers. Am J Epidemiol 126: 280–291, 1987

47. McCarty R, Gold PE: Catecholamines, stress, and disease: A psychobiological perspective. Psychosom Med 58: 590–597, 1996

48. Mittleman MA, Maclure M, Sherwood JB et al: Triggering of acute myocardial infarction onset by episodes of anger. Circulation 92: 1720–1725, 1995

49. Moser DK, Dracup K: Is anxiety after myocardial infarction associated with subsequent ischemic and arrhythmic events? Psychosom Med 58: 395–401, 1996

50. Nunes EV, Frank KA, Kornfeld DS: Psychologic treatment for the type A behavior pattern and for coronary heart disease: A meta-analysis of the literature. Psychosom Med 48: 159–173, 1987

51. Friedman M, Rosenman RH: Type A behavior pattern: its association with cornary heart disease. Ann Clin Res 3(6): 300–312, 1971.

52. Rosenman RH, Brand RJ, Jenkins CD et al: Coronary heart disease in the Western Collaborative Group Study: Final follow-up experience of 8.5 years. JAMA 233: 872–877, 1975

53. Rozanski A, Bairy CN, Krantz DS et al: Mental stress and the induction of myocardial ischemia in patients with coronary artery disease. N Engl J Med 318: 1005–1012, 1988

54. Scheier M, Bridges M: Person variables and health: Personality predispositions and acute psychological states as shared determinants of disease. Psychosom Med 57: 255–268, 1995

55. Scherwitz LW, Perkins LL, Chesney MA et al: Hostility and health behaviors in young adults: The CARDIA Study—Coronary Artery Risk Development in Young Adults Study. Am J Epidemiol 136: 136–145, 1992

56. Schwartz J, Pieper C, Krarasek RA: A procedure for linking psychosocial job characteristics data to health surveys. Am J Public Health 78: 904–909, 1988

57. Selye H: The Stress of Life. New York, McGraw-Hill, 1956

58. Shekelle RB, Hulley SB, Neaton JD: The MRFIT behavior pattern study: Type A behavior and the incidence of coronary heart disease. Am J Epidemiol 122: 559–570, 1985

59. Smith CE, Fernengel K, Holcroft C et al: Meta-analysis of the associations between social support and health outcomes. Ann Behav Med 16: 352–362, 1994

60. Smith TW: Hostility and health: Current status of a psychosomatic hypothesis. Health Psychol 11: 139–150, 1992

61. Spielberg C, Falkenhaln D, Willich S et al: Circadian, day-of-week, and seasonal variability in myocardial infarction: Comparison between working and retired patients. Am Heart J 132: 579–585, 1996

62. Spitzer R, Williams JB, Linzer M et al: Utility of a new procedure for diagnosing mental disorders in primary care: The PRIME-MD 1000 Study. JAMA 272: 1749–1756, 1994

63. Suzuki S, Sakamotot S, Koide M et al: Hanshi-Awaji earthquake as a trigger for acute myocardial infarction. Am Heart J 134: 974–977, 1997

64. Taylor CB, Bandura A, Ewart C et al: Exercise testing to enhance wives confidence in their husbands cardiac capacity soon after clinically uncomplicated myocardial infarction. Am J Cardiol 55: 635–638, 1985

65. Taylor CB, Houston-Miller N, DeBusk RF: The effect of a home-based case-managed, multifactor risk-reduction program on psychological distress in patients with cardiovascular disease. J Cardiopulm Rehabil 17: 157–162, 1997

66. Yeung AC, Vekshtein VI, Krantz DS et al: The effect of atherosclerosis on the vasomotor responses of coronary arteries to mental stress. N Engl J Med 325: 1551–1556, 1991

31

Smoking Cessation: A Systematic Approach to Managing Patients With Coronary Heart Disease

KIRSTEN MARTIN
NANCY HOUSTON MILLER
ERIKA S. SIVARAJAN FROELICHER

With a yearly death toll of more than 400,000 Americans, cigarette smoking remains the number one cause of premature death in the United States. It is a known cause of cardiovascular disease, stroke, cancer, and obstructive pulmonary disease.[1] In particular, smoking alone causes nearly one fifth of all cardiovascular deaths.[2] In addition to the human costs of smoking, 50 billion dollars are spent yearly on direct medical care, and 47 billion dollars in wages and productivity are lost every year because of smoking-related disabilities.[1] In fact, one fourth of the approximately 33 million hospital admissions annually involve smokers.[3] Therefore, health and policy experts have made cigarette smoking a major focus of risk factor modification; for example, the Agency for Health Care Policy and Research (AHCPR) has published a clinical practice guideline titled *Smoking Cessation*.[1] In addition, smoking cessation has been included as a national health goal in *Healthy People 2000: National Health Promotion and Disease Prevention Objectives*.[4]

Although nurses know that smoking has a negative impact on health, especially cardiovascular health, most fail to provide a smoking cessation intervention. Successful smoking cessation interventions usually have behavior modification as a core component. Behavioral modification skills include identifying areas of concern for patients, teaching patients strategies to cope with difficult situations, and role playing strategies with patients to allow them to practice their new coping strategies. These behavioral modification skills usually are not part of most nursing school curricula.

Even when they are taught, there is rarely an opportunity for practice, feedback, and development of confidence in performing these skills. This chapter focuses on the important steps in smoking cessation interventions that should be provided to patients with cardiovascular disease, with an emphasis on behavioral as well as pharmacologic approaches. After completing this chapter, the nurse, no matter what setting he or she practices in—intensive care unit, cardiac care unit, medical-surgical, labor and delivery, outpatient care—will posses the necessary knowledge to provide a smoking cessation intervention to every patient who smokes, every time the patient is encountered.

Permanent smoking cessation should be the goal for every intervention and every person who smokes. Achievement of this goal is difficult, however, because the nicotine in tobacco products is an addictive substance.[5] Smokers are physically and emotionally compelled to continue smoking even in the face of serious adverse health consequences. In addition, multiple quit attempts and failure to quit smoking despite high levels of motivation are common. The presence of withdrawal symptoms is another indicator of the addictive properties of nicotine. The criteria for diagnosis of nicotine withdrawal are met when any four of the following symptoms commence within 24 hours of the abrupt cessation of nicotine use: dysphoric or depressed mood; insomnia; irritability, frustration, or anger; anxiety; difficulty concentrating; restlessness; decreased heart rate; or increased appetite or weight gain.[6] Rapid identification of these withdrawal symptoms and prompt intervention are important skills for all nurses, particularly hospital-based nurses, because these withdrawal symptoms may be so intense for a given patient that he or she is unable to make rational health care decisions and may leave the hospital against medical advice to relieve them with a cigarette.

HARMFUL EFFECTS OF SMOKING

Cigarette smoking, hypercholesterolemia, hypertension, and physical inactivity are considered the four major risk factors for cardiovascular disease. What makes cigarette smoking unique among these is that it interacts synergistically with hypercholesterolemia and hypertension to increase greatly the risk for coronary heart disease (CHD). For example, in people who smoke and have hypercholesterolemia or hypertension, the risk for CHD is doubled. For people who have all three risk factors, the risk for CHD is quadrupled.[7]

In general, cigarette smoking accelerates atherosclerosis throughout the body, but this effect is most important in the coronary arteries, the aorta, and the carotid and cerebral arteries. Several mechanisms have been described to explain how cigarette smoking leads to atherosclerosis. These include (1) adverse effects on lipid profiles, (2) endothelial damage or dysfunction, (3) hemodynamic stress, (4) oxidant injury, (5) neutrophil activation, (6) enhanced thrombosis, and (7) increased blood viscosity.[8]

Although the acceleration of atherosclerosis is a major contributor to cardiovascular morbidity (e.g., aggravation of stable angina pectoris, vasospastic angina, intermittent claudication), a major focus in the population of smokers with cardiovascular disease is how smoking mediates acute cardiovascular events (e.g., myocardial infarction [MI], sudden death, stroke) that lead to hospitalization. The smoking-related mechanisms thought to contribute to these events are (1) induction of a hypercoagulable state, (2) increased myocardial workload, (3) reduced oxygen-carrying capacity of the blood, (4) coronary vasoconstriction, and (5) catecholamine release.[8]

Nicotine and carbon monoxide, although only 2 of the more than 4,000 chemicals in cigarette smoke, are generally considered to be the major contributors to atherosclerotic disease.[9] Nicotine disrupts lipid metabolism, resulting in an increased level of low-density lipoprotein and a decreased level of high-density lipoprotein. Nicotine is also responsible for the increased platelet aggregation and hypercoagulability found in smokers. In addition, it leads to increased production of catecholamines, which in turn increase blood pressure, heart rate and contractility, and systemic vascular resistance, all of which result in increased myocardial oxygen demand.[8,10] Unfortunately, meeting this demand is difficult because cigarette smoking constricts large and small epicardial arteries and coronary resistance vessels, leading to a decrease in coronary blood flow.[11] In fact, in a study of patients with established CHD, Barry and colleagues[12] found that continued cigarette smoking was related to a

12-fold increase in the amount of total ischemia daily. Episodes of ischemic ST segment depression occurred 3 times as often, and the duration was 12 times longer in smokers compared with nonsmokers (median duration of 24 min/24 h, vs. 2 min/24 h). This increased ischemia may be related to the increased probability of recurrent coronary events in people who smoke. The increase in heart rate may also lead to endothelial injury, myocardial ischemia and MI, arrhythmias, and sudden death.[8]

Carbon monoxide interferes with oxygen transport, leading to a reduced supply of oxygen to the tissues and, more important, to the myocardium at a time when the demand is high because of a higher heart rate.[9] Carbon monoxide interferes with the oxygen-carrying capacity of red blood cells by binding to hemoglobin, thereby reducing the amount of hemoglobin available for binding with oxygen, and by impeding oxygen release from hemoglobin.[8] Carbon monoxide also increases the permeability of endothelial membranes, resulting in increased uptake of cholesterol that leads to atherogenesis.[10]

When the number of cigarettes smoked daily, the total number of years of smoking, the degree of inhalation, and the age of smoking initiation are considered, the risk for development of CHD is found to increase with increasing exposure to cigarette smoke. Overall, cigarette smokers have a two- to fourfold greater incidence of CHD than do nonsmokers, and cigarette smokers have a 70% greater death rate due to CHD than nonsmokers. Cigarette smokers also experience a two- to fourfold greater risk of sudden death than nonsmokers.[10]

The damage caused by cigarette smoking is not restricted to the heart alone. Cigarette smokers have a higher incidence of arteriosclerotic peripheral vascular disease and more severe atherosclerosis of the aorta than nonsmokers,[9] as well as an increased rate of stroke and cerebrovascular disease.[10]

BENEFITS OF SMOKING CESSATION

The health benefits of smoking cessation on the cardiovascular system are well documented. The increased tendency to thrombus formation, coronary artery spasm, arrhythmias, and reduced oxygen supply are likely to reverse in a short time.[13] For example, evidence suggests that quitting smoking after an initial MI decreases a person's risk of death from CHD by at least 50% in the first year after quitting.[14] This decline in risk appears to be independent of the severity of the MI.[15] In addition, reports from the Coronary Artery Surgery Study (CASS) indicate that smoking cessation significantly improves survival for people of all ages, including those older than 70 years of age.[16] In fact, after 1 year of abstinence from smoking, the excess risk of CHD related to smoking is cut in half, and then gradually continues to decline over time. After 15 years of abstinence, the former smoker has achieved a risk level similar to that of a person who has never smoked. Smoking cessation also lowers the overall risk for stroke to that of a nonsmoker within 5 to 15 years of abstinence.[9]

Because the overall death rate and rate of reinfarction is higher in patients with established CHD, intensive smoking intervention should be directed to this population. Nurses who provide care for patients with cardiovascular disease in all practice settings must not miss the opportunity to encourage smokers to quit at every encounter. In addition to the smoking cessation efforts of public education, commercial programs, and worksite health promotion, primary care efforts to assist patients who have manifestations of CHD are worthwhile.

THEORETICAL FRAMEWORK FOR SMOKING CESSATION

The Transtheoretical Model classifies smokers into four categories or stages based on their desire to quit smoking and their smoking status. The stages include precontemplation, contemplation, action, and maintenance. Smokers in the precontemplation stage are not seriously considering quitting within the next 6 months. Smokers in the contemplation stage are seriously considering quitting within the next 6 months.[17] Those in the action stage have been continuously abstinent for less than 6 months, and those in the maintenance stage have continuously abstained from smoking for longer than 6 months.[18]

Research on the processes of change in people who quit on their own without intervention from health care providers has shown that subjects in the precontemplation stage have fewer negative emotional reactions to their smoking and do little to change their focus on smoking. On the other hand, smokers who are in the contemplation stage are more open to information about smoking and to responding to feedback and education as sources of information about smoking. Once in the action stage, subjects use both counter-conditioning, such as doing something else when the urge to smoke strikes them, and stimulus-control procedures, such as removing ash trays and other reminders of smoking from their environment to take active part in changing their smoking behaviors. These subjects are also more likely to use self- and social reinforcement and to rely on helping relationships to maintain their nonsmoking status. These same characteristics are true of subjects in the maintenance stage.[19]

Research has identified a strong correlation between the stage a subject is in and his or her beliefs regarding the ratio between the pros and cons of smoking. Precontemplators anticipate more cons than pros related to smoking cessation. Contemplators see the pros and cons as being more balanced. Those in the action stage anticipate more pros than cons.[17,20-22]

Research has also identified a strong correlation between the stage a patient is in and his or her self-efficacy expectations. Self-efficacy is defined as the smoker's level of confidence that he or she could refrain from smoking in various challenging situations such as social situations (with friends in a cafe, when someone offers them a cigarette), emotional situations (when feeling tense or depressed), and habitual-addictive situations (when desiring a cigarette or when they are experiencing withdrawal symptoms).[20] Smokers in the action and maintenance stages had significantly higher levels of confidence across the various situations compared with those in the contemplation or precontemplation stages.[17,20,21] DiClemente and colleagues[17] also found that contemplators had significantly higher self-efficacy than precontemplators.

SMOKING CESSATION INTERVENTIONS IN THE CORONARY HEART DISEASE POPULATION

Few randomized clinical trials of smoking cessation intervention have been conducted in patients with established CHD. Most of the studies have been observational or cross-sectional, using primarily physician advice, education, or group counseling to help patients quit smoking. Studies have usually been limited by small sample size, lack of uniformity regarding the definition of abstinence, and reliance on self-report data for confirmation of smoking status.[23] Finally, no randomized clinical trials have been conducted in women with CHD.

In spite of these limitations, some studies do suggest that physicians and other health care professionals can have a positive impact on smoking behavior.[24-26] The expected cessation rate in the general population is approximately 6% per year when simple advice is provided by physicians,[27] whereas group programs using behavioral methods may achieve yearly cessation rates as high as 26% to 40%.[28] In the CHD population in particular, the strong stimulus provided by a CHD event results in rates of smoking cessation that are higher than in most studies conducted in the general population.[25,29,30] In particular, studies on those patients having coronary artery bypass graft surgery show smoking cessation rates of approximately 50%,[31,32] whereas those undergoing coronary arteriography have smoking cessation rates of up to 62%.[33] Finally, studies of patients with an MI or angina pectoris reported smoking cessation rates of between 20% and 70%.[25,26,29,30,34,35]

A significant body of research has also focused on nurse-managed smoking cessation interventions that begin in the hospital and then continue with telephone follow-up after discharge from the hospital. The effectiveness of this type of intervention has been demonstrated in patients after MI[25] and cancer surgery,[36] and in patients admitted to the hospital.[37]

In general, research indicates that those patients with high motivation or strong intention to quit,[32,33] more severe disease,[33] who were given strong advice to quit by their physician,[25,38] who have cardiovascular disease,[38] have made fewer attempts to quit in the past, and who had no difficulty refraining from smoking while in the hospital[32] achieved the highest smoking cessation rates. Patients with CHD who continue to smoke are in general younger, female, unmarried/not living with a partner,[39] belong to a lower socioeconomic and educational level, have a less negative attitude about smoking, smoke a greater number of cigarettes, and are more likely to be anxious or depressed.[40] Whereas effective interventions have been conducted to address some of these characteristics, interventions aimed at people of lower educational and socioeconomic status are still lacking.

GENERAL TRENDS IN SMOKING CESSATION INTERVENTIONS

The public health approach to smoking cessation that has predominated in the smoking literature in the 1990s has primarily targeted populations or high-risk groups in their natural environments, such as worksites. Public health interventions are usually brief, low cost, and often provided by laypeople or through automated means (e.g., mail, contests).

Clinical approaches, on the other hand, are targeted to people who are self-referred or recruited, are most commonly applied in a medical or group setting, use trained professionals, and provide intensive multisession interventions. Because patients with CHD are at risk for recurrent cardiac events, such as another MI, a clinical approach is more cost effective for this population—it is cheaper to help patients quit smoking than to hospitalize them for a repeat MI.[41]

Many intensive group smoking cessation programs are offered, but most smokers prefer to quit on their own or with individualized support.[42] For example, in a study of cardiovascular patients admitted to the hospital who were smoking at the time of admission, 86% expressed an interest in quitting. However, of the 86% who were interested in quitting, 79% stated they were interested in quitting on their own, with 50% expressing interest in the use of self-help materials. Fewer than 10% of patients endorsed a formal treatment program.[43] The literature also supports the fact that 90% of all smokers eventually quit on their own, normally after three to four unsuccessful attempts.[44] It therefore behooves nurses to consider methods that may be individualized to patient needs, combining a clinical approach with multicomponent strategies without requiring patients to attend a formal treatment program.

AGENCY FOR HEALTH CARE POLICY AND RESEARCH SMOKING CESSATION CLINICAL PRACTICE GUIDELINE

As the body of knowledge about the health consequences of smoking and the health benefits of smoking cessation grows, smoking cessation interventions play an even greater role in decreasing smoking-related cardiovascular morbidity and mortality. After a thorough, evidence-based review of the available literature, the AHCPR concluded

that tobacco use is a serious health threat and that effective smoking cessation interventions are available, but that health care providers do not provide these interventions consistently. To address these issues, the AHCPR convened an expert panel and charged it with identifying effective, experimentally validated smoking cessation treatments and practices through a systematic review and analysis of available scientific research. The result, the AHCPR *Smoking Cessation Clinical Practice Guideline*,[1] provides recommendations for primary care clinicians, smoking cessation specialists, and health care administrators, insurers, and purchasers. These recommendations are pertinent to the cardiovascular nurse as well, especially because one of the primary roles of the cardiovascular nurse is risk factor modification.

The five primary recommendations of the AHCPR are (1) systematically identify tobacco users and document their smoking status; (2) strongly urge all smokers to quit; (3) identify smokers willing to make a quit attempt; (4) aid the smoker in quitting by using a variety of interventions; and (5) schedule follow-up contact. Examples of how to implement a smoking cessation intervention consistent with AHCPR guidelines follow.

Step 1: ASK—Systematically Identify All Tobacco Users at Every Visit

To identify every smoker every time he or she is seen by a clinician, a system-wide structure must be put in place. It can be as simple as adding assessment of smoking status to the routine vital signs (heart rate, blood pressure, respiratory rate, temperature) at every visit. To ensure that the smoking status question is asked every time, preprinted progress notes can be used, vital sign stamps can be made, special stickers indicating smoking status can be placed on the outside of charts, and for those with computer charting, a query of smoking status can be inserted into the data collection tool. To obtain this information on patients who are hospitalized, smoking status must be asked as part of the routine admission questionnaire or, as in the outpatient setting, assessed with initial vital signs. It is especially important to identify hospitalized smokers because hospitalization causes them to become ex-smokers owing to no-smoking policies. If not identified, these patients may go through severe nicotine withdrawal unnecessarily, which may lead to noncompliance with treatments and, in the extreme case, a patient leaving against medical advice.

Even though surveys indicate that physicians believe they have a responsibility to help smokers, only half of all physicians provide such advice.[45] In addition, half of the nurses surveyed by Kviz and colleagues[46] believe that the responsibility for advising patients 50 years of age or older is equally divided between nurses and physicians. These statistics show how easily a smoker can slip through the cracks. Often, if a responsibility is shared, it never gets done because one person assumes the other person did it. Therefore, the roles of the nurse and the physician need to be clearly identified in each setting. However, in one study,

---

DISPLAY 31-1

How to Ask About Smoking Status

INITIAL ASSESSMENT

"We're interested in knowing about your lifestyle and habits as they relate to your health. Have you ever smoked in your life? Are you still smoking?" or

"Over the course of a lifetime, many people pick up the smoking habit. Have you ever smoked? Do you still smoke?"

FOLLOW-UP

If the patient was not ready to quit at the last visit: "I'm sure it must be difficult, but have you seriously considered making an attempt to quit smoking since your last visit?"

If the patient was in the precontemplation stage at the last visit: "At your last visit, you were seriously thinking about quitting smoking. Were you able to cut down on the number of cigarettes you smoke, or were you successful at quitting since your last visit?"

If the patient was in the action stage at the last visit: "Have you had any problems in refraining from smoking since your last visit?"

43% of nurses reported that they did not know how to counsel patients, 27% claimed it was not rewarding, 8% thought it was too time consuming, and only 14% reported ever receiving formal training in smoking cessation counseling.[47] In addition, Faulkner and Ward[48] found that nurses' knowledge of the effects of smoking was limited because they were on average able to name only two physiologic effects and three disease processes related to smoking, even when given cues to correct answers. Lack of knowledge is not the only problem; attitudes and opinions must also be altered. For example, nurses in general believe that patients who smoke are not concerned about the health consequences of smoking and do not have a strong desire to stop smoking. Furthermore, nurses believe that if they do advise a patient to stop smoking, the likelihood of the patient actually stopping is not very high.[46] It is thus critically important that physicians and nurses, as well as all other health care professionals, assess their level of comfort in offering advice and, if necessary, receive training on how to counsel people. Simply bringing up the subject may seem overwhelming to health care professionals. Simple ways to introduce the subject are shown in Display 31-1.

Step 2: ADVISE—Strongly Urge All Smokers to Quit

Smokers tend to deny anything but the most direct advice and clear-cut message about quitting. Therefore, the first step in the process of providing help to a smoker is to give him or her a clear, strong, and personalized message about quitting, such as "Your smoking is harming your health. As your nurse, I need to tell you that smoking is your major risk factor for cardiovascular disease. Continuing to smoke will lead to further cardiovascular disease and possibly death. Together, we must figure out how to help you become a non-smoker." Clear and strong, however, is not enough. The message must be personalized. Make your message relevant to the smoker's current concerns about his or her health, disease status, family or social situation, age, sex, and past smoking behaviors. For example, if a patient is hospitalized for a coronary angioplasty, it is necessary for him or her to know that continued smoking is associated with an increased restenosis rate. Follow this with information about the health risks associated with continuing to smoke (see section on Harmful Effects of Smoking) and the health and social benefits of smoking cessation (see section on Benefits of Smoking Cessation). The following examples illustrate how a smoker may interpret an inadequate message.

If you say:	The smoker may think:
You probably should stop smoking.	I guess I don't have to stop smoking.
You are older, but stopping smoking may help any way.	I don't have much time to live, so why stop smoking now?
The surgery has restored your circulation to normal.	Good. Now I don't have to quit smoking.

Step 3: ASSESS—Identify Smokers Willing to Make a Quit Attempt

After providing advice, it is important to determine if the patient is willing to quit smoking at this time. Willingness to quit can be measured through a simple yes–no question, "Are you willing to quit smoking now?" Another measure of a patient's willingness to quit smoking can be assessed using an intention question: "Do you intend to stay off cigarettes or other tobacco products in the next month?" A response scale is shown below.

1	2	3	4	5	6	7
Definitely No	Probably No	Possibly No	Maybe	Possibly Yes	Probably Yes	Definitely Yes

Patients who score a three or less usually are not interested or ready to quit.[26] (See scale on the previous page.)

If patients are unwilling to quit, it is important to determine why. In some cases, patients may not have been given enough information about associated risks. Whatever the barrier, providing help or solutions to anticipated problems may encourage the patient to think further about quitting, moving him or her from the precontemplation stage to the contemplation or action stage.

If the patient is willing to quit, move to step 4. If not, provide a motivational intervention. The best way to provide a motivational intervention is to remember the four Rs: relevance, risks, rewards, and repetition.[1] To make an intervention relevant and meaningful to a patient, discuss smoking cessation in light of the patient's disease status, family or social situation, age, sex, and other characteristics unique to the patient. Three types of risks should be addressed with the patient. Acute risks include shortness of breath and exacerbation of asthma. Long-term risks include heart attack, stroke, cancer, and chronic obstructive pulmonary disease. Environmental risks include risks that put the patient's children and other family members at risk for lung cancer, sudden infant death syndrome, and asthma.[1] The rewards of smoking cessation should also be discussed with the patient. These include improved health, sense of smell and taste, and self-esteem, as well as freedom from worry about the effect the patient's smoking has on his or her children and other family members. Finally, repetition is included because the relevance, risks, and rewards need to be reviewed with the patient every time he or she is seen— on any given visit, the patient may finally be receptive to a smoking cessation intervention.

Step 4: ASSIST—Aid the Patient in Quitting

SETTING A QUIT DATE AND PLANNING FOR AN INTERVENTION

The first phase of assisting the patient ready to quit smoking involves setting a quit date. If a patient is motivated, setting a quit date within 2 weeks of meeting with the health care provider is most appropriate. Some patients, however, prefer to quit suddenly, or "cold turkey." If the smoker is identified in the hospital, setting a quit date is not necessary because the patient has become an ex-smoker owing to the hospital smoking ban. Some programs have patients monitor the situations that cause them to smoke before they quit, or reduce the number of cigarettes in the weeks before quitting. These techniques, however, although helpful to some, may simply prolong the process of quitting.

Signing a contract at this point is a behavioral technique that has proved effective in helping patients to quit smoking. This process helps to formalize the smoker's commitment to quitting and can serve as a method by which the nurse extends support to the patient in this process. Con-

tracts must be simple and explicitly written so that both parties agree with the stated terms, and they should specify the consequences of not adhering to the expected behavior (see Harmful Effects of Smoking), as well as the rewards of successful adherence (see Benefits of Smoking Cessation).[49]

When planning a smoking cessation intervention, the nurse should take into account the patient's desire for formal help. Literature on compliance suggests that when the patient participates in developing a personalized plan of action, greater follow-through is achieved. Because most people choose individual methods for cessation, providing self-help materials is a low-cost method of intervention. When combined with strong advice by the nurse, these materials often double success rates. For the cardiac patient, the American Heart Association's "An Active Partnership for the Health of Your Heart" offers effective multimedia materials, including a videotape, audiotape, and workbook. Other self-help materials, like those from the American Cancer Society and the American Lung Association, along with information for the nurse, are listed at the end of this chapter, before the References.

Although most patients choose to quit on their own with minimal help, some patients prefer, and may benefit from, a group program that provides 8 to 10 weeks of behavior modification. Knowing available community resources and making them available to patients by providing them with a list of programs to choose from, including the intervention methods, costs, and a contact person, ensures that patients are adequately informed. The patient may also be encouraged to address the issue with his or her employer because many larger employers offer smoking cessation programs as an employee benefit.

Occasionally, patients may decide that acupuncture or hypnosis is a viable alternative. The success rates of these types of smoking cessation interventions are unknown because of a lack of randomized clinical trials. Some patients, however, anecdotally report being helped. If a patient chooses a group cessation program or an alternative intervention, referral should be made and follow-up scheduled to determine the success of the chosen intervention.

The AHCPR's expert panel[1] found that effective smoking cessation interventions include three components, which are (1) provider support, (2) skills training for relapse prevention, and (3) nicotine replacement therapy (NRT). The most common elements of supportive smoking cessation treatments include providing basic information, encouragement, displaying concern, and providing the patient with an opportunity to discuss his or her fears, concerns, difficulties, and successes.

RELAPSE PREVENTION

The second component of successful smoking cessation interventions is relapse prevention training,[50] which involves (1) identifying the patient's high-risk situations, (2) providing skills training to help the patient cope with

		YES	NO
1.	Have you ever felt you ought to CUT DOWN on your drinking?	☐	☐
2.	Have people ANNOYED you by criticizing your drinking?	☐	☐
3.	Have you ever felt GUILTY about your drinking?	☐	☐
4.	Have you ever had a drink first thing in the morning (EYE OPENER) to steady your nerves or get rid of a hangover?	☐	☐

FIGURE 31-1 The CAGE questionnaire. (From Ewing JA: Detecting alcoholism: The CAGE questionnaire. JAMA 252:1905–1907, 1984)

these situations, and (3) rehearsing the coping mechanisms. Two useful ways to help patients identify their personal high-risk situations are self-monitoring and self-efficacy scales. Through self-monitoring, patients keep a record of each cigarette smoked, noting the time of day, situation during which they smoke, and a rating of mood. A thorough examination of this record can be used to identify patterns of smoking behavior. Self-efficacy scales, on the other hand, measure a patient's confidence to resist the urge to smoke in a variety of situations. Studies have shown that self-efficacy ratings in smoking are predictive of subsequent outcome, and, when smoking is resumed, specific situations are frequently predictive of a relapse episode.[51] A 14-item self-efficacy scale, which is a shorter version of the scale by Condiotte and Lichtenstein,[51] is illustrated in Figure 31-1. In one study,[26] less than 70% confidence for a given efficacy item denoted a high-risk situation for which patients may require help. Patients are taught to work on those situations in which they show the least confidence to resist smoking.

After identification of high-risk situations, skills training helps people mobilize their resources by developing cognitive and behavioral strategies to cope with the situation. Tsoh and colleagues[52] recommend teaching patients to cope with urges to smoke by using the ACE (Avoid, Cope, Escape) strategies. For example, if a patient does not feel ready to handle a risky situation, encourage the patient to avoid it until the patient's confidence in his or her ability to handle that particular risky situation improves. If a patient routinely watches football at a smoke-filled sports bar, have him or her invite some nonsmoking friends over to his or her home to watch the game. Or, if a patient is going to a restaurant, he or she can ask to sit in the nonsmoking section, thereby avoiding the option to smoke.

If a patient cannot avoid a risky situation, then coping with it is the next step. Possible coping strategies include distraction, incompatible behaviors, and positive self-talk. Distraction from the urge to smoke can be achieved by going for a walk, telephoning a friend, reading, or any other activity that gets the patient's mind off smoking. Behaviors that are incompatible with smoking include chewing gum, snacking on low-calorie, low-fat foods, or engaging in tasks that occupy the hands, like knitting, sewing, woodworking, or crossword puzzles. Positive self-talk involves the patient telling himself or herself that he or she can continue to be a nonsmoker. For example, a patient may say, "I can do this. I am capable of remaining a nonsmoker. I have the power to improve my health by remaining a nonsmoker." Other things a patient can do include reminding himself or herself about the health risks of cigarette smoking, the health benefits of quitting, and the monetary savings.

If the patient cannot avoid or cope with a risky situation, escape is the next option. "Escape" means getting out of a risky situation without a puff. For example, if the patient is at a party with friends, the patient can socialize with nonsmokers in attendance instead of stepping outside with smokers. When dining out with others, escape can mean stepping outside while the others smoke their after-dinner cigarette. It is important to stress to the patient that a combination of strategies (ACE) is essential. By having many strategies, the patient decreases the risk of being caught in a situation he or she is not prepared to handle.

The last step in relapse prevention training is practicing the coping response through rehearsal. Even though an urge may occur, if the patient is prepared to handle the situation, it decreases the likelihood that he or she will pick up a cigarette. One nursing responsibility includes practicing the different strategies to strengthen coping responses by role playing with the patient a solution to handle the high-risk situation.

In addition to the strategies developed for specific situations, relapse prevention training focuses on general lifestyle modifications that help to enhance the patient's self-control.[50] Exercise and relaxation techniques are two such strategies that have been used successfully to help patients develop a greater sense of self-control. In a study of patients after MI, smokers participating in an exercise training program combined with smoking cessation had greater cessation rates and smoked significantly fewer cigarettes than those who did not participate in such a program.[53] Exercise may also help reduce weight gain after quitting smoking and may minimize some withdrawal symptoms. For these reasons, patients should be encouraged to increase their activity levels through walking or other forms of exercise.

NICOTINE REPLACEMENT THERAPY (NRT)

The third component of successful smoking cessation interventions is NRT, a pharmacologic therapy that most often takes the form of a nicotine patch or gum. Patients who have had severe withdrawal symptoms in the past on making an attempt to quit are likely to be highly addicted to nicotine. The Fagerstrom Tolerance Tool[54] (Fig. 31-2) is an eight-item tool commonly used to measure addiction to nicotine. Patients can administer this self-test to identify their degree of dependence. In a study of cardiovascular patients, Taylor and coworkers[26] noted that patients who smoke more than 25 cigarettes per day, who smoke as soon as they get up in the morning, and who smoke when they are so ill they are in bed, are highly addicted to nicotine. Patients who meet the criteria for nicotine dependence or who have experienced particularly troublesome withdrawal

Questions	Answers	Points
1. How soon after you wake up do you smoke your first cigarette?	Within 30 min	1
	After 30 min	0
2. Do you find it difficult to refrain from smoking in places where it is forbidden? (church, libraries)	Yes	1
	No	0
3. Which cigarette would you hate most to give up?	First one in the A.M.	1
	Any other	0
4. How many cigarettes a day do you smoke?	15 or less	0
	16–25	1
	26 or more	2
5. Do you smoke more frequently during the first hours after waking than the rest of the day?	Yes	1
	No	0
6. Do you smoke if you are so ill that you are in bed most of the day?	Yes	1
	No	0
7. What is the tar content (nicotine level) of your usual brand of cigarettes?	Low	0
	Medium	1
	High	2
8. Do you inhale?	Never	0
	Sometimes	1
	Always	2

SCORE   0 to 6   = Low to moderate dependence;   **TOTAL** _____
7 to 11 = High dependence

FIGURE 31-2 The Fagerstrom tolerance test. (Fagerstrom KO: Measuring degree of physical dependence to tobacco smoking with reference to individualization of treatment. Addict Behav 3: 235–241, 1978)

symptoms may be more successful in quitting if they are provided NRT in the form of a nicotine patch or gum. In fact, studies have shown that NRT alone leads to a smoking cessation rate of 8.8%, and 15.2% when combined with provider support.[52]

The AHCPR's expert panel,[1] however, concluded that NRT is contraindicated in patients who have had an MI within 4 weeks, have serious arrhythmias, or have worsening angina pectoris. Although the presence of cardiovascular disease is a relative contraindication to NRT, physicians and patients must weigh the advantages of stopping smoking against the risks of using a medication that releases nicotine into the blood. Blood levels obtained during the use of 2-mg nicotine gum average 12 mg/mL during smoking, compared with peak levels without the gum of 35 to 54 mg/mL during smoking.[55] Moreover, in assessing the effects of transdermal nicotine in cardiac patients, no increase in complications or symptoms such as angina or arrhythmias was observed in 156 patients using 14- to 21-mg patches.[56] A review found that NRT constricts coronary arteries and alters hemodynamic profiles, leading to increased myocardial workload and oxygen demand. Cigarette smoking, on the other hand, precipitates acute cardiac events by three mechanisms, which are (1) it produces a hypercoagulable state and promotes thrombosis; (2) it delivers carbon monoxide, which limits oxygen delivery to the heart; and (3) it alters hemodynamic profiles. The reviewers also concluded that the alterations in hemodynamic profiles caused by NRT were less hazardous than those produced by cigarette smoking.[8] Therefore, it appears that the effects of NRT on the cardiovascular system are no greater and are probably less than the effects of cigarette smoking.[9]

Both nicotine gum and patches appear to result in similar cessation rates.[57–59] Choice of which agent to use can be made by determining patient preference; whether the patient wears dentures, which precludes the use of nicotine gum; and whether the smoking habit is associated with oral gratification, which may favor the gum. Both agents and their use are described in Display 31-2.

An alternative form of NRT that has not been widely used is the nicotine nasal spray. Widespread use may be prohibited by the common adverse effects of nicotine nasal spray, including headache, burning sensations in the nose or throat, watery eyes, nasal and throat irritation, sneezing, runny nose, cough, and sleep disturbances. These adverse effects usually begin on the first day of use but diminish over time.[60] Nicotine nasal spray, however, may be especially helpful for the highly addicted smoker because of its rapid onset of action.[61] Another alternative to NRT is bupropion (Zyban, Wellbutrin SR [GlaxoWellcome, Research Triangle Park, NC]), an oral medication that comes in tablet form. This pharmacologic aid for smoking cessation has been used for many years to treat depression. The exact mechanism that promotes smoking cessation is unknown. Bupropion does, however, affect levels of dopamine and norepinephrine. It appears to result in cessation rates similar to those with NRT at the completion of the 7- to 12-week treatment period. Long-term follow-up has not been conducted, however. It is contraindicated in patients at high risk for seizure due to previous head trauma, central nervous system tumor, anorexia nervosa, bulimia, previous seizure, or concomitant use with another medication that lowers the seizure threshold. The most common side effects are insomnia and dry mouth.[62]

DISPLAY 31-2

Nicotine Replacement Therapy (NRT)

NICOTINE GUM

Nicotine chewing gum has been available in the United States since 1984, and has been available over the counter since 1997. It comes in 2- and 4-mg doses. It is a resin-based gum that releases nicotine into the bloodstream through the buccal mucosa inside the mouth. The success of nicotine gum is highly dependent on its proper use. It has been shown to be highly ineffective when dispensed without proper chewing instruction. Moreover, when nicotine gum is prescribed without any counseling or strong advice, it has been shown to produce very low cessation rates.[73,74]

The gum should be prescribed immediately after the patient stops smoking. Although nicotine gum was originally prescribed to be taken on an as-needed basis, studies suggest that a regular schedule of taking the gum, normally one piece every 60 minutes during waking hours, ensures constant blood nicotine levels.[75] Side effects are also minimal and transient if the gum is administered properly. Most often, these side effects are limited to local mouth irritation, some gastrointestinal distress such as nausea and heartburn, palpitations, and jaw ache from excessive chewing.

An acidic environment in the mouth blocks nicotine absorption. Because the use of beverages such as colas, coffee, tea, and juices changes the oral pH to an acidic environment, these agents should not be used within 15 minutes of using the gum or during the first 15 minutes of chewing the gum.[76] Because nicotine gum is now available over the counter, it is imperative that teaching be done by the nurse or, alternatively, the patient should be encouraged to discuss proper use with a pharmacist.

Nicotine chewing gum is normally used for a period of 3 to 6 months. A tapering schedule of at least 1 month is recommended. Weaning can be accomplished by decreasing the dosage, cutting gum pieces in half, and substituting sugarless gum for some of the doses. Nurses should also be aware that 8% to 25% of nicotine gum users who successfully quit smoking use the gum beyond the 6 months recommended for maximal use. Habitual use of the gum to deal with negative emotional states is often the cause of this prolonged use.[77]

NICOTINE PATCH

The transdermal nicotine patch is a relatively new pharmacologic aid. Available in the United States by prescription since 1991 and over the counter since 1997, the nicotine patch produces a therapeutic effect by releasing a controlled amount of nicotine through the skin that is absorbed through the capillary bed. Although few studies have been conducted in patients with coronary heart disease, the success of treatment in the general population varies widely, from as high as 71% at 6 weeks[78] after cessation to as low as 18% at 3 weeks after cessation.[79] Higher success rates have been achieved in patients who receive supportive counseling or therapy,[56,78,80–83] but these rates decrease to approximately half of the initial rates 6 to 12 months after beginning treatment.

Nicotine patches ameliorate some aspects of tobacco withdrawal but not all cravings or urges. Some studies have shown that self-reported cravings have been reduced,[58,84] and negative affect and lethargic feelings are decreased.[79] However, the nicotine patch has little effect on body weight or habit-based urges.[79]

The nicotine patch is designed to be worn for a period of 16 to 24 hours depending on the brand, with a recommended dose of 21 mg/24 h, or 15 mg/16 h. Lower doses (10–14 mg) are recommended for the cardiovascular patient. Patches are designed to be changed daily and are normally recommended to be used for 8 weeks, with weaning beginning at 4 weeks. During the weaning period, the dose is reduced in a stepwise manner (i.e., 21, 14, 7 mg) to 7 mg/24 h, or 5 mg/16 h, and finally discontinued.[1]

The most frequent side effect of the nicotine patch is local skin redness, which occurs in approximately 35% to 54% of patients using the patch.[85–88] Severe skin reactions, which include rashes or eczema, have led to discontinuation of therapy in less than 7% of patients.[79,83] Other side effects reported, which occur much less frequently, include gastrointestinal problems of dyspepsia, abdominal pain, and diarrhea; muscle and limb weakness; paresthesia; nervousness; and vivid or disturbing dreams.[80]

Step 5: ARRANGE—Schedule Follow-up Contact

A meta-analysis conducted by Kottke and colleagues[27] concluded that reinforcement by numerous contacts and health care professionals leads to greater smoking cessation rates. Ideally, follow-up contact should occur shortly after the established quit date, preferably within the first week and then again within the first month. Follow-up can be done in person or by telephone. Important components of follow-up include congratulations on success, support, reinforcement, and problem solving. If the patient slipped or relapsed, follow-up provides the opportunity to review the circumstances that led to the slip or relapse, create a new plan to deal with a similar situation in the future, and estab-

lish a new quit date. Follow-up also allows the clinician to review and trouble-shoot any problems associated with the use of NRT. Finally, those patients who do not choose to quit initially may benefit from being reminded about the hazards of continuing to smoke, which may move them into the contemplation or action stage.

SPECIAL AREAS ON WHICH TO FOCUS

Stress

Patients may often relapse to smoking during stressful times, especially those involving emotional circumstances, such as arguments or a crisis situation with a spouse, family members, or coworkers.[63] The frequency and severity of distressing demands during everyday life have also been shown to be predictors of later relapse to smoking in both men and women.[64,65] Although some patients may need in-depth counseling to help them with such problems, simple relaxation training may produce a sense of increased control, which may in turn affect the patient's confidence to withstand the urge to smoke. Many patients can benefit from the use of inexpensive relaxation audiotapes that use simple instructions on how to use muscle tension and deep-breathing exercises to achieve relaxation.

Alcohol Use

Social situations that involve alcohol use are another predictor of relapse to smoking.[63] For this reason, nurses need to determine whether the smoker attempting to quit consumes excessive alcohol regularly. This information can be ascertained while taking a smoking history by using the simple four-item CAGE questionnaire[66] (see Fig. 31-1), which is a screening tool for alcohol abuse. If a diagnosis of alcoholism is made, patients should be encouraged to seek treatment for alcoholism and smoking cessation simultaneously. Patients who are heavy social drinkers should also be encouraged to avoid alcohol or decrease their consumption substantially until they feel successful in their smoking cessation efforts.

Loss

For many patients, giving up smoking is like "losing a best friend." Nurses must help patients to recognize and understand the magnitude of this loss. Helping patients acknowledge how they feel about their loss and working with them to select new activities that provide immediate gratification is important. For example, patients should be encouraged to focus on old, or select new hobbies. They can also develop reward systems for their daily success in remaining nonsmokers. Nurses should also encourage patients to build new activities into their daily schedules that also increase confidence as their focus shifts to new behaviors.

Weight Gain

The average weight gain after smoking cessation is approximately 6 to 10 pounds, much of which is due to metabolic changes that occur with cessation.[67] It appears weight gain is more often associated with those who smoke more cigarettes, have a history of weight problems.[68] In addition, those who quit smoking often crave sweet-tasting foods.[69] Encouraging patients to be more active through daily exercise and helping them to identify low-calorie snacks and sweets can help patients avoid excessive weight gain. Patients must also be aware that the risks of continued smoking far outweigh the risks of gaining a few pounds.

Weight gain cannot be treated lightly because up to 75% of women and 35% of men have reported an unwillingness to gain 5 or more pounds as a result of stopping smoking. In particular, more than half of women younger than 25 years of age and 39% of women older than 40 years stated that they were unwilling to gain any weight.[52] Providers must therefore openly discuss the possibility of weight gain, but stress to the patient that the amount of weight gained is usually limited and that a program of exercise can reduce it to precessation levels, and possibly more.

Social Support

Support from a spouse or family members is directly related to quitting smoking and short-term maintenance of the nonsmoking behavior.[70] If family members or close friends smoke, it is important to initiate a plan to help the patient resist the temptation to smoke when around others who are smoking. It is imperative to prepare the patient for this situation if the family member or friend who smokes lives with the patient. The ideal situation, of course, is when the family member or friend attempts to quit at the same time the patient does. If this is not feasible, the nurse should counsel the family member or friend to (1) not smoke in the presence of the patient if possible, (2) remove all cigarettes and other tobacco products from the household, and (3) refrain from offering cigarettes to the patient who is trying to quit. Family members and friends should also be encouraged to provide daily positive reinforcement for patients successful at quitting. It may also be appropriate for the nurse to teach the patient some basic assertiveness skills, so that the patient is prepared to ask assertively that the family member or friend not smoke in his or her presence, not offer him or her cigarettes, and so forth.

Women

Research has shown that women are less likely to quit smoking than men.[33] Some possible explanations are differences in physiology, and behavioral and psychological factors. For example, the menstrual cycle may play a role in smoking cessation. The symptoms of menstrual distress include depression, irritability, anxiety, tension, decreased ability to concentrate, and weight changes, all of which are also symptoms of nicotine withdrawal. Withdrawal has been shown to be greater when the quit date is set during the luteal phase (ovulation to day before menses) of the menstrual cycle as opposed to the follicular phase (day 1 of menses to day 15). Therefore, it may be valuable to asses the menstrual cycle pattern before setting a quit date to reduce compounding withdrawal with normal menstrual distress.[71] Behavioral and psychological factors that play a large role in smoking cessation for women are fear of weight gain, low social support, reliance on cigarettes for control of negative affect or stress management, and self-efficacy in quitting.[65] These areas must be addressed when implementing a smoking cessation intervention with a woman. As always, it is best to tailor the intervention to the individual patient. Specific benefits of smoking cessation we have found helpful to discuss with women include improved complexion, fewer wrinkles, no odor of cigarettes on their breath or in their hair or clothes, and better health for children and family members. Given the lack of information on characteristics predictive of smoking cessation success in women and the limited number of women-only smoking cessation studies, the information on how specifically to support the female smoker in quitting is limited. The Women's Initiative For Non-Smoking (WINS)[72] study is studying the efficacy of a smoking cessation intervention specifically tailored to women with cardiovascular disease to improve the care of patients in this significantly large and understudied population.

In summary, a systematic approach to smoking cessation leads to better outcomes. The measure of success should be based on the frequency with which the nurse asks about a patient's smoking status. Multicomponent strategies that include strong physician and nurse advice, self-help materials, behavioral counseling, pharmacologic therapy when necessary, and follow-up can be used to help the general population and those with CHD.

PATIENT AND NURSING REFERENCES

Patient Materials

"Calling it Quits" and "An Active Partnership for the Health of your Heart"
American Heart Association
1-800-AHA-USA1 (242-8721)

"I Quit Kit"
American Cancer Society
1599 Clifton Road NE
Atlanta, GA 30026
(or call your local chapter of the American Cancer Society)

"A Lifetime of Freedom from Smoking"
American Lung Association
1740 Broadway
New York, NY 10019
(or call your local chapter of the American Lung Association)

"You Can Quit Smoking"
Agency for Health Care Policy and Research
1-800-358-9295
AHCPR Publication No. 96-0695

Materials for Nurses

"Nurses: Help Your Patients Stop Smoking"
National Heart, Lung, and Blood Institute
Smoking Education Program
P.O. Box 30105
Bethesda, MD 20824-0105
NIH publication no. 92-2962

Smoking Cessation: Information for Specialists
Quick Reference Guide to Clinical Practice Guideline #18
Agency for Health Care Policy and Research
1-800-358-9295
AHCPR publication no. 96-0694

"Helping Smokers Quit"
A Guide for Primary Care Clinicians
Agency for Health Care Policy and Research
1-800-358-9295
AHCPR publication no. 96-0693

REFERENCES

1. Agency for Health Care Policy and Research: U.S. Department of Health and Human Services Clinical Practice Guideline: Smoking Cessation. Publication no. 96-0692. Washington, DC, Government Printing Office, 1996
2. American Heart Association: Heart and Stroke Facts: Statistical Supplement. Dallas, American Heart Association, 1996
3. Britton R, McMahon M, Bryant D: Smoking in hospitalized patients. Addict Behav 16: 79–81, 1991
4. U.S. Department of Health and Human Services: Healthy People 2000: National Health Promotion and Disease Prevention Objectives. Washington, DC, Government Printing Office, 1991
5. U.S. Department of Health and Human Services: The Health Consequences of Smoking: Nicotine Addiction. A Report of the Surgeon General. DHHS Publication no. (CDC) 88-8406. Washington, DC, Government Printing Office, 1988
6. American Psychiatric Association: Diagnostic and Statistical Manual of Mental Disorders, 4th ed. Washington, DC, American Psychiatric Association, 1994
7. U.S. Department of Health and Human Services: Reducing The Health Consequences of Smoking: 25 Years of Progress. A Report of the Surgeon General. DHHS Publication no. (CDC) 89-8411. Washington, DC, Government Printing Office, 1989
8. Benowitz N, Gourlay S: Cardiovascular toxicity of nicotine: Implications for nicotine replacement therapy. J Am Coll Cardiol 29: 1422–1431, 1997
9. Stillman FA: Smoking cessation for the hospitalized cardiac patient: Rationale for and report of a model program. J Cardiovasc Nurs 9: 25–36, 1995
10. U.S. Department of Health and Human Services: The Health Consequences of Smoking: Cardiovascular Disease. A Report of the Surgeon General. Washington, DC, Government Printing Office, 1983
11. Quillen JE, Rossen JD, Oskarsson HJ et al: Acute effect of cigarette smoking on the coronary circulation: Constriction of epicardial and resistance vessels. J Am Coll Cardiol 22: 642–647, 1993
12. Barry J, Mead K, Nabel E et al: Effect of smoking on the activity of ischemic heart disease. JAMA 261: 398–402, 1989
13. Samet J: Health benefits of smoking cessation. Clin Chest Med 12: 669–679, 1991
14. Sparrow D, Dawber T, Colton T: The influence of cigarette smoking on prognosis after a first myocardial infarction. Journal of Chronic Disease 31: 425–432, 1978
15. Wilhelmsson L, Elmfeldt D, Vedin JA et al: Smoking and myocardial infarction. Lancet 1: 415–420, 1975
16. Hermanson B, Omenn G, Krommel R et al: Beneficial six-year outcome of smoking cessation in older men and women with coronary artery disease: Results from the CASS registry. N Engl J Med 319: 1365–1368, 1988
17. DiClemente C, Prochaska J, Fairhurst et al: The process of smoking cessation: An analysis of precontemplation, contemplation, and preparation stages of change. J Consult Clin Psychol 59: 295–304, 1991
18. Velicer W, Fava J, Prochaska et al: Distribution of smokers by stage in three representative samples. Prev Med 24: 401–411, 1995
19. Prochaska J, DiClemente C: Stages and processes of self-change of smoking: Toward an integrative model of change. J Consult Clin Psychol 51: 390–395, 1983

20. Dijkstra A, DeVries H, Bakker M: Pros and cons of quitting, self-efficacy, and the stages of change in smoking cessation. J Consult Clin Psychol 64: 758–763, 1996

21. King T, Marcus B, Pinto B et al: Cognitive-behavioral mediators of changing multiple behaviors: Smoking and a sedentary lifestyle. Prev Med 25: 684–691, 1996

22. Prochaska JO, Velicer WF, Rossi JS et al: Stages of change and decisional balance for 12 problem behaviors. Health Psychol 13: 39–46, 1994

23. Burling TA, Singleton EG, Bigelow GE et al: Smoking following myocardial infarction: A critical review of the literature. Health Psychol 3: 83–96, 1984

24. Pozen MW, Stockmuller JA, Harris W et al: A nurse rehabilitator's impact on patients with myocardial infarction. Med Care 15: 830–836, 1977

25. Burt A, Thornley R, Illingworth D et al: Stopping smoking after myocardial infarction. Lancet 1: 304–306, 1974

26. Taylor CB, Miller NH, Killen JD et al: Smoking cessation after myocardial infarction: Effects of a nurse-managed intervention. Ann Int Med 113: 118–123, 1990

27. Kottke TE, Battista RN, DeFriese GH et al: Attributes of successful smoking cessation interventions in medical practice: A meta-analysis of 39 controlled trials. JAMA 259: 2883–2998, 1988

28. Schwartz JL: Review and evaluation of smoking cessation methods: The United States and Canada, 1978–1985. DHHS publication No. (NIH) 87-2940. Washington, DC, Department of Health and Human Services, Public Health Service, 1987

29. Mulcahy R: Influence of cigarette smoking on morbidity and mortality after myocardial infarction. Br Heart J 49: 410–415, 1983

30. Baile NF, Bigelow GE, Gottlieb SH et al: Rapid resumption of cigarette smoking following myocardial infarction: Inverse relation to myocardial infarction severity. Addict Behav 7: 373–380, 1982

31. Crouse J, Hagaman A: Smoking cessation in relation to cardiac procedures. Am J Prev Med 7: 131–135, 1991

32. Rigotti NA, McKool KM, Shiffman S: Predictors of smoking cessation after coronary bypass graft surgery: Results of a randomized trial with 5-year follow-up. Ann Intern Med 120: 287–293, 1994

33. Ockene J, Kristeller J, Goldberg R et al: Smoking cessation and severity of disease: The coronary artery smoking intervention study. Health Psychol 11: 119–126, 1992

34. Havik OE, Maeland JG: Changes in smoking behavior after a myocardial infarction. Health Psychol 7: 403, 1988

35. Scott RR, Lamparski D: Variables related to long-term smoking status following cardiac events. Addict Behav 10: 257–264, 1985

36. Stanislaw AE, Wewers ME: A smoking cessation intervention with hospitalized surgical cancer patients: A pilot study. Cancer Nurs 17: 81–86, 1993

37. Miller NH, Smith PM, DeBusk RF et al: Smoking cessation in hospitalized patients: Results of a randomized trial. Arch Intern Med 157: 409–415, 1997

38. Miller NH, Smith PM, DeBusk RF et al: Smoking cessation in hospitalized patients: Results of a randomized trial. Arch Intern Med 157: 409–415, 1997

39. Glasgow RE, Stevens VJ, Vogt TM et al: Changes in smoking associated with hospitalization: Quit rates, predictive variables, and intervention implications. American Journal of Health Promotion 6(1): 24–29, 1991

40. Ockene JK, Hosmer D, Rippe J et al: Factors affecting cigarette smoking status in patients with ischemic heart disease. Journal of Chronic Disease 38: 985–994, 1985

41. Krumholz HM, Cohen BJ, Tsevat J et al: Cost-effectiveness of a smoking cessation program after myocardial infarction. J Am Coll Cardiol 22: 1697–1702, 1993

42. Fiore MC, Novotny TF, Pierce JP et al: Methods used to quit smoking in the United States: Do cessation programs help? JAMA 263: 2760–2765, 1990

43. Emmons KM, Goldstein MG: Smokers who are hospitalized: A window of opportunity for cessation interventions. Prev Med 21: 262–269, 1992

44. Pechacek TF: Modification of smoking behavior. In Smoking and Health: A Report of the Surgeon General. Washington, DC, Government Printing Office, 1984

45. Frank E, Winkleby MA, Altman DG et al: Predictors of physician's smoking cessation advice. JAMA 266: 3139–3144, 1991

46. Kviz F, Clark M, Prohaska T et al: Attitudes and practices for smoking cessation counseling by provider type and patient age. Prev Med 24: 201–212, 1995

47. Goldstein AO, Hellier A, Fitzgerald S et al: Hospital nurse counseling of patients who smoke. Am J Public Health 77: 1333–1334, 1987

48. Faulkner A, Ward L: Nurses as health educators in relation to smoking. Nursing Times 79(8): 47–48, 1983

49. Taylor CB, Houston Miller N, Flora J: Principles of health behavior change. In Resource Manual for Guidelines for Exercise Testing and Prescription, pp 323–328. Philadelphia, Lea & Febiger, 1988

50. Marlatt AG: Relapse prevention: A self control program for the treatment of addictive behaviors. In Stuart RB (ed): Adherence, Compliance and Generalization in Behavioral Medicine, pp 329–378. New York, Brunnel/Mazel, 1982

51. Condiotte MM, Lichtenstein E: Self-efficacy and relapse in smoking cessation programs. J Consult Clin Psychol 49: 648–658, 1981

52. Tsoh JY, McClure JB, Skaar KL et al: Smoking cessation 2: Components of effective intervention. Behav Med 23: 15–27, 1997

53. Taylor CB, Miller NH, Haskell WL et al: Smoking cessation after acute myocardial infarction: The effects of exercise training. Addict Behav 13: 331–335, 1988

54. Fagerstrom KO: Measuring degree of physical dependence to tobacco smoking with reference to individualization of treatment. Addict Behav 3: 235–241, 1978

55. Benowitz NL: Pharmacological aspects of cigarette smoking and nicotine addiction. N Engl J Med 319: 1318–1329, 1988

56. Rennard S, Draughton D, Fortman SP et al: Transdermal nicotine enhances smoking cessation in coronary artery disease patients (Abstract). Chest 100: 5S, 1991

57. Lam W, Sze PC, Sacks HS et al: Meta-analysis of randomized controlled trials of nicotine chewing gum. Lancet 2: 27–30, 1987

58. Abelin T, Buehler A, Miller P et al: Controlled trial of transdermal nicotine patch in tobacco withdrawal. Lancet 1: 7–10, 1989

59. Tönneson P, Fryd V, Hansen M, et al: Effect of nicotine chewing gum in combination with group counseling and the cessation of smoking. N Engl J Med 318: 15–18, 1988

60. Hurt RD, Lowell CD, Croghan GA et al: Nicotine nasal spray for smoking cessation: Patterns of use, side effects, relief of withdrawal symptoms, and cotinine levels. Mayo Clin Proc 73: 118–125, 1998

61. Schneider NG, Lunell E, Olmstead RE, Fagerstrom KO: Clinical pharmacokinetics of nasal nicotine delivery. Clin Pharmacokinet 31: 65–80, 1996

62. The Medical Letter: Bupropion (Zyban) for smoking cessation. Medical Letter 39: 77–80, 1997

63. Shiffman S: A cluster-analytic classification of relapse episodes. Addict Behav 11: 295–307, 1986

64. Romano PS, Bloom J, Syme SL: Smoking, social support, and hassles in an urban African American community. Am J Public Health 81: 1415–1422, 1991

65. Gritz ER, Nielsen IR, Brooks LA: Smoking cessation and gender: The influence of physiological, psychological, and behavioral factors. Journal of the American Medical Women's Association 51: 35–42, 1996

66. Ewing JA: Detecting alcoholism: The CAGE questionnaire. JAMA 252: 1905–1907, 1984

67. Wack JT, Rodin J: Smoking and its effects on body weight and systems of caloric regulation. Am J Clin Nutr 35: 366–380, 1982

68. Hall SM, Ginsburg D, Jones RT: Smoking cessation and weight gain. J Consult Clin Psychol 54: 342–346, 1986

69. Grunberg NE: The effects of nicotine and cigarette smoking on food consumption and taste preferences. Addict Behav 7: 317–331, 1982

70. Cohen S, Lichtenstein E, Mermelstein R et al: Social support interventions for smoking cessation. In BH Gottlieb (ed): Marshaling Social Support: Formats, Processes, and Effects, pp 211–240. Newbury Park, CA, Sage, 1988

71. O'Hara P, Portser SA, Anderson BP: The influence of menstrual cycle changes on the tobacco withdrawal syndrome in women. Addict Behav 14: 595–600, 1989

72. Women's Initiative for Non-Smoking (WINS) NIH-NHLBI RO1-HL50749-01A3

73. Cummings SR, Hansen B, Richard RJ et al: Internists and nicotine gum. JAMA 260: 1565–1569, 1988

74. Sachs DL: Nicotine polacrilex: Practical use requirements. Current Pulmonology 10: 141–158, 1989

75. Killen JD, Fortmann SP, Newman B et al: Evaluation of a treatment approach combining nicotine gum and self-guided treatment for smoking relapse prevention. J Consult Clin Psychol 58: 85–92, 1990

76. Henningfield JE, Radizius A, Cooper TM, Clayton RR: Drinking coffee and carbonated beverages blocks absorption of nicotine from nicotine polacrilex gum. JAMA 264: 1560–1564, 1990

77. Hajek P, Jackson P, Belcher M: Long term use of nicotine chewing gum. JAMA 260: 1593–1596, 1988

78. Hurt RD, Lauger GG, Offord KP et al: Nicotine replacement therapy with the use of a transdermal nicotine patch: A randomized double-blind placebo-controlled trial. Mayo Clin Proc 65: 1529–1537, 1990

79. Rose JE, Levin ED, Behm FM et al: Transdermal nicotine facilitates smoking cessation. Clin Pharmacol Ther 47: 323–330, 1990

80. Transdermal Nicotine Study Group: Transdermal nicotine for smoking cessation: Six-month results from two multicenter controlled clinical trials. JAMA 266: 3133–3138, 1991

81. Krumpe P, Malani N, Adler J et al: Effects of transdermal nicotine administration as an adjunct for smoking cessation in heavily addicted smokers (Abstract). American Review of Respiratory Diseases 139: 337, 1989

82. Mulligan SC, Masterson JG, Devane JG et al: Clinical and pharmacokinetics of transdermal nicotine patch. Clin Pharmacol Ther 47: 331–337, 1990

83. Draughton DM, Heatley SA, Prendergast JJ et al: Effect of transdermal nicotine delivery as an adjunct to low intervention smoking cessation therapy. Arch Intern Med 151: 749–752, 1991

84. Tönnesen P, Nörregaard J, Simonsen K et al: A double blind trial of a 16 hour transdermal nicotine patch in smoking cessation. N Engl J Med 325: 311–315, 1991

85. Ciba-Geigy Corporation: Habitrol (nicotine transdermal therapeutic system) prescribing information. Edison, NJ, Ciba-Geigy, 1992

86. Marion Merrell Dow, Inc: Nicoderm (nicotine transdermal system) prescribing information. Kansas City, MO, Marion Merrell Dow, Inc., 1991

87. Lederele Laboratories: PROSTEP (nicotine transdermal system) prescribing information. Wayne, NJ, Lederele Laboratories, 1992

88. Parke-Davis: Nicotrol (nicotine transdermal system) prescribing information. Morris Plains, NJ, Parke-Davis, 1992

32

High Blood Pressure

SUSANNA CUNNINGHAM

High blood pressure (BP) is the most common risk factor for cardiovascular disease in developed and developing countries. Since the late 1960s, in Europe and the United States, there has been a dramatic decline in the mortality rate from hypertensive heart disease, primarily due to the development of several classes of antihypertensive drugs. At least 43 million Americans have hypertension, and an additional large number have BPs at the upper level of the normal range, which puts them at greater risk for development of hypertension than people with lower BPs.

High BP is also known as *hypertension*. The National High Blood Pressure Program since its inception in 1972 has intentionally used the phrase *high blood pressure* instead of the word *hypertension*. This choice was made because of the misconceptions that occur when the word *hypertension* is used. People think that because they are neither "tense" nor "hyper" that they will be unlikely to have hypertension. Among health care professionals, it is useful to use the word *hypertension,* but it is important to remember that because this word can be confusing, *high blood pressure* is a better term to use when communicating with the public.

High BP can be considered as a sign, a risk factor, and a disease. Because BP is a continuous variable, one of the challenging aspects is deciding the boundaries between normal and abnormal for the two components of BP: systolic and diastolic BP.

DATABASE FOR MANAGEMENT

Definitions

One problem with setting specific definitions of normal and high BP is that systolic and diastolic BPs are both continuous variables. In addition, elevations of either systolic or diastolic pressure increase a person's risk of having a clinical event. Because some of the early clinical trials investigating the efficacy of drug treatment of hypertension used diastolic BP as their main outcome variable, the myth has arisen that elevations in diastolic BP are more serious than elevations in systolic pressure.[254, 255] The truth is that elevations in either diastolic or systolic pressure are associated with increased risk. The greater the elevation, the greater the risk. Con-

versely, it is generally true that the lower the pressures, the lower the risk of morbidity and mortality, except in the relatively uncommon situations of sympathetic nervous system dysfunction or hypovolemia. The risks associated with elevations in systolic BP have been documented in the White-hall Study as well as among the approximately 360,000 men screened for the Multiple Risk Factor Intervention Study.[148,236]

ADULTS

As new research has become available, many countries have established guidelines on the detection, evaluation, and treatment of high BP.[241] The two best known guidelines defining normal and elevated BP levels were developed by The Joint National Committee of the National High Blood Pressure Education Program (JNC), and the Guidelines Subcommittee of the World Health Organization and the International Society of Hypertension (WHO/ISH). Since 1977, the JNCs have produced six reports, the most recent in 1997 (JNC VI).[243] The most recent set of WHO/ISH guidelines was issued in 1999.[87] These committees agree that a systolic BP of greater than 140 mm Hg and a diastolic BP greater than 90 mm Hg should be defined as hypertensive, and use identical terminology for all levels of BP. Both reports agree that BP should be considered together with other risk factors for atherosclerotic cardiovascular disease when making decisions about when to initiate treatment.

To reflect the curvilinear nature of the relationship between systolic and diastolic BP and risk, JNC VI has defined three levels of BP within a "normal" range and three stages of hypertension, as shown in Table 32-1.[243] The three levels of normal pressure are optimal, normal, and high-normal. These terms were chosen to communicate the increasing risk associated with increasing pressures even though the pressures have not risen to a level that would be considered hypertensive. Above the level of 140/90 mm Hg, there are three stages of hypertension, with defined ranges for systolic and diastolic pressures. The JNC has chosen to use *stages* rather than the previously used terms of *mild, moderate,* and *severe* because they hoped to convey the seriousness of BP elevations by using terminology mirroring

TABLE 32-1	Classification of Blood Pressure for Adults Age 18 Years and Older*		
Category	**Systolic (mm Hg)**		**Diastolic (mm Hg)**
Optimal†	<120	and	<80
Normal	<130	and	<85
High normal	130–139	or	85–89
Hypertension‡			
Stage 1	140–159	or	90–99
Stage 2	160–179	or	100–109
Stage 3	≥180	or	≥110

*Not taking antihypertensive drugs and not acutely ill. When systolic and diastolic blood pressures fall into different categories, the higher category should be selected to classify the person's blood pressure status. For example, 160/92 mm Hg should be classified as stage 2 hypertension, and 174/120 mm Hg should be classified as stage 3 hypertension. Isolated systolic hypertension is defined as SBP of 140 mm Hg or greater and diastolic blood pressure below 90 mm Hg and staged appropriately (e.g., 170/82 mm Hg is defined as stage 2 isolated systolic hypertension). In addition to classifying stages of hypertension on the basis of average blood pressure levels, clinicians should specify presence or absence of target organ disease and additional risk factors. This specificity is important for risk classification and treatment.

†Optimal blood pressure with respect to cardiovascular risk is below 120/80 mm Hg. However, unusually low readings should be evaluated for clinical significance.

‡Based on the average of two or more readings taken at each of two or more visits after an initial screening.

that used in other chronic diseases such as cancer. Isolated systolic hypertension is defined as the occurrence of a systolic BP greater than 140 mm Hg with a diastolic pressure less than 90 mm Hg. The incidence of isolated systolic hypertension increases with age and thus is predominantly a problem of the elderly.[180]

Previous classifications of high BP such as labile, benign, or malignant (accelerated) were confusing and often misleading.[136] The term *benign* has a false association with lower morbidity, and "malignant" hypertension, often reversible with proper treatment, is not always fatal. The development of the JNC and WHO/ISH classification schemes as well as advances in the detection and treatment of high BP have made most of these terms obsolete. Types of high BP are classified as (1) systolic and diastolic hypertension (either primary or secondary) and (2) isolated systolic hypertension caused by increased cardiac output or increasing rigidity of the aorta.

CHILDREN

Criteria used for categorizing BP in adults are not applicable to children. The level of BP considered normal increases gradually from infancy to adulthood. Systolic and diastolic BP levels correlate with height and weight, as well as age.[258] BP for children is considered normal if it is less than the 90th percentile for age, sex, and height.[182] High-normal BP refers to that pressure, measured on at least three occasions, that falls between the 90th and 95th percentiles for age, height, and sex. Tables 32-2 and 32-3 show the current BP levels for the 90th and 95th percentiles for boys and girls. Hypertension is defined as systolic or diastolic BP, or both, above the 95th percentile for age, height, and sex. Data from the longitudinal Bogalusa Heart Study indicate that in children (up to age 13 years), the fourth Korotkoff sound may be a more reliable predictor of the risk of development of hypertension in adulthood than the fifth Korotkoff sound.[60]

Epidemiology

INCIDENCE AND PREVALENCE OF HIGH BLOOD PRESSURE

Based on the results of the third National Health and Nutrition Examination Survey conducted in the United States between 1988 and 1991, it is estimated that approximately 24%, or just over 43 million Americans have hypertension.[29] For the survey, a person was considered to be hypertensive if the measured BP was 140/90 mm Hg or more, or if the person reported taking antihypertensive medications. Other sources have estimated the prevalence to be closer to 50 million.[7] Overall, 69% of the people who were found to have an elevated BP were aware of their condition, and 53% were taking medications to control their blood pressure. Of those taking medications, only 45% had their BPs under control, which was defined as having a BP less than 140/90 mm Hg.[29] Using the BP categories from JNC VI, it was estimated that 47% of Americans had an optimal BP level, 21% a normal level, and 13% a high-normal level, whereas 14% had stage 1 hypertension, 4% stage 2, and 1% stage 3 (see Table 32-1 for definitions of each category). In Americans between 30 and 69 years of age, the incidence of high BP has been estimated to be 1.8 million cases per year.[196]

AGE, WEIGHT, AND SEX

The evidence suggests that hypertension begins in childhood, perhaps even *in utero*.[143, 228] Because hypertension in children is defined as a pressure greater than the 95th percentile for a child of any given age and height, the initial incidence of hypertension in children is automatically 5%. However, because the recommendations suggest that before a child is diagnosed as having high BP the measurement should be repeated for a total of three consecutive examinations, the true incidence is usually found to be lower.[182] In a study of junior high school students it was found that, even by the second examination, the prevalence of persistent ele-

TABLE 32-2	Blood Pressure Levels for the 90th and 95th Percentiles of Blood Pressure for Boys Aged 1 to 17 Years by Percentiles of Height[182]

Age (y)	Blood Pressure Percentile*	Systolic Blood Pressure by Percentile of Height† (mm Hg)							Diastolic Blood Pressure by Percentile of Height† (mm Hg)						
		5%	10%	25%	50%	75%	90%	95%	5%	10%	25%	50%	75%	90%	95%
1	90th	94	95	97	98	100	102	102	50	51	52	53	54	54	55
	95th	98	99	101	102	104	106	106	55	55	56	57	58	59	59
2	90th	98	99	100	102	104	105	106	55	55	56	57	58	59	59
	95th	101	102	104	106	108	109	110	59	59	60	61	62	63	63
3	90th	100	101	103	105	107	108	109	59	59	60	61	62	63	63
	95th	104	105	107	109	111	112	113	63	63	64	65	66	67	67
4	90th	102	103	105	107	109	110	111	62	62	63	64	65	66	66
	95th	106	107	109	111	113	114	115	66	67	67	68	69	70	71
5	90th	104	105	106	108	110	112	112	65	65	66	67	68	69	69
	95th	108	109	110	112	114	115	116	69	70	70	71	72	73	74
6	90th	105	106	108	110	111	113	114	67	68	69	70	70	71	72
	95th	109	110	112	114	115	117	117	72	72	73	74	75	76	76
7	90th	106	107	109	111	113	114	115	69	70	71	72	72	73	74
	95th	110	111	113	115	116	118	119	74	74	75	76	77	78	78
8	90th	107	108	110	112	114	115	116	71	71	72	73	74	75	75
	95th	111	112	114	116	118	119	120	75	76	76	77	78	79	80
9	90th	109	110	112	113	115	117	117	72	73	73	74	75	76	77
	95th	113	114	116	117	119	121	121	76	77	78	79	80	80	81
10	90th	110	112	113	115	117	118	119	73	74	74	75	76	77	78
	95th	114	115	117	119	121	122	123	77	78	79	80	80	81	82
11	90th	112	113	115	117	119	120	121	74	74	75	76	77	78	78
	95th	116	117	119	121	123	124	125	78	79	79	80	81	82	83
12	90th	115	116	117	119	121	123	123	75	75	76	77	78	78	79
	95th	119	120	121	123	125	126	127	79	79	80	81	82	83	83
13	90th	117	118	120	122	124	125	126	75	76	76	77	78	79	80
	95th	121	122	124	126	128	129	130	79	80	81	82	83	83	84
14	90th	120	121	123	125	126	128	128	76	76	77	78	79	80	80
	95th	124	125	127	128	130	132	132	80	81	81	82	83	84	85
15	90th	123	124	125	127	129	131	131	77	77	78	79	80	81	81
	95th	127	128	129	131	133	134	135	81	82	83	83	84	85	86
16	90th	125	126	128	130	132	133	134	79	79	80	81	82	82	83
	95th	129	130	132	134	136	137	138	83	83	84	85	86	87	87
17	90th	128	129	131	133	134	136	136	81	81	82	83	84	85	85
	95th	132	133	135	136	138	140	140	85	85	86	87	88	89	89

*Blood pressure percentile was determined by a single measurement.
†Height percentile was determined by standard growth curves.

vations in pressure was approximately 1%.[229] Both height and weight directly influence children's BPs. It has been found that after infancy, people whose birth weight was lower had higher systolic BPs up to age 70 years.[143]

Normally, BP increases in children at a rate of between 1 and 4 mm Hg per year for both systolic and diastolic BP, and then levels off after 18 to 20 years of age. Children whose BP consistently falls above the 95th percentile for height, sex, and age are at risk for development of sustained hypertension and should be evaluated and possibly treated.[182]

In adults, BP tends to increase with age.[29, 45, 115] Overall, men have a higher prevalence of hypertension than women. The age-adjusted incidence for men is 25.9%, and for women, 22.2%. When examined by decade, however, men have more hypertension than women up to the seventh decade, from which point on there is a greater prevalence in women.[29] JNC VI states that preventing the increase in BP that usually occurs with age is one of the public health challenges of the new millennium.[243]

Data from the Framingham Heart Study and other epidemiologic studies have shown that as body weight

TABLE 32-3 — Blood Pressure Levels for the 90th and 95th Percentiles of Blood Pressure for Girls Aged 1 to 17 Years by Percentiles of Height

Age (y)	Blood Pressure Percentile*	Systolic Blood Pressure by Percentile of Height† (mm Hg)							Diastolic Blood Pressure by Percentile of Height† (mm Hg)						
		5%	10%	25%	50%	75%	90%	95%	5%	10%	25%	50%	75%	90%	95%
1	90th	97	98	99	100	102	103	104	53	53	53	54	55	56	56
	95th	101	102	103	104	105	107	107	57	57	57	58	59	60	60
2	90th	99	99	100	102	103	104	105	57	57	58	58	59	60	61
	95th	102	103	104	105	107	108	109	61	61	62	62	63	64	65
3	90th	100	100	102	103	104	105	106	61	61	61	62	63	63	64
	95th	104	104	105	107	108	109	110	65	65	65	66	67	67	68
4	90th	101	102	103	104	106	107	108	63	63	64	65	65	66	67
	95th	105	106	107	108	109	111	111	67	67	68	69	69	70	71
5	90th	103	103	104	106	107	108	109	65	66	66	67	68	68	69
	95th	107	107	108	110	111	112	113	69	70	70	71	72	72	73
6	90th	104	105	106	107	109	110	111	67	67	68	69	69	70	71
	95th	108	109	110	111	112	114	114	71	71	72	73	73	74	75
7	90th	106	107	108	109	110	112	112	69	69	69	70	71	72	72
	95th	110	110	112	113	114	115	116	73	73	73	74	75	76	76
8	90th	108	109	110	111	112	113	114	70	70	71	71	72	73	74
	95th	112	112	113	115	116	117	118	74	74	75	75	76	77	78
9	90th	110	110	112	113	114	115	116	71	72	72	73	74	74	75
	95th	114	114	115	117	118	119	120	75	76	76	77	78	78	79
10	90th	112	112	114	115	116	117	118	73	73	73	74	75	76	76
	95th	116	116	117	119	120	121	122	77	77	77	78	79	80	80
11	90th	114	114	116	117	118	119	120	74	74	75	75	76	77	77
	95th	118	118	119	121	122	123	124	78	78	79	79	80	81	81
12	90th	116	116	118	119	120	121	122	75	75	76	76	77	78	78
	95th	120	120	121	123	124	125	126	79	79	80	80	81	82	82
13	90th	118	118	119	121	122	123	124	76	76	77	78	78	79	80
	95th	121	122	123	125	126	127	128	80	80	81	82	82	83	84
14	90th	119	120	121	122	124	125	126	77	77	78	79	79	80	81
	95th	123	124	125	126	128	129	130	81	81	82	83	83	84	85
15	90th	121	121	122	124	125	126	127	78	78	79	79	80	81	82
	95th	124	125	126	128	129	130	131	82	82	83	83	84	85	86
16	90th	122	122	123	125	126	127	128	79	79	79	80	81	82	82
	95th	125	126	127	128	130	131	132	83	83	83	84	85	86	86
17	90th	122	123	124	125	126	128	128	79	79	79	80	81	82	82
	95th	126	126	127	129	130	131	132	83	83	83	84	85	86	86

*Blood pressure percentile was determined by a single reading.
†Height percentile was determined by standard growth curves.

increases, so does systolic and diastolic BP in both adults and children.[78,115,123,182] It has been estimated that in people who are obese, the prevalence of hypertension is approximately 50%.[140] This relationship between weight and BP is thought to be one of the reasons that BP increases with age.

FAMILY HISTORY AND GENETIC FACTORS

Family history of hypertension has been used as an indicator of the influence of genetics on the epidemiology of hypertension. With progress on the human genome project, it is possible that we may be able to predict risk with more precision, although expense and issues of privacy must also be considered. Depending on how a positive family history of hypertension is defined, a person with a positive history has a relative risk of development of hypertension of between 2.4 and 5.0.[104] The risks are greater the more family members there are who have high BP, and if these family members were diagnosed as hypertensive before age 55. The risk associated with a positive family history is slightly greater for women than for men. The influence of family history is seen in children as well as adults.[222]

ETHNIC AND GEOGRAPHIC DIFFERENCES

Data from the third National Health and Nutrition Examination Survey show that for almost every age group, non-Hispanic black men and women have higher crude and age-adjusted prevalence rates of high BP than non-Hispanic white and Mexican-American men and women.[29] The same analysis also found that non-Hispanic black men and women have the highest systolic and diastolic BPs in almost all age groups.

Geographic differences in the prevalence of high BP have been described for different parts of the world as well as in the United States. Worldwide, the prevalence of hypertension is lowest in rural Africa and southern China and highest in Finland, Russia, and parts of the United States.[35] In the United States, a group of states in the southeast has been designated as "the stroke belt" because of the high incidence of hypertension and strokes.[91,137] It is not clear whether these geographic variations are due to any genetic or environmental factors. The stroke belt is also an area with dietary, physical activity, low–birth-weight, and obesity patterns that may account for most or all of the excess prevalence of hypertension.[91]

INCOME AND EDUCATION

An inverse relationship between socioeconomic status, including educational level and income, and prevalence of high BP has been documented in many studies.[47,99,107,237] The impact of socioeconomic status on BP is thought to be related to both social and financial barriers to health care and to the more frequent adoption of low-risk lifestyles by those of higher socioeconomic lifesyles.[112]

Hemodynamics of High Blood Pressure

Blood pressure is the product of the amount of blood pumped by the heart each minute (cardiac output) and the degree of dilation or constriction of the arterioles (systemic vascular resistance). Arterial BP is controlled over short periods by the arterial baroreceptors that sense pressure changes in the major arteries, and then through neurohumoral feedback mechanisms that vary heart rate, myocardial contractility, and vascular smooth muscle contraction to maintain the BP within normal limits. Over longer periods (hours to days), neurohumoral and direct renal regulation of vascular volume also play an important role in maintaining a normal BP. Baroreceptors in the low-pressure components of the cardiovascular system, such as the veins, atria, and pulmonary circulation, play a role in the neurohumoral regulation of vascular volume.

For a person to have hypertension, there must be an increase in cardiac output or systemic vascular resistance.[113,155] It may be that either one is elevated or that both are elevated. Because BP can be measured relatively easily and because it is not easy to measure cardiac output or systemic vascular resistance, we identify dysfunction of these variables as disorders of BP regulation. As discussions in several chapters of this text reveal, each of these variables, cardiac output and systemic vascular resistance, are themselves influenced by many factors. Given all the factors that can influence it, BP needs to be considered as an extremely complex variable.

Two investigators, Stevo Julius[113] and Per Lund-Johansen,[155] are known for their studies of the hemodynamics of hypertension. In a longitudinal prospective study of a relatively small group of hypertensive men, Lund-Johansen[156] found variability in hemodynamics. In the younger men, hypertension was due to an increase in either cardiac output or systemic vascular resistance. Over 20 years of follow-up, he found that all subjects who were hypertensive at baseline, regardless of their initial hemodynamic pattern, acquired an increase in systemic vascular resistance plus a decrease in cardiac index and stroke index. Even subjects whose BP had been controlled with medications showed a significant increase in resistance. Similarly, Julius[113] found that most people with borderline hypertension had an elevated cardiac output. Over time, the hypertension remained but transitioned from a high cardiac output state to a state of elevated total peripheral resistance. Therefore, the data indicate that initially an elevated pressure may be secondary to either an elevated cardiac output or systemic vascular resistance—or to elevations in both. In long-established hypertension, the usual hemodynamic finding is an elevated systemic vascular resistance.

Etiology

Despite years of research and countless publications, the underlying cause of most cases of high BP is unknown. To distinguish between hypertension with a known cause and that whose cause is unknown, the terminology of *primary* and *secondary* hypertension or high BP is used. *Primary* or *idiopathic high BP* is the term used to indicate those cases of hypertension for which no cause can be identified. Approximately 90% to 95% of cases of hypertension fall in this category.[44,230] The term *secondary hypertension* describes the 5% to 10% of cases of high BP for which a cause can be identified.

PRIMARY HIGH BLOOD PRESSURE

Medical professionals originally thought that if no cause for a person's hypertension could be determined, a higher BP must be necessary, or "essential" for getting blood through narrowed arteries and arterioles. It was thought that any attempt to lower that pressure would result in inadequate tissue perfusion. It has subsequently been demonstrated that this hypothesis was in error; lowering BP does reduce morbidity and mortality rates, even in the elderly.[9,105,215,254,255]

The cause or causes of primary hypertension remain in question. BP is a complex variable involving mechanisms that influence cardiac output, systemic vascular resistance, and blood volume. Hypertension is caused by one or several abnormalities in the function of these mechanisms or the failure of other factors to compensate for these malfunctioning mechanisms. The current revolution in genetics and molecular biology has begun to shed light on some causes of high BP and to raise the hope that the more complex polygenic and environmental interactions that contribute to high BP will soon be understood.[149,261]

A genetic predisposition; environmental factors such as stress, obesity, and excess sodium (Na^+) intake; and sympathetic nervous system dysfunction may all contribute to high BP. Several explanations regarding the etiology of primary hypertension are being investigated. These explanations are not mutually exclusive, and it is likely that the eventual understanding of hypertension's etiology will involve the integration of more than one of these hypotheses. Some of the hypotheses include:

1. *Dysfunction of the autonomic nervous system*—Autonomic nervous system imbalance may be due to inheritance of genes related to an exaggerated defense reaction resulting in increased sympathetic nervous system output.[6]
2. *Genetic variations in renal sodium reabsorption*—Identification of several genes involved in rare inherited forms of hypertension support the hypothesis that primary hypertension may be related to mutations in several genes that increase a person's susceptibility to disorders of renal reabsorption of sodium, chloride, and water.[149]
3. *Dysfunction of the renin–angiotensin–aldosterone (RAA) system*—Increased RAA system activity results in elevated extracellular fluid volume expansion and systemic vascular resistance. Family studies have identified variations in the gene coding for angiotensinogen as having a role in the development of high BP.[110]
4. *Impaired vascular responsiveness*—Research has revealed impairments in vascular dilation and increased vascular contraction related to the function of the endothelium in people with hypertension. It is not clear whether these changes in vascular reactivity and endothelial function precede or follow the onset of high BP.[66,73,98,133]
5. *Insulin resistance as a causative factor in hypertension*—Hypertension and diabetes frequently occur together. It has been hypothesized that insulin resistance may be a common factor that links hypertension, type II diabetes, and other metabolic abnormalities.[65,74,175,210] This clustering of cardiovascular risk factors has been called syndrome X, insulin resistance syndrome, and "the deadly quartet." The term *quartet* refers to the clustering of upper body obesity, glucose intolerance, hypertriglyceridemia, and hypertension.[119]

SECONDARY HIGH BLOOD PRESSURE

Although secondary hypertension affects less than 10% of all hypertensive adults, most of the hypertension that occurs in children younger than 10 years of age is secondary to a specific physiologic condition.[228] In children younger than 10 years, the most common causes of persistent hypertension are renal disease and vascular problems such as coarctation of the aorta. In adults, chronic renal disease, renovascular disease, primary aldosteronism, and use of oral contraceptives are the most common causes of secondary high BP.[44,230] In one study of 3,783 people referred to a specialty hypertension clinic in Scotland, these causes of secondary hypertension accounted for 7.8% of all cases of high BP, with all other secondary causes accounting for only 0.1%.[230] Display 32-1 summarizes many of the secondary causes of hypertension in children and adults. The newest additions to this list are the relatively rare, but fascinating, genetic mutations that cause hypertension.[149]

Chronic Renal Disease. The relationship between the kidneys and hypertension is circular: chronic renal disease causes hypertension and hypertension contributes to the development of chronic renal disease. Chronic renal disease causes between 2.5% and 5.6% of all hypertension and is the most common type of primary high BP.[44,230] In chronic renal disease, there are three major factors that contribute to the development of high BP: loss of nephrons leading to retention of sodium, chloride, and water; decreased release of vasodilator substances such as nitric oxide; and activation of the RAA system. Research has shown that treatment of hypertension with a low-protein diet and antihypertensive medications reduces the progression of chronic renal disease to end-stage renal disease.[144,198,246]

Renovascular Disorders. Renovascular hypertension occurs when there is disease of the renal arteries leading to decreased perfusion of one or both the kidneys. The most common causes of renal artery stenosis are atherosclerosis, which can proceed to occlusion, and fibromuscular hyperplasia, which rarely causes occlusion.[200] Hypertension initially is due to activation of the RAA system, resulting in retention of sodium, chloride, and water. Renovascular hypertension is treated by angioplasty, revascularization, or drug therapy with either angiotensin-converting enzyme (ACE) inhibitors or calcium channel blockers. The longer the underlying stenosis is not treated, the greater the secondary damage to the vasculature caused by the hypertension. In one study of 110 patients with renovascular hypertension, it was found that surgery on those with high BP for less than 5 years resulted in a 78% success rate, whereas those with hypertension for longer than 5 years had only a 25% success rate.[102]

Primary Aldosteronism. Primary aldosteronism, a disease characterized by excess secretion of aldosterone, is most commonly caused by an adrenocortical adenoma.[76] Two other causes are adrenal hyperplasia and, rarely, adrenal carcinoma. With high circulating levels of aldosterone there is retention of sodium, chloride, and water, resulting in an expanded extracellular fluid volume. Common signs and symptoms of primary aldosteronism include hypokalemia, metabolic alkalosis, a high or elevated serum sodium, and a daily urinary potassium excretion exceeding 30 mmol even though the person has hypokalemia.[76] Primary aldosteronism caused by adrenocortical adenoma is treated by surgical removal of the tumor, if possible. If there is no tumor, treatment with spironolactone, an aldosterone antagonist, is usually effective.

Use of Oral Contraceptives. Before the development of the new low-dose oral contraceptives, hypertension related to the use of oral contraceptives accounted for approximately 1% of cases of secondary hypertension.[44,230] An analysis of the data from the Nurses' Health Study found the rate of hypertension in users of low-dose contraceptive pills to be 41.5 cases per 10,000 years of follow-up.[30] The data indicated that cessation of the use of the pills resulted in a return to normal BP. Even though the low-dose pills do not cause hypertension, analysis of the circadian rhythm of BP of 20 women taking oral contraceptives and 20 women who were not showed that the women using oral contraceptives had significantly higher BPs.[96]

DISPLAY 32-1

Secondary Causes of High Blood Pressure in Order of Frequency

KIDNEY DISORDERS

Renal artery stenosis
Unilateral
  Tumor
  Hypoplasia
  Renal tuberculosis
  Pyelonephritis
  Hydronephrosis
  Single cysts
Bilateral
  Acute or chronic renal failure
  Polycystic disease
  Pyelonephritis
  Glomerulonephritis
  Nephropathy from gout, diabetes, and phenacetin
    abuse
  Lupus erythematosus
  Progressive systemic sclerosis
  Periarteritis nodosa
  Amyloidosis
  Radiation nephritis
Renin-secreting tumors
  Wilms' tumor
    Nephroblastoma
    Paraganglioma
  Hemangiopericytoma
  Renin-producing pulmonary carcinoma

ENDOCRINE DISORDERS

Adrenal cortex
  Primary aldosteronism
  Secondary aldosteronism
  Cushing's syndrome
  Excess deoxycortisol
  Congenital adrenal hyperplasia
  Adenoma
Adrenal medulla
  Pheochromocytoma
Hypothyroidism
Hyperparathyroidism
Acromegaly

CARDIOVASCULAR DISORDERS

Coarctation of the aorta
Patent ductus arteriosus
Polycythemia hypertonica

NEUROLOGIC DISORDERS

Autonomic hyperreflexia
Excessive rapid-eye-movement sleep
Increased intracranial pressure
Ganglioneuromas, neuroblastomas, and tumors
  of the posterior fossa
Sleep apnea syndrome

SURGICAL PROCEDURES INVOLVING THE CARDIOVASCULAR SYSTEM

PREGNANCY

Preeclampsia
Eclampsia

EXOGENOUS COMPOUNDS

Sympathomimetic agents
  Amphetamine
  Caffeine
  Adrenalin
  Dopamine
  Nicotine
  Methyldopa
  Tyramine
Tricyclic antidepressants
Phenacetin-containing analgesics
Licorice
Chewing tobacco
Steroid therapy
Monoamine oxidase inhibitors
  Isocarboxazid [Marplan]
  Isoniazid
  Nialamide (Niamid)
  Pargyline (Eutonyl)
  Phenelzine (Nardil)
  Procarbazine
  Tranylcypromine (Parnate)
Tryptophan- and tyramine-containing foods
  Chicken liver
  Pickled herring
  Yeast extract
  Broad beans
  Matured cheeses (especially cheddar)
  Beer
  Wines (especially Chianti)
Oral contraceptives
Trace metals, minerals, and electrolytes
  Cadmium
  Zinc
  Lead
  Selenium
  Mercury
  Calcium
  Magnesium
  Potassium
  Sodium
Cocaine
Cyclosporine
Erythropoietin

GENETIC DISORDERS—SINGLE-GENE MUTATIONS

Glucocorticoid-remediable aldosteronism
Syndrome of apparent mineralocorticoid excess
Liddle's syndrome

Coarctation of the Aorta. Coarctation, or narrowing of the lumen, of the aorta is a rare cause of hypertension in adults, although it is relatively common in children.[228] The narrowing most commonly occurs distal to the origin of the left subclavian artery.[48] People with coarctation of the aorta have hypertension above the lesion and reduced pressure beyond the lesion. If untreated, coarctation can cause left ventricular hypertrophy. The longer the coarctation is untreated, the worse the prognosis. Treatment is usually with surgical repair of the lesion or angioplasty.[48]

Clinical Manifestations of High Blood Pressure

SIGNS AND SYMPTOMS

Unfortunately, there are few signs and no symptoms of hypertension until it becomes very severe and target organ damage has occurred. The major sign, obviously, is the presence of elevated arterial BP based on the criteria for the definition and measurement of high BP (see Table 32-1). Other signs and symptoms are described in the following section on complications of hypertension.

The morbidity and mortality associated with elevations in BP are predominantly a consequence of damage to a selected set of organs known as *target organs*. These target organs are the blood vessels, heart, brain, kidneys, and eyes. When the influence of hypertension is manifested in any of these organs, it is called *target organ disease*. Assessment of a client with an elevated BP includes examining for evidence of damage in one of these target organs. Evidence of target organ disease is considered a serious prognostic sign in a person with hypertension. The JNC VI recognized the importance of target organ disease, risk factors for athero-

---

DISPLAY 32-2

Components of Cardiovascular Risk Stratification in Patients With Hypertension[243]

MAJOR RISK FACTORS

Smoking
Dyslipidemia
Diabetes mellitus
Age older than 60 years
Sex (men and postmenopausal women)
Family history of cardiovascular disease: women younger than age 65 or men younger than age 55 years

TARGET ORGAN DAMAGE/CLINICAL CARDIOVASCULAR DISEASE

Heart diseases

◆ Left ventricular hypertrophy
◆ Angina/prior myocardial infarction
◆ Prior coronary revascularization
◆ Heart failure

Stroke or transient ischemic attack
Nephropathy
Peripheral arterial disease
Retinopathy

---

sclerotic disease, and clinical cardiovascular disease by integrating them into risk groups that can be used to stratify patients as a basis for therapeutic decision making.[243] A list of these components of cardiovascular risk plus the classification scheme are shown in Display 32-2 and Table 32-4.

TABLE 32-4 **Risk Stratification and Treatment*[243]**

Blood Pressure Stages (mm Hg)	Risk Group A (No Risk Factors; no TOD/CCD)[†]	Risk Group B (At Least 1 Risk Factor, Not Including Diabetes; no TOD/CCD)	Risk Group C (TOD/CCD or Diabetes, With or Without Other Risk Factors)
High normal (130–139/85–89)	Lifestyle modification	Lifestyle modification	Drug therapy[§]
Stage 1 (140–159/90–99)	Lifestyle modification (up to 12 mo)	Lifestyle modification[‡] (up to 6 mo)	Drug therapy
Stages 2 and 3 (≥160/≥100)	Drug therapy	Drug therapy	Drug therapy

For example, a patient with diabetes and a blood pressure of 142/94 mm Hg plus left ventricular hypertrophy should be classified as having stage 1 hypertension with target organ disease (left ventricular hypertrophy) and with another major risk factor (diabetes). This patient would be categorized as **Stage 1, Risk Group C,** and recommended for immediate initiation of pharmacologic treatment.

*Lifestyle modification should be adjunctive therapy for all patients recommended for pharmacologic therapy.
[†]TOD/CCD indicates target organ disease/clinical cardiovascular disease.
[‡]For patients with multiple risk factors, clinicians should consider drugs as initial therapy plus lifestyle modifications.
[§]For those with heart failure, renal insufficiency, or diabetes.

VASCULAR CHANGES ASSOCIATED WITH HIGH BLOOD PRESSURE

The blood vessels, specifically the arteries, are unique in that they are both a separate target organ as well as a part of the other major target organs. Hypertension can influence the endothelium, vascular smooth muscle, extracellular matrix, and connective tissue of the arteries. In addition, hypertension contributes to the rate at which atherosclerosis accumulates in the large elastic arteries and the intermediate-sized muscular arteries and arterioles.

In a normal artery, the intima is composed of the endothelium, a smooth-surfaced inner lining and the potential space between the endothelial cells and the internal elastic lamina. The media or middle layer consists of the internal elastic lamina, smooth muscle cells, elastin, collagen, and extracellular matrix. The smooth muscle cells control the beat-to-beat adjustment of vascular diameter by contracting and relaxing to dilate and constrict the vessel. The adventitia or outer layer is made up of connective tissue, fibroblasts, and a few smooth muscle cells. Its major role is thought to be anchoring the vessel to surrounding structures. In the early stages of hypertension, hypertrophy of the large arteries and the arterioles is observed. This medial thickening results in a narrower vessel lumen and hence, higher vascular resistance.[151] Under conditions of sustained hypertension, the layers of the normal artery change. The following sections discuss changes in endothelial function and then changes in artery structure, including atherosclerosis, arteriosclerosis, and fibrinoid arteriolar necrosis.

Changes in the Vascular Endothelium.

Some experts consider the vascular endothelium to be the largest organ in the body.[232] The designation of the endothelium as a separate organ reflects the recognition that the endothelium is a highly dynamic interface between the blood and the rest of the body, not simply the smooth lining of the blood vessels. The endothelium regulates vasomotion; coagulation and fibrinolysis; the traffic of inflammatory and immune cells between the blood, lymph, and tissues; the movement of nutrients and waste products between the blood and tissues; and secretion of a wide variety of cytokines and growth factors.[52]

Impaired endothelial vasodilation has been identified in people with hypertension and even in the normotensive children of hypertensive parents.[193,242] Preliminary work with 33 subjects found evidence that the degree of endothelial impairment was negatively correlated with mean BP.[98] This result indicates that the higher the BP, the greater the impairment in vascular dilation. Investigation has not yet revealed what aspect of the nitric oxide vasodilation system is dysfunctional in hypertension. Other factors that cause endothelial dysfunction include aging, hypercholesterolemia, diabetes, smoking, physical inactivity, and homcysteinemia.[15,193,232] Researchers hope that understanding the molecular basis for endothelial dysfunction in hypertension will be the pathway to developing new therapies to reduce the impact of hypertension. It is not yet known whether endothelial dysfunction is truly a precursor of hypertension or a sequel. It is also not known whether improving endothelial function will improve hypertension, but researchers are hypothesizing that it will.

Atherosclerosis.

Hypertension is one of the major modifiable risk factors for atherosclerosis. Atherosclerosis affects primarily the aorta and large to medium-sized arteries. It develops in areas where pressure is high, such as the bronchial arteries, particularly at branch points, and not in areas where pressure is low, as in the pulmonary arteries. It is the most common vascular lesion associated with cerebral infarction, renovascular hypertension, and systolic hypertension in the elderly. The pathogenesis of atherosclerosis is discussed in Chapter 20.

Arteriosclerosis.

Arteriosclerosis refers to the changes in the artery wall that occur as a result of aging.[153,185] The literature on the subject reflects confusion in the use of this term because sometimes it is clearly used to mean atherosclerosis, whereas in other situations the authors make a clear differentiation between arteriosclerosis and atherosclerosis.[219,268] O'Rourke[185] states that arteriosclerosis differs from atherosclerosis because it results in lesions that are concentric and dilated, whereas atherosclerosis results in eccentric and constricting lesions. Arteries with arteriosclerosis are stiff because of loss of elastin and an increase in collagen. In addition, hyaline, which is glycoprotein plus a small amount of lipid, is found beneath the internal elastic lamina as a component of the arteriosclerotic lesion. In the kidney, arteriosclerosis occurs most commonly in the afferent arterioles.[151]

Fibrinoid Arteriolar Necrosis.

Fibrinoid necrosis occurs in the small arterioles in people with accelerated (malignant) hypertension. The primary lesion in fibrinoid necrosis is accumulation of deposits of fibrin, fibrinogen, and other plasma proteins within the vessel wall. In addition, there is evidence of cell death within the vessel wall. This lesion is most frequently seen in the kidney and may also be called *malignant nephrosclerosis*.[151]

HEART

The cardiac sequelae of hypertension include left ventricular hypertrophy, heart failure, coronary artery disease, and myocardial infarction. Data from the Framingham Heart Study indicate that people with hypertension have at least a twofold greater risk of coronary disease and heart failure than people who are normotensive.[114] Chapters 20 and 22 discuss coronary heart disease and heart failure, respectively. Although left ventricular hypertrophy is most commonly seen in adults, it has also been found in children with hypertension.[43,218]

There is a positive correlation between cardiovascular morbidity and mortality and left ventricular hypertrophy. The greater the left ventricular mass, the greater the risk of dying of heart disease.[116] This risk is intensified if the person also has hypertension, glucose intolerance, or dyslipidemia, or is a cigarette smoker.

Although the mechanisms contributing to left ventricular hypertrophy are not well understood, studies have implicated angiotensin, aldosterone, and the atrial natriuretic peptides as potential causative factors.[177,209] Other growth factors and cytokines are probably also involved in the development of hypertrophy.[240] Rossi and colleagues[211] found increases in collagen, extracellular matrix, and myocyte diameter in hypertrophied human hearts studied at autopsy. The putative role of the RAA system in the development of left ventricular hypertrophy is supported by the finding that treatment of hypertension with ACE inhibitors is associated with regression of the hypertrophy.[82,220] Other interventions that have been associated with regression of left ventricular hypertrophy include weight loss, physical activity, and treatment with angiotensin II receptor blocking agents, calcium channel antagonists, beta blockers, and diuretics.[82,130,160,188,220,245] It is assumed, but not yet demonstrated, that regression of left ventricular hypertrophy will be associated with reduced morbidity and mortality.

KIDNEY

There is a vicious, circular relationship between hypertension and renal disease. Patients with kidney disease and hypertension have a worse prognosis than those who are normotensive. In a follow-up study of the 332,544 middle-aged, high-risk men screened for the Multiple Risk Factor Intervention Trial, a strong positive relationship was found between baseline BP and end-stage renal disease.[126] Compared with men with BPs less than 120/80 mm Hg, those with pressures from high normal to severe hypertension had significantly elevated adjusted relative risks of end-stage renal disease, ranging from 1.9 in the high-normal subjects to 22.1 for those with pressures exceeding 210/120 mm Hg. Several studies have demonstrated that BP control, often using ACE inhibitors, can slow the progression of renal insufficiency.[13,79,147,163]

In a healthy kidney, contraction of the afferent arterioles prevents variations in pressure from being transmitted to the glomerulus and thus influencing filtration. In people with chronic renal failure or prolonged hypertension, it is thought that the afferent arterioles may fail to protect the glomerulus from elevated systemic arterial pressure. Pro-teinuria is a clinical manifestation of elevated glomerular filtration pressure. Microalbuminuria, defined as a daily urinary protein excretion greater than 20 mg, is found in approximately 15% of people with essential hypertension.[10]

Pathologists describe the renal lesions associated with hypertension as arteriosclerotic with patches of hyaline sclerosis. In addition, atherosclerosis of the renal arteries can have a contributing role, as is seen in renovascular hypertension.[10,121]

EYE

The retina is the only part of the body where arteries and arterioles can be seen easily without invasive methods. Evidence of vessel damage in the retina indicates blood vessel damage elsewhere.

Hypertensive changes in the retina include changes in the diameter of the arteries, focal spasms, hemorrhages, formation of exudates, local infarctions, and edema of the optic fundus. Various combinations of these changes have been used over the years to classify the condition of the retina as either normal or as one of several grades of hypertensive retinopathy. One classification is shown in Table 32-5.[194] In this classification, the major criteria used to grade retinopathy are the ratio of the retinal artery diameter to the retinal vein diameter; the presence or absence of focal spasm of the retinal arteries; and the presence or absence of hemorrhages, exudates, and papilledema. Grades I and II differ only in the degree of arterial narrowing. If either retinal hemorrhages or exudates are present, it is grade III retinopathy. The presence of edema of the optic fundus indicates grade IV.

Some criteria that are included in other classifications are the arterial light reflex and what is known as *A-V nicking*. The arterial light reflex is an indicator of the amount of thickening of the walls of the retinal arteries. With moderate thickening, the arteries have a "copper-wire" appear-

TABLE 32-5	**Classification of Hypertensive Retinopathy**[194]				
	Vasculopathy		**Neuroretinal Changes**		
Grade	Arterial Narrowing AV Ratio*	Focal Spasm[†]	Hemorrhage	Exudates	Papilledema
Normal	>3:4 (>75%)	None	0	0	0
Grade I	3:4–1:2 (75%–50%)	None	0	0	0
Grade II	<1:2–1:3 (49%–33%)	<1:1–2:3 (>66%)	0	0	0
Grade III	<1:3–1:4 (32%–25%)	<2:3–1:3 (66%–33%)	+	+	0
Grade IV	<1:4 (<25%) Thread-like	<1:3 (<33%) Fibrous cords	+	+	+

*Retinal artery diameter to vein diameter ratio.
[†]Arterial focal spasm diameter to proximal artery ratio.

ance, and with severe narrowing the arteries are thought to resemble silver wire. A-V nicking, which occurs at locations where arteries and veins cross, is an indentation in the outer contour of a vein secondary to compression caused by thickening of the walls of the crossing retinal artery.

Diagrams of the optic fundus and the changes associated with hypertension are included in Chapter 10. Research on pigs and rhesus monkeys has revealed that cotton-wool spots result from retinal ischemia and infarction.[95,166,176] Infarction blocks axonal transport, and the accumulation of material in the axon is seen as the whitish patches known as cotton-wool spots. The swelling of the optic nerve head that occurs with hypertension needs to be differentiated from the papilledema that occurs with increased intracranial pressure.[194] Some authorities refer to the optic nerve edema in accelerated hypertension as papilledema, whereas others are careful to use terms like disc edema.[120,194] There is controversy over both the ability of clinicians to identify papilledema and whether it is a useful prognostic indicator.[3,71,165] In a 10-year follow-up of 96 people with hypertension, McGregor and colleagues[165] found that those with grades III and IV retinopathy had survival rates of 46% and 48%, respectively. Unfortunately, the sample size was small, making the clinical implications of these results uncertain.

BRAIN

Two changes occur in the cerebral arteries in response to chronic elevations in BP: remodeling and hypertrophy. Remodeling is a reduction in the outer diameter of an arteriole, whereas hypertrophy results in an increase in the thickness of the vessel wall. Both changes promote vasoconstriction and inhibit vasodilation, and they also support cerebral autoregulation. Autoregulation is a property of vascular beds that allows them to maintain a constant blood flow in response to a relatively wide range of perfusion pressure. With autoregulation, blood flow in an organ is held almost constant except at very low or high perfusion pressures. In hypertension, it has been demonstrated that cerebral autoregulation is maintained but the pressure–flow relationship is shifted to the right of that seen with normotension.[16]

Stroke. Hypertension is a clearly identifiable risk factor for strokes and their precursors, transient ischemic attacks.[125] Research has documented the positive relationship between stroke and high BP as well as the reduction in stroke with BP control.[34,77,86,158] Stroke is the leading cause of marked disability and the third leading cause of death in the United States.[2]

Ischemic injury to the brain is caused by decreased cerebral perfusion as a consequence of thrombosis, embolism, or a decreased blood supply to an area. It is now recognized that small strokes can occur without complete occlusion of the cerebral arteries.[207] Emboli from the left ventricle or from the peripheral veins through a patent foramen ovale cause approximately 20% of strokes. Another source of emboli may be atherosclerotic plaques in the carotid arteries. Hypertension increases the risk of stroke and transient ischemic attacks because it contributes to the formation and

growth of atherosclerotic plaque. Hypertension also causes hypertrophy in arteriolar walls, luminal narrowing, and, therefore, decreased cerebral perfusion and ischemia. The accumulation of hyaline in cerebral arteries secondary to hypertension contributes to occlusion of the cerebral arteries. Hypertension also contributes to both the rupture of cerebral arteries, leading to hemorrhage, and to the formation of aneurysms.[207]

Hypertensive Encephalopathy. Cerebral encephalopathy is a consequence of accelerated or malignant hypertension. Encephalopathy occurs when BP levels exceed the upper limit of autoregulation so that the cerebral arteries become dilated and the blood–brain barrier in the cerebral venules is disrupted.[16] This disruption of the blood–brain barrier is thought to contribute to the formation of cerebral edema; local changes in ion and cytokine concentrations; or alteration in neural function. Although rare, hypertensive encephalopathy occurs in children as well as in adults.[267]

MANAGEMENT OF HIGH BLOOD PRESSURE

Assessment and Diagnosis

DIAGNOSIS

Hypertension is relatively easy to diagnose. The fact that people with hypertension usually have no symptoms presents the greatest problem in establishing the diagnosis. Partly because of the lack of symptoms, in 1991 to 1994, approximately 30% of the hypertensive population in the United States were unaware of their condition.[243] The awareness, treatment, and control rates for hypertension in the United States between 1976 and 1994 are shown in Table 32-6. The hypertension control rate in 1991 to 1994 of 27% indicates a need for increased efforts on the part of health care professionals to manage the treatment of hypertension successfully.

Blood Pressure Measurement. The diagnosis of hypertension cannot be made from a single measurement because BP can vary markedly over weeks, days, and even minutes. In both hypertensive and normotensive people, there is diurnal variation in BP, with the highest pressures occurring between 8:00 and 11:00 AM, and lowest during sleep between 2:00 and 6:00 AM.[172] There can be a marked variation in BP during rapid eye movement sleep and a substantial elevation when a person first awakens.[49,150] Furthermore, a person's BP can be elevated during an office visit because of apprehension, pain, or preexisting illness. In view of the normal lability and biologic variations in BP, JNC VI has established guidelines for the detection and follow-up of high BP.[243] A diagnosis can be established only on the basis of an average of two or more BPs taken on two or more subsequent occasions. Follow-up criteria to be used after the first measurement for adults aged 18 years and older can be found in Table 32-7. The reliability and accuracy of BP readings depend on good technique and

TABLE 32-6 Trends in the Awareness, Treatment, and Control of High Blood Pressure in Adults: United States, 1976 to 1994*[243]

	NHANES II (1976–80)	NHANES III (Phase 1, 1988–91)	NHANES III (Phase 2, 1991–94)
Awareness	51%	73%	68.4%
Treatment	31%	55%	53.6%
Control[†]	10%	29%	27.4%

NHANES, National Health and Nutrition Examination Survey.
*Data are for adults 18 to 74 years of age with systolic BP of 140 mm Hg or greater, diastolic BP of 90 mm Hg or greater, or taking antihypertensive medication.
†Systolic BP below 140 mm Hg and diastolic BP below 90 mm Hg.
From Burt V et al. and unpublished NHANES III, phase 2, data provided by the Centers for Disease Control and Prevention, National Center for Health Statistics.

standardization of the procedure. The American Heart Association's *Recommendations for Human BP Determination by Sphygmomanometers*[195] and the American Society of Hypertension's *Recommendations for Routine BP Measurement by Indirect Cuff Sphygmomanometry*[8] contain current national standards for BP measurement.

Clinical Evaluation. The objectives of the medical assessment for hypertension are to determine if there is (1) target organ involvement, (2) other cardiovascular risk factors, (3) cardiovascular disease and any response to its treatment, (4) an identifiable cause for the elevated pressure, and (5) comorbid conditions. The assessment should include a careful history and physical examination. Display 32-3 lists many of the important variables to assess during the history and physical examination. It is also important to ask the client about any nontraditional remedies he or she may be using, including herbs, vitamins, and other supplements. Display 32-4 lists the basic and optional laboratory tests recommended by JNC VI for assessment of target organ damage.

Although secondary hypertension is rare (<10% of all hypertension), practitioners should nevertheless attempt to rule out secondary causes. Additional evaluation is recommended in patients whose age, severity of hypertension, history, physical examination, or laboratory findings are suggestive of secondary hypertension. Poor response to antihypertensive drug therapy, accelerated or malignant hypertension, or an accelerated phase of previously well controlled hypertension also indicates a need for further investigation.[243]

PROGNOSIS

The Veterans Administration Cooperative Group Study on Antihypertensive Agents[255] documented a morbidity rate of 55% in people with an untreated diastolic pressure of 90 to 114 mm Hg. With untreated diastolic pressures above 115 mm Hg, the morbidity rate was 80%.[254] In patients with diastolic pressure above 115 mm Hg, there were four deaths in the placebo group compared with none in the

TABLE 32-7 Recommendations for Follow-up Based on Initial Blood Pressure Measurements for Adults[243]

Initial Blood Pressure (mm Hg)*		Follow-up Recommended[†]
Systolic	Diastolic	
<130	<85	Recheck in 2 y
130–139	85–89	Recheck in 1 y[‡]
140–159	90–99	Confirm within 2 mo
160–179	100–109	Evaluate or refer to source of care within 1 mo
≥180	≥110	Evaluate to refer to source of care immediately or within 1 wk, depending on clinical situation

*If systolic and diastolic categories are different, follow recommendations for shorter follow-up (e.g., 160/86 mm Hg should be evaluated or referred to source of care within 1 mo).
†Modify the scheduling of follow-up according to reliable information about past blood pressure measurements, other cardiovascular risk factors, or target organ disease.
‡Provide advice about lifestyle modifications.

DISPLAY 32-3

Important Aspects of the History and Physical Examination[120]

HISTORY

Duration of the hypertension
　Last known normal blood pressure
　Course of the blood pressure
Prior treatment of the hypertension
　Drugs: types, doses, side effects
Intake of agents that may cause hypertension
　Oral contraceptives
　Sympathomimetics
　Adrenal steroids
　Excessive sodium intake
Family History
　Hypertension
　Premature cardiovascular disease or death
　Familial diseases: pheochromocytoma, renal disease,
　　diabetes, gout
Symptoms of secondary causes
　Muscle weakness
　Spells of tachycardia, sweating, tremor
　Thinning of the skin
　Flank pain
Symptoms of target organ damage
　Headaches
　Transient weakness or blindness
　Loss of visual acuity
　Chest pain
　Dyspnea
　Claudication

Presence of other risk factors
　Smoking
　Diabetes
　Dyslipidemia
　Physical inactivity
Dietary history
　Sodium
　Alcohol
　Saturated fats
Psychosocial factors
　Family structure
　Work status
　Educational level
Sexual function
Features of sleep apnea
　Early morning headaches
　Daytime somnolence
　Loud snoring
　Erratic sleep

PHYSICAL EXAMINATION

Accurate measurement of blood pressure
General appearance: distribution of body fat, skin lesions,
　muscle strength, alertness
Funduscopy
Neck: palpation and auscultation of carotids, thyroid
Heart: size, rhythm, sounds
Lungs: rhonchi, rales
Abdomen: renal masses, bruits over aorta or renal arteries,
　femoral pulses
Extremities: peripheral pulses, edema
Neurologic assessment

DISPLAY 32-4

Recommended and Optional Laboratory Tests and Diagnostic Procedures[243]

RECOMMENDED

Urinalysis
Complete blood cell count
Blood chemistries
　Sodium, potassium, creatinine, fasting glucose, total
　　and high-density lipoprotein cholesterol
12-Lead electrocardiogram

OPTIONAL

Creatinine clearance
Microalbuminuria
24-Hour urinary protein
Blood chemistries
　Calcium, uric acid, fasting triglycerides, low-density
　　lipoprotein cholesterol, glycosylated hemoglobin,
　　thyroid-stimulating hormone
Limited echocardiogram to assess for left ventricular
　hypertrophy

---

treatment group. This and other studies have documented that treatment can prevent morbidity and mortality in people with elevated BPs.[106,168]

The strong, graded, independent, and continuous relationships between systolic BP, diastolic BP, and cardiovascular risk were clearly illustrated by the analysis of 6 years of follow-up data from the screenings for the Multiple Risk Factor Intervention Trial (MRFIT).[236] Data from the 361,662 men screened for the study from 1973 to 1975 showed that relative risk of cardiovascular disease began increasing above a SBP of 120 mm Hg and a diastolic pressure of 90 mm Hg. Mortality rates were two to three times higher for men with systolic pressures greater than 120 mm Hg. Two meta-analyses by MacMahon, Peto, Collins, and associates[34,158] explored the data documenting the nature and strength of the relationships between BP control, stroke incidence, and coronary heart disease.

Treatment Options

Answers to a series of questions outline progress in the treatment of high BP. In the 1950s, the initial question was whether any treatment would reduce morbidity and mortality. Once clinical trials revealed that treatment was beneficial in reducing both morbid and mortal events, the following questions became relevant. Did the benefits extend to people different from those included in the initial clinical trials? What was the risk/benefit profile of different medications? How low should BP be lowered? Did the benefits extend to the elderly? Can high BP be prevented? What lifestyle or nonpharmacologic interventions are most effective? What is the best way to support people in following the prescribed therapy, both in changing their lifestyles to reduce risk and in taking medications routinely? The current state of knowledge relating to these questions is discussed in the following sections, beginning with prevention of hypertension and then moving to lifestyle and pharmacologic management, and then finally to management of hypertension in special populations.

The goal of therapy for patients with hypertension is the prevention of morbidity and mortality related to the elevated pressure, specifically the prevention of target organ damage and progression of atherosclerotic cardiovascular disease. In recognition of this goal, the JNC VI report has developed a table to guide clinicians in their choice of therapy. Information about a client's major cardiovascular risk factors, presence of target organ disease, and clinical signs of cardiovascular disease are used to assign the client to one of three risk groups designated A, B, or C. As shown in Table 32-4, the health care provider is then guided to the appropriate type of intervention by the client's risk group and actual BP stage. Such a classification is always used in concert with the clinician's clinical judgment. Other factors to consider in making treatment choices are any comorbid conditions, cost of treatment, client preference, and potential impacts on the client's quality of life.

An important tool in the management of high BP is the concept of setting a "goal BP" for each client. This pressure is usually less than 140/90 mm Hg, although for patients with diabetes mellitus or renal disease a lower goal is recommended. (See section on special populations for specific information on people with renal disease and diabetes mellitus.) The clinician may choose lower or higher goals depending on the individual client. The concept of goal BP has been demonstrated to be an effective tool in client management.[105,144]

PREVENTION OF HIGH BLOOD PRESSURE

The concept of hypertension prevention is relatively new. JNC VI for the first time included the word *prevention* in its title.[243] The information in JNC VI was based on a 1993 report on the primary prevention of hypertension.[179]

Of the 12 interventions that have been studied in 5 major clinical trials of hypertension prevention, only 4 have been demonstrated to be effective.[40,108,238,247,248] The four interventions that have been shown to delay or prevent the onset of high BP are weight loss, sodium restriction, a reduction in alcohol intake, and exercise. The interventions that were not shown to be effective were supplements of potassium, calcium, magnesium, fiber, and fish oil given in pill form; stress management; and alterations in macronutrients such as protein, carbohydrates, and fats.[40,179] It is possible that some of these apparently ineffective interventions may be shown to have an impact in the future because there

have been relatively few studies, and the studies that have been done have been of relatively short duration using selected middle-aged populations.

A short-term dietary study has provided evidence that a diet high in fruits and vegetables combined with low-fat dairy products and a reduction in saturated and total fat may be helpful in preventing high BP.[11] After 8 weeks on the diet, the 326 normotensive subjects had significantly greater reductions in their systolic and diastolic pressures (3.5 and 2.1 mm Hg, respectively, $P < 0.003$) than the control group. The key question is whether such reductions could be maintained for longer periods. In the Trial of Hypertension Prevention, one important finding was that the subjects had difficulty maintaining their changes in weight and sodium intake over prolonged periods.[248] Reductions in BP were greatest at 6 months and declined over the 3-year follow-up period.

NONPHARMACOLOGIC MANAGEMENT OF HIGH BLOOD PRESSURE

The most effective nonpharmacologic or lifestyle measures to prevent hypertension are three nutritional measures and exercise or increased physical activity. The nutritional measures that have been demonstrated to be most effective are weight loss, sodium restriction, and a diet high in fruits and vegetables. Physical activity/exercise is effective alone as well as being an important component of weight management and weight loss. In addition, people with high BP are encouraged to modify other risk factors for cardiovascular disease such as dyslipidemia and smoking because of their additive impact on the rate of development and progression of atherosclerosis.

Weight Control. The results of many studies indicate a direct relationship between hypertension and obesity.[78,101,115] JNC IV defines obesity as a body mass index (weight in kilograms/height in meters²) greater than 27.[243] There is also a correlation between the presence of excess abdominal adiposity (defined as a waist-to-hip ratio of over 0.85 in women and 0.95 in men) and the development of hypertension, diabetes, dyslipidemia, and increased coronary heart disease mortality.[23,51,68,88,189] Studies in Framingham, Massachusetts, and Evans County, Georgia reveal that overweight people have from two to three times the risk for development of hypertension than people who are not overweight.[115,239] The exact mechanism by which obesity contributes to hypertension is unclear. However, the influence of weight may be related to alterations in cardiovascular, endocrine, and metabolic factors caused by obesity. These alterations include increased cardiac output, increased blood volume, and sodium retention. There is also evidence that hyperinsulinemia, insulin resistance, decreased carbohydrate tolerance, and decreased insulin sensitivity occur in conjunction with obesity.[162,175] Research also indicates that endothelial function is altered with obesity.[175]

Weight loss has consistently been demonstrated to reduce BP more effectively than any other lifestyle measure.[108,142,247,248,260,264] Langford and associates,[142] studying a group of subjects whose BP had been controlled with medications for 5 years, found that an average weight loss of

10 pounds prevented 60% of the overweight subjects from having to return to taking medications. In addition, weight loss has been found to complement pharmacologic management of mild high BP.[183,186] Counseling hypertensive, overweight patients about weight reduction is important, both as a preventive measure as well as an independent or complementary treatment for high BP. The challenge for both clinicians and clients is supporting maintenance of weight loss, because longitudinal studies have shown that subjects who lose weight initially tend to gain back the weight over time.[264] In a study of male health professionals, Coakley and associates[32] found that vigorous physical activity was associated with weight loss, whereas eating between meals and watching television were associated with weight gain.

Sodium Restriction. The role of sodium in the development of hypertension, and the efficacy of reduced sodium intake as an intervention to treat or prevent high BP, are controversial topics. It is clear that some, but not all, hypertensive people respond to a reduction in sodium intake with a fall in BP. Ferri and colleagues[66] found a possible relationship between damage to the vascular endothelium and salt sensitivity. What has been even more controversial is whether a public health approach that lowered the sodium intake of all members of a population would result in lower morbidity and mortality related to high BP.[41,154,171]

Clinical trials of nonpharmacologic approaches to the treatment of hypertension have consistently shown that reduction of sodium intake is effective in reducing BP.[41,108,142,171,247,248] In two separate meta-analyses of randomized trials of reduced sodium intake in people with high BP, it was found that for a 100 mmol/d decrease in sodium intake, there was a 3.7 to 5.8 mm Hg decrease in systolic BP and a 0.9 to 2.5 mm Hg decrease in diastolic pressure.[41,171] The impact of reducing sodium intake was greater in people who were older and who had higher levels of BP.

The JNC VI recommends a goal sodium intake of no more than 100 mmol per day, which is equivalent to approximately 6 g of sodium chloride or 2.4 g of sodium per day.[243] In many of the clinical trials of sodium reduction, the goals levels of sodium intake were between 70 and 100 mmol per day although the average intake for most subjects ranged between 104 and 124 mmol per day. The apparent difficulty in achieving the goal sodium intake underscores the challenge of reducing sodium intake. It is estimated that the average adult man uses approximately 3.9 g of sodium daily, whereas women take in approximately 2.8 g.[61] It may help clients to know that it takes 8 to 12 weeks to adjust one's sense of taste to a lower sodium intake.[164]

Sodium restriction has also been shown to be a beneficial adjunct to the pharmacologic treatment of high BP.[56,262] Weinberger and colleagues[262] found that subjects who decreased their intake of sodium to between 50 and 100 mmol/d were able to decrease their doses of diuretics and potassium-sparing agents significantly. Salt intake also influences the plasma concentration of medications such as verapamil.[46] Plasma levels of verapamil were lower when subjects ingested 400 mEq/d compared with 10 mEq/d of sodium. Sodium restriction (1 to 3 g/d) has been shown to restore

the typical circadian rhythm of BP in people with both essential hypertension and primary aldosteronism.[252,253]

The variability of individual BP responses to the level of sodium intake has been called *salt sensitivity*.[74,81] Although it is known that some people experience a fall in BP when sodium intake is reduced, whereas others have no change, there is no test that allows the clinician to identify who is susceptible. Analysis of participants in the Trial of Hypertension Prevention study found differences in angiotensinogen genotype between those who were salt sensitive and those who were not.[103] Until there is a test for sodium sensitivity, clinicians can do an "N of 1" study by trying a period of salt restriction with a client and measuring BP before and after to determine the person's response. A useful measure of a client's sodium intake is a 24-hour urine sample analyzed for sodium content.

Diet High in Fruits and Vegetables. The Dietary Approaches to Stop Hypertension (DASH) study examined the effects of an 8-week dietary intervention on BP in both normotensive and hypertensive subjects.[11] In the 133 hypertensive subjects, the investigators found that adherence to a diet high in fruits, vegetables, and low-fat dairy products and low in saturated and total fat resulted in a marked decline in both systolic and diastolic BP. Compared with normotensive control subjects, those with a systolic pressure between 140 and 160 mm Hg or a diastolic pressure between 90 and 95 mm Hg had decreases in BP of 11.4/5.5 mm Hg. There was no significant change in weight during the study in any of the study groups. The DASH diet included 8 to 10 servings per day of fruits and vegetables and 2.7 servings of low-fat dairy products. The subjects were either fed at the research center or were given their meals in coolers to eat at home or work. Clearly, the diet can work, but the challenge will be in finding a way to support adoption of the diet in a manner that fits with the patient's daily life. A description of the DASH diet is provided in Table 32-8, and a sample menu is shown in Table 32-9. Information on the DASH diet is available on the World Wide Web at http://dash.bwh.harvard.edu. Further research is also needed to look at the impact of the DASH diet over extended periods.

Physical Activity. A sedentary lifestyle is one of the risk factors for hypertension.[12,24,100,145,263] The results of a meta-analysis of 36 studies of the effect of physical activity on hypertension concluded that aerobic training does reduce BP.[63] The data indicated that physical fitness training had a graded influence on BP, from a small influence on normotensive people to a larger impact on those with hypertension. The respective decreases in systolic and diastolic pressures were 3/3 mm Hg for normotensive people, 6/7 mm Hg for those with borderline hypertension, and 10/8 mm Hg for people with hypertension. Additional studies have supported the conclusions of the meta-analysis.[130,170] Other analyses of research data indicate that people who are physically active experience reduced cardiovascular and all-cause mortality rates.[25,59,62,69,72,90,134,135,191,216,217,225,226]

Physical activity is known to have a variety of metabolic and other effects that may partially explain its beneficial

TABLE 32-8	The Dietary Approaches to Stop Hypertension (DASH) Diet*[243]			
Food Group	**Daily Servings**	**Serving Sizes**	**Examples and Notes**	**Significance of Each Food Group to the DASH Diet Pattern**
Grains and grain products	7–8	1 slice bread 1/2 C dry cereal 1/2 C cooked rice, pasta, or cereal	Whole-wheat bread, English muffin, pita bread, bagel, cereals, grits, oatmeal	Major sources of energy and fiber
Vegetables	4–5	1 C raw leafy vegetable 1/2 C cooked vegetable 6 oz vegetable juice	Tomatoes, potatoes, carrots, peas, squash, broccoli, turnip greens, collards, kale, spinach, artichokes, beans, sweet potatoes	Rich sources of potassium, magnesium, and fiber
Fruits	4–5	6 oz fruit juice 1 medium fruit 1/4 C dried fruit 1/2 C fresh, frozen, or canned fruit	Apricots, bananas, dates, grapes, oranges, orange juice, grapefruit, grapefruit juice, mangoes, melons, peaches, pineapples, prunes, raisins, strawberries, tangerines	Important sources of potassium, magnesium, and fiber
Low-fat or nonfat dairy foods	2–3	8 oz milk 1 C yogurt 1.5 oz cheese	Skim or 1% milk, skim or low-fat buttermilk, nonfat or low-fat yogurt, part-skim mozzarella cheese, nonfat cheese	Major sources of calcium and protein
Meats, poultry, and fish	2 or less	3 oz cooked meats, poultry, or fish	Select only lean; trim away visible fats; broil, roast, or boil, instead of frying; remove skin from poultry	Rich sources of protein and magnesium
Nuts, seeds, and legumes	4–5 per week	1.5 oz or 1/3 C nuts 1/2 oz or 2 Tbsp seeds 1/2 C cooked legumes	Almonds, filberts, mixed nuts, peanuts, walnuts, sunflower seeds, kidney beans, lentils	Rich sources of energy, magnesium, potassium, protein, and fiber

*The DASH eating plan shown is based on 2,000 calories a day. Depending on an individual's caloric needs, the number of daily servings in a food group may vary from those listed.

effects on BP. One confounding factor in some of these studies is that sometimes the physical activity intervention is combined with weight loss.[50] Another problem is that the studies usually enroll a small number of subjects because of the cost and complexity of doing invasive measurements. In a study of nine hypertensive and obese men with an average age of 62 years, it was found that a 6-month period of physical training improved both glucose and lipid metabolism. The men lost 9% of their body weight and improved their exercise capacity ($\dot{V}O_2$max) by 16%. A study of 18 African-American men with both high BP and left ventricular hypertrophy found that after 32 weeks of exercising three times a week, the men had significant decreases in left ventricular mass and left ventricular mass index.[130] The 1996 Surgeon General's Report[251] on physical activity and health documents the extent of the known benefits of physical activity for chronic disease prevention.

The 1996 Surgeon General's Report[251] recommends that all Americans engage in moderate physical activity most days of the week. JNC VI uses the Surgeon General's recommendation that people with high BP should exercise moderately for 30 to 45 minutes almost every day of the week.[243] The report states that a thorough physical examination is not required for a program of brisk walking unless the client has other major health problems in addition to high BP. However, no patient with high BP, or any other major cardiovascular risk factor, should leave the care of their health provider without instructions on the signs and symptoms of heart attack and stroke—and a discussion of what to do if symptoms occur (i.e., call 911 or its local equivalent).

Reduction of Alcohol Intake. The data from epidemiologic studies clearly indicate that an alcohol intake of greater than three to four standard drinks per day is associated with high BP.[17,39,128,244] A standard drink has been defined as approximately 14 g of alcohol, which is the amount contained in 12 ounces of beer, 5 ounces of wine, or 1.5 ounces of distilled liquor such as vodka, gin, or scotch.[39] There is some dispute over whether people who have a modest intake of alcohol (i.e., one to two drinks per day) may have a lower BP than nondrinkers. A case–control study of adults older than 40 years of age found a lower incidence of ischemic stroke in people with an alcohol intake of one to two drinks per day compared with abstainers.[214] Some research has found a higher rate of hypertension and mortality in nondrinkers than in those who report one to two drinks a day. However, nondrinkers differ significantly from people who drink in relation to factors such as educational level and body weight.[201]

Intervention studies have found that reducing alcohol intake results in lower systolic and diastolic pressures.[39,40,206] Unfortunately, most of these studies have been of short duration (2 to 18 weeks), whereas the two longest studies (52 and 104 weeks) were able to demonstrate only marginally significant reductions in BP.[40,259] The authors of the

TABLE 32-9   Dietary Approaches to Stop Hypertension (DASH) Diet Sample Menu (Based on 2,000 Kcal/d)[243]

Food	Amount	Servings Provided
Breakfast		
Orange juice	6 oz	1 fruit
1% Low-fat milk	8 oz (1 C)	1 dairy
Corn flakes (with 1 tsp sugar)	1 C	2 grains
Banana	1 medium	1 fruit
Whole-wheat bread (with 1 Tbsp jelly)	1 slice	1 grain
Soft margarine	1 tsp	1 fat
Lunch		
Chicken salad	3/4 C	1 poultry
Pita bread	1/2, large	1 grain
Raw vegetable medley:		
Carrot and celery sticks	3–4 sticks each	
Radishes	2	1 vegetable
Loose-leaf lettuce	2 leaves	
Part-skim mozzarella cheese	1.5 slice (1.5 oz)	1 dairy
1% Low-fat milk	8 oz (1 C)	1 dairy
Fruit cocktail in light syrup	1/2 C	1 fruit
Dinner		
Herbed baked cod	3 oz	1 fish
Scallion rice	1 C	2 grains
Steamed broccoli	1/2 C	1 vegetable
Stewed tomatoes	1/2 C	1 vegetable
Spinach salad:		
Raw spinach	1/2 C	
Cherry tomatoes	2	1 vegetable
Cucumber	2 slices	
Light Italian salad dressing	1 Tbsp	1/2 fat
Whole-wheat dinner roll	1 small	1 grain
Soft margarine	1 tsp	1 fat
Melon balls	1/2 C	1 fruit
Snacks		
Dried apricots	1 oz (1/4 C)	1 fruit
Mini-pretzels	1 oz (3/4 C)	1 grain
Mixed nuts	1.5 oz (1/3 C)	1 nuts
Diet ginger ale	12 oz	0

Total number of servings in 2,000 kcal/d menu:

Food Group	Servings
Grains	= 8
Vegetables	= 4
Fruits	= 5
Dairy foods	= 3
Meats, poultry, and fish	= 2
Nuts, seeds, and legumes	= 1
Fats and oils	= 2.5

Tips on Eating the DASH Way

- Start small. Make gradual changes in your eating habits.
- Center your meal around carbohydrates, such as pasta, rice, beans, or vegetables.
- Treat meat as one part of the whole meal, instead of the focus.
- Use fruits or low-fat, low-calorie foods such as sugar-free gelatin for desserts and snacks.

REMEMBER! If you use the DASH diet to help prevent or control high blood pressure, make it part of a lifestyle that includes choosing foods lower in salt and sodium, keeping a healthy weight, being physically active, and, if you drink alcohol, doing so in moderation

To learn more about high blood pressure, call 1-800-575-WELL or visit the NHLBI web site at http://www.nhlbi.nih.gov/nhlbi/nhlbi.htm. DASH is also on-line at http://dash.bwh.harvard.edu.

most recent of these studies, the Prevention and Treatment of Hypertension Study (PATHS), believed the most reasonable explanation for this small impact of reduced drinking was that the reported intake difference was only 1.3 drinks per day between the treatment and control groups.[40] They also discussed the difficulty of motivating subjects to reduce alcohol intake.

The JNC VI recommends that people with hypertension should not consume more than 24 ounces of beer, 2 ounces of 100-proof distilled spirits, or 10 ounces of wine per day.[243] The report also recommends that the assessment of people with high BP include an in-depth history of the person's current alcohol intake and habits.

Other Potential Interventions. A number of other interventions that may have the potential to reduce BP have been studied but have not been found in large clinical trials to be effective.[5,132,179,243,247] Some of the interventions that have been suggested include stress reduction; reduced caffeine intake; increased garlic or onion intake; and increased intake of potassium, magnesium or calcium. Even though clinical trials have not shown calcium to be very beneficial for BP reduction, it is important for the prevention of osteoporosis. Further research on these factors may show any one or more of them to have a role in the management of high BP, especially when more is learned about the causes of hypertension.

Control of Other Risk Factors. Any person who has an elevated systolic or diastolic BP has an increased risk of atherosclerotic cardiovascular disease. In addition, longitudinal epidemiologic studies have shown that the major risk factors have an additive effect on the probability that a person will have a morbid or mortal event.[117,146,157,190] Therefore, even though quitting smoking and improving dyslipidemia do not improve a client's BP, these interventions reduce the risk of morbidity and mortality from atherosclerotic cardiovascular disease.[54,85,92,97,124,138,224]

PHARMACOLOGIC MANAGEMENT

Since the 1960s, randomized, placebo-controlled clinical trials have provided evidence that pharmacologic treatment of high BP reduces mortality and morbidity. The Veterans Administration Cooperative Group Studies on Antihypertensive Agents were the first studies in the United States demonstrating that drug treatment was extremely beneficial in people with moderate and severe hypertension.[254,255] Subsequent clinical trials have explored the benefits of treatment in more representative populations as well as at lower BP levels. The Hypertension Detection and Follow-up Program (HDFP), with a study population of 10,940, was one of the first to demonstrate the benefits of hypertension treatment extended to people with diastolic BPs between 90 and 105 mm Hg.[105,106] Studies with varying approaches and in different countries have strengthened the conclusion that hypertension treatment reduces both morbidity and mortality in men and women across the age span.[42,131,161,168,174,205]

Two issues remain controversial in the treatment of high BP. The first is how far BP should be lowered in the treatment of hypertension, and the second concerns the relative risks and benefits of the different classes of antihypertensive medications. Some specialists in the field of BP management have been concerned that excessive lowering of BP may increase the risk of cardiovascular mortality.[37,67,93] The Hypertension Optimal Treatment (HOT) Study was designed to examine the optimal target diastolic pressure for people with hypertension.[94] The HOT randomized trial enrolled 18,790 men and women between 50 and 80 years of age from 20 countries. One third of the subjects were randomized to one of three target diastolic pressures, 80, 85, and 90 mm Hg. Initial drug treatment was with felodipine, a calcium channel antagonist, and other agents were added as needed according to a protocol. In the last 6 months of the study, the mean achieved BPs for the three target groups were, 81, 83, and 85 mm Hg respectively. When the relationships between achieved BPs and the study outcomes were examined, the lowest risk for major cardiovascular events was at a pressure of 138.5/82.6 mm Hg, for stroke 142.2/<80 mm Hg, and for cardiovascular mortality, 138.8/86.5 mm Hg. In hypertensive patients, lowering the BP below 140/85 mm Hg showed neither added risk nor benefit. Because the BPs achieved by the three groups in this study were so close, additional research is needed to determine if lowering the BP further than 80 mm Hg

would be beneficial or harmful.[118] In diabetes and renal disease, data support a lower target BP, as discussed later in the section on special populations.

The relative benefits and risks associated with the major classes of medications used to treat hypertension have also been very controversial. Some experts have advocated the use of diuretics and beta blockers because they are the drugs that were used in the major randomized, controlled trials that demonstrated reduced cardiovascular and all-cause mortality.[75,205] Questions have been raised about the risks associated with the use of calcium channel antagonists.[4,28,75,167,204] The Syst-Eur Trial, which compared nitrendipine with placebo in the treatment of isolated systolic hypertension, found no evidence of a harmful effect of calcium channel blockers.[234] In addition, a follow-up analysis found that nitrendipine was particularly effective in the subjects who also had diabetes mellitus.[250] Variables that need to be considered in analyzing this controversy are the type of calcium channel antagonist, the dose used, and the length of action of the drug. The short-acting dihydropyridine calcium channel antagonists are thought to be associated with adverse outcomes.[167] Ultimately, the answers about the effectiveness of the various antihypertensive agents will come from clinical trials comparing the drugs and evaluating the risks and benefits of each.

Individualized Stepped Care. A systematic approach to the treatment of hypertension, known as *stepped care,* was suggested in the early 1970s by a task force of the National Heart, Lung, and Blood Institute and revised in each of the subsequent JNC reports. The current algorithm for hypertension management is shown in Figure 32-1. With the advent of new classes of antihypertensive medications and the recognition that coexisting conditions influence the appropriateness of an individual medication, the suggestions of the best drug for initial therapy have broadened. Table 32-10 lists the comorbid conditions that need to be considered when selecting medications for the person with hypertension. Other factors that need to be considered in choosing therapy include cost, convenience, duration of action, frequency of adverse effects, client preference, quality of life, and other medications the client is taking, both those available over the counter and those prescribed by a health care provider. Table 32-11 lists some of the known interactions between antihypertensive agents and other medications plus selected foods.

Six classes of drugs are available for the treatment of hypertension: (1) diuretics; (2) adrenergic inhibitors, of which there are ß-adrenergic blocking agents, centrally acting inhibitors, central α-adrenergic agonists, α-adrenergic blockers, and combined α- and ß-adrenergic blockers; (3) vasodilators; (4) calcium channel blocking agents; (5) ACE inhibitors; and (6) angiotensin II receptor blockers. Table 32-12 lists the generic and trade names, usual dose ranges, and selected side effects of most of the common antihypertensive agents. Some of the most commonly used combination medications are listed in Table 32-13. These combinations can be very useful in simplifying therapy once the clinician has titrated the dose of each medica-

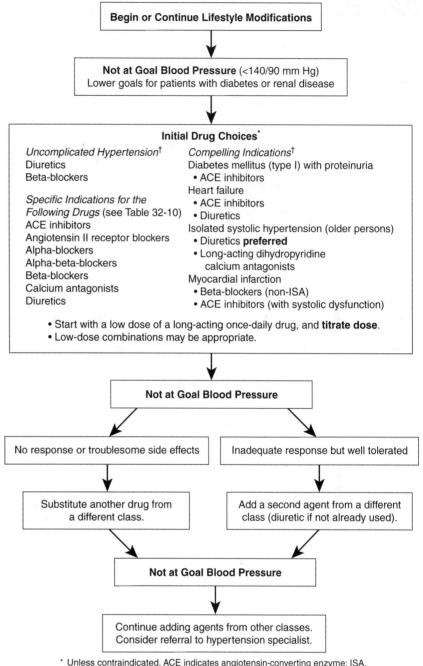

FIGURE 32-1 Algorithm for the treatment of hypertension.

* Unless contraindicated. ACE indicates angiotensin-converting enzyme; ISA, intrinsic sympathomimetic activity.

† Based on randomized controlled trials.

tion for effectiveness in the individual client. An endothelin receptor antagonist, bosentan, has been shown to be effective in lowering BP, but is not yet commercially available.[18,133] Once an initial drug has been chosen, it is recommended that the client begin with a low dose, and then either the dose is increased or a new drug is added if the goal BP is not achieved after 1 to 2 months.[243]

Hypertensive Crisis. Acute hypertensive crises are rare situations in which patients require immediate intervention to reduce BP. Hypertensive crises have been classified into two types: hypertensive emergencies and urgencies. A *hypertensive emergency* has been defined as occuring when end-organ damage is acute or imminent and immediate reduction in BP, usually by intravenous medication in an intensive

TABLE 32-10	Considerations for Individualizing Antihypertensive Drug Therapy[243]
Indication	**Drug Therapy**

Compelling Indications Unless Contraindicated	
Diabetes mellitus (type I) with proteinuria	ACE I
Heart failure	ACE I, diuretics
Isolated systolic hypertension (older patients)	Diuretics (preferred), CA (long-acting DHP)
Myocardial infarction	Beta blockers (non-ISA), ACE I (with systolic dysfunction)

May Have Favorable Effects on Comorbid Conditions*	
Angina	Beta blockers, CA
Atrial tachycardia and fibrillation	Beta blockers, CA (non-DHP)
Cyclosporine-induced hypertension (caution with the dose of cyclosporine)	CA
Diabetes mellitus (types I and II) with proteinuria	ACE I (preferred), CA
Diabetes mellitus (type II)	Low-dose diuretics
Dyslipidemia	Alpha blockers
Essential tremor	Beta blockers (non-CS)
Heart failure	Carvedilol, losartan potassium
Hyperthyroidism	Beta blockers
Migraine	Beta blockers (non-CS), CA (non-DHP)
Myocardial infarction	Diltiazem hydrochloride, verapamil hydrochloride
Osteoporosis	Thiazides
Preoperative hypertension	Beta blockers
Prostatism (BPH)	Alpha blockers
Renal insufficiency (caution in renovascular hypertension and creatinine ≥265.2 µmol/L [3 mg/dL])	ACE I

May Have Unfavorable Effects on Comorbid Conditions*†	
Bronchospastic disease	Beta blockers[‡]
Depression	Beta blockers, central alpha agonists, reserpine[‡]
Diabetes mellitus (types I and II)	Beta blockers, high-dose diuretics
Dyslipidemia	Beta blockers (non-ISA), diuretics (high-dose)
Gout	Diuretics
Second- or third-degree heart block	Beta blockers,[‡] CA (non-DHP)[‡]
Heart failure	Beta blockers (except carvedilol), CA (except amlodipine besylate, felodipine)
Liver disease	Labetalol hydrochloride, methyldopa[‡]
Peripheral vascular disease	Beta blockers
Pregnancy	ACE I,[‡] angiotensin II receptor blockers[‡]
Renal insufficiency	Potassium-sparing agents
Renovascular disease	ACE I, angiotensin II receptor blockers

ACE I angiotensin-converting enzyme inhibitors; BPH, benign prostatic hyperplasia; CA, calcium antagonists; DHP, dihydropyridine; ISA, intrinsic sympathomimetic activity; MI, myocardial infarction; non-CS, noncardioselective.

   *Conditions and drugs are listed in alphabetical order.
   †These drugs may be used with special monitoring unless contraindicated.
   ‡Contraindicated.

care unit, is required. A *hypertensive urgency* has been defined as occuring when the BP is critically high with signs such as edema of the optic disc; there is but less evidence of target organ damage, so that BP reduction can be achieved over a longer period using oral antihypertensive medications.[243] Clearly there is a continuum from emergencies to urgencies, and excellent assessment and judgment are required. Acute elevations of BP may occur after certain medications such as clonidine are discontinued, or the client either forgets to take or runs out of medication.[184]

TABLE 32-11 **Selected Drug Interactions with Antihypertensive Therapy**[243]

Class of Agent	Increase Efficacy	Decrease Efficacy	Effect on Other Drugs
Diuretics	• Diuretics that act at different sites in the nephron (e.g., furosemide + thiazides)	• Resin-binding agents • NSAIDs • Steroids	• Diuretics raise serum lithium levels. • Potassium-sparing agents may exacerbate hyperkalemia due to ACE inhibitors.
Beta blockers	• Cimetidine (hepatically metabolized beta blockers) • Quinidine (hepatically metabolized beta blockers) • Food (hepatically metabolized beta blockers)	• NSAIDs • Withdrawal of clonidine • Agents that induce hepatic enzymes, including rifampin and phenobarbital	• Propranolol hydrochloride induces hepatic enzymes to increase clearance of drugs with similar metabolic pathways. • Beta blockers may mask and prolong insulin-induced hypoglycemia. • Heart block may occur with nondihydropyridine calcium antagonists. • Sympathomimetics cause unopposed α-adrenoceptor-mediated vasoconstriction. • Beta blockers increase angina-inducing potential of cocaine.
ACE inhibitors	• Chlorpromazine or clozapine	• NSAIDs • Antacids • Food decreases absorption (moexipril)	• ACE inhibitors may raise serum lithium levels. • ACE inhibitors may exacerbate hyperkalemic effect of potassium-sparing diuretics.
Calcium antagonists	• Grapefruit juice (some dihydropyridines) • Cimetidine or ranitidine (hepatically metabolized calcium antagonists)	• Agents that induce hepatic enzymes, including rifampin and phenobarbital	• Cyclosporine levels increase* with diltiazem hydrochloride, verapamil hydrochloride, mibefradil dihydrochloride, or nicardipine hydrochloride (but not felodipine, isradipine, or nifedipine). • Nondihydropyridines increase levels of other drugs metabolized by the same hepatic enzyme system, including digoxin, quinidine, sulfonylureas, and theophylline. • Verapamil hydrochloride may lower serum lithium levels.
Alpha blockers			• Prazosin may decrease clearance of verapamil hydrochloride.
Central α_2-agonists and peripheral neuronal blockers		• Tricyclic antidepressants (and probably phenothiazines) • Monoamine oxidase inhibitors • Sympathomimetics or phenothiazines antagonize guanethidine monosulfate or guanadrel sulfate • Iron salts may reduce methyldopa absorption	• Methyldopa may increase serum lithium levels. • Severity of clonidine hydrochloride withdrawal may be increased by beta blockers. • Many agents used in anesthesia are potentiated by clonidine hydrochloride.

NSAIDs, nonsteroidal anti-inflammatory drugs; ACE, angiotensin-converting enzyme.

*This is a clinically and economically beneficial drug–drug interaction because it both retards progression of accelerated atherosclerosis in heart transplant recipients and reduces the required daily dose of cyclosporine.

TABLE 32-12 **Oral Antihypertensive Drugs***

Drug	Trade Name	Usual Dose Range, Total mg/d* (Frequency per Day)	Selected Side Effects and Comments*
Diuretics (partial list)			Short term: increases cholesterol and glucose levels; biochemical abnormalities: decreases potassium, sodium, and magnesium levels, increases uric acid and calcium levels; rare: blood dyscrasias, photosensitivity, pancreatitis, hyponatremia
Chlorthalidone (G)†	Hygroton	12.5–50 (1)	
Hydrochlorothiazide (G)	HydroDIURIL, Microzide, Esidrix	12.5–50 (1)	
Indapamide	Lozol	1.25–5 (1)	(Less or no hypercholesterolemia)
Metolazone	Mykrox	0.5–1.0 (1)	
	Zaroxolyn	2.5–10 (1)	
LOOP DIURETICS			
Bumetanide (G)	Bumex	0.5–4 (2–3)	(Short duration of action, no hypercalcemia)
Ethacrynic acid	Edecrin	25–100 (2–3)	(Only nonsulfonamide diuretic, ototoxicity)
Furosemide (G)	Lasix	40–240 (2–3)	(Short duration of action, no hypercalcemia)
Torsemide	Demadex	5–100 (1–2)	
POTASSIUM-SPARING AGENTS			Hyperkalemia
Amiloride hydrochloride (G)	Midamor	5–10 (1)	
Spironolactone (G)	Aldactone	25–100 (1)	(Gynecomastia)
Triamterene (G)	Dyrenium	25–100 (1)	
Adrenergic Inhibitors			
PERIPHERAL AGENTS			
Guanadrel sulfate	Hylorel	10–75 (2)	(Postural [orthostatic] hypotension, diarrhea)
Guanethidine monosulfate	Ismelin	10–150 (1)	(Postural [orthostatic] hypotension, diarrhea)
Reserpine (G)[11]	Serpasil	0.05–0.25 (1)	(Nasal congestion, sedation, depression, activation of peptic ulcer)
CENTRAL ALPHA AGONISTS			Sedation, dry mouth, bradycardia, withdrawal hypertension
Clonidine hydrochloride (G)	Catapres	0.2–1.2 (2–3)	(More withdrawal)
Guanabenz acetate (G)	Wytensin	8–32 (2)	
Guanfacine hydrochloride (G)	Tenex	1–3 (1)	(Less withdrawal)
Methyldopa (G)	Aldomet	500–3,000 (2)	(Hepatic and "autoimmune" disorders)
ALPHA BLOCKERS			Postural (orthostatic) hypotension
Doxazosin mesylate	Cardura	1–16 (1)	
Prazosin hydrochloride (G)	Minipress	2–30 (2–3)	
Terazosin hydrochloride	Hytrin	1–20 (1)	
BETA BLOCKERS			Bronchospasm, bradycardia, heart failure, may mask insulin-induced hypoglycemia; less serious: impaired peripheral circulation, insomnia, fatigue, decreased exercise tolerance, hypertriglyceridemia (except agents with intrinsic sympathomimetic activity)
Acebutolol§‡	Sectral	200–800 (1)	
Atenolol (G)§	Tenormin	25–100 (1–2)	
Betaxolol§ hyperchloride	Kerlone	5–20 (1)	
Bisoprolol fumarate§	Zebeta	2.5–10 (1)	
Carteolol hydrochloride‡	Cartrol	2.5–10 (1)	
Metoprolol tartrate (G)§	Lopressor	50–300 (2)	
Metoprolol succinate§	Toprol XL	50–300 (1)	
Nadolol (G)	Corgard	40–320 (1)	
Penbutolol sulfate‡	Levatol	10–20 (1)	
Pindolol (G)‡	Visken	10–60 (2)	
Propranolol hydrochloride (G)	Inderal	40–480 (2)	
	Inderal LA	40–480 (1)	
Timolol maleate (G)	Blocadren	20–60 (2)	

(continued)

TABLE 32-12	Oral Antihypertensive Drugs* *(Continued)*

Drug	Trade Name	Usual Dose Range, Total mg/d* (Frequency per Day)	Selected Side Effects and Comments*
COMBINED ALPHA AND BETA BLOCKERS			Postural hypotension, bronchospasm
Carvedilol	Coreg	12.5–50(2)	
Labetalol hydrochloride (G)	Normodyne, Trandate	200–1,200 (2)	
Direct Vasodilators			*Headaches, fluid retention, tachycardia*
Hydralazine hydrochloride (G)	Apresoline	50–300 (2)	(Lupus syndrome)
Minoxidil (G)	Loniten	5–100 (1)	(Hirsutism)
Calcium antagonists			
NONDIHYDROPYRIDINES			Conduction defects, worsening of systolic dysfunction, gingival hyperplasia
Diltiazem hydrochloride	Cardizem SR	120–360 (2)	(Nausea, headache)
	Cardizem CD, Dilacor XR, Tiazac	120–360 (1)	
Mibefradil dihydrochloride (T-channel calcium antagonist)	Posicor	50–100 (1)	(No worsening of systolic dysfunction; contraindicated with terfenadine [Seldane], astemizole [Hismanal], and cisapride [Propulsid])
Verapamil hydrochloride	Isoptin SR, Calan SR	90–480 (2)	(Constipation)
	Verelan, Covera HS	120–480 (1)	
DIHYDROPYRIDINES			Edema of the ankle, flushing, headache, gingival hypertrophy
Amlodipine besylate	Norvasc	2.5–10 (1)	
Felodipine	Plendil	2.5–20 (1)	
Isradipine	DynaCirc	5–20 (2)	
	DynaCirc CR	5–20 (1)	
Nicardipine	Cardene SR	60–90 (2)	
Nifedipine	Procardia XL, Adalat CC	30–120 (1)	
Nisoldipine	Sular	20–60 (1)	
Angiotensin-Converting Enzyme Inhibitors			Common: cough; rare: angioedema, hyperkalemia, rash, loss of taste, leukopenia
Benazepril hydrochloride	Lotensin	5–40 (1–2)	
Captopril (G)	Capoten	25–150 (2–3)	
Enalapril maleate	Vasotec	5–40 (1–2)	
Fosinopril sodium	Monopril	10–40 (1–2)	
Lisinopril	Prinivil, Zestril	5–40 (1)	
Moexipril	Univasc	7.5–15 (1–2)	
Quinapril hydrochloride	Accupril	5–80 (1–2)	
Ramipril	Altace	1.25–20 (1–2)	
Trandolapril	Mavik	1–4 (1)	
Angiotensin II Receptor Blockers			*Angioedema (very rare), hyperkalemia*
Losartan potassium	Cozaar	25–100 (1–2)	
Valsartan	Diovan	80–320 (1)	
Irbesartan	Avapro	150–300 (1)	

*These dosages may vary from those listed in the *Physicians' Desk Reference* (51st edition), which may be consulted for additional information. The listing of side effects is not all-inclusive and side effects are for the class of drugs except where noted for individual drugs (in parentheses); clinicians are urged to refer to the package insert for a more detailed listing.

†(G) indicates generic available.

‡Has intrinsic sympathomimetic activity.

§Cardioselective.

¹¹Also acts centrally.

TABLE 32-13 Combination Drugs for Hypertension	
Drug	**Trade Name**
ß-Adrenergic Blockers and Diuretics	
Atenolol, 50 or 100 mg/chlorthalidone, 25 mg	Tenoretic
Bisoprolol fumarate, 2.5, 5, or 10 mg/hydrochlorothiazide, 6.25 mg	Ziac*
Metoprolol tartrate, 50 or 100 mg/hydrochlorothiazide, 25 or 50 mg	Lopressor HCT
Nadolol, 40 or 80 mg/bendroflumethiazide, 5 mg	Corzide
Propranolol hydrochloride, 40 or 80 mg/hydrochlorothiazide, 25 mg	Inderide
Propranolol hydrochloride (extended release), 80, 120, or 160 mg/hydrochlorothiazide, 50 mg	Inderide LA
Timolol maleate, 10 mg/hydrochlorothiazide, 25 mg	Timolide
ACE Inhibitors and Diuretics	
Benazepril hydrochloride, 5, 10, or 20 mg/hydrochlorothiazide, 6.25, 12.5, or 25 mg	Lotensin HCT
Captopril, 25 or 50 mg/hydrochlorothiazide, 15 or 25 mg	Capozide*
Enalapril maleate, 5 or 10 mg/hydrochlorothiazide, 12.5 or 25 mg	Vaseretic
Lisinopril, 10 or 20 mg/hydrochlorothiazide, 12.5 or 25 mg	Prinzide, Zestoretic
Angiotensin II Receptor Antagonists and Diuretics	
Losartan potassium, 50 mg/hydrochlorothiazide, 12.5 mg	Hyzaar
Calcium Antagonists and ACE Inhibitors	
Amlodipine besylate, 2.5 or 5 mg/benazepril hydrochloride, 10 or 20 mg	Lotrel
Diltiazem hydrochloride, 180 mg/enalapril maleate, 5 mg	Teczem
Verapamil hydrochloride (extended release), 180 or 240 mg/trandolapril, 1, 2, or 4 mg	Tarka
Felodipine, 5 mg/enalapril maleate, 5 mg	Lexxel
Other Combinations	
Triamterene, 37.5, 50, or 75 mg/hydrochlorothiazide, 25 or 50 mg	Dyazide, Maxzide
Spironolactone, 25 or 50 mg/hydrochlorothiazide, 25 or 50 mg	Aldactazide
Amiloride hydrochloride, 5 mg/hydrochlorothiazide, 50 mg	Moduretic
Guanethidine monosulfate, 10 mg/hydrochlorothiazide, 25 mg	Esimil
Hydralazine hydrochloride, 25, 50, or 100 mg/hydrochlorothiazide, 25 or 50 mg	Apresazide
Methyldopa, 250 or 500 mg/hydrochlorothiazide, 15, 25, 30, or 50 mg	Aldoril
Reserpine, 0.125 mg/hydrochlorothiazide, 25 or 50 mg	Hydropres
Reserpine, 0.10 mg/hydralazine hydrochloride, 25 mg/hydrochlorothiazide, 15 mg	Ser-Ap-Es
Clonidine hydrochloride, 0.1, 0.2, or 0.3 mg/chlorthalidone, 15 mg	Combipres
Methyldopa, 250 mg/chlorothiazide, 150 or 250 mg	Aldoclor
Reserpine, 0.125 or 0.25 mg/chlorthalidone, 25 or 50 mg	Demi-Regroton
Reserpine, 0.125 or 0.25 mg/chlorothiazide, 250 or 500 mg	Diupres
Prazosin hydrochloride, 1, 2, or 5 mg/polythiazide, 0.5 mg	Minizide

ACE, angiotensin-converting enzyme.
*Approved for initial therapy.

The parenteral drugs recommended for use in hypertensive emergencies are listed in Table 32-14. One drug that is not recommended because of the high rate of adverse events that accompanies its use is sublingual nifedipine.[84] The oral medications recommended for use in urgencies are ones with a fast onset of action, such as loop diuretics, beta blockers, calcium antagonists, α_2-agonists, and ACE inhibitors.[243] The guidelines for the management of hypertensive emergencies specify that during the first treatment period of up to 2 hours, the initial mean BP should not be lowered by more than 25% of its initial value. A subsequent target BP is approximately 160/100 mm Hg. The goal is to reduce the pressure so that target organ damage is prevented or minimized while preventing the cerebral or myocardial ischemia that could result from too rapid a reduction in pressure.[256]

BLOOD PRESSURE MANAGEMENT IN SPECIAL POPULATIONS

The management of hypertension is modified based on the characteristics of the individual patient as well as additional knowledge about care in specific groups. The following sections outline some additional information that guides the

TABLE 32-14   Parenteral Drugs for Treatment of Hypertensive Emergencies*

Drug	Dose	Onset of Action	Duration of Action	Adverse Effects‡	Special Indications
Vasodilators					
Sodium nitroprusside	0.25–10 µg/kg/min as IV infusion‡ (maximal dose for 10 min only)	Immediate	1–2 min	Nausea, vomiting, muscle twitching, sweating, thiocyanate and cyanide intoxication	Most hypertensive emergencies; caution with high intracranial pressure or azotemia
Nicardipine hydrochloride	5–15 mg/h IV	5–10 min	1–4 h	Tachycardia, headache, flushing, local phlebitis	Most hypertensive emergencies except acute heart failure; caution with coronary ischemia
Fenoldopam mesylate	0.1–0.3 µg/kg/min IV infusion	<5 min	30 min	Tachycardia, headache, nausea, flushing	Most hypertensive emergencies; caution with glaucoma
Nitroglycerin	5–100 µg/min as IV infusion§	2–5 min	3–5 min	Headache, vomiting, methemoglobinemia, tolerance with prolonged use	Coronary ischemia
Enalaprilat	1.25–5 mg every 6 h IV	15–30 min	6 h	Precipitous fall in pressure in high-renin states; response variable	Acute left ventricular failure; avoid in acute myocardial infarction
Hydralazine hydrochloride	10–20 mg IV 10–50 mg IM	10–20 min 20–30 min	3–8 h	Tachycardia, flushing, headache, vomiting, aggravation of angina	Eclampsia
Diazoxide	50–100 mg IV bolus repeated, or 15–30 mg/min infusion	2–4 min	6–12 h	Nausea, flushing, tachycardia, chest pain	Now obsolete; when no intensive monitoring available
Adrenergic Inhibitors					
Labetalol hydrochloride	20–80 mg IV bolus every 10 min 0.5–2.0 mg/min IV infusion	5–10 min	3–6 h	Vomiting, scalp tingling, burning in throat, dizziness, nausea, heart block, orthostatic hypotension	Most hypertensive emergencies except acute heart failure
Esmolol hydrochloride	250–500 µg/kg/min for 1 min, then 50–100 µg/kg/min for 4 min; may repeat sequence	1–2 min	10–20 min	Hypotension, nausea	Aortic dissection, perioperative
Phentolamine mesylate	5–15 mg IV	1–2 min	3–10 min	Tachycardia, flushing, headache	Catecholamine excess

IV, intravenous; IM, intramuscular.
*These doses may vary from those in the *Physicians' Desk Reference* (51st edition).
†Hypotension may occur with all agents.
‡Require special delivery system.

management of high BP in the elderly, in pregnancy, and in people with other conditions such as diabetes, renal disease, and hyperlipidemia.

The Elderly. The elderly experience both systolic diastolic hypertension as well as isolated systolic hypertension. Isolated systolic hypertension is defined as a systolic BP greater than 160 mm Hg with a diastolic pressure less than 90 mm Hg.[243] Borderline isolated systolic hypertension is a systolic BP of 140 to 159 mm Hg with a diastolic pressure below 90 mm Hg.[215] In Europe, the upper limit of diastolic pressure in isolated systolic hypertension is 95 mm Hg.[9,234]

The incidence of isolated systolic hypertension increases with age. One study reported an incidence of 7% in people older than 70 years of age, and in people older than 80 years of age the incidence was over 25%.[233] Analysis of data from the Framingham Heart Study reveals that even borderline systolic hypertension is associated with significant morbidity and mortality.[215] People with borderline isolated systolic pressure had increased risks for all cardiovascular disease, coronary heart disease, stroke, transient ischemic attack, heart failure, and mortality from cardiovascular disease. The hazard ratios for each of these were significant, ranging from 1.42 to 1.60 after the data had been adjusted for sex, decade of age, cholesterol level, body mass index, cigarette smoking, and glucose intolerance. In a community study of BP in 3,657 elderly people in East Boston, a linear relationship between systolic BP and mortality was identified. A person's risk of cardiovascular and total mortality increased with his or her systolic BP.[80]

Several large, randomized trials have demonstrated the benefits of BP control in the elderly.[9,42,174,223,234] A meta-analysis of five clinical trials on people older than 60 years of age found that treatment reduced the incidence of coronary heart disease by 19% and stroke by 34%.[159] The largest study, the Systolic Hypertension in the Elderly Program (SHEP), had a population of 4,736 men and women older than age 60 years with a mean baseline BP of 170/70 mm Hg.[223] The goal of this clinical trial was to determine drug efficacy, side effects, and long-term outcomes related to morbidity and mortality from cardiovascular disease. With the 17 mm Hg reduction in mean systolic pressure in the treatment group compared with the control group, there was a significant decrease in the incidence of stroke. No serious short-term side effects occurred as a result of treatment. The Swedish Trial in Old Patients with Hypertension (STOP-Hypertension) studied a group of 1,627 subjects with both systolic and diastolic hypertension (mean entry BP, 195/102 mm Hg). In the group treated with diuretics or beta blockers, there was a mean drop in BP of 27/9 mm Hg, with statistically significant declines in both fatal and nonfatal strokes and congestive heart failure. This study showed the benefit of treating elderly patients with both systolic and diastolic hypertension.

Treatment of the elderly is similar to that of younger clients. More emphasis can be put on lifestyle management, including weight loss, sodium restriction, and exercise, because of the multiple benefits to the older person.[22] Physical activity, for example, offers not only reduction of BP but weight management, reduced disability, and decreased mortality.[139,257] The same medications are used in the elderly, but smaller initial doses are recommended and there may be more comorbid conditions that make one medication a better choice than another. Cost is also a factor because many elderly people have a limited income. Because the elderly have an increased sensitivity to orthostatic hypotension, caution is required with drugs that may cause dizziness on standing, such as diuretics in large doses, peripheral adrenergic blockers, and alpha blockers.[243]

Hypertension in Pregnancy. High BP occurs in pregnancy either because of preexisting chronic high BP or because of the development of pregnancy-induced hypertension, including gestational hypertension, preeclampsia, and eclampsia. Elevated BP (>140/90 mm Hg) in a woman before she becomes pregnant, that develops before the 20th week of pregnancy, or that persists more than six weeks after delivery, is considered chronic hypertension.[181] Gestational hypertension is defined as an elevated BP that usually occurs in the third trimester and is not accompanied by other signs and symptoms.[227] In preeclampsia and eclampsia, the elevated BP is considered one of several signs and symptoms of an underlying disorder of organ perfusion. Edema and proteinuria usually occur with pregnancy-induced hypertension. Although there has been controversy over whether the fourth or fifth Korotkoff sound should be used to indicate diastolic pressure in pregnant women, research now indicates that the fifth sound is closer to actual intra-arterial pressure and should therefore be used.[27]

Table 32-15 lists the JNC VI recommendations about drugs to be used to treat high BP in pregnant women. Neither the ACE inhibitors nor the angiotensin II receptor blocking agents or atenolol should be used in pregnancy.[227] Methyldopa is considered the drug of choice because of the long experience with its use and the lack of adverse impact on mother and infant.[243]

Diabetes Mellitus and Hypertension. Risk factor clustering is found in patients with diabetes mellitus.[19,33,50,169,249] In one study, 57% of people with non–insulin-dependent diabetes were found to have hypertension.[26] Because of reductions in mortality and progression to end-stage renal disease, JNC VI has set the goal BP for people with both diabetes and hypertension at less than 130/85 mm Hg.[144,243] Lifestyle interventions, including weight control and exercise, are crucial to BP control in people with diabetes.[109,197] Because of their lack of adverse effects on blood glucose levels, serum lipids, and renal function, the recommended medications are ACE inhibitors, alpha blockers, calcium antagonists, and low-dose diuretics.[13,147]

Renal Disease and Hypertension. Control of hypertension has been shown to be extremely effective in preventing the progression of renal failure in people with renal disease.[126,127,144] JNC VI has set the goal BP for people with renal disease at a minimum of 130/85 mm Hg and suggested an even lower goal of 125/75 mm Hg for people with proteinuria of more than 1 g of protein per 24-hour period.[243] The lifestyle interventions that have been shown to be effective in controlling BP in people with renal disease are restriction of sodium intake to less than 100 mmol/d and restriction of dietary protein. One small study of 15 subjects with hypertensive diabetic nephropathy demonstrated that calcium channel antagonist therapy with long-acting diltiazem was effective in reducing albuminuria only when sodium intake was also restricted to 50 mmol/d.[14] When the BP was lowered equivalently but the subjects were on a high-sodium (250 mmol/d) diet, there was no decrease in albuminuria. JNC VI recommends use of ACE inhibitors in treating people with hypertension and renal

TABLE 32-15   Antihypertensive Drugs Used in Pregnancy*[243]

The report of the NHBPEP Working Group on High Blood Pressure in Pregnancy[181] permits continuation of drug therapy in women with chronic hypertension (except for ACE inhibitors). In addition, angiotensin II receptor blockers should not be used during pregnancy. In women with chronic hypertension with diastolic levels of 100 mm Hg or greater (lower when end-organ damage or underlying renal disease is present), and in women with acute hypertension when levels are 105 mm Hg or greater, the following agents are suggested.

Suggested Drug	Comments
Central α-agonists	Methyldopa (C) is the drug of choice recommended by the NHBPEP Working Group.[181]
Beta blockers	Atenolol (C) and metoprolol (C) appear to be safe and effective in late pregnancy. Labetalol (C) also appears to be effective (alpha and beta blockers).
Calcium antagonists	Potential synergism with magnesium sulfate may lead to precipitous hypotension. (C)
ACE inhibitors, angiotensin II receptor blockers	Fetal abnormalities, including death, can be caused, and these drugs should not be used in pregnancy. (D)
Diuretics	Diuretics (C) are recommended for chronic hypertension if prescribed before gestation or if patients appear to be salt sensitive. They are not recommended in preeclampsia.
Direct vasodilators	Hydralazine (C) is the parenteral drug of choice based on its long history of safety and efficacy. (C)

ACE, angiotensin-converting enzyme; NHBPEP, National High Blood Pressure Education Program.
*There are several other antihypertensive drugs for which there are very limited data. The U.S. Food and Drug Administration classifies pregnancy risk as follows: C, adverse effects in animals; no controlled trials in humans; use if risk appears justified; D, positive evidence of fetal risk.
Adapted from Lindheimer MD: Pre-clampsia-eclampsia 1996: preventable? Have disputes on its treatment been resolved? Current opinion in Nephrology and Hypertension5: 452–458, 1996.

disease because there have been several clinical trials demonstrating their effectiveness.[79,163]

Hyperlipidemia and Hypertension. Dyslipidemia is another of the cardiovascular risk factors that clusters with hypertension.[33] The dyslipidemia includes a low high-density lipoprotein cholesterol level and high levels of low-density lipoprotein cholesterol and triglycerides. In people with hypertension, this clustering is important because some antihypertensive medications, particularly higher doses of both thiazide and loop diuretics and beta blockers are known to have adverse effects on serum lipids.[122] Weight loss and physical activity are lifestyle interventions that have been shown both to lower BP and improve dyslipidemia.[83,235]

Achieving Blood Pressure Control

Despite the impressive array of lifestyle and pharmacologic treatments for high BP and the existence of the National High Blood Pressure Education Program since 1972, the awareness, treatment, and control rates of hypertension are low. Table 32-6 shows the levels of these factors that have been measured in the National Health and Nutrition Examination Surveys three times since 1976 in the United States. In 1991 to 1994, only slightly over half of the people with

hypertension were treated, and only 27% had their BPs controlled to less than 140/90 mm Hg. A survey of 56,026 patients in The Netherlands found that BP was not controlled in 30% of the women and 47% of the men with hypertension.[129] This lack of success in managing high BP has many contributing factors.[57,212] These are explored by looking at the groups that influence the management of hypertension and focusing on what each group can do to improve BP control. Some of the actions that care providers, patients, and health care organizations can take to improve BP control are listed in Table 32-16. Although the terms *adherence* and *compliance* are often used in discussions of BP control, they are not used here because their use implies that the patient is mainly responsible for poor BP control.

ROLE OF HEALTH CARE PROFESSIONALS

Health care providers in partnership with clients hold the keys to BP control. The provider's responsibilities range from knowing and using the latest guidelines for BP control to motivating the client to follow the treatment plan. At a minimum, the challenges to a provider include correctly diagnosing the client's condition; communicating the importance of BP as both a disease and as a risk factor for atherosclerosis; prescribing an effective treatment plan that

TABLE 32-16	Actions to Increase Compliance With Prevention and Treatment Recommendations
Actions	**Specific Strategies**

Actions by Patients

Actions	Specific Strategies
Patients must engage in essential prevention and treatment behaviors.	
Decide to control risk factors.	Understand rationale, importance of commitment.
Negotiate goals with provider.	Develop communication skills.
Develop skills for adopting and maintaining recommended behaviors.	Use reminder systems.
Monitor progress toward goals.	Use self-monitoring skills.
Resolve problems that block achievement of goals.	Develop problem-solving skills, use social support networks.
	Define own needs on basis of experience.
Patients must communicate with providers about prevention and treatment services.	
	Validate rationale for continuing to follow recommendations.

Actions by Providers

Actions	Specific Strategies
Providers must foster effective communication with patients.	
Provide clear, direct messages about importance of a behavior or therapy.	Provide oral and written instruction, including rationale for treatments.
	Develop skills in communication/counseling.
Include patients in decisions about prevention and treatment goals and related strategies.	Use tailoring and contracting strategies.
	Negotiate goals and a plan.
	Anticipate barriers to compliance and discuss solutions.
Incorporate behavioral strategies into counseling.	Use active listening.
	Develop multicomponent strategies (ie., cognitive and behavioral).
Providers must document and respond to patient's progress toward goals.	
Create an evidence-based practice.	Determine methods of evaluating outcomes.
Assess patient's compliance at each visit.	Use self-report or electronic data.
Develop a reminder system to ensure identification and follow-up of patient status.	Use telephone follow-up.

Actions by Health Care Organizations

Actions	Specific Strategies
Develop an environment that supports prevention and treatment interventions.	Develop training in behavioral science, office set-up for all personnel.
	Use preappointment reminders.
	Use telephone follow-up.
	Schedule evening/weekend office hours.
	Provide group/individual counseling for patients and families.
Provide tracking and reporting systems.	Develop computer-based systems (electronic medical records).
Provide education and training for providers.	Require continuing education courses in communication, behavioral counseling.
Provide adequate reimbursement for allocation of time for all health care professionals.	Develop incentives tied to desired patient and provider outcomes.
Adopt systems to incorporate innovations rapidly and efficiently into medical practice.	Incorporate nursing case management.
	Implement pharmacy patient profile and recall review systems.
	Use of electronic transmission storage of patient's self-monitored data.
	Obtain patient data on lifestyle behavior before visit.
	Provide continuous quality improvement training.

Adapted from Miller NH, Hill MN, Kottke T, Ockene IS: The multilevel compliance challenge: Recommendations for a call to action. Circulation 95: 1085–1090, 1997. Reprinted with permission.

DISPLAY 32-5

Preventing, Monitoring, and Addressing Problems of Adherence

EDUCATE ABOUT CONDITIONS AND TREATMENT

◆ Assess patient's understanding and acceptance of the diagnosis and expectations of being in care.
◆ Discuss patient's concerns and clarify misunderstandings.
◆ Inform patient of blood pressure level.
◆ Agree with patient on a goal blood pressure.
◆ Inform patient about recommended treatment and provide specific written information.
◆ Elicit concerns and questions and provide opportunities for patient to state specific behaviors to carry out treatment recommendations.
◆ Emphasize need to continue treatment, that patient cannot tell if blood pressure is elevated, and that control does not mean cure.

INDIVIDUALIZE THE REGIMEN

◆ Include patient in decision making.
◆ Simplify the regimen.
◆ Incorporate treatment into patient's daily lifestyle.
◆ Set, with the patient, realistic short-term objectives for specific components of the treatment plan.
◆ Encourage discussion of side effects and concerns.
◆ Encourage self-monitoring.
◆ Minimize cost of therapy.
◆ Indicate you will ask about adherence at next visit.
◆ When weight loss is established as a treatment goal, discourage quick weight loss regimens, fasting, or unscientific methods, because these are associated with weight cycling which may increase cardiovascular morbidity and mortality.

PROVIDE REINFORCEMENT

◆ Provide feedback regarding blood pressure level.
◆ Ask about behaviors to achieve blood pressure control.
◆ Give positive feedback for behavioral and blood pressure improvement.
◆ Hold exit interviews to clarify regimen.
◆ Make appointment for next visit before patient leaves the office.
◆ Use appointment reminders and contact patients to confirm appointments.
◆ Schedule more frequent visits to counsel nonadherent patients.
◆ Contact and follow up patients who missed appointments.
◆ Consider clinician–patient contracts.

PROMOTE SOCIAL SUPPORT

◆ Educate family members to be part of the blood pressure control process and provide daily reinforcement.
◆ Suggest small group activities to enhance mutual support and motivation.

COLLABORATE WITH OTHER PROFESSIONALS

◆ Draw on complementary skills and knowledge of nurses, pharmacists, dietitians, optometrists, dentists, and physician assistants.
◆ Refer patients for more intensive counseling.

National High Blood Pressure Education Program: The Fifth Report of the Joint National Committee on Detection, Evaluation, and Treatment of High Blood Pressure. NIH publication no. 93–1088. Bethesda, MD, US Department of Health and Human Services National Institutes of Health, 1994.

fits the client's lifestyle and economic situation; and evaluating the results of the therapy. To achieve these goals, the care provider needs skills in assessment, diagnosis, communication, and behavioral counseling. The care provider has the responsibility of ensuring that the client is educated about his or her condition and the treatment plan. Display 32-5 summarizes strategies that health care providers can use to improve BP control. Some medical and nursing schools include courses in risk factor management and health promotion in their curricula and offer students clinical opportunities to practice the skills required to support clients in effective disease prevention and risk factor management.[187] There remains a need for more research on effective methods to promote behavior change, because the traditional professional approaches of screening, patient education, and counseling have had little impact on secondary risk factors such as obesity.[141]

The adequacy of the care of 800 hypertensive veterans with an average age of 65.5 years was evaluated over a two-year period.[20] The researchers found that less than 25% of the patients had pressures under 140/90 mm Hg, and 40% had pressures over 160/90 mm Hg despite 2 years of treatment for high BP with an average of five medical-clinic visits yearly. The patients who received the most intensive or aggressive treatment were most likely to have their BPs con-

trolled. The researchers interpreted their findings as indicating that physicians need to be more aggressive in their management of high BP. The clinical trials of BP control have demonstrated the potential impact of BP reduction on morbidity and mortality, but if health care providers do not prescribe adequate therapy to lower BP, this potential will never be realized.

ROLE OF CLIENTS

The challenge for clients in achieving BP control is to modify their lives in ways that support their treatment plan. Making the decision to control BP is the critical client factor that precedes lifestyle modification and BP control.[266] Based on their Transtheoretical Model of Behavior Change, Prochaska and DiClemente[202,203] have developed a set of questions that the health care provider can use to stage where the client is in the process of making the decision to change (Display 32-6). The Transtheoretical Model postulates that people go through a series of stages in the process of changing behavior. The stages are precontemplation, contemplation, preparation, action, and maintenance. The actual decision to change comes between preparation and action. A relapse can occur at any time and sends a person back to an earlier stage, usually either precontemplation or

---

DISPLAY 32-6

Determining a Client's Stage of Change Based on the Transtheoretical Model of Change

STEP ONE

Ask the client to respond to the following true/false statements. (Note: these statements are for exercise; the clinician can replace the word *exercise* with whatever behavior is the topic of discussion.)

1. I currently do not exercise.
2. I intend to exercise in the next 6 months.
3. I currently exercise regularly.
4. I have exercised regularly for the past 6 months.

STEP TWO

Use the following scoring system to determine where your client is in the process of change.

Precontemplation: 1 = true, 2 = false
Contemplation: 1 = true, 2 = true
Preparation: 1 = false, 2 = true, 3 = false
Action: 3 = true, 4 = false
Maintenance: 3 = true, 4 = true

STEP THREE

Once the client's stage of change for the behavior of interest has been determined, use the suggestions in Table 32-17 as a guide for planning an intervention to help the client move toward the next change stage. If the client is in the maintenance or termination stages, support their healthy choice.

Adapted from Prochaska JO, DiClemente CC: Stages and processes of self-change of smoking: Toward integrative model of change. J Consult Clin Psychol 51: 310–395, 1983.

---

contemplation. Use of the questions and the Transtheoretical Model allows clinicians to tailor their interventions to the patient's stage of change—and prevents them from wasting time developing a detailed plan of action for the person who is not yet ready to change. Table 32-17 lists the stages of change and some suggested strategies appropriate to each stage.

ROLE OF HEALTH CARE ORGANIZATIONS

Some of the actions that health care organizations can take to improve BP control are listed in Display 32-5. Health-System Minnesota (Minneapolis, Minnesota) has implemented a hypertension services program using a team approach, with nurse coordinators delivering primary care in partnership with patients and physicians.[31] Health care organizations have the opportunity to provide education for both providers and patients; set standards of care; implement computerized data systems; document the impact of care on patient outcomes; and determine which types of care are cost effective while maintaining quality of life.[21]

ROLE OF PUBLIC HEALTH FOR THE COMMUNITY

Community-based interventions in the United States and Europe have demonstrated that community action can reduce the risks of cardiovascular disease.[64,208] Data collected using a nationwide, yearly telephone survey of adults' risk factors and preventive practices indicate that there are geographic/regional variations in the prevalence of risk factors. It is believed that this regional variability is related to the local sociocultural environment, which may or may not promote risk factor reduction.[89] Such variability of risk, and the evidence that community programs can affect risk, challenges

---

TABLE 32-17 **The Stages of Change With Definitions, Interventions Appropriate to Each Step, and the Goal of Care at Each Stage**

Stage	Definition	Interventions	Goal of Care
Precontemplation	No intention to change	Information on risk Support, "I'm here when you are ready." Clear message	Move to contemplation
Contemplation	Considering change No commitment	Targeted information on benefits of change	Move to preparation
Preparation	Ready to change Some commitment	Skill development Self-monitoring	Move to action
Action	Made change within last 6 mo More committed	Set realistic goals Select strategies to support change	Maintain action Move to maintenance
Maintenance	Made change >6 mo ago Committed	Relapse prevention Management of high-risk situations Planned relapse	Maintain change Move to termination
Termination	Change is now part of regular lifestyle	Support Provide latest information	Maintain

Adapted from Prochaska JO, DiClemente CC: Stages and processes of self-change of smoking: Toward an integrative model of change. J Consult Clin Psychol 51: 390–395, 1983.

communities to initiate projects that promote healthy lifestyles. Kalamazoo, Michigan and the state of Kansas have developed programs to reduce chronic disease risk by promoting healthy diets and exercise.[53,192] The National High Blood Pressure Program suggests that community programs should have the goals of promoting the intake of foods lower in calorie and sodium content and higher in potassium; increased physical activity; and moderation in alcohol intake.[179] Other suggested roles for community programs are increasing awareness of risk factors, supporting entry into the health care system, and supporting people in following their treatment plans.[58] The National High Blood Pressure Education Program also has resources to support the development of community programs in schools, churches, sporting events, and workplaces as well as in rural, suburban, urban, and inner-city settings.[243]

In the early years of community programs, the emphasis was on screening to identify people with hypertension.[111] In subsequent years, the emphasis of community programs was shifted toward integrated cardiovascular risk factor management, and screening was recommended only for populations considered to be at high risk for having large numbers of people with undetected high BP.[1,178] BP screenings may be done as part of local events such as health fairs. If a BP screening is included in such an event, it is important that there be mechanisms for following up any person found to have an elevated pressure and that the screeners have the latest recommendations on follow-up, as shown in Table 32-7.

ROLE OF POLICY

The impressive impact of legislation to reduce smoking in public places, such as airplanes, highlights the powerful role of policy in the reduction of cardiovascular risk. In the area of hypertension, national policy makers can encourage the food manufacturing and marketing industries to reduce the sodium, calorie, and saturated fat content of processed foods as well as make information about diet and risk available at points of food purchase.[179] Another important policy arena is assurance of the provision of health care and payment for medications for people without health insurance.[55] Finally, continuation of the policy of funding basic and applied research related to cardiovascular disease is important to unraveling the causes of primary hypertension.

TEAM APPROACH TO BLOOD PRESSURE MANAGEMENT

The optimal management of high BP requires the collaboration of health care professionals.[36,173] Team members include the client, health educator, nurse, nutritionist, pharmacist, and physician. The Mayo Clinic has documented its successful use of a hypertension clinic that uses the team approach. In this setting, the patient's care is managed by the nurse clinician. Successful teams require expertise in communication and coordination, and an appreciation of the skills of each team member.[36]

The Role of Nursing in Blood Pressure Management

Nurses and nursing have a role in all aspects of hypertension management, from taking BPs, to research, to setting national policy. The role of the individual nurse depends on that person's preparation and work experience. The successful use of nurses to manage patients with hypertension has been reported in the literature since the 1970s.[38,152,199,221,231] The current era of cost containment and advanced preparation for nurse practitioners creates a climate for further development of the nurse's role in hypertension management.

NURSING DIAGNOSES

The nursing diagnoses for the person with hypertension are derived from data collected to formulate a complete and accurate nursing assessment. These diagnoses may include the following:

1. Knowledge deficit about the disease process of high BP, its consequences, and treatment, related to lack of effective teaching as manifested by verbal acknowledgement of a deficiency in knowledge, expressions of an inaccurate perception of health status, or incorrect performance of the desired or prescribed health behavior
2. Potential ineffective management of therapeutic regimen: noncompliance, related to knowledge deficit, failure to follow a prescribed regimen, inadequate support system, or lack of involvement in the treatment plan
3. Potential ineffective coping related to the lack of motivation to respond, depression in response to the stress of a chronic disease, or unsatisfactory support system
4. Potential fluid volume deficit related to abnormal fluid loss due to use of diuretics
5. Potential alteration in tissue perfusion: cardiovascular, related to hypertension and cerebrovascular blood flow

Nursing Care Plan 32-1 summarizes care for two of the most important nursing diagnoses.

GOALS

General goals for people who have hypertension are the following:

1. Achievement and maintenance of goal BP
2. Understanding, participating in, and implementing the prescribed treatment plan
3. Movement toward adapting to a chronic condition that increases the risk of atherosclerotic cardiovascular disease and stroke
4. Confidence in ability to cope with hypertension within the demands of daily life

NURSING CARE PLAN 32-1 ◆ The Patient With Hypertension

Nursing Diagnosis 1:	Knowledge deficit about the disease process, its consequences and treatment related to lack of effective teaching as manifested by verbal acknowledgment of knowledge deficit, inaccurate perception of health care status, and failure to perform the desired or prescribed health behaviors
Nursing Goal:	To detect early and reduce signs and symptoms of knowledge deficit
Outcome Criteria:	The patient will be able to ◆ Describe the disease process and the causes and factors contributing to the course of the disease ◆ Describe the procedure for hypertension control ◆ Actively participate in health behaviors prescribed or desired ◆ Experience less anxiety related to fear of loss of control, misconceptions, or misinformation Blood pressure will be maintained within normal limits

NURSING INTERVENTION

1. Assess, document, and report factors contributing to knowledge deficit.
   a. Level of knowledge
   b. Emotional readiness for learning
   c. Stage of change (Display 32–6)
   d. Support system
   e. Health beliefs
2. Provide patient with additional information regarding pathology, general well-being (dietary habits, weight control, alcohol, exercise, caffeine, smoking, stress management), and risks of uncontrolled high blood pressure.
3. Develop an individualized teaching plan based on patient's knowledge, habits, and experience.
4. Initiate behavior modification methods.
   a. Have patient keep written diary of activities, diet, and medication over a week's time.
   b. Ask patient to recall activities, dietary intake, and medication over a 2-day period.
   c. Teach patient to take and record own blood pressure, and to record factors of concern.
   d. Explore patient's beliefs in relation to his or her identified behaviors.
5. Discuss drug actions, interactions, and side effects.

   a. Discuss potential for sexual dysfunction.

   b. Discuss replacing oral contraceptives with other birth control methods.
   c. Provide information about possibility of interactions with over-the-counter drugs such as cough or cold medications.
   d. Discuss general side effects of drugs: light-headedness, lethargy, orthostatic hypotension.

   e. Teach patient to increase large muscle activity or lie down briefly if hypotensive effects occur.

RATIONALE

1. Learning needs differ depending on the dispositions and conditions that influence patient's health behavior. Assessment before developing a teaching plan ensures greater efficiency, appropriateness, and success of teaching and learning process.

2. Enables patient to make choices about lifestyle changes and adherence to medical regimen.

3. Same rationale as no. 1 above.

4. Patient education and opportunities to make voluntary adaptions of behavior will improve or maintain health. This implies active involvement of the patient in his or her own care and assumes that the patient takes responsibility for learning.[266]

5. Knowledge, attitudes, and skills of the four critical patient behaviors are essential to taking medication and ultimately to achievement of long-term blood pressure control.[266]
   a. Antihypertensive medications affect the autonomic nervous system, which plays a part in libidinal reactions. Change in drug or dosage may relieve signs and symptoms.
   b. Oral contraceptives may increase renin production by the kidney and increase BP.
   c. May contain sympathomimetic agents, which may increase BP or counteract antihypertensive effects.
   d. Upright position produces decrease in venous return because of decreased BP, decreased systemic vascular resistance, and decreased cardiac output.

(continued)

NURSING CARE PLAN 32-1 ◆ The Patient With Hypertension (Continued)

Nursing Diagnosis 2: Potential ineffective management of therapeutic regimen: noncompliance to long-term disease management, related to the chronic nature of the disease, knowledge deficit, inability to follow treatment regimens, lack of social support, or a lack of active involvement in self-care as manifested by verbalization of nonparticipation, missed appointments, partially used or unused medications, persistence of symptoms, or progression of the disease process

Nursing Goal: To promote development of a treatment plan acceptable to the patient and understanding of disease control

Outcome Criteria: The patient will
  ◆ Assume responsibility for self-care as able
  ◆ Develop personal and health care goals that contribute to following the treatment plan and control of high blood pressure

NURSING INTERVENTION	RATIONALE
1. Assess patient's perception of his illness and its treatment.	1. Inaccurate perceptions held by the patient about his or her disease and its treatment must be identified and corrected. Misunderstandings of the nature and seriousness of the illness and susceptibility to complications can greatly affect compliance.

2. Assess patient's self-care performance.
  a. Determine baseline actions regarding medications, diet, weight, exercise, stress management, smoking, and alcohol.
  b. Monitor and record improvement in following the treatment plan.
	2. Assessment of patient participation is best accomplished by asking patients in a nonjudgmental way if they have problems in following the prescribed regimen.

3. Develop a system for patient tracking.
  a. Patient contact system—mail, telephone, and personal contact
  b. Record-keeping system—patient outcomes, teaching plan, patient education, prescription refills, progress in adherence
  c. Alert system to signal need for patient contact (missed appointments, laboratory results, and so forth)
	3. A tracking system improves adherence and consequently BP control. Increased contact between the patient and the health care provider is essential to participation, communication, and learning.

4. Encourage the patient to express any fears or frustrations he or she has related to health needs.	4. Fears and frustrations about prescribed treatment (whether valid or not) can interfere with following the treatment plan and must be discussed openly for effective problem solving to take place.

5. Explain the regimen to the patient.
  a. Discuss benefits, problems, or inconvenience.
  b. Assist patient to incorporate regimen into everyday life (written medication schedule, diet, lifestyle modification, appointment keeping, multimedia information).
	5. Patient participation and satisfaction is enhanced when patient–clinician interaction is good and when patient is actively involved in decisions about self-care. Explicit instructions and focusing on one task or skill at a time help to ensure mastery of critical behaviors for BP control.[266]

6. Provide continual feedback and reinforcement of treatment plan.	6. Same rationale as diagnosis no. 1, rationale no. 1.

7. Simplify the therapeutic regimen.
  a. Provide written instructions on medication dosage, schedule side effects, and goals of therapy.
  b. Schedule medication taking in association with daily activities.
  c. Stress not stopping or changing medication without calling clinician.
	7. Same rationale as no. 5 above.

(continued)

NURSING CARE PLAN 32-1 ◆ The Patient With Hypertension (Continued)

NURSING INTERVENTION	RATIONALE

8. Encourage active participation by the patient and his or her family.
   a. Identify desirable self-care behaviors (make decision to control BP, follow treatment plan, monitor progress toward goal BP, resolve barriers blocking BP control).
   b. Take home BP measurements.
   c. Keep a graphic record of BP and medication schedule, dosage, and side effects.
   d. Assist in planning menus, shopping for and preparation of meals.
9. Devise a verbal or written contract with the patient specifying each particular behavior to be changed.
	8. People are more likely to take an active role in their care if they believe that they have control over treatment outcomes. Helps the patient to be more aware of BP and treatment trends and places emphasis on therapeutic goals. The focus is on the outcome as well as the problems encountered.[266]
	
	9. Contracting increases patient participation in care and encourages behavior modification.

CLIENT EDUCATION

The nurse shares the responsibility for client teaching with other members of the care team. In individual situations, it may be either the nurse or health educator who assumes responsibility for ensuring that the client does learn about his or her high BP. Some of the barriers to successful client education are low literacy, lack of understanding of the importance of treating a condition without apparent symptoms, language differences, and great variability in health beliefs, perceptions, and priorities.[70,265] The National High Blood Pressure Education Program and the American Heart Association are good sources for patient education materials in English. The American Heart Association also has some materials in Spanish. Both agencies maintain web sites with directions for downloading or acquiring their materials.

EVALUATION

Evaluation of goal achievement is based on whether the goal BP has been attained, whether the patient's participation in the treatment regimen is improved, and whether the teaching goals for the patient with high BP are met. In essence, goal achievement consists of adaptation to, and the ability to cope with, a chronic, lifelong condition.

Another aspect of evaluation is the nurse's evaluation of her performance as a care provider to people with high BP. Is the nurse measuring BP according to the recognized standards? Is the nurse explaining to every client the meaning of the systolic and diastolic BP numbers? Does the nurse see every encounter with the client as an opportunity to learn and teach? The encounter can be an opportunity to learn how the client is managing, whether he or she is experiencing side effects, and whether the educational materials are in the relevant language and at the correct literacy level. If the nurse is running a hypertension clinic—what is the control rate for high BP in her clinic? Are all clients leaving with a clear understanding of what they should do when they get home or what types of medications they are taking? Because all clients with high BP have at least one risk factor for atherosclerotic cardiovascular disease, do all clients know the signs and symptoms for heart attacks and stroke, and what to do if they have these signs or symptoms?

REFERENCES

1. The Fifth Report of the Joint National Committee on Detection, Evaluation, and Treatment of High Blood Pressure (JNC V). Arch Intern Med 153: 154–183, 1993
2. Stroke (Brain Attack) Page. American Heart Association World Wide Web site. Available: http://www.american-heart.org/statistics/05stroke.html, February 2, 1999
3. Ahmed ME, Walker JM, Beevers DG et al: Lack of difference between malignant and accelerated hypertension. BMJ 292: 235–237, 1986
4. Alderman MH, Cohen H, Roqué R et al: Effect of long-acting and short-acting calcium antagonists on cardiovascular outcomes in hypertensive patients. Lancet 349: 594–598, 1997
5. Allender SP, Cutler JA, Follmann D et al: Dietary calcium and blood pressure: A meta-analysis of randomized clinical trials. Ann Intern Med 124: 825–831, 1996
6. Amerena J, Julius S: The role of the autonomic nervous system in hypertension. Hypertens Res 18: 99–110, 1995
7. American Heart Association: 1998 Heart and Stroke Statistical Update. Dallas, American Heart Association, 1997
8. American Society for Hypertension: Recommendations for routine blood pressure measurement by indirect cuff sphygmomanometry. Am J Hypertens 5: 207–209, 1992
9. Amery A, Birkenhäger W, Brixko P et al: Mortality and morbidity results from the European working party on high blood pressure in the elderly trial. Lancet 1: 1349–1354, 1985
10. Anderson S: Pathogenesis of hypertensive renal damage. In Izzo JL Jr, Black HR (eds): Hypertension Primer, pp 190–193. Philadelphia, Lippincott Williams & Wilkins, 1999
11. Appel LJ, Moore TJ, Obarzanek E et al: A clinical trial of the effects of dietary patterns on blood pressure. N Engl J Med 336: 1117–1124, 1997

12. Arakawa K: Hypertension and exercise. Clin Exp Hypertens 15: 1171–1179, 1993

13. Bakris GL, Mangrum A, Copley JB et al: Effect of calcium channel or beta-blockade on the progression of diabetic nephropathy in African Americans. Hypertension 29: 744–750, 1997

14. Bakris GL, Smith A: Effects of sodium intake on albumin excretion in patients with diabetic nephropathy treated with long-acting calcium antagonists. Ann Intern Med 125: 201–204, 1996

15. Bataineh A, Raij L: Angiotensin II, nitric oxide, and end-organ damage in hypertension. Kidney Int Suppl 68: S14–S19, 1998

16. Baumbach GL, Heistad DD: Cerebrovascular disease: Cerebrovascular disease in experimental models of hypertension. In Swales JD (ed): Textbook of hypertension, pp 682–690. Oxford, Blackwell, 1994

17. Beilin LJ, Puddey IB: Alcohol and hypertension. Clinical and Experimental Hypertension: Part A, Theory and Practice 14: 119–138, 1992

18. Benigni A, Remuzzi G: Endothelin antagonists. Lancet 353: 133–138, 1999

19. Berenson GS, Srinivasan SR, Bao W: Precursors of cardiovascular risk in young adults from a biracial (black-white) population: The Bogalusa Heart Study. Ann N Y Acad Sci 817: 189–198, 1997

20. Berlowitz DR, Ash AS, Hickey EC et al: Inadequate management of blood pressure in a hypertensive population. N Engl J Med 339: 1957–1963, 1998

21. Bernard DB, Townsend RR, Sylvestri MF: Health and disease management: What is it and where is it going? What is the role of health and disease management in hypertension? Am J Hypertens 11: 103S–108S, 1998

22. Black HR: Management of hypertension in older persons. In Izzo JL Jr, Black HR (eds): Hypertension Primer, pp 430–432. Philadelphia, Lippincott Williams & Wilkins, 1999

23. Blair D, Habicht J-P, Sims EA et al: Evidence for an increased risk for hypertension with centrally located body fat and the effect of race and sex on this risk. Am J Epidemiol 119: 526–540, 1984

24. Blair SN, Goodyear NN, Gibbons LW et al: Physical fitness and incidence of hypertension in healthy normotensive men and women. JAMA 252: 487–490, 1984

25. Blair SN, Kohl HW, Paffenbarger RS et al: Physical fitness and all-cause mortality: A prospective study of healthy men and women. JAMA 262: 2395–2401, 1989

26. Bog-Hansen E, Lindblad U, Bengtsson K et al: Risk factor clustering in patients with hypertension and non–insulin-dependent diabetes mellitus: The Skaraborg Hypertension Project. J Intern Med 243: 223–232, 1998

27. Brown MA, Buddle ML, Farrell T et al: Randomised trial of management of hypertensive pregnancies by Korotkoff phase IV or phase V. Lancet 352: 777–781, 1998

28. Buring JE, Glynn RJ, Hennekens CH: Calcium channel blockers and myocardial infarction: A hypothesis formulated but not yet tested. JAMA 274: 654–655, 1995

29. Burt VL, Whelton P, Roccella EJ et al: Prevalence of hypertension in the US adult population: Results from the Third National Health and Nutrition Examination Survey, 1988–1991. Hypertension 25: 305–313, 1995

30. Chasan-Taber L, Willett WC, Manson JE et al: Prospective study of oral contraceptives and hypertension among women in the United States. Circulation 94: 483–489, 1996

31. Christianson JB, Pietz L, Taylor R et al: Implementing programs for chronic illness management: The case of hypertension services. Joint Commission Journal on Quality Improvement 23: 593–601, 1997

32. Coakley EH, Rimm EB, Colditz G et al: Predictors of weight change in men: Results from the Health Professionals Follow-up Study. Int J Obes Relat Metab Disord 22: 89–96, 1998

33. Cobbe SM: Lipids in hypertensive patients. Am J Hypertens 11: 887–889, 1998

34. Collins R, Peto R, MacMahon S et al: Blood pressure, stroke, and coronary heart disease: Part 2. Short-term reductions in blood pressure: Overview of randomised drug trials in their epidemiological context. Lancet 335: 827–838, 1990

35. Cooper RS: Geographic patterns of hypertension: A global perspective. In Izzo JL Jr, Black HR (eds): Hypertension Primer, pp 224–225. Philadelphia, Lippincott Williams & Wilkins, 1999

36. Coordinating Committee of the National High Blood Pressure Education Program: Collaboration in high blood pressure control: Among professionals and with the patient. Ann Intern Med 101: 393–395, 1984

37. Cruickshank JM, Thorp JM, Zacharias FJ: Benefits and potential harm of lowering high blood pressure. Lancet 1: 581–584, 1987

38. Curzio JL, Rubin PC, Kennedy SS et al: A comparison of the management of hypertensive patients by nurse practitioners compared with conventional hospital care. J Hum Hypertens 4: 665–670, 1990

39. Cushman WC: Alcohol use and blood pressure. In Izzo JL Jr, Black HR (eds): Hypertension Primer, pp 263–265. Philadelphia, Lippincott Williams & Wilkins, 1999

40. Cushman WC, Cutler JA, Hanna E et al: Prevention and treatment of hypertension study (PATHS): Effects of an alcohol treatment program on blood pressure. Arch Intern Med 158: 1197–1207, 1998

41. Cutler JA, Follmann D, Allender PS: Randomized trials of sodium reduction: An overview. Am J Clin Nutr 65: 643S–651S, 1997

42. Dahlof B, Lindholm LH, Hansson L et al: Morbidity and mortality in the Swedish Trial in Old Patients with Hypertension (STOP-Hypertension). Lancet 338: 1281–1285, 1991

43. Daniels SR, Loggie JM, Khoury P et al: Left ventricular geometry and severe left ventricular hypertrophy in children and adolescents with essential hypertension. Circulation 97: 1907–1911, 1998

44. Danielson M, Dammstrom B: The prevalence of secondary and curable hypertension. Acta Medica Scandinavica 209: 451–455, 1981

45. Dannenberg AL, Garrison RJ, Kannel WB: Incidence of hypertension in the Framingham Study. Am J Public Health 78: 676–679, 1988

46. Darbar D, Fromm MF, Dell'Orto S et al: Modulation by dietary salt of verapamil disposition in humans. Circulation 98: 2702–2708, 1998

47. Daugherty SA: Hypertension detection and follow-up: Description of the enumerated and screened population. Hypertension 5(Suppl IV): IV1–IV43, 1983

48. de Leeuw PW, Birkenhäger WH: Coarctation of the aorta. In Swales JD (ed): Textbook of Hypertension, pp 969–979. Oxford, Blackwell, 1994

49. de Leeuw PW, van Leeuwen SJ, Birkenhager WH: Effect of sleep on blood pressure and its correlates. Clinical and Experimental Hypertension: Part A, Theory and Practice 7: 179–186, 1985

50. Dengel DR, Hagberg JM, Pratley RE et al: Improvements in blood pressure, glucose metabolism, and lipoprotein lipids after aerobic exercise plus weight loss in obese, hypertensive middle-aged men. Metabolism 47: 1075–1082, 1998

51. Despres JP, Moorjani S, Lupien PJ et al: Regional distribution of body fat, plasma lipoproteins, and cardiovascular disease. Arteriosclerosis 10: 497–511, 1990

52. DiCorleto PE, Gimbrone Jr MA: Vascular endothelium. In Fuster V, Ross R, Topol EJ (eds): Atherosclerosis and Coronary Artery Disease, pp 387–399. Philadelphia, Lippincott–Raven, 1996

53. Diehl HA: Coronary risk reduction through intensive community-based lifestyle intervention: The Coronary Health Improvement Project (CHIP) experience. Am J Cardiol 82: 83T–87T, 1998

54. Doll R, Peto R: Mortality in relation to smoking: 20 years' observations on male British doctors. BMJ 2: 1525–1536, 1976

55. Dustan HP, Francis CW, Allen HD et al: Principles of access to health care: Access to Health Care Task Force, American Heart Association. Circulation 87: 657–658, 1993

56. Dustan HP, Schneckloth RE, Corcoran AC et al: The effectiveness of long-term treatment of malignant hypertension. Circulation 18: 644–651, 1958

57. Ebrahim S: Detection, adherence and control of hypertension for the prevention of stroke: a systematic review. Health Technol Assess 2: 1–78, 1998

58. Egan BM, Lackland DT: Strategies for cardiovascular disease prevention: Importance of public and community health programs. Ethn Dis 8: 228–239, 1998

59. Ekelund L, Haskell WL, Johnson JL et al: Physical fitness as a predictor of cardiovascular mortality in asymptomatic North American men. N Engl J Med 319: 1379–1384, 1988

60. Elkasabany AM, Urbina EM, Daniels SR et al: Prediction of adult hypertension by K4 and K5 diastolic blood pressure in children: The Bogalusa Heart Study. J Pediatr 132: 687–692, 1998

61. Engstrom A, Tobelmann RC, Albertson AM: Sodium intake trends and food choices. Am J Clin Nutr 65: 704S–707S, 1997

62. Erikssen G, Liestol K, Bjornholt J et al: Changes in physical fitness and changes in mortality. Lancet 352: 759–762, 1998

63. Fagard RH: Physical fitness and blood pressure. J Hypertens 11(Suppl 5): S47–S52, 1993

64. Farquhar JW, Fortmann SP, Flora JA et al: Effects of communitywide education on cardiovascular disease risk factors: The Stanford Five-City Project. JAMA 265: 359–365, 1990

65. Ferrannini E, Natali A: Essential hypertension, metabolic disorders, and insulin resistance. Am Heart J 121: 1274–1282, 1991

66. Ferri C, Bellini C, Desideri G et al: Clustering of endothelial markers of vascular damage in human salt-sensitive hypertension: Influence of dietary sodium load and depletion. Hypertension 32: 862–868, 1998

67. Fletcher AE, Bulpitt CJ: How far should blood pressure be lowered? N Engl J Med 326: 251–254, 1992

68. Folsom AR, Prineas RJ, Kaye SA et al: Incidence of hypertension and stroke in relation to body fat distribution and other risk factors in older women. Stroke 21: 701–706, 1990

69. Ford ES, DeStefano F: Risk factors for mortality from all causes and from coronary heart disease among persons with diabetes. Am J Epidemiol 133: 1220–1230, 1991

70. Fouad MN, Kiefe CI, Bartolucci AA et al: A hypertension control program tailored to unskilled and minority workers. Ethn Dis 7: 191–199, 1997

71. Frank RN: The eye in hypertension. In Izzo JL Jr, Black HR (eds): Hypertension Primer, pp 194–196. Philadelphia, Lippincott Williams & Wilkins, 1999

72. Fried LP, Kronmal RA, Newman AB et al: Risk factors for 5-year mortality in older adults: The Cardiovascular Health Study. JAMA 279: 585–592, 1998

73. Frostegard J, Wu R, Gillis-Haegerstrand C et al: Antibodies to endothelial cells in borderline hypertension. Circulation 98: 1092–1098, 1998

74. Fuenmayor N, Moreira E, Cubeddu LX: Salt sensitivity is associated with insulin resistance in essential hypertension. Am J Hypertens 11: 397–402, 1998

75. Furberg CD, Psaty BM, Meyer JV: Nifedipine: Dose-related increase in mortality in patients with coronary heart disease. Circulation 92: 1326–1331, 1995

76. Ganguly A: Primary aldosteronism. N Engl J Med 339: 1828–1834, 1998

77. Garraway WM, Whisnant JP: The changing pattern of hypertension and the declining incidence of stroke. JAMA 258: 214–217, 1987

78. Garrison RJ, Kannel WB, Stokes III J et al: Incidence and precursors of hypertension in young adults: The Framingham Offspring Study. Prev Med 16: 235–251, 1987

79. Giatras I, Lau J, Levey AS: Effect of angiotensin-converting enzyme inhibitors on the progression of nondiabetic renal disease: A meta-analysis of randomized trials. Angiotensin-Converting-Enzyme Inhibition and Progressive Renal Disease Study Group. Ann Intern Med 127: 337–345, 1997

80. Glynn RJ, Field TS, Rosner B et al: Evidence for a positive linear relation between blood pressure and mortality in elderly people. Lancet 345: 825–829, 1995

81. Gonzalez-Albarran O, Ruilope LM, Villa E et al: Salt sensitivity: Concept and pathogenesis. Diabetes Res Clin Pract 39(Suppl): S15–S26, 1998

82. Gottdiener JS, Reda DJ, Massie BM et al: Effect of single-drug therapy on reduction of left ventricular mass in mild to moderate hypertension: Comparison of six antihypertensive agents. The Department of Veterans Affairs Cooperative Study Group on Antihypertensive Agents. Circulation 95: 2007–2014, 1997

83. Grimm RH, Jr., Flack JM, Grandits GA et al: Long-term effects on plasma lipids of diet and drugs to treat hypertension: Treatment of Mild Hypertension Study (TOMHS) Research Group. JAMA 275: 1549–1556, 1996

84. Grossman E, Messerli FH, Grodzicki T et al: Should a moratorium be placed on sublingual nifedipine capsules given for hypertensive emergencies and pseudoemergencies? JAMA 276: 1328–1331, 1996

85. Grover SA, Paquet S, Levinton C et al: Estimating the benefits of modifying risk factors of cardiovascular disease: A comparison of primary vs secondary prevention [published erratum appears in Arch Intern Med 158: 1228, 1998]. Arch Intern Med 158: 655–662, 1998

86. Gueyffier F, Boutitie F, Boissel JP et al: Effect of antihypertensive drug treatment on cardiovascular outcomes in women and men: A meta-analysis of individual patient data from randomized, controlled trials. The INDANA Investigators. Ann Intern Med 126: 761–767, 1997

87. Guidelines Subcommittee: 1999 World Health Organization-International Society of Hypertension guidelines for the management of hypertension. J Hypertens 11: 905–918, 1999

88. Haarbo J, Hassager C, Riis BJ et al: Relation of body fat distribution to serum lipids and lipoproteins in elderly women. Atherosclerosis 80: 57–62, 1989

89. Hahn RA, Heath GW, Chang MH: Cardiovascular disease risk factors and preventive practices among adults—United States, 1994: A behavioral risk factor atlas. Behavioral Risk Factor Surveillance System State Coordinators. MMWR Morb Mortal Wkly Rep 47: 35–69, 1998

90. Hakim AA, Petrovitch H, Burchfiel CM et al: Effects of walking on mortality among nonsmoking retired men. N Engl J Med 338: 94–99, 1998

91. Hall WD: Geographic patterns of hypertension in the United States. In Izzo JL Jr, Black HR (eds): Hypertension Primer, pp 226–228. Philadelphia, Lippincott Williams & Wilkins, 1999

92. Hallstrom AP, Cobb LA, Ray R: Smoking as a risk factor for recurrence of sudden cardiac arrest. N Engl J Med 314: 271–275, 1986

93. Hansson L: How far should blood pressure be lowered? What is the role of the J-curve? Am J Hypertens 3: 726–729, 1990

94. Hansson L, Zanchetti A, Carruthers SG et al: Effects of intensive blood-pressure lowering and low-dose aspirin in patients with hypertension: Principal results of the Hypertension Optimal Treatment (HOT) randomised trial. Lancet 351: 1755–1762, 1998

95. Hayreh SS, Servais GE, Virdi PS: Cotton-wool spots (inner retinal ischemic spots) in malignant arterial hypertension. Ophthalmologica 198: 197–215, 1989

96. Heintz B, Schmauder C, Witte K et al: Blood pressure rhythm and endocrine functions in normotensive women on oral contraceptives. J Hypertens 14: 333–339, 1996

97. Hermanson B, Omenn GS, Kronmal RA et al: Beneficial six-year outcome of smoking cessation in older men and women with coronary artery disease. N Engl J Med 319: 1365, 1988

98. Higashi Y, Oshima T, Ozono R et al: Aging and severity of hypertension attenuate endothelium-dependent renal vascular relaxation in humans. Hypertension 30: 252–258, 1997

99. Holme I, Helgeland A, Hjermann I et al: Coronary risk factors and socioeconomic status: The Oslo Study. Lancet 2: 1396–1398, 1976

100. Horan MJ, Lenfant C: Epidemiology of blood pressure and predictors of hypertension. Hypertension 15: I20–24, 1990

101. Huang Z, Willett WC, Manson JE et al: Body weight, weight change, and risk for hypertension in women. Ann Intern Med 128: 81–88, 1998

102. Hughes JS, Dove HG, Gifford RW Jr et al: Duration of blood pressure elevation in accurately predicting surgical cure of renovascular hypertension. Am Heart J 101: 408–413, 1981

103. Hunt SC, Cook NR, Oberman A et al: Angiotensinogen genotype, sodium reduction, weight loss, and prevention of hypertension: Trials of hypertension prevention, phase II. Hypertension 32: 393–401, 1998

104. Hunt SC, Williams RR: Genetics and family history of hypertension. In Izzo JL Jr, Black HR (eds): Hypertension Primer, pp 218–221. Philadelphia, Lippincott Williams & Wilkins, 1999

105. Hypertension Detection and Follow-up Program Cooperative Group: Five-year findings of the Hypertension Detection and Follow-up Program: I. Reduction in mortality of persons with high blood pressure, including mild hypertension. JAMA 242: 2562–2571, 1979

106. Hypertension Detection and Follow-up Program Cooperative Group: The effect of treatment on mortality in "mild" hypertension: Results of the Hypertension Detection and Follow-up Program. N Engl J Med 307: 976–980, 1982

107. Hypertension Detection and Follow-up Program Cooperative Group: Educational level and 5-year all-cause mortality in the hypertension detection and follow-up program. Hypertension 9: 641–646, 1987

108. Hypertension Prevention Trial Research Group: The Hypertension Prevention Trial: Three-year effects of dietary changes on blood pressure. Arch Intern Med 150: 153–162, 1990

109. Ikeda T, Gomi T, Hirawa N et al: Improvement of insulin sensitivity contributes to blood pressure reduction after weight loss in hypertensive subjects with obesity. Hypertension 27: 1180–1186, 1996

110. Jeunemaitre X, Soubrier F, Kotelevtsev YV et al: Molecular basis of human hypertension: Role of angiotensinogen. Cell 71: 169–180, 1992

111. Joint National Committee on Detection Evaluation and Treatment of High Blood Pressure: The 1984 Report of the Joint National Committee on Detection, Evaluation, and Treatment of High Blood Pressure. Arch Intern Med 144: 1045–1057, 1984

112. Jones DW: Socioeconomic status and blood pressure. In Izzo JL Jr, Black HR (eds): Hypertension Primer, pp 242–243. Philadelphia, Lippincott Williams & Wilkins, 1999

113. Julius S: Transition from high cardiac output to elevated vascular resistance in hypertension. Am Heart J 116: 600–606, 1988

114. Kannel WB: Blood pressure as a cardiovascular risk factor: Prevention and treatment. JAMA 275: 1571–1576, 1996

115. Kannel WB, Brand N, Skinner JJ Jr et al: The relation of adiposity to blood pressure and development of hypertension: The Framingham Study. Ann Intern Med 67: 48–59, 1967

116. Kannel WB, Cobb J: Left ventricular hypertrophy and mortality: Results from the Framingham Study. Cardiology 81: 291–298, 1992

117. Kannel WB, McGee D, Gordon T: A general cardiovascular risk profile: The Framingham Study. Am J Cardiol 38: 46–51, 1976

118. Kaplan N: J-curve not burned off by HOT study. Lancet 351: 1748–1749, 1998

119. Kaplan NM: The deadly quartet: Upper-body obesity, glucose intolerance, hypertriglyceridemia, and hypertension. Arch Intern Med 149: 1514–1520, 1989

120. Kaplan NM: Clinical Hypertension, 7th ed. Baltimore, Williams & Wilkins, 1998

121. Kashgarian M: Hypertensive disease and kidney structure. In Laragh JH (ed): Hypertension: Pathophysiology, Diagnosis and Management, pp 389–398. New York, Raven Press, 1990

122. Kasiske BL, Ma JZ, Kalil RS et al: Effects of antihypertensive therapy on serum lipids. Ann Intern Med 122: 133–141, 1995

123. Kaufman JS, Owaje EE, James SA et al: The determinants of hypertension in West Africa: Contribution of anthropometric and dietary factors to urban-rural and socio-economic gradients. Am J Epidemiol 143: 1203–1218, 1996

124. Kawachi I, Colditz GA, Stampfer MJ et al: Smoking cessation in relation to total mortality rates in women: A prospective study. Ann Intern Med 119: 992–1000, 1993

125. Khaw KT: Epidemiology of stroke. J Neurol Neurosurg Psychiatry 61: 333–338, 1996

126. Klag MJ, Whelton PK, Randall BL et al: Blood pressure and end-stage renal disease in men. N Engl J Med 334: 13–18, 1996

127. Klag MJ, Whelton PK, Randall BL et al: End-stage renal disease in African-American and white men: 16-year MRFIT findings. JAMA 277: 1293–1298, 1997

128. Klatsky AL, Friedman GD, Siegelaub AB et al: Alcohol consumption and blood pressure Kaiser-Permanente Multiphasic Health Examination data. N Engl J Med 296: 1194–1200, 1977

129. Klungel OH, de Boer A, Paes AH et al: Undertreatment of hypertension in a population-based study in The Netherlands. J Hypertens 16: 1371–1378, 1998

130. Kokkinos PF, Narayan P, Colleran JA et al: Effects of regular exercise on blood pressure and left ventricular hypertrophy in African-American men with severe hypertension. N Engl J Med 333: 1462–1467, 1995

131. Kostis JB, Davis BR, Cutler J et al: Prevention of heart failure by antihypertensive drug treatment in older persons with isolated systolic hypertension: SHEP Cooperative Research Group. JAMA 278: 212–216, 1997

132. Kotchen TA, McCarron DA: Dietary electrolytes and blood pressure: A statement for healthcare professionals from the American Heart Association Nutrition Committee. Circulation 98: 613–617, 1998

133. Krum H, Viskoper RJ, Lacourciere Y et al: The effect of an endothelin-receptor antagonist, bosentan, on blood pressure in patients with essential hypertension. N Engl J Med 338: 784–790, 1998

134. Kujala UM, Kaprio J, Sarna S et al: Relationship of leisure-time physical activity and mortality: The Finnish Twin Cohort. JAMA 279: 440–444, 1998

135. Kushi LH, Fee RM, Folsom AR et al: Physical activity and mortality in postmenopausal women. JAMA 277: 1287–1292, 1997

136. Labarthe DR: Problems in definition of mild hypertension. Ann NY Acad Sci 304: 3–14, 1978

137. Lackland DT, Bachman DL, Carter TD et al: The geographic variation in stroke incidence in two areas of the southeastern stroke belt: The Anderson and Pee Dee Stroke Study. Stroke 29: 2061–2068, 1998

138. LaCroix AZ, Lang J, Scherr P et al: Smoking and mortality among older men and women in three communities. N Engl J Med 324: 1619–1625, 1991

139. Lakka TA, Venalainen JM, Rauramaa R et al: Relation of leisure-time physical activity and cardiorespiratory fitness to the risk of acute myocardial infarction in men. N Engl J Med 330: 1549–1554, 1994

140. Landsberg L: Obesity. In Izzo JL Jr, Black HR (eds): Hypertension Primer, pp 118–120. Philadelphia, Lippincott Williams & Wilkins, 1999

141. Langeluddecke PM: The role of behavioral change procedures in multifactorial coronary heart disease prevention programs. Prog Behav Modif 20: 199–225, 1986

142. Langford HG, Blaufox MD, Oberman A et al: Dietary therapy slows the return of hypertension after stopping prolonged medication. JAMA 253: 657–664, 1985

143. Law CM, M. de Swiet, Osmond C et al: Initiation of hypertension in utero and its amplification throughout life. BMJ 306: 24–27, 1993

144. Lazarus JM, Bourgoignie JJ, Buckalew VM et al: Achievement and safety of a low blood pressure goal in chronic renal disease: The Modification of Diet in Renal Disease Study Group. Hypertension 29: 641–650, 1997

145. Ledoux M, Lambert J, Reeder BA et al: Correlation between cardiovascular disease risk factors and simple anthropometric measures: Canadian Heart Health Surveys Research Group. CMAJ 157(Suppl 1): S46–S53, 1997

146. Lerner DJ, Kannel WB: Patterns of coronary heart disease morbidity and mortality in the sexes: A 26-year follow-up of the Framingham population. Am Heart J 111: 383–390, 1986

147. Lewis EJ, Hunsicker LG, Bain RP et al: The effect of angiotensin-converting-enzyme inhibition on diabetic nephropathy: The Collaborative Study Group. N Engl J Med 329: 1456–1462, 1993

148. Lichtenstein MJ, Shipley MJ, Rose G: Systolic and diastolic blood pressures as predictors of coronary heart disease mortality in the Whitehall Study. BMJ 291: 243–245, 1985

149. Lifton RP: Molecular genetics of human blood pressure variation. Science 272: 676–680, 1996

150. Lightman SL, James VH, Linsell C et al: Studies of diurnal changes in plasma renin activity, and plasma noradrenaline, aldosterone and cortisol concentrations in man. Clin Endocrinol (Oxf) 14: 213–223, 1981

151. Lindop GBM: The effects of hypertension on the structure of human resistance vessels. In Swales JD (ed): Textbook of Hypertension, pp 663–669. Oxford, Blackwell, 1994

152. Logan AG, Milne BJ, Achber C et al: Work-site treatment of hypertension by specially trained nurses: A controlled trial. Lancet 2: 1175–1178, 1979

153. London GM, Guerin AP, Pannier B et al: Large artery structure and function in hypertension and end-stage renal disease. J Hypertens 16: 1931–1938, 1998

154. Luft FC: Salt and hypertension at the close of the millennium. Wien Klin Wochenschr 110: 459–466, 1998

155. Lund-Johansen P: Central haemodynamics in essential hypertension. Acta Medica Scandinavica 603(Suppl 1): 35–42, 1977

156. Lund-Johansen P: Twenty-year follow-up of hemodynamics in essential hypertension during rest and exercise. Hypertension 18(Suppl III): III-54–III-61, 1991

157. Luria MH, Erel J, Sapoznikov D et al: Cardiovascular risk factor clustering and ratio of total cholesterol to high-density lipoprotein cholesterol in angiographically documented coronary artery disease. Am J Cardiol 67: 31–36, 1991

158. MacMahon S, Peto R, Cutler J et al: Blood pressure, stroke, and coronary heart disease: Part 1. Prolonged differences in blood pressure: Prospective observational studies corrected for dilution bias. Lancet 335: 765–774, 1990

159. MacMahon S, Rodgers A: The effects of blood pressure reduction in older patients: An overview of five randomized controlled trials in elderly hypertensives. Clin Exp Hypertens 15: 967–978, 1993

160. MacMahon SW, Wilcken DEL, MacDonald GJ: The effect of weight reduction on left ventricular mass: A randomized controlled trial in young, overweight hypertensive patients. N Engl J Med 314: 334–339, 1986

161. Management Committee of the Australian Therapeutic Trial in Mild Hypertension: Untreated mild hypertension. Lancet 1: 185–190, 1982

162. Manolio TA, Savage PJ, Burke GL et al: Correlates of fasting insulin levels in young adults: The CARDIA study. J Clin Epidemiol 44: 571–578, 1991

163. Maschio G, Alberti D, Janin G et al: Effect of the angiotensin-converting-enzyme inhibitor benazepril on the progression of chronic renal insufficiency: The Angiotensin-Converting-Enzyme Inhibition in Progressive Renal Insufficiency Study Group. N Engl J Med 334: 939–945, 1996

164. Mattes RD: The taste for salt in humans. Am J Clin Nutr 65: 692S–697S, 1997

165. McGregor E, Isles CG, Jay JL et al: Retinal changes in malignant hypertension. BMJ 292: 233–234, 1986

166. McLeod D, Marshall J, Kohner EM et al: The role of axoplasmic transport in the pathogenesis of retinal cotton-wool spots. Br J Ophthalmol 61: 177–191, 1977

167. McMurray J, Murdoch D: Calcium-antagonist controversy: The long and short of it? Lancet 349: 585–586, 1997

168. Medical Research Council Working Party: MRC trial of treatment of mild hypertension: Principal results. BMJ 291: 97–104, 1985

169. Meigs JB, D'Agostino RB Sr, Wilson PW et al: Risk variable clustering in the insulin resistance syndrome: The Framingham Offspring Study. Diabetes 46: 1594–1600, 1997

170. Melby CL, Goldflies DG, Hyner GC: Blood pressure and anthropometric differences in regularly exercising and nonexercising black adults. Clinical and Experimental Hypertension: Part A, Theory and Practice 13: 1233–1248, 1991

171. Midgley JP, Matthew AG, Greenwood CM et al: Effect of reduced dietary sodium on blood pressure: A meta-analysis of randomized controlled trials. JAMA 275: 1590–1597, 1996

172. Millar-Craig MW, Bishop CN, Raftery EB: Circadian variation of blood-pressure. Lancet 1: 795–797, 1978

173. Miller NH, Hill M, Kottke T et al: The multilevel compliance challenge: Recommendations for a call to action. A statement

for healthcare professionals. Circulation 95: 1085–1090, 1997

174. MRC Working Party: Medical Research Council trial of treatment of hypertension in older adults: principal results. BMJ 304: 405–412, 1992

175. Muller-Wieland D, Kotzka J, Knebel B et al: Metabolic syndrome and hypertension: Pathophysiology and molecular basis of insulin resistance. Basic Res Cardiol 93: 131–134, 1998

176. Murata M, Yoshimoto H: Morphological study of the pathogenesis of retinal cotton wool spot. Jpn J Ophthalmol 27: 362–379, 1983

177. Muscholl MW, Schunkert H, Muders F et al: Neurohormonal activity and left ventricular geometry in patients with essential arterial hypertension. Am Heart J 135: 58–66, 1998

178. National Heart, Lung, and Blood Institute: 1988 Report of the Joint National Committee on Detection, Evaluation, and Treatment of High Blood Pressure. Arch Intern Med 148: 1023–1038, 1988

179. National High Blood Pressure Education Program: National High Blood Pressure Education Program Working Group Report on Primary Prevention of Hypertension. NIH publication no. 93-2669. Bethesda, MD, U.S. Department of Health and Human Services, National Institutes of Health, 1993

180. National High Blood Pressure Education Program Working Group: National High Blood Pressure Education Program Working Group report on hypertension in the elderly. Hypertension 23: 275–285, 1994

181. National High Blood Pressure Education Program Working Group on High Blood Pressure in Pregnancy: National High Blood Pressure Education Program Working Group report on high blood pressure in pregnancy. Am J Obstet Gynecol 163: 1691–1712, 1990

182. National High Blood Pressure Education Program Working Group on Hypertension Control in Children and Adolescents: Update on the 1987 task force report on high blood pressure in children and adolescents: A working group report from the National High Blood Pressure Education Program. Pediatrics 98: 649–658, 1996

183. Neaton JD, Grimm RH, Prineas RJ et al: Treatment of Mild Hypertension Study: Final results. JAMA 270: 713–724, 1993

184. Neusy AJ, Lowenstein J: Blood pressure and blood pressure variability following withdrawal of propranolol and clonidine. J Clin Pharmacol 29: 18–24, 1989

185. O'Rourke MF: Arterial stiffness and hypertension. In Izzo JL Jr, Black HR (eds): Hypertension Primer, pp 160–162. Philadelphia, Lippincott Williams & Wilkins, 1999

186. Oberman A, Wassertheil-Smoller S, Langford HG et al: Pharmacologic and nutritional treatment of mild hypertension: Changes in cardiovascular risk status. Ann Intern Med 112: 89–95, 1990

187. Ockene JK, Ockene IS: Training program. In Ockene IS, Ockene JK (eds): Prevention of Coronary Heart Disease, pp 567–579. Boston, Little, Brown, 1992

188. Ofili EO, Cohen JD, St. Vrain JA et al: Effect of treatment of isolated systolic hypertension on left ventricular mass. JAMA 279: 778–780, 1998

189. Ostlund RE, Staten M, Kohrt WM et al: The ratio of waist-to-hip circumference, plasma insulin level, and glucose intolerance as independent predictors of the HDL2 cholesterol level in older adults. N Engl J Med 322: 229–234, 1990

190. Otten MW, Teutsch SM, Williamson DF et al: The effect of known risk factors on the excess mortality of black adults in the United States. JAMA 263: 845–850, 1990

191. Paffenbarger RS Jr, Hyde RT, Wing AL et al: Physical activity, all-cause mortality, and longevity of college alumni. N Engl J Med 314: 605–613, 1986

192. Paine-Andrews A, Harris KJ, Fawcett SB et al: Evaluating a statewide partnership for reducing risks for chronic diseases. J Community Health 22: 343–359, 1997

193. Panza JA: Endothelial dysfunction in essential hypertension. Clin Cardiol 20: II-26–II-33, 1997

194. Patel V, Kohner EM: The eye in hypertension. In Swales JD (ed). Textbook of Hypertension, pp 1015–1025. Oxford, Blackwell, 1994

195. Perloff D, Grim C, Flack J et al: Human blood pressure determination by sphygmomanometry. Circulation 88: 2460–2470, 1993

196. Perneger TV, Klag MJ, Feldman H et al: Projections of hypertension-related renal disease in middle-aged residents of the United States. JAMA 269: 1272–1277, 1993

197. Perseghin G, Price TB, Petersen KF et al: Increased glucose transport-phosphorylation and muscle glycogen synthesis after exercise training in insulin-resistant subjects. N Engl J Med 335: 1357–1362, 1996

198. Peterson JC, Adler S, Burkart JM et al: Blood pressure control, proteinuria, and the progression of renal disease: The Modification of Diet in Renal Disease Study. Ann Intern Med 123: 754–762, 1995

199. Pheley AM, Terry P, Pietz L et al: Evaluation of a nurse-based hypertension management program: Screening, management, and outcomes. J Cardiovasc Nurs 9: 54–61, 1995

200. Pickering TG: Renovascular hypertension: Etiology and pathophysiology. Semin Nucl Med 19: 79–88, 1989

201. Potter JD: Hazards and benefits of alcohol. N Engl J Med 337: 1763–1764, 1997

202. Prochaska JO, DiClemente CC: Stages and processes of self-change of smoking: Toward an integrative model of change. J Consult Clin Psychol 51: 390–395, 1983

203. Prochaska JO, Goldstein MG: Process of smoking cessation: Implications for clinicians. Clin Chest Med 12: 727–735, 1991

204. Psaty BM, Heckbert SR, Koepsell TD et al: The risk of myocardial infarction associated with antihypertensive drug therapies. JAMA 274: 620–625, 1995

205. Psaty BM, Smith NL, Siscovick DS et al: Health outcomes associated with antihypertensive therapies used as first-line agents: A systematic review and meta-analysis. JAMA 277: 739–745, 1997

206. Puddey IB, Parker M, Beilin LJ et al: Effects of alcohol and caloric restrictions on blood pressure and serum lipids in overweight men. Hypertension 20: 533–541, 1992

207. Pullicino P: Pathogenesis of stroke. In Izzo JL Jr, Black HR (eds): Hypertension Primer, pp 183–185. Philadelphia, Lippincott Williams & Wilkins, 1999

208. Puska P, Tuomilehto J, Nissinen A et al: The North Karelia project: 15 years of community-based prevention of coronary heart disease. Ann Med 21: 169–173, 1989

209. Ramirez-Gil JF, Delcayre C, Robert V et al: In vivo left ventricular function and collagen expression in aldosterone/salt-induced hypertension. J Cardiovasc Pharmacol 32: 927–934, 1998

210. Reaven GM, Lithell H, Landsberg L: Hypertension and associated metabolic abnormalities: The role of insulin resistance and the sympathoadrenal system. N Engl J Med 334: 374–381, 1996

211. Rossi MA: Pathologic fibrosis and connective tissue matrix in left ventricular hypertrophy due to chronic arterial hypertension in humans. J Hypertens 16: 1031–1041, 1998

212. Roter DL, Hall JA, Merisca R et al: Effectiveness of interventions to improve patient compliance: A meta-analysis. Med Care 36: 1138–1161, 1998

213. Ruggiero L, Prochaska JO: From research to practice: Introduction. Diabetes Spectrum 6: 22–24, 1993

214. Sacco RL, Elkind M, Boden-Albala B et al: The protective effect of moderate alcohol consumption on ischemic stroke. JAMA 281: 53–60, 1999

215. Sagie A, Larson MG, Levy D: The natural history of borderline isolated systolic hypertension. N Engl J Med 329: 1912–1917, 1993

216. Salonen JT, Slater JS, Tuomilehto H et al: Leisure time and occupational physical activity: Risk of death from ischemic heart disease. Am J Epidemiol 127: 87–94, 1988

217. Sandvik L, Erikssen J, Thaulow E et al: Physical fitness as a predictor of mortality among healthy, middle-aged Norwegian men. N Engl J Med 328: 533–537, 1993

218. Schieken RM, Clarke WR, Lauer RM: Left ventricular hypertrophy in children with blood pressures in the upper quintile of the distribution: The Muscatine Study. Hypertension 3: 669–675, 1981

219. Schmahl FW, Kahle PF: Screening for risk factors of arteriosclerosis in occupational medicine with special consideration of serum lipids: Implications for health policy. Int J Occup Med Environ Health 9: 93–101, 1996

220. Schmieder RE, Martus P, Klingbeil A: Reversal of left ventricular hypertrophy in essential hypertension: A meta-analysis of randomized double-blind studies. JAMA 275: 1507–1513, 1996

221. Schultz JF, Sheps SG: Management of patients with hypertension: A hypertension clinic model. Mayo Clin Proc 69: 997–999, 1994

222. Shear CL, Burke GL, Freedman DS et al: Value of childhood blood pressure measurements and family history in predicting future blood pressure status: Results from 8 years of follow-up in the Bogalusa Heart Study. Pediatrics 77: 25–29, 1986

223. SHEP Cooperative Research Group: Prevention of stroke by antihypertensive drug treatment in older persons with Isolated Systolic Hypertension: Final results of the Systolic Hypertension in the Elderly Program (SHEP). JAMA 265: 3255–3264, 1991

224. Shepherd J, Cobbe SM, Ford I et al: Prevention of coronary heart disease with pravastatin in men with hypercholesterolemia. N Engl J Med 333: 1301–1307, 1995

225. Sherman SE, D'Agostino RB, Cobb JL et al: Does exercise reduce mortality rates in the elderly? Experience from the Framingham Heart Study. Am Heart J 128: 965–972, 1994

226. Sherman SE, D'Agostino RB, Cobb JL et al: Physical activity and mortality in women in the Framingham Heart Study. Am Heart J 128: 879–884, 1994

227. Sibai BM: Treatment of hypertension in pregnant women. N Engl J Med 335: 257–265, 1996

228. Sinaiko AR: Current concepts: Hypertension in children. N Engl J Med 335: 1968–1973, 1996

229. Sinaiko AR, Gomez-Marin O, Prineas RJ: Prevalence of "significant" hypertension in junior high school-aged children: The Children and Adolescent Blood Pressure Program. J Pediatr 114: 664–669, 1989

230. Sinclair AM, Isles CG, Brown I et al: Secondary hypertension in a blood pressure clinic. Arch Intern Med 147: 1289–1293, 1987

231. Smith ED, Merritt SL, Patel MK: Church-based education: An outreach program for African Americans with hypertension. Ethn Health 2: 243–253, 1997

232. Sowers JR, Izzo JL Jr: Endothelial dysfunction. In Izzo JL Jr, Black HR (eds): Hypertension Primer, pp 167–169. Philadelphia, Lippincott Williams & Wilkins, 1999

233. Staessen J, Amery A, Fagard R: Isolated systolic hypertension in the elderly. J Hypertens 8: 393–405, 1990

234. Staessen JA, Fagard R, Thijs L et al: Randomised double-blind comparison of placebo and active treatment for older patients with isolated systolic hypertension. Lancet 350: 757–764, 1997

235. Stamler J, Briefel RR, Milas C et al: Relation of changes in dietary lipids and weight, trial years 1–6, to changes in blood lipids in the special intervention and usual care groups in the Multiple Risk Factor Intervention Trial. Am J Clin Nutr 65: 272S–288S, 1997

236. Stamler J, Stamler R, Neaton JD: Blood pressure, systolic and diastolic, and cardiovascular risks. Arch Intern Med 153: 982–988, 1993

237. Stamler R, Shipley M, Elliott P et al: Higher blood pressure in adults with less education: Some explanations from INTERSALT. Hypertension 19: 237–241, 1992

238. Stamler R, Stamler J, Gosch FC et al: Primary prevention of hypertension by nutritional-hygienic means: Final report of a randomized, controlled trial [published erratum appears in JAMA 262: 3132, 1989]. JAMA 262: 1801–1807, 1989

239. Stamler R, Stamler J, Riedlinger WF et al: Weight and blood pressure: Findings in hypertension screening of 1 million Americans. JAMA 240: 1607–1610, 1978

240. Susic D, Nunez E, Frohlich ED: Reversal of hypertrophy: An active biologic process. Curr Opin Cardiol 10: 466–472, 1995

241. Swales JD: Guidelines on guidelines. J Hypertens 11: 899–903, 1993

242. Taddei S, Virdis A, Mattei P et al: Defective L-arginine-nitric oxide pathway in offspring of essential hypertensive patients. Circulation 94: 1298–1303, 1996

243. The Joint National Committee on Prevention Detection Evaluation and Treatment of High Blood Pressure and the National High Blood Pressure Education Program Coordinating Committee: The Sixth Report of the Joint National Committee on Prevention, Detection, Evaluation, and Treatment of High Blood Pressure. Arch Intern Med 157: 2413–2446, 1997

244. Thun MJ, Peto R, Lopez AD et al: Alcohol consumption and mortality among middle-aged and elderly U.S. adults. N Engl J Med 337: 1705–1714, 1997

245. Thurmann PA, Kenedi P, Schmidt A et al: Influence of the angiotensin II antagonist valsartan on left ventricular hypertrophy in patients with essential hypertension. Circulation 98: 2037–2042, 1998

246. Toto RD, Mitchell HC, Smith RD et al: "Strict" blood pressure control and progression of renal disease in hypertensive nephrosclerosis. Kidney Int 48: 851–859, 1995

247. Trials of Hypertension Prevention Collaborative Research Group: The effects of nonpharmacologic interventions on blood pressure of persons with high normal levels: Results of the Trials of Hypertension Prevention, phase I. JAMA 267: 1213–1220, 1992

248. Trials of Hypertension Prevention Collaborative Research Group: Effects of weight loss and sodium reduction intervention on blood pressure and hypertension incidence in overweight people with high-normal blood pressure: The Trials of Hypertension Prevention, phase II. Arch Intern Med 157: 657–667, 1997

249. Tsao PS, Niebauer J, Buitrago R et al: Interaction of diabetes and hypertension on determinants of endothelial adhesiveness. Arterioscler Thromb Vasc Biol 18: 947–953, 1998

250. Tuomilehto J, Rastenyte D, Birkenhager WH et al: Effects of calcium-channel blockade in older patients with diabetes and systolic hypertension. N Engl J Med 340: 677–684, 1999

251. U.S. Department of Health and Human Services: Physical activity and health: A Report of the Surgeon General. Atlanta, U.S. Department of Health and Human Services, Centers for Disease Control and Prevention, National Center for Chronic Disease Prevention and Health Promotion, 1996

252. Uzu T, Ishikawa K, Fujii T et al: Sodium restriction shifts circadian rhythm of blood pressure from nondipper to dipper in essential hypertension. Circulation 96: 1859–1862, 1997

253. Uzu T, Nishimura M, Fujii T et al: Changes in the circadian rhythm of blood pressure in primary aldosteronism in response to dietary sodium restriction and adrenalectomy. J Hypertens 16: 1745–1748, 1998

254. Veterans Administration Cooperative Study Group on Antihypertensive Agents: Effects of treatment on morbidity in hypertension: Results in patients with diastolic blood pressures averaging 115 through 129 mm Hg. JAMA 202: 116–122, 1967

255. Veterans Administration Cooperative Study Group on Antihypertensive Agents: Effects of treatment on morbidity in hypertension: II. Results in patients with diastolic blood pressure averaging 90 through 114 mm Hg. JAMA 213: 1143–1152, 1970

256. Vidt DG: Management of hypertensive emergencies and urgencies. In Izzo JL Jr, Black HR (eds): Hypertension Primer, pp 437–440. Philadelphia, Lippincott Williams & Wilkins, 1999

257. Vita AJ, Terry RB, Hubert HB et al: Aging, health risks, and cumulative disability. N Engl J Med 338: 1035–1041, 1998

258. Voors AW, Webber LS, Berenson GS: Relationship of blood pressure levels to height and weight in children. J Cardiovasc Med 3: 911–918, 1978

259. Wallace P, Cutler S, Haines A: Randomised controlled trial of general practitioner intervention in patients with excessive alcohol consumption. BMJ 297: 663–668, 1988

260. Wassertheil-Smoller S, Oberman A, Blaufox MD et al: The Trial of Antihypertensive Interventions and Management (TAIM) Study: Final results with regard to blood pressure, cardiovascular risk, and quality of life. American Journal of Hypertension 5: 37–44, 1992

261. Weder AB: Pathogenesis of hypertension: Genetic and environmental factors. In Hollenberg NK (ed): Hypertension: Mechanisms and Therapy, pp 1.1–1.28. Philadelphia, Current Medicine, 1998

262. Weinberger MH, Cohen SJ, Miller JZ et al: Dietary sodium restriction as adjunctive treatment of hypertension. JAMA 259: 2561–2565, 1988

263. Westheim A, Os I: Physical activity and the metabolic cardiovascular syndrome. J Cardiovasc Pharmacol 20: S49–S53, 1992

264. Whelton PK, Appel LJ, Espeland MA et al: Sodium reduction and weight loss in the treatment of hypertension in older persons: A randomized controlled trial of nonpharmacologic interventions in the elderly (TONE). JAMA 279: 839–846, 1998

265. Williams MV, Baker DW, Parker RM et al: Relationship of functional health literacy to patients' knowledge of their chronic disease: A study of patients with hypertension and diabetes. Arch Intern Med 158: 166–172, 1998

266. Working Group to Define Critical Patient Behaviors in High Blood Pressure Control: Critical patient behaviors in high blood pressure control: Guidelines for professionals. JAMA 241: 2534–2537, 1979

267. Wright RR, Mathews KD: Hypertensive encephalopathy in childhood. J Child Neurol 11: 193–196, 1996

268. Zou Y, Hu Y, Metzler B et al: Signal transduction in arteriosclerosis: Mechanical stress-activated MAP kinases in vascular smooth muscle cells. International Journal of Molecular Medicine 1: 827–834, 1998

33

Lipid Management and Coronary Heart Disease

JOAN M. FAIR
KATHLEEN A. BERRA

Coronary heart disease (CHD), the leading cause of death for American women and men, is responsible for approximately one in three deaths.[55] Serum cholesterol and, particularly, low-density lipoprotein (LDL) cholesterol is a significant and modifiable risk factor associated with the development and progression of CHD. More than 97 million (52%) Americans have a total blood cholesterol above the desirable level of 200 mg/dL.[2] Furthermore, more than 38 million (20%) Americans have a blood cholesterol above 240 mg/dL, a level at which current treatment guidelines recommend the initiation of dietary or pharmacologic interventions.[61] There is a large body of evidence, including animal studies,[4] observational studies,[3] and more than 50 clinical trials, that consistently points to a relationship between high blood lipids and CHD. Table 33-1 summarizes the results of the more recent, large cholesterol-lowering primary and secondary prevention trials.[27,88,92] Meta-analyses of the cholesterol-lowering clinical trials estimated that a 10-mg reduction in total cholesterol results in a 22% reduction in CHD incidence after 2 years of intervention, and a 25% reduction after 5 years.[44,71] This information shows that both the incidence of high blood cholesterol and the benefits of treatment are substantial. Cardiovascular nurses need to understand hyperlipidemia and actively participate in its treatment and management.

BLOOD LIPIDS: STRUCTURE AND FUNCTIONS

The complex relationships between genetic and metabolic mechanisms and the molecular interactions within the cell wall help explain the association between lipid abnormalities and CHD. The major lipid particles, cholesterol and triglycerides, both have important func-

tions in the body. Cholesterol is an essential component of cell membranes, functioning to provide stability while permitting membrane transport; it is a precursor to adrenal steroids, sex hormones, and bile and bile acids. Triglycerides are the major source of energy for the body. Both cholesterol and triglycerides are insoluble molecules and must be transported in the circulation as lipoproteins.

Lipoproteins are complexes of nonpolar lipid cores (triglycerides and cholesterol esters) surrounded by a surface coat of polar lipids (phospholipids and free cholesterol) and specific proteins called apoproteins. Total cholesterol, for example, is composed of 18 different lipid and lipoprotein particles.[19] Lipoproteins can be classified according to their density, their migration on an electrophoretic field, or their lipid and apoprotein composition.[89]

During the 1980s, significant advances were made in determining the function of the apoproteins, the lipid-processing enzymes, and lipoprotein receptors. Apoproteins function as more than transport vehicles; they have variant properties that activate enzyme systems or receptor sites to promote the catabolism or removal of lipoproteins from the circulation.[43] The functions of nine apoproteins in the lipid metabolic cascade have been identified: apo A-I, apo A-II, apo B-100, apo B-48, apo C-I, apo C-II, apo C-III, apo E2, apo E3, apo E4, and lipoprotein(a) (Lp[a]). In addition, the actions of several lipoprotein-processing enzymes (lipoprotein lipase [LPL], hepatic lipase, lecithin cholesterol acyltransferase [LCAT], and cholesterol ester transfer protein) and the function of cell receptors, including the LDL and chylomicron remnant receptor, are now established. These advances permit an understanding of lipid metabolism, as well as the abnormalities leading to elevated blood cholesterol.

819

TABLE 33-1	Large, Randomized Clinical Trials Using Statin Therapy to Lower Cholesterol					
Trial	Number of Patients	Age (y)	Lipids (mean, mg/dL)	Length of Follow-up	Mean Lipid Reduction	Outcomes
Primary Prevention						
West of Scotland (WOSCOPS)	6,595 men	45–64	TC: 272 LDL: 192	4.9 y	TC: 20% LDL: 26%	Nonfatal MI and CHD death: 31%
AFCAPS/TEXCAPS	5,608 men, 997 women		TC: 221 LDL: 150	5.2 y	TC: 18% LDL: 25%	Major coronary events (MI, unstable angina, or sudden cardiac death: 37%)
Secondary Prevention						
Scandinavian Simvastatin Survival Study (4S)	3,617 men, 427 women	35–70	TC LDL: 188	5.4 y	TC: 28% LDL: 38%	CHD deaths: 42% Nonfatal MI and CHD death: 37%

CHD, coronary heart disease; LDL, low-density lipoprotein; MI, myocardial infarction; TC, total cholesterol.

LIPID METABOLISM AND TRANSPORT

The gut and liver are responsible for the production of the six principal lipoproteins. Exogenous lipoproteins are formed in the mucosa of the small intestine after digestion of dietary fats. The endogenous lipid transport system originates in the liver. During the digestive process, hydrolyzed products of ingested fats enter epithelial cells of the small intestine, where they are converted into triglycerides and cholesterol esters. These products are then aggregated into the lipoprotein complexes known as chylomicrons. Chylomicrons pass into small lymph vessels and reach the circulatory system through the thoracic duct. In the peripheral capillaries, chylomicrons are hydrolyzed by the enzyme LPL, located on the capillary endothelium. Free fatty acids and glycerol then enter adipose tissue cells. A cholesterol-rich chylomicron remnant (a second lipoprotein complex) is released into the circulation when lipolysis is nearly complete. Chylomicron remnants are cleared rapidly by the liver[45,46] (Fig. 33-1).

In the liver, the endogenous lipoprotein cascade begins with the production of very-low-density lipoproteins (VLDL). Triglycerides are resynthesized from chylomicrons and packaged with specific apoproteins, apo B-100, apo C-I, apo C-II, and apo E, to form VLDL. Once VLDL is released into the circulation, intermediate-density lipoproteins (IDL) and VLDL remnants are formed from VLDL lipolysis. This process takes place in the capillary endothelium and is mediated by LPL, the same enzyme responsible for the hydrolysis of chylomicrons. Apo C-II also acts as a cofactor in these processes.[12]

Low-density lipoprotein receptors in the liver recognize and bind with apo E on the IDL particle and remove approximately half of the IDL from the circulation. The

remainder is converted by hepatic lipase into smaller, cholesterol-rich lipoproteins, known as LDLs. Apo B-100 is the remaining protein left on the surface coat of LDL particles. The LDL receptors on cells of the liver and other organs that require cholesterol for structural and metabolic functions bind with apo B-100 and facilitate the removal of LDL from the blood. Figure 33-2 illustrates the endogenous pathway.

The LDL particle is the major cholesterol-carrying lipoprotein in the blood and, consequently, the most atherogenic lipoprotein.[89] Under normal conditions, more than 93% of the cholesterol in the body is located in the cells, and only 7% circulates in the blood. Two thirds of the

EXOGENOUS PATHWAY

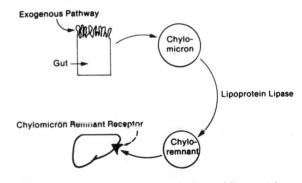

FIGURE 33-1 The exogenous metabolism of lipoproteins and the transport of chylomicrons to the tissues and chylomicron remnants to the liver. (From American Heart Association: Professional Cholesterol Education Program. Dallas, American Heart Association, 1987. Reproduced by permission of the American Heart Association, Inc.)

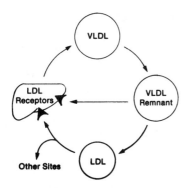

FIGURE 33-2 The endogenous lipid transport system originates in the liver. Low-density lipoproteins provide essential cholesterol to the tissue cells. (From American Heart Association: Professional Cholesterol Education Program. Dallas, American Heart Association, 1987. Reproduced by permission of the American Heart Association, Inc.)

blood cholesterol is carried by LDL. Increased cellular uptake of cholesterol through the LDL receptor pathway suppresses the cell's own synthesis of cholesterol by inhibiting the hydroxymethylglutaryl coenzyme-A (HMG-CoA) reductase enzyme. This enzyme determines the rate of cholesterol synthesis. As cellular cholesterol levels increase, the activity of the LDL receptor is downregulated, and synthesis of new LDL receptors is inhibited.[38] These feedback control mechanisms serve as the rationale for determining the treatment of elevated blood cholesterol.

Several metabolic and genetic disorders can be related to elevated LDL cholesterol levels. Habitually high dietary intakes of saturated fats and cholesterol beyond that needed for cell functions result in blood levels of LDL beyond normal and result in inhibited LDL receptor activity. High LDL levels also can result from a decrease in clearance of LDL due to a deficiency in LDL receptors. This deficiency may be caused by genetic abnormalities in the structure of the receptor binding sites (where apolipoproteins bind), or by a decrease in LDL receptors on the surface of cells. In addition, genetic mutation in apoproteins, particularly apo E and apo B-100, can result in decreased cholesterol clearance. The metabolic consequence is an increased blood level of this atherogenic lipoprotein and the synthesis of cholesterol within cells, a process normally suppressed by LDL uptake.

REVERSE CHOLESTEROL TRANSPORT

The intestine and liver are responsible for synthesizing the precursors for the sixth lipoprotein, high-density lipoprotein (HDL). HDL and its major apoproteins facilitate the transport of excess cholesterol from tissues to the liver. The major apolipoprotein components of HDL are apo A-I, A-II, C-II, C-III, and E. The apolipoprotein components, primarily apo A-I and phospholipid constituents, such as lecithin, form incomplete (or nascent) HDL precursors. The precursors are converted to a stable, spherical particle

through the action of the blood enzyme, LCAT, which converts free cholesterol in the tissues into a cholesteryl ester core.[42,99] Apo A-I has been shown to activate LCAT and may influence the activity of the cholesteryl ester transfer protein.[98] Apo C-II is a cofactor for LPL. In the presence of circulating triglycerides, apo C-II moves from HDL to the triglyceride particle, activating LPL and promoting the catabolism of VLDL.[80] This mechanism, in part, explains the clinical observation of an inverse association between high triglycerides and low HDL levels. A third apoprotein, apo E, is thought to facilitate direct transfer of cholesterol esters to hepatocyte receptors.[80] Cholesterol esters are then excreted in bile or bile acids.[87]

Although the protective effect of HDL has been linked to its role in the reverse transport of cholesterol, it is clear that other factors, particularly genetic factors, determine coenzyme, apoprotein, and receptor activity. There are two major subclasses of HDL based on density and apoprotein composition. HDL_3 is richer in apo A-II than HDL_2, which has a higher concentration of apo A-I.[28] Production of apo A-I is higher in women than in men and is increased by alcohol consumption and estrogen administration.[89] Premenopausal women have more than three times the concentration of HDL_2 than do men. Studies have also suggested that HDL may act as an antioxidant, preventing the oxidation of LDL.[13,98]

High-density lipoproteins are not atherogenic; rather, increased circulating levels of HDL may well be antiatherogenic.[45] High HDL has been associated with a reduced risk of CHD.[40,88,101] It has been suggested that the protective effect of HDL is greater than the atherogenic effect of LDL cholesterol. For men in the Framingham Heart Study, a 50% reduction in coronary risk was found with every 10-mg/dL increment in HDL.[63] Studies have indicated that increased apo A-I levels may also be inversely related to CHD.[28] Given the protective role of HDL, lipid disorders of combined elevated blood LDL and decreased levels of protective HDL present the major risk for CHD.[63]

LOW-DENSITY LIPOPROTEIN VARIANTS

Low-Density Lipoprotein Particle Size

Mounting evidence suggests that the size of the LDL particle plays an important role in its atherogenicity. Particle size is determined by flotation rates after ultracentrifugation procedures. LDL can be separated into a small, dense LDL particle (phenotype B) and a larger, less dense LDL particle (phenotype A).[6] Clinical trial evidence suggests that people with a predominance of small, dense LDL particles have a higher incidence of CHD and more accelerated progression of coronary lesions.[36] The exact mechanism of the negative influence of the small, dense LDL particle is not completely understood. One possible explanation is that the smaller, denser particles have a greater ability to penetrate the endothelial space and participate fully in the subendothelial atherosclerotic process. Small LDL particles also appear to be more susceptible to oxidation than larger LDL particles.[26] In addition, the small, dense LDL particle is most commonly found in conjunction with a constellation of other factors, including hypertriglyceridemia, low HDL cholesterol, and insulin resistance.[86] Research also suggests that it is possible to increase (alter) the size of the LDL particle to the larger (phenotype A) size by reducing triglycerides and normalizing insulin sensitivity. In addition, lipid-lowering drugs such as bile acid binding resins, niacin, and the fibrates are reported to alter particle size favorably.[6]

Oxidized Low-Density Lipoprotein

Ongoing research in lipid metabolism is investigating the issue of oxidation. Molecular biologists have established that modified or oxidized LDL is taken up more rapidly *in vitro* by monocytes and macrophages than is native LDL.[7,96] Oxidized LDL has been found to be cytotoxic, and it is postulated that this facilitates endothelial injury, leading to the development of fatty streaks and atherosclerotic lesions. Oxidative inhibitors can block the modification of LDL; thus, it is speculated that natural antioxidants, such as vitamins C and E, may protect against the development of atherosclerotic lesions.

The Role of Lipoprotein(a)

Genetic researchers investigating variant LDL particles uncovered a lipoprotein, Lp(a), that is similar to LDL except for the addition a large protein linked to apo B-100. Elevated levels of Lp(a) have been shown to be an independent risk factor for CHD, conferring a sixfold increase in risk. Lp(a) has also been detected in atherosclerotic plaques.[73] Gene cloning allowed researchers to determine that the Lp(a) protein is similar in DNA sequence to plasminogen, a substance that breaks up blood clots. It is hypothesized that this variant LDL evolved at a time when our ancestors had markedly lower levels of blood cholesterol, and that it would assist in wound healing, bringing needed cholesterol to repair cell membranes.[73] More research is needed to provide a full understanding of the role of Lp(a).

CHOLESTEROL AND ENDOTHELIAL FUNCTION

Serum cholesterol levels and diets high in fat have been associated with impairments in endothelial functioning. The endothelium acts to regulate vascular tone, platelet adhesion, thrombosis, and growth factors.[30] Studies have demonstrated that elevated cholesterol results in a reduced vasodilation response. Furthermore, when cholesterol is lowered, vasodilation responses improve.[103] Elevated cholesterol also increases platelet aggregation and monocyte adhesion, factors that lead to thrombus formation and plaque rupture.[75] Continuing research suggests that the lipids influence a variety of endothelial responses that appear to contribute to the atherosclerotic process.

DYSLIPIDEMIC DISORDERS

Although the metabolic processes related to blood lipids are complex and influenced by both genetic and environmental factors, the management of dyslipidemias has been well characterized. National recommendations have been developed based on scientific evidence and taking into account the need for both primary and secondary prevention of CHD.[82] In general, lipid disorders can be characterized by the specific lipid abnormalities observed (Table 33-2).

HYPERCHOLESTEROLEMIA

Hypercholesterolemia is the most common dyslipidemia and, in most people, decreased LDL clearance is responsible for the observed abnormality. A high intake of dietary cholesterol and saturated fatty acids downregulates LDL receptor activity and receptor synthesis, resulting in decreased LDL clearance.[15]

Familial (Severe) Hypercholesterolemia

Severe hypercholesterolemia is caused most commonly by a genetic disorder and is known as familial hypercholesterolemia (FH). There are two types of FH, heterozygous and homozygous. Plasma LDL cholesterol normally binds to cell membrane receptors and is taken into the cell for sev-

TABLE 33-2	Lipid Abnormalities and Associated Mechanisms
Lipid Abnormality	**Mechanisms**
Elevated total cholesterol	High dietary intake of saturated fat and cholesterol
	LDL receptor deficiency or down regulation
Elevated LDL-cholesterol	LDL receptor deficiency
	Apoprotein B-100 genetic defect
	High dietary intake of saturated fat and cholesterol
Elevated triglycerides	Deficiency in lipoprotein lipase
	Obesity, physical inactivity
	Insulin resistance, glucose intolerance
	Excessive alcohol intake
	Estrogen replacement
Low HDL	Apoprotein A-I deficiency
	Estrogen replacement
	Reduced VLDL clearance
	Cigarette smoking, physical inactivity
Combined dsylipidemias Small, dense LDL, high triglycerides, low HDL Elevated LDL and triglycerides	Defects in VLDL and LDL receptor activities coexisting with environmental influences such as obesity, physical inactivity, diet high in saturated fat, and cigarette smoking

HDL, high-density lipoprotein; LDL, low-density lipoprotein; VLDL, very–low-density lipoprotein.

eral biologic functions. In heterozygous FH, there is one normal gene and one abnormal gene for the LDL receptor. Because only half the normal number of LDL receptors are synthesized, LDL is removed from the blood occurs at two-thirds the normal rate.[38] The result is a two- to threefold increase in blood LDL levels. One person in 500 is thought to have this genetic disorder, which eventually results in an increased risk for myocardial infarction (MI).[82] The homozygous form of FH develops when two abnormal genes are inherited. The 1 in 1 million people who have this disorder have LDL levels six times normal and may have an MI as early as 5 to 15 years of age.[38,82] In addition, a genetic defect related to apo B-100 results in marked elevations in LDL cholesterol.

Hypertriglyceridemia

The relationship between triglycerides and CHD is not clear. Elevated serum triglyceride levels have been associated with CHD. However, the strength of the association is diminished when other CHD risks are accounted for, leading some to suggest that elevated triglycerides are a marker for other atherogenic factors.[47] Chylomicrons and VLDL are lipoprotein carriers of triglyceride, and, whereas chylomicrons are not considered to be atherogenic, the remnants of VLDL catabolism are smaller particles that are richer in cholesterol esters.[47] These remnant particles, or IDL, are considered more atherogenic.[68] Elevated triglycerides are frequently observed in people who also have low HDL levels and small, dense LDL particles. This combination of lipid abnormalities is considered an atherogenic phenotype.[47] In addition, elevated triglycerides commonly exist with insulin resistance, glucose intolerance, hypertension, and obesity, a metabolic quartet linked to increased CHD risk. It is this association that suggests elevated triglycerides may be a marker for other CHD risks. Diabetes also results in increased plasma triglyceride levels because of increased VLDL. HDL is often low in diabetic patients as a result of increased hepatic lipase triglyceride activity. LDL cholesterol is more glycated in diabetic patients compared with nondiabetic subjects. Glycated LDL particles have increased oxidative susceptibility.[50] High triglyceride levels are also related to high carbohydrate and alcohol intake. As a marker for CHD risk, the reduction of plasma triglyceride levels to less than 200 mg/dL is a desirable goal.[82]

Hypoalphalipoproteinemia

A familial HDL deficiency state, hypoalphalipoproteinemia, has been linked to premature CHD. Whereas high HDL levels may mobilize cholesterol from arterial luminal surfaces and return it to the liver, low HDL usually reflects an enzymatic or apoprotein abnormality affecting the catabolism of LDL or VLDL. Alterations of the human apo A-I gene have been found in those with familial HDL deficiency and premature CHD.[83] This suggests that low HDL may represent a genetic marker for identifying those at risk for CHD. The abnormalities related to VLDL catabolism explain the common coexistence of low HDL with elevated triglycerides. Furthermore, when triglycerides are lowered, increases in HDL are observed. In the absence of a genetic deficiency, lower HDL levels are related to environmental factors such as cigarette smoking and physical inactivity.

Combined Dyslipidemias

Combined dyslipidemias usually represent a combination of genetic lipoprotein or apoprotein defects and environmental effects. The specific lipid abnormalities observed provide clues to the genetic disorders. Table 33-2 summarizes observed lipid abnormalities and associated mechanisms. An understanding of these mechanisms guides the management of lipid abnormalities.

THE MANAGEMENT OF HIGH BLOOD CHOLESTEROL

Since the late 1980s, a large and convincing body of evidence has associated elevated blood lipids with CHD. Furthermore, clinical trials have demonstrated that reducing blood cholesterol is effective for both the primary and secondary prevention of CHD. This research has prompted groups such as the National Institutes of Health, American Heart Association, and the American College of Cardiology to establish health policy guidelines for the detection and treatment of lipid disorders.[1,48,82,93]

Recommendations for Detection of High Blood Cholesterol

Health policy recommendations for detection of high cholesterol include the measurement of total cholesterol and HDL cholesterol in all adults aged 20 years and older, with repeat measurement within 5 years. Nonfasting measurements are deemed acceptable. Total cholesterol below 200 mg/dL is considered desirable, levels between 200 mg/dL to 239 mg/dL are classified as borderline high, and those above 240 mg/dL are considered high blood cholesterol. Measures of HDL below 35 mg/dL are considered low and constitute a risk factor for CHD. Other, nonlipid factors that contribute to CHD risk status also should be assessed, including cigarette smoking, hypertension, diabetes mellitus, a family history of premature heart disease, and sex and age (men older than 45 years and women older than 55 years of age). Table 33-3 provides target levels for modifiable CHD risk factors. If total cholesterol is greater than 200 mg/dL or HDL is less than 35 mg/dL, a full lipoprotein analysis is required and treatment is based on LDL levels. Risk factor reduction, including dietary therapy and increased physical activity, are major therapies for CHD prevention in patients at low risk and a major component of the therapeutic management of those at high risk or those with established CHD.

Recommended Goals for the Treatment of High Blood Cholesterol

The goal for cholesterol management is the achievement of ideal LDL levels. If CHD and cardiovascular risk factors are

TABLE 33-3	Risk Factors and Target Goal Levels for the Prevention of Coronary Heart Disease
CHD Risk Factors	**Target Level for Modifiable Risk Factors**

Age
  Men: ≥45 y
  Women: ≥55 y or premature menopause without hormone replacement	

Family history of premature CHD
  Mother or sister <65 y
  Father or brother <55 y	

TC >200 mg/dL HDL cholesterol <35 mg/dL HDL cholesterol >60 mg/dL is a negative risk factor for CHD	TC <200 and HDL >35 mg/dL. In the presence of CHD or with two or more CHD risk factors, LDL levels as targeted for goal levels.*
Cigarette smoking	Complete cessation
Hypertension ≥140/90 mm Hg or on hypertensive medication	≤140/85 mm Hg†
Diabetes mellitus	Fasting blood sugar <127 mg/dL‡

*CHD, coronary heart disease; HDL, high-density lipoprotein; LDL, low-density lipoprotein; TC, total cholesterol.
†Joint National Commission on the Identification and Treatment of Hypertension VI. NIH Publication no. 93–1088. March, 1998.
‡American Diabetes Association: Clinical practice recommendations 1997. Diabetes Care 20 (Suppl 1): S1–S70.

absent, an ideal LDL level is less than 130 mg/dL. Because LDL levels of 130 and 160 mg/dL correspond reasonably well to total cholesterol levels of 200 mg/dL and 240 mg/dL, respectively, the screening cholesterol levels and the person's risk profile can be used to determine evaluation and treatment. If CHD and/or multiple risk factors are present, an ideal LDL is a level less than 100 mg/dL. Health policy guidelines strongly encourage consideration of risk status for both the evaluation and the treatment of elevated cholesterol. Table 33-4 provides an overview of LDL goals, treatment considerations, and follow-up recommendations.

EVALUATION OF THE PATIENT WITH ELEVATED CHOLESTEROL

It is appropriate that the patient with high blood cholesterol receive a thorough clinical evaluation in addition to a lipoprotein analysis. Several other medical diagnoses have been associated with high cholesterol (Table 33-5). Abnormal lipid profiles may be the first clue to undiagnosed endocrine disorders such as hypothyroidism or diabetes. A careful family history is also important. Genetic forms of hypercholesterolemia are relatively common in the general population; for example, FH has an estimated frequency of

1 in 500[89]; it is therefore advisable that first-degree relatives be screened for lipid disorders.

Hyperlipidemia, like hypertension, is a relatively asymptomatic disorder and is usually first recognized by abnormal laboratory findings. Subcutaneous or tendinous lipid deposits, called xanthoma, are the one physical finding that may be prominent in severe lipid disorders. Xanthelasma palpebrarum are seen in the inner corner of eyelids and are associated with FH in approximately half of patients with this finding. Tendinous xanthomas often are found in extensor tendons of the hands and Achilles tendon. Planar xanthomas are lipid deposits in the webs of the hand and occur in children with FH. Corneal arcus is caused by cholesterol deposition within the corneal rim and can be seen as a white band around the cornea. This finding may be indicative of FH in younger people but may not be meaningful in the older adult.[41]

Certain types of hyperlipoproteinemia are characterized by abdominal pain. Possible causes for the abdominal pain include pancreatitis and hepatosplenomegaly. Abdominal pain of unknown cause also has been documented as a physical finding. This pain may be associated with ischemic bowel and is related to increased blood viscosity, macrophage ingestion of fat particles, or the effect of the size of the lipid particles on abdominal tissue.[41] Patients with chylomicronemia, or markedly elevated triglycerides levels, have a high risk of pancreatitis.

LIPOPROTEIN MEASUREMENT

The measurement of plasma lipids and lipoproteins is essential for the diagnosis of lipid abnormalities and for the identification of those at risk for CHD. These measurements also provide important feedback to the patient modifying his or her risk profile. The most common lipid analysis includes measurement of total cholesterol, total triglycerides, and HDL cholesterol. This allows calculation of LDL using the following equation: LDL = total cholesterol minus (triglycerides/5) minus HDL.[35] This indirect assessment of LDL can be used if triglycerides are less than 400 mg/dL. If triglycerides are above 400 mg/dL, LDL must be directly measured using the more complex and costly ultracentrifugation procedure.

To interpret the results of lipid measurements, some knowledge of the accuracy and precision of the measure is useful. One of the common scenarios encountered in lipid management is a laboratory report with values extremely different from previously measured values, and the patient protests, "I haven't been doing anything differently." Intraindividual cholesterol measurements have been shown to vary by 4% to 11% over a 1-year period.[104] Although there are several sources for variability or error in cholesterol measures, the most obvious is analytic variability, or laboratory error, which has been estimated to contribute one third to one half of the intraindividual variability. Laboratories must make their standardization criteria available, and should strive to achieve less than 3% measurement variability. Biologic and physiologic factors constitute the other major source for measurement variability.

TABLE 33-4 National Cholesterol Education Program (NCEP) Evaluation and Treatment Guidelines for High Blood Cholesterol in Adults

Screening Measure	Risk Factors	Actions	LDL Goal	Repeat Testing
TC<200 mg/dL	+/-	Provide diet and exercise information for general population	TC <200 mg/dL	TC in 5 y
TC >200 mg/dL or HDL <35 mg/dL	+/-	Lipoprotein analysis to calculate LDL	TC <200 mg/dL	According to LDL goal

Evaluation Measure	Risk Factors	Actions	LDL Goal	Repeat Testing
Desirable LDL <130 mg/dL	No CHD +/-	Provide diet and exercise information	TC <200 mg/dL	TC in 5 y
Borderline LDL 130–159 mg/dL	No CHD and < 2 risk factors	Provide diet and exercise information appropriate for general population	TC <200 mg/dL	TC in 1 y
Borderline LDL 130–159 mg/dL	NO CHD and ≥ 2 risk factors	Clinical evaluation, diet assessment. Instruct on Step I diet, weight control, and exercise. If diet at Step I, move to Step II diet.	LDL <130 mg/dL	TC 4–6 wk and 3 mo. If TC <200 mg/dL, reconfirm LDL. Follow long-term monitoring plan: 4 times/y and 2 times/y thereafter.
Borderline LDL 130–159 mg/dL	CHD	Step II diet, weight control, exercise, and risk factor modification. If LDL>130 mg/dL after maximum dietary effort of 6 mo, consider medication therapy.	LDL <100 mg/dL	
High LDL >160 mg/dL	No risk factors	Step II diet and exercise instruction. Caution re: medication.	TC <240 or LDL <160 mg/dL	Drug therapy monitoring plan LDL at 4–6 wk LDL at 3 mo, then every 4 mo unless closer monitoring required.
High LDL >160 mg/dL	≥ 2 Risk factors or CHD	Step II diet and risk factor education. If LDL >190 mg/dL consider medication therapy. If LDL >130 mg/dL after maximum dietary effort of 6 mo, consider medication therapy. If LDL >220 mg/dL consider medication earlier.	LDL <100 mg/dL	

CHD, coronary heart disease; HDL, high-density lipoprotein; LDL, low-density lipoprotein; TC, total cholesterol.

TABLE 33-5	Factors that Influence Low-Density Lipoprotein (LDL) and High-Density Lipoprotein (HDL) Levels
Increased with	**Decreased with**
LDL Levels	
Diets high in cholesterol	Low-cholesterol diet
Diets high in saturated fat	Low-fat diet
Hypothyroidism	Exercise
Obstructive liver disease	
Nephrosis	
Thiazide diuretics	
β-Adrenergic blocking agents	
Progestins and anabolic steroids	
HDL Levels	
Not smoking	Cigarette smoking
Lean body mass	Obesity
Estrogen	
Vigorous exercise	Male gender
Diet low in sucrose and starch	Sedentary lifestyle
Increased clearance of very–low-density lipoprotein (triglyceride)	Non–insulin-dependent diabetes mellitus
	Hypertriglyceridemia
Alcohol	Progesterone
	Anabolic steroids
	Starvation
	β-Adrenergic blocking agents

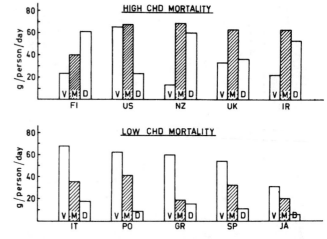

FIGURE 33-3 A comparison of the daily intake (in grams) of the major food fats in countries with high and low coronary heart disease (CHD)-related deaths. V, vegetable fats; M, meat fats; D, dairy fats; FI, Finland; US, United States; NZ, New Zealand; UK, United Kingdom; IR, Ireland; IT, Italy; PO, Portugal; GR, Germany; SP, Spain; JA, Japan. (From Turpienen O: Effect of cholesterol-lowering diet on mortality from coronary heart disease and other causes. Circulation 59:3, 1979. Used with permission of the American Heart Association, Inc.)

To minimize measurement variability, the National Cholesterol Education Laboratory Standardization Panel[104] recommends the following standards of practice:

◆ A stable lifestyle, including health status, diet, medication, and activity level, should be followed for at least 2 weeks before measurement.
◆ Cholesterol measures should be made no sooner than 8 weeks after an MI, surgical procedure, trauma, or an acute bacterial or viral infection.
◆ Blood collection procedures should include a 12-hour fast (except for water and usual medications) before sampling if lipid measures other than total cholesterol are to be performed.
◆ The patient should sit quietly for 5 minutes before the venipuncture.
◆ The sample should be obtained within 1 minute of tourniquet application.
◆ Standardized procedures for processing and transporting samples should be followed.

DIETARY MANAGEMENT OF HYPERLIPIDEMIA

Evidence of the relationship between dietary intake, plasma cholesterol, and CHD has been steadily accumulating. Population studies have shown that countries with the highest incidence of CHD and elevated blood cholesterol levels also have high dietary intakes of saturated fats.[5,64,71,78] Developing countries with a mean cholesterol level below 150 mg/dL have a very low incidence of CHD and also have diets low in total fat, saturated fatty acids, and cholesterol.[64] Figure 33-3 illustrates the relationship of CHD mortality to types of fat intake. Animal studies have demonstrated that high-fat diets result in increased total and LDL cholesterol and lead to the development of atherosclerotic vascular lesions.[4] Metabolic ward studies also support the relationship between saturated fat consumption and plasma cholesterol,[53,65] and have demonstrated that lowering fat intake can achieve as much as a 30% reduction in plasma cholesterol. Clinical trials have used angiography to demonstrate slower rates of CHD progression in subjects adhering to low-fat and low-cholesterol diets.[84,91,105] Blankenhorn and colleagues[9] examined the relationship of new lesion development and diet in the placebo-plus-diet group of the Cholesterol Lowering Atherosclerosis Study (CLAS); they observed that the dietary fat intake in the subset not acquiring new lesions was 27% of calories, compared with 34% in the subset acquiring new lesions. It is the evidence that LDL receptor synthesis and activity are decreased in response to diets high in saturated fat that lends ultimate support to the inclusion of dietary therapy as the cornerstone for lipid management.[15]

Dietary Recommendations

The goal of diet therapy is to reduce LDL cholesterol to desirable levels predicated by the person's CHD risk status while maintaining a nutritionally sound eating pattern. The initial dietary intervention recommended by the National Cholesterol Education Program (NCEP) is the Step I diet.[82] This diet plan includes reduction in total fat intake to 30% of total caloric intake. Saturated fats should be no more than 10% of total caloric intake and cholesterol intake should not exceed 300 mg/d. If the LDL goal is not achieved within 3 months or the patient is already adhering to a Step I diet, it is recommended that the Step II diet be implemented. This diet plan recommends that saturated fat intake be further reduced to 7% of calories and that dietary cholesterol be reduced to less than 200 mg/d.[82]

Before initiating any dietary change, an assessment of the patient's current dietary pattern and usual eating habits is necessary. Dietary assessments are based on subjective reports and are predisposed to problems of recall accuracy and reliability. Review articles on dietary assessment issues suggest that food frequency inventories or careful diet history provide the most accurate information on usual eating patterns.[33,34] Assessment tools are reported in the literature[21] or can be obtained from agencies such as the American Dietetic Association, American Heart Association, or the NCEP, or from product manufacturers.

Dietary surveys of Americans between 1976 and 1980 showed that the average American intake of dietary fat was 37% of total calories, saturated fat intake was 13% of total calories, and cholesterol consumption averaged 260 and 430 mg/d for women and men, respectively.[10] When these same data were analyzed by comparing those who reported following a "low-fat diet" with "nondieters," the intake pattern of the dieters averaged 33% of total calories from fat, 11% of calories from saturated fat, and an average cholesterol intake of 287 mg/d. Extensive professional and public attention has been given to the issue of cholesterol, such that the most recent dietary survey (from 1988 to 1991) in the U.S. population shows a significant 6- to 8-mg/dL decrease in serum cholesterol levels.[61] The data from these surveys and from clinical trials on CHD progression[51] suggest that people with established CHD or with CHD risk factors are likely to have adopted a Step I diet without the intervention and support of health care professionals. The NCEP guidelines note that a Step I diet involves reduction in the major and obvious sources of saturated fat and cholesterol, whereas a Step II diet requires careful attention to the whole diet, and implementation may require the services of a nutritionally qualified professional.[82]

Several aspects related to a lipid-lowering diet remain controversial. Although most experts recommend reducing intake of saturated fats, there is disagreement over what nutrients should replace the reduction in fat. Is the ideal lipid-lowering diet a low-fat, high-carbohydrate diet, or a diet that replaces saturated fats with unsaturated fats? Saturated fatty acids, with the exception of stearic acid, raise total and LDL cholesterol, probably through a mechanism decreasing LDL receptor synthesis.[11] Studies suggest that diets high in monounsaturated fat relative to saturated fat convey a desirable plasma lipid profile, with lowering of total and LDL cholesterol and no reduction in HDL.[49] The major criticism of these studies has been that the addition only of unsaturated fats to the diet is not practical among free-living individuals. For example, food items high in stearic acid usually contain other highly saturated fatty acids as well. Second, studies have yet to determine whether such diets are associated with beneficial outcomes beyond

changes to the lipid profile. Low-fat, high-carbohydrate diets produce lower LDL levels than high-fat diets, but such diets may result in higher triglyceride and lower HDL levels. A 1-year study comparing four fat-restricted diets (30%, 26%, 22%, and 18% of calories from fat) found significant reductions in LDL ranging from 5% to 13%.[66] Triglycerides increased significantly in the two most fat-restricted diets (18% and 22% of calories from fat). These authors concluded that moderate reduction in fat is beneficial but that more severe restrictions may produce undesirable effects. The marked increase in obesity of the U.S. population that some attribute to increased carbohydrate consumption has further added to this controversy. In an effort to reduce dietary fat, Americans frequently select low-fat manufactured products containing sugar rather than choosing plant-based carbohydrate foods. This is evident in that the consumption of refined sugar has increased from 120 lbs/person in 1970 to 150 lbs/person in 1995, and fiber intake remains low.[31] Even those researchers who advocated diets high in monounsaturated fats also recommend increased consumption of fruits and vegetables.[23]

The omega-3 fatty acids, primarily found in fish and fish oils, have also been shown to affect plasma lipids, primarily triglycerides.[22,74] The response is dose related and is sufficiently high that it is unlikely to be achieved using food choices only or without supplemental use. The omega-3 fatty acids are postulated to decrease VLDL synthesis and thereby reduce triglycerides. They also exert antithrombotic effects through the thromboxane-prostaglandin pathways, resulting in decreases in both platelet aggregation and vasoconstriction. Although the safety of consumption of large amounts of fish oils is an issue, most researchers agree that the inclusion of fish several times each week is a safe and prudent alternative.

The response to dietary intervention is variable and appears related not only to the specific fatty acid composition of the diet but to the level of plasma lipids. People with the higher lipid levels usually experience the greatest response to dietary interventions.[69] (See reviews[37,69,79] for more detailed discussion of the specific effects of fatty acids.) The most practical recommendations are to reduce the total quantity of fat in the diet, change the quality of fat by replacing food items high in saturated fat with foods containing monounsaturated or polyunsaturated fatty acids, and increase the quantities of fruits, vegetables, and fiber.

Dietary Change Strategies

For most patients, recommendations for dietary change are not sufficient to effect dietary change. Substantial knowledge must be acquired and specific behavior skills must be learned and practiced. Required knowledge should include an understanding of the relationship between dietary fat, dietary cholesterol, and blood cholesterol; defining reasonable expectations for dietary change; understanding the differences in the quality of fats; ability to read and interpret food labels; sufficient knowledge about food items to estimate fat content of unlabeled items; and knowledge of food preparation methods that affect fat content. Because eating is a part of our social environment, the behavioral skills must be adapted to a variety of social settings, such as travel, eating out, celebrations, and the work environment. Patients should practice label reading and menu selections, and questioning food preparers or waiters. Anticipatory responses for avoiding high-fat foods in social situations should be explicitly identified. Adapting recipes and developing grocery shopping lists that include brand-name selections are also useful skills to learn.

Several studies have examined patterns of food and food group changes occurring during adoption of low-fat diets.[16,39,70,77,90,94] In general, patients were successful in reducing their consumption of eggs, high-fat meats, and fried-food items; substituting lower-fat items for high-fat items, such as skim milk for milk or low-calorie spreads and salad dressings in place of high-fat dressings; and in replacing high-fat items with low-fat items, such as replacing sour cream with yogurt. Although patients were successful at selecting less saturated fats, they were less successful at decreasing their consumption of total and added fats. The most difficult food items to reduce or replace included cheese and snack foods, such as crackers. Until more adequate products become available from food manufacturers, substitution for these areas of difficult change may be a practical strategy.

Computer modeling techniques have been used to examine the effect of dietary fat reduction strategies to determine the most effective strategy for meeting Step I dietary goals.[94] The strategies included substitution of low-fat counterparts for high-fat items, reduction in quantity of high-fat foods, replacement of high-fat foods with other types of foods (e.g., beans for meat), and modifying preparation techniques (e.g., broiling instead of frying). For men, the strategy of replacement was the single strategy that met the dietary goals. No single strategy was effective for women. The results suggest that the most significant changes occur using combinations of dietary strategies.

Education alone is unlikely to facilitate dietary change. Studies examining educational interventions have found only a small relationship between knowledge, attitudes, and dietary behavior.[7] When behavioral interventions were combined with educational strategies, more positive dietary outcomes were observed.[24,32,39] Behavioral strategies are based on the principles of social learning theory.[8] Social learning theory principles include examining the antecedents of the behavior (expectations and values placed on the behavior outcome), the skills and knowledge needed to perform the behavior, and the reinforcement contingencies associated with the behavior (rewards, feedback, and evaluation). Many behavioral techniques, such as self-monitoring, goal setting, defining alternatives and choices, evaluation, rewards, and feedback can be used to assist patients in the change process.[29,77]

Daily logs of food patterns, eating habits, environmental setting, and self-efficacy measures provide an opportunity for the patient to evaluate his or her own behavior and to receive feedback on specific successes or assistance in identifying undesirable patterns or trends. The antecedents to the behavior can be examined for positive or negative influences on dietary behavior. Small, portable computers are available that can record dietary intake and give an immediate nutrient analysis. This type of device incorporates the techniques of self-monitoring, evaluation, and feedback and, in some cases, can supply alternative choices. Less sophisticated written records that detail the food item, amount, and type of

preparation have also been shown to be adequate for the purposes of monitoring and changing behavior. It is not unusual for record keeping alone to lead to altered behavior.

Record analysis can also be useful in determining appropriate goals. Many behaviorists view goal setting as a key element. The goal should be defined by the patient and should be one that is small, specific, and measurable. Nurses can assist the patient through the process, ensuring that these key goal attributes exist.

A variety of aids have been developed to assist personal monitoring and evaluation of food choices.[16,20] Booklets listing the grams of fat for typical portions of commonly consumed foods have been successfully used for this purpose.[85] A daily fat gram goal for both total and saturated fat can be established based on usual daily caloric intake. If daily intake is 2,000 calories, a diet with less than 20% of calories from fat would restrict fat intake to 44 g (2,000 kcal × 20% = 400 kcal; 400 kcal/[9 kcal/g] = 44 g). Recall that 1 g of fat equals 9 kcal. These booklets usually are pocket sized and are easily carried grocery shopping or to restaurants, and usually include a diary for recording personal daily intake.

Behavior can be reinforced using evaluation and feedback techniques. Feedback can be provided through analysis of food records and by measurement of blood lipids. It is possible to achieve plasma cholesterol reductions of 15% to 20% with adherence to a low-fat and low-cholesterol diet. However, given the individual variability of response, caution should be used in providing feedback based totally on plasma cholesterol measures. Feedback and rewards based on dietary behaviors are likely to provide more positive and long-lasting reinforcement.

WEIGHT CONTROL AND LIPID MANAGEMENT

The prevalence of obesity in the United States has increased since the late 1970s. It is estimated that more than one third (65 million) of adults have a body mass index (weight in kilograms divided by height [in meters squared]) greater than 31 and would be considered severely obese.[54] Because both LDL and the incidence of CHD are reduced in people who maintain a normal body weight, these data are alarming. Studies examining weight loss have reported varying effects on lipid profiles. A meta-analysis of 70 studies examining the effect of weight reduction on lipoproteins found that a 1-kg reduction in weight was associated with a 0.05-mmol/L decrease in total cholesterol (1 mmol/L = 38.67 mg/dL).[25] Significant decreases in LDL and triglycerides were also found. The effect of weight loss on HDL varies, decreasing during the active weight loss period and increasing after a period of stable reduced weight. The mechanisms postulated to account for these alterations in lipoproteins include decreased HMG-CoA reductase activity and enhanced cholesterol excretion in bile acids. The release of cholesterol from adipose tissues is also thought to inhibit hepatic synthesis of cholesterol.

For all patients with dyslipidemia, the secondary goal of diet intervention is weight reduction. Patients with dyslipidemia should be counseled to expect an initial reduction in HDL during active weight loss. Increased levels of physical activity may minimize the HDL reduction and facilitate weight loss.[106]

ALCOHOL AND LIPOPROTEINS

Moderate alcohol intake has been reported to be protective for CHD. France, a country with a low rate of CHD, has a markedly higher per capita consumption of alcohol, particularly of wine.[76] One possible mechanism for this protective effect may be related to the increase in HDL observed with alcohol intake. Researchers have established that moderate alcohol intake increases HDL_3, apo A-I, and apo A-II.[17,52] Alcohol may also alter platelet aggregation and lower fibrinogen levels. Alcohol also increases catabolism of VLDL, the triglyceride-carrying lipoprotein. Patients with elevated triglyceride levels may have dramatic improvements in triglyceride levels with cessation of alcohol. Most researchers agree that the inverse association between alcohol intake and CHD risk is a consistent but weak association.[95] Recommendations to consume alcohol must therefore be considered cautiously, given the potential side effects of impaired judgment, decreased motor coordination, and possible addiction associated with alcohol use.

PHYSICAL ACTIVITY AND LIPOPROTEINS

The American Heart Association has added physical inactivity to dyslipidemia, smoking, and hypertension as the fourth major modifiable risk factor for coronary artery and other vascular diseases.[93] Physical activity works through a variety of mechanisms to lower coronary risk. Regular physical activity aids in weight loss by increasing caloric output. Weight loss decreases serum triglylcerides, which can result in increased levels of HDL cholesterol. Exercise improves glycemic control in type II diabetes by lessening insulin resistance and improving insulin sensitivity. In some people, exercise also lowers LDL cholesterol, although LDL reductions usually are modest. Regular physical activity has a positive influence on endothelial function. Research has shown that regular exercise can improve vasodilation responses and reduce platelet adhesion.[30] Given these beneficial effects, regular physical activity should be a part of the multifactorial intervention program used to manage dyslipidemia.

HORMONES AND LIPOPROTEINS

Clinical heart disease develops in women almost a decade later in life than in men, likely because of the protective effects of estrogen. Several mechanisms have been suggested to account for this beneficial effect. Estrogen decreases LDL and increases HDL and apo A-I levels.[18] Estrogen use has been associated with lower Lp(a), reduced LDL oxidative susceptibility, and improved endothelial vasodilation responses.[18,97] Several clinical trials are examining the effect of hormone replacement therapy (HRT) for primary and secondary coronary artery disease prevention. The Heart and Estrogen-progestin Replacement Study (HERS) evaluated the infuence of premarin plus medroxyprogesterone acetate versus placebo in 2,763 women with CHD at baseline. After an average follow-up of 4.1 years, no differences were detected in acute myocardial infarction and coronary death between the two groups. In addition, there was a pattern of early increased risk of CHD and thrombotic events with a pattern of late benefit in the women randomized to HRT. As a result of this trial, the role of HRT as a treatment for women with CHD is being questioned. Until there is more data from ongoing randomized trials, such as the Women's Health Initiative, the HERS investigators do not recommend that women with CHD begin HRT as a secondary prevention therapy. If, however, they are currently on HRT, it is appropriate to continue HRT. [57]

PHARMACOLOGIC MANAGEMENT OF HYPERLIPIDEMIA

The primary rationale for the treatment of hyperlipidemia is the reduction of CHD morbidity and mortality. Studies using hypolipidemic drug therapy to achieve LDL reductions have demonstrated lower CHD morbidity and mortality and lower overall mortality rates.[88,92] Angiographic studies using lipid-lowering drugs have demonstrated less progression of angiographically determined CHD with reduction of LDL.[14,51,62,105] The rate of progression of CHD appears to be a dose-related response, with slower rates of progression associated with greater LDL lowering. Angiographic studies have been of sufficiently short duration and lack long-term follow-up data such that the effect on total and CHD mortality cannot be determined.

Until very–long-term studies have been conducted, the safety and efficacy of hypolipidemic drug therapy will be questioned. Meta-analytic techniques have been used to analyze lipid-lowering studies and suggest that the decrease in CHD mortality is offset by increased death rates from other causes, particularly cancer deaths and non–illness-related deaths such as injury deaths and suicides.[58,60,81] These meta-analyses did not include data from the more recent, very large clinical trials investigating lipid-lowering drugs (4S, WOSCOPS, AFCAPS/TEXCAPS). These studies did not observe any increase in cancer or non–illness-related deaths. Although the explanations for these findings remain controversial, the consensus of experts is that hypolipidemic drug therapy should always be instituted with nonpharmacologic interventions, including a low-fat, low-cholesterol diet, regular exercise, weight control, smoking cessation, control of hypertension, and control of blood glucose in patients with diabetes. Hypolipidemic drug therapy requires careful consideration of individual risks as well as the benefits of such drug therapy.

Lipid Criteria and Goals for Drug Therapy

Consideration of hypolipidemic drug therapy for primary prevention (i.e., in people without existing CHD) is indicated in those without CHD risk factors but with LDL levels greater than 190 mg/dL, or in people with two or more CHD risk factors and LDL levels greater than 160 mg/dL. The target goals of treatment should be to achieve LDL levels of less than 160 or 130 mg/dL, respectively. In secondary prevention (i.e., in patients with established CHD), drug therapy can be considered if LDL levels are at least 130 mg/dL. The goal for patients with CHD is an LDL of less than 100 mg/dL[100] (see Table 33-4).

Classes of Hypolipidemic Drugs

The major classes of hypolipidemic drugs include the bile acid binding resins, nicotinic acid, and the HMG-CoA reductase inhibitors (statins). Other drug classes that can be considered in selected circumstances include fibric acid derivatives, antioxidants, and estrogen replacement therapy. Individual response to each of these agents is variable, and each of the agents has potential side effects. Nursing can play a major role in the management of patients by assisting the patient to minimize side effects, while promoting adherence to the regimen that achieves the desired lipid profile. In this section, the action, indications for use, and specific adherence strategies for each of the classes of hypolipidemic drugs are reviewed (Table 33-6).

BILE ACID BINDING RESINS

Actions and Indications for Use.   Bile acid binding resins are insoluble in water and are not absorbed from the intestine. These agents bind with bile acids in the intestine, forming an insoluble complex. The enterohepatic circulation of bile acids is interrupted and fecal excretion of bile acids is increased. This results in increased synthesis of bile acids from hepatic cholesterol stores. Reduced hepatic cholesterol stimulates LDL receptor formation and increases HMG-CoA reductase activity, resulting in increased extrac-tion of LDL from the bloodstream and a lower plasma concentration of LDL. Hepatic production of VLDL is also enhanced, resulting in increased triglyceride levels. The expected response to resin therapy is seen in 2 to 4 weeks and may result in a 20% to 25% reduction in LDL.[89]

Strategies for Increased Efficacy and Adherence.   The major side effect of the bile acid binding resins is constipa-tion; the resins can be unpalatable, which may affect com-pliance. Resins come in both powder and tablet formula-tions. In powder form, the resins must be mixed with water. Because they are insoluble, they form a gritty solution. It is helpful to demonstrate the mixing process and allow the patient to taste the drug as part of the prescription process. If constipation develops, instruct the patient in the use of fiber, stool softeners, and other hygienic measures, such as increased fluid intake. Bile acid binding resins should be taken with meals, particularly with the largest meal of the day, because intestinal bile acids are greatest during that time. Because these drugs are binding agents, they have the potential to bind and interfere with the absorption of other medications. Consequently, the patient should be instructed to take other medications 1 hour before or 4 hours after taking the resin. Reviewing the mechanism of action with the patient promotes adherence and a better understanding of the rationale for these instructions.

TABLE 33-6 **Pharmacologic Approach to Dyslipidemia**

Lipid-Lowering Drug	Lipid Effects	Mechanism	Major Side Effects

Bile acid binding resins
  Cholestyramine
  Colestipol
	LDL 15%–25%
	HDL 5%
	Triglycerides
		Binds bile acids
		Stimulates LDL receptor
		  synthesis
		Increases extraction of LDL from
		  the plasma
			Constipation, bloating
			Nausea
			Decreased absorption of fat-soluble
			  vitamins and other drugs

Nicotinic acid
  Niacin
  Niacor
  Nicolar
  Niaspan
	LDL 15%–25%
	HDL 15%–30%
	Triglycerides 20%–50%
	Lp (a)
		Decreases hepatic production of
		  VLDL
		Blocks release of free fatty acids
		  from adipose stores, leading to
		  decreased triglycerides
			Cutaneous flushing, pruritus, or dry
			  skin
			Gastrointestinal discomfort
			Reversible elevations in liver
			  function enzymes

HMG-CoA reductase
  inhibitors
  Lovastatin,
  Pravastatin,
  Simvastatin,
  Fluvastatin,
  Atorvastatin,
  Cerivastatin
	Agent and dose dependent
	  LDL 25%–40%
	  HDL 5%–10%
	  Triglycerides
		Inhibits rate-limiting enzyme in
		  cholesterol synthesis
		Increase LDL receptor synthesis
			Gastrointestinal distress, headache,
			  insomnia
			Elevations in liver enzymes
			Myopathies, rare rhabdomyolysis
			Interactions with gemfibrozil, niacin,
			  and immunosuppressants

Fibrates
  Gemfibrozil
  Fenofibrate
	Triglycerides 20%–50%
	LDL—may increase with
	  triglyceride lowering
		Stimulates lipoprotein lipase
		  production
		Enhances VLDL catabolism
			Dyspepsia, nausea, abdominal pain

Estrogen	LDL 15%–20%
	HDL 10%–15%
	Triglycerides
	Lp (a)
		Reduces migration of oxidized
		  LDL into arterial wall
		Affects thrombotic and
		  endothelial functions
			Increases uterine cell proliferation,
			  countered by progesterone
			  administration
			Menstruation symptoms—breast
			  tenderness, cyclic bleeding

HDL, high-density lipoprotein; HMG-CoA, hydroxymethylglutaryl coenzyme-A; LDL, low-density lipoprotein; VLDL, very-low-density lipoprotein. Lp(a), lipoprotein(a).

NICOTINIC ACID (NIACIN)

Actions and Indications for Use.   Nicotinic acid, or niacin, is a vitamin B_3 derivative that in large doses blocks the release of free fatty acids from adipose tissues, resulting in less hepatic conversion of free fatty acids into triglycerides.[89] The hepatic production of VLDL is also decreased. Because VLDL is converted to IDL and LDL, decreased VLDL levels lead to favorable reductions in these lipoproteins as well.

Contraindications to use include active liver disease and peptic ulcer disease, and caution is needed when it is used in patients with diabetes and atrial arrhythmias.

Strategies for Increased Efficacy and Adherence.   The most common side effect of nicotinic acid use is cutaneous flushing caused by a prostaglandin-mediated vasodilation effect on vascular smooth muscle. This effect can be minimized with the use of aspirin taken 30 minutes before the nicotinic acid dose. Other, less common side effects include abdominal discomfort; nausea; elevations in glucose, uric acid, and liver enzymes; reversible hepatotoxicity; and potentiation of atrial arrhythmias. Abdominal side effects are reduced if niacin is taken with meals.

Niacin use must be monitored by a health professional, with liver enzymes measured before, and periodically during, therapy. Side effects can be minimized by starting at low doses and increasing the dose gradually. Written instructions, including a suggested dosage schedule, should be provided to the patient. The patient should be informed of the various side effects and instructed to contact a health professional if hepatotoxic side effects, such as flu-like symptoms and malaise, occur.

HMG-CoA REDUCTASE INHIBITORS (STATINS)

The statins inhibit HMG-CoA reductase, the rate-limiting enzyme in cholesterol synthesis. Reduced cholesterol synthesis in the hepatocytes stimulates increased LDL receptor activity, thereby promoting clearance of VLDL and LDL from the bloodstream.[102]

Strategies for Increased Efficacy and Adherence.   The statins in general are well tolerated. Single daily doses may be sufficient to achieve lipid goals. If single-day dosage is used, lipid response has been shown to be greatest with evening use. Mild gastrointestinal complaints and headaches are the most common side effects. Liver enzyme elevations occur in 1% to 2% of users and resolve with discontinuation of the drug. Myopathies (muscle aching, soreness, or weakness) associated with elevations in creatine kinase greater than three times normal occur in 0.5% of users, but the incidence is increased when statins are used in combination with immunosuppressants, gemfibrozil, and niacin.[43] Patients should be instructed to report muscle aching. If such symptoms are present, liver aminotransferases and creatine kinase should be measured and the drug stopped.

OTHER HYPOLIPIDEMIC THERAPIES

Fibric acid derivatives, have been used as hypolipidemic agents. They act primarily to increase LPL activity, which enhances catabolism of VLDL and thereby reduces triglyceride levels.[43] Because of their limited LDL effect, these drugs are not considered first-line therapy.

Observational studies suggest that estrogen replacement therapy provides a protective effect from CHD in postmenopausal women. Oral estrogens have a favorable impact on LDL and HDL, reducing LDL and increasing HDL by up to 15% each.[67] Triglyceride levels are also increased, however, and the effect of cyclic progesterones may counter the lipid benefit conveyed by estrogen. Until experimental evidence is available, recommendations for use of estrogen replacement therapy must be made on an individual basis.

General Adherence Strategies

It is estimated that 50% of patients discontinue drug therapy after 1 year[59] and only one third adhere to dietary interventions beyond 1 year.[56] Factors related to nonadherence include lack of knowledge, misconceptions, beliefs and attitudes about the therapy, complexity of the regime, side effects, and the strength of the relationship between the patient and the health care provider.[59] Patient education should include information about the specific drug regime, how the drug works, when and how to take the drug, and how to minimize potential side effects. Barriers to medication adherence include faulty health perceptions. Beliefs and attitudes may interfere with adherence. Social and environmental barriers may include such problems as difficulty taking medication in social settings or restaurants and lack of equipment for mixing medication. It is appropriate to explore common beliefs, attitudes, and difficulties with the patient and develop strategies together to address these issues. Anticipation of potential side effects should also be explored. Studies indicate that adverse side effects and therapeutic ineffectiveness were the major reasons cited for discontinuing lipid-lowering drugs.[59]

Cues to action are important determinants of adherence to medication regimes. Ideal cues are ones that are a part of the patient's habitual routine. Because such cues are habitual, the patient may need assistance in recognizing possible cues. Monitoring and recording medication as it is taken can be useful in identifying potential cues.

Feedback is a powerful reinforcer of behavior. Procedures for rapid lipid analysis should be used when possible. Communicating changes in blood lipid response and responding to side effect issues are essential components of lipid management and can often be accomplished by telephone. Consideration should be give to routine telephone contacts to promote adherence and increase the effectiveness of lipid management. Nursing case-managed intervention studies have demonstrated that adherence to lifestyle changes and lipid-lowering drug therapies can be achieved, perhaps due in part to the strength of the relationship between the nurse and the patient.[51]

The nurse is in an excellent position to promote adherence. The focus of the intervention should include the concept of dyslipidemia as a "silent disease," one that is present for life but one for which treatment has been proven effective.

REFERENCES

1. 27th Bethesda Conference: Matching the intensity of risk factor management with the hazard for coronary disease events. J Am Coll Cardiol 27: 957–1047, 1996
2. American Heart Association: Heart and Stroke Statistical Update. Dallas, American Heart Association, 1998
3. Anderson KM, Castelli WP, Levy D: Cholesterol and mortality: 30 years of follow-up from the Framingham Study. JAMA 257: 2176–2180, 1987
4. Armstrong ML, Warner ED, Connor WE: Regression of coronary atheromatosis in rhesus monkeys. Circ Res 27: 59–67, 1970
5. Arntzenius AC et al: Diets, lipoproteins, and the progression coronary atherosclerosis: The Lieden Intervention Trial. N Engl J Med 312: 805–811, 1985
6. Austin MD, Hokanson JE, Brunzell JD: Characterization of low-density lipoprotein subclasses: Methodologic approaches and clinical relevance. Curr Opin Lipidol 5: 395–403, 1994
7. Axelson ML, Federline TL, Brinberg D: A meta-analysis of food- and nutrition-related research. Journal of Nutrition Education 17: 51–54, 1985
8. Bandura A: Social Learning Theory. Englewood Cliffs, NJ, Prentice-Hall, 1977
9. Blankenhorn DH et al: The influence of diet on the appearance of new lesions in human coronary arteries. JAMA 263: 1646–1652, 1990
10. Block G, Rosenberger WF, Patterson BH: Calories, fat and cholesterol: Intake patterns in the US population by race, sex, and age. Am J Public Health 78: 1150–1155, 1988
11. Bonanome A, Grundy SM: Effect of stearic acid on plasma cholesterol and lipoprotein levels. N Engl J Med 318: 1244–1248, 1988
12. Breslow JL: The genetic basis of lipoprotein disorders: Introduction and review. J Intern Med 231: 627–631, 1992
13. Brown BG et al: Lipid altering or antioxidant vitamins for patients with coronary disease and very low HDL cholesterol? The HDL-Atherosclerosis Treatment Study design. Can J Cardiol 14: 6A–13A, 1998
14. Brown G et al: Regression of coronary artery disease as a result of intensive lipid-lowering therapy in men with high levels of apolipoprotein B. N Engl J Med 323: 1289–1298, 1990
15. Brown MS, Goldstein JL: A receptor-mediated pathway for cholesterol homeostasis. Science 232: 34–47, 1986
16. Buzzard IM et al: Diet intervention methods to reduce fat intake: Nutrient and food group composition of self-selected low-fat diets. J Am Diet Assoc 90: 42–50, 53, 1990
17. Camargo CA et al: The effect of moderate alcohol intake on serum apolipoproteins A-I and A-II. JAMA 253: 2854–2857, 1985
18. Campos H et al: Differences in apolipoproteins and low-density lipoprotein subfractions in postmenopausal women on and off estrogen therapy: Results from the Framingham Offspring Study. Metabolism 39: 1033–1038, 1990
19. Castelli WP: Lipids, risk factors and ischaemic heart disease. Atherosclerosis 124(Suppl): S1–S9, 1996
20. Connor SL, Gustafson Jr, Arthud-Wild SM et al: The cholesterol/saturated-fat index: An indication of the hypercholesterolemic and atherogenic potential of food. Lancet 1 (8492) 18492: 1229–1232, 1986
21. Connor SL, Gustafson Jr, Sexton R et al: The diet habit survey: A new method of dietary assessment that relates to plasma cholesterol. J Am Diet Assoc 92: 41–47, 1992
22. Connor WE, Connor SL, Connor SL: Diet, atherosclerosis, and fish oil. Adv Intern Med 35: 135–172, 1990
23. Connor WE, Connor SL, Katan MB et al: Should a low-fat, high-carbohydrate diet be recommended for everyone? A clinical debate. N Engl J Med 337: 562–567, 1997
24. Crouch SJF, Farquhar JW, Haskell WL et al: Personal and mediated health counseling for sustained dietary reduction of hypercholesterolemia. Prev Med 15: 282–291, 1986
25. Dattilo AM, Kris-Etherton PM: Effects of weight reduction on blood lipids and lipoproteins: A meta-analysis. Am J Clin Nutr 56: 320–328, 1992
26. deGraaf J, Hak-Lemmers H, Hector P et al: Enhanced susceptibility to in vitro oxidation of the low-density lipoprotein subfractions in healthy subjects. Arteriosclerosis and Thrombosis 11: 298–306, 1991
27. Downs JR, Clearfield M, Weis S et al: Primary prevention of acute coronary events with lovastatin in men and women with average cholesterol levels. JAMA 279: 1615–1622, 1998
28. Eisenberg S: High-density lipoprotein metabolism. J Lipid Res 25: 1017–1054, 1984
29. Ewart CK: Changing dietary behavior: A social action theory approach. Clin Nutr 8: 9–16, 1989
30. Fair JM, Berra KA: Endothelial function and coronary risk reduction: Mechanisms and influences of nitric oxide. Cardiovascular Nursing 32: 17–22, 1996
31. Food Surveys Research Group and Agricultural Research Services: Data Tables: Results from USDA's 1995 Continuing Survey of Food Intakes by Individuals and 1995 Diet and Health Knowledge Survey: CSFI/DHKS, 1995. Riverdale, MD, Department of Agriculture, 1995
32. Fraser GE, Schneider LE, Mattison S et al: Behavioral interventions from an office setting in patients with cardiac disease. J Cardiopulm Rehabil 8: 50–57, 1988
33. Freudenheim JL: A review of study designs and methods of dietary assessment in nutritional epidemiology of chronic disease. J Nutr 123: 401–405, 1993
34. Friedenreich CM, Slimani N, Riboli E: Measurement of past diet: Review of previous and proposed methods. Epidemiol Rev 14: 177–196, 1992
35. Friedewald WT, Levy RI, Fredrickson DS: Estimation of the concentration of low-density lipoprotein cholesterol in plasma, with the use of preparative ultracentrifuge. Clin Chem 18: 499–502, 1972
36. Gardner CD, Fortmann SP, Krauss RM: Small low-density lipoprotein particles are associated with the incidence of coronary artery disease in men and women. JAMA 276: 875–881, 1996
37. Gardner CD, Kraemer HC: Monounsaturated versus polyunsaturated dietary fat and serum lipids: A meta-analysis. Arterioscler Thromb Vasc Biol 15: 1917–1927, 1995
38. Goldstein JL, Brown MS: Regulation of low-density lipoprotein receptors: Implication for pathogenesis and therapy of hypercholesterolemia and atherosclerosis. Circulation 76: 505–507, 1987
39. Gorder D, Dolecek TA, Coleman GG et al: Dietary intake in the Multiple Risk Factor Intervention Trial (MRFIT): Nutrient and food group changes over 6 years. J Am Diet Assoc 86: 744–751, 1986
40. Gordon DJ, Probstfield JL, Garrison RJ: High density lipoprotein cholesterol and cardiovascular disease: Four prospective studies. Circulation 79: 8–15, 1989
41. Gotto AM: Clinical diagnosis of hyperlipoproteinemia. Am J Med 74(5A): 5–9, 1983
42. Gotto AM: High-density lipoproteins: Biochemical and metabolic factors. Am J Cardiol 54(4): 2B–8B, 1983
43. Gotto AM, Pownall HJ: Manual of Lipid Disorders. Baltimore, Williams & Wilkins, 1992
44. Gould AL et al: Cholesterol reduction yields clinical benefit: A new look at old data. Circulation 91: 2274–2282, 1995
45. Grundy SM: Hyperlipoproteinemia: Metabolic basis and rationale for therapy. Am J Cardiol 54: 20C–26C, 1984

46. Grundy SM: Pathogenesis of hyperlipoproteinemia. J Lipid Res 25: 1611–1618, 1984

47. Grundy SM: Hypertriglyceridemia, atherogenic dyslipidemia, and the metabolic syndrome. Am J Cardiol 81(4A): 18B–25B, 1998

48. Grundy SM et al: Guide to the primary prevention of cardiovascular diseases. Circulation 95: 2329–2331, 1997

49. Grundy SM, Vega GL: Plasma cholesterol responsiveness to saturated fatty acids. Am J Clin Nutr 47: 822–824, 1983

50. Hafner SM: Management of dyslipidemia in adults with diabetes. Diabetes Care 21: 160–178, 1998

51. Haskell WL et al: Effects of intensive multiple risk reduction on coronary atherosclerosis and clinical cardiac events in men and women with coronary artery disease. Circulation 89: 975–990, 1994

52. Haskell WL et al: The effect of cessation and resumption of moderate alcohol intake on serum high-density-lipoprotein subfractions. N Engl J Med 310: 805–810, 1984

53. Hegsted DM et al: Quantitative effects of dietary fat on serum cholesterol in man. Am J Clin Nutr 17: 281–295, 1965

54. Heini AF, Weinsier RL: Divergent trends in obesity and fat intake patterns: The American paradox. Am J Med 102: 259–264, 1997

55. Hennekens CH: Increasing burden of cardiovascular disease: Current knowledge and future directions for research on risk factors. Circulation 97: 1095–1102, 1998

56. Houston Miller N: Compliance with treatment regimens in chronic asymptomatic diseases. Am J Med 102: 43–49, 1997

57. Hulley SB, Grady D, Bush T et al. Randomized trial of estrogen plus progestin for secondary prevention of coronary heart disease in post menopausal women JAMA 280 (1998): 605–613.

58. Hulley SB, Herman TB, Grady D et al: Should we be measuring blood cholesterol levels in young adults? JAMA 269: 1416–1419, 1993

59. Insull W: The problem of compliance to cholesterol altering therapy. J Intern Med 241: 317–325, 1997

60. Jacobs D, Blackburn H, Higgins M et al: The Conference on Low Cholesterol: Mortality associations. Circulation 86: 1046–1060, 1992

61. Johnson CL, Rifkind BM, Sempos CT 26; 81(4A): 138–178 Rifkind BM, Sempos CT et al: Declining serum total cholesterol levels among US adults: The National Health and Nutrition Examination Surveys. JAMA 269: 3002–3008, 1993

62. Kane JP, Malloy MJ, Ports TA et al: Regression of coronary atherosclerosis during treatment of familial hypercholesterolemia with combined drug regimes. JAMA 264: 3007–3012, 1990

63. Kannel WB, High-density lipoproteins: Epidemiologic profile and risks of coronary artery disease. Am J Cardiol 52(4): 9B–12B, 1983

64. Keys A: Coronary heart disease in seven countries. Circulation 41(Suppl I): 1–211, 1970

65. Keys A, Parlin RW: Cholesterol response to changes in dietary lipids. Am J Clin Nutr 19: 175–181, 1966

66. Knopp RH, Walden CE, Retzlaff BM et al: Long-term cholesterol-lowering effects of 4 fat-restricted diets in hypercholesterolemic and combined hyperlipidemic men. JAMA 278: 1509–1515, 1997

67. Krauss RM: Effects of commonly used sex steroid hormones on plasma lipoprotein levels in women. In Eaker ED, Packard B, Wenger NK et al (eds): Coronary Heart Disease in Women, pp 177–180. New York, Haymarket Doyma, 1987

68. Krauss RM: Atherogenicity of triglyceride-rich lipoproteins. Am J Cardiol 26; 81(4A): 138–178: 81(4A): 13B–17B, 1998

69. Kris-Etherton P et al: The effect of diet on plasma lipids, lipoproteins, and coronary heart disease. J Am Diet Assoc 88: 1373–1400, 1988

70. Kristal AR, Shattuck AL, Henry HJ: Patterns of dietary behavior associated with selecting diets low in fat: Reliability and validity of a behavioral approach to dietary assessment. J Am Diet Assoc 90: 214–220, 1990

71. Kushi LH et al: Diet and 20 year mortality from coronary heart disease. N Engl J Med 312: 811–818, 1985

72. Law MR, Wald NJ, Thompson SG: By how much and how quickly does reduction in serum cholesterol concentration lower risk of ischaemic heart disease? BMJ 308: 367–373, 1994

73. Lawn RM: Lipoprotein (a) in heart disease. Sci Am 92(6): 54–60, 1992

74. Leaf A, Weber PC: Cardiovascular effects of n-3 fatty acids. N Engl J Med 318: 549–557, 1988

75. Levine GN, Keaney JF, Vita JA: Cholesterol reduction in cardiovascular disease. N Engl J Med 332: 512–521, 1995

76. Marmot MG: Alcohol and coronary disease. Int J Epidemiol 13: 160–167, 1984

77. McCann BS et al: Promoting adherence to low-fat, low-cholesterol diets: Review and recommendations. J Am Diet Assoc 90: 1414–1417, 1990

78. McGee DL, Reed DM, Yano KAJE: Ten-year incidence of coronary heart disease in the Honolulu Heart Program: Relationship to nutrient intake. Am J Epidemiol 119: 667–676, 1984

79. Mensink RP, Katan MB: Effect of dietary fatty acids on serum lipids and lipoproteins: A meta-analysis of 27 trials. Arteriosclerosis and Thrombosis 12: 911–919, 1992

80. Miller NE: HDL metabolism and its role in lipid transport. Eur Heart J 11: H1–H3, 1990

81. Muldoon MF, Manuck SB, Matthews KA: Lowering cholesterol concentrations and mortality: A quantitative review of primary prevention trials. BMJ 301: 309–314, 1990

82. National Institutes of Health, National Cholesterol Education Program: Second Report for the Expert Panel on Detection, Evaluation and Treatment of High Blood Cholesterol in Adults. NIH Publication no. 93-3095. Bethesda, MD, U.S. Department of Health and Human Services, 1993

83. Ordovas JM et al: Apoprotein A-I gene polymorphism associated with premature coronary artery disease and familial hypoalphalipoproteinemia. N Engl J Med 314: 671–677, 1986

84. Ornish D et al: Can lifestyle changes reverse coronary heart disease? Lancet 336: 129–133, 1990

85. Pope-Cordle J, Katahn ME: The T-factor Fat Gram Counter. New York, Norton, 1991

86. Reaven GM et al: Insulin resistance and hyperinsulinemia in individuals with small, dense, low-density lipoprotein particles. J Clin Invest 92: 141–146, 1993

87. Rifkind BM: Drug Treatment of Hyperlipidemia. New York, Marcel Dekker, 1991

88. Scandinavian Simvastatin Survival Study Group: Randomised trial of cholesterol lowering in 4444 patients with coronary heart disease: The Scandinavian Simvastatin Survival Study (4S). Lancet 344: 1383–1389, 1995

89. Schaefer EJ, Levy RI: Pathogenesis and management of lipoprotein disorders. N Engl J Med 312: 1300–1310, 1985

90. Schectman G et al: Dietary intake of Americans reporting adherence to low cholesterol diet (NHANES II). Am J Public Health 80: 698–703, 1990

91. Schuler G et al: Regular physical exercise and low fat diet: Effects on progression of coronary artery disease. Circulation 86: 1–11, 1992

92. Shepherd J et al: Prevention of coronary heart disease with pravastatin in men with hypercholesterolemia. N Engl J Med 333: 1301–1307, 1995

93. Smith SC et al: Preventing heart attack and death in patients with coronary disease. Circulation 92: 2–4, 1995

94. Smith-Schneider LM, Sigman-Grant MJ, Kris-Etherton PM: Dietary fat reduction strategies. J Am Diet Assoc 92: 34–38, 1992

95. Stampfer MJ et al: A prospective study of moderate alcohol consumption and the risk of coronary disease and stroke in women. N Engl J Med 319: 267–273, 1988

96. Steinberg D et al: Beyond cholesterol: Modification of low-density lipoprotein that increase its atherogenicity. N Engl J Med 320: 915–924, 1989

97. Sullivan MJ: Estrogen replacement. Circulation 94: 2699–2702, 1996

98. Tall AR: Overview of reverse cholesterol transport. Eur Heart J 19: A31–35, 1998

99. Tall AR, Small DM: Current concepts: Plasma high-density lipoproteins. N Engl J Med 299: 1232–1236, 1978

100. The Expert Panel: Summary of the second report of the National Cholesterol Education Program Expert Panel on Detection, Evaluation, and Treatment of High Blood Cholesterol in Adults (Adult Treatment Panel II). JAMA 269: 3015–3023, 1993

101. The Lipid Research Clinic Investigators: The Lipid Research Clinics Primary Prevention Trials results. JAMA 251: 351–364, 1984

102. Tobert JA: New developments in lipid-lowering therapy: The role of inhibitors of hydroxymethylglutaryl-coenzyme A reductase. Circulation 76: 534–538, 1987

103. Treasure CB et al: Beneficial effects of cholesterol-lowering therapy on the coronary endothelium in patients with coronary artery disease. N Engl J Med 332: 481–487, 1995

104. U.S. Department of Health and Human Services: Recommendations for Improving Cholesterol Measurement: A Report from the Laboratory Standardization Panel of the National Cholesterol Education Program. Bethesda, MD, U.S. Department of Health and Human Services, 1990

105. Watts GF et al: Effects on coronary artery disease of lipid-lowering diet, or diet plus cholestyramine, in the St. Thomas Arteriosclerosis Regression Study (STARS). Lancet 339: 563–569, 1992

106. Wood PD, Stefanick ML, Haskell WL: The effects on plasma lipoproteins of a prudent weight reducing diet with and without exercise in overweight men and women. N Engl J Med 325: 461–466, 1991

Exercise and Activity

DEANNA E. RITCHIE
JONATHAN N. MYERS

Since the late 1950s, numerous scientific reports have examined the relationships between physical activity, physical fitness, and cardiovascular health. Expert panels convened by organizations such as the Centers for Disease Control and Prevention (CDC), American College of Sports Medicine (ACSM), American Association of Cardiovascular and Pulmonary Rehabilitation (AACVPR), and the American Heart Association (AHA),[1-6] along with the 1996 U.S. Surgeon General's report on physical activity and health,[7] have reinforced scientific evidence linking regular physical activity to various measures of cardiovascular health. The prevailing view in these reports is that more active or fit people tend to experience less coronary heart disease (CHD) than their sedentary counterparts, and when they do acquire CHD, it occurs at a later age and tends to be less severe.[1,4,8,9] Cardiac rehabilitation, as an industry, has evolved in large part owing to the abundance of scientific evidence indicating that regular exercise improves physical function, and reduces the risk of reinfarction and sudden death in patients with known CHD.[5,9-12] Despite this evidence, however, most adults in the United States remain effectively sedentary,[4] and more than 80% of patients who sustain a myocardial infarction (MI) are not referred to a cardiac rehabilitation program.[12] It is therefore incumbent on the nurse or other health care provider to encourage patients to become more physically active, to appreciate the role of rehabilitation in cardiac care, and to develop strategies that promote the adoption of physically active lifestyles in all their patients.

This chapter describes the scientific evidence linking physical activity and health, summarizes the physiologic changes that occur with a program of regular exercise, and provides an outline for cardiac rehabilitation in the modern treatment era.

ROLE OF EXERCISE IN CARDIOVASCULAR HEALTH

Epidemiologic Evidence Supporting Physical Activity

It has been estimated that as many as 250,000 deaths per year in the United States are attributable to lack of regular physical activity.[13,14] Ongoing longitudinal studies have provided consistent evidence of varying strength documenting the protective effects of activity for a number of chronic diseases, including CHD,[3-11] non–insulin-dependent diabetes,[15-17] hypertension,[18] osteoporosis,[19] and colon cancer.[20] In contrast, low levels of physical fitness are consistently associated with higher cardiovascular and all-cause mortality rates.[3,4,7,8] Midlife increases in physical activity, through change in occupation or recreational activities, are associated with a decrease in mortality rates.[21]

The landmark work of Paffenbarger and associates[9,20,21] has been particularly persuasive in the epidemiology of physical activity, and thus the development of the CDC, AHA, and ACSM guidelines. Table 34-1 illustrates the rates and relative risks of death over a 9-year period among 11,864 Harvard alumni by patterns of physical activity assessed in 1977. These subjects had self-reported the absence of CHD on each of two mail questionnaires returned either in 1962 or 1966 and in 1977. Several findings in Table 34-1 are particularly noteworthy. The largest benefits in terms of mortality appear to accrue through engaging in moderate activity levels; *moderate* has been defined as activity performed at an intensity of 3 to 6 METs (a multiple of the resting metabolic rate), roughly equivalent to brisk walking for most adults.[23] Note also that regular, moderate walking or sportsplay is associated with a 30% to 40% reduction in mortality (relative risk of death 0.60 to 0.70). Likewise, the physical activity index, expressed as kilocalories per week (the sum of walking, stair climbing, and sports play) suggests that a 40% reduction in mortality occurs by engaging in modest levels of activity (1,000 to 2,000 kcal/week, equivalent to three to five 1-hour sessions of activity), whereas only minimal additional benefits are achieved by engaging in greater-intensity activity. These findings agree closely with earlier results among 16,936 Harvard alumni (including some of the same men) assessed in the early 1960s and followed for all-cause mortality until 1978.[24] Similar results have been reported from large studies that have followed people for CHD morbidity and mortality in the range of 10 to 20 years among British civil servants,[25,26] U.S. railroad workers,[27] San Francisco longshoremen,[28] and other cohorts (for review, see Powell and colleagues[29] or Lee and Paffenbarger[30]). Clearly, the evidence linking a physically active lifestyle and cardiovascular health is substantial.

TABLE 34-1	Rates and Relative Risks of Death* Among Harvard Alumni, 1977 to 1985, by Patterns of Physical Acivity				
Physical Activity (weekly)		Man-Years (%)	No. of Deaths	Deaths per 10,000 Man-Years	Relative Risk of Death	p Value of Trend
Walking (km)	<5	26	228	86.2	1.00 ⎫	
	5–14	42	275	67.4	0.78 ⎬	<0.001
	15+	32	194	57.7	0.67 ⎭	
Stair climbing (floors)	<20	37	341	80.0	1.00 ⎫	
	20–54	48	293	62.9	0.79 ⎬	0.001
	55+	15	80	59.6	0.75 ⎭	
All sportsplay	None	12	156	88.9	1.00 ⎫	
	Light only[†]	10	152	97.4	1.10 ⎬	<0.001
	Light and moderate	36	208	59.7	0.67 ⎬	
	Moderate only[‡]	42	178	56.4	0.63 ⎭	
Moderate sportsplay (h)	<1	30	308	92.9	1.00 ⎫	
	1–2	41	126	58.2	0.63 ⎬	<0.001
	3+	29	64	43.6	0.47 ⎭	
Index (kcal)[§]	<500	12 ⎫	197	110.3 ⎫	1.00 ⎫	
	500–999	18 ⎬	135	69.1 ⎬	0.63 ⎬	
	1,000–1,499	15 ⎬ 58	111	68.9 ⎬ 78.9	0.62 ⎬ 1.00	
	1,500–1,999	13 ⎭	73	61.4 ⎭	0.56 ⎭	
	2,000–2,499	10 ⎫	51	52.4 ⎫	0.48 ⎫	<0.001
	2,500–2,999	8 ⎬	44	64.6 ⎬	0.59 ⎬	
	3,000–3,499	6 ⎬ 42	36	74.7 ⎬ 55.4	0.68 ⎬ 0.70	
	3,500+	18 ⎭	82	48.1 ⎭	0.44 ⎭	

METs, metabolic equivalents.
*Age-adjusted.
[†]<4.5 METs intensity.
[‡]4.5+ METs intensity.
[§]Sum of walking, stair climbing, and all sportsplay.
From Paffenbarger RS, Hyde RT, Wing AL et al: Some interrrelations of physical activity, physical fitness, health, and longevity. In Bouchard C, Shephard RJ, Stephens T (eds): Physical Activity Fitness, and Health, pp. 119–133. Champaign, IL, Human Kinetics, 1994.

Physiologic Fitness and Health

Several studies have been published in which physical fitness, determined by standardized exercise testing, was determined among large samples of asymptomatic men and women and who were followed for the incidence of CHD morbidity and mortality for up to 9 years.[27,31,32] Each of these studies demonstrated that higher levels of fitness were associated with lower rates of CHD or all-cause mortality. Importantly, these associations appear to be independent of other CHD risk factors. Moreover, the low levels of fitness in these studies did not appear to be associated with subclinical disease. In general, fitness levels have also been associated with physical activity status assessed by questionnaire.[33]

Blair and associates[31] assessed fitness by treadmill performance in 10,244 men and 3,120 women and followed them for 110,482 person years (averaging >8 years) for all-cause mortality. These results are presented in Table 34-2. Mortality rates were lowest (18.6 per 10,000 man-years) among the most fit and highest (64.0) among the least fit men, with the corresponding rates among the women 8.5 and 39.5 per 10,000 man-years, respectively. These findings closely parallel the results from studies relating physical activity levels and mortality.[20–30] Although physical activity status and physiologic fitness are clearly linked, the latter carries an important genetic component; that is, some peo-

ple remain comparatively fit without engaging in a great deal of physical activity. The findings of Blair and colleagues[31] and others[34] imply that the benefits of physical activity on health and survival are mediated largely through fitness status.

Surgeon General's Report on Physical Activity and Health

This document, published in 1996, is the strongest policy statement ever made by the U.S. Government concerning physical activity.[7] It represented a historic turning point redefining exercise as a key component to health promotion and disease prevention. The federal government is mounting a multiyear educational campaign based on this report. In this report, the epidemiologic evidence supporting physical activity in the prevention of CHD morbidity and mortality is reviewed in detail. The document also outlines how much exercise is necessary to achieve these benefits. It is suggested that each person perform a moderate amount of activity daily, with the amount of activity emphasized rather than the intensity. The idea is that this offers people more opportunities for activities that fit into their daily lives. It is suggested that people perform this moderate amount of activity for 30 minutes or more on most, and preferably all,

TABLE 34-2	Rates and Relative Risks of Death* Among 10,244 Men and 3,120 Women in an 8-Year Follow-up, by Gradients of Physical Fitness					
	Men			**Women**		
Quintiles of Fitness†	No. of Deaths	Deaths per 10,000 Man-Years	Relative Risk of Death‡	No. of Deaths	Deaths per 10,000 Woman-Years	Relative Risk of Death‡
1 (low)	75	64.0	1.00	18	39.5	1.00
2	40	25.5	0.40	11	20.5	0.52
3	47	27.1	0.42	6	12.2	0.31
4	43	21.7	0.34	4	6.5	0.15
5 (high)	35	18.6	0.29	4	8.5	0.22

*Age adjusted.
†Quintiles of fitness determined by maximal exercise testing.
‡p Value for trend <0.05.
From Blair SN, Kohl III HW, Paffenbarger Jr. RS, et al: Physical fitness and all-cause mortality: A prospective study of healthy men and women. JAMA 262: 2395–2401, 1989.

days of the week. These activities can take the form of brisk walking, yardwork or other household chores, jogging, or a wide variety of recreational activities.

Within the Surgeon General's report, the National Institutes of Health (NIH) Consensus Conference Statement on Physical Activity and Cardiovascular Health is quoted.[35] This report more specifically outlines the cardiovascular benefits of exercise and states what is required for these benefits. The NIH document underscores the recommendation that all children and adults should set a long-term goal to accumulate at least 30 minutes or more of moderate-intensity physical activity on most days of the week. Repeated intermittent or shorter bouts of activity (≥ 10 minutes), including occupational, nonoccupational, or tasks of daily living, have similar cardiovascular and health benefits if performed at a level of moderate intensity (e.g., brisk walking, cycling, swimming, home repair, and yardwork) with an accumulated duration of at least 30 minutes per day. People who already meet these standards receive additional benefits from increasing this to more vigorous activity.

"Health" versus "Fitness" Benefits of Exercise

A noteworthy theme that is consistent in each of the aforementioned documents is that considerable health benefits are derived from moderate levels of activity; it is in general not necessary to engage in vigorous activity to derive these benefits. Until recently, an exercise program was thought to be effective only if an improvement in some measure of cardiopulmonary function was observed. During the last few years, the philosophy on exercise recommendations as a means to this end ("fitness" measured by exercise capacity) has changed significantly. It is now appreciated that substantial health benefits can be achieved through minimal amounts of regular exercise, regardless of whether exercise results in a measurable improvement in exercise capacity. Epidemiologic studies have shown that death rates from cardiovascular causes are considerably lower even among people who engage in modest amounts of exercise, less than the threshold that was generally thought necessary to increase exercise capacity.[1-5,7,31] It is important for health professionals to be aware of the distinction between "health" and "fitness" when making activity recommendations to patients with cardiovascular disease, those at high risk for its development, and healthy adults. Under the umbrella of "health" should be included, in addition to cardiopulmonary fitness, measures of fat and lean weight, bone density, glucose and insulin metabolism, blood lipid and lipoprotein metabolism, and quality of life. A favorable profile for these variables represents a clear advantage in terms of health outcomes as assessed by morbidity and mortality statistics.

Role of Exercise in Secondary Prevention

During the 1970s and 1980s, numerous controlled trials addressed whether participation in a rehabilitation program influenced morbidity or mortality in patients with CHD. Although the results of these trials independently were inconclusive, most demonstrated a favorable trend for a lower mortality rate among patients who exercised compared with control subjects. For example, the National Exercise and Heart Disease Project was a controlled, randomized trial in the United States on the effects of prescribed supervised exercise involving 651 men with acute MI.[36] The cumulative 3-year total mortality rates in this study were 7.3% and 4.6% for the control and exercise groups, respectively, whereas the rates for recurrent MI were 7.0% and 5.4%, respectively. Although this represented 37% and 24% reductions in mortality and reinfarction rates, respectively, for the exercise groups, more than twice as many patients would have been necessary in the study for these differences to be statistically significant. The lack of adequate sample size in this study is typical of the secondary prevention trials that have assessed mortality; although the trends are generally

TABLE 34-3	Meta-Analysis of Controlled Exercise Trials in Patients With Coronary Heart Disease			
	No. of Events (%)	No. of Patients	Pooled Odds Ratio (95% Confidence Interval)	p Value
	Treatment	Control		
All-cause death	236/1823 (12.9)	289.1791 (16.1)	0.76 (0.63–0.92)	0.004
Cardiovascular death	204/2051 (9.9)	252/1993 (12.6)	0.75 (0.62–0.93)	0.006

From Oldridge NB, Guyatt GH, Fischer ME, et al: Cardiac rehabilitation with exercise after myocardial infarction. JAMA 260: 945–950, 1988.

favorable, few have independently demonstrated that patients randomized to an exercise program have a significantly lower mortality compared with control subjects.

Two cardiac rehabilitation trials in Europe were noteworthy for their favorable morbidity and mortality outcomes. Vermeulen and associates,[37] in a study involving fewer than 100 patients, found that a 6-week rehabilitation program, including comprehensive risk factor reduction and exercise, resulted in a 50% lower rate of combined CHD morbidity and mortality in the "rehabilitated" compared with the control patients over a 5-year follow-up period. In the second of these multiple risk factor intervention trials, Kallio and colleagues[38] studied 375 consecutive male and female patients post-MI younger than 65 years of age in two clinical centers in Finland. After 3 years of follow-up, the cumulative CHD mortality rate was significantly lower in the intervention group compared with the control group (18.6% vs. 29.4%). This difference primarily reflected a reduction in sudden death in the intervention group during the first 6 months after an MI. A favorable trend toward reduction in nonfatal reinfarctions also was observed in the intervention group.

An alternate but less rigorous scientific approach, in the absence of a definitive clinical trial, is to pool data from existing long-term, randomized, secondary prevention trials in which exercise training was a component. A number of such meta-analyses have been published in which data from 6 to 22 randomized, long-term clinical trials were pooled using the intention-to-treat principle.[10,11,39] In the trials included in these meta-analyses, intervention consisted of either a formal exercise program or simply exercise advice generally in combination with multiple risk factor management, making it impossible to determine the independent contribution of exercise to subsequent morbidity and mortality. Nevertheless, patients randomized to active cardiac rehabilitation programs after an MI had statistically significant reductions of approximately 25% in 1- to 3-year rates of fatal cardiovascular events and total mortality compared with control patients (Table 34-3). However, significant differences in general were not found in the rate of nonfatal recurrent reinfarctions in patients undergoing intervention compared with control patients. The reduction in mortality attributed to cardiac rehabilitation by these pooled data is similar in extent to that associated with beta-blocking drugs in clinical trials after a MI.[39]

Rehabilitation in Patients With Chronic Heart Failure

In the mid-1980s and earlier, stable congestive heart failure (CHF) was considered by many authorities to be a contraindication to participation in an exercise program. Today, it is known that selected patients with CHF derive considerable benefits from cardiac rehabilitation. With improvements in therapy (i.e., thrombolytics, angiotensin-converting enzyme inhibitors), survival among patients with CHF has improved considerably, and more of these patients are available as candidates for rehabilitation. The incidence of CHF is approximately 500,000 per year in the United States. Since the late 1980s, studies performed in the United States and Europe have consistently demonstrated that training is safe and provides both physiologic and quality-of-life benefits for patients with CHF.[40] The major physiologic benefit from training in CHF appears to occur in the skeletal muscles rather than in the heart itself.[41,42] Special considerations for the patient with CHF participating in rehabilitation are discussed later in the section on outpatient rehabilitation.

Physiologic Benefits of Exercise Training

Regular exercise increases work capacity; hundreds of studies have been performed cross-sectionally that document higher maximum oxygen consumption ($\dot{V}O_2$max) values among active versus sedentary people, or between groups after a period of training. The magnitude of improvement in $\dot{V}O_2$max with training varies widely, usually ranging from 5% to 25%, but increases as large as 50% have been reported. The degree of change in exercise capacity depends primarily on initial state of fitness and intensity of training. Training increases exercise capacity by increasing both maximal cardiac output and the ability to extract oxygen from the blood.

The physiologic benefits of a training program can be classified as *morphologic*, *hemodynamic*, and *metabolic* (Display 34-1). Many animal studies have demonstrated significant morphologic changes with training, including myocardial hypertrophy with improved myocardial function, increases in coronary artery size, and increases in the myocardial capillary-to-fiber ratio. However, such changes have been difficult to demonstrate in humans.[6,43] The major

---

DISPLAY 34-1

Physiologic Adaptations to Physical Training in Humans

MORPHOLOGIC ADAPTATIONS
Myocardial hypertrophy

HEMODYNAMIC ADAPTATIONS
Increased blood volume
Increased end-diastolic volume
Increased stroke volume
Increased cardiac output
Reduced heart rate for any submaximal workload

METABOLIC ADAPTATIONS
Increased mitochondrial volume and number
Greater muscle glycogen stores
Enhanced fat utilization
Enhanced lactate removal
Increased enzymes for aerobic metabolism
Increased maximal oxygen uptake

DISPLAY 34-2

Physiologic Consequences of Prolonged Bed Rest

1. Loss of muscle mass, strength, and endurance
2. Decreased plasma and blood volume
3. Decreased ventricular volume
4. Increased hematocrit and hemoglobin
5. Diuresis and natriuresis
6. Venous stasis
7. Bone demineralization
8. Increased heart rate at rest and submaximal levels of activity
9. Decreased resting and maximum stroke volume
10. Decreased maximum cardiac output
11. Decreased maximal oxygen uptake
12. Increased venous compliance
13. Increased risk of venous thrombosis and thromboembolism
14. Decreased orthostatic tolerance
15. Increased risk of atelectasis, pulmonary emboli

From Myers J: Physiologic adaptations to exercise and immobility. In Woods SL, Sivarajan Froelicher ES, Halpenny CJ, Underhill Motzer S (eds): Cardiac Nursing, 3rd ed, pp 147–162. Philadelphia, JB Lippincott, 1995.

---

morphologic outcome of a training program in humans is probably an increase in cardiac size; however, this adaptation also appears to occur mainly in younger, healthy people, and is an unlikely outcome in patients with heart disease. However, significant hemodynamic changes have been well documented among patients with heart disease after training. These include reductions in heart rate (HR) at rest and any matched submaximal workload, which is beneficial in that it results in a reduction in myocardial oxygen demand during activities of daily living (ADLs). Other hemodynamic changes that have been demonstrated after training include reductions in blood pressure, increases in blood volume, and increases in maximal oxygen uptake. The most important physiologic benefits of training among patients with heart disease occur in the skeletal muscle. The metabolic capacity of the skeletal muscle is enhanced through increases in mitochondrial volume and number, capillary density, and oxidative enzyme content. These adaptations enhance perfusion and the efficiency of oxygen extraction.[6,43]

Cardiovascular Effects of Immobility

The deleterious physiologic effects of prolonged bed rest have been studied extensively, and since the late 1960s, these studies have been an important stimulus for cardiac rehabilitation. Although these effects are commonly attributed simply to the absence of regular physical activity, an additional, important factor underlying the deconditioning of bed rest is the absence of normal hydrostatic pressure due to orthostatic stress (i.e., due to gravity). Thus, even short periods of bed rest (2 to 5 days) are accompanied not only by a reduced exercise capacity but by reductions in muscle mass and strength, alterations in body fluid distribution, and orthostatic intolerance (Display 34-2). The importance of the absence of orthostatic stress on the deconditioning

response has been documented by studies demonstrating that exercise training during bed rest is only partially effective or fails to maintain $\dot{V}O_2$max.[44,45]

In the early 1900s, patients were almost completely immobilized in bed for 6 to 8 weeks after an MI. As recently as the 1960s, extended periods of bed rest were thought to facilitate myocardial healing for patients recovering from an MI. Today, the converse is true: carefully prescribed and supervised physical activity is recommended as soon as 1 day after the event to counteract the many negative physiologic effects of bed rest. In addition to a cardiovascular event, patients may be subjected to long periods of immobilization because of severe pain; musculoskeletal or nervous system impairment, including paralysis; generalized weakness; psychosocial problems such as severe depression; and infectious disease. The extensive literature available on the deleterious effects of immobility has been reviewed elsewhere.[44,45]

Agency for Health Care Policy and Research Guidelines

In 1995, the Agency for Health Care Policy and Research (AHCPR) published clinical practice guidelines on cardiac rehabilitation.[12] These guidelines have had a major impact on substantiating the value of cardiac rehabilitation for patients with heart disease. The guidelines thoroughly review and categorize existing studies evaluating the efficacy of training and the role of rehabilitation in reducing risk factors for coronary artery disease. In the guidelines, the following components of rehabilitation are rated in terms of strength of evidence: exercise tolerance, strength training, exercise habits, symptoms, smoking, lipids, body weight, blood pressure, psychosocial well-being, social adjustment and functioning, return to work, morbidity and safety issues, mortality, pathophysiology, atherosclerosis extent, hemodynamics, myocardial perfusion or evolution of myocardial ischemia, myocardial contractility/ventricular wall motion abnormalities, occurrence of cardiac arrhythmias, CHF, transplants, and the elderly. Exercise tolerance, return to work, morbidity and safety issues, and CHF symptoms all received an "A" rating in terms of strength of evidence, this means that "scientific evidence provided by well-designed, well-conducted, controlled trials (randomized and nonrandomized) with statistically significant results that consistently support the guideline recommendation."

Body weight received a "C" rating, which was defined as "expert opinion suggesting that the available scientific evidence did not present consistent results, or controlled trials are lacking." The issue of body weight has been studied further since the guidelines were published, and therefore further analysis may be needed to assess accurately the relationship between exercise tolerance and body weight as it affects CHD. All of the other issues listed received a "B" rating for strength of evidence. This was defined as "scientific evidence provided by observational studies or by controlled trials with less consistent results to support the guideline recommendation."

The AHCPR Cardiac Rehabilitation Guidelines have had a positive impact on the implementation of exercise and other cardiac rehabilitation interventions in treatment plans for patients with cardiovascular disease. It has given health care providers the data to substantiate the inclusion of risk factor reduction as a vital part of all cardiac care. Other chapters in the document speak to the other CHD risk factors, and a second core content reviews the effects of cardiac rehabilitation education, counseling, and behavioral interventions. The guidelines also stress the importance of cardiac rehabilitation services for people having undergone other interventions, such as angioplasty, valve replacement, and transplantation, and those with CHF. The guidelines broaden the scope for cardiac rehabilitation in several important areas for patients and health care providers. First, there is a preponderant theme of keeping the individual patient at the center of all cardiac rehabilitation endeavors. Second, the rigid phases of cardiac rehabilitation in the hospital or other health care facility are not the only avenues for providing the needed exercise training, education, counseling, and behavioral interventions. The concept is more global and descriptive of an atmosphere of individualized programs for patients based on their individual risk factors and risk stratification.

CARDIAC REHABILITATION

The AHCPR Guidelines define cardiac rehabilitation as follows:

Cardiac rehabilitation services are comprehensive, long-term programs involving medical evaluation, prescribed exercise, cardiac risk factor modification, education, and counseling. These programs are designed to limit the physiologic and psychological effects of cardiac illness, reduce the risk for sudden death or reinfarction, control cardiac symptoms, stabilize or reverse the atherosclerotic process, and enhance the psychosocial and vocational status of selected patients. Cardiac rehabilitation services are prescribed for patients who: 1) have had an MI; 2) have had coronary artery bypass surgery (CABS); or 3) have chronic stable angina pectoris. The services are in three phases beginning during hospitalization, followed by a supervised ambulatory outpatient program lasting 3–6 months, and continuing in a lifetime maintenance stage in which physical fitness and risk factor reduction are accomplished in a minimally supervised or unsupervised setting.[12]

Cardiac rehabilitation is most commonly initiated at the time of a cardiac event, such as acute MI, CABS, percutaneous transluminal coronary angioplasty or atherectomy (PTCA), stent placement, or diagnostic confirmation of coronary artery disease by coronary angiography. In addition, it is often instituted after valvular replacement, cardiac transplantation, and pacemaker implantation. Even though most patients are referred to cardiac rehabilitation in the context of acute MI, CABS, and, more recently, PTCA, we are seeing more referrals for the other diagnoses and procedures listed as well. A common goal for all these patients is achieving a better quality and sometimes quantity of life through a healthier lifestyle. The addition of exercise and increased activity is the positive action for beginning to achieve this goal.

Cardiac rehabilitation as a whole is aimed at improving the cardiac patient's quality of life through reduction of risk factors for cardiac disease or another cardiac event. Although the emphasis and examples in this chapter pertain to cardiac rehabilitation, many of the concepts and principles also apply to primary prevention in the healthy population. *Primary prevention* refers to the ability of a factor (e.g., exercise) to prevent the initiation of a disease process, such as atherosclerosis.[46] *Secondary prevention* refers to the role a factor can play in arresting a developing disease while the patient is still asymptomatic.[46] *Tertiary prevention* deals with minimization of disability, morbidity, and mortality once the disease is clinically manifest. The CDC and AHA now list inactivity as a major risk factor, with an overall weight in terms of prevention similar to high blood pressure, smoking, and increased blood cholesterol.[47] Although exercise exerts an independent preventive effect, some of its value is related to associated improvements in other risk factors (Display 34-3).

Opinions have differed over how much exercise is needed for this beneficial effect. However, as discussed previously, there is now a growing consensus about how much is needed. With cardiac patients, it is crucial to find leisure activities, occupational activities, and ADLs that are safe and are likely to be performed regularly by an individual patient.[3] Clearly, these activities will be different in terms of type and intensity for different patients. Today, the rigid phases of cardiac rehabilitation are emphasized less because it is recognized that every patient may not need to progress through "phases." More emphasis is placed on risk stratifi-

---

DISPLAY 34-3

Changes in Risk Factors Influenced by Exercise Training

Decrease in blood pressure
Increase in high-density lipoprotein cholesterol level
Augmented weight reduction efforts
Psychological effects
   Less depression
   Reduced anxiety
Improved glucose tolerance

From Fletcher GF, Balady G, Froelicher VF et al: Exercise Standards: A Statement for Healthcare Professionals from the American Heart Association, p 23. Dallas, American Heart Association, 1995.

cation and risk factor analysis in defining a program for the individual patient.

Thus, prescribing exercise and activity is discussed as it relates to the in-hospital course followed by the rehabilitation course after the patient is discharged. As mentioned earlier, the acute in-hospital length of stay has changed significantly; the average in-hospital stay is now 3 to 7 days for the patient with uncomplicated acute MI and CABS. For other interventions, the stay may be as little as 1 to 2 days. Only high-risk, complicated patients are staying for longer periods.

The convalescent stage after hospital discharge varies depending on the intervention and the individual patient. Referrals to cardiac rehabilitation occur within a few days to weeks. All patients are not treated the same on entry to cardiac rehabilitation, as was true in the past. Cardiac rehabilitation professionals are making an effort to evaluate patients individually for the particular program that will best meet the patient's needs. We have become more proficient in evaluating people using risk stratification. The patient who has had PTCA, for example, may not always need the traditional monitored program. Often, such patients may be low risk and need primarily to learn to exercise safely, and therefore do not need to be monitored. However, some programs still start all new cardiac rehabilitation patients by monitoring them. Most insurance companies and Medicare have either a time or session number limit for this modality. Currently, Medicare pays for the allowable 12 weeks or 36 sessions, and many insurance companies do the same. Some are for more and some are for less allotted time. They also vary according to the amount they pay. In addition, several insurance companies specifically exclude cardiac rehabilitation from coverage. This presents problems for both the patient and the health care provider, and partially explains why so many (>80%) eligible patients do not receive cardiac rehabilitation. The nurse often has a critical role in assessing patient needs and insurance issues, and in finding creative ways of providing patients with the information and guidance they need to obtain reimbursement for this important service.

When patients enter into cardiac rehabilitation, they may start in the hospital or they may be referred later. Whenever a patient is referred for cardiac rehabilitation, the following process takes place:[3]

- ◆ Assess previous activity and exercise habits.
- ◆ Initiate gradual progression of activity and exercise.
- ◆ Evaluate and monitor response to activity and exercise.
- ◆ Prescribe increases in activity and exercise.
- ◆ Teach the patient the ability to monitor his or her own response to activity and exercise.

The extended outpatient program for patients who need to continue with some health care supervision was traditionally called phase III or IV, and lasts from 3 to 6 months or longer. It is also referred to as the transitional or maintenance phase.

Formal cardiac rehabilitation programs typically consist of an interdisciplinary team to ensure a thorough approach to rehabilitation. Whether working independently with the patient in a hospital or medical center or in a cardiac rehabilitation program, the nurse has a pivotal role in assisting the patient to resume and increase his or her exercise and activity. Commonly, the nurse is the program director or coordinator of the cardiac rehabilitation program, the primary care provider in the cardiac rehabilitation process, or both.

Definition of Terms

Activity refers to movements that are accomplished in the course of meeting human physiologic needs, including ADLs such as shaving, bathing, dressing, eating, walking, and driving a car.[48]

Exercise refers to physical exertion at a prescribed frequency, duration, and intensity to prevent deconditioning, improve health, correct physical deformity or disability, and provide cardiovascular conditioning.[48]

Isometric exercise is constant muscular contraction without movement that imposes a greater pressure than volume load on the left ventricle in relation to the body's ability to supply oxygen (e.g., handgrip).[3]

Isotonic exercise is muscular contraction resulting in movement, primarily providing a volume load to the left ventricle and the cardiovascular response, and is proportional to the intensity of the exercise.[3]

Stretching refers to exercise that increases or maintains flexibility and joint range of motion.

Calisthenics refers to dynamic exercises that are designed to develop muscular tone and strength.

Warm-up periods are designed gradually to increase the metabolic rate from the resting level of 1 MET to the MET level required for conditioning. They usually last 5 to 10 minutes and may include walking or slow jogging, light stretching exercises, and calisthenics or other types of muscle-conditioning exercises.

Cool-down periods or cool-downs include exercises of diminishing intensity, such as slower walking or jogging, stretching, and, in some cases, relaxation activities.

In-Hospital Phase

ASSESSMENT

The assessment that occurs before beginning activities in the hospital and that which occurs when the patient is ready to begin an exercise program as an outpatient are somewhat different. With the inpatient, the nurse assesses the acute response to increasing activities, whereas in the outpatient program, the acute response as well as the responses the patient reports since discharge are assessed. The assessment is discussed under the overall discussion for inpatient and outpatient cardiac rehabilitation.

Because of shorter hospital stays for cardiac surgery and MI, early assessment is important so that activity and education can begin in a timely manner once the patient is medically stable. Patients with cardiac surgery or MI can at least begin assisted range of motion 24 to 48 hours after the event. In general, cardiac surgery patients without complications progress somewhat faster than those with MI. However, a patient with an uncomplicated MI, or one who has been admitted days after the MI occurred, may progress more rapidly than a patient with a complicated MI (Display 34-4).

For the cardiac surgery patient, a presurgery assessment is most desirable. This is usually possible if the surgery is elective or planned. Obviously, if it is emergent, this is not feasible. Assessing the patient before surgery obtains information about the patient's premorbid lifestyle and evaluates function and mobility without the complexities of incisions and other postoperative discomforts. This information then serves as a valuable baseline for postoperative function and mobility. This is particularly useful in the older patient (>65 years of age) who may have neuromuscular and orthopedic problems before surgery. The preoperative assessment also introduces the patient to the activity he or she will be expected to perform after surgery. By introducing the patient to staff and cardiac rehabilitation activity plans before surgery, the course of phase I runs smoother and the patient's anxiety about resuming activity may be decreased.

Assessment of the patient with MI obviously is not possible before the event, but this assessment should take place as soon as the diagnosis of an acute MI has been confirmed. This may not be possible if there are complications, but baseline data can be gathered from the chart and from staff discussion and collaboration. Because of the short hospital stay, patients with PTCA often do not have a full inpatient activity course, but instead are introduced to the outpatient program or receive risk factor counseling.

How the in-hospital phase is initiated and who carries it out may vary in different medical centers. Many centers no longer put as much emphasis on inpatient cardiac rehabilitation. Instead, nurses are guiding the patient to increased activity. In many programs, a physical therapist, occupational therapist, or clinical exercise physiologist have an important role in guiding the patient's activity after a cardiac event. The order to begin inpatient cardiac rehabilitation is often a standing order as part of the admission for cardiac surgery or MI. However, it may take a day or two to confirm the diagnosis of MI, so initiation of activities would not take place until then. Different team members (physical therapist and occupational therapist) often assist with initial evaluation and assessment before ambulating the patient. However, in most instances, the nurse is the one who first assesses the patient. A risk stratification model is often used. One adaptation of this typical outpatient model is shown in Display 34-5. Based on this risk stratification, activity can then be started according to the activity guidelines in Display 34-6.

The actual assessment of the patient before initiating the inpatient rehabilitation program includes a careful evaluation of disease stability, other clinical factors, and issues that may be more difficult to measure, such as the patient's psychological status and motivation to begin the program. Each of these issues is addressed in the following sections.

Age. The patient's age is becoming more of an issue in cardiac rehabilitation because of the aging of the population in general and the concomitant increase in heart disease in the elderly. Elderly people are receiving cardiac interventions much more frequently than they did previously. An important part of their care is to get them active as soon as possible because they are more prone to the hazards of immobility.

Elderly patients with MI differ from younger patients in several important ways. They are more likely to be admitted with silent ischemia or a presentation of CHF, and the MI may be days to weeks old. Silent ischemia occurs more often because of a decreased sympathetic response or the combination of diabetes mellitus and neuropathy, and may complicate the initial presentation. The diagnosis of MI may also be less clear because the three main diagnostic criteria may be altered: (1) decreased presentation of pain; (2) electrocardiographic (ECG) changes normal for the elderly may mask MI changes[49]; and (3) total creatinine phosphokinase

---

DISPLAY 34-4

Criteria for Classification of Complicated* Myocardial Infarction

Continued cardiac ischemia (pain, late enzyme rise)
Left ventricular failure (congestive heart failure, new murmurs, roentgenographic changes)
Shock (blood pressure drop, pallor, oliguria)
Important cardiac dysrhythmias (premature ventricular contractions greater than six per minute, atrial fibrillation)
Conduction disturbances (bundle-branch block, atrioventricular block, hemiblock)
Severe pleurisy or pericarditis
Complication illnesses
Marked creatinine kinase rise without a noncardiac explanation or after thrombolysis

*One or more criteria classify a myocardial infarction as complicated.
(From Froelicher VF: Cardiac rehabilitation. In Chatterjee K, Cheitlin MD, Karliner J et al (eds): Cardiology: An Illustrated Text/Reference, vol 2, p 7,208. Philadelphia, JB Lippincott, 1991.)

DISPLAY 34-5

Risk Stratification

LOW RISK

- No significant LV dysfunction (i.e., EF >50%).
- Has had successful reperfusion of myocardium (e.g., PTCA, CABG).
- No resting or activity-induced myocardial ischemia manifested as angina or ST segment displacement on the telemetry monitor or from stress test.
- No resting or activity-induced complex arrhythmias.
- No orthostatic BP changes causing patient to become symptomatic.
- Patient followed a regular exercise program or had an "active" lifestyle before hospitalization.
- No other current health problems that would potentially complicate activity regime (e.g., PVD, orthopedic problems, moderate to severe COPD/emphysema, pericarditis).

INTERMEDIATE RISK

- Mild to moderately depressed LV function (e.g., EF 31%–49%).
- Has had successful reperfusion of myocardium (e.g., PTCA, CABG).
- No activity-induced myocardial ischemia (1–2 mm ST segment depression on stress test) or reversible ischemic defects (echo or nuclear radiography).
- May have orthostatic BP changes but is not symptomatic.
- Patient did not participate in a regular exercise program before hospitalization but may have had an "active" lifestyle.
- No other current health problems that would potentially complicate activity regime (e.g., PVD, orthopedic problems, moderate to severe COPD/emphysema, pericarditis).

HIGH RISK

- Severely depressed LV function (i.e., EF <30%).
- Complex ventricular arrhythmias at rest or appearing or increasing with exercise.
- Decrease in systolic blood pressure >20 mm Hg during activity or failure to rise with increasing activity workloads.
- Survivor of sudden cardiac death.
- Myocardial infarction complicated by congestive heart failure, cardiogenic shock, or complex ventricular arrhythmias.
- Severe coronary artery disease and marked activity-induced myocardial ischemia (>2-mm ST segment depression on stress test).
- Orthostatic BP changes and is symptomatic.
- Patient did not participate in a regular exercise program and did not have an "active" lifestyle before hospitalization.

BP, blood pressure; CABG, coronary artery bypass grafting; COPD, chronic obstructive pulmonary disease; EF, ejection fraction; LV, left ventricular; PTCA, percutaneous transluminal angioplasty; PVD, peripheral vascular disease. From Saint Luke's Shawnee Mission Health System, Kansas City, MO, Mid America Heart Institute 1997. Courtesy of Jan E. Foresman, RN, MS, Cardiac Rehabilitation Specialist.

(CPK) elevations are often normal or lower, whereas CPK isoenzyme levels are elevated.[50] This is a particular problem in medical centers where, for cost reasons, only total CPKs in the higher range are tested for isoenzymes. For cardiac rehabilitation, this means the patient's initial diagnosis of MI may come late in the course, after complications have stabilized (i.e., CHF). The tendency is to discharge patients quickly before they have been assessed for mobility and safety issues. Also, elderly patients may have to make more compromises to their previous activities because of the deconditioning that occurs with bed rest of any duration; it takes elderly people longer to regain strength.

Gender. The differences between men and women returning to activity do not necessarily depend on gender. This is discussed more in the section on Immediate Outpatient Cardiac Rehabilitation.

Weight. Weight strongly influences activity and exercise, but probably more in the long term, as an outpatient, than in the short term, in the hospital. Patients who are overweight often have more difficulty transferring and mobilizing after surgery.

Physique. Physique probably influences the patient's level of exercise more than his or her ability to return to ADLs, which is addressed during the inpatient phase.

Motivation. This is an extremely important element to assess for the inpatient. How motivated the patient is after the cardiac event determines how rapidly and successfully he or she returns to his or her previous activity level. Acutely, the lack of motivation may be closely related to fear or depression about the condition. If the patient has a high motivation to return to previous activities, inpatient education and activity

---

DISPLAY 34-6

Activity Guidelines

LOW RISK

◆ Chair with meals.

◆ Up in room and bathroom privileges as tolerated (if gait is steady)

◆ Ambulate two to four times per day.
  Initial ambulation with a nurse (a resting HR and BP, either lying or sitting, and BP standing followed by a HR and BP on immediate return to room). Initial ambulation is determined by how well the patient is tolerating the activity (i.e., no dyspnea, dizziness, chest discomfort). The length of time spent during the initial ambulation must be noted.
  All subsequent ambulation will have 1 minute added per day.

◆ For those patients who are stratified as a low risk but may have "other special situation" such as orthopedic problems, severe claudication, paraplegia, and so forth, or who cannot ambulate for their activity, the cardiac rehabilitation specialist or physical therapist should be consulted.

INTERMEDIATE RISK

◆ Chair with meals.

◆ Ambulate two to three times per day (see ambulation information for low-risk patients).

◆ For those patients who are stratified as intermediate risk but may have "other special situations" such as orthopedic problems, severe claudication, paraplegia, and so forth, or who cannot ambulate for their activity, the cardiac rehabilitation specialist or physical therapist should be consulted.

HIGH RISK

◆ The cardiac rehabilitation specialist will be called to assist in designing an activity program for this classification of patient.

BP, blood pressure; HR, heart rate. From Saint Luke's Shawnee Mission Health System, Kansas City, Mo, Mid America Heart Institute 1997. Courtesy of Jan E. Foresman, RN, MS, Cardiac Rehabilitation Specialist.

---

may assist the overzealous cardiac patient from becoming too active too quickly and increasing the oxygen demand of the healing myocardium. On the other hand, guidance during hospitalization aimed at gradual return to activities assists less motivated patients to reach realistic goals that they may not have been able to set on their own. Both types of patient benefit from a structured approach to increasing activity. The approach by the care provider may be different for each person, but the same protocol can be used.

Previous Activity Level.   The assessment of the patient's lifestyle should begin with an evaluation of the living situation: one- or two-story home, private home versus apartment or trailer, steps to front or back door, stairs to bedroom and bathroom, lives alone or with spouse or others. Who does most of the household chores, both inside and outside? Who does the cleaning, cooking, and so forth? When this basic information is obtained, vocational, recreational, and desirable activity can be assessed and reasonable goals can be set. Is the patient employed or retired, and in what type of work? Is he or she sedentary or active; does he or she do much walking or lifting; is there stress with work? What are the patient's desires to return to work? What are the current plans, or are they uncertain? What are his or her recreational or leisure-time activities?

This is an introductory inpatient assessment. It is not meant to solve activity issues, but to evaluate the patient's previous lifestyle and hopes for the future after the cardiac event. Another approach to questioning the patient is to have him or her fill out a questionnaire such as the one depicted in Figure 34-1. This particular questionnaire was used in a study of 258 patients recuperating from MI and was found to be both reliable and valid.[51] Other questionnaires deal with evaluating the patient's self-efficacy about returning to previous activities. This type of questionnaire is useful because it can be given again in the outpatient phases.[52,53] By assessing the previous activity level, the nurse can assist patients in deciding what activities they can resume immediately, what needs to be modified, and what needs to be changed completely. Also, this initial assessment provides information to pass along to the outpatient cardiac rehabilitation nurse about the patient's previous exercise pattern in work and leisure.

Cardiovascular History.   The patient undergoing CABS, PTCA, or stent placement, or experiencing an MI has usually had a physical examination by the physician and nurse on admission, and daily since admission. Because the nurse caring for the patient makes most of the decisions regarding the patient's activity level, the nurse usually does the patient's daily cardiovascular examination. If there is a specific cardiac rehabilitation nurse, the admitting examination can be referred to in the cardiac rehabilitation assessment. In addition, a detailed knowledge of the duration of cardiovascular impairment before the event is essential. Specifically, information about previous MI, angiography, thrombolytic therapy, PTCA, valvular disease, exercise-induced arrhythmia, chest discomfort of any kind, or other cardiac problems should be obtained. The details of the current hospitalization should be outlined and taken into consideration as the

ACTIVITY SUMMARY QUESTIONNAIRE

Week of _____ to _____ Name _____

As a participant in the Cardiac Rehabilitation Project, your help is needed in providing us with information about how much activity you are doing now. Try to estimate the *average* number of *minutes* you spent on each activity in a day. In the next column, write down how many *days* you did that activity this week. Include even those activities you did only once or twice. You may not be doing every activity, so put a 0 next to those activities you did not do this week. Where it says "specify," tell exactly what you did.

Activity	Approximate No.	
	Min per day	Days per week
1. Walking (shopping, doing errands, etc.)		
2. Walking for exercise distance: time:		
3. Climbing stairs number of floors: how often each day:		
4. Calisthenics (please specify)		
5. Housekeeping light: (dishes, dusting, sweeping, etc.) heavy: (laundry, mopping, ironing, etc.)		
6. Visiting at-home visitors: visiting away: (parties, movies, friends, etc.)		
7. Sports/Recreation (please specify) (golf, bowling, sailing, cycling, etc.)		
8. Gardening light: (riding mower, planting, etc.) heavy: (pushing mower, digging, hoeing, etc.)		
9. Hobbies (please specify)		
10. Driving car		
11. Repair and maintenance light: (basic car tune-up, fixing appliances, etc.) heavy: (woodworking, plumbing, painting, etc.)		
12. If not retired, have you returned to work? No_____ Yes_____ If yes, Full time_____ Part time_____ hours per week_____		
13. Have you resumed sexual activity? Yes_____ No_____		
14. Other activities (please specify)		
15. Was this more or less activity than last week?		
16. If different from last week, what was the reason?		

Thank you very much for your help in answering these questions

FIGURE 34-1 A questionnaire used to determine a patient's activity level for a cardiac rehabilitation program. (Reprinted with permission from Lindskog BD, Sivarajan ES: A method of evaluation of activity and exercise in a controlled study of early cardiac rehabilitation. J Cardiac Rehabil 2–3: 156–165, 1982.)

*As noted, the subjective patient response of RPE is incorporated. It is also extremely important that the nurse is alert to subtle signs and symptoms of mood or attitude as patients come to each exercise session. Patients may be experiencing physical or psychological changes that can make a particular exercise session difficult. A personal approach to each patient is extremely important, even though the patients are being seen in a group. If adverse physical changes have occurred during the exercise session, or are reported as occurring since the last session, the referring physician should be notified so that medical intervention can occur.

inpatient activity level is prescribed. For instance, in the case of an MI, it is important to note the following:

Site: inferior, anterior, posterior, lateral, septal, or a combination

Type: transmural or nontransmural

Treatment: thrombolytic therapy, heparin, nitroglycerin, antiarrhythmics, PTCA, stent

Complications: CHF, shock, arrhythmias, ongoing angina

Diagnostic information: ECG changes, enzymes, patient presentation, coronary angiogram, gated blood pool study, low-level exercise tolerance test (LLETT), other previous exercise tolerance tests (ETTs), echocardiogram, significant laboratory results, cholesterol levels

Coronary artery disease risk factors pertinent to patient: hypertension, smoking, elevated cholesterol, sedentary lifestyle, obesity, stress

Typical anginal pattern: mid-chest, radiation pattern to throat, arms, jaw

Medications: past and current

ECG rhythm: any arrhythmias during this hospitalization or in the past

The same information is important to gather for the patient undergoing CABS and PTCA, in addition to any complications from the intervention and the treatment.

As mentioned earlier, at the time of the initial assessment, it is also important to obtain information to stratify the patient's levels of risk. Risk stratification has typically been used to guide the cardiac rehabilitation practitioner concerning the duration of supervision and the type and frequency of monitoring for outpatient cardiac rehabilitation. The levels of risk are delineated using the patient's medical history, clinical course, physiologic variables, and other test results. An inpatient risk stratification model is shown in Display 34-5. The outpatient levels of risk are listed in Table 34-4 and are discussed further in the section on outpatient rehabilitation.[3,54-58]

Other Health Problems. Other health problems that would influence, limit, or contraindicate the normal inpatient activity progression should be assessed in each patient. Patients with chronic renal failure who are on dialysis are usually anemic and may not be able to increase their activity level. Tolerance to increases in activity may also be diminished in patients with chronic respiratory disease due to hypoxia. For a diabetic patient, the stress of hospitalization and an acute cardiac event can often increase the need for insulin or oral glucose-lowering medications. Patients with severe psychological disturbances may have difficulty increasing their activity at a normal pace and following instruction. Patients with upper or lower extremity weakness or mobility limitations are also of special concern when increasing activity in the hospital in preparation for discharge.

INITIATION OF INPATIENT ACTIVITY

The objectives for inpatient activity and education are as follows:

◆ To educate the patient and family about the particular cardiac event and diagnostic tests and to prepare them for the stages of cardiac rehabilitation and returning to life at home.

◆ To offset the deleterious physiologic and psychological effects of bed rest.

◆ To return the patient to ADLs.

◆ To provide additional medical surveillance of the patient.

◆ To introduce the patient to risk factor behavior modification.

◆ To stratify the patient's risk for future cardiac rehabilitation[59] (see Table 34-4).

The patient experiencing an MI, CABS, or PTCA is usually transferred from the cardiac or intensive care unit to a telemetry unit and sometimes to a general medicine or surgical unit. However, with decreased length of stays, many are discharged directly from the telemetry or step-down unit. The nurses on each of these units are usually the ones who orient and explain to the patient the processes involved in diagnosis and treatment of the specific cardiovascular event. This information is discussed elsewhere in this text (see Chapters 29 to 33 and 35 to 37). Education about risk factor reduction and the important aspects of medical observation of the patient are discussed in Chapters 29 to 33 and 35 to 37. This chapter addresses the activity and exercise preparation for the inpatient time period.

As mentioned earlier, before 1960, patients were relegated to strict bed rest after an acute MI. It was thought that any physical activity could lead to complications such as ventricular aneurysm formation, cardiac rupture, CHF, dysrhythmias, reinfarction, or sudden death.[58] Numerous studies disputed this, and it was subsequently shown that there was no increase in complications when early ambulation was used compared with bed rest. The detrimental physiologic effects of strict bed rest can occur after just a few days. In addition to decreased cardiorespiratory fitness, there is a decrease in blood volume, red blood cell count, nitrogen and protein balance, and strength and flexibility. Orthostatic hypotension and thromboembolism can also occur. Upright posture shifts, ambulation, and range-of-motion exercise help alleviate all of these problems. Early postoperative physical activity has been found to decrease postsurgical stiffness and prevent postsurgical atelectasis in patients undergoing CABS. It has the added benefits of decreasing depression and reducing anxiety, improving self-esteem, and reducing type A behavior characteristics, such as hostility and anger.[61]

In 1973, Wenger established the concept of patients progressing through systematic steps to increase activity in the hospital. This approach included early mobilization, range-of-motion exercises, and progressive activity. This step concept is not used as often as previously. If a step protocol is used, the steps are seen more as guidelines rather than mandating that patients stay within the particular steps. The emphasis is much more on individually evaluating and stratifying the patient for increased activity. A sample step program is shown in Table 34-5.

While carrying out a program of education and increasing activity for the inpatient, measurable objectives should be established that are both general and specific to each patient. Some examples of these objectives might include having the patient:

◆ Ambulate 1,000 feet around the unit two to three times per day before discharge.

◆ Take pulse and relate rating of perceived exertion to activities performed.

TABLE 34-4 Comparison of ACSM/ACP, AACVPR, and AHA Risk Stratification Criteria

Risk	ACSM/ACP	AACVPR	AHA
Low Risk			
Functional capacity	≥8 METS	≥7 METS	>6 METS
LV function	No LV dysfunction	EF >50%	No evidence of heart failure NYHA class 1 or 2
Myocardial ischemia	No ischemia	No evidence of myocardial ischemia	Free of ischemia or angina at rest or on GXT <6 METS
Resting ECG	No complex dysrhythmias	Absence of significant ventricular ectopy	No sequential PVCs
Hospital complications	Uncomplicated MI or bypass surgery	Uncomplicated course in hospital	No specific guidelines
Exterional blood pressure	No specific guidelines	No specific guidelines	Appropriate rise in systolic blood pressure during exercise
Self-monitoring	No specific guidelines	No specific guidelines	Ability satisfactorily to self-monitor intensity of activity
Intermediate/Moderate Risk			
Functional capacity	<8 METS	No specific guidelines	The AHA has combined moderate and high-risk categories; AHA moderate risk guidelines are listed under high risk
LV function	No specific guidelines	EF = 35%–49%	
Myocardial ischemia	Exercise induced ischemia of <2 mm ST segment depression	Changing pattern or new development of angina Reversible thallium defects	
Exercise ECG ST segment changes	Exercise induced ischemia of <2 mm ST segment depression	ST segment depression ≥2 mm flat or downsloping	
Hospital complications	Shock or CHF during recent MI (<6 mo)	No specific guidelines	
Self-monitoring	Inability to self-monitor HR Failure to comply with exercise prescription	No specific guidelines	
High Risk			
Functional capacity	No specific guidelines	<5 METS with hypotensive blood pressure response	<6 METS
LV function	EF <30%	EF <35%	EF <30% NYHA class 3 or greater
Resting ECG	Resting complex ventricular dysrhythmias	High-grade ventricular ectopy	No specific guidelines
Exercise ECG ST segment changes	Exercise ischemia >2 mm ST depression	≥2 mm ST segment depression at HR ≤135 bpm, or ≥1 mm ST segment depression with functional capacity <5 METS	Horizontal/downsloping ST segment depression ≥4 mm
Exercise ECG dysrhythmias	PVCs appearing or increasing with exercise	No specific guidelines	Ventricular tachycardia at workload <6 METS
Exertional blood pressure response	Exertional hypotension (≥15 mm Hg)	Fall in systolic blood pressure or failure to rise more than 10 mm Hg on GXT	Fall in systolic blood pressure with exercise
Cardiac pathology	Recent MI (<6 mo) with serious dysrhythmias	Previous MI involving ≥35% of left ventricle	Two or more MIs; three-vessel or left main disease
Hospital complications	No specific guidelines	Persistent/recurrent ischemic pain ≥24 h after hospital admission	No specific guidelines; states "A medical problem that a physician believes may be life-threatening"
Previous cardiac arrest	Survivors of cardiac arrest	No specific guidelines	Previous episode of ventricular fibrillation or arrest that did not occur in the presence of acute ischemic event/procedure; previous episode of primary cardiac arrest

ACSM, American College of Sports Medicine; ACP, American College of Physicians; AACVPR, American Association of Cardiovascular and Pulmonary Rehabilitation; AHA, American Heart Association.

LV, left ventricular; EF, ejection fraction; NYHA, New York Heart Association; GXT, graded exercise test; MI, myocardial infarction; ECG, electrocardiogram; HR, heart rate; CHF, congestive heart failure; METs, metabolic equivalents; PVCs, premature ventricular contractions.

From Verril D, Bergey D, McElveen G et al: Recommended guidelines for cardiac maintenance (phase IV) programs: A position paper by the North Carolina Cardiopulmonary Rehabilitation Association. J Cardiopulm Rehabil 13:87–95, 1993.

TABLE 34-5	Seattle VA Medical Center Rehabilitation Medicine Cardiac Rehabilitation (CR) Protocol for Phase I (Inpatient)			
Step	**Nursing**	**Physical Therapy**	**Occupational Therapy**	**Dietary**
Step 1 (bed rest)* 1 MET	Orient patient to cardiac care unit, use of commode (1.5); arms supported for upper extremity (UE) activities, decrease anxiety, advise patient of activity limitations	Lower extremity (LE), active range of motion (AROM), and evaluation	UE, AROM, and evaluation, intro to sternal precautions and CR progress	
Step 2 (in room) 2 METs	Sit in chair for meals, and 20 min at a time, three–four times a day, personal activities of daily living (ADLs) at bedside or sink, answer patient questions as they arise	Walking in room, or 50 ft (2.0), warm-ups (WU) and cool-downs (CD) (2.5–3.0)	UE activity with shoulder flexion 45 degrees, 10 reps, education: activity guidelines and risk factor introduction	Diet survey
Step 3 (short walking) 3 METs	Sitting shower (3.5), continue risk factor education	Walking 100–250 ft with WU and CD, instruction in independent walking	Increasing abduction to 90 degrees and 15 reps, continue energy conservation and showering guidelines	Introduction to heart, healthy eating
Step 4 (long walking) 4 METs	Independent in ADLs and walking on ward, standing shower (3.7); discharge instruction: Meds, appts, emergencies, review plans for risk factor reduction efforts	Walking 250–1000 ft three–four times a day, one flight of stairs (12 steps) (3.5–4.0). Given and taught home exercise program	Review of ADLs at home, work, and leisure (postsurgery and postmyocardial infarction activity precautions, sex, driving)	Review of dietary follow-up as needed

*All metabolic equivalent (MET) determinations are in parentheses.
From Seattle Veterans Affairs Medical Center, Seattle, Washington.

◆ Climb a flight of stairs without distress.
◆ Relate upper extremity activity guidelines (sternal guidelines) after cardiac surgery.
◆ Perform self-care ADLs.
◆ Relate plans for resuming other ADLs (i.e., driving, sexual relations, and other strenuous life activities).
◆ Relate plan to carry out walking or biking exercise program.

Physical and occupational therapists carry out many formal inpatient activity programs. Physical therapists often do the warm-up and cool-down exercises and ambulation with the patient. The occupational therapist works with patients to educate them about ADLs, upper extremity activity, and energy conservation techniques. Physical therapists and occupational therapists are valuable members of a cardiac rehabilitation team, for whom function and mobility are key issues in patient recovery.

Approaches to increasing activity can differ considerably. As mentioned previously, the progressive, stepped concept has become widespread. However, more recently there has been interest in adapting the inpatient phase to common activities the patient performs, as well as walking. For example, it might be deduced that when patients can walk 250 feet, they are ready to take a sitting shower. At 500 feet, they are ready to choose either a sitting or standing shower. Showering has been studied independently for its effect on patients following a MI. Sitting versus standing has no difference in physiologic effect.[61] Other activities such as dressing can also be used as indicators for progression.

We no longer hold back patients from moving to the next step. Just because they are at a specific step does not mean that they cannot do activities in the next step if they feel ready and physiologically able. Because hospital stays have become shorter (3 to 5 days), we need to find methods to modify the inpatient program. There is no time for all 14 steps, or even 8 steps, at 1 step per day. If indications for advancement are used, patients with uncomplicated MI and those undergoing cardiac surgery can be progressed more quickly.

EVALUATION DURING THE INPATIENT STAY

Continuing evaluation of the patient in the hospital is crucial to the patient's progress and permits early recognition of complications. The important issues on which to focus include subjective and objective responses and ECG changes.

Subjective Responses. Some of the adverse subjective responses, due either to limited tolerance or to overexertion, include fatigue, shortness of breath, chest pain, dizziness, and palpitations. All complaints of symptoms by the patient should be assessed carefully. Fatigue, a symptom often reported by patients, is usually overlooked as being too vague. However, fatigue is a reliable symptom that correlates well with objective measurements of the patient's exercise capacity.[63] The location, radiation, intensity, and duration of chest pain, if present, should be noted. The circumstances that precipitated the chest pain should be examined so that preventive steps can be taken in the future. Dizziness is indicative of reduced cerebral perfusion as a result of a decrease in cardiac output with or without hyperventilation from anxiety. Palpitations may be due either to rapid HRs or to premature contractions, indicating myocardial irritability. After surgery, many patients have supraventricular arrhythmias. The patient's description of irregularities or changes in pulse should be assessed through such objective measurements as systolic blood pressure (SBP), HR, and ECG.

Objective Responses. Skin color, temperature, and perspiration provide information about the relative stress of a given activity. Flushing accompanied by warm sweating means that the effort put forth by the patient is sufficient to increase heat production. The body's compensatory mechanism of vasodilatation in the skin to dissipate heat is a normal response to exercise. In contrast, pale or cyanotic skin that is cool and clammy indicates that the exercise represents either an excessive strain, resulting in a fall in cardiac output with compensatory vasoconstriction, or patient anxiety, which also results in vasoconstriction to the skin.

Respiratory rate should be noted and recorded. Any shortness of breath that does not subside with cessation of exercise should be further evaluated to determine presence of heart failure. HR should be measured (1) at rest, (2) in response to activity and exercise, and (3) during the recovery period after activity or exercise. Because increases in HR increase myocardial oxygen requirements, a resting tachycardia (<100 beats/min) indicates that exercise should be postponed. The common reasons for resting tachycardia in patients with acute MI are anxiety, fever produced by myocardial injury, and heart failure. HR increases during activity and exercise in direct proportion to the workload until it reaches a peak that coincides with exercise capacity. Maximal attainable HR decreases with age. However, in normal elderly people, the stroke volume increases to provide adequate cardiac output[49] (Display 34-7).

Blood pressure is an important objective response to activity and exercise that should be assessed in all patients. When the patient is allowed to resume activity after a prolonged period of bed rest, there is a decreased adaptability to change in posture. The loss of normal postural vasomotor reflexes and hypovolemia often cause the patient to be unable to maintain sufficient blood pressure on sitting or standing, leading to symptoms of weakness and fainting. This orthostatic hypotension can be detected before ambulating the patient by measuring the blood pressure while the patient is supine, sitting, and standing (see Chapters 10 and 32 for techniques and criteria). SBP rises with an increase in the activity level. Diastolic blood pressure provides an indication of peripheral resistance and normally remains the same or decreases with prolonged activity and exercise. A diastolic blood pressure that increases with exercise to above 100 mm Hg is considered abnormal.

DISPLAY 34-7

Structural Alterations in the Cardiovascular System That Occur with Age

NORMAL CHANGES (AT REST)

Thickening and stiffening of large and medium-sized arteries
Concentric left ventricular hypertrophy
Modest left atrial enlargement
Modest aortic root dilation
Variable degree of fibrosis of left cardiac skeleton

DURING STRESS OF EXERCISE

Maximal aerobic capacity ($\dot{V}O_2$max) is maintained

1. Less increase in exercise heart rate
2. Less decrease in end-systolic volume
3. Increase in end-diastolic volume (Frank-Starling mechanism)

Maximal A-$\dot{V}O_2$ difference declines but can be improved
Decreased responsiveness to β-adrenergic stimulation

Adapted from Fleg JL, Gerstenblith G, Lakatta EG: Pathophysiology of the aging heart and circulation. In Messerli FH (ed): Cardiovascular Disease in the Elderly, 3rd ed. Boston, Kluwer, 1993.

Pressure–rate product is an indirect indication of myocardial oxygen consumption and is easily calculated by multiplying SBP and HR.[64] Pressure–rate product increases with exercise, indicating increasing myocardial oxygen consumption. In patients with CHD, when the increased myocardial oxygen demand cannot be met, signs of ischemia such as angina and ECG changes appear. If the pressure–rate product at which ischemic signs occur is known, measures can be taken to reduce either HR or SBP by modifying the activity and exercise intensity. Beta blockers or calcium blockers often are prescribed; these agents can help delay the ischemic response by lowering HR and SBP, reducing myocardial oxygen demand. Biofeedback techniques and relaxation exercises can also be taught to the patient to help keep the pressure–rate product below the critical level.

Electrocardiographic Responses. Both heart rhythm and changes in the ST segment should be assessed using the ECG. When arrhythmias are present, the time of their occurrence and whether they increase or decrease in response to activity should be recorded.

A rehabilitation program should have preestablished criteria or use the ACSM criteria[2] in regard to exercise prescription in the presence of arrhythmias (Display 34-8).

Lown and Wolf[65] have developed a grading system, shown in Table 34-6, that designates patients according to severity of risk for sudden death due to arrhythmias. Grades 4 and 5 are considered the most significant. Although the use of such grading systems to predict risk of sudden death is controversial, it is recognized that patients with significant (complex) arrhythmias and left ventricular dysfunction

---

DISPLAY 34-8

Clinical Indications and Contraindications for Inpatient and Outpatient Cardiac Rehabilitation

- Unstable angina
- Resting systolic blood pressure >200 mm Hg or diastolic >110 mm Hg
- Blood pressure drop of >20 mm Hg with symptoms
- Moderate to severe aortic stenosis
- Acute systemic illness or fever
- Uncontrolled atrial or ventricular arrhythmias
- Uncontrolled tachycardia (>100 bpm)
- Uncompensated congestive heart failure
- Third-degree heart block (without pacemaker)
- Active pericarditis or myocarditis
- Recent embolism
- Thrombophlebitis
- Resting ST displacement (>2 mm)
- Uncontrolled diabetes
- Orthopedic problems prohibiting exercise
- Other metabolic problems

From the American College of Sports Medicine: *Guidelines for Exercise Testing and Prescription*, 5th ed, p 179. Philadelphia, Lea & Febiger, 1995.

(ejection fraction <50%) are at higher risk than patients who have either alone. Whenever significant ECG responses to exercise are observed, communication of these findings to the patient's nurse and physician is imperative. Often medications can be adjusted to ameliorate the frequency of arrhythmias.

PRESCRIPTION FOR INCREASING ACTIVITY FOR THE INPATIENT

Following the assessment, initiation, and evaluation of response to activity, inpatients are ready to proceed with guidelines for home activity and beginning exercise. Some practitioners do a low level exercise tolerance test (LLETT) for acute MI patients before discharge. This is useful because it provides a monitored testing environment for patients in whom it is uncertain if these are still ischemia, serious arrhythmias, or symptoms, which might contraindicate exercise.

One MET is defined as the energy equivalent for a person at rest in a sitting position. It represents the consumption of 3.5 mL of oxygen per kilogram of body weight per minute. A patient's exercise capacity is often expressed as a multiple of the resting metabolic rate (i.e., number of METs). For instance, the low-level Bruce protocol requires approximately 4 METs at completion of 12 minutes[65] (Table 34-7). This amount of energy is roughly the upper limit for most ADLs.

Most patients progress in a phase I cardiac rehabilitation protocol to walking, showering, and so forth by discharge. These activities are equivalent to 3 to 5 METs. It can then be safely assumed that these patients are ready to resume ADLs at home without always doing a LLETT. If there is any uncertainty or if the patient is sent home before completing the phase I protocol, a LLETT should be done. MET tables for activities to be resumed should be discussed with the patient before discharge (Fig. 34-2).

As mentioned earlier, the risk stratification of inpatients, particularly those with MIs, is important. The AHA guidelines[3] provide a useful tool for physicians and nurses in prescribing the type of activity or exercise program. The data for risk stratifying of patients need to be collected from inpatient records. There are several different risk stratification lists. The widely circulated work by DeBusk and colleagues[55] identified patients largely based on ejection fraction and ETT results. This was expanded to include other criteria. Table 34-4 lists the various risk stratification methods. Because there can be substantial differences in these methods, the most conservative approach should be used when stratifying patients after an MI.

The patient who is stratified as low risk, or class B of the AHA list, should be able to return home and start a walking program of 10 minutes at a slow, regular pace. This should increase as tolerated up to 1 hour. With this type of walking schedule, patients usually progress to 50% to 70%

TABLE 34-6   The Lown and Wolf Grading System

Lown Grade	Definition
0	No premature ventricular contractions (PVCs)
1	Fewer than 30 PVCs/h
2	30 or more PVCs/h
3	Multiform PVCs
4A	Paired PVCs
4B	Ventricular tachycardia
5	R-on-T PVCs

Data from Lown B: Sudden cardiac death: The major challenge confronting contemporary cardiology. Am J Cardiol 43: 313–328, 1979; and Lown B, Wolf M: Approaches to sudden death from coronary heart disease. Circulation 44: 130–142, 1971.

TABLE 34-7   Protocol for Low-Level Exercise Testing

Level	Speed (mph)	Gradient (%)	Time (min)	MET*
I	1.2	0	3	2.1 ± 0.4
II	1.2	3	3	2.4 ± 0.3
III	1.2	6	3	2.7 ± 0.3
IV	1.7	6	3	3.9 ± 0.5

*One MET is defined as the energy equivalent for an individual at rest in sitting position; represents the consumption of 3.5–4.0 mL of oxygen per kilogram of body weight per minute.

From Sivarajan ES, Bruce RA: Early exercise testing after MI, Cardiovascular Nursing 17: 1–5, 1981.

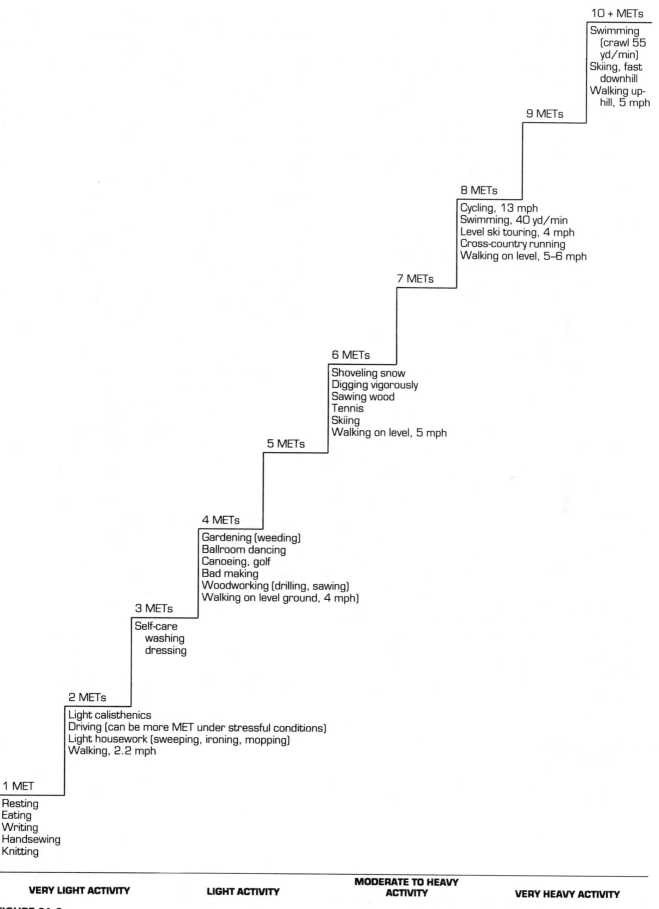

FIGURE 34–2

Energy cost (in METs [metabolic equivalents]) of activity and exercise.

of their $\dot{V}O_2$max.[58] Warm-ups and cool-downs should precede and conclude the exercise, respectively. Within 2 to 3 weeks of the event, patients should begin an outpatient cardiac rehabilitation program and have a symptom-limited exercise tolerance test (SLETT) done for the exercise prescription. The AHA recommends that activity be monitored, if possible, and that the exercise prescription be based on a SLETT. However, if an outpatient program is unavailable, dynamic exercise can be prescribed for a home program (e.g., walking or stationary bike). Range-of-motion exercises and light calisthenics can also be performed in the unmonitored setting.[3]

INPATIENT EDUCATION

The activity and exercise component of inpatient education involves teaching patients about activities they can do, as well as those they should be more cautious in doing, during the first few weeks of their rehabilitation. This differs somewhat for patients having cardiac surgery versus those with MI. The activity limitations after cardiac surgery involve sternal precautions and psychological adjustment to a major surgery. Those activities that put stress on the sternal incision are listed in Display 34-9. It is advisable for cardiac surgery patients to wait at least 4 to 6 weeks before driving a vehicle, partly because the sternal incision would be at risk in an impact. There is also some cognitive adjustment that needs to take place after a major surgery before the patient's reflexes are fully intact.

Patients with MI have slightly different reasons for activity limitations. They need to return to activities gradually because of the added work placed on the healing myocardium. As mentioned earlier, early mobilization of the patient with acute MI is now well accepted; however, there are important reasons not to cause a sudden increase in oxygen demand on the heart during the first few weeks of rehabilitation. In addition, those patients who have undergone both a PTCA and a stent placement are often cautioned to refrain from strenuous activity for at least 6 weeks. A SLETT is usually postponed until that time as well.

There should also be a gradual conditioning program for patients after MI and surgery. Patients in a walking program are usually instructed to continue the walking they have been doing in the hospital. In addition to the walking program, patients are also educated about the MET category they fit into when they go home. They are often given an MET list to help determine in which activities they can safely engage (see Fig. 34-2). They should be shown how to take their pulse and taught about the rating of perceived exertion (RPE) scale. This scale has proven to be highly correlated with patient's pulse and, when given a range of RPE, the patient can then objectively judge his or her level of exercise exertion (Table 34-8).

Patients should also be taught that the medications they are taking might have an effect on their HR and blood pressure (i.e., beta blockers, calcium channel blockers, and acetylcholinesterase inhibitors). Patients also should be reinstructed on when and how to take nitroglycerin and when to call for medical assistance. This cannot be overemphasized. Inpatients' retention of information is low, and therefore it is important to repeat certain guidelines several times and also to provide written information. Patients should have a written walking or biking program that includes mode, frequency, and duration of exercise. They should have a copy of the warm-up and cool-down exercises, preferably the same ones they were taught as an inpatient. Patients should be provided with their target HR (THR; usually 20 beats/min above the standing resting HR); the RPE scale noting the intensity they should be at when exercising (3 to 4 at the beginning); and a place to record HR, RPE, and symptoms. There should also be a list of precautions about exercise (Display 34-10).

At the time of discharge, some method of contacting the patient for outpatient cardiac rehabilitation follow-up should be established to continue the patient's education about exercise and to develop the appropriate continuation of an exercise program. Appointments should be made for follow-up in outpatient cardiac rehabilitation within 1 to 3 weeks after discharge.

TABLE 34-8	**Original and Revised Scales for Ratings of Perceived Exertion**		
Original Scale		**Revised Scale**	
6		0	Nothing
7	Very, very light	0.5	Very, very weak
8		1	Very weak
9	Very light	2	Weak
10		3	Moderate
11	Fairly light	4	Somewhat strong
12		5	Strong
13	Somewhat hard	6	
14		7	Very strong
15	Hard	8	
16		9	
17	Very hard	10	Very, very strong
18			Maximal
19	Very, very hard		
20			

In ACSM's Guidelines for Exercise Testing and Prescription pp 68. From Noble BJ, Borg GAV, Jacobs I et al: A category-ratio perceived exertion scale: Relationship to blood and muscle lactates and heart rate. Med Sci Sports Exerc 15: 523–528, 1983.

DISPLAY 34-9

Sternal Precautions and Activity Guidelines (for at least 6 Weeks After Cardiac Surgery)

Do not lift more than 10 pounds.
Do not push **up** as if getting out of bed or **out** as if pushing a cart.
No pulling.
No arm activities above the level of the heart.

Immediate Outpatient Cardiac Rehabilitation

As mentioned earlier, this phase of cardiac rehabilitation should be started within 3 weeks of the cardiac event. Usually the patient is scheduled for an initial interview, where baseline data are gathered and information about the program is given to the patient. At this initial interview, the nurse should have reviewed the inpatient chart so that the patient's risk stratification level is known. The objectives of the outpatient program include the following:

- Increase activity level and functional capacity
- Increase regular exercise participation
- Improve the patient's psychosocial status, depression, or anxiety through participation in exercise, education, or counseling when appropriate.
- Educate and support patients in other risk factor reduction efforts (i.e., stop smoking, control hypertension, normalize lipid values, and maintain healthy weight)

ASSESSMENT

When the patient is being considered for outpatient rehabilitation, it is important to take into account the patient's clinical condition, previous exercise history, motivation, and other health problems. All of these factors can influence the exercise prescription developed for an individual patient.

Age.　As mentioned previously, age is an important factor in developing an exercise program for cardiac patients. Older patients entering a program may have social as well as physical issues to address. They may need assistance with transportation to and from the cardiac program. They often live alone. Physically, they may be more deconditioned than younger patients. It has been shown that the traditional 12-week cardiac rehabilitation often is not long enough to produce a conditioning effect in elderly patients after a cardiac event. Medicare and most insurance companies pay 80% of only 12 weeks (36 visits) for an outpatient cardiac rehabilitation program. The benefits of exercise for people older than 65 years of age are essentially the same as for younger people. The elderly should exercise at a consistent intensity for longer periods of time before increasing the intensity.

Gender.　There are physiologic differences in the work capacities of men and women. These differences seem to be related to the size of the contracting muscle mass, and not necessarily to an inherent gender-related difference in oxygen transport and utilization.[67] Because of the larger proportion of muscle mass in men, they tend to have a higher work capacity than women. Historically, women have not been as accustomed to exercising, particularly recreationally. It has been shown that, after CABS, although women do not engage in heavy activity compared with men, they do return to household activity sooner.[68]

Weight.　It is important to know the patient's pattern of weight gain and loss throughout life.[69] The age at which a person has been at his or her highest and lowest weights should be recorded. Current assessment of weight in relation to body composition should be made to establish whether the patient has a normal percentage range of body fat. Estimations of body fat can be made using several methods.[60] Measurement of skinfold thickness using calipers specifically designed for this purpose is one method that is relatively inexpensive and quick and does not inconvenience the patient. Frequent measurements can be made to provide valuable feedback and reinforcement for the patient. Once fat weight is estimated, a desired body weight can be determined. (The equations used to determine ideal body weight are given by Pollock and colleagues.[60]) Men are considered obese if they carry 25% or more of their weight as fat. Women are considered obese if they carry more than 35% of their weight as fat (see Chapter 35).

Physique.　Posture, flexibility, equilibrium, and agility should be directly observed and assessed because these factors are related to ease of movement, safety, and risk of injury. The need for physical therapy referrals to prescribe specific exercises for neuromuscular or orthopedic problems should be assessed. Often the exercises prescribed in physical therapy can be performed as part of the cardiac rehabilitation program.

Motivation. It is important to assess the patient's attitude toward exercise, his or her diagnosis, and the prescription for an exercise program. Patients who have not exercised in the past may lack the motivation necessary to comply with the activity and exercise prescription. Sedentary patients may do well in a supervised cardiac rehabilitation setting, which provides motivation and an environment that gives the patient a feeling of greater safety. The patient who is overzealous about exercise and is always testing the limits of the exercise prescription should be identified and counseled on the importance of adhering to prescribed limits. A supervised exercise program is advised for this type of patient. Usually patients making the effort to participate in an outpatient cardiac rehabilitation are well motivated.

Previous Activity. As patients enter the program, it is important to gather all information about their past activity level. This includes all data from their inpatient stay. Also, it is important to determine how much they have been exercising (e.g., following the walking program instructions they might have been given) since discharge and their tolerance of this exercise. Knowledge of the patient's activity level before the cardiac event gives the cardiac rehabilitation care provider a frame of reference for the patient when prescribing his or her beginning level of exercise. Because people vary in their response to a cardiac event, patients may be overzealous or extremely frightened to perform any type of exercise. Therefore, it is important to start every patient gradually and be certain of his or her physical and psychological responses.

Cardiovascular History. Gathering all medical data for risk stratification is very important for outpatient cardiac rehabilitation. This enables the cardiac practitioner to establish accurate monitoring and supervision guidelines.[3] The cardiovascular history should include all of the elements of the inpatient assessment. In addition, because much of the outpatient program deals with teaching patients to exercise on their own, it is useful to get a general sense of what the patients know about their cardiac history. This is discussed further in the section on Patient Education in Outpatient Cardiac Rehabilitation.

Other Health Problems. All pulmonary, metabolic, neurologic, orthopedic, and muscular problems need to be identified so that the exercise mode and stimulus can be modified if necessary. Of special note in the outpatient program are patients with diabetes. Glucose levels should be checked before and at the conclusion of several sessions (approximately six sessions) to note changes in pre-exercise and postexercise glucose levels. Also, having juice on hand for hypoglycemic episodes is advisable.

EVALUATION IN OUTPATIENT CARDIAC REHABILITATION

Evaluation of the patient's response to exercise is crucial to the outpatient program. During outpatient rehabilitation, a progress report should be sent to the patient's physician periodically. An initial confirmation note and plan for intervention should also be sent. If the outpatient cardiac rehabilitation is a 12-week program, follow-up evaluation reports should be done at least at 6 weeks and at the program conclusion. If the patient has a physician's appointment coming up, it is also recommended that a progress report be sent to the physician at this time. A typical outpatient session progresses as follows:

1. Patient weighs self, and puts on the telemetry monitor (if indicated from risk stratification). Most patients are monitored for at least six sessions and then taught to take their pulse. If there is any question about arrhythmias or ischemic changes, monitoring should continue for a longer period. Specific criteria for monitoring have been outlined by the AHA[3] and AACVPR.[61]
2. Patient is asked his or her weight, and the attendant records it on flow sheet or in the computerized monitoring system.
3. A resting blood pressure is taken and recorded.
4. A resting rhythm strip is run on telemetry, or the patient is asked to report the resting pulse. With the new computerized telemetry monitoring systems, rhythm strips are automatically obtained during each mode of rest and exercise.
5. Patient is asked about his or her home exercise program, and it is recorded.
6. The attendant leads patient in warm-up exercises or, if the patient has been oriented to them, he or she can do them independently with prompting as necessary.
7. Patient is told the mode, intensity, and duration of his or her first exercise.
8. At least halfway into some modes of exercise, the patient's blood pressure is taken, along with a telemetry rhythm strip or pulse, and the patient is asked for the Rating of Perceived Exertion (RPE) (see Table 34–8).
9. After the first dynamic exercise, the patient goes to the defibrillator monitor for a quick look at the rhythm strip if he or she is not wearing a telemetry unit. This is then attached to the flow sheet.
10. After the first dynamic exercise (usually lower extremity), the patient may walk around and get a drink of water.
11. The second exercise is some type of upper extremity exercise (e.g., arm ergometer or theraband exercises). This is usually done for about 10 minutes.
12. An appropriate weight-lifting program is initiated.[60] Surgical patients less than 6 weeks after surgery should not lift over 2 pounds, and overhead movements should be limited.
13. Usually three or four different strengthening and aerobic modes of exercise are done to complete the approximately 1-hour session. The patient can again walk around and get a drink.
14. The attendant then leads cool-down stretches or, again, the patient may have been oriented to these and can perform them with prompting as necessary.
15. The patient can sit and rest. After 2 minutes, a resting blood pressure and pulse, or resting rhythm strip, are recorded.

Several additional considerations are appropriate for the elderly patient:

1. Longer warm-up and cool-down sessions.
2. Shorter times on different modes of exercise.
3. A THR of 40% to 60% of the HR reserve, or 20 beats/min above the standing resting HR if no ETT is done. (RPE may be a better indicator because the HR does not increase in the same manner as in the younger population, even though the same cardiac output is attained.[49])
4. When using weights for strengthening, start with small hand weights of no more than 1 to 5 pounds or use the lowest weight on a pulley system. Specific guidelines for weight lifting should be adhered to.[61]

REHABILITATION OF THE PATIENT WITH CONGESTIVE HEART FAILURE

As mentioned earlier, an increasing number of patients with CHF are surviving longer, and a greater number participate in rehabilitation.

The clinical approach to the patient with CHF who is considered for rehabilitation is similar to that for the patient post-MI, although there are several important differences. The risk for sudden cardiac death is higher in patients with CHF than in patients with normal left ventricular function. This is the population in whom sudden, fatal arrhythmias occur most often.[70] There are a greater number of medications to be considered that can influence exercise responses, including vasoactive, antiarrhythmic, inotropic, and, in more recent years, beta blocking agents. Exercise capacity tends to be significantly lower than in the typical patient with CHD. Numerous hemodynamic abnormalities underlie the reduced exercise capacity commonly observed in CHF, including impaired HR responses, inability to distribute cardiac output normally, abnormal arterial vasodilatory capacity, abnormal cellular metabolism in the skeletal muscle, higher-than-normal systemic vascular resistance, higher-than-normal pulmonary pressures, and ventilatory abnormalities that increase the work of breathing and cause exertional dyspnea. Newer imaging technologies such as magnetic resonance imaging and spectroscopy suggest that some of these abnormalities can be improved by exercise training.[41,70]

Many patients with reduced left ventricular function who are clinically stable and have reduced exercise tolerance are candidates for exercise programs. It is often necessary to exclude patients with signs and symptoms of right-sided failure or to treat them judiciously before entry into a program. An exercise test is particularly important before initializing the program to ensure safety of participation. Rhythm abnormalities, exertional hypotension, or other signs of instability should be ruled out. Expired gas exchange measurements are particularly informative in this group because they provide an improvement in accuracy and permit an assessment of ventilatory abnormalities that are common in this condition.[71] ECG monitoring during exercise is more often indicated in this group. Attention should be paid to daily changes in body weight, rhythm status, and symptoms.

There are increasing numbers of patients who have undergone cardiac transplantation for end-stage heart failure, and today approximately 90% of these patients remain alive after 3 years.[72] The question has been raised as to whether these patients can also benefit from exercise training. A growing body of evidence suggests that post-transplantation patients derive substantial benefits from training. These studies have demonstrated increases in peak oxygen uptake, reductions in resting and submaximal HRs, and improved ventilatory responses to exercise.[73] Because the transplant recipient's heart is denervated, some intriguing hemodynamic responses to exercise are observed. The heart is not responsive to the normal actions of the parasympathetic and sympathetic systems. The absence of vagal tone explains the high resting HRs in these patients (100 to 110 bpm) and the relatively slow adaptation of the heart to a given amount of submaximal work.[74] This slows the delivery of oxygen to the working tissue, contributing to an earlier-than-normal metabolic acidosis and hyperventilation during exercise. Maximal HR (MHR) is lower in transplant recipients than in normal people, which contributes to a reduction in cardiac output and exercise capacity. Whether the major physiologic adaptation to exercise is improved cardiac function, changes in skeletal muscle metabolism, or simply an improvement in strength remains to be determined. Psychosocial studies of rehabilitation in transplant recipients are lacking, as are studies of the effects of regular exercise on survival.

PRESCRIPTION FOR INCREASING ACTIVITY IN OUTPATIENT CARDIAC REHABILITATION

The typical patient starts out with an initial session as follows. A telemetry strip, blood pressure, and RPE are obtained during most modes of exercise.

- ◆ Resting heart rate and rhythm from telemetry
- ◆ Resting blood pressure
- ◆ Weight
- ◆ Warm-up exercises
- ◆ A 5- to 10-minute session on the treadmill at 1 to 1.5 mph and 0% grade (speed may be less for elderly or patients with lower extremity impairments)
- ◆ A 5-minute session of arm exercise
- ◆ A 5-minute session on the cycle ergometer (0 watts) or airdyne bike (0.8 to 1.0 intensity level)
- ◆ A 2- to 5-minute session of weight lifting (free weights or arm pulley at 1, 2, or 3 pounds, depending on patient)
- ◆ Cool-down stretches
- ◆ Resting heart rate and rhythm strip from telemetry
- ◆ Resting blood pressure

The prescribed exercise is increased in duration and intensity by small increments at each session until the patient reaches the THR of 20 beats/min above standing resting HR. If a SLETT has been done, the THR calculated from the test is used. The patient finally works up to 20 minutes on the treadmill, airdyne, or cycle ergometer for his or her lower extremity dynamic exercise. As the patient progresses, it is usually preferable to alternate modes of exercise using different lower extremity devices (e.g., cycle, treadmill, stepping), along with a session of upper arm exercise until the patient can exercise for 40 to 45 continuous minutes. This may be followed by 5 to 10 minutes of upper extremity strengthening with free weights, arm pulley, or resistance machines. All intensities are increased gradually along with duration. Intensity is increased as the blood pressure, HR, rhythm, and RPE tolerate.

Often the patient has a SLETT and the THR can be calculated. Most commonly, the HR reserve method is used to calculate the THR. When calculating the THR from the HR reserve, two percentages are obtained. Most commonly, 50% and 80% are used. This provides a range of THRs instead of one number. The MHR is the highest attained HR during the SLETT or when the patient stops due to angina, fatigue, or other signs or symptoms. Likewise, if the patient is stopped by the person administering the test because of blood pressure, arrhythmias, or ST segment changes (indicative of ischemia), the HR at which these changes resulted in stopping the test is used as the MHR for calculating the THR. Therefore, it is extremely important that the cardiac nurse obtain a copy of the entire ETT, so that the point of ischemic changes can be noted as the MHR for accurate calculation of the THR. The HR reserve is calculated as follows: ([MHR achieved – resting HR] × % exercise intensity desired) + resting HR.

A SLETT is done anywhere from 3 to 6 weeks after the cardiac event. It is often advisable to have the patient start cardiac rehabilitation and get used to the mode he or she will be tested on, such as treadmill, bike, arm ergometer, or airdyne. Often a final ETT is done at the 3-month conclusion of the program to assess progress and to revise the exercise prescription.

PATIENT EDUCATION IN OUTPATIENT CARDIAC REHABILITATION

The education component in an outpatient rehabilitation program usually focuses on modifying risk factors for heart disease. Chapters 29 to 33 and 35 to 37 address risk factor modification in detail. Exercise, as mentioned previously, is the main focus of cardiac rehabilitation. However, exercise affects other alterable risk factors such as hypertension, elevated cholesterol, obesity, smoking, and diabetes. During exercise, opportunities arise to teach informally about risk factor modification in all these areas.

Teaching the patient about exercise is done formally, through presentations, and informally as each patient progresses with exercise and as the home program is defined and discussed. Other issues can be addressed in formal classroom sessions, in short sessions after the exercise training periods, or by passing out educational materials. The home exercise prescription should be given to the patient soon after starting outpatient cardiac rehabilitation. Patients should be asked to exercise at home on the days they do not come to cardiac rehabilitation. The aim is gradually to have them exercising three to five times per week for 20 to 60 minutes of dynamic exercise each time, as recommended by the AHA, Surgeon General's, and ACSM guidelines. If they attempt to do it every day, they will be most likely to achieve the recommended three to five times per week. When patients walk for exercise, they can often increase this up to 60 minutes. Walking is the most common home exercise, but if the patient has access to other forms of exercise, then prescriptions should be given for these modes. Two excellent home exercise references for patients are the *ACSM Fitness Book* and *Exercise for Heart and Health*.[75,76]

Continuation Programs

In several instances, a continuing program is provided following the immediate Outpatient Cardiac Rehab. These programs may be for the purpose of transition to independent exercise or maintenance of exercise for the cardiac patient. As mentioned earlier, these programs are sometimes referred to as Phase III and IV. The transitional program is often a 3-month program following the immediate outpatient progrm. The maintenance program may be of any length or perhaps indefinite.

ASSESSMENT FOR A CONTINUATION PROGRAM

The goals of the maintenance program are often much the same as those for the initial outpatient cardiac rehabilitation program, except that patients are taught to initiate and monitor their own response to exercise.[57–59,61] The assessment for the maintenance program is actually a review of the last 12 weeks of progress. As the nurse is writing the initial outpatient program summary, he or she is assessing the entrance into the maintenance program. This is, of course, simpler if the programs are in the same medical center or clinic area. Some maintenance programs are held in gyms, YMCAs, and other community facilities. If the initial program is in a medical center environment and the maintenance program is run by a different organization, a new assessment of the patient is needed. This assessment would include a physical examination, history of the patient's cardiovascular disease and other related diagnoses, previous activity level (obtained from the initial program), and the patient's knowledge of his or her cardiovascular history and exercise prescription.

INITIATION OF THE CONTINUATION PROGRAM

The objectives for the maintenance program are[57]:

- ◆ Continued exercise training
- ◆ Therapeutic fitness outings
- ◆ Risk factor modification
- ◆ Health promotion activities
- ◆ Exercise prescription based on initial and periodic graded exercise testing
- ◆ ECG telemetry monitoring for intermediate or high-risk patients, if indicated
- ◆ Work evaluation, testing, and counseling, if indicated

The transition from the initial program to the maintenance program usually depends on the patient's desire to continue attending a formalized exercise program. Most insurance companies and Medicare do not reimburse for the maintenance program, and therefore the patient does need to agree to attend and pay the expenses, which are usually minimal compared with the initial program because of less monitoring. Patients may be moved into a maintenance program or an extended supervised stage for several reasons other than length of time in the initial program: (1) their desired cardiovascular and physiologic responses to exercise have been obtained, (2) the desired objectives have been achieved, or (3) no additional progress is evident. Patients may be moved back and forth between the programs because of changes in cardiac status.[60,61]

EVALUATION FOR A CONTINUATION PROGRAM

Patients who are stratified as moderate and high risk may still need telemetry monitoring or a quick look with the defibrillator monitor periodically if the clinician observes symptoms or changes in their condition. Patient evaluation in the maintenance program involves a transition to assist patients toward evaluating their own response to exercise and finding the adequate level of exercise for themselves. The nurse guides the patient with an exercise prescription, but the patient should be able to remember this prescription and adhere to it. The primary goal of this program is to instill in the patient self-monitoring skills for exercise.

PRESCRIPTION FOR EXERCISE IN THE CONTINUATION PROGRAM

The exercise prescription for the phase III patient is based on either the last SLETT or a new one done at the conclusion of the initial program. As the patient maintains a consistent response to exercise, or as more work is needed to gain the same response, the intensity of exercise can be increased.

PATIENT EDUCATION IN THE CONTINUATION PROGRAM

Teaching patients independence in their exercise is the main goal of the maintenance program. The aim is for patients to exercise several times at home in addition to the times they attend the program. By this time, they should know their THR and be able to take their pulse and readily assess RPE. Some patients have difficulty monitoring their pulse and may need to purchase a pulse monitor. Patients should be encouraged to venture out and try different forms of exercise. Perhaps a sport they thought was no longer possible can be done in moderation to give them a sense of achievement. In addition, patients should be encouraged to reduce other cardiac risk factors.

Many patients prefer to come to the often self-pay maintenance program in cardiac rehabilitation instead of exercising independently at home. This is a decision the cardiac rehabilitation team members and patient should discuss before graduation from the initial outpatient program. The patient should have a plan about how he or she is going to keep working on all risk factors, including continuing to exercise.

Many programs now include follow-up process to monitor outcomes. The patient comes back to the program periodically, usually every 3 months, for perhaps 2 years. At these visits, risk factor and other outcomes such as quality of life, readmissions, and the like are assessed. This allows the program to monitor how well it is doing in meeting patients' needs for risk factor reduction. It also offers the patient an opportunity to renew his or her health goals with the health care team.

This chapter has discussed traditional cardiac rehabilitation. However, there are many alternative ways that nurses can have an impact in helping people reduce the risks associated with a sedentary life. Many home exercise programs are now offered by many centers. In these programs, people perform their exercise at home, and they may be telemonitored or they may record their HRs and blood pressures and phone them in. Alternatively, they may come into a program occasionally to be evaluated and provided feedback as to how they are doing with their exercise and other risk factors. The important fact for nurses to remember is that we need to assist our patients individually to reduce their risk factors to prevent the progression of cardiovascular disease.

REFERENCES

1. Centers for Disease Control and Prevention: Prevalence of sedentary lifestyle-behavioral risk factor surveillance system, United States: 1991. MMWR 42: 576–579, 1993
2. American College of Sports Medicine: Position stand on the recommended quantity and quality of exercise for developing and maintaining cardiorespiratory and muscular fitness in healthy adults. Med Sci Sports Exerc 22: 265–274, 1990
3. Fletcher GF, Balady G, Froelicher VF et al: Exercise Standards: A Statement for Healthcare Professionals from the American Heart Association. Dallas, American Heart Association, 1995
4. Pate RR, Pratt MP, Blair SN et al: Physical activity and public health: A recommendation from the Centers for Disease Control and Prevention and the American College of Sports Medicine. JAMA 273: 402–407, 1995
5. Leon AS, Certo C, Comoss P et al: Position paper of the American Association of Cardiovascular and Pulmonary Rehabilitation: Scientific evidence of the value of cardiac rehabilitation services with emphasis on patients following myocardial infarction. Section 1: Exercise conditioning component. J Cardiopulm Rehabil 10: 79–87, 1990
6. American College of Sports Medicine: Guidelines for Exercise Testing and Prescription, 5th ed. Philadelphia, Lea & Febiger, 1995
7. U.S. Public Health Service, Office of the Surgeon General: Physical Activity and Health: A Report of the Surgeon General. Atlanta, U.S. Department of Health and Human Services, Centers for Disease Control and Prevention, National Center for Chronic Disease Prevention and Health Promotion, 1996
8. Haskell WL, Leon AS, Caspersen CJ et al: Cardiovascular benefits and assessment of physical activity and physical fitness in adults. Med Sci Sports Exerc 24: 5201–5220, 1992
9. Paffenbarger RS, Hyde RT, Wing AL et al: Physical activity, all-cause mortality, and longevity of college alumni. N Engl J Med 314: 605–613, 1986
10. O'Conner GT, Buring JE, Yusaf S et al: An overview of randomized trials of rehabilitation with exercise after myocardial infarction. Circulation 80: 234–244, 1989
11. Oldridge NB, Guyatt GH, Fischer ME et al: Cardiac rehabilitation with exercise after myocardial infarction. JAMA 260: 945–950, 1988
12. Wenger NK, Froelicher ES, Smith LK, et al: Cardiac Rehabilitation: Clinical Practice Guideline No. 17. AHCOR Publication no. 96-0672. Rockville, MD, U.S. Department of Health and Human Services, Public Health Service, Agency for

Health Care Policy and Research and the National Heart, Lung, and Blood Institute, October, 1995

13. Hahn RA, Teutsh SM, Rothenberg RB et al: Excess deaths from nine chronic diseases in the United States. JAMA 264: 2654–2659, 1986

14. McGinnis JM, Foege WH: Actual causes of death in the United States. JAMA 270: 2207–2212, 1993

15. Helmrich SP, Ragland DR, Leung RW et al: Physical activity and reduced occurrence of non-insulin-dependent diabetes mellitus. N Engl J Med 325: 147–152, 1991

16. Manson JE, Nathan DM, Kroleski AS et al: A prospective study of exercise and incidence of diabetes among US male physicians. JAMA 268: 63–67, 1992

17. Manson JE, Rimm EB, Stampfer MJ et al: Physical activity and incidence of non-insulin-dependent diabetes mellitus in women. Lancet 338: 774–775, 1991

18. Hagberg JM: Exercise, fitness, and hypertension. In Bouchard C, Shephard RJ, Stephens T et al (eds): Exercise, Fitness, and Health, pp 455–566. Champaign, IL, Human Kinetics, 1990

19. Marcus R, Drinkwater B, Dalsky G et al: Osteoporosis and exercise in women. Med Sci Sports Exerc 24(Suppl): S301–S307, 1992

20. Lee I, Paffenbarger RS, Hsieh C: Physical activity and risk of developing colorectal cancer among college alumni. J Natl Cancer Inst 83: 1324–1329, 1991

21. Paffenbarger RS, Hyde RT, Wing AL et al: The association of changes in physical-activity level and other lifestyle characteristics with mortality among men. N Engl J Med 328: 538–545, 1993

22. Paffenbarger RS, Hyde RT, Wing AL et al: Some interrelations of physical activity, physiological fitness, health, and longevity. In Bouchard C, Shephard RJ, Stephens T (eds): Physical Activity, Fitness, and Health, pp 119–133. Champaign, IL, Human Kinetics, 1994

23. Ainsworth BE, Haskell WL, Leon AS et al: Compendium of physical activities: Classification of energy costs of human physical activities. Med Sci Sports Exerc 25: 71–80, 1993

24. Paffenbarger RS Jr, Hyde RT, Wing AL et al: Chronic disease in former college students: XXV. A natural history of athleticism and cardiovascular health. JAMA 252: 491–495, 1984

25. Morris JN, Kagan A, Pattison DC et al: Incidence and prediction of ischaemic heart disease in London busmen. Lancet 2: 552–559, 1966

26. Morris JN, Everitt MG, Pollard R et al: Vigorous exercise in leisure-time: Protection against coronary heart disease. Lancet 2: 1207–1210, 1980

27. Slattery ML, Jacobs DR Jr, Nichaman MZ: Leisure time physical activity and coronary heart disease death: The U.S. railroad study. Circulation 79: 304–311, 1989

28. Paffenbarger RS Jr, Laughlin ME, Gima AS et al: Work activity of longshoreman as related to death from coronary heart disease and stroke. N Engl J Med 282: 1109–1114, 1970

29. Powell KE, Thompson PD, Caspersen CJ et al: Physical activity and the incidence of coronary heart disease. Annu Rev Public Health 8: 253–287, 1987

30. Lee IM, Paffenbarger RS: Do physical activity and physical fitness avert premature mortality? Exerc Sport Sci Rev 24: 135–172, 1996

31. Blair SN, Kohl HW III, Paffenbarger RS Jr et al: Physical fitness and all-cause mortality: A prospective study of healthy men and women. JAMA 262: 2395–2401, 1989

32. Ekelund LG, Haskell WL, Johnson JL et al: Physical fitness as a predictor of cardiovascular mortality in asymptomatic North American men: The Lipid Research Clinics Mortality Follow-up Study. N Engl J Med 319: 1379–1384, 1988

33. Paffenbarger RS, Blair SN, Lee I et al: Measurement of physical activity to assess health effects in free-living populations. Med Sci Sports Exerc 25: 60–70, 1993

34. Arraiz GA, Wigle DT, Mao Y: Risk assessment of physical activity and physical fitness in the Canada health survey mortality follow-up study. J Clin Epidemiol 45: 419–428, 1992

35. NIH Consensus Development Panel on Physical Activity and Cardiovascular Health: Physical activity and cardiovascular health. JAMA 27: 241–246, 1996

36. Shaw L: Effects of a prescribed supervised exercise program on mortality and cardiovascular morbidity in patients after myocardial infarction. Am J Cardiol 48: 39–44, 1981

37. Vermeulen A, Lie K, Durber D: Effects of cardiac rehabilitation after myocardial infarction: Changes in coronary risk factors and long term prognosis. Am Heart J 105: 798–801, 1983

38. Kallio V, Lamalainen H, Hakkila J et al: Reduction of sudden deaths by a multifactorial intervention programme after acute myocardial infarction. Lancet 2: 1091–1094, 1979

39. May GS, Eberlein KA, Furberg CD et al: Secondary prevention after myocardial infarction: A review of long-term trials. Prog Cardiovasc Dis 24: 331–362, 1982

40. McKelvie RS, Teo KK, McCartney N et al: Effects of exercise training in patients with congestive heart failure: A critical review. J Am Coll Cardiol 25: 789–796, 1995

41. Dubach P, Myers J, Dziekan G et al: Effect of exercise training on myocardial remodeling in patients with reduced left ventricular function after myocardial infarction: Application of magnetic resonance imaging. Circulation 95: 2060–2067, 1997

42. Clark AL, Poole-Wilson PA, Coats AJ: Exercise limitation in chronic heart failure: Central role of the periphery. Department of Cardiac Medicine, National Heart and Lung Institute. J Am Coll Cardiol 28: 1092–1102, 1996

43. Froelicher VF, Myers J, Follansbee W et al: Exercise and the Heart. St. Louis, Mosby-Year Book, 1993

44. Myers J: Physiologic adaptations to exercise and immobility. In Woods SL, Sivarajan Froelicher ES, Halpenny CJ, Underhill Motzer S Cardiac Nursing, 3rd ed, pp 147–162. Philadelphia, JB Lippincott, 1995

45. Rousseau P: Immobility in the aged. Department of Geriatrics, Veterans Affairs Medical Center, Phoenix, Arizona. Arch Fam Med 2: 169–177, 1993

46. Mausner JS, Bahn AK (eds): Epidemiology: An Introductory Text, pp 9–11. Philadelphia, WB Saunders, 1979

47. CDC: Protective effect of physical activity on coronary heart disease. MMWR 36: 426–430, 1987

48. Mansfield LW, Sivarajan ES, Bruce RA: Exercise testing of myocardial infarction patients prior to hospital discharge: A quantitative basis for exercise prescription. Cardiac Rehabil 8: 17–20, 1978

49. Fleg JL, Gerstenblith G, Lakatta EG: Pathophysiology of the aging heart and circulation. In Messerli FH (ed): Cardiovascular Disease in the Elderly, 2nd ed, pp 17–43. Boston, Martinus Nijhoff, 1988

50. Wenger NK, Marcus FI, O'Rourke RA: Cardiovascular disease in the elderly. J Am Coll Cardiol 9: 80A–87A, 1987

51. Lindskog BD, Sivarajan ES: A method of evaluation of activity and exercise in a controlled study of early cardiac rehabilitation. J Cardiac Rehabil 23: 156–165, 1982

52. Gortner S, Miller NH, Jenkins L: Self-efficacy: A key to recovery. In Rossman-Jillings C (ed): Cardiac Rehabilitation Nursing, pp 89–101. Rockville, MD, Aspen, 1988

53. Gulanick M, Kim M, Holm K: Resumption of home activities. Prog Cardiovasc Nurs 6: 21–28, 1991

54. Chang JA, Froelicher VF: Clinical and exercise test markers of prognosis in patients with stable coronary artery disease. Curr Probl Cardiol 19: 533–588, 1994

55. Beller GA, Gibson RS: Risk stratification after myocardial infarction. Modern Concepts of Cardiovascular Disease 55: 5–10, 1986

56. DeBusk RF, Blomqvist CG, Kouchoukos NT et al: Identification and treatment of low-risk patients after acute myocardial infarction and coronary artery bypass graft surgery. N Engl J Med 314: 161–166, 1986

57. Department of Veterans Affairs: Strategic planning, Chapter 9: Criteria and standards and program planning factors, Appendix 9O: Criteria and standards for cardiology continuum of care, pp 19–23. In Veterans Health Administration Manual M-9. Washington, DC, Department of Veterans Affairs, 1992

58. Froelicher VF: Cardiac rehabilitation. In Chatterjee K, Cheitlin MD, Karliner J et al (eds): Cardiology: An Illustrated Text/Reference, Vol 2, pp 7.204–7.216. Philadelphia, JB Lippincott, 1991

59. Verril D, Bergey D, McElveen G et al: Recommended guidelines for cardiac maintenance (phase IV) programs: A position paper by the North Carolina Cardiopulmonary Rehabilitation Association. J Cardiopulm Rehabil 13: 87–95, 1993

60. Pollock ML, Wilmore JL: Exercise in Health and Disease, 2nd ed, pp 128–138. Philadelphia, WB Saunders, 1990

61. American Association of Cardiovascular and Pulmonary Rehabilitation: Guidelines for Cardiac Rehabilitation Programs. Champaign, IL, Human Kinetics, 1998

62. Robichaud-Ekstrand S: Shower versus sink bath: Evaluation of heart rate, blood pressure, and subjective response of the patient with myocardial infarction. Heart Lung 20: 375–382, 1991

63. Noble BJ, Borg GAV, Jacobs I et al: A category-ratio perceived exertion scale: Relationship to blood and muscle lactates and heart rate. Med Sci Sports Exerc 15: 523–528, 1983

64. Kitamura K, Jorgensen CR, Gobel FL et al: Hemodynamic correlates of myocardial oxygen consumption during upright exercise. J Appl Physiol 32: 516–522, 1972

65. Lown B, Wolf M: Approaches to sudden death from coronary heart disease. Circulation 44: 130–142, 1971

66. Sivarajan ES, Snydsman A, Smith B et al: Low-level treadmill testing of 41 patients with acute myocardial infarction prior to discharge from hospital. Heart Lung 6: 975–980, 1977

67. Wilmore JH, Thomas EL. Importance of differences between men and woman for exercise testing and exercise prescription. In Skinner JS (ed): Exercise Testing and Exercise Prescription for Special Cases, pp 31–48. Philadelphia, Lea & Febiger, 1987

68. Penckofer SM, Holm K: Women undergoing coronary artery bypass surgery: Physiological and psychosocial perspectives. Cardiovasc Nurs 26: 13–17, 1990

69. Thomas AE, McKay DA, Cutlip MB: A nomograph method for assessing body weight. Am J Clin Nutr 29: 302–304, 1976

70. Stratton JR, Dunn JF, Adamopoulos S et al: Training partially reverses skeletal muscle metabolic abnormalities during exercise in heart failure. J Appl Physiol 76: 1575–1582, 1994

71. Myers J: Essentials of Cardiopulmonary Exercise Testing. Champaign, IL, Human Kinetics, 1996

72. Lin HM, Kauffman HM, McBride MA et al: Center-specific graft and patient survivals rates: 1997 United Network for Organ Sharing (UNOS) report. JAMA 280: 1153–1160, 1998

73. Shephard RJ: Responses of the cardiac transplant patient to exercise and training. Exerc Sport Sci Rev 20: 297–320, 1992

74. Stinson EB, Grieep RL, Schroeder JS et al: Hemodynamic observations one and two years after cardiac transplantation in man. Circulation 14: 1181–1193, 1972

75. American College of Sports Medicine: ACSM Fitness Book. Champaign, IL, Leisure Press, 1992

76. Fletcher BJ, Cantwell JD, Fletcher GF: Exercise for heart and health. Atlanta, Pritchutt & Hull, 1985

Obesity: An Overview of Assessment and Treatment

LORA E. BURKE*

Obesity is a multifactorial disease involving complex interactions among genetic, metabolic, environmental, cultural, and psychosocial factors. In the United States today, obesity is described as an epidemic, the most common nutritional problem, a significant contributor to increased health care costs, and the second leading cause of preventable death.[1-3] In the 1990s, the prevalence of obesity and overweight has escalated in the United States and in several other countries, underscoring the seriousness of the problem. These trends affect women more than men, ethnic women more than white, non-Latino women, and those with lower educational levels more than those with higher educational attainment.[3-5]

Obesity has been linked to a host of chronic disorders associated with heart disease, including type II diabetes, dyslipidemia, and hypertension. It is associated with deleterious effects on the heart and circulatory system, contributing to an increased risk of arrhythmia, sudden death, congestive heart failure, and ischemic heart disease.[6] Moreover, several physiologic parameters that affect cardiovascular risk factors are associated with obesity, such as lipoprotein oxidizability, arterial blood pressure, and hemostatic or fibrinolytic abnormalities.[7] In June, 1998, obesity was added to the list of major risk factors for coronary heart disease (CHD).[8]

In the midst of the mounting evidence demonstrating the deleterious effects of obesity on health in general, and the cardiovascular system in particular, research has demonstrated numerous benefits to health by as little as a 10% reduction in initial weight. A modest weight loss, such as a 20-pound weight loss in a 200-pound male, can ameliorate

several of the previously described complications.[7] However, reports in the literature indicate that patients regain one third of their weight loss during the first year after cessation of active treatment, and that most regain the full amount by the fifth year.[9] These facts underscore the importance of identifying the patient at risk and implementing an early treatment course that may prevent the development of complications.

This major health problem has not gone unnoticed by the scientific community. Several organizations and policy-making groups have joined forces to evaluate the existing obesity treatment programs and to develop guidelines for the identification and treatment of the disorder. More specifically, in 1995, the Institute of Medicine published an extensive report that provided criteria for evaluating three categories of weight-management programs: "do it yourself," nonclinical, and clinical programs.[10] A year later, the Shape Up America! Organization and the American Obesity Association joined forces to develop and publish *Guidance for Treatment of Adult Obesity*,[11] and in 1998, the National Heart, Lung, and Blood Institute (NHLBI) issued the *Evidence Report*,[3] which provided empirically based guidelines for the identification, evaluation, and treatment of overweight and obesity in adults.

This chapter, drawing on these works and an extensive literature, provides an overview of treatment for overweight and obesity. It begins with a review of the process of identification and evaluation of a patient's risk status and the selection of appropriate treatment. The major components of treatment are covered: lifestyle modification, which includes dietary, exercise, and behavioral therapy; drug therapy; and surgical therapy. Finally, maintenance strategies to enhance long-term adherence to the lifestyle changes that facilitated the weight loss are reviewed.

*The author was supported by grant HL07560, National Institute of Health, National Heart, Lung, and Blood Institute.

IDENTIFICATION AND ASSESSMENT OF THE OVERWEIGHT OR OBESE PATIENT

Weight Status

Until recently, the United States used cutoff points for the classification of overweight and obese based on body mass index (BMI) distribution in the National Health and Nutrition Examination Survey I (NHANES I) study, whereas most other countries used the classification developed by the World Health Organization (WHO).[5] In 1998, criteria in the United States were changed to be consistent with the WHO, defining normal weight as a BMI range of 18.50 to 24.99, overweight as a BMI of 25.00 to 29.99, and obese as a BMI of 30 or more.[3,12]

BODY MASS INDEX (BMI) MEASUREMENT PROCEDURE

Weight and height measurements, required for the BMI determination, should be taken with the patient wearing undergarments and no shoes. Using the height and weight values, the BMI can be calculated or determined by available normograms.[3,13]
The BMI is calculated as follows:
BMI = weight (kg)/height/squared (m²)
    The BMI can be estimated from pounds and inches as follows: [*weight(pounds)/height (inches)²*] × 704.5

Waist (Abdominal) Circumference

Visceral obesity is an excess of fat in the abdomen that is out of proportion to total body fat.[3,14] Upper body or abdominal obesity is considered more sensitive and specific than BMI as a predictor of obesity-related morbidity and mortality.[14] Visceral obesity can be measured more accurately by computed tomography or magnetic resonance imaging, but these are expensive and impractical for clinical assessment in a practitioner's office.[15-17] Waist circumference measurement is a clinically acceptable method to assess the patient's visceral or abdominal fat content from baseline through weight loss treatment. Sex-specific cutoffs have been established to identify relative risk for development of obesity-associated risks factors. Men with a waistline circumference greater than 40 inches (102 cm) and women with greater than 35 inches (88 cm) are at high risk for development of obesity-related morbidity (e.g., type II diabetes, dyslipidemia, and cardiovascular disease).[3] Patients of normal weight with increased waist circumference measurements may be at increased cardiovascular risk. Because patients with a BMI in excess of 35 exceed the waist circumference cutoffs, these indicators of relative risk lose their predictive power, making it unnecessary to measure waist circumference in this group.[3] See Table 35-1 for the classification of overweight and obesity with waist circumference incorporated in the relative risk assessment.

WAIST (ABDOMINAL) CIRCUMFERENCE MEASUREMENT PROCEDURE

The patient should be dressed in undergarments or in an examining gown. Standing to the right of the patient, palpate the upper hip bone to locate the right iliac crest and draw a horizontal mark just above the upper border of the iliac crest. Cross that line with a vertical mark on the mid-axillary line. Place the measuring tape in a horizontal plane (parallel to the floor) around the abdomen at the level of the marked point and hold the tape snug to, but not compressing the skin. Take the measurement at a normal minimal respiration.[18]

TABLE 35-1	**Classification of Overweight and Obesity by Body Mass Index, Waist Circumference, and Associated Risk***			
	Body Mass Index (Kg/m²)	**Obesity Class**	**Disease Risk* Relative to Normal Weight and Waist Circumference**	
			Men ≤102 cm (≤40 in.) Women ≤88 cm (≤35 in.)	Men >102 cm (>40 in.) Women >88 cm (>35 in.)
Underweight	<18.5		—	—
Normal†	18.5–24.9		—	—
Overweight	25.0–29.9		Increased	High
Obesity	30.0–34.9	I	High	Very high
	35.0–39.9	II	Very high	Very high
Extreme Obesity	≥40	III	Extremely high	Extremely high

*Disease risk for type II diabetes, hypertension, and cardiovascular disease.
    †Increased waist circumference can be a marker for increased risk even in people of normal weight.
    Original source: World Health Organization (WHO): Preventing and Managing the Global Epidemic of Obesity: Report of the World Health Organization Consultation of Obesity. Geneva, WHO, June 1997; adapted from original source for National Heart, Lung, and Blood Institute Expert Panel: Clinical Guidelines on the Identification, Evaluation, and Treatment of Overweight and Obesity in Adults: The Evidence Report. Bethesda, MD, National Institutes of Health, 1998.

Assessment of Cardiovascular Disease Risk Factors

Having established the patient's relative risk based on the overweight/obesity and abdominal obesity criteria, the third part of the assessment is determination of the patient's absolute risk status in terms of comorbid conditions or risk factors for cardiovascular disease.

VERY HIGH ABSOLUTE RISK

Patients who are overweight or obese or have abdominal obesity are considered at very high risk if they have the following disease conditions: established CHD, presence of other atherosclerotic diseases (peripheral arterial disease, abdominal aortic aneurysm, or symptomatic carotid disease), type II diabetes, sleep apnea, or target organ damage in the hypertensive patient.[3] People meeting these profiles require aggressive treatment to reduce their cardiovascular disease risk profiles (e.g., cholesterol-lowering therapy, blood pressure control).[3]

HIGH ABSOLUTE RISK

Obese patients who have three or more of the following risk factors can be considered at high absolute risk for obesity-related comorbid conditions: cigarette smoking; hypertension; low-density lipoprotein of 160 mg/dL or more, or 130 to 159 mg/dL in the presence of two or more other risk factors; high-density lipoprotein (HDL) less than 35 mg/dL; impaired fasting glucose; family history of premature CHD; and male sex, 45 years of age or older, or female sex, 55 years of age or older, or postmenopausal status. The provider should follow the established guidelines in estimating absolute risk status and in treating the identified risk factors,[19–21] which are discussed in detail in other chapters.

OTHER RISK FACTORS

The presence of additional risk factors (e.g., physical inactivity and elevated triglycerides) can increase a patient's absolute risk to a level higher than that estimated from the preceding categories.[3,22,23] A sedentary lifestyle in the presence of obesity heightens the risk for associated disorders. Elevated triglycerides in the obese patient may represent a common manifestation of a lipoprotein phenotype that includes elevated triglycerides, low HDL levels, and small low-density lipoprotein particles, a pattern considered atherogenic.[23]

INCREASED RISK

Obese patients who have osteoarthritis, gallstones, gynecologic abnormalities, and stress incontinence are not facing life-threatening consequences, but require appropriate management.[3] The provider needs to address these conditions and make the patient aware that these conditions are influenced by his or her weight.

SUBGROUPS

Two groups that providers may be reluctant to treat are patients who are older than 65 years of age and smokers. However, weight reduction improves functional status and reduces concomitant risk factors in the older population in a way similar to that in the younger adult, and therefore this subgroup should at least receive intervention to prevent weight gain, if not achieve weight reduction.[3,24] The overweight or obese smoker carries excess risk from obesity-associated risk factors.[3] This patient should be advised to quit and prevention of weight gain should be addressed through lifestyle approaches, with the emphasis on smoking abstinence.[3]

CLINICAL EVALUATION AND TREATMENT STRATEGIES

Baseline assessment of the cardiac patient includes the BMI, waist circumference, and cardiovascular risk profile, as well as the noncardiovascular conditions noted. The NHLBI *Evidence Report*[3] includes an algorithm that addresses the assessment and treatment decisions based on that assessment (Fig. 35-1). This algorithm is focused on weight-related assessment and treatment and does not include evaluation for other disorders for which the patient may be seeing a health care provider. As noted in Figure 35-1, if the patient's BMI and waist circumference are in the normal range, these parameters should be measured again in 2 years.

For the patient whose parameters are not normal, assessment needs to include the patient's history, including prior excess weight or weight fluctuations. If not done previously, a physical examination and laboratory measurements to assess lipid profile, glucose level, and related parameters need to be performed. Detection of existing cardiovascular disease and end-organ damage needs to be determined and treated. Obesity needs to be treated in the context of the patient's risk profile and existence of comorbid conditions.[3] Weight loss frequently ameliorates risks by reducing blood pressure and triglycerides and raising HDL. Therefore, risk factors should be addressed through weight loss treatment.[3,25]

A nutritional and physical activity assessment provides additional information that can be used in the treatment plan. This can be done by having the patient complete a 3-day food and activity diary, which should include 2 work and 1 nonwork or leisure-type days. When using a 3-day food and activity diary, the patient needs to be instructed on completion of the diary and the detail that needs to be included (e.g., exact amount of foods eaten and inclusion of recipes or package labels if the food is unusual).[13,17] Food frequency and activity questionnaires are another means of assessing past year food consumption, or current level of physical activity, such as the Willet[26,27] or Block[28] Food Frequency Questionnaires or the Paffenbarger Physical Activity Questionnaire.[29] These questionnaires can be scored by the health care professional.

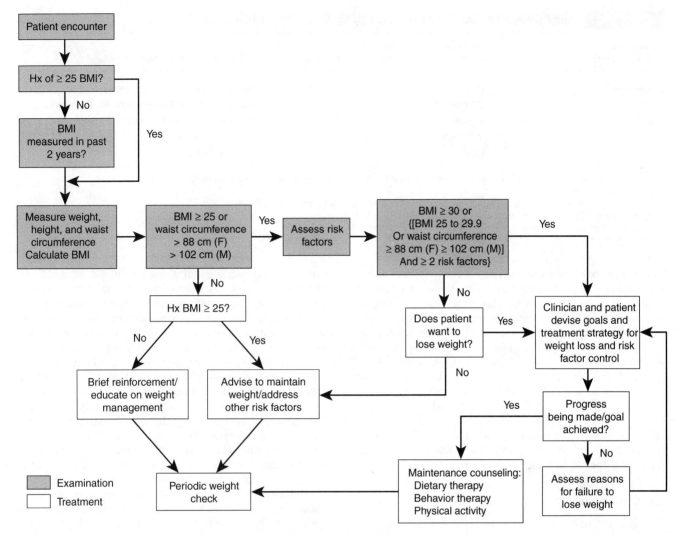

FIGURE 35-1 Treatment algorithm. This algorithm applies only to assessment for overweight and obesity and decisions based on that assessment. It does not reflect any initial overall assessment for other conditions and diseases that the physician may wish to do. (Adapted from NHLBI Clinical Guidelines on the Identification, Evaluation, and Treatment of Overweight and Obesity in Adults, The Evidence Report, US Department of Health and Human Service, NIH, NHLBI. 1998)

Before considering treatment options, the patient's motivation for engaging in weight loss treatment needs to be assessed. Embarking on a weight loss and maintenance program requires a commitment to a change in lifestyle and an investment of the patient's and provider's resources. Moreover, the change is not for a limited time, but rather lifelong. Factors to consider in the initial assessment include the patient's attitude toward weight loss, prior treatment failures and successes, support system, comprehension of risk posed by weight status, willingness to initiate an exercise program, self-efficacy for achieving weight loss, time commitment, barriers to behavior change, and financial issues if the treatment is not covered by insurance.[3] If the patient is not motivated, the provider needs to review the risks of excess weight and the benefits of initiating treatment and discuss how this treatment may be different and

how the patient will be assisted. If the patient remains uninterested in treatment, the provider needs to address coexisting risk factors and initiate management of these, including weight gain prevention.[3,25] Having completed the assessment, a treatment plan needs to be considered.

TREATMENT OF OVERWEIGHT AND OBESITY

Treatment Approach

Treatment for obesity can be approached through lifestyle modification, which includes dietary and exercise programs, pharmacotherapy, or surgical treatment. The latter two approaches are adjunctive to lifestyle therapy (Table 35-2).

TABLE 35-2	Approaches to Treatment of Obesity by Severity and Disease Risk	
Body Mass Index (Kg/m²)	Comorbid Conditions or Cardiovascular Disease Risk Factors	Treatment Approaches[1,8,9]
25–30	Absent	Lifestyle modification*/prevention of weight gain
27–30	≥2 Present[†]	Lifestyle modification + pharmacotherapy[‡]
>30	Absent	Lifestyle modification + pharmacotherapy[‡]
>35	≥2 Present	Consider surgical therapy[‡]
>40	Absent	Surgical therapy[†]

*Lifestyle modification includes caloric restriction (400 kcal/d deficit), <30% fat diet, exercise at least 5 days/wk, and behavioral therapy.

[†]Comorbid conditions warranting drug therapy: hypertension, coronary heart disease, type II diabetes, congestive heart failure, and sleep apnea.

[‡]Pharmacotherapy and surgical therapy are adjunctive to lifestyle modification.

The severity of obesity and presence of comorbidities determine the approach to treatment (e.g., the coexistence of non–insulin-dependent diabetes, hypertension, or congestive heart failure).[25,30] In the absence of comorbid conditions, patients with a BMI between 25 and 30 can achieve adequate weight reduction through lifestyle approaches. Pharmacotherapy is usually limited to those with a BMI greater than 30 or, in the presence of comorbidities, to those with a BMI between 27 and 30. Surgical therapy is considered for a BMI in excess of 35 with comorbid conditions, or when the BMI exceeds 40. Pharmacologic or surgical therapy are never used in isolation, but rather are adjunctive to lifestyle modification, which needs to be maintained indefinitely after the use of these other treatment modalities.

Goal of Treatment

The goal of weight loss is not to achieve some cosmetic standard of attractiveness, but rather to reduce morbidity and increase mobility. The recommended initial weight loss goal is 10% of baseline weight, a weight loss that can be maintained for at least a year or longer.[1,3,30] The rate of loss should be approximately 0.5 to 1 pound per week for the moderately obese and 1 to 2 pounds per week in the severely obese.

It is important to discuss treatment strategies and goals with the patient because these have to be arrived at through mutual decision making, and there could be a discrepancy between the provider's and the patient's goal.[3,31–33] An example would be a 65-year-old woman who has lower body obesity and no additional risk factors but may wish to lose a certain amount of weight. This patient may achieve the loss and feel better about her appearance, but if she is unable to sustain this loss, she will regain and be frustrated. This person may benefit from guidance for a lower weight loss goal and exercise or a plan for stability of current weight. However, if this same woman had upper body weight or presence of risk factors, she should be counseled for achieving a 10% weight reduction. A middle-aged woman may wish to achieve a body weight that is significantly below her current weight and one she has not had since she was in her twenties. Not only is achievement of the goal unlikely, but so is maintenance of the weight. This patient may benefit from an initial

goal of 10% reduction, and if this is achieved, an additional goal can be established. Other patients may have no desire to reduce and may benefit from a discussion regarding their risk profile and the benefits of weight reduction. If the person is unmotivated to change, a plan of weight gain prevention may be appropriate for the time.[3,30,32]

Furthermore, the provider needs to discuss with the patient what other goals she has for weight loss. A patient may think that improved personal relationships or professional opportunities will result from achieving the weight loss goal, but this is rarely the case because more than weight loss usually is necessary for such goals to be realized. The provider needs to emphasize to the patient the health benefits resulting from a 10% loss, and assist the patient in being realistic about weight loss outcomes.[30,32,33]

Once the patient and provider have agreed on the treatment approach and the initial goals, it is time to prepare the patient for the course of treatment. Orienting the patient to the active participation required for successful weight loss facilitates cooperation and adherence. Patients need to be oriented to self-monitoring food and caloric intake and expenditure. Conveying to the patient understanding and support during the challenging course and providing reinforcement for behavioral change can go a long way in sustaining the person's motivation.[3,31]

TREATMENT COMPONENTS

Lifestyle Modification

Lifestyle therapy includes three components: nutritional or dietary therapy, exercise and daily activity, and behavioral therapy. The changes in the patient's dietary and activity habits are facilitated and reinforced through the behavioral strategies used in weight loss treatment. The following sections describe the three components.

DIETARY THERAPY

During weight loss treatment, the strongest determinant of the rate and amount of weight loss that will occur is the extent of the negative energy balance.[34] A key component of dietary therapy is a reduction in total caloric intake by 500 to 1,000 kilocalories (kcal)/d, resulting in the patient consuming 800 to 1,500 kcal/d. This is referred to as a low-calorie diet and has been shown to reduce weight by 8% over 6 months. A deficit of 500 kcal/d results in a 1 pound per week weight loss (1 pound is the equivalent of 3,500 kcal). Depending on the patient's baseline weight and the amount of weight loss desired, the patient may follow a diet ranging from 800 to 1,500 kcal/d.[3,9]

An important component of dietary therapy is addressing both fat and caloric restriction. Studies have evaluated the restriction of either one alone and have demonstrated less weight loss, especially when fat is restricted in the absence of caloric limitations.[35] In general, a 20% to 30% fat diet is recommended and the patient is provided a daily fat gram goal along with the calorie goal.[9] The recommended diet composition is consistent with the Adult Treatment Panel Step I Diet[36] (Table 35-3), although many programs use a 20% fat eating plan.[9]

Very–low-calorie diets, which are restricted to less than 800 kcal/d, are no longer recommended for several reasons. They provide inadequate nutrition unless supplemented, require medical supervision to monitor the patient's nutritional and electrolyte status, and increase the risk for development of gallstones. Furthermore, studies have shown that the rapid weight loss is followed by a rapid regain, and at 1 year, the percentage of weight loss retained with the very–low-calorie diets is less than with the low-calorie diet.[9,30,37]

Programs using the lifestyle approach include nutritional education.[9,30] The focus of the instruction includes the energy value of foods (e.g., fat contains 9 calories per gram compared to protein and carbohydrates, which contain

TABLE 35-3 Low-Calorie Step I Diet

Nutrient	Recommended Intake
Calories	Approximately 500–1,000 kcal/d reduction from usual intake
Total fat	≤30% of total calories
Saturated fatty acids	8–10% of total calories
Monounsaturated fatty acids	Up to 15% of total calories
Polyunsaturated fatty acids	Up to 10% of total calories
Cholesterol	<300 mg/d
Protein	Approximately 15% of total calories
Carbohydrate	≥55% of total calories
Sodium chloride	≤100 mmol/d (approximately 2.4 g of sodium or 6 g of sodium chloride)
Calcium	1,000–1,500 mg/d
Fiber	20–30 g/d

From National Heart, Lung, and Blood Institute Expert Panel: Clinical Guidelines on the Identification, Evaluation, and Treatment of Overweight and Obesity in Adults: The Evidence Report. Bethesda, MD, National Institutes of Health, 1998.

4 calories per gram), how to read labels, the three types of fat and the recommended distribution of these in the diet, methods to reduce fat and increase fiber and complex carbohydrate intake, and how to prepare foods to reduce the addition of calories. Patients also are instructed on recipe modification and ordering from a restaurant menu.[9,38]

EXERCISE AND PHYSICAL ACTIVITY

Patients are allowed to focus on changes in eating patterns during the initial weeks of a program and then introduced to weekly exercise goals at around the third week. The goals are gradually increased so that behavior can be shaped to include an exercise routine, eventually reaching a caloric expenditure goal of 1,000 kcal/wk, which can be reached by walking 2 miles a day on 5 days. Some programs provide supervised exercise and thus allow modeling of exercise behavior,[39] whereas others have tested the use of short versus long bouts of exercise.[40] However, the first study demonstrated improved adherence and weight loss in the group that exercised at home rather than attending group exercise,[39] and the short-bout (10 minutes) exercise group achieved better weight loss and greater total exercise time than those who exercised for 20- to 40-minute bouts.[40] Trials examining weight loss with and without exercise have consistently demonstrated improved weight loss with the combined diet and exercise components.[9,41] The single best predictor of weight loss maintenance is exercise.[42] Daily activity is also addressed in weight loss. Patients are encouraged to use the stairs and walk more through daily activities. Another approach is to decrease the amount of sedentary activities (i.e., TV viewing or computer use), and replace them with activities such as gardening or recreational sports.

Depending on the patient's age, risk factor profile, and concomitant conditions and symptoms, exercise testing to assess cardiopulmonary function and presence of disease may be indicated. This needs to be determined before initiating an exercise program. Patients also require instruction on injury prevention, how to initiate and maintain an exercise program, proper attire, and weather conditions. The kind of activity or exercise and the amount of time spent engaged in it are recorded in the patients' diaries. Lists of activities and their caloric expenditure are provided to patients so they can monitor progress toward their exercise goals.

BEHAVIORAL THERAPY

Behavioral therapy, based on the earlier work of Stuart,[43] has at its core the functional analysis of behavior.[9] Eating and exercise behaviors are analyzed to delineate their association with environmental events, including times, people, places, thoughts, and emotions.[9,30] Patients record their eating and exercise behaviors and use these self-monitoring data to determine specific problem areas. The environment controlling the problem areas is then restructured and the problem behaviors modified.[9]

Among the distinguishing features of behavioral therapy is its goal orientation. The objectives of treatment are clearly defined, specific, and measurable. In addition, behavioral therapy attempts to change behavior and, finally, it is a process-oriented approach in that it is a method of learning about one's behavior. Behaviors are broken down into a series of small events, and acquisition of behavior shaped through small steps.[30]

Behavioral treatment programs usually use a multidisciplinary approach and may include a psychologist, nutritionist, exercise physiologist, nurse, or physician.[3,44] No studies have been performed evaluating the different health care professionals delivering the intervention, but it is suggested that providers avail themselves of the expertise offered by professionals who have counseled patients in this area.[3] Duration of treatment is 16 to 24 weeks of either weekly or a combination of weekly and biweekly contacts. More recently, programs are extending treatment to 12 months and use biweekly or monthly meetings during the second 6-month period.[9] Behavioral therapy is usually delivered in a closed-group context, that is, the group is formed at the initiation of treatment and no new members are permitted to join thereafter. This approach facilitates the development of group cohesiveness and reduces attrition.[9] The group approach also offers economic benefits.

Behavioral therapy may use numerous strategies to facilitate behavior change. Specific strategies are as follows:

◆ *Self-monitoring*—often considered the *sine qua non* of behavioral treatment.[9] It entails instructing patients to record their food intake, calories, fat grams, and exercise caloric expenditure or time spent in programmed activity. This requires patients to look up these values in books provided and makes them aware not only of their behavior but of the caloric and fat content of foods eaten.

◆ *Goal setting*—patients are given goals for total calories, fat grams and percent of total calories, and energy expenditure through exercise; goals need to be proximal, specific, and attainable.

◆ *Stimulus control*—considered the hallmark of behavioral therapy.[43] It is based on the assumption that environmental antecedents control behaviors, and that changing the environment to include positive cues for appropriate eating and exercise behaviors leads to desired behavior—for example, remove high-fat foods and replace them with attractive fruits that are ready to eat, store other tempting foods out of sight, restrict places of eating.[9]

◆ *Problem solving*—using the approach described by D'Zurilla and Goldfried,[45] patients are taught four specific steps: identify the problem situation leading to inappropriate eating or exercise behavior, generate solutions, select one solution to test, and evaluate the use of the solution in resolving the problem.

◆ *Relapse prevention*—patients are taught that lapses are a natural occurrence and should be anticipated and planned for with strategies that can be used in coping with the situation, and thereby prevent relapses.[46]

◆ *Cognitive restructuring*—entails teaching patients about negative thoughts, rationalizations, comparisons with others, and all-or-none thinking, and how these thoughts serve the patient; patients are taught how to counter these thoughts with more positive thinking and self-statements.[9]

Other strategies that can be used include contingency management, reinforcement, dealing with high-risk situations, stress management, and enlisting and providing social support. The best results for treatment success are attained through a combination of dietary therapy, exercise and physical activity, and use of behavioral therapy.[3,9,30] This regimen should be continued for at least 6 months, followed by maintenance strategies.

Pharmacotherapy

Drug therapy for the treatment of obesity has had a tumultuous history.[47] This was accentuated by the withdrawal in 1997 of two drugs, fenfluramine and dexfenfluramine, after cardiac valvular abnormalities were noted on echocardiograms in women receiving the popular drugs.[48] Subsequently, the approval of other antiobesity agents has been delayed.[49] Numerous drugs are under study for future treatment. It is beyond the scope of this chapter to explore each category of agents, but the interested reader is referred to detailed reviews.[47,50–52]

Pharmacologic therapy for treatment of obesity has limited indications, such as for treatment of patients with a BMI of at least 30 in the absence of comorbid conditions, or for patients with a BMI of 27 or more with concomitant morbidity. Drug therapy needs to be instituted in combination with a program of lifestyle modification. One drug available for long-term use, sibutramine, is a specific reuptake inhibitor for norepinephrine and serotonin.[49,53,54] A second drug, orlistat, is pending Food and Drug Administration approval.[3,49] Orlistat, which does not act through the central nervous system, inhibits gastric and pancreatic lipases, which are essential for effective digestion of fats, and thereby decreases fat absorption.[47,54]

The limited effectiveness of antiobesity agents in producing weight loss emphasizes their necessarily adjunctive role. Most weight loss occurs within the first 6 months of treatment and averages 5% to 10% of the baseline weight,[54,55] which translates to 2 to 10 kg.[3] People who lose weight during the initial 6 months of therapy and maintain that loss without side effects may be considered successful and maintained on the drug with periodic follow-up to monitor progress, side effects, weight, blood pressure, and laboratory values, and provide reinforcement.[3] There are limited data on the use of these agents beyond 1 year.[47] However, short-term treatment in this chronic condition is not helpful because weight gain often occurs with discontinuation of drug therapy.

Adverse effects of sibutramine include increases in blood pressure and heart rate. It is contraindicated in patients with hypertension, CHD, arrhythmias, congestive heart failure, or history of stroke.[53,55] Side effects that may occur with orlistat include oily or loose stools or malabsorption of fat-soluble vitamins, requiring supplementation.[54]

Surgical Therapy

Surgical approaches, which are primarily for the purpose of reducing food intake, are indicated only for patients with severe obesity (BMI ≥40) or a BMI of 35 to 40 and concomitant morbidity, such as sleep apnea, uncontrolled type II diabetes, cardiovascular disease, or weight-related problems interfering with daily functioning. Surgical procedures include gastroplasty, which reduces the size of the stomach through vertical gastric banding, and gastric bypass with the Roux-en-Y procedure, which also reduces intestinal absorption.[1,37] Substantial weight loss can result from these procedures. Patients undergoing these procedures require ongoing medical follow-up and lifelong treatment with behavior modification that includes diet and exercise therapy.[3]

Maintenance of Weight Loss

Approximately 1 year after treatment, patients maintain 60% of their initial weight loss, but return to their baseline weight within 3 to 5 years.[9] Thus, the greatest challenge facing health care professionals who treat these patients is identifying the means to assist patients to sustain the initial weight loss. Several strategies have been investigated for their efficacy in improving weight loss maintenance.[56-62] Those that have most consistently demonstrated improved weight loss maintenance include ongoing contact with the provider,[60,63] inclusion of aerobic exercise,[59] and provision of social support.[64] Use of the chronic disease model to treat obesity, an important advance, can facilitate ongoing follow-up and reinforcement beyond the point of reaching the weight loss goal. National Weight Control Registry data reveal that people who are successful in maintaining a weight loss of 13.6 kg (30 lb) or more for at least 1 year report expending 11,830 kJ/wk through physical activity, an amount equivalent to 2,800 kcal/wk, or walking 28 miles.[65] This finding underscores the importance of exercise as a maintenance strategy. However, adherence to exercise remains a problem.[66] Maintenance of weight loss is the ultimate form of compliance because it requires long-term adherence to the numerous changes in lifestyle that created the initial weight loss.[67] Therefore, the provider needs to implement strategies to enhance adherence throughout the treatment and maintenance phases; these are detailed elsewhere in the text.[66]

SUMMARY

Obesity is a chronic medical condition with numerous adverse effects on the cardiovascular system. The goal of treatment is reduced morbidity and improved health. Current treatment consists of lifestyle interventions and, increasingly, pharmacotherapy. For the first time, we have evidence-based guidelines for use in the identification, evaluation, and treatment of overweight and obese patients in the clinical setting.[3] These guidelines emphasize multidisciplinary approaches to the treatment of this chronic disorder. Practitioners can teach patients strategies for self-management, following the precedent established in treating similar conditions (e.g., hypertension, dyslipidemia, and diabetes).[68,69] Similar to the role nurses play in the treatment of these chronic conditions, nurses need to take the lead in addressing the needs of this ever-growing subgroup of the population. Two important areas to address are prevention of further weight gain and sustaining the weight loss achieved initially.

REFERENCES

1. Rosenbaum M, Leibel RL, Hirsch J: Obesity. N Engl J Med 337: 396–407, 1997
2. Quesebberry CJ, Caan B, Jacobson A: Obesity, health services use, and health care costs among members of a health maintenance organization. Arch Intern Med 158: 466–472, 1998
3. National Heart, Lung, and Blood Institute Obesity Education Initiative Expert Panel on the Identification, Evaluation, and Treatment of Overweight and Obesity: Clinical Guidelines on the Identification, Evaluation, and Treatment of Overweight and Obesity in Adults: The Evidence Report. Bethesda, MD, National Institutes of Health, 1998
4. Flegal KM, Carroll MD, Kuczmarski RJ et al: Overweight and obesity in the United States: prevalence and trends 1960–1994. International Journal of Obesity 22: 39–47, 1998
5. Seidell JC, Rissanen AM: Time trends in the worldwide prevalence of obesity. In Bray GA, Bourchard C, James WPT (eds): Handbook of Obesity, pp 79–91. New York, Marcel Dekker, 1998
6. Saltzman E, Benotti PN: The effects of obesity on the cardiovascular system. In Bray GA, Bourchard C, James WPT (eds). Handbook of Obesity, pp 637–649. New York, Marcel Dekker, 1998
7. Van Gaal LF, Wauters MA, Leeuw IH: The beneficial effects of modest weight loss on cardiovascular risk factors. International Journal of Obesity 21(Suppl 1): S5–S9, 1997
8. Eckel RH, Krauss RM: American Heart Association call to action: Obesity as a major risk factor of coronary heart disease. Circulation 97 (21): 2099–2100, 1998
9. Wing RR: Behavioral approaches to the treatment of obesity. In Bray GA, Bourchard C, James WPT (eds). Handbook of Obesity, pp 855–877. New York, Marcel Dekker, 1998
10. Institute of Medicine: Weighing the Options Criteria for Evaluating Weight-Management Programs. Washington, DC, National Academy Press, 1995
11. Shape Up America! and American Obesity Association: Guidance for Treatment of Adult Obesity. Bethesda, MD, Shape Up America!, 1996
12. World Health Organization: Preventing and Managing the Global Epidemic of Obesity: Report of the World Health Organization Consultation of Obesity. Geneva, WHO, 1997
13. Gibson RS: Principles of Nutritional Assessment, pp 170–195. New York, Oxford University Press, 1990
14. VanItallie TB, Lew EA: Estimation of the effect of obesity on health and longevity. In Stunkard AJ, Wadden TA (eds): Obesity: Theory and Therapy, 2nd ed, pp 219–230. New York, Raven Press, 1993
15. Abate N, Garg A, Peshock RM et al: Relationship of generalized and regional adiposity to insulin sensitivity in men with NIDDM. Diabetes 45: 1684–1693, 1996
16. Lean ME, Han TS, Morrison CE: Waist circumference as a measure for indicating need for weight management. BMJ 311: 158–161, 1995
17. Allison DB, ed: Handbook of Assessment Methods for Eating Behaviors and Weight Related Problems: Measures, Theory, and Research. Thousand Oaks, CA, Sage, 1995
18. U.S. Department of Health and Human Services: NHANES III Anthropometric Procedures Video. Washington, DC, U.S. Government Printing Office Stock Number 017-022-01335-5, 1996
19. National Cholesterol Education Program: Summary of the Second Report of the National Cholesterol Education Program Expert Panel on Detection, Evaluation, and Treatment of High Blood Cholesterol in Adults (Adult Treatment Panel II). JAMA 269: 3015–3023, 1993
20. Joint National Committee on Prevention, Detection, Evaluation, and Treatment of High Blood Pressure: The Sixth Report of the Joint National Committee on Prevention, Detection, Evaluation, and Treatment of High Blood Pressure (JNCVI). Arch Intern Med 157: 2413–2446, 1997
21. Fiore MC, Bailey WC, Cohen SJ: Smoking Cessation: Clinical Practice Guidelines No. 18. Bethesda, MD, U.S. Department of Health and Human Services, Public Health Service, Agency for Health Care Policy and Research, 1996

22. Paffenbarger RS Jr, Hyde RT, Wing AL et al: The association of changes in physical-activity level and other lifestyle characteristics with mortality among men. N Engl J Med 328: 538–545, 1993

23. NIH Consensus Conference: Triglyceride, high-density lipoprotein, and coronary heart disease. NIH Consensus Development Panel on Triglyceride, High-Density Lipoprotein, and Coronary Heart Disease. JAMA 269: 505–510, 1993

24. Schwartz RS: Obesity in the elderly. In Bray GA, Bourchard C, James WPT (eds): Handbook of Obesity, pp 103–114. New York, Marcel Dekker, 1998

25. Eckel RH, Krauss RM: Obesity and heart disease. Circulation 96: 3248–3250, 1997

26. Willet W: Nutritional Epidemiology, pp 52–126. New York, Oxford University Press, 1990

27. Willett WC, Sampson L, Stampfer MJ et al: Reproducibility and validity of a semiquantitative food frequency questionnaire. Am J Epidemiol 122: 51–65, 1985

28. Block G: Human dietary assessment: Methods and issues. Prev Med 18: 643–660, 1989

29. Pereira MA, FitzGerald SJ, Gregg EW et al: A Collection of Physical Activity Questionnaires for Health-Related Research. Med Sci Sports Exerc 29(Suppl): S1–S205, 1997

30. Wadden TA: The treatment of obesity. In Stunkard AJ, Wadden TA (eds): Obesity: Theory and Therapy, 2nd ed, pp 197–217. New York, Raven Press, 1993

31. Stunkard AJ: Talking with patients. In Stunkard AJ, Wadden TA (eds): Obesity: Theory and Therapy, 2nd ed, pp 355–363. New York, Raven Press, 1993

32. Foster GD, Wadden TA, Vogt RA et al: What is a reasonable weight loss? Patients' expectations and evaluations of obesity treatment outcome. J Consult Clin Psychol 65: 79–85, 1997

33. Williamson DF, Serdula MK, Anada RF et al: Weight loss attempts in adults: Goals, duration, and rate of weight loss. Am J Public Health 82: 1251–1257, 1992

34. Hill JO, Drougas H, Peters JC: Obesity treatment: Can diet composition play a role? Ann Intern Med 119: 694–697, 1993;

35. Harvey-Berino J: The efficacy of dietary fat vs. total energy restriction for weight loss. Obes Res 6: 202, 1998

36. National Cholesterol Education Program: Second Report of the Expert Panel on Detection, Evaluation, and Treatment of High Blood Cholesterol in Adults. National Institutes of Health, National Heart, Lung, and Blood Institute, 1993

37. Glenny A-M, O'Meara S, Melville A et al: The treatment and prevention of obesity: A systematic review of the literature. International Journal of Obesity 21: 715–737, 1997

38. Brownell KD: The LEARN Program for Weight Control, 7th ed. Dallas, American Health Publishing Company, 1997

39. Perri MG, Martin DA, Leermaker EA et al: Effects of group-versus home-based exercise in the treatment of obesity. Journal of Consulting and Clinical Cardiology 65: 278–285, 1997

40. Jakicic JM, Wing RR, Butler BA et al: Prescribing exercise in multiple short bouts versus one continuous bout: Effects on adherence, cardiorespiratory fitness, and weight loss in overweight women. International Journal of Obesity 19: 893–901, 1995

41. Pavlou KN, Krey S, Steffe WP: Exercise as an adjunct to weight loss and maintenance in moderately obese subjects. Am J Clin Nutr 49: 1115–1123, 1989

42. Anderson JT, Grande FKA: Cholesterol-lowering diets. J Am Diet Assoc 62: 133–142, 1973

43. Stuart RB: Behavioral control of overeating. Behav Res Ther 5: 357–365, 1967

44. Perri MG: Improving maintenance of weight loss following treatment by diet and lifestyle modification. In Wadden TA, Van Itallie TB (eds): Treatment of the Seriously Obese Patient New York, The Guilford Press. 456–477, 1992

45. D'Zurilla TJ, Goldfried MR: Problem solving and behavior modification. J Abnorm Psychol 78: 107–126, 1971

46. Marlatt GA, Gordon JR: Determinants of relapse: Implications for the maintenance of behavior change. In Davidson PO, Davidson SM (eds): Behavioral Medicine: Changing Health Lifestyles, pp 410–452. New York, Brunner/Mazel, 1980

47. Bray GA: Pharmacological treatment of obesity. In Bray GA, Bourchard C, James WPT (eds): Handbook of Obesity, pp 953–975. New York, Marcel Dekker, 1998

48. Connolly HM, Crary JL, McGoon MD: Valvular heart disease associated with fenfluramine-phentermine. N Engl J Med 337: 581–588, 1997

49. Bray G: Drug treatment of obesity: Don't throw the baby out with the bath water. Am J Clin Nutr 67: 1–4, 1998

50. Weiser M, Fishman WH, Michaelson MD et al: The pharmacologic approach to the treatment of obesity. J Clin Pharmacol 37: 453–473, 1997

51. Finer N: Present and future pharmacological approaches. Br Med Bull 53: 409–432, 1997

52. National Task Force on the Prevention and Treatment of Obesity: Long-term pharmacotherapy in the management of obesity. JAMA 276: 1907–1915, 1996

53. Lean MEJ: Sibutramine: A review of clinical efficacy. International Journal of Obesity 21: S30–S36, 1997

54. James WPT, Avenell A, Broom J et al: A one-year trial to assess the value of orlistat in the management of obesity. International Journal of Obesity 21: S24–S30, 1997

55. Ryan DH, Kaiser P, Bray GA: Sibutramine: A novel new agent for obesity treatment. Obes Res 3: 553S–559S, 1995

56. Wing RR, Jeffery RW, Hellerstedt WL et al: Effect of frequent phone contacts and optional food provision on maintenance of weight loss. Ann Behav Med 18: 172–176, 1996

57. Perri MG, Shapiro RM, Ludwig WW et al: Maintenance strategies for the treatment of obesity: An evaluation of relapse prevention training and posttreatment contact by mail and telephone. J Consult Clin Psychol 52: 404–413, 1984

58. Perri MG, McAllister DA, Gange JJ et al: Effects of four maintenance programs on the long-term management of obesity. J Consult Clin Psychol 56: 529–534, 1988

59. Perri MG, McAdoo WG, McAllister DA et al: Enhancing the efficacy of behavior therapy for obesity: Effects of aerobic exercise and a multicomponent maintenance program. J Consult Clin Psychol 54: 670–675, 1986

60. Perri MG, McAdoo WG, Spevak PA et al: Effect of a multicomponent maintenance program on long-term weight loss. J Consult Clin Psychol 52: 480–481, 1984

61. Perri MG, McAdoo GW, McAllister DA et al: Effects of peer support and therapist contact on long-term weight loss. J Consult Clin Psychol 55: 615–617, 1987

62. Perri MG, Nezu AM, Patti ET et al: Effect of length of treatment on weight loss. J Consult Clin Psychol 57: 450–452, 1989

63. King AC, Frey-Hewitt B, Dreon DM et al: Diet vs exercise in weight maintenance. Arch Intern Med 149: 2741–2746, 1989

64. Wing RR, Jeffery RW: Benefits of recruiting participants with friends and increasing social support for weight loss and maintenance. Journal of Consulting and Clinical Psychology 67(1): 132–138, 1999

65. Klem ML, Wing RR, McGuire MT et al: A descriptive study of individuals successful at long-term maintenance of substantial weight loss. Am J Clin Nutr 66: 239–246, 1997

66. Burke LE, Dunbar-Jacob J, Hill MN: Compliance to cardiovascular risk reduction strategies: Review of the research. Ann Behav Med 19: 239–263, 1997

67. Burke LE: Strategies to enhance compliance to weight loss treatment. In Fletcher G, Grundy S, Hayman L (eds): Obesity: Impact on Cardiovascular Disease. Armonk, NY, Futura 1999

68. Keller C, Oveland D, Hudson S: Strategies for weight control success in adults. Nurse Pract 22: 33–54, 1997

69. Simkin-Silverman L, Wing RR. Management of obesity in primary care. Obes Res 5: 603–612, 1997

Diabetes Mellitus

MARGARET I. WALLHAGEN

Diabetes mellitus is a major risk factor for numerous complications, including cardiovascular disease,[2,7,34] yet data increasingly suggest that many of these risks can be minimized through intensive management.[49,71] In addition, a greater understanding of the pathophysiologic processes involved in diabetes has led to revisions in the criteria for its diagnosis and promoted the development of targeted interventions.[2,21,58] The purposes of this chapter are to discuss (1) the new criteria for diagnosing diabetes, (2) the pathophysiology of type I and type II diabetes, (3) the pathophysiology of major complications, and (4) current treatment recommendations. This discussion builds on and emphasizes the importance of understanding and referring to the other topics discussed in this section of the text: coronary heart disease, hypertension, hyperlipidemia, activity and exercise, obesity, and issues related to adherence. Knowledge of these data allows cardiovascular specialists to provide appropriate and comprehensive assessment of people with diabetes and to minimize long-term complications.

DEFINITION, PREVALENCE, AND ECONOMIC CONSEQUENCES

Diabetes mellitus describes a heterogeneous group of metabolic disorders characterized by elevated blood glucose levels; disturbances in carbohydrate, protein and fat metabolism; and relative or absolute deficiencies in insulin secretion or action.[2,12,67] Since the 1980s, diabetes has been classified according to criteria that recognized two major forms: insulin-dependent diabetes mellitus (IDDM or type I) and non–insulin-dependent diabetes mellitus (NIDDM or type II).[2] In acknowledgment that diabetes is a syndrome that incorporates disorders with different etiologies and clinical presentations, several additional, less common types were also categorized: gestational, malnutrition related, and other, a category that included a diverse group of etiologies ranging from pancreatic disease to drug-induced glucose abnormalities.

This classification was based on both treatment requirements and pathogenesis, and often led to confusion.[45] Thus,

both the American Diabetes Association (ADA) and the World Health Organization reviewed these criteria in light of current data.[2] New recommendations were derived from the reports of these two groups. The new classification system (Table 36-1) is based on the current understanding of the pathophysiologic processes involved in the various causes of diabetes. The new diagnostic criteria (Display 36-1) are based on increasing awareness of the negative consequences of hyperglycemia. A fasting plasma glucose level of 126 mg/dL is approximately equivalent to a 2-hour glucose tolerance test level of 200 mg/dL, and both levels are associated with an increased risk of both microvascular and macrovascular disease and correlate with a dramatic rise in the prevalence of retinopathy.[2,45,46]

The emphasis on minimizing confusion in diagnosis and on promoting early recognition of diabetes is significant. In 1997, 10.3 million people in the United States reported they had diabetes, whereas another 5.4 million were estimated to have undiagnosed diabetes.[17] The prevalence of combined diagnosed and undiagnosed diabetes in the United States in those 40 to 74 years of age increased from 8.9% in 1976 to 1980 to 12.3% in 1988 to 1994.[33] Worldwide, 124 million people were estimated to have diabetes in 1997.[6]

Of all cases of diabetes, 90% to 97% are classified as NIDDM or type II.[6,17] And although type I diabetes is more prevalent in people of northern European descent,[8] type II diabetes is especially prominent in minority populations. Compared with whites, African Americans, Latinos, and Native Americans all have significantly higher prevalence rates of type II diabetes and experience significantly more complications.[17,33]

Both type I and type II diabetes are associated with negative health outcomes. People with type I diabetes have a two- to fourfold greater risk of dying in young adulthood and middle age than age-matched peers,[30] and people with either type I or type II diabetes are at significant risk for complications, including retinopathy, neuropathy, amputations, nephropathy, and cardiovascular disease.[2,11] Diabetes also exerts multiple demands on the patient and his or her family that change across time.[52,61] Responses to these demands can influence glycemic control and long-term outcomes.

TABLE 36-1	New Classifications for Diabetes Mellitus
Classification	**Description**
I. Type I	Beta-cell destruction and absolute insulin deficiency.
II. Type II	A state of insulin resistance with a relative lack of insulin. The primary problem may be either insulin resistance or insufficient insulin secretion. Treatment may include the use of insulin, oral agents, or diet and exercise.
III. Other specific types	Includes diabetes related to specific genetic defects and secondary causes such as other endocrinopathies, drugs, or infections.
IV. Gestational	Includes any degree of glucose intolerance that is first recognized during pregnancy.
VI. Impaired glucose tolerance and impaired fasting glucose	Although not specifically included in the etiologic classification schema, impaired glucose tolerance and fasting glucose are considered a metabolic stage intermediate between normal glucose homeostasis and clinically defined diabetes. These are considered indicators of risk for future diabetes as well as cardiovascular disease.

Adapted from Lorber DL: Redefining diabetes. Practical Diabetology 16: 19–24, 1997; and American Diabetes Association: Clinical practice recommendations 1998. Diabetes Care 21(3)(Suppl): 53–590, 1998.

Diabetes also has a significant impact on health care costs. Direct medical expenditures attributable to diabetes in 1997 totaled $44.1 billion, whereas indirect costs amounted to $54.1 billion.[3] Most of the direct costs were for inpatient care (62%), and two thirds were incurred by elderly patients. Of the six chronic complications that accounted for 35% of all hospitalizations resulting from diabetes, cardiovascular disease ranked highest (24.7%).

DISPLAY 36-1

Diagnostic Criteria

1. Diabetes: the presence of any of the following*:
   a. The presence of symptoms (e.g., polyuria, polydipsia, polyphagia, weight loss) along with a casual (random—without regard to meals) blood glucose reading of ≥200 mg/dL (11.1 mmol/L).
   b. A fasting (≥8 h) glucose level of ≥126 mg/dL (7.0 mmol/L).
   c. A 2-hour plasma glucose reading of ≥200 mg/dL (11.1 mmol/L) during an oral glucose tolerance test. The glucose tolerance test has to be based on World Health Organization criteria and involve the use of a 75-g anhydrous glucose.
2. Impaired glucose tolerance: a 2-hour plasma glucose reading of ≥140 mg/dL (7.8 mmol/L) but <200 mg/dL (11.1 mmol/L).
3. Impaired fasting glucose: a fasting plasma glucose of ≥110 mg/dL (6.1 mol/L) but <126 mg/dL (7.0 mmol/L).

*Must be confirmed on a subsequent day unless there is unequivocal hyperglycemia with acute metabolic decompensation.
Adapted from Lorber DL: Redefining diabetes. Practical Diabetology 16: 19–24, 1997; and American Diabetes Association: Clinical practice recommendations 1998. Diabetes Care 21(3)(Suppl): 53–590, 1998.

PATHOPHYSIOLOGY OF DIABETES MELLITUS

Insulin Action and Glucose Metabolism

As a heterogeneous group of diseases, the various forms of diabetes mellitus have no single unifying etiology. However, an overview of glucose metabolism and the actions of insulin facilitates an understanding of the multiple sites where alterations may occur. Complex metabolic processes maintain plasma glucose concentrations within narrow limits while ensuring a consistent supply of substrate for central nervous system function, maintaining a supply of carbohydrate for emergency energy use, and preserving adequate protein for structural integrity and enzyme function.[64,67] Maintenance of this fuel homeostasis involves the interplay of numerous neurohormones, with insulin playing a central role.

Insulin is a protein hormone produced and secreted by the beta cells of the islets of Langerhans through a series of steps; preproinsulin is changed to proinsulin, which is then cleaved to form insulin and a C-peptide fragment.[23] Insulin and C-peptide are then stored in granules, with small amounts of basal insulin released every hour.[20] An abrupt increase in glucose levels after food ingestion stimulates a rapid burst of insulin release, termed the first- or acute-phase response, that lasts approximately 10 minutes and prevents postprandial hyperglycemia.[20,21] A second-phase insulin response then occurs that lasts until glucose stimulation ceases. First-phase insulin may be from granules that are close to the cell membrane, whereas second-phase insulin appears to be from more internal granules or newly formed hormone.[20]

Released insulin binds to its receptor on cells throughout the body, activating tyrosine kinase and initiating a series of phosphorylation reactions that are essential to its various actions.[58] Insulin's actions are anabolic: it is primarily responsible for activating the transport systems and enzymes that promote the uptake, storage, and use of glucose, amino acids, and fatty acids; and for limiting hepatic glucose production by inhibiting gluconeogenesis and the breakdown of glycogen, protein, and fat. Insulin also acts as a vasodilator, thus promoting its own delivery to target tissues.[58]

In the fasting state, insulin levels drop, the aforementioned processes are reversed, and glucagon, which is released from the alpha cells of the pancreas, promotes the release of glucose from the liver to maintain an adequate supply for neurologic function. Other catabolic counterregulatory neurohormones that promote the breakdown of stored supplies for energy use when needed include catecholamines, cortisol, and growth hormone. Data suggest that the kidney may also be important in this homeostatic process, with renal production of glucose accounting for as much as 25% of systemic glucose production.[70] Because diabetes is characterized by an absolute or relative deficiency of insulin, metabolism in diabetes has been described as a "runaway fasting state."[67]

Type I Diabetes Mellitus

The most common etiology of type I diabetes mellitus is cell-mediated autoimmune destruction of the beta cells of the pancreas.[2] This may occur rapidly or slowly, but the ultimate outcome is an absolute lack of insulin, necessitating lifelong replacement therapy. The underlying cause of the autoimmune response appears to involve an interplay of a genetic predisposition interacting with environmental factors that promote an immune response, such as exposure to a viral or dietary antigen.[8,30] Although most commonly presenting during childhood or adolescence, it can occur at any age, and late-onset type I diabetes may be more common than previously appreciated.[5]

Type II Diabetes Mellitus

Type II diabetes encompasses conditions characterized by varying degrees of insulin resistance, beta cell failure, and increased hepatic glucose release.[2,21,39,67] Its occurrence requires some form of genetic susceptibility interacting with environmental factors.[2,55] Although the pathogenesis of the various defects found in type II diabetes are still not fully understood, the overt presentation of the disease is usually preceded by a long period of impaired glucose tolerance (insulin resistance), a condition associated with increased risk for macrovascular complications. Thus, patients often already have long-term complications at the time of diagnosis. This may be less true in the future given the new criteria for diagnosis.

Insulin resistance is a state of decreased responsiveness to the effects of insulin, resulting in a plasma glucose level that is higher than would be expected for a given level of plasma insulin.[21,63] The cause of insulin resistance remains unresolved. As noted previously, when insulin binds to its receptor it activates tyrosine kinase, which initiates a series of phosphorylation reactions that are essential to its action. Thus, insulin resistance could be related to alterations in insulin binding to its receptor, alterations in signal transmission, or alterations in the intracellular processes involved in initiating a response.[1] Although research continues to

explore each of these possible mechanisms, data suggest that insulin binding is not specifically altered in type II diabetes, but that defects occur in postbinding processes.[5,21,48]

Multiple factors can, however, influence one or more of the steps noted previously. For example, obesity, inactivity, hyperglycemia, hyperinsulinemia, and aging each are associated with altered cellular responsivity and insulin resistance. These are considered a risk factor for diabetes, as is "syndrome X." The latter term describes the concurrence of a number of physiologic abnormalities, including hypertension; hyperinsulinemia; a dyslipidemia characterized by elevated triglycerides, decreased high-density lipoproteins and increased small, dense, low-density lipoprotein (LDL) particles; obesity; and cardiovascular disease.[56,63] Aside from aging, most of these risk factors are modifiable and are targets for therapy.

In addition to insulin resistance, patients with type II diabetes also evidence altered beta cell function.[39] One of the first deficits to occur is loss of the first-phase or rapid-response secretion of insulin.[21,39,58] This results in diminished suppression of hepatic glucose production in the immediate period after food ingestion.[5] Other deficits include a change in the characteristic pulsatile secretion of insulin and an increase in the ratio of proinsulin to insulin.[21,58] Over time, both the first phase and second phase become impaired.

Hyperglycemia also depresses beta cell function (glucose toxicity), further diminishing the ability of the body to respond to a glucose load.[5] In addition, loss of insulin's inhibitory effect on lipolysis and fatty acid oxidation results in elevated levels of free fatty acid, which contribute to tissue insulin resistance, stimulate hepatic gluconeogenesis (increased precursor products), and further diminish beta cell function.[21,56]

COMPLICATIONS OF DIABETES MELLITUS

The complications of diabetes can be classified as acute or chronic. Acute complications include episodes of hypoglycemia in patients treated with glucose-lowering medications, diabetic ketoacidosis (DKA), and hyperosmolar hyperglycemic nonketotic syndrome (HHNS).[4,5,47] Chronic complications are categorized as microvascular or macrovascular. Although chronic complications are the main focus of this chapter, a few points are important in relation to acute events.

Acute Complications

Acute complications are the result of acute changes in glucose levels, are often life threatening, and require immediate intervention. Symptoms of hypoglycemia, generally defined as a blood sugar of less than 50 to 60 mg/dL, occur when insufficient glucose is available for cerebral functioning. This is usually the result of excess insulin (either from injection or oral hypoglycemic stimulation), decreased or delayed carbohydrate intake, or increased utilization, as through exercise.[4] Hypoglycemia is a major limiting factor in the management of diabetes, especially type I. Because the incidence of hypoglycemia is increased in those undergoing intensive control, it influences the decision-making process regarding diabetes management.[2]

Both DKA and HHNS are the result of insufficient insulin and represent the extreme of the diabetic state. DKA is more common in type I diabetes, whereas HHNS is most common in older people with type II diabetes. These conditions can be precipitated by multiple factors, including acute infections (pneumonia, influenza, urinary tract), therapeutic procedures (surgery), or acute events (myocardial infarction, trauma).[4,5] It is therefore always important to look for an underlying problem.

Microvascular Complications

Common microvascular complications include retinopathy, neuropathy, and nephropathy. Retinopathy is directly related to the duration of diabetes and blood glucose levels; almost all patients with type I diabetes and more than 60% of those with type II experience some degree of retinopathy after 20 years.[2] Macular edema is also associated with duration of diabetes, and cataracts appear earlier and progress more rapidly in people with diabetes than in the general population.[41] Ongoing ophthalmologic evaluations are essential. In general, yearly dilated examinations should occur after the initial evaluation, or more frequently if retinopathy is detected and is progressing.[2]

Diabetic nephropathy is known to be the preeminent cause of end-stage renal disease in the United States.[43] The prevalence of end-stage renal disease is greater in type I diabetes, reaching approximately 40%. However, because of the numbers of people with type II diabetes, there are more people with type II on dialysis than type I. Diabetic nephropathy is also a major cause of elevated blood pressure in type I diabetes, and can be a cause in type II.[9]

Overt nephropathy is preceded by a phase in which most laboratory values are normal but the excretion of albumin is increased to approximately 0.03 to 0.3 g/24 hours (30 to 300 mg).[43] This microalbuminuria is not detected on routine dipstick until it reaches approximately 150 mg/L, so more refined tests are needed. These include either 24-hour urine collections, which also allow for quantification of glomerular filtration rate, or the assessment of urinary to creatinine ratio in an early morning collection.

Neuropathy is another common problem. Fedele and Giugliano[26] note that data indicate that the prevalence of neuropathy does not differ between type I and type II diabetes. The major factors involved appear to be the duration of the disease, the age of the patient, and metabolic control. Although comprising a wide range of clinical patterns, neuropathy is usually classified as somatic (sensorimotor peripheral neuropathy) and autonomic.[18] Dejgaard[22] adds central neuropathy as a category that has not received much attention in the past.

Peripheral neuropathy is an important risk factor for multiple complications as well as a cause of significant disability and pain.[2,31,73] Neuropathic foot ulcers secondary to trauma occur frequently and are a leading cause of amputa-

tions. Neuroarthropathy or Charcot's joint is also thought to be related to recurrent trauma to the joints and surrounding bony structures of the feet that go unnoticed by the person.[31] The resulting deformity contributes to significant morbidity and immobility. Autonomic neuropathies can cause altered sweating patterns, postural hypotension, neuropathic bladders, altered sexual function, and diabetic gastroparesis.[31,73] Altered sweating patterns can increase the risk for decreased thermoregulatory capacity, whereas diabetic gastroparesis can influence metabolic control. The latter may also go unnoticed. Enck and Frieling[25] note that silent gastroparesis, the occurrence of altered gastrointestinal function without symptoms, may result in the inappropriate assumption that patients are not following their treatment regimen.

Macrovascular Complications

Steinberg[68] observed that people with diabetes frequently have microvascular disease but die more commonly from macrovascular (cardiovascular and cerebrovascular) diseases. He also noted that even those who are well controlled and who do not have significant lipid abnormalities experience higher risk for premature coronary heart disease, for reasons that are not totally clear. Although macrovascular disease does not correlate strongly with the duration and severity of disease, both type I and type II diabetes appear to confer as much as 75% to 90% excess risk for coronary heart disease and increase the negative effects of other major risk factors such as smoking, dyslipidemia, and hypertension.[29] The risk for cardiovascular disease in women with type II diabetes is three to four times greater than in women without the condition; diabetes effectively eliminates the protection afforded premenopausal women.[5] In general, approximately 35% of people with type I diabetes and 75% of those with type II die from cardiovascular disease.[29]

PATHOPHYSIOLOGY OF COMPLICATIONS

Hypoglycemic Unawareness

Repeated episodes of hypoglycemia, although not the only cause, are related to hypoglycemic unawareness, a situation where the normal warning signs of hypoglycemia (neuroglycopenic and neurogenic) do not occur until the blood sugar is so low the person passes out or has a seizure.[19,69,74] This may occur because of impaired counterregulatory neurohormone response or brain adaptation through facilitated uptake at below-normal blood glucose levels. The normal glucagon secretory response to hypoglycemia is lost in people with type I diabetes within a few years of disease onset, and the threshold for epinephrine secretion is altered so that lower levels of glucose have to occur for its release.[19] People with hypoglycemic unawareness need to monitor blood sugar levels carefully. Preventing episodes of hypoglycemia can often reestablish appropriate physiologic responses to hypoglycemic events.

Chronic Complications

Chronic macrovascular or microvascular complications are the result of long-standing metabolic disturbances created by the underlying pathophysiologic processes that precede and result in increased hyperglycemia as well as the hyperglycemia itself. Microvascular complications appear to be especially related to chronic hyperglycemia, which causes alterations in the polyol or sorbitol pathway, formation of advanced glycation end products (AGE), and increased formation of free radicals.[14,27,28,59,72]

The polyol or sorbitol pathway is a series of metabolic processes involving a family of enzymes capable of reducing sugar-derived compounds to their sugar alcohols or polyols. This pathway converts glucose to sorbitol and galactose to galactitol. It is found in many tissues that do not require insulin to take up glucose, such as nerves, the retina and lens, the glomerulus of the kidney, and blood vessels.[14,28] Hyperglycemia increases intracellular glucose and its substrates, which leads to the accumulation of metabolic products of the polyol pathway, including sorbitol, that can directly or indirectly contribute to tissue damage or the development of cataracts. Another outcome of enhanced polyol pathway activity is a decrease in myoinositol, a substance that is important to neuronal and vascular function. The sorbitol–myoinositol derangements have been implicated in glomerular hyperfiltration, increased permeability of the blood–retinal barrier, and hypertension.

Chronic hyperglycemia is also associated with increased formation of glycosylated proteins.[14,28] Glucose rapidly attaches to the amino groups of proteins through a nonenzymatic process to form what are termed *Schiff base adducts.*[42] This process is the basis of the glycosylated hemoglobin test that is used to assess blood glucose control across the previous 3 to 4 months. Although a normally occurring process, excessive glycated proteins can adversely affect tissue function, possibly enhance the uptake of LDL cholesterol into the vascular wall, and create free radicals that in turn can damage tissues. Although some of the components that are formed are reversible, others undergo continued chemical rearrangement and become highly stable AGE. The level of AGE has been shown to predict changes in kidney morphology of patients with IDDM,[13] and to be associated with glycemic control.[49]

A third and interrelated process involves the formation of excess free radicals. A free radical is an atom or molecule that has an unpaired or free electron in an outer orbit, a state that renders it highly reactive and predisposed to interact with almost any biologic substrate.[42,51] Formed normally during oxidative metabolism, free radicals are counteracted by a complex intrinsic antioxidant defense system. When excessive amounts of free radicals are formed, the biologic antioxidant supply can become depleted and tissue damage can occur. Data suggest that free radicals increase the formation of glycated proteins and contribute to both microvascular and macrovascular abnormalities.[75]

The etiology of the macrovascular complications is multifactorial. There is no difference in the atheromatous lesions in people with diabetes compared with those without, although they may be more extensive and severe.[29] People with type I diabetes who have good glycemic control also are noted to have lipid profiles similar to those of nondiabetic people.[36] Further, the level of glycemia, at least in patients with type II diabetes, is less clearly related to macrovascular than to microvascular complications.[2] However, increased insulin concentrations, insulin resistance, and defective blood coagulation have each been suggested as potential etiologic factors.[29] There also may be interrelationships between the underlying causes of macrovascular and microvascular problems; for example, increased AGE formation has been noted to induce thrombosis-promoting changes by stimulating AGE receptors on endothelial cells.[14]

NURSING MANAGEMENT OF DIABETES

Management of diabetes involves a comprehensive, multidisciplinary effort that is highly dependent on assisting the patient with diabetes and his or her family to establish a regimen that will fit their life situation. Types of diabetes differ, occur at different points in the life span, and are associated with varying risk factors. Thus, although the ADA publishes an update of its clinical practice recommendations each year,[2] all regimens must be tailored to the individual patient's desires, goals, and concurrent physiologic status. Because type II diabetes is especially common in older people, alterations that occur with age are important to consider in discussing treatment options and monitoring response to therapies (Table 36-2).

In addition, because the management of diabetes often involves many lifestyle changes, patients with diabetes not only need to understand their condition and be prepared to make often complex decisions about their care,[52] but to develop strategies that facilitate self-care. Reichard[57] described the role of the health professional in this relationship as teacher, tutor, and professional friend. In this model, both the health professional and the person with diabetes enter the exchange as "experts" who learn together by experiencing and trying different approaches to address issues encountered in everyday life. Being a professional friend involves being "someone who cares, never accuses and who is engaging in a mutual practice to make life with diabetes easier while metabolic control is acceptable."[57] This model emphasizes the importance of avoiding blame when clients are unable to attain specific goals, and focuses on developing a problem-solving approach to issues that arise.

In general, management of diabetes involves controlling blood sugar, minimizing risk factors, and preventing or treating complications. This includes appropriate screening, monitoring, and intervention. Of major importance is a complete assessment of each person (Table 36-3) with an emphasis on the identification of complications, concurrent physiologic states that alter glucose control, risk factors, and level of knowledge. Data from the other chapters in this section discuss approaches to facilitate behavior change and risk factor reduction. Thus, as much as possible, only aspects of care specific to people with diabetes are included here.

TABLE 36-2	Age-Related Factors Influencing Care of Older Adults With Diabetes

Change With Age	Implications
Altered renal function	
Decreased glomerular filtration rate	Decreased renal excretion of many drugs
Decreased capacity to concentrate/dilute urine	Assess renal function, especially before use of metformin
Altered body composition	
Decreased lean body mass	Increased concentration of water-soluble drugs
	Serum creatinine unreliable as measure of renal function; use creatinine clearance
Increased proportion of adipose tissue	Deposition and storage of lipid-soluble drugs and long half-life
Decreased liver size and blood flow and alterations in phase I metabolism	Decreased hepatic metabolism and first-pass metabolism
Decreased total body fluids	Greater concentration of drug for given dose
	Assess/monitor drug response and side effects
	Start dose low, go slow with titration
Altered sensory perception	
Vision	Altered ability to recognize color, hear instructions (especially high frequencies)
Hearing	Use vision and hearing aids; assess perception and need for special aids
Increased prevalence of comorbidities	Increased potential for drug interactions and use of drugs that alter diabetes control (antihypertensives, antilipemics, nonsteroidal anti-inflammatory drugs)
	Consider concurrent cardiovascular disease in prescribing exercise
Altered neuromuscular functioning	
Slower central nervous system processing	Possible need for repetition of materials and longer periods of reinforcement; possible need for family member assistance
Decreased delayed recall	
Possible altered number/sensitivity of receptors	Increased sensitivity to side effects of drugs
Decreased fine motor coordination	Difficulty manipulating syringes, meters
Altered mobility	Decreased ease of access to health care
	Dependence on family/friends for transportation
	Assess social support, community support, safety of setting for exercise
Long-established lifestyle patterns; often highly motivated with regard to health	Assess goals, life patterns; assist with strategies to incorporate behavior change

TABLE 36-3	Nursing Assessment

Assessment	Comment
History	
Knowledge level and previous education	Many older adults are diagnosed after being admitted for an acute event or HHNS.
	People with diabetes may need review and updates of new data, but also come with extensive personal knowledge of how they respond to treatment.
Concurrent chronic conditions	
Recent stressful life events	Stress increases blood sugar.
Medications; prescribed over the counter	Many medications influence blood glucose.
Physical examination	
Cardiovascular/peripheral vascular status	Cardiovascular events such as myocardial infarction can precipitate DKA or HHNS.
Neurologic	Autonomic neuropathy can impair the response to hypoxia.[50]
	High blood glucose levels can impair immune response and wound healing.
Signs of infection	Infections can precipitate DKA or HHNS.
Skin (cellulitis), feet, oral, urinary tract	Confusion/altered mental status can be the presenting sign of infection in older adults.
Renal status	Influences drug dosing, use of metformin.
Laboratory evaluation	
Blood glucose; lipids; hemoglobin A_{1c}	Plasma glucose values are 10% to 15% higher than whole-blood glucose values.
	Many meters measure whole-blood glucose.
	Glycosylated hemoglobin assay methods vary; it is important to know laboratory norms and factors that interfere with accurate results.

General Goals and Recommendations

GLYCEMIC CONTROL

Maintaining an average hemoglobin A_{1c} of 7.2% has been shown to reduce the development of microvascular complications by 50% to 75% in patients with type I diabetes.[71] Other data suggest that similar benefits might accrue in type II diabetes.[65] The goal is to maintain as near euglycemic levels as possible; blood glucose goals for intensive management are (1) 80 to 120 mg/dL before meals; (2) 100 to 140 mg/dL at bedtime; and (3) a hemoglobin A_{1c} of less than 7% (or <1% above the normal for a given laboratory).[2] Treatment modification is considered when these ranges are not established or maintained.

Because intensive therapy is associated with higher rates of hypoglycemic events, certain people may not be candidates for tight control; such factors as comorbid disease, age (very young or very old), and other life circumstances must be considered.[2] Older adults with severe cardiovascular or cerebrovascular disease who are at risk for a stroke or myocardial infarction may need different glycemic goals.

Blood glucose monitoring is necessary to achieve or maintain glycemic control. It allows people to assess the impact of various foods and life events. Since July, 1998, Medicare has covered the cost of a glucose meter and limited numbers of strips and lancets regardless of whether insulin is being used.[16] Assessment of glycosylated hemoglobin at 3- to 6-month intervals is also recommended to provide data on metabolic control over the last 2 to 3 months.

CARDIOVASCULAR RISK AND LIPID CONTROL

In general, goals for the treatment of dyslipidemia, specifically related to LDL, are similar to those established by the National Cholesterol Education Program (see Chapter 33). Because macrovascular complications are common and significant in diabetes, aggressive lipid management is recommended. In those with coronary heart disease, peripheral vascular disease, and cardiovascular disease, drug therapy is initiated if, after diet and blood glucose lowering interventions, LDL remains over 100 mg/dL. In those without these concurrent problems, drug therapy is initiated if the LDL level remains over 130 mg/dL, with a goal of less than 130 mg/dL. When patients have clinical coronary vascular disease or very high LDL levels (≥200 mg/dL), drug therapy may be started along with nutrition and exercise interventions.[2]

BLOOD PRESSURE CONTROL

Hypertension is discussed in Chapter 32. In diabetes, aggressive treatment of blood pressure is considered of utmost importance to minimize cardiovascular and renal impairment. The goal for blood pressure control in adults with diabetes is less than 130/85 mm Hg.[2] For patients with isolated systolic hypertension in excess of 180 mm Hg, the goal is initially less than 160 mm Hg, whereas for those with systolic blood pressures between 160 and 179 mm Hg, the goal is initially to work toward a reduction of 20 mm Hg. Further reductions are based on individual assessment and how well any regimen is tolerated.

Because there have not been any large population-based, randomized clinical trials of hypertension specifically in people with diabetes, the best approach to management has not been clearly identified, although some drugs are considered less desirable because of their potential side effects in this group of patients. β-Adrenergic blocking agents can mask the symptoms of hypoglycemia, impair insulin release, and have a negative affect on blood lipids.[40] Thiazide diuretics are also known adversely to affect blood glucose and lipid levels, but usually at doses higher than 25 mg. Angiotensin-converting enzyme (ACE) inhibitors, alpha blocking agents, calcium channel blockers, or low-dose thiazide diuretics are often preferred.[3] ACE inhibitors may be particularly beneficial because they have been shown to provide renal protection.[5,40] However, an individualized approach that takes into account other factors that influence drug choice is still recommended.[40]

FOOT CARE/NEUROLOGIC ASSESSMENT

Foot ulcers, foot problems, and neurologic dysfunction are major causes of morbidity, mortality, and disability. Minor foot trauma in an insensate foot can initiate a process that ultimately leads to amputation. Performing a foot screen at least annually that includes a vascular, neurologic, musculoskeletal, skin, and soft tissue assessment is essential.[2] The neurologic examination should include an assessment of sensation; this can be done using a 10-g (5.07) Semmes-Weinstein monofilament. Loss of the ability consistently to feel the touch of this monofilament is equated with loss of protective sensation, places the person at risk, and evidences the need for a comprehensive program to prevent foot trauma.

As noted previously, several other neurologic abnormalities can influence the well-being of people with diabetes, including orthostatic hypotension, sexual dysfunction, and gastroparesis. Each of these needs careful assessment at ongoing intervals and usually requires a multidisciplinary approach to treatment. Orthostatic hypotension places the person at risk for falls and thus requires assessment of environmental safety features. This symptom is often difficult to manage. Sexual dysfunction may not be openly discussed by many patients but needs to be addressed because there are a number of treatment options. And gastroparesis may need to be considered in those people who have difficulty controlling their blood sugars even when following an active treatment program.

Interventions to Achieve Metabolic Control

DIET AND EXERCISE

Diet and exercise remain the cornerstones of treatment for diabetes. Obesity is discussed in Chapter 35, and exercise and diet for hyperlipidemia are discussed in Chapters 34 and 33 respectively. In diabetes, approaches to nutritional management have evolved with increased emphasis on individualizing each regimen and incorporating the expertise of a registered dietitian who is knowledgeable about medical nutrition therapy into any diabetes care team.[2] Overall recommendations related to carbohydrates have been liberalized so that simple sugars are no longer proscribed and total grams of carbohydrates consumed are emphasized. Thus, actual amounts of specific foods depend on an assessment of each person's food habits, weight, lipid levels, and management regimen (insulin, oral hypoglycemic, diet).[2] There is debate, however, regarding the most appropriate distribution of carbohydrate versus fat for people with increased levels of triglycerides and very–low-density lipoprotein, especially in those who are obese. Some recommend a moderate increase in monounsaturates with more limited carbohydrates because a high-carbohydrate, low-fat diet may elevate postprandial blood glucose levels and both postprandial and fasting triglyceride levels while diminishing high-density lipoprotein levels in insulin-resistant people.[2] Limiting carbohydrates to as low as 40% of total calories while increasing total fat intake to as much as 45% may improve lipid levels and blood glucose control.[5]

Exercise remains a key aspect of therapy but needs to be adapted to individual needs. In people with type I diabetes and in people with type II diabetes who are being treated with insulin or glucose-lowering agents, exercise can lead to either hyperglycemia or hypoglycemia.[2] Hyperglycemia may occur when insulin levels are inadequate because counterregulatory hormones are produced, elevating glucose and ketone levels. On the other hand, if exogenous insulin is present, it may attenuate counterregulatory forces and hypoglycemia may occur. Thus, exercise must be carefully adapted to the insulin and dietary regimen.

In type II diabetes, exercise can improve insulin sensitivity and lower the need for medication. Precautions must be taken in people who have been sedentary for many years, have insensate feet or peripheral vascular insufficiency, proliferative retinopathy, or hypertension.[5] People with insensate feet need special shoes and should avoid high-impact sports.

MEDICATIONS

Approaches to drug therapy in patients with diabetes have expanded dramatically in the 1990s and allow for a more targeted approach to therapy, especially in people with type II diabetes. Hyperglycemia can be the result of not enough insulin or insulin resistance. The latter can include decreased glucose uptake and loss of inhibition of gluconeogenesis, glycogenolysis, and lipolysis. Drug therapy can now be targeted to the underlying pathologic process. A brief review of these agents is provided in the following sections. By combining agents, adequate glycemic control often can be achieved more readily and with fewer side effects.

Insulin. Insulin is essential in type I diabetes and a frequent approach to achieving glycemic control in type II. A range of insulins is available, although Eli Lilly and Company stopped making Iletin I, mixed beef–pork insulin, in late 1998.[24] Thus, human insulin has become the main source of insulin.

With intensive management, people with type I diabetes use frequent injections or an insulin pump, which allows for adjustments to fit more closely each person's lifestyle. The newest form of insulin, Lispro, is a short-acting insulin (onset 5 minutes, peak 0.5 to 1 hour, duration 3 hours) that can be taken immediately before eating.[4] The advantage of this short-acting insulin in adults is greater flexibility regarding eating because it can be taken immediately rather than one half-hour before a meal, results in a postprandial insulin pattern resembling that seen in nondiabetic people, and leaves less insulin systemically between meals to cause hypoglycemia. Lispro is not indicated for everyone; in people with gastroparesis and delayed food absorption or in those who eat very slowly, a rapidly acting insulin can cause hypoglycemia.

Oral Glucose-Lowering Drugs.

SULFONYLUREAS. Sulfonylureas continue to play an important role in the treatment of type II diabetes and work mainly by stimulating the release of second-phase insulin from the pancreas. They exert their effect by closing adenosine triphosphate (ATP)-sensitive potassium channels in the beta-cell membrane, causing depolarization and the influx of calcium, which in turn triggers the release of insulin.[32,37] Both first-generation (chlorpropamide, tolbutamide) and second-generation (glyburide, glipizide) agents have similar actions. Selection of an agent should be based on its individual profile and the needs of a given patient. Long-acting agents, especially chlorpropamide, should be avoided in the elderly.[37] Scheen[62] notes that the maximum effect of these agents is usually reached at lower doses than previously assumed.

Major side effects of sulfonylureas are related to their insulin-stimulating properties and include hypoglycemia and weight gain, the latter of which can be a problem in patients whose condition is strongly related to their weight. There is concern that sulfonylureas have negative cardiovascular effects because of an early study using tolbutamide. There may be a physiologic basis for a negative effect because these agents close the ATP-sensitive potassium channel nonspecifically, thus affecting those channels in the cardiovascular system as well as the pancreas.[66] Opening of these channels during ischemia is considered cardioprotective, and thus their closure could potentially prevent a normal vasodilatory response. However, there appear to be few clinical data supporting a negative effect, and other data suggest positive cardioprotective benefits.[32,54] In addition, a newer sulfonylurea derivative, glimepiride (Amaryl; Hoechst-Marion Roussel, Kansas City, MO), influences receptors only in the pancreas.[54,66]

BIGUINIDES. The only biguinide available for use, metformin (Glucophage; Bristol-Myers Squibb, Princeton, NJ), lowers glucose mainly through its effect on hepatic glucose production; it is not effective in the absence of insulin.[32,62] It may also influence gut absorption of glucose and peripheral resistance, but these actions do not appear to be its main benefit. Metformin usually has a positive effect on weight and lipid levels and may be the drug of choice in obese patients. As monotherapy, metformin does not cause hypoglycemia, but it can when used concurrently with other glucose-lowering drugs. Side effects of metformin are mainly gastrointestinal complaints, including dyspepsia, anorexia, diarrhea, and a metallic taste.

Of greatest concern is the rare occurrence of lactic acidosis. This, although infrequent, can be fatal. It usually occurs in people who have contraindications to metformin's use: diminished renal or hepatic function, respiratory or cardiac failure, and alcohol abuse.[32,62] Metformin should not be used in people with serum creatine levels of 1.3mg/dL in women or 1.5mg/dL for men. However, serum creatinine is less reliable in older people because of a decrease in lean body mass (less creatinine production) that is concurrent with a decline in renal function. Thus, the creatinine clearance, an assessment of glomerular filtration rate, is a better tool to assess renal function in the elderly before considering the use of this drug. Metformin is not recommended when the glomerular filtration rate is less than 60 mL/min.[44]

Metformin is also usually contraindicated in conditions that predispose to acidosis, such as decreased circulation, and should be withheld before surgery or studies involving the use of iodinated contrast materials.[53,62] The manufacturer recommends that metformin be withheld 48 hours before any radiologic procedures using iodinated contrast materials and not resumed until 48 hours after the procedure and after renal function has been reevaluated.[53] However, guidelines proposed by Laboratory Performance Standards Committee of the Society for Cardiac Angiography and Interventions suggest that if renal function is normal and metformin has been taken within the past 48 hours, the study may not necessarily have to be postponed, but the patient should be well hydrated with intravenous fluids to minimize the likelihood of renal failure.[35] After the procedure, renal function should be reassessed before metformin is resumed. In people with abnormal renal function, elective procedures should be postponed, whereas emergent or urgent cases require individual assessment of the risks and benefits and, if the procedure is done, adequate precautions must be used.[35] The assessment of renal function is thus essential in all cases.

α-GLUCOSIDASE INHIBITORS. Acarbose (Precose; Bayer Corporation, West Haven, CT), and the recently released Miglitol (Glyset, Pharmacia & Upjohn, Bridgewater, NJ) are relatively new additions to the therapeutic approaches to diabetes management. α-Glucosidase inhibitors delay the absorption of carbohydrates in the gut by inhibiting enzymes that lead to their breakdown into monosaccharides.[5,62] This effectively decreases the postprandial rise in blood sugar levels. Like metformin, these agents would not cause hypoglycemia when used as monotherapy, but have less of a glucose-lowering effect by themselves than other agents.

The major side effects of α-glucosidase inhibitors are gastrointestinal and include flatulence and diarrhea. Starting at very low doses and increasing gradually facilitates adaptation. Although generally safe if used in conjunction with other agents that can lead to hypoglycemia, treatment of hypoglycemia must include glucose and not sucrose, because the latter is blocked by the drug's action.[10,53] In addition, over-the-counter agents such as Beano, an α-glucosidase that is used for relief of flatulence, effectively replaces the substance that is being inhibited. In addition, these agents are usually contraindicated in people with inflammatory bowel disease, colonic ulceration, or partial intestinal obstruction.[5,53] Additional agents in this class will soon be marketed.

THIAZOLIDINEDIONES. Troglitazone (Rezulin; Parke-Davis, Morris Plains, NJ), another recently released substance, works by increasing insulin sensitivity in skeletal muscle, liver tissue, and adipose tissue.[38] Troglitazone is generally well tolerated, with fluid retention and weight gain the main adverse effects in human trials.[5] However, a more serious adverse reaction that has caused greater concern since its release is liver toxicity, which, although apparently occurring in only a small number of people, has resulted in cases of liver failure and death.[38] Thus, new guidelines emphasize that liver function (liver enzymes and bilirubin) should be assessed before starting troglitazone, then every month for 6 months, then every other month for the remainder of the first year, and then periodically thereafter.[3,38] In addition, findings that related drugs may cause cardiac changes in animals and increased plasma volume in humans have led some to recommend caution in the use of this medication in people with cardiac disease, especially New York Heart Association class III or IV heart failure.[3,38] A potentially safer alternative, Rosiglitazone maleate (Avandia, SmithKline Beecham, Philadelphia, PA) was just released.

MEGLITINIDES. Repaglinide (Prandin; Novo/Nordisk Pharmaceuticals, Princeton, NJ), a member of a new class of oral beta-cell stimulators, the meglitinides, is another very recent addition.[15] Considered a nonsulfonylurea hypoglycemic,[60] repaglinide stimulates insulin release by attaching to a different part of the ATP-sensitive potassium channel. Repaglinide is also more glucose dependent than other agents; that is, it augments the secretion of insulin in a glucose-dependent fashion, but not when insulin is absent.[15] Its onset of action is rapid and its half-life is short (<1 hour), so it is taken with each meal. This may promote more flexibility and limit the risk of hypoglycemia between meals. In addition, because it is excreted mainly through the gastrointestinal system as a bile product and not through the kidneys, it may be a safer agent in people with renal insufficiency.[15] However, because it is metabolized by the cytochrome P-450 enzyme system 34A, it has the potential to interact with agents using the same pathway.[15] Because it is newly available, there are few data on its long-term effects, although data reported from clinical trials suggest that the adverse events are comparable with those associated with sulfonylureas.[15]

HEALTH SCREENING AND MONITORING

Because diabetes is a chronic condition that increases the risk for many complications, ongoing health care maintenance and diabetes monitoring are key elements in therapy. Routine health maintenance activities, including immunizations and health screening, should be addressed. In addition to using aspirin therapy as a secondary prevention strategy in people with macrovascular disease, low-dose aspirin therapy is recommended as a primary prevention strategy in both men and women with diabetes who have cardiac risk factors.[2] The use of the antioxidant vitamin E is also supported. In women, estrogen therapy should be discussed with perimenopausal and postmenopausal women.

SUMMARY

Diabetes mellitus is a complex, heterogeneous chronic condition that contributes significantly to individual morbidity and mortality as well as to health care costs. At the same time, data are continuing to accumulate that support the positive benefits of glycemic control and cardiovascular risk reduction, and new treatment modalities allow a more targeted approach to the underlying pathophysiologic abnormalities. Because diabetes can occur at any time across the life span, may require many lifestyle changes, and involves multiple organ systems, its management necessitates a comprehensive multidisciplinary approach that includes the patient and his or her family.

REFERENCES

1. Alzaid A, Rizza RA: Insulin resistance and its role in the pathogenesis of impaired glucose tolerance and non-insulin dependent diabetes mellitus. In Moller DE (ed): Insulin Resistance, pp 143–186. New York, John Wiley & Sons, 1993
2. American Diabetes Association: Clinical practice recommendations 1998. Diabetes Care 21 (Suppl 1): 53–590, 1998
3. American Diabetes Association: Economic consequences of diabetes mellitus in the U.S. in 1997. Diabetes Care 21: 296–309, 1998
4. American Diabetes Association: Medical Management of Type 1 Diabetes, 3rd ed. Alexandria, VA, American Diabetes Association, 1998
5. American Diabetes Association: Medical Management of Type 2 Diabetes, 4th ed. Alexandria, VA, American Diabetes Association, 1998
6. Amos AF, McCarty DJ, Zimmet P: The rising global burden of diabetes and its complications: Estimates and projections to the year 2020. Diabet Med 14 (Suppl 5): S1–S5, 1997
7. Atherogenesis in Diabetes: The Clinical Benefit of Lipid-Lowering Therapy. Houston, TX, Baylor College of Medicine, December, 1997
8. Atkinson MA, Maclaren NK: The pathogenesis of insulin-dependent diabetes mellitus. N Engl J Med 331: 1428–1436, 1994
9. Baba T, Neugebauer S, Watanabe T: Diabetic nephropathy: Its relationship to hypertension and means of pharmacological intervention. Drugs 54: 197–234, 1997
10. Balfour JA, McTavish D: Acarbose: An update of its pharmacology and therapeutic use in diabetes mellitus. Drugs 46: 1025–1054, 1993
11. Bennett PH, Rewers MJ, Knowler WC: Epidemiology of diabetes mellitus. In Porte D, Sherwin RS (eds): Ellenberg and Rifkin's Diabetes Mellitus, 5th ed, pp 373–400. Stamford, CT, Appleton & Lange, 1997
12. Bennett PH: Definition, diagnosis, and classification of diabetes mellitus and impaired glucose tolerance. In Kahn CR, Weir, GC (eds): Joslin's Diabetes Mellitus, 13th ed, pp 193–200. Philadelphia, Lea & Febiger, 1994
13. Berg TJ, Bangstad HJ, Torjesen PA et al: Advanced glycation end products in serum predict changes in kidney morphology of patients with insulin dependent diabetes mellitus. Metabolism: Clinical and Experimental 46: 661–665, 1997
14. Brownlee M: Advanced products of nonenzymatic glycosylation and the pathogenesis of diabetic complications. In Porte D, Sherwin RS (eds): Ellenberg and Rifkin's Diabetes Mellitus, 5th ed, pp 229–245. Stamford, CT, Appleton & Lange, 1997
15. Brodows R: Repaglinide (Prandin): A new therapy for type 2 diabetes. Practical Diabetology 17(2): 32–36, 1998

16. Carter M: New Medicare law will help seniors pay for supplies and education. Diabetes Forecast 51(8): 43–45, 1998
17. Centers for Disease Control and Prevention: Diabetes Surveillance. Atlanta, U.S. Department of Health and Human Services, 1997
18. Cohen JA, Jeffers BW, Faldut D et al: Risks for sensorimotor peripheral neuropathy and autonomic neuropathy in non-insulin-dependent diabetes mellitus (NIDDM). Muscle Nerve 21: 72–80, 1998
19. Cryer PE, Gerich JE: Hypoglycemia in insulin dependent diabetes mellitus. In Porte D, Sherwin RS (eds): Ellenberg and Rifkin's Diabetes Mellitus, 5th ed, pp 745–760. Stamford, CT, Appleton & Lange, 1997
20. Cook DL, Taborsky GJ: B-cell function and insulin secretion. In Porte D, Sherwin RS (eds): Ellenberg and Rifkin's Diabetes Mellitus, 5th ed, pp 49–73. Stamford, CT, Appleton & Lange, 1997
21. Dagogo-Jack S, Santiago JV: Pathophysiology of type 2 diabetes and modes of action of therapeutic interventions. Arch Intern Med 157: 1802–1917, 1997
22. Dejgaard A: Pathophysiology and treatment of diabetic neuropathy. Diabet Med 15: 97–112, 1998
23. Docherty K, Steiner DF: Molecular and cellular biology of the beta cell. In Porte D, Sherwin RS (eds): Ellenberg and Rifkin's Diabetes Mellitus, 5th ed, pp 29–48. Stamford, CT, Appleton & Lange, 1997
24. Eli Lilly and Company: Deletion of all Iletin I (mixed beef–pork insulins) (Letter). May 15, 1998
25. Enck P, Frieling T: Pathophysiology of diabetic gastroparesis. Diabetes 46 (Suppl 2): S77–S81, 1997
26. Fedele D, Giugliano D: Peripheral diabetic neuropathy: Current recommendations and future prospects for its prevention and management. Drugs 54: 414–421, 1998
27. Forrester JV, Knott M: Pathogenesis of diabetic retinopathy and cataract. In Pickup JC, Williams G (eds): Textbook of Diabetes, vol 2, 2nd ed, pp 45.1–45.19. Oxford, Blackwell, 1997
28. Giardino I, Brownlee M: The biochemical basis of microvascular disease. In Pickup JC, Williams G (eds): Textbook of Diabetes, vol 1, 2nd ed, pp 42.1–42.16. Oxford, Blackwell, 1997
29. Gray RP, Yudkin JS: Cardiovascular disease in diabetes mellitus. In Pickup JC, Williams G (eds): Textbook of Diabetes, vol 2, 2nd ed, pp 57.1–55.22. Oxford, Blackwell, 1997
30. Green A, Sjolie AK, Eshoj O: Insulin-dependent diabetes mellitus. In Pickup JC, Williams G (eds): Textbook of Diabetes, vol 1, 2nd ed, pp 3.1–3.16. Oxford, Blackwell, 1997
31. Greene DA, Feldman EL, Stevens MJ et al: Diabetic neuropathy. In Porte D, Sherwin RS (eds): Ellenberg and Rifkin's Diabetes Mellitus, 5th ed, pp 1009–1076. Stamford, CT, Appleton & Lange, 1997
32. Groop LC: Drug treatment of non-insulin-dependent diabetes mellitus. In Pickup JC, Williams G (eds): Textbook of Diabetes, vol 1, 2nd ed, pp 38.1–38.18. Oxford, Blackwell, 1997
33. Harris MI, Flegal KM, Cowie CC et al: Prevalence of diabetes, impaired fasting glucose, and impaired glucose tolerance in U.S. adults. Diabetes Care 21: 518–524, 1998
34. Hennekens CH: Risk factors for coronary heart disease in women. Cardiol Clin 16: 1–8, 1998
35. Heupler FA: Guidelines for performing angiography in patients taking Metformin. Cathet Cardiovasc Diagn 43: 121–123, 1998
36. Iltz JL, White JR: Clinical management of hyperlipidemia in diabetic patients. Diabetes Spectrum 11(2): 88–93, 1998
37. Jennings PE: Oral antihyperglycaemics: Considerations in older patients with non-insulin-dependent diabetes mellitus. Drugs Aging 10: 323–331, 1997

38. Johnson MD, Campbell LK, Campbell RK: Troglitazone: Review and assessment of its role in the treatment of patients with impaired glucose tolerance and diabetes mellitus. Ann Pharmacother 32: 337–348, 1998

39. Kahn SE, Porte D: The pathophysiology of type II (non-insulin-dependent diabetes mellitus): Implications for treatment. In Porte D, Sherwin RS (eds): Ellenberg and Rifkin's Diabetes Mellitus, 5th ed, pp 487–512. Stamford, CT, Appleton & Lange, 1997

40. Kaplan NM: Hypertension and diabetes. In Porte D, Sherwin RS (eds): Ellenberg and Rifkin's Diabetes Mellitus, 5th ed, pp 1097–1104. Stamford, CT, Appleton & Lange, 1997

41. Klein R: Epidemiology of diabetic eye disease. In Pickup JC, Williams G (eds): Textbook of Diabetes, vol 2, 2nd ed, pp 44.1–44.9. Oxford, Blackwell, 1997

42. Kristal BS, Yu BP: An emerging hypothesis: Synergistic induction of aging by free radicals and Maillard reactions. J Gerontol Biol Sci 47: B107–B114, 1992

43. Lapuz MHS: Diabetic nephropathy. Med Clin North Am 81: 679–688, 1997

44. Lorber DL: Metformin: A "new" drug for type II diabetes. Practical Diabetology 14(2): 8–12, 1995

45. Lorber DL: Redefining diabetes. Practical Diabetology 16(3): 19–24, 1997

46. McCance DR, Hanson RL, Pettitt DJ et al: Diagnosing diabetes mellitus: Do we need new criteria? Diabetologia 40: 247–255, 1997

47. Molitch ME: Complications of diabetes mellitus and implications for nutrition therapy. In Powers MA(ed): Handbook of Diabetes Medical Nutrition, pp 15–30. Gaithersburg, MD, Aspen Publishers, Inc., 1996

48. National Diabetes Education Initiative: How important is insulin resistance? Issues 2(1): 1, 3–4, 1998

49. Odetti P, Traverso N, Cosso L et al: Good glycaemic control reduces oxidation and glycation end-products in collagen of diabetic rats. Diabetologia 39: 1440–1447, 1996

50. Ouellette SM: Diabetes mellitus: Overview and current concepts in anesthetic management. AANA 66: 65–76, 1998

51. Pacifici RE, Davies KJA: Protein, lipid and DNA repair systems in oxidative stress: The free-radical theory of aging revisited. Gerontology 37: 166–180, 1991

52. Peragallo-Dittko V: A Core Curriculum for Diabetes Education, 2nd ed. Chicago, American Association of Diabetes Educators, 1993

53. Physician's Desk Reference. Montvale, NJ, Medical Economics, 1998

54. Pogátsa G: What kind of cardiovascular alterations could be influenced positively by oral antidiabetic agents? Diabetes Res Clin Pract 31(Suppl): S27–S31, 1996

55. Raffel LJ, Scheuner MT, Rotter JI: Genetics of diabetes. In Porte D, Sherwin RS (eds): Ellenberg and Rifkin's Diabetes Mellitus, 5th ed, pp 401–454. Stamford, CT, Appleton & Lange, 1997

56. Reaven GM: Pathophysiology of insulin resistance in human disease. Physiol Rev 75: 473–486, 1995

57. Reichard P: To be a teacher, a tutor and a friend: The physician's role according to the Stockholm Diabetes Intervention Study (SDIS). Patient Education and Counseling 29: 231–235, 1996

58. Reusch JE-B: Focus on insulin resistance in type 2 diabetes: Therapeutic implications. Diabetes Educator 24: 188–193, 1998

59. Trevisan R, Barnes DJ, Gian Carlo V: Pathogensis of diabetic nephropathy. In Pickup JC, Williams G (eds): Textbook of Diabetes, 2nd ed, vol 2, pp 52.1–52.12, Cambridge, MA, Blackwell Science, Inc., 1997

60. Rodeen LM, Baker DE, Campbell RK: New treatments for patients with diabetes. Diabetes Spectrum 11(1): 18–25, 1998

61. Ryan CM: Psychological factors and diabetes mellitus. In Pickup JC, Williams G (eds): Textbook of Diabetes, vol 2, 2nd ed, pp 66.1–66.17. Oxford, Blackwell, 1997

62. Scheen AJ: Drug treatment of non-insulin-dependent diabetes mellitus in the 1990s. Drugs 54: 355–368, 1997

63. Seely BL, Olefsky JM: Potential cellular and genetic mechanisms for insulin resistance in the common disorders of diabetes and obesity. In Moller DE (ed): Insulin Resistance, pp 187–252. New York, John Wiley & Sons, 1993

64. Kruszynska, YT: Normal metabolism: The physiology of fuel homeostatis. In Pickup JC, Williams G (eds): Textbook of Diabetes, 2nd ed, Vol 1, pp 11.1–11.37. Cambridge, MA, Blackwell Science, Inc., 1997

65. Skyler JS: Relationship of glycemic control to diabetic complications. In Porte D, Sherwin RS (eds): Ellenberg and Rifkin's Diabetes Mellitus, 5th ed, pp 1235–1254. Stamford, CT, Appleton & Lange, 1997

66. Smits P, Bijlstra PJ, Russel FGM et al: Cardiovascular effects of sulfonylurea derivatives. Diabetes Res Clin Pract 31(Suppl): S55–S59, 1996

67. Stachura ME: Pathophysiology. In Powers MA (ed): Handbook of Diabetes Medical Nutrition Therapy, pp 3–14. Gaithersburg, MD, Aspen, 1996

68. Steinberg D: Diabetes and atherosclerosis. In Porte D, Sherwin RS (eds): Ellenberg and Rifkin's Diabetes Mellitus, 5th ed, pp 193–206. Stamford, CT, Appleton & Lange, 1997

69. Stowig S, Raskin P: Intensive management of insulin-dependent diabetes mellitus. In Porte D & Sherwin RS (eds), Ellenberg and Rifkin's Diabetes Mellitus, 5th ed, pp 709–743. Stamford, CT, Appleton & Lange, 1997

70. Stumvoll M, Meyer C, Mitrakou A et al: Renal glucose production and utilization: New aspects in humans. Diabetologia 40: 749–757, 1997

71. The Diabetes Control and Complications Trail Research Group: The effect of intensive treatment of diabetes on the development and progression of long-term complications in insulin-dependent diabetes mellitus. N Engl J Med 329: 977–986, 1993

72. Ward JD, Tesfaye S: Pathogenesis of diabetic neuropathy. In Pickup JC, Williams G (eds): Textbook of Diabetes, vol 2, 2nd ed, pp 49.1–49.19. Oxford, Blackwell, 1997

73. Watkins PJ, Edmonds ME: Clinical features of diabetic neuropathy. In Pickup JC, Williams G (eds): Textbook of Diabetes, vol 2, 2nd ed, pp 50.1–50.20. Oxford, Blackwell, 1997

74. Williams G, Wilding J: The central nervous system in diabetes mellitus. In Pickup JC, Williams G (eds): Textbook of Diabetes, vol 2, 2nd ed, pp 65.1–65.30. Oxford, Blackwell, 1997

75. Ying W: Deleterious network hypothesis of aging. Med Hypothesis 48: 143–148, 1997

37

Adherence
to Cardiovascular
Treatment Regimens

LORA E. BURKE*

The terms *adherence* and *compliance* are used interchangeably in the literature, and are used similarly in this chapter. Traditionally, the definition of compliance given by Sackett and Haynes[1] in 1976 has been used, which is "the extent to which patient's behavior (in terms of taking medications, following diets, or exercising other life-style changes) coincides with the clinical prescription." More recently, adherence was defined as a partnership between the health care provider and patient, the goal of this relationship being to ensure that the patient is as self-sufficient in managing his or her health as possible.[2] The latter definition emphasizes the mutual responsibility of the patient and provider and reinforces the provider's commitment to enable the patient to implement the recommended treatment.[3]

This chapter reviews the problem of nonadherence and its significance in the management of the cardiac patient. Methods used to assess adherence across the behaviors of medication taking, dietary self-management, following an exercise program, and smoking cessation are reviewed. Strategies to enhance adherence are discussed and guidelines for implementing educational and behavioral strategies are provided.

SIGNIFICANCE OF NONADHERENCE

A number of pharmacologic therapies are used in the acute and chronic management of cardiovascular disease. However, the extent to which these therapies are effective can be influenced by the patient's adherence to the treatment regimen.[4] Because of increased awareness and treatment of high blood pressure, improved management of hypertension has been demonstrated. However, because of poor

adherence, only one fifth of known hypertensive patients are controlled.[5] An earlier report suggested that it would be more cost effective to remediate the poor adherers than to identify new cases of hypertension.[6,7] Similarly, inadequate adherence is a factor in not realizing the benefits demonstrated in clinical trials of lipid-lowering therapy. Andrade and colleagues[8] reported a 15% discontinuation rate with lovastatin and a 37% discontinuation rate with gemfibrozil, whereas Simons and colleagues[9] reported that 56% of those prescribed HMG CoA reductase inhibitors and 78% of those prescribed gemfibrozil had discontinued the drugs within 12 months. Rates of adherence to cholestyramine or niacin are lower, with approximately 20% using the drugs at 12 months.[5,8] These examples illustrate how medication nonadherence is a major health problem, the magnitude of which is underscored by a report that 50% of the 3 billion prescriptions written each year are followed incorrectly.[10] Despite ongoing research on medication compliance, this figure has not improved since the 1980s.[11] Nonadherence is observed in regimens affecting lifestyle as well.

Compliance with structured exercise programs has been low, and approximately 50% of patients discontinue participation in cardiac rehabilitation within the first year.[12,13] Smoking cessation rates at 1 year are still low at 62%, but with the addition of nicotine replacement therapy, increase to 67%.[14,15] Wing[16] reported that participants regain approximately one third of their achieved weight loss at 1 year post-treatment, and most return to their baseline weight at 3 years, suggesting an abandonment of the behaviors that facilitated the weight loss. These early rates of adherence are predictive of adherence behavior over the long term.[4,17,18]

The duration of treatment is usually a factor influencing compliance, with an initial decline in adherence observed in the first year followed by a gradual decline over time.[4,19] This pattern was observed in the dietary changes made by participants in the Lipid Research Clinic–Coronary Primary Prevention Trial (LRC-CPPT).[20,21] Moreover, it is observed

*The author was supported by grant Hl07560.

repeatedly among those participating in cardiac rehabilitation programs and in the maintenance phase of weight loss programs.[4] The prevention and treatment of cardiovascular disease requires ongoing management of lifestyle habits and, increasingly, inclusion of pharmacologic therapy such as aspirin, hypolipidemic agents, and hormone replacement therapy. In the absence of sustained adherence, the benefits of prevention or treatment cannot be realized.

In the clinical arena, nonadherence at any point in the treatment continuum poses a threat to satisfactory outcomes. Medication noncompliance has been associated with increased risk of coronary heart disease, precipitated episodes of heart failure, and late organ rejection among heart transplant recipients.[11,22,23] These reports emphasize the mediating effects of compliance on clinical outcome, and the impact nonadherence can have on morbidity and mortality associated with cardiovascular disease regardless of when it occurs in the treatment continuum.

In the research arena, noncompliance affects therapy evaluation before its introduction into the clinical setting. Incomplete adherence to the treatment under study underestimates its efficacy, and the diminished effect observed reduces the study's power.[4] Furthermore, nonadherence to the treatment protocol may mask side effects or result in an overestimation of optimal dosage.[4] Finally, intermittent or varying adherence to the study protocol may reflect varying adherence to concomitantly prescribed therapeutic modalities, which may affect study outcomes.[24]

A review of international studies indicated that rates of compliance are similar across countries.[4] Moreover, compliance threatens effective prevention of heart disease as well as clinical outcomes across the disease continuum. Because the aggregate sample of the 45 studies of adults included in the review was 90% white and 85% male, little is known about women's and minorities' adherence behavior. Differences in sex are seldom reported. One study reported that women had better dietary adherence,[25] which has also been shown in cross-sectional studies.[26] In the Multiple Risk Factor Intervention Trial (MRFIT), black participants' rates of attendance, smoking cessation, and dietary change were comparable with those of white participants.[27] Clearly, much needs to be learned about adherence behavior across cultures, sex, and age groups.

METHODS OF MEASUREMENT

Assessment of adherence needs to be incorporated into each clinical encounter.[3] It is important that the clinician separate adherence from therapeutic or clinical outcome, which can be affected by a myriad of variables besides adherence. For example, inadequate control of blood pressure or cholesterol may be due to inadequate drug dosage, individual variation in pharmacokinetic factors of different drugs, daytime or seasonal variations in measurement values, or personal factors.[3,28,29] Conversely, the absence of symptoms or achievement of goal does not confirm adherence. Clinical outcomes are indirect measures of adherence, whereas patient behavior (e.g., weight loss, exercise, taking the medication) are direct measures of adherence. Both direct and indirect measures have inherent advantages and disadvantages.[29] Unfortunately, it is difficult to measure behavior directly, and thus there is a great reliance on self-reported behavior. Table 37-1 summarizes the numerous measurement methods and the advantages and disadvantages to their use.

Adherence assessment can be conducted through numerous methods. However, a weakness common to all forms of measurement is a bias toward overestimation of adherence.[3] One of the reasons for this measurement error is that the period being measured is usually not representative of the patient's usual behavior. Research has shown that patients' adherence varies in relation to the clinical appointment, with adherence increasing immediately before and after the visit.[30] Thus, when the patient is asked to report on his or her behavior, the report may be influenced by the recall of most recent behavior and overestimate adherence for the longer period.[3,28] A variety of measurement methods are available for clinical use. These include self-report, biologic and electronic measures, pill counts, and records such as pharmacy refills.

Self-Report Measures

Self-report measures consist of interviews, structured questionnaires, and diaries. This form of adherence assessment is used most frequently, which is probably explained by its ease of administration and low cost.

Interviews, often used in the research setting to assess adherence behavior at each contact, can easily be conducted in the clinical setting. Two brief interview scales were developed to assess global medication compliance among hypertensive patients. The four-item scale developed by Morisky and colleagues[31] pertains to areas of omission, such as forgetting, being careless, and stopping the medication when feeling better or when feeling worse. This scale, for which adequate psychometric properties have been reported, has been used in minority and general populations to assess patient understanding as well as medication adherence.[31] Shea and colleagues[32] adapted Morisky's scale by making minor modifications in the wording and adding a fifth item, which asked if the blood pressure medication was ever missed for any reason. Again, adequate psychometric properties were demonstrated in a sample comprising predominantly blacks and Hispanics.

Adherence can also be ascertained through a 7-day recall interview by asking the patient to report the number of pills and the times at which these were taken for each day of the week before the visit. However, these tend to provide an overestimation of adherence.[33,34] When comparing self-reported interview adherence to electronic measured adherence, Dunbar-Jacob and colleagues[33] found 97% adherence reported in the interview compared with 84% adherence measured by an unobtrusive electronic event monitor.

Dietary behavior may be assessed through 24-hour recall interviews or through the lengthier diet history interview. Assessing dietary adherence requires a determination of what the person eats and the degree to which the food intake approximates the recommended diet.[3] The interview allows more exact descriptions of foods (e.g., brands, degree of fat modification). It also requires interviewer skill at eliciting detail and cooperation on the part of the patient.

TABLE 37-1	Methods of Adherence Measurement and Features of Their Use		
Measurement Method	**Behavior***	**Advantages**	**Disadvantages**
Self-report			
Interview	All behaviors	Inexpensive, provides details	Overreports adherence
24-Hour recall	All behaviors	Increased accuracy because of short recall period	Underrepresentation of time may increase bias if recall day is atypical
Questionnaire	All behaviors	Numerous scales available, does not influence behavior	Requires literacy, may be lengthy, needs to be sensitive and appropriate to age, sex and ethnic group
Diaries	All behaviors	Provides detail of circumstances of behavior	May influence the behavior, may under- or overreport, requires cooperation of patient
Biologic outcomes (serum, urine, or saliva level of drug or its metabolite)	All behaviors	May provide a validation of behavior	Are indirect measures of adherence; measure adherence only close to time of measurement
Electronic monitors (electronic event monitors, heart rate monitors, accelerometers, diaries)	Medication taking, exercise, smoking cessation, pain control	Provides detailed pattern of adherence, provides data on unsupervised exercise; diaries provide data on adherence to recording protocol	Cost prohibits widespread use, use of the device may influence behavior
Pill counts	Medication taking	Inexpensive, easy to conduct	Overestimates, does not provide pattern of adherence
Pharmacy records	Medication taking	Provides another source of adherence data	Not available universally, requires use of pharmacy, does not provide adherence pattern

*Medication taking, eating, exercise, smoking cessation.

A benefit of the 24-hour recall is that there is increased accuracy because of the shortened recall period, but a disadvantage is that there may be increased bias if the recall is conducted for days on which the eating pattern may vary, such as a weekend or the day before a clinic visit.[35] The 24-hour recall is usually limited to population-based studies because 1 day's intake is unlikely to be representative of a person's usual intake.[36,37] The purpose of the food history is to obtain a detailed description of food consumption over an extended period, including an assessment of normative as well as divergent eating patterns.[38] Validity of this method is threatened by the potential of generalizing recent behavior to long-term behavior, and the person's faulty ability to recall food intake.[3] Dietary interviews in the Framingham Study, separated by 2 years, showed close agreement across macronutrients.[39] A good example of a food history format is the Block Health Habits and History Questionnaire, for which software for analysis purposes is available.[38]

Adherence to exercise regimens may also be assessed through interviews. Unlike medication adherence, when 7-day recall interviews for exercise were compared with electronically monitored heart rate and motion detector data, there was 94% agreement between the measures.[40] However, Dishman and colleagues[41] reported that self-reports of free-living physical activity and social cognitive variables did not generalize to physical activity estimated by electromechanical accelerometer. Exercise poses an additional challenge because of the multiple dimensions to measure (e.g., aerobic capacity, strength, flexibility, and caloric expenditure).[3]

Questionnaires are available to assess adherence across multiple behaviors. Although there are numerous scales available for assessment of eating and exercise behaviors, few exist for medication-taking behavior. The Morisky scale was used as a questionnaire among patients treated for hypercholesterolemia. Used in this format, the scale demonstrated adequate psychometric properties.[42]

Dietary adherence can be measured by several established questionnaires, including the Connor Diet Habit Survey,[43] the Eating Pattern Questionnaire,[44] a Dietary and Risk Factor Questionnaire,[45] and the Willett[46,47] or Block Food Frequency Questionnaires.[48] The first two questionnaires focus on fat intake and have reported psychometric properties when used in cardiac and general populations.[43,44] Food frequency questionnaires, which typically have precoded forms, are usually used in epidemiologic studies, for which they are extremely practical and inexpensive to score.[47] They are best used for averaging long-term diet and for ranking intake of particular food or food groups.[49] Their limitation is the number and types of items listed, which reduces their utility among ethnic groups.[3,46] Good reliability and validity of the questionnaires have been established.[49]

Measurement of physical activity has received the most attention in the public health field, which has relied primarily on the questionnaire.[13,41] The exercise assessment questionnaires, which are subjective measures, have been validated by objective measures of physical activity, such as measures of total energy expenditure (doubly labeled water), estimates of physical fitness (heart rate), or measures of physical motion by accelerometers.[50] A beneficial trait of the questionnaire is that it does not influence the behavior being measured, and although less precise than the objective measures, it estimates activity in relative to others in the population. The questionnaire may range from one item to an array of questions covering a wide range of occupational and leisure activities, and may cover varying time intervals. A compilation of physical activity questionnaires and a review of their psychometric properties has been published, providing an excellent resource for anyone wishing to measure exercise adherence.[51] In selecting a questionnaire, the investigator must consider characteristics of the population, such as sex, age, culture, and the outcome of interest. Most of the activity questionnaires were developed with men's activities in mind, so they may be less sensitive to differences in physical activity levels in women.[50]

In summary, questionnaires with a shorter time interval are less vulnerable to recall bias and easier to validate with objective measures. However, using a shorter time frame reduces the likelihood of obtaining a picture of usual behavior, because eating and exercise patterns may vary by season. Reliability and validity are affected by the person's ability to store and retrieve information, and by potential influence of the interviewer or respondent bias.[50]

Diaries

Daily diaries for food intake or exercise circumvent the bias of recall, but require training and cooperation of the patient or study participant. Little data are available on the utility or acceptability of diaries as assessment tools. Food and exercise diaries are often used periodically and cover a 3- or 7-day period, including one nonwork or leisure day. Recording for extended periods (i.e., over 3 days) may reduce accuracy, and the recording may begin to influence the recorder's behavior.

To summarize, self-report measures are common, easy to use, and inexpensive. Moreover, they provide information on the circumstances surrounding the good or poor adherence. Issues of concern with self-report measures include deliberate and nondeliberate errors in recall or reporting; for example, one study reported that a group of obese subjects underreported their food consumption and overreported their energy expenditure.[52] Staff should be trained on how to teach participants to record the information, and potential problems with memory and social desirability need to be reduced.[3,53] For example, recording the behavior immediately reduces forgetting and conveying an expectation of a full range of behaviors may help reduce less than truthful reports.

Biologic Measures

Adherence is often reported in terms of biologic end points, such as serum cholesterol or glycosylated hemoglobin level. Other biologic assays frequently used include serum, urine, or saliva level of a drug or its metabolites. Examples include medication adherence measured by serum digoxin level, dietary adherence measured by urine sodium, smoking cessation by serum or saliva thiocyanate or cotinine, and exercise by direct or indirect calorimetry and maximal oxygen uptake.[3,4] Doubly labeled water, a procedure that requires the subject to ingest water enriched with ^{18}O and ^2H isotopes, is the most accurate measurement of total energy expenditure available, but is too costly to be used on a widespread basis.[49] A limitation of biologic assays is that daily variability in compliance cannot be detected. Instead, they indicate if the person has been adherent close to the time of assessment and may serve as a validation of the behavior. Moreover, biologic assays may be influenced by many other factors.[4,54]

Electronic Monitoring

Technology has provided tools for ongoing and detailed assessment of adherence behavior. Electronic methods consist of bar code scanners[55] and unobtrusive electronic monitors[30] for medication use, heart rate monitors[56] and electronic motion detectors[57-59] for exercise, and electronic diaries[60-62] for symptom reporting or answering a set of programmed questions on a daily basis. Use of the bar code scanner requires that the patient scan the bottle once for each pill ingested. This allows an indication of the dose taken but requires active participation by the patient, which may influence behavior, and also depends on the patient remembering to use the scanner. The electronic or medication event monitor, which consists of an electronic chip housed inside the medication bottle cap, provides data on the day and time the medication bottle was opened, but does not provide information on the number of pills taken.[63,64] Neither of these methods guarantees the medication was consumed. Additional applications of the electronic monitor include blister pill packs, eye drop solutions, and aerosol spray nebulizers.

Exercise adherence can be measured by several devices. Heart rate monitors such as the Vitalog Corporation (Mountain View, CA), an ambulatory microprocessor that measures and sequentially stores average heart rate values, provides data on adherence to the exercise prescription.[56] In a comparison of self-reports of daily exercise with Vitalog activity recording, there was a 99% agreement rate in men and 87% in women.[56] Electronic accelerometers are motion sensors that register body accelerations and decelerations, and thus provide a direct and objective measure of movement intensity and frequency during physical activity. A correlation of 0.95 between total energy expenditure and the sum of motion from three directions[57] and a correlation of 0.88 between the accelerometer output and total daily energy expenditure as determined with doubly labeled water was reported.[65,66] Jakicic and colleagues[58] reported the first use of the Tri-Trac (Professional Products, Madison, WI) (an accelerometer that uses three planes of motion) in a clinical study and suggested there was some discrepancy in the number of exercise bouts reported by the participants and the number recorded by the accelerometer. These measures can provide patterns of exercise adherence in an unsupervised setting.

Electronic hand-held diaries are available to answer a set of programmed questions, or report symptoms or cravings *ad lib* or when prompted by a sound.[61,62,67] These monitoring devices provide the possibility of objectively measuring adherence to a recording schedule under naturalistic conditions.[61] An added benefit is that the data are directly entered by the person and later downloaded on a computer for analysis.[67] Acceptability of the hand-held computers has been reported as comparable with that of paper-and-pencil diaries. The number of days the diary was completed was 92% for the written diary and 89% for the electronic format. However, assessment times were more accurate in 92% of the electronic diaries, compared with 78% of the written diaries.[67] Innovative approaches include the use of web sites for patients to log onto and report their eating and exercise behaviors (Deborah Aaron, personal communication, 1998).

In summary, electronic monitors provide a detailed picture of the temporal pattern of adherence, from medication taking to self-reporting of symptoms. However, because of cost, the technology has limited application. In the evaluation of intervention strategies or therapeutic "failures," consideration needs to be given to the precise approximation of adherence these devices provide.[3,68]

Pill Counts and Pharmacy Refills

Unique to the assessment of medication-taking compliance, these measures provide opportunities for alternative or concurrent measurement methods. The pill count is done by tabulating pills remaining from a previous dispensing for a specific interval, and comparing that number with what should have been remaining. An adherence rate is calculated by dividing the number that should have been taken by the number prescribed and multiplying by 100. These methods tend to overestimate adherence; in one study, the pill count rate of adherence was 94%, compared with 84% for the medication event monitor.[33] In the age of managed care and large organizations filling prescriptions, pharmacy refill records are becoming commonplace.[4] The disadvantage with the pill count and pharmacy record is that they do not provide information on the pattern of adherence, which may vary in relation to several factors.[4]

In summary, ongoing assessment of adherence is important, primarily because adherence varies over time. An example is the variability of adherence in relation to the medical appointment, with adherence during the 5 days preceding the appointment averaging 88%, and 5 days after the appointment 86%, with a decline to 67% 1 month later.[69] Compliance cannot be assumed, nor can the clinician make a clinical judgment that adherence is present. Use of one or more of these various methods provides the clinician or researcher some indication of adherence and possibly some information regarding the circumstances surrounding it. In general, it is recommended that more than one method be used concurrently.

DISPLAY 37-1

Determinants of Adherence

Patient-related factors

- ◆ Prior adherence behavior
- ◆ Efficacy expectancy—perceived confidence in capability to perform behavior
- ◆ Presence of social support
- ◆ Knowledge and comprehension of treatment regimen
- ◆ Skills to implement treatment regimen
- ◆ Satisfaction with provider and care received
- ◆ Barriers to regimen implementation

Regimen-related factors

- ◆ Regimen complexity (e.g., number and frequency of medications taken, extent of lifestyle change required)
- ◆ Regimen duration

Provider-related factors

- ◆ Communication style of provider
- ◆ Attitude of provider
- ◆ Provider's teaching skills

Process-oriented factors

- ◆ Ease of arranging/receiving care (e.g., availability of appointments, waiting room time, distance and convenience of reaching clinic, parking costs, continuity of care)

DETERMINANTS OF ADHERENCE

A myriad of factors have been suggested and investigated for their association with adherence, including sociodemographic traits, psychological distress, health beliefs, benefits, and barriers.[70–72] However, many have been inconsistent in their association with adherence, and their predictive power is at best modest.[70,73] Moreover, sociodemographic factors are not remedial. However, there are several factors that are usually identified as related to adherence, and, most important, these factors can be addressed through interventions.[3] They can be divided into categories: patient-related, regimen-related, provider-related, and process-oriented factors. The salient factors affecting compliance are summarized in Display 37-1. These need to be kept in mind as interventions to improve adherence are reviewed.

MODELS OF BEHAVIOR CHANGE

Improving adherence to treatment regimens is one of the greatest challenges facing health care professionals. The general level of adherence to medication is less than ideal and needs improvement. However, assisting patients with lifestyle changes and, most important, maintaining those changes poses the greatest challenge. Lifestyle modification for the cardiac patient may include adopting a physical activity program, consuming a diet low in fat, cholesterol, and sodium, and possibly adjusting caloric intake to reduce or maintain a healthy weight. In addition, smoking cessation and drug therapy may be added to an already complex regimen.

Various models of behavior change have guided studies investigating determinants of adherence or evaluating strategies to improve adherence. Earlier models included operant learning, which focused on the environment and used stimulus control strategies to restructure the environment. More recently, cognitive–motivational models have focused on beliefs, intentions, and self-efficacy, and most recently, readiness to change. Intervention strategies used today have arisen from research based on these models of behavior change, which have been predominantly based on social cognitive theory.[74] Social cognitive theory, formerly known as social learning theory, is based on an underlying assumption that behavior, the environment, and cognition function as interacting determinants with a bidirectional influence on each other.[74]

Using the cognitive–motivational models, studies have examined the role of health beliefs, susceptibility, barriers, and intentions in the explanation of adherence behavior change.[75] However, these constructs explained little variance of behavior change in modifying cardiac risk factors.[70,72,76–78] More recently, the social cognitive models have included self-efficacy. There is evidence that judgments of perceived efficacy predict subsequent performance across a variety of domains, including regaining functional status after an MI or cardiac surgery, smoking cessation, weight loss, and exercise and dietary adherence.[42,79–83]

Self-efficacy is defined as a person's perceived capacity for exerting control over his or her motivation, cognition, behavior, and environmental demands.[84] It is concerned not with a person's skills, but with the person's judgments of what he or she can do with those skills.[42] Self-efficacy is behavior specific, that is, a person's self-efficacy for exercise may be different from self-efficacy for maintaining a healthy diet. There are four sources of efficacy: (1) mastery experience—the most powerful source comes from achievement of a series of sub-goals; (2) modeling or vicarious learning—observing another perform a task; (3) physiologic cues—making inferences from autonomic arousal or other symptoms; and (4) verbal or social persuasion—convincing others they possess the capability to achieve their goal.[74,84]

Kristeller and colleagues[85] used the transtheoretical model of behavior change. This model suggests that people fall along a continuum of change comprising five stages: (1) precontemplation—uninterested in changing behavior; (2) contemplation—thinking about and making plans to change; (3) action—actively modifying behavior; (4) maintenance—sustaining the behavior; and (5) relapse—reverting to previous behavior. People may relapse and work their way through the cycles repeatedly. This theory has been applied to adoption of exercise, altering diet to reduce fat intake, and smoking cessation.[85,86]

Based on research guided by the models of behavior change, a list of strategies for use in assisting patients to improve adherence to behavior change follows. These strategies are summarized in Display 37-2.

DISPLAY 37-2

Adherence-Enhancing Strategies

Self-monitoring—record behavior for analysis
Stimulus control—arrange environment to be supportive to goals
Goal setting—have patient set specific, proximal, attainable goals
Reinforcement—focus on positive change or behavior,
Modeling behavior—credible person demonstrating/performing behavior
Self-efficacy enhancement—provide opportunities for mastery, positive feedback, convince patient he or she is capable of doing, interpret physiological cues or symptoms
Social support provision—enlisting support of others, having a "buddy"
Cuing—set up system of reminder
Habit building—pair a new behavior with an established behavior
Contracting—written plan for what, when, how behavior goal will be reached
Problem solving—problem identification, definition, solution generation, selecting trial of one solution, evaluation of solution strategy
Relapse prevention—identify high-risk situation, identify/rehearse coping strategies to deal with situation
Tailoring the regimen—develop regimen plan realistic for patient, address cultural sensitivity
Assessing readiness for change—use strategy appropriate for patient readiness phase, may be providing reading material or plan of action
Use of frequent, short exercise bouts—exercise in five to six 10-minute bouts per day
Home-based exercise—teach patients how and where to exercise independently
Ongoing contact—continued contact by mail, telephone, or internet
Use of internal cognitive aids—use of appointment schedules, cards, medication schedule card
Nurse-managed care—serving as case managers, nurses provide clinic follow-up, ongoing contact, and behavior change counseling
Supplementary education and training—teach patient about the regimen to be performed, use return demonstration, provide practice opportunities for skill development, provide pertinent reading material as appropriate
Skill development—provide opportunities for return demonstration and practice by patient

---

ADHERENCE-ENHANCING STRATEGIES

SELF-MONITORING

A key technique in approaches to behavioral change, self-monitoring requires the patient to record behavior (e.g., eating, exercise, or smoking behaviors) and use this information for behavioral analysis (i.e., the patient and provider can identify problem behaviors that could be altered). The provider reviews the self-monitoring record and provides reinforcement for progress.

STIMULUS CONTROL

Using information recorded in the diary on the circumstances of the behavior allows identification of the antecedent or trigger for problem behaviors.[4,16,42,87] The patient is counseled to remove the stimuli and to restructure the environment to minimize the will power needed to overcome strong stimuli.[16]

GOAL SETTING

Goal setting entails working with the patient in developing realistic and attainable goals that are specific and proximal. The goal should include what will be done, when, and how: for example, "will walk for 15 minutes three times a week for the next 2 weeks." As each sub-goal is reached, the duration, frequency, or intensity of the next goal is increased.[84]

REINFORCEMENT

Giving positive feedback to the patient on progress made, supporting self-motivation by highlighting accomplishments, encouraging continued progress, and instilling confidence in the person's capability of meeting a goal all constitute reinforcement. When providing positive feedback, focus on the behavior rather than on the clinical outcome.

MODELING BEHAVIOR

The patient can observe a credible model perform a task or have an activity demonstrated, which may be done by watching a video or live action. It is important that the patient find the model credible and the activity feasible, such as observing fellow patients exercising in cardiac rehabilitation programs.

SELF-EFFICACY ENHANCEMENT

Self-efficacy enhancement strategies are based on the sources of self-efficacy and include providing opportunities for successful performance or mastery. Provide feedback and praise for progress and achieving specific behavioral goals, convince the person he or she is capable of performing the activity, and interpret symptoms of physiologic response, such as breathlessness due to inactivity and diminished symptoms after a program of regular exercise.

SOCIAL SUPPORT

Social support includes enlisting others to assist the patient through the behavior change process, and inclusion of supportive others from various aspects of the patient's life (e.g., family, friends, coworker, community).[3] The purpose of this strategy is to have supportive allies in place during successes and failures. This may take the form of enlisting a "buddy" for exercise or eating behavior change, or having someone there for reinforcement. Social support has been shown to be important in most behavior change, but particularly in programs of dietary change.[88-90]

CUING

Cuing consists of setting up a system of reminders or cues to perform certain activities (e.g., a sticker to remind the person to take a medication, or setting out exercise shoes as a prompt to exercise on a busy day).

HABIT BUILDING

Habit building is derived from the stimulus control model and is based on the premise that a large amount of behavior is automatic and responsive to stimuli.[91] It further suggests that behavior can be modified by establishing a relationship between the behavior stimulus and the target behavior, such as pairing a new behavior (medication taking) with an established behavior (brushing teeth). Using cues, as described previously, is a related strategy. These techniques may be particularly helpful when in an unusual environment (e.g., traveling). Pairing the medication bottle with the toothpaste or adding a note to the travel alarm clock may prevent an episode of nonadherence.

CONTRACTING

A form of public commitment, contracting involves the patient in the development of the plan and clearly specifies in writing what is expected, the time frame, and any conditions for a reward if the goal is achieved. The contract needs to specify a behavior rather than the health outcome, and should specify the incremental steps necessary to achieve a goal that is attainable and valued by the patient.[3] A contingency reward may be included for achievement of the goal. This needs to be a reward valued by the person and reinforcing to the healthier behavior, such as a new outfit for someone in a weight reduction program, but not dinner at their favorite restaurant.

PROBLEM SOLVING

Problem solving involves several steps, beginning with identification or acknowledgment of a problem, defining the problem, generating potential solutions, selecting one solution or set of actions to resolve the problem, and then evaluating the success of the attempt to resolve the problem.[92,93] This technique is integral to maintenance of behavior change and is facilitated by reviewing self-monitoring records and identifying high-risk situations. Anticipatory problem solving can help a patient prepare for an upcoming situation, such as a major social event or vacation.[3]

RELAPSE PREVENTION

Based on the work of Marlatt and Gordon,[94] the relapse prevention technique emphasizes that slips or lapses are natural occurrences in the process of behavior change. Patients are taught to anticipate high-risk situations and to identify ways to cope with the situation.[95] When possible, patients should practice problem solving to develop these skills better and rehearse the strategies they would use to resolve the threat to adherence or maintenance.

TAILORING THE REGIMEN

Tailoring the regimen addresses the patient's capability to carry out the plan, that is, what is realistic for the patient to achieve in behavior change. It includes accommodating the patient's schedule for appointments, being sensitive to cultural issues in recommending dietary change or other behavior, and being sensitive to financial constraints in general. It is an important consideration in medication-taking compliance (e.g., considering the costs, memory requirements, and schedule when prescribing a drug that may be available in numerous dosing forms).

MATCHING THE INTERVENTION TO THE PERSON'S STAGE OF READINESS FOR CHANGE

The patient's readiness for behavior change is assessed, and the intervention planned accordingly.[96] If the patient is in the precontemplation phase, then talking to the patient and raising his or her awareness of the problem is appropriate, with follow-up at subsequent visits to determine if he or she has moved into the action phase.[97] The intervention needs to fit the stage of readiness, such as providing the patient an informational pamphlet in the contemplative stage and directing behavior change strategies during the active stage.

USE OF FREQUENT, SHORT BOUTS AND HOME-BASED EXERCISE SESSIONS

This gives patients the option of exercising for 10-minute periods five to six times per day, as well as the standard 30- to 45-minute exercise session. Jakicic and coworkers[58] reported that a sample of overweight women had greater total exercise time and lost more weight when assigned to frequent, short bouts compared with those in the standard exercise group. Perri and colleagues[98] also reported that patients who were allowed to exercise at home adhered better than those who were required to travel to a clinic facility.

ONGOING CONTACT

Continued contact, either through mail or telephone follow-up, has consistently demonstrated improved adherence in maintaining behavior change, including adherence to medication taking, cholesterol-lowering dietary therapy, smoking cessation, exercise maintenance, weight loss maintenance, and general cardiac risk factor reduction.[4,42,87,99–105]

The mail can be used as a method of ongoing contact by having patients return preprinted postcards periodically on which they record their exercise or eating behavior, followed by a brief phone call to provide feedback.[103,104] Patients may also return eating and exercise diaries; for example, patients can self-monitor their ongoing behavior 1 week of each month, or during difficult times, and send this record in to the provider. This technique adds the accountability factor and encourages ongoing communication with the provider.

Similarly, the telephone provides ongoing support and assistance with problem solving.[42,103,105] A brief phone call to a patient can provide encouragement that may help the patient sustain the behavior during a challenging period. Regular telephone contacts need to have a structure in terms of purpose, what is to be accomplished, approximate time allowed, and a schedule of when the calls should occur. Scripting or outlining the main steps to follow in the contact can help maintain a focus and ensure that each point is addressed. When considering initiating a telephone follow-up system, the nurse needs to consider the purpose or goal of the system, if these can be met given the frequency and duration of the planned contacts, and the costs in terms of staff time.[42]

USE OF EXTERNAL COGNITIVE AIDS

External cognitive aids include appointment reminder letters, follow-up letters for missed appointments, reminder cards for medication refill, medication calendars or reminder charts, and unit-of-use packaging of pills. Any of these strategies can enhance adherence to appointment keeping and to medication taking.[4,55,106–109]

NURSE-MANAGED CARE

Serving as case managers, nurses provide clinic and telephone follow-up, initiate therapy for risk reduction, and provide counseling for behavior change (e.g., smoking cessation, dietary change). Use of this treatment model demonstrated improved clinical outcome in two studies of patients with coronary heart disease in which several of the previously described strategies were incorporated into the treatment plan.[100,101]

EDUCATIONAL STRATEGIES TO IMPROVE ADHERENCE

Didactic, cognitive interventions may be used to transmit information about the disease process or the treatment regimen. Often a behavior change requires educating the patient about the regimen, such as how to follow a low-fat diet or initiate an exercise program. The underlying aim may be to increase the person's knowledge in the expectation that behavior change will follow. However, the association between knowledge and behavior is small.[110] Educational interventions alone have not yielded positive results.[4,111–114] The literature suggests that supplementing educational interventions with behavioral strategies increases the effectiveness of the teaching intervention.[3] A list of guidelines for delivering educational interventions is presented in Display 37-3. It is important to incorporate in the intervention the behavioral strategies previously described.

DISPLAY 37-3

Guidelines to Follow in Delivering Educational Interventions

♦ Keep instructions specific to the activity
♦ Assess the reading level of material; make sure it is understandable, accurate, and appropriate
♦ Deliver informational material over time
♦ Provide verbal instructions in small amounts
♦ Use printed materials to reinforce verbal instructions
♦ Provide printed materials in small amounts over time
♦ Encourage questions of patient and ask patient questions to determine level of comprehension
♦ Focus on the regimen, not the disease
♦ Use a variety of media formats (videotapes, interactive computer programs, visual illustrations)
♦ Provide demonstrations to augment verbal instructions
♦ Provide for return demonstrations and practice opportunities (e.g., mixing medications, taking nitroglycerin, completing diaries, counting pulse)
♦ Use community resources (e.g., American Heart Association, local hospital for health classes, cardiac rehabilitation programs)
♦ Provide patients information on additional appropriate resources (e.g., web sites, lay organizations, and lay literature)

QUESTIONNAIRES RELEVANT TO ADHERENCE-ENHANCING INTERVENTIONS

Most interventions to improve adherence focus on one or more of the constructs of social cognitive theory (i.e., barriers, self-efficacy, or readiness to change). Research has produced several psychometrically sound instruments to measure the constructs that may influence adherence across several behavioral domains. Hill and Berk[115] reported on an instrument developed to measure attitudes and perceived risks and benefits related to blood pressure control and treatment. A preliminary report suggested the instrument has sound psychometric properties.[115] Because of their behavioral specificity, several self-efficacy scales have been developed, including for following a general cardiac diet and exercise program,[116,117] for adhering to a cholesterol-lowering diet,[118–121] for following a weight-loss diet,[71,79,122] for smoking cessation,[123] and for medication taking.[124] More recently, instruments have been developed that apply the processes of change to risk reduction behavior, including an instrument that measures readiness for change to a low-fat diet[86] and one to measure future success in smoking cessation.[85] These represent just a few of the self-administered scales that can be used in the clinical or research setting.

BUILDING A THERAPEUTIC RELATIONSHIP WITH THE PATIENT

Working with a patient to ensure adequate adherence at the initiation of treatment, and over the long term either to enhance compliance or remediate poor adherence, requires good rapport and clear communication lines between the patient and provider. Having a good therapeutic relationship allows ongoing assessment of the patient's adherence and also provides an environment conducive to the patient confiding in the provider when barriers to adherence arise. The patient needs to be queried regularly if he or she has any concerns about the condition or the treatment, and should be commended for seeking and following through on the treatment process.[125]

Communication can be facilitated by listening reflectively to the patient and being supportive. The provider should try to listen more than talk. Encourage the patient to express problems he or she anticipates having or has encountered in implementing the treatment. Listen with interest. Acknowledge how difficult the new, possibly complex, treatment is and the demands it places on the patient—for example, "I am sure all of this is overwhelming to you. What concerns you the most about your treatment?" Assist the patient to identify barriers to implementing or following the treatment, such as no available time or place where he or she can exercise safely, or, for the patient who needs to quit smoking, a spouse who smokes and has no intentions of quitting. Determine what the patient's view of the treatment is, and clarify what the patient's responsibilities will be in carrying out the treatment.[125] If possible, give priority to the patient's goal in the treatment plan.[126]

When it is time to begin working on the treatment plan, the nurse may begin by acknowledging the challenge, "I know how difficult it is to make changes in long-established eating habits. We are asking you to make changes gradually over time and will work with you in making those changes. What may we do to assist you with this?" and "What would you like to focus on first?" Express confidence in the patient's ability to implement the treatment, and in the treatment having a beneficial effect if it is followed. Assist the patient gradually to assume responsibility for the treatment. Involve the patient in development and implementation of the treatment.[126] Before the close of the session, review with the patient exactly what will be done: "Now let's go over this plan once more just to make sure I have given you all the information you need. What is the medication you're going to be taking?" Or, to avoid putting the patient in an awkward position: "The name of the drug is . . . Now please tell me how many pills you plan to take and when. Are there any symptoms you should report to us?"

In follow-up sessions, acknowledge each time how difficult it is take medications or follow whatever treatment regimen has been recommended (e.g., smoking cessation, dietary change, or regular exercise) and assess how the patient is doing. The nurse may say, "I know it can be difficult to remember to take your pills each time. Do you find that you forget to take your pills sometime?" or "Sometimes when patients feel better, they skip their medications. Do you ever skip taking your pills when you feel good?" A general question may also be asked, such as "Tell me about your medicines and how you are taking them." Ask the patient to go through each medication and describe how many pills are being taken and when. The same general questions can be applied to other activities.[125]

An important part of follow-up is providing encouragement and reinforcement. The nurse needs to acknowledge the difficulties the patient faces, but also must be firm regarding the importance of the treatment and continue to instill confidence in the patient. Reinforcement should be given for the behavior change made, not for the clinical outcome. Providing information on clinical outcomes (e.g., blood cholesterol levels) can be an additional reinforcement to the patient, showing the progress he or she has made in changing behavior and its positive effects on health.[125]

The greatest challenge in compliance is to assist the patient to maintain the behavioral changes for the long term. As noted previously, there is a decline in adherence during the first year of treatment, with a continued erosion over time. This decline is usually accelerated in the absence of any contact with the health care professional. Thus, adherence needs to be addressed at each visit with the previously suggested questions. If there is an indication the patient is lapsing, additional attention needs to be provided. It may take the form of periodic telephone contacts and or mail contact. This may include the patient reporting on progress made toward a goal, or the nurse assisting with problem solving in difficult situations, correcting any further problems, providing reinforcement for attempts and progress, and helping the patient set new goals, if appropriate. It may help to have the patient self-monitor behavior for a period and have these records returned before each phone call, or have the patient bring them in at each visit. It is important that these be reviewed and used in pointing out positive behaviors and making suggestions for healthier behaviors.[4,125]

SUMMARY

Inadequate adherence to the recommended treatment plan remains a significant problem facing health care professionals in all settings and populations. Progress has been made in the measurement of adherence and in identifying strategies that may enhance adherence. However, these measurement methods or intervention strategies are not applied in the clinical setting often enough to affect adherence significantly.[4,73] Furthermore, the nurse faces additional challenges because of the changing health care environment, including shortened length of hospital stay, increased level of acuity of patients during their hospitalization and at discharge, reduced number of visits after acute events, and increasingly complex treatment regimens that patients need to learn how to implement. However, the nurse is often in

the best position to address adherence. As nursing assumes an expanded role in an array of settings, the nurse often assumes responsibility for patient education, ensuring that the patient understands the regimen, and for arranging needed follow-up.

Just as the nursing profession has shown leadership in promoting patient education in past decades, nursing needs again to take the lead in improving adherence. This requires looking at how health care is provided and determining where in the system interventions need to be directed (i.e., at the level of the provider; the preventive, acute, or chronic treatment regimen; or the patient). Most likely, all three components of the system need to be addressed when making changes to facilitate improved adherence.[127] Moreover, the changes need to be addressed over the continuum of care provision, particularly during the maintenance phase, when nonadherence is most likely to become an issue.

ADDITIONAL READING

Brownell KD: The LEARN Manual for Weight Control. Dallas: American Health Publishing Company, 1997

Dishman RK (ed): Advances in Exercise Adherence. Champaign, IL: Human Kinetics, 1994

Helm KK, Klawitter B: Nutrition Therapy: Advanced Counseling Skills. Lake Dallas, TX: Helm Seminars, 1995

Kris-Etherton PM (ed): Cardiovascular Disease: Nutrition for Prevention and Treatment. Chicago: American Dietetic Association, 1990

Miller NH, Taylor CB: Lifestyle Management for Patients with Coronary Heart Disease. Champaign, IL: Human Kinetics, 1995

REFERENCES

1. Sackett DL, Haynes RB: Introduction. In Sackett DL, Haynes RB (eds): Compliance with Therapeutic Regimens, pp 1–5. Baltimore, The Johns Hopkins University Press, 1976

2. American Hospital Association and the Centers for Disease Control Health Education Project: Strategies to Promote Self Management of Chronic Disease. Chicago, American Hospital Association, 1982

3. Burke LE, Dunbar-Jacob J: Adherence to medication, diet, and activity recommendations: From assessment to maintenance. J Cardiovasc Nurs 9: 62–79, 1995

4. Burke LE, Dunbar-Jacob J, Hill MN: Compliance to cardiovascular risk reduction strategies: Review of the research. Ann Behav Med 19: 239–263, 1997

5. Pearson TA, Feinberg W: Behavioral issues in the efficacy versus effectiveness of pharmacologic agents in the prevention of cardiovascular disease. Ann Behav Med 19: 230–238, 1997

6. Stason WB, Weinstein MC: Allocation of resources to manage hypertension. N Engl J Med 296: 732–739, 1977

7. Stason WB: Opportunities to improve the cost-effectiveness of treatment for hypertension. Hypertension 18: 1161–1166, 1991

8. Andrade SE, Walker AM, Gottlieb LK et al: Discontinuation of antihyperlipidemic drugs: Do rates reported in clinical trials reflect rates in primary care settings? N Engl J Med 332: 1125–1131, 1995

9. Simons LA, Levis G, Simon J: Apparent discontinuation rates in patients prescribed lipid-lowering drugs. Med J Aust 164: 208–211, 1996

10. Berg JS, Dischler J, Wagner DJ et al: Medication compliance: A health care problem. Ann Pharmacother 27(Suppl): S2–S22, 1993

11. Ghali JK, Kadakia S, Cooper R et al: Precipitating factors leading to decompensation of heart failure. Arch Intern Med 148: 2013–2016, 1988

12. Oldridge NB: Compliance and dropout in cardiac exercise rehabilitation. J Cardiac Rehabil 4: 166–177, 1984

13. Miller TD, Balady GJ, Fletcher GF: Exercise and its role in the prevention and rehabilitation of cardiovascular disease. Ann Behav Med 19: 220–229, 1997

14. Burt A, Thornley P, Illingworth D et al: Stopping smoking after myocardial infarction. Lancet 1: 304–306, 1974

15. Dale LC, Hurt RD, Offord KP et al: High-dose nicotine patch therapy: Percentage of replacement and smoking cessation. JAMA 274: 1353–1391, 1995

16. Wing RR: Behavioral approaches to the treatment of obesity. In Bray G, Bourchard C, James PT (eds): Handbook of Obesity, pp 855–877. New York, Marcel Dekker, 1997

17. Sherbourne CD, Ilays RD, Ordway L et al: Antecedents of adherence to medical recommendations: Results from the Medical Outcomes Study. J Behav Med 15: 447–468, 1992

18. Dew MA, Roth LH, Thompson ME et al: Medical compliance and its predictors in the first year after heart transplantation. J Heart Lung Transplant 14: S70, 1995

19. Haynes RB: A critical review of the determinants of patient compliance with therapeutic regimens. In Sackett DL, Haynes RB (eds): Compliance with Therapeutic Regimens, pp 26–50. Baltimore: The Johns Hopkins University Press, 1976

20. Lipid Research Clinics Program: The Lipid Research Clinics Coronary Primary Prevention Trial results: I. Reduction in incidence of coronary heart disease. JAMA 251: 351–364, 1984

21. Lipid Research Clinics Program: The Lipid Research Clinics Coronary Primary Prevention Trial results: II. The relationship of reduction in incidence of coronary heart disease to cholesterol lowering. JAMA 251: 365–374, 1984

22. Psaty BM, Koepsell TD, Wagner EH et al: The relative risk of incident coronary heart disease associated with recently stopping the use of beta-blockers. JAMA 263: 1653–1657, 1990

23. De Geest S, Abraham I, Vanhaecke J: Clinical risk differentiation associated with subclinical noncompliance with cyclosporine-therapy: A cluster analytic study in heart transplant recipients. Presented at the Fifth International Transplant Nurses Society Symposium and General Assembly, May 16–18, 1996, New Orleans, Louisiana

24. Urquhart J: Patient compliance as an explanatory variable in four selected cardiovascular studies. In Cramer JA, Spilker B (eds). Patient Compliance in Medical Practice and Clinical Trials, pp 301–322. New York, Raven Press, 1991

25. Mojonnier ML, Hall Y, Berkson DM et al: Experience in changing food habits of hyperlipidemic men and women. J Am Diet Assoc 77: 140–148, 1980

26. Schuster PM, Wright C, Tomich P: Gender differences in the outcomes of participants in home program compared to those in structured cardiac rehabilitation programs. Rehabilitation Nursing 30: 93–101, 1995

27. Connett JE, Stamler J: Responses of black and white males to the special intervention program of the Multiple Risk Factor Intervention Trial. Am Heart J 108: 839–848, 1984

28. Dunbar-Jacob J, Burke LE, Puczynski S: Clinical assessment and management of adherence to medical regimens. In Nicassio P, Smith T (eds): Managing Chronic Illness: A Biopsychosocial Perspective, pp 313–349. Washington, DC, American Psychological Association, 1995

29. Morris LS, Schulz RM: Patient compliance: An overview. J Clin Pharm Ther 17: 283–295, 1992

30. Cramer JA, Mattson RH, Prevey ML et al: How often is medication taken as prescribed? A novel assessment technique. JAMA 261: 3273–3277, 1989

31. Morisky DE, Green LW, Levine DM: Concurrent and predictive validity of a self-reported measure of medication adherence. Med Care 24: 67–74, 1986

32. Shea S, Misra D, Ehrlich MH et al: Correlates of nonadherence to hypertension treatment in an inner-city minority population. Am J Public Health 82: 1607–1611, 1992

33. Dunbar-Jacob J, Burke LE, Rohay JM et al: Comparability of self-report, pill count, and electronically monitored adherence data. Control Clin Trials 7: 80S, 1996

34. Dunbar-Jacob J, Burke LE, Rohay JM et al: How comparable are self-report, pill count, and electronically monitored adherence data? Circulation 96(8): Suppl I-738, 1997

35. Block G: A review of validations of dietary assessment methods. Am J Epidemiol 115: 492–504, 1982

36. Dolocek TA, Milas NC, Van Horn LV et al: A long-term nutrition intervention experience: Lipid responses and dietary adherence patterns in the Multiple Risk Factor Intervention Trial. J Am Diet Assoc 86: 752–758, 1986

37. Wylie-Rosett J, Wassertheil-Smoller S, Elmer P: Assessing dietary intake for patient education planning and evaluation. Patient Education and Counseling 15: 217–227, 1990

38. Wolper C, Heshka S, Heymsfield SB: Measuring food intake: An overview. In Allison DB (ed): Handbook of Assessment Methods for Eating Behaviors and Weight Related Problems, pp 215–240. Thousand Oaks, CA, Sage, 1995

39. Dawber TR, Pearson G, Anderson P et al: Dietary assessment in the epidemiologic study of coronary heart disease: The Framingham Study. Am J Clin Nutr 11: 226–234, 1962

40. Taylor CB, Coffey T, Berra K et al: Seven day activity recall compared to a direct measure of physical activity. Am J Epidemiol 120: 818–824, 1984

41. Dishman RK (ed): Advances in Exercise Adherence. Champaign, IL, Human Kinetics, 1994

42. Burke LE: Improving Adherence to a Cholesterol-Lowering Diet: A Behavioral Intervention Study. Unpublished doctoral dissertation. Pittsburgh, PA, University of Pittsburgh, 1997.

43. Connor SL, Gustafson JR, Sexton G et al: The Diet Habit Survey: A new method of dietary assessment that relates to plasma cholesterol changes. J Am Diet Assoc 92: 41–47, 1992

44. Kristal AR, Shattuck AL, Henry HJ: Patterns of dietary behavior associated with selecting diets low in fat: Reliability and validity of a behavioral approach to dietary assessment. J Am Diet Assoc 90: 214–220, 1990

45. Smucker R, Block G, Coyle L et al: A dietary and risk factor questionnaire and analysis system for personal computers. Am J Epidemiol 129: 445–449, 1989

46. Willett WC, Sampson L, Stampfer MJ: Reproducibility and validity of a semi-quantitative food frequency questionnaire. Am J Epidemiol 122: 51–65, 1985

47. Willet W: Nutritional Epidemiology, pp 52–126. New York, Oxford University Press, 1990

48. Block G, Hartman AM, Dresser CM et al: A data-based approach to diet questionnaire and testing. Am J Epidemiol 124: 453–469, 1986

49. Allison DB (ed): Handbook of Assessment Methods for Eating Behaviors and Weight Related Problems: Measures, Theory, and Research, pp 231–235. Thousand Oaks, CA, Sage, 1995

50. Kriska AM, Caspersen CJ: Introduction to a collection of physical activity questionnaires. Med Sci Sports Exerc 29: S5–S9, 1997

51. Pereira MA, FitzGerald SJ, Gregg EW et al: A collection of physical activity questionnaires for health-related research. Med Sci Sports Exerc 29(Suppl): S1–S205, 1997

52. Lichtman SW, Pisarska K, Berman ER et al: Discrepancy between self-reported and actual caloric intake and exercise in obese subjects. N Engl J Med 327: 1893–1898, 1992

53. Gibson RS: Measurement errors in dietary assessment. In Gibson RS (ed): Principles of Nutritional Assessment, pp 85–96. New York, Oxford University Press, 1990

54. Epstein LH, Koeske R, Wing RR: Adherence to exercise in obese children. J Cardiac Rehabil 4: 185–195, 1984

55. Park DC, Morrell RW, Frieske D et al: Medication adherence behaviors in older adults: Effects of external cognitive supports. Psychol Aging 7: 252–256, 1992

56. Rogers F, Juneau M, Taylor CB et al: Assessment by a microprocessor of adherence to home-based moderate-intensity exercise training in healthy, sedentary middle-aged men and women. Am J Cardiol 60: 71–75, 1987

57. Bouten CV, Westerterp KR, Verduin M et al: Assessment of energy expenditure for physical activity using a triaxial accelerometer. Med Sci Sports Exerc 26: 1516–1523, 1994

58. Jakicic JM, Wing RR, Butler BA et al: Prescribing exercise in multiple short bouts versus one continuous bout: Effects on adherence, cardiorespiratory fitness, and weight loss in overweight women. International Journal of Obesity 19: 893–901, 1995

59. Pambianco G, Wing RR, Robertson R: Accuracy and reliability of the Caltrac accelerometer for estimating energy expenditure. Med Sci Sports Exerc 22: 858–862, 1990

60. Bengtsson K: Rehabilitation after myocardial infarction. Scand J Rehabil Med 15: 1–9, 1983

61. Hermann C, Peters ML, Blanchard EB: Use of hand-held computers for symptom-monitoring: The case of chronic headache. Mind and Body Medicine 1: 59–71, 1995

62. McGuire WJ: Attitudes and attitude change. In Lindzey G, Aronson E (eds): Handbook of Social Psychology, vol II: Special Fields and Applications, 3rd ed, pp 233–346. New York, Random House, 1985

63. Urquhart J: Electronic monitoring of patient compliance. Pharmaceutical Manufacturing Technology International '91. 1991.

64. Dunbar-Jacob J, Sereika S, Rohay JB et al: Electronic methods in: Assessing adherence to medical regimens. In Krantz DS (ed): Perspectives in Behavioral Medicine: Technological and Methodological Innovations pp 95–113. New Jersey, Erlbaum, 1998

65. Meijer GAL: Physical Activity: Implications for Human Energy Metabolism. Doctoral thesis. Maastricht, The Netherlands, Riijksuniversiteit Limburg, 1990

66. Meijer GAL, Westerterp KR, Koper HBM et al: Assessment of energy expenditure by recording heart rate and body acceleration. Med Sci Sports Exerc 21: 343–347, 1989

67. Donova S, Mills J, Goulder MA et al: Electronic patient diaries: A pilot study. Applied Clinical Trials 4(70): 40–48, 1996

68. Urquhart J, Chevalley C: Impact of unrecognized dosing errors on the cost and effectiveness of pharmaceuticals. Drug Information Journal 22: 363–378, 1988

69. Cramer JA, Scheyer RD, Mattson RH: Compliance declines between clinic visits. Arch Intern Med 150: 1509–1510, 1990

70. Dunbar-Jacob J, Schlenk EA, Burke LE et al: Predictors of patient adherence: Patient characteristics. In Schumaker SA, Schron E, Ockene J et al (eds): Handbook of Health Behavior Change, 2nd ed, pp 491–511. New York, Springer-Verlag, 1998

71. Stotland S, Zuroff DC: Relations between multiple measures of dieting self-efficacy and weight change in a behavioral weight control program. Behavior Therapy 22: 47–59, 1991

72. Caggiula AW, Watson JE: Characteristics associated with compliance to cholesterol lowering eating patterns. Patient Education and Counseling 19: 33–41, 1992

73. Hill MN, Houston Miller N: Compliance enhancement: A call for multidisciplinary team approaches. Circulation 93: 4–6, 1996

74. Bandura A: Social Foundations of Thought and Action: A Social Cognitive Theory. Englewood Cliffs, NJ, Prentice-Hall, 1986

75. Fleury J: The application of motivational theory to cardiovascular risk reduction. Image 24: 229–239, 1992

76. Miller PS, Wikoff R, McMahon M: Personal adjustments and regimen compliance one year after myocardial infarction. Heart Lung 18: 339–346, 1989

77. Miller SP, Wikoff R, Garrett MJ et al: Regimen compliance two years after myocardial infarction. Nurs Res 39: 333–336, 1990

78. Naslund GK, Fredrikson M, Hellenius M-L et al: Determinants of compliance in men enrolled in a diet and exercise intervention trial: A randomized, controlled study. Patient Education and Counseling 29: 247–256, 1996

79. Bernier M, Avard J: Self-efficacy, outcome, and attrition in a weight-reduction program. Cognitive Therapy and Research 10: 319–338, 1986

80. Condiotte MM, Lichtenstein E: Self-efficacy and relapse in smoking cessation programs. J Consult Clin Psychol 49: 648–658, 1981

81. Ewart CK, Stewart KJ, Gillilan RE: Usefulness of self-efficacy in predicting overexertion during programmed exercise in coronary artery disease. Am J Cardiol 57: 557–561, 1986

82. Weinberg RS, Hughes HH, Critelli JW et al: Effects of preexisting and manipulated self-efficacy on weight loss in a self-control program. Journal of Research in Personality 18: 352–358, 1984

83. Allen JK: Coronary risk factor modification in women after coronary artery bypass surgery. Nurs Res 45: 260–265, 1996

84. Bandura A. Self-efficacy. In Social Foundations of Thought and Action: A Social Cognitive Theory, pp 390–450. Englewood Cliffs, NJ, Prentice-Hall, 1986

85. Kristeller JK, Rossi JS, Ockene JK et al: Processes of change in smoking cessation: A cross-validation study in cardiac patients. J Subst Abuse 4: 263–276, 1992

86. Bowen DJ, Meischke H, Tomoyasu N: Preliminary evaluation of the processes of changing to a low-fat diet. Health Education Research Theory and Practice 9: 85–94, 1994

87. King AC, Taylor CB, Haskell WL et al: Strategies for increasing early adherence to and long-term maintenance of home-based exercise training in healthy middle-aged men and women. Am J Cardiol 61: 628–632, 1988

88. Bovbjerg VE, McCann BS, Brief DJ et al: Spouse support and long-term adherence to lipid-lowering diets. Am J Epidemiol 141: 451–460, 1995

89. Wing RR, Jeffery RW: Benefits of recruiting participants with friends and increasing social support for weight loss and maintenance. Journal of Consulting and Clinical Psychology 67(1): 132–138, 1999

90. Dunbar-Jacob J, Dwyer K, Dunning EJ: Compliance with antihypertensive regimen: A review of the research in the 1980's. Ann Behav Med 13: 31–39, 1991

91. Bandura A: Principles of Behavior Modification. New York, Holt, Rhinehart & Winston, 1969

92. Bedell JR, Archer RP, Marlowe HA: A description and evaluation of a problem-solving skills training program. In Upper D, Ross SM (eds): Behavioral Group Therapy: An Annual Review, pp 32–40. Champaign, IL, Research Press, 1980

93. D'Zurilla TJ, Goldfried MR: Problem solving and behavior modification. J Abnorm Psychol 78: 107–126, 1971

94. Marlatt GA, Gordon JR: Determinants of relapse: Implications for the maintenance of behavior change. In Davidson PO, Davidson SM (eds): Behavioral Medicine: Changing Health Lifestyles, pp 410–452. New York, Brunner/Mazel, 1980

95. Ryder RE, Hayes TM, Mulligan IP et al: How soon after myocardial infarction should plasma lipid values be assessed? BMJ 289(6459) 1651–1653, 1984

96. Prochaska JO, Velicer WF, Rossi JS et al: Stages of change and decisional balance for 12 problem behaviors. Health Psychol 13: 39–46, 1994

97. Glanz K: Nutritional intervention: A behavioral and educational perspective. In Ockene IS, Ockene JK (eds): Prevention of Coronary Heart Disease, pp 231–260. Boston, Little, Brown, 1992

98. Perri MG, Martin DA, Leermakers EA et al: Effects of group-versus home-based exercise in the treatment of obesity. Journal of Consulting and Clinical Cardiology 65: 278–285, 1997

99. Dunbar-Jacob J, Sereika S, Burke LE et al: Can poor adherence be improved? Ann Behav Med 17(Suppl): S061, 1995

100. DeBusk RF, Miller NH, Superko HR et al: A case-management system for coronary risk factor modification after acute myocardial infarction. Ann Intern Med 120: 721–729, 1994

101. Haskell WL, Alderman EL, Fair JM et al: Effects of intensive multiple risk factor reduction on coronary atherosclerosis and clinical cardiac events in men and women with coronary artery disease. Circulation 89: 975–990, 1994

102. Taylor CB, Houston-Miller N, Killen JD et al: Smoking cessation after acute myocardial infarction: Effects of a nurse-managed intervention. Ann Intern Med 113: 118–123, 1990

103. Perri MG, Shapiro RM, Ludwig WW et al: Maintenance strategies for the treatment of obesity: An evaluation of relapse prevention training and posttreatment contact by mail and telephone. J Consult Clin Psychol 52: 404–413, 1984

104. King AC, Frey-Hewitt B, Dreon DM et al: Diet vs exercise in weight maintenance. Arch Intern Med 149: 2741–2746, 1989

105. Burke LE, Dunbar-Jacob J, Orchard TJ et al: Improving adherence to a cholesterol-lowering diet: A behavioral intervention study. 1998 (submitted for publication)

106. Saunders LD, Irwig LM, Gear JSS et al: A randomized controlled trial of compliance improving strategies in Soweto hypertensives. Med Care 29: 669–678, 1991

107. Skaer TL, Sclar DA, Markowski DJ et al: Effect of value-added utilities on prescription refill compliance and health-care expenditures for hypertension. J Hum Hypertens 7: 515–518, 1993

108. Raynor DK, Booth TG, Blenkinsopp A: Effects of computer generated reminder charts on patients' compliance with drug regimens. BMJ 306: 1158–1161, 1993

109. Marcharia WM, Leon G, Rowe BH et al: An overview of intervention to improve appointment keeping for medical services. JAMA 267: 1813–1817, 1992

110. Burke LE, Dunbar-Jacob J, Orchard TJ et al: Is there an association between self-reported dietary adherence and nutrition knowledge? Ann Behav Med 20: Suppl 199, 1998

111. Mazzuca SA: Does patient education in chronic disease have therapeutic value. Journal of Chronic Diseases 35: 521–529, 1982

112. Mullen PD, Green LW, Persinger GS: Clinical trials of patient education for chronic conditions: A comparative meta-analysis of intervention types. Prev Med 14: 753–781, 1985

113. Van Horn L, Kavey RE: Diet and cardiovascular disease prevention: What works? Ann Behav Med 19: 197–212, 1997

114. Mullen PD, Simons-Morton DG, Ramirez G et al: A meta-analysis of trials evaluating patient education and counseling for three groups of preventive health behaviors. Patient Education and Counseling 32: 157–173, 1997

115. Hill MN, Berk RA: Psychological barriers to hypertension therapy adherence: Instrument development and preliminary psychometric evidence. Cardiovascular Nursing 31: 37–43, 1995

116. Hickey ML, Owen SV, Froman RD: Instrument development: Cardiac diet and exercise self-efficacy. Nurs Res 41: 347–351, 1992

117. Sallis JF, Pinski RB, Grossman RM et al: The development of self-efficacy scales for health-related diet and exercise behaviors. Health Education Research 3: 283–292, 1988

118. Burke LE, Ewart CK, Thompson PD et al: Psychometric evaluation of the Cholesterol-Lowering Diet Self-Efficacy Scale. Circulation Suppl I 92: 66, 1995

119. Burke LE, Dunbar-Jacob J, Sereika S et al: The Cholesterol-Lowering Diet Self-Efficacy Scale: Development and validation. 1998 (submitted for publication)

120. McCann BS, Retzlaff BM, Dowdy AA et al: Promoting adherence to low-fat, low-cholesterol diets: Review and recommendations. J Am Diet Assoc 90: 1408–1414, 1417, 1990

121. Glynn SM, Ruderman AJ: The development and validation of an eating self-efficacy scale. Cognitive Therapeutic Research 10: pp 403–420, 1986

122. Clark MM, Abrams DB, Niaura RS et al: Self-efficacy in weight management. J Consult Clin Psychol 59: 739–744, 1991

123. Baer JS, Holt CS, Licktenstein E: Self-efficacy and smoking reexamined: Construct validity and clinical utility. J Consult Clin Psychol 54: 846–852, 1986

124. De Geest S, Abraham I, Gemoets H et al: Development of the long-term medication behaviour self-efficacy scale: Qualitative study for item development. J Adv Nurs 19: 233–238, 1994

125. Oka RK, Sivarajan Froelicher ES, Burke LE: Health promotion and behavioral interventions. In Wood SL, Froelicher ESS, Halpenny CJ et al (eds): Cardiac Nursing, 3rd ed, pp 690–707. Philadelphia, JB Lippincott, 1995

126. Kanfer FH, Schefft BK: Guiding the Process of Therapeutic Change. Champaign, IL, Research Press, 1988

127. Miller NH, Hill MN, Kottke T et al: The multilevel compliance challenge: Recommendations for a call to action. A statement for healthcare professionals. Circulation 95: 1085–1090, 1997

Index

Page numbers followed by *f* indicate figures, *t* tables, *d* displays, and *ncp* nursing care plans

A

Abciximab, use of after coronary stent placement, 550

Abdomen, physical assessment of, 223–225, 224*f*–225*f*

Abdominal obesity, 861, 861*t*

Abdominojugular reflux, 202

Aberrancy, *vs.* ventricular atopy, 338–346, 339*f*–346*f*, 339*t*. *See also* Ventricular atopy, *vs.* aberrancy

Acarbose, 877

Accelerated idioventricular rhythm, 323, 323*f*

Accessory pathways, in Wolff-Parkinson-White syndrome, 330, 330*f*–331*f*

ACE inhibitors. *See* Angiotensin-converting enzyme (ACE) inhibitors

Acetylcholine
in blood pressure regulation, 88
and electrical activity, 29–30, 30*f*

Acid-base balance
processes in, 153
terminology related to, 153

Acid-base imbalances, 155–160, 156*d*–159*d*, 158*t*, 160*t*
arterial blood gases in, 159–160
metabolic acidosis and, 156–157, 157*d*, 158*t*
metabolic alkalosis and, 158–159, 159*d*
mixed, 160, 160*t*
respiratory acidosis and, 155–156, 156*d*
respiratory alkalosis and, 158, 158*d*
vascular effects of, 158*t*

Acid buffers, 153–154, 154*t*–155*t*

Acidosis, 155–159, 156*d*–157*d*, 158*t*
and electrical activity, 30
metabolic, 156–157, 157*d*, 158*t*
respiratory, 155–156, 156*d*

Acids
definition of, 153
excretion of, 154, 155*t*
production of, 153

ACT (activated clotting time), 242

Action potential, 22–27, 23*f*–26*f*, 23*t*
of atrioventricular node cells, 26, 26*f*
of bundle of His cells, 26
early repolarization phase of, 24–25
interim between, 25
late rapid repolarization phase of, 25
of myocardial cells, 23–25, 24*f*
myocardial ischemia and, 499–500, 500*f*
phases of, 23–24
plateau, 25
upstroke, 24, 24*f*

of Purkinje cells, 23*f*–24*f*, 26
refractory period in, 26*f*, 26–27
of sinus node cells, 23*f*, 25

Activated clotting time (ACT), 242

Activated partial thromboplastin time (aPTT), 242

Activity
after myocardial infarction, 527
in control of hypertension, 791–792
definition of, 841
and hyperlipidemia, 829
increased, during cardiac rehabilitation, 850, 850*t*, 851*f*, 852
in prevention of coronary heart disease, 743*f*–744*f*, 743–745
previous level of, and cardiac rehabilitation, 844, 845*f*, 854
for treatment of obesity, 865

Activity-exercise functional pattern, assessment of, 194

Activity intolerance, after cardiac transplantation, 608*d*

Acute marginal branch, of right coronary artery, 14–15

Adaptive atrioventricular delay, 664*d*

Adenosine
properties of, 303*t*
for tachyarrhythmias, 311*t*

Adenosine diphosphate (ADP), in hemostasis, 112

Adenosine triphosphate (ATP), and myocardial metabolism, 42

ADH. *See* Antidiuretic hormone (ADH)

Adherence, 38–39, 39*f*, 92
with antihyperlipidemic therapy, 831–832
with antihypertensive therapy, 804*t*, 805*d*, 809*d*–810*d*
behavior change for, models of, 884–885, 885*d*
definition of, 880
factors affecting, 884, 884*d*
measurement of, 881–884, 882*t*
biologic methods of, 882*t*, 883
electronic monitoring in, 882*t*, 883–884
pill counts in, 884
self-report in, 881–883, 882*t*
patient/family education about, 887–888, 888*d*
strategies for enhancing, 885*d*, 885–887
questionnaires for, 887–888, 888*d*
therapeutic relationship and, 888–889

ADP. *See* Adenosine diphosphate (ADP)

Adrenergic inhibitors
for antihypertensive therapy, 798*t*

parenteral, for hypertensive crisis, 801*t*

Adrenergic nerves, distribution of, 83*f*

Adrenergic stimulation, of vascular system, 58–59, 59*f*

Adrenergic substances, and electrical activity, 29*f*–30*f*, 29–30

α-Adrenergic system, and control of venous system, 96*f*, 96–97

Adrenoreceptors, function of, 84, 86, 86*t*, 87*f*

Adult respiratory distress syndrome (ARDS), radiographic imaging of, 260*f*–261*f*

Advanced cardiac life support, 642–646, 644*f*

Adventitia, morphology of, 482, 482*f*

Adventitious breath sounds, 223, 223*f*

Afterdepolarization, triggered activity from, 298*f*, 298–299

Afterload, 36–37, 37*f*
and cardiac output, 91–92
decrease in, ventricular function curve in, 456*f*
force-velocity relationship and, 39*f*, 39–40
as hemodynamic index, 460*t*

Age, and cardiac rehabilitation, 842–843, 853

Agency for Health Care Policy and Research (AHCPR)
algorithm for management of heart failure, 571*f*
guidelines for cardiac rehabilitation, 839–840
smoking cessation clinical practice guidelines of, 767–772, 768*d*, 770*f*–771*f*, 772*d*

Aging
and cardiovascular function, 183–184, 849*d*
changes related to, classification of, 183
and chronic illness, 182, 182*f*
demographics of, 181, 181*f*
and drug absorption, 185–186
and drug distribution, 186
and drug metabolism, 186
and hepatic function, 185
and renal function, 185
and respiratory function, 184*f*, 184–185
and sleep, 166*f*, 166–167
theories of, 182

AHCPR. *See* Agency for Health Care Policy and Research

AH interval, in electrophysiology studies, 363, 365*f*

AICDs. *See* Implantable cardioverter-defibrillators (ICDs)

893

Air embolism
from arterial pressure monitoring, 434
from pulmonary artery pressure
monitoring, 449t
Airway, aging and, 184–185
Alcohol, and hyperlipidemia, 829
Alcohol use
reduction of, in control of hypertension,
792–793
and smoking cessation, 773
Aldosterone, and urinary excretion, 134t
Aldosteronism, and hypertension, 782
Alkaline phosphatase, levels of, 245
Alkalosis, 157–159, 158d–159d
and electrical activity, 30
metabolic, 158–159, 159d
respiratory, 158, 158d
Allografts
atherosclerosis in, 600
for prosthetic valves, 706
Alpha blockers
for antihypertensive therapy, 798t–799t
drug interactions with, 797t
Amiodarone, properties of, 303t–304t
Ammonia, and acid-base balance, 154
Amrinone, for heart failure, 572
Anaerobic metabolism
in myocardial ischemia, 498, 498f
in shock, 617
Anaphylactic shock. See Shock, anaphylactic
Anemia, 240
Aneroid manometers, 204, 205f
Aneurysms
aortic
ascending, repair of, 588–589
dissecting, radiographic imaging
of, 257f
left ventricular
from myocardial infarction, 520–521
radiographic imaging of, 259f
ANF (atrial natriuretic factor), in heart
failure, 564
Anger, and coronary heart disease,
759–761
Angina
classification of, 506, 507d,
507t–509t, 508f
diagnosis of, 506–510, 509d–510d
cardiac catheterization in, 510
cardiac imaging in, 509–510
coronary angiography in, 510
electrocardiography in, 509
history in, 506–509, 510d
physical assessment in, 508–509
stress testing in, 509
differential diagnosis of, 190t
during exercise testing, 399, 400d
medical management of, 510–511
nursing management of, 511–512
prognosis in, 511
during sleep, 169–170
stable
classification of, 506, 508f
medical management of, 510–511
unstable
classification of, 506, 507t–509t
medical management of, 511

variant
classification of, 506
medical management of, 511
Angiography
in myocardial ischemia, 510
quantitative, 417, 417f
radioisotope, 382f
Angioplasty, laser, 549
Angiotensin-converting enzyme
(ACE) inhibitors
with calcium antagonists, for
antihypertensive therapy, 800t
with diuretics, for antihypertensive
therapy, 800t
drug interactions with, 797t
for heart failure, 570–571, 573t
and hyperkalemia, 140
for myocardial infarction, 531
Angiotensin II, function of, 89, 89f
Angiotensin II receptor blockers, for
antihypertensive therapy, 799t
Anion gap, calculation of, 245t
Anions, superoxide, vascular effects of, 57
Anisotropic reentry, 301
Anisoylated plasminogen streptokinase
activator complex, 541–542
Ankle–brachial systolic pressure index, 210
ANP. See Atrial natriuretic peptide (ANP)
Antegrade conduction, through accessory
pathway, in Wolff-Parkinson-White
syndrome, 330, 331f
Antiarrhythmic agents
classification of, 302t
for heart failure, 574
for hypertrophic cardiomyopathy, 726
properties of, 303t
Antibiotics, for infectious endocarditis, 731
Anticoagulants
for deep venous thrombosis prophylaxis,
125, 127d
for pulmonary embolism, 129
Antidiuretic hormone (ADH)
in blood pressure regulation, 90
and urinary excretion, 134t
Antidromic circus movement tachycardia,
335, 335f
Antioxidants, and risk of coronary heart
disease, 749–750
Antiplatelet agents, use of after coronary
stent placement, 550–551
Antitachycardia pacing, 667
Antithrombin, functions of, 114
Antithymocyte preparations, side effects of,
602t, 603
Anxiety
and coronary heart disease, 760–762
during interventional cardiology
procedures, 555
from myocardial infarction, 536–537
Aortic aneurysms
ascending, repair of, 588–589
dissecting, radiographic imaging of, 257f
Aortic ejection sound, 216
Aortic impedance, in heart failure, 563
Aortic insufficiency, 715–716, 716t
imaging studies of, 385, 386f
new-onset, auscultation of, 217

Aortic pressure, changes in, during cardiac
cycle, 63f
Aortic root, echocardiography of, 380
Aortic stenosis, 713–715, 714f
imaging studies of, 385
Aortic valve
anatomy of, 8–9
echocardiography of, 380
replacement of, 587, 715, 716
Apoproteins, function of, 819
Aprotinin, for postoperative bleeding from
cardiac surgery, 591
aPTT (activated partial thromboplastin
time), 242
ARDS. See Adult respiratory distress
syndrome (ARDS)
Arginine vasopressin. See Antidiuretic
hormone (ADH)
Arm circumference, in assessment of blood
pressure, 204t
Arrhythmias, 297–359. See also specific type
and Conduction disorders
after cardiac catheterization, 420
assessment of blood pressure during,
208–209
basic, 302–328, 314f–328f
originating in sinus node, 302,
310f–317f, 314–317
complex, 329f–346f, 329–346
preexcitation syndromes and,
329f–332f, 329–333
supraventricular tachycardia and,
333–335, 334f–335f
ventricular tachycardia and, 335–338,
336f–337f
during exercise testing, 399
hypercalcemia and, 143
hyperkalemia and, 141
hypokalemia and, 139–140
hypomagnesemia and, 145
from interventional cardiology procedures,
556–557
malignant, electrical therapy for, 642–643
in mitral valve prolapse, 711
in myocardial infarction, 519–520
myocardial ischemia and, 500–501
originating in atria, 317f–320f, 317–321
originating in atrioventricular junction,
321f, 321–322
originating in ventricles, 322f–325f,
322–325
pathophysiology of, 297–301,
298f–301f
abnormal impulse conduction in,
299–301, 300f–301f
abnormal impulse initiation in,
297–299, 298f
postoperative, 592f–593f, 592–593
sinus, 91, 315, 315f
during sleep, 170
sleep apnea and, 171
ventricular, pacing and, 685
Arterial baroreceptors, in blood pressure
regulation, 82, 83f
Arterial blood gases, 243
in heart failure, 568
interpretation of, 159–160

Arterial blood pressure, in shock, 616
Arterial circulation, assessment of, 210
Arterial dilators, for heart failure, 573
Arterial line, drawing blood from, 436, 436*d*
Arterial occlusion, acute, 122*f*,
    122–123, 123*t*
Arterial oxygen partial pressure (PaO₂),
    factors influencing, 74
Arterial oxygen saturation (SaO₂), 243
  and oxygen delivery, 79
Arterial pressure, 62
  baroreceptor response to, 101*f*–102*f*,
    101–102
  monitoring of, 433–436, 434*f*–435*f*, 436*d*
    catheter placement in, 433
    complications of, 433–434
    interpretation of data from,
      434–435, 435*f*
    vs. cuff pressure, 436
Arterial pressure wave, 62–63, 63*f*
Arterial pulse, assessment of, 199–202,
    200*f*–201*f*
Arterial thrombosis
  from arterial pressure monitoring, 434
  from cardiac catheterization, 420
  from coronary stents, 554
Arterial wall, morphology of,
    481–482, 482*f*
Arterial waveforms, during cardiac cycle,
    435*f*, 435–436
Arteries
  anatomy of, 52, 52*f*
  distensibility of, 62
Arteriography, coronary, 415–416, 416*f*
  in heart failure, 568–569
Arteriolar sclerosis, definition of, 481
Arterioles
  resistance in, local regulation of, 94
  structure of, 52
Arteriosclerosis
  definition of, 481
  hypertension and, 785
Arteriovenous fistulas, from coronary
    stents, 554
Ascending aortic aneurysm, repair of,
    588–589
Ashman's phenomenon, 343
Aspartate aminotransferase, 238*t*, 239
Aspirin, for myocardial infarction, 528
Assessment
  history-taking in, 190*t*, 190–195, 195*t*. *See
    also* History-taking
  physical, 195–225. *See also*
    Physical assessment
Asynchronous pacing, 663*d*, 669–670
Asystole
  management of, 647, 650*f*
  treatment of, 313*t*
  ventricular, 325, 325*f*
Atelectasis, radiographic imaging of, 256*f*
Atenolol, properties of, 304*t*
Atherectomy, 546–549, 547*f*–548*f*
  complications of, 548–549
  directional, 547, 547*f*
  rotational ablation in, 547*f*, 547–548
  transluminal extraction, 548, 548*f*
Atheroma, morphology of, 489*f*

Atherosclerosis
  in allograft, 600
  classification of, 545*d*
  definition of, 481
  hypertension and, 785
  hypomagnesemia and, 146
  pathogenesis of, inflammatory response
    hypothesis in, 489–491
  peripheral, 210
  smoking and, 765
Atherosclerotic plaques
  components of, 482–487, 483*f*–485*f*
    cytokines as, 486–487
    endothelial cells as, 482, 483*f*, 491
    extracellular matrix as, 486
    growth factors as, 485–487
    lymphocytes as, 485, 485*f*
    macrophages as, 484–485, 485*f*
    monocytes as, 484–485, 485*f*
    platelets as, 485–486
    vasa vasorum as, 486
    vascular smooth muscle cells as,
      482–484, 484*f*
  distribution of, 487
  evolution of, 488*f*
  morphologic classification of, 487–489,
    488*f*–489*f*
    complicated, 489
    fatty, 488
    fatty streaks in, 487–488
    fibrous, 488, 489*f*
    stable, 489, 590*d*
    vulnerable, 489, 490*f*
  vascular remodeling of, 489, 490*f*
Atria, arrhythmias originating in, 317*f*–320*f*,
    317–321
Atrial arrhythmias
  postoperative, 592–593, 593*f*
  treatment of, radiofrequency catheter
    ablation in, 370
Atrial capture, evaluation of, 680–681
Atrial conduction, 30–31, 31*t*
Atrial contraction, 45*f*, 46–47
Atrial electrocardiography, 592*f*
Atrial electrogram, in differential diagnosis of
    ventricular atopy *vs.* aberrancy,
    344–346, 345*f*
Atrial enlargement, electrocardiography in,
    288–289, 289*f*
Atrial escape interval, 678
Atrial fibrillation, 319–320, 320*f*
  with aberrancy, 344*f*–345*f*
  through accessory pathway, in Wolff-
    Parkinson-White syndrome,
    330, 331*f*
  treatment of, 311*t*–312*t*
    radiofrequency catheter ablation in,
      369–370
Atrial flutter, 319, 319*f*
  with aberrancy, 344*f*
  treatment of, radiofrequency catheter
    ablation in, 369–370
  with Wenckebach exit block,
    353, 354*f*
Atrial natriuretic factor (ANF)
  in blood pressure regulation, 83
  in heart failure, 564

Atrial natriuretic peptide (ANP), and urinary
    excretion, 134*t*
Atrial overdrive pacing, 667
Atrial pacing state, 679, 680*f*–681*f*
Atrial parasystole, 357, 357*f*
Atrial pressure, monitoring of, phlebostatic
    axis for, 428, 429*f*–430*f*
Atrial refractory period, 664*d*
Atrial sensing, evaluation of, 681
Atrial tachycardia
  multifocal, 318, 318*f*
  treatment of, 311*t*–312*t*
  with Wenckebach conduction, 349*f*
Atrial tracking, 664*d*
Atrial tracking state, 679, 680*f*–681*f*
Atrioventricular block
  first-degree, 325, 325*f*
  high-grade, 328, 328*f*
  multilevel, 351–353, 352*f*–354*f*
  second-degree, 325–327, 326*f*–327*f*
    2:1 conduction in, 327, 327*f*
    treatment of, 313*t*
    type I (Wenckebach), 326, 326*f*
    type II, 326*f*, 326–327
  third-degree (complete), 328, 328*f*
    with atrioventricular dissociation,
      354, 355*f*
    treatment of, 313*t*
  Wenckebach, treatment of, 313*t*. *See also*
    Wenckebach conduction
Atrioventricular delay
  adaptive, 664*d*, 678
  nonphysiologic, 684, 685*f*
Atrioventricular dissociation, 209, 354,
    355*f*–356*f*
Atrioventricular interval, in dual-chamber
    pacing, 664*d*
Atrioventricular junction, arrhythmias
    originating in, 321*f*, 321–322
Atrioventricular nodal branch, of right
    coronary artery, 15
Atrioventricular nodal reentrant tachycardia
    (AVNRT), 333, 334*f*
  treatment of, 311*t*–312*t*
    radiofrequency catheter ablation in,
      368, 369*f*
Atrioventricular node, 263
  anatomy of, 10–11, 12*f*
  cells in, action potential of, 26, 26*f*
Atrioventricular reciprocating tachycardia,
    335, 335*f*
Atrioventricular reentrant tachycardia,
    treatment of, radiofrequency
    catheter ablation in,
    368–369, 370*f*
Atrioventricular sequential pacing state, 679,
    680*f*–681*f*
Atrioventricular sulcus, 5
Atrioventricular valves, anatomy of, 8, 8*f*
Atrium, right, anatomy of, 5
Atropine
  for bradyarrhythmias, 313*t*
  properties of, 304*t*
Auscultation
  in assessment of abdomen, 224
  in assessment of blood pressure, 205–207,
    206*f*, 206*t*

Auscultation (*continued*)
in assessment of heart, 212–219, 213*f*–217*f*, 213*t*–218*t*
in assessment of lungs, 221–223, 224*f*
dynamic, 217–219, 218*t*
of murmurs, 216*f*, 216*t*, 215–216
of normal heart sounds, 213*f*–214*f*, 213–214
technique of, 213, 213*t*
use of stethoscope in, 212–213
Auscultatory gap, 206*f*, 206–207
Autacoids, and vascular resistance, 55, 92–93
Automated exercise testing report, 395*d*–396*d*
Automatic implantable carioverter-defibrillators (AICDs). *See* Implantable cardioverter-defibrillators (ICDs)
Automatic interval, 663*d*
Automaticity, 18
abnormal, 297–298
enhanced normal, 297, 298*f*
myocardial ischemia and, 501
normal, 297
Autonomic nervous system
in blood pressure regulation, 84–88, 85*f*, 86*t*, 87*f*–88*f*
cardiovascular effects of, 86*t*
Autoregulation, 94–96, 95*f*
metabolic hypothesis of, 95
myogenic hypothesis of, 94–95
tissue pressure hypothesis of, 95–96
AV. *See* Atrioventricular *entries*
AVNRT. *See* Atrioventricular nodal reentrant tachycardia (AVNRT)
Axes, determination of, on electrocardiography, 273*f*–276*f*, 273–275
Azathioprine, side effects of, 602*t*, 603

B

Background outward current, 27*t*, 28
Backward heart failure, 560–561
Bacterial endocarditis, imaging of, 387
Balke treadmill test, 393
Balloon-expandable coronary stents, 552, 552*t*, 554*f*
Baroreceptors
arterial, in blood pressure regulation, 82, 83*f*, 101*f*–102*f*, 101–102
cardiopulmonary, in blood pressure regulation, 82–83
left ventricular, in blood pressure regulation, 83–84
Barrel chest, 222*f*
Basal tone, and regulation of blood pressure, 93–94
Base rate, in pacing, 663*d*
Bases, definition of, 153
Basophils, properties of, 111
B cells, properties of, 111
Bed rest
cardiovascular effects of, 839, 839*d*
and orthostatic hypotension, 99
Behavioral therapy, for treatment of obesity, 865–866
Behavior change, models of, 884–885, 885*d*

Benzodiazepines, for sleep, 174
Beta blockers
for antihypertensive therapy, 798*t*–799*t*
contraindications to, 530
with diuretics, for antihypertensive therapy, 800*t*
for heart failure, 570, 573–574
for hypertrophic cardiomyopathy, 726
for myocardial infarction, 529–530
parenteral, for hypertensive crisis, 801*t*
properties of, 302*t*
for tachyarrhythmias, 311*t*
Bezold-Jarisch reflex, 83–84
Biatrial enlargement, electrocardiography in, 289
Bicarbonate, excretion of, 154
Bicarbonate buffer system, 153, 154*t*–155*t*
Bicarbonate concentration, interpretation of, 159
Bicycle ergometry, after cardiac transplantation, 603
Bifascicular block, electrocardiography in, 281–282, 282*f*
Bigeminal pulses, 200, 200*f*
Biguanides, 876–877
Bile acid binding agents, for hyperlipidemia, 830, 830*t*
Bileaflet valves, 705
Bilirubin, levels of, 245–246
Bioimpedance cardiac output measurement, 461–462
Biologic membranes, characteristics of, 18*t*, 18–19, 19*f*
Bipolar leads, for electrocardiography, placement of, 269, 270*f*
Bipolar pacing, 663*d*, 668–669, 670*f*
Bladder distention, assessment of, 224–225
Blanking period, 664*d*, 678, 684, 685*f*
Bleeding
after cardiac surgery, 591
in disseminated intravascular coagulation, 119*d*
from thrombolytic therapy, 543
Bleeding disorders, 115*d*, 115–118, 117*t*–118*t*, 119*d*–121. *See also* Disseminated intravascular coagulation (DIC)
Block response, in dual-chamber pacing, 682, 682*f*
Blood
functions of, 109
hydrostatic pressure of, 133
oxygen content of, 79
pH of, 153
Blood chemistries, 244–247, 245*t*, 247*t*
after cardiac surgery, 246
of serum electrolytes, 244–245, 245*t*
specimen collection for, 246
Blood cultures, 241
Blood flow
blood pressure and, 61, 61*f*
to brain, during sleep, 168
coronary
alterations in, 497
control of, 43*f*, 43–44
definition of, 60
determinants of, 61–62

impaired, and thrombosis, 122
local metabolic control of, 57–58, 58*f*
nonturbulent, 61
in stenotic vessels, 497
through cardiac chambers, 8*f*
through microvascular system, 64
Blood gases
arterial, 243
in heart failure, 568
interpretation of, 159–160
reference values for, 238*t*
Blood glucose, monitoring of, in diabetes mellitus, 875
Blood lipids, 246–247, 247*t*
structure and function of, 819
Blood pressure
arterial, in shock, 616
assessment of, 203–209, 204*t*–206*t*, 205*f*–208*f*, 787–788, 788*t*
arm position in, 205
during arrhythmias, 208–209
auscultation in, 205–207, 206*f*, 206*t*
in community settings, 209
diastolic, 206
follow-up after, 788*t*
obesity and, 209
palpation in, 205
paradoxical, 208, 208*f*
postural, 207–208
in shock, 209
systolic, 205–206
on thigh, 209
use of sphygmomanometer in, 203–205, 204*t*, 205*f*
during cardiac rehabilitation, 849
decreased, sympathetic response to, 101*f*, 101–102
during exercise testing, 396–397
invasive monitoring of, equipment for, 427*f*
physiology of, 61, 61*f*
postural, extracellular fluid volume deficit and, 135
regulation of
acetylcholine in, 88
antidiuretic hormone in, 90
arterial baroreceptors in, 82, 83*f*
atrial natriuretic factor in, 83
autonomic nervous system in, 84–88, 85*f*, 86*t*, 87*f*–88*f*
parasympathetic, 87–88
sympathetic, 84–87, 85*f*, 86*t*, 87*f*–88*f*
baroreceptors in, 101*f*–102*f*, 101–102
cardiopulmonary receptors in, 82–83
central nervous system in, 84
cotransmitters in, 88
epinephrine in, 88–89
left ventricular baroreceptors in, 83–84
long-term, 93
neurotransmitters in, 86–87, 88*f*
renin-angiotensin-aldosterone system in, 89, 89*f*
respiration and, 99–100
sleep and, 167
Blood reservoir, 75
Blood specimens
collection of, 227–230, 228–229

from arterial line, 436, 436*d*
patient preparation for, 227
positioning for, 229
from pulmonary artery catheter, 228
timing of, 229
universal precautions for, 227
contamination of, 228
hemolysis in, 229
results of, interpretation of, 229–230
Blood studies, reference values for, 229
Blood transfusions, and hyperkalemia, 140
Blood urea nitrogen (BUN), 246
Blood vessels
classification of, 51
injury to, and thrombosis, 121*f*, 121–122
structure of, 51*f*–54*f*, 51–55
Blood volume, peripheral, increased,
maintenance of end-diastolic
volume with, 98–99
BMI. *See* Body mass index (BMI)
Body fluid compartments, 132
Body fluids
distribution of, 133
excretion of, 133, 134*f*
extracellular. *See* Extracellular fluid (ECF)
intracellular. *See* Intracellular fluid (ICF)
loss of, abnormal means of, 134
Body mass index (BMI)
calculation of, 861, 861*t*
and coronary heart disease, 746–748, 747*f*
Body temperature
after cardiac catheterization, 420
assessment of, 196–197
during sleep, 168
Body weight. *See* Weight
Brachial plexus injury, from cardiac
surgery, 594
Bradyarrhythmias
in myocardial infarction, 520
treatment of, 313*t*
Bradycardia
sinus, 314, 314*f*
during sleep, 170
treatment of, 313*t*
symptomatic, management of, 653, 654*f*
treatment of, by implantable cardioverter-
defibrillator, 693
Brady-tachy syndrome, 316*f*, 316–317
Brain, blood flow to, during sleep, 168
Breath sounds, adventitious, 223, 223*f*
Bretylium, properties of, 305*t*
Bronchial sounds, 223
Bronchovesicular sounds, 223
Bruce treadmill test, 393
Bruits, 201–202
Buffer systems, 153–154, 154*t*–155*t*
BUN. *See* Blood urea nitrogen (BUN)
Bundle branch block
electrocardiography in, 276–278, 278*f*
left, QRS morphology in, 340–341, 342*f*
right, QRS morphology in, 340,
341*f*–342*f*
Bundle branches, 264
Wenckebach conduction in, 349–350, 350*f*
Bundle branch reentrant tachycardia,
treatment of, radiofrequency
catheter ablation in, 370

Bundle of His, 263
anatomy of, 11, 11*f*
cells in, action potential of, 26

C
CABG. *See* Coronary artery bypass
graft (CABG)
CAGE questionnaire, 770*f*
Caged-ball valves, 705–706
Calcium
balance of, 138*t*, 141–144, 142*d*–143*d*
equilibrium potential of, 21
in excitation-contraction coupling, 32*f*,
32–33
serum levels of, 244, 245*t*
sources of, 59
and vascular system, 59–60, 60*f*
Calcium antagonists
with angiotensin-converting enzyme
inhibitors, for antihypertensive
therapy, 800*t*
drug interactions with, 797*t*
Calcium channel blockers, 302*t*
for heart failure, with systolic
dysfunction, 570
for hypertrophic cardiomyopathy, 726
for myocardial infarction, 530
for tachyarrhythmias, 311*t*
Calcium concentration, sarcoplasmic,
modulation of, 35–36
Calcium currents, 27*t*, 28
Calcium signaling, 59–60, 60*f*
cAMP. *See* Cyclic adenosine
monophosphate (cAMP)
Canadian Cardiovascular Society, classification
of angina, 509*d*
Capillaries, structure of, 52–53
Capillary filtration coefficient, 65
Capillary pressure, mean, 66
Capillary refill time, 210
Captopril, for heart failure, 571, 573*t*
Capture, 670
evaluation of, 674–675, 676*f*, 680–681
Capture beats, in ventricular atopy, *vs.*
aberrancy, 341, 342*f*–343*f*, 343
Carbon dioxide
alveolar-capillary transfer of, 76*f*–77*f*, 76–77
diffusion of, 78
Carbon dioxide partial pressure (PCO$_2$),
factors influencing, 74
Carbonic acid, production of, 153
Carbon monoxide
adverse effects of, smoking and, 765
thoracic electrical bioimpedance
measurement of, 461–462
Cardiac arrest
impending, management of, 647–653,
654*f*–656*f*
with ventricular tachycardia, 647–653,
652*f*–656*f*
management of, 642–653, 644*f*–652*f*,
646*d*–647*d*
advanced cardiac life support in,
642–646, 644*f*
defibrillation in, 642–646, 644*f*–646*f*
medical management of, 653–656, 655*f*

cerebral resuscitation in, 653–655
immediate goals in, 653
ongoing care in, 655, 655*f*
reduction of ischemia in, 655–656
pathophysiology of, 639–642, 640*d*, 641*f*
abnormal ventricular function in, 641
initiating mechanisms in, 641*f*, 641–642
structural abnormalities in,
639–641, 640*d*
ventricular fibrillation in, 642
patient/family education about, 656–657
prognosis after, 653
recurrent, risk factors for, 642
survivors of, electrophysiology studies in,
364–365
Cardiac catheterization, 409–424
in aortic insufficiency, 716
in aortic stenosis, 713
approaches to, 412*f*, 412–413
complications of, 419*t*, 420–421
contraction abnormalities on, 424*f*
contraindications to, 410
contrast agents for, 418
coronary. *See* Coronary arteriography
for determination of cardiac output,
416–418, 417*f*
discharge planning in, 420*t*
history of, 409
indications for, 409–410
of left heart, 413*f*–414*f*, 413–415
results of, 423*f*
outpatient, 411
patient/family education about, 410–411,
419–420, 420*t*
patient preparation for, 410–411
percutaneous, 412*f*, 412–413
postprocedure care in, 419*t*, 419–420
results of
interpretation of, 421*t*, 421–423,
422*f*–424*f*
reference values for, 421*t*, 421–422,
422*f*–424*f*
of right heart, 413, 413*f*
results of, 422*f*
ventricular. *See* Ventriculography
Cardiac catheterization laboratory, 411–412
role of nurse in, 418–421, 419*t*–420*t*
Cardiac cells
hyperpolarization of. *See* Hyperpolarization
mechanical properties of, 33–36, 34*f*–36*f*.
See also Contraction; Relaxation
Cardiac conduction. *See* Conduction
Cardiac cycle, 44–48, 45*f*, 46*t*
arterial waveforms during, 435*f*, 435–436
atrial contraction in, 45*f*, 46–47
changes in arterial pressure during, 63*f*
diastolic events in, 48
left ventricular, 45*f*, 45–46, 46*t*
right ventricular, 47
systolic events in, 47
valvular, 47
waves, complexes, and intervals of, 264*f*,
264–266, 265*t*–266*t*
Cardiac enzymes, 231–239, 232*f*–237*f*,
232*t*, 235*t*–238*t*. *See also*
specific enzymes
elevation of, after atherectomy, 548

Cardiac fibers, stretching of, and electrical
activity, 30
Cardiac impulse, propagation of, 30–33,
31t, 32f
Cardiac impulse conduction velocity, 29
Cardiac index, in heart failure, 569
Cardiac muscle
contractility of, 40, 40f
relaxation of, molecular basis of, 35
Cardiac nerves, anatomy of, 16–17
Cardiac output
afterload and, 91–92
and central venous pressure, 97f–98f,
97–99
clinically important changes in, 456–459,
457t–460t
decreased
after cardiac transplantation, 605d–606d
in myocardial infarction, 538d–539d
in patient with intra-aortic balloon
pump, 631d
in shock, 618, 618f, 636
in heart failure, 575–576
heart rate and, 91
maximization of, for cardiogenic shock,
621–622
measurement of, 452f–453f, 452–459,
454d, 456f
bioimpedance, 461–462
calibration constant for, 453
catheter position and, 452
closed injectate system for, 456
complications of, 457t–458t
concomitant infusions and, 455
continuous, 460–461, 461f
injection port for, 453
injection technique for, 454d, 454–455
positioning for, 455
respiratory effects on, 455
and oxygen delivery, 78
preload and, 91
respiration and, 99–100
studies of, 416–418, 417f
Cardiac perforation, from electrophysiology
studies, 364
Cardiac plexus, anatomy of, 16
Cardiac rehabilitation
Agency for Health Care Policy and
Research guidelines on, 839–840
and cardiac risk factors, 841d
in chronic heart failure, 838
continuation programs for, 856–857
definition of, 840
goals of, 840
inpatient, 842d–852d, 842–852, 845f,
847t–852t, 851f
assessment in, 842d–844d, 842–846,
845f, 847t
concurrent health problems and, 846
educational component of, 852,
852d–853d, 852t
electrocardiography during, 849–850,
850f, 850t
evaluation during, 848–850,
849d–850d
increasing activity during, 850, 850t,
851f, 852

indications for, 850t
initiation of, 846–848, 848t
risk stratification in, 843d–844d, 847t
outpatient, 853–856
assessment in, 853–854
educational component of, 856, 857
evaluation during, 854–855
increasing activity in, 855–856
for patient with congestive heart
failure, 855
terms related to, 841
Cardiac reserve, 41, 41f, 81
Cardiac rhythm. See also Arrhythmias
on electrocardiography, 268
Cardiac surgery. See also specific procedures
coagulation studies after, 243
complications of
early, 591–595, 592f–593f
gastrointestinal, 594
neuropsychological, 594
pulmonary, 593
renal, 593–594
late, 595, 595f
minimally invasive, 581f–582f, 581–584
myocardial protection during, 583
preoperative assessment in, 580–581
sleep after, 169
trends in, 580
Cardiac tamponade, 723
paradoxical blood pressure during,
208, 208f
postoperative, 591, 595
Cardiac tissue, anatomy of, 9f–12f, 9–12, 13t
Cardiac transplantation, 595–610
contraindications to, 597t
for dilated cardiomyopathy, 725
discharge planning in, 604
dyspnea index for, 604t
evaluation of candidates for,
596–597, 597t
evaluation of donor for, 597
exercise testing after, 405
exercise training after, 603–604, 604f, 604t
medical management of, 599t–602t,
599–603, 600f
cardiac function and, 599, 599t
hemodynamic monitoring in,
599, 599t
monitoring for immunosuppressant side
effects in, 601–603, 602t
monitoring for infection in, 601
monitoring for rejection in, 600f, 600t,
600–601
preoperative status and, 599
nursing management of, 605, 605d–715d
patient/family education about, 604,
609d–610d
procedure for, 597–598, 598f
progress in, 596
sexual dysfunction after, 603
surgical procedure for, 597–598, 598f
Cardiac valves. See also specific valves
anatomy of, 12f
in cardiac cycle, 47
prosthetic. See Prosthetic valves
Cardiogenic pulmonary edema, 258, 258f
Cardiogenic shock. See Shock, cardiogenic

Cardiomyopathy, 724d, 724–729
classification of, 724, 724d
dilated
clinical manifestations of, 724–725
etiology of, 724, 724d
medical management of, 725
nursing management of, 728
hypertrophic
clinical manifestations of, 726
etiology of, 725
imaging studies of, 385
medical management of, 726
nursing management of, 729
pathophysiology of, 725
prognosis in, 726
imaging studies in, 384–385
restrictive, 727
Cardiomyoplasty, dynamic, 588
for dilated cardiomyopathy, 725
Cardioplegia, 583
Cardiopulmonary bypass (CPB), 581f–582f,
581–583
Cardiopulmonary receptors, in blood
pressure regulation, 82–83
Cardiovascular disease
diabetes and, 872
history of. See also History-taking
and cardiac rehabilitation, 844, 846
and hypertension, 783d
sleep and, 168–169
Cardiovascular function
aging and, 183–184, 849d
sleep and, 167
Cardiovascular system, pressure changes
in, 64f
Cardioversion, 647–653, 651f–652f
energy requirements for, 652f, 652–653
for tachyarrhythmias, 311t
urgent synchronized, 653
Care plan. See Nursing care plan
Carotid pulse, assessment of, 201
Carotid sinus massage, for tachycardia, 346
Carotid sinus test, 366
Carvedilol, for heart failure, 570, 574
Catecholamines
and electrical activity, 29f–30f, 29–30
and hypokalemia, 137
levels of, 246
Catheterization, cardiac. See Cardiac
catheterization
Catheters
for arterial pressure monitoring, placement
of, 433
for directional atherectomy, 547, 547f
dynamic response characteristics of,
430–432, 433f
for electrophysiology studies, placement of,
363, 364f
for hemodynamic monitoring
radiographic imaging of, 259f–260f
removal of, 436
pulmonary artery. See Pulmonary
artery catheters
right ventricular ejection, 449, 451f
for rotational ablation, 547f, 547–548
for transluminal extraction atherectomy,
548, 548f

Catheter site dressings, replacement of, frequency of, 428*t*

Caval interruption, 125–126
  for pulmonary embolism, 129

CBC. *See* Complete blood count (CBC)

CCU. *See* Coronary intensive care unit (CICU)

CD4 cells, in atherosclerotic plaques, 485, 485*f*

CD8 cells, in atherosclerotic plaques, 485, 485*f*

CDH. *See* Coronary heart disease (CHD)

Cell morphology, laboratory studies of, 240–241

Central cyanosis, 196

Central nervous system (CNS), in blood pressure regulation, 84

Central sleep apnea, 171

Central venous pressure, cardiac output and, 97*f*–98*f*, 97–99

Central venous pressure (CVP), monitoring of, 436–438, 437*f*, 438*t*
  catheters for, radiographic imaging of, 259*f*

Centrifugal-kinetic energy pump, 633*f*–634*f*, 633–635

Cerebral function, shock and, 618

Cerebral resuscitation, after cardiac arrest, 653–655

CFUs. *See* Colony-forming units (CFUs)

Chemokines, in atherosclerotic plaques, 487

Chemosensor reflexes, 90

Chest, configuration of, 219, 222*f*

Chest leads, for electrocardiography, placement of, 268*f*, 269, 270*f*

Chest pain
  in angina, 508–510, 510*f*, 512*d*
  differential diagnosis of, 190*t*, 190–191, 512*d*
  during exercise testing, 399*d*
  in myocardial infarction, 517*f*
    nursing management of, 531, 534–535
  during myocardial ischemia, 502
    management of, 523*f*
  in pericarditis, 721
  in pulmonary embolism, 128

Chest radiography, 252–262. *See also* specific conditions
  in aortic insufficiency, 716
  directed-search, 253*f*–254*f*, 253–254
  interpretation of, 253*f*–254*f*, 253–254
  positioning for, 252*f*
  principles of, 252*f*–253*f*, 252–253
  structures visible on, 253*f*

Cheyne-Stokes respiration, during sleep, 171

CHF. *See* Congestive heart failure (CHF)

Chin electromyography, 163, 164*f*

Chloride
  equilibrium potential of, 21
  serum levels of, 244

Cholesterol
  and endothelial function, 822
  levels of, factors affecting, 247, 247*t*
  reverse transport of, 821

Cholinergic nerves, distribution of, 83*f*

Cholinergic receptors, in blood pressure regulation, 87–88

Cholinergic substances, and electrical activity, 29–30, 30*f*

Christa supraventricularis, 6

Chronic illness, aging and, 182, 182*f*

Chronic obstructive pulmonary disease (COPD), sleep and, 170

Chronic renal disease, and hypertension, 782, 783*d*

Chronic venous insufficiency, 211

Chylomicrons, transport of, in lipid metabolism, 821, 821*f*

CICU. *See* Coronary intensive care unit (CICU)

Cigarette smoking. *See* Smoking; Smoking cessation

Circadian rhythm, and myocardial infarction, 170

Circulation
  collateral, 44
  coronary
    anatomy of, 12–16, 13*f*–16*f*
    physiology of, 42–44, 43*f*
    vessel dominance in, 14
  microvascular
    blood flow through, 64
    transport mechanisms in, 64–66, 67*f*
  peripheral, assessment of, 201, 201*f*
  pulmonary, 73–75, 74*t*
    anatomy of, 75
    carbon dioxide in, 78
    gas exchange in, 73, 74*t*
    nonpulmonary functions of, 73–74
    oxygen in, 78
    ventilation-perfusion matching in, 74–75
  regional, 92
  shock and, 619–620
  systemic. *See also* Vascular system
    neurohumoral stimulation of, 58–59, 59*f*

Circulatory arrest, deep hypothermic, 583–584

Circulatory assist devices, 624*d*, 624–636, 625*f*–628*f*, 633*f*–636*f*, 656*d*–659*d*. *See also* Intra-aortic balloon pump (IABP); Left ventricular assist device (LVAD)

Circumflex artery, anatomy of, 15

Circus movement tachycardia, 335, 335*f*

CK. *See* Creatine kinase (CK)

CK-MR, in myocardial infarction, 518

Clots, formation of, 121*f*, 121–122

Clotting factors, 112, 113*t*

Clubbing, 210, 210*f*

Coagulation, 112–114, 113*f*, 113*t*
  disorders of, 121–130
  extrinsic and intrinsic pathways of, 113*f*, 113–114
  shock and, 619

Coagulation studies, 241–243
  after cardiac surgery, 243
  reference values for, 238*t*
  specimen collection for, 243

Cocaine, and myocardial infarction, 496–497

Cognitive aids, for enhancement of adherence, 887

Cognitive-motivational model of behavior change, 885

Cognitive-perceptual functional pattern, assessment of, 194

Collagen, in atherosclerotic plaques, 486

Collateral circulation, 44

Collateral vessels, blood flow in, 497

Colloid osmotic pressure, 65

Colony-forming units (CFUs), differentiation of, 109

Color Doppler echocardiography, 377–378

Complete blood count (CBC), 239–241
  after cardiac surgery, 241

Compliance. *See* Adherence; Nonadherence

Computed tomography (CT), electron beam, 383

Conduction
  antegrade, through accessory pathway, in Wolff-Parkinson-White syndrome, 330, 331*f*
  atrial, 30–31, 31*t*
  concealed, 357–359, 358*f*–359*f*
    affecting subsequent impulse conduction, 357–358, 358*f*
    affecting subsequent impulse formation, 358, 359*f*
  decremental, 299–300
  junctional, 31
  ventricular, 31–32, 32*f*

Conduction abnormalities, intraventricular, electrocardiography in, 276–282, 277*f*–282*f*

Conduction block, 299–301, 300*f*–301*f*
  decremental, 299–301, 300*f*
  hyperkalemia and, 141
  phase 3, 300, 300*f*
  phase 4, 300*f*, 300–301
  reentry, 301, 301*f*

Conduction disorders
  atrioventricular block, 351–353, 352*f*–354*f*
  atrioventricular dissociation, 354, 355*f*–356*f*
  parasystole, 356*f*–357*f*, 356–357
  Wenckebach, 346–351, 347*f*–352*f*. *See also* Wenckebach conduction

Conduction ratio, 2:1, in second-degree atrioventricular block, 327, 327*f*

Conduction system, 263*f*, 263–264
  anatomy of, 10–12, 11*f*–12*f*, 13*t*

Conductivity, hydraulic, 65

Congestive cardiomyopathy, imaging studies of, 384

Congestive heart failure (CHF), and cardiac rehabilitation, 855

Constrictive pericarditis, 721–722

Continuous cardiac output monitoring, 460–461, 461*f*

Continuous endothelium, 53

Continuous-flow left ventricular assist device, 633*f*–634*f*, 633–635

Continuous positive airway pressure (CPAP), 171

Contour II implantable cardioverter-defibrillator, 691*t*

Contraceptives, oral
  and hypertension, 782
  and risk of coronary heart disease, 748

Contractility, 40, 40*f*, 92
decrease in, ventricular function curve in, 456*f*, 458
metabolic acidosis and, 157
and oxygen consumption, 43
respiratory acidosis and, 155
Contracting, for enhancement of adherence, 886
Contraction
cross-bridge theory of, 34, 36*f*
isometric, 33, 34*f*
isotonic, 33, 34*f*–35*f*
principles of, 33, 34*f*–35*f*
Contrast agents, for cardiac catheterization, 418
Cool-down period, 841
COPD. *See* Chronic obstructive pulmonary disease (COPD)
Coping, by family, ineffective, in patient with intra-aortic balloon pump, 633*ncp*
Coping-stress functional pattern, assessment of, 194
Core sleep, 167
Coronary arteriography, 415–416, 416*f*
in heart failure, 568–569
Coronary artery
anatomy of, 12–15, 13*f*–14*f*
revascularization of
postoperative care in, 589, 590*t*
procedures for, 584*f*–586*f*, 584–587.
See also Coronary artery bypass graft (CABG)
transmyocardial laser, 587
spasm of, hypomagnesemia and, 145–146
Coronary artery bypass graft (CABG), 584*f*–585*f*, 584–586
conduits for, 584*f*, 584–585
contraindications to, 584
indications for, 584
minimally invasive, 586, 586*f*
for myocardial ischemia, 513
off-pump, 586
results of, 585–586
Coronary artery disease (CAD)
in allograft, 600
diagnosis of, exercise testing in, 389–405.
See also Exercise testing
with segmental wall motion abnormalities of, imaging of, 387
sleep and, 169
with ventricular tachycardia, radiofrequency catheter ablation in, 371
Coronary atherectomy, 546–549, 547*f*–548*f*.
See also Atherectomy
Coronary blood flow
alterations in, 497
competitive redistribution of, in myocardial ischemia, 497
Coronary capillaries, anatomy of, 16
Coronary heart disease (CHD)
epidemiology of, 737–739, 738*f*–739*f*, 738*t*
psychosocial interventions in, 760–762
risk factors for, 737–750
activity level as, 743*f*–744*f*, 743–745
antioxidants and, 749–750
anxiety as, 760

depression as, 760
diabetes mellitus as, 745*f*, 745–746
family history as, 739–740
folate and, 749
homocysteine and, 749
hyperlipidemia as, 741–743, 742*t*
hypertension as, 741, 742*f*
obesity as, 746–748, 747*f*
personality as, 759–760
reproductive hormones as, 748–749
smoking as, 740*f*, 740–741
stress as, 757–758
smoking cessation and. *See* Smoking cessation
and sudden cardiac arrest, 639–640
Coronary intensive care unit (CICU)
management of myocardial infarction in, 524–526, 525*f*
postoperative protocol in, 590*t*
sleep in, 169, 173
Coronary laser angioplasty, 549
Coronary stents, 549*f*–554*f*, 549–554, 552*t*
balloon-expandable, 552, 552*t*, 554*f*
clinical trials of, 549–551, 551*f*–554*f*, 552*t*
complications of, 552–553, 557
future research on, 554–555
GFX, 553*f*
Gianturco-Roubin Flex-Stent, 549*f*
history of, 549
NIR, 553*f*
Palmaz-Schatz, 550*f*, 552
placement of
antiplatelet therapy after, 550–551
intravascular ultrasonography before, 549–550, 551*f*
self-expanding, 552, 552*t*, 554*f*
sheath removal after, 553–554, 554*f*
technological advances in, 551–552, 552*t*, 553*f*–554*f*
Coronary veins, anatomy of, 16, 16*f*
Corpuscle indices, 240
reference values for, 238*t*
Corticosteroids, side effects of, 602*t*, 603
Cough, assessment of, 219
CPAP (continuous positive airway pressure), 171
CPB. *See* Cardiopulmonary bypass (CPB)
Crackles, 223
Creatine kinase (CK), 231–237, 232*f*–236*f*, 232*t*–238*t*
after cardiac surgery, 236*f*
after myocardial infarction, 231–232, 232*f*
after valvuloplasty, 235
factors affecting, in healthy subjects, 233
function of, 231
isoenzymes of, 232, 232*t*
reference values for, 236*t*, 238*t*
specimen collection of, 236–237
tissue distribution of, 232*t*
Creatine kinase-BB (CK-BB), 233
tissue distribution of, 232*t*
Creatine kinase-MB (CK-MB)
after myocardial infarction, 233–235, 234*f*, 235*t*
isoforms of, 236
mass concentration of, 236
noncardiac disorders and, 235, 235*t*

reference values for, 236*t*
tissue distribution of, 232*t*
Creatine kinase-MM (CK-MM), 233
tissue distribution of, 232*t*
Creatinine, levels of, 246
Creatinine clearance, calculation of, 185
Cross-bridge theory of contraction, 34, 36*f*
Crosstalk, 664*d*, 683–684
Cuing, for enhancement of adherence, 886
CVP. *See* Central venous pressure (CVP)
Cyanosis, 196
Cycle ergometer test, 394
Cyclic adenosine monophosphate (cAMP)
receptors dependent on, 86, 87*f*
in vasodilation, 59, 59*f*
Cyclosporine
and prognosis after cardiac transplantation, 596
side effects of, 601, 602*t*
Cytokines
in atherosclerotic plaques, 486–487
properties of, 109–110

D

Decremental conduction, 299–300
Deep hypothermic circulatory arrest, 583–584
Deep venous thrombosis (DVT), 124–126, 127*d*–128*d*
clinical manifestations of, 124
diagnosis of, 124–125
medical management of, 124–126
nursing management of, 126, 127*d*–128*d*
risk factors for, 124
Defibrillation
for cardiac arrest, 642–646, 644*f*–646*f*
early, 643, 644*f*
electrode position for, 643–646, 646*f*
energy requirements for, 643, 645*f*
equipment for, 643
procedure for, 646
transthoracic resistance for, 643
Delirium, postcardiotomy, 594
Demand pacing, 663*d*, 670
Depolarization, 18
diastolic, hypokalemia and, 139
on electrocardiography, 269*f*, 271–273, 272*f*
factors affecting, 28–30, 29*f*–30*f*
hyperkalemia and, 141
Depression, and coronary heart disease, 760–762
Diabetes mellitus, 869–878
classification of, 869, 870*t*
complications of, 871–872
chronic, 873
and coronary heart disease, 745*f*, 745–746
definition of, 869
diagnostic criteria for, 870*d*
and hypertension, 802
insulin-dependent, 869, 870*t*, 871
management of, 873–877, 874*t*
blood pressure control in, 875
diet in, 875–876
exercise in, 875–876

foot care in, 875
glycemic control in, 875
lipid control in, 875
neurologic assessment in, 875
in older adults, 874*t*
pharmacologic, 876–877
non–insulin-dependent, 869, 870*t*, 871
nursing management in, 874*t*
pathophysiology of, 870–871
patient/family education about, 873
screening for, 877
Diabetic nephropathy, 872
Diabetic neuropathy, 872
Diapedesis, 111
Diaphragm, air under, radiographic imaging of, 257*f*
Diaries, for improvement of adherence, 882*t*, 883
Diastole
clinical applications of, 48
ventricular, 45*f*, 46
Diastolic blood pressure, assessment of, 205–206
Diastolic depolarization, hypokalemia and, 139
Diastolic dysfunction, in heart failure, 561, 564–565, 565*f*
treatment of, 570–571
Diastolic heart sounds, extra, 214–215, 215*f*
Diastolic reserve, 41
Diazoxide, parenteral, for hypertensive crisis, 801*t*
Diet
adherence to, assessment of, 881–883, 882*t*
after myocardial infarction, 527
for control of hypertension, 791, 792*t*–793*t*
for diabetes mellitus, 875–876
for hyperlipidemia, 826*f*, 826–828
low-calorie, 865*t*
for obesity, 864–865, 865*t*
Diffusion, 64–65
of carbon dioxide, 78
of gases, 73
of oxygen, 78
Diffusional force, 19
Digitalis
for heart failure, 572
toxicity of, hypomagnesemia and, 145
Digoxin
for heart failure, 573*t*
properties of, 305*t*
Dihydropyridines, for antihypertensive therapy, 799*t*
Dilated cardiomyopathy. *See* Cardiomyopathy, dilated
Diltiazem, properties of, 305*t*
Directed-search chest radiography, 253*f*–254*f*, 253–254
Direct Fick method, for determination of cardiac output, 417–418
Directional atherectomy, 547, 547*f*
Discharge planning
after cardiac catheterization, 420*t*
after implantable cardioverter-defibrillator insertion, 695, 696*t*
for cardiac transplantation patient, 604

Discontinuous endothelium, 53
Disopyramide, properties of, 305*t*
Dissecting aortic aneurysm
radiographic imaging of, 257*f*
repair of, 588–589
Disseminated intravascular coagulation (DIC), 115–118, 117*t*–118*t*, 119*d*–121*d*
assessment in, 117, 118*t*
clinical manifestations of, 116–117, 117*d*, 118*t*
definition of, 115
etiology of, 115–116, 116*f*, 117*d*
medical management of, 117–118, 118*t*
nursing management of, 118, 119*ncp*
pathology of, 116, 116*f*
Diuretics
with angiotensin-converting enzyme inhibitors, for antihypertensive therapy, 800*t*
for antihypertensive therapy, 798*t*
with beta blockers, for antihypertensive therapy, 800*t*
drug interactions with, 797*t*
for heart failure, 570–571, 573*t*
and hypokalemia, 137, 139
potassium-sparing
for antihypertensive therapy, 798*t*
for heart failure, 573*t*
DO₂. *See* Oxygen delivery (DO₂)
Dobutamine, for heart failure, 572
Dominance, 14
Dominant pacemaker, 297
Doppler echocardiography, 376–378, 377–380*f*. *See also* Echocardiography, Doppler entires
Doppler principle, 376
Doppler ultrasonography, for assessment of arterial blood flow, 201, 201*f*
Dreaming, 165
Dressings, catheter site, frequency of, 428*t*
Dressler's syndrome, 521–522, 722
Drugs. *See also* specific types
absorption of, aging and, 185–186
auscultatory response to, 219
distribution of, aging and, 186
metabolism of, aging and, 186
reference valuues for, 247–248, 248*t*
"Dry" pericarditis, 720
Dual-chamber pacing
block response in, 682, 682*f*
fall-back response in, 682, 683*f*
rate smoothing in, 682, 683*f*
Dynamic auscultation, 217–219, 218*t*
Dynamic cardiomyoplasty, 588
Dynamic response, of monitoring systems, 430–432, 433*f*
Dyslipidemia, 822*t*, 822–823. *See also* Hyperlipidemia
Dyspnea, during exercise testing, 399, 400*d*
Dyspnea index, for cardiac transplantation patient, 604*t*

E

Early ejection sounds, 215–216, 216*f*
ECF. *See* Extracellular fluid (ECF)

ECG. *See* Electrocardiography (ECG)
Echocardiography, 375–381. *See also* specific structures
in aortic insufficiency, 716
in aortic stenosis, 713
diagnostic, 378*f*–380*f*, 378–381
Doppler, 376–378, 377–380*f*
color, 377–378
pulsed, 376
with exercise testing, 403–404
in heart failure, 568
in mitral stenosis, 703
in myocardial infarction, 519
in myocardial ischemia, 512
positioning for, 375*f*
principles of, 375*f*–379*f*, 375–378
stress, 381
transducers for, 375*f*–376*f*, 375–376
transesophageal, 381
in infectious endocarditis, 730
transthoracic, in mitral insufficiency, 709
two-dimensional, 376
Ectopic focus, exit block from, Wenckebach conduction with, 350–351, 351*f*–352*f*
Edema
assessment of, 210–211
formation of, 67*f*, 67–68, 133
of optic disc, 198
peripheral, in heart failure, 562, 566
EDHF (endothelium-derived hyperpolarizing factors), 55*t*, 56
EDRF (endothelium-derived relaxing factors), 56, 56*f*
Education, patient/family. *See* Patient/family education
EEG. *See* Electroencephalography (EEG)
Ejection fraction, 47
calculation of, 417
measurement of, 446*f*
Elderly persons. *See* Older adults
Electrical activity
aging and, 183
factors modifying, 28–30, 29*f*–30*f*
of ions, 21
Electrical current, 19–21, 20*f*
Electrical impulse, spread of, 264
Electrocardiography (ECG), 263–295. *See also* specific conditions
atrial, 592*f*
in atrial enlargement, 288–289, 289*f*
axis determination in, 273*f*–276*f*, 273–275
during cardiac rehabilitation, 849–850, 850*f*, 850*t*
cardiac rhythm on, 268
depolarization on, 269*f*, 271–273, 272*f*
designation of time on, 267*f*
designation of voltage on, 267*f*
in electrolyte imbalances, 140–144, 291–295, 293*f*–295*f*
in exercise testing, 398*f*, 398–399
preparation for, 391*f*, 391–392
in heart failure, 568*t*
heart rate on, 267, 267*f*
in intraventricular conduction abnormalities, 276–282, 277*f*–282*f*

Electrocardiography (ECG), (*continued*)
in ischemia/infarction, 282*f*–288*f*,
282–288, 283*d*, 286*d*, 286*t*
principles of, 266–268, 267*f*
in pulmonary embolism, 129
twelve-lead, 268*f*–273*f*, 268–273
hexaxial reference system in, 269, 271*f*
normal, 273, 273*f*
normal waveform configurations
on, 265*t*
placement of bipolar leads in, 269, 270*f*
placement of chest leads in, 268*f*,
269, 270*f*
placement of limb leads in, 268*f*,
268–269
placement of posterior leads in,
269, 270*f*
placement of unipolar leads in,
269, 270*f*
twelve views of heart on, 271–273, 272*f*
in ventricular enlargement, 289–291, 290*f*,
291*t*, 292*d*, 292*f*
Electrodes
Mason-Likar placement system for,
391, 391*f*
for pacemakers, 663*d*
placement of, for monitoring after
myocardial infarction, 525*f*,
525–526
Electroencephalography (EEG), during sleep,
163, 164*f*–165*f*
Electrogram, intra-atrial, in differential
diagnosis of ventricular atopy *vs.*
aberrancy, 344–346, 345*f*
Electrolytes. *See also* specific type
balance of, 137, 138*t*
excretion of, 137
during sleep, 168
imbalance of, 137–148
serum, 244–245, 245*t*
after cardiac surgery, 245
reference values for, 238*t*
Electromagnetic interference
with implantable cardioverter-
defibrillator, 694
in single-chamber pacing, 663*d*
Electromyography (EMG), chin, 163, 164*f*
Electron beam computed tomography, 383
Electronic monitoring, for assessment of
adherence, 882*t*, 883–884
Electrophysiology studies, 363–371
diagnostic, 363–368, 364*f*–365*f*,
366*d*–367*d*
in cardiac arrest survivors, 364–365
complications of, 364
indications for, 364–368, 366*d*–367*d*
patient preparation for, 363
in syncope, 365–366, 367*d*
technique of, 363–365, 364*f*–365*f*
in wide-complex tachycardia, 365
interventional, 368–371, 369*f*–370*f*. *See
also* Radiofrequency catheter
ablation
nursing care in, 371
Elimination functional pattern, assessment
of, 194
Embolectomy, 123

Embolism
air. *See* Air embolism
arterial, 122*f*, 122–123, 123*t*
intracardiac sources of, imaging of, 387
from prosthetic valves, 707
pulmonary. *See* Pulmonary embolism
Emergency cardiac care, algorithm for, 648*f*
EMG. *See* Electromyography (EMG)
Emotional stress, and chest pain, 509
Emotional support, for survivors of sudden
death, 656
Enalapril
for heart failure, 571, 573*t*
parenteral, for hypertensive crisis, 801*t*
Encephalopathy, hypertensive, 787
Endarteritis, from coronary stents, 554
End-diastolic volume, maintenance of, with
increased peripheral blood volume,
98–99
Endless-loop tachycardia, 664*d*
Endocarditis
bacterial, imaging of, 387
infective, 729*d*, 729–732, 731*t*
clinical manifestations of, 699*t*,
730–731, 731*t*
diagnosis of, 700, 700*f*
epidemiology of, 729
indications for surgery in, 701*d*
medical management of, 731
nursing management of, 732
pathophysiology of, 730
prevention of, 731–732
risk factors for, 701*d*, 729*d*
types of, 729–730
and valvular heart disease, 700*t*,
700–701, 701*d*
from prosthetic valves, 707
Endocardium, anatomy of, 10
Endocrine disorders, and
hypertension, 783*d*
Endocrine function, during sleep, 168
Endothelial cells
in atherosclerotic plaques, 482, 483*f*, 491
and vascular smooth muscle cells, 60*f*
Endothelin-1, vascular effects of, 57
Endothelium
of exchange vessels, 53, 54*f*
function of, cholesterol and, 822
pulmonary, anatomy of, 75
vascular, and vasomotor function, 55*t*
Endothelium-derived contracting factors, 55*t*,
56–57, 57*f*
Endothelium-derived hyperpolarizing factors
(EDHF), 55*t*, 56
Endothelium-derived mediators, of vascular
resistance, 96
Endothelium-derived relaxing factors
(EDRF), 56, 56*f*
Endothelium-derived vasoactive substances,
and vascular resistance, 55*t*, 55–58,
56*f*–58*f*
Endotracheal tubes, radiographic imaging
of, 259*f*
Environmental management, for sleep
disorders, 173
Environmental smoke, and coronary heart
disease, 741

Enzymes, cardiac, 231–239, 232*f*–237*f*, 232*t*,
235*t*–238*t*. *See also* specific enzymes
Eosinophils, properties of, 111
Epicardial pacing, 666, 666*f*
initiation of, 671
Epicardial wires, for temporary pacemakers,
care of, 673
Epicardium, anatomy of, 9
Epinephrine
in blood pressure regulation, 88–89
for bradyarrhythmias, 313*t*
properties of, 306*t*
Epochs, during sleep, 163
Eptifibatide, use of after coronary stent
placement, 551
Equilibrium potentials, of ions, 20*f*, 20–21
Ergometer tests, cycle, 394
Erythrocyte count, 239–240
reference values for, 238*t*
Erythrocyte sedimentation rate, 241
Erythrocytes. *See* Red blood cells (RBCs)
Escape interval, 663*d*, 678
Esmolol, properties of, 306*t*
Esophageal leads, in differential diagnosis of
ventricular atopy *vs.* aberrancy,
344–346, 345*f*
Estrogen replacement therapy
and deep venous thrombosis, 124
for hyperlipidemia, 831
and risk of coronary heart disease, 748–749
Ethnicity, and high blood pressure, 781
Exchange vessels, endothelium of, 53, 54*f*
Excitation, myocardial, 18*t*, 18–19, 19*f*
Excitation-contraction coupling, 32*f*, 32–33
Excretion, 133, 134*f*
of electrolytes, 137
Exercise
after cardiac transplantation, 603–604,
604*f*, 604*t*, 608*d*
and cardiovascular health, 835–840,
836*t*–838*t*, 839*d*
epidemiologic evidence of, 835,
836*t*–837*t*
Surgeon General's report on, 836–837
and creatine kinase-MM levels, 233
definition of, 841
for diabetes mellitus, 875–876
and fitness, *vs.* health, 837
home-based, and adherence to
program, 887
and hyperlipidemia, 829
isometric, 841
isotonic, 841
physiologic benefits of, 838–839, 839*d*
in prevention of coronary heart disease,
10*f*, 743*f*, 743–745
in secondary prevention, 837–838, 838*t*
short bouts of, and adherence to
program, 887
for treatment of obesity, 865
Exercise capacity, determination of, 397*f*,
397–398
Exercise programs, adherence to, 882
Exercise testing, 389–406
accuracy of, 401–402, 402*d*
after transplantation, 405
ancillary methods with, 402–404

angina during, 399, 400*d*
in aortic stenosis, 713
arrhythmias during, 399
benefits of, 389
blood pressure during, 396–397
contraindications to, 390*d*
determination of exercise capacity during, 397*f*, 397–398
echocardiography in, 381, 403–404
electrocardiographic response to, 398*f*, 398–399
electrocardiography in, preparation for, 391*f*, 391–392
false-positive/false-negative responses to, 402, 402*d*
with gas exchange techniques, 404
guidelines for, 390*d*
heart rate during, 8*f*, 394
indications for, 389
isometric, 392
medications affecting, 391, 391*t*
metabolic equivalents in, 392–393
modalities for, 392
in older adults, 405
with pharmacologic stress techniques, 404
and prediction of disease prognosis, 404
pretest considerations in, 390–392, 391*t*
protocols for, 392–394, 393*f*
Balke treadmill, 393
Bruce treadmill, 393
cycle ergometer, 394
Naughton treadmill, 393–394
ramp, 394
recovery period after, 401
reports of, 394, 395*d*–396*d*
safety of, 389–390, 390*d*
subjective response to, 399–400, 400*d*
submaximal, 394
termination of, 400*d*–401*d*, 400–401
with ventricular function studies, 403
in women, 404–405
Expiration, auscultatory effects of, 218*t*
Extracellular fluid (ECF), 132
deficit of, 134–135, 135*d*
excess of, 135, 135*d*
imbalance of, with osmolality imbalance, 137
osmolality of, 133
potassium concentration of, 137
volume of, balance of, 134–135, 135*d*
Extracellular matrix (ECM), in atherosclerotic plaques, 486
Extremities, physical assessment of, 209–211, 210*f*
Extrinsic coagulation pathway, 113*f*, 113–114
Eyes, physical assessment of, 197*f*–199*f*, 197–198

F

Facial characteristics, assessment of, 196
Fagerstrom Tolerance Tool, 770, 771*f*
Fall-back response, in dual-chamber pacing, 682, 683*f*
Familial hypercholesterolemia, 822–823
Family, education of. *See* Patient/family education

Family coping, ineffective, in patient with intra-aortic balloon pump, 633*ncp*
Family history, 192–193
Family process, altered, shock and, 637
Fascicular block, electrocardiography in, 278–281, 281*f*–282*f*
Fast-response cells, 22–23, 23*f*
Fast sodium current, 27*t*, 27–28
Fatty acids, and hyperlipidemia, 827
Fatty plaques, classification of, 488
Fatty streaks, in atherosclerotic plaques, 487–488
FDPs (fibrin degradation products), 115
Fear, from myocardial infarction, 536–537
Fenestrated vascular endothelium, 53
Fenoldopam mesylate, parenteral, for hypertensive crisis, 801*t*
Fiberoptic pulmonary artery catheters, 463*f*, 463–464
Fibrin degradation products (FDPs), 115
Fibrinogen, levels of, 242
Fibrinoid arteriolar necrosis, hypertension and, 785
Fibrinolysis, 114*f*, 114–115
Fibrous plaques, 488, 489*f*
Fibrous skeleton, anatomy of, 6, 6*f*
Filtration, 133
physiology of, 65
Fistulas, arteriovenous, from coronary stents, 554
Fitness, *vs.* health, 837
Flaccid heart, 499
Flecainide, properties of, 306*t*
Fluid balance
intake and, 132–133
principles of, 132–134, 134*d*
Fluids. *See also* Body fluids
intake of, 132–133
Fluid therapy
for hypovolemic shock, 621
for septic shock, 623
Fluid volume deficit
in disseminated intravascular coagulation, 119*d*–346*d*
from interventional cardiology procedures, 555–556
Fluid volume excess, in heart failure, 577
Folate, and risk of coronary heart disease, 749
Foot care, in diabetes mellitus, 875
Force of contraction, as hemodynamic index, 460*t*
Force-velocity relationship, afterload and, 39*f*, 39–40
Foreign bodies, imaging of, 387
Forward heart failure, 560–561
Frank-Starling law, 563, 563*f*
Free radicals, excess, in diabetes mellitus, 873
Fremitus, 221
Friction rub
pericardial, 217, 217*f*
in pericarditis, 721
Functional patterns, in history-taking, 193–194
Funduscopic assessment, 197, 197*f*–199*f*

Fusion beats, 663*d*
in ventricular atopy, *vs.* aberrancy, 341, 342*f*–343*f*, 343

G

Gas exchange, 73, 74*t*
impaired, in pulmonary embolism, 129–130
measurement of, with exercise testing, 404
Gastric tonometry, 462
Gastroepiploic artery, bypass grafts using, 585
Gastrointestinal function
after cardiac surgery, 594
shock and, 619
Gated blood pool radionuclide scans, in aortic stenosis, 714
Gem implantable cardioverter-defibrillator, 691*t*
Gender, and cardiac rehabilitation, 843, 853
Genetic disorders, and hypertension, 783*d*
GFX coronary stent, 553*f*
Gianturco-Roubin Flex-Stent, 549*f*
Glucose
intravenous, and hypophosphatemia, 147
levels of, 246
metabolism of, in diabetes mellitus, 870–871
α-Glucosidase inhibitors, for diabetes mellitus, 877
Glycolysis, anaerobic, in myocardial ischemia, 498
Glycoprotein IIB/IIIA receptor inhibitors, use of after coronary stent placement, 550–551
Glycoproteins, in atherosclerotic plaques, 486
Goal setting, for enhancement of adherence, 886
Graft atherosclerosis, 600
Great vessels, echocardiography of, 377*f*
Growth factors
in atherosclerotic plaques, 485–487
properties of, 110*t*

H

Habit building, for enhancement of adherence, 886
HDLs. *See* High-density lipoproteins (HDLs)
Head, physical assessment of, 196–198, 197*f*–198*f*
Health, *vs.* fitness, 837
Health care providers
role of, in management of hypertension, 803, 804*t*, 805*d*, 805–806
sleep in, 174
Health history. *See* History-taking
Health perception–health management, assessment of, 194
Heart
anatomy of, 3–6, 4*f*–5*f*
aging and, 183
fibrous structures, 6*f*–8*f*, 6–9
left, 7–8, 8*f*
right, 6–7, 7*f*–8*f*
autonomic innervation of, 86*t*
chambers of, 6–8, 7*f*–8*f*
blood flow through, 8*f*

Heart (*continued*)
  denervated, exercise and, 603–604, 604*f*
  flaccid, 499
  innervation of, 16–17
  physical assessment of, 211*f*–217*f*,
      211–219, 213*t*, 218*t*. *See also*
      Physical assessment
  position of, 3, 4*f*
  radioisotope scanning of, 382*f*, 382–383
  stiff, 499
  surfaces of, 3, 4*f*–5*f*
  topographic anatomy of, 211*f*–217*f*,
      211–219, 213*t*, 218*t*
  twelve views of, on electrocardiography,
      271–273, 272*f*
  valves of, 8*f*, 8–9
Heart biopsy, 600, 600*f*
Heart failure
  acute *vs.* chronic, 561
  backward *vs.* forward, 560–561
  classification of, 570
  clinical manifestations of, 565–566,
      566*f*, 567*t*
    in left-sided failure, 565–566,
        566*f*, 567*t*
    in right-sided failure, 566, 566*f*, 567*t*
  decompensated, management of,
      622*f*, 623*d*
  diagnosis of, 567–570, 568*t*–569*t*
    laboratory studies in, 567–569,
        568*t*–569*t*
    physical examination in, 567
  diastolic dysfunction in, 564–565, 565*f*
  etiology of, 560*t*
  high-output *vs.* low-output, 561
  hypocalcemia and, 142
  incidence of, 560
  length-tension relationship in, 38
  medical management of, 567–574
    acute, 570
    AHCPR algorithm for, 571*f*
    chronic, 570–571, 571*f*–572*f*, 573*t*
    physical examination in, 567
  nursing management of, 574–577, 575*d*
  pathophysiology of, 561–565, 562*f*–565*f*
    left ventricular function in, 563, 563*f*
    myocardial hypertrophy in, 563–564
    neurohumoral, 564
    renal function in, 562
    sympathetic nervous system in, 562
    tissue oxygen extraction in, 564
  patient/family education about, 575*d*
  prognosis in, 574
  rehabilitation in, 838
  right-sided *vs.* left-sided, 561
  surgical techniques for, 588, 588*f*
  systolic dysfunction in, 561
Heartmate ventricular assist device, 636
Heart murmurs. *See* Murmurs
Heart rate
  after cardiac catheterization, 420
  and cardiac output, 91
  on electrocardiography, 267, 267*f*
  during exercise testing, 394, 396*f*
  in heart failure, 567
  and myocardial oxygen consumption, 42
  regulation of, 90–91

sleep and, 167
  target, in cardiac rehabilitation, 855–856
Heart sounds
  diastolic, extra, 214–215, 215*f*
  first, 213*f*, 213–214
  fourth, 215, 215*f*
  in heart failure, 567
  normal, 47, 213*f*–214*f*, 213–214
  second, 213*f*, 213–214
    splitting of, 214, 214*f*
  systolic, extra, 215–216, 216*f*
  in ventricular atopy, *vs.* aberrancy,
      346, 346*f*
Heart transplantation. *See* Cardiac
      transplantation
Hematocrit, 240
  reference values for, 238*t*
Hematologic studies, 239–243
  nursing care after, 243
Hematoma, from coronary stents, 554
Hematopoiesis
  platelets in, 112
  red blood cells in, 110–111
  regulation of, 109–110
  stem cells in, 109
  steps in, 109, 110*f*
  white blood cells in, 111–112
Hemiblock, electrocardiography in,
      278–281, 281*f*
Hemodynamic function, myocardial ischemia
      and, 499
Hemodynamic monitoring, 427–466. *See also*
      specific type
  after cardiac transplantation, 599*t*
  after myocardial infarction, 525*f*, 525–527
  catheters for
    radiographic imaging of, 259*f*–260*f*
    removal of, 436
  equipment for, 427*f*, 427–428
  in heart failure, 569*t*, 569–570
  in myocardial infarction, 519
  in shock, 620
  technical aspects of, 427*f*–433*f*, 427–432,
      428*t*, 431*d*–432*d*
    dynamic response characteristics as,
        430–432, 433*f*
    reference level in, 428–429, 429*f*–430*f*
    zeroing as, 430, 431*d*–432*d*
Hemoglobin, 240
  and oxygen delivery, 78–79
Hemolysis, in blood specimen, 229
Hemopump, 634*f*, 634–635
Hemorrhage, from antifibrinolytic
      agents, 123
Hemostasis, 112–114, 113*f*, 113*t*
  coagulation phase of, 112–114, 113*f*, 113*t*
  platelet phase of, 112
  vascular phase of, 112
Henry-Gauer reflex, 90
Heparin
  for acute arterial thrombosis, 123
  for disseminated intravascular
      coagulation, 118
  low molecular weight, for deep venous
      thrombosis prophylaxis, 125
  for myocardial infarction, 528–529
  for pulmonary embolism, 129

Hepatic function, aging and, 185
Hexaxial reference system, 269, 271*f*
High blood pressure. *See* Hypertension
High-density lipoproteins (HDLs)
  and coronary heart disease, 741, 742*t*, 743
  levels of
    factors affecting, 247*t*
    factors influencing, 826*t*
  in reverse cholesterol transport, 821
His bundle, anatomy of, 11, 11*f*
History-taking, 190*t*, 190–195, 195*t*
  cardiovascular, 189
  chief complaint in, 190–191
  family history in, 192–193
  functional patterns in, 193–194
  history of present illness in, 191–192
  identifying information in, 190
  New York Heart Association Functional
      and Therapeutic Classification in,
      194–195, 195*t*
  past history in, 192
  patient's perceptions of illness in, 193
  review of systems in, 193
  social history in, 193
HMG-CoA reductase inhibitors, for
      hyperlipidemia, 830*t*, 831
Homans' sign, 124
Home-based exercise, and adherence to
      program, 887
Homocysteine, and risk of coronary heart
      disease, 749
Homografts, for prosthetic valves, 706
Hormone replacement therapy, and risk of
      coronary heart disease, 748–749
Hormones
  in blood pressure regulation, 88–89
  reproductive, and risk of coronary heart
      disease, 748–749
  secretion of, during sleep, 168
  and urinary excretion, 134*t*
Hostility, and coronary heart disease,
      759–761
HV interval, in electrophysiology studies,
      363, 365*f*
Hydralazine
  for heart failure, 573
  parenteral, for hypertensive crisis, 801*t*
Hydraulic conductivity, 65
Hydrostatic column, 54
Hydrostatic pressure, 133
  and fluid transport, 65
Hypercalcemia, 143*d*, 143–144
  causes of, 143*d*
  electrocardiography in, 292, 295*f*
Hypercholesterolemia, statin therapy
      for, 820*t*
Hypercoagulability, 122
Hyperglycemia
  chronic, 873
  management of, 875
Hyperkalemia, 140*d*, 140–141
  cardiac effects of, 141
  causes of, 140*d*
  electrocardiography in, 291–292, 294*f*
  vascular effects of, 141
Hyperlipidemia, 822*t*, 822–823
  and coronary heart disease, 741–743, 742*t*

diagnosis of, 823, 824*t*
evaluation of, 824, 825*t*
and hypertension, 803
management of, 823–824, 824*t*–825*t*
    activity in, 829
    adherence issues in, 831–832
    alcohol in, 829
    in diabetes mellitus, 875
    dietary, 826*f*, 826–828
    pharmacologic, 829–832, 830*t*
        bile acid binding agents in, 830, 830*t*
        goals of, 829
        HMG-CoA reductase inhibitors in, 830*t*, 831
        nicotinic acid in, 830*t*, 831
    weight control in, 828–829
Hyperlipoproteinemia, clinical features of, in eyes, 197, 197*f*
Hypermagnesemia, 146, 146*d*
Hypernatremia, 136*d*, 136–137
Hyperpolarization, hypokalemia and, 139
Hypertension, 777–810
    after revascularization, 589
    and atherosclerosis, 785
    in children, 778–779, 779*f*–780*f*
    classification of, 777–778, 778*t*–780*t*
    clinical features of, in eyes, 198, 198*f*
    clinical manifestations of, 784*d*, 784*t*, 784–787, 786*t*
        cardiac, 785–786
        neurologic, 787
        ocular, 786*t*, 786–787
        renal, 786
        vascular, 785
    and coronary heart disease, 741, 742*f*
    definition of, 777
    diagnosis of, 787–788, 788*t*, 789*d*
    epidemiology of, 778–781
        ethnicity and, 781
        family history and, 780
    etiology of, 781–784, 783*d*
        primary, 781–782
        secondary, 782, 783*d*, 784
    hemodynamics of, 781
    management of
        adherence issues in, 804*t*, 805*d*, 808*d*–809*d*
        in diabetes mellitus, 802, 875
        in hyperlipidemia, 803
        nonpharmacologic, 790–794, 792*t*–793*t*
            diet in, 791, 792*t*–793*t*
            physical activity in, 791–792
            reduction of alcohol intake in, 792–793
            sodium restriction in, 791
            weight control in, 790–791
        nursing care plan for, 808*ncp*–810*ncp*
        in older adults, 801–802
        pharmacologic, 794–800, 795*f*, 796*t*–800*t*
            combination therapy in, 800*t*
            drug interactions in, 797*t*
            for hypertensive crisis, 795–796, 800, 801*t*
            stepped care in, 794–795, 795*f*, 796*t*–800*t*

in pregnancy, 802, 803*t*
public health programs in, 806–807
in renal disease, 802–803
role of client in, 805–806, 806*d*, 806*t*
role of health care organizations in, 806
role of health care professionals in, 803, 804*t*, 805*d*, 805–806
role of nursing in, 807, 808*d*–810*d*
team approach to, 807
patient/family education about, 810
prevention of, 790
prognosis in, 788–789
public awareness of, 788*t*
renovascular, 782
risk stratification in, 784*d*, 784*t*
sleep apnea and, 171
systolic, aging and, 184
Hypertensive crisis, management of, 795–796, 800, 801*t*
Hypertriglyceridemia, 823
Hypertrophic cardiomyopathy. *See* Cardiomyopathy, hypertrophic
Hypoalphalipoproteinemia, 823
Hypocalcemia, 142–143
    causes of, 142*d*
    electrocardiography in, 292, 295*f*
    vascular effects of, 143*d*
Hypoglycemia, diabetes mellitus and, 871–872
Hypoglycemia unawareness, 872
Hypoglycemics, oral, 876–877
Hypokalemia, 137, 139*d*, 139–140
    cardiac effects of, 139–140
    causes of, 139*d*
    electrocardiography in, 291, 293*f*
    vascular effects of, 140
Hypomagnesemia, 144*d*, 144–146
    cardiac effects of, 145
    causes of, 144*d*
    electrocardiography in, 292
    vascular effects of, 145–146
Hyponatremia, 136, 136*d*
Hypophosphatemia, 147*d*, 147–148
Hypotension
    after revascularization, 589
    from cardiac catheterization, 420
    hypocalcemia and, 143
    orthostatic, bed rest and, 99
Hypothermic circulatory arrest, 583–584
Hypoventilation
    in chronic obstructive pulmonary disease, sleep and, 170
    during sleep, 167
Hypovolemic shock. *See* Shock, hypovolemic
Hypoxic vasoconstriction, 74
Hysteresis, 663*d*

I

IABP. *See* Intra-aortic balloon pump (IABP)
Ibutilide
    properties of, 307*t*
    for tachyarrhythmias, 312*t*
Iced injectate, for thermodilution measurement of cardiac output, 454–455
ICF (intracellular fluid), 132

Idioventricular rhythm, accelerated, 323, 323*f*
Illness, chronic, aging and, 182, 182*f*
Immobility, cardiovascular effects of, 839, 839*d*
Immune function, shock and, 619
Immunosuppressants, side effects of, 601–603, 602*t*, 726*d*–727*d*
Implantable cardioverter-defibrillators (ICDs), 656, 686–697
    complications of, 693–694, 694*t*
    development of, 686
    follow-up care of, 695–696
    indications for, 686–688, 687*d*
    insertion of, 693
        discharge planning after, 695, 696*t*
        interaction with pacemaker, 694
        nursing care for, 694–695
    operation of, 690–693, 691*t*, 692*f*–693*f*
    properties of, 688–690, 689*f*
    sensing and detection by, 689–690, 690*f*, 692*f*
    troubleshooting for, 696–697, 697*f*
    types of, 686*f*
Impulse conduction
    abnormal, 299–301, 300*f*–301*f*
    concealed conduction affecting, 357–358, 358*f*
Impulse formation, concealed conduction affecting, 358, 359*f*
Impulse generation, and electrical activity, 29
Impulse initiation, abnormal, 297–299, 298*f*
Indicator dilution technique, for determination of cardiac output, 417
Infections. *See also* specific types
    after cardiac transplantation, 601
    from arterial pressure monitoring, 433–434
    immunosuppressants and, 606*d*–607*d*
    from intra-aortic balloon pump, 628–629
    and pericarditis, 719
    from pulmonary artery pressure monitoring, 449*t*
Infective endocarditis. *See* Endocarditis, infective
Infiltrative cardiomyopathy, imaging studies of, 385
Inflammatory response hypothesis, in formation of atherosclerotic plaques, 489–491
Inhibited response, 663*d*
Inhibited state, in dual-chamber pacing, 679–680, 680*f*–681*f*
Inotropic agents
    action of, 87*f*
    and contractility, 40, 40*f*
    for heart failure, 571–572
Inoue's technique, of mitral valvuloplasty, 712, 712*f*
INR (International Standard Ratio), and prothrombin time, 242
Insomnia, management of, 173–174
Inspiration, auscultatory effects of, 218*t*, 218–219
Insulin
    action of, in diabetes mellitus, 870–871
    for diabetes mellitus, 876

Insulin-dependent diabetes mellitus. *See*
Diabetes mellitus, insulin-dependent
Insulin resistance, and hypertension, 782
Intake, and fluid balance, 132–133
Intensive care unit. *See* Coronary intensive
care unit (CICU)
Intercalated discs, 17
Internal mammary artery (IMA), bypass
grafts using, 584–585, 585*f*
International Standard Ratio (INR), and
prothrombin time, 242
Interstitial fluid, osmotic pressure of, 133
Interventional cardiology, 541–557
coronary atherectomy in, 546–549,
547*f*–548*f*. *See also* Atherectomy
coronary stents in, 549*f*–554*f*,
549–554, 552*t*
laser angioplasty in, 549
percutaneous transluminal coronary
angioplasty in, 544–546,
545*d*, 546*f*
procedures for
altered tissue perfusion from, 556–557
anxiety from, 555
arrhythmias from, 556–557
fluid volume deficit from, 555–556
thrombolytic therapy in, 541–544, 542*d*.
See also Thrombolytic therapy
Interventricular septum, echocardiography
of, 380
Intima, morphology of, 481–482, 482*f*
Intra-aortic balloon pump (IABP),
624*d*–626*d*, 624–629, 630*d*–633*d*
complications of, 628–629
contraindications to, 626–627
indications for, 624*d*
insertion of, 624–625, 625*f*
timing of, 627*f*–628*f*, 627–628
nursing care plan for, 629, 630*ncp*–633*ncp*
physiologic principles of, 625*f*–626*f*,
625–626, 626*d*
positioning of, 261*f*
Intra-atrial electrogram, in differential
diagnosis of ventricular atopy *vs.*
aberrancy, 344–346, 345*f*
Intracardiac masses, imaging of, 387
Intracellular fluid (ICF), 132
Intramyocardial tension, and oxygen
consumption, 42
Intravascular devices, replacement of,
frequency of, 428*t*
Intravascular ultrasonography, before
coronary stent placement,
549–550, 551*f*
Intraventricular conduction abnormalities,
electrocardiography in, 276–282,
277*f*–282*f*
Intraventricular septum, blood supply to, 13*t*
Intrinsic coagulation pathway, 113*f*, 113–114
Inward currents, 27*t*, 27–28
Ion currents, sarcolemmal, 27*t*, 27–28
Ions
electrical activity of, 21
equilibrium potential of, 20*f*, 20–21
movement of, across myocardial cell
membrane, 21–22
myocardial distribution of, 19–22, 20*f*

Ischemia, distal, from arterial pressure
monitoring, 434
Isometric contraction, 33, 34*f*
Isometric exercise, 841
auscultatory effects of, 219
testing with, 392
Isorhythmic dissociation, 354, 356*f*
Isosorbide dinitrate, for heart failure, 573*t*
Isotonic contraction, 33, 34*f*–35*f*
Isotonic exercise, 841
Isotonic twitch, 42–43
Isovolumic ventricular relaxation, 45*f*, 46

J

Job stress, and coronary heart disease, 758
Judkins technique, for coronary
arteriography, 415–416, 416*f*
Jugular venous pulse, assessment of,
202*f*–203*f*, 202–203
Junctional conduction, 31
Junctional rhythm, 321*f*, 311–321
Junctional tachycardia, 321*f*, 311–321

K

Kent bundles, 11
Kidneys
excretion of acids by, 154, 155*t*
sodium chloride excretion by, 93
Knowledge deficit
after cardiac transplantation,
609*ncp*–610*ncp*
in hypertension, 808*ncp*
in myocardial infarction, 537
in pulmonary embolism, 130
Korotkoff sounds, 205–206, 206*t*
Krogh model, of cardiac output/central
venous pressure relationship,
98, 98*f*
Kyphoscoliosis, 222*f*

L

Laboratory studies, 227–248. *See also*
specific types
of cardiac enzymes, 231–239, 232*f*–236*f*,
232*t*–238*t*. *See also* specific
enzymes
hematologic, 239–243
nursing care after, 243
during sleep, 163, 164*f*
using blood
interpreting results of, 229–230
reference values for, 229
specimen collection for, 227–230. *See
also* Blood specimens
Lactate, and oxygen supply and demand,
462–463
Lactate dehydrogenase (LDH), 237,
237*f*, 239
after cardiac surgery, 239
isoenzymes of, 237, 237*f*, 239
sample collection for, 239
Laplace equation, 44, 91–92
Laser angioplasty, 549
Latent pacemaker, 297
LDH. *See* Lactate dehydrogenase (LDH)

LDLs. *See* Low-density lipoproteins (LDLs)
Leads
for electrocardiography
for monitoring after myocardial
infarction, 525*f*, 525–526
placement of, 268*f*–270*f*, 268–269
for implantable cardioverter-defibrillator,
688, 689*f*
for pacemakers, 663*d*, 668, 669*f*
perforation by, 684–685
Left anterior descending artery, anatomy
of, 15
Left anterior fascicular block,
electrocardiography in, 281,
281*f*–282*f*
Left atrial enlargement, electrocardiography
in, 288–289, 289*f*
Left atrium, reference point for,
428–429, 430*f*
Left axis deviation, 273, 273*f*, 275, 276*f*
Left bundle branch, anatomy of, 12
Left bundle-branch block,
electrocardiography in, 278, 280*f*
Left coronary artery, anatomy of, 15
Left heart, catheterization of, 413*f*–414*f*,
413–415
results of, 423*f*
Left posterior fascicular block,
electrocardiography in, 281
Left ventricle
aneurysms of, radiographic imaging
of, 259*f*
baroreceptors in, and blood pressure
regulation, 83–84
blood supply to, 13*t*
cardiac cycle in, 45*f*, 45–46, 46*t*
compliance of, 38–39, 39*f*
echocardiography of, 377*f*, 378, 378*f*–379*f*
enlargement of, electrocardiography in,
289, 290*f*, 291*t*
stiffness of, 39*f*
Left ventricular aneurysm, from myocardial
infarction, 520–521
Left ventricular assist device (LVAD),
629–636, 633*f*–636*f*
indications for, 629
principles of, 629, 633
pulsatile, 635*f*–636*f*, 635–636
types of, 633*f*–634*f*, 633–635
Left ventricular failure
hemodynamic response to, 459*t*
in myocardial infarction, 520
Left ventricular function
after myocardial infarction, radioisotope
angiography of, 382*f*
in heart failure, 563, 563*f*
Left ventricular hypertrophy, and sudden
death, 640–641
Left ventricular preload, pulmonary artery
wedge pressure and, 441*f*
Left ventricular remodeling, from myocardial
infarction, 520–521
Length-tension relationship, preload and,
37–39, 38*f*–39*f*
Leukocyte count, 240
reference values for, 238*t*
Lidocaine, properties of, 307*t*

Life span, phases of, 181
Limb leads, for electrocardiography, placement of, 268f, 268–269
Lipids
blood levels of, 246–247, 247t
metabolism of, 820f–821f, 820–821
structure and function of, 819
Lipoproteins
measurement of, 824, 826
role of, 822
Liver, size of, measurement of, 224f–225f, 224–225
Liver function, shock and, 619
Long-cycle aberrancy, 300f, 300–301
Loop diuretics, for heart failure, 573t
Loss, smoking cessation and, 773
Low-calorie diet, 865t
Low-density lipoproteins (LDLs)
in atherosclerotic plaques, 482, 483f
and coronary heart disease, 741, 742t, 743
levels of, factors affecting, 247t, 826t
in lipid metabolism, 821–822, 822f
oxidized, 822
particle size of, 821–822
Low molecular weight heparin, for deep venous thrombosis prophylaxis, 125
Lown and Wolf grading system, for cardiac rehabilitation, 850t
Lown-Ganong-Levine syndrome, 332, 332f
Lung capacity, 74t
Lung lobes, radiographic imaging of, 254f
Lung pressure, effects of, 75–76, 76f
Lungs. See also Pulmonary entries
excretion of acids by, 154, 155t
gas exchange by, 73, 74t
physical assessment of, 219–223, 220f–222f, 221f
zones of, 75–76, 76f
Lung volume, aging and, 184, 184f
LVAD. See Left ventricular assist device (LVAD)
Lymphatics, structural characteristics of, 53, 54f
Lymphatic system, 66–67
anatomy of, 16
Lymphocytes
in atherosclerotic plaques, 485, 485f
properties of, 111
Lymphoid cells, types of, 109

M

Macrophages
in atherosclerotic plaques, 484–485, 485f
properties of, 111
Magnesium
balance of, 138t, 144d, 144–146, 146d
properties of, 307t
serum levels of, 244–245
Magnetic resonance imaging (MRI), 383–384
Magnet mode, 663d
Malignancy, and disseminated intravascular coagulation, 115–116
Manometer, use of, 204, 205f
MAP. See Mean arterial pressure (MAP)

Mason-Likar electrode placement, for exercise testing, 391, 391f
Matrix metalloproteinases (MMPs)
in atherosclerotic plaques, 487
function of, 485
Maximum tracking rate (MTR), 664t, 678
Mean arterial pressure (MAP)
calculation of, 62, 434–435
in shock, 619–620
Mean capillary pressure, 66
Mechanical ventilation, pulmonary artery pressure monitoring during, 447–448
Media, morphology of, 482, 482f
Medial calcific sclerosis, definition of, 481
Medications. See Drugs; specific classes
Meglitinides, 877
Melatonin, therapeutic use of, 168
Membrane resting potential, 18
calculation of, 21
Mercury manometers, 204
Metabolic acidosis, 156–157, 157d, 158t
Metabolic acids, production of, 153
Metabolic alkalosis, 158–159, 159d
Metabolic equivalents (METs), 850, 850t, 851f
and exercise capacity, 397f, 397–398
in exercise testing, 392–393
Metabolic hypothesis, of autoregulation, 95
Metabolism
anaerobic, in shock, 617
myocardial, 42
Metformin, 876–877
Metoprolol, properties of, 308t
METs. See Metabolic equivalents (METs)
Mexiletine, properties of, 308t
Micro Jewel II implantable cardioverter-defibrillator, 691t
Microvascular beds
structure of, 52–53
systemic, local regulation of, 94–96, 95f
Microvascular circulation
blood flow through, 64
transport mechanisms in, 64–66, 67f
Milrinone
for dilated cardiomyopathy, 725
for heart failure, 572
Minckeberg's sclerosis, definition of, 481
Mini III implantable cardioverter-defibrillator, 691t
Minute ventilation, during sleep, 167
Mitochondria, 17
Mitral insufficiency, 708t, 708–710, 710f
clinical manifestations of, 708–709
diagnosis of, 709
etiology of, 708, 708t
medical management of, 709–710, 710f
pathophysiology of, 708
Mitral pressure half-time, 385
Mitral regurgitation
hemodynamic response to, 459t
imaging studies of, 385
from myocardial infarction, 521
Mitral stenosis, 702–704, 703t, 704f
clinical manifestations of, 702
diagnosis of, 702–703, 703t
echocardiography in, 380f

etiology of, 702
hemodynamic monitoring in, 444f
imaging studies of, 385
medical management of, 703–704, 704f
pathology of, 702
Mitral valve
anatomy of, 8
echocardiography of, 378f–379f, 380
replacement of, 587, 710, 710f
surgical replacement of, 703–704
Mitral valve prolapse, 710–712, 711f–712f
clinical manifestations of, 711
diagnosis of, 711f–712f, 711–712
etiology of, 710
imaging studies of, 385
management of, 712, 712f
pathophysiology of, 710–711
Mitral valvuloplasty, Inoue's technique of, 712, 712f
Mixed venous oxygen saturation, 463f, 463–464
MMPs. See Matrix metalloproteinases (MMPs)
Modeling behavior, for enhancement of adherence, 886
Monitoring, hemodynamic. See Hemodynamic monitoring
Monocytes
in atherosclerotic plaques, 484–485, 485f
properties of, 111
Monomorphic ventricular tachycardia, 335–336, 336f
Motivation, and cardiac rehabilitation, 843–844, 854
MRI. See Magnetic resonance imaging (MRI)
MTR. See Maximum tracking rate (MTR)
Multifocal atrial tachycardia, 318, 318f
Murmurs
auscultation of, 216f, 216t, 215–216
classification of, 216f
configuration of, 216f
innocent, 217
intensity of, grading of, 216t, 217
from papillary muscle dysfunction, 217
Muscarinic receptors, in blood pressure regulation, 88
Muscle pump, and upright posture, 99
Mycophenolate mafetii, 603
Myeloid cells, types of, 109
Myocardial cells
action potential of, 23–25, 24f
aging and, 183
electrical properties of, 18t, 18–22, 19f–20f
automaticity as, 18
excitation as, 18t, 18–19, 19f
ion distribution as, 19–22, 20f
ion concentrations in, 18t
structure of, 17, 17f
Myocardial depression, postoperative, 591–592
Myocardial hypertrophy, in heart failure, 563–564
Myocardial infarction (MI). See also Myocardial ischemia
anterior, 515
electrocardiography in, 284f, 285, 287f

Myocardial infarction (MI) (*continued*)
    chest radiography in, 254*f*–257*f*, 254–258
    circadian rhythm and, 170
    classification of, 515–516
    cocaine and, 496–497
    complicated, diagnostic criteria for, 842*d*
    complications of, 519–522
        arrhythmias as, 519–520
        left ventricular aneurysms as, 521
        left ventricular failure as, 520
        mechanical, 521
        pericarditis as, 521–522
        radiographic imaging of, 258,
            258*f*, 258*t*
    creatine kinase after, 231–232, 232*f*
    creatine kinase-MB after, 233–235,
        234*f*, 235*t*
    diagnosis of, 516–519, 517*d*,
        517*f*–518*f*, 518*t*
        cardiac imaging in, 519
        echocardiography in, 519
        electrocardiography in, 518, 518*f*
        hemodynamic monitoring in, 519
        history in, 516
        physical assessment in, 517*d*,
            517–518, 518*t*
        serum markers in, 518–519
    differential diagnosis of, 255*t*
    electrocardiography in, 282*f*–288*f*,
        282–288, 283*d*, 286*d*, 286*t*
        location of, 284–285, 286*t*, 287*f*
    hypomagnesemia after, 145
    inferior, 515
        electrocardiography in, 285, 288*f*
    lateral, 515–516
        electrocardiography in, 286*f*
    left ventricular, 515–516
        vs. right ventricular, 518*t*
    left ventricular function after, radioisotope
        angiography of, 382*f*
    medical management of, 23*f*, 522*d*, 525*f*
        in coronary intensive care unit,
            524–526, 525*f*
        diet in, 527
        in emergency department, 524
        hemodynamic monitoring in, 525*f*,
            525–527
        interventional cardiology in, 522
        limitation of infarct size in, 526–528
        pacemakers in, 527
        pain control in, 526–527
        physical activity in, 527
        prehospital, 522, 524
    non–Q-wave, 516
    nursing management of, 531–540,
        532*d*–534*d*, 538*d*–539*d*
        for chest pain, 531, 534–535
        for decreased tissue perfusion
            myocardial, 532*ncp*–534*ncp*, 535–536
            systemic, 536
        for fear/anxiety, 536–537
        for knowledge deficit, 537
    pathologic phases of, 495–496, 496*f*
    pathophysiology of, failure of contraction
        in, 498–499
    pericarditis after, 722
    pharmacologic management of, 528–531

angiotensin-converting enzyme
        inhibitors in, 531
    aspirin in, 528
    beta blockers in, 529–530
    calcium channel blockers in, 530
    heparin in, 528–529
    nitrates in, 529
    warfarin in, 531
posterior, 515
    electrocardiography in, 286–287, 288*f*
postoperative, 592
Q-wave, 516
right ventricular, 516
    complications of, 521
    electrocardiography in, 287, 288*f*
    hemodynamic monitoring in, 519
    medical management of, 527–528
    nursing management of, 537,
        538*ncp*–539*ncp*, 540
    thrombolytic therapy for, 542*d*–543*d*,
        542–543
Myocardial injury, electrocardiography in,
        283, 283*f*
Myocardial ischemia
    from arterial reocclusion after stenting, 557
    circadian variations in, 502
    cocaine and, 496–497
    diagnosis of, 506–510, 509*d*–510*d*
        cardiac catheterization in, 510
        cardiac imaging in, 509–510
        coronary angiography in, 510
        electrocardiography in, 509
        history in, 506–508, 510*d*
        physical assessment in, 508–509
        stress testing in, 509
    electrocardiography in, 282*f*–288*f*,
        282–288, 283*d*, 286*d*, 286*t*
    epidemiology of, 508
    in heart failure, 564
    localization of, electrocardiography in, 287*f*
    medical management of, 512–513
    nursing issues in, 503
    nursing management of, 513–514
    pathophysiology of
        altered coronary blood flow in, 497
        altered metabolism in, 498, 498*f*
        arrhythmias in, 500–501
        electrophysiologic, 499–501, 500*f*
        endothelial–blood cell interactions in,
            497–498
        hemodynamic function in, 499
        and pain, 502
        parasympathetic, 501–502
        sympathetic, 501
        ventricular function in, 499
    prognosis in, 511
    reocclusion after, 503
    reperfusion after, consequences of, 498*f*,
        502–503
    restenosis after, 503
    shock and, 618–619
    silent, 502
Myocardial metabolism scanning, 383
Myocardial perfusion
    imaging of
        with exercise testing, 403
        radioisotope, 383

inadequate, in myocardial infarction,
        532*d*–534*d*, 535–536
Myocardial protection, during cardiac
        surgery, 583
Myocardial proteins, 230–231
Myocarditis, 727*d*, 727–728
    clinical manifestations of, 728
    etiology of, 727*d*
    medical management of, 728
    nursing management of, 729
    pathophysiology of, 728
Myocardium
    anatomy of, 9*f*–10*f*, 9–10
    function of, radioisotope evaluation of,
        382*f*, 382–383
    mechanical properties of, 36–42, 37*f*–41*f*
        afterload, 36–37, 37*f*
        cardiac reserve, 41, 41*f*
        contractility, 40, 40*f*
        force-velocity relationship, 39*f*, 39–40
        preload, 36, 37*f*
        pump performance, 41–42
        treppe, 40, 40*f*
    metabolism in, 42
    oxygen balance in, 495, 496*f*
    oxygen consumption in, 42–43
    oxygen supply to, 43*f*, 43–44
    proteins in, 19
    stunned, 503
Myocytes, necrosis of, in myocardial
        infarction, 495
Myofibrils, 17
Myogenic hypothesis, of autoregulation,
        94–95
Myoglobin, 231
Myopotential, 663*d*
Myosin, and contraction, 33–34

N

Nasogastric tubes, radiographic imaging
        of, 259*f*
National Cholesterol Education Program,
        treatment guidelines of, 825*t*
Native valve endocarditis, 730
Naughton treadmill test, 393–394
NBTE lesions, 730
Nephropathy, diabetic, 872
Nernst equation, 20*f*, 20–21
Netherlands clues, in ventricular atopy, *vs.*
        aberrancy, 342*f*
Neurogenic shock. *See* Shock, neurogenic
Neurohumoral stimulation, of vascular
        system, **58–59**, **59*f***
Neurologic disorders, and
        hypertension, 783*d*
Neurologic function, after cardiac surgery,
        594–595
Neuropathy, diabetic, 872
Neurotransmitters, and blood pressure
        regulation, 86–87, 88*f*
Neutrophils, function of, 111
New-onset aortic insufficiency, auscultation
        of, 217
New York Heart Association Functional and
        Therapeutic Classification,
        194–195, 195*t*

Nicardipine, parenteral, for hypertensive crisis, 801*t*

Nicotine, adverse effects of, 765

Nicotine replacement therapy, 770–771, 772*d*

Nicotine withdrawal, diagnostic criteria for, 764

Nicotinic acid, for hyperlipidemia, 830*t*, 831

Nicotinic receptors, in blood pressure regulation, 88

NIR coronary stent, 553*f*

Nitrates, for myocardial infarction, 529

Nitric oxide, and vasodilation, 56, 56*f*

Nodal cells, function of, 10

Nonadherence. *See also* Adherence significance of, 880–881

Nonbacterial thrombotic endocarditis (NBTE) lesions, 730

Noncompliance. *See* Adherence; Nonadherence

Noninvasive studies, scope of, 374–375

Non–rapid eye movement (NREM) sleep, 163, 165*f*–166*f*

Nonturbulent blood flow (Q), 61

Norepinephrine
    and regulation of blood pressure, 86–87, 88*f*
    spillover of, 90
    stimulation of vascular system by, 58

Normal sinus rhythm, 302, 314, 314*f*

Novacor pump, 635*f*–636*f*, 635–636

NREM (non–rapid eye movement) sleep, 163, 165*f*–166*f*

Nucleus tractus solitarius, in blood pressure regulation, 84

Nurses
    role of, in hypertension management, 807, 808*d*–810*d*
    sleep in, 174

Nursing care plan
    for cardiac transplantation, 605, 605*ncp*–610*ncp*
    for deep venous thrombosis, 127*ncp*–128*ncp*
    for disseminated intravascular coagulation, 119*ncp*–121*ncp*
    for hypertension management, 808*ncp*–810*ncp*
    for intra-aortic balloon pump, 629, 630*ncp*–633*ncp*
    for myocardial infarction, 532*ncp*–534*ncp*, 538*ncp*–539*ncp*
    for shock, 636*ncp*–637*ncp*

Nutrition. *See also* Diet
    altered, in heart failure, 577

Nutritional assessment, in evaluation of obesity, 862–863

Nutrition-metabolism functional pattern, assessment of, 194

O

Obesity
    adverse effects of, 860
    and blood pressure assessment, 209
    and cardiovascular disease, classification of risk in, 862
    and coronary heart disease, 746–748, 747*f*
    evaluation of, 862–863, 863*f*
    identification of, 861*t*, 861–862
    scope of, 860
    treatment of
        algorithm for, 863*f*
        approach to, 863–864, 864*t*
        behavioral therapy in, 865–866
        diet in, 864–865, 865*t*
        exercise in, 865
        goals of, 864
        pharmacologic, 866
        surgical, 866–867

Obstructive sleep apnea, 171

Off-pump coronary artery bypass graft, 586

OFRs. *See* Oxygen free radicals (OFRs)

Older adults
    diabetes management in, 874*t*
    exercise testing in, 405
    management of hypertension in, 801–802

Oncotic pressure, and fluid transport, 65

Opening snap, 215, 215*f*

Opsonization, 111

Optic disc, edema of, 198

Oral contraceptives
    and hypertension, 782
    and risk of coronary heart disease, 748

Organ donors, for cardiac transplantation, evaluation of, 597

Orlistat, 866

Orthoclone OKT3, side effects of, 602*t*, 603

Orthodromic circus movement tachycardia, 335, 335*f*

Orthostatic hypotension, bed rest and, 99

Orthotopic cardiac transplantation. *See* Cardiac transplantation

Osmolality, 132
    balance of, 135–137, 136*d*
    serum, calculation of, 245, 245*t*

Osmotic pressure, 133

Output, in single-chamber pacing, 663*d*

Outward currents, 27*t*, 28

Overdrive suppression, 297

Oversensing, 663*d*, 677–678

Overwedging, of pulmonary artery catheter, 451*t*

Oxygen
    alveolar-capillary transfer of, 76*f*–77*f*, 76–77
    content in blood, 79
    diffusion of, 78
    tissue extraction of, in heart failure, 564

Oxygen affinity, factors affecting, 77

Oxygenation
    red blood cells and, 110–111
    of tissue, monitoring of, 80–81, 462

Oxygen balance, myocardial, 495, 496*f*

Oxygen consumption (VO_2), 78
    measurement of, 79–80
    myocardial, 42–43
    relationship with oxygen delivery, 80
    systemic, 464, 465*t*
    clinical applications of, 465*t*, 465–466

Oxygen delivery (DO_2), 78–79
    alterations in, response to, 464–465
    relationship with oxygen consumption, 80

Oxygen extraction ratio, 81, 465

Oxygen free radicals (OFRs), production of, during reperfusion, 502–503

Oxygen saturation (SaO_2)
    arterial, 243
    and oxygen delivery, 79
    normal ranges of, 76*f*

Oxygen supply, myocardial, 43*f*, 43–44

Oxygen supply and demand
    global indicators of, 462–464, 463*f*, 464*t*
    local indicators of, 462

Oxygen therapy
    for cardiogenic shock, 621
    for myocardial infarction, 526

Oxyhemoglobin dissociation curve, 76–77, 77*f*

P

P_2, 214, 214*f*

Pacemaker cells, resting potential of, factors affecting, 298

Pacemaker currents, 27*t*, 28

Pacemaker-mediated tachycardia, 665*d*, 683, 684*f*

Pacemakers, 661–686. *See also* Pacing
    classification of, 667*t*, 667–668
    components of, 668
    dominant, 297
    firing of, factors affecting, 297, 298*f*
    five-letter code for, 667*t*, 667–668
    function of, assessment of, 674–678, 675*f*–677*f*
    interaction with implantable cardioverter-defibrillator, 694
    leads for, 663*d*, 668, 669*f*
        perforation by, 684–685
    permanent, 665
        insertion of, nursing's role in, 672–673
    right ventricular, electrodes for, positioning of, 261*f*–262*f*
    subsidiary, 297
        acceleration of, and atrioventricular dissociation, 354, 355*f*
    temporary, 665–667
        epicardial wire care for, 673
        insertion site care for, 673
        pulse generators for, 668, 668*f*
    types of, 662–667
    wandering atrial, 317, 317*f*

Pacemaker syndrome, 663*d*, 685

Pacing. *See also* Pacemakers
    antitachycardia, 667
    asynchronous, 663*d*, 669–670
    atrial overdrive, 667
    bipolar, 663*d*, 668–669, 670*f*
    blanking period in, 664*d*, 678, 684, 685*f*
    for bradyarrhythmias, 313*t*
    capture in, 670
    complications of, 684–686
    crosstalk in, 664*d*, 683–684
    demand, 670
    dual-chamber, 667
        evaluation of, 678–680, 680–681
        four states of, 679–680, 680*f*–681*f*
        for hypertrophic cardiomyopathy, 727
        temporary, 671–672
        terminology related to, 664*d*–665*d*

Pacing, dual-chamber (*continued*)
  timing cycles in, 678
    upper-rate behavior in, 681–682, 682f
  epicardial, 666, 666f
    initiation of, 671
  external, after myocardial infarction, 528
  indications for, 661–662, 662t
  nursing issues in, 672–674
  rate-adaptive, 667
  sensing in, 670–671
  single-chamber, 667
    terminology related to, 663d–664d
  temporary
    initiation of, 671–672
    transvenous, 665f–666f, 665–666
    transcutaneous, 666f, 666–667
  unipolar, 669–670, 670f
  VVI
    intermittent loss of capture in, 676f
    intermittent loss of sensing in, 676f
    normal function in, 675f
    timing cycles in, 679f
Pacing interval, 663d
Pacing spike, 663d
PaCO₂, interpretation of, 159
PACs (premature atrial complexes),
    317, 317f
PAEDP. *See* Pulmonary artery end-diastolic
    pressure (PAEDP)
Pain management, for myocardial infarction,
    526–527
Pallor, 196
Palmaz-Schatz coronary stent, 550f, 552
Palpation
  in assessment of abdomen, 225, 225f
  in assessment of blood pressure, 205
  in assessment of heart, 212
  in assessment of lungs, 219–221, 222f, 223
Pancoast tumor, radiographic imaging
    of, 257f
PaO₂. *See* Arterial oxygen partial
    pressure (PaO₂)
Papillary muscle dysfunction, murmurs
    from, 217
Papillary muscles, anatomy of, 8
Papilledema, 199f
Paradoxical blood pressure, assessment of,
    208, 208f
Paradoxical pulse, from cardiac
    catheterization, 420
Paraspecific fibers of Mahaim, 11
Parasympathetic nervous system
  in blood pressure regulation, 87–88
  myocardial ischemia and, 501–502
Parasystole, 356f–357f, 356–357
Paroxysmal atrial tachycardia, 318f,
    318–319
Partial pressure of oxygen (PO₂), and oxygen
    delivery, 79
Partial thromboplastin time (PTT), 242
  blood collection for, 228
Passive vasodilation, 86, 94
Patient/family education
  about adherence, 887–888, 888d
  about cardiac arrest, 656–657
  about cardiac catheterization, 410–411,
    419–420, 420t

about cardiac transplantation, 604,
    609d–610d
about diabetes mellitus, 873
about dilated cardiomyopathy, 728
about heart failure, 575d
about hypertension, 810
about infectious endocarditis, 732
about low-cholesterol diet, 827–828
about myocardial infarction, 537
during cardiac rehabilitation
  inpatient, 852, 852d–853d, 852t
  outpatient, 856, 857
PAWP. *See* Pulmonary artery wedge
    pressure (PAWP)
PCO₂. *See* Carbon dioxide partial
    pressure (PCO₂)
Pectinate muscles, 6
PEEP. *See* Positive end-expiratory
    pressure (PEEP)
Percussion
  in assessment of abdomen, 224f–225f,
    224–225
  in assessment of lungs, 221, 221t,
    222f–223f, 223
Percutaneous aortic catheter balloon
    valvuloplasty, 714–715
Percutaneous cardiac catheterization, 412f,
    412–413
Percutaneous mitral catheter balloon
    valvuloplasty, 703, 704f
Percutaneous transluminal coronary
    angioplasty (PTCA), 544–546,
    545d, 546f
  creatine kinase-MB after, 234, 234f
  efficacy of, 544–545, 546f
  limitations of, 546
  for myocardial infarction, 522
  for myocardial ischemia, 513
  patient selection for, 544, 545d
  pre- and postprocedure management in,
    545–546
  procedure for, 544–545, 546f
  restenosis after, 545
Perfusion, 73
Pericardial constriction, hemodynamic
    response to, 459t
Pericardial disease. *See also* Pericarditis
  etiology of, 720t
  imaging of, 387
  nursing management of, 723–724
Pericardial effusion, 722–723
  myocardial infarction and, 258f
  radiographic imaging of, 255f
Pericardial friction rub, 217, 217f
Pericardial tamponade
  hemodynamic response to, 459t
  pulmonary artery waveform in, 444f
Pericarditis
  acute
    after myocardial infarction, 722
    noneffusive, 720
  clinical manifestations of, 721
  constrictive, 721–722
  etiology of, 719–720, 720d
  medical management of, 721–722
  from myocardial infarction, 521–522
  myocardial infarction and, 258f

Pericardium
  anatomy of, 9, 719
  echocardiography of, 381
  physiology of, 719
  restrictive effects of, 92
Peripheral arteries, in assessment of
    pulse, 201f
Peripheral atherosclerosis, 210
Peripheral circulation, assessment of, 201,
    201f
Peripheral edema, in heart failure, 562, 566
Peripheral neuropathy, diabetic, 872
Peripheral vascular resistance, respiratory
    acidosis and, 156
Peripheral vascular system, physical
    assessment of, 209–211, 210f
Personality, and coronary heart disease,
    759–760
Perspiration, 133
PET. *See* Positron emission
    tomography (PET)
pH, 153
  interpretation of, 159
  in metabolic acidosis, 157
  in metabolic alkalosis, 159
  in respiratory acidosis, 155
  in respiratory alkalosis, 157–158
Phagocytes, properties of, 111
Pharmacologic stress testing, 404
Phasic vascular smooth muscle, 58
Phlebostatic axis, 428, 429f–430f
Phonocardiography, 384, 384f
Phosphate, balance of, 138t, 147d, 147–148
Phosphodiesterase inhibitors, for heart
    failure, 572
Physical activity. *See* Activity; Exercise
Physical assessment, 195–225
  of abdomen, 223–225, 224f–225f
  of blood pressure, 203–209, 204t–206t,
    205f–208f
  cardiac, components of, 195
  before cardiac catheterization, 410–411
  general appearance in, 196
  of head, 196–198, 197f–199f
  of heart, 211f–217f, 211–219, 213t, 218t
    auscultation in, 212–219, 213f–217f,
      213t–218t. *See also* Auscultation
    inspection in, 212
    palpation in, 212
  of lungs, 219–223, 220f–222f, 221t
    auscultation in, 221–223, 224f
    inspection in, 219, 221f
    palpation in, 219–221, 222f, 223
    percussion in, 221, 221t,
      222f–224f, 223
  of peripheral vascular system,
    209–211, 210f
  precordial, 211f
Physical fitness, in prevention of coronary
    heart disease, 743f–744f, 743–745
Physical therapy, after cardiac transplantation,
    603–604, 604f, 604t, 608d
Pill counts, for measurement of
    adherence, 884
Plaques. *See* Atherosclerotic plaques
Plasma, functions of, 109
Plasminogen, in fibrinolysis, 114f, 114–115

Platelet count, 241–242
Platelets
    in atherosclerotic plaques, 485–486
    properties of, 112
Pleural effusion
    after cardiac surgery, 595*f*
    radiographic imaging of, 255*f*
Pneumonia, radiographic imaging of, 256*f*
Pneumothorax
    pacing and, 684
    radiographic imaging of, 257*f*
PO_2. *See* Partial pressure of oxygen (PO_2)
Point of maximal impulse, 3
Poiseuille's law, 62
Polymorphic ventricular tachycardia,
    336, 336*f*
Polysomnography, 163, 164*f*–165*f*
Position, changes in, auscultatory effects of,
    218*t*, 219
Positioning
    for chest radiography, 252*f*
    for measurement of cardiac output, 455
    for pulmonary artery catheter insertion,
        445, 446*f*–447*f*
Positive end-expiratory pressure (PEEP),
    pulmonary artery pressure
    monitoring during, 447–448
Positron emission tomography (PET), 383
    in myocardial ischemia, 511
Postcardiotomy syndrome, 595
Posterior leads, for electrocardiography,
    placement of, 269, 270*f*
Postextrasystolic beats, 219
Postganglionic fibers, function of, 84, 85*f*
Postural blood pressure
    extracellular fluid volume deficit and, 135
    measurement of, 207–208
Posture, muscle pump and, 99
Postventricular atrial refractory period
    (PVARP), 665*d*, 678
Potassium
    balance of, 137–141, 138*t*, 139*d*–140*d*
    equilibrium potential of, 20, 20*f*
    serum levels of, 244
Potassium channel blockers, properties
    of, 302*t*
Potassium currents, 27*t*, 28
Potassium-sparing diuretics
    for antihypertensive therapy, 798*t*
    for heart failure, 573*t*
Potential difference, in myocardial cells,
    18, 19
Prazosin, for heart failure, 573
Precordial examination, 211*f*
Precordial leads, for electrocardiography,
    placement of, 270*f*
Preexcitation syndromes, 329*f*–332*f*,
    329–333
    Lown-Ganong-Levine syndrome,
        332, 332*f*
    treatment of, 332–333
    Wolff-Parkinson-White syndrome,
        329*f*–331*f*, 329–331
Preganglionic fibers, function of,
    84, 85*f*
Preload, 36, 37*f*
    and cardiac output, 91

decrease in, ventricular function curve in,
    456*f*, 456–459
    as hemodynamic index, 460*t*
    increase in, ventricular function curve in,
        456*f*, 456–459
    length-tension relationship and, 37–39,
        38*f*–39*f*
Premature atrial complexes (PACs),
    317, 317*f*
Premature ectopic beats, 209
Premature junctional complexes, 321, 321*f*
Premature ventricular contractions (PVCs),
    322*f*, 322–323
    in cardiac arrest, 639, 640
    during sleep, 170
Pressure-volume curves, 441*f*
PR interval, 266
    in Wenckebach conduction, 338,
        348*f*–349*f*
Prinzmetal angina. *See* Variant angina
Problem-solving, for enhancement of
    adherence, 886
Probucol, for hyperlipidemia, 831
Procainamide
    for preexcitation syndromes, 333
    properties of, 308*t*
    for tachyarrhythmias, 312*t*
Propafenone, properties of, 308*t*
Propranolol, properties of, 309*t*
Prostanoids, vascular effects of, 57
Prosthetic valve endocarditis, 730
Prosthetic valves, 703*f*, 704–708, 705*t*, 706*f*
    complications of, 707–708
    degeneration of, 708
    imaging of, 386–387
    insertion of, minimally invasive surgery for,
        706–707, 707*f*
    mechanical, 705–706
    selection of, 705*t*
    tissue, 706, 706*f*
Protamine, for postoperative bleeding from
    cardiac surgery, 591
Protein, levels of, 246
Protein(s), myocardial, 230–231
Proteins, myocardial, 19
Proteoglycans, in atherosclerotic plaques, 486
Prothrombin time (PT), 242
    blood collection for, 228
Pseudoaneurysm, from coronary stents, 554
Pseudofusion beat, 663*d*, 665*d*
Pseudohypertension, 209
Psychosocial interventions, 760–762
PT. *See* Prothrombin time (PT)
PTCA. *See* Percutaneous transluminal
    coronary angioplasty (PTCA)
PTT. *See* Partial thromboplastin time (PTT)
Public health programs, role of in
    hypertension management,
    806–807
Pulmonary. *See also* Lung *entries*
Pulmonary arterial pressure, in heart
    failure, 567
Pulmonary artery, perforation of, from
    pulmonary artery pressure
    monitoring, 448*t*
Pulmonary artery catheters
    collection of blood from, 228

complications of, 448, 448*t*–451*t*
    features of, 438, 439*f*–440*f*
    fiberoptic, 463*f*, 463–464
    functioning of, assessment of,
        445–447, 447*f*
    insertion of, 438–439, 457*t*–458*t*
        positioning for, 445, 446*f*–447*f*
    radiographic imaging of, 259*f*–260*f*
Pulmonary artery end-diastolic pressure
    (PAEDP), 442*f*
Pulmonary artery end-diastolic pressure
    (PAEDP)–pulmonary artery wedge
    pressure (PAWP) gradient, 446–447
Pulmonary artery pressure
    measurement of, procedure for,
        431*d*–432*d*
    monitoring of, 438–452
        complications of, 448, 448*t*–451*t*
        indications for, 438
        during spontaneous *vs.* mechanical
            ventilation, 447–448
        technical aspects of, 444–448, 445*d*,
            446*f*–447*f*
    relationship to electrocardiographic
        findings, 438*t*
    waveforms from, 439, 440*f*
        interpretation of, 441–444, 442*f*–444*f*
Pulmonary artery systolic pressure, 442*f*
Pulmonary artery wedge pressure
    (PAWP), 438*t*
    measurement of, procedure for,
        431*d*–432*d*
    waveforms from, 439–441, 441*f*
        interpretation of, 442*f*–444*f*,
            443–444
Pulmonary artery wedge pressure–pulmonary
    artery end-diastolic pressure
    (PAEDP) gradient, 446–447
Pulmonary circulation, 73–75, 74*t*. *See also*
    Circulation, pulmonary
Pulmonary edema, cardiogenic, 258, 258*f*
    management of, 622*d*, 623
Pulmonary embolism, 126*f*, 126–130
    clinical manifestations of, 128
    hemodynamic response to, 459*t*
    medical management of, 128–129
    nursing management of, 129–130
    pathology of, 126*f*
    pathophysiology of, 128
    postoperative, 593
    prognosis in, 129
Pulmonary endothelium, anatomy of, 75
Pulmonary function, shock and, 619–620
Pulmonary infarction, from pulmonary artery
    pressure monitoring, 449*f*
Pulmonary pressure, effects of, 75–76, 76*f*
Pulmonary respiration, 76, 76*f*
Pulmonary valves, anatomy of, 8–9
Pulmonary vascular bed, physiology of, 75
Pulmonary vascular resistance (PVR), 61–62
Pulmonary vessels, anatomy of, 75
Pulmonic insufficiency, imaging studies of,
    385–386
Pulmonic valve, echocardiography of, 380
Pulse
    assessment of, 199–202, 200*f*–201*f*
    in heart failure, 567

Pulse (*continued*)
paradoxical, from cardiac catheterization, 420
Pulsed Doppler echocardiography, 376
Pulse generator, 664*d*
for implantable cardioverter-defibrillator, 688
Pulse generators, for temporary pacemakers, 668, 668*f*
Pulseless electrical activity, management of, 647, 649*f*
Pulse oximetry, 80–81
Pulse pressure, 62
measurement of, 207, 207*f*
Pulsus alternans, 200, 200*f*
Pulsus bisferiens, 200, 200*f*
Pulsus paradoxus, 200, 200*f*, 723
Pulsus parvus et tardus, 200, 200*f*
Pump performance, assessment of, 41–42
Purkinje cells
action potential of, 23*f*–24*f*, 26
in ventricular conduction, 31–32
function of, 10
Purkinje fibers, 264
PVARP (postventricular atrial refractory period), 665*d*, 678
PVCs. *See* Premature ventricular contractions (PVCs)
PVR (pulmonary vascular resistance), 61–62
P wave, 264, 264*f*, 268
in left atrial enlargement, 288, 289*f*
normal configuration of, 265*t*
in ventricular atopy, *vs.* aberrancy, 338, 340, 340*f*–341*f*

Q

Q (nonturbulent blood flow), 61
QRS axis, on electrocardiography, 273*f*–276*f*, 273–275
QRS complex, 264*f*, 264–265, 266*f*
morphology of, in ventricular atopy, *vs.* aberrancy, 340–341, 341*f*–342*f*
wide, differential diagnosis of, 339*t*, 340*f*
QT interval, 266*t*
Quadruple rhythm, 215, 215*f*
Quality of life, with implantable cardioverter-defibrillator, 695
Quantitative angiography, 417, 417*f*
Questionnaires
for assessment of adherence, 882*t*, 882–883
for enhancement of adherence, 887–888, 888*d*
Quinidine, properties of, 309*t*

R

Radial artery, bypass grafts using, 585
Radiofrequency catheter ablation, 368–371, 369*f*–370*f*
for atrial arrhythmias, 370
for atrial fibrillation/flutter, 369–370
for atrioventricular nodal reentrant tachycardia, 368, 369*f*
for atrioventricular reentrant tachycardia, 368–369, 370*f*
for tachyarrhythmias, 312*t*

technique of, 368
for ventricular tachycardia, 370–371
for Wolff-Parkinson-White syndrome, 368–369, 370*f*
Radiography, of chest. *See* Chest radiography
Radioisonuclides, risks of, 383
Radioisotope scans, of heart, 382*f*, 382–383
Radionuclide scanning
gated blood pool, in aortic stenosis, 714
in myocardial ischemia, 511
Radius Stent, 552, 554*f*
Ramp exercise testing, 394
Rapid eye movement (REM) sleep, 163, 165*f*–166*f*
in chronic obstructive pulmonary disease, 170
Rapid ventricular ejection, in cardiac cycle, 45*f*, 46, 46*t*
Rate-adaptive atrioventricular delay, 664*d*
Rate-adaptive pacing, 667
Rate modulation, 664*d*
in single-chamber pacing, 664*d*
Rate response, 665*d*
Rate smoothing, 665*d*
in dual-chamber pacing, 682, 683*f*
Rating of perceived exertion (RPE), 401*d*, 852, 852*t*
RBCs. *See* Red blood cells (RBCs)
Rectifying current, outward, 27*t*, 28
Red blood cell (RBC) count, 239–240
reference values for, 238*t*
Red blood cells (RBCs), properties of, 110–111
Reduced ventricular ejection, in cardiac cycle, 45*f*, 46
Reduction ventriculoplasty, 588, 588*f*
Reentrant pathways, Wenckebach conduction in, 350, 350*f*
Reentry, 301, 301*f*
myocardial ischemia and, 501
Reference level, in hemodynamic monitoring, 428–429, 429*f*–430*f*
Reference values, for blood studies, 229
Reflection coefficient, 66
Refractory period
in action potential, 26*f*, 26–27
in dual-chamber pacing, 664*d*–665*d*, 678
in ventricular atopy, *vs.* aberrancy, 338, 339*f*
Rehabilitation. *See* Cardiac rehabilitation
Reinforcement, for enhancement of adherence, 886
Rejection, after cardiac transplantation, 600*f*, 600*t*, 600–601
Relapse prevention, for enhancement of adherence, 886–887
Relaxation, of cardiac muscle, molecular basis of, 35
Relaxation techniques, for sleep disorders, 174
REM. *See* Rapid eye movement (REM) sleep
Renal disease, and hypertension, 782, 783*d*, 786
management of, 802–803
Renal function
after cardiac surgery, 593–594
aging and, 185

diabetes and, 872
in heart failure, 562
shock and, 619–620
Renin-angiotensin-aldosterone system, 89, 89*f*
impairment of, and hypertension, 782
Renovascular hypertension, 782
Reocclusion, 503
Repaglinide, 877
Reperfusion, consequences of, 498*f*, 502–503
Reperfusion injury, 502–503
Repolarization
factors affecting, 28–30, 29*f*–30*f*
ventricular, 32
Reproductive hormones, and risk of coronary heart disease, 748–749
Resistance, calculation of, 62
Respiration
assessment of, 219, 221*f*
and blood pressure, 99–100
and cardiac output, 99–100
Cheyne-Stokes, during sleep, 171
muscles of, 75
pulmonary, 76, 76*f*
and stroke volume, 99–100
in tissue, 76, 77*f*
Respiratory acidosis, 155–156, 156*d*
Respiratory alkalosis, 158, 158*d*
Respiratory excursion, assessment of, 222*f*
Respiratory function
aging and, 184*f*, 184–185
altered, in heart failure, 576
sleep and, 167–168
Respiratory pump, 99
Res-Q Micron implantable cardioverter-defibrillator, 691*t*
Restenosis, 503
after percutaneous transluminal coronary angioplasty, 545
Resting potential, factors affecting, 298
Restrictive cardiomyopathy, 727
Retinopathy, hypertensive, 786*t*, 786–787
Revascularization
of coronary artery, procedures for, 584*f*–586*f*, 584–587
for myocardial ischemia, 513
postoperative care in, 589, 590*t*
transmyocardial laser, 587
Reverse cholesterol transport, 821
Rheumatic heart disease, 699*f*, 699–700
Right atrial enlargement, electrocardiography in, 289
Right atrial pressure, monitoring of, 436–438, 437*f*, 438*t*
Right axis deviation, 273, 273*f*
Right bundle branch, anatomy of, 11–12
Right bundle-branch block, electrocardiography in, 277–278, 279*f*, 282*f*
Right coronary artery, anatomy of, 14–15
Right heart, catheterization of, 413, 413*f*
results of, 422*f*
Right heart function, variables in, 452*t*
Right ventricle
blood supply to, 13*t*
cardiac cycle in, 47
echocardiography of, 378*f*, 380

Right ventricular enlargement, electrocardiography in, 289–291, 292*d*, 292*f*
Right ventricular infarction, hemodynamic response to, 459*t*
Right ventricular volume, measurement of, 449–452, 451*f*, 452*t*
Roles and relationships, assessment of, 194
Ross procedure, 706, 706*f*
Rotational ablation, 547*f*, 547–548
RPE (rating of perceived exertion), 401*d*, 852, 852*t*
"Rule of bigeminy," 343
R wave
  normal configuration of, 265*t*
  in right ventricular enlargement, 289, 291, 292*f*

S

S₁, 213*f*, 213–214
S₂, 213*f*, 213–214
  splitting of, 214, 214*f*
S₄, 215, 215*f*
Safety pacing, 665*d*, 684, 685*f*
San Francisco clues, in ventricular atopy, *vs.* aberrancy, 342*f*
SaO₂. *See* Oxygen saturation (SaO₂)
Saphenous vein bypass graft, 584*f*, 585
Sarcolemma
  ion currents in, 27*t*, 27–28
  structure of, 17–19
Sarcomeres, properties of, 33
Sarcoplasm, calcium concentration in, modulation of, 35–36
Second-hand smoke, and coronary heart disease, 741
Second wind phenomenon, 509
Sedatives, for sleep, 174
Seldinger technique, of cardiac catheterization, 412*f*, 412–413
Self-care deficit, shock and, 636–637
Self-concept, disturbance in, after cardiac transplantation, 609*d*
Self-efficacy, and behavior change, 885–886
Self-expanding coronary stents, 552, 552*t*, 554*f*
Self-monitoring, for enhancement of adherence, 885–886
Self-perception, assessment of, 194
Semilunar valves, anatomy of, 8–9
Sensing, 670–671
  evaluation of, 675, 676*f*
  by implantable cardioverter-defibrillator, 689–690, 690*f*, 692*f*
Sensing threshold, 664*d*
Sensitivity threshold, test of, 674
Sensory-perceptual alteration, in patient with intra-aortic balloon pump, 632*d*
Septic shock, hemodynamic response to, 459*t*
Serum, drug levels in, 247–248, 248*t*
Serum electrolytes, 244–245, 245*t*
  after cardiac surgery, 245
  reference values for, 238*t*
Serum lactate, and oxygen supply and demand, 462–463

Serum osmolality, calculation of, 245, 245*t*
Sex hormones, reproductive, and risk of coronary heart disease, 748–749
Sexual dysfunction, after cardiac transplantation, 603
Sexuality, assessment of, 194
Shock, 614–637
  anaphylactic, pathophysiology of, 615
  assessment of blood pressure in, 209
  cardiogenic
    diagnosis of, 620*f*, 620–621
    from myocardial infarction, 520
    pathophysiology of, 615
    treatment of, 621–623, 622*d*–623*d*
  classification of, 614, 614*d*
  clinical manifestations of, 618–619
  compensatory mechanisms in, 615–619, 616*f*–618*f*
    in initial stage, 616*f*, 616–617
    in intermediate stage, 617*f*, 617–618
    in irreversible stage, 618, 618*f*
  definition of, 561
  distributive, 615
  hypovolemic
    diagnosis of, 620
    pathophysiology of, 615
    treatment of, 621–624, 622*d*–623*d*, 622*f*
  neurogenic, pathophysiology of, 615
  nursing care plan for, 636*ncp*–637*ncp*
  pathophysiology of, 614–615
  physical assessment in, 619–620
  prognosis in, 621
  septic
    diagnosis of, 621
    hemodynamic response to, 459*t*
    management of, 623–624
    pathophysiology of, 615
Short-cycle aberrancy, 300, 300*f*
Shunt, physiologic, 74
Sibutramine, 866
Sick sinus syndrome, 316*f*, 316–317
Single-chamber pacing. *See* Pacing, single-chamber
Sinus arrest, 315, 315*f*
Sinus arrhythmia, 91, 315, 315*f*
Sinus bradycardia. *See* Bradycardia, sinus
Sinus exit block, 316, 316*f*
Sinus node, 263
  anatomy of, 10
  arrhythmias originating in, 302, 310*f*–317*f*, 314–317
  Wenckebach conduction in, 348–349, 349*f*
Sinus node artery, anatomy of, 14–15
Sinus node cells, action potential of, 23*f*, 25
Sinus rhythm, normal, 302, 314, 314*f*
Sinus tachycardia, 314, 314*f*
  with Wenckebach exit block, 352, 353*f*
Skin
  assessment of, in shock, 619
  examination of, in heart failure, 567
SLE. *See* Systemic lupus erythematosus (SLE)
Sleep, 163–173
  after cardiac surgery, 169
  aging and, 166*f*, 166–167
  angina during, 169–170
  arrhythmias during, 170

  assessment of, 171, 172*t*
  and cardiovascular disease, 168–169
  cardiovascular responses to, 167
  and chronic obstructive pulmonary disease, 170
  in coronary care unit, 169, 173
  definition of, 163
  duration of, 165
  function of, 167
  in health care providers, 174
  laboratory studies during, 163, 164*f*
  medications promoting, 174
  nature of, 163–167, 164*f*–166*f*
  respiratory function during, 167–168
  stages of, 163–165, 165*f*
Sleep apnea, 171
Sleep cycle, 165, 166*f*
Sleep disorders, nursing management of, 171–174, 172*t*
Sleep hygiene, 173
Sleepiness, 166, 166*f*
Sleep latency, 166*f*
Sleep-rest functional pattern, assessment of, 194
Slow myocytes. *See* Sinus node cells
Slow-response cells, 22–23, 23*f*
Smoking
  adverse effects of, 765
  and coronary heart disease, 740*f*, 740–741
  societal impact of, 764
Smoking cessation, 764–774
  alcohol use and, 773
  benefits of, 765–766
  resource materials for, 774
  and sense of loss, 773
  social support and, 773
  stress and, 772–773
  and weight gain, 773
  in women, 773–774
Smoking cessation interventions
  of Agency for Health Care Policy and Research, 767–772, 768*d*, 770*f*–771*f*, 772*d*
  for assistance in quitting, 769–771, 770*f*–771*f*
  in coronary heart disease patients, 766–767
  for encouraging smokers to quit, 768
  for follow-up, 772
  for identification of smokers willing to quit, 768–769
  for identification of tobacco users, 767–768, 768*d*
  for relapse prevention, 769–770, 770*f*
  theoretical basis of, 766
  trends in, 767
Smooth muscle, vascular
  endothelial cells and, 60*f*
  properties of, 58
Snoring, 171
Social history, 193
Social support
  for enhancement of adherence, 886
  nursing interventions for, 760–761
  and smoking cessation, 773
Sodium
  equilibrium potential of, 21
  restriction of, in control of hypertension, 791

Sodium (*continued*)
  retention of, in heart failure, 562
  serum concentration of, 135–137, 136*d*
Sodium-calcium exchange, 22
Sodium channel, activity of, 22
Sodium channel blockers, properties of, 302*t*
Sodium chloride, renal excretion of, 93
Sodium current, fast, 27*t*, 27–28
Sodium homeostasis, aging and, 185
Sodium-potassium adenosine triphosphatase
    pump, 22
Sodium reabsorption, and hypertension, 782
Solutes, diffusion of, 64–65
Sones technique, for coronary arteriography,
    415–416, 416*f*
Sonographers, role of, 375
Sotalol, properties of, 309*t*
Sphygmomanometer, use of, 203–205,
    204*t*, 205*f*
Sputum, assessment of, 219
SR, in myocardial cells, 17
Staircase phenomenon, 40, 40*f*
Standard precautions, 227
Starling's equation, 66, 67*f*
Starling's law, 37–39, 38*f*–39*f*
Statin therapy, for hypercholesterolemia, 820*t*
Stem cells, properties of, 109
Stenotic vessels, blood flow in, 497
Stent Restenosis Trial (STRESS), 549
Stents, 549*f*–554*f*, 549–554, 552*t*. *See also*
    Coronary stents
Stepped care, in management of
    hypertension, 794–795, 795*f*,
    796*t*–800*t*
Stethoscope, use of, 212–213
Stiff heart, 499
Stimulation threshold, 664*d*
Stimulation threshold test, 673
Stimulus control, for enhancement of
    adherence, 886
Stimulus release, evaluation of, 674, 675*f*
Streptokinase, for thrombolytic therapy, 541
Stress
  and coronary heart disease, 757–758
  emotional, and chest pain, 509
  physiologic effects of, 757, 758*f*
  and smoking cessation, 772–773
STRESS (Stent Restenosis Trial), 549
Stress echodardiography, 381
Stress testing, in angina, 511
Stretching, of cardiac fibers, and electrical
    activity, 30
Stroke, hypertension and, 787
Stroke volume, 47
  definition of, 561
  respiration and, 99–100
Stroke volume index (SVI), 460*t*
ST segment
  exercise testing and, 398*f*–399*f*,
    398–399
  in myocardial infarction, 285*f*, 518, 518*f*
    anterolateral, 287*f*
    posterior, 288*f*
    right ventricular, 287, 288*f*
  in myocardial ischemia, 283*d*, 284
  normal configuration of, 265*t*, 266
Subsidiary pacemaker, 297

Sudden death
  causes of, 640*d*
  definition of, 639
  survivors of
    nursing management of, 656–657
    use of implantable cardioverter-
        defibrillators in, 687–688
Sulfonylureas, 876
Summation gallop, 215*f*
Superoxide anions, vascular effects of, 57
Supraventricular tachycardia (SVT), 320*f*,
    320–321, 333–335, 334*f*–335*f*
  management of, 647–653, 651*f*–652*f*
SVI. *See* Stroke volume index (SVI)
SVR. *See* Systemic vascular resistance (SVR)
SVT. *See* Supraventricular tachycardia (SVT)
Swan-Ganz catheters, radiographic imaging
    of, 259*f*
Swan-Ganz ejection fraction catheter,
    449, 451*f*
S wave
  in left ventricular enlargement, 289, 290*f*
  normal configuration of, 265*t*
Sympathetic nervous system
  in blood pressure regulation, 84–87, 85*f*,
    86*t*, 87*f*–88*f*
  heart failure and, 562
  increased response of, decreased blood
    pressure and, 101*f*, 101–102
  myocardial ischemia and, 501
Synchronized cardioversion, 653
Syncope
  classification of, 367*d*
  electrophysiology studies in,
    365–366, 367*d*
  left ventricular baroreceptors in, 84
  of unknown origin, implantable
    cardioverter-defibrillators for, 688
Systemic lupus erythematosus (SLE)
  clinical features of, 196
  and pericarditis, 720
Systemic oxygen consumption, 464, 465*t*
  clinical applications of, 465*t*, 465–466
Systemic vascular resistance (SVR), 62
  in heart failure, 569
  vs. afterload, 91
Systole
  clinical applications of, 47
  ventricular, 45*f*, 45–46, 46*t*
Systolic blood pressure, assessment of,
    205–206
Systolic click, 216, 216*f*
Systolic compression, and coronary blood
    flow, 43, 43*f*
Systolic dysfunction, in heart failure, 561,
    564, 564*f*–565*f*
  treatment of, 570, 571*f*, 572*f*, 573*t*
Systolic heart sounds, extra, 215–216, 216*f*
Systolic hypertension. *See* Hypertension,
    systolic
Systolic reserve, 41

T

Tachyarrhythmias
  in myocardial infarction, 519–520
  treatment of, 311*t*–312*t*

Tachycardia
  atrial, 318*f*–319*f*, 318–319
  atrioventricular nodal reentry, 333, 334*f*
  circus movement, 335, 335*f*
  endless-loop, 664*d*
  junctional, 321*f*, 321–322
  management of, 651*f*
  pacemaker-mediated, 665*d*, 683, 684*f*
  sinus, 314, 314*f*
  supraventricular, 320*f*, 320–321, 333–335,
    334*f*–335*f*
    management of, 647–653, 651*f*–652*f*
  ventricular. *See* Ventricular tachycardia
  wide-complex, electrophysiology studies
    in, 365
Tacrolimus, side effects of, 601, 602*t*
Target heart rate (THR), in cardiac
    rehabilitation, 855–856
TARP (total atrial refractory period),
    665*d*, 678
T cells
  in atherosclerotic plaques, 485, 485*f*
  properties of, 111
  types of, 111–112
Technetium-99m sestamibi, for myocardial
    perfusion imaging, 403
Temperature, body. *See* Body temperature
TER. *See* Thoracic electrical
    bioimpedance (TER)
Thallium-201, for myocardial perfusion
    imaging, 403
Therapeutic relationship, for enhancement of
    adherence, 888–889
Thermodilution technique, for determination
    of cardiac output, 417, 452*f*–456*f*,
    452–459, 454*d*. *See also* Cardiac
    entries output, measurement of
Thiazide diuretics, for heart failure, 573*t*
Thiazolidinediones, 877
Thick filaments
  in contraction, 33
  and length-tension relationship, 38*f*
Thigh, blood pressure measurement on, 209
Thin filaments
  in contraction, 34
  and length-tension relationship, 38*f*
Thirst, physiology of, 132–133
Thoracic cavity, structures in, 4*f*
Thoracic electrical bioimpedance (TER),
    461–442
Thoratec pump, 635, 635*f*
Thrombin time, 242–243
Thromboembolism, venous, 123–130, 126*f*,
    127*d*–128*d*. *See also* Deep venous
    thrombosis (DVT); Pulmonary
    embolism
Thrombolytic therapy, 541–544, 542*d*
  anisoylated plasminogen streptokinase
    activator complex for, 541–542
  efficacy of, 543–544
  for myocardial infarction, 522
  patient selection for, 542*d*–543*d*,
    542–543
  protocols for, 544
  for pulmonary embolism, 129
  streptokinase for, 541
  tissue-type plasminogen activator for, 542

Thrombophlebitis, physical examination in, 210
Thrombosis
    arterial
        from arterial pressure monitoring, 434
        from cardiac catheterization, 420
        from coronary stents, 554
        from coronary stents, 552–553
        from prosthetic valves, 707
        venous, from electrophysiology studies, 364
Thromboxane A, vascular affects of, 57
Thrombus, formation of, 121*f*, 121–122
Tight-junction endothelium, 53
Tilting-disk valve, 705
Tilt test, 366
TIMPs. *See* Tissue inhibitors of metalloproteinases (TIMPs)
Tirofiban, use of after coronary stent placement, 551
Tissue factor, and coagulation, 113, 113*f*
Tissue inhibitors of metalloproteinases (TIMPs), function of, 485
Tissue oxygenation, monitoring of, 80–81, 462
Tissue oxygen extraction, in heart failure, 564
Tissue perfusion
    altered
        in deep venous thrombosis, 127*d*
        in disseminated intravascular coagulation, 120*ncp*
        from interventional cardiology procedures, 556–557
        in myocardial infarction, 532*ncp*–534*ncp*, 535–536
    decreased
        in patient with intra-aortic balloon pump, 630*d*
        shock and, 636
Tissue pressure hypothesis, of autoregulation, 95–96
Tissue respiration, 76, 77*f*
Tissue-type plasminogen activator (tPA), 114, 114*f*
    for thrombolytic therapy, 542
Tobacco smoking. *See* Smoking; Smoking cessation
Tobacco users, identification of, 768
Tocainide, properties of, 309*t*
Tonic vascular smooth muscle, 58
Tonometry, gastric, 462
Torsades de pointes, 336, 337*f*, 338
Total atrial refractory period (TARP), 665*d*, 678
Total-body magnesium depletion, 144–146
Tourniquet, use of, for blood specimen collection, 227–228
tPA. *See* Tissue-type plasminogen activator (tPA)
Tracheostomy tubes, radiographic imaging of, 259*f*
Transcutaneous pacing, 666*f*, 666–667
    for bradyarrhythmias, 313*t*
Transducers, for echocardiography, function of, 375*f*–376*f*, 375–376
Transesophageal echocardiography, 381
    in infectious endocarditis, 730

Transfusions, and hyperkalemia, 140
Transient diastolic inward currents, 27*t*, 28
Transluminal extraction atherectomy, 548, 548*f*
Transmembrane resting potential (TRP), 297–298, 298*f*
Transmitted voice sounds, auscultation of, 223
Transmyocardial laser revascularization, 587
Transplantation. *See* Cardiac transplantation
Transseptal left heart catheterization, 414*f*, 414–415
Transtheoretical model of behavior change, 885
    for smoking cessation, 766
Transthoracic echocardiography, in mitral insufficiency, 709
Transthoracic resistance, for defibrillation, 643
Transvenous pacing, 665*f*–666*f*, 665–666
    initiation of, 671
    temporary, for bradyarrhythmias, 313*t*
Treadmill tests
    Balke, 393
    Bruce, 393
    Naughton, 393–394
Treppe, 40, 40*f*
Tricuspid regurgitation, imaging studies of, 386
Tricuspid valve
    anatomy of, 6, 7*f*, 8
    echocardiography of, 380
Tricuspid valve disease, 704, 705*t*
Troglitazone, 877
Troponins, 230–231
    in myocardial infarction, 519
TRP (transmembrane resting potential), 297–298, 298*f*
T-tubule system, 17
Tumors, intracardiac, imaging of, 387
T wave
    changes in, differential diagnosis of, 283*d*
    normal configuration of, 265, 265*t*
24-hour diet recall, 881–882
Twiddler's syndrome, 685
2:1 conduction ratio, in second-degree atrioventricular block, 327, 327*f*
Type A personality, and coronary heart disease, 759–761

U

Ulnar neuropathy, from cardiac surgery, 594–595
Ultrafiltration, 65–66, 67*f*
Ultrasonography
    Doppler, for assessment of arterial blood flow, 201, 201*f*
    intravascular, before coronary stent placement, 549–550, 551*f*
Undersensing, 664*d*, 677, 677*f*
Unipolar, definition of, 664*d*
Unipolar leads, for electrocardiography, placement of, 269, 270*f*
Unipolar pacing, 669–670, 670*f*
Universal precautions, 227
Upper-rate behavior, in dual-chamber pacing, 681–682, 682*f*

Upright posture, muscle pump and, 99
Upstroke phase, of action potential, 24, 24*f*
Urea nitrogen, levels of, 246
Uremia, and pericarditis, 719–720
Uric acid, levels of, 246
Urine, volume of, 133, 134*t*
Urine flow, during sleep, 168
Urine output, after cardiac catheterization, 420
U wave, 265

V

Vagal maneuvers, for tachycardia, 346
Vagal stimulation, and heart rate, 90
Valsalva maneuver, 219
    hemodynamic response to, 100*f*, 100–101
Values-beliefs, assessment of, 194
Valvular heart disease. *See also* specific valves
    acquired, 699–716
        diagnosis of, 702
        murmurs associated with, 705*t*
        valvular repair for, 587
        valvular replacement for, 587
    classification of, 699
    epidemiology of, 699
    etiology of, 699*f*, 699–702, 700*t*, 701*d*
    imaging studies of, 385–387
Valvuloplasty
    creatine kinase levels after, 235
    percutaneous aortic catheter balloon, 714–715
Variant angina
    classification of, 508
    medical management of, 513
    during sleep, 170
Varicose veins, assessment of, 211
Vasa vasorum, in atherosclerotic plaques, 486
Vascular bed, pulmonary, physiology of, 75
Vascular endothelium
    fenestrated, 53
    and vasomotor function, 55*t*
Vascular injury, from intra-aortic balloon pump, 628
Vascular resistance
    autacoids and, 55
    control of, 92–93
    endothelium-derived vasoactive substances and, 55*t*, 55–58, 56*f*–58*f*
    local metabolic control of, 57–58, 58*f*
    local regulation of, 94–96, 95*f*
    mediators of, endothelium-derived, 96
Vascular responsiveness, impaired, and hypertension, 782
Vascular sheath, removal of, after coronary stent placement, 553–554, 554*f*
Vascular smooth muscle, properties of, 58
Vascular smooth muscle cells, in atherosclerotic plaques, 482–484, 484*f*
Vascular spasm, from atherectomy, 548
Vascular system
    aging and, 183–184
    autonomic innervation of, 86
    blood flow in, 60–62
    calcium and, 59–60, 60*f*
    neurohumoral stimulation of, 58–59, 59*f*

Vascular system (*continued*)
  peripheral, physical assessment of, 209–211, 210*f*
  smooth muscle cells in, endothelial cells and, 60*f*
  volume distribution in, 60, 61*f*
Vascular tone, maintenance of, 78
Vasoactive substances, endothelium-derived, and vascular resistance, 55*t*, 55–58, 56*f*–58*f*
Vasoconstriction
  hypercalcemia and, 144
  hypoxic, 74
  passive *vs.* active, 94
Vasoconstrictors, action of, 57*f*
Vasodilation, passive, 86, 94
Vasodilators
  action of, 87*f*
  for antihypertensive therapy, 799*t*
  for heart failure, 572–573, 574*t*
  parenteral, for hypertensive crisis, 801*t*
Vasomotor function, vascular endothelium and, 55*t*
Vasopressin, increased levels of, in heart failure, 564
Veins
  constriction of, 54–55
  structure of, 53–55
  valves of, 54
Venous circulation, assessment of, 210–211
Venous compliance, 64
Venous dilators, for heart failure, 573
Venous insufficiency, chronic, 211
Venous pressure, 63–64, 64*f*
Venous pulse, assessment of, 202*f*–203*f*, 202–203
Venous system, neurohumoral control of, 96*f*, 96–97
Venous thromboembolism, 123–130, 126*f*, 127*d*–128*d*. *See also* Deep venous thrombosis (DVT); Pulmonary embolism
  from electrophysiology studies, 364
Ventak AV III DR implantable cardioverter-defibrillator, 691*t*
Ventilation, 73
  during sleep, 167
Ventilation-perfusion (VQ) matching, 74–75
Ventilation-perfusion (VQ) mismatch, in pulmonary embolism, 128
Ventricles
  anatomy of, 6–8, 7*f*–8*f*
  arrhythmias originating in, 322*f*–325*f*, 322–325
  left. *See* Left ventricle
  muscle fibers of, 9, 9*f*
  right. *See* Right ventricle
Ventricular arrhythmias, pacing and, 685
Ventricular asystole, 325, 325*f*
Ventricular atopy, *vs.* aberrancy, 338–346, 339*f*–346*f*, 339*t*
  capture beats in, 341, 342*f*–343*f*, 343
  clinical features of, 346, 346*f*
  cycle length variations in, 343–344, 344*f*–345*f*
  esophageal leads in, 344–346, 345*f*
  fusion beats in, 341, 342*f*–343*f*, 343

intra-atrial electrogram in, 49*f*, 344–346
  mechanisms of aberration in, 338, 339*f*
  P wave in, 338, 340, 340*f*–341*f*
  QRS morphology in, 340–341, 341*f*–342*f*
  refractory period in, 338, 339*f*
Ventricular conduction, 31–32, 32*f*
Ventricular diastole, 45*f*, 46
Ventricular dilatation, in heart failure, 563, 563*f*
Ventricular ejection, in cardiac cycle, 45*f*, 46, 46*t*
Ventricular enlargement, electrocardiography in, 289–291
Ventricular fibrillation, 324*f*, 324–325
  in cardiac arrest, 639, 640*f*, 642
  management of, 645*f*, 646–647
  treatment of, by implantable cardioverter-defibrillator, 692, 692*f*
Ventricular filling, 45*f*, 46
Ventricular flutter, 324, 324*f*
Ventricular function curves, 456*f*, 456–459
Ventricular function studies, with exercise testing, 403
Ventricular parasystole, 356*f*, 356–357
Ventricular preload, in heart failure, 562
Ventricular refractory period, 665*d*, 678
Ventricular remodeling, in heart failure, 563*f*, 563–564
Ventricular repolarization, 32
Ventricular septal defect (VSD)
  hemodynamic response to, 459*t*
  repair of, 588
Ventricular septal rupture, from myocardial infarction, 521
Ventricular systole, 45*f*, 45–46, 46*t*
Ventricular tachycardia, 323–324, 324*f*, 335–338, 336*f*–337*f*
  management of, 647–653, 651*f*–652*f*
  monomorphic, 335–336, 336*f*
  polymorphic, 336, 336*f*
  pulseless, management, 645*f*, 646–647
  sustained, implantable cardioverter-defibrillators in, 688
  torsades de pointes, 336, 337*f*, 338
  treatment of, 311*t*–312*t*
    by implantable cardioverter-defibrillator, 692, 692*f*
    radiofrequency catheter ablation in, 370–371
    with Wenckebach exit block, 352*f*
Ventriculography, 415, 415*f*
  in heart failure, 569*t*
  radioisotope, 382*f*
Ventriculoplasty, reduction, 588, 588*f*
Venules, structure of, 53
Verapamil, properties of, 310*t*
Very low-density lipoprotein (VLDL), production of, 821
Viral infections, and myocarditis, 728
Virchow's triad, 121*f*, 121–122
Visceral obesity, 861, 861*t*
Vision, assessment of, 197
Vitalog, 883
VLDL. *See* Very low-density lipoprotein (VLDL)
VO₂. *See* Oxygen consumption (VO₂)
Voice sounds, auscultation of, 223

Voltage, on electrocardiography, designation of, 267*f*
Volume-pressure curve, in veins, 96*f*, 96–97
VQ mismatch. *See* Ventilation-perfusion (VQ) mismatch
VSD. *See* Ventricular septal defect (VSD)
V wave, on pulmonary artery wedge pressure tracing, 443, 443*f*

W

Waist circumference, measurement of, 861
Wakefulness, stages of, 163–165, 165*f*
Wandering atrial pacemaker, 317, 317*f*
Warfarin
  for myocardial infarction, 531
  and prothrombin time, 242
Warm-up period, 841
Water
  filtration of, endothelium and, 53, 54*f*
  transport of, 64–66, 67*f*
Waveforms
  arterial, during cardiac cycle, 435*f*, 435–436
  pulmonary artery, 439, 440*f*
  pulmonary artery wedge, 439–441, 441*f*
WBCs. *See* White blood cells (WBCs)
Weight
  and cardiac rehabilitation, 843, 853
  and coronary heart disease, 746–748, 747*f*
Weight gain, smoking cessation and, 773
Weight loss, maintenance of, 867
Weight management
  in control of hypertension, 790–791
  and hyperlipidemia, 828–829
Wenckebach atrioventricular block, 326, 326*f*
  treatment of, 313*t*
Wenckebach conduction, 346–351, 347*f*–352*f*
  alternating, 351
  atrioventricular, 347*f*–349*f*, 347–348
  in bundle branches, 349–350, 350*f*
  with exit block from ectopic focus, 350–351, 351*f*–352*f*
  in reentrant pathways, 350, 350*f*
  in sinus node, 348–349, 349*f*
Wenckebach upper-rate response, 682, 682*f*
Wheezes, 223
White blood cell (WBC) count, 240
  reference values for, 238*t*
White blood cell (WBC) differential, 240
White blood cells (WBCs), properties of, 111–112
Wide-complex tachyardia, electrophysiology studies in, 365
Wolff-Parkinson-White (WPW) syndrome, 329*f*–331*f*, 329–331
  treatment of, radiofrequency catheter ablation in, 368–369, 370*f*
Wound infections, after cardiac surgery, 595
WPW syndrome. *See* Wolff-Parkinson-White (WPW) syndrome

X

X-rays, principles of, 252*f*, 252–253

Z

Zeroing, 430, 431*d*–432*d*